NURSE'S HANDBOOK OF DRUG THERAPY

Springhouse Corporation
Springhouse, Pennsylvania

STAFF

Executive Director, Editorial
Stanley Loeb

Editorial Director
Helen Klusek Hamilton

Clinical Director
Barbara F. McVan, RN

Art Director
John Hubbard

Drug Information Editor
George J. Blake, RPh, MS

Clinical Project Editor
Judith A. Schilling McCann, RN, BSN

Clinical Editors
Roseann Barrett, RN, BSN; Sherri Izes Becker, RN, MBA, CCRN; June Breit, RN; Marlene Ciranowicz, RN, MSN, CDE; Susan B. Fralick, RN, MSN; Mary C. Gyetvan, RN, BSEd; Eileen E. Jaskuta, RN, BSN; Galene Sellers, LPN; Julie N. Tackenberg, RN, MA, CNRN; Beverly Ann Tscheschlog, RN; Eileen M. Wenckus, RN, MSN, CS

Copy Editors
Jane V. Cray (supervisor), Mary T. Durkin, Traci A. Ginnona, Jennifer Mintzer, Christina A. Price, Nancee Vogel, Doris Weinstock

Designers
Stephanie Peters (associate art director), Lorraine Lostracco Carbo (book designer)

Typography
David C. Kosten (director), Diane Paluba (manager), Elizabeth Bergman, Joyce Rossi Biletz, Phyllis Marron, Robin Mayer, Valerie Rosenberger

Manufacturing
Deborah C. Meiris (manager), T.A. Landis

Production Coordination
Colleen M. Hayman

Editorial Assistants
Maree DeRosa, Beverly Lane, Mary Madden, Margaret A. Rastiello

Indexer
Barbara Hodgson

AGDH-010993
ISBN 0-87434-527-8

Nurse's handbook of drug therapy.
p. cm.
Includes index.
1. Pharmacology—Handbooks, manuals, etc.
2. Nursing—Handbooks, manuals, etc.
I. Springhouse Corporation.
[DNLM: 1. Drug Therapy—handbooks.
2. Drug Therapy—nurses' instruction. 3. Drugs—handbooks. 4. Drugs—nurses' instruction.
QV 39 N97345]
RM301.12.N88 1992
615'.1—dc20
DNLM/DLC 92-2338
ISBN 0-87434-527-8 CIP

CONTENTS

Generic drugs and pharmacologic classes

CLINICAL CONSULTANTS AND PHARMACY REVIEWERS

At the time of publication, the clinical consultants and pharmacy reviewers held the following positions.

Clinical Consultants

Michael J. Booth, RN, MA, CRNA, Co-Director, Graduate Program of Nurse Anesthesia; Assistant Professor, Department of Anesthesiology, Medical College of Pennsylvania and Medical College of Pennsylvania Hospital, Philadelphia

Mary Ann Cali-Ascani, RNC, MSN, OCN, Oncology Nurse Manager, Easton (Pa.) Hospital

Sandy R. Conover, RN, MS, GNP-C, Associate Professor of Nursing, Cerritos College, Norwalk, Calif.

Charmaine J. Cummings, RN, MSN, Director, Nursing Education, National Institutes of Health, Clinical Center, Bethesda, Md.

Nancy G. Evans, RN, BSN, CGRN, Nurse Manager, Gastroenterology Department, Daniel Freeman Memorial and Marina Hospitals, Inglewood, Calif.

Walter Carl Faubion, RN, MHSA, Manager, Parenteral and Enteral Nutrition Team, University of Michigan Medical Center, Ann Arbor

Terry Matthew Foster, RN, BSN, CEN, CCRN, Director, Mercy Hospital–Anderson, Cincinnati

Betty M. Hanson, RN, MN, Coordinator, First Year Associate of Science in Nursing Program, Santa Fe Community College, Gainesville, Fla.

Jeannine L. Hayduk, RN, PhD, CS, Director of Nursing and Allied Health, Southern Illinois Collegiate Common Market, Carterville, Ill.

Roseann Hendrickson, RN, Nursing Consultant, Emergency Physician Associates, P.A., Woodbury, N.J.

Marcia Jo Hill, RN, MSN, Manager, Dermatology Therapeutics, The Methodist Hospital, Houston; Clinical Assistant Professor, Department of Dermatology, Baylor College of Medicine, Houston

Sandra S. Huddleston, RN, MSN, CCRN, Assistant Professor of Nursing, Berea (Ky.) College

Karen Landis, RN, MS, CCRN, Pulmonary Clinical Nurse Specialist, Lehigh Valley Hospital Center, The Allentown (Pa.) Hospital

Meredith Ann McCord, RN, MS, Assistant Professor, Oregon Health Sciences University School of Nursing, Portland

Chris Platt Moldovanyi, RN, MSN, CDE, Endocrinology Clinical Specialist; Staff Nurse, Gynecology Operating Room, Cleveland (Ohio) Clinic Foundation

Rita S. Monahan, RN, MSN, EdD, Associate Professor, Oregon Health Sciences University School of Nursing, Eastern Oregon State College, LaGrande

Mary D. Naylor, RN, PhD, FAAN, Associate Dean and Director of Undergraduate Studies, University of Pennsylvania, School of Nursing, Philadelphia

Deborah P. Nelson, RN, MS, CCRN, Cardiovascular Clinical Specialist, LaGrange, Ill.

C. Lynne Ostrow, RN, EdD, Associate Professor, West Virginia University School of Nursing, Morgantown

Sandra C. Pendergraft, RN, MSN, Professor of Nursing, Valencia Community College, Orlando, Fla.

Patricia Peschman, RN, MS, CNN, Renal Clinical Nurse Specialist, Abbott Northwestern Hospital, Minneapolis

Lois Piano, RN, C, MSN, Assistant Professor, Gwynedd-Mercy College, Gwynedd Valley, Pa.

Margaret A. Smellie-Belfield, RN, BSN, CCRN, Clinical Services Director, SICU/PACU, Veterans Administration Medical Center, San Diego

Marilyn Sawyer Sommers, RN, PhD, CCRN, Assistant Professor, College of Nursing and Health, University of Cincinnati

Sue Svoboda, RN, MEd, Coordinator of Non-Traditional Programs, St. John's School of Nursing, Springfield, Mo.

Dolores Vaz, RN, MSN, MEd, Professor of Nursing, Bristol Community College, Fall River, Mass.

Anita L. Wynne, RN, PhD, Associate Professor, School of Nursing, University of Portland (Ore.)

Pharmacy Reviewers

Paula Castor, RPh, MHA, Director of Pharmacy Services, Moss Rehabilitation Hospital, Philadelphia

Bruce M. Frey, RPh, PharmD, Assistant Professor of Clinical Pharmacy, Philadelphia College of Pharmacy and Science; Clinical Pharmacist in Pediatrics and Neonatology, Thomas Jefferson University Hospital, Philadelphia

Jill A. Hoffman, RPh, BS, Staff Pharmacist, Presbyterian Medical Center of Philadelphia

Susanne P. Mulligan, RPh, BS, Staff Pharmacist, Presbyterian Medical Center, Philadelphia

Kathleen A. Piontkowski, RPh, BS, Staff Pharmacist, Cooper Hospital University Medical Center, Camden, N.J.

David R. Pipher, RPh, PharmD, Assistant Director for Clinical Services, Forbes Regional Health Center, Monroeville, Pa.

Joseph F. Steiner, RPh, PharmD, Professor of Clinical Pharmacy, University of Wyoming, Casper

HOW TO USE THIS BOOK

The Nurse's Handbook of Drug Therapy is an authoritative drug reference that offers nurses comprehensive drug information about virtually all clinically significant drugs and pharmacologic classes in an easy-to-use encyclopedic format.

Generic entries

Arranged alphabetically by generic name, each drug entry begins with the generic name (with alternate generic names following in parentheses) followed by a phonetic guide to pronunciation and an alphabetically arranged list of current trade names. A single dagger (†) identifies drugs available only in Canada; a double dagger (‡), drugs available only in Australia; an open diamond (◇), drugs available without a prescription. A single asterisk (*) identifies drugs whose liquid formulation may contain alcohol. This is particularly important for persons taking disulfiram (Antabuse) as part of a treatment program for alcoholism; it is also important for persons taking drugs that may elicit a disulfiram-like adverse reaction (such as metronidazole). A double asterisk (**) identifies drugs that contain tartrazine dye (FD&C Yellow No. 5), a coloring agent that can provoke a severe allergic reaction in susceptible persons. Although the incidence of tartrazine sensitivity is low (about 1 in 10,000 persons), persons with asthma or aspirin sensitivity may be at higher risk. Several drugs available solely as combinations (for example, pyrimethamine with sulfadoxine) are listed according to the first generic in the combination.

Controlled substance identifies any drug the Food and Drug Administration (FDA) lists as a controlled substance and specifies the DEA schedule of control as II, III, IV, or V. *Classification* identifies the drug's pharmacologic group.

Pregnancy risk category identifies the potential risk to the fetus. These categories, labeled A, B, C, D, or X, define a drug's potential to cause birth defects or fetal death. They are listed and explained below. Drugs in category A are usually considered safe to use in pregnancy; drugs in category X are contraindicated.

A: Adequate studies in pregnant women have failed to show a risk to the fetus in the first trimester of pregnancy, and there is no evidence of risk in later trimesters.

B: Animal studies have not shown an adverse effect on the fetus, but there are no adequate clinical studies in pregnant women.

C: Animal studies have shown an adverse effect on the fetus, but there are no adequate studies in humans. Or there are no adequate studies in animals or humans. Pregnancy risk is unknown.

D: There is evidence of risk to the human fetus, but the potential benefits of use in pregnant women may be acceptable despite potential risks.

X: Studies in animals or humans show fetal abnormalities, or adverse reaction reports indicate evidence of fetal risk. The risks involved clearly outweigh potential benefits.

How supplied lists the preparations available for each drug (for example, tablets, capsules, solution, or injection), specifying available dosage forms and strengths.

Action summarizes the drug's pharmacodynamics and pharmacokinetics. As available, information in this section includes *Mechanism, Absorption, Distribution, Metabolism, Excretion, Half-life,* and *Onset, peak, and duration.*

Indications and dosage presents all approved indications for use, with dosage recommendations for adults and children. Specific recommendations for infants, elderly patients, or other special patient groups are included when appropriate.

Contraindications and precautions lists conditions that are associated with special risks in patients who receive the drug and includes rationales for warnings.

Interactions specifies the clinically significant additive, synergistic, or antagonistic effects that result from combined use of the drug with other drugs.

Effects on diagnostic tests lists significant interference with a diagnostic test or its result by direct effects on the test itself or by systemic drug effects that lead to misleading test results.

Adverse reactions lists the undesirable effects that may follow use of the drug; these effects are arranged by body system: blood, central nervous system (CNS), cardiovascular (CV), eyes, ears, nose, throat (EENT), gastrointestinal (GI), genitourinary (GU), hepatic, metabolic, respiratory, skin, local, and other. Local effects occur at the site of drug administration (by application, infusion, or injection); adverse reactions not specific to a single body system (for example, the effects of hypersensitivity) are listed under "Other." For easy identification by the reader, common reactions are listed in italic type; life-threatening reactions, in boldface italic.

Nursing considerations follow. For special convenience to nursing students, these are organized strictly according to the nursing process—from assessment to evaluation—and include selected nursing diagnoses, detailed recommendations for supportive care, and patient teaching. Selected nursing diagnoses exemplify those most commonly applied to drug therapy. In actual use, nursing diagnoses must be relevant to an individual patient; therefore, they may not include the selected examples and may include others not listed. The Planning and Implementation section contains action-oriented recommendations for monitoring the effects of drug therapy; for preventing and treating adverse reactions; for promoting patient comfort; for preparing, administering, and storing the drug; and for teaching patients. Special instructions for drug administration—especially for I.V. use—are graphically highlighted. Nursing considerations emphasize drug-specific recommendations and, therefore, omit the repetition in each entry of the well-known universal recommendations, such as "assess the five rights of drug therapy (patient, drug, dose, time, and route) before administration" and "assess the patient's compliance with drug therapy," which apply to all drugs.

Pharmacologic class entries

Interwoven alphabetically among the generic drug entries, each pharmacologic class entry begins with a complete list of generic drugs that fall into a major pharmacologic group (for example, benzodiazepines or phenothiazines). A brief overview of pharmacology follows. Next, *Clinical indications and actions* summarizes therapeutic applications of drugs in the class. *Overview of adverse reactions* summarizes the clinically significant reactions associated with drugs in the class.

Representative combinations lists major combinations of generic drugs in the class with other generics of the same or of another class, followed by trade names of products that contain each combination of generics.

As appropriate, selected class entries include charted comparisons of dosage, uses, and adverse reactions of generic drugs in the class.

GUIDE TO ABBREVIATIONS

The following abbreviations are used repeatedly in this book:

AIDS . . . . . . acquired immunodeficiency syndrome
ALT . . . . alanine aminotransferase
AST . . . . asparate aminotransferase
ATP . . . . adenosine triphosphate
AV . . . . atrioventricular
b.i.d. . . . . . . twice daily
BUN . . . . blood urea nitrogen
cAMP . . . . . cyclic 3′,5′ adenosine monophosphate
CBC . . . . complete blood count
CHF . . . . congestive heart failure
CMV . . . . . . cytomegalovirus
CNS . . . . central nervous system
COPD . . . . . chronic obstructive pulmonary disease
CPK . . . . creatine phosphokinase
CPR . . . . cardiopulmonary resuscitation
CSF . . . . cerebrospinal fluid
CV . . . . cardiovascular
CVA . . . . cerebrovascular accident
CVP . . . . central venous pressure
DNA . . . . . . deoxyribonucleic acid
ECG . . . . electrocardiogram
EEG . . . . electroencephalogram
EENT . . . . . . eyes, ears, nose, throat
FDA . . . . Food and Drug Administration
g . . . . gram
G . . . . gauge
GI . . . . gastrointestinal
GFR . . . . glomerular filtration rate
GU genitourinary
G6PD . . . . . glucose-6-phosphate dehydrogenase
h.s. . . . . at bedtime
I.M. . . . . intramuscular
IND . . . . investigational new drug
IPPB . . . . intermittent positive-pressure breathing
ID . . . . intradermal
IU . . . . international unit
I.V. . . . . intravenous
kg . . . . kilogram
L . . . . liter
M . . . . molar
m^2 . . . . square meter
mm^3 . . . . . . cubic millimeter
MAO . . . . . . monoamine oxidase
mcg or μg . . microgram
mEq . . . . . . milliequivalent
mg . . . . milligram
MI . . . . myocardial infarction
ml . . . . milliliter
Na . . . . sodium
NaCl . . . . . . sodium chloride
ng . . . . nanogram (millimicrogram)
NSAID . . . . . nonsteroidal anti-inflammatory drug
OTC . . . . over the counter
PABA . . . . . . para-aminobenzoic acid
P.O. . . . . by mouth
P.R. . . . . by rectum
p.r.n. . . . . . . as needed
q . . . . every
q.d. . . . . every day
q.i.d. . . . . . . four times daily
RBC . . . . red blood cell
RDA . . . . recommended daily allowance
REM . . . . . . rapid eye movement
RNA . . . . . . ribonucleic acid
RSV . . . . respiratory syncytial virus
SA . . . . sinoatrial
S.C. . . . . subcutaneous
SGOT . . . . . . serum glutamic oxaloacetic transaminase
SGPT . . . . . . serum glutamic pyruvic transaminase
SHBG . . . . . . sex hormone-binding globulin
SIADH . . . . . syndrome of inappropriate antidiuretic hormone
S.L. . . . . sublingual
t.i.d. . . . . . . three times daily
UCE . . . . urea cycle enzymopathy
USP . . . . United States Pharmacopeia
WBC . . . . . . white blood cell

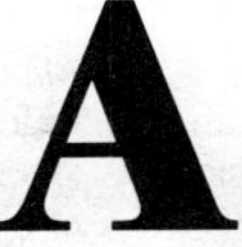

acebutolol

(a se byoo´ toe lole)
Monitan†, Sectral

• *Classification:* antihypertensive, antiarrhythmic (beta-adrenergic blocking agent)
• *Pregnancy Risk Category:* B

HOW SUPPLIED

Capsules: 200 mg, 400 mg

ACTION

Mechanism: Decreases heart rate and myocardial contractility. It has mild intrinsic sympathomimetic activity.
Absorption: Well absorbed after oral administration, but undergoes extensive first-pass metabolism in the liver.
Distribution: About 26% is protein-bound; minimal quantities are detected in CSF.
Metabolism: In the liver to active and inactive metabolites.
Excretion: From 30% to 40% of a dose is excreted in urine; the remainder in feces and bile. Half-life: Of acebutolol, about 3 to 4 hours; diacetolol, 8 to 13 hours.
Onset, peak, duration: Peak plasma levels occur at about 2½ hours. Peak levels of diacetolol, the major active metabolite, occur at about 3½ hours.

INDICATIONS & DOSAGE

Treatment of hypertension–
Adults: 400 mg P.O. either as a single daily dosage or divided b.i.d. Patients may receive as much as 1,200 mg daily.
Ventricular arrhythmias–
Adults: 400 mg P.O. daily divided b.i.d. Dosage is then increased to provide an adequate clinical response. Usual dosage is 600 to 1,200 mg daily.

CONTRAINDICATIONS & PRECAUTIONS

Contraindicated in patients with hypersensitivity to the drug; in patients with persistent severe bradycardia or overt cardiac failure because drug may worsen these conditions; and in patients with second- or third-degree atrioventricular block or cardiogenic shock.

Use cautiously in patients with impaired hepatic or renal function (decrease dosage if creatinine clearance falls below 50 ml/minute); coronary insufficiency because beta-adrenergic blockade may precipitate congestive heart failure; diabetes mellitus or hyperthyroidism because acebutolol may mask tachycardia (but not dizziness or sweating) caused by hypoglycemia or hyperthyroidism; and, bronchospastic diseases, such as asthma or emphysema, because higher doses of the drug may inhibit bronchodilating effects of endogenous catecholamines.

ADVERSE REACTIONS

Common reactions are in italics; life-threatening reactions are in bold italics.
CNS: *fatigue,* headache, dizziness, insomnia.
CV: chest pain, edema, bradycardia, CHF, *hypotension.*
GI: nausea, constipation, diarrhea, dyspepsia.
Metabolic: hypoglycemia without tachycardia.
Respiratory: dyspnea, ***bronchospasm.***
Skin: rash.
Other: fever.

INTERACTIONS

Digitalis glycosides: excessive bradycardia and increased depressant effect on myocardium. Use together cautiously.
Indomethacin: decreased antihypertensive effect. Monitor blood pressure and adjust dosage.
Insulin, hypoglycemic drugs (oral): can alter dosage requirements in previously stabilized diabetics. Observe patient carefully.

EFFECTS ON DIAGNOSTIC TESTS

ANA: positive titers

NURSING CONSIDERATIONS

Besides those related universally to drug therapy (see "How to use this book"), consider the following specific recommendations:

Assessment

• Obtain a baseline assessment of the patient's blood pressure before therapy.
• Be alert for adverse reactions and drug interactions throughout therapy.
• Evaluate the patient's and family's knowledge about acebutolol therapy.

Nursing Diagnoses

• High risk for injury related to the patient's underlying condition.
• Fatigue related to acebutolol induced CNS adverse reaction.
• Knowledge deficit related to acebutolol therapy.

Planning and Implementation

Preparation and Administration

• Be aware that dosage should be reduced in patients with decreased renal function and that elderly patients may require lower doses. For such patients, dosage should not exceed 800 mg daily.
• Always check patient's apical pulse before giving this drug; if slower than 60 beats/minute, hold drug and call doctor.
• Do not discontinue abruptly; can exacerbate angina and myocardial infarction.

Monitoring

• Monitor effectiveness by regularly assessing the patient's blood pressure and pulse rate.
• Monitor thyroid function studies and blood glucose levels in patients with hyperthyroidism and diabetes mellitus (especially insulin-dependent patients) respectively as drug may mask the signs of hyperthyroidism and hyperglycemia, and potentiate insulin-induced hypoglycemia.

Supportive Care

• Keep glucagon and a source of rapid-acting carbohydrate nearby. Be prepared to treat insulin-induced hypoglycemia immediately. Follow treatment with a complex carbohydrate snack and notify doctor so that appropriate dosage adjustment can be made.
• Schedule patient's activities to provide frequent rest periods if the patient experiences fatigue.
• Before surgery, notify anesthesiologist that patient is receiving this drug.

Patient Teaching

• Teach patient how to take his pulse and instruct him to withhold the dose and notify doctor if pulse rate is below 60 beats/minute.
• Warn patient that drug may cause dizziness. Instruct patient to avoid sudden postural changes and to sit down immediately if he feels dizzy.
• Explain the importance of taking this drug as prescribed, even when feeling well.
• Warn patient not to discontinue drug suddenly, but to notify the doctor of unpleasant adverse reactions.
• Instruct the patient to check with the doctor or pharmacist before taking any OTC medications.
• Warn patient that drug may cause fatigue and instruct patient how to prevent fatigue.

Evaluation
In patients receiving acebutolol, appropriate evaluation statements may include:
• Patient's blood pressure is within normal limits.
• Patient does not experience fatigue throughout acebutolol therapy.
• Patient and family state an understanding of acebutolol therapy.

acetaminophen (paracetamol)
(a set a mee´ noe fen)
Acephen◇, Aceta*◇, Ace-Tabs†◇, Acetaminophen Unicerts◇, Actamin◇, Actamin Extra◇, Anacin-3◇, Anacin-3 Maximum Strength◇, Anuphen◇, Apacet◇, Apacet Extra Strength◇, Apacet Oral Solution◇, APAP◇, Apo-Acetaminophen†◇, Atasol†◇, Atasol Forte†◇, Banesin◇, Campain†◇, Ceetamol‡, Children's Anacin-3◇, Children's Apacet◇, Children's Genapap◇, Children's Panadol◇, Children's Tylenol◇, Children's Ty-PAP◇, Children's Ty-Tabs◇, Dapa◇, Datril◇, Datril Extra Strength◇, Dolanex*◇, Dymadon‡, Exdol†◇, Exdol Strong†◇, Genapap◇, Genebs◇, Genebs Extra Strength◇, Gentabs◇, Halenol◇, Infant's Anacin-3◇, Infant's Apacet◇, Infant's Tylenol◇, Infant's Ty-PAP◇, Junior Disprol‡, Liquiprin◇, Meda Cap◇, Meda Tab◇, Myapap◇, Neopap◇, Oraphen-PD◇, Panadol◇, Panadol Junior Strength◇, Panamax‡, Panex◇, Paraphen†◇, Parmol‡, Pedric*◇, Phenaphen◇, Robigesic†◇, Rounox†◇, Suppap◇, Tapanol◇, Tapanol Extra Strength◇, Tempra◇, Tenol◇, Ty Caplets◇, Ty Caps◇, Tylenol*, Tylenol Extra Strength◇, Ty Tabs◇, Valadol*◇, Valorin◇

• *Classification:* nonnarcotic analgesic, antipyretic agent (para-aminophenol derivative)
• *Pregnancy Risk Category:* B

HOW SUPPLIED
Tablets: 160 mg◇, 325 mg◇, 500 mg◇, 650 mg◇
Tablets (chewable): 80 mg◇
Capsules: 325 mg◇, 500 mg◇
Oral solution: 100 mg/ml◇
Oral suspension: 120 mg/5 ml‡
Oral liquid: 160 mg/5 ml◇, 500 mg/15 ml◇
Elixir: 120 mg/5 ml◇*, 160 mg/5 ml◇*, 320 mg/5 ml◇*
Wafers: 120 mg◇
Effervescent granules: 325 mg/capful◇
Suppositories: 120 mg◇, 125 mg◇, 135 mg◇, 650 mg◇

ACTION
Mechanism: Produces analgesia by inhibition of prostaglandin synthesis, and possible inhibition of the synthesis or action of other substances that sensitize pain receptors to stimulation. Relieves fever by central action in the hypothalamic heat-regulating center.
Absorption: Rapidly and completely absorbed from the GI tract.
Distribution: The drug is 25% protein-bound. Plasma concentrations correlate well with toxicity but not with analgesic effect.
Metabolism: Approximately 90% to 95% is metabolized in the liver.
Excretion: Excreted in urine. Half-life: 1 to 4 hours. In acute overdose, half-life is prolonged and correlated with toxic effects; half-life over 4 hours is associated with hepatic necrosis; over 12 hours with coma.
Onset, peak, duration: Peak plasma concentrations occur in 30 minutes to 2 hours, slightly faster for liquid preparations.

INDICATIONS & DOSAGE
Mild pain or fever—
Adults and children over 11 years: 325 to 650 mg P.O. or rectally q 4 hours; or 1 g P.O. q.i.d. p.r.n. Maximum dosage should not exceed 4 g

daily. Dosage for long-term therapy should not exceed 2.6 g daily.
Children 11 years: 480 mg/dose.
Children 9 to 10 years: 400 mg/dose.
Children 6 to 8 years: 320 mg/dose.
Children 4 to 5 years: 240 mg/dose.
Children 2 to 3 years: 160 mg/dose.
Children 12 to 23 months: 120 mg/dose.
Children 4 to 11 months: 80 mg/dose.
Children up to 3 months: 40 mg/dose.

CONTRAINDICATIONS & PRECAUTIONS

Contraindicated in patients with hypersensitivity to this compound. Use drug cautiously in patients with anemia or hepatic or renal disease because it has been known to induce these disorders; and in patients with a history of GI disease, increased risk of GI bleeding, or decreased renal function. May mask the signs and symptoms of acute infection (fever, myalgia, erythema); patients with high infection risk (such as those with diabetes) should be carefully evaluated.

ADVERSE REACTIONS

Common reactions are in italics; life-threatening reactions are in bold italics.
Hepatic: ***severe liver damage with toxic doses.***
Skin: rash, urticaria.

INTERACTIONS

Diflunisal: increases acetaminophen blood levels. Don't use together.
Ethanol: increased risk of hepatic damage.
Warfarin: increased hypoprothrombinemic effect with chronic acetaminophen use.

EFFECTS ON DIAGNOSTIC TESTS

Urine 5-HIAA: false-positive results.

NURSING CONSIDERATIONS

Besides those related universally to drug therapy (see "How to use this book"), consider the following specific recommendations:

Assessment
- Obtain a baseline assessment of the patient's pain, temperature, or cardiovascular condition before therapy.
- Be alert for adverse reactions and drug interactions throughout therapy.
- Evaluate the patient's and family's knowledge about acetaminophen therapy.

Nursing Diagnoses
- Pain related to the patient's underlying condition.
- High risk for injury related to acetaminophen-induced liver damage with toxic doses.
- Knowledge deficit related to acetaminophen therapy.

Planning and Implementation

Preparation and Administration
- ***P.O. use:*** Administer the liquid form to children and other patients who have difficulty swallowing.

Monitoring
- Monitor effectiveness by regularly evaluating relief of pain or fever.
- Monitor liver function studies regularly in the patient receiving large doses of the drug.
- Observe closely for liver toxicity (change in mental status, jaundice) in patients with liver disease or history of alcohol abuse.

Supportive Care
- Hold drug and notify the doctor if the patient develops skin rash, urticaria, or any sign of liver damage (jaundice, change in mental status).

Patient Teaching
- Warn the patient that high dosage, unsupervised chronic use, or excessive ingestion of alcoholic beverages can lead to liver damage.
- Advise the patient not to self-medicate for marked pain or fever (over 103.1° F [39.5° C]), pain or fever that persists longer than 3 days, or recurrent fever unless directed by doctor.
- Tell the patient to notify the doctor

*Liquid form contains alcohol. **May contain tartrazine.

if acetaminophen fails to relieve pain or fever.

• Tell the patient that many OTC medications contain acetaminophen. If taking such medications, patient must consider this when calculating total daily dosage of the acetaminophen.

Evaluation

In patients receiving acetaminophen, appropriate evaluation statements may include:

• Patient reports relief of pain after acetaminophen use.

• Patient's liver function studies remain normal.

• Patient and family state an understanding of acetaminophen therapy.

acetazolamide

(a set a zole´ a mide)

Acetazolam†, Ak-Zol, Apo-Acetazolamide†, Dazamide, Diamox, Diamox Sequels, Storzolamide

acetazolamide sodium

Diamox Parenteral, Diamox Sodium†

• *Classification:* adjunctive treatment for open-angle glaucoma, perioperative treatment for acute angle-closure glaucoma, anticonvulsant, management of edema, prevention and treatment of high-altitude sickness (carbonic anhydrase inhibitor)

• *Pregnancy Risk Category:* C

HOW SUPPLIED

Tablets: 125 mg, 250 mg

Capsules (extended-release): 500 mg

Injection: 500 mg/vial

ACTION

Mechanism: Blocks the action of carbonic anhydrase, an enzyme that catalyzes the formation of hydrogen and bicarbonate ions from carbon dioxide and water. It promotes the renal excretion of sodium, potassium, bicarbonate, and water; bicarbonate ion excretion makes the urine alkaline. May promote the development of metabolic acidosis. Also decreases secretion of aqueous humor in the eye, thereby lowering intraocular pressure. Anticonvulsant effects may be related to metabolic acidosis or inhibition of carbonic anhydrase in the CNS. Elevating carbon dioxide tension in the CNS may decrease abnormal neuronal discharge.

Absorption: Well absorbed from the GI tract after oral administration.

Distribution: Throughout body tissues.

Metabolism: None.

Excretion: Primarily in urine via tubular secretion and passive reabsorption.

Onset, peak, duration: Peak plasma levels are seen in 1 to 3 hours after an oral dose.

INDICATIONS & DOSAGE

Narrow-angle glaucoma–

Adults: 250 mg q 4 hours; or 250 mg P.O., I.M., or I.V. b.i.d. for short-term therapy.

Edema in congestive heart failure–

Adults: 250 to 375 mg P.O., I.M., or I.V. daily in a.m.

Children: 5 mg/kg daily in a.m.

Open-angle glaucoma–

Adults: 250 mg daily to 1 g P.O., I.M., or I.V. divided q.i.d.

Prevention or amelioration of acute mountain sickness–

Adults: 250 mg P.O. q 8 to 12 hours.

Myoclonic, refractory generalized tonic-clonic (grand mal) or absence (petit mal), or mixed seizures–

Adults: 375 mg P.O., I.M., or I.V. daily up to 250 mg q.i.d. Alternatively, use sustained-release form 250 to 500 mg P.O. daily or b.i.d. Initial dosage when used with other anticonvulsants usually is 250 mg daily.

Children: 8 to 30 mg/kg P.O. daily, divided t.i.d. or q.i.d. Maximum dosage is 1.5 g daily, or 300 to 900 mg/ m^2 daily.

CONTRAINDICATIONS & PRECAUTIONS

Contraindicated in patients with hepatic insufficiency because the drug may precipitate hepatic coma; low potassium or sodium concentration level or hyperchloremic acidosis because it may worsen electrolyte imbalance; and severe renal impairment because nephrotoxicity has been reported.

Use cautiously in patients with respiratory acidosis or other severe respiratory problems because the drug may produce acidosis; diabetes because it may cause hyperglycemia and glycosuria; in patients taking cardiac glycosides because they are more susceptible to digitalis toxicity from acetazolamide-induced hypokalemia; and in patients taking diuretics.

ADVERSE REACTIONS

Common reactions are in italics; life-threatening reactions are in bold italics.

Blood: ***aplastic anemia,*** hemolytic anemia, leukopenia.

CNS: drowsiness, paresthesias, confusion.

EENT: transient myopia.

GI: nausea, vomiting, anorexia.

GU: crystalluria, renal calculi, hematuria.

Metabolic: *hyperchloremic acidosis,* hypokalemia, asymptomatic hyperuricemia.

Skin: rash.

Local: *pain at injection site,* sterile abscesses.

INTERACTIONS

None significant.

EFFECTS ON DIAGNOSTIC TESTS

Thyroid function tests: decreased iodine uptake.

Urine protein: false-positive proteinuria (with Albutrix or Albutest).

NURSING CONSIDERATIONS

Besides those related universally to drug therapy (see "How to use this book"), consider the following specific recommendations:

Assessment

- Obtain a baseline assessment of patient's underlying condition, including, as appropriate, eye discomfort and intraocular pressure in patients with glaucoma; edema in patient with signs and symptoms of CHF; neurological status in patient with seizures, before initiating acetazolamide therapy.
- Be alert for adverse reactions and drug interactions throughout therapy.
- Evaluate the patient's and family's knowledge about acetazolamide therapy.

Nursing Diagnoses

- Fluid volume excess related to the patient's underlying condition.
- Altered urinary elimination related to diuretic action (frequency, urgency) of drug.
- Knowledge deficit related to acetazolamide therapy.

Planning and Implementation

Preparation and Administration

- Give P.O. or I.M. preparations early in the morning to avoid nocturia. Give second doses in early afternoon.
- Be aware that diuretic effect is decreased when acidosis occurs but can be reestablished by withdrawing drug as prescribed for several days and then restarting, or by using intermittent administration schedule as ordered.
- Reconstitute 500-mg vial with at least 5 ml sterile water for injection. Use within 24 hours of reconstitution.
- ***P.O. use:*** To make an oral liquid, soften 1 tablet in 2 teaspoons of very warm water and add to 2 teaspoons honey or syrup (chocolate or cherry). Don't use fruit juice.
- ***I.M. use:*** Be aware that I.M. injec-

*Liquid form contains alcohol. **May contain tartrazine.

tion is painful because of alkalinity of solution.
• ***I.V. use:*** Administer direct I.V. using a 21G or 23G needle, inject 100 to 500 mg/minute into a large vein. Intermittent or continuous infusion is not recommended.

Monitoring

• Monitor effectiveness by regularly assessing patient for signs of improvement.
• Monitor urine output, blood pressure, presence of peripheral edema, and quality of breath sounds when drug is used to treat CHF.
• Monitor weight daily. Be aware that rapid or excessive fluid loss causes weight loss and hypotension.
• Monitor elderly patients closely because they are especially susceptible to excessive diuresis.
• Monitor for signs of hypokalemia (muscle weakness and cramping).
• Monitor serum electrolytes, especially potassium, and BUN levels.
• Monitor vital signs: hypotension, dyspnea, tachycardia, and fever may indicate dehydration.
• In the patient with gout, monitor serum uric acid.
• Monitor skin turgor and mucous membranes for signs of fluid volume depletion.

Supportive Care

• Hold drug and notify the doctor if hypersensitivity or adverse reactions occur.
• Keep accurate record of intake and output.
• Elevate the patient's legs to aid decrease of peripheral edema if present.
• Encourage diet low in sodium and high in potassium.
• Provide frequent skin and mouth care to relieve dryness due to diuretic therapy.
• Answer the patient's call bells promptly; make sure patient's bathroom or bed pan are easily accessible.
• Use safety precautions to avoid risk of falls due to hypotension.

Patient Teaching

• Teach the patient to monitor fluid volume by daily weight and intake and output.
• Encourage the patient to avoid foods high in sodium and to choose foods high in potassium.
• Advise the patient to take drug early in the day to avoid interruption of sleep by nocturia.
• Instruct patient how to recognize signs and symptoms of fluid and electrolyte imbalance and to notify doctor if they occur.

Evaluation

In patients receiving acetazolamide, appropriate evaluation statements may include:
• Patient is free of edema.
• Patient demonstrates adjustment of life-style to deal with altered patterns of urinary elimination.
• Patient and family state an understanding of acetazolamide therapy.

acetohexamide

(a set oh hex′ a mide)
Dimelor†, Dymelor

• *Classification:* antidiabetic agent (sulfonylurea)
• *Pregnancy Risk Category:* D

HOW SUPPLIED

Tablets: 250 mg, 500 mg

ACTION

Mechanism: A sulfonylurea that lowers blood glucose by stimulating insulin release from the pancreatic beta cells and reducing glucose output by the liver. An extrapancreatic effect increases peripheral sensitivity to insulin.
Absorption: Rapidly absorbed from the GI tract.
Distribution: Not fully understood,

but is probably similar to that of the other sulfonylureas; drug is highly protein-bound.
Metabolism: In the liver, primarily to a potent active metabolite.
Excretion: Primarily (80%) in urine. Half-life: Approximately 6 hours.
Onset, peak, duration: Onset of action within 1 hour, with a maximum decrease in serum glucose levels within 2 hours; duration of action is 12 to 24 hours.

INDICATIONS & DOSAGE

Adjunct to diet to lower the blood glucose in patients with non-insulin-dependent diabetes mellitus (type II)–
Adults: initially, 250 mg P.O. daily before breakfast; may increase dosage q 5 to 7 days (by 250 to 500 mg) as needed to maximum of 1.5 g daily, divided b.i.d. to t.i.d. before meals.
To replace insulin therapy–
Adults: if insulin dosage is less than 20 units daily, insulin may be stopped and oral therapy started with 250 mg P.O. daily, before breakfast, increased as above if needed. If insulin dosage is 20 to 40 units daily, start oral therapy with 250 mg P.O. daily, before breakfast, while reducing insulin dosage 25% to 30% daily or every other day, depending on response to oral therapy.

CONTRAINDICATIONS & PRECAUTIONS

Contraindicated in patients with hypersensitivity to sulfonylureas or thiazides; burns, acidosis, diabetic coma, severe infection, ketosis, severe trauma, or major surgery because such conditions of severe physiologic stress require insulin for adequate control of serum glucose levels; and nonfunctioning beta cells.

Use with caution in patients with hepatic or renal insufficiency because it is metabolized in the liver and excreted in urine; and in those with adrenal, pituitary, or thyroid dysfunction.

ADVERSE REACTIONS

Common reactions are in italics; life-threatening reactions are in bold italics.
GI: nausea, heartburn, vomiting.
Metabolic: sodium loss, *hypoglycemia.*
Skin: rash, pruritus, facial flushing.
Other: hypersensitivity reactions.

INTERACTIONS

Anabolic steroids, chloramphenicol, clofibrate, guanethidine, MAO inhibitors, oral anticoagulants, phenylbutazone, salicylates, sulfonamides: increased hypoglycemic activity. Monitor blood glucose level.
Beta blockers, clonidine: prolonged hypoglycemic effect and masked symptoms of hypoglycemia. Use together cautiously.
Corticosteroids, glucagon, rifampin, thiazide diuretics: decreased hypoglycemic response. Monitor blood glucose level.

EFFECTS ON DIAGNOSTIC TESTS

Serum uric acid concentration, cholesterol, alkaline phosphatase, bilirubin, and BUN: altered levels.

NURSING CONSIDERATIONS

Besides those related universally to drug therapy (see "How to use this book"), consider the following specific recommendations:

Assessment

- Obtain a baseline assessment of the patient's blood glucose level before initiating acetohexamide therapy.
- Be alert for adverse reactions and drug interactions throughout therapy.
- Evaluate the patient's and family's knowledge about acetohexamide therapy.

Nursing Diagnoses

- Altered nutrition: More than body requirements related to the patient's inability to release sufficient insulin

to maintain normal blood glucose levels.
• High risk for injury related to acetohexamide-induced hypoglycemia.
• Knowledge deficit related to acetohexamide therapy.

Planning and Implementation

Preparation and Administration
• Consider that some patients taking drug may be controlled effectively on a once-daily regimen, whereas others show better response with divided dosing.
• ***P.O. use:*** Administer once-daily doses with breakfast; divided doses are usually given before the morning and evening meals.

Monitoring
• Monitor effectiveness by regularly checking patient's blood glucose levels. Monitor blood glucose levels more frequently if the patient is under stress, having difficulty controlling blood glucose levels or is newly diagnosed.
• Monitor for signs and symptoms of both hyperglycemia and hypoglycemia; note time and circumstances of each reaction.
• Monitor the patient's hemoglobin A1C regularly as ordered.
• Monitor the patient for cardiovascular dysfunction because sulfonylureas have been associated with an increased risk of cardiovascular mortality as compared to diet or diet and insulin therapy.

Supportive Care
• Notify the doctor if blood glucose levels remain elevated or frequent episodes of hypoglycemia occur.
• Treat a hypoglycemic reaction with an oral form of rapid-acting glucose if the patient is awake or with glucagon or I.V. glucose if the patient cannot be aroused. Follow up treatment with a complex carbohydrate snack when patient is awake, and determine cause of reaction.
• Be sure other treatment measures, such as diet and exercise programs, are being used appropriately.
• Discuss with the doctor how to deal with noncompliance.
• Patients transferring from insulin therapy to an oral antidiabetic requires blood glucose monitoring at least t.i.d. before meals. Patient may require hospitalization during transition.

Patient Teaching
• Emphasize the importance of following the prescribed diet, exercise, and medical regimens.
• Tell the patient to take the medication at the same time each day. If a dose is missed, it should be taken immediately, unless it's almost time for the next dose. Instruct the patient not to take double doses.
• Advise the patient to avoid alcohol while taking drug. Remind him that many foods and nonprescription medications contain alcohol.
• Encourage the patient to wear a medical alert bracelet or necklace.
• Tell the patient to take drug with food; once-daily dosage should be taken with breakfast.
• Teach the patient how to monitor blood glucose levels as prescribed.
• Teach the patient how to recognize the signs and symptoms of hyperglycemia and hypoglycemia and what to do if they occur.
• Stress the importance of compliance and close follow-up with drug therapy.

Evaluation

In patients receiving acetohexamide, appropriate evaluation statements may include:
• Patient's blood glucose level is normal.
• Patient recognizes hypoglycemia early and treats hypoglycemic episodes effectively before injury occurs.
• Patient and family express an understanding of acetohexamide therapy.

acetylcysteine
(a se teel sis´ tay een)
Airbron†, Mucomyst, Mucosol, Parvolex†‡

• *Classification:* mucolytic agent, antidote for acetaminophen overdose (amino acid)
• *Pregnancy Risk Category:* B

HOW SUPPLIED
Solution: 10%, 20%
Injection: 200 mg/ml†‡

ACTION
Mechanism: Increases production of respiratory tract fluids to help liquefy and reduce the viscosity of thick, tenacious secretions. Also restores liver stores of glutathione in the treatment of acetaminophen toxicity.
Absorption: Most inhaled acetylcysteine acts directly on the mucus in the lungs; the remainder is absorbed by pulmonary epithelium. After oral administration, the drug is absorbed from the GI tract.
Metabolism: In the liver.
Onset, peak, duration: Mucolytic effect begins within 1 minute after inhalation, and immediately upon direct intratracheal instillation; peak effect occurs within 5 to 10 minutes.

INDICATIONS & DOSAGE
Pneumonia, bronchitis, tuberculosis, cystic fibrosis, emphysema, atelectasis (adjunct), complications of thoracic surgery and CV surgery–
Adults and children: 1 to 2 ml 10% to 20% solution by direct instillation into trachea as often as every hour; or 3 to 5 ml 20% solution, or 6 to 10 ml 10% solution, by mouthpiece t.i.d. or q.i.d.
Acetaminophen toxicity–
Adults and children: 140 mg/kg initially P.O., followed by 70 mg/kg q 4 hours for 17 doses (a total of 1,330 mg/kg).

CONTRAINDICATIONS & PRECAUTIONS
Contraindicated in patients with hypersensitivity to the drug; however, it may be given to hypersensitive patients to treat acetaminophen overdose if the allergic symptoms are controlled. Use cautiously in patients with asthma because bronchospasm may occur; if it does, discontinue immediately. Also use cautiously in elderly or debilitated patients with respiratory insufficiency because it may increase airway obstruction; and in all patients with inadequate cough because secretions may occlude airways.

ADVERSE REACTIONS
Common reactions are in italics; life-threatening reactions are in bold italics.
EENT: *rhinorrhea, hemoptysis.*
GI: *stomatitis, nausea.*
Other: ***bronchospasm*** *(especially in asthmatics).*

INTERACTIONS
Activated charcoal: don't use together in treating acetaminophen toxicity. Limits acetylcysteine's effectiveness.

EFFECTS ON DIAGNOSTIC TESTS
None reported.

NURSING CONSIDERATIONS
Besides those related universally to drug therapy, (see "How to use this book"), consider the following specific recommendations:
Assessment
• Obtain a baseline assessment of the patient's respiratory secretions before initiating therapy.
• Be alert for adverse reactions and drug interactions throughout therapy.
• Evaluate the patient's and family's knowledge about acetylcysteine therapy.

Nursing Diagnoses
• Ineffective airway clearance related to the patient's underlying condition.
• Altered oral mucous membrane related to acetylcysteine-induced stomatitis.
• Knowledge deficit related to acetylcysteine therapy.

Planning and Implementation
Preparation and Administration
• ***Nebulization:*** Use plastic, glass, stainless steel, or another nonreactive metal when administering the medication by nebulization. Hand bulb nebulizers are not recommended because output is too small and particle size too large. Before aerosol administration, instruct the patient to clear the airway by coughing. Be aware that acetylcysteine may have a foul taste or smell that the patient may find distressing.
• After opening acetylcysteine, store it in the refrigerator and use it within 96 hours.
• Have suction equipment available for the patient, who may have difficulty effectively clearing his air passages.
• ***P.O. use:*** Dilute oral doses with cola, fruit juice, or water before administering. If patient vomits within 1 hour of administration, repeat the dose.
Monitoring
• Monitor effectiveness by regularly evaluating sputum production and characteristics.
• Monitor respiratory function closely for bronchospasms.
• Monitor hydration status; record intake and output.
• Monitor the patient's oral mucous membranes for signs of stomatitis (swollen gums, ulcers in mouth and throat).
Supportive Care
• Provide necessary tissues and waste receptacles for disposal of expectorated respiratory secretions.
• Provide for good oral hygiene for the patient receiving acetylcysteine. If stomatitis develops, alert the doctor and provide supportive care: warm water mouth rinses (antiseptic mouthwashes are contraindicated because they are irritating), application of a topical anesthetic to relieve mouth ulcer pain, and a bland or liquid diet.
• Alert the doctor if patient's respiratory secretions thicken or become purulent, or if bronchospasms occur.
• Obtain an order for an antiemetic if nausea is severe.
Patient Teaching
• Instruct the patient to follow the directions on the medication label exactly. Explain the importance of not taking more of the drug than directed.
• Tell the patient to monitor the type and frequency of his cough and to notify his doctor if the medication has not improved his condition within 10 days. This drug should not be used for prolonged periods unless the patient is under direct medical supervision.
• Tell the patient to increase fluid intake to at least 8 full (8-oz) glasses of fluid per day.
• Encourage the patient to do deep-breathing exercises. The patient should sit properly in a straight chair, take several deep breaths, and then attempt to cough.
• Advise the patient to avoid sources of respiratory irritants, such as fumes, smoke, and dust.
• Teach patient correct use of the nebulizer.
• Warn the patient of unpleasant odor (rotten egg odor of hydrogen sulfide) and explain that increased amounts of liquefied bronchial secretion plus unpleasant odor may cause nausea and vomiting; have the patient rinse mouth with water after nebulizer treatment because it may leave a sticky coating on the oral cavity.

Evaluation
In patients receiving acetylcysteine, appropriate evaluation statements may include:
• Patient's lung sounds are clear with decreased respiratory secretions and decreased frequency and severity of cough.
• Patient's oral mucous membranes remain unchanged with acetylcysteine therapy.
• Patient and family state an understanding of acetylcysteine therapy.

activated charcoal

Actidose-Aqua◇, Charcoaide◇, Charcocaps◇, Liqui-Char◇, Superchar◇

• *Classification:* antidote, antidiarrheal, antiflatulent (adsorbent)
• *Pregnancy Risk Category:* C

HOW SUPPLIED

Tablets: 200 mg‡◇, 300 mg‡◇, 325 mg◇, 650 mg◇
Capsules: 260 mg◇
Powder: 30 g◇, 50 g◇
Oral suspension: 0.625 g/5 ml◇, 0.83 g/5 ml◇, 1 g/5 ml◇,1.25 g/5 ml◇

ACTION

Mechanism: Adsorbs many drugs and chemicals, inhibiting their absorption from the GI tract.
Absorption: Not absorbed from the GI tract.
Excretion: In feces.

INDICATIONS & DOSAGE

Flatulence or dyspepsia–
Adults: 600 mg to 5 g P.O. t.i.d. or q.i.d.
Poisoning–
Adults: initially, 1g/kg (30 to 100 g) P.O. or 5 to 10 times the amount of poison ingested as a suspension in 180 to 240 ml of water.
Children: 5 to 10 times estimated weight of drug or chemical ingested. Minimum dose is 30 g P.O. in 250 ml water to make a slurry. Give orally, preferably within 30 minutes of poisoning. Larger dose is necessary if food is in the stomach. For treating poisoning or overdosage with acetaminophen, amphetamines, aspirin, antimony, atropine, arsenic, barbiturates, camphor, cocaine, cardiac glycosides, glutethimide, ipecac, malathion, morphine, poisonous mushrooms, opium, oxalic acid, parathion, phenol, phenothiazines, potassium permanganate, propoxyphene, quinine, strychnine, sulfonamides, or tricyclic antidepressants.

CONTRAINDICATIONS & PRECAUTIONS

Contraindicated in patients with poisoning resulting from ingestion of cyanide, mineral acids, strong bases, methanol, and ethanol because it is relatively ineffective. It may produce vomiting, or may obstruct endoscopic evaluation of GI lesions.

ADVERSE REACTIONS

Common reactions are in italics; life-threatening reactions are in bold italics.
GI: black stools, nausea.

INTERACTIONS

Acetylcysteine, ipecac: rendered ineffective. Don't administer together or lavage stomach until all charcoal is removed.

EFFECTS ON DIAGNOSTIC TESTS

None reported.

NURSING CONSIDERATIONS

Besides those related universally to drug therapy (see "How to use this book"), consider the following specific recommendations:
Assessment
• Obtain a baseline assessment of circumstances surrounding situation,

substance reportedly ingested, mental and respiratory status before therapy.
• Be alert for adverse reactions and drug interactions throughout therapy.
• Evaluate the patient's and family's knowledge about activated charcoal therapy.

Nursing Diagnoses
• High risk for injury related to ingestion of poisonous substance.
• High risk for fluid volume deficit related to activated charcoal-induced nausea.
• Knowledge deficit related to activated charcoal therapy.

Planning and Implementation

Preparation and Administration
• ***P.O. use:*** Powder form is most effective. Mix with tap water to form consistency of thick syrup. May add small amount of fruit juice or flavoring to make more palatable.
• Do not give in ice cream, milk, or sherbet. Reduces absorptive capacity.
• Repeat dose if patient vomits shortly after administration.
• Space doses at least 1 hour apart from other drugs if activated charcoal is being used for any indication other than poisoning.

Monitoring
• Monitor effectiveness by observing the patient for toxic effects.
• Observe for signs of respiratory difficulty.
• Monitor vital signs frequently until stable.
• Monitor intake and output.
• Monitor neurological status.

Supportive Care
• Do not give to semiconscious or unconscious persons unless airway is protected. Can be given by nasogastric tube after lavage.
• Because activated charcoal absorbs and inactivates syrup of ipecac, give only after emesis is complete.
• Keep an airway, oxygen, and suction equipment nearby.

Patient Teaching
• Instruct patient and family to report respiratory difficulty or changes in mental status immediately.
• If patient is alert, encourage sufficient fluid intake to prevent fluid volume deficit.
• Warn patient that feces will be black after administration of activated charcoal.

Evaluation
In patients receiving activated charcoal, appropriate evaluation statements may include:
• Patient remains free from adverse effects of substance ingested.
• Patient exhibits no signs of fluid volume deficit.
• Patient and family state an understanding of activated charcoal therapy.

acyclovir sodium (systemic)

(ay sye´ kloe ver)
Zovirax

• *Classification:* antiviral agent
• *Pregnancy Risk Category:* C

HOW SUPPLIED

Capsules: 200 mg
Injection: 500 mg/vial

ACTION

Mechanism: Becomes incorporated into viral DNA and inhibits viral multiplication.
Absorption: Slow and incomplete with oral administration; not affected by food.
Distribution: Widely distributed to organ tissues and body fluids. CSF concentrations equal approximately 50% of serum concentrations. About 9% to 33% of a dose binds to plasma proteins.
Metabolism: Metabolized inside the viral cell to its active form. Approxi-

mately 10% of a dose is metabolized extracellularly.
Excretion: Up to 92% of systemically absorbed acyclovir is excreted as unchanged drug by the kidneys by glomerular filtration and tubular secretion. Half-life: In patients with normal renal function, half-life is 2 to 3½ hours. Renal failure may extend half-life to 19 hours.
Onset, peak, duration: Peak concentrations occur in 1½ to 2 hours.

INDICATIONS & DOSAGE

Treatment of initial and recurrent episodes of mucocutaneous herpes simplex virus (HSV-1 and HSV-2) infections in immunocompromised patients; severe initial episodes of herpes genitalis in patients who are not immunocompromised–
Adults and children over 11 years: 5 mg/kg, given at a constant rate over a period of 1 hour by I.V. infusion q 8 hours for 7 days (5 days for herpes genitalis).
Children under 12 years: 250 mg/m², given at a constant rate over a period of 1 hour by I.V. infusion q 8 hours for 7 days (5 days for herpes genitalis).
Treatment of initial genital herpes–
Adults: 200 mg P.O. q 4 hours while awake (a total of 5 capsules daily). Treatment should continue for 10 days.
Intermittent therapy for recurrent genital herpes–
Adults: 200 mg P.O. q 4 hours while awake (a total of 5 capsules daily). Treatment should continue for 5 days. Initiate therapy at the first sign of recurrence.
Chronic suppressive therapy for recurrent genital herpes–
Adults: 200 mg P.O. t.i.d. for up to 6 months.
Treatment of varicella-zoster (chicken pox) infections–
Children under age 13: 20 mg/kg P.O. four times a day for 5 days.
Adolescents 13 and over and adults: 800 mg P.O. q.i.d. for 5 days.

CONTRAINDICATIONS & PRECAUTIONS

Contraindicated in patients with hypersensitivity to the drug. Use cautiously in patients with dehydration, renal dysfunction, or preexisting neurologic dysfunction, because drug may aggravate these disorders. Risk of neurologic abnormalities may increase in patients who experience neurologic reactions to interferon or intrathecal methotrexate.

ADVERSE REACTIONS

Common reactions are in italics; life-threatening reactions are in bold italics.
CNS (associated with I.V. dosage): *headache,* ***encephalopathic changes (lethargy, obtundation, tremors, confusion, hallucinations, agitation, seizures, coma).***
CV: hypotension.
GI (associated with P.O. dosage): *nausea, vomiting,* diarrhea.
GU: *transient elevations of serum creatinine,* hematuria.
Skin: rash, itching.
Local: *inflammation, vesicular eruptions and phlebitis at injection site.*

INTERACTIONS

Probenecid: increased acyclovir blood levels. Monitor for possible toxicity.

EFFECTS ON DIAGNOSTIC TESTS

Serum creatinine, BUN: levels may increase.

NURSING CONSIDERATIONS

Besides those related universally to drug therapy (see "How to use this book"), consider the following specific recommendations:
Assessment
- Obtain a baseline assessment of infection before therapy.
- Be alert for adverse reactions and drug interactions throughout therapy.

• Evaluate the patient's and family's knowledge about acyclovir sodium therapy.

Nursing Diagnoses

• High risk for injury related to ineffectiveness of acyclovir to eradicate the infection.

• High risk for fluid volume deficit related to adverse GI reactions to oral acyclovir.

• Knowledge deficit related to acyclovir.

Planning and Implementation

Preparation and Administration

• Be aware that patient must be adequately hydrated throughout therapy.

• ***I.V. use:*** Reconstitute in 10 ml of sterile water for injection or in a combination of bacteriostatic water with benzyl alcohol. If refrigerated, the reconstituted solution may form a precipitate, which dissolves when warmed to room temperature. Once reconstituted, the drug should be used within 12 hours.

• Infusion must be administered over at least 1 hour to prevent renal tubular damage. Do not administer by bolus injection.

Monitoring

• Monitor effectiveness by regularly assessing for improvement in the infection.

• Be aware that bolus injection, dehydration, preexisting renal disease, and the concomitant use of other nephrotoxic drugs increase the risk of renal toxicity.

• Monitor patient's mental status when administering drug I.V. Encephalopathic changes are more likely in patients with neurologic disorders or in those who have had neurologic reactions to cytotoxic drugs.

• Monitor renal function.

• Monitor patient's hydration status if adverse GI reactions occur with oral administration of the drug.

Supportive Care

• Obtain an order for an antiemetic or antidiarrheal agent as needed.

• Keep patient adequately hydrated throughout acyclovir therapy.

• Notify the doctor if serum creatinine level does not return to normal within a few days. Patient may need increased hydration, dosage adjustment, or discontinuation of acyclovir.

Patient Teaching

• Encourage patient to drink adequate amounts of fluid throughout acyclovir therapy.

• Teach patient that oral drug is effective in managing herpes virus infection but does not eliminate or cure it.

• Instruct patient that acyclovir will not prevent spread of infection to others.

• Urge patient to recognize the early symptoms of recurring infection (tingling, itching, or pain) so he can take acyclovir before the infection fully develops.

• Tell patient to alert the nurse if pain or discomfort occurs at the site of I.V. injection.

Evaluation

In patients receiving acyclovir, appropriate evaluation statements may include:

• Patient's infection remains controlled.

• Patient maintains adequate hydration throughout acyclovir therapy.

• Patient and family state an understanding of acyclovir therapy.

acyclovir (topical)

(ay sye´ kloe ver)

Zovirax

• *Classification:* antiviral (synthetic purine nucleoside)

• *Pregnancy Risk Category:* C

HOW SUPPLIED

Ointment: 5%

INDICATIONS & DOSAGE

Initial herpes genitalis; limited, non–life-threatening mucocutaneous herpes simplex virus infections in immunocompromised patients–
Adults and children: apply sufficient quantity to adequately cover all lesions q 3 hours six times daily for 7 days.

CONTRAINDICATIONS & PRECAUTIONS

Contraindicated in patients with hypersensitivity to the drug.

Use cautiously in patients with dehydration, renal dysfunction, or preexisting neurologic dysfunction because it may aggravate these disorders. The risk of neurologic abnormalities may increase in patients who experience neurologic reactions to interferon or intrathecal methotrexate.

ADVERSE REACTIONS

Common reactions are in italics; life-threatening reactions are in bold italics.
Skin: transient burning and stinging, rash, pruritus.

INTERACTIONS

None reported.

EFFECTS ON DIAGNOSTIC TESTS

Serum creatinine and BUN: increased levels.

NURSING CONSIDERATIONS

Besides those related universally to drug therapy (see "How to use this book"), consider the following specific recommendations:

Assessment

- Obtain a baseline assessment of lesions before therapy.
- Be alert for adverse reactions and drug interactions throughout therapy.
- Evaluate the patient's and family's knowledge about topical acyclovir therapy.

Nursing Diagnoses

- Impaired tissue integrity related to the patient's mucocutaneous lesions.
- High risk for impaired skin integrity related to rash as adverse reaction.
- Knowledge deficit related to topical acyclovir therapy.

Planning and Implementation

Preparation and Administration

- ***Cutaneous use:*** Apply ½" ribbon of ointment on each 4" square of surface area; dosage will vary depending upon the total lesion area. Don't apply to the eye. Apply with finger cot or rubber glove to prevent autoinoculation of other body sites and transmission of infection to other persons. Cover all lesions thoroughly with ointment.

Monitoring

- Monitor effectiveness by assessing the patient's lesions.
- Monitor the patient for adverse reactions and drug interactions by assessing the patient's skin regularly for rashes.

Supportive Care

- Be aware therapy should begin as soon as possible after onset of signs and symptoms of herpes.
- Notify the doctor if skin rash occurs.

Patient Teaching

- Emphasize importance of compliance for successful therapy.
- Inform patient that he may transmit the virus even during treatment.
- Teach patient how to apply medication.

Evaluation

In patients receiving topical acyclovir, appropriate evaluation statements may include:

- Patient reports decrease or absence of lesions.
- Patient does not develop a rash.
- Patient and family state an understanding of topical acyclovir therapy.

adenosine

(a den´ oh seen)
Adenocard

- *Classification:* antiarrhythmic (nucleoside)
- *Pregnancy Risk Category:* C

HOW SUPPLIED

Injection: 3 mg/ml in 2-ml vials

ACTION

Mechanism: A naturally occurring nucleoside that acts on the atrioventricular (AV) node to slow conduction and inhibit reentry pathways.
Absorption: Administered by rapid I.V. injection; enters circulation immediately.
Distribution: Rapidly taken up by erythrocytes and vascular endothelial cells.
Metabolism: Metabolized to inosine and adenosine monophosphate.
Excretion: Half-life: Plasma half-life is less than 10 seconds.
Onset, peak, duration: Drug effects appear within 1 to 2 minutes of injection.

INDICATIONS & DOSAGE

Conversion of PSVT to sinus rhythm–
Adults: 6 mg I.V. by rapid bolus injection (over 1 to 2 seconds). If PSVT is not eliminated in 1 to 2 minutes, give 12 mg by rapid I.V. push. Repeat 12-mg dose if necessary. Single doses over 12 mg are not recommended.

CONTRAINDICATIONS & PRECAUTIONS

Contraindicated in patients with atrial flutter, atrial fibrillation, and ventricular tachycardia because the drug is ineffective in treating these arrhythmias; and in patients allergic to the drug.

Because it decreases conduction through the AV node, adenosine may produce a transient first-, second-, or third-degree heart block, it is therefore contraindicated in patients with second- or third-degree heart block or sick sinus syndrome, unless the patient has an artificial pacemaker. Because the drug has a short half-life, these effects are usually transient; however, patients who develop significant block after receiving adenosine should not receive additional doses.

Inhaled adenosine will cause bronchoconstriction in asthmatic patients.

According to some experimental evidence, high concentrations of adenosine may induce chromosomal damage. The clinical significance of this effect is unknown.

ADVERSE REACTIONS

Common reactions are in italics; life-threatening reactions are in bold italics.
CNS: apprehension, back pain, blurred vision, burning sensation, dizziness, heaviness in arms, lightheadedness, neck pain, numbness, tingling in arms.
CV: chest pain, *facial flushing,* headache, hypotension, palpitations, sweating.
GI: metallic taste, nausea.
Respiratory: *chest pressure, dyspnea, shortness of breath,* hyperventilation.
Other: *tightness in throat, groin pressure.*

INTERACTIONS

Carbamazepine: higher degrees of heart block may occur.
Dipyridamole: may potentiate the drug's effects. Smaller doses may be necessary.
Methylxanthines: antagonism of the drug's effects. Patients receiving theophylline or caffeine may require higher doses or may not respond to adenosine therapy.

EFFECTS ON DIAGNOSTIC TESTS

None reported.

NURSING CONSIDERATIONS

Besides those related universally to drug therapy (see "How to use this book"), consider the following specific recommendations:

Assessment

• Obtain a baseline assessment of the patient's heart rate and rhythm before adenosine therapy.
• Be alert for adverse reactions and drug interactions throughout therapy.
• Evaluate the patient's and family's knowledge about adenosine therapy.

Nursing Diagnoses

• Decreased cardiac output related to ineffectiveness of adenosine therapy.
• Altered protection related to adenosine-induced proarrhythmias.
• Knowledge deficit related to adenosine therapy.

Planning and Implementation

Preparation and Administration

• ***I.V. use:*** Administer rapidly for effective drug action. Administer directly into a vein if possible; if an I.V. line is used, employ the most proximal port and follow with a rapid saline flush to ensure that the drug reaches the systemic circulation quickly.
• Check solution for crystals, which may occur if solution is cold. If crystals are visible, gently warm solution to room temperature. Do not use solutions that aren't clear.
• Discard any unused drug because it contains no preservative.

Monitoring

• Monitor effectiveness by evaluating continuous ECG recordings.
• Monitor ECG for new arrhythmias. In clinical trials, more than half of the patients exhibited new arrhythmias when adenosine was used to convert to normal sinus rhythm. They are usually transient but may include sinus bradycardia or tachycardia, atrial premature contractions, various degrees of AV block, premature ventricular contractions, and skipped beats.

Supportive Care

• If ECG disturbances occurs, withhold the drug, obtain a rhythm strip, and notify the doctor immediately.
• Have emergency equipment and drugs on hand to treat new arrhythmias.
• Institute safety precautions if CNS adverse reactions occur.

Patient Teaching

• Teach the patient about his disease and therapy.
• Stress the importance of alerting nurse if chest pain or dyspnea occurs.

Evaluation

In patients receiving adenosine, appropriate evaluation statements may include:

• Patient's ECG reveals arrhythmia has been corrected.
• Patient does not experience proarrhythymias with adenosine use.
• Patient and family state an understanding of adenosine therapy.

PHARMACOLOGIC CLASS

adrenergics, direct and indirect acting

albuterol sulfate
bitolterol mesylate
dobutamine hydrochloride
dopamine hydrochloride
ephedrine
ephedrine hydrochloride
ephedrine sulfate
epinephrine
epinephrine bitartrate
epinephrine hydrochloride
epinephryl borate
isoetharine hydrochloride
isoetharine mesylate
isoproterenol
isoproterenol hydrochloride
isoproterenol sulfate
metaproterenol sulfate
metaraminol bitartrate
metaxalone
naphazoline hydrochloride
norepinephrine bitartrate

phenylephrine hydrochloride
pirbuterol
pseudoephedrine hydrochloride
pseudoephedrine sulfate
terbutaline sulfate
tetrahydrozoline
xylometazoline

OVERVIEW

Adrenergic drugs may mimic the naturally occurring catecholamines norepinephrine, epinephrine, and dopamine, or they may function indirectly by stimulating the release of norepinephrine.

Over the years, more specific alpha- and beta-receptor agonists and antagonists have been synthesized and studied, and these agents have permitted the subclassification of these receptors. $Alpha_1$ receptors are located on smooth muscle and glands and are excitatory; $alpha_2$ receptors are prejunctional regulatory receptors in the CNS and postjunctional receptors in many peripheral tissues. $Beta_1$ receptors are located in cardiac tissues and are excitatory; $beta_2$ receptors are located primarily on smooth muscle and glands and are inhibitory.

Most of the actions of the clinically useful adrenergic agents involve peripheral excitatory actions on glands and vascular smooth muscle; cardiac excitatory actions; CNS excitatory actions; peripheral inhibitory actions on smooth muscle of the bronchial tree, blood vessels supplying skeletal muscle, and gut; and metabolic and endocrine effects. Because different tissues respond in varying degrees to adrenergic agonists, differences in the actions of catecholamines are attributed to the presence of different receptor types within the tissues (alpha and beta).

CLINICAL INDICATIONS AND ACTIONS

Hypotension

Alpha agonists (norepinephrine, metaraminol, phenylephrine, and pseudoephedrine) cause arteriolar and venous constriction, resulting in increased blood pressure. This action is useful in supporting blood pressure in hypotensive states and in management of various serious allergic conditions. Topical formulations are used to induce local vasoconstriction (decongestion), to arrest superficial hemorrhage (styptic), to stimulate radial smooth muscle of the iris (mydriasis), and in combination with local anesthetics to localize anesthesia and prolong duration of action.

Cardiac stimulation

The $beta_1$ agonists (dobutamine) act primarily in the heart, producing a positive inotropic effect. Because they increase heart rate, enhance atrioventricular (AV) conduction, and increase the strength of the heartbeat, $beta_1$ agonists may be used to restore heartbeat in cardiac arrest and for heart block in syncopal seizures (not treatment of choice), or to treat acute heart failure and cardiogenic or other types of shock. Their use in shock is somewhat controversial, because $beta_1$ agonists induce lipolysis (increase of free fatty acids in plasma), which promotes a metabolic acidosis, and because they favor arrhythmias, which pose a special threat in cardiogenic shock.

Bronchodilation

$Beta_2$ agonists (albuterol, bitolterol, isoetharine, metaproterenol, and terbutaline) act primarily on smooth muscle of the bronchial tree, vasculature, intestine, and uterus. They also induce hepatic and muscle glycogenolysis, which results in hyperglycemia (sometimes useful in insulin overdose) and hyperlactic acidemia.

Some are used as bronchodilators; some as vasodilators. They are also used to relax the uterus and delay delivery in premature labor and for dysmenorrhea. Some degree of cardiostimulation may occur, because all $beta_2$ agonists have some degree of $beta_1$ activity.

Shock

Dopamine is currently the only commercially available sympathomimetic with significant dopaminergic activity, although some other sympathomimetics appear to act on dopamine receptors in the CNS. Dopamine receptors are prominent in the periphery (splanchnic and renal vasculature), where they mediate vasodilation, which is useful in treating shock and acute heart failure. Renal vasodilation may induce diuresis.

OVERVIEW OF ADVERSE REACTIONS

As expected, the multiple activities of sympathomimetics can produce numerous adverse reactions. However, certain precautions apply to all. Patients known to be more sensitive to the effects of these drugs include elderly persons, infants, and patients with thyrotoxicosis or cardiovascular disease.

The alpha agonists commonly produce cardiovascular reactions. An excessive increase in blood pressure is a major adverse reaction of systemically administered alpha agonists. Exaggerated pressor response may occur in hypertensive or elderly patients, which may evoke vagal reflex responses resulting in bradycardia and various degrees of AV block. Alpha agonists also interfere with lactation and may cause nausea, vomiting, sweating, piloerection, rebound congestion, rebound miosis, difficult urination, and headache. Ophthalmic use may cause mydriasis and photophobia.

The beta agonists most frequently cause tachycardia, palpitations, and other arrhythmias. Their other effects include premature atrial and ventricular contraction; tachyarrhythmias, and myocardial necrosis. Reflex tachycardia and palpitations occur with $beta_2$ agonists because of decreased blood pressure.

Metabolic reactions to beta agonists include hyperglycemia, increased metabolic rate, hyperlactic acidosis, local and systemic acidosis (decreases bronchodilator response).

Respiratory reactions include increased perfusion of nonfunctioning portions of lungs (in chronic obstructive pulmonary disease); mucus plugs may develop as a result of increased mucus secretion.

Other reactions include tremors, vertigo, insomnia, sweating, headache, nausea, vomiting, and anxiety.

The centrally acting adrenergics have similar effects, which may also be associated with dry mouth, flushing, diarrhea, impotence, hyperthermia (excessive doses), agitation, anorexia, dizziness, dyskinesia, and changes in libido. Chronic use of adrenergics in children may cause endocrine disturbances that arrest growth; however, growth usually rebounds after withdrawal of drug.

REPRESENTATIVE COMBINATIONS

Ephedrine sulfate with guaifenesin and theophylline: Bronkaid, Bronkolixir; with guaifenesin, theophylline, and phenobarbital: Bronkotabs; with belladonna extract, boric acid, zinc oxide, bismuth oxyiodide, bismuth subcarbonate, balsam peru, beeswax, and cocoa butter: Wyanoids.

Epinephrine with lidocaine: Ardecaine; with benzalkonium chloride: Mytrate, Glaucon; with pilocarpine: E-Pilo, Epicar, E-Carpine.

Isoproterenol hydrochloride with phenylephrine bitartrate: Duo-Medihaler.

Naphazoline with antazoline phosphate, boric acid, phenylmercuric acetate, carbonate anhydrous:

*Liquid form contains alcohol.

**May contain tartrazine.

Vasocon-A Ophthalmic; with antazoline and polyvinyl alcohol: Albalon-A Liquifilm; with methapyrilene hydrochloride, cetylpyridinium chloride, and thimerosal: Vapocyn II Nasal Spray; with pheniramine maleate: Naphcon A; with phenylephrine hydrochloride, pyrilamine maleate, and phenylpropanolamine hydrochloride: 4-Way Nasal Spray; with polyvinyl alcohol: Albalon Ophthalmic Solution.

Phenylephrine and pilocarpine: Pilofrin.

Pseudoephedrine with chlorpheniramine: Chlor-trimeton; with codeine phosphate and guaifenesin: Alamine Expectorant, Bazhistine Expectorant, C-Tussin, Deproist Expectorant with Codeine, Isoclar Expectorant, Novohistine Expectorant, Robitussin-DAC; with dextromethorphan: Contac Cough, Mediquell Decongestant, Sudafed DM; with dextromethorphan and acetaminophen: Viro-Med Liquid; with dextromethorphan, acetaminophen, and guaifenesin: Day-Care, Vicks Formula 44M; with dextrompheniramine: Disophrol, Drixoral; with dexchlorpheniramine: Polaramine; with guaifenesin: Robitussin-P.E., Sudafed Expectorant*, Zephrex, Pseudo-Bid, Head and Chest; with hydrocordone bitartrate: Bay Cotussend Liquid, De-Tuss, Detussin Liquid, Entuss-D, Tussend; with triprolidine: Actacin, Actagen, Actamine, Actifed, Actihist, Allerfrin OTC, Aprodine, Cerafed Plus, Norafed, Trifed, Triphed, Tripodrine, Triposed.

See also antihistamines, barbiturates, xanthines.

albumin, normal serum 5%
(al byoo´ min)
Albuminar 5%, Albutein 5%, Buminate 5%, Plasbumin 5%

albumin, normal serum 25%
Albuminar 25%, Albumisol 25%, Buminate 25%, Plasbumin 25%

- *Classification:* plasma volume expander (blood derivative)
- *Pregnancy Risk Category:* C

HOW SUPPLIED
albumin 5%
Injection: 5%, in 50-ml, 250-ml, 500-ml, 1,000-ml bottles
albumin 25%
Injection: 25%, in 10-ml, 20-ml, 50-ml, 100-ml vials.

ACTION
Mechanism: Normal serum albumin 25% provides intravascular oncotic pressure in a 5:1 ratio, which causes a shift of fluid from interstitial spaces to the circulation and slightly increases plasma protein concentration. Normal serum albumin 5% supplies colloid to the blood and expands plasma volume.
Absorption: Destroyed within the GI tract.
Distribution: Albumin accounts for approximately 50% of plasma proteins; it is distributed into the intravascular space and extravascular sites, including skin, muscle, and lungs. In patients with reduced circulating blood volume, hemodilution secondary to albumin administration persists for many hours; in patients with normal blood volume, excess fluid and protein are lost.
Metabolism: Although synthesized in the liver, the liver is not involved in clearance of albumin from plasma in healthy individuals.
Excretion: Little is known about excretion in healthy individuals. Administration of albumin decreases hepatic albumin synthesis and increases albumin clearance if plasma oncotic pressure is high. In certain pathologic states, the liver, kidneys, or intestines

may provide elimination mechanisms for albumin.

INDICATIONS & DOSAGE

Shock–
Adults: initially, 500 ml (5% solution) by I.V. infusion, repeat q 30 minutes, p.r.n. Dosage varies with patient's condition and response.
Children: 25% to 50% adult dose in nonemergency.
Hypoproteinemia–
Adults: 1,000 to 1,500 ml 5% solution by I.V. infusion daily, maximum rate 5 to 10 ml/minute; or 25 to 100 g 25% solution by I.V. infusion daily, maximum rate 3 ml/minute. Dosage varies with patient's condition and response.
Burns–
Adults: dosage varies according to extent of burn and patient's condition. Usually maintain plasma albumin at 2 to 3 g/100 ml.
Hyperbilirubinemia–
Infants: 1 g albumin (4 ml 25%)/kg before transfusion.

CONTRAINDICATIONS & PRECAUTIONS

Contraindicated in patients with severe anemia and heart failure because of potential for fluid overload.

Use cautiously in patients without albumin deficiency or in those with low cardiac reserve, severely restricted salt intake, hepatic or renal failure, dehydration, or pulmonary disease because of potential for hypervolemia.

ADVERSE REACTIONS

Common reactions are in italics; life-threatening reactions are in bold italics.
CV: ***vascular overload after rapid infusion,*** hypotension, altered pulse rate.
GI: increased salivation, nausea, vomiting.
Skin: urticaria.
Other: chills, fever, altered respiration.

INTERACTIONS

None significant.

EFFECTS ON DIAGNOSTIC TESTS

Plasma albumin: increased levels.
Serum alkaline phosphatase: levels increased by albumin derived from placental tissue.

NURSING CONSIDERATIONS

Besides those related universally to drug therapy, (see "How to use this book"), consider the following specific recommendations:

Assessment
- Obtain a baseline assessment of vital signs before therapy.
- Be alert for adverse reactions and drug interactions throughout therapy.
- Evaluate the patient's and family's knowledge about serum albumin therapy.

Nursing Diagnoses
- Fluid volume deficit related to the patient's underlying condition.
- Fluid volume excess related to the adverse effects of normal serum albumin.
- Knowledge deficit related to normal serum albumin therapy.

Planning and Implementation
Preparation and Administration
- Available in sterile, nonpyrogenic vials packed with infusion kits. Store below 99° F (37° C), but do not freeze. Discard unused portion after 4 hours.
- ***Intermittent infusion:*** Infuse at a rate appropriate to the patient's condition, usually over 15 to 30 minutes. When albumin is used for plasma volume expansion, don't exceed rate of 2 to 4 ml/minute with 5% solution and 1 ml/minute with 25% solution. In hypoproteinemia, don't exceed 5 to 10 ml/minute of 5% solution or 2 to 3 ml/minute of 25% solution. In hypertension or mild-to-moderate

cardiac failure, infuse 10% solution slowly.

• ***Continuous infusion:*** Infuse diluted solution slowly just according to patient response and changes in blood pressure.

• ***Direct injection:*** Not recommended.

Monitoring

• Monitor effectiveness by checking the vital signs carefully.

• Monitor serum albumin, total protein, hemoglobin, hematocrit, and electrolyte levels.

• Check the patient for signs of circulatory overload or pulmonary edema. If signs occur, discontinue infusion, keep vein open with ordered solution and notify the doctor.

• Monitor intake and output, report changes. Increased colloid pressure mobilizes extracellular fluid, causing diuresis for 3 to 20 hours.

• Monitor patients with cerebral edema. Withhold fluids for 8 hours after infusion to avoid fluid overload.

Supportive Care

• Remember that allergic reactions may be minimized by giving antihistamines, as ordered, before infusion and by slowing infusion rate.

Patient Teaching

• Tell the patient to report chills, fever dyspnea, nausea rash, or tachycardia immediately.

Evaluation

In patients receiving normal serum albumin, appropriate evaluation statements may include:

• Patient's vital signs are within normal parameters.

• Patient has not experienced problems with circulatory overload or pulmonary edema during therapy.

• Patient and family state an understanding of normal serum albumin therapy.

albuterol (salbutamol)

(al byoo´ ter ole)

Proventil, Respolin‡

albuterol sulfate (salbutamol sulphate)

Proventil, Proventil Repetabs, Respolin Inhaler‡, Respolin Inhaler Solution‡, Ventolin Obstetric Injection‡

• *Classification:* bronchodilator (adrenergic)

• *Pregnancy Risk Category:* C

HOW SUPPLIED

albuterol

Aerosol inhaler: 90 mcg/metered spray, 100 mcg/metered spray‡

albuterol sulfate

Tablets (extended-release): 4 mg

Syrup: 2 mg/5 ml

Aqueous solution (for respirator): 5 mg/ml‡

Injection: 1 mg/ml‡

ACTION

Mechanism: Relaxes bronchial smooth muscle by acting on beta$_2$-adrenergic receptors.

Absorption: After oral administration, drug is rapidly absorbed from the GI tract; after inhalation, acts directly on receptors in the respiratory tract, and appears to be absorbed into the bloodstream gradually (over several hours) from the respiratory tract. However, most of the dose is swallowed and absorbed through the GI tract.

Distribution: Does not cross the blood-brain barrier; however, crosses the placenta.

Metabolism: Extensively metabolized in the liver to inactive compounds.

Excretion: In urine and feces. After inhalation, 70% of a dose is excreted in urine (as drug and metabolites) within 24 hours; 10% in feces. After ingestion, 75% of a dose is excreted

in urine within 72 hours (mostly as metabolites); 4% in feces. Half-life: About 4 hours following either route of administration.
Onset, peak, duration: After inhalation, onset of action occurs within 5 to 15 minutes, peaks in 30 minutes to 2 hours, and lasts 3 to 6 hours. After ingestion, onset occurs within 30 minutes, peaks in 2 to 3 hours, and lasts 4 hours or longer.

INDICATIONS & DOSAGE

Prevention and treatment of bronchospasm in patients with reversible obstructive airway disease–
Adults and children over 13 years: 1 to 2 inhalations q 4 to 6 hours. More frequent administration or a greater number of inhalations is not recommended.

Usual dosage range is 10 to 50 mcg/minute.
*Oral tablets–*2 to 4 mg t.i.d. or q.i.d. Maximum dosage is 8 mg q.i.d.
*Extended-release tablets–*4 to 8 mg q 12 hours. Maximum dosage is 16 mg b.i.d.
Children 6 to 13 years: 2 mg (1 teaspoonful) P.O. t.i.d. or q.i.d.
Children 2 to 5 years: 0.1 mg/kg P.O. t.i.d., not to exceed 2 mg (1 teaspoonful) t.i.d.
Adults over 65 years: 2 mg P.O. t.i.d. or q.i.d.
To prevent exercise-induced asthma–
Adults: 2 inhalations 15 minutes before exercise.
Prevention of premature labor‡–
Adults: initially, 10 mcg/minute by continuous I.V. infusion (use an infusion pump). Dosage should be increased in 10-minute intervals until the desired response is achieved.

CONTRAINDICATIONS & PRECAUTIONS

Contraindicated in patients with hypersensitivity to the drug. Use cautiously in patients with hyperthyroidism, diabetes mellitus, cardiovascular disorders (coronary insufficiency or hypertension), or sensitivity to sympathomimetic amines, as drug may worsen these conditions.

ADVERSE REACTIONS

Common reactions are in italics; life-threatening reactions are in bold italics.
CNS: *tremor, nervousness,* dizziness, insomnia, headache.
CV: tachycardia, palpitations, hypertension.
EENT: drying and irritation of nose and throat (with inhaled form).
GI: heartburn, nausea, vomiting.
Other: muscle cramps.

INTERACTIONS

MAO inhibitors, tricyclic antidepressants: increased adverse cardiovascular effects.
Propranolol and other beta blockers: mutual antagonism. Monitor patient carefully.

EFFECTS ON DIAGNOSTIC TESTS

Spirometry (for diagnosis of asthma): decreased sensitivity.

NURSING CONSIDERATIONS

Besides those related universally to drug therapy (see "How to use this book"), consider the following specific recommendations.

Assessment

- Obtain a baseline assessment of the patient's respiratory status by taking vital signs and evaluating breathe sounds.
- Be alert for adverse reactions and drug interactions throughout therapy.
- Evaluate the patient's and family's knowledge about albuterol therapy.

Nursing Diagnoses

- Ineffective airway clearance related to patient's underlying condition.
- High risk for injury related to the albuterol-induced adverse reactions.
- Knowledge deficit related to albuterol therapy.

*Liquid form contains alcohol.

**May contain tartrazine.

Planning and Implementation

Preparation and Administration

- Check that patient has not received recent theophylline therapy before giving loading dose.
- ***P.O. use:*** Pleasant tasting syrup may be taken by children as young as age 2 years. This form contains no alcohol or sugar.
- ***I.V. use:*** Prepare infusion using sodium chloride injection, dextrose injection, or sodium chloride and dextrose injection. The drug should never be administered without dilution. Do not mix with any other medication. Discard any unused portion after 24 hours.
- ***I.V. use during premature labor:*** After uterine contractions have ceased, the drip rate of the drug should be maintained for 1 hour, then gradually tapered at 50% increments in six hourly intervals. Infusions should not continue for more than 48 hours. If therapy will continue over 48 hours, the doctor may prescribe 4 to 8 mg P.O. q.i.d.
- ***Inhalation:*** Wait at least 2 minutes between inhalation doses, if more than one inhalation dose is ordered. If a steroid inhaler is also used, first use the bronchodilator, wait 5 minutes and then use the steroid inhaler. This permits the bronchodilator to open air passages for maximum effectiveness.
- Store in light-resistant container.
- Patients may use tablets and aerosols concomitantly.
- Expect elderly patients to receive a lower dosage.

Monitoring

- Monitor effectiveness by regularly checking breath sounds, respiratory rate and laboratory study results, such as arterial blood gases.
- Monitor closely for toxicity, particularly in elderly patients.
- When used to prevent premature labor, monitor maternal heart rate closely. It should not exceed 140 beats/minute.
- Monitor the patient closely for tremor, nervousness, and other adverse reactions.
- Remember that albuterol may be prescribed for use 15 minutes before exercise to prevent exercise-induced bronchospasm.

Supportive Care

- Be aware that albuterol reportedly produces less cardiac stimulation than other sympathomimetics, especially isoproterenol.
- Institute safety precautions, such as continuous use of side rails, if CNS adverse reactions occur.

Patient Teaching

- Warn the patient about the possibility of paradoxical bronchospasm. If this occurs, instruct the patient to discontinue the drug immediately.
- Instruct the patient to perform oral inhalation correctly as follows: Clear nasal passages and throat. Breathe out, expelling as much air from the lungs as possible. Place the mouthpiece well into the mouth as the dose from the inhaler is released, and inhale deeply. Hold breath for several seconds, remove the mouthpiece, and exhale slowly. If more than one inhalation is ordered, the patient should wait at least 2 minutes before repeating the procedure for a second dose.
- Explain why it is necessary to use the bronchodilator first if other inhalants, such as a steroid inhaler, are prescribed (This allows the bronchodilator to open air passages for maximum effectiveness.) Tell the patient to allow 5 minutes between the inhalant treatments.
- Warn the patient to avoid accidentally spraying the inhalant into the eyes, which may cause temporary blurring of vision.
- Tell the patient to reduce the intake of foods containing caffeine, such as coffee, colas, and chocolates, when taking a bronchodilator.

• Show the patient how to check the pulse. Instruct the patient to check his pulse before and after using a bronchodilator and to call the doctor if his pulse increases more than 20 to 30 beats/minute.

Evaluation

In patients receiving albuterol, appropriate evaluation statements may include:

• Patient's respiratory signs and symptoms are improved with albuterol.
• Injury did not occur; patient did not experience CNS adverse reactions to albuterol.
• Patient and family state an understanding of albuterol therapy.

alclometasone dipropionate

(al kloe met´ a sone)

Alclovate, Logoderm‡

• *Classification:* topical anti-inflammatory (adrenocorticoid)
• *Pregnancy Risk Category:* C

HOW SUPPLIED

Cream: 0.05%
Ointment: 0.05%

ACTION

Mechanism: Produces local anti-inflammatory, vasoconstrictor, and antipruritic actions. Drug diffuses across cell membranes to form complexes with specific cytoplasmic receptors, influencing cellular metabolism. Corticosteroids stabilize leukocyte lysosomal membranes, inhibit local actions and accumulation of macrophages, decrease local edema, and reduce the formation of scar tissue.

Absorption: Amount absorbed depends on the amount applied and on the nature of the skin at the application site. Absorption ranges from about 1% in areas with thick stratum corneum (on the palms, soles, elbows, and knees) to as high as 36% in thinner areas (face, eyelids, and genitals). Absorption increases in areas of skin damage, inflammation, or occlusion. Some systemic absorption of topical steroids may occur, especially through the oral mucosa.

Distribution: After topical application, distributed throughout the local skin. If absorbed into the circulation, drug is rapidly removed from the blood and distributed into muscle, liver, skin, intestines, and kidneys.

Metabolism: After topical administration, metabolized primarily in the skin. The small amount that is absorbed into systemic circulation is metabolized primarily in the liver to inactive compounds.

Excretion: Inactive metabolites are excreted by the kidneys, primarily as glucuronides and sulfates, but also as unconjugated products. Small amounts of the metabolites are also excreted in feces.

INDICATIONS & DOSAGE

Inflammation of corticosteroid-responsive dermatoses–

Adults: apply a thin film to affected areas b.i.d. or t.i.d. Gently massage until the medication disappears.

CONTRAINDICATIONS & PRECAUTIONS

Contraindicated in patients who are hypersensitive to any component of the preparation and in patients with viral, fungal, or tubercular skin lesions. Use with extreme caution in patients with impaired circulation because it may increase the risk of skin ulceration.

ADVERSE REACTIONS

Common reactions are in italics; life-threatening reactions are in bold italics.

Skin: burning, itching, irritation, dryness, folliculitis, striae, acneiform eruptions, perioral dermatitis, hypopigmentation, hypertrichosis, allergic contact dermatitis. With occlusive dressings: *secondary infection, maceration, atrophy, striae, miliaria.*

INTERACTIONS

None significant.

EFFECTS ON DIAGNOSTIC TESTS

None significant.

NURSING CONSIDERATIONS

Besides those related universally to drug therapy (see "How to use this book"), consider the following specific recommendations:

Assessment

- Obtain a baseline assessment of inflamed skin before therapy.
- Be alert for adverse reactions and drug interactions throughout therapy.
- Evaluate the patient's and family's knowledge about alclometasone dipropionate therapy.

Nursing Diagnoses

- Impaired skin integrity related to patient's underlying condition.
- High risk for infection related to alclometasone dipropionate-induced secondary infection.
- Knowledge deficit related to alclometasone dipropionate therapy.

Planning and Implementation

Preparation and Administration

- ***Topical use:*** Before applying, wash skin gently. To prevent damage to skin, rub medication in gently, leaving a thin coat. When treating hairy sites, part hair and apply directly to lesion.
- ***For an occlusive dressing:*** Apply cream, then cover with a thin, pliable, nonflammable plastic film; seal adjacent normal skin with hypoallergenic tape. To minimize adverse reactions, use occlusive dressing intermittently. Don't leave in place longer than 16 hours each day. Occlusive dressings should not be used in presence of infections or with weeping or exudative lesions.

Monitoring

- Monitor effectiveness by regularly assessing skin of affected area.
- Observe for signs of systemic absorption, skin irritation or ulceration, hypersensitivity, or infection. If they develop, discontinue drug and notify doctor. (If antifungals or antibiotics are being use concurrently, and infection does not respond immediately, corticosteroids should be discontinued until infection is controlled.)
- Check patient's temperature regularly and remove occlusive dressing if fever develops. Notify doctor.
- Monitor for adverse reactions by inspecting the patient's skin for infection, striae, and atrophy.

Supportive Care

- Change the patient's dressings as ordered by the doctor. Be prepared to discontinue drug and notify doctor if infection, striae, or atrophy occur.
- Use cautiously in viral skin diseases, such as varicella, vaccinia, and herpes simplex; in fungal infections.
- Be aware that systemic absorption is especially likely with occlusive dressings, prolonged treatment, or application to extensive body surface.
- Remember that treatment should be continued for a few days after clearing of lesions to prevent recurrence.

Patient Teaching

- Teach patient to apply medication.
- Warn patient not to use for more than 14 consecutive days because of the potential for systemic absorption and suppression of hypothalamic-pituitary-adrenal axis.
- Instruct patient to avoid application near eyes or mucous membranes. Do not apply to face, armpits, groin, or under breasts unless specifically ordered.
- Inform patient that repeated application can result in diminished effectiveness.

Evaluation
In patients receiving alclometasone dipropionate, appropriate evaluation statements may include:
- Patient states his lesions are healing.
- Patient does not develop secondary infection.
- Patient and family state an understanding of alclometasone dipropionate therapy.

alfentanil hydrochloride
(al fen´ ta nill)
Alfenta

- Controlled Substance Schedule II
- *Classification:* analgesic, anesthetic (opioid)
- *Pregnancy Risk Category:* B (D for prolonged use or use of high doses at term)

HOW SUPPLIED
Injection: 500 mcg/ml

ACTION
Mechanism: Binds with opiate receptors at many sites in the CNS (brain, brain stem, and spinal cord), altering both perception of and emotional response to pain through an unknown mechanism.
Distribution: Highly (>90%) protein-bound.
Metabolism: Hepatic.
Excretion: In urine. Half-life: About 1½ hours.
Onset, peak, duration: Immediate onset of action; duration is variable.

INDICATIONS & DOSAGE
Adjunct to general anesthetic–
Adults: initially, 8 to 50 mcg/kg I.V., then give increments of 3 to 15 mcg/kg I.V.
As a primary anesthetic–
Adults: initially, 130 to 245 mcg/kg I.V., then give 0.5 to 1.5 mcg/kg/minute I.V.

CONTRAINDICATIONS & PRECAUTIONS
Contraindicated in patients with hypersensitivity to any phenylpiperidine (diphenoxylate, fentanyl, meperidine, or sufentanil). Use with extreme caution in patients with supraventricular arrhythmias; avoid, or use with extreme caution in patients with head injury or increased intracranial pressure because drug obscures neurologic parameters; or during pregnancy and labor because drug readily crosses placenta (premature infants are especially sensitive to respiratory and CNS depressant effects of narcotic agonists).

Use cautiously in patients with renal or hepatic dysfunction because drug accumulation or prolonged duration of action may occur; pulmonary disease (asthma, chronic obstructive pulmonary disease) because drug depresses respiration and suppresses cough reflex; and seizure disorders because drug may precipitate seizures; in those undergoing biliary tract surgery because drug may cause biliary spasm; and in elderly or debilitated patients, who are more sensitive to both therapeutic and adverse drug effects; and in patients prone to physical or psychological addiction because of the high risk of addiction to this drug.

In patients weighing more than 20% above their ideal body weight, determine dosage based on ideal body weight.

Alfentanil may produce bradycardia (which may be treated with atropine); use with particular caution in patients with preexisting bradyarrhythmias.

ADVERSE REACTIONS

Common reactions are in italics; life-threatening reactions are in bold italics.
CV: hypotension, hypertension, bradycardia, tachycardia.
GI: nausea, vomiting.
Skin: itching.
Other: chest wall rigidity, intraoperative muscle movement, ***respiratory depression.***

INTERACTIONS

Alcohol, CNS depressants: additive effects. Use together cautiously.

EFFECTS ON DIAGNOSTIC TESTS

None reported.

NURSING CONSIDERATIONS

Besides those related universally to drug therapy (see "How to use this book"), consider the following specific recommendations:

Assessment

- Obtain a baseline assessment of the patient's cardiovascular and respiratory status before therapy.
- Be alert for adverse reactions and drug interactions throughout therapy.
- Evaluate the patient's and family's knowledge about alfentanil therapy.

Nursing Diagnoses

- Decreased cardiac output related to adverse cardiac effects of therapy.
- Ineffective breathing pattern related to alfentanil-induced respiratory depression.
- Knowledge deficit related to alfentanil therapy.

Planning and Implementation

Preparation and Administration

- Should be administered only by persons specifically trained in the use of I.V. anesthetics.
- Keep in mind that as a primary anesthetic, alfentanil may be prescribed for induction of anesthesia for general surgery requiring endotracheal intubation and mechanical ventilation.
- Discontinue infusion at least 10 to 15 minutes before the end of surgery.
- To administer small volumes of alfentanil accurately, use a tuberculin syringe.
- Reduce dosage, as ordered, for elderly and debilitated patients.

Monitoring

Closely monitor respiratory, cardiovascular, and neurologic systems during and after surgery. Keep in mind that alfentanil induces a shorter period of respiratory depression than other fentanyl derivatives. Respiratory depression may cause carbon dioxide retention, increasing CSF pressure.

Supportive Care

- Administer analgesics as ordered shortly after surgery.
- Notify the doctor immediately if vital signs deteriorate.
- ***Treatment of overdose:*** Reverse effects with naloxone, then give symptomatic care. For apnea, administer oxygen and provide mechanical ventilation. Use positive-pressure ventilation via bag or mask. For hypotension, give I.V. fluids and vasopressors. For muscle rigidity, give a neuromuscular blocking drug.
- Recognize that the patient who develops tolerance to other opioids may become intolerant to alfentanil as well.

Patient Teaching

- Explain the anesthetic effect of alfentanil as well as preoperative and postoperative care measures.
- Inform the patient that another analgesic will be available to relieve pain after effects of alfentanil have worn off.

Evaluation

In patients receiving alfentanil, appropriate evaluation statements may include:

- Cardiac status is within normal limits.
- Respiratory status is within normal limits.

• Patient and family state an understanding of alfentanil therapy.

PHARMACOLOGIC CLASS

alkylating agents

altretamine
busulfan
carboplatin
carmustine
chlorambucil
cisplatin
cyclophosphamide
dacarbazine
ifosfamide
lomustine
mechlorethamine
melphalan
streptozocin
thiotepa
uracil mustard

OVERVIEW

Alkylating antineoplastic agents appear to act independently of the specific phase of the cell cycle. Varying degrees of specificity exist among the different agents. They are polyfunctional compounds which can be divided chemically into five groups: nitrogen mustards, ethylenimines, alkylsulfonates, triazenes, and nitrosoureas. Alkylating agents are highly reactive, primarily targeting nucleic acids. They are often effective against tumors with large volumes and slow cell turnover rate.

CLINICAL INDICATIONS AND ACTIONS

Alkylating agents are useful alone or in combination with other types of antineoplastic agents for the treatment of a variety of tumors. See individual agents for specific uses.

OVERVIEW OF ADVERSE REACTIONS

The most frequent adverse reactions include bone marrow depression, leukopenia, thrombocytopenia, fever, chills, sore throat, nausea, vomiting, diarrhea, flank or joint pain, anxiety, swelling of feet or lower legs, loss of hair, and redness or pain at injection site.

REPRESENTATIVE COMBINATIONS

None.

allopurinol

(al oh pure´ i nole)
Alloremed‡, Capurate‡, Lopurin, Zyloprim

• *Classification:* antigout (xanthine oxidase inhibitor)
• *Pregnancy Risk Category:* C

HOW SUPPLIED

Tablets (scored): 100 mg, 300 mg
Capsules: 100 mg‡, 300 mg‡

ACTION

Mechanism: Blocks the enzyme xanthine oxidase, an enzyme that converts hypoxanthine to xanthine and xanthine to uric acid. Reduces serum uric acid levels.
Absorption: After oral administration, approximately 80% to 90% of a dose of allopurinol is absorbed.
Distribution: Widely distributed throughout the body except in the brain, where concentrations of the drug are 50% of those found in the rest of the body. Allopurinol and oxypurinol are not bound to plasma proteins.
Metabolism: Metabolized to oxypurinol by xanthine oxidase.
Excretion: 5% to 7% excreted in urine unchanged within 6 hours of ingestion. After this, it is excreted by the kidneys as oxypurinol, allopurinol, and oxypurinol ribonucleosides. About 70% of the administered daily dose is excreted in urine as oxypurinol and an additional 2% appears in feces as unchanged drug within 48 to

72 hours. Half life: Allopurinol is 1 to 2 hours; oxypurinol, approximately 15 hours.
Onset, peak, duration: Peak concentrations of allopurinol are achieved 2 to 6 hours after an oral dose.

INDICATIONS & DOSAGE

Gout, primary or secondary to hyperuricemia; secondary to diseases such as acute or chronic leukemia, polycythemia vera, multiple myeloma, and psoriasis–
Dosage varies with severity of disease; can be given as single dose or divided, but doses larger than 300 mg should be divided.
Adults: mild gout, 200 to 300 mg P.O. daily; severe gout with large tophi, 400 to 600 mg P.O. daily. Same dosage for maintenance in secondary hyperuricemia.
Hyperuricemia secondary to malignancies–
Children 6 to 10 years: 300 mg P.O. daily or divided t.i.d.
Children under 6 years: 50 mg P.O. t.i.d.
Impaired renal function–
Adults: 200 mg P.O. daily if creatinine clearance is 10 to 20 ml/minute; 100 mg P.O. daily if creatinine is less than 10 ml/minute; 100 mg P.O. more than 24 hours apart if clearance is less than 3 ml/minute.
To prevent acute gouty attacks–
Adults: 100 mg P.O. daily; increase at weekly intervals by 100 mg without exceeding maximum dose (800 mg), until serum uric acid falls to 6 mg/100 ml or less.
To prevent uric acid nephropathy during cancer chemotherapy–
Adults: 600 to 800 mg P.O. daily for 2 to 3 days, with high fluid intake.
Recurrent calcium oxalate calculi–
Adults: 200 to 300 mg P.O. daily in single dose or divided doses.

CONTRAINDICATIONS & PRECAUTIONS

Contraindicated in patients with hypersensitivity to the drug and in those with idiopathic hemochromatosis. Use cautiously in pregnant and breast-feeding women. Patients with impaired renal function must be carefully monitored while receiving allopurinol. Dosage adjustments may be necessary in patients with bone marrow depression, lower GI tract disease, and impaired renal function.

ADVERSE REACTIONS

Common reactions are in italics; life-threatening reactions are in bold italics.
Blood: ***agranulocytosis,*** anemia, ***aplastic anemia.***
CNS: drowsiness, headache.
EENT: cataracts, retinopathy.
GI: nausea, vomiting, diarrhea, abdominal pain.
Hepatic: altered liver function studies, hepatitis.
Skin: *rash, usually maculopapular; exfoliative,* urticarial, and purpuric lesions; erythema multiforme; severe furunculosis of nose; ichthyosis, ***toxic epidermal necrolysis.***

INTERACTIONS

Alcohol, bumetanide, diazoxide, ethacrynic acid, furosemide, triamterene, mecamylamine, pyrazinamide: increased serum acid concentration; adjust dosage of allopurinol.
Ampicillin, bacampicillin, hetacillin: increased possibility of skin rash.
Anticoagulants: potentiation of anticoagulant effect. Dosage adjustments may be necessary.
Antineoplastic agents: increased potential for bone marrow suppression. Monitor patient carefully.
Chlorpropamide: possible increased hypoglycemic effect.
Uricosuric agents: additive effect; may be used to therapeutic advantage.
Urinary acidifying agents (ammo-

nium chloride, ascorbic acid, potassium or sodium phosphate): may increase the possibility of kidney stone formation.
Xanthines: increased serum theophylline. Adjust dosage of theophyllines.

EFFECTS ON DIAGNOSTIC TESTS

Alkaline phosphatase, AST (SGOT), and ALT (SGPT): increased levels.

NURSING CONSIDERATIONS

Besides those related universally to drug therapy (see "How to use this book"), consider the following specific recommendations:

Assessment

- Obtain a baseline assessment of patient's uric acid results, joint stiffness, and pain.
- Be alert for adverse reactions and drug interactions throughout therapy.
- Evaluate the patient's and family's knowledge about allopurinol therapy.

Nursing Diagnoses

- Pain (joint) related to patient's underlying condition.
- High risk for infection related to allopurinol-induced agranulocytosis.
- Knowledge deficit related to allopurinol therapy.

Planning and Implementation

Preparation and Administration

- Administer with meals or immediately after meals to minimize GI adverse reactions.
- Discontinue at first sign of rash, which may precede severe hypersensitivity reaction, or any other adverse reaction.
- If ordered, administer colchicine concurrently with allopurinol. This will prophylactically treat the acute gout attacks that may occur in the first 6 weeks of therapy.

Monitoring

- Monitor effectiveness by noting serum uric acid levels and assessing patient's complaints of discomfort.
- Monitor CBC with differential results for abnormalities. Monitor for elevated temperature and observe for other signs of infection.
- Observe for adverse skin reactions.
- Monitor intake and output; daily urine output of at least 2 liters and maintenance of neutral or slightly alkaline urine is desirable.

Supportive Care

- If the patient develops persistent signs of GI distress, notify the doctor.
- Remember, if renal insufficiency exists at any time during treatment, allopurinol dosage will be reduced.
- Periodically check CBC and hepatic and renal function, especially at start of therapy.
- If patient develops a headache, obtain an order for a mild analgesic, such as acetaminophen.

Patient Teaching

- Tell the patient to report any adverse reactions immediately.
- Advise patients who are taking allopurinol for treatment of recurrent calcium oxalate stones, to reduce dietary intake of animal protein, sodium, refined sugars, oxalate-rich foods, and calcium.
- Advise patient to avoid driving a car and other hazardous activities requiring mental alertness until CNS effects of the drug are known because allopurinol has been known to cause drowsiness.
- Inform the patient that allopurinol may predispose him to an ampicillin-induced rash. Allopurinol may cause a rash even weeks after discontinuation. Note that skin reactions are more common in patients taking diuretics and in those with renal disorders.
- Encourage the patient to drink plenty of fluids while taking this drug unless otherwise indicated.
- Tell the patient with gout to avoid alcohol because it will increase the urate level.
- Advise the patient to avoid all medications that contain aspirin because

they may precipitate gout. Acetaminophen may be used for pain.

Evaluation

In patients receiving allopurinol, appropriate evaluation statements may include:

- Patient expresses relief of joint pain.
- Patient does not develop infection.
- Patient and family state an understanding of allopurinol.

PHARMACOLOGIC CLASS

alpha-adrenergic blocking agents

dihydroergotamine mesylate
doxazosin mesylate
ergotamine tartrate
phenoxybenzamine hydrochloride
phentolamine mesylate
prazosin hydrochloride
terazosin hydrochloride
tolazoline hydrochloride

OVERVIEW

Drugs that block the effects of neurohormonal transmitters (norepinephine, epinephrine, and related sympathomimetic amines) on adrenergic receptors in various effector systems are designated as adrenergic blocking agents. As adrenoreceptors are classified into two subtypes—alpha and beta—so too are the blocking agents. Essentially, those agents that antagonize mydriasis, cause vasoconstriction, nonvascular smooth muscle excitation, and other adrenergic responses due to alpha receptor stimulation are termed alpha-adrenergic blocking agents.

Nonselective alpha antagonists

Ergotamine, phentolamine, and phenoxybenzamine antagonize both $alpha_1$ and $alpha_2$ receptors. Generally, alpha blockade results in tachycardia, palpitations, and increased secretion of renin.

Selective alpha antagonists

$Alpha_1$ blockers have readily observable effects and are currently the only alpha-adrenergic agents with known clinical uses. They decrease vascular resistance and increase venous capacitance, thereby lowering blood pressure. In theory, $alpha_1$ blockers should be useful in the same conditions as nonselective alpha blockers; however, doxazosin, prazosin, and terazosin are approved only for treating hypertension. Prazosin also has proven useful in refractory heart failure because of its ability to decrease cardiac afterload.

$Alpha_2$ blockers produce more subtle physiologic effects and currently have no therapeutic applications. Yohimbine is one such agent.

CLINICAL INDICATIONS AND ACTIONS

Peripheral vascular disorders

Alpha-adrenergic blocking agents are indicated for treating peripheral vascular disorders including Raynaud's disease, acrocyanosis, frost bite, acute atrial occlusion, phlebitis, and diabetic gangrene. Dihydroergotamine and ergotamine have been used to treat vascular headaches. Prazosin has been used to treat Raynaud's disease. Phentolamine is indicated to treat dermal necrosis caused by extravasation of norepinephrine.

Hypertension

Phenoxybenzamine is used to treat pheochromocytoma. Tolazoline is indicated to treat persistent pulmonary hypertension in neonates. Prazosin and terazosin are used in managing essential hypertension. Phentolamine is used to control hypertension and is a useful adjunct in surgical treatment of pheochromocytoma.

OVERVIEW OF ADVERSE REACTIONS

Nonselective alpha antagonists typically cause postural hypotension, tachycardia, palpitations, fluid retention (from excess renin secretion), nasal and ocular congestion, and aggravation of the signs and symptoms of respiratory infection. Use of these agents is contraindicated in patients with severe cerebral and coronary atherosclerosis and in those with renal insufficiency.

Selective alpha antagonists typically cause severe postural hypotension and syncope, especially during early treatment, which are the most common side effects of $alpha_1$ blockade. Excessive tachycardia, stroke volume, and plasma renin levels may result from $alpha_2$ blockade.

REPRESENTATIVE COMBINATIONS
None.

---

alprazolam
(al pray´ zoe lam)
Xanax

- Controlled Substance Schedule IV
- *Classification:* anxiolytic agent (benzodiazepine)
- *Pregnancy Risk Category:* D

HOW SUPPLIED
Tablets: 0.25 mg, 0.5 mg, 1 mg

ACTION
Mechanism: Depresses the CNS at the limbic and subcortical levels of the brain.
Absorption: Well absorbed after oral administration.
Distribution: Widely distributed; highly (80% to 90%) bound to plasma proteins.
Metabolism: In the liver to inactive metabolites.
Excretion: In urine. Half-life: 12 to 15 hours.
Onset, peak, duration: Onset of action within 15 to 30 minutes; peak action in 1 to 2 hours.

INDICATIONS & DOSAGE
Anxiety and tension–
Adults: usual starting dose is 0.25 to 0.5 mg P.O. t.i.d. Maximum total daily dosage is 4 mg in divided doses. In elderly or debilitated patients, usual starting dose is 0.25 mg b.i.d. or t.i.d.

CONTRAINDICATIONS & PRECAUTIONS
Contraindicated in patients with hypersensitivity to the drug; in patients with acute narrow-angle glaucoma or untreated open-angle glaucoma because of possible anticholinergic effects; in patients in coma; and in patients with acute alcohol intoxication who have depressed vital signs, because the drug will worsen CNS depression.

Use cautiously in patients with psychoses because the drug is rarely beneficial in such patients and may induce paradoxical reactions; myasthenia gravis or Parkinson's disease, because it may exacerbate the disorder; in patients with impaired renal or hepatic function, which prolongs elimination of the drug; and in elderly or debilitated patients, who are usually more sensitive to the drug's CNS effects. Abrupt withdrawal may precipitate seizures in some patients. Alprazolam may produce additive CNS depression in patients with acute alcohol intoxication.

Use cautiously in individuals prone to addiction or drug abuse.

ADVERSE REACTIONS
Common reactions are in italics; life-threatening reactions are in bold italics.
CNS: *drowsiness, light-headedness,* headache, confusion, hostility.
CV: transient hypotension, tachycardia.
EENT: dry mouth.
GI: nausea, vomiting, constipation, discomfort.

INTERACTIONS

Alcohol, other CNS depressants: increased CNS depression. Avoid concomitant use.
Cimetidine: increased sedation. Monitor carefully.
Tricyclic antidepressants: increased plasma levels of tricyclic antidepressants.

EFFECTS ON DIAGNOSTIC TESTS

EEG: minor changes (low-voltage, fast activity) during and after therapy.
Liver function tests: elevated results.

NURSING CONSIDERATIONS

Besides those related universally to drug therapy (see "How to use this book") consider the following specific recommendations:

Assessment

- Obtain a baseline assessment of the patient's anxiety level before therapy.
- Be alert for adverse reactions and drug interactions throughout therapy.
- Evaluate the patient's and family's knowledge about alprazolam therapy.

Nursing Diagnoses

- Anxiety related to the patient's underlying condition.
- High risk for injury related to alprazolam-induced CNS reactions.
- Knowledge deficit related to alprazolam therapy.

Planning and Implementation

Preparation and Administration

- When administering alprazolam, make sure the patient has swallowed the tablets before leaving the bedside.
- Expect to administer lower doses at longer intervals in elderly or debilitated patients.

Monitoring

- Monitor effectiveness by regularly asking the patient about feelings of anxiety and by evaluating the patient's behavior.
- Monitor the patient for adverse drug reactions by frequently monitoring his vital signs for hypotension or tachycardia.
- Monitor bowel patterns to detect constipation before it becomes severe.

Supportive Care

- Provide encouragement and support with supplementary measures prescribed to augment alprazolam therapy, such as counseling and problem identification with professionals.
- If drowsiness, light-headedness, or confusion occurs, institute safety measures, such as supervising patient activities. Reorient patient as needed and ensure a safe environment.
- Provide frequent sips of water or ice chips for dry mouth.
- If not contraindicated, increase the patient's fluid intake and dietary fiber to prevent constipation.
- Be aware that drug should not be prescribed for everyday stress or for long-term use (more than 4 months).
- Do not withdraw drug abruptly. Abuse or addiction is possible and withdrawal symptoms may occur.

Patient Teaching

- Warn the patient not to combine drug with alcohol or other CNS depressants and to avoid driving and other hazardous activities that require alertness and psychomotor coordination until CNS adverse reactions are known.
- Caution the patient against giving medication to others.
- Warn the patient to take this drug only as directed and not to discontinue drug without the doctor's approval. Inform the patient of the drug's potential for dependence if taken longer than directed.
- Recommend sugarless chewing gum, hard candy, or ice chips to relieve dry mouth.
- Tell the patient to increase fluid and fiber intake to prevent constipation.

Evaluation

In the patient receiving alprazolam, appropriate evaluation statements may include:
- Patient states he is less anxious.
- Patient does not experience injury as a result of adverse CNS reactions.
- Patient and family state an understanding of alprazolam therapy.

alprostadil

(al pross´ ta dil)

Prostin VR Pediatric

- *Classification:* ductus arteriosus patency adjunct (prostaglandin)
- *Pregnancy risk category:* C

HOW SUPPLIED

Injection: 500 mcg/ml

ACTION

Mechanism: Relaxes the smooth muscle of the ductus arteriosus.
Distribution: Rapidly distributed throughout the body.
Metabolism: 68% of a dose is metabolized in one pass through the lung, primarily by oxidation; 100% is metabolized within 24 hours.
Excretion: All metabolites are excreted in urine within 24 hours.

INDICATIONS & DOSAGE

Palliative therapy for temporary maintenance of patency of ductus arteriosus until surgery can be performed–

Infants: 0.05 to 0.1 mcg/kg/minute by I.V., intraarterial, or intraaortic infusion. When therapeutic response is achieved, reduce infusion rate to give lowest dosage that will maintain response. Maximum dosage is 0.4 mcg/kg/minute. Alternatively, administer through umbilical artery catheter placed at ductal opening.

CONTRAINDICATIONS & PRECAUTIONS

Contraindicated in infants with respiratory distress syndrome because of the potential for adverse cardiovascular effects. Use cautiously in infants with bleeding tendencies because it inhibits platelet aggregation.

ADVERSE REACTIONS

Common reactions are in italics; life-threatening reactions are in bold italics.
Blood: ***disseminated intravascular coagulation.***
CNS: ***seizures.***
CV: *flushing,* bradycardia, hypotension, tachycardia.
GI: diarrhea.
Other: ***apnea,*** *fever, sepsis.*

INTERACTIONS

None reported.

EFFECTS ON DIAGNOSTIC TESTS

None reported.

NURSING CONSIDERATIONS

Besides those related universally to drug therapy (see "How to use this book"), consider the following specific recommendations:

Assessment
- Obtain a baseline assessment of cardiopulmonary status before therapy.
- Be alert for adverse reactions and drug interactions throughout therapy.
- Evaluate the patient's and family's knowledge about alprostadil therapy.

Nursing Diagnoses
- Altered tissue perfusion (cardiopulmonary) related to underlying condition.
- Altered tissue perfusion (cerebral) related to adverse effects of medication.
- Knowledge deficit related to alprostadil therapy.

Planning and Implementation
Preparation and Administration
• Alprostadil is administered via the intravenous, intra-arterial, or intra-aortic routes only.
• Drug must be diluted before being administered. Do not use diluents containing benzyl alcohol. Fresh solutions must be prepared daily. Discard any solution more than 24 hours old.
• Set rate once therapeutic response has been achieved.
• ***I.V. use:*** This drug is not recommended for direct injection or intermittent infusion. Administer by continuous infusion using a constant rate pump. Infuse through a large peripheral or central vein or through an umbilical artery catheter placed at the level of the ductus arteriosus.
Monitoring
• Monitor effectiveness by evaluating cardiopulmonary status.
• Monitor arterial blood pressure by umbilical artery catheter, auscultation, or Doppler transducer.
• Monitor drug effectiveness with blood pH as well as systemic blood pressure in infants with restricted systemic blood flow.
• Monitor blood oxygenation in the infant with restrictive pulmonary blood flow.
• Monitor for signs of drug overdose such as apnea and bradycardia.
• Observe the infant weighing less than 2 kg or receiving the infusion for longer than 48 hours for increased susceptibility to CNS adverse reactions.
• Observe the infant for flushing as an indication to reposition the catheter.
Supportive Care
• Observe the neonate with bleeding tendencies during the infusion for disseminated intravascular coagulation.
• Titrate infusion rate according to therapeutic response, for example, slow rate of infusion if arterial pressure falls significantly.
• Keep respiratory support available.
• If apnea or bradycardia occur, stop the infusion immediately and notify the doctor. These signs may reflect drug overdose.
• Reduce infusion rate if fever or significant hypotension occurs.
• Notify the doctor of significant changes in cardiopulmonary status.
Patient Teaching
• Keep parents informed of the infant's status.
• Explain to the parents that they will be allowed as much time and physical contact with the infant as feasible.

Evaluation
In patients receiving alprostadil, appropriate evaluation statements may include:
• Patient demonstrates a stable and effective cardiopulmonary status as indicated by adequate cardiac and pulmonary parameters, and peripheral systemic perfusion.
• Patient is seizure-free during and immediately after infusion of the medication.
• Patient and family state an understanding of alprostadil therapy.

---

alteplase (tissue plasminogen activator, recombinant; t-PA)
(al´ ti plase)
Actilyse‡, Activase

• *Classification:* thrombolytic (enzyme)
• *Pregnancy Risk Category:* C

HOW SUPPLIED
Injection: 20-mg (11.6 million–IU), 50-mg (29 million–IU) vials

ACTION
Mechanism: Genetically engineered human tissue plasminogen activator

(t-PA). Binds to fibrin in a thrombus, and locally converts plasminogen to plasmin, which initiates local fibrinolysis and dissolves the clot.
Distribution: Rapidly cleared from the plasma by the liver; 80% of a dose is cleared within 10 minutes after infusion is discontinued.
Metabolism: Primarily hepatic.
Excretion: Over 85% of drug is excreted in the urine, 5% in the feces. Half-life: Plasma half-life is less than 10 minutes.
Onset, peak, duration: Most patients experience reperfusion of the coronary artery within 1½ hours of the start of the infusion. Significant improvements in ejection fraction and survival are evident for several months following treatment.

INDICATIONS & DOSAGE

Lysis of thrombi obstructing coronary arteries in acute myocardial infarction–
Adults: 100 mg I.V. infusion over 3 hours as follows: 60 mg in the first hour, of which 6 to 10 mg is given as a bolus over the first 1 to 2 minutes. Then 20 mg/hr infusion for 2 hours. Smaller adults (< 65 kg) should receive a dose of 1.25 mg/kg in a similar fashion (60% in the first hour, with 10% as a bolus; then 20% of the total dose per hour for 2 hours).
Management of acute massive pulmonary embolism–
Adults: 100 mg I.V. infusion over 2 hours. Begin heparin at the end of the infusion when the partial thromboplastin time or thrombin time returns to twice normal or less.

CONTRAINDICATIONS & PRECAUTIONS

Contraindicated in patients with active internal bleeding, bleeding diathesis, aneurysm, arteriovenous malformation, history of cerebrovascular accident, recent intraspinal or intracranial surgery or trauma, brain tumor, or severe uncontrolled hypertension because of the potential for uncontrolled bleeding. Use with extreme caution in patients with acute pericarditis, cerebrovascular disease, diabetic hemorrhagic retinopathy, significant hepatic disease, marked hypertension, subacute bacterial endocarditis, septic thrombophlebitis, or in patients who are at risk for left heart thrombi (mitral stenosis with atrial fibrillation), because bleeding problems (the most common adverse effects of alteplase therapy) may pose a substantial risk to these patients.

ADVERSE REACTIONS

Common reactions are in italics; life-threatening reactions are in bold italics.
Blood: ***severe, spontaneous bleeding (cerebral, retroperitoneal, GU, GI).***
CNS: ***cerebral hemorrhage,*** fever.
CV: hypotension, arrhythmias.
GI: nausea, vomiting.
Local: bleeding at puncture sites.
Other: hypersensitivity, urticaria.

INTERACTIONS

Aspirin, dipyridamole, heparin, coumarin anticoagulants: increased risk of bleeding. Monitor patient carefully.

EFFECTS ON DIAGNOSTIC TESTS

Coagulation studies: altered results. Addition of aprotinin (150 to 200 units/ml) to the blood sample may attenuate this interference.

NURSING CONSIDERATIONS

Besides those related universally to drug therapy (see "How to use this book"), consider the following specific recommendations:

Assessment

- Obtain a baseline assessment of ECG and vital signs before therapy.
- Be alert for adverse reactions and drug interactions throughout therapy.
- Evaluate the patient's and family's knowledge about alteplase therapy.

Nursing Diagnoses
• Altered tissue perfusion (cardiopulmonary) related to the patient's underlying condition.
• High risk for injury related to the adverse effects of alteplase.
• Knowledge deficit related to alteplase therapy.

Planning and Implementation
Preparation and Administration
• ***I.V. use:*** Administer as continuous infusion: Available as a lyophilized powder in 20-mg and 50-mg vials. Store at room temperature or refrigerate. Reconstitute just before injection. Using an 18G needle, reconstitute to 1 mg/ml by adding 20 or 50 ml of preservative-free, sterile water for injection, provided by manufacturer. (Don't use bacteriostatic water for injection). Aim diluent at lyophilized cake and expect slight foaming. Let vial stand for several minutes. If necessary, dilute drug to 0.5 mg/ml in glass bottles or PVC bag. For 20 ml vial, add 20 ml of 0.9% sodium chloride or dextrose 5% in water; for 50-ml vial, add 50 ml. Avoid undue agitation. Dilute solution remains stable at room temperature for 8 hours. Infuse at recommended rate. Heparin infusion may be ordered before or during therapy to prevent new clot formation. Drug must be given within 6 hours after the onset of symptoms.
• Direct injection or intermittent infusion is recommended.

Monitoring
• Monitor effectiveness by regularly checking the patient's ECG, blood pressure, pulse, and respirations.
• Monitor ECG because transient arrhythmias result from reperfusion after coronary thrombolysis. Keep atropine or lidocaine available to treat arrhythmias.
• Obtain coagulation studies before therapy. Watch the patient for bleeding. If severe bleeding occurs and doesn't stop with local pressure, discontinue alteplase and heparin infusions.

Supportive Care
• Remember to avoid IM injections, venipuncture, and arterial puncture during therapy because of the increased risk of bleeding. If arterial puncture is necessary, select a site on an arm and apply pressure for 30 minutes afterward. Also use pressure dressings, sand bags, or ice packs on recent puncture sites to prevent bleeding.
• Try to avoid turning and moving the patient excessively during infusion.

Patient Teaching
• Tell the patient to report chest pain, dyspnea, changes in heart rate or rhythm, nausea, or bleeding immediately.

Evaluation
In patients receiving alteplase, appropriate evaluation statements may include:
• Patient's ECG and vital signs demonstrate improvement in perfusion.
• Patient has not experienced injury during therapy; significant blood loss or arrhythmias related to the adverse effects of alteplase did not occur.
• Patient and family state an understanding of alteplase therapy.

altretamine (hexamethylmelamine; HMM)
(al tree´ tah meen)
Hexalen

• *Classification:* antineoplastic (alkylating agent)
• *Pregnancy Risk Category:* D

HOW SUPPLIED
Capsules: 50 mg

ACTION
Mechanism: Unknown. Structurally similar to the alkylating agent trieth-

ylenemelamine, but neither the drug nor its metabolites are alkylating agents. Metabolism is known to be important for antitumor activity.
Absorption: Well-absorbed from the GI tract after oral administration; however, rapid and extensive demethylation in the liver causes variations in plasma levels.
Distribution: Does not cross the blood-brain barrier to a significant extent. The drug and its metabolites show binding to plasma proteins.
Metabolism: Rapid and extensive demethylation in the liver; major metabolites are pentamethylmelamine and tetramethylmelamine.
Excretion: Metabolites are excreted primarily in the urine. A small amount is eliminated through the lungs in expired air; trace amounts are excreted in feces. Half-life: Terminal elimination half-life ranges from 4.7 to 10.2 hours.

INDICATIONS & DOSAGE

Palliative treatment of patients with persistent or recurrent ovarian cancer after first-line therapy with cisplatin or alkylating agent–based combination therapy–
Adults: 260 mg/m² P.O. daily in four divided doses with meals and h.s. for 14 or 21 consecutive days in a 28-day cycle.

CONTRAINDICATIONS & PRECAUTIONS

Contraindicated in patients with hypersensitivity to the drug and in patients with preexisting severe bone marrow depression or severe neurologic toxicity. Unresponsive GI intolerance, WBC count below 2,000/mm³ or granulocytes below 1,000/mm³, platelets below 7,500/mm³, and progressive neurotoxicity require temporary discontinuation for 14 days or more and a dosage reduction to 200 mg/m²/day when restarted.

ADVERSE REACTIONS

Common reactions are in italics; life-threatening reactions are in bold italics.
Blood: leukopenia, ***thrombocytopenia,*** anemia.
CNS: *sensory neuropathy,* anorexia, fatigue, seizures.
GI: *nausea and vomiting.*
Other: increased serum creatinine and elevated BUN levels.

INTERACTIONS

Cimetidine: may increase the half-life and toxicity of altretamine. Monitor closely for toxicity.
MAO inhibitors: severe orthostatic hypotension. Avoid concomitant use.

EFFECTS ON DIAGNOSTIC TESTS

Blood and urine uric acid: increased concentrations.
Serum creatinine and BUN levels: altered results.

NURSING CONSIDERATIONS

Besides those related universally to drug therapy (see "How to use this book"), consider the following specific recommendations:

Assessment
- Obtain a baseline assessment of patient's underlying condition before initiating therapy.
- Be alert for adverse reactions and drug interactions throughout therapy.
- Evaluate the patient's and family's knowledge about altretamine therapy.

Nursing Diagnoses
- High risk for fluid volume deficit related to drug-induced adverse reactions.
- High risk for infection related to drug-induced adverse reactions.
- Knowledge deficit related to altretamine therapy.

Planning and Implementation
Preparation and Administration
- Obtain baseline CBC, platelet count, and kidney and liver function before initiating therapy.
- ***P.O. use:*** If drug is given continu-

ously, administer with antiemetics. Drug dosage may have to be altered if nausea and vomiting are severe.

Monitoring

• Monitor effectiveness by checking tumor size and rate of growth through appropriate studies; by noting the results of follow-up diagnostic tests and overall physical status.
• Monitor CBC and platelet count between each course of therapy and monthly thereafter.
• Monitor for signs of bleeding (hematuria, ecchymosis, petechiae, epistaxis, melena).
• Monitor for signs of infection (temperature elevation, sore throat, malaise).
• Monitor neurologic functioning daily. Continuous high-dose daily treatment is associated with mild-to-moderate neurotoxicity. It appears to be reversible when the drug is discontinued.
• Monitor the patient's hydration status if nausea and vomiting is severe.

Supportive Care

• Therapy should be started after a careful neurologic assessment.
• Provide the patient with fluids if severe nausea and vomiting occur.
• Obtain an order for an antiemetic if the patient develops nausea and vomiting.
• Be prepared to alter drug dosage, as ordered, if nausea and vomiting are severe.
• Be prepared to discontinue the drug for at least 14 days if laboratory tests indicate a platelet count below 75,000/mm^3, WBC count below 2,000/mm^3, or granulocyte count below 1,000/mm^3. Drug should be discontinued if neurologic symptoms fail to stabilize. Unconfirmed reports suggest that pyridoxine may be useful to decrease neurotoxicity.

Patient Teaching

• Inform patients that nausea, vomiting, and sensory neuropathy may occur.
• Advise the patient to use a barrier contraception during treatment because drug may cause fetal harm.
• Tell the patient that he may have to discontinue drug temporarily for at least 14 days if laboratory tests show a lowered platelet count.

Evaluation

In patients receiving altretamine, appropriate evaluation statements may include:

• Patient does not develop fluid volume loss.
• Patient remains infection-free.
• Patient and family state an understanding of altretamine therapy.

aluminum carbonate

(a loo´ mi num)

Basaljel◇

• *Classification:* antacid, hypophosphatemia agent (inorganic aluminum salt)
• *Pregnancy Risk Category:* C

HOW SUPPLIED

Tablets or capsules: aluminum hydroxide equivalent 500 mg◇
Oral suspension: aluminum hydroxide equivalent 400 mg/5 ml◇, 1 g/5 ml◇

ACTION

Mechanism: An antacid that reacts with hydrochloric acid in the GI tract to form aluminum chloride, water, and carbon dioxide. Reduces total acid load and elevates gastric pH to reduce pepsin activity. Also forms aluminum phosphate with phosphate in the intestinal lumen; if dietary phosphate is limited, phosphate absorption is decreased and calcium absorption is enhanced.
Absorption: Largely unabsorbed; small amounts may be absorbed systemically.
Distribution: None.
Metabolism: None.

Excretion: In feces; some may be excreted in breast milk.

INDICATIONS & DOSAGE

As antacid–
Adults: suspension: 5 to 10 ml P.O., p.r.n. Extra-strength suspension: 2.5 to 5 ml, p.r.n. Tablets: 1 to 2, p.r.n. Capsules: 1 to 2, p.r.n.
To prevent formation of urinary phosphate stones (with low-phosphate diet)–
Adults: suspension: 15 to 30 ml suspension in water or juice P.O. 1 hour after meals and h.s.; 5 to 15 ml extra-strength suspension in water or juice 1 hour after meals and h.s.; 2 to 6 tablets or capsules 1 hour after meals and h.s.

CONTRAINDICATIONS & PRECAUTIONS

Contraindicated in patients with hypophosphatemia, appendicitis, impaired renal function, undiagnosed rectal or GI bleeding, constipation, fecal impaction, chronic diarrhea, gastric outlet obstruction, and intestinal obstruction because the drug may exacerbate these conditions.

Use cautiously in patients with hemorrhoids because constipation associated with drug use may be irritating; and in patients with decreased GI motility, such as elderly patients and those receiving anticholinergics or antidiarrheals.

ADVERSE REACTIONS

Common reactions are in italics; life-threatening reactions are in bold italics.
GI: anorexia, *constipation,* intestinal obstruction.
Metabolic: hypophosphatemia.

INTERACTIONS

Allopurinol, antibiotics (including quinolones and tetracyclines), corticosteroids, diflunisal, digoxin, iron, isoniazid, penicillamine, phenothiazines, ranitidine: decreased pharmacologic effect because absorption may be impaired. Separate administration times.

EFFECTS ON DIAGNOSTIC TESTS

Gastric acid secretion tests: antagonism of pentagastrin's effect.
Imaging techniques using sodium pertechnetate Tc 99m: test interference.
Serum gastrin: increased levels.
Serum phosphate: decreased levels.

NURSING CONSIDERATIONS

Besides those related universally to drug therapy (see "How to use this book"), consider the following specific recommendations:

Assessment
- Obtain a baseline assessment of the patient's pain or discomfort before beginning therapy.
- Be alert for adverse reactions and drug interactions throughout therapy.
- Evaluate the patient's and family's knowledge about aluminum carbonate therapy.

Nursing Diagnoses
- Pain related to gastric hyperacidity.
- Constipation related to aluminum carbonate-induced adverse reactions.
- Knowledge deficit related to aluminum carbonate therapy.

Planning and Implementation
Preparation and Administration
- ***P.O. use:*** Administer drug 1 hour after meals and at bedtime if the drug is administered for the ulcer treatment. Do not give other oral medications within 1 to 2 hours of antacid administration. May cause premature release of enteric-coated drugs in stomach. Suspension: Shake suspension well; give with small amount of water or juice to ensure passage to stomach. When administering through nasogastric tube, make sure tube is placed correctly and is patent. After instilling antacid, flush tube with water.

Monitoring
• Monitor effectiveness by regularly assessing pain relief.
• Monitor long-term, high-dose use in patients on restricted sodium intake.
• Monitor the patient's bowel pattern. Watch for development of constipation, especially in the elderly patient.
• Periodically monitor serum calcium and phosphate levels; decreased serum phosphate levels may lead to increased serum calcium levels. Watch for symptoms of hypophosphatemia (anorexia, muscle weakness, and malaise) in patients taking the drug for a prolonged time.
Supportive Care
• If the patient develops constipation, notify the doctor and obtain an order for a laxative or stool softener and monitor its effectiveness. Also, if not contraindicated, encourage the patient to eat a high-fiber diet and to drink 8 to 13 8-oz glasses (2 to 3 liters) of water per day to help prevent constipation. Alternate this drug with magnesium-containing antacids (if the patient does not have renal disease).
• Encourage patient to discuss any emotional factors or dietary habits that may be contributing to the patient's GI problems.
• Keep in mind that aluminum carbonate therapy may interfere with imaging techniques using sodium pertechnetate Tc 99m and thus impair evaluation of Meckel's diverticulum. It may also interfere with reticuloendothelial imaging of liver, spleen, and bone marrow using technetium Tc 99m sulfur colloid. Drug may antagonize pentagastrin's effect during gastric acid secretion tests. Aluminum hydroxide may elevate serum gastrin levels and reduce serum phosphate levels.
Patient Teaching
• Caution the patient to take aluminum carbonate only as directed, to shake suspension well, and to follow with sips of water or juice.
• As indicated, instruct the patient to restrict sodium intake, drink plenty of fluids, or follow a low-phosphate diet.
• Advise the patient not to switch to another antacid without consulting the doctor.
• Teach the patient how to prevent constipation during therapy.
• Explain the importance of taking these medications as prescribed, and not taking other medications simultaneously.
• Warn the patient that drug may color his stool white or cause white streaks. Advise the patient to contact the doctor immediately if his stool becomes black.
• Explain to the patient whose sodium intake is restricted that long-term, high-dose usage of aluminum carbonate is not recommended.

Evaluation

In patients receiving aluminum carbonate, appropriate evaluation statements may include:
• Patient's pain subsides or is relieved.
• Patient experiences no constipation and maintains normal bowel function during therapy.
• Patient and family state an understanding of aluminum carbonate therapy.

aluminum hydroxide

(a loo´ mi num)

ALternaGEL◇, Alu-Cap◇, Alu-Tab◇, Amphojel◇, Amphotabs‡, Dialume◇, Nephrox◇

• *Classification:* antacid, hypophosphotemic agent, adsorbent (aluminum salt)
• *Pregnancy Risk Category:* C

HOW SUPPLIED

Tablets: 300 mg◇, 600 mg◇
Capsules: 475 mg◇, 500 mg◇

Oral suspension◇: 320 mg/5 ml◇, 600 mg/5 ml◇

ACTION

Mechanism: Aluminum hydroxide reacts with hydrochloric acid in the stomach to form aluminum chloride and water. Reduces total acid load and elevates gastric pH to reduce pepsin activity. Also forms aluminum phosphate with phosphate in the intestinal lumen; if dietary phosphate is limited, phosphate absorption is decreased and calcium absorption is enhanced.
Absorption: Minimally absorbed; small amounts may be absorbed systemically.
Distribution: None.
Metabolism: None.
Excretion: In feces; some drug may be excreted in breast milk.

INDICATIONS & DOSAGE

Antacid–
Adults: 600 mg P.O. (5 to 10 ml of most products) 1 hour after meals and h.s.; 300- or 600-mg tablet, chewed before swallowing, taken with milk or water 5 to 6 times daily after meals and h.s.
Hyperphosphatemia in renal failure–
Adults: 500 mg to 2 g P.O. b.i.d. to q.i.d.

ADVERSE REACTIONS

Common reactions are in italics; life-threatening reactions are in bold italics.
GI: anorexia, *constipation,* intestinal obstruction.
Metabolic: hypophosphatemia.

INTERACTIONS

Allopurinol, antibiotics (including quinolones and tetracyclines), corticosteroids, diflunisal, digoxin, iron, isoniazid, penicillamine, phenothiazines, ranitidine: decreased pharmacologic effect because absorption may be impaired. Separate administration times.

CONTRAINDICATIONS & PRECAUTIONS

Contraindicated in patients with hypophosphatemia, appendicitis, impaired renal function, undiagnosed rectal or GI bleeding, constipation, fecal impaction, chronic diarrhea, gastric outlet obstruction, or intestinal obstruction because the drug may exacerbate these symptoms.

Use cautiously in patients with hemorrhoids and in patients with decreased GI motility, such as elderly patients and those receiving anticholinergics or antidiarrheals, because constipation associated with drug use may be irritating.

EFFECTS ON DIAGNOSTIC TESTS

Gastric acid secretion tests: antagonism of pentagastrin's effect.
Imaging techniques using sodium pertechnetate Tc 99m: test interference.
Serum gastrin: elevated levels.
Serum phosphate: reduced levels.

NURSING CONSIDERATIONS

Besides those related universally to drug therapy (see "How to use this book"), consider the following specific recommendations:

Assessment
- Obtain a baseline assessment of the patient's discomfort before beginning therapy.
- Be alert for adverse reactions and drug interactions throughout therapy.
- Evaluate the patient's and family's knowledge about aluminum hydroxide therapy.

Nursing Diagnoses
- Pain related to gastric hyperacidity.
- Constipation related to binding effect of aluminum hydroxide.
- Knowledge deficit related to aluminum hydroxide therapy.

Planning and Implementation
Preparation and Administration
- ***P.O. use:*** Administer drug 1 hour after meals and at bedtime if the

*Liquid form contains alcohol. **May contain tartrazine.

drug is administered for ulcer treatment. Do not give other oral medications within 1 to 2 hours of antacid administration. May cause enteric-coated drugs to be released prematurely in stomach.

• ***Suspension:*** Shake suspension well; give with small amount of water or juice to ensure passage to stomach. When administering through nasogastric tube, make sure tube is placed correctly and is patent. After instilling antacid, flush tube with water.

• ***Chewable tablets:*** Ensure that this form of the medication is chewed completely before swallowing and is followed by a glass of water or milk.

Monitoring

• Monitor effectiveness by regularly assessing reduction or relief of the patient's pain or, if the drug is used in patients with renal failure to control hyperphosphatemia, monitor serum phosphate levels.

• Monitor long-term, high-dose use in patients on restricted sodium intake.

• Monitor the patient's bowel pattern. Watch for development of constipation, especially in the elderly patient.

• Periodically monitor serum calcium and phosphate levels; decreased serum phosphate levels may lead to increased serum calcium levels. Watch for symptoms of hypophosphatemia (anorexia, muscle weakness, and malaise) in patients taking the drug for a prolonged time.

Supportive Care

• If the patient develops constipation, notify the doctor and obtain an order for a laxative or stool softener and monitor its effectiveness. Also, if not contraindicated, encourage the patient to eat a high-fiber diet and to drink 8 to 13 8-oz glasses (2 to 3 liters) of water per day to help prevent constipation. Alternate this drug with magnesium-containing antacids (if the patient does not have renal disease).

• Encourage patient to discuss any emotional factors or dietary habits that may be contributing to the patient's GI problems.

• Keep in mind that aluminum hydroxide therapy may interfere with imaging techniques using sodium pertechnetate Tc 99m and thus impair evaluation of Meckel's diverticulum. It may interfere with reticuloendothelial imaging of liver, spleen, and bone marrow using technetium Tc 99m sulfur colloid; antagonize pentagastrin's effect during gastric acid secretion tests; elevate serum gastrin levels; and reduce serum phosphate levels.

Patient Teaching

• Caution the patient to take aluminum hydroxide only as directed, to shake suspension well, and to follow with sips of water or juice. Tell the patient receiving the chewable tablet form of the drug to chew the tablets completely before swallowing and, after swallowing, to drink a glass of milk or water.

• As indicated, instruct the patient to restrict sodium intake, drink plenty of fluids, or follow a low-phosphate diet.

• Advise the patient not to switch to another antacid without consulting the doctor.

• Teach the patient how to prevent constipation during therapy.

• Explain the importance of taking these medications as prescribed and not taking other medications simultaneously.

• Warn the patient that these drugs may color his stool white or cause white streaks. Advise the patient to contact the doctor immediately if his stool becomes black.

• Explain to the patient whose sodium intake is restricted that long-term, high-dose usage of aluminum hydroxide is not recommended.

Evaluation

In patients receiving aluminum hydroxide, appropriate evaluation statements may include:

• Patient's pain subsides or is relieved.
• Patient experiences no constipation; maintains normal bowel function during therapy.
• Patient and family state an understanding of aluminum hydroxide therapy.

aluminum phosphate

(a loo´ mi num)
Phosphaljel◇

• *Classification:* antacid (aluminum salt)
• *Pregnancy Risk Category:* C

HOW SUPPLIED

Oral suspension: 233 mg/5 ml◇

ACTION

Mechanism: An antacid that reacts with hydrochloric acid in the stomach to form aluminum chloride, phosphoric acid, and water. Reduces total acid load in the GI tract and elevates gastric pH to reduce pepsin activity.
Absorption: Small amounts may be absorbed systemically.
Distribution: None.
Metabolism: None.
Excretion: In feces; some may be excreted in breast milk.

INDICATIONS & DOSAGE

Antacid–
Adults: 15 to 30 ml undiluted P.O. q 2 hours between meals and h.s.

CONTRAINDICATIONS & PRECAUTIONS

Contraindicated in patients with impaired renal function, appendicitis, constipation, fecal impaction, undiagnosed rectal or GI bleeding, chronic diarrhea, gastric outlet obstruction, or intestinal obstruction because drug may exacerbate these conditions.

Use cautiously in patients who must restrict sodium intake because of the sodium content of the suspension; in patients who have hemorrhoids; and in patients with decreased GI motility, such as elderly patients and those receiving anticholinergics or antidiarrheals, because it may cause constipation and increase irritation.

ADVERSE REACTIONS

Common reactions are in italics; life-threatening reactions are in bold italics.
GI: *constipation,* intestinal obstruction.

INTERACTIONS

Ciprofloxacin, quinolone antibiotics, tetracyclines: decreased antibiotic effect. Separate administration times.

EFFECTS ON DIAGNOSTIC TESTS

Gastric acid secretion tests: antagonism of pentagastrin's effect.
Imaging techniques using sodium pertechnetate Tc 99m: test interference.
Serum gastrin: increased levels.
Serum phosphate: decreased levels.

NURSING CONSIDERATIONS

Besides those related universally to drug therapy (see "How to use this book"), consider the following specific recommendations:

Assessment
• Obtain a baseline assessment of the patient's pain or discomfort before beginning therapy.
• Be alert for adverse reactions and drug interactions throughout therapy.
• Evaluate the patient's and family's knowledge about aluminum phosphate therapy.

Nursing Diagnoses
• Pain related to gastric hyperacidity.
• Constipation related to aluminum carbonate-induced adverse reactions.
• Knowledge deficit related to aluminum phosphate therapy.

Planning and Implementation

Preparation and Administration

• ***P.O. use:*** Administer drug 1 hour after meals and at bedtime if the drug is administered for ulcer treatment. Do not give other oral medications within 1 to 2 hours of antacid administration. May cause premature release of enteric-coated drugs in stomach. Shake suspension well; give with small amount of water or milk to ensure passage to stomach. When administering through nasogastric tube, make sure tube is placed correctly and is patent. After instilling antacid, flush tube with water to facilitate passage to stomach and to maintain tube patency.

Monitoring

• Monitor effectiveness by regularly assessing reduction or relief of the patient's pain.

• Monitor long-term, high-dose use in patients on restricted sodium intake.

• Monitor the patient's bowel pattern. Watch for development of constipation, especially in elderly patients.

Supportive Care

• If the patient develops constipation, notify the doctor and obtain an order for a laxative or stool softener and monitor its effectiveness. Also, if not contraindicated, encourage the patient to eat a high-fiber diet and to drink 8 to 13 8-oz glasses (2 to 3 liters) of water per day to help prevent constipation. Alternate this drug with magnesium-containing antacids (if the patient does not have renal disease).

• Encourage patient to discuss any emotional factors or dietary habits that may be contributing to the patient's GI problems.

• Remember that this drug may interfere with imaging techniques using sodium pertechnetate Tc 99m and thus impair evaluation of Meckel's diverticulum; interfere with reticuloendothelial imaging of liver, spleen, and bone marrow using technetium Tc 99m sulfur colloid; antagonize pentagastrin's effect during gastric acid secretion tests; elevate serum gastrin levels; and reduce serum phosphate levels.

• Keep in mind that this drug can reverse hypophosphatemia induced by aluminum hydroxide.

Patient Teaching

• Caution the patient to take aluminum phosphate only as directed, to shake suspension well, and to follow with sips of water or juice.

• Advise the patient not to switch to another antacid without consulting the doctor.

• Teach the patient how to prevent constipation during therapy.

• Explain the importance of taking these medications as prescribed and not taking other medications simultaneously.

• Warn the patient that drug may color his stool white or cause white streaks. Advise the patient to contact the doctor immediately if his stool becomes black.

• Explain to the patient whose sodium intake is restricted that long-term, high-dose usage of aluminum phosphate is not recommended.

Evaluation

In patients receiving aluminum phosphate, appropriate evaluation statements may include:

• Patient's pain subsides or is relieved.

• Patient experiences no constipation; maintains normal bowel function during therapy.

• Patient and family state an understanding of aluminum phosphate therapy.

amantadine hydrochloride

(a man´ ta deen)

Antadine‡, Symadine, Symmetrel

• *Classification:* antiviral, antiparkinsonian agent

• *Pregnancy Risk Category:* C

HOW SUPPLIED

Capsules: 100 mg
Syrup: 50 mg/5 ml

ACTION

Mechanism: Interferes with penetration of influenza A virus into susceptible cells. Action in parkinsonism is largely unknown, but the drug may directly stimulate dopamine receptors.
Absorption: With oral administration, well absorbed from the GI tract.
Distribution: Distributed widely throughout the body and crosses the blood-brain barrier.
Metabolism: About 10% of dose is metabolized.
Excretion: About 90% of dose is excreted unchanged in urine, primarily by renal tubular secretion; some may be excreted in breast milk. Excretion rate depends on urine pH (acidic pH enhances excretion). Half-life: In patients with normal renal function, elimination half-life is approximately 24 hours. In patients with renal dysfunction, may be prolonged to 10 days.
Onset, peak, duration: Peak serum levels occur in 1 to 8 hours; usual serum level is 0.2 to 0.9 mcg/ml. (Neurotoxicity may occur at levels exceeding 1.5 mcg/ml.)

INDICATIONS & DOSAGE

Prophylaxis or symptomatic treatment of influenza type A virus, respiratory tract illnesses–
Adults to 64 years and children 10 years and over: 200 mg P.O. daily in a single dose or divided b.i.d.
Children 1 to 9 years: 4.4 to 8.8 mg/kg P.O. daily, divided b.i.d. or t.i.d. Don't exceed 150 mg daily.
Adults over 64 years: 100 mg P.O. once daily.

Treatment should continue for 24 to 48 hours after symptoms disappear. Prophylaxis should start as soon as possible after initial exposure and continue for at least 10 days after exposure. May continue prophylactic treatment up to 90 days for repeated or suspected exposures if influenza vaccine unavailable. If used with influenza vaccine, continue dose for 2 to 3 weeks until protection from vaccine develops.
To treat drug-induced extrapyramidal reactions–
Adults: 100 mg P.O. b.i.d., up to 300 mg daily in divided doses. Patient may benefit from as much as 400 mg daily, but dosages over 200 mg must be closely supervised.
To treat idiopathic parkinsonism, parkinsonian syndrome–
Adults: 100 mg P.O. b.i.d.; in patients who are seriously ill or receiving other antiparkinsonism drugs, 100 mg daily for at least 1 week, then 100 mg b.i.d., p.r.n.

CONTRAINDICATIONS & PRECAUTIONS

Contraindicated in patients with hypersensitivity to the drug. Administer cautiously to patients with a history of hepatic disease, seizures, psychosis, renal disease, recurrent eczematoid dermatitis, epilepsy, cardiovascular disease (especially CHF), peripheral edema, or orthostatic hypotension, because the drug may exacerbate these disorders. Do not administer to pregnant women or women of childbearing age without adequate contraceptive measures because animal studies have demonstrated embryotoxic and teratogenic potential.

ADVERSE REACTIONS

Common reactions are in italics; life-threatening reactions are in bold italics.
CNS: depression, fatigue, confusion, dizziness, psychosis, hallucinations, anxiety, *irritability,* ataxia, *insomnia,* weakness, headache, light-headedness, difficulty concentrating.

*Liquid form contains alcohol. **May contain tartrazine.

CV: peripheral edema, orthostatic hypotension, CHF.
GI: anorexia, nausea, constipation, vomiting, dry mouth.
GU: urine retention.
Skin: *livedo reticularis* (with prolonged use).

INTERACTIONS
None reported.

EFFECTS ON DIAGNOSTIC TESTS
None reported.

NURSING CONSIDERATIONS
Besides those related universally to drug therapy (see "How to use this book"), consider the following specific recommendations:

Assessment
- Obtain a baseline assessment of infection before therapy.
- Be alert for adverse reactions and drug interactions throughout therapy.
- Evaluate the patient's and family's knowledge about amantadine therapy.

Nursing Diagnoses
- High risk for injury related to ineffectiveness of amantadine to eradicate the infection.
- High risk for fluid volume deficit related to adverse GI reactions to oral amantadine.
- Knowledge deficit related to amantadine.

Planning and Implementation

Preparation and Administration
- ***P.O. use:*** Administer drug after meals for best absorption.

Monitoring
- Monitor effectiveness by regularly assessing for improvement in the infection.
- Be aware that elderly patients are more susceptible to neurologic adverse reactions.
- Monitor patient's hydration status if adverse GI reactions occur.

Supportive Care
- Obtain an order for an antiemetic agent as needed.
- If patient develops neurologic adverse reactions, notify the doctor. Dividing the drug into b.i.d. doses may reduce incidence of adverse reactions.
- If insomnia occurs, administer the drug several hours before bedtime.

Patient Teaching
- Tell patient to take drug after meals to enhance absorption.
- Instruct patient to report adverse reactions to the doctor, especially dizziness, depression, anxiety, nausea, and urine retention.
- If orthostatic hypotension occurs, instruct patient not to stand or change positions too quickly.
- Instruct patient to take drug several hours before bedtime if it causes insomnia.
- When drug is prescribed for parkinsonism, warn patient against discontinuing it abruptly because this could provoke a parkinsonian crisis.

Evaluation
In patients receiving amantadine, appropriate evaluation statements may include:
- Patient is free of infection.
- Patient's maintains adequate hydration throughout amantadine therapy.
- Patient and family state an understanding of amantadine therapy.

---

amcinonide
(am sin´ oh nide)
Cyclocort

- *Classification:* anti-inflammatory (adrenocorticoid)
- *Pregnancy Risk Category:* C

HOW SUPPLIED
Cream: 0.1%
Ointment: 0.1%

ACTION
Mechanism: Produces local anti-inflammatory, vasoconstrictor, and

antipruritic actions. Drug diffuses across cell membranes to form complexes with specific cytoplasmic receptors, influencing cellular metabolism. Corticosteroids stabilize leukocyte lysosomal membranes, inhibit local actions and accumulation of macrophages, decrease local edema, and reduce the formation of scar tissue.
Absorption: Amount absorbed depends on the amount applied and on the nature of the skin at the application site. It ranges from about 1% in areas with thick stratum corneum (on the palms, soles, elbows, and knees) to as high as 36% in thinner areas (face, eyelids, and genitals). Absorption increases in areas of skin damage, inflammation, or occlusion. Some systemic absorption of topical steroids may occur, especially through the oral mucosa.
Distribution: After topical application, distributed throughout the local skin. If absorbed into the circulation, drug is rapidly removed from the blood and distributed into muscle, liver, skin, intestines, and kidneys.
Metabolism: After topical administration, metabolized primarily in the skin. The small amount absorbed into systemic circulation is metabolized primarily in the liver to inactive compounds.
Excretion: Inactive metabolites are excreted by the kidneys, primarily as glucuronides and sulfates, but also as unconjugated products. Small amounts of the metabolites are also excreted in feces.

INDICATIONS & DOSAGE

Inflammation of corticosteroid-responsive dermatoses–
Adults and children: apply a light film to affected areas b.i.d. or t.i.d. Cream should be rubbed in gently and thoroughly until it disappears.

CONTRAINDICATIONS & PRECAUTIONS

Contraindicated in patients who are hypersensitive to any component of the preparation and in patients with viral diseases of the skin, such as varicella or herpes simplex, because it suppresses the patient's immune response.

Use with extreme caution in patients with impaired circulation because it may increase the risk of skin ulceration.

Avoid applying to the face or genital area because increased absorption may result in striae.

ADVERSE REACTIONS

Common reactions are in italics; life-threatening reactions are in bold italics.
Skin: burning, itching, irritation, dryness, folliculitis, striae, acneiform eruptions, perioral dermatitis, hypopigmentation, hypertrichosis, allergic contact dermatitis. With occlusive dressings: *secondary infection, maceration, atrophy, striae, miliaria.*

INTERACTIONS

None significant.

EFFECTS ON DIAGNOSTIC TESTS

None significant.

NURSING CONSIDERATIONS

Besides those related universally to drug therapy (see "How to use this book"), consider the following specific recommendations:

Assessment
- Obtain a baseline assessment of skin in the affected area before therapy.
- Be alert for adverse reactions and drug interactions throughout therapy.
- Evaluate the patient's and family's knowledge about amcinonide therapy.

Nursing Diagnoses
- Impaired skin integrity related to the patient's underlying condition.
- High risk for impaired skin integ-

rity related to amcinonide-induced maceration.
• Knowledge deficit related to amcinonide therapy.

Planning and Implementation

Preparation and Administration

• ***Topical use:*** Before applying, gently wash skin. Rub medication in gently, leaving a thin coat, to prevent damage to skin. When treating hairy sites, part hair and apply directly to lesion.
• To apply an occlusive dressing (if ordered): apply cream, then cover with a thin, pliable nonflammable plastic film; seal to adjacent normal skin with hypoallergenic tape. Don't leave in place longer than 16 hours each day. Occlusive dressings should not be used in presence of infections or with weeping or exudative lesions. Hold dressings in place with gauze, elastic bandages, stockings or stockette, for a patient with eczematous dermatitis who may develop irritation with adhesive material.

Monitoring

• Monitor effectiveness by regularly examining patient's skin.
• Monitor for signs of systemic absorption, skin irritation or ulceration, hypersensitivity, or infection; if they develop, stop drug and notify doctor. (If antifungals or antibiotics are being used with corticosteroids and infection does not respond immediately, corticosteroids should be stopped until infection is controlled.)
• Check patient's temperature regularly for fever; if it develops, remove occlusive dressing and notify doctor.
• Monitor for adverse reactions and interactions by frequently inspecting his skin for infection, striae, and atrophy.

Supportive Care

• Change dressings as ordered by doctor. Be prepared to discontinue the drug and notify the doctor if infection, straie, or atrophy occur.
• Be aware that treatment should be continued for a few days after clearing of lesions to prevent recurrence.
• Use cautiously in patients with viral skin diseases, such as varicella, vaccinia, or herpes simplex; fungal infections; or bacterial skin infections.
• Remember, systemic absorption especially likely with occlusive dressings, prolonged treatment, or extensive body-surface treatment.
• Avoid the use of plastic pants or tight-fitting diapers in treated areas, when used in young children.
• Minimize adverse reactions by using occlusive dressing intermittently.

Patient Teaching

• Teach patient how to apply medication.
• Instruct patient to avoid application near eyes or mucous membranes. Do not use on face, armpits, groin, in ear canal, or under breasts unless specifically ordered. Tell patient to discontinue drug and notify doctor if maceration occurs.

Evaluation

In patients receiving amcinonide, appropriate evaluation statements may include:
• Patient states his dermatoses has resolved.
• Patient did not develop drug-induced maceration.
• Patient and family state an understanding of amcinonide therapy.

amikacin sulfate

(am i kay´ sin)
Amikin

• *Classification:* aminoglycoside antibiotic
• *Pregnancy Risk Category:* C

HOW SUPPLIED

Injection: 50 mg/ml, 250 mg/ml

ACTION

Mechanism: Becomes incorporated into viral DNA and inhibits viral multiplication.
Absorption: Slow and incomplete with oral administration; not affected by food.
Distribution: Widely distributed to organ tissues and body fluids. CSF concentrations equal approximately 50% of serum concentrations. About 9% to 33% of a dose binds to plasma proteins.
Metabolism: Metabolized inside the viral cell to its active form. Approximately 10% of a dose is metabolized extracellularly.
Excretion: Up to 92% of systemically absorbed acyclovir is excreted as unchanged drug by the kidneys by glomerular filtration and tubular secretion. Half-life: In patients with normal renal function, half-life is 2 to 3½ hours. Renal failure may extend half-life to 19 hours.
Onset, peak, duration: Peak concentrations occur in 1½ to 2 hours.

INDICATIONS & DOSAGE

Serious infections caused by sensitive Pseudomonas aeruginosa, Escherichia coli, Proteus, Klebsiella, Serratia, Enterobacter, Acinetobacter, Providencia, Citrobacter, Staphylococcus–
Adults and children with normal renal function: 15 mg/kg/day divided q 8 to 12 hours I.M. or I.V. infusion (in 100 to 200 ml dextrose 5% in water run in over 30 to 60 minutes). May be given by direct I.V. push if necessary.
Neonates with normal renal function: initially, 10 mg/kg I.M. or I.V. infusion (in dextrose 5% in water run in over 1 to 2 hours), then 7.5 mg/kg q 12 hours I.M. or I.V. infusion.
Meningitis–
Adults: systemic therapy as above; may also use up to 20 mg intrathecally or intraventricularly daily.
Children: systemic therapy as above; may also use 1 to 2 mg intrathecally daily.
Uncomplicated urinary tract infections–
Adults: 250 mg I.M. or I.V. b.i.d.
Adults with impaired renal function: initially, 7.5 mg/kg. Subsequent doses and frequency determined by blood amikacin levels and renal function studies.

CONTRAINDICATIONS & PRECAUTIONS

Contraindicated in patients with hypersensitivity to amikacin or any aminoglycoside.

Use cautiously in patients with decreased renal function; tinnitus, vertigo, or high-frequency hearing loss, who are susceptible to ototoxicity; dehydration, because of increased risk of nephrotoxicity with decreased urine output; myasthenia gravis, parkinsonism, and hypocalcemia, because the drug may exacerbate associated symptoms; in neonates or other infants; and in elderly patients.

ADVERSE REACTIONS

Common reactions are in italics; life-threatening reactions are in bold italics.
CNS: headache, lethargy, ***neuromuscular blockade.***
EENT: *ototoxicity (tinnitus, vertigo, hearing loss).*
GU: *nephrotoxicity (cells or casts in urine, oliguria, proteinuria, decreased creatinine clearance, increased BUN and serum creatinine levels).*
Other: ***hypersensitivity reactions, hepatic necrosis.***

INTERACTIONS

Cephalothin: increased nephrotoxicity. Use together cautiously.
Dimenhydrinate: may mask symptoms of ototoxicity. Use with caution.
General anesthetics, neuromuscular blocking agents: may potentiate neuromuscular blockade.

I.V. loop diuretics (e.g., furosemide): increase ototoxicity. Use cautiously.
Other aminoglycosides, amphotericin B, cisplatin, methoxyflurane: increases nephrotoxicity. Use together cautiously.
Parenteral penicillins (e.g., carbenicillin, ticarcillin): amikacin inactivation in vitro. Don't mix together in I.V.

EFFECTS ON DIAGNOSTIC TESTS

BUN, nonprotein nitrogen, serum creatinine: increased levels.
Urinalysis: increased excretion of casts.

NURSING CONSIDERATIONS

Besides those related universally to drug therapy (see "How to use this book"), consider the following specific recommendations:

Assessment

- Obtain a baseline assessment of infection before therapy.
- Be alert for adverse reactions and drug interactions throughout therapy.
- Evaluate the patient's and family's knowledge about amikacin therapy.

Nursing Diagnoses

- High risk for injury related to ineffectiveness of amikacin to eradicate the infection.
- Altered urinary elimination related to amikacin-induced nephrotoxicity.
- Knowledge deficit related to amikacin.

Planning and Implementation

Preparation and Administration

- Obtain specimen for culture and sensitivity tests before first dose. Therapy may begin pending test results.
- Weigh patient and obtain baseline renal function studies before therapy begins.
- Ensure adequate hydration during therapy to minimize chemical irritation of the renal tubules.
- Potency of drug is not affected if solution turns light yellow.
- ***I.V. use:*** Drug may be administered direct I.V. push if necessary and prescribed. After I.V. administration, flush line with 0.9% sodium chloride solution or dextrose 5% in water.

Monitoring

- Monitor effectiveness by regularly assessing patient for improvement in infectious process.
- Monitor serum amikacin level. Draw blood for peak amikacin level 1 hour after I.M injection and 30 minutes to 1 hour after infusion ends; for trough levels, draw blood just before next dose. Don't collect blood in a heparinized tube because heparin is incompatible with aminoglycosides.
- Peak blood levels over 35 mcg/ml and trough levels over 10 mcg/ml may be associated with higher incidence of toxicity.
- Monitor renal function, including intake and output, specific gravity, urinalysis, BUN, and creatinine levels and creatinine clearance.

Supportive Care

- Notify doctor of signs of decreasing renal function.
- Encourage the patient to maintain fluid intake of at least 2,000 ml/day (unless contraindicated).
- If patient complains of tinnitus, vertigo, or hearing loss, notify doctor of suspected ototoxicity and prepare the patient for audiometric testing.
- Notify the doctor if amikacin peak or trough level exceeds normal limits.
- Usual duration of therapy is 7 to 10 days. If no response after 3 to 5 days, therapy may be discontinued and new specimens obtained for culture and sensitivity.

Patient Teaching

- Instruct the patient to notify the doctor immediately of changes in hearing or changes in appearance or elimination pattern of urine. Teach patient how to measure his intake and output.
- Instruct the patient to notify the

doctor if the infection worsens or does not improve.
• Stress the importance of recommended laboratory tests to monitor amikacin level, renal function, and toxicity.
• Emphasize the need to drink 2,000 ml of fluid each day, not including coffee, tea, or other caffeinated beverages.
• Teach patient to watch for and promptly report signs of superinfection (continued fever and other signs of new infections, especially of upper respiratory tract).

Evaluation

In patients receiving amikacin, appropriate evaluation statements may include:
• Patient is free of infection.
• Patient's renal function studies remain normal throughout amikacin therapy.
• Patient and family state an understanding of amikacin therapy.

amiloride hydrochloride

(a mill´ oh ride)

Kaluril‡, Midamor

• *Classification:* diuretic, antihypertensive (potassium-sparing diuretic)
• *Pregnancy Risk Category:* B

HOW SUPPLIED

Tablets: 5 mg

ACTION

Mechanism: A potassium-sparing diuretic that inhibits sodium reabsorption and potassium excretion by direct action on the distal tubule.
Absorption: About 50% of an amiloride dose is absorbed from the GI tract. Food decreases absorption to 30%.
Distribution: Wide extravascular distribution.
Metabolism: Insignificant.
Excretion: Primarily in urine. Half-life: 6 to 9 hours in patients with normal renal function.
Onset, peak, duration: Diuresis usually begins in 2 hours and peaks in 6 to 10 hours.

INDICATIONS & DOSAGE

Hypertension; edema associated with congestive heart failure, usually in patients who are also taking thiazide or other potassium-wasting diuretics—

Adults: usual dosage is 5 mg P.O. daily. Dosage may be increased to 10 mg daily, if necessary. As much as 20 mg daily can be given.

CONTRAINDICATIONS & PRECAUTIONS

Contraindicated in patients with serum potassium levels over 5.5 mEq/liter or who are receiving other potassium-sparing diuretics or potassium supplements; anuria, acute or chronic renal insufficiency, or diabetic nephropathy because of the potential for hyperkalemia; and hypersensitivity to the drug.

Use cautiously in patients with severe hepatic insufficiency because electrolyte imbalance may precipitate hepatic encephalopathy, and in patients with diabetes, who are at increased risk of hyperkalemia.

ADVERSE REACTIONS

Common reactions are in italics; life-threatening reactions are in bold italics.
CNS: *headache,* weakness, dizziness.
CV: orthostatic hypotension.
GI: *nausea, anorexia, diarrhea, vomiting,* abdominal pain, constipation.
GU: impotence.
Metabolic: hyperkalemia.

INTERACTIONS

ACE inhibitors, potassium-sparing diuretics, potassium supplements:

possible hyperkalemia. Avoid concomitant use.
NSAIDs: decreased diuretic effectiveness. Avoid concomitant use.

EFFECTS ON DIAGNOSTIC TESTS

Glucose tolerance testing: interference; discontinue amiloride at least 3 days before testing.
Renal and hepatic function tests: transient abnormal results.
Serum potassium: severe hyperkalemia in diabetic patients after I.V.

NURSING CONSIDERATIONS

Besides those related universally to drug therapy (see "How to use this book"), consider the following specific recommendations:

Assessment

• Obtain a baseline assessment of blood pressure, urine output, weight, serum electrolytes, and peripheral edema before initiating drug therapy.
• Be alert for adverse reactions and drug interactions throughout therapy.
• Evaluate the patient's and family's knowledge about amiloride therapy.

Nursing Diagnoses

• Fluid volume excess related to the patient's underlying condition as evidenced by edema.
• High risk for injury related to hyperkalemia due to amiloride therapy.
• Knowledge deficit related to amiloride therapy.

Planning and Implementation

Preparation and Administration

• ***P.O. use:*** Give drug with meals to prevent nausea and early in the day to prevent nocturia.

Monitoring

• Monitor effectiveness by regularly checking urine output, blood pressure, weight, and evidence of edema.
• Monitor BUN levels and serum electrolytes, especially potassium. Be aware that risk of hyperkalemia is greater when a potassium-wasting drug is not taken concurrently. When amiloride is taken this way, be sure to monitor daily potassium.
• Monitor for signs of hyperkalemia: muscle weakness and cramps, paresthesia, diarrhea, and cardiac arrhythmias.
• Monitor skin turgor and mucous membranes for signs of fluid volume depletion.

Supportive Care

• Hold drug and notify the doctor if hyperkalemia or dehydration occurs. Discontinue drug immediately if potassium level exceeds 6.5 mEq/liter.
• Keep accurate record of intake and output, and blood pressure.
• Weigh the patient daily.
• Provide frequent skin and mouth care to relieve dryness due to diuretic therapy.
• Answer the patient's call bells promptly; make sure patient's bathroom or bedpan is easily accessible.
• Use safety precautions to prevent the risk of injury due to falls.
• Elevate the patient's legs to reduce peripheral edema.

Patient Teaching

• Teach the patient and family to identify and report signs of hyperkalemia.
• Teach the patient and family to monitor the patient's fluid volume by recording daily weight and intake and output.
• Advise the patient to avoid excessive intake of high-potassium foods and of potassium-containing sodium substitutes.
• Instruct the patient to avoid concomitant use of potassium supplements.
• Advise the patient to change positions slowly, especially when rising to a standing position, to avoid dizziness and fainting due to orthostatic hypotension.
• Tell the patient to take drug with meals and, if possible, early in the day to avoid interruption of sleep by nocturia.

Evaluation

In patients receiving amiloride, appropriate evaluation statements may include:

• Patient is free of edema.
• Patient's serum potassium remains within normal range.
• Patient and family state an understanding of amiloride therapy.

amino acid injection

FreAmine HBC, HepatAmine

amino acid solution (crystalline amino acid solution)

Aminosyn II, FreAmine III, Novamine, Travasol

• *Classification:* nutritional and caloric agent (protein substrates)
• *Pregnancy Risk Category:* C

HOW SUPPLIED

amino acid injection

Injection: sulfur-containing amino acid–10-ml additive syringe (50 mg/ml)
Injection (with electrolytes): 1,000 ml (3%, 3.5%); 500 ml (3.5%, 5.5%, 7%, 8%, 8.5%)
Injection (without electrolytes): 1,000 ml (3.5%, 5%, 8.5%, 10%, 11.4%); 500 ml (5%, 5.5%, 7%, 8.5%, 10%, 11.4%); 250 ml (5%, 10%, 11.4%)

amino acid solution

Injection: sulfur-containing amino acid–10-ml additive syringe (50 mg/ml)
Injection (with electrolytes): 1,000 ml (3%, 3.5%); 500 ml (3.5%, 5.5%, 7%, 8%, 8.5%)
Injection (without electrolytes): 1,000 ml (3.5%, 5%, 8.5%, 10%, 11.4%); 500 ml (5%, 5.5%, 7%, 8.5%, 10%, 11.4%); 250 ml (5%, 10%, 11.4%)

ACTION

Mechanism: Prevents nitrogen loss by the body when enteral nutrition is not possible by acting as a substrate for protein synthesis or by enhancing conservation of existing body protein. Usually mixed with dextrose, electrolyte, or vitamins before administration.
Distribution: Widely distributed throughout the body.
Metabolism: Catabolized by the liver to form carbohydrates and energy. Branched-chain amino acids (valine, leucine, and isoleucine) are mainly catabolized by skeletal muscles. During catabolism, amino groups are removed and the alpha-keto acid is used to form carbohydrates or fats, or is converted into energy by oxidation. Amino groups form urea.
Excretion: By the kidneys.

INDICATIONS & DOSAGE

Treatment of hepatic encephalopathy in patients with cirrhosis or hepatitis; nutritional support–
Adults: 80 to 120 g of amino acids (12 to 18 g of nitrogen)/day. Typically, 500 ml is mixed with 500 ml dextrose 50% in water and administered over a 24-hour period. Add electrolytes, vitamins, and trace elements p.r.n.
Total, supportive, or supplemental and protein-sparing parenteral nutrition when gastrointestinal system must rest during healing, or when patient can't, shouldn't, or won't eat at all or eat enough to maintain normal nutrition and metabolism–
Adults: 1 to 1.5 g/kg amino acid solution I.V. daily.
Children: 2 to 3 g/kg amino acid solution I.V. daily. Individualize dosage to metabolic and clinical response as determined by nitrogen balance and body weight corrected for fluid balance. Add electrolytes, vitamins, and nonprotein caloric solutions as needed.

CONTRAINDICATIONS & PRECAUTIONS

Contraindicated in patients with decreased circulating blood volume, inborn errors of amino acid metabolism, or hypersensitivity to any component. General amino acid formulations are contraindicated in patients with severe renal failure, severe liver disease, hepatic coma, hepatic encephalopathy, or hyperammonemia. Renal failure formulations are contraindicated in patients with severe electrolyte and acid-base imbalance and hyperammonemia. Hepatic failure and hepatic encephalopathy formulations are contraindicated in patients with anuria. High metabolic stress formulations are contraindicated in patients with anuria, hepatic coma, or severe electrolyte or acid-base imbalances.

Electrolytes should be administered cautiously in patients with cardiac insufficiency, renal impairment, or pulmonary disease. Administering sodium to patients with chronic heart failure, renal failure, or edema with sodium retention requires special precautions. Administering potassium requires caution in patients with hyperkalemia, severe renal failure, or potassium retention. Acetate must be used cautiously in patients with alkalosis or hepatic insufficiency.

Amino acid infusions should be used with special caution in patients with elevated BUN levels, which usually result from increased protein intake; discontinue infusion if BUN levels continue to rise. Renal failure or GI bleeding may also increase BUN levels; use should be avoided in patients with azotemia unless total nitrogen concentration is considered.

When used as protein-sparing therapy, if daily BUN levels increase for more than 3 days, protein-sparing therapy should be discontinued and a nonprotein regimen substituted. Circulatory overload should be avoided in patients with cardiac dysfunction. Amino acids should always be administered with dextrose in patients with myocardial infarction.

Hypertonic solutions containing more than 12.5% dextrose should not be administered peripherally. Hyperosmolar solutions should not be used in dehydrated patients with intracranial or intraspinal hemorrhage or delirium tremens.

Patients should be monitored carefully for glucose imbalance; glucose intolerance is quite common, especially in septic or hypermetabolic patients and in patients with renal failure. Metabolic adaptation to a large glucose load takes up to 72 hours. Reducing the administration rate may help prevent glucose intolerance. Excessive carbohydrates may cause fatty infiltration of the liver. Excessive glucose may precipitate respiratory failure. Abrupt discontinuation of concentrated dextrose solutions may result in rebound hypoglycemia; a dextrose 5% solution should be administered during gradual withdrawal.

Intravenous nutritional therapy requires continuous monitoring. Amino acid metabolism may result in hyperchloremic metabolic acidosis; therefore, chloride content must be minimized. Conservative doses of amino acid injection must be administered to patients with impaired liver function. Hyperammonemia requires discontinuation and reevaluation of amino acid therapy. This occurs most often in children or adults with renal or hepatic disease with a diminished ability to handle the protein load. Hyperammonemia is particularly significant in infants, who may develop mental retardation as a result.

ADVERSE REACTIONS

Common reactions are in italics; life-threatening reactions are in bold italics.

CNS: mental confusion, unconsciousness, headache, dizziness.

CV: hypervolemia, *CHF* (in susceptible patients), ***pulmonary edema,*** exacerbation of hypertension (in predisposed patients).
GI: nausea, vomiting.
GU: glycosuria, osmotic diuresis.
Hepatic: fatty liver.
Metabolic: *rebound hypoglycemia* (when long-term infusions are abruptly stopped), *hyperglycemia,* metabolic acidosis, alkalosis, hypophosphatemia, *hyperosmolar nonketotic syndrome,* hyperammonemia, *electrolyte imbalances,* dehydration (if hyperosmolar solutions are used).
Skin: chills, flushing, feeling of warmth.
Local: tissue sloughing at infusion site due to extravasation, *catheter sepsis, thrombophlebitis,* thrombosis.
Other: allergic reactions.

INTERACTIONS
None significant.

EFFECTS ON DIAGNOSTIC TESTS
None reported.

NURSING CONSIDERATIONS
Besides those related universally to drug therapy (see "How to use this book"), consider the following specific recommendations:

Assessment
- Obtain a baseline assessment of patient's underlying condition before therapy.
- Be alert for adverse reactions and drug interactions throughout therapy.
- Evaluate the patient's and family's knowledge about amino acid injection therapy.

Nursing Diagnoses
- Altered nutrition: Less than body requirements, related to the patient's underlying condition.
- High risk for fluid volume deficit related to adverse drug reaction.
- Knowledge deficit related to therapy with amino acid injections.

Planning and Implementation
Preparation and Administration
- ***I.V. use:*** Control infusion rate carefully with an infusion pump. Direct injection and intermittent infusion are not recommended.
- If infusion rate falls behind, do not attempt to catch up. Notify doctor.
- Peripheral infusions should be limited to 2.5% amino acids and dextrose 10%.
- If a subclavian catheter is used, the solution is administered into the midsuperior vena cava.

Monitoring
- Monitor for adverse reactions by assessing serum electrolytes, and glucose, BUN, and renal and hepatic function.
- Monitor diabetic patients closely during administration. To prevent hyperglycemia, insulin may be required.
- Monitor patients with cardiac insufficiency during administration. May cause circulatory overload. Patients with fluid restrictions may only tolerate 1 to 2 liters.
- Monitor for extraordinary electrolyte losses, which may occur from nasogastric suctioning, vomiting, or drainage from GI fistula.
- Check infusion site frequently for erythema, inflammation, irritation, tissue sloughing, necrosis, and phlebitis.
- Check fractional urine every 6 hours for glycosuria initially, then every 12 to 24 hours in stable patients. Abrupt onset of glycosuria may be an early sign of impending sepsis or infection.

Supportive Care
- Change peripheral I.V. sites routinely to prevent irritation and infection.
- If patient has chills, fever, or other signs of sepsis, replace I.V. tubing and bottle, and send them to the laboratory to be cultured.

Patient Teaching
• Tell the patient to report discomfort at the injection site.

Evaluation

In patients receiving amino acid injections, appropriate evaluation statements may include:
• Patient's nutritional status is improving.
• Patient does not develop drug-induced nausea and vomiting.
• Patient and family state an understanding of therapy with amino acid injections.

aminocaproic acid

(a mee noe ka proe´ ik)
Amicar

• *Classification:* fibrinolysis inhibitor (carboxylic acid derivative)
• *Pregnancy Risk Category:* C

HOW SUPPLIED

Tablets: 500 mg
Syrup: 250 mg/ml
Injection: 5 g/20 ml for dilution, 24 g/96 ml for infusion

ACTION

Mechanism: Inhibits plasminogen activator substances. To a lesser degree, it blocks antiplasmin activity by inhibiting fibrinolysis.
Absorption: Rapidly and completely absorbed from the GI tract.
Distribution: Readily permeates human blood cells and other body cells. It is not protein-bound.
Metabolism: Insignificant.
Excretion: 40% to 60% of a single oral dose is excreted unchanged in urine in 12 hours.
Onset, peak, duration: Plasma peak level occurs in 2 hours; sustained plasma levels are achieved by repeated oral doses or continuous I.V. infusion. Duration of action of a single parenteral dose is less than 3 hours.

INDICATIONS & DOSAGE

Excessive bleeding resulting from hyperfibrinolysis–
Adults: initially, 5 g P.O. or slow I.V. infusion, followed by 1 to 1.25 g hourly until bleeding is controlled. Maximum dosage is 30 g daily.

CONTRAINDICATIONS & PRECAUTIONS

Contraindicated in patients with active intravascular clotting; in patients with disseminated intravascular coagulation (DIC) without concomitant heparin therapy, because aminocaproic acid may induce thrombus formation; in neonates because it contains benzyl alcohol, which has been associated with toxicity.

Administer cautiously to patients with thrombophlebitis or cardiac disease because of potential for clotting abnormalities, and to patients with hepatic or renal disease because of potential for drug accumulation.

ADVERSE REACTIONS

Common reactions are in italics; life-threatening reactions are in bold italics.
Blood: generalized thrombosis.
CNS: dizziness, malaise, headache.
CV: hypotension, bradycardia, arrhythmias (with rapid I.V. infusion).
EENT: tinnitus, nasal stuffiness, conjunctival suffusion.
GI: nausea, cramps, diarrhea.
Skin: rash.
Other: malaise.

INTERACTIONS

Oral contraceptives, estrogens: increased probability of hypercoagulability. Use together cautiously.

EFFECTS ON DIAGNOSTIC TESTS

Creatinine phosphokinase (CPK), ALT (SGOT), and AST(SGPT): increased levels.

Serum potassium: elevated level in some patients with decreased renal function.

NURSING CONSIDERATIONS

Besides those related universally to drug therapy (see "How to use this book"), consider the following specific recommendations:

Assessment

• Obtain a baseline assessment of history of blood loss, coagulation studies, blood pressure, and heart rhythm before therapy.
• Be alert for adverse reactions and drug interactions throughout therapy.
• Evaluate the patient's and family's knowledge about aminocaproic acid therapy.

Nursing Diagnoses

• Fluid volume deficit related to excessive bleeding.
• Altered tissue perfusion (venous) related to aminocaproic acid-induced generalized thrombosis.
• Knowledge deficit related to aminocaproic acid therapy.

Planning and Implementation

Preparation and Administration

• ***I.V. use:*** Dilute solution with sterile water for injection, normal saline injection, dextrose 5% in water, or Ringer's injection.
• Infuse slowly. Do not give direct or intermittent injection.

Monitoring

• Monitor effectiveness by checking the patient's coagulation studies.
• Monitor vital signs frequently until stable.
• Observe cardiac rhythm especially when giving I.V. dose.
• Monitor hemoglobin, hematocrit, and WBC.
• Monitor fluid and electrolyte balance. Test urine specific gravity.
• Monitor skin color, temperature, and turgor.
• Weigh patient daily until stable.
• Observe for changes in mental and neurologic status.
• Observe for development of emboli: auscultate lungs regularly; observe for dyspnea, cough, hemoptysis; check peripheral pulses; check for peripheral edema.

Supportive Care

• Do not give in active intravascular clotting.
• Use with caution in patients with thrombophlebitis and cardiac, renal, or hepatic disease.
• Keep oxygen and resuscitation equipment nearby.
• Administer fluids, blood, and blood products as ordered.
• Elevate lower extremities to aide venous return. Apply antiemboli stockings.
• Cover patient lightly; keep patient warm but avoid overheating.
• Relieve anxiety and pain. Offer emotional support and reassurance.
• Drug is sometimes helpful as an adjunct in treating hemophilia.
• Also used as antidote for streptokinase or urokinase toxicity; not beneficial in treating thrombocytopenia.

Patient Teaching

• Explain all procedures to patient and family.
• Instruct patient and family to report respiratory difficulty, pain, or changes in mental status immediately.

Evaluation

In patients receiving aminocaproic acid, appropriate evaluation statements may include:

• Patient exhibits decrease of absence of fluid volume deficit due to bleeding.
• Patient maintains demonstrates no signs of impaired venous tissue perfusion.
• Patient and family state an understanding of aminocaproic acid therapy.

aminoglutethimide

(a mee noe gloo teth´ i mide)
Cytadren

- *Classification:* antineoplastic (antiadrenal hormone)
- *Pregnancy Risk Category:* D

HOW SUPPLIED

Tablets: 250 mg

ACTION

Mechanism: Blocks conversion of cholesterol to delta-5-pregnenolone in the adrenal cortex, inhibiting the synthesis of glucocorticoids, mineralocorticoids, and other steroids.
Absorption: Well absorbed across the GI tract after oral administration.
Distribution: Widely distributed into body tissues.
Metabolism: In the liver by acetylation. Genetic factors influence a patient's ability to metabolize the drug. Acetylated metabolites are about 20% as active as the parent compound.
Excretion: Drug and its metabolites are primarily eliminated through the kidneys, mostly as unchanged drug. Half-life: Initially 11 to 16 hours, but over 1 to 2 weeks of daily administration, half-life decreases to 5 to 9 hours.

INDICATIONS & DOSAGE

Suppression of adrenal function in Cushing's syndrome and adrenal cancer; metastatic breast cancer–
Adults: 250 mg P.O. q.i.d. at 6-hour intervals. Dosage may be increased in increments of 250 mg daily every 1 to 2 weeks to a maximum daily dosage of 2 g.

CONTRAINDICATIONS & PRECAUTIONS

Contraindicated in patients with a history of hypersensitivity to the drug or to glutethimide, as cross-sensitivity may exist. Use cautiously in elderly patients because these patients may be more sensitive to the CNS adverse effects of this drug, and in those with serious infections or hypothyroidism because the drug may worsen the symptoms of these disorders.

ADVERSE REACTIONS

Common reactions are in italics; life-threatening reactions are in bold italics.
Blood: transient leukopenia, ***severe pancytopenia.***
CNS: *drowsiness,* headache, dizziness.
CV: hypotension, tachycardia.
Endocrine: adrenal insufficiency, masculinization, hirsutism.
GI: nausea, anorexia.
Skin: *morbilliform skin rash,* pruritus, urticaria.
Other: fever, myalgia.

INTERACTIONS

Alcohol: may potentiate the effects of aminoglutethimide.
Dexamethasone, medroxyprogesterone, digitoxin, theophylline: aminoglutethimide increases hepatic metabolism of these agents.
Oral anticoagulants: decreased anticoagulant effect.

EFFECTS ON DIAGNOSTIC TESTS

Plasma cortisol, serum thyroxine, and urine aldosterone: decreased levels.
Serum alkaline phosphatase, ALT (SGOT), and thyroid-stimulating hormone: increased levels.

NURSING CONSIDERATIONS

Besides those related universally to drug therapy (see "How to use this book"), consider the following specific recommendations:
Assessment
- Obtain a baseline assessment of the patient's underlying condition before initiating drug therapy.

• Be alert for adverse reactions and drug interactions throughout therapy.
• Evaluate the patient's and family's knowledge about aminoglutethimide therapy.

Nursing Diagnoses

• High risk for injury related to drug-induced drowsiness.
• High risk for impaired skin integrity related to drug-induced rash.
• Knowledge deficit related to aminoglutethimide therapy.

Planning and Implementation

Preparation and Administration

• When used to treat breast or prostatic cancer, dosage may be combined with 40 mg hydrocortisone per day usually 10 mg in the morning and at 5 p.m. and 20 mg at bedtime.)

Monitoring

• Monitor effectiveness by noting results of follow-up diagnostic tests and overall physical status; by performing baseline hematologic studies; and by monitoring CBC periodically.
• Monitor blood pressure frequently.
• Monitor thyroid function tests during therapy; this drug may cause a decrease in thyroid hormone production.
• Monitor for morbilliform skin rash.
• Monitor for signs of bleeding (hematuria, ecchymosis, petechiae, epistaxis, melena).
• Monitor for pancytopenia and drowsiness, common side effects of drug therapy.
• Monitor for adrenal hypofunction, especially under stressful conditions, such as surgery, trauma, or acute illness.
• Monitor for signs of infection (temperature elevation, sore throat, malaise).

Supportive Care

• Be prepared to terminate therapy if rash persists more than 5 to 8 days.
• Know that anticoagulants and aspirin products should be used with extreme caution.
• Assist the patient with ambulation and institute safety precautions if patient develops drowsiness and dizziness.
• Obtain baseline CBC, adrenal and thyroid function tests before initiating therapy.

Patient Teaching

• Warn patients to watch for signs of infection (sore throat, fever, fatigue), and for signs of bleeding (easy bruising, nosebleeds, bleeding gums). Take temperature daily.
• Teach patient to avoid the use of all OTC products containing aspirin.
• Advise patient to minimize orthostatic hypotension by rising slowly to standing position.
• Warn patient that drowsiness and dizziness may occur. Advise patient to avoid activities that require alertness and good psychomotor coordination until CNS effects of the drug are known.
• Ask patient to report any skin rash that persists more than 8 days.
• Reassure patient that drowsiness, nausea, and loss of appetite will diminish within 2 weeks after start of drug therapy.

Evaluation

In patients receiving aminoglutethimide, appropriate evaluation statements may include:
• Patient does not develop drug-induced drowsiness.
• Patient does not develop impaired skin integrity.
• Patient and family state an understanding of aminoglutethimide therapy.

PHARMACOLOGIC CLASS

aminoglycosides

amikacin sulfate
gentamicin sulfate
kanamycin sulfate
neomycin sulfate
netilmicin sulfate
streptomycin sulfate

tobramycin sulfate

OVERVIEW

Aminoglycoside antibiotics were discovered during the search for drugs to treat serious penicillin-resistant gram-negative infections. Streptomycin, derived from soil actinomycetes, was the first therapeutically useful aminoglycoside. Bacterial resistance to this prototype and adverse reactions soon led to the development of kanamycin, gentamicin, neomycin, netilmicin, tobramycin, and amikacin.

The basic structure of aminoglycosides is a hexose nucleus joined to at least two amino sugars by glycosidic linkage—hence the name aminoglycosides.

The aminoglycosides share certain pharmacokinetic properties, such as poor oral absorption, poor CNS penetration, and renal excretion, as well as serious adverse reactions and toxicity; their clinical use requires close monitoring of serum levels.

Aminoglycosides are bactericidal. They are active against many aerobic gram-negative organisms and some aerobic gram-positive organisms; they do not kill fungi, viruses, or anaerobic bacteria.

Gram-negative organisms susceptible to aminoglycosides include *Acinetobacter, Citrobacter, Enterobacter, Escherichia coli, Klebsiella,* indole-positive and indole-negative *Proteus, Providencia, Pseudomonas aeruginosa, Salmonella, Serratia,* and *Shigella.* Streptomycin is active against *Brucella, Calymmatobacterium granulomatis, Pasteurella multocida,* and *Yersinia pestis.*

Susceptible aerobic gram-positive organisms include *Staphylococcus aureus* and *S. epidermidis.* Streptomycin is active against *Nocardia, Erysipelothrix,* and some mycobacteria, including *Mycobacterium tuberculosis, M. marinum,* and certain strains of *M. kansasii* and *M. leprae.*

Aminoglycosides are not systemically absorbed after oral administration to patients with intact GI mucosa and, with few exceptions, are used parenterally for systemic infections; intraventricular or intrathecal administration is necessary for CNS infections. Kanamycin and neomycin are given orally for bowel sterilization.

Aminoglycosides are distributed widely throughout the body after parenteral administration; CSF concentrations are minimal even in patients with inflamed meninges. Over time, aminoglycosides accumulate in body tissue, especially the kidney and inner ear, causing drug saturation. The drug is released slowly from these tissues. Most aminoglycosides are minimally protein-bound, and are not metabolized. They don't penetrate abscesses well.

Aminoglycosides are excreted primarily in urine, chiefly by glomerular filtration; neomycin is chiefly excreted unchanged in feces when taken orally. Elimination half-life ranges between 2 and 4 hours and is prolonged in patients with decreased renal function.

CLINICAL INDICATIONS AND ACTIONS

Infection caused by susceptible organisms

Aminoglycosides are used as sole therapy for:

• infections caused by susceptible aerobic gram-negative bacilli, including septicemia; postoperative, pulmonary, intra-abdominal, and urinary tract infections; and infections of skin, soft tissue, bones, and joints
• infections from aerobic gram-negative bacillary meningitis (not susceptible to other antibiotics); because of poor CNS penetration, drugs are

AMINOGLYCOSIDES: RENAL FUNCTION AND HALF-LIFE

As the chart shows, the aminoglycosides, which are excreted by the kidneys, have significantly prolonged half-lives in patients with end-stage renal disease. Knowing this can help you assess the patient's potential for drug accumulation and toxicity. Nephrotoxicity, a major hazard of therapy with aminoglycosides, is clearly linked to serum concentrations that exceed the therapeutic concentrations listed in the chart below. Therefore, monitoring peak and trough levels is essential for safe use of these drugs.

	HALF-LIFE		THERAPEUTIC CONCENTRATIONS (mcg/ml)	
DRUG AND ADMINISTRATION	NORMAL RENAL FUNCTION	END-STAGE RENAL DISEASE	PEAK	TROUGH
amikacin I.M., I.V.	2 to 3 hr	30 to 86 hr	15 to 30	<5
gentamicin I.M., I.V., topical	2 to 3 hr	24 to 60 hr	4 to 10	<2
kanamycin I.M., I.V., topical	2 to 4 hr	27 to 80 hr	8 to 16	<5
neomycin oral, topical	2 to 3 hr	12 to 24 hr	Not applicable	Not applicable
netilmicin I.M., I.V.	2 to 2½ hr	18 to 30 hr	0.5 to 10	<4
streptomycin I.M., I.V.	2 to 3 hr	4 to 110 hr	5 to 25	1 to 5
tobramycin I.M., I.V., topical	2 to 3 hr	24 to 60 hr	4 to 8	<2

given intrathecally or intraventricularly (in ventriculitis).

Aminoglycosides are combined with other antibacterials in many other types of infection, including:
• serious staphylococcal infections (with an anti-staphylococcal penicillin)
• serious *P. aeruginosa* infections (with such drugs as an antipseudomonal penicillin or cephalosporin)
• enterococcal infections, including endocarditis (with such drugs as penicillin G, ampicillin, or vancomycin)
• as initial empiric therapy in febrile, leukopenic compromised host (with an antipseudomonal penicillin and/or cephalosporin)
• serious *Klebsiella* infections (with a cephalosporin)
• nosocomial pneumonia (with a cephalosporin)
• anaerobic infections involving *Bacteroides fragilis* (with such drugs as clindamycin, metronidazole, cefoxitin, doxycycline, chloramphenicol, or ticarcillin)
• tuberculosis (concomitant use of parenteral kanamycin or streptomycin with other antitubercular agents).

OVERVIEW OF ADVERSE REACTIONS

• *Systemic reactions:* Ototoxicity and nephrotoxicity are the most serious complications of aminoglycoside therapy. Ototoxicity involves both vestibular and auditory functions and usually is related to persistently high serum drug levels. The number of affected sensory hair cells determines the degree of permanent dysfunction; cumulative hair cell destruction can cause permanent deafness. Elderly patients, patients taking other ototoxic drugs, and those with preexisting auditory loss are most susceptible as are patients taking other potentially ototoxic drugs. In addition, tobramycin, gentamicin, and streptomycin primarily affect vestibular function; amikacin, kanamycin, and neomycin are primarily audiotoxic. Damage is reversible only if detected early and if drug is discontinued promptly.

Any aminoglycoside may cause usually reversible nephrotoxicity; the incidence of reported reactions ranges from 2% to 10%. The damage results in tubular necrosis. Mild proteinuria and granular cylindruria are early signs of declining renal function; elevated serum creatinine levels follow several days after the decline has begun. Nephrotoxicity usually begins on the 4th to 7th day of therapy and appears to be dose-related. The best management is preventive monitoring of urinary cast excretion and serum drug levels, especially in patients at maximum risk: elderly patients, patients with hypovolemia or preexisting renal dysfunction, and patients requiring extended therapy.

Neuromuscular blockade results in skeletal weakness and respiratory distress similar to that seen with the use of neuromuscular blocking agents like tubocurarine and succinylcholine. It is most likely to occur in patients receiving those blocking agents; in patients with preexisting neuromuscular disease such as myasthenia gravis; in patients receiving general anesthetics; and in patients with hypocalcemia.

Oral aminoglycoside therapy most often causes nausea, vomiting, and diarrhea. Less common adverse reactions include hypersensitivity reactions (ranging from mild rashes, fever, and eosinophilia to fatal anaphylaxis); hematologic reactions include hemolytic anemia, transient neutropenia, leukopenia, and thrombocytopenia. Transient elevations of liver function values also occur.

• *Local reactions:* Parenterally administered forms of aminoglycosides may cause vein irritation, phlebitis, and sterile abscess.

REPRESENTATIVE COMBINATIONS

Neomycin with polymixin B sulfates and bacitracin: Neosporin, Mycitracin, Foille, Neo-Polycin; with polymixin B sulfates and gramicidin: Neosporin; with polymixin B sulfates and hydrocortisone: Corticosporin, Drotic, Octicair, Ortega Otic-M, Otocart, Otoreid-HC; with dexomethasone sodium phosphate: Neodecadron; with flurandrenolide: Cordron-N.

See also adrenocorticoids, topical.

aminophylline (theophylline ethylenediamine)

(am in off´ i lin)

Aminophyllin, Cardophyllin‡, Corophyllin†, Phyllocontin, Somophyllin-DF

• *Classification:* bronchodilator (xanthine derivative)
• *Pregnancy Risk Category:* C

HOW SUPPLIED

Tablets: 100 mg, 200 mg
Tablets (controlled-release): 225 mg
Oral liquid: 105 mg/5 ml
Injection: 250 mg/10 ml, 500 mg/20 ml, 500 mg/2 ml, 100 mg/100 ml in 0.45% sodium chloride, 200 mg/100 ml in 0.45% sodium chloride
Rectal solution: 300 mg/5 ml
Rectal suppositories: 250 mg, 500 mg

ACTION

Mechanism: Releases free theophylline, which is responsible for the pharmacologic actions of the drug. Theophylline inhibits phosphodiesterase, the enzyme that degrades cyclic 3', 5' adenosine monophosphate (cyclic AMP). Increased cyclic AMP levels alter intracellular calcium movement resulting in relaxation of smooth muscle of the bronchial tree, bronchodilation and increased pulmonary blood flow.
Absorption: Dissolution of the drug into free theophylline in the stomach is the rate-limiting step in oral absorption. Food alters the rate but not the extent of absorption. After I.M. administration, absorption is erratic. Absorption of the rectal suppository is also unreliable and slow.
Distribution: In all tissues and extracellular fluids except fatty tissue.
Metabolism: Metabolized to inactive compounds.
Excretion: Small amounts (8% to 12%) are excreted in the urine; only about 10% is excreted unchanged in the feces. Half-life: Variable; averages 7 to 9 hours in healthy adults, 1½ to 9½ hours in children, and 15 to 58 hours in neonates. The half-life in smoking adults is shorter (4 to 5 hours); it is longer in adults with CHF, cor pulmonale, chronic obstructive pulmonary disease, or liver disease.
Onset, peak, duration: Dependent on serum concentration of drug; serum theophylline concentrations of 10 to 20 mcg/ml are usually required for optimum response.

INDICATIONS & DOSAGE

Symptomatic relief of bronchospasm–
Patients not currently receiving theophylline who require rapid relief of symptoms: loading dose is 6 mg/kg (equivalent to 4.7 mg/kg anhydrous theophylline) I.V. slowly (less than or equal to 25 mg/minute), then maintenance infusion.
Adults (nonsmokers): 0.7 mg/kg/hour for 12 hours; then 0.5 mg/kg/hour.
Otherwise healthy adult smokers: 1 mg/kg/hour for 12 hours; then 0.8 mg/kg/hour.
Older patients and adults with cor pulmonale: 0.6 mg/kg/hour for 12 hours; then 0.3 mg/kg/hour.
Adults with CHF or liver disease: 0.5 mg/kg/hour for 12 hours; then 0.1 to 0.2 mg/kg/hour.
Children 9 to 16 years: 1 mg/kg/hour for 12 hours; then 0.8 mg/kg/hour.
Children 6 months to 9 years: 1.2 mg/kg/hour for 12 hours; then 1 mg/kg/hour.
Patients currently receiving theophylline: aminophylline infusions of 0.63 mg/kg (0.5 mg/kg anhydrous theophylline) will increase plasma levels of theophylline by 1 mcg/ml. Some clinicians recommend a dose of 3.1 mg/kg (2.5 mg/kg anhydrous theophylline) if no obvious signs of theophylline toxicity are present.
Chronic bronchial asthma–
Adults: 600 to 1,600 mg P.O. daily divided t.i.d. or q.i.d.
Children: 12 mg/kg P.O. daily divided t.i.d. or q.i.d.

CONTRAINDICATIONS & PRECAUTIONS

Contraindicated in patients with hypersensitivity to xanthines or ethylenediamine. Use cautiously in patients with compromised cardiac or circulatory function, diabetes, glaucoma, hypertension, hyperthyroidism, peptic ulcer, or gastroesophageal reflux because drug may worsen these conditions.

ADVERSE REACTIONS

Common reactions are in italics; life-threatening reactions are in bold italics.
CNS: *restlessness, dizziness,* headache, *insomnia,* light-headedness, *seizures,* muscle twitching.

CV: *palpitations, sinus tachycardia,* extrasystoles, flushing, marked hypotension, increase in respiratory rate.
GI: *nausea, vomiting, anorexia,* bitter aftertaste, dyspepsia, heavy feeling in stomach, diarrhea.
Skin: urticaria.
Local: *rectal suppositories may cause irritation.*

INTERACTIONS

Alkali-sensitive drugs: reduced activity. Do not add to I.V. fluids containing aminophylline.
Barbiturates, phenytoin, rifampin: enhanced metabolism and decreased theophylline blood levels. Monitor for decreased aminophylline effect.
Beta-adrenergic blockers: antagonism. Propranolol and nadolol, especially, may cause bronchospasm in sensitive patients. Use together cautiously.
Influenza virus vaccine, oral contraceptives, troleandomycin, erythromycin, cimetidine: decreased hepatic clearance of theophylline; elevated theophylline levels. Monitor for signs of toxicity.

EFFECTS ON DIAGNOSTIC TESTS

Plasma-free fatty acids: increased.
Uric acid assay: altered results depending on method.

NURSING CONSIDERATIONS

Besides those related universally to drug therapy (see "How to use this book"), consider the following specific recommendations:

Assessment

- Obtain a baseline assessment of the patient's cardiopulmonary status by assessing vital signs, ECG results, and auscultating the heart and lungs.
- Be alert for any adverse reactions and drug interactions throughout therapy.
- Evaluate the patient's and family's knowledge about aminophylline therapy.

Nursing Diagnoses

- Ineffective airway clearance related to patient's underlying condition.
- High risk for fluid volume deficit related to aminophylline-induced GI adverse reactions.
- Knowledge deficit related to aminophylline therapy.

Planning and Implementation

Preparation and Administration

- Check that the patient has not had recent theophylline therapy before giving loading dose.
- ***P.O. use:*** Take oral drug with a full glass of water to help relieve GI symptoms, although food in stomach delays absorption. Enteric-coated tablets may also delay and impair absorption.
- ***Rectal use:*** Use rectal preparations if patient cannot take the drug orally. Schedule after evacuation, if possible, and before a meal because they may be better retained. Be sure patient remains recumbent for 15 to 20 minutes after insertion. Suppositories are slowly and erratically absorbed; retention enemas may be absorbed more rapidly.
- ***I.V. use:*** Dilute with 5% dextrose in water solution as I.V. drug administration can cause burning.

Monitoring

- Monitor effectiveness by regularly auscultating lungs and noting respiratory rate and results of laboratory studies, such as arterial blood gases.
- Monitor vital signs; expected clinical effects include improvement in quality of pulse and respirations.
- Measure intake and output.
- Monitor for GI adverse reactions especially nausea and vomiting and dizziness. Dizziness is common at the start of therapy and occurs often in elderly patients.
- Monitor patient response to and tolerance of the drug, pulmonary function studies, and serum theophylline levels. Because individuals metabolize xanthines at different rates,

the doctor may want to adjust the dosage. Theophylline concentrations should range from 10 to 20 mcg/ml: toxicity has been reported with levels above 20 mcg/ml.
• Monitor plasma clearance because abnormal results may require dosage adjustment. It may be decreased in patients with CHF, hepatic dysfunction, or pulmonary edema; smokers may show accelerated clearance.
Supportive Care
• Notify the doctor if GI adverse reactions occur. Keep in mind that there is no evidence that antacids reduce GI adverse reactions.
Patient Teaching
• Tell patients taking the drug orally to take it with a full glass of water to reduce GI adverse reactions. If a suppository is used, teach the patient how to administer it. Tell him to use the suppository after a bowel evacuation and before a meal because it will be easier to retain the suppository. Tell the patient to remain recumbent for at least 15 minutes after inserting the suppository.
• Supply instructions for home care and dosage schedule. Some patients require an around-the-clock dosage schedule. Be sure the patient understands his dosage schedule.
• Tell the patient to check with the doctor or pharmacist before taking any other medications, as OTC remedies may contain ephedrine in combination with theophylline salts and excessive CNS stimulation may result.
• Warn patients with allergies that exposure to allergens may exacerbate bronchospasm.

Evaluation

In patients receiving aminophylline, appropriate evaluation statements may include:
• Patient's respiratory signs and symptoms are improved with aminophylline.
• Patient maintains normal fluid and electrolyte balance.
• Patient and family state an understanding of aminophylline therapy.

amiodarone hydrochloride

(a mee´ oh da rone)
Cordarone, Cordarone X‡

• *Classification:* antiarrhythmic agent (benzofuran derivative)
• *Pregnancy Risk Category:* C

HOW SUPPLIED

Tablets: 100 mg†‡, 200 mg

ACTION

Mechanism: A class III antiarrhythmic that prolongs the refractory period and duration of action potential and decreases repolarization.
Absorption: Slow, variable absorption. Bioavailability estimates range from 22% to 86%.
Distribution: Widely distributed; it accumulates in adipose tissue and in highly perfused organs, such as the lungs, liver, and spleen; highly protein-bound (96%). The therapeutic serum level probably ranges from 1 to 2.5 mcg/ml.
Metabolism: Extensive hepatic conversion to an active metabolite, desethyl amiodarone.
Excretion: Mainly hepatic, through the biliary tree (with enterohepatic recirculation). Because no renal excretion occurs, impaired renal function does not require dosage reduction. Half-life: Terminal elimination half-life – 25 to 110 days – is the longest of any antiarrhythmic; in most patients, half-life ranges from 40 to 50 days.
Onset, peak, duration: Peak plasma levels occur 3 to 7 hours after oral administration; onset of action may be delayed from 2 to 3 days to 2 to 3 months – even with loading doses.

INDICATIONS & DOSAGE

Ventricular and supraventricular arrhythmias, including recurrent supraventricular tachycardia (Wolff-Parkinson-White syndrome), atrial fibrillation and flutter, and ventricular tachycardia refractory to other antiarrhythmics–

Adults: loading dose is 5 to 10 mg/kg by I.V. infusion via central line, followed by I.V. infusion of 10 mg/kg/day for 3 to 5 days. (*Note:* I.V. use of amiodarone is investigational.) Or, give loading dose of 800 to 1,600 mg P.O. daily for 1 to 3 weeks until initial therapeutic response occurs. Maintenance dosage is 200 to 600 mg P.O. daily.

CONTRAINDICATIONS & PRECAUTIONS

Contraindicated in patients with preexisting sinus-node dysfunction and bradycardia causing syncope or second- or third-degree heart block (except if patient has artificial pacemaker), because of its potent effects on the atrioventricular conduction system. Use with caution in patients with CHF because of the potential for adverse hemodynamic effects; in patients with liver disease because metabolism may be reduced; and in patients with hypokalemia, because drug may be ineffective.

ADVERSE REACTIONS

Common reactions are in italics; life-threatening reactions are in bold italics.

CNS: peripheral neuropathy, extrapyramidal symptoms, headache, *malaise, fatigue.*

CV: bradycardia, hypotension, ***arrhythmias,*** *CHF.*

EENT: *corneal microdeposits,* visual disturbances.

Endocrine: hypothyroidism, hyperthyroidism, gynecomastia.

GI: *nausea, vomiting,* constipation.

Hepatic: *altered liver enzymes,* hepatic dysfunction.

Respiratory: ***severe pulmonary toxicity (pneumonitis/alveolitis).***

Skin: *photosensitivity,* blue-gray skin pigmentation.

Other: muscle weakness.

INTERACTIONS

Antiarrhythmic agents: use with amiodarone may induce torsade de pointes; amiodarone may reduce the hepatic or renal clearance of flecainide, procainamide, and quinidine.

Antihypertensives: increased hypotensive effect. Use together cautiously.

Beta blockers, calcium channel blockers: increased cardiac depressant effects; may potentiate slowing of sinus node and AV conduction. Use together cautiously.

Digitalis glycosides: increased serum digoxin levels.

Phenytoin: phenytoin metabolism may be decreased.

Warfarin: increased anticoagulant effect. Monitor patient closely.

EFFECTS ON DIAGNOSTIC TESTS

Serum thyroxine (T_4): increased levels.

Triiodothyronine (T_3): decreased levels.

NURSING CONSIDERATIONS

Besides those related universally to drug therapy (see "How to use this book"), consider the following specific recommendations:

Assessment

- Obtain a baseline assessment of the patient's heart rate and rhythm before amiodarone therapy.
- Be alert for adverse reactions and drug interactions throughout therapy.
- Evaluate the patient's and family's knowledge about amiodarone therapy.

Nursing Diagnoses

- Decreased cardiac output related to ineffectiveness of amiodarone therapy.
- Impaired gas exchange related to

amiodarone-induced pulmonary toxicity.
• Knowledge deficit related to amiodarone.

Planning and Implementation

Preparation and Administration

• ***P.O. use:*** Divide oral loading dose into three equal doses and give with meals to decrease GI intolerance. Maintenance dosage may be given once daily, but may be divided into two doses taken with meals if GI intolerance occurs.

Monitoring

• Monitor effectiveness by regularly evaluating the patient's ECG. Monitor blood pressure and heart rate and rhythm frequently. Continuous ECG monitoring should be performed during initiation and adjustment of dosage.
• Monitor pulmonary function studies and chest X-ray. Also monitor patient for signs and symptoms of respiratory dysfunction.
• Monitor patient for pulmonary toxicity, which can be fatal. Incidence rises in patients receiving more than 400 mg/day.
• Monitor serum electrolyte levels, particularly potassium and magnesium levels.
• Monitor closely for visual disturbances. These occur in only 2% to 3% of patients. However, most patients treated show corneal microdeposits on slit-lamp ophthalmologic examination. Onset of this effect occurs from 1 to 4 months after beginning amiodarone therapy.

Supportive Care

• If ECG disturbances occur, withhold the drug, obtain a rhythm strip, and notify the doctor immediately. Also notify doctor of respiratory dysfunction.
• Institute safety precautions if CNS or visual disturbances occur.
• Schedule activities to allow frequent rest periods if patient experiences fatigue.
• Obtain an order for a mild analgesic if the patient develops a headache.
• Obtain an order for an antiemetic if nausea and vomiting occur.
• Assist the patient with daily activities if muscle weakness occurs.
• To minimize corneal microdeposits, recommend instillation of methylcellulose ophthalmic solution during amiodarone therapy.

Patient Teaching

• Stress importance of taking the drug exactly as prescribed.
• Emphasize the importance of close follow-up and regular diagnostic studies to monitor drug action and assess for adverse reactions.
• Warn the patient that amiodarone may cause a blue-gray skin pigmentation.
• Advise the patient to use a sunscreen to prevent photosensitivity.
• Tell the patient to schedule activities to provide frequent rest periods if fatigue occurs.
• Teach the patient appropriate skin and foot care if peripheral neuropathy is present.
• Warn the patient to avoid hazardous activities that require manual dexterity or good vision if extrapyramidal symptoms or visual disturbances occur.
• Warn male patients about the possibility of gynecomastia.
• Tell the patient to limit fluid and sodium intake if fluid retention develops.

Evaluation

In patients receiving amiodarone, appropriate evaluation statements may include:
• Patient's ECG reveals arrhythmia has been corrected.
• Patient's respiratory status remains unchanged throughout amiodarone therapy.
• Patient and family state an understanding of amiodarone therapy.

amitriptyline hydrochloride

(a mee trip´ ti leen)

Amitril, Apo-Amitriptylene†, Elavil, Emitrip, Endep, Enovil, Laroxyl‡, Levate†, Meravil†, Novo-Triptyn†

- *Classification:* tricyclic antidepressant
- *Pregnancy Risk Category:* D

HOW SUPPLIED

Tablets: 10 mg, 25 mg, 50 mg, 75 mg, 100 mg, 150 mg
Injection: 10 mg/ml

ACTION:

Mechanism: Increases the amount of norepinephrine or serotonin, or both, in the synapse by blocking their reuptake by presynaptic neurons. This prolongs the action of these neurotransmitters.
Absorption: Rapidly absorbed from the GI tract after oral administration and from muscle tissue after I.M. administration.
Distribution: Widely distributed and is 96% protein-bound. Drug is found in breast milk.
Metabolism: By the liver to the active metabolite nortriptyline; a significant first-pass effect may account for variability of serum concentrations in different patients taking the same dosage.
Excretion: Mainly in urine. Half-life: Variable; ranges from 10 to 50 hours.
Onset, peak, duration: Peak levels are seen 2 to 12 hours after a dose. Steady state is reached after 4 to 10 days of daily administration. Antidepressant effect may not occur for 4 weeks or more.

INDICATIONS & DOSAGE

Treatment of depression–
Adults: 50 to 100 mg P.O. h.s., increasing to 200 mg daily; maximum dosage is 300 mg daily if needed; or 20 to 30 mg I.M. q.i.d. Alternatively, the entire dosage can be given at bedtime.
Elderly patients and adolescents: 30 mg P.O. daily in divided doses. May be increased to 150 mg.

CONTRAINDICATIONS & PRECAUTIONS

Contraindicated in patients with hypersensitivity to tricyclic antidepressants, trazodone, and related compounds; in the acute recovery phase of myocardial infarction because of drug's arrhythmogenic potential; in patients in coma or with severe respiratory depression because of additive depressant effects on CNS; and during or within 14 days of therapy with monoamine oxidase (MAO) inhibitors.

Use cautiously in patients with other cardiac disease (arrhythmias, CHF, angina pectoris, valvular disease, or heart block); respiratory disorders; alcoholism, seizure disorders; scheduled electroconvulsive therapy; bipolar disease; glaucoma; hyperthyroidism, or in those taking thyroid replacement; Type I and Type II diabetes; prostatic hypertrophy, paralytic ileus, or urinary retention; hepatic or renal dysfunction; Parkinson's disease; and in those having general anesthesia.

ADVERSE REACTIONS

Common reactions are in italics; life-threatening reactions are in bold italics.
CNS: *drowsiness, dizziness,* excitation, tremors, weakness, confusion, headache, nervousness.
CV: *orthostatic hypotension, tachycardia, ECG changes,* hypertension.
EENT: *blurred vision,* tinnitus, mydriasis.
GI: *dry mouth, constipation,* nausea, vomiting, anorexia, paralytic ileus.
GU: *urine retention.*
Skin: rash, urticaria.
Other: *sweating,* allergy.
After abrupt withdrawal of long-term

therapy: nausea, headache, malaise. (Does not indicate addiction.)

INTERACTIONS

Barbiturates: decrease tricyclic antidepressant (TCA) blood levels. Monitor for decreased antidepressant effect.
Cimetidine, methylphenidate: increases TCA blood levels. Monitor for enhanced antidepressant effect.
Epinephrine, norepinephrine: increase hypertensive effect. Use with caution.
MAO inhibitors: may cause severe excitation, hyperpyrexia, or seizures, usually with high dosage. Use together cautiously.

EFFECTS ON DIAGNOSTIC TESTS

CBC: decreased WBC counts.
ECG: elongated Q-T and PR intervals; flattened T waves.
Liver function test: elevated results.
Serum glucose: decreased or increased levels.

NURSING CONSIDERATIONS

Besides those related universally to drug therapy (see "How to use this book"), consider the following specific recommendations:

Assessment
- Obtain a baseline assessment of the patient's depression before therapy.
- Be alert for adverse reactions and drug interactions throughout therapy.
- Evaluate the patient's and family's knowledge about amitriptyline therapy.

Nursing Diagnoses
- Ineffective individual coping related to the patient's underlying condition.
- High risk for injury related to adverse CNS reactions to amitriptyline.
- Knowledge deficit related to amitriptyline therapy.

Planning and Implementation
Preparation and Administration
- Whenever possible, patient should take full dose at bedtime.
- Expect reduced dosage in elderly or debilitated patients and adolescents.

Monitoring
- Monitor effectiveness by having the patient discuss his feelings (ask broad, open-ended questions) and by evaluating his behavior.
- Monitor blood pressure (supine and standing) for alterations in heart rate and ECG for tachycardia.
- Watch for signs of oversedation, especially in elderly patients.
- Monitor bowel patterns for constipation.
- Monitor for suicidal tendencies.

Supportive Care
- Discuss alternative therapy or changes in regimen with doctor if drug is ineffective.
- Institute safety precautions if CNS adverse reactions occur.
- Do not withdraw drug abruptly.
- If psychotic signs increase, notify doctor and expect reduction of dosage.
- If not contraindicated, increase the patient's fluid and fiber intake to prevent constipation; if needed, obtain an order for a laxative.
- Assist the patient in changing positions slowly to minimize orthostatic hypotension.

Patient Teaching
- Tell the patient that dry mouth may be relieved with sugarless hard candy or gum. Explain that saliva substitutes may be necessary.
- Teach the patient to increase fluid intake to lessen constipation. Suggest stool softener or high-fiber diet, if needed.
- Warn the patient to avoid driving and other hazardous activities that require alertness and good psychomotor coordination until CNS effects of the drug are known. Tell the patient that drowsiness and dizziness usually subside after first few weeks. Inform the patient that drug has strong sedative effects; warn against combining

it with alcohol or other CNS depressants.
• Tell the patient to expect delay of 2 weeks or more before noticeable effect. Full effect may take 4 weeks or more. Encourage the patient to continue to take medication until it achieves its full therapeutic effect.
• Advise the patient not to take any other drugs (prescription or OTC) without first consulting the doctor.
• Warn the patient about the possibility of morning orthostatic hypotension. Instruct the patient to rise slowly and to sit for several minutes before standing up.

Evaluation

In patients receiving amitriptyline, appropriate evaluation statements may include:
• Patient behavior and communication indicate improvement of depression.
• Patient has not experienced injury from CNS adverse reactions.
• Patient and family state an understanding of amitriptyline therapy.

---

amobarbital
(am oh bar´ bi tal)
Amytal

amobarbital sodium
Amytal Sodium

• Controlled Substance Schedule II
• *Classification:* sedative-hypnotic, anticonvulsant (barbiturate)
• *Pregnancy Risk Category:* B

HOW SUPPLIED

amobarbital
Tablets: 50 mg
amobarbital sodium
Capsules: 200 mg
Powder for injection: 500 mg

ACTION

Mechanism: Interferes with transmission of impulses from the thalamus to the cortex of the brain.
Absorption: Well absorbed after oral administration; 100% absorption after I.M. administration.
Distribution: Widespread throughout body tissues and fluids.
Metabolism: In the liver by oxidation to a tertiary alcohol.
Excretion: Less than 1% of a dose is excreted unchanged in the urine; the rest is excreted as metabolites. Half-life: Biphasic, with a first phase about 40 minutes and a second phase about 20 hours.
Onset, peak, duration: Onset of action is 45 to 60 minutes. Duration of action is 6 to 8 hours.

INDICATIONS & DOSAGE

Sedation–
Adults: usually 50 mg P.O. b.i.d. or t.i.d.
Children: 3 to 6 mg/kg P.O. daily in four equally divided doses.
Insomnia–
Adults: 50 to 200 mg P.O. or deep I.M. h.s.; I.M. injection not to exceed 5 ml in any one site. Maximum dosage is 500 mg.
Children: 3 to 5 mg/kg deep I.M. h.s.; I.M. injection not to exceed 5 ml in any one site.
Preanesthetic sedation–
Adults and children: 200 mg P.O. or I.M. 1 to 2 hours before surgery.
Manic reactions, as an adjunct in psychotherapy, anticonvulsant–
Adults and children over 6 years: 65 to 500 mg slow I.V.; rate not to exceed 100 mg/minute. Maximum dosage is 1 g.
Children under 6 years: 3 to 5 mg/kg slow I.V. or I.M.

CONTRAINDICATIONS & PRECAUTIONS

Contraindicated in patients with hypersensitivity to barbiturates and in patients with bronchopneumonia, status asthmaticus, or other severe respiratory distress because of the potential for respiratory depression. Amobarbital should not be used in patients who are depressed or suicidal because the drug can worsen depression; in patients with uncontrolled acute or chronic pain because paradoxical excitement can occur; or in patients with porphyria because this drug can trigger symptoms of this disease.

Use cautiously in patients who must perform hazardous tasks requiring mental alertness because the drug causes drowsiness. Administer parenteral amobarbital slowly and with extreme caution to patients with hypotension or severe pulmonary or cardiovascular disease because of potential adverse hemodynamic effects. Because tolerance and physical or psychological dependence may occur, prolonged use of high doses should be avoided.

Use cautiously in patients with renal or hepatic disease, as drug accumulation may occur. CNS depression may be exacerbated in patients with shock or uremia. Use parenteral amobarbital cautiously in patients with cardiovascular disease. Prenatal exposure to barbiturates is associated with an increased incidence of fetal abnormalities and possibly brain tumors. Use of barbiturates in the third trimester may be associated with physical dependence in neonates.

ADVERSE REACTIONS

Common reactions are in italics; life-threatening reactions are in bold italics.

CNS: *drowsiness, lethargy, hangover,* paradoxical excitement in elderly patients.

GI: nausea, vomiting.

Skin: rash, urticaria.

Local: pain, irritation, sterile abscess at injection site.

Other: ***Stevens-Johnson syndrome,*** angioedema, exacerbation of porphyria.

INTERACTIONS

Alcohol or other CNS depressants, including narcotic analgesics: excessive CNS and respiratory depression. Use together cautiously.

Griseofulvin: decreased absorption of griseofulvin.

MAO inhibitors: inhibit metabolism of barbiturates; may cause prolonged CNS depression. Reduce barbiturate dosage.

Oral anticoagulants, estrogens and oral contraceptives, doxycycline, corticosteroids: amobarbital may enhance the metabolism of these drugs. Monitor for decreased effect.

Rifampin: may decrease barbiturate levels. Monitor for decreased effect.

EFFECTS ON DIAGNOSTIC TESTS

Cyanocobalamin ^{57}Co: impaired absorption.

EEG: altered patterns with a change in low-voltage, fast activity.

Phentolamine test: false-positive results.

Serum bilirubin: decreased concentrations in neonates, epileptic patients, and in patients with congenital nonhemolytic unconjugated hyperbilirubinemia.

NURSING CONSIDERATIONS

Besides those related universally to drug therapy (see "How to use this book"), consider the following specific recommendations:

Assessment

- Obtain a baseline assessment of sleeping patterns and mental status before therapy.
- Be alert for adverse reactions and drug interactions throughout therapy.
- Evaluate the patient's and family's knowledge about amobarbital therapy.

Nursing Diagnoses

- Sleep pattern disturbance related to underlying patient problem.

• High risk for trauma related to adverse CNS reactions caused by amobarbital.
• Knowledge deficit related to amobarbital therapy.

Planning and Implementation

Preparation and Administration

• Use injectable solution within 30 minutes after opening container to minimize deterioration. Don't use cloudy or precipitated solution. Don't shake solution; mix with sterile water only.
• Expect to reduce dosage during labor because barbiturates potentiate the effects of opiates.
• ***I.V. use:*** Reserve I.V. injection for emergency treatment. Give only to hospitalized patients under close observation. Be prepared to give artificial respiration. Administer I.V. slowly; do not exceed 100 mg/minute.
• ***I.M. use:*** Give I.M. injection deeply. Superficial injection may cause pain, sterile abscess, and sloughing.
• ***P.O. use:*** Before leaving the bedside, make sure the patient has swallowed tablet or capsule.

Monitoring

• Monitor effectiveness by regularly evaluating the patient's ability to sleep after administration.
• Monitor the patient's CNS status after initiating therapy for evidence of adverse reactions.
• Closely monitor the elderly patients' responses to the drug as these patients are more sensitive to CNS adverse reactions.
• Monitor for signs of barbiturate toxicity: coma, pupillary constriction, cyanosis, clammy skin, and hypotension. Overdose can be fatal.
• Monitor the neonate's respiratory status closely if the mother received drug during labor because excessive dosage may cause neonatal respiratory depression.
• Monitor respiratory status closely following I.V. administration.
• After drug discontinuation, be alert for withdrawal symptoms.

Supportive Care

• After administration, institute safety precautions, such as: remove cigarettes; keep bed rails up, and supervise or assist ambulations.
• Withhold the drug if barbiturate toxicity is suspected.
• Do not discontinue the drug abruptly after prolonged use. The drug may cause dependence and severe withdrawal symptoms. Withdraw gradually over 5 to 6 days.
• Take precautions to prevent hoarding or self-overdosing, especially by patients who are depressed, suicidal, or have histories of drug abuse.
• If the patient has pain, consult with the patient's doctor to obtain an analgesic order. Barbiturates have no analgesic effect and may cause restlessness or delirium in presence of pain.
• Be aware that amobarbital may be used in psychiatric settings as an "Amytal interview" to elicit information that patient can't or won't offer when fully conscious. May be used in Wada testing to help determine language and memory function.
• ***With I.V. use:*** If overdose occurs, maintain airway, and if needed, provide ventilatory support. Monitor vital signs and fluid balance. For shock, give fluids and follow standard care measures; for hypotension give vasopressors, as ordered. In normal renal function, forced diuresis may help remove drug; hemodialysis or hemoperfusion may enhance removal.

Patient Teaching

• Explain that morning hangover is common after hypnotic dose. Encourage the patient to report severe hangover or oversedation so the doctor can be consulted for change of dose or drug.
• Explain that hypnotic drugs suppress rapid eye movement sleep. The patient may experience increased

dreaming after the drug is discontinued.
- Instruct the patient to remain in bed after taking drug and to call for assistance to use the bathroom.
- Warn the patient that drug may cause physical dependence.
- Warn the patient to avoid hazardous activities that require mental alertness if CNS adverse reactions are present after awakening.
- Tell the patient to notify the nurse or doctor if sleep pattern disturbances persist despite continued therapy.

Evaluation

In the patient receiving amobarbital, appropriate evaluation statements may include:
- Patient states drug was effective in inducing sleep.
- Patient's safety is maintained.
- Patient and family state an understanding of amobarbital therapy.

amoxapine
(a mox´ a peen)
Asendin

- *Classification:* tricyclic antidepressant (dibenzoxapine)
- *Pregnancy Risk Category:* C

HOW SUPPLIED
Tablets: 25 mg, 50 mg, 100 mg, 150 mg

ACTION
Mechanism: Blocks the reuptake of norepinephrine or serotonin, or both, into presynaptic neurons, prolonging their action.
Absorption: Rapidly and completely absorbed from the GI tract after oral administration.
Distribution: Widely distributed, with highest concentrations in the heart, lungs, kidneys, spleen, and brain. Both parent compound and active metabolite are present in breast milk. Proposed therapeutic plasma levels (parent drug and metabolite) range from 200 to 400 ng/ml.
Metabolism: By the liver to the active metabolite 8-hydroxyamoxapine; a significant first-pass effect may explain variability of serum concentrations in different patients taking the same dosage.
Excretion: In urine and feces (7% to 18%); about 60% of a given dose is excreted as the conjugated form within 6 days. Half-life: About 8 hours.
Onset, peak, duration: Peak plasma levels occur 8 to 10 hours after dosing; steady-state levels are reached within 2 to 7 days of daily administration. Onset of antidepressant effect may take several weeks.

INDICATIONS & DOSAGE
Treatment of depression—
Adults: initial dose 50 mg P.O. t.i.d. May increase to 100 mg t.i.d. on third day of treatment. Increases above 300 mg daily should be made only if 300 mg daily has been ineffective during a trial period of at least 2 weeks. When effective dosage is established, entire dosage (not exceeding 300 mg) may be given at bedtime. Maximum dosage is 600 mg in hospitalized patients.

CONTRAINDICATIONS & PRECAUTIONS
Contraindicated in patients with hypersensitivity to tricyclic antidepressants, trazodone, or related compounds; in the acute recovery phase of myocardial infarction because of potential arrhythmogenic effects; in patients in coma or severe respiratory depression because of additive CNS depression; and during or within 14 days of monoamine oxidase (MAO) therapy.

Use cautiously in patients with other cardiac disease (arrhythmias,

CHF, angina pectoris, valvular disease, or heart block); respiratory disorders; seizure disorders; scheduled electroconvulsive therapy; bipolar disease; glaucoma; hyperthyroidism or in those taking thyroid replacement; Type I and Type II diabetes; prostatic hypertrophy, paralytic ileus, or urine retention; hepatic or renal dysfunction; Parkinson's disease; and in those having general anesthesia. Caution also is recommended in patients with tardive dyskinesia, because amoxapine may induce or exacerbate this disorder.

ADVERSE REACTIONS

Common reactions are in italics; life-threatening reactions are in bold italics.
CNS: *drowsiness, dizziness,* excitation, tremors, weakness, confusion, headache, nervousness, *tardive dyskinesia* (especially in elderly women).
CV: *orthostatic hypotension, tachycardia, ECG changes,* hypertension.
EENT: *blurred vision,* tinnitus, mydriasis.
GI: *dry mouth, constipation,* nausea, vomiting, anorexia, paralytic ileus.
GU: *urine retention, **acute renal failure.***
Skin: rash, urticaria.
Other: *sweating,* weight gain and craving for sweets, allergy.
After abrupt withdrawal of long-term therapy: nausea, headache, malaise. (Does not indicate addiction.)

INTERACTIONS

Barbiturates: decrease tricyclic antidepressant (TCA) blood levels. Monitor for decreased antidepressant effect.
Cimetidine: may increase amoxapine serum levels. Monitor for increased adverse effects.
Epinephrine, norepinephrine: increase hypertensive effect. Use with caution.
MAO inhibitors: may cause severe excitation, hyperpyrexia, or seizures, usually with high dose. Use together cautiously.
Methylphenidate: increases TCA blood levels. Monitor for enhanced antidepressant effect.

EFFECTS ON DIAGNOSTIC TESTS

CBC: decreased WBC.
ECG: elongated Q-T and PR intervals; flattened T waves.
Liver function tests: elevated results.
Serum glucose levels: increased or decreased levels.

NURSING CONSIDERATIONS

Besides those related universally to drug therapy (see "How to use this book"), consider the following specific recommendations:

Assessment
- Obtain a baseline assessment of pain before therapy.
- Be alert for adverse reactions and drug interactions throughout therapy.
- Evaluate the patient's and family's knowledge about amoxapine therapy.

Nursing Diagnoses
- Ineffective individual coping related to the patient's underlying condition.
- High risk for injury related to amoxapine-induced adverse reactions.
- Knowledge deficit related to amoxapine therapy.

Planning and Implementation

Preparation and Administration
- Whenever possible, patient should take full dose at bedtime.
- Expect reduced dosage in elderly or debilitated patients and adolescents.

Monitoring
- Monitor effectiveness by encouraging patient to discuss his feelings (ask broad, open-ended questions) and by evaluating his behavior.
- Monitor blood pressure (supine and standing) for changes in heart rate and ECG for tachycardia.
- Watch for signs of oversedation, especially in the elderly patient.
- Monitor for signs of tardive dyskinesia especially in elderly women.

• Monitor bowel patterns for constipation.
• Monitor for suicidal tendencies.

Supportive Care
• Institute safety precautions if adverse CNS reactions occur.
• Do not withdraw drug abruptly.
• If psychotic signs increase, notify doctor and expect reduction of dosage.
• If not contraindicated, increase the patient's fluid and fiber intake to prevent constipation; if needed, obtain an order for a laxative.
• Assist the patient in changing positions slowly to minimize orthostatic hypotension.

Patient Teaching
• Tell the patient to relieve dry mouth with sugarless hard candy or gum; explain that saliva substitutes may be necessary.
• Advise the patient to increase fluid intake to lessen constipation. Suggest stool softener or high-fiber diet, if needed.
• Warn the patient to avoid driving and other hazardous activities that require alertness and good psychomotor coordination until CNS effects of the drug are known. Tell the patient that drowsiness and dizziness usually subside after first few weeks. Inform the patient that drug has strong sedative effects; warn against combining it with alcohol or other CNS depressants.
• Tell the patient to expect delay of 2 weeks or more before noticeable effect. Full effect may take 4 weeks or more. Encourage the patient to continue to take medication until it achieves its full therapeutic effect.

Evaluation

In patients receiving amoxapine, appropriate evaluation statements may include:
• Patient behavior and communication indicate improvement of depression.
• Patient has not experienced injury from adverse CNS reactions.
• Patient and family state an understanding of amoxapine therapy.

amoxicillin/clavulanate potassium (amoxycillin/clavulanate potassium)

(a mox i sill′ in)/(klav′ yoo la nate)
Augmentin, Clavulin†

• *Classification:* aminopenicillin and beta-lactamase inhibitor
• *Pregnancy Risk Category:* B

HOW SUPPLIED

Tablets (chewable): 125 mg amoxicillin trihydrate, 31.25 mg clavulanic acid; 250 mg amoxicillin trihydrate, 62.5 mg clavulanic acid
Tablets (film-coated): 250 mg amoxicillin trihydrate, 125 mg clavulanic acid; 500 mg amoxicillin trihydrate, 125 mg clavulanic acid
Oral suspension: 125 mg amoxicillin trihydrate and 31.25 mg clavulanic acid/5 ml (after reconstitution); 250 mg amoxicillin trihydrate and 62.5 mg clavulanic acid/5 ml (after reconstitution)

ACTION

Mechanism: Amoxicillin prevents bacterial cell wall synthesis during active replication. Clavulanic acid increases amoxicillin effectiveness by inactivating beta-lactamases, which destroy amoxicillin.
Absorption: Well absorbed after oral administration.
Distribution: Amoxicillin and clavulanate distribute into pleural fluid, lungs, and peritoneal fluid; high urine concentrations are attained. Amoxicillin also distributes into synovial fluid, liver, prostate, muscle, and gallbladder and penetrates into middle ear effusions, maxillary sinus secretions, tonsils, sputum, and bron-

chial secretions. Both drugs cross the placenta; low concentrations occur in breast milk. Amoxicillin and clavulanate have minimal protein-binding of 17% to 20% and 22% to 30%, respectively.
Metabolism: Amoxicillin is metabolized only partially. The metabolic fate of clavulanate is not completely known, but it appears to undergo extensive metabolism.
Excretion: Amoxicillin is excreted principally in urine by renal tubular secretion and glomerular filtration; also excreted in breast milk. Clavulanate is excreted by glomerular filtration. Half-life: Elimination half-life of amoxicillin in adults is 1 to 1½ hours, prolonged to 7½ hours in severe renal impairment. Half-life of clavulanate in adults is about 1 to 1½ hours, prolonged to 4½ hours in severe renal impairment.
Onset, peak, duration: Peak serum levels occur at 1 to 2½ hours.

INDICATIONS & DOSAGE

Lower respiratory infections, otitis media, sinusitis, skin and skin structure infections, and urinary tract infections caused by susceptible strains of gram-positive and gram-negative organisms–
Adults: 250 mg (based on the amoxicillin component) P.O. q 8 hours. For more severe infections, 500 mg q 8 hours.
Children: 20 to 40 mg/kg (based on the amoxicillin component) P.O. daily given in divided doses q 8 hours.

CONTRAINDICATIONS & PRECAUTIONS

Contraindicated in patients with hypersensitivity to any penicillin or cephalosporin. Drug should not be used in patients with mononucleosis because many patients develop a rash during therapy.

Use cautiously in patients with renal impairment because drug is excreted by kidneys; decreased dosage is required in moderate to severe renal failure.

ADVERSE REACTIONS

Common reactions are in italics; life-threatening reactions are in bold italics.
Blood: anemia, thrombocytopenia, thrombocytopenic purpura, eosinophilia, leukopenia.
GI: *nausea,* vomiting, *diarrhea.*
Other: *hypersensitivity (erythematous maculopapular rash, urticaria,* ***anaphylaxis),*** overgrowth of nonsusceptible organisms.

INTERACTIONS

Allopurinol: increased incidence of skin rash.
Probenecid: increases blood levels of amoxicillin and other penicillins. Probenecid may be used for this purpose.

EFFECTS ON DIAGNOSTIC TESTS

Aminoglycoside serum levels: falsely decreased concentrations.
Coombs' tests: possible false-positive results.
Urine glucose tests with copper sulfate (Benedict's reagent or Clinitest): false-positive results. Use glucose enzymatic methods (Clinistix or Tes-Tape).

NURSING CONSIDERATIONS

Besides those related universally to drug therapy (see "How to use this book"), consider the following specific recommendations:

Assessment

- Obtain a baseline assessment of patient's infection before amoxicillin therapy.
- Be alert for adverse reactions and drug interactions throughout therapy.
- Evaluate the patient's and family's knowledge about amoxicillin therapy.

Nursing Diagnoses
• High risk for injury related to ineffectiveness of amoxicillin to eradicate the infection.
• High risk for fluid volume deficit related to amoxicillin-induced adverse GI reactions.
• Knowledge deficit related to amoxicillin therapy.

Planning and Implementation

Preparation and Administration
• Obtain specimen for culture and sensitivity tests before first dose. Therapy may begin pending test results.
• Before first dose, ask the patient about previous allergic reactions to this drug or other penicillins. However, a negative history of penicillin allergy does not guarantee future safety.
• Give amoxicillin at least 1 hour before bacteriostatic antibiotics.
• ***P.O. use:*** Administer with food to prevent GI distress.
• Be aware that both the "250" and "500" tablets contain the same amount of clavulanic acid (125 mg). Therefore, two "250" tablets are not equivalent to one "500" tablet.

Monitoring
• Monitor effectiveness by regularly assessing for improvement of infection.
• Monitor the patient's hydration status if adverse GI reactions occur. This combination produces higher incidence of diarrhea than amoxicillin alone.
• Monitor patient closely for a bacterial or fungal superinfection during prolonged or high-dose therapy, especially in elderly, debilitated, or immunosuppressed patients.

Supportive Care
• Obtain an order for an antiemetic or antidiarrheal agent as needed.

Patient Teaching
• Advise the patient who becomes allergic to amoxicillin to wear medical alert identification stating this information.
• Tell the patient to take drug exactly as prescribed and to complete the entire prescription even after he feels better.
• Tell the patient to call the doctor if rash develops. A rash is a sign of an allergic reaction.
• Instruct patient to take amoxicillin with food to prevent GI distress.

Evaluation
In patients receiving amoxicillin, appropriate evaluation statements may include:
• Patient is free of infection.
• Patient maintains adequate hydration throughout amoxicillin therapy.
• Patient and family state an understanding of amoxicillin therapy.

---

amoxicillin trihydrate (amoxycillin trihydrate)

(a mox i sill′ in)

Alphamox‡, Amoxil, Apo-Amoxi†, Axicillin†, Cilamox‡, Ibiamox‡, Moxacin‡, Novamoxin†, Polymox†, Trimox, Utimox, Wymox

• *Classification:* antibiotic (aminopenicillin)
• *Pregnancy Risk Category:* B

HOW SUPPLIED
Tablets (chewable): 125 mg, 250 mg
Capsules: 250 mg, 500 mg
Oral suspension: 50 mg/5 ml (pediatric drops), 125 mg/5 ml, 250 mg/5 ml (after reconsititution)

ACTION
Mechanism: Bactericidal against microorganisms by inhibiting cell wall synthesis during active multiplication. Bacteria resist amoxicillin by producing penicillinases—enzymes that hydrolyze amoxicillin.
Absorption: Approximately 80% is absorbed after oral administration.

Distribution: Distributed into pleural, peritoneal, and synovial fluids, and into the lungs, prostate, muscle, liver, and gallbladder. Also penetrates middle ear, maxillary sinus and bronchial secretions; tonsils; and sputum; readily crosses the placenta. Drug is 17% to 20% protein-bound.
Metabolism: Metabolized only partially.
Excretion: Mainly excreted in urine by renal tubular secretion and glomerular filtration; also excreted in breast milk. Half-life: Elimination half-life in adults is 1 to 1½ hours, prolonged to 7½ hours in severe renal impairment.
Onset, peak, duration: Peak serum concentrations occur 1 to 2½ hours after an oral dose.

INDICATIONS & DOSAGE

Systemic infections, acute and chronic urinary tract infections caused by susceptible strains of gram-positive and gram-negative organisms–
Adults: 750 mg to 1.5 g P.O. daily in divided doses given q 8 hours.
Children: 20 to 40 mg/kg P.O. daily in divided doses given q 8 hours.
Uncomplicated gonorrhea–
Adults: 3 g P.O. with 1 g probenecid given as a single dose.
Uncomplicated urinary tract infections caused by susceptible organisms–
Adults: 3 g P.O. given as a single dose.

CONTRAINDICATIONS AND PRECAUTIONS

Contraindicated in patients with hypersensitivity to any penicillin or cephalosporin. Amoxicillin should not be used in patients with infectious mononucleosis, because many patients develop a rash during therapy.

Use cautiously in patients with renal impairment because drug is excreted by the kidneys; decreased dosage is required in moderate to severe renal failure.

ADVERSE REACTIONS

Common reactions are in italics; life-threatening reactions are in bold italics.
Blood: anemia, thrombocytopenia, thrombocytopenic purpura, eosinophilia, leukopenia.
GI: *nausea,* vomiting, *diarrhea.*
Other: *hypersensitivity (erythematous maculopapular rash, urticaria,* ***anaphylaxis****),* overgrowth of nonsusceptible organisms.

INTERACTIONS

Allopurinol: increased incidence of skin rash.
Probenecid: increases blood levels of amoxicillin and other penicillins. Probenecid may be used for this purpose.

EFFECTS ON DIAGNOSTIC TESTS

Aminoglycoside levels: falsely decreased concentrations.
Urine glucose tests with copper sulfate (Benedict's reagent or Clinitest): false-positive results. Use glucose enzymatic methods (Clinistix or Tes-Tape).

NURSING CONSIDERATIONS

Besides those related universally to drug therapy (see "How to use this book"), consider the following specific recommendations:
Assessment
- Obtain a baseline assessment of patient's infection before therapy.
- Be alert for adverse reactions and drug interactions throughout therapy.
- Evaluate the patient's and family's knowledge about amoxicillin therapy.

Nursing Diagnoses
- High risk for injury related to ineffectiveness of amoxicillin to eradicate the infection.
- High risk for fluid volume deficit

related to amoxicillin-induced adverse GI reactions.
• Knowledge deficit related to amoxicillin therapy.

Planning and Implementation

Preparation and Administration

• Obtain specimen for culture and sensitivity tests before first dose. Therapy may begin pending test results.
• Before first dose, ask the patient about previous allergic reactions to this drug or other forms of penicillin. However, a negative history of penicillin allergy does not guarantee future safety.
• Give amoxicillin at least 1 hour before bacteriostatic antibiotics.
• ***P.O. use:*** Administer with food to prevent GI distress.
• Trimox oral suspension may be stored at room temperature for up to 2 weeks. Check individual product labels for storage information.

Monitoring

• Monitor effectiveness by regularly assessing for improvement of infectious process.
• Monitor the patient's hydration status if adverse GI reactions occur.
• Monitor patient closely for a bacterial or fungal superinfection during prolonged or high-dose therapy, especially in elderly, debilitated, or immunosuppressed patients.

Supportive Care

• Obtain an order for an antiemetic or antidiarrheal agent as needed.
• Be aware that drug may cause false-positive urine glucose determinations with copper sulfate tests (Clinitest); drug does not affect glucose enzymatic tests (Clinistix, Tes-Tape).

Patient Teaching

• Advise the patient who becomes allergic to amoxicillin to wear medical alert identification stating this information.
• Tell the patient to take drug exactly as prescribed and to complete the entire prescription even after he feels better.
• Tell the patient to call the doctor if rash, fever, or chills develop. A rash is the most common allergic reaction.
• Instruct patient to take amoxicillin with food to prevent GI distress.
• Warn patient never to use leftover amoxicillin for a new illness or to share it with others.

Evaluation

In patients receiving amoxicillin, appropriate evaluation statements may include:
• Patient is free of infection.
• Patient maintains adequate hydration throughout amoxicillin therapy.
• Patient and family state an understanding of amoxicillin therapy.

PHARMACOLOGIC CLASS

amphetamines

amphetamine sulfate
benzphetamine hydrochloride
dextroamphetamine sulfate
diethylpropion hydrochloride
fenfluramine hydrochloride
methamphetamine hydrochloride
phendimetrazine hydrochloride
phenmetrazine hydrochloride
phentermine hydrochloride

OVERVIEW

Amphetamines were the first drugs widely prescribed as anorexigenics. They no longer are used for this purpose because dependence can develop. The Food and Drug Administration has found no advantage to their use as compared with other, safer anorexigenics.

Amphetamines are sympathomimetic amines with CNS stimulant activity; in children with hyperkinesia, they have a paradoxical calming effect. Their mechanisms of action for narcolepsy, attention deficit disorder, and appetite control are unknown; anorexigenic effects are thought to occur in the hypothalamus, where decreased smell and taste acuity decreases appetite.

CLINICAL INDICATIONS AND ACTIONS

Narcolepsy; attention deficit disorders
Amphetamines may be used to treat narcolepsy and as adjuncts to psychosocial measures in attention deficit disorder in children.
Adjuncts in managing obesity
Amphetamines may be tried for short-term control of refractory obesity, with caloric restriction and behavior modification; anorexigenic effects persist only a few weeks, and patient must be encouraged to learn modification of eating habits rapidly.

OVERVIEW OF ADVERSE REACTIONS

Adverse reactions to the amphetamines reflect excessive sympathomimetic and CNS stimulation and commonly include insomnia, tremor, and restlessness; toxic dosage levels can induce psychosis, mydriasis, hypertension, arrhythmias, coma, circulatory collapse, and death.

Tolerance to amphetamines can occur within a few weeks, necessitating increased dosages to produce desired effects; abusers take an average of 1 to 2 g/day. Both physical tolerance and psychological dependence may occur. Symptoms of chronic abuse include mental impairment, loss of appetite, somnolence, social withdrawal, and occupational and emotional problems; prolonged abuse may cause schizoid syndromes and hallucinations.

REPRESENTATIVE COMBINATIONS

Amphetamine sulfate with dextroamphetamine sulfate: Biphetamine, Obetrol.

Methamphetamine hydrochloride with amobarbital and homatropine: Obe-Slim; with dl-methamphetamine and butabarbital: Span-RD; with Pamabrom, pyrilamine, homatropine, hyoscyamine sulfate, and scopolamine hydrobromide: Aridol; with pentobarbital; Fetamin; with phenobarbital and ascorbic acid: Obetrim-T.

See also barbiturates.

amphetamine sulfate
(am fet´ a meen)

- Controlled Substance Schedule II
- *Classification:* CNS stimulant, adjunctive anorexigenic agent, sympathomimetic amine (amphetamine)
- *Pregnancy Risk Category:* C

HOW SUPPLIED

Tablets: 5 mg, 10 mg
Capsules: 5 mg, 10 mg

ACTION

Mechanism: Main site of activity appears to be the cerebral cortex and the reticular activating system. Promotes nerve impulse transmission by releasing stored norepinephrine from nerve terminals in the brain. In children with hyperkinesia, amphetamines have a paradoxical calming effect.
Absorption: Completely absorbed within 3 hours of oral administration.
Distribution: Widely distributed throughout the body, with high concentrations in the brain.
Metabolism: Hepatic.
Excretion: Drug and metabolites are excreted in urine.
Onset, peak, duration: Therapeutic effects persist for 4 to 24 hours.

INDICATIONS & DOSAGE

Attention deficit disorder with hyperactivity (ADDH)–
Children 6 years and older: 5 mg P.O. daily, with 5-mg increments weekly, p.r.n.

Children 3 to 5 years: 2.5 mg P.O. daily, with 2.5-mg increments weekly, p.r.n.
Narcolepsy–
Adults: 5 to 60 mg P.O. daily in divided doses.
Children over 12 years: 10 mg P.O. daily, with 10-mg increments weekly, p.r.n.
Children 6 to 12 years: 5 mg P.O. daily, with 5-mg increments weekly, p.r.n.
Short-term adjunct in exogenous obesity–
Adults: single 10- or 15-mg long-acting capsule daily, or 2 if needed, up to 30 mg daily; or 5 to 30 mg daily in divided doses 30 to 60 minutes before meals. Not recommended for children under 12 years.

CONTRAINDICATIONS & PRECAUTIONS

Contraindicated in patients with hypersensitivity or idiosyncratic reaction to sympathomimetic amines; in those with symptomatic cardiovascular disease, hyperthyroidism, nephritis, angina pectoris, hypertension, glaucoma, advanced arteriosclerosis, or agitated states; and in patients with a history of drug or alcohol abuse; also contraindicated for concomitant use with monoamine oxidase (MAO) inhibitors or within 14 days of discontinuing MAO inhibitors.

Use cautiously in patients with diabetes mellitus; in elderly, debilitated, or hyperexcitable patients; and in children with Gilles de la Tourette's syndrome. Avoid long-term therapy, when possible, because of the risk of psychological or physical dependence.

ADVERSE REACTIONS

Common reactions are in italics; life-threatening reactions are in bold italics.
CNS: *restlessness,* tremor, *hyperactivity, talkativeness, insomnia,* irritability, dizziness, headache, chills, overstimulation, dysphoria.
CV: *tachycardia, palpitations,* hypertension, hypotension.
GI: nausea, vomiting, cramps, dry mouth, diarrhea, constipation, metallic taste, anorexia, weight loss.
Other: urticaria, impotence, altered libido.

INTERACTIONS

Ammonium chloride, ascorbic acid: observe for decreased amphetamine effect.
Antacids, sodium bicarbonate, acetazolamide: increased renal reabsorption. Monitor for enhanced effect.
MAO inhibitors: severe hypertension; possible hypertensive crisis. Don't use together.
Phenothiazines, haloperidol: observe for decreased amphetamine effect.

EFFECTS ON DIAGNOSTIC TESTS

Plasma corticosteroids: elevated levels.
Urinary steroid determinations: test interference.

NURSING CONSIDERATIONS

Besides those related universally to drug therapy (see "How to use this book"), consider the following specific recommendations:

Assessment
- Obtain a baseline assessment of the patient's CNS status, behavior, or weight, depending on underlying disorder.
- Be alert for adverse reactions and drug interactions throughout therapy.
- Evaluate the patient's and family's knowledge about amphetamine sulfate therapy.

Nursing Diagnoses
- Ineffective individual coping related to patient's underlying disorder.
- Sleep pattern disturbance related to amphetamine sulfate-induced insomnia.
- Knowledge deficit related to amphetamine sulfate therapy.

Planning and Implementation

Preparation and Administration

• Administer drug at least 6 hours before bedtime to avoid interference with sleep.

• When used for obesity, administer drug 30 minutes to 1 hour before meals.

• Avoid prolonged administration because psychological dependence may occur, especially in patients with a history of drug addiction. When used long-term, reduce dosage gradually to prevent acute rebound depression.

Monitoring

• Monitor effectiveness by observing the patient's CNS status and behavior or assessing the patient's weight.

• Monitor vital signs for evidence of tachycardia or blood pressure changes; question the patient regularly about palpitations. Keep in mind that this drug may reverse beneficial effects of antihypertensives.

• Monitor sleeping pattern, and observe for signs of excessive stimulation.

• Monitor blood glucose levels in diabetic patients because drug may alter daily insulin needs.

• Monitor dietary intake, when used for obesity.

Supportive Care

• Provide frequent rest periods and assistance with activities as needed; fatigue may result as drug's effects wear off.

• Institute safety precautions by making environment safe and providing supervision of patient's activities.

• When used for obesity, make sure the patient is also on a weight-reduction program. Do calorie counts, if necessary. Be aware that this drug is not recommended for first-line treatment of obesity. Use as an anorexigenic agent is prohibited in some states.

• Be aware that this drug should not be used to overcome fatigue. Also use as an analeptic is usually discouraged, since CNS stimulation superimposed on CNS depression can lead to neuronal instability and seizures.

Patient Teaching

• Warn the patient to avoid activities that require alertness or good psychomotor coordination until CNS effects of the drug are known.

• Tell the patient to avoid beverages containing caffeine, which increase the stimulant effects of amphetamines and related amines.

• Have the patient report signs of excessive stimulation.

• Tell the patient to weigh himself weekly in the same clothes at the same time of day to evaluate effectiveness in obesity therapy.

• Tell the diabetic patient to monitor blood glucose levels closely.

• Teach the patient how to take the drug to minimize insomnia and enhance effectiveness.

• Tell the patient that, when tolerance to anorexigenic effect develops, dosage should not be increased, but drug discontinued. Patient should call the doctor to report decreased effectiveness of drug. Warn the patient against stopping drug abruptly.

• Tell the patient to notify the nurse or doctor if severe insomnia develops.

Evaluation

In patients receiving amphetamine sulfate, appropriate evaluation statements may include:

• Patient demonstrates clinical improvement and related improved coping ability.

• Patient is able to sleep without difficulty.

• Patient and family state an understanding of amphetamine sulfate therapy.

amphotericin B (topical)

(am foe ter´ i sin)
Fungizone

- *Classification:* antifungal (macrolide)
- *Pregnancy Risk Category:* B

HOW SUPPLIED

Cream: 3%
Lotion: 3%
Ointment: 3%

ACTION

Mechanism: Probably acts by binding to sterols in the fungal cell membrane. Has mainly fungistatic action but may be fungicidal in high concentrations.
Absorption: Rapidly absorbed after topical administration.

INDICATIONS & DOSAGE

Cutaneous or mucocutaneous candidal infections–
Adults and children: apply liberally b.i.d., t.i.d., or q.i.d. for 1 to 3 weeks; up to several months for interdigital lesions and paronychias.

CONTRAINDICATIONS & PRECAUTIONS

Contraindicated in patients with hypersensitivity to the drug, unless no other therapy is effective. Use cautiously in patients taking other nephrotoxic drugs.

ADVERSE REACTIONS

Common reactions are in italics; life-threatening reactions are in bold italics.
Skin: possible drying, contact sensitivity, erythema, burning, pruritus.

INTERACTIONS

None significant.

EFFECTS ON DIAGNOSTIC TESTS

BUN, serum creatinine, alkaline phosphatase, and bilirubin: increased levels.
CBC: decreased WBC, RBC, and platelet counts.
Serum electrolyte levels: hypokalemia and hypomagnesemia.

NURSING CONSIDERATIONS

Besides those related universally to drug therapy (see "How to use this book"), consider the following specific recommendations:

Assessment
- Obtain a baseline assessment of infected lesions before therapy.
- Be alert for adverse reactions and drug interactions throughout therapy.
- Evaluate the patient's and family's knowledge about amphotericin B therapy.

Nursing Diagnoses
- Impaired tissue integrity related to infected lesions.
- High risk for impaired skin integrity related to drug-induced erythema and drying.
- Knowledge deficit related to amphotericin B therapy.

Planning and Implementation
Preparation and Administration
- ***Topical use:*** Clean area before applying. Use cream or lotion for areas such as folds of groin, armpit, and neck creases. Avoid occlusive dressings. Be aware that cream can cause skin discoloration. Lotion may stain nail lesions. Store at room temperature.

Monitoring
- Monitor effectiveness by assessing the patient's infected lesions.
- Monitor for adverse reactions by frequently assessing the skin for signs of local irritation. Cream may have a drying effect on the skin; ointment may irritate if applied to moist, hairy areas.

Supportive Care
• Keep in mind, topical amphotericin B therapy is well tolerated, even by infants, for long periods.
• Notify the doctor if erythema or drying occurs.
Patient Teaching
• Teach patient to apply medication.
• Tell patient to continue using medication for full length of time prescribed, even if condition has improved.
• Inform patient that discoloration of fabric caused by cream or lotion can usually be removed by ordinary washing; discoloration caused by ointment requires removal with cleaning fluid.
Evaluation
In patients receiving amphotericin B, appropriate evaluation statements may include:
• Patient states his lesions are healed.
• Patient does not develop erythema and dryness.
• Patient and family state an understanding of amphotericin B therapy.

amphotericin B (systemic)
(am foe ter´ i sin)
Fungilin Oral‡, Fungizone

• *Classification:* antifungal (macrolide)
• *Pregnancy Risk Category:* B

HOW SUPPLIED
Tablets: 100 mg‡
Oral suspension: 100 mg/ml‡
Lozenges: 10 mg‡
Injection: 50-mg lyophilized cake

ACTION
Mechanism: Probably acts by binding to sterols in the fungal cell membrane, altering cell permeability and allowing leakage of intracellular components.
Absorption: Poorly absorbed from the GI tract. Must be given parenterally to treat systemic fungal infections; oral amphotericin is only used to treat local fungal infections in the GI tract. Note that oral formulations are not available in the U.S.
Distribution: After I.V. administration, the drug distributes well into inflamed pleural cavities and joints; in low concentrations into aqueous humor, bronchial secretions, pancreas, bone, muscle, and parotids. CSF concentrations reach about 3% of serum concentrations. Drug is 90% to 95% bound to plasma proteins. It reportedly crosses the placenta.
Metabolism: Not well defined.
Excretion: After I.V. administration, about 2% to 5% of the drug is excreted unchanged in urine. Amphotericin B is not readily removed by hemodialysis. Half-life: Elimination is biphasic; elimination half-life is about 15 days.
Onset, peak, duration: Peak plasma concentrations range from approximately 0.5 to 2 mcg/ml. After a rapid initial fall, plasma concentrations plateau at about 0.5 mcg/ml. Drug can be detected in the urine for at least 7 weeks after discontinuation because of slow elimination.

INDICATIONS & DOSAGE
Systemic fungal infections (histoplasmosis, coccidioidomycosis, blastomycosis, cryptococcosis, disseminated moniliasis, aspergillosis, phycomycosis), meningitis–
Adults: initially, 1 mg in 250 ml of dextrose 5% in water infused over 2 to 4 hours; or 0.25 mg/kg daily by slow infusion over 6 hours. Increase daily dosage gradually as patient tolerance develops to maximum 1 mg/kg daily. Therapy must not exceed 1.5 mg/kg. If drug is discontinued for 1 week or more, administration must resume with initial dose and again increase gradually.
Intrathecal: 25 mcg/0.1 ml diluted with 10 to 20 ml of cerebrospinal

fluid and administered by barbotage 2 or 3 times weekly. Initial dose should not exceed 100 mcg.
Treatment of Candida albicans *infections involving the GI tract*–
Adults: 100 mg P.O. q.i.d. for 2 weeks.
Oral and perioral candidal infections–
Adults: 1 lozenge q.i.d. for 7 to 14 days. The lozenge should be sucked and allowed to dissolve slowly in the mouth.

CONTRAINDICATIONS & PRECAUTIONS

Contraindicated in patients with hypersensitivity to the drug, unless no other therapy is effective. Use with caution in patients taking other nephrotoxic drugs.

ADVERSE REACTIONS

Common reactions are in italics; life-threatening reactions are in bold italics.
Blood: normochromic, normocytic anemia.
CNS: headache, peripheral neuropathy; with intrathecal administration–peripheral nerve pain, paresthesias.
CV: hypotension, ***cardiac arrhythmias, asystole.***
GI: *anorexia, weight loss, nausea,* vomiting, dyspepsia, diarrhea, epigastric cramps.
GU: abnormal renal function with *hypokalemia, azotemia, hyposthenuria,* renal tubular acidosis, nephrocalcinosis; with large doses–permanent renal impairment, anuria, oliguria.
Local: burning, stinging, irritation, tissue damage with extravasation, *thrombophlebitis,* pain at site of injection.
Other: arthralgia, myalgia, muscle weakness secondary to hypokalemia, *fever, chills,* malaise, generalized pain.

INTERACTIONS

Other nephrotoxic antibiotics: may cause additive renal toxicity. Administer very cautiously.

EFFECTS ON DIAGNOSTIC TESTS

Alkaline phosphatase, bilirubin: increased levels.
BUN, serum creatinine: increased levels.
Electrolytes: hypokalemia and hypomagnesemia.
RBC, WBC, platelet counts: decreased.

NURSING CONSIDERATIONS

Besides those related universally to drug therapy (see "How to use this book"), consider the following specific recommendations:

Assessment
- Obtain a baseline assessment of fungal infection and appropriate samples to identify fungi before therapy.
- Be alert for adverse reactions and drug interactions throughout therapy.
- Evaluate the patient's and family's knowledge about amphotericin B therapy.

Nursing Diagnoses
- High risk for injury related to ineffectiveness of amphotericin B to eradicate the infection.
- Altered health maintenance related to amphotericin B-induced adverse reactions.
- Knowledge deficit related to amphotericin B.

Planning and Implementation
Preparation and Administration
- Remember that cultures and histologic and sensitivity testing must be completed and diagnosis confirmed before starting therapy in nonimmunocompromised patient.
- ***P.O. use:*** Oral form is not available in the U.S.
- ***I.V. use:*** Prepare infusion as manufacturer directs with strict aseptic technique using only 10 ml of sterile water to reconstitute. To avoid precip-

itation, do not mix or piggyback with solutions containing sodium chloride, other electrolytes, antibiotics, or bacteriostatic agents, such as benzyl alcohol. The I.V. solution appears compatible with small amounts of heparin sodium, hydrocortisone sodium succinate, and methylprednisolone sodium succinate.
• Use an in-line filter with a mean pore diameter larger than 1 micron for I.V. infusion. Infuse *slowly* over 3 to 4 hours because rapid infusion may cause CV collapse. Administer in distal veins.
• Store at room temperature. Solution is stable at room temperature and indoor light for 24 hours or in refrigerator for 1 week.

Monitoring
• Monitor effectiveness by regularly assessing for improvement of infection.
• Monitor I.V. site for discomfort or thrombosis.
• Monitor vital signs every 30 minutes for at least 4 hours after start of I.V. infusion; fever may appear in 1 to 2 hours but should subside within 4 hours after discontinuing drug.
• Monitor intake and output.
• Monitor potassium levels closely; monitor calcium and magnesium levels twice weekly; perform liver and renal function studies and CBC weekly as prescribed.
• Monitor ECG for arrhythmias.

Supportive Care
• Notify doctor immediately if changes in urine appearance or volume occur. Renal damage may be reversible if drug is discontinued at earliest sign of dysfunction.
• Be aware that the severity of some adverse reactions can be reduced by premedication with aspirin, acetaminophen, antihistamines, antiemetics, or small doses of corticosteroids; by addition of phosphate buffer to the solution; and by alternate-day dosing. Severe reactions may require discontinuation of drug for varying periods.
• Notify doctor if thrombosis occurs. Alternate-day therapy may be necessary.
• Obtain an order for an antiemetic or antidiarrheal agent as needed.

Patient Teaching
• Teach the patient signs and symptoms of hypersensitivity, and stress importance of reporting them immediately.
• Warn patient that therapy may take several months; teach personal hygiene and other measures to prevent spread and recurrence of lesions.
• Urge compliance with prescribed regimen and recommended follow-up.

Evaluation

In patients receiving amphotericin B, appropriate evaluation statements may include:
• Patient's infection is alleviated.
• Patient does not experience serious adverse reactions associated with amphotericin B.
• Patient and family state an understanding of amphotericin B therapy.

ampicillin
(am pi sill′ in)
Amcill, Ampicin†, Ampilean†, Apo-Ampi†, Novo Ampicillin†, Omnipen, Penbritin†, Principen

ampicillin sodium
Ampicyn Injection‡, Omnipen-N, Polycillin-N, Totacillin-N

ampicillin trihydrate
Amcill, Ampicyn Oral‡, D-Amp, Omnipen, Penamp-250, Penamp-500, Penbritin‡, Polycillin, Principen-250, Principen-500, Totacillin

• *Classification:* antibiotic (aminopenicillin)
• *Pregnancy Risk Category:* B

HOW SUPPLIED

Capsules: 250 mg, 500 mg
Oral suspension: 100 mg/ml (pediatric drops), 125 mg/5 ml, 250 mg/5 ml, 500 mg/5 ml (after reconstitution)
Injection: 125 mg, 250 mg, 500 mg, 1 g, 2 g
Infusion: 500 mg, 1 g, 2 g
Pharmacy bulk package: 10-g vial

ACTION

Mechanism: Bactericidal against microorganisms by inhibiting cell wall synthesis during active multiplication. Bacteria resist ampicillin by producing penicillinases—enzymes that hydrolyze ampicillin.
Absorption: Approximately 30% to 55% of an oral dose of ampicillin is absorbed. After I.M. administration, peak serum levels are higher and occur sooner.
Distribution: Into pleural, peritoneal, and synovial fluids, lungs, prostate, liver, and gallbladder; also penetrates middle ear effusions, maxillary sinus and bronchial secretions, tonsils, and sputum and readily crosses the placenta; drug is minimally protein-bound at 15% to 25%.
Metabolism: Metabolized only partially.
Excretion: Excreted in urine by renal tubular secretion and glomerular filtration; also excreted in breast milk. Half-life: Elimination half-life is about 1 to 1½ hours; 10 to 24 hours in patients with extensive renal impairment.
Onset, peak, duration: Peak serum concentrations occur at 1 to 2 hours after oral administration; at 1 hour after I.M. administration.

INDICATIONS & DOSAGE

Systemic infections, acute and chronic urinary tract infections caused by susceptible strains of gram-positive and gram-negative organisms—
Adults: 1 to 4 g P.O. daily, divided into doses given q 6 hours; 2 to 12 g I.M. or I.V. daily, divided into doses given q 4 to 6 hours.
Children: 50 to 100 mg/kg P.O. daily, divided into doses given q 6 hours; or 100 to 200 mg/kg I.M. or I.V. daily, divided into doses given q 6 hours.
Meningitis—
Adults: 8 to 14 g I.V. daily for 3 days, then I.M. divided q 3 to 4 hours.
Children: up to 300 mg/kg I.V. daily for 3 days, then I.M. divided q 4 hours.
Uncomplicated gonorrhea—
Adults: 3.5 g P.O. with 1 g probenecid given as a single dose.

CONTRAINDICATIONS & PRECAUTIONS

Contraindicated in patients with hypersensitivity to any penicillin or cephalosporin. Drug should not be used in patients with infectious mononucleosis because many patients develop a rash during therapy.

Use cautiously in patients with renal impairment because drug is excreted by kidneys; decreased dosage is required in moderate to severe renal failure.

ADVERSE REACTIONS

Common reactions are in italics; life-threatening reactions are in bold italics.
Blood: anemia, thrombocytopenia, thrombocytopenic purpura, eosinophilia, leukopenia.
GI: *nausea,* vomiting, *diarrhea,* glossitis, stomatitis.
Local: pain at injection site, vein irritation, thrombophlebitis.
Other: *hypersensitivity (erythematous maculopapular rash, urticaria, **anaphylaxis**),* overgrowth of nonsusceptible organisms.

INTERACTIONS

Allopurinol: increased incidence of skin rash.
Probenecid: increases blood levels of ampicillin and other penicillins. Pro-

*Liquid form contains alcohol.

**May contain tartrazine.

benecid may be used for this purpose.

EFFECTS ON DIAGNOSTIC TESTS

Aminoglycoside levels: falsely decreased concentrations.
Urine glucose tests that use copper sulfate (Benedict's reagent or Clinitest): false-positive results. Use glucose determinations with glucose enzymatic methods (Clinistix or Tes-Tape).

NURSING CONSIDERATIONS

Besides those related universally to drug therapy, (see "How to use this book"), consider the following specific recommendations:

Assessment

- Obtain a baseline assessment of patient's infection before ampicillin therapy.
- Be alert for adverse reactions and drug interactions throughout therapy.
- Evaluate the patient's and family's knowledge about ampicillin therapy.

Nursing Diagnoses

- High risk for injury related to ineffectiveness of ampicillin to eradicate the infection.
- High risk for fluid volume deficit related to ampicillin-induced adverse GI reactions.
- Knowledge deficit related to ampicillin therapy.

Planning and Implementation

Preparation and Administration

- Obtain specimen for culture and sensitivity tests before first dose. Therapy may begin pending test results.
- Before first dose, ask the patient about previous allergic reactions to this drug or other penicillins. However, a negative history of penicillin allergy does not guarantee future safety.
- Give ampicillin at least 1 hour before bacteriostatic antibiotics.
- Expect to reduce dosage of ampicillin for a patient with reduced renal function.
- In pediatric meningitis, may be given concurrently with parenteral chloramphenicol for 24 hours pending results of cultures.
- ***P.O. use:*** Drug may cause GI disturbances. Because food may interfere with absorption, give 1 to 2 hours before meals or 2 to 3 hours after.
- ***I.V. use:*** Do not add or mix other drugs with I.V. infusions; they may be chemically and physically incompatible. If other drugs must be given I.V., temporarily stop infusion.
- Infuse intermittently (over 30 minutes) to prevent vein irritation.
- Mix with dextrose 5% in water or a sodium chloride solution. Initial dilution in vial is stable for 1 hour. Follow manufacturer's directions for stability after further dilution for I.V. infusion.

Monitoring

- Monitor effectiveness by regularly assessing for improvement of infection.
- Allergic reactions are the major adverse reactions to ampicillin, especially with large doses, parenteral administration, or prolonged therapy. Keep in mind that the previously nonallergic patient may become sensitized during therapy.
- Monitor hydration status if adverse GI reactions occur.

Supportive Care

- Discontinue the drug immediately if the patient develops signs of anaphylactic shock (rapidly developing dyspnea and hypotension). Notify the doctor and prepare to administer immediate treatment, such as epinephrine, corticosteroids, antihistamines, and other resuscitative measures as indicated.
- Change I.V. infusion site every 48 hours.
- Obtain an order for an antiemetic or antidiarrheal agent as needed. If GI reactions are severe, expect to dis-

continue the oral drug or replace it with a parenteral form.
• If the patient develops a rash, notify the doctor and expect to discontinue the drug.

Patient Teaching
• Advise the patient who becomes allergic to ampicillin to wear medical alert identification stating this information.
• Tell the patient to take drug exactly as prescribed and to complete the entire prescription even after he feels better.
• Tell the patient to call the doctor if rash, fever, or chills develop. A rash is the most common allergic reaction.
• Warn the patient never to use leftover ampicillin for a new illness or to share it with others.
• Advise the diabetic patient that drug may cause false-positive urine glucose determinations with copper sulfate tests (Clinitest); it does not affect glucose enzymatic tests (Clinistix, Tes-Tape).
• Tell the patient to take oral ampicillin 1 hour before or 2 hours after meals for best absorption.

Evaluation
In patients receiving ampicillin, appropriate evaluation statements may include:
• Patient is free of infection.
• Patient maintains adequate hydration throughout ampicillin therapy.
• Patient and family state an understanding of ampicillin therapy.

---

ampicillin sodium/sulbactam sodium
(am pi sill′ in)/(sul bak′ tam)
Unasyn

• *Classification:* antibiotic (aminopenicillin and beta-lacatamse inhibitor)
• *Pregnancy Risk Category:* C

HOW SUPPLIED
Injection: vials and piggyback vials containing 1.5 g (1 g ampicillin sodium with 500 mg sulbactam sodium) and 3 g (2 g ampicillin sodium with 1 g sulbactam sodium)

ACTION
Mechanism: Ampicillin inhibits cell wall synthesis during active multiplication. Sulbactam inactivates bacterial beta-lactamase, the enzyme that inactivates ampicillin and provides bacterial resistance to it.
Absorption: Both components are well absorbed after I.M. administration, but peak serum levels are higher after I.V. administration.
Distribution: Distributed into pleural, peritoneal and synovial fluids, lungs, prostate, liver, and gallbladder; also penetrate middle ear effusions, maxillary sinus and bronchial secretions, tonsils, and sputum. Ampicillin readily crosses the placenta; it is minimally protein-bound at 15% to 25%; sulbactam is about 38% bound.
Metabolism: Only 15% to 25% of both drugs is metabolized.
Excretion: Both components are excreted in the urine by renal tubular secretion and glomerular filtration; also excreted in breast milk. Half-life: Elimination half-life is 1 to 1½ hours; range is 10 to 24 hours in patients with severe renal impairment.
Onset, peak, duration: Peak plasma levels occur immediately after I.V. infusion and within 1 hour after I.M. injection.

INDICATIONS & DOSAGE
Intra-abdominal, gynecologic, and integumentary infections caused by susceptible strains of bacteria –
Adults: dosage expressed as total drug (each 1.5-g vial contains 1 g ampicillin sodium and 0.5 g sulbactam sodium): 1.5 to 3 g I.M. or I.V. q 6 hours. Maximum daily dose is 4 g

*Liquid form contains alcohol. **May contain tartrazine.

sulbactam (12 g of the combined drugs).

CONTRAINDICATIONS AND PRECAUTIONS

Contraindicated in patients with a history of hypersensitivity to any penicillin because this combination may cause a serious anaphylactoid reaction. Avoid use in patients with mononucleosis because they may develop a skin rash after treatment with ampicillin.

ADVERSE REACTIONS

Common reactions are in italics; life-threatening reactions are in bold italics.
CNS: fatigue, malaise, headache, chills.
CV: edema, erythema.
GI: diarrhea, nausea, vomiting, flatulence, abdominal distention.
GU: dysuria, urine retention.
Local: pain at injection site, thrombophlebitis.
Other: rash, itching, candidiasis, ***anaphylaxis.***

INTERACTIONS

Allopurinol: increased incidence of skin rash.
Probenecid: increased levels of ampicillin. Probenecid may be used for this purpose.

EFFECTS ON DIAGNOSTIC TESTS

Estrogens in pregnant women: transient decreases in serum estradiol, conjugated estrone, conjugated estriol, and estriol glucuronide.
Urine glucose tests with copper sulfate (Benedict's reagent or Clinitest): false-positive results. Use glucose enzymatic methods (Clinistix or Tes-Tape).

NURSING CONSIDERATIONS

Besides those related universally to drug therapy, (see "How to use this book"), consider the following specific recommendations:

Assessment
- Obtain a baseline assessment of patient's infection before therapy.
- Be alert for adverse reactions and drug interactions throughout therapy.
- Evaluate the patient's and family's knowledge about ampicillin therapy.

Nursing Diagnoses
- High risk for injury related to ineffectiveness of ampicillin to eradicate the infection.
- High risk for fluid volume deficit related to ampicillin-induced adverse GI reactions.
- Knowledge deficit related to ampicillin therapy.

Planning and Implementation
Preparation and Administration
- Obtain specimen for culture and sensitivity tests before first dose. Therapy may begin pending test results.
- Before first dose, ask the patient about previous allergic reactions to this drug or other penicillins. However, a negative history of penicillin allergy does not guarantee future safety.
- Give ampicillin at least 1 hour before bacteriostatic antibiotics.
- Expect to reduce dosage in patients with impaired renal function.
- ***I.M. use:*** Administer drug deep I.M. Drug may be reconstituted with sterile water for injection, or 0.5% or 2% lidocaine hydrochloride injection. Add 3.2 ml to a 1.5-g vial (or 6.4 ml to a 3-g vial) to yield a concentration of 375 mg/ml.
- ***I.V. use:*** Do not add or mix other drugs with I.V. infusions, they may be chemically and physically incompatible. If other drugs must be given I.V. temporarily stop infusion. When preparing I.V. injection, reconstitute powder with any of the following diluents: 0.9% sodium chloride solution, dextrose 5% in water, lactated Ringer's injection, 1/6 M sodium lactate, dextrose 5% and 0.45% saline injection, and 10% invert sugar. Stability

varies with diluent, temperature, and concentration of solution. After reconstitution, allow vials to stand for a few minutes while foam dissipates to permit visual inspection of contents for particles.
• Give I.V. dose by slow injection (over 10 to 15 minutes), or dilute in 50 to 100 ml of a compatible diluent and infuse over 15 to 30 minutes. If permitted, give by intermittent I.V. infusion to prevent vein irritation.
Monitoring
• Monitor effectiveness by regularly assessing for improvement of infection.
• Allergic reactions are the major adverse reactions to ampicillin, especially with large doses, parenteral administration, or prolonged therapy. Keep in mind that the previously nonallergic patient may become sensitized during therapy.
• Monitor the patient's hydration status if adverse GI reactions occur.
• Monitor closely for bacterial and fungal superinfections during prolonged or high-dose therapy especially in elderly, debilitated, or immunosuppressed patients.
Supportive Care
• Discontinue the drug immediately if the patient develops signs of anaphylactic shock (rapidly developing dyspnea and hypotension). Notify the doctor and prepare to administer immediate treatment, such as epinephrine, corticosteroids, antihistamines, and other resuscitative measures as indicated.
• Obtain an order for an antiemetic or antidiarrheal agent as needed.
• If the patient develops a rash, notify the doctor and expect to discontinue the drug.
• Change I.V. infusion site every 48 hours.
Patient Teaching
• Advise the patient who becomes allergic to ampicillin to wear medical alert identification stating this information.
• Tell the patient to call the doctor if rash, fever, or chills develop. A rash is the most common allergic reaction.
• Advise the diabetic patient that drug may cause false-positive urine glucose determinations with copper sulfate tests (Clinitest); drug does not affect glucose enzymatic tests (Clinistix, Tes-Tape).
Evaluation
In patients receiving ampicillin, appropriate evaluation statements may include:
• Patient is free of infection.
• Patient maintains adequate hydration throughout ampicillin therapy.
• Patient and family state an understanding of ampicillin therapy.

amrinone lactate
(am´ ri none)
Inocor

• *Classification:* inotropic, vasodilator (bipyridine derivative)
• *Pregnancy Risk Category:* C

HOW SUPPLIED
Injection: 5 mg/ml

ACTION
Mechanism: Increases cardiac output by a direct inotropic effect and by causing vasodilation, reducing afterload. Produces inotropic action by increasing levels of cyclic adenosine monophosphate (cyclic AMP) in myocardial cells, resulting in increased calcium availability for muscle contraction. Produces vasodilation by directly relaxing vascular smooth muscle.
Absorption: Rapidly absorbed after oral administration, but is usually adminstered I.V.
Distribution: Volume of distribution is 1.2 liters/kg. Protein binding esti-

mated at 10% to 49%. Therapeutic steady-state serum levels range from 0.5 to 7 mcg/ml (ideal concentration: 3 mcg/ml).
Metabolism: In the liver to several metabolites of unknown activity.
Excretion: In normal patients, excreted in the urine. Half-life: Terminal elimination half-life of about 4 hours may be prolonged slightly in patients with CHF.
Onset, peak, duration: With I.V. administration, onset of action in 2 to 5 minutes; peak effects in about 10 minutes. Cardiovascular effects may persist for 1 to 2 hours.

INDICATIONS & DOSAGE

Short-term management of CHF–
Adults: initially, 0.75 mg/kg I.V. bolus over 2 to 3 minutes. Then begin maintenance infusion of 5 to 10 mcg/kg/minute. Additional bolus of 0.75 mg/kg may be given 30 minutes after start of therapy. Total daily dosage should not exceed 10 mg/kg.

CONTRAINDICATIONS & PRECAUTIONS

Contraindicated in patients with hypersensitivity to amrinone or sulfites (because sodium metabisulfite is used as a preservative). In patients with severe aortic or pulmonary valvular disease, amrinone should not be used in place of surgery. Use with caution in patients with hypertrophic subaortic stenosis because it may exacerbate outflow tract obstruction; in patients recovering from acute phase of myocardial infarction (in acute phase) because it may be arrhythmogenic; in patients with hepatic disease because it may be hepatotoxic; and in patients with renal impairment, because of the potential for drug accumulation.

ADVERSE REACTIONS

Common reactions are in italics; life-threatening reactions are in bold italics.
Blood: *thrombocytopenia* (dose dependent).
CV: ***arrhythmias,*** hypotension.
GI: nausea, vomiting, cramps, dyspepsia, diarrhea.
Hepatic: elevated enzymes, rarely hepatotoxicity.
Local: burning at site of injection.
Other: hypersensitivity (pericarditis, ascites, myositis vasculitis, pleuritis).

INTERACTIONS

Digitalis glycosides: Enhanced inotropic effect. Beneficial drug interaction.
Disopyramide: excessive hypotension. Don't administer concurrently.

EFFECTS ON DIAGNOSTIC TESTS

Hepatic enzymes: increased levels.
Serum potassium: decreased levels.

NURSING CONSIDERATIONS

Besides those related universally to drug therapy (see "How to use this book"), consider the following specific recommendations:

Assessment
- Obtain a baseline assessment of degree of CHF present before amrinone therapy.
- Be alert for adverse reactions and drug interactions throughout therapy.
- Evaluate the patient's and family's knowledge about amrinone therapy.

Nursing Diagnoses
- Fluid volume excess related to ineffectiveness of amrinone to relieve CHF.
- Decreased cardiac output related to amrinone-induced arrhythmias.
- Knowledge deficit related to amrinone.

Planning and Implementation
Preparation and Administration
- Be aware that dosage should be based on clinical response, including assessment of pulmonary artery pressures and cardiac output.
- ***I.V. use:*** Administer undiluted or dilute in 0.45% or 0.9% sodium chlo-

ride to a concentration of 1 to 3 mg/ml. Don't dilute with solutions containing dextrose because a slow chemical reaction occurs over 24 hours. (However amrinone can be injected into running dextrose infusions through a Y connector or directly into the tubing.) Diluted solution remains stable for 24 hours. When administering as direct injection give over 2 to 3 minutes into vein or I.V. tubing containing a free-flowing, compatible solution. Avoid extravasation. After injection, flush tubing and cannula with 0.9% sodium chloride. When administering as a continuous infusion may be piggybacked into line close to insertion site containing dextrose 5% in water. Infusion rate should be controlled by pump at 5 to 10 mcg/kg/minute.
• Don't mix other drug into amrinone solution. For example, furosemide will form a precipitate with amrinone solutions.

Monitoring
• Monitor effectiveness by frequently assessing cardiopulmonary status for improvement, including assessment of patient's pulmonary artery pressures and cardiac output.
• Monitor patient's blood pressure and heart rate throughout the infusion.
• Monitor platelet count. Platelet count below 150,000/mm³ usually requires a decreased dosage.
• Monitor ECG for arrhythmias.

Supportive Care
• Slow or stop infusion if patient's blood pressure falls and notify the doctor.
• Alert doctor if an arrhythmia develops and be prepared to treat with appropriate supportive therapy.
• Obtain an order for an antiemetic or antidiarrheal agent as needed.

Patient Teaching
• Warn the patient that burning may occur at the site of injection.

Evaluation
In patients receiving amrinone, appropriate evaluation statements may include:
• Patient's breath sounds are clear; heart rate is normal, and no evidence of edema is present.
• Patient's ECG exhibits no new arrhythmias.
• Patient and family state an understanding of amrinone therapy.

amyl nitrite
(am´ il nye´ trite)

• *Classification:* vasodilator, cyanide poisoning adjunct (nitrate)
• *Pregnancy Risk Category:* C

HOW SUPPLIED
Ampules (crushable): 0.18 ml, 0.3 ml

ACTION
Mechanism: Reduces cardiac oxygen demand by decreasing left ventricular end-diastolic pressure (preload) and systemic vascular resistance (afterload). Increases blood flow through the collateral coronary vessels. Converts hemoglobin to methemoglobin (which binds cyanide) to treat cyanide poisoning.
Absorption: Inhaled amyl nitrite is absorbed readily through the respiratory tract.
Metabolism: By the liver to form inorganic nitrites, which are much less potent vasodilators than the parent drug.
Excretion: One-third of the inhaled dose is excreted in urine. Half-life: Unknown.
Onset, peak, duration: Action begins in 30 seconds and lasts 3 to 5 minutes.

INDICATIONS & DOSAGE

Relief of angina pectoris; relief of renal or gallbladder colic–
Adults and children: 0.2 to 0.3 ml by inhalation (one glass ampule inhaler), p.r.n.
Antidote for cyanide poisoning–
0.2 or 0.3 ml by inhalation for 30 to 60 seconds q 5 minutes until conscious.

CONTRAINDICATIONS & PRECAUTIONS

Contraindicated in patients with severe anemia or hypersensitivity, head trauma, or cerebral hemorrhage because it dilates the meningeal vessels. Use cautiously in patients with hypotension or glaucoma. Because it reduces maternal blood pressure and blood flow to the placenta, use in pregnancy could harm the fetus.

ADVERSE REACTIONS

Common reactions are in italics; life-threatening reactions are in bold italics.
Blood: methemoglobinemia.
CNS: *headache, sometimes with throbbing;* dizziness; weakness.
CV: *orthostatic hypotension, tachycardia,* flushing, palpitations, fainting.
GI: nausea, vomiting.
Skin: cutaneous vasodilation.
Other: hypersensitivity.

INTERACTIONS

None significant.

EFFECTS ON DIAGNOSTIC TESTS

Serum cholesterol: falsely decreased levels with Zlatkis-Zak color reaction.

NURSING CONSIDERATIONS

Besides those related universally to drug therapy (see "How to use this book"), consider the following specific recommendations:

Assessment
- Obtain a baseline assessment of the patient's pain as related to underlying condition before drug therapy.
- Be alert for adverse reactions and drug interactions throughout therapy.
- Evaluate the patient's and family's knowledge about amyl nitrite therapy.

Nursing Diagnoses
- Pain related to the patient's underlying condition.
- High risk for injury related to amyl nitrite–induced drug reaction.
- Knowledge deficit related to amyl nitrite therapy.

Planning and Implementation
Preparation and Administration
- Wrap ampule in cloth and crush. Hold near the patient's nose and mouth so the vapor is inhaled.
- Extinguish all cigarettes before use, or ampule may ignite.
- Drug is effective within 30 seconds but has a short duration of action (3 to 5 minutes).
- Drug is often abused for alleged aphrodisiac benefits. Street names include "Amy" and "Poppers."
- Drug is rarely used for treatment of angina because it is expensive, inconvenient, and frequently causes adverse reactions.
- Sometimes used to induce changes in heart murmurs. Patient inhales the drug until reflex tachycardia is induced, then discontinues.
- Store drug away from light.

Monitoring
- Watch for orthostatic hypotension. Have the patient sit and avoid rapid position changes while inhaling the drug.
- Monitor the patient for drug-induced headache.

Supportive Care
- Make sure the patient does not have any burning cigarettes nearby while inhaling the vapor. Ampule may ignite.
- If orthostatic hypotension develops, have the patient keep his head low,

take deep breaths, and move his extremities to relieve dizziness, syncope, or weakness.
• Obtain an order for a mild analgesic if patient experiences a headache.

Patient Teaching
• Instruct the patient to wrap the ampule in cloth to crush and then hold near his nose and mouth to inhale the vapor.
• Teach patient to sit and avoid any position changes while inhaling the drug to prevent orthostatic hypotension.
• Tell the patient to take a mild analgesic for drug-induced headache.

Evaluation
In patients receiving amyl nitrite, appropriate evaluation statements may include:
• Patient's pain is relieved.
• No injury occurs while patient is on amyl nitrite therapy.
• Patient and family state an understanding of amyl nitrite therapy.

PHARMACOLOGIC CLASS

angiotensin-converting enzyme inhibitors
captopril
enalapril maleate
fosinopril sodium
lisinopril
ramipril

OVERVIEW
Angiotensin-converting enzyme (ACE) inhibitors are relatively new therapeutic agents used to manage hypertension and congestive heart failure.

ACE inhibitors prevent the conversion of angiotensin I to angiotensin II, a potent vasoconstrictor. Besides decreasing vasoconstriction, and thus reducing peripheral arterial resistance, inhibition of angiotensin II decreases adrenocortical secretion of aldosterone. This results in decreased sodium and water retention and extracellular fluid volume.

CLINICAL INDICATIONS AND ACTIONS
Hypertension, CHF
ACE inhibitors are used to treat hypertension; their antihypertensive effects are secondary to decreased sodium and water retention.

Captopril and enalapril are used to manage congestive heart failure; they decrease systemic vascular resistance (afterload) and pulmonary capillary wedge pressure (preload). ACE inhibitors may also increase cardiac output.

OVERVIEW OF ADVERSE REACTIONS
The most common adverse effects of therapeutic doses of ACE inhibitors are headache, fatigue, tachycardia, dysgeusia, proteinuria, hyperkalemia, rash, cough, and angioedema of the face and extremities. Severe hypotension usually occurs at toxic drug levels. ACE inhibitors should be used cautiously in patients with impaired renal function or serious autoimmune disease, and in patients taking other drugs known to depress white blood cell (WBC) count or immune response. Proteinuria and nephrotic syndrome may occur; reevaluate therapy if proteinuria is persistent or exceeds 1 g/day.

REPRESENTATIVE COMBINATIONS
Captopril with hydrochlorothiazide: Capozide.
Enalapril with hydrochlorothiazide: Vaseretic.

anistreplase (anisoylated plasminogen-streptokinase activator complex; APSAC)

(an eye´ strep lase)
Eminase

- *Classification:* thrombolytic (enzyme)
- *Pregnancy Risk Category:* C

HOW SUPPLIED

Injection: 30 units/vial

ACTION

Mechanism: Anistreplase is derived from Lys-plasminogen and streptokinase. The active Lys-plasminogen-streptokinase activator complex is progressively formed in the bloodstream or within the thrombus. It converts plasminogen to plasmin, which initiates local fibrinolysis and dissolves the clot.
Distribution: Not fully characterized; the formation of plasmin from plasminogen takes place both in the bloodstream and within the thrombus.
Metabolism: Unknown; the active drug is spontaneously activated within the bloodstream.
Excretion: Half-life: In vitro half-life is about 2 hours. The half-life of fibrinolytic activity of the circulating anistreplase is 70 to 120 minutes.
Onset, peak, duration: Reperfusion occurs between 45 minutes and 2 hours after administration.

INDICATIONS & DOSAGE

Lysis of coronary artery thrombi following acute myocardial infarction–
Adults: 30 units I.V. over 2 to 5 minutes. Administer by direct injection.

CONTRAINDICATIONS & PRECAUTIONS

Contraindicated in patients with history of hypersensitivity to streptokinase; with confirmed or suspected dissecting or intracranial aneurysm, or both; arteriovenous malformation; active bleeding; brain tumor or neoplasm metastatic to CNS; history of cerebrovascular accident; recent thoracic, intracranial, or intraspinal surgery; recent trauma to CNS; or severe uncontrolled hypertension.

Use cautiously in patients with history of mild allergic reaction to anistreplase or streptokinase or in use of either drug within past 5 days to 6 months; recent streptococcal infection; childbirth within past 10 days; uncontrolled coagulation defects; subacute bacterial endocarditis; severe GI bleeding within past 10 days; history of GI ulcer or other lesion; hemorrhagic ophthalmic conditions; neurosurgical procedure within past 2 months; organ biopsy within past 10 days; mitral stenosis with atrial fibrillation; and acute pericarditis and in patients age 75 and older.

Observe patient closely for bleeding. Fibrin deposits are lysed wherever they exist because the drug promotes conversion of plasminogen to plasmin within or upon the thrombus or embolus as well as in circulating blood. Lysis of fibrin deposits responsible for homeostasis is also promoted.

ADVERSE REACTIONS

Common reactions are in italics; life-threatening reactions are in bold italics.
Blood: bleeding.
CNS: ***intracranial hemorrhage.***
CV: arrhythmias, conduction disorders, hypotension.
EENT: hemoptysis, gum/mouth hemorrhage.
GI: *bleeding.*
GU: hematuria.
Skin: hematomas, urticaria, itching, flushing, delayed (2 weeks after therapy) purpuric rash.
Local: bleeding at puncture sites.
Other: ***anaphylactoid reactions*** *(rare).*

INTERACTIONS

Heparin, oral anticoagulants, and drugs that alter platelet function (including aspirin and dipyridamole): may increase the risk of bleeding. Use together cautiously.

EFFECTS ON DIAGNOSTIC TESTS

Activated partial thromboplastin time, prothrombin time, and thrombin time: prolonged. Drug can cause degradation of fibrinogen in blood samples drawn for analysis; addition of aproteinuria or aminocaproic acid to the sample may reduce this effect.
Alpha$_2$-antiplasmin activity, Factor V activity, Factor VIII activity, fibrinogen activity, and plasminogen activity: decreased.
Fibrinogen- and fibrin-degradation products: increased concentrations.
Hematocrit and hemoglobin: moderate reductions.

NURSING CONSIDERATIONS

Besides those related universally to drug therapy (see "How to use this book"), consider the following specific recommendations:

Assessment

• Obtain a baseline assessment of ECG and vital signs before therapy.
• Be alert for adverse reactions and drug interactions throughout therapy.
• Evaluate the patient's and family's knowledge about anistreplase therapy.

Nursing Diagnoses

• Altered tissue perfusion related to the patient's underlying condition.
• High risk for injury related to the adverse effects of anistreplase.
• Knowledge deficit related to anistreplase therapy.

Planning and Implementation

Preparation and Administration

• Direct injection: Store the drug in the refrigerator at 36° F to 46° F (2° C to 8° C). Reconstitute by slowly adding 5 ml of sterile water for injection. Direct the stream at the side of the vial not the drug itself. Gently roll the vial to mix the dry powder and water. To avoid excess foaming, don't shake the vial. The reconstituted solution should be colorless to pale yellow. Inspect for particulate matter. Do not dilute reconstituted solution. Do not mix with other drugs. Discard the drug if not administered within 30 minutes after reconstitution. Inject the drug over 2 to 5 minutes into an I.V. line or vein. Heparin may be ordered for administration during or after infusion to prevent new clot formation. Anistreplase must be given within 6 hours after onset of symptoms.
• ***Intermittent or continuous infusion:*** Not recommended.

Monitoring

• Monitor effectiveness by carefully checking ECG and vital signs.
• Monitor the patient for reperfusion arrhythmias, including sinus bradycardia, accelerated idioventricular rhythm, ventricular tachycardia, or premature ventricular contractions. Have emergency treatment readily available.
• Monitor the patient for bleeding, which may occur internally or externally at puncture sites. Avoid I.M. injections, venipuncture, and arterial puncture during therapy because of increased risk of bleeding. If arterial puncture is necessary, select a compressible site (such as an arm) and apply pressure for 30 minutes afterward. Also use pressure dressings, sandbags, or ice packs on recent puncture sites to prevent bleeding.

Supportive Care

• Remember that although anistreplase is derived from human plasma, no cases of hepatitis or human immunodeficiency virus have been reported to date. The manufacturing process is designed to purify the plasma used in the preparation of the drug.
• Try to avoid turning and moving

the patient excessively during therapy.

Patient Teaching

• Teach the patient signs of internal bleeding (including hematemesis, hematuria, and black tarry stools). Tell him to report these immediately.

• Teach the patient dental care techniques to avoid excessive gum trauma.

Evaluation

In patients receiving anistreplase, appropriate evaluation statements may include:

• Patient's ECG and vital signs reflect improvement in cardiopulmonary perfusion.

• Patient has not experienced injury from excessive bleeding or arrhythmias related to the adverse effects of anistreplase.

• Patient and family state an understanding of anistreplase therapy.

PHARMACOLOGIC CLASS

antibiotic antineoplastics

bleomycin sulfate
dactinomycin
daunorubicin hydrochloride
doxorubicin hydrochloride
idarubicin
mitomycin
mitoxantrone
plicamycin
procarbazine hydrochloride
streptozocin

OVERVIEW

Although classified as antibiotics, these agents exert cytotoxic effects, ruling out their use as antimicrobial agents. These agents interfere with proliferation of malignant cells through several mechanisms. Their action may be cycle-phase nonspecific, cycle-phase specific, or both. Some even demonstrate activity resembling alkylating agents or antimetabolites; for example, streptozocin is considered an alkylating agent because of its therapeutic activity.

By binding to or complexing with DNA, antineoplastic antibiotics inhibit DNA and RNA synthesis.

CLINICAL INDICATIONS AND ACTIONS

Antibiotic antineoplastics are useful alone or in combination with other types of antineoplastics for treating various tumors. See individual agents for specific uses.

OVERVIEW OF ADVERSE REACTIONS

The most frequent adverse reactions include nausea, vomiting, diarrhea, fever, chills, sore throat, anxiety, confusion, flank or joint pain, swelling of feet or lower legs, loss of hair, redness or pain at injection site, bone marrow depression, and leukopenia.

REPRESENTATIVE COMBINATIONS

None.

PHARMACOLOGIC CLASS

anticholinergics

Belladonna alkaloids

atropine sulfate
belladonna leaf
hyoscyamine sulfate
levorotatory alkaloids of belladonna

Semisynthetic belladonna derivative

methscopolamine bromide

Synthetic quaternary anticholinergics

anisotropine methylbromide
clidinium bromide
hexocyclium methylsulfate
isopropamide iodide
mepenzolate bromide
methantheline bromide
oxyphenonium bromide
propantheline bromide

†Available in Canada only. ‡Available in Australia only. ◇Available OTC.

Tertiary synthetic (antispasmodic) derivatives
dicyclomine hydrochloride
oxyphencyclimine hydrochloride

Antiparkinsonism agents
benztropine mesylate
biperiden hydrochloride
biperiden lactate
glycopyrrolate
procyclidine hydrochloride
scopolamine
scopolamine hydrobromide
trihexyphenidyl hydrochloride

OVERVIEW

Belladonna alkaloids are naturally occurring anticholinergics that have been used for centuries. Many semisynthetic alkaloids and synthetic anticholinergic compounds are available; however, most offer few advantages over naturally occurring alkaloids.

Anticholinergics competitively antagonize the actions of acetylcholine and other cholinergic agonists within the parasympathetic nervous system. Lack of specificity for site of action increases the hazard of adverse effects in association with therapeutic effects.

Antispasmodics are structurally similar to anticholinergics; however, their anticholinergic activity usually occurs only at high doses. They are believed to directly relax smooth muscle.

CLINICAL INDICATIONS AND ACTIONS

Hypersecretory conditions
Many anticholinergics (anisotropine, atropine, belladonna leaf, clidinium, glycopyrrolate, hexocyclium, hyoscyamine, isopropamide, levorotatory alkaloids of belladonna, mepenzolate, and methantheline) are used therapeutically for their antisecretory properties; these properties derive from competitive blockade of cholinergic receptor sites, causing decreased gastric acid secretion, salivation, bronchial secretions, and sweating.

GI tract disorders
Some anticholinergics (atropine, belladonna leaf, glycopyrrolate, hexocyclium, hyoscyamine, isopropamide, levorotatory alkaloids of belladonna, mepenzolate, methantheline, and propantheline), as well as the antispasmodics dicyclomine and oxyphencyclimine, treat spasms and other GI tract disorders. These drugs competitively block acetylcholine's actions at cholinergic receptor sites. Antispasmodics presumably act by a nonspecific, direct spasmolytic action on smooth muscle. These agents are useful in treating peptic ulcer disease, pylorospasm, ileitis, and irritable bowel syndrome.

Sinus bradycardia
Atropine is used to treat sinus bradycardia caused by drugs, poisons, or sinus node dysfunction. It blocks normal vagal inhibition of the SA node and causes an increase in heart rate.

Dystonia and parkinsonism
Benztropine, biperiden, and procyclidine are used to treat acute dystonic reactions and drug-induced extrapyramidal adverse effects. They act centrally by blocking cholinergic receptor sites, balancing cholinergic activity.

Perioperative use
Atropine, glycopyrrolate, and hyoscyamine are used postoperatively with anticholinesterase agents to reverse nondepolarizing neuromuscular blockade. These agents block muscarinic effects of anticholinesterase agents by competitively blocking muscarinic receptor sites.

Atropine, glycopyrrolate, and scopolamine are used preoperatively to decrease secretions and block cardiac vagal reflexes. They diminish secretions by competitively inhibiting muscarinic receptor sites; they block cardiac vagal reflexes by preventing nor-

*Liquid form contains alcohol.

**May contain tartrazine.

mal vagal inhibition of the sinoatrial node.

Motion sickness

Scopolamine is effective in preventing nausea and vomiting associated with motion sickness. Its exact mechanism of action is unknown, but it is thought to affect neural pathways originating in the labyrinth of the ear.

OVERVIEW OF ADVERSE REACTIONS

Dry mouth, decreased sweating or anhidrosis, headache, mydriasis, blurred vision, cycloplegia, urinary hesitancy and retention, constipation, palpitations, and tachycardia most commonly occur with therapeutic doses and usually disappear once the drug is discontinued. Signs of drug toxicity include CNS signs resembling psychosis (disorientation, confusion, hallucinations, delusions, anxiety, agitation, and restlessness) and such peripheral effects as dilated, nonreactive pupils; blurred vision; hot, dry, flushed skin; dry mucous membranes; dysphagia; decreased or absent bowel sounds; urinary retention; hyperthermia; tachycardia; hypertension; and increased respiration.

REPRESENTATIVE COMBINATIONS

Atropine with meperidine: Atropine/Demerol injection; with scopolamine hydrobromide (hyoscine hydrobromide), hyoscyamine sulfate, and phenobarbital: Atrosed, Barbella, Barbeloid, Brobella-P.B., Belbutal, Bellaphen, Donnacin, Donnatal, Haponal, Hyatal, Hybephen, Kinesed, Nilspasm, Sedamine, Sedapar, Sedralex, Seds, Spasdel, Spasidon, Spasloids, Spasmolin, Spastolate, Stannitol; with scopolamine hydrobromide (hyoscine hydrobromide), hyoscyamine sulfate, kaolin, pectin, sodium benzoate, alcohol, and powdered opium: Donnagel PB; with scopolamine hydrobromide (hyoscine hydrobromide), hyoscyamine sulfate, and pentobarbital sodium: Eldonal; with hyoscyamine hydrobromide, scopolamine hydrobromide; acetaminophen, chlorpheniramine maleate, phenylephrine hydrochloride, and phenylpropanolamine: Koryza; with phenazopyridine, hyoscyamine, and scopolamine: Urogesic; with hyoscyamine sulfate, scopolamine hydrobromide (hyoscine hydrobromide) and butabarbital: Zemarine; with hyoscyamine, methenamine, phenyl salicylate, methylene blue, and benzoic acid: Urised.

Anisotropine methylbromide with phenobarbital: Valpin 50 PB.

Belladonna alkaloids with phenylpropanolamine, chlorpheniramine maleate, and pheniramine maleate: Decobel Lanacaps, Fitacol Stankaps; with ergotamine tartrate, caffeine, and phenacetin: Wigraine.

Belladonna Extract with ephedrine, boric acid, zinc oxide, bismuth subcarbonate, peruvian balsam, and cocoa butter in a suppository: Wyanoids; with amobarbital: Amobell; with phenobarbital: Belap; with phenobarbital and activated charcoal: Bellachar; with phenylephrine hydrochloride, pyrilamine maleate, and chlorpheniramine maleate: Bellafedrol; with butabarbital: Butibel.

Dicyclomine with phenobarbital: Bentyl with phenobarbital, Dicyclon No.2, Dicyclon No.3; with pyrilamine maleate and pyridoxine hydrochloride: Dicyclon-M.

---

antihemophilic factor (AHF)

(an tee hee moe fill´ ik)

Hemofil M, Koate-HS, Koate-HT, Monoclate

- *Classification:* antihemophilic (blood derivative)
- *Pregnancy Risk Category:* C

HOW SUPPLIED

Injection: vials, with diluent. Number of units on label.

A new porcine product is now available for patients with congenital hemophilia A who have antibodies to human factor VIII:C.

ACTION

Mechanism: Directly replaces deficient clotting factor.
Absorption: Must be given parenterally for systemic effect.
Distribution: Equilibrates intravascular and extravascular compartments; it does not readily cross placenta.
Metabolism: Rapidly cleared from plasma.
Excretion: Consumed during blood clotting. Half-life: Ranges from 4 to 24 hours (average 12 hours).

INDICATIONS & DOSAGE

Prophylaxis of spontaneous hemorrhage in patients with hemophilia A (factor VIII deficiency)–
Adults and children: dosage must be calculated using the formula:

$$\text{AHF required (IU)} = \text{body weight (kg)} \times \text{desired factor VIII increase (\% of normal)} \times 0.5$$

To prevent spontaneous hemorrhage, the desired level of factor VIII is 5% of normal. Following trauma and surgery, the desired level is 30%.
Treatment of bleeding in patients with hemophilia A (factor VIII deficiency)–
Adults and children: 15 to 25 units/kg by slow I.V. injection or I.V. infusion, followed by 8 to 15 units/kg q 8 to 12 hours for 3 to 4 days as necessary.

CONTRAINDICATIONS & PRECAUTIONS

Use cautiously in patients with hepatic disease and in neonates and infants because of susceptibility to hepatitis, which it may transmit.

The risk potential for viral transmission has been considerably reduced by heat treatment of all available AHF products, using a newer method similar to pasteurization.

Monoclonal antibody–derived AHF is contraindicated in patients with hypersensitivity to mouse protein.

ADVERSE REACTIONS

Common reactions are in italics; life-threatening reactions are in bold italics.
CNS: headache, paresthesias, clouding or loss of consciousness.
CV: tachycardia, hypotension, ***possible intravascular hemolysis in patients with blood type A, B, or AB.***
EENT: visual disturbances.
GI: nausea, vomiting.
Skin: erythema, *urticaria.*
Other: *chills, fever, backache, flushing,* chest constriction; ***hypersensitivity.***

INTERACTIONS

None significant.

EFFECTS ON DIAGNOSTIC TESTS

None reported.

NURSING CONSIDERATIONS

Besides those related universally to drug therapy (see "How to use this book"), consider the following specific recommendations:

Assessment

- Obtain a baseline assessment of patients underlying condition (include hematocrit, coagulation studies, and vital signs) before therapy.
- Be alert for adverse reactions and drug interactions throughout therapy.
- Evaluate the patient's and family's knowledge about factor VIII concentrate (AHF) therapy.

Nursing Diagnoses

- Altered tissue perfusion related to the patient's underlying condition.
- High risk for altered body tempera-

ture related to the adverse side effects of AHF.
• Knowledge deficit related to factor VIII concentrate (AHF) therapy.

Planning and Implementation

Preparation and Administration

• ***Direct injection:*** If refrigerated, warm concentrate to room temperature before use. Reconstitute with diluent, using sterile technique and following manufacturer's directions. Don't refrigerate reconstituted drug. Use within 3 hours. Using the filter needle provided, draw reconstituted drug into a plastic syringe (don't use glass; drug may adhere to ground glass surfaces). Inject about 5 ml/minute, using a 21G or 23G winged infusion set. To minimize adverse reactions, reduce rate if ordered. I.V. administration of 1 IU/kg increases plasma antihemophilic activity by about 2%.
• ***Continuous infusion:*** Using an infusion pump, complete administration within 3 hours of reconstitution. Intermittent infusion is not recommended.

Monitoring

• Monitor effectiveness by carefully checking vital signs.
• Monitor hematocrit in persons with type A, B, or AB blood who require large doses for a prolonged period. Hemolysis is possible. Factor VIII concentrate contains naturally occurring blood-group–specific antibodies. Alternative therapy includes administration of a concentrate that is blood-group specific, if circulating isohemagglutinins are positive. If RBC replacement is necessary, use compatible type O packed RBCs.
• Check liver function tests and screen for hepatitis if the patient has received multiple infusions.
• Monitor therapy carefully, especially if surgery is necessary. About 5% to 8% of patients develop inhibitors to factor VIII, requiring larger doses or alternative therapy.

Supportive Care

• Remember that factor VIII concentrate carries a risk of transmitting severe infection especially non-A, non-B hepatitis. Its benefits and risks should be weighed against those of using single donor cryoprecipitate.
• Keep in mind that new factor VIII concentrates use a monoclonal antibody purification method. Although still made from human blood products, these highly purified concentrates may further reduce the risk of viral transmission and protein exposure.

Patient Teaching

• Educate the patient about human immunodeficiency virus (HIV) and AIDS. Explain that the risk of infection with HIV is low in patients receiving heat-treated factor VIII concentrates from screened donors.
• Inform the patient about hepatitis and encourage immunization against hepatitis B in HBsAg-negative patients.

Evaluation

In patients receiving factor VIII concentrate (AHF), appropriate evaluation statements may include:
• Patient's vital signs and blood studies are within normal parameters, and he has not experienced continued bleeding.
• Patient's temperature has remained stable, and he has not experienced symptoms of anaphylaxis.
• Patient and family state an understanding of factor VIII concentrate (AHF) therapy.

PHARMACOLOGIC CLASS

antihistamines

astemizole
azatadine maleate
brompheniramine maleate
buclizine hydrochloride
carbinoxamine maleate
chlorpheniramine maleate
clemastine fumarate

cyclizine hydrochloride
cyclizine lactate
cyproheptadine hydrochloride
dexchlorpheniramine maleate
dimenhydrinate
diphenhydramine hydrochloride
meclizine hydrochloride
methdilazine
methdilazine hydrochloride
promethazine hydrochloride
pyrilamine maleate
terfenadine
trimeprazine tartrate
tripelennamine citrate
tripelennamine hydrochloride
triprolidine hydrochloride

OVERVIEW

Antihistamines, synthetically produced histamine H_1-receptor antagonists, were discovered in the late 1930s and proliferated rapidly during the next decade. They have many applications related specifically to chemical structure, their widespread use testifying to their versatility and relative safety.

Antihistamines are structurally related chemicals that compete with histamine for histamine H_1-receptor sites on the smooth muscle of the bronchi, GI tract, uterus, and large blood vessels, binding to the cellular receptors and preventing access and subsequent activity of histamine. They do not directly alter histamine or prevent its release.

CLINICAL INDICATIONS AND ACTIONS

Allergy

Most antihistamines (azatadine, brompheniramine, carbinoxamine, chlorpheniramine, clemastine, cyproheptadine, dexchlorpheniramine, diphenhydramine, promethazine, terfenadine, tripelennamine, and triprolidine) are used to treat allergic symptoms, such as rhinitis and urticaria. By preventing access of histamine to H_1-receptor sites, they suppress histamine-induced allergic symptoms.

Pruritus

Cyproheptadine, hydroxyzine, methdilazine, tripelennamine, and trimeprazine are used systemically. It is believed that these drugs counteract histamine-induced pruritus by a combination of peripheral effects on nerve endings and local anesthetic and sedative activity.

Tripelennamine and diphenhydramine are used topically to relieve itching associated with minor skin irritation. Structurally related to local anesthetics, these compounds prevent initiation and transmission of nerve impulses.

Vertigo; nausea and vomiting

Buclizine, cyclizine, dimenhydrinate, and meclizine are used only as antiemetic and antivertigo agents; their antihistaminic activity has not been evaluated. Diphenhydramine and promethazine are used as antiallergic and antivertigo agents and as antiemetics and antinauseants. Although the mechanisms are not fully understood, antiemetic and antivertigo effects probably result from central antimuscarinic activity.

Sedation

Diphenhydramine and promethazine are used for their sedative action; the mechanism of antihistamine-induced CNS depression is unknown.

Suppression of cough

Diphenhydramine syrup is used as an antitussive. The cough reflex is suppressed by a direct effect on the medullary cough center.

Dyskinesia

The central antimuscarinic action of diphenhydramine reduces drug-induced dyskinesia and parkinsonism via inhibition of acetylcholine (anticholinergic effect).

*Liquid form contains alcohol. **May contain tartrazine.

OVERVIEW OF ADVERSE REACTIONS

At therapeutic dosage levels, all antihistamines except astemizole and terfenadine are likely to cause drowsiness and impaired motor function during initial therapy. Also, their anticholinergic action usually causes dry mouth and throat, blurred vision, and constipation. Antihistamines that are also phenothiazines, such as promethazine, may cause other adverse effects, including cholestatic jaundice (thought to be a hypersensitivity reaction) and may predispose patients to photosensitivity; patients taking such drugs should avoid prolonged exposure to sunlight.

Toxic doses elicit a combination of CNS depression and excitation as well as atropine-like symptoms, including sedation, reduced mental alertness, apnea, cardiovascular collapse, hallucinations, tremors, convulsions, dry mouth, flushed skin, and fixed, dilated pupils. Toxic effects reverse when medication is discontinued. Used appropriately, in correct dosages, antihistamines are safe for prolonged use.

REPRESENTATIVE COMBINATIONS

Carbinoxamine maleate with acetaminophen: Clistin-D; with ammonium chloride: Clistin Expectorant; with pseudoephedrine and dextromethorphan: Baydec DM Drops, Carbodec DM, Pseudocar DM, Rondec-DM, Tussafed; with pseudoephedrine hydrochloride: Rondec, Rondec-TR; with pseudoephedrine and guaifenesin: Brexin.

Chlorpheniramine with atropine: Histunex; with phenylephrine and phenylpropanolamine: Naldecon; with phenylephrine, analgesics, and vitamin C: Corico; with dextromethorphan: "Vicks Formula 44" Cough Mixture; with dextromethorphan and acetaminophen: Remcol-C; with codeine and guaifenesin: Tussar-2 Cough, Tussar SF; with acetaminophen: Remcol-C; with pseudoephedrine and dextromethorphan: Cremacoat, Histolet DM, Novahistine, Pediacare, Rhinosyn DM; with pseudoephedrine, dextromethorphan, and acetaminophen: Co-Apap, Contac Severe Cold Formula, CoTylenol, Dristan Ultra Colds Formula; with phenylpropanolamine: Contac 12-hour Caplets, Oragest, Ornade, Resaid S.R., Triaminic-12, Duravent, Rta-Tuss II.

Cyclizine with ergotamine tartrate and caffeine: Migral.

Dexchlorpheniramine maleate with pseudoephedrine sulfate: Anafed, Anamine, Brexin L.A., Chlorafed, Chlor-Trimeton, Codimal-L.A., Co-Pyronil, Deconamine, Fedahist, Histalet, Isoclor, Novafed A Novahistex*, Pseudo-Hist, Sudafed Plus.

Diphenhydramine with codeine and ammonium chloride: Benylin with Codeine*, Calmylin with Codeine*; with dextromethorphan and ammonium chloride: Benlin-DM*; with pseudoephedrine: Benadryl Decongestant, Benylin D.

Promethazine with codeine: Phenergan with codeine; with dextromethorphan: Phenergan with Dextromethorphan; with phenylephrine: My-K, Phenergan VC; with phenylephrine and codeine: Phenergan VC with codeine; with pseudoephedrine: Phenergan-D.

Pyrilamine maleate with codeine and terpin hydrate: Tricodene; with phenylephrine and codeine; Codimal; with phenylephrine and dextromethorphan: Codimal DM; with phenylephrine, dextromethorphan, and acetaminophen: Robitussin Night Relief Colds Formula; with phenylephrine and hydrocodone: Codimal; with phenylephrine, hydrocodone, and ammonium chloride: Hycomine*, Hycomine-S Pediatric*; with phenylpropanolamine, dextromethorphan, and sodium salicylate: Kolephrin NN Liquid.

Triprolidine with pseudoephedrine and codeine: Actifed with Codeine Cough, CoActifed*, Pseudodine C Cough; with pseudoephedrine: Actacin, Actagen, Actamine, Actifed, Actahist, Allerfrin, Norafed, Pseudodine, Rofed, Tagafed, Triacin, Triafed, Trifed, Tri-fed, Trilitron, Triphed, Triprodrine, Triposed.

PHARMACOLOGIC CLASS

antimetabolites

cytarabine
floxuridine
fluorouracil
hydroxyurea
mercaptopurine
methotrexate
thioguanine
trimetrexate

OVERVIEW

Antimetabolites are structural analogs of normally occurring metabolites and can be divided into three subcategories: purine analogs, pyrimidine analogs, and folinic acid analogs. Most of these agents interrupt cell reproduction at a specific phase of the cell cycle and are most effective against tumors that have high numbers/proportion of cells dividing at any one time.

The mechanism of action of each subcategory differs according to function with which the drug interferes. The purine analogs are incorporated into DNA and RNA, interfering with nucleic acid synthesis (via miscoding) and replication. Pyrimidine analogs interfere with the biosynthesis of uridine and thymine. Folinic acid analogs prevent conversion of dehydrofolate to tetrahydrofolate.

Antimetabolites may slow the entry of some cells into the "S" phase, thus sparing these cells from the drug's cytotoxic effects. As most antimetabolites act in the "S" phase of the cell cycle, this slowing effect may limit their cytotoxicity.

CLINICAL INDICATIONS AND ACTIONS

Antimetabolites are useful alone or in combination with other types of antineoplastic agents for treating various tumors. See individual agents for specific uses.

OVERVIEW OF ADVERSE REACTIONS

The most frequent adverse effects include nausea, vomiting, diarrhea, fever, chills, possible loss of hair, flank or joint pain, redness or pain at injection site, anxiety, bone marrow depression, leukopenia, and swelling of feet or lower legs.

REPRESENTATIVE COMBINATIONS

None.

asparaginase (L-asparaginase)

(a spare´ a gi nase)
Elspar, Kidrolase†

- *Classification:* antineoplastic (enzyme, cell cycle-phase specific, G_1 phase)
- *Pregnancy Risk Category:* C

HOW SUPPLIED

Injection: 10,000-IU vials

ACTION

Mechanism: An enzyme derived from *Escherichia coli* that metabolizes the amino acid asparagine to aspartic acid and ammonia. Asparagine is needed for DNA and protein synthesis. Certain leukemic cells, especially in patients with acute lymphocytic leukemia (ALL), cannot synthesize asparagine. This leads to death of the leukemic cell.
Absorption: Not absorbed across the

GI tract after oral administration; therefore the drug must be given I.V. or I.M.
Distribution: A large molecule that doesn't diffuse out of capillaries, asparaginase distributes primarily within the intravascular space, with detectable concentrations in the thoracic and cervical lymph. Minimal amounts of the drug cross the blood-brain barrier.
Metabolism: Hepatic sequestration by the reticuloendothelial system may occur.
Excretion: Only trace amounts of the drug appear in the urine. Half-life: Ranges from 8 to 30 hours. Not affected by dose, sex, age, or hepatic or renal function.
Onset, peak, duration: In some patients, plasma levels of the drug plateau after several days of therapy and persist for up to 22 days following discontinuation of the drug.

INDICATIONS & DOSAGE

Acute lymphocytic leukemia (when used along with other drugs) –
Adults and children: 1,000 IU/kg I.V. daily for 10 days, injected over 30 minutes or by slow I.V. push; or 6,000 IU/m^2 I.M. at intervals specified in protocol.
Sole induction agent for acute lymphocytic leukemia –
200 IU/kg I.V. daily for 28 days.

CONTRAINDICATIONS & PRECAUTIONS

Contraindicated in patients with a history of anaphylactoid reactions to the drug or in patients with pancreatitis or a history of pancreatitis. Use cautiously in patients with impaired liver function, infections, or recent therapy with antineoplastics or radiation because of risk of increased adverse effects.

ADVERSE REACTIONS

Common reactions are in italics; life-threatening reactions are in bold italics.
Blood: ***hypofibrinogenemia*** and depression of other clotting factors, thrombocytopenia, *leukopenia,* depression of serum albumin.
CNS: lethargy, somnolence.
GI: *vomiting (may last up to 24 hours), anorexia, nausea,* cramps, weight loss.
GU: *azotemia,* renal failure, uric acid nephropathy, glycosuria, polyuria.
Hepatic: elevated AST (SGOT), ALT (SGPT), *hepatotoxicity.*
Metabolic: elevated alkaline phosphatase and bilirubin (direct and indirect); increase or decrease in total lipids; *hyperglycemia; increased blood ammonia.*
Skin: *rash, urticaria.*
Other: ***hemorrhagic pancreatitis*** *and* ***anaphylaxis (relatively common),*** chills, fever.

INTERACTIONS

Methotrexate: decreased methotrexate effectiveness.
Vincristine, prednisone: concurrent use is associated with increased toxicity.

EFFECTS ON DIAGNOSTIC TESTS

Thyroid function tests: altered results by decreasing concentrations of serum thyroxine-binding globulin.

NURSING CONSIDERATIONS

Besides those related universally to drug therapy (see "How to use this book"), consider the following specific recommendations:
Assessment
• Obtain a baseline assessment of the patient's underlying condition before therapy.
• Be alert for adverse reactions and drug interactions throughout therapy.
• Evaluate the patient's and family's knowledge about asparaginase therapy.

Nursing Diagnoses
- High risk for fluid volume deficit related to drug-induced adverse reactions.
- High risk for infection related to drug-induced adverse reactions.
- Knowledge deficit related to asparaginase therapy.

Planning and Implementation
Preparation and Administration
- ***I.M. use:*** Limit dose at single injection site to 2 ml. Avoid all I.M. injections when the platelet count is less than 100,000/mm³.
- ***I.V. use:*** Exercise caution when preparing and administering this drug to avoid mutagenic, teratogenic, and carcinogenic risks. Use a biological containment cabinet, use gloves and mask, and avoid contaminating work surfaces. Give over 30 minutes through a running solution of dextrose 5% in water or normal saline solution.
- Expect to administer lower doses in renal, hepatic, or hematopoietic impairment.
- Antiemetics may be given preceding or during infusion of this drug to decrease severe nausea and vomiting. Increased fluids may also be administered to decrease these effects.
- Reconstitute with 2 to 5 cc sterile water for injection or sterile saline.
- Reconstituted solution is stable for 6 hours at room temperature or 24 hour refrigerated. Optimally, use within 8 hours of preparation. Refrigerate unopened dry powder.
- Don't shake vial; may cause loss of potency. Don't use cloudy solution.
- Administer only under the supervision of a doctor who is experienced with the use of chemotherapeutic agents.

Monitoring
- Obtain baseline CBC, clotting factors, bone marrow, serum albumin, hepatic function, renal function, uric acid, alkaline phosphatase, bilirubin, glucose, amylase and ammonia levels before initiating therapy.
- Monitor effectiveness by noting the results of follow-up diagnostic tests and overall physical status; and by regularly checking tumor size and rate of growth through appropriate studies.
- Monitor for signs of bleeding (hematuria, ecchymosis, petechiae, epistaxis, melena).
- Monitor for signs of infection (temperature elevation, sore throat, malaise). Take temperature daily.
- Monitor serum uric acid level.
- Monitor blood and urine glucose before and during therapy. Watch for signs of hyperglycemia, such as glycosuria and polyuria.
- Monitor CBC, bone marrow function, hepatic and renal function.
- Monitor frequent serum amylase to watch for impending pancreatitis. Drug should be discontinued if levels rise.
- Monitor vital signs frequently during I.V. infusion of this drug.
- Monitor intake and output during drug therapy.

Supportive Care
- Anticoagulants and aspirin products should be used with extreme caution.
- Provide the patient with fluids since nausea and vomiting occur in almost all patients.
- Increase the patients fluid intake to prevent uric acid nephropathy which can result from tumor lysis.
- Be prepared to administer, as ordered, allopurinol to prevent hyperuricemia with resulting uric acid nephropathy. Adequate hydration is needed with administration of allopurinol.
- Be prepared to administer epinephrine, corticosteroids, or antihistamines, as ordered, to treat anaphalactoid reactions. Response is usually immediate with treatment.
- Know that patients who are allergic to this drug may be able to tolerate

Erwinia asparaginase, available from the National Cancer Institute.
• Know that therapeutic effects are often accompanied by toxicity.
Patient Teaching
• Warn patients to watch for signs of infection (sore throat, fever, fatigue), and for signs of bleeding (easy bruising, nosebleeds, bleeding gums). Suggest that they take their temperature daily.
• Teach patient to avoid the use of all OTC products containing aspirin.
• Encourage the patient to increase his fluid intake daily and to void as often as possible.
Evaluation
In patients receiving asparaginase, appropriate evaluation statements may include:
• Patient does not develop fluid volume loss.
• Patient does not develop infection.
• Patient and family state an understanding of asparaginase therapy.

---

aspirin (acetylsalicylic acid)

(as´ pir in)
Ancasal† ◇, Arthrinol† ◇, Artria SR ◇, ASA ◇, ASA Enseals ◇, Aspergum ◇, Aspro‡, Astrin† ◇, Bayer Aspirin ◇, Bex‡, Coryphen† ◇, Easprin ◇, Ecotrin ◇, Empirin ◇, Entrophen† ◇, Measurin ◇, Norwich Aspirin ◇, Novasen† ◇, Riphen-10† ◇, Sal-Adult† ◇, Sal-Infant† ◇, Solprin‡, Supasa† ◇, Triaphen-10† ◇, Vincent's Powders‡, Winsprin Capsules‡, ZORprin ◇

• *Classification:* nonnarcotic analgesic, antipyretic, anti-inflammatory, antiplatelet agent (salicylate)
• *Pregnancy Risk Category:* C (D in 3rd trimester)

HOW SUPPLIED

Tablets ◇*:* 65 mg, 75 mg, 81 mg, 300 mg, 325 mg, 500 mg, 600 mg, 650 mg
Tablets (chewable): 81 mg ◇
Tablets (enteric-coated): 325 mg ◇, 500 mg ◇, 650 mg ◇, 975 mg
Tablets (extended-release): 800 mg
Tablets (timed-release): 650 mg ◇
Capsules: 325 mg ◇, 500 mg ◇
Powder: 500 mg
Chewing gum: 227.5 mg ◇
Suppositories: 60 to 120 mg ◇

ACTION

Mechanism: Produces antipyretic effects by an ill-defined effect on the hypothalamus. Produces analgesia by an unknown central action and by blocking generation of pain impulses in the periphery. Peripheral action may result from anti-inflammatory effects that involve inhibition of prostaglandin synthesis.
Absorption: Rapidly and completely absorbed from the GI tract. Therapeutic blood salicylate concentrations for analgesia and anti-inflammatory effect are 15 to 50 mg/100 ml.
Distribution: Widely distributed into most body tissues and fluids. Protein-binding to albumin is concentration dependent, ranges from 75% to 90%, and decreases as serum concentration increases; severe toxic effects may occur at serum concentrations over 400 mcg/ml.
Metabolism: Hydrolyzed partially in the GI tract to salicylic acid with almost complete metabolism in the liver.
Excretion: In urine as salicylate and its metabolites. Half-life: Ranges from 15 to 20 minutes.
Onset, peak, duration: With immediate-release tablets, onset is less than 1 hour; enteric-coated and sustained-action forms are variable. Peak levels occur in 45 minutes with regular release tablets, about 4 hours with extended-release tablets, 8 to 14

hours with enteric-coated tablets, and about 4 hours with suppositories.

INDICATIONS & DOSAGE

Adults: *Arthritis*—2.6 to 5.4 g P.O. daily in divided doses.
Mild pain or fever—325 to 650 mg P.O. or rectally q 4 hours, p.r.n.
Thromboembolic disorders—325 to 650 mg P.O. daily or b.i.d.
Transient ischemic attacks in men—650 mg P.O. b.i.d. or 325 mg q.i.d.
To reduce the risk of heart attack in patients with previous myocardial infarction or unstable angina—325 mg P.O. once daily.
Children: *Arthritis*—90 to 130 mg/kg P.O. daily divided q 4 to 6 hours.
Fever—40 to 80 mg/kg P.O. or rectally daily divided q 6 hours, p.r.n.
Mild pain—65 to 100 mg/kg P.O. or rectally daily divided q 4 to 6 hours, p.r.n.

CONTRAINDICATIONS & PRECAUTIONS

Contraindicated in patients with hypersensitivity to aspirin or other nonsteroidal anti-inflammatory drugs (NSAIDs). Aspirin-induced bronchospasm is commonly associated with asthma, nasal polyps, and chronic urticaria. Patients sensitive to yellow tartrazine dye should avoid aspirin. Children or teenagers who have chicken pox or flu symptoms should avoid aspirin and salicylates because they have been associated with Reye's syndrome, a rare but life-threatening condition. Also contraindicated in patients with GI ulcer or GI bleeding because the drug's irritant effects may worsen these conditions. Patients should avoid aspirin during pregnancy, especially during the third trimester, because of potential adverse maternal and fetal effects.

Use cautiously in patients with hypoprothrombinemia, vitamin K deficiency, bleeding disorders, renal impairment, or liver disease because the drug may cause bleeding.

ADVERSE REACTIONS

Common reactions are in italics; life-threatening reactions are in bold italics.
Blood: *prolonged bleeding time.*
EENT: *tinnitus and hearing loss.*
GI: *nausea, vomiting, GI distress, occult bleeding.*
Hepatic: abnormal liver function studies, hepatitis.
Skin: *rash,* bruising.
Other: ***hypersensitivity manifested by anaphylaxis and/or asthma.***

INTERACTIONS

Ammonium chloride (and other urine acidifiers): increased blood levels of aspirin products. Monitor for aspirin toxicity.
Antacids in high doses (and other urine alkalinizers): decreased levels of aspirin products. Monitor for decreased aspirin effect.
Corticosteroids: enhance salicylate elimination. Monitor for decreased salicylate effect.
Oral anticoagulants, heparin: increased risk of bleeding. Avoid using together if possible.
Oral hypoglycemic agents: increased hypoglycemic effect.

EFFECTS ON DIAGNOSTIC TESTS

Bleeding time: prolonged.
Serum uric acid: falsely increased levels.
Urine acetoacetic acid (Gerhardt's test): interference.
Urine glucose analysis: interference with Clinistix, Tes-Tape, Clinitest, and Benedict's solution.
Urine 5-HIAA and VMA tests: interference.

NURSING CONSIDERATIONS

Besides those related universally to drug therapy (see "How to use this book"), consider the following specific recommendations:

*Liquid form contains alcohol. **May contain tartrazine.

Assessment

• Obtain a baseline assessment of the patient's pain before therapy.
• Be alert for adverse reactions and drug interactions throughout therapy.
• Evaluate the patient's and family's knowledge about aspirin therapy.

Nursing Diagnoses

• Pain related to the patient's underlying condition.
• Altered nutrition: Less than body requirements, related to adverse GI reactions to salicylate therapy.
• Knowledge deficit related to aspirin therapy.

Planning and Implementation

Preparation and Administration

• ***P.O. use:*** Give aspirin with food, milk, antacid, or large glass of water to reduce GI adverse reactions. For the patient who has difficulty swallowing, crush aspirin, combine it with soft food, or dissolve it in liquid. After mixing aspirin with a liquid, administer it immediately because the drug doesn't stay in solution. Don't crush enteric-coated aspirin.
• Remember that enteric-coated products are slowly absorbed and are not suitable for acute effects. They cause less GI bleeding and may be more suited for long-term therapy, for example, of arthritis.

Monitoring

• Monitor effectiveness by regularly reevaluating the patient's pain level.
• During chronic therapy, monitor blood salicylate level. Therapeutic level in arthritis is 10 to 30 mg/dl. With chronic therapy, mild toxicity may occur at plasma levels of 20 mg/dl. Tinnitus may occur at plasma levels of 30 mg/dl and above, but does not reliably indicate toxicity, especially in very young patients and those over age 60.
• Monitor serum levels of AST (SGOT), ALT (SGPT), alkaline phosphatase, and bilirubin. Aspirin can cause an increase in these levels.
• Ask the patient if GI adverse reactions have occurred and if they have affected nutrition.
• Inspect the patient's skin regularly for bruising and ask about bleeding from gums, spontaneous epistaxis, or GI bleeding; test all emesis and stool for occult blood.
• Regularly ask the patient about tinnitus or hearing changes.

Supportive Care

• Hold dose and notify the doctor if the patient develops bleeding, salicylism (tinnitus, hearing loss), or GI adverse reactions.
• If possible, discontinue aspirin dosage 5 to 7 days before elective surgery.

Patient Teaching

• Advise the patient receiving high-dose prolonged treatment to watch for petechiae, bleeding gums, and signs of GI bleeding and to maintain adequate fluid intake. Encourage the use of a soft toothbrush.
• Because of the many possible drug interactions involving aspirin, warn the patient taking prescription drugs to check with the doctor or pharmacist before taking OTC combinations containing aspirin.
• Explain that concomitant use with alcohol, steroids, or other NSAIDs may increase the risk of GI bleeding.
• Explain that various OTC preparations contain aspirin and warn patient to read labels carefully to avoid overdosage.
• Instruct the patient to take aspirin with food or milk.
• Instruct the patient not to chew enteric-coated products.
• Emphasize safe storage of medications in the home. Teach the patient to keep aspirin and other drugs out of children's reach. Aspirin is a leading cause of poisoning in children. Encourage use of child-resistant containers in households that include children, even if only as occasional visitors.

Evaluation
In patients receiving aspirin, appropriate evaluation statements may include:
- Patient states aspirin has relieved pain.
- Patient's nutritional status is unaffected by GI adverse reactions.
- Patient and family state an understanding of aspirin therapy.

astemizole
(as stem´ mi zole)
Hismanal

- *Classification:* antiallergy agent (histamine$_1$, receptor antagonist)
- *Pregnancy Risk Category:* C

HOW SUPPLIED
Tablets: 10 mg
Oral suspension: 2 mg/ml‡

ACTION
Mechanism: Blocks the effects of histamine at H_1 receptors. Astemizole is a nonsedating antihistamine because its chemical structure prevents entry into the CNS.
Absorption: Rapidly absorbed from the GI tract.
Distribution: About 96% of the drug is bound to plasma proteins.
Metabolism: Hepatic.
Excretion: Primarily in the feces. Half-life: Elimination half-life is 1 to 2½ days.
Onset, peak, duration: Peak plasma levels occur within 1 hour.

INDICATIONS AND DOSAGE
Relief of symptoms associated with chronic idiopathic urticaria and seasonal allergic rhinitis–
Adults and children over 12 years: 10 mg P.O. daily. A loading dose may be given in order to achieve steady-state plasma levels quickly. Begin therapy at 30 mg on the first day, followed by 20 mg on the second day, and 10 mg daily thereafter.

CONTRAINDICATIONS & PRECAUTIONS
Contraindicated in patients hypersensitive to astemizole. Use cautiously in patients with hepatic or renal disease.

Because antihistamines may possess anticholinergic effects, use cautiously in patients with lower airway diseases, including asthma, to avoid excessive drying and formation of bronchial mucus plug.

ADVERSE REACTIONS
Common reactions are in italics; life-threatening reactions are in bold italics.
CNS: headache, nervousness, dizziness, drowsiness.
EENT: dry mouth, pharyngitis, conjunctivitis.
GI: nausea, diarrhea, abdominal pain, increased appetite.
Other: arthralgia, weight gain.

INTERACTIONS
None significant.

EFFECTS ON DIAGNOSTIC TESTS
None reported.

NURSING CONSIDERATIONS
Besides those related universally to drug therapy (see "How to use this book"), consider the following specific recommendations.

Assessment
- Obtain a baseline assessment of the patient's underlying condition before astemizole therapy.
- Be alert for adverse reactions and drug interactions throughout therapy.
- Evaluate the patient's and family's knowledge about astemizole therapy.

Nursing Diagnoses
- Ineffective airway clearance related to the patient's underlying condition.
- High risk for injury related to astemizole-induced CNS adverse reactions.

• Knowledge deficit related to astemizole therapy.

Planning and Implementation

Preparation and Administration

• ***P.O. use:*** Give patient this drug on an empty stomach at least 2 hours after a meal and be sure patient avoids eating for at least 1 hour after dosing.

Monitoring

• Monitor effectiveness by regularly assessing the patient's condition for relief of symptoms.

• Monitor respiratory status, noting rate and breath sounds.

• Observe the patient for CNS adverse reactions including drowsiness, nervousness, and dizziness.

Supportive Care

• Institute safety measures if drowsiness, nervousness or dizziness occurs.

Patient Teaching

• Tell the patient to take the drug on an empty stomach (at least 2 hours after a meal) and not to eat for at least 1 hour after taking the drug.

• Warn patient to discontinue astemizole 4 days before allergy skin testing to preserve the accuracy of the tests.

• Tell patient to notify the doctor if dizziness or nervousness occur.

Evaluation

In patients receiving astemizole, appropriate evaluation statements may include:

• Patient's allergic symptoms are relieved with astemizole.

• Patient has not experienced astemizole-induced CNS adverse reactions.

• Patient and family state an understanding of astemizole therapy.

atenolol

(a ten´ oh lole)

Noten‡, Tenormin

• *Classification:* antihypertensive, antianginal (beta-adrenergic blocking agent)

• *Pregnancy Risk Category:* C

HOW SUPPLIED

Tablets: 50 mg, 100 mg

Injection: 5 mg/10 ml

ACTION

Mechanism: Blocks response to beta stimulation and depresses renin secretion.

Absorption: About 50% to 60% of a dose is absorbed.

Distribution: Into most tissues and fluids except the brain and CSF; approximately 5% to 15% protein-bound.

Metabolism: Minimal hepatic metabolism.

Excretion: Approximately 40% to 50% of a given dose is excreted unchanged in urine; remainder in feces as unchanged drug and metabolites. Half-life: In patients with normal renal function, plasma half-life is 6 to 7 hours; half-life increases as renal function decreases.

Onset, peak, duration: An effect on heart rate usually occurs within 60 minutes, with peak effect at 2 to 4 hours. Antihypertensive effect persists for about 24 hours.

INDICATIONS & DOSAGE

Treatment of hypertension—

Adults: initially, 50 mg P.O. daily as a single dose. Dosage may be increased to 100 mg once daily after 7 to 14 days. Dosages greater than 100 mg are unlikely to produce further benefit. Dosage adjustment is necessary in patients with creatinine clearance below 35 ml/minute.

Angina pectoris—

Adults: 50 mg P.O. once daily. May increase to 100 mg daily after 7 days for optimal effect. May give as much as 200 mg daily.

To reduce cardiovascular mortality

and risk of reinfarction in patients with acute myocardial infarction—
Adults: 5 mg I.V. over 5 minutes, followed by another 5 mg I.V. 10 minutes later. After an additional 10 minutes, administer 50 mg P.O., followed by 50 mg P.O. in 12 hours. Thereafter, give 100 mg P.O. daily (as a single dose or 50 mg b.i.d.) for at least 7 days.
To reduce the incidence of supraventricular tachycardia in patients undergoing coronary artery bypass—
Adults: 50 mg P.O. daily starting 3 days before surgery.

CONTRAINDICATIONS & PRECAUTIONS

Contraindicated in patients with hypersensitivity to the drug; and in patients with overt cardiac failure, second- or third-degree atrioventricular block, or cardiogenic shock, because the drug may worsen these conditions.

Use cautiously in patients with impaired renal function because drug elimination may be impaired; coronary insufficiency because beta-adrenergic blockade may precipitate CHF; diabetes mellitus or hyperthyroidism because atenolol may mask tachycardia (but not dizziness or sweating) caused by hypoglycemia or hyperthyroidism; and bronchospastic diseases, such as asthma or emphysema, because dosages exceeding 100 mg/day may inhibit bronchodilating effects of endogenous catecholamines.

ADVERSE REACTIONS

Common reactions are in italics; life-threatening reactions are in bold italics.
CNS: fatigue, lethargy.
CV: *bradycardia, hypotension,* ***congestive heart failure,*** peripheral vascular disease.
GI: nausea, vomiting, diarrhea.
Respiratory: dyspnea, ***bronchospasm.***
Skin: rash.
Other: fever.

INTERACTIONS

Antihypertensives: enhanced hypotensive effect. Use together cautiously.
Digitalis glycosides: excessive bradycardia and increased depressant effect on myocardium. Use together cautiously.
Indomethacin: decrease in antihypertensive effect. Monitor blood pressure and adjust dosage.
Insulin, hypoglycemic drugs (oral): can alter dosage requirements in previously stablilized diabetics. Observe patient carefully.

EFFECTS ON DIAGNOSTIC TESTS

ECG: changes in exercise tolerance.
Platelet count: increased.
Serum glucose: increased or decreased levels in diabetic patients.
Serum potassium, uric acid, transaminase, alkaline phosphatase, lactate dehydrogenase, creatinine, and BUN: increased levels.

NURSING CONSIDERATIONS

Besides those related universally to drug therapy (see "How to use this book"), consider the following specific recommendations:

Assessment
- Obtain a baseline assessment of patient's blood pressure before drug therapy.
- Be alert for adverse reactions and drug interactions throughout therapy.
- Evaluate the patient's and family's knowledge about atenolol therapy.

Nursing Diagnoses
- High risk for injury related to patient's underlying condition.
- Decreased cardiac output related to atenolol-induced cardiovascular adverse reactions.
- Knowledge deficit related to atenolol therapy.

Planning and Implementation

Preparation and Administration

• Expect reduced dosage if patient has renal insufficiency. Hemodialysis patients should receive 50 mg of drug after each dialysis session.

• Always check patient's apical pulse before giving this drug; if slower than 60 beats/minute, hold drug and call doctor.

• Don't discontinue drug abruptly; can exacerbate angina and myocardial infarction (MI). Drug should be withdrawn gradually over a 2-week period.

• ***I.V. use:*** I.V. doses may be mixed with 5% dextrose, sodium chloride injection, or dextrose and sodium chloride injection. The solution is stable for 48 hours after mixing. Administer by direct I.V. into a large vein over at least 5 minutes.

Monitoring

• Monitor effectiveness by frequently checking blood pressure if prescribed for hypertension, frequency and severity of anginal pain if prescribed for angina pectoris, heart rate and rhythm if prescribed for selected patients with supraventricular tachycardia, and signs of reinfarction if prescribed to reduce cardiovascular mortality and risk of reinfarction after acute MI.

• Monitor for conditions that may cause decreased cardiac output as a result of drug therapy, such as bradycardia, hypotension, or congestive heart failure.

• Monitor dialysis patient closely for marked decreases in blood pressure.

Supportive Care

• Be aware that full antihypertensive effect may not appear for 1 to 2 weeks after initiating therapy.

• Be prepared to treat shock or hypoglycemia as this drug masks common signs of these conditions. However, atenolol doesn't potentiate insulin-induced hypoglycemia or delay recovery of blood glucose to normal levels.

• Institute safety measures if lethargy occurs.

• Notify doctor immediately if patient shows signs of decreased cardiac output: hypotension, bradycardia, or changes in level of consciousness. Be prepared to provide supportive measures as prescribed.

Patient Teaching

• Advise patient to take the orally prescribed drug at the same time every day. Drug can be dispensed in a 28-day calendar pack.

• Inform the patient that full hypertensive effect may not appear for 1 to 2 weeks after initiating therapy.

• Explain the importance of taking this drug as prescribed, even when feeling well. Tell patient not to discontinue drug suddenly, but to call the doctor if unpleasant adverse reactions occur.

• Teach patient how to take his pulse. Tell patient to withhold drug and call the doctor if pulse rate is below 60 beats/minute.

• Instruct patient to check with doctor or pharmacist before taking OTC medications.

Evaluation

In patients receiving atenolol, appropriate evaluation statements may include:

• Patient's blood pressure is within normal limits.

• Patient's cardiac output remains unchanged throughout drug therapy.

• Patient and family state an understanding of atenolol therapy.

atropine sulfate (systemic)

(a´ troe peen)

• *Classification:* antiarrhythmic, vagolytic (anticholinergic, belladonna alkaloid)

• *Pregnancy Risk Category:* C

HOW SUPPLIED

Tablets: 0.4 mg, 0.6 mg, 0.6 mg
Injection: 0.05 mg/ml, 0.1 mg/ml, 0.3 mg/ml, 0.4 mg/ml, 0.5 mg/ml, 0.6 mg/ml, 0.8 mg/ml, 1 mg/ml, 1.2 mg/ml

ACTION

Mechanism: An anticholinergic that inhibits acetylcholine at the parasympathetic neuroeffector junction, blocking vagal effects on the sinoatrial (SA) node; this increases depolarization rate of the SA node, enhances conduction through the atrioventricular node, and speeds heart rate.
Absorption: Well absorbed after P.O. and I.M. administration. After endotracheal administration, well absorbed from the bronchial tree (used in 1-mg doses in acute bradyarrhythmia when an I.V. line has not been established).
Distribution: Well distributed throughout the body, including the CNS. Only 18% of the drug binds with plasma protein (clinically insignificant).
Metabolism: In the liver to several metabolites.
Excretion: About 30% to 50% of a dose is excreted by the kidneys as unchanged drug. Small amounts may be excreted in the feces and expired air. Half-life: Biphasic, with an initial 2-hour phase followed by a terminal half-life of about 12½ hours.
Onset, peak, duration: Effects on heart rate peak within 2 to 8 minutes after I.V. administration. Peak inhibitory effects on salivation occur in 30 minutes to 1 hour after oral or I.M. administration. Drug effects persist for about 4 to 6 hours.

INDICATIONS & DOSAGE

Symptomatic bradycardia, bradyarrhythmia (junctional or escape rhythm)–
Adults: usually 0.5 to 1 mg I.V. push; repeat q 5 minutes, to maximum of 2 mg. Lower doses (less than 0.5 mg) can cause bradycardia.
Children: 0.01 mg/kg I.V. dose up to maximum of 0.4 mg; or 0.3 mg/m² dose; may repeat q 4 to 6 hours.
Antidote for anticholinesterase insecticide poisoning–
Adults and children: 2 mg I.M. or I.V. repeated hourly until muscarinic symptoms disappear. Severe cases may require up to 6 mg I.M. or I.V. q 1 hour.
Preoperatively for diminishing secretions and blocking cardiac vagal reflexes–
Adults: 0.4 to 0.6 mg I.M. 45 to 60 minutes before anesthesia.
Children: 0.01 mg/kg I.M. up to a maximum dose of 0.4 mg 45 to 60 minutes before anesthesia.
Adjunctive treatment of peptic ulcer disease; treatment of functional GI disorders such as irritable bowel syndrome–
Adults: 0.4 to 0.6 mg P.O. q 4 to 6 hours.
Children: 0.01 mg/kg or 0.3 mg/m² (not to exceed 0.4 mg) q 4 to 6 hours.

CONTRAINDICATIONS & PRECAUTIONS

Use cautiously in patients with acute myocardial infarction because it may promote arrhythmias, including ventricular fibrillation and tachycardia as well as atrial fibrillation; the resulting increase in heart rate may increase myocardial oxygen consumption and worsen myocardial ischemia.

Also use cautiously in patients with narrow-angle glaucoma, obstructive uropathy, obstructive GI tract disease, myasthenia gravis, paralytic ileus, intestinal atony, unstable cardiovascular status from acute hemorrhage, and toxic megacolon because the drug may worsen these symptoms or disorders.

ADVERSE REACTIONS

Common reactions are in italics; life-threatening reactions are in bold italics.
Blood: leukocytosis.
CNS: *headache, restlessness,* ataxia, disorientation, hallucinations, delirium, ***coma,*** *insomnia, dizziness;* excitement, agitation, and confusion (especially in elderly patients).
CV: 1 to 2 mg–*tachycardia, palpitations; greater than 2 mg–extreme tachycardia, angina.*
EENT: 1 mg–*slight mydriasis,* photophobia; 2 mg–*blurred vision, mydriasis.*
GI: *dry mouth (common even at low doses),* thirst, *constipation,* nausea, vomiting.
GU: urine retention.
Skin: hot, flushed skin.

INTERACTIONS

Methotrimeprazine: may produce extrapyramidal symptoms. Monitor patient carefully.

EFFECTS ON DIAGNOSTIC TESTS

None reported.

NURSING CONSIDERATIONS

Besides those related universally to drug therapy (see "How to use this book"), consider the following recommendations:

Assessment
- Review the patient's history for a condition that contraindicates the use of atropine.
- Obtain a baseline assessment of the patient's heart rate and rhythm before atropine therapy.
- Be alert for adverse reactions and drug interactions throughout therapy.
- Evaluate the patient's and family's knowledge about atropine therapy.

Nursing Diagnoses
- Decreased cardiac output related to ineffectiveness of atropine therapy.
- Altered protection related to atropine-induced tachycardia.
- Knowledge deficit related to atropine.

Planning and Implementation

Preparation and Administration
- ***I.V. use:*** Inject prescribed amount of undiluted drug into vein or I.V. tubing over 1 to 2 minutes; monitor patient closely during administration for paradoxical bradycardia, which usually disappears within 2 minutes.

Monitoring
- Monitor effectiveness by evaluating continuous ECG recordings when used to treat an arrhythmia.
- Monitor for tachycardia, especially in the cardiac patient because it may precipitate ventricular fibrillation.
- Monitor patient for anticholinergic effects such as dry mouth, constipation, or urine retention.

Supportive Care
- If ECG disturbances occurs, withhold the drug, obtain a rhythm strip, and notify the doctor immediately.
- Have emergency equipment and drugs on hand to treat new arrhythmias. Be aware that other anticholinergic drugs may increase vagal blockage.
- Have physostigmine salicylate readily available as the antidote for atropine.
- Institute safety precautions if CNS adverse reactions occur.
- Encourage patient to void before receiving drug because drug may cause urine retention and hesitancy, especially in elderly men with benign prostatic hypertrophy.

Patient Teaching
- Teach the patient about his disease and therapy.
- Instruct patient to ask for assistance with activities if CNS adverse reactions occur.
- Teach patient how to handle distressing anticholinergic effects.

Evaluation

In patients receiving atropine, appropriate evaluation statements may include:

• Patient's ECG reveals arrhythmia has been corrected.
• Patient does not experience tachycardia with atropine use.
• Patient and family state an understanding of atropine therapy.

---

atropine sulfate (ophthalmic)

(a´ troe peen)
Atropisol, Atropt‡, BufOpto Atropine, Isopto Atropine

• *Classification:* mydriatric; cycloplegic (cholinergic blocker)
• *Pregnancy Risk Category:* C

HOW SUPPLIED

Ophthalmic ointment: 0.5%, 1%
Ophthalmic solution: 1%, 2%, 3%

ACTION

Mechanism: Blocks muscarinic acetylcholine receptors in the eye. Anticholinergic action leaves the pupil under unopposed adrenergic influence, causing it to dilate. Causes mydriasis and cycloplegia.
Absorption: Readily absorbed across the conjunctival mucosa.
Distribution: In animal studies, highest concentrations are found in the aqueous and vitreous humors and the cornea.
Onset, peak, duration: Peak mydriasis occurs in 30 to 40 minutes, and persists for 7 to 12 days. Peak cycloplegia occurs in 1 to 3 hours, and recovery is seen in 6 to 12 days.

INDICATIONS & DOSAGE

Treatment of acute iritis; treatment of uveitis–
Adults and children: instill 1 drop of 1% solution or small amount of ointment q.d. to b.i.d.
Cycloplegic refraction–
Adults: instill 1 to 2 drops of 1% solution 1 hour before refracting.
Children: instill 1 to 2 drops of 0.5% to 1% solution in each eye b.i.d. for 1 to 3 days before eye examination and 1 hour before refraction, or instill small amount of ointment daily or b.i.d. 2 to 3 days before examination.

CONTRAINDICATIONS & PRECAUTIONS

Contraindicated in patients hypersensitive to belladonna alkaloids or any component of the formulation. Also contraindicated in children under age 3 months; in patients with glaucoma or a tendency toward glaucoma (including patients with a narrow anterior chamber angle). Usually contraindicated in elderly patients because of the risk of undiagnosed elevated intraocular pressure.
Avoid use in breast-feeding women because the drug may be absorbed systemically; atropine is detectable in breast milk.

ADVERSE REACTIONS

Common reactions are in italics; life-threatening reactions are in bold italics.
Eye: ocular congestion in long-term use, conjunctivitis, contact dermatitis, edema, *blurred vision,* eye dryness, *photophobia.*
Systemic: flushing, dry skin and mouth, fever, tachycardia, abdominal distention in infants, ataxia, irritability, confusion, somnolence.

INTERACTIONS

None significant.

EFFECTS ON DIAGNOSTIC TESTS

Intraocular pressure: may be increased.

NURSING CONSIDERATIONS

Besides those related universally to drug therapy (see "How to use this book"), consider the following specific recommendations:
Assessment
• Obtain a baseline assessment of the patient's vision and pupil size.

• Be alert for adverse reactions and drug interactions throughout therapy.
• Evaluate the patient's and family's knowledge about atropine therapy.

Nursing Diagnoses

• Sensory/perceptual alterations (visual) related to the patient's underlying condition.
• High risk for poisoning related to the drug's systemic adrenergic effects.
• Knowledge deficit related to atropine therapy.

Planning and Implementation

Preparation and Administration

• Apply thin strip of ointment to conjunctival sac; avoid touching applicator to any surface. Wipe tip with clean tissue or gauze before recapping.
• Instill solution in lacrimal sac; remove excess solution around eyes with clean tissue or gauze and apply light finger pressure to lacrimal sac for 1 minute.

Monitoring

• Monitor effectiveness by assessing the patient's visual status and pupil size.
• Monitor for drug-induced glaucoma by assessing intraocular pressure.
• Monitor for systemic adrenergic effects, especially in children and the elderly.

Supportive Care

• Notify the doctor if changes in the patient's health status occur.
• Keep physostigmine salicylate (I.M. or I.V.) on hand to reverse systemic adrenergic effects.

Patient Teaching

• Teach the patient how to apply the ointment or drops and advise him to wash his hand before and after administering the drug.
• Warn the patient to avoid hazardous activities, such as driving, until the temporary visual impairment caused by the drug wears off.
• Advise the patient that dark glasses will ease any discomfort from photophobia.
• Advise the patient to carry hard candy or gum to ease dry mouth.

Evaluation

In patients receiving atropine, appropriate evaluation statements may include:
• Patient experiences therapeutic mydriasis.
• Patient remains free of systemic adrenergic effects.
• Patient and family state an understanding of atropine therapy.

auranofin

(au rane´ oh fin)
Ridaura

• *Classification:* antirheumatic (gold derivative)
• *Pregnancy Risk Category:* C

HOW SUPPLIED

Capsules: 3 mg

ACTION

Mechanism: Unknown. Anti-inflammatory effects in rheumatoid arthritis are probably caused by inhibition of sulfhydryl systems, which alters cellular metabolism. May also alter enzyme function and immune response and suppress phagocytic activity.
Absorption: When administered P.O., 25% is absorbed through the GI tract.
Distribution: 60% protein-bound and widely distributed in body tissues. Oral gold from auranofin is more highly bound to plasma proteins than the injectable form. Synovial fluid levels are approximately 50% of blood concentrations. No correlation between blood gold concentrations and safety or efficacy has been determined.
Metabolism: Drug is not believed to be broken down into elemental gold.
Excretion: 60% of the absorbed au-

ranofin (15% of the administered dose) is excreted in the urine; the remainder in the feces. Half-life: Average plasma half-life is 26 days.
Onset, peak, duration: Time to peak plasma concentration is 1 to 2 hours.

INDICATIONS & DOSAGE

Rheumatoid arthritis–
Adults: 6 mg P.O. daily, administered either as 3 mg b.i.d. or 6 mg once daily. After 6 months, may be increased to 9 mg daily.

CONTRAINDICATIONS & PRECAUTIONS

Contraindicated in patients with hypersensitivity to gold or other heavy metals or with a history of blood dyscrasias, because the drug may induce blood dyscrasias; in patients with severe diabetes, congestive heart failure, hemorrhagic conditions, systemic lupus erythematosus, tuberculosis, or exfoliative dermatitis because it may exacerbate these conditions; in patients with colitis, because the drug can precipitate GI distress; and in patients with impaired renal or hepatic function.

Use cautiously in patients with decreased cerebral or cardiovascular circulation, a history of drug rash, a history of hepatic or renal disease, or severe hypertension.

ADVERSE REACTIONS

Common reactions are in italics; life-threatening reactions are in bold italics.
Blood: *thrombocytopenia* (with or without purpura), *aplastic anemia, agranulocytosis,* leukopenia, eosinophilia.
GI: *diarrhea, abdominal pain, nausea, vomiting, stomatitis, enterocolitis,* anorexia, metallic taste, dyspepsia, flatulence.
GU: *proteinuria,* hematuria, nephrotic syndrome, glomerulonephritis.
Hepatic: jaundice, elevated liver enzymes.
Respiratory: ***interstitial pneumonitis.***
Skin: *rash, pruritus, dermatitis,* ***exfoliative dermatitis.***

INTERACTIONS

Phenytoin: auranofin may increase phenytoin blood levels. Monitor for toxicity.

EFFECTS ON DIAGNOSTIC TESTS

Serum protein-bound iodine test (chloric acid digestion method): false readings during and for several weeks after therapy.

NURSING CONSIDERATIONS

Besides those related universally to drug therapy (see "How to use this book"), consider the following specific recommendations:

Assessment
- Obtain a baseline assessment of the patient's joint pain and stiffness before initiating auranofin therapy.
- Be alert for adverse reactions and drug interactions throughout therapy.
- Evaluate the patient's and family's knowledge about auranofin therapy.

Nursing Diagnoses
- Pain (arthritic) related to patient's underlying condition.
- High risk for fluid volume deficit related to adverse GI reactions to auranofin.
- Knowledge deficit related to auranofin therapy.

Planning and Implementation

Preparation and Administration
- Store at controlled room temperature and in a light-resistant container.
- Administer concomitant drug therapy such as NSAIDs, as ordered.

Monitoring
- Monitor effectiveness by regularly assessing the status of the patient's rheumatoid arthritis.
- Monitor the patient's CBC and

platelet counts for adverse blood reactions.
• Monitor hydration status if adverse GI reactions occur.
• Monitor renal and hepatic function studies for abnormalities.
• Monitor diagnostic test results. Limited data suggest that auranofin may enhance the patient's reaction to tuberculin skin tests.
• Monitor results of urinalysis regularly. If proteinuria or hematuria is detected, discontinue drug because it can produce a nephrotic syndrome or glomerulonephritis.
Supportive Care
• Notify the doctor and expect to discontinue the drug if the patient's platelet count falls below 100,000/mm³; if hemoglobin drops suddenly; if granulocytes are below 1,500/mm³, and if leukopenia (WBC count below 4,000/mm³) or eosinophilia (eosinophils greater than 75%) occurs.
• If the patient develops mild diarrhea, notify the doctor and obtain an order for an antidiarrheal agent. Diarrhea is the most common adverse reaction to this drug. If the patient develops blood in his stool, notify the doctor immediately.
Patient Teaching
• Emphasize the importance of monthly follow-up to monitor patient's platelet count.
• Reassure the patient that beneficial drug effect may be delayed as long as 3 months. However, if response is inadequate after 3 months and maximum dosage has been reached, the doctor will probably discontinue auranofin.
• Encourage the patient to take the drug as prescribed and not to alter the dosage schedule.
• Tell the patient to continue taking this drug if he experiences mild diarrhea, the most common adverse reaction; however, if he notes blood in his stool, he should contact the doctor immediately.
• Tell the patient to continue taking concomitant drug therapy, such as NSAIDs, if prescribed.
• Advise the patient to report any rashes or other skin problems immediately. Pruritus often precedes dermatitis and should be considered a warning of impending skin reactions. Any pruritic skin eruption while a patient is receiving auranofin should be considered a reaction to this drug until proven otherwise. Therapy is discontinued until the reaction subsides.
• Advise the patient to immediately report a metallic taste as this symptom often precedes stomatitis. Recommend careful oral hygiene during therapy.
• Warn the patient not to give the drug to others as auranofin is prescribed only for selected rheumatoid arthritis patients.
• Give the patient a copy of the patient information insert supplied by the manufacturer.

Evaluation

In patients receiving auranofin, appropriate evaluation statements may include:
• Patient expresses that his arthritic pain is relieved.
• Patient maintains fluid volume balance.
• Patient and family state an understanding of auranofin therapy.

---

aurothioglucose
(aur oh thee oh gloo´ kose)
Gold-50‡, Solganal

gold sodium thiomalate
Myochrysine

• *Classification:* antirheumatic (gold derivative)

• *Pregnancy Risk Category:* C

HOW SUPPLIED

aurothioglucose
Injection (suspension): 50 mg/ml in sesame oil with aluminum monostearate 2% and propylparaben 0.1% in a 10 ml container
gold sodium thiomalate
Injection: 10 mg/ml, 50 mg/ml with benzyl alcohol

ACTION

Mechanism: Unknown. Anti-inflammatory effects in rheumatoid arthritis are probably caused by inhibition of sulfhydryl systems, which alters cellular metabolism. Gold salts may also alter enzyme function and immune response and suppress phagocytic activity.
Absorption: After I.M. injection, absorption is slow and erratic because it is in oil suspension.
Distribution: Widely distributed throughout the body in lymph nodes, bone marrow, kidneys, liver, spleen, and tissues. About 85% to 90% is protein-bound. Higher tissue concentrations occur with parenteral as compared to orally administered gold salts, with a mean steady-state plasma level of 1 to 5 mcg/ml. No correlation between blood gold concentrations and safety or efficacy has been determined.
Metabolism: Not broken down into elemental gold.
Excretion: About 70% of the drug is excreted in the urine, 30% in the feces. Half-life: With cumulative dosing, 14 to 40 days.
Onset, peak, duration: Peak levels occur 3 to 6 hours after injection.

INDICATIONS & DOSAGE

Rheumatoid arthritis—
Adults: initially, 10 mg (aurothioglucose) I.M., followed by 25 mg for second and third doses at weekly intervals. Then, 50 mg weekly until 1 g has been given. If improvement occurs without toxicity, continue 25 to 50 mg at 3- to 4-week intervals indefinitely as maintenance therapy.
Children 6 to 12 years: ¼ usual adult dosage. Alternatively, 1 mg/kg I.M. once weekly for 20 weeks.
Rheumatoid arthritis—
Adults: initially, 10 mg (gold sodium thiomalate) I.M., followed by 25 mg in 1 week. Then, 50 mg weekly until 14 to 20 doses have been given. If improvement occurs without toxicity, continue 50 mg q 2 weeks for 4 doses; then, 50 mg q 3 weeks for 4 doses; then, 50 mg q month indefinitely as maintenance therapy. If relapse occurs during maintenance therapy, resume injections at weekly intervals.
Children: 1 mg/kg I.M. weekly for 20 weeks. If response is good, may be given q 3 to 4 weeks indefinitely.

CONTRAINDICATIONS & PRECAUTIONS

Contraindicated in patients with uncontrolled diabetes mellitus, systemic lupus erythromatosus, Sjögren's syndrome, agranulocytosis, or blood dyscrasias; in patients who recently received radiation therapy; in breast-feeding patients, because the drug distributes into breast milk; and in patients with a history of sensitivity to gold compounds.

Use cautiously in patients with marked hypertension, compromised cerebral or cardiovascular function, or renal or hepatic dysfunction, because gold may exacerbate these conditions. Use cautiously in women of childbearing age, because gold compounds are teratogenic in high doses in animals.

ADVERSE REACTIONS

Common reactions are in italics; life-threatening reactions are in bold italics.

Adverse reactions to gold are considered severe and potentially life-threatening. Report any side effects to the doctor at once.

Blood: *thrombocytopenia* (with or without purpura), *aplastic anemia,* ***agranulocytosis,*** leukopenia, eosinophilia.

CNS: *dizziness,* syncope, sweating.

CV: bradycardia, hypotension.

EENT: corneal gold deposition, corneal ulcers.

GI: *metallic taste, stomatitis,* difficulty swallowing, nausea, vomiting.

GU: *albuminuria, proteinuria,* ***nephrotic syndrome,*** nephritis, acute tubular necrosis.

Hepatic: hepatitis, jaundice.

Skin: *rash and dermatitis in 20% of patients. (If drug is not stopped, may lead to* ***fatal exfoliative dermatitis.****)*

Other: ***anaphylaxis,*** angioneurotic edema.

INTERACTIONS

None significant.

EFFECTS ON DIAGNOSTIC TESTS

Serum protein-bound iodine test (chloric acid digestion method): false readings during and for several weeks after therapy.

NURSING CONSIDERATIONS

Besides those related universally to drug therapy (see "How to use this book"), consider the following specific recommendations:

Assessment

- Obtain a baseline assessment of the patient's comfort level before beginning therapy.
- Be alert for adverse reactions and drug interactions throughout therapy.
- Evaluate the patient's and family's knowledge about aurothioglucose therapy.

Nursing Diagnoses

- Pain (joint) related to patient's underlying condition.
- Alteration in oral mucous membrane related to aurothioglucose-induced adverse reaction.
- Knowledge deficit related to aurothioglucose therapy.

Planning and Implementation

Preparation and Administration

- Administer only under constant supervision of a doctor who is thoroughly familiar with the drug's toxicities and benefits.
- Administer all gold salts I.M. , preferably intragluteally. Aurothioglucose is pale yellow; do not use if it darkens.
- Observe the patient for 30 minutes after administration because of possible anaphylactic reaction.
- Aurothioglucose is a suspension. Immerse vial in warm water and shake vigorously before injecting.
- Have the patient lie down and remain incumbent for 10 to 20 minutes after gold sodium thiomalate injection to minimize hypotension.
- Keep dimercaprol on hand to treat acute toxicity.

Monitoring

- Monitor effectiveness by evaluating joint mobility and stiffness as well as patient's complaints of discomfort.
- Monitor CBC, including platelet count results after every second injection. Monitor platelet count results when patient develops purpura or ecchymoses.
- Monitor urinalysis results for protein and sediment changes before each injection.
- Observe for complaints of oral discomfort, difficulty chewing, and swallowing as well as signs of bleeding and inflammation of the oral mucosa.

Supportive Care

- Be aware that gold therapy may alter results of liver function studies.
- Remember that most adverse reactions are readily reversible if the drug is discontinued immediately.
- Notify the doctor if skin rash develops and obtain an order for antipruritic when necessary.
- Provide good oral hygiene and administer analgesics for stomatitis, as

ordered. Stomatitis is the second most common adverse reaction to gold therapy.

Patient Teaching

• Advise patient to report any skin rashes or problems immediately. Dermatitis is the most common adverse reaction to gold salts. Pruritus often precedes dermatitis and should be considered a warning of impending skin reactions. Any pruritic skin eruption while a patient is receiving gold therapy should be considered a reaction unless proven otherwise. Expect therapy to be stopped until reaction subsides.

• Inform the patient that benefits of therapy may not appear for 3 to 4 months or longer.

• Tell the patient to minimize exposure to sunlight or artificial ultraviolet light.

• Advise the patient to notify the doctor if he suspects stomatitis. Tell him that it is often preceded by a metallic taste. Encourage good oral hygiene and dental visits.

• Tell the patient that increased joint pain may occur 1 to 2 days after injection. This usually subsides after a few injections.

• Inform the patient that most adverse reactions are readily reversible if drug is discontinued immediately and that if adverse effects are mild, some rheumatologists resume gold therapy after 2 to 3 weeks of rest.

• Advise the patient of the importance of close medical follow-ups and the need for frequent blood and urine tests during therapy.

Evaluation

In patients receiving aurothioglucose, appropriate evaluation statements may include:

• Patient expresses relief of joint stiffness and pain.

• Patient maintains good oral hygiene.

• Patient and family state an understanding of aurothioglucose therapy.

azatadine maleate

(a za´ ta deen)

Optimine, Zadine‡

• *Classification:* antiallergy (piperidine antihistamine)

• *Pregnancy Risk Category:* B

HOW SUPPLIED

Tablets: 1 mg

Syrup: 0.5 mg/5 ml‡

ACTION

Mechanism: Blocks the effects of histamine at H_1 receptors. Prevents but does not reverse histamine-mediated responses.

Absorption: Well absorbed from the GI tract.

Distribution: Not fully known; apparently crosses the blood-brain barrier resulting in CNS effects; minimally protein-bound.

Metabolism: 80% is metabolized by the liver.

Excretion: Drug and metabolites are excreted in urine; about 20% of drug is excreted unchanged. Half-life: About 9 to 12 hours.

Onset, peak, duration: Its effects begin in 15 to 30 minutes, and peak effect occurs at about 4 hours.

INDICATIONS & DOSAGE

Rhinitis, allergy symptoms, chronic urticaria –

Adults: 1 to 2 mg P.O. b.i.d. Maximum dosage is 4 mg daily.

Not intended for children under 12 years.

CONTRAINDICATIONS & PRECAUTIONS

Contraindicated in patients with hypersensitivity to this drug or antihistamines with similar chemical structures (cyproheptadine); in patients experiencing asthmatic attacks because azatadine thickens bronchial secretions; and in patients who have taken monoamine oxidase (MAO) inhibitors within the previous 2 weeks because these drugs prolong and intensify sedative and anticholinergic effects of antihistamines.

Use cautiously in patients with narrow-angle glaucoma; in those with pyloroduodenal obstruction or urinary bladder obstruction from prostatic hypertrophy or narrowing of the bladder neck because of their marked anticholinergic effects; in patients with cardiovascular disease, hypertension, or hyperthyroidism because of the risk of palpitations and tachycardia; and in patients with renal disease, diabetes, bronchial asthma, urine retention, or stenosing peptic ulcers.

Pregnant women should avoid antihistamines, especially in the third trimester, as should breast-feeding women; although most antihistamines have not been studied in such patients, seizures have occurred in premature infants and other neonates.

ADVERSE REACTIONS

Common reactions are in italics; life-threatening reactions are in bold italics.
Blood: thrombocytopenia.
CNS: (especially in elderly patients) *drowsiness, dizziness,* vertigo, disturbed coordination.
CV: hypotension, palpitations.
GI: anorexia, nausea, vomiting, *dry mouth and throat,* epigastric distress.
GU: urine retention.
Skin: urticaria, rash.
Other: thick bronchial secretions.

INTERACTIONS

CNS depressants: increased sedation. Use together cautiously.
MAO inhibitors: increased anticholinergic effects. Don't use together.

EFFECTS ON DIAGNOSTIC TESTS

Diagnostic skin tests: interference with positive reactions.

NURSING CONSIDERATIONS

Besides those related universally to drug therapy (see "How to use this book"), consider the following specific recommendations:

Assessment

- Obtain a baseline assessment of the patient's underlying condition before azatadine therapy.
- Be alert for adverse reactions and drug interactions throughout therapy.
- Evaluate the patient's and family's knowledge about azatadine therapy.

Nursing Diagnoses

- Ineffective airway clearance related to the patient's underlying condition.
- High risk for injury related to azatadine maleate-induced CNS adverse reactions.
- Knowledge deficit related to azatadine maleate therapy.

Planning and Implementation

Preparation and Administration

- ***P.O. use:*** Reduce GI distress by giving with food or milk.

Monitoring

- Monitor effectiveness by frequently checking the patient's respiratory status and, if the drug was given for urticaria, by checking the condition of the patient's rash and severity of itching.
- Monitor blood counts during long-term therapy; watch for signs of blood dyscrasias.

Supportive Care

- If you notice that the patient is developing a tolerance for the drug, discuss this with the doctor. It may be necessary to substitute another antihistamine.
- Institute safety measures, such as assisting the patient when out of bed and using side rails continuously, if CNS adverse reactions (dizziness, severe drowsiness) occur.

Patient Teaching

- Tell the patient that coffee or tea may reduce drowsiness and that sugarless gum, sour hard candy, or ice chips may relieve dry mouth.

• Warn patient to avoid drinking alcoholic beverages during therapy and avoid hazardous activities that require alertness until CNS response to drug is determined.
• Advise patient to discontinue azatadine 4 days before allergy skin testing to preserve the accuracy of the tests.
• Tell the patient to notify the doctor if CNS reactions occur.

Evaluation
In patients receiving azatadine maleate, appropriate evaluation statements may include:
• Patient's allergic symptoms are relieved with azatadine maleate.
• Patient has not experienced significant CNS adverse effects.
• Patient and family state an understanding of azatadine maleate therapy.

---

azathioprine
(ay za thye´ oh preen)
Imuran, Thioprine‡

• *Classification:* immunosuppressive (purine antagonist)
• *Pregnancy Risk Category:* D

HOW SUPPLIED
Tablets: 50 mg
Injection: 100 mg

ACTION
Mechanism: A purine analogue that mainly exhibits immunosuppressive activity. Blocks T-cell–mediated rejection in patients undergoing renal allotransplantation; drug has variable effects on antibody formation.
Absorption: Well absorbed orally.
Distribution: Azathioprine and its major metabolite, mercaptopurine, are distributed throughout the body; both are 30% protein-bound. Drug is rapidly cleared from the plasma. Azathioprine and its metabolites cross the placenta.
Metabolism: Metabolized to mercaptopurine, which is then oxidized and methylated to several derivatives.
Excretion: Small amounts of azathioprine and mercaptopurine are excreted in urine unchanged; most of a given dose is excreted in urine as secondary metabolites.
Onset, peak, duration: The effect of azathioprine and its metabolite mercaptopurine may not be evident until several days after the start of therapy. Drug effects persist for several days after termination of therapy.

INDICATIONS & DOSAGE
Immunosuppression in renal transplants–
Adults and children: initially, 3 to 5 mg/kg P.O. or I.V. daily usually beginning on the day of transplantation. Maintain at 1 to 3 mg/kg daily (dosage varies considerably according to patient response).
Treatment of severe, refractory rheumatoid arthritis–
Adults: initially, 1 mg/kg P.O. taken as a single dose or as two doses. If patient response is not satisfactory after 6 to 8 weeks, dosage may be increased by 0.5 mg/kg daily (up to a maximum of 2.5 mg/kg daily) at 4-week intervals.

CONTRAINDICATIONS & PRECAUTIONS
Contraindicated in patients with hypersensitivity to the drug and in pregnant patients. Use cautiously in patients with hepatic or renal dysfunction; in patients receiving cadaveric kidneys, who may have decreased elimination; and in rheumatoid arthritis patients previously treated with alkylating agents (cyclophosphamide, chlorambucil, or melphalan) who are at increased risk of neoplasia.

ADVERSE REACTIONS

Common reactions are in italics; life-threatening reactions are in bold italics.
Blood: ***leukopenia, bone marrow suppression,*** anemia, ***pancytopenia,*** thrombocytopenia.
GI: nausea, vomiting, anorexia, *pancreatitis,* steatorrhea, mouth ulceration, esophagitis.
Hepatic: hepatotoxicity, jaundice.
Skin: rash.
Other: ***immunosuppression*** *(possibly profound),* arthralgia, muscle wasting, alopecia.

INTERACTIONS

Allopurinol: impaired inactivation of azathioprine. Decrease azathioprine dose to ¼ or ⅓ normal dose.
Nondepolarizing neuromuscular blocking agents: azathioprine may reverse the neuromuscular blockade.

EFFECTS ON DIAGNOSTIC TESTS

CBC and differential: altered results.
Liver enzyme tests: elevated results.
Serum uric acid: decreased levels.

NURSING CONSIDERATIONS

Besides those related universally to drug therapy (see "How to use this book"), consider the following specific recommendations:

Assessment
- Obtain a baseline assessment of the patient's immune status before therapy.
- Be alert for adverse reactions and drug interactions throughout therapy.
- Evaluate the patient's and family's knowledge about azathioprine therapy.

Nursing Diagnoses
- Altered protection related to the threat of organ rejection.
- High risk for infection related to azathioprine-induced immunosuppression.
- Knowledge deficit related to azathioprine therapy.

Planning and Implementation
Preparation and Administration
- In renal homotransplants, start drug 1 to 5 days before surgery.
- ***I.V. use:*** Only used in patients unable to tolerate oral medications.

Monitoring
- Monitor effectiveness by observing for signs of organ rejection.
- Watch for clay-colored stools, dark urine, pruritus, and yellow skin and sclera, which may indicate hepatotoxicity.
- Monitor for increased alkaline phosphatase, bilirubin, AST (SGOT), and ALT (SGPT).
- Hemoglobin, WBC, and platelet counts should be done at least once a month; more often at the beginning of treatment.
- Observe for signs of bleeding.

Supportive Care
- Use with caution in patients with hepatic or renal dysfunction.
- Avoid I.M. injections of any drug in patients with severely depressed platelet counts (thrombocytopenia) to prevent injury.
- The drug should be discontinued immediately when WBC count is less than 3,000/mm^3 to prevent irreversible bone marrow suppression.
- Obtain orders for antiemetics as needed.
- Provide frequent mouth care to alleviate azathioprine-induced mouth ulceration.

Patient Teaching
- Warn the patient to report even mild infections (colds, fever, sore throat, and malaise) because of the drug's potent immunosuppressive abilities.
- Caution patients to avoid conception during therapy and up to 4 months after stopping therapy.
- Warn patients that some thinning hair is possible.
- Advise patients taking azathioprine for refractory rheumatoid arthritis

that it may take up to 12 weeks to be effective.

Evaluation

In patients receiving azathioprine, appropriate evaluation statements may include:

• Patient exhibits no signs of organ rejection.

• Patient demonstrates no signs and symptoms of infection.

• Patient and family state an understanding of azathioprine therapy.

aztreonam

(az´ tree oh nam)

Azactam

• *Classification:* antibiotic (monobactam)

• *Pregnancy Risk Category:* B

HOW SUPPLIED

Injection: 500-mg, 1-g, 2-g vials

ACTION

Mechanism: Inhibits bacterial cell wall synthesis, promoting osmotic instability. Bactericidal.

Absorption: Poor from the GI tract after oral administration; rapid and complete after I.M. administration. Peak levels after I.M. injection are slightly lower than those after I.V. administration.

Distribution: Distributed rapidly and widely to all body fluids and tissues, including bile, breast milk, and CSF. Drug crosses the placenta and is found in fetal circulation.

Metabolism: From 6% to 16% is metabolized in inactive metabolites by nonspecific hydrolysis of the beta-lactam ring; 56% to 60% is protein-bound, less if renal impairment is present.

Excretion: Primarily in urine as unchanged drug by glomerular filtration and tubular secretion; 1.5% to 3.5% is excreted in feces as unchanged drug; also excreted in breast milk. Half-life: Averages 1.7 hours.

Onset, peak, duration: Peak serum concentrations after I.M. injection occur within 60 minutes.

INDICATIONS & DOSAGE

Treatment of urinary tract infections, lower respiratory tract infections, septicemia, skin and skin structure infections, intra-abdominal infections, and gynecologic infections caused by various gram-negative organisms–

Adults: 500 mg to 2 g I.V. or I.M. q 8 to 12 hours. For severe systemic or life-threatening infections, 2 g q 6 to 8 hours may be given. Maximum dosage is 8 g daily.

CONTRAINDICATIONS & PRECAUTIONS

Contraindicated in patients with hypersensitivity to the drug.

Use cautiously in patients with a history of hypersensitivity or allergic reactions to other beta-lactam antibiotics and in those with impaired hepatic or renal function (reduced dosage may be required).

ADVERSE REACTIONS

Common reactions are in italics; life-threatening reactions are in bold italics.

Blood: neutropenia, anemia.

CNS: seizures, headache, insomnia.

CV: hypotension.

GI: diarrhea, nausea, vomiting.

Hepatic: transient elevations of AST (SGOT) and ALT (SGPT).

Local: thrombophlebitis at I.V. site, discomfort and swelling at I.M. injection site.

Other: hypersensitivity, ***anaphylaxis,*** altered taste, halitosis.

INTERACTIONS

Furosemide, probenecid: increased serum aztreonam levels.

EFFECTS ON DIAGNOSTIC TESTS

ALT (SGPT), AST (SGOT), LDH, and serum creatinine: transiently increased levels.
Coombs' test: may become positive.
Prothrombin time, partial thromboplastin time: may be prolonged.
Urine glucose with copper sulfate (Clinitest or Benedict's reagent): false-positive results. Use glucose enzymatic methods (Diastix, Tes-Tape).

NURSING CONSIDERATIONS

Besides those related universally to drug therapy (see "How to use this book"), consider the following recommendations.

Assessment

- Obtain a baseline assessment of infection before therapy.
- Be alert for adverse reactions and drug interactions throughout therapy.
- Evaluate the patient's and family's knowledge about aztreonam therapy.

Nursing Diagnoses

- High risk for injury related to ineffectiveness of aztreonam to eradicate the infection.
- High risk for fluid volume deficit related to adverse GI reactions to aztreonam.
- Knowledge deficit related to aztreonam.

Planning and Implementation

Preparation and Administration

- Obtain specimen for culture and sensitivity tests before first dose. Therapy may begin pending test results.
- ***I.M. use:*** Administer deeply into a large muscle mass, such as the upper outer quadrant of the gluteus maximus or the lateral part of the thigh.
- ***I.V. use:*** To administer a bolus, inject drug slowly (over 3 to 5 minutes) directly into a vein or I.V. tubing.

Monitoring

- Monitor effectiveness by regularly assessing for improvement of infection.
- Monitor hepatic function.
- Monitor patient's hydration status if adverse GI reactions occur.

Supportive Care

- Obtain an order for an antiemetic or antidiarrheal agent as needed.

Patient Teaching

- Warn patient receiving the drug I.M. that pain and swelling at the injection site may occur.
- Tell patient to inform the nurse of pain or discomfort at the I.V. site.

Evaluation

In patients receiving aztreonam, appropriate evaluation statements may include:

- Patient is free from infection.
- Patient's maintains adequate hydration throughout aztreonam therapy.
- Patient and family state an understanding of aztreonam therapy.

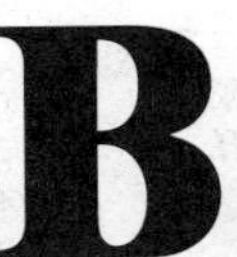

bacampicillin hydrochloride

(ba kam pi sill´ in)
Penglobe†, Spectrobid

- *Classification:* antibiotic (aminopenicillin)
- *Pregnancy Risk Category:* B

HOW SUPPLIED

Tablets: 400 mg
Oral suspension: 125 mg/5 ml (after reconstitution)

ACTION

Mechanism: Converted to ampicillin in vivo, each mg of bacampicillin yields 623 to 727 mcg ampicillin. Bactericidal against microorganisms by inhibiting cell wall synthesis during active multiplication. Bacteria resist bacampicillin by producing penicillinases—enzymes that hydrolyze its active form (ampicillin).
Absorption: Hydrolyzed rapidly to ampicillin, ethanol, carbon dioxide, and acetaldehyde after oral administration. Hydrolysis occurs both in GI tract and plasma. About 80% to 100% of a dose is absorbed.
Distribution: No unchanged bacampicillin is found in serum after oral administration; ampicillin distributes into pleural, peritoneal, and synovial fluids, lungs, prostate, muscle, liver, and gallbladder; it penetrates middle ear effusions, maxillary sinus and bronchial secretions, tonsils, and sputum; and crosses the placenta. Drug is 15% to 25% protein-bound.
Metabolism: Ampicillin (the active component) is metabolized partially.
Excretion: Ampicillin and metabolites are excreted in urine by renal tubular secretion and glomerular filtration; they are also excreted in breast milk. Half-life: Elimination half-life in adults is 1 to 1½ hours; 7½ hours in severe renal impairment.
Onset, peak, duration: Peak plasma concentrations occur 30 to 90 minutes after an oral dose.

INDICATIONS & DOSAGE

Upper and lower respiratory tract infections due to streptococci, pneumococci, staphylococci, and Hemophilus influenzae; *urinary tract infections due to* Escherichia coli, Proteus mirabilis, *and* Streptococcus faecalis; *skin infections due to streptococci and susceptible staphylococci*–
Adults and children weighing more than 25 kg: 400 to 800 mg P.O. q 12 hours.
Gonorrhea–
Usual dosage is 1.6 g plus 1 g probenecid given as a single dose.

Not recommended for children under 25 kg.

CONTRAINDICATIONS & PRECAUTIONS

Contraindicated in patients with hypersensitivity to any other penicillin or cephalosporin. Bacampicillin should not be used in patients with infectious mononucleosis because many patients develop a rash during therapy.

Use cautiously in patients with renal impairment, because drug is excreted by the kidneys; decreased dosage is required in moderate to severe renal failure.

ADVERSE REACTIONS

Common reactions are in italics; life-threatening reactions are in bold italics.

Blood: anemia, thrombocytopenia, thrombocytopenic purpura, eosinophilia, leukopenia.
GI: *nausea,* vomiting, *diarrhea,* glossitis, stomatitis.
Other: *hypersensitivity (erythematous maculopapular rash, urticaria,* ***anaphylaxis***), overgrowth of nonsusceptible organisms.

INTERACTIONS

Allopurinol: increased incidence of skin rash.
Probenecid: increases blood levels of bacampicillin or other penicillins. Probenecid may be used for this purpose.

EFFECTS ON DIAGNOSTIC TESTS

Aminoglycoside serum levels: falsely decreased concentrations.
Urine glucose tests with copper sulfate (Benedict's reagent or Clinitest): false-positive results. Use glucose enzymatic methods (Clinistix or Tes-Tape).

NURSING CONSIDERATIONS

Besides those related universally to drug therapy (see "How to use this book"), consider the following specific recommendations:

Assessment
- Obtain a baseline assessment of infection before therapy.
- Be alert for adverse reactions and drug interactions throughout therapy.
- Evaluate the patient's and family's knowledge about bacampicillin therapy.

Nursing Diagnoses
- High risk for injury related to ineffectiveness of bacampicillin to eradicate the infection.
- High risk for fluid volume deficit related to bacampicillin-induced adverse GI reactions.
- Knowledge deficit related to bacampicillin therapy.

Planning and Implementation
Preparation and Administration
- Obtain specimen for culture and sensitivity tests before first dose. Therapy may begin pending test results.
- Before first dose, ask the patient about previous allergic reactions to this drug or other penicillins. However, a negative history of penicillin allergy does not guarantee future safety.
- Give bacampicillin at least 1 hour before bacteriostatic antibiotics.
- ***P.O. use:*** Administer tablets with food to prevent GI distress. However, bacampicillin suspension should be taken on an empty stomach.
- Be aware that bacampicillin is especially formulated to produce high blood levels of antibiotic when administered twice daily.

Monitoring
- Monitor effectiveness by regularly assessing for improvement of infection.
- Monitor hydration status if adverse GI reactions occur.
- Monitor for bacterial or fungal superinfections during prolonged or high-dose therapy, especially in elderly, debilitated, or immunosuppressed patients.
- Periodically evaluate patient's and family's knowledge about bacampicillin.

Supportive Care
- Obtain an order for an antiemetic or antidiarrheal agent as needed.
- If the patient develops a rash, notify the doctor and expect to discontinue the drug.

Patient Teaching
- Advise the patient who becomes allergic to bacampicillin to wear medical alert identification stating this information.
- Tell the patient to take drug exactly as prescribed and to complete the entire prescription even after he feels better.

• Tell the patient to call the doctor if rash, fever, or chills develop. A rash is the most common allergic reaction.
• Warn the patient never to use leftover bacampicillin for a new illness or to share it with others.
• Tell the patient to take bacampicillin tablets with food to prevent GI distress, but to take bacampicillin suspension on an empty stomach.

Evaluation

In patients receiving bacampicillin, appropriate evaluation statements may include:

• Patient is free of infection.
• Patient maintains adequate hydration throughout bacampicillin therapy.
• Patient and family state an understanding of bacampicillin therapy.

bacillus Calmette-Guérin (BCG), live intravesical

(kal met´ geh rang´)

TheraCys, TICE BCG

• *Classification:* antineoplastic (bacterial agent)
• *Pregnancy Risk Category:* C

HOW SUPPLIED

TheraCys

Suspension (freeze-dried) for bladder instillation: 27 mg/vial

TICE BCG

Suspension (freeze-dried) for bladder instillation: approximately 50 mg/ampule

ACTION

Mechanism: Exact mechanism unknown. Instillation of the live bacterial suspension causes a local inflammatory response. Local infiltration of histiocytes and leukocytes is followed by a decrease in the superficial tumors within the bladder.

Pharmacokinetics: Unknown.

INDICATIONS & DOSAGE

Treatment of in situ carcinoma of the urinary bladder (primary and relapsed) –

Adults: Administer 3 reconstituted and diluted vials intravesically once weekly for 6 weeks (induction) followed by additional treatments at 3, 6, 12, 18, and 24 months (TheraCys); 1 bladder instillation (1 ampule suspended in 50 ml sterile, preservative-free saline solution) once weekly for 6 weeks, then once monthly for 6 to 12 months (TICE BCG).

CONTRAINDICATIONS & PRECAUTIONS

Because of the risk of bacterial infection, contraindicated in patients with compromised immune systems; in patients receiving immunosuppressive therapy; in patients with fever of unknown origin. If the fever is caused by an infection, the drug should be withheld until the patient has recovered. Also contraindicated in patients with urinary tract infection because of the risk of increased bladder irritation or disseminated BCG infection. Persons with immune deficiency should not handle the product.

Patients with a small bladder capacity may experience increased local irritation with the usual dose of BCG live.

ADVERSE REACTIONS

Common reactions are in italics; life-threatening reactions are in bold italics.

Blood: anemia, leukopenia, thrombocytopenia.

GI: nausea, vomiting, anorexia, diarrhea, mild abdominal pain.

GU: *dysuria, urinary frequency, hematuria,* cystitis, urinary urgency, urinary incontinence, urinary tract infection, cramps, pain, decreased bladder capacity, tissue in urine, local infection, renal toxicity, genital pain.

Other: malaise, *fever above 101° F*

(38.3° C), chills, myalgia, arthralgia, elevated liver enzymes.

INTERACTIONS

Antibiotics: antimicrobial therapy for other infections may attenuate the response to BCG intravesical. Avoid concomitant use.

Immunosuppressants, bone marrow depressants, and radiation therapy: may impair the response to BCG intravesical because these treatments can decrease the patient's immune response and may also increase the risk of osteomyelitis or disseminated BCG infection. Avoid concomitant use.

EFFECTS ON DIAGNOSTIC TESTS

Tuberculin sensitivity: positive results. Patient's reactivity to tuberculin should be determined before therapy.

NURSING CONSIDERATIONS

Besides those related universally to drug therapy (see "How to use this book"), consider the following specific recommendations:

Assessment

- Obtain a baseline assessment of patient's underlying condition before initiating therapy.
- Be alert for adverse reactions or drug interactions during therapy.
- Evaluate the patient's and family's knowledge about BCG therapy.

Nursing Diagnoses

- High risk for fluid volume deficit related to drug-induced adverse reactions.
- Altered renal tissue perfusion related to bladder instillation of drug.
- Knowledge deficit related to BCG therapy.

Planning and Implementation

Preparation and Administration

- Use strict aseptic technique to administer the drug to minimize trauma to GU tract and to prevent introducing other contaminants to the area.
- To administer TICE BCG, use thermosetting plastic or sterile glass containers and syringes. Draw 1 ml of sterile, preservative-free 0.9% sodium chloride solution into a 3-ml syringe. Add to one ampule of the drug; gently expel back into the ampule three times to ensure thorough mixing. Dispense the cloudy suspension into the top end of a catheter-tipped syringe that contains 49 ml 0.9% sodium chloride solution. Gently rotate the syringe.
- To administer TheraCys, reconstitute the drug with only 1 ml of the provided diluent per vial, just before use. Do not remove the rubber stopper to prepare the solution. The contents of the three reconstituted vials are to be added to 50 ml of sterile, preservative-free 0.9% sodium chloride solution (final volume 53 ml). A urethral catheter is placed into the bladder, the bladder is drained, and the 53 ml of prepared solution is infused by gravity. The catheter is then removed.
- Handle the drug and all materials used for the instillation of drug as infectious material because it contains live attenuated mycobacteria. Dispose of all associated materials as biohazardous waste.
- If there is evidence of traumatic catheterization, do not administer the drug. Subsequent treatment may resume after 1 week as if no interruption occurred.
- Know that this drug should not be used as an immunizing agent for the prevention of cancer. Do not use to prevent tuberculosis because the drug should not be confused with BCG vaccine.
- BCG intravesical should not be administered within 7 to 14 days of transurethral resection or biopsy. Fatal disseminated BCG infection has occurred after traumatic catheterization.

Monitoring
• Monitor effectiveness by regularly checking tumor size and rate of growth through appropriate studies; and by noting results of follow-up diagnostic tests and overall physical status.
• Monitor for signs of bleeding (hematuria, ecchymosis, petechiae, epistaxis, melena).
• Monitor for signs of systemic BCG infection (temperature elevation, sore throat, malaise). Take temperature daily. BCG infections are rarely detected by positive culture. Withhold therapy if systemic infection is suspected (short-term fever > 103° F; persistent fever > 101° F over 2 days with severe malaise).
• Monitor CBC, hepatic and renal function, and serum uric acid level.
• Monitor vital signs frequently during infusion of this drug.
• Monitor the patient's hydration status if nausea, vomiting, and diarrhea occur.
• Monitor intake and output because the drug causes inflammation of the bladder. It has been associated with bacterial urinary tract infection, hematuria, dysuria, and frequency.
• Monitor for hypersensitivity reactions. Tuberculin sensitivity may be rendered positive by BCG intravesical treatment.
Supportive Care
• Be prepared to treat bladder irritation with phenazopyridine, acetaminophen, and propantheline. Systemic hypersensitivity reactions can be treated with diphenhydramine (Benadryl).
• Patients with a small bladder capacity may experience increased local irritation with the usual dose of BCG intravesical.
• Provide the patient with fluids if nausea, vomiting, and diarrhea occur.
Patient Teaching
• Tell the patient to retain the drug in the bladder for 2 hours after instillation. Change of lying position should occur every 15 minutes for the first hour. Sitting position is allowed for the second hour.
• Instruct patient to sit when voiding.
• Teach patient to disinfect urine for 6 hours after instillation of the drug. Add equal volume of undiluted household bleach to voided urine in toilet, and allow to stand 15 minutes before flushing.
• Tell the patient to call if symptoms worsen or if any of the following develop: blood in urine, chills, fever, frequent urge to urinate, painful urination, nausea, vomiting, joint pain, or rash.
• Tell the patient that a cough that develops after therapy could indicate a life-threatening BCG infection and should be reported to the doctor immediately.

Evaluation
In patients receiving BCG, appropriate evaluation statements may include:
• Patient does not develop fluid volume deficit.
• Renal tissue perfusion remains adequate for normal functioning.
• Patient and family state an understanding of BCG therapy.

bacitracin (ophthalmic)
(bass i tray´ sin)

• *Classification:* ophthalmic antibiotic (polypeptide)
• *Pregnancy Risk Category:* C

HOW SUPPLIED
Ophthalmic ointment: 500 units/g

ACTION
Mechanism: Inhibits bacterial cell wall synthesis by blocking the incorporation of amino acids and nucleotides into the cell wall. Bactericidal or bacteriostatic, depending on con-

centration and infection. Active against staphylococci (including some penicillin-resistant strains), streptococci, anaerobic cocci, clostridia, and corynebacteria.
Absorption: Not significantly absorbed after topical ophthalmic administration.

INDICATIONS & DOSAGE

Ocular infections–
Adults and children: apply small amount of ointment into conjunctival sac several times daily or p.r.n. until favorable response is observed.

CONTRAINDICATIONS & PRECAUTIONS

Contraindicated in patients with hypersensitivity or previous toxic reactions to the agent. Use cautiously (if at all) in patients with preexisting renal dysfunction because it is nephrotoxic.

ADVERSE REACTIONS

Common reactions are in italics; life-threatening reactions are in bold italics.
Eye: slowed corneal wound healing, temporary visual haze.
Other: overgrowth of nonsusceptible organisms.

INTERACTIONS

Heavy metals (e.g., silver nitrate): inactivate bacitracin. Do not use together.

EFFECTS ON DIAGNOSTIC TESTS

Serum creatinine and blood urea nitrogen (BUN): increased levels.
Urinary sediment tests: increased protein and cast excretion.

NURSING CONSIDERATIONS

Besides those related universally to drug therapy (see "How to use this book"), consider the following specific recommendations:

Assessment
- Obtain a baseline assessment of the patient's allergies before therapy.
- Be alert for adverse reactions or drug interactions during therapy.
- Evaluate the patient's and family's knowledge about bacitracin.

Nursing Diagnoses
- Altered protection related to ocular infection.
- Sensory/perceptual alteration (visual) related to ointment-induced visual blurring.
- Knowledge deficit related to bacitracin.

Planning and Implementation
Preparation and Administration
- Store in tightly closed, light-resistant container.
- Always wash hands before and after applying ointment.
- Cleanse eye area of excessive exudate before application.
- Solution is not commercially available but may be prepared by the pharmacy. Store up to 3 weeks in refrigerator.

Monitoring
- Monitor effectiveness by checking for presence of microorganism by culturing the eye.
- Observe character, amount, and location of exudate.
- Check patient's vision.

Supportive Care
- Apply warm soaks to eyes to aid in removal of dried exudate.
- Use cautiously in patients with hereditary predisposition to antibiotic hypersensitivity.
- Use safety precautions if patient's vision is impaired. Assist with activities.

Patient Teaching
- Teach the patient how to apply ointment. Advise him to wash hands before and after application and not to touch tip of tube or dropper to the eye or surrounding tissue.
- Instruct the patient that only a small amount of ointment is needed;

excess ointment may cause visual blurring.
• Stress the importance of compliance with recommended therapy.
• Instruct the patient to watch for signs of sensitivity (itching lids, swelling, constant burning). If they occur, stop the drug and notify the doctor immediately.
• Warn patients to avoid sharing washcloths and towels with family members during infection.
• Advise the patient not to share eye medication with family members. A family member who develops the same symptoms should contact the doctor.

Evaluation
In patients receiving bacitracin, appropriate evaluation statements may include:
• Patient remains free of signs and symptoms of infection.
• Patient reports decrease or absence of visual blurring.
• Patient and family state an understanding of bacitracin ointment therapy.

bacitracin (topical)

(bass i tray´ sin)
Baciguent◇, Bacitin†

• *Classification:* topical antibiotic (polypeptide)
• *Pregnancy Risk Category:* C

HOW SUPPLIED

Ointment: 500 units/g

ACTION

Mechanism: Inhibits bacterial cell-wall synthesis. Effective mainly against gram-positive organisms, such as staphylococci and streptococci.
Pharmacokinetics: Unknown.

INDICATIONS & DOSAGE

Topical infections, impetigo, abrasions, cuts, and minor burns or wounds–
Adults and children: apply thin film b.i.d. or t.i.d. or more often, depending on severity of condition.

CONTRAINDICATIONS & PRECAUTIONS

Contraindicated in patients with hypersensitivity or previous toxic reactions to the agent. Administer cautiously (if at all) to patients with preexisting renal dysfunction because it is nephrotoxic. Topical ointment is contraindicated for application in external ear canal if eardrum is perforated.

ADVERSE REACTIONS

Common reactions are in italics; life-threatening reactions are in bold italics.
Skin: stinging, rashes, and other allergic reactions; itching, burning, swelling of lips or face.
Other: *possible systemic adverse reactions when used over large areas for prolonged periods: potentially* ***nephrotoxic*** *and ototoxic; allergic reactions;* tightness in chest, hypotension.

INTERACTIONS

None significant.

EFFECTS ON DIAGNOSTIC TESTS

Serum creatinine and BUN: increased levels.
Urinary sediment tests: increased protein and cast excretion.

NURSING CONSIDERATIONS

Besides those related universally to drug therapy (see "How to use this book"), consider the following specific recommendations:

Assessment
• Obtain a baseline assessment of wounds before therapy.

*Liquid form contains alcohol. **May contain tartrazine.

• Be alert for adverse reactions and drug interactions throughout therapy.
• Evaluate the patient's and family's knowledge about bacitracin therapy.

Nursing Diagnoses

• Impaired skin integrity related to patient's underlying condition.
• Altered urinary elimination related to bacitracin-induced nephrotoxicity.
• Knowledge deficit related to bacitracin therapy.

Planning and Implementation

Preparation and Administration

• ***Cutaneous use:*** Cleanse area before applying, especially in areas with crusted or suppurative lesions.
• Be aware that application in the external ear canal is contraindicated if the eardrum is perforated.

Monitoring

• Monitor effectiveness by regularly examining patient's wounds.
• Observe patient. If patient's condition does not improve or worsens, discontinue drug.
• Monitor renal function study results.
• Monitor for adverse reactions and interactions by frequently assessing the patient's urinary elimination pattern.

Supportive Care

• Consider alternative treatment for burns that cover more than 20% of body surface, especially if patient suffers impaired renal function.
• Prolonged use may cause overgrowth of nonsusceptible organisms.
• Be prepared to discontinue the drug and notify the doctor if patient's condition worsens.

Patient Teaching

• Inform patient that allergy to neomycin may be associated with allergy to bacitracin.
• Teach patient how to apply medication.

Evaluation

In patients receiving bacitracin, appropriate evaluation statements may include:

• Patient's wounds are healing.
• Patient did not develop nephrotoxicity.
• Patient and family state an understanding of bacitracin therapy.

baclofen

(bak´ loe fen)
Lioresal, Lioresal DS

• *Classification:* skeletal muscle relaxant (chlorophenyl derivative)
• *Pregnancy Risk Category:* C

HOW SUPPLIED

Tablets: 10 mg, 20 mg, 25 mg‡

ACTION

Mechanism: A centrally acting muscle relaxant that reduces transmission of impulses from the spinal cord to skeletal muscle.
Absorption: Rapidly and extensively absorbed from the GI tract but is subject to individual variation. Also, as dose increases, rate and extent of absorption decreases.
Distribution: Widely distributed throughout the body, with small amounts crossing the blood-brain barrier; about 30% plasma protein-bound.
Metabolism: About 15% is metabolized in the liver via deamination.
Excretion: Half-life: 2½ to 4 hours.
Onset, peak, duration: Onset of therapeutic effect may not be immediately evident; varies from hours to weeks. Peak effect is seen at 2 to 3 hours. Peak plasma levels occur in 2 to 3 hours.

INDICATIONS & DOSAGE

Spasticity in multiple sclerosis, spinal cord injury–
Adults: initially, 5 mg P.O. t.i.d. for 3 days, 10 mg t.i.d. for 3 days, 15 mg t.i.d. for 3 days, 20 mg t.i.d. for 3

days. Increase according to response up to maximum of 80 mg daily.

CONTRAINDICATIONS & PRECAUTIONS

Contraindicated in patients with hypersensitivity to the drug. Use cautiously in patients with impaired renal function, peptic ulcer disease, cerebral lesions, cerebrovascular accident (increased risk of CNS, respiratory, or cardiac depression), diabetes (may increase blood glucose levels), epilepsy (may cause deterioration of seizure control and EEG), or in patients who need spasticity to maintain upright posture and balance.

ADVERSE REACTIONS

Common reactions are in italics; life-threatening reactions are in bold italics.
CNS: *drowsiness, dizziness,* headache, *weakness, fatigue,* confusion, insomnia, dysarthria, *seizures.*
CV: hypotension.
EENT: nasal congestion, blurred vision.
GI: *nausea,* constipation.
GU: urinary frequency.
Hepatic: increased AST (SGOT) and alkaline phosphatase.
Metabolic: hyperglycemia.
Skin: rash, pruritus.
Other: ankle edema, excessive perspiration, weight gain.

INTERACTIONS

Alcohol, CNS depressants: increased CNS depression.

EFFECTS ON DIAGNOSTIC TESTS

Blood glucose, SGOT, and alkaline phosphatase: increased levels.

NURSING CONSIDERATIONS

Besides those related universally to drug therapy (see "How to use this book"), consider the following specific recommendations:

Assessment
- Obtain a baseline assessment of the patient's pain and muscle spasms related to his underlying condition before drug therapy.
- Be alert for adverse reactions and drug interactions throughout therapy.
- Evaluate the patient's and family's knowledge about baclofen therapy.

Nursing Diagnoses
- Pain related to the patient's underlying condition.
- Injury related to high risk for drug-induced drowsiness.
- Knowledge deficit related to baclofen therapy.

Planning and Implementation

Preparation and Administration
- Give with meals or milk to prevent GI distress.
- Amount of relief determines if amount of dosage (and drowsiness) can be reduced.

Monitoring
- Monitor effectiveness by regularly assessing the severity and frequency of muscle spasms.
- Monitor the patient for adverse reactions by frequently checking the patient's vital signs for hypotension.
- Monitor for changes in bowel or bladder function, especially constipation or urine retention.
- Monitor for drowsiness.
- Watch for increased incidence of seizures in epileptics.
- Watch for sensitivity reactions, such as fever, skin eruptions, and respiratory distress.
- Evaluate the patient's vision by asking if he has blurred vision.
- Monitor for hallucinations and rebound spasticity if drug is withdrawn.

Supportive Care
- Obtain an order for a mild laxative if he develops constipation.
- Institute safety precautions if he develops blurred vision, confusion, or dizziness.
- Do not withdraw the drug abruptly

unless required by severe adverse reactions.
• Know that treatment of overdose is entirely supportive; do not induce emesis or use a respiratory stimulant in obtunded patients.
• Know that this drug is used investigationally for treatment of unstable bladder.
• To reduce GI distress, give the drug with milk or meals.

Patient Teaching
• Advise the patient to report urinary frequency.
• If constipation is troublesome, advise patient to increase fluid intake and use a stool softener.
• Warn the patient to avoid driving and other hazardous activities that require alertness until CNS effects of drug are known.
• Advise the patient not to suddenly stop taking the drug.
• Advise the patient to follow the doctor's recommendations for rest and physical therapy.
• Advise the patient to take the drug with food or milk to prevent GI distress.

Evaluation
In patients receiving baclofen, appropriate evaluation statements may include:
• Patient reports pain and muscle spasms have ceased.
• Patient does not experience injury as a result of drug-induced drowsiness.
• Patient and family state an understanding of baclofen therapy.

PHARMACOLOGIC CLASS

barbiturates
amobarbital
amobarbital sodium
aprobarbital
butabarbital
mephobarbital
metharbital
pentobarbital sodium
phenobarbital
phenobarbital sodium
primidone
secobarbital sodium

OVERVIEW
Barbituric acid was compounded over 100 years ago in 1864. The first hypnotic barbiturate, barbital, was introduced into medicine in 1903. Although barbiturates have been used extensively as sedative-hypnotics and antianxiety agents, benzodiazepines are the current drugs of choice for these effects. Phenobarbital remains a cornerstone of anticonvulsant therapy. A few short-acting barbiturates are used as general anesthetics.

Barbiturates are structurally related compounds that act throughout the CNS. The exact mechanism(s) of action of barbiturates at the presynaptic and postsynaptic membrane is not known, nor is it clear which cellular and synaptic actions result in sedative-hypnotic effects. Barbiturates can produce all levels of CNS depression, from mild sedation to coma to death. The principal anticonvulsant mechanism of action is reduction of nerve transmission and decreased excitability of the nerve cell. Barbiturates also raise the seizure threshold. After oral or rectal administration all barbiturates act within 20 to 60 minutes.

CLINICAL INDICATIONS AND ACTIONS
Seizure disorders
Phenobarbital is used in the prophylactic treatment of seizure disorders. It is used mainly in tonic-clonic (grand mal) and partial seizures. At anesthetic doses, all barbiturates have anticonvulsant activity.

Barbiturates suppress the spread of seizure activity produced by epileptogenic foci in the cortex, thalamus, and limbic systems by enhancing the effects of GABA.

Sedation, hypnosis
All currently available barbiturates are used as sedative-hypnotics for short-term (up to 2 weeks) treatment of insomnia because of their nonspecific CNS effects.

Barbiturates are not used as routinely as sedatives because of excess sedation, short-term efficacy, and the potential for severe adverse reactions upon withdrawal or overdose; they have been replaced for such use by benzodiazepines and nonspecific sedatives. Barbiturate-induced sleep differs from physiologic sleep by decreasing the rapid-eye-movement (REM) sleep cycles.

OVERVIEW OF ADVERSE REACTIONS

Drowsiness, lethargy, vertigo, headache, and CNS depression are common with barbiturates. After hypnotic doses, a hangover effect, subtle distortion of mood, and impairment of judgment or motor skills may continue for many hours. After a decrease in dosage or discontinuation of barbiturates used for hypnosis, rebound insomnia or increased dreaming or nightmares may occur. Barbiturates cause hyperalgesia in subhypnotic doses. Hypersensitivity reactions (rash, fever, serum sickness) are not common, and are more likely to occur in patients with a history of asthma or allergies to other drugs; reactions include urticaria, rash, angioedema, and Stevens-Johnson syndrome. Barbiturates can cause paradoxical excitement at low doses, confusion in elderly patients, and hyperactivity in children. High fever, severe headache, stomatitis, conjunctivitis, or rhinitis may precede skin eruptions. Because of the potential for fatal consequences, discontinue barbiturates if dermatologic reactions occur.

Withdrawal symptoms may occur after as little as 2 weeks of uninterrupted therapy. Symptoms of abstinence usually occur within 8 to 12 hours after the last dose, but may be delayed up to 5 days. They include weakness, anxiety, nausea, vomiting, insomnia, hallucinations, and possibly seizures.

REPRESENTATIVE COMBINATIONS

Amobarbital with ephedrine hydrochloride, theophylline, and chlorpheniramine maleate: Theo-Span; with secobarbital: Amsc, Compobarb, Dusotal, Lanabarb, Tuinal; with dextroamphetamine: Amodex.

Butabarbital with acetaminophen: Constalgesic, G-3, Sedapap, Sedapap 10, Amino-Bar, Minotal; with acetaminophen and mephenesin: T-caps; with acetaminophen, phenacetin, and caffeine: Windolor; with aminophylline, phenylpropanolamine hydrochloride, chlorpheniramine maleate, aluminum hydroxide, and magnesium hydrobromide: Pedo-Sol; with acetaminophen, salicylamide, d-amphetamine Sedragesic; with amphetamine sulfate: Bontril; with belladonna: Butibel, Quiebel; with secobarbital and phenobarbital: Tri-Barbs.

Pentobarbital sodium with acetaminophen, salicylamide, and codeine: Tega-Code; with adiphenine hydrochloride: Spasmasorb; with atropine sulfate, hyoscine hydrobromide, and hyoscyamine: Eldonal; with carbromal: Carboprent; with ephedrine: Ephedrine and Nembutal; with ergotamine tartrate, caffeine, and bellafoline: Cafergot-P.B.; with homatropine methylbromide, dehydrocholic acid, and ox bile extract: Homachol; with phenobarbital: Penotal; with pyrilamine maleate: A-N-R, Rectorette; with secobarbital, butabarbital, and phenobarbital: Quadrabarb; with vitamin compounds and d-methamphetamine hydrochloride: Fetamin.

Phenobarbital with CNS stimulants: Amodrine, Aristrate, Asminyl, Belka-

*Liquid form contains alcohol.

**May contain tartrazine.

tal, Bellophen, Bowdrin, Bronkolixir, Bronkatab, Duovent, Ephenyllin, Luasmin, Phelantin, Phyldrox, Quadrinal, Sedamine, Spabelin, Synophedal, T.E.P.; with mannitol hexanitrate: Hyrunal, Manotensin, Ruhexatal, Vascused, Vermantin; with veratrum viride: Hyperlon, Hyrunal, Verabar; with theobromine: Harbolin, Theocardone, T.P.K.I.; with hyoscyamus: Anaspaz PB, Elixiral, Floramine, Gylanphenb, Neoquess, Nevrotose, Restophen, Sedajen.

See also anticholinergics (belladonna alkaloids), salicylates, xanthine derivatives.

beclomethasone dipropionate (oral inhalation)

(be kloe meth´ a sone)

Aldecin Inhaler‡, Becloforte Inhaler‡, Beclovent, Beclovent Rotacaps†, Vanceril

- *Classification:* anti-inflammatory, antiasthmatic agent (glucocorticord)
- *Pregnancy Risk Category:* C

HOW SUPPLIED

Oral inhalation aerosol: 42 mcg/metered spray, 50 mcg/metered spray‡, 250 mcg/metered spray‡

ACTION

Mechanism: Decreases inflammation, mainly by stabilizing leukocyte lysosomal membranes. Also suppresses the immune response, stimulates bone marrow, and influences protein, fat, and carbohydrate metabolism.
Absorption: After oral inhalation, the drug is rapidly absorbed from the lungs and GI tract. Greater systemic absorption is associated with oral inhalation, but systemic effects do not occur at usual doses because of rapid metabolism in the liver and local metabolism of drug that reaches the lungs.
Distribution: No evidence of tissue storage of beclomethasone or its metabolites. About 10% to 25% of orally inhaled dose is deposited in the respiratory tract. The remainder, deposited in the mouth and oropharynx, is swallowed. When absorbed, it is 87% bound to plasma proteins.
Metabolism: Rapidly metabolizes in the liver or GI tract; Some metabolites are pharmacologically active. The portion that is inhaled into the respiratory tract is partially metabolized before absorption into systemic circulation.
Excretion: Excretion of inhaled form has not been described; however, after systemic administeration metabolites are excreted mainly in feces via biliary elimination and to a lesser extent in urine. Half-life: Average, 15 hours.
Onset, peak, duration: Onset of action usually occurs in a few days but may take as long as 3 weeks in some patients.

INDICATIONS & DOSAGE

Steroid-dependent asthma –
Adults: 2 to 4 inhalations t.i.d. or q.i.d. Maximum dosage is 20 inhalations daily.
Children 6 to 12 years: 1 to 2 inhalations t.i.d. or q.i.d. Maximum dosage is 10 inhalations daily.

CONTRAINDICATIONS & PRECAUTIONS

Contraindicated in patients with acute status asthmaticus and in patients who are hypersensitive to any component of the preparation.

Use cautiously in patients receiving systemic corticosteroids because of increased risk of hypothalamic-pituitary-adrenal axis suppression; when substituting inhalation for oral systemic administration because withdrawal symptoms may occur; and in patients with tuberculosis, healing nasal septal ulcers, oral or nasal surgery or trauma, or bacterial, fungal, or viral respiratory infection.

ADVERSE REACTIONS

Common reactions are in italics; life-threatening reactions are in bold italics.
EENT: hoarseness, fungal infections of mouth and throat, throat irritation.
GI: dry mouth.

INTERACTIONS

None significant.

EFFECTS ON DIAGNOSTIC TESTS

None reported.

NURSING CONSIDERATIONS

Besides those related universally to drug therapy (see "How to use this book"), consider the following specific recommendations:

Assessment

• Obtain a baseline assessment of the patient's asthmatic condition before initiating drug therapy.
• Be alert for adverse reactions and drug interactions throughout therapy.
• Evaluate the patient's and family's knowledge about beclomethasone therapy.

Nursing Diagnoses

• Ineffective airway clearance related to the patient's underlying condition.
• Altered oral mucous membranes related to drug-induced fungal infections.
• Knowledge deficit related to beclomethasone therapy.

Planning and Implementation

Preparation and Administration

• Never administer the drug to relieve an emergency asthmatic attack because onset of action is too slow.
• Be aware that oral glucocorticoid therapy should be tapered slowly as acute adrenal insufficiency and death have occurred in asthmatics who changed abruptly from oral corticosteroids to beclomethasone.
• Expect to administer systemic corticosteroids during times of physiologic stress (trauma, surgery, infection) to prevent adrenal insufficiency in previously steroid-dependent patients.
• Always administer prescribed bronchodilators several minutes before beclomethasone.
• ***Inhalation:*** Have patient rest 1 minute between puffs and to hold breath for a few seconds after each puff to enhance drug action. Use of a spacer device with the Becloforte Inhaler is not recommended.

Monitoring

• Monitor effectiveness by regularly assessing the patient's respiratory status for improvement.
• Monitor the patient's oral mucous membranes for early signs of a fungal infection.

Supportive Care

• Notify doctor if decreased response is noted after administration of drug.
• Have patient drink a glass of water following inhalations to help prevent oral fungal infections.
• Keep inhaler clean and unobstructed by washing it with warm water and drying it thoroughly after each use.

Patient Teaching

• Instruct the patient on how to administer the drug and care for the inhaler device.
• Be sure that the patient understands the need to take the drug as prescribed. Give the patient instructions on what to do if a dose is inadvertently missed.
• Stress the importance of never using the drug to alleviate an acute asthmatic attack because drug takes too long to work.
• Warn the patient not to discontinue the drug abruptly or without the doctor's approval nor to exceed the recommended dose.
• Instruct the patient to contact doc-

tor if he notices a decreased response or if symptoms don't improve within 3 weeks after start of therapy.
• Tell patient to drink a glass of water following inhalations to help prevent oral fungal infections.
• Tell the patient to carry a medical alert card indicating the need for supplemental adrenocorticoids during stress.

Evaluation

In the patient receiving beclomethasone, appropriate evaluation statements may include:
• Patient's lungs are clear and breathing and skin color are normal.
• Patient does not exhibit an oral fungal infection during therapy.
• Patient and family state an understanding of beclomethasone therapy.

beclomethasone dipropionate (nasal)

(be kloe meth´ a sone)

Aldecin Aqueous Nasal Spray, Beconase AQ Nasal Spray, Beconase Nasal Inhaler, Vancenase AQ Nasal Spray, Vancenase Nasal Inhaler

• *Classification:* local anti-inflammatory (glucocorticoid)
• *Pregnancy Risk Category:* C

HOW SUPPLIED

Nasal aerosol: 42 mcg/metered spray, 50 mcg/metered spray‡
Nasal spray: 0.042%, 50 mcg/metered spray‡

ACTION

Mechanism: Produces local anti-inflammatory, vasoconstrictor, and antipruritic actions. Diffuses across cell membranes to form complexes with specific cytoplasmic receptors, influencing cellular metabolism. Corticosteroids stabilize leukocyte lysosomal membranes, inhibit local actions and accumulation of macrophages, decrease local edema, and reduce the formation of scar tissue.
Absorption: Minimal systemic absorption. After nasal inhalation, acts topically on the nasal mucosa.
Distribution: No evidence of tissue storage of beclomethasone or its metabolites. About 10% to 25% of a nasal dose is deposited in the respiratory tract. The remainder, deposited in the mouth and oropharynx, is swallowed. When absorbed, it is 87% bound to plasma proteins.
Metabolism: Swallowed drug undergoes rapid metabolism in the liver or GI tract to a variety of metabolites, some of which have minor glucocorticoid activity. Inhaled portion is partially metabolized before absorption into systemic circulation. Most of the drug is metabolized in the liver.
Excretion: Excretion of inhaled drug has not been described; however, when administered systemically, metabolites are excreted mainly in feces via biliary elimination and to a lesser extent in urine. Half-life: Systemically administered drug, averages 15 hours.
Onset, peak, duration: Usually occurs in a few days but may take as long as 3 weeks in some patients.

INDICATIONS & DOSAGE

Relief of symptoms of seasonal or perennial rhinitis; prevention of recurrence of nasal polyps after surgical removal–
Adults and children over 12 years: usual dosage is 1 spray (42 mcg) in each nostril two to four times daily (total dosage 168 to 336 mcg daily). Most patients require 1 spray in each nostril t.i.d. (252 mcg daily).

Not recommended for children under 12 years.

CONTRAINDICATIONS & PRECAUTIONS

Contraindicated in patients with acute status asthmaticus and in those with hypersensitivity to any component of the preparation. Use with caution in patients receiving systemic corticosteroids, because of increased risk of hypothalamic-pituitary-adrenal axis suppression; when substituting inhalation for oral systemic administration, because withdrawal symptoms may occur; and in patients with tuberculosis, healing nasal septal ulcers, oral or nasal surgery or trauma, or bacterial, fungal, or viral respiratory infection.

ADVERSE REACTIONS

Common reactions are in italics; life-threatening reactions are in bold italics.

CNS: headache.

EENT: *mild transient nasal burning and stinging,* nasal congestion, sneezing, epistaxis, watery eyes.

GI: nausea and vomiting.

Other: development of nasopharyngeal fungal infections.

INTERACTIONS

None reported.

EFFECTS ON DIAGNOSTIC TESTS

None reported.

NURSING CONSIDERATIONS

Besides those related universally to drug therapy (see "How to use this book"), consider the following specific recommendations:

Assessment

- Obtain a baseline assessment of the patient's breathing pattern and degree of nasal congestion.
- Be alert for adverse reactions and drug interactions throughout therapy.
- Evaluate the patient's and family's knowledge about beclomethasone therapy.

Nursing Diagnoses

- Ineffective airway clearance related to the patient's underlying condition.
- Altered oral mucous membrane related to beclomethasone-induced nasopharyngeal fungal infections.
- Knowledge deficit related to beclomethasone therapy.

Planning and Implementation

Preparation and Administration

- ***Nasal use:*** Shake container and invert. Patient should first clear nasal passages, then tilt head back. Insert nozzle into nostril (pointed away from septum), holding other nostril closed. Deliver spray while patient inspires. Repeat in other nostril.

Monitoring

- Monitor effectiveness by assessing the patient's breathing pattern and degree of nasal congestion.
- Monitor compliance. Beclomethasone is not effective for active exacerbation, because effects are not immediate. Most patients achieve a benefit in a few days, but some may need to continue the drug for 2 to 3 weeks before achieving maximum benefit.
- Observe for signs of fungal infection.

Supportive Care

- Obtain a culture, as ordered, if signs of nasal infection occur.
- Notify the doctor if relief is not obtained or if signs of infection appear.

Patient Teaching

- Teach the patient how to administer the spray and tell him that the medicine should be used by one person only.
- Teach the patient good nasal and oral hygiene.
- Warn the patient that administration of drug may cause mild, transient nasal burning.
- Advise the patient to discontinue the drug and notify the doctor if symptoms do not improve after 3 weeks, if irritation persists, or if symptoms of nasal or oral infection occur. Explain that the drug may be discontinued if infection occurs.
- Advise the patient to use the drug regularly, as prescribed. Tell him that effectiveness depends on regular use.

Evaluation
In patients receiving beclomethasone, appropriate evaluation statements may include:
• Patient achieves relief from nasal congestion.
• Patient remains free of fungal infection.
• Patient and family state an understanding of beclomethasone therapy.

benzonatate
(ben zoe´ na tate)
Tessalon

• *Classification:* nonnarcotic antitussive agent (local anesthetic)
• *Pregnancy Risk Category:* C

HOW SUPPLIED
Capsules: 100 mg

ACTION
Mechanism: Suppresses the cough reflex by direct action on the cough center in the medulla (brain). Also has local anesthetic action.
Pharmacokinetics: Unknown.
Onset, peak, duration: Action begins within 15 to 20 minutes and lasts for 3 to 8 hours.

INDICATIONS & DOSAGE
Nonproductive cough–
Adults and children over 10 years: 100 mg P.O. t.i.d.; up to 600 mg daily.
Children under 10 years: 8 mg/kg P.O. in 3 to 6 divided doses.

CONTRAINDICATIONS & PRECAUTIONS
Contraindicated in patients with hypersensitivity to the drug or to related compounds, such as tetracaine.

ADVERSE REACTIONS
Common reactions are in italics; life-threatening reactions are in bold italics.
CNS: dizziness, drowsiness, headache.
EENT: nasal congestion, sensation of burning in eyes.
GI: nausea, constipation.
Skin: rash.
Other: chills.

INTERACTIONS
None significant.

EFFECTS ON DIAGNOSTIC TESTS
None reported.

NURSING CONSIDERATIONS
Besides those related universally to drug therapy (see "How to use this book"), consider the following specific recommendations:
Assessment
• Obtain a baseline assessment of the patient's cough (type and frequency) before initiating therapy.
• Be alert for common adverse reactions and drug interactions.
• Evaluate the patient's and family's knowledge about benzonatate therapy.
Nursing Diagnoses
• Ineffective airway clearance related to underlying condition producing nonproductive cough.
• High risk for injury related to adverse CNS reactions to benzonatate.
• Knowledge deficit related to benzonatate therapy.
Planning and Implementation
Preparation and Administration
• ***P.O. use:*** Instruct patient not to chew capsules or leave in mouth to dissolve; local anesthesia will result. If capsules dissolve in mouth, CNS stimulation may cause restlessness, tremors, and possibly seizures.
• Do not use when cough is a valuable diagnostic sign or is beneficial (as after thoracic surgery).
Monitoring
• Monitor effectiveness by regularly evaluating relief of patient's cough.
• Monitor hydration status; record intake and output.
• Monitor for dizziness and drowsiness.

Supportive Care
• Notify the doctor if cough is unrelieved with benzonatate.
• Encourage the patient to take 2,000 to 3,000 ml of liquids daily, if not contraindicated.
• Institute safety precautions if adverse CNS reactions occur.
• Obtain an order for an antiemetic if nausea persists or becomes severe.
• Perform percussion and chest vibration, as ordered.

Patient Teaching
• Instruct the patient to follow the directions on the medication bottle exactly; explain the importance of not taking more of the drug than directed.
• Tell the patient to call the doctor if cough persists more than 7 days.
• Suggest sugarless throat lozenges to decrease throat irritation and resulting cough.
• Advise the patient to use a humidifier to filter out dust, smoke, and air pollutants.
• Tell the patient to avoid sources of respiratory irritants, such as fumes, smoke, and dust.
• Advise caution regarding driving or other hazardous activities that require alertness until CNS effects of the drug are known; drug may cause drowsiness or dizziness.
• Explain the importance of maintaining fluid intake to help liquefy sputum.

Evaluation
In the patient receiving benzonatate, appropriate evaluation statements may include:
• Patient's lungs are clear and cough is decreased.
• Patient does not suffer injury as a result of benzonatate therapy.
• Patient and family state an understanding of benzonatate therapy.

PHARMACOLOGIC CLASS

benzodiazepines

alprazolam
chlordiazepoxide hydrochloride
clonazepam
clorazepate dipotassium
diazepam
estazolam
flurazepam hydrochloride
halazepam
lorazepam
midazolam
oxazepam
prazepam
quazepam
temazepam
triazolam

OVERVIEW

Benzodiazepines, synthetically produced sedative-hypnotics, gained popularity in the early 1960s, replacing barbiturates as the treatment of choice for anxiety, convulsive disorders, and sedation. These drugs are preferred over barbiturates because therapeutic doses produce less drowsiness and impairment of motor function and toxic doses are less likely to be fatal.

Benzodiazepines are a group of structurally related chemicals that selectively act on polysynaptic neuronal pathways throughout the CNS. Their precise sites and mechanisms of action are not completely known. However, the benzodiazepines enhance or facilitate the action of gamma-aminobutyric acid (GABA), an inhibitory neurotransmitter in the CNS. All of the benzodiazepines have CNS-depressant activities; however, individual derivatives act more selectively at specific sites, allowing them to be subclassified into five categories based on their predominant clinical use.

CLINICAL INDICATIONS AND ACTIONS

Seizure disorders

Four of the benzodiazepines (diazepam, clonazepam, clorazepate, and · parenteral lorazepam) are used as anticonvulsants. Their anticonvulsant properties are derived from an ability to suppress the spread of seizure activity produced by epileptogenic foci in the cortex, thalamus, and limbic systems by enhancing presynaptic inhibition. Clonazepam is particularly useful in the adjunctive treatment of petit mal variant (Lennox-Gastaut syndrome), myoclonic, or akinetic seizures. Parenteral diazepam is indicated to treat status epilepticus.

Anxiety, tension, and insomnia

Most benzodiazepines (alprazolam, chlordiazepoxide, clorazepate, diazepam, estazolam, flurazepam, halazepam, lorazepam, oxazepam, prazepam, temazepam, and triazolam) are useful as antianxiety agents and sedative-hypnotic agents. They have a similar mechanism of action: they are believed to facilitate the effects of GABA in the ascending reticular activating system, increasing inhibition and blocking both cortical and limbic arousal.

They are used to treat anxiety and tension that occur alone or as a side effect of a primary disorder. They are not recommended for tension associated with everyday stress. The choice of a specific benzodiazepine depends on individual metabolic characteristics of the drug. For instance, in patients with depressed renal or hepatic function, alprazolam, lorazepam, or oxazepam may be selected because they have a relatively short duration of action and have no active metabolites. The sedative-hypnotic properties of chlordiazepoxide, clorazepate, diazepam, lorazepam, and oxazepam make these the drugs of choice as preoperative medication and as an adjunct in the rehabilitation of alcoholics.

Surgical adjuncts for conscious sedation or amnesia

Diazepam, midazolam, and lorazepam have amnesic effects. The mechanism of such action is not known. Parenteral administration before such procedures as endoscopy or elective cardioversion causes impairment of recent memory and interferes with the establishment of memory trace, producing anterograde amnesia.

Skeletal muscle spasm, tremor

Because oral forms of diazepam and chlordiazepoxide have skeletal muscle relaxant properties, they are often used to treat neurologic conditions involving muscle spasms and tetanus. The mechanism of such action is unknown, but they are believed to inhibit spinal polysynaptic and monosynaptic afferent pathways.

OVERVIEW OF ADVERSE REACTIONS

Therapeutic dosage of the benzodiazepines usually causes drowsiness and impaired motor function, which should be monitored early in treatment. It may or may not be persistent. GI discomfort, such as constipation, diarrhea, vomiting, and changes in appetite, with urinary alterations also have been reported. Visual disturbances and cardiovascular irregularities also are common. Continuing problems with short-term memory, confusion, severe depression, shakiness, vertigo, slurred speech, staggering, bradycardia, shortness of breath or difficulty breathing, and severe weakness usually indicate a toxic dose level. Prolonged or frequent use of benzodiazepines can cause physical dependency and withdrawal syndrome when use is discontinued.

REPRESENTATIVE COMBINATIONS

Chlordiazepoxide with amitriptyline hydrochloride: Limbitrol, Mylan; with clidinium bromide: Librax; with esterified estrogens: Menrium.

---

benzquinamide hydrochloride

(benz kwin´ a mide)
Emete-Con

- *Classification:* antiemetic (benzoquinolizine derivative)
- *Pregnancy Risk Category:* C

HOW SUPPLIED

Injection: 50 mg/vial

ACTION

Mechanism: Exact mechanism unknown; drug blocks acetylcholine, serotonin, and histamine receptors, and is also a depressant. Probably depresses the chemoreceptor trigger zone to inhibit nausea and vomiting.
Absorption: Rapidly absorbed after oral, I.M., or rectal administration.
Distribution: Distributed rapidly in body tissues, with highest concentration in the liver and kidneys. About 55% to 60% of the drug is plasma protein-bound.
Metabolism: In the liver.
Excretion: About 5% to 10% is excreted unchanged in urine. Metabolites are excreted in urine, bile, and feces. Half-life: 40 minutes.
Onset, peak, duration: Onset of action occurs in about 15 minutes, and duration of action is 3 to 4 hours.

INDICATIONS & DOSAGE

Nausea and vomiting associated with anesthesia and surgery–
Adults: 50 mg I.M. (0.5 mg/kg to 1 mg/kg). May repeat in 1 hour, and thereafter q 3 to 4 hours, p.r.n.; or 25 mg (0.2 mg/kg to 0.4 mg/kg) I.V. as single dose, administered slowly.

CONTRAINDICATIONS & PRECAUTIONS

Contraindicated in patients who are hypersensitive to this drug and in patients receiving drugs that cause arrhythmias or that increase heart rate or blood pressure because the drug may exacerbate these symptoms. I.V. administration is contraindicated in patients with cardiovascular disease and within 15 minutes of preanesthetics or cardiovascular drugs because it may cause premature atrial or ventricular contractions or a sudden rise in blood pressure.

Drug may mask signs of overdose of toxic agents or of intestinal obstruction or brain tumor.

ADVERSE REACTIONS

Common reactions are in italics; life-threatening reactions are in bold italics.
CNS: *drowsiness,* fatigue, insomnia, restlessness, headache, excitation, tremors, twitching, dizziness.
CV: sudden rise in blood pressure and transient arrhythmias (premature atrial and ventricular contractions, atrial fibrillation) after I.V. administration; hypertension; hypotension.
EENT: dry mouth, salivation, blurred vision.
GI: anorexia, nausea.
Skin: urticaria, rash.
Other: muscle weakness, flushing, hiccups, sweating, chills, fever. May mask symptoms of ototoxicity, brain tumor, or intestinal obstruction.

INTERACTIONS

None significant.

EFFECTS ON DIAGNOSTIC TESTS

Free serum fatty acid: increased levels.

NURSING CONSIDERATIONS

Besides those related universally to drug therapy (see "How to use this

*Liquid form contains alcohol. **May contain tartrazine.

book"), consider the following specific recommendations:

Assessment

• Obtain a baseline assessment of cardiovascular status and blood pressure.

• Be alert for adverse reactions or drug interactions throughout therapy.

• Evaluate the patient's and family's knowledge about benzquinamide therapy.

Nursing Diagnoses

• High risk for aspiration related to nausea and vomiting induced by anesthesia and surgery.

• Altered cardiopulmonary tissue perfusion related to benzquinamide-induced cardiac arrhythmias.

• Knowledge deficit related to benzquinamide therapy.

Planning and Implementation

Preparation and Administration

• ***I.V. use:*** Contraindicated in cardiovascular disease. Don't give I.V. within 15 minutes of preanesthetic or cardiovascular drugs.

• ***I.M. use:*** Administer in large muscle mass. Use deltoid area only if well developed. Be sure to aspirate syringe for I.M. injection to avoid inadvertent I.V. injection.

• Do not reconstitute with 0.9% sodium chloride; precipitation occurs.

• Reconstituted solution is stable for 14 days at room temperature. Store reconstituted solution in a light-resistant container.

Monitoring

• Monitor effectiveness by observing the patient for nausea and vomiting.

• Monitor blood pressure frequently.

• Monitor for signs of adverse CNS reactions (restlessness, drowsiness, excitation, tremors).

• Monitor for cardiac arrhythmia after I.V. administration.

Supportive Care

• Position patient on side. Keep an airway and suction equipment nearby in case of aspiration.

• Use safety precautions if adverse CNS reactions develop.

• Excellent alternative if prochlorperazine is contraindicated.

Patient Teaching

• Warn patient that drowsiness usually follows administration.

Evaluation

In patients receiving benzquinamide, hydrochloride, appropriate evaluation statements may include:

• Patient demonstrates no signs of aspiration induced by anesthesia or surgery.

• Patient exhibits no signs of impaired cardiopulmonary tissue perfusion.

• Patient and family state an understanding of benzquinamide therapy.

benztropine mesylate

(benz´ troe peen)

Apo-Benztropine†, Bensylate†, Cogentin, PMS Benztropine†

• *Classification:* antiparkinsonian agent (anticholinergic)

• *Pregnancy Risk Category:* C

HOW SUPPLIED

Tablets: 0.5 mg, 1 mg, 2 mg

Injection: 1 mg/ml in 2-ml ampules

ACTION

Mechanism: Blocks central cholinergic receptors, helping to balance cholinergic activity in the basal ganglia.

Distribution: Largely unknown; however, the drug crosses the blood-brain barrier and may cross the placenta.

Excretion: Like other muscarinics, excreted in the urine as unchanged drug and metabolites. After oral therapy, small amounts are probably excreted in feces as unabsorbed drug.

INDICATIONS & DOSAGE

Acute dystonic reaction–
Adults: 1 to 2 mg I.V. or I.M. followed by 1 to 2 mg P.O. b.i.d. to prevent recurrence.
Parkinsonism–
Adults: 0.5 to 6 mg P.O. daily. Initial dose is 0.5 mg to 1 mg. Increase 0.5 mg q 5 to 6 days. Adjust dosage to meet individual requirements. Usual dose is 1 to 2 mg per day.

CONTRAINDICATIONS & PRECAUTIONS

Contraindicated in patients with narrow-angle glaucoma because drug-induced cycloplegia and mydriasis may increase intraocular pressure.

Use cautiously in patients with prostatic hypertrophy because the drug may exacerbate urine retention; tachycardia because the drug may block vagal inhibition of the sinoatrial node pacemaker and exacerbate tachycardia; and in elderly patients and young children because they may be more susceptible to the drug's effects.

ADVERSE REACTIONS

Common reactions are in italics; life-threatening reactions are in bold italics.
CNS: disorientation, restlessness, irritability, incoherence, hallucinations, headache, sedation, depression, muscular weakness.
CV: palpitations, tachycardia, paradoxical bradycardia.
EENT: dilated pupils, blurred vision, photophobia, difficulty swallowing.
GI: *constipation, dry mouth,* nausea, vomiting, epigastric distress.
GU: urinary hesitancy, urine retention.
Skin: warming, dry, flushing.
Note: Some adverse reactions may be due to pending atropine-like toxicity and are dose related.

INTERACTIONS

Amantadine, phenothiazines, tricyclic antidepressants: additive anticholinergic adverse reactions, such as confusion and hallucinations. Reduce dosage before administering amantadine.

EFFECTS ON DIAGNOSTIC TESTS

None reported.

NURSING CONSIDERATIONS

Besides those related universally to drug therapy (see "How to use this book"), consider the following specific recommendations:

Assessment
- Obtain a baseline assessment of the patient's parkinsonian signs and symptoms before therapy.
- Be alert for adverse reactions and drug interactions throughout therapy.
- Evaluate the patient's and family's knowledge about benztropine therapy.

Nursing Diagnoses
- Impaired physical mobility related to underlying parkinsonism.
- Altered oral mucous membranes related to dry mouth, an adverse reaction to drug therapy.
- Knowledge deficit related to benztropine therapy.

Planning and Implementation
Preparation and Administration
- ***P.O. use:*** To help prevent GI distress, administer after meals.
- Never discontinue this drug abruptly. Dosage must be reduced gradually.
- If patient is to receive single daily dose, give at bedtime.
- ***I.V use:*** Rarely used because of small difference in onset time compared to I.M. route.

Monitoring
- Monitor effectiveness by regularly checking body movements for signs of improvement; full effect of drug may take 2 to 3 days.
- Monitor vital signs carefully. Watch closely for adverse reactions, espe-

cially in elderly or debilitated patients.
• Monitor for intermittent constipation, distention, and abdominal pain, which may signal onset of paralytic ileus.
• Regularly check oral mucous membranes for dryness.
• Monitor mental status and behavior closely.
• Monitor GU status for urinary hesitancy or urine retention.

Supportive Care
• Give the patient fluids, ice chips, sugarless gum, or hard candy to relieve dry mouth.
• Assist the patient with activities as needed, and institute safety precautions.

Patient Teaching
• Warn the patient to avoid hazardous activities that require alertness until CNS effects of the drug are known.
• Explain that drug may take 2 to 3 days to exert full effect.
• Advise the patient to report signs of urinary hesitancy and urine retention.
• Advise the patient to limit activities during hot weather because drug-induced anhydrosis may result in hyperthermia.
• Tell the patient to take the drug after meals to minimize GI discomfort.
• Warn the patient not to discontinue drug abruptly.
• Tell the patient how to manage troublesome adverse reactions, such as dry mouth.

Evaluation
In patients receiving benztropine, appropriate evaluation statements may include:
• Patient exhibits improved mobility with reduction in muscle rigidity, akinesia, and tremor.
• Patient maintains integrity of oral mucous membranes.
• Patient and family state an understanding of benztropine therapy.

bepridil hydrochloride
(be´ pri dil)
Vascor

• *Classification:* antianginal (calcium channel blocker)
• *Pregnancy Risk Category:* C

HOW SUPPLIED
Tablets: 200 mg, 300 mg, 400 mg

ACTION
Mechanism: A calcium channel blocking agent that inhibits calcium ion influx across cardiac and smooth muscle cells.
Absorption: Rapidly and completely absorbed after oral administration. Food does not impair absorption.
Distribution: Highly (more than 99%) bound to plasma proteins.
Metabolism: Hepatic.
Excretion: Over a 10-day period, approximately 70% of a single dose is excreted in urine and 22% in feces, as metabolites. Half-life: Biphasic with a distribution half-life of about 2 hours; terminal elimination half-life after multiple dosing averages 42 hours (range, 26 to 64 hours.)
Onset, peak, duration: Peak plasma levels occur 2 to 3 hours after an oral dose.

INDICATIONS & DOSAGE
Treatment of chronic stable angina in patients intolerant of or who fail to respond to other agents—
Adults: initially, 200 mg P.O. daily. After 10 days, increase dosage based on response. Maintenance dosage in most patients is 300 mg/day. Maximum daily dosage is 400 mg.

CONTRAINDICATIONS & PRECAUTIONS
Contraindicated in patients with hypersensitivity to the drug and in patients with a history of serious ven-

tricular arrhythmias, sick sinus syndrome, second- or third-degree atrioventricular block (except those with a functioning ventricular pacemaker), hypotension (below 90 mm Hg systolic), uncompensated cardiac insufficiency, congenital QT interval prolongation, and in patients who are taking other drugs that prolong the QT interval.

Use cautiously in patients with left bundle branch block or sinus bradycardia and serious renal or hepatic disorders.

ADVERSE REACTIONS

Common reactions are in italics; life-threatening reactions are in bold italics.
Blood: ***agranulocytosis.***
CNS: dizziness.
CV: edema, flushing, palpitations, tachycardia, ***ventricular arrhythmias.***
GI: nausea, diarrhea.
Skin: rash.
Other: dyspnea.

INTERACTIONS

Fentanyl anesthesia: severe hypotension has been reported with concomitant use of a beta blocker and a calcium channel blocker. Be sure to inform anesthesiologist that the patient is taking a calcium channel blocker.

EFFECTS ON DIAGNOSTIC TESTS

ALT (SGPT): increased levels.
Liver function tests: abnormal results.

NURSING CONSIDERATIONS

Besides those related universally to drug therapy (see "How to use this book"), consider the following specific recommendations:

Assessment
- Obtain a baseline assessment of the patient's anginal status before bepridil therapy.
- Be alert for adverse reactions and drug interactions throughout therapy.
- Evaluate the patient's and family's knowledge about bepridil therapy.

Nursing Diagnoses
- Pain related to ineffectiveness of bepridil therapy.
- Altered protection related to bepridil-induced ventricular arrhythmia.
- Knowledge deficit related to bepridil.

Planning and Implementation

Preparation and Administration
- ***P.O. use:*** Administer drug following usual protocol for oral drug administration.

Monitoring
- Monitor effectiveness by regularly evaluating the severity and frequency of the patient's anginal pain.
- Monitor patient's ECG, heart rate, and rhythm regularly.
- Monitor patient for unusual bruising or bleeding or any persistent infections.

Supportive Care
- Consult the doctor if the patient does not experience pain relief.
- Maintain safety precautions if dizziness occurs; assist the patient with daily activities to minimize energy expenditure.
- Restrict the patient's fluid and sodium intake to minimize edema.
- Obtain an order for an antiemetic or antidiarrheal agent as needed.

Patient Teaching
- Stress importance of taking the drug exactly as prescribed even when feeling well.
- Tell the patient to schedule activities to allow adequate rest.
- Encourage the patient to restrict fluid and sodium intake to minimize edema.

Evaluation

In patients receiving bepridil, appropriate evaluation statements may include:
- Patient states anginal pain relief occurs with bepridil therapy.
- Patient's ECG, heart rate, and

COMPARING BETA-ADRENERGIC BLOCKING AGENTS

DRUG	HALF-LIFE (HR)	LIPID SOLUBILITY	MEMBRANE-STABILIZING ACTIVITY	INTRINSIC SYMPATHOMIMETIC ACTIVITY
Nonselective				
carteolol	6	low	0	+ +
labetalol	6 to 8	moderate	0	0
metipranolol	4	low to moderate	0	0
nadolol	20	low	0	0
penbutolol	5	high	0	+
pindolol	3 to 4	moderate	+	+ + +
propranolol	4	high	+ +	0
timolol	4	low to moderate	0	0
Beta$_1$-selective				
acebutolol	3 to 4	low	+	+
atenolol	6 to 7	low	0	0
betaxolol	14 to 22	low	+	0
esmolol	0.15	low	0	0
metoprolol	3 to 7	moderate	*	0

* = only in higher-than-usual doses

rhythm are unchanged with bepridil therapy.

• Patient and family state an understanding of bepridil therapy.

PHARMACOLOGIC CLASS

beta-adrenergic blockers

beta$_1$ blockers
acebutolol
atenolol
metoprolol tartrate

beta$_1$ and beta$_2$ blockers
betaxolol hydrochloride
carteolol hydrochloride
esmolol
labetalol
levobunolol
metipranolol hydrochloride
nadolol
penbutolol
pindolol
propranolol
timolol maleate

OVERVIEW

Beta-adrenergic blocking agents were first used clinically in the early 1960s. They are chemicals that compete with beta agonists for available beta-receptor sites; individual agents differ in their ability to affect beta receptors. Most available agents are considered nonselective; that is, they block both beta$_1$ receptors in cardiac muscle and beta$_2$ receptors in bronchial and vascular smooth muscle. Several agents are cardioselective and in lower doses primarily inhibit beta$_1$ receptors. Some beta blockers have intrinsic sympathomimetic activity and simultaneously stimulate and block beta receptors, decreasing cardiac output; still others also have membrane-stabilizing activity, which affects cardiac action potential.

CLINICAL INDICATIONS AND ACTIONS

Hypertension

All currently available beta blockers are used to treat hypertension. Although the exact mechanism of their antihypertensive effect is unknown, the action is thought to result from decreased cardiac output, decreased sympathetic outflow from the CNS, and suppression of renin release.

Angina

Propranolol and nadolol are used to treat angina pectoris; they decrease myocardial oxygen requirements via blockade of catecholamine-induced increases in heart rate, blood pressure, and the extent of myocardial contraction.

Arrhythmia

Propranolol, acebutolol, and esmolol are used to treat arrhythmias; they prolong the refractory period of the atrioventricular (AV) node and slow AV conduction.

Glaucoma

The mechanism by which betaxolol, levobunolol, metipranolol, and timolol reduce intraocular pressure is unknown, but the drug effect is at least partially caused by decreased production of aqueous humor.

Myocardial infarction

Timolol, propranolol, and metoprolol are used to prevent myocardial infarction (MI) in susceptible patients; the mechanism of this protective effect is unknown.

Migraine prophylaxis

Propranolol is used to prevent recurrent attacks of migraine and other vascular headaches. The exact mechanism by which propranolol decreases the incidence of migraine headache attacks is unknown, but it is thought to result from inhibition of vasodilation of cerebral vessels.

Other uses

Beta blockers have been used as antianxiety agents, as adjunctive therapy of bleeding esophageal varices, and to treat portal hypertension.

OVERVIEW OF ADVERSE REACTIONS

Therapeutic doses of beta-adrenergic blockers usually cause bradycardia, fatigue, and dizziness; some may cause other CNS disturbances such as nightmares, depression, memory loss, and hallucinations. Impotence, cold extremities, and elevated serum cholesterol levels have been reported. Severe hypotension, bradycardia, heart failure, or bronchospasm usually indicates toxic dosage levels.

REPRESENTATIVE COMBINATIONS

Atenolol with chlorthalidone: Tenoretic.

Metoprolol with hydrochlorothiazide: Lopressor HCT.

Nadolol with bendroflumethiazide: Corzide.

Pindolol with hydrochlorothiazide: Viskazide.

Propranolol with hydrochlorothiazide: Inderide, Inderide LA.

Timolol with hydrochlorothiazide: Timolide.

---

betamethasone benzoate

(bay ta meth´ a sone)

Benisone, Uticort

betamethasone dipropionate

Alphatrex, Diprolene, Diprolene AF, Diprosone

betamethasone valerate

Betatrex, Beta-Val, Betnovate†‡, Valisone

- *Classification:* anti-inflammatory (topical glucocorticoid)
- *Pregnancy Risk Category:* C

HOW SUPPLIED

benzoate

Cream: 0.025%
Gel: 0.025%
Lotion: 0.025%
Ointment: 0.025%

dipropionate

Aerosol: 0.1%
Cream: 0.05%

Lotion: 0.05%
Ointment: 0.05%
valerate
Aerosol: 0.1%
Cream: 0.01%, 0.1%
Lotion: 0.1%
Ointment: 0.1%

ACTION

Mechanism: Produces local anti-inflammatory, vasoconstrictor, and antipruritic actions. Drug diffuses across cell membranes to form complexes with specific cytoplasmic receptors, influencing cellular metabolism. Corticosteroids stabilize leukocyte lysosomal membranes, inhibit local actions and accumulation of macrophages, decrease local edema, and reduce the formation of scar tissue.
Absorption: Amount absorbed depends on the amount applied and on the nature of the skin at the application site. Absorption ranges from about 1% in areas with thick stratum corneum (on the palms, soles, elbows, and knees) to as high as 36% in thinner areas (face, eyelids, and genitals). Absorption increases in areas of skin damage, inflammation, or occlusion. Some systemic absorption of topical steroids may occur, especially through the oral mucosa.
Distribution: After topical application, distributed throughout the local skin. If absorbed into the circulation, drug is rapidly removed from the blood and distributed into muscle, liver, skin, intestines, and kidneys.
Metabolism: After topical administration, metabolized primarily in the skin. The small amount absorbed into systemic circulation is metabolized primarily in the liver to inactive compounds.
Excretion: Inactive metabolites are excreted by the kidneys, primarily as glucuronides and sulfates, but also as unconjugated products. Small amounts of the metabolites are also excreted in feces.

INDICATIONS & DOSAGE

Inflammation of corticosteroid-responsive dermatoses–
Adults and children: clean area; apply cream, lotion, spray, or gel sparingly daily to q.i.d.

CONTRAINDICATIONS & PRECAUTIONS

Contraindicated in patients who are hypersensitive to any component of the preparation and in patients with viral, fungal, or tubercular skin lesions. Use with extreme caution in patients with impaired circulation, because it may increase the risk of skin ulceration.

ADVERSE REACTIONS

Common reactions are in italics; life-threatening reactions are in bold italics.
Skin: burning, itching, irritation, dryness, folliculitis, striae, acneiform eruptions, perioral dermatitis, hypopigmentation, hypertrichosis, allergic contact dermatitis. With occlusive dressings: *secondary infection, maceration, atrophy, striae, miliaria.*

INTERACTIONS

None significant.

EFFECTS ON DIAGNOSTIC TESTS

None reported.

NURSING CONSIDERATIONS

Besides those related universally to drug therapy (see "How to use this book"), consider the following specific recommendations:
Assessment
- Obtain a baseline assessment of skin in affected area before therapy.
- Be alert for adverse reactions and drug interactions throughout therapy.
- Evaluate the patient's and family's knowledge about topical betamethasone therapy.

Nursing Diagnoses
- Impaired skin integrity related to the patient's underlying condition.

• High risk for infection related to betamethasone-induced secondary infection.
• Knowledge deficit related to topical betamethasone therapy.

Planning and Implementation

Preparation and Administration

• ***Topical use:*** Before applying, gently wash skin. To prevent damage to skin, rub medication in gently, leaving a thin coat. When treating hairy sites, part hair and apply directly to lesion.
• To apply an occlusive dressing (if ordered): Apply cream, then cover with a thin, pliable nonflammable plastic film; seal to adjacent normal skin with hypoallergenic tape. Hold dressing in place with gauze, elastic bandages, stockings or stockinette, for patient with eczematous dermatitis who may develop irritation with adhesive material.

Monitoring

• Monitor effectiveness by regularly checking skin of affected area.
• Check patient's temperature; if fever occurs, notify doctor and remove occlusive dressing.
• Monitor for adverse reactions or interactions by frequently inspecting the patient's skin for infection, striae, and atrophy.
• Monitor for signs of systemic absorption, skin irritation or ulceration, hypersensitivity, or infection; if they occur, discontinue drug and notify doctor. (If antifungals or antibiotics are being used with corticosteroids, they should be stopped until infection is controlled.)

Supportive Care

• Change the patient's dressings as ordered by the doctor. Be prepared to discontinue drug and notify doctor if striae, atrophy, or infection occur.
• Expect treatment to continue for a few days after clearing of lesions to prevent recurrence.
• Note that Diprolene and Diprolene AF may not be substituted generically because other products have different potencies.
• Keep in mind that systemic absorption is especially likely with occlusive dressings, prolonged treatment, or extensive body-surface treatment.
• Use cautiously in viral skin diseases, such as varicella or herpes simplex; fungal infections and bacterial skin infections.
• When treating diaper area in young children, avoid the use of plastic pants or tight-fitting diaper.

Patient Teaching

• Teach patient how to apply medication.
• Instruct patient to avoid application near eyes, mucous membranes, or in ear canal.
• Inform patient that due to alcohol content of vehicle, gel preparations may cause mild, transient stinging, especially if used on or near excoriated skin.
• Tell patient to discontinue drug if fever or irritation occur and to notify the doctor.

Evaluation

In patients receiving topical betamethasone benzoate, appropriate evaluation statements may include:
• Patient states that his dermatoses is healing.
• Patient did not develop secondary infection.
• Patient and family state an understanding of topical betamethasone therapy.

betamethasone (systemic)

(bay ta meth´ a sone)

Betnelan†, Celestone*

betamethasone acetate and betamethasone sodium phosphate
Celestone Chronodose‡, Celestone Soluspan

betamethasone sodium phosphate
Betameth, Betnesol†, B.S.P., Celestone Phosphate, Cel-U-Jec, Prelestone, Selestoject

• *Classification:* anti-inflammatory agent (glucocorticoid)
• *Pregnancy Risk Category:* C

HOW SUPPLIED

betamethasone
Tablets: 600 mcg
Tablets (extended-release): 1 mg
Syrup: 600 mcg/5 ml
betamethasone acetate and betamethasone sodium phosphate
Injection: betamethasone acetate 3 mg and betamethasone sodium phosphate (equivalent to 3-mg base)/ml.
betamethasone sodium phosphate
Effervescent tablets: 500 mcg*
Injection: 4 mg (3-mg base)/ml in 5-ml vials

ACTION

Mechanism: Decreases inflammation, mainly by stabilizing leukocyte lysosomal membranes. Also suppresses the immune response, stimulates bone marrow, and influences protein, fat, and carbohydrate metabolism.
Absorption: Absorbed rapidly after oral administration. Systemic absorption occurs slowly following intra-articular injections.
Distribution: Rapidly removed from the blood and distributed to muscle, liver, skin, intestines, and kidneys; weakly bound to plasma proteins (transcortin and albumin). Only the unbound portion is active. Adrenocorticoids are distributed into breast milk and through the placenta.
Metabolism: In the liver to inactive glucuronide and sulfate metabolites.
Excretion: The inactive metabolites and small amounts of unmetabolized drug are excreted by the kidneys. Insignificant amounts are also excreted in feces. Half-life: 36 to 54 hours.
Onset, peak, duration: After oral and I.V. administration, peak effects occur in 1 to 2 hours. Onset and duration of action of the suspensions for injection vary, depending on whether they are injected into an intra-articular space or a muscle, and on the local blood supply.

INDICATIONS & DOSAGE

Severe inflammation or immunosuppression–
Adults: 0.6 to 7.2 mg P.O. daily; or 0.5 to 9 mg (sodium phosphate) I.M., I.V., or into joint or soft tissue daily; or 1.5 to 12 mg (sodium phosphate-acetate suspension) into joint or soft tissue q 1 to 2 weeks, p.r.n.
Prevention of neonatal respiratory distress syndrome–
Adults (pregnant women): 12 mg I.M. Celestone Soluspan 36 to 48 hours before premature delivery. Repeat in 24 hours.

CONTRAINDICATIONS & PRECAUTIONS

Contraindicated in patients with hypersensitivity to ingredients of adrenocorticoid preparations or with systemic fungal infections. Patients who are receiving betamethasone should not be given live virus vaccines because betamethasone suppresses the immune response.

Use with extreme caution in patients with GI ulceration, renal disease, hypertension, osteoporosis, diabetes mellitus, thromboembolic disorders, idiopathic thrombocytopenic purpura, seizures, myasthenia gravis, CHF, tuberculosis, hypoalbuminemia, hypothyroidism, cirrhosis of the liver, emotional instability, psychotic tendencies, hyperlipidemias, glaucoma, or cataracts because the drug may exacerbate these conditions.

Because adrenocorticoids increase susceptibility to and mask symptoms of infection, betamethasone should not be used (except in life-threatening situations) in patients with viral or bacterial infections not controlled by anti-infective agents.

ADVERSE REACTIONS

Common reactions are in italics; life-threatening reactions are in bold italics.

Most adverse reactions of corticosteroids are dose- or duration-dependent.

CNS: *euphoria, insomnia,* psychotic behavior, pseudotumor cerebri.
CV: *CHF,* hypertension, edema.
EENT: cataracts, glaucoma.
GI: *peptic ulcer,* GI irritation, increased appetite.
Metabolic: *possible hypokalemia, hyperglycemia and carbohydrate intolerance,* growth suppression in children.
Skin: delayed wound healing, acne, various skin eruptions.
Other: muscle weakness, pancreatitis, hirsutism, susceptibility to infections.
Acute adrenal insufficiency may follow increased stress (infection, surgery, or trauma) or abrupt withdrawal after long-term therapy.
Withdrawal symptoms: rebound inflammation, fatigue, weakness, arthralgia, fever, dizziness, lethargy, depression, fainting, orthostatic hypotension, dyspnea, anorexia, hypoglycemia. ***Sudden withdrawal may be fatal.***

INTERACTIONS

Barbiturates, phenytoin, rifampin: decreased corticosteroid effect. Corticosteroid dose may need to be increased.
Indomethacin, aspirin: increased risk of GI distress and bleeding. Give together cautiously.

EFFECTS ON DIAGNOSTIC TESTS

Diagnostic skin tests: suppressed reaction.
Glucose and cholesterol: increased levels.
Nitroblue tetrazolium tests: false-negative results.
Serum potassium, calcium, thyroxine, and triiodothyronine: decreased levels.
Thyroid function tests: decreased ^{131}I uptake and protein-bound iodine concentrations.
Urine glucose and calcium: increased levels.

NURSING CONSIDERATIONS

Besides those related universally to drug therapy (see "How to use this book"), consider the following specific recommendations:

Assessment
- Obtain a baseline assessment of the patient's condition before initiating drug therapy.
- Be alert for adverse reactions and drug interactions throughout drug therapy.
- Evaluate the patient's and family's knowledge about betamethasone therapy.

Nursing Diagnoses
- Impaired tissue integrity related to the patient's underlying condition.
- High risk for injury related to betamethasone-induced adverse reactions.
- Knowledge deficit related to betamethasone therapy.

Planning and Implementation
Preparation and Administration
- Do not use for alternate-day therapy.
- Gradually reduce drug dosage after long-term therapy. Never abruptly discontinue therapy as sudden withdrawal can be fatal.
- Always titrate to lowest effective dose as prescribed.
- Give a daily dosage in the morning for better results and less toxicity.

• Expect to increase dosage as prescribed during times of physiological stress (surgery, trauma, or infection).
• *P.O. use:* Give with food when possible to avoid GI upset.
• *I.M. use:* Give injection deep into gluteal muscle. Rotate injection sites to prevent muscle atrophy.
• *I.V. use:* When administering as direct injection, inject diluted dose directly into vein or into an I.V. line containing a free-flowing compatible solution over 5 to 10 minutes. When administering as an intermittent infusion, dilute solution according to manufacturer's instructions and give over 20 to 30 minutes. Not recommended for continuous infusion.

Monitoring

• Monitor effectiveness by regularly assessing for improvement of signs and symptoms of the underlying condition.
• Monitor the patient for adverse drug reactions as drug can cause serious or even life-threathening multisystem dysfunction.
• Monitor the patient's weight, blood pressure, blood glucose level, and serum electrolyte levels regularly.
• Monitor the patient for infection. Drug may mask or exacerbate infections.
• Monitor the patient's stress level. Stress (fever, trauma, surgery, or emotional problems) may increase adrenal insufficiency. Dose may have to be increased.
• Monitor growth in infants and children on long-term therapy.
• Monitor patients receiving immunizations for decreased antibody response.
• Monitor for early signs of adrenal insufficiency or cushingoid symptoms.

Supportive Care

• Notify the doctor immediately if serious adverse drug reactions occur, and be prepared to administer supportive care.
• Unless contraindicated, give the patient a low-sodium diet high in potassium and protein. Potassium supplement may be needed.

Patient Teaching

• Be sure that the patient understands the need to take the drug as prescribed. Give the patient instructions on what to do if a dose is inadvertently missed.
• Warn the patient not to discontinue the drug abruptly or without the doctor's approval.
• Advise the patient to take oral form with meals to minimize GI adverse reactions.
• Inform the patient of the possible therapeutic and adverse effects of the drug, so that he may report complications to the doctor as soon as possible.
• Tell the patient to carry a medical alert card indicating the need for supplemental adrenocorticoids during stress.
• Teach the patient to recognize signs of early adrenal insufficiency (fatigue, muscular weakness, joint pain, fever, anorexia, nausea, dyspnea, dizziness, and fainting) and to notify the doctor promptly if they occur.
• Warn patients on long-term therapy about cushingoid symptoms, which may develop regardless of route of administration.
• Tell patient to eat a low-sodium diet that is high in potassium and protein unless contraindicated.

Evaluation

In patients receiving betamethasone, appropriate evaluation statements may include:
• Patient's condition being treated with betamethasone therapy shows improvement.
• Patient injury did not occur; patient did not experience serious adverse reactions associated with betamethasone.
• Patient and family state an understanding of betamethasone therapy.

betaxolol hydrochloride (ophthalmic)

(be tax´ oh lol)
Betoptic

• *Classification:* antiglaucoma agent (beta-adrenergic blocking agent)
• *Pregnancy Risk Category:* C

HOW SUPPLIED

Ophthalmic solution: 5 mg/ml (0.5%) in 5-ml, 10-ml dropper bottles

ACTION

Mechanism: Selectively blocks $beta_1$-adrenergic receptors. Reduces formation of aqueous humor, and possibly increases its outflow from the eye.
Absorption: Minimal after ophthalmic use.
Excretion: Primarily renal (about 80%). Half-life: Elimination half-life is prolonged in patients with hepatic disease, but clearance is not affected, so dosage adjustment is unnecessary. Plasma half-life is 14 to 22 hours.
Onset, peak, duration: Onset, about 30 minutes; peak effect, about 2 hours; duration, about 12 hours.

INDICATIONS & DOSAGE

Chronic open-angle glaucoma and ocular hypertension—
Adults: instill 1 drop of 0.5% solution in eyes b.i.d.

CONTRAINDICATIONS & PRECAUTIONS

Contraindicated in patients hypersensitive to any ingredient in the formulation.

Use cautiously in patients with angle-closure glaucoma (use with miotic), or muscle weakness (myasthenic-like symptoms).

ADVERSE REACTIONS

Common reactions are in italics; life-threatening reactions are in bold italics.
CNS: insomnia, confusion.
Eye: *stinging upon instillation,* occasional tearing, photophobia.

INTERACTIONS

Calcium channel blocking agents: AV conduction disturbances, ventricular failure, hypotension if significant systemic absorption occurs.
Cocaine: may inhibit betaxolol's effects.
Digitalis glycosides: excessive bradycardia; may require ECG monitoring if significant systemic absorption occurs.
Dipivefrin, ophthalmic epinephrine: may produce mydriasis.
Inhalational hydrocarbon anesthetics: prolonged severe hypotension if significant systemic absorption occurs.
Insulin, oral hypoglycemics: dosage adjustments or hypoglycemic medication may be necessary because of the risk of hypoglycemia or hyperglycemia if significant systemic absorption occurs.
Phenothiazines: additive hypotensive effects, increased risk of side effects if significant systemic absorption occurs.
Reserpine: excessive beta blockade.
Systemic beta blockers: additive effects.

EFFECTS ON DIAGNOSTIC TESTS

None reported.

NURSING CONSIDERATIONS

Besides those related universally to drug therapy (see "How to use this book"), consider the following specific recommendations:

Assessment
• Obtain a baseline assessment of the patient's visual status, ocular pressure, and vital signs.
• Be alert for adverse reactions and drug interactions throughout therapy.
• Evaluate the patient's and family's knowledge about betaxolol hydrochloride therapy.

Nursing Diagnoses
• Sensory/perceptual alterations (visual) related to the patient's underlying condition.
• Altered sleep patterns related to possible CNS adverse effects.
• Knowledge deficit related to betaxolol hydrochloride therapy.

Planning and Implementation

Preparation and Administration
• Instill in lacrimal sac; remove excess solution from around eyes with a clean tissue or gauze and apply light finger pressure to lacrimal sac for 1 minute.

Monitoring
• Monitor effectiveness by assessing the patient's visual status and intraacular pressure. Some patients may require a few weeks to stabilize their response. Determine intraocular pressure after 4 weeks of treatment.
• Monitor blood pressure and apical rate for drug-induced hypotension and bradycardia; obtain EKG as indicated especially if patient has underlyinq cardiac disease.

Supportive Care
• Notify the doctor immediately if changes in the patient's health status occur.
• Encourage the patient to try relaxation techniques if insomnia occurs. Notify the doctor if patient feels insomnia is a serious problem.

Patient Teaching
• Teach the patient how to instill the solution and advise him to wash his hands before and after administering the drug.
• Warn the patient not to exceed the recommended dosage and encourage compliance with the prescribed regimen (usually BID).
• Advise the patient to continue with regular medical supervision during therapy.
• Warn the patient that transient stinging may follow instillation.
• Advise the patient to wear dark glasses in bright weather to ease discomfort from photophobia.
• Warn diabetic patients that betaxolol may require adjustments of insulin or hypoglycemic dosage, and close monitoring of blood glucose.

Evaluation

In patients receiving betaxolol hydrochloride, appropriate evaluation statements may include:
• Patient experiences therapeutic reduction in ocular pressure.
• Patient remains free of insomnia.
• Patient and family state an understanding of betaxolol hydrochloride therapy.

betaxolol hydrochloride (systemic)

(be tax´ oh lol)
Kerlone

• *Classification:* antihypertensive (beta-adrenergic blocking agent)
• *Pregnancy Risk Category:* C

HOW SUPPLIED

Tablets: 10 mg, 20 mg

ACTION

Mechanism: A $beta_1$-selective blocking agent that decreases blood pressure, probably by slowing heart rate and decreasing cardiac output.
Absorption: Essentially complete after oral administration; minimal after ophthalmic use. A small first-pass effect reduces bioavailability by about 10%. Absorption is not affected by food.
Distribution: About 50% bound to plasma proteins.
Metabolism: Hepatic; about 85% of the drug is recovered in the urine as metabolites.
Excretion: Primarily renal (about 80%). Half-life: 14 to 22 hours; prolonged in patients with hepatic dis-

ease, but clearance is not affected, so dosage adjustment in unnecessary.
Onset, peak, duration: Peak concentrations in plasma occur about 3 hours (range, 1.5 to 6 hours) after a single oral dose.

INDICATIONS & DOSAGE

Management of hypertension (used alone or with other antihypertensives) –
Adults: initially, 10 mg P.O. once daily. After 7 to 14 days, full antihypertensive effect should be seen. If necessary, may double dosage to 20 mg P.O. once daily.

CONTRAINDICATIONS & PRECAUTIONS

Contraindicated in patients with bronchial asthma, a history of bronchial asthma, or severe chronic obstructive pulmonary disease, sinus bradycardia, second- or third-degree atrioventricular block, CHF, cardiac failure, or cardiogenic shock because the drug may worsen these symptoms or conditions and in hypersensitivity to any components of the preparation.

Use cautiously in patients with angle-closure glaucoma (use with miotic), muscle weakness (myasthenic-like symptoms), or a history of heart failure or restricted pulmonary function because the drug may worsen these symptoms or conditions; or in patients with diabetes mellitus because the drug may mask some signs of hypoglycemia, such as tachycardia.

Use cautiously in patients with CHF controlled by digitalis and diuretics because beta-adrenergic blocking agents do not block the inotropic effects of digitalis. Patients with a history of CHF but no overt symptoms may exhibit signs of cardiac decompensation with oral beta blocker therapy.

Patients with bronchospastic disease (asthma, chronic bronchitis, emphysema) should avoid beta-blocker-receptor antagonism from cardioselective agents, such as betaxolol. However, some clinicians prescribe them for such patients who cannot tolerate other antihypertensives. Patients with unrecognized coronary artery disease may exhibit signs of angina pectoris upon rapid withdrawal of the drug.

Beta blockade may block the signs and symptoms of hypoglycemia (such as tachycardia and blood pressure changes) and may inhibit glycogenolysis. Beta blocking agents may mask tachycardia associated with hyperthyroidism. In patients suspected of having thyrotoxicosis, beta blocker therapy should be withdrawn gradually to avoid thyroid storm.

The anesthesiologist should be informed that the patient is receiving a beta blocking agent so that isoproterenol or dobutamine is made readily available for the reversal of the drug's cardiac effects.

ADVERSE REACTIONS

Common reactions are in italics; life-threatening reactions are in bold italics.
CV: bradycardia, chest pain, hypotension, worsening of angina, peripheral vascular insufficiency, ***CHF,*** edema, syncope, postural hypotension, conduction disturbances.
CNS: dizziness, fatigue, headache, lethargy, anxiety.
GI: flatulence, constipation, nausea, diarrhea, dry mouth, vomiting, anorexia.
Respiratory: dyspnea, wheezing, ***bronchospasm.***
Skin: rash.

INTERACTIONS

Calcium channel blocking agents: increased risk of hypotension, left ventricular failure, and AV conduction disturbances. I.V. calcium antagonists should be used with caution.

General anesthetics: increased hypotensive effects. Observe carefully for excessive hypotension or bradycardia, or orthostatic hypotension.
Lidocaine: beta blockers may increase the effects of lidocaine.
Reserpine, catecholamine-depleting drugs: may have an additive effect when administered with a beta blocker.

EFFECTS ON DIAGNOSTIC TESTS

Glucose tolerance tests: altered results.
Serum glucose: decreased levels.

NURSING CONSIDERATIONS

Besides those related universally to drug therapy (see "How to use this book"), consider the following specific recommendations:

Assessment

- Obtain a baseline assessment of patient's blood pressure before drug therapy.
- Be alert for adverse reactions and drug interactions throughout therapy.
- Evaluate the patient's and family's knowledge about betaxolol therapy.

Nursing Diagnoses

- High risk for injury related to patient's underlying condition.
- Decreased cardiac output related to betaxolol-induced cardiovascular adverse reactions.
- Knowledge deficit related to betaxolol therapy.

Planning and Implementation

Preparation and Administration

- Don't discontinue abruptly in patients with suspected thyrotoxicosis; withdraw gradually to avoid thyroid storm.
- Be aware that withdrawal of beta blocker therapy before surgery is controversial. Some clinicians advocate withdrawal to prevent any impairment of cardiac responsiveness to reflex stimuli and decreased responsiveness to administration of catecholamines.

Monitoring

- Monitor effectiveness by frequently checking patient's blood pressure.
- Monitor patient for conditions, such as bradycardia, hypotension, or CHF, that may cause decreased cardiac output as a result of drug therapy.
- Regularly monitor patient for signs of angina pectoris upon withdrawal of drug.
- Regularly monitor serum potassium level as hyperkalemia may occur.
- Regularly monitor for abnormalities of CBC and renal function studies.
- Closely monitor diabetic patient's blood glucose level. Drug may mask glycogenolysis and the signs and symptoms of hypoglycemia (such as tachycardia and blood pressure changes).
- Monitor hyperthyroid patient closely for signs of thyroid storm. Remember that drug may mask tachycardia associated with hyperthyroidism.

Supportive Care

- Be prepared to treat thyroid storm or hypoglycemia because drug masks common signs of thyroid storm and hypoglycemia.
- Inform the anesthesiologist that the patient is receiving a beta blocking agent so that isoproterenol or dobutamine is made readily available for reversal of the cardiac effects of the drug.
- Institute safety measures if lethargy occurs.
- Notify doctor immediately if patient shows signs of decreased cardiac output, such as hypotension, bradycardia, or changes in level of consciousness, and be prepared to provide supportive measures as prescribed.
- Assist patient with activities and provide frequent rest periods if patient experiences fatigue.

Patient Teaching

- Explain the importance of taking this drug as prescribed, even when feeling well. Tell patient not to dis-

continue drug suddenly but to call the doctor if unpleasant adverse reactions occur.
• Emphasize the importance of promptly reporting shortness of breath or difficulty breathing, unusually fast heartbeat, cough, or fatigue with exertion.
• Warn patient that drug may cause loss of taste.
• Stress importance of regular blood and urine studies as ordered to detect adverse drug reactions.
Evaluation
In patients receiving betaxolol, appropriate evaluation statements may include:
• Patient's blood pressure is within normal limits.
• Patient's cardiac output remains unchanged throughout drug therapy.
• Patient and family state an understanding of betaxolol therapy.

bethanechol chloride
(be than´ e kole)
Duvoid, Urabeth, Urecholine, Urocarb Liquid‡, Urocarb Tablets‡

• *Classification:* urinary tract and GI tract stimulant (cholinergic agonist)
• *Pregnancy Risk Category:* C

HOW SUPPLIED
Tablets: 5 mg, 10 mg, 25 mg, 50 mg
Liquid: 1 mg/5 ml‡
Injection: 5 mg/ml

ACTION
Mechanism: Binds to cholinergic (muscarinic) receptors, mimicking the action of acetylcholine.
Absorption: Poorly absorbed from the GI tract (absorption varies considerably among patients).
Distribution: Largely unknown; however, therapeutic doses do not penetrate the blood-brain barrier.
Onset, peak, duration: After oral administration, action usually begins in 30 minutes to 1½ hours; after S.C. administration, in 5 to 15 minutes. Usual duration of effect after oral administration is 1 hour; after S.C. administration, up to 2 hours.

INDICATIONS & DOSAGE
Acute postoperative and postpartum nonobstructive (functional) urine retention, neurogenic atony of urinary bladder with retention, abdominal distention, megacolon, or reflux esophagitis caused by low esophageal sphincter pressure–
Adults: 10 to 30 mg P.O. b.i.d. to q.i.d. Or, 2.5 to 10 mg S.C. Never give I.M. or I.V. When used for urine retention, some patients may require 50 to 100 mg P.O. per dose. Use such doses with extreme caution.

Test dose is 2.5 mg S.C. repeated at 15- to 30-minute intervals to total of 4 doses to determine the minimal effective dose; then use minimal effective dose q 6 to 8 hours. All doses must be adjusted individually.

CONTRAINDICATIONS & PRECAUTIONS
Contraindicated in patients with uncertain bladder wall strength or integrity; conditions in which increased muscular activity of the GI or urinary tract poses a risk; mechanical obstruction of the GI or urinary tract because of drug's stimulatory effect on smooth muscle; bradycardia, vagotonia, hyperthyroidism, hypotension, or Parkinson's disease because the drug may exacerbate these conditions; seizure disorders because of the drug's possible CNS stimulatory effects; cardiac or coronary artery disease because of stimulatory effects on the cardiovascular system; peptic ulcer because drug may stimulate gastric acid secretion; and asthma because the drug may precipitate asthma attacks.

Use cautiously in patients with hypertension and vasomotor instability because of its stimulatory effects and in patients with peritonitis or other acute GI inflammatory conditions because the drug may aggravate these conditions.

ADVERSE REACTIONS

Common reactions are in italics; life-threatening reactions are in bold italics.
Dose-related:
CNS: headache, malaise.
CV: bradycardia, hypotension, *cardiac arrest,* reflex tachycardia.
EENT: lacrimation, miosis.
GI: *abdominal cramps, diarrhea,* salivation, nausea, vomiting, belching, borborygmus, esophageal spasms.
GU: urinary urgency.
Skin: flushing, sweating.
Other: ***bronchoconstriction,*** increased bronchial secretions.

INTERACTIONS

Atropine, anticholinergic agents, procainamide, quinidine: may reverse cholinergic effects. Observe for lack of drug effect.

EFFECTS ON DIAGNOSTIC TESTS

Serum amylase, lipase, bilirubin, and AST (SGOT): increased levels.
Sulfobromophthalein retention time: increased.

NURSING CONSIDERATIONS

Besides those related universally to drug therapy (see "How to use this book"), consider the following specific recommendations:

Assessment

- Obtain a baseline assessment of the patient's underlying condition before drug therapy.
- Be alert for adverse reactions and drug interactions throughout therapy.
- Evaluate the patient's and family's knowledge about bethanechol chloride therapy.

Nursing Diagnoses

- Altered urinary elimination related to patient's underlying condition.
- Ineffective breathing pattern related to adverse drug reactions.
- Knowledge deficit related to bethanechol chloride therapy.

Planning and Implementation

Preparation and Administration

- Drug should never be given I.M. or I.V.; could cause circulatory collapse, hypotension, severe abdominal cramping, bloody diarrhea, shock, or cardiac arrest.
- ***P.O. use:*** Larger doses may be required due to poor and variable oral absorption. Oral and S.C. doses are not interchangeable.
- Drug is usually effective 5 to 15 minutes after injection and 30 minutes to 1½ hours after oral use.
- Give on an empty stomach; if taken after meals, may cause nausea and vomiting.
- Discontinue all other cholinergics before giving this drug.

Monitoring

- Monitor closely for adverse reactions that may indicate drug toxicity, especially with S.C. administration, by frequently checking vital signs, especially respirations.
- Monitor intake and output frequently.
- Monitor for lack of drug effect if the patient is also receiving atropine, anticholinergic agents, procainamide, or quinidine.
- Monitor for diarrhea; if present, assess hydration status frequently.

Supportive Care

- Provide respiratory support, if adverse reactions occur.
- Be prepared to insert a rectal tube to help passage of gas, if ordered, when the drug is used to prevent abdominal distention and GI distress.
- Provide the patient with a bedpan if the drug is used to treat urine retention.
- Have atropine injection readily

available and be prepared to give atropine 0.5 mg subcutaneously or slow I.V. push, as ordered.

Patient Teaching

• Advise the patient to take oral dose on an empty stomach.

• Tell the patient drug is usually effective 30 minutes to 1½ hours after oral use and 5 to 15 minutes after injection.

Evaluation

In patients receiving bethanechol, appropriate evaluation statements may include:

• The patient is able to void without urine retention.

• The patient's respiratory function remains normal.

• Patient and family state an understanding of bethanechol therapy.

biperiden hydrochloride

(bye per´ i den)

Akineton

biperiden lactate

Akineton Lactate

• *Classification:* antiparkinsonian agent (anticholinergic)

• *Pregnancy Risk Category:* C

HOW SUPPLIED

Tablets: 2 mg

Injection: 5 mg/ml in 1-ml ampules

ACTION

Mechanism: Blocks central cholinergic receptors, helping to balance cholinergic activity in the basal ganglia.

Excretion: In the urine as unchanged drug and metabolites. After oral therapy, small amounts are probably excreted as unabsorbed drug.

INDICATIONS & DOSAGE

Extrapyramidal disorders–

Adults: 2 to 6 mg P.O. daily, b.i.d., or t.i.d., depending on severity. Usual dose is 2 mg daily, or 2 mg I.M. or I.V. q half hour, not to exceed 4 doses or 8 mg total daily.

Parkinsonism–

Adults: 2 mg P.O. t.i.d. to q.i.d. Some patients may require as much as 16 mg per day.

CONTRAINDICATIONS & PRECAUTIONS

Use cautiously in patients with prostatic hypertrophy because the drug may exacerbate urine retention; cardiac arrhythmias because it may block vagal inhibition of the sinoatrial node pacemaker; or narrow-angle glaucoma because drug-induced cycloplegia and mydriasis may increase intraocular pressure.

ADVERSE REACTIONS

Common reactions are in italics; life-threatening reactions are in bold italics.

CNS: disorientation, euphoria, restlessness, irritability, incoherence, dizziness, increased tremor.

CV: transient postural hypotension (with parenteral use).

EENT: blurred vision.

GI: *constipation, dry mouth,* nausea, vomiting, epigastric distress.

GU: urinary hesitancy, urine retention.

Note: Adverse reactions are dose-related and may resemble atropine toxicity.

INTERACTIONS

Phenothiazines, tricyclic antidepressants: excessive CNS anticholinergic effects.

EFFECTS ON DIAGNOSTIC TESTS

None reported.

NURSING CONSIDERATIONS

Besides those related universally to drug therapy (see "How to use this book"), consider the following specific recommendations:

Assessment
• Obtain a baseline assessment of the patient's parkinsonian signs and symptoms before therapy.
• Be alert for adverse reactions and drug interactions throughout therapy.
• Evaluate the patient's and family's knowledge about biperiden therapy.
Nursing Diagnoses
• Impaired physical mobility related to underlying parkinsonism or other extrapyramidal disorders.
• High risk for injury related to biperiden's adverse effect on the CNS.
• Knowledge deficit related to biperiden therapy.
Planning and Implementation
Preparation and Administration
• ***P.O. use:*** Give oral doses with or after meals to decrease GI adverse reactions.
• ***I.V. use:*** Inject I.V. drug slowly.
• ***Parenteral use:*** Keep patient supine for parenteral injections. Parenteral administration may cause transient postural hypotension and coordination disturbances.
• Keep in mind that tolerance may develop and require increased dosage.
Monitoring
• Monitor effectiveness by regularly checking body movements for signs of improvement. However, be aware that in severe parkinsonism, tremors may increase as spasticity is relieved.
• Monitor vital signs carefully. Watch closely for adverse reactions, especially in elderly or debilitated patients.
• Regularly check oral mucous membranes for dryness.
• Monitor mental status and behavior closely.
• Monitor GU status for urinary hesitancy or urine retention.
Supportive Care
• Notify the doctor if the patient develops serious adverse reactions that may require dosage reduction.
• Give the patient fluids, ice chips, sugarless gum, or hard candy to relieve dry mouth.
• Assist the patient with activities as needed, and institute safety precautions. Because of possible dizziness, help patient when he gets out of bed.
Patient Teaching
• Warn the patient to avoid hazardous activities that require alertness until CNS effects of the drug are known.
• Advise the patient to report signs of urinary hesitancy or urine retention.
• Suggest measures for relieving dry mouth.
• Tell the patient to take the drug after meals to minimize GI discomfort.
• Tell the family to notify the nurse or doctor if CNS adverse reactions develop.
Evaluation
In patients receiving biperiden, appropriate evaluation statements may include:
• Patient exhibits improved mobility with reduction in muscle rigidity and tremor.
• Patient's safety is maintained and no adverse CNS reactions occur.
• Patient and family state an understanding of biperiden therapy.

bisacodyl
(bis a koe´ dill)
Bisacolax†◇, Bisalax‡, Bisco-Lax**◇, Dacodyl◇, Deficol◇, Dulcolax◇, Durolax‡, Fleet Bisacodyl◇, Laxit†◇, Theralax◇

• *Classification:* stimulant laxative (diphenylmethane derivative)
• *Pregnancy Risk Category:* C

HOW SUPPLIED
Tablets (enteric-coated): 5 mg◇
Enema: 33 mg/dl◇, 10 mg/5 ml (microenema)‡
Powder for rectal solution (bisacodyl

tannex): 1.5 mg bisacodyl and 2.5 g tannic acid
Suppositories: 5 mg◇, 10 mg◇

ACTION

Mechanism: A stimulant laxative that increases peristalsis by direct effect on the smooth muscle of the intestine. Thought either to irritate the musculature or to stimulate the colonic intramural plexus. Also promotes fluid accumulation in the colon and small intestine.
Absorption: Minimal.
Distribution: Locally distributed.
Metabolism: Up to 15% of an oral dose may enter the enterohepatic circulation.
Excretion: Primarily in feces; some in urine.
Onset, peak, duration: Action begins 6 to 8 hours after oral administration and 15 minutes to 1 hour after rectal administration.

INDICATIONS & DOSAGE

Chronic constipation; preparation for delivery, surgery, or rectal or bowel examination–
Adults: 10 to 15 mg P.O. in evening or before breakfast. Up to 30 mg may be used for thorough evacuation needed for examinations or surgery.
Children 6 years and older: 5 to 10 mg P.O.
Adults and children over 2 years: 10 mg rectally.
Children under 2 years: 5 mg rectally.

CONTRAINDICATIONS & PRECAUTIONS

Contraindicated in patients with fluid and electrolyte disturbances, appendicitis, any abdominal condition necessitating immediate surgery, ulcerative colitis, rectal fissures, ulcerated hemorrhoids, fecal impaction, and intestinal obstruction because the drug may exacerbate these conditions.

Chronic use may decrease serum potassium levels.

Bisacodyl tannex should not be used if multiple enemas are to be administered because significant absorption of tannic acid may result in hepatotoxicity.

ADVERSE REACTIONS

Common reactions are in italics; life-threatening reactions are in bold italics.
CNS: muscle weakness in excessive use.
GI: *nausea, vomiting, abdominal cramps,* diarrhea with high doses, *burning sensation in rectum with suppositories.*
Metabolic: alkalosis, hypokalemia, tetany, protein-losing enteropathy in excessive use, fluid and electrolyte imbalance.
Other: laxative dependence in long-term or excessive use.

INTERACTIONS

None significant.

EFFECTS ON DIAGNOSTIC TESTS

None reported.

NURSING CONSIDERATIONS

Besides those related universally to drug therapy (see "How to use this book"), consider the following specific recommendations:

Assessment

- Obtain a baseline assessment of history of bowel disorder, GI status, fluid intake, nutritional status, exercise habits, and normal pattern of elimination.
- Be alert for adverse reactions or drug interactions throughout therapy.
- Evaluate the patient's and family's knowledge about bisacodyl.

Nursing Diagnoses

- Constipation related to interruption of normal pattern of elimination characterized by infrequent or absent stools.

• Pain related to bisacodyl-induced abdominal cramps.
• Knowledge deficit related to bisacodyl therapy.

Planning and Implementation

Preparation and Administration

• Read order carefully; determine correct form of bisacodyl required.
• Store tablets and suppositories at temperature below 86° F (30° C).
• Do not give within 30 minutes of milk or antacid intake.
• Schedule administration of drug to avoid interfering with scheduled activities or sleep.
• Insert suppositories as high as possible into the rectum, and try to position the suppository against the rectal wall. Avoid embedding in fecal material because this may delay onset of action.
• Tablets and suppositories may be used together to cleanse colon before and after surgery and before barium enema.

Monitoring

• Monitor effectiveness by checking frequency and characteristics of stools.
• Auscultate bowel sounds at least once a shift. Assess pain and cramping.
• Monitor nutritional status and fluid intake.

Supportive Care

• Do not give to patients with abdominal pain, nausea, vomiting, or other symptoms of appendicitis or acute surgical abdomen, or in rectal fissures or ulcerated hemorrhoids.
• Oral preparation begins to act 6 to 12 hours after administration.
• Soft, formed stool is usually produced 15 minutes to 1 hour after rectal administration.
• Be aware that bisacodyl is for short-term treatment. This type of laxative—that is, a stimulant laxative—is the most commonly abused.
• Unless contraindicated, encourage fluid intake of 2500 ml a day.
• Consult with dietitian to modify diet to increase fiber and bulk.

Patient Teaching

• Warn the patient that bisacodyl works by increasing GI peristalsis and is likely to cause cramping. Reassure patient that cramps diminish as the colon empties.
• Tell patient to swallow enteric-coated tablets whole to avoid GI irritation.
• Discourage excessive use of laxatives.
• Teach patients about the relationship between fluid intake, exercise, dietary fiber, and constipation. Assist them to develop a plan to incorporate these elements into their lifestyle.
• Inform the patient about good sources of dietary fiber; bran and other cereals, fresh fruit and vegetables.

Evaluation

In patients receiving bisacodyl, appropriate evaluation statements may include:
• Patient reports return of normal pattern of elimination.
• Patient is free from abdominal pain and cramping.
• Patient and family state an understanding of bisacodyl therapy.

bismuth subgallate

(bis´ meth)

Devrom◇

bismuth subsalicylate

Maximum Strength Pepto-Bismol Liquid◇, Pepto-Bismol◇

• *Classification:* antidiarrheal (adsorbent)
• *Pregnancy Risk Category:* C (D in third trimester)

HOW SUPPLIED

subgallate
Tablets (chewable): 200 mg◇
subsalicylate
Tablets (chewable): 262 mg◇
Oral suspension: 262 mg/15 ml◇, 525 mg/15 ml◇

ACTION

Mechanism: Has water-binding capacity; also may adsorb toxins and provide protective coating for mucosa.
Absorption: Poorly absorbed; significant salicylate absorption may occur after using bismuth subsalicylate.
Distribution: Locally distributed in the gut.
Metabolism: Minimally metabolized.
Excretion: Salicylate is excreted in urine.

INDICATIONS & DOSAGE

Mild, nonspecific diarrhea –
Adults: 1 to 2 tablets P.O. chewed or swallowed whole t.i.d. (subgallate).
Adults: 30 ml or 2 tablets P.O. q ½ to 1 hour up to a maximum of 8 doses and for no longer than 2 days (subsalicylate).
Children 9 to 12 years: 20 ml or 1 tablet P.O.
Children 6 to 9 years: 10 ml or ⅔ tablet P.O.
Children 3 to 6 years: 5 ml or ⅓ tablet P.O.
Prevention and treatment of traveler's diarrhea (turista) –
Adults: prophylactically, 60 ml (bismuth subsalicylate) P.O. q.i.d. during the first 2 weeks of travel. During acute illness, 30 to 60 ml P.O. q 30 minutes for a total of 8 doses. Alternatively, 2 tablets P.O. q.i.d. for up to 3 weeks.

CONTRAINDICATIONS & PRECAUTIONS

Contraindicated in patients with hypersensitivity to salicylates. Use with caution in patients who are taking aspirin.

ADVERSE REACTIONS

Common reactions are in italics; life-threatening reactions are in bold italics.
GI: temporary darkening of tongue and stools.
Other: salicylism (high doses).

INTERACTIONS

Oral anticoagulants, oral hypoglycemic agents: theoretical risk of increased effects of these agents following high doses of bismuth subsalicylate. Monitor patient closely.
Probenecid: theoretical risk of decreased uricosuric effects following high doses of bismuth subsalicylate. Monitor patient closely.

EFFECTS ON DIAGNOSTIC TESTS

Radiologic GI examination: interference because bismuth is radiopaque.

NURSING CONSIDERATIONS

Besides those related universally to drug therapy (see "How to use this book"), consider the following specific recommendations:

Assessment
- Obtain a baseline assessment of history of bowel disorder, GI status, and frequency of loose stools before therapy.
- Be alert for adverse reactions or drug interactions throughout therapy.
- Evaluate the patient's and family's knowledge about bismuth subgallate or bismuth subsalicylate therapy.

Nursing Diagnoses
- Diarrhea related to interruption of normal pattern of elimination characterized by frequent loose stools.
- Sensory/perceptual alteration (auditory) related to bismuth subsalicylate-induced salicylism.
- Knowledge deficit related to bismuth subgallate or bismuth subsalicylate therapy.

Planning and Implementation
Preparation and Administration
- ***P.O. use:*** Liquid and tablet forms available.

• Read label carefully because dosage varies with form of drug.

Monitoring

• Monitor effectiveness by checking the frequency and characteristics of stools.

• Auscultate bowel sounds at least once a shift. Assess for pain and cramping.

• Monitor fluid and electrolyte balance.

• Weigh patient daily until diarrhea is controlled to detect fluid loss or retention.

• Check skin daily to detect and prevent breakdown in the perianal area.

• Check hearing if patient is taking bismuth subsalicylate in large doses.

Supportive Care

• Encourage patient to drink fluids to prevent fluid loss.

• Provide good skin care especially in the perianal area; apply soothing powders and lotion.

• Consult with dietitian to modify diet to help control diarrhea.

• Discontinue if tinnitus occurs.

• Consult with doctor before giving bismuth subsalicylate to children or teenagers during or after recovery from the flu or chicken pox.

Patient Teaching

• Warn the patient that bismuth subsalicylate contains a large amount of salicylate (each tablet provides 102 mg salicylate; the regular strength liquid provides 130 mg/15 ml).

• Instruct the patient to chew the tablets well.

• Advise the patient that both the liquid and tablet forms of Pepto-Bismol are effective against traveler's diarrhea. Tablets may be more convenient to carry.

• Inform the patient that the drug may cause temporary darkening of the tongue and stools.

• Instruct the patient to report changes in hearing or ringing in ears immediately.

Evaluation

In patients receiving bismuth subgallate or bismuth subsalicylate, appropriate evaluation statements may include:

• Patient reports decrease or absence in loose stools.

• Patient remains free from signs and symptoms of salicylism.

• Patient and family state an understanding of bismuth subgallate or bismuth subsalicylate therapy.

bitolterol mesylate

(bye tole´ ter ole)

Tornalate

• *Classification:* bronchodilator ($beta_2$-adrenergic agonist)

• *Pregnancy Risk Category:* C

HOW SUPPLIED

Aerosol inhaler: 370 mcg/metered spray

ACTION

Mechanism: Relaxes bronchial smooth muscle by acting on $beta_2$-adrenergic receptors.

Absorption: After oral inhalation, bronchodilation results from local action on the bronchial tree, with most of the inhaled dose being swallowed.

Distribution: Concentrates in lung tissue; also found in kidneys, liver, heart, spleen and bile; lower levels in the brain.

Metabolism: Hydrolyzed by esterases to active metabolite colterol. Colterol is metabolized to inactive compounds.

Excretion: After oral administration, bitolterol and its metabolites are excreted primarily in urine; only 10% found in feces within 48 hours of a dose.

Onset, peak, duration: Onset of action occurs within 3 to 5 minutes, peaks in 30 minutes to 2 hours, and lasts 4 to 8 hours.

INDICATIONS & DOSAGE

To prevent and treat bronchial asthma and bronchospasm–
Adults and children over 12 years: to treat bronchospasm, two inhalations at an interval of at least 1 to 3 minutes followed by a third inhalation, if needed. To prevent bronchospasm, the usual dose is two inhalations q 8 hours. In either case, dose should never exceed three inhalations q 6 hours or two inhalations q 4 hours.

CONTRAINDICATIONS & PRECAUTIONS

Contraindicated in patients with hypersensitivity to the drug. Use cautiously in patients with cardiovascular disorders (ischemic heart disease, hypertension, or cardiac arrhythmias), hyperthyroidism, diabetes, seizure disorders, or sensitivity to other sympathomimetic amines.

ADVERSE REACTIONS

Common reactions are in italics; life-threatening reactions are in bold italics.
CNS: *tremors,* nervousness, headache, dizziness, light-headedness.
CV: palpitations, chest discomfort, tachycardia.
EENT: throat irritation, cough.
GI: nausea.
Other: dyspnea, ***hypersensitivity.***

INTERACTIONS

None significant.

EFFECTS ON DIAGNOSTIC TESTS

AST (SGOT): increased levels.
CBC: decreased platelet and WBC count.
Spirometry (for diagnosis of asthma): test insensitivity.
Urinalysis: proteinuria.

NURSING CONSIDERATIONS

Besides those related universally to drug therapy (see "How to use this book"), consider the following specific recommendations:

Assessment

- Obtain a baseline assessment of the patient's cardiopulmonary status by taking vital signs, performing an EKG (if ordered), and auscultating lung fields.
- Be alert for any adverse reactions and drug interactions throughout therapy.
- Evaluate the patient's and family's knowledge about bitolterol therapy.

Nursing Diagnoses

- Ineffective airway clearance related to the patient's underlying condition.
- High risk for injury related to adverse effects of bitolterol mesylate therapy.
- Knowledge deficit related to use of bitolterol mesylate.

Planning and Implementation

Preparation and Administration

- ***Inhalation:*** If more than one inhalation is ordered, have the patient wait at least 2 minutes before repeating the procedure for a second dose. If the patient is also using a steroid inhaler, be sure that he uses the bronchodilator first and then waits about 5 minutes before using the steroid. This allows the bronchodilator to open air passages for maximum effectiveness.

Monitoring

- Monitor effectiveness by regularly auscultating the lungs, taking the respiratory rate, and noting results of laboratory studies, such as arterial blood gases. When monitoring the effectiveness of the drug, remember that bitolterol mesylate has a rapid onset of action, about 3 to 4 minutes. Peak effect occurs in 30 minutes to 1 hour.
- Monitor blood pressure regularly.

Supportive Care

- Institute safety precautions until CNS effects are known or if adverse reactions, such as tremors, dizziness, or light-headedness, occur.

Patient Teaching
• Instruct the patient to perform oral inhalation correctly using the following procedure: Clear nasal passages and throat. Breathe out, expelling as much air from the lungs as possible. Place the mouthpiece well into the mouth as the dose from the inhaler is released, and inhale deeply. Hold breath for several seconds, remove the mouthpiece, and exhale slowly.
• If more than one inhalation is ordered, tell the patient to wait at least 2 minutes before repeating the procedure for a second dose. Explain why it is necessary to use the bronchodilator first if other inhalants, such as a steroid inhaler, are prescribed. Tell the patient that this allows the bronchodilator to open air passages for maximum effectiveness. Allow 5 minutes between the inhalant treatments.
• Advise patients not to exceed recommended dose. Explain that too frequent usage may cause tachycardia.
• Remind the patient that beneficial effects last up to 8 hours, longer than most other similar bronchodilators.

Evaluation
In patients receiving bitolterol mesylate, appropriate evaluation statements may include:
• Patient's respiratory signs and symptoms are improved with bitolterol mesylate.
• Injury did not occur; patient tolerates therapy well.
• Patient and family state an understanding of bitolterol mesylate therapy.

bleomycin sulfate
(blee oh mye´ sin)
Blenoxane

• *Classification:* antineoplastic (antibiotic, cell-cycle-phase specific, G_2 and M phase)
• *Pregnancy Risk Category:* D

HOW SUPPLIED
Injection: 15-unit vials (1 unit = 1 mg)

ACTION
Mechanism: An antineoplastic antibiotic that probably acts by inhibiting the incorporation of thymidine into DNA. Inhibits DNA synthesis and causes scission of single- and double-stranded DNA. Also active against gram-negative and gram-positive bacteria and fungi, but toxicity prohibits its use as an antimicrobial.
Absorption: Poorly absorbed across the GI tract following oral administration. I.M. administration results in lower serum levels than those occurring after equivalent I.V. doses; systemic absorption also follows intrapleural or intraperitoneal administration.
Distribution: Mainly into skin, lungs, kidneys, peritoneum, and lymphatic tissue. Low concentrations in bone marrow, probably because of the presence of degradative enzymes.
Metabolism: Tissue inactivation occurs in the bone marrow, liver and kidney and much less in the skin and lungs.
Excretion: Primarily in urine, with 60% to 70% as active drug. Half-life: Terminal elimination half-life is 2 hours.

INDICATIONS & DOSAGE
Dosage and indications may vary. Check patient's protocol with doctor.
Cervical, esophageal, head, neck, and testicular cancer–
Adults: 10 to 20 units/m² I.V., I.M., or S.C. 1 or 2 times weekly to total 300 to 400 units.
Hodgkin's disease–
Adults: 10 to 20 units/m² I.V., I.M., or S.C. 1 or 2 times weekly. After 50% response, maintenance 1 unit

I.M. or I.V. daily or 5 units I.M. or I.V. weekly.
Lymphomas–
Adults: first two doses should be 2 units or less, and patient should be monitored for any allergic reaction. If no reaction occurs, then follow above dosing schedule.

CONTRAINDICATIONS & PRECAUTIONS

Contraindicated in patients with a history of hypersensitivity or idiosyncratic reaction to the drug. Use cautiously in patients with renal impairment because drug accumulation may occur; also use cautiously in patients with pulmonary impairment and monitor the patient carefully for signs of pulmonary toxicity because pulmonary fibrosis may occur. Patient should have chest X-rays every 1 to 2 weeks during therapy and evaluation of pulmonary diffusion capacity for carbon dioxide every month.

ADVERSE REACTIONS

Common reactions are in italics; life-threatening reactions are in bold italics.
CNS: hyperesthesia of scalp and fingers, headache.
GI: *stomatitis, prolonged anorexia in 13% of patients, nausea, vomiting,* diarrhea.
Skin: *erythema, vesiculation, and hardening and discoloration of palmar and plantar skin in 8% of patients;* desquamation of hands, feet, and pressure areas; *hyperpigmentation; acne.*
Other: *reversible alopecia,* swelling of interphalangeal joints, *pulmonary fibrosis in 10% of patients, pulmonary adverse reactions (fine crackles, fever, dyspnea), leukocytosis and nonproductive cough, allergic reaction (fever up to 106° F. [41.1° C.] with chills up to 5 hours after injection;* ***anaphylaxis*** *in 1% to 6% of patients).*

INTERACTIONS

Digitalis glycosides: combination therapy that includes bleomycin may result in decreased serum digoxin levels.

EFFECTS ON DIAGNOSTIC TESTS

Blood and urine uric acid: increased concentrations.

NURSING CONSIDERATIONS

Besides those related universally to drug therapy (see "How to use this book"), consider the following specific recommendations:
Assessment
- Obtain a baseline assessment of the patient's overall physical status, especially respiratory status; CBC; pulmonary function and renal function tests before initiating therapy.
- Be alert for adverse reactions or drug interactions during therapy.
- Evaluate the patient's and family's knowledge about bleomycin therapy.

Nursing Diagnoses
- Hyperthermia related to allergic reaction to bleomycin.
- Ineffective airway clearance related to bleomycin-induced adverse pulmonary reactions.
- Knowledge deficit related to bleomycin therapy.

Planning and Implementation
Preparation and Administration
- Follow institutional policy to avoid mutagenic, teratogenic, and carcinogenic risks.
- Be aware that due to an increased risk of anaphylactoid reactions, the first two doses in patients with lymphoma should be limited to 2 units or less.
- Refrigerate unopened vials containing powder.
- Keep in mind that refrigerated, reconstituted solution is stable for 4 weeks; at room temperature it is stable for 2 weeks.
- ***I.V. use:*** Be aware that bleomycin may adsorb to plastic (PVC) I.V.

bags. For prolonged stability, use glass containers.

Monitoring

• Monitor effectiveness by noting results of follow-up diagnostic tests and patient's overall physical status.

• Closely monitor the patient during infusion and for 1 hour after.

• Auscultate lungs for basilar rales; monitor for nonproductive cough, dyspnea, and tachypnea.

• Monitor chest X-ray, pulmonary function tests, BUN, and creatinine clearance. Expect to stop the drug if tests show marked deterioration.

• Monitor injection site for signs of irritation.

• Monitor for indications of allergic or anaphylactoid reactions. Keep in mind that allergic reactions may be delayed for several hours, especially in lymphoma. Also be aware that bleomycin-induced fever is common. Take patient's temperature during and following therapy. Fever ususally occurs within 3 to 6 hours of administration.

Supportive Care

• Be aware that pulmonary adverse reactions are common in patients older than age 70. Fatal pulmonary fibrosis occurs in 1% of patients, especially when cumulative dose exceeds 400 units. Report pulmonary signs and symptoms promptly.

• Keep in mind that drug concentrates in keratin of squamous epithelium. To prevent linear streaking, don't use adhesive dressing on skin.

• In patients prone to post-treatment fever, give acetaminophen, as ordered, before treatment and for 24 hours after it.

• If ordered, after treatment give supplemental oxygen at an FIO_2 no higher than 25% to avoid potential lung damage.

Patient Teaching

• Be certain that patient understands the risks associated with therapy, especially the potential for serious pulmonary reactions in high-risk patients.

• Explain the necessity for monitoring and the type of monitoring necessary.

• Advise patient that alopecia is common, but often reversible.

Evaluation

In patients receiving bleomycin, appropriate evaluation statements may include:

• Patient's temperature is within normal range or slightly elevated.

• Airway remains clear without evidence of pulmonary fibrosis.

• Patient and family state an understanding of bleomycin therapy.

boric acid (ophthalmic)

Blinx◇, Collyrium◇, Neo-Flo◇

• *Classification:* ophthalmic anti-infective (acid)
• *Pregnancy Risk Category:* C

HOW SUPPLIED

Ophthalmic ointment: 5%◇, 10%◇
Ophthalmic solution: 30 ml◇, 120 ml◇, 180 ml◇

ACTION

Mechanism: Unknown. However, drug has fungistatic and bacteriostatic properties.
Pharmacokinetics: Unknown.

INDICATIONS & DOSAGE

For irrigation following tonometry, gonioscopy, foreign body removal, or use of fluorescein; used to soothe and cleanse the eye–
Adults: apply 5% or 10% ointment, p.r.n.

CONTRAINDICATIONS & PRECAUTIONS

Contraindicated in patients with hypersensitivity to any components of the preparations. Ophthalmic preparation is contraindicated in patients with eye lacerations or abraded cornea.

ADVERSE REACTIONS

Common reactions are in italics; life-threatening reactions are in bold italics.
Ear: irritation or itching.
Skin: urticaria.
Other: overgrowth of nonsusceptible organisms.

INTERACTIONS

Idoxuridine, polyvinyl alcohol (Liquifilm): may form insoluble complex. Check with pharmacy on contents in other eye drugs and contact lens wetting solutions.

EFFECTS ON DIAGNOSTIC TESTS

None reported.

NURSING CONSIDERATIONS

Besides those related universally to drug therapy (see "How to use this book"), consider the following specific recommendations:

Assessment
- Obtain a baseline assessment of history of eye condition and allergies before therapy.
- Be alert for adverse reactions or drug interactions during therapy.
- Evaluate the patient's and family's knowledge about boric acid.

Nursing Diagnoses
- Altered protection related to ocular infection.
- High risk for injury related to boric acid-induced toxicity.
- Knowledge deficit related to boric acid therapy.

Planning and Implementation
Preparation and Administration
- Wash hands before and after instilling solution or ointment.
- Avoid contaminating solution container.

Monitoring
- Monitor effectiveness by observing the eye for signs of inflammation or infection.
- Check the eye area for abraded skin areas or granulating wounds.

Supportive Care
- Do not apply to abraded cornea or eye laceration.
- Not for use with soft contact lenses.

Patient Teaching
- Instruct the patient not to share eye solutions with family members.
- Teach the patient good hand washing technique and tell patient to wash hands before and after administering solution.

Evaluation
In patients receiving boric acid, appropriate evaluation statements may include:
- Patient remains free from signs and symptoms of infection.
- Patient demonstrates no signs of boric acid toxicity.
- Patient and family state an understanding of boric acid therapy.

bretylium tosylate

(bre til´ ee um)
Bretylate†‡, Bretylol

- *Classification:* antiarrhythmic (adrenergic blocking agent)
- *Pregnancy Risk Category:* C

HOW SUPPLIED

Injection: 50 mg/ml

ACTION

Mechanism: A class III antiarrhythmic that initially exerts transient adrenergic stimulation through release of norepinephrine. Subsequent depletion of norepinephrine causes adrenergic blocking actions to predominate. Repolarization is prolonged; duration of action potential and effective refractory period are increased.

Absorption: Incompletely and erratically absorbed from the GI tract; well absorbed after I.M. administration.
Distribution: Widely distributed throughout the body. It does not cross the blood-brain barrier. Only about 1% to 10% is plasma protein-bound.
Metabolism: No metabolites have been identified.
Excretion: Mainly in the urine mostly as unchanged drug. Half-life: Ranges from 5 to 10 hours (longer in patients with renal impairment).
Onset, peak, duration: After I.M. administration, the drug's antiarrhythmic (ventricular tachycardia and ectopy) action begins within about 20 to 60 minutes but may not reach maximal level for 6 to 9 hours; therefore, I.M. administration is not recommended for treating life-threatening ventricular fibrillation.

With I.V. administration, antifibrillatory action begins within a few minutes. However, suppression of ventricular tachycardia and other ventricular arrhythmias occurs more slowly–usually within 20 minutes to 2 hours; peak antiarrhythmic effects may not occur for 6 to 9 hours. Duration of effect ranges from 6 to 24 hours and may increase with continued dosage increases. (Patients with ventricular fibrillation may require continuous infusion to maintain desired effect.)

INDICATIONS & DOSAGE

Ventricular fibrillation–
Adults: 5 mg/kg by I.V. push over 1 minute. If necessary, increase dose to 10 mg/kg and repeat q 15 to 30 minutes until 30 mg/kg have been given.
Children: safety and efficacy have not been established, but some clinicians use 2 to 5 mg/kg I.M. as a single dose, or 5 mg/kg I.V. followed by 10 mg/kg I.V. if fibrillation persists.
Other ventricular arrhythmias–
Adults: initially, 500 mg diluted to 50 ml with dextrose 5% in water or normal saline solution and infused I.V. over more than 8 minutes at 5 to 10 mg/kg. Dose may be repeated in 1 to 2 hours. Thereafter, repeat q 6 to 8 hours.
I.V. maintenance–
Adults: infused in diluted solution of 500 ml dextrose 5% in water or normal saline solution at 1 to 2 mg/minute.
I.M. injection–
Adults: 5 to 10 mg/kg undiluted. Repeat in 1 to 2 hours if needed. Thereafter, repeat q 6 to 8 hours.

CONTRAINDICATIONS & PRECAUTIONS

Contraindicated in patients with digitalis-induced arrhythmias, because the resulting release of norepinephrine may aggravate digitalis toxicity.

Use with extreme caution in patients with aortic stenosis or pulmonary hypertension because these patients may be unable to compensate for the fall in blood pressure; and in patients with fixed cardiac output, aortic stenosis, and pulmonary hypertension, because the drug may cause sudden severe hypotension.

ADVERSE REACTIONS

Common reactions are in italics; life-threatening reactions are in bold italics.
CNS: *vertigo, dizziness, lightheadedness, syncope* (usually secondary to hypotension).
CV: *severe hypotension (especially orthostatic), bradycardia,* anginal pain, transient arrhythmias.
GI: severe nausea, vomiting (with rapid infusion).

INTERACTIONS

All antihypertensives: may potentiate hypotension. Monitor blood pressure.
Other antiarrhythmics: additive or

antagonistic antiarrhythmic effects. Monitor for additive toxicity.

EFFECTS ON DIAGNOSTIC TESTS

None reported.

NURSING CONSIDERATIONS

Besides those related universally to drug therapy (see "How to use this book"), consider the following specific recommendations:

Assessment

• Obtain a baseline assessment of the patient's heart rate and rhythm before bretylium therapy.
• Be alert for adverse reactions and drug interactions throughout therapy.
• Evaluate the patient's and family's knowledge about bretylium therapy.

Nursing Diagnoses

• Decreased cardiac output related to ineffectiveness of bretylium therapy.
• Altered tissue perfusion (cerebral) related to bretylium-induced severe hypotension.
• Knowledge deficit related to bretylium therapy.

Planning and Implementation

Preparation and Administration

• Expect to decrease dosage in patients with renal impairment.
• Follow dosage directions carefully to avoid nausea and vomiting.
• ***I.M. use:*** Administer undiluted following usual protocol for intramuscular administration. Rotate injection sites to prevent tissue damage, and don't exceed 3-ml volume in any one site.
• ***I.V. use:*** Infuse in diluted solution of 500 ml dextrose 5% in water or normal saline solution at 1 to 2 mg/minute; however, patients who are hypersensitive to corn or corn products should not receive the commerically available preparation mixed in dextrose 5% in water. Administer continuous infusion at a rate of 1 to 2 mg/min. When infusing drug intermittently, infuse ordered dose over 10 to 30 minutes. When administering as a direct I.V. injection, use a 20G to 22G needle and inject over about 1 minute into vein or into I.V. line containing a free-flowing, compatible solution.

Monitoring

• Monitor effectiveness by evaluating continuous ECG recordings as well as blood pressure and heart rate.
• Monitor ECG for new arrhythmias.
• Monitor for increased anginal pain in susceptible patients.
• Monitor fluid and electrolyte balance if patient experiences adverse GI reactions.

Supportive Care

• If ECG disturbances occurs, withhold the drug, obtain a rhythm strip, and notify the doctor immediately.
• Have emergency equipment and drugs on hand to treat new arrhythmias and hypotension. If supine systolic blood pressure falls below 75 mm Hg, notify doctor, who may order norepinephrine, dopamine, or volume expanders to raise blood pressure. However, monitor patient carefully if pressor amines (sympathomimetics) are given to correct hypotension, because bretylium potentiates pressor amines.
• Keep patient supine until tolerance to hypotension develops.
• Be aware that drug is given along with other cardiopulmonary resuscitative measures, such as CPR, countershock, epinephrine, sodium bicarbonate, and lidocaine.
• Institute safety precautions if adverse CNS reactions occur.

Patient Teaching

• Stress the importance of alerting nurse if chest pain or dyspnea occurs.
• Tell patient to avoid sudden position changes.

Evaluation

In patients receiving bretylium, appropriate evaluation statements may include:

• Patient's ECG reveals arrhythmia has been corrected.
• Patient's blood pressure remains normal throughout bretylium therapy.
• Patient and family state an understanding of bretylium therapy.

bromocriptine mesylate

(broe moe krip´ teen)
Parlodel

• *Classification:* antiparkinsonian agent, inhibitor of prolactin release, inhibitor of growth hormone release (dopamine receptor antagonist, ergot alkaloid)
• *Pregnancy Risk Category:* C

HOW SUPPLIED

Tablets: 2.5 mg
Capsules: 5 mg

ACTION

Mechanism: Acts as a dopamine-receptor agonist by activating postsynaptic dopamine receptors. Inhibits secretion of prolactin.
Absorption: 28% of an oral dose is absorbed from the GI tract; however, because of extensive first-pass metabolism, only 6% of the absorbed dose reaches the systemic circulation unchanged.
Distribution: 90% to 96% bound to serum albumin.
Metabolism: Completely metabolized in the liver before excretion. Substantial first-pass metabolism occurs.
Excretion: Primarily in the feces via the bile. Almost all (89.6%) is excreted in the feces in 120 hours. Only 2.5% to 5.5% of the dose is excreted in the urine. Half life: About 3 hours.
Onset, peak, duration: Peak levels are reached in 1 to 3 hours. Prolactin secretion remains suppressed for 14 hours.

INDICATIONS & DOSAGE

To treat amenorrhea and galactorrhea associated with hyperprolactinemia; treatment of female infertility–
Women: 1.25 to 2.5 mg P.O. daily. Increase dosage by 2.5 mg daily at 3- to 7-day intervals until desired effect is achieved. Safety and efficacy of doses greater than 100 mg daily have not been established.
Prevention of postpartum lactation–
Women: 2.5 mg P.O. b.i.d. with meals for 14 days. Treatment may be extended for up to 21 days, if necessary.
Treatment of Parkinson's disease–
Adults: 1.25 mg P.O. b.i.d. with meals. Dosage may be increased q 14 to 28 days, up to 100 mg daily.
Treatment of acromegaly–
Adults: 1.25 to 2.5 mg P.O. for 3 days. An additional 1.25 to 2.5 mg may be added q 3 to 7 days until patient receives therapeutic benefit.

CONTRAINDICATIONS & PRECAUTIONS

Contraindicated in patients with a sensitivity to any ergot alkaloids and in those with severe ischemic heart disease or peripheral vascular disease because of the cardiovascular effects of the drug. Because bromocriptine prevents lactation, it should not be used by breast-feeding women.

Use cautiously in patients with Raynaud's disease, which may be exacerbated; hepatic and renal dysfunction or with a history of psychiatric disorders because the drug may worsen these disorders; and a history of myocardial infarction with residual arrhythmias because the drug may induce arrhythmias.

ADVERSE REACTIONS

Common reactions are in italics; life-threatening reactions are in bold italics.
CNS: confusion, hallucinations, uncontrolled body movements, *dizziness, headache,* fatigue, mania, delu-

sions, nervousness, insomnia, depression.
CV: *hypotension,* syncope.
EENT: nasal congestion, tinnitus, blurred vision.
GI: *nausea,* vomiting, *abdominal cramps,* constipation, diarrhea.
GU: urine retention, urinary frequency.
Other: *pulmonary infiltration and pleural effusion,* coolness and pallor of fingers and toes.

INTERACTIONS

Antihypertensive drugs: increased hypotensive effects. Adjust dosage of antihypertensive agent.
Haloperidol, loxapine, phenothiazines, methyldopa, metoclopramide, MAO inhibitors, reserpine: may interfere with bromocriptine's effects.
Levodopa: additive effects. Adjust dosage of levodopa.
Oral contraceptives, estrogens, progestins: interfere with effects of bromocriptine. Concurrent use not recommended.

EFFECTS ON DIAGNOSTIC TESTS

BUN, ALT (SGPT), AST (SGOT), CPK, alkaline phosphatase, and uric acid: transiently elevated levels.

NURSING CONSIDERATIONS

Besides those related universally to drug therapy (see "How to use this book"), consider the following specific recommendations:

Assessment

- Obtain a baseline assessment of the patient's signs and symptoms related to hormonal malfunctioning or parkinsonism before beginning therapy.
- Be alert for adverse reactions or drug interactions throughout therapy.
- Evaluate the patient's and family's knowledge about bromocriptine therapy.

Nursing Diagnoses

- Impaired mobility related to Parkinson's disease.
- High risk for injury related to adverse CNS or cardiovascular effects of drug therapy.
- Knowledge deficit related to bromocriptine therapy.

Planning and Implementation

Preparation and Administration

- Adjust dosage, if ordered, for patients with impaired renal functioning.
- Administer with meals to minimize GI distress.
- When used to treat Parkinson's disease, expect to administer with either levodopa alone or levodopa-carbidopa combination.
- Gradually titrate doses to effective levels to minimize adverse reactions.

Monitoring

- Monitor effectiveness by regularly checking body appearance or movements, or menstrual and lactation status for signs of improvement. Keep in mind recurrence rates are high (70% to 80%) when used to treat amenorrhea or galactorrhea associated with hyperprolactinemia.
- Monitor for adverse reactions, particularly at the beginning of therapy. Orthostatic hypotension is common. Incidence of adverse reactions is high (68%); but most reactions are mild to moderate, and only 6% of patients discontinue drug for this reason. Check for nausea which is the most common reaction.
- Be especially diligent in monitoring patient's with Parkinson's disease because they commonly develop adverse reactions.
- Monitor blood pressure closely in women who receive bromocriptine for suppression of postpartum lactation. In such patients, transient hypotension is common; however, hypertension, seizures, and stroke have also been reported.
- Test for pregnancy every 4 weeks or whenever patient misses period after menses are reinitiated. May lead to early postpartum conception.

Supportive Care
• Assist the patient with activities as needed, and institute safety precautions.
• Be aware that patient should be examined carefully for pituitary tumor (Forbes-Albright syndrome). Use of bromocriptine will not affect tumor size but may alleviate amenorrhea or galactorrhea.
Patient Teaching
• Warn the patient to avoid hazardous activities that require alertness until CNS and cardiovascular effects of the drug are known.
• Tell the patient to take the drug with meals to minimize GI distress.
• Advise patients to avoid dizziness and fainting by rising slowly to an upright position and avoiding sudden position changes.
• Advise patient to use contraceptive methods other than oral contraceptives during treatment.
• Advise the patient that it may take 6 to 8 weeks or longer for menses to be reinstated and galactorrhea to be suppressed.
• Explain that patient may experience mild-to-moderate rebound breast secretion, congestion, or engorgement when therapy is discontinued.
Evaluation
In patients receiving bromocriptine, appropriate evaluation statements may include:
• Patient exhibits improved mobility.
• Patient's safety is maintained; CNS and cardiovascular status is unaffected by drug therapy.
• Patient and family state an understanding of bromocriptine therapy.

brompheniramine maleate

(brome fen ir´ a meen)
Brombay◇, Bromphen*◇, Chlorphed◇, Codimal-A, Conjec-B◇, Cophene-B, Dehist, Diamine TD, Dimetane*◇, Dimetane Extentabs◇, Dimetane-Ten◇, Histaject Modified, Nasahist B, ND-Stat Revised, Oraminic II, Sinusol-B, Veltane

• *Classification:* antihistamine (histamine 1-receptor antagonist, alkylamine)
• *Pregnancy Risk Category:* C

HOW SUPPLIED

Tablets: 4 mg◇
Tablets (timed-release): 8 mg◇, 12 mg◇
Elixir: 2 mg/5 ml*◇
Injection: 10 mg/ml◇

ACTION

Mechanism: Blocks the effects of histamine at H_1 receptors. Prevents but does not reverse histamine-mediated responses.
Absorption: Readily absorbed from the GI tract.
Distribution: Widely distributed; apparent volume of distribution is 11.7 L/kg.
Metabolism: Hepatic.
Excretion: Drug and metabolites are excreted primarily in urine; a small amount in feces. About 5% to 10% of an oral dose of brompheniramine is excreted unchanged in urine. Half-life: About 12 to 34½ hours.
Onset, peak, duration: Action begins within 15 to 30 minutes and peaks in 2 to 5 hours. A second lower peak effect apparently exists, possibly from drug reabsorption in the distal small intestine.

INDICATIONS & DOSAGE

Rhinitis, allergy symptoms—
Adults: 4 to 8 mg P.O. t.i.d. or q.i.d.; or (timed-release) 8 to 12 mg P.O. b.i.d. or t.i.d.; or 5 to 20 mg q 6 to 12 hours I.M., I.V., or S.C. Maximum dosage is 40 mg daily.
Children over 6 years: 2 to 4 mg P.O. t.i.d. or q.i.d.; or (timed-release) 8 to 12 mg q 12 hours; or 0.5 mg/kg I.M.,

I.V., or S.C. daily divided t.i.d. or q.i.d.
Children under 6 years: 0.5 mg/kg P.O., I.M., I.V., or S.C. daily divided t.i.d. or q.i.d.

Note: Children under 12 years should use only as directed by a doctor.

CONTRAINDICATIONS & PRECAUTIONS

Contraindicated in patients with hypersensitivity to this drug and in those taking antihistamines with similar chemical structures (chlorpheniramine, dexchlorpheniramine, and triprolidine); in patients experiencing asthmatic attacks because brompheniramine thickens bronchial secretions; and in patients who have taken monoamine oxidase (MAO) inhibitors within the previous 2 weeks.

Use cautiously in patients with narrow-angle glaucoma; pyloroduodenal obstruction or urinary bladder obstruction from prostatic hypertrophy or narrowing of the bladder neck because of their marked anticholinergic effects; cardiovascular disease, hypertension, or hyperthyroidism because of the risk of palpitations and tachycardia; and renal disease, diabetes, bronchial asthma, urinary retention, prostatic hypertrophy, or stenosing peptic ulcers.

Do not use during pregnancy (especially in the third trimester) or during breast-feeding. Antihistmines have caused seizures and other severe reactions in premature infants and other neonates.

ADVERSE REACTIONS

Common reactions are in italics; life-threatening reactions are in bold italics.

Blood: thrombocytopenia, ***agranulocytosis.***
CNS: (especially in elderly patients) dizziness, tremors, irritability, insomnia, *drowsiness, stimulation.*
CV: hypotension, palpitations.
GI: anorexia, nausea, vomiting, *dry mouth and throat.*
GU: urine retention.
Skin: urticaria, rash.
After parenteral administration: local reaction, sweating, syncope.

INTERACTIONS

CNS depressants: increased sedation. Use together cautiously.
MAO inhibitors: increased anticholinergic effects. Don't use together.

EFFECTS ON DIAGNOSTIC TESTS

Diagnostic skin tests: reduced or masked positive response.

NURSING CONSIDERATIONS

Besides those related universally to drug therapy (see "How to use this book"), consider the following specific recommendations:

Assessment
- Obtain a baseline assessment of the patient's underlying condition before therapy.
- Be alert for adverse reactions or drug interactions throughout therapy.
- Evaluate the patient's and family's knowledge about brompheniramine maleate therapy.

Nursing Diagnoses
- Altered protection related to allery symptoms.
- Hyperthermia related to potential brompheniramine maleate-induced agranulocytosis.
- Knowledge deficit related to brompheniramine maleate therapy.

Planning and Implementation

Preparation and Administration
- ***I.V. use:*** Administer injectable form containing 10 mg/ml diluted or undiluted very slowly I.V. Do not administer the 100 mg/ml injection I.V.
- ***P.O. use:*** Reduce GI distress by giving with food or milk.

Monitoring
- Monitor blood counts during long-term therapy; watch for signs of blood dyscrasias.

• Monitor vital signs frequently. Note fever.

Supportive Care

• Notify the doctor if you notice that the patient is developing a tolerance for this drug. He may substitute another antihistamine.

• Remember that brompheniramine maleate causes less drowsiness than some other antihistamines. Protect the patient from injury if drowsiness does occur.

Patient Teaching

• Warn patient to avoid drinking alcoholic beverages during therapy and to avoid hazardous activities that require alertness until adverse CNS effects are known.

• Suggest that patient drink coffee or tea to reduce drowsiness; sugarless gum, sour hard candy, or ice chips may relieve dry mouth.

• Warn patient to discontinue brompheniramine maleate 4 days before allergy skin testing to preserve the accuracy of the tests.

Evaluation

In patients receiving brompheniramine maleate, appropriate evaluation statements may include:

• Patient's allergic symptoms are relieved with brompheniramine maleate therapy.

• Patient does not experience hyperthermia; agranulocytosis did not occur.

• Patient and family state an understanding of brompheniramine maleate therapy.

buclizine hydrochloride

(byoo´ kli zeen)

Bucladin-S**

• *Classification:* antiemetic, antivertigo agent (piperazine derivative antihistamine)

• *Pregnancy Risk Category:* C

HOW SUPPLIED

Tablets: 50 mg

ACTION

Mechanism: An antihistamine that also blocks acetylcholine receptors; drug also has antispasmotic, local anesthetic, and CNS depressant effects. May affect neural pathways originating in the labyrinth to inhibit nausea and vomiting, but the exact mechanism of action is unknown.

Pharmacokinetics: Unknown.

Onset, peak, duration: Duration of action is 4 to 6 hours.

INDICATIONS & DOSAGE

Motion sickness (prevention)–

Adults: 50 mg P.O. at least one half hour before beginning travel. If needed, may repeat another 50 mg P.O. after 4 to 6 hours.

Vertigo–

Adults: 50 mg P.O., up to 150 mg P.O. daily in severe cases. Maintenance dose is 50 mg b.i.d.

CONTRAINDICATIONS & PRECAUTIONS

Contraindicated in patients with hypersensitivity to this drug or other antiemetic antihistamines with a similar chemical structure, such as cyclizine, meclizine, or dimenhydrinate; and in pregnancy because it is teratogenic in animals. Use cautiously in patients with narrow-angle glaucoma, asthma, prostatic hypertrophy (particularly elderly men), or GU or GI obstruction because of its anticholinergic effects; drug may mask signs of intestinal obstruction or brain tumor. Bucladin-S Softabs contain tartrazine (FD&C yellow #5 dye), which may cause bronchial asthma or other allergic reactions in patients who are sensitive to tartrazine or aspirin.

ADVERSE REACTIONS

Common reactions are in italics; life-threatening reactions are in bold italics.

CNS: *drowsiness,* headache, dizziness, jitters.
EENT: blurred vision, dry mouth.
GU: urine retention.
Other: may mask symptoms of ototoxicity, intestinal obstruction, or brain tumor.

INTERACTIONS
None significant.

EFFECTS ON DIAGNOSTIC TESTS
None reported.

NURSING CONSIDERATIONS
Besides those related universally to drug therapy (see "How to use this book"), consider the following specific recommendations:

Assessment
- Obtain a baseline assessment of mental status and fluid balance before therapy.
- Be alert for adverse reactions or drug interactions throughout therapy.
- Evaluate the patient's and family's knowledge about buclizine therapy.

Nursing Diagnoses
- High risk for fluid volume deficit related to motion-sickness–induced nausea and vomiting.
- Altered thought processes related to buclizine-induced drowsiness.
- Knowledge deficit related to buclizine therapy.

Planning and Implementation

Preparation and Administration
- Tablets may be placed in mouth and allowed to dissolve without water, or chewed or swallowed whole.

Monitoring
- Monitor effectiveness by observing the patient for nausea and vomiting.
- Monitor fluid balance.
- Observe for signs of CNS adverse reaction (drowsiness, headache, jitters, dizziness).

Supportive Care
- Use safety precautions in patients with CNS adverse reactions.
- Encourage patient to maintain adequate fluid intake to prevent fluid volume deficit.
- Be aware that buclizine is an antihistamine.

Patient Teaching
- Inform patient that buclizine should be taken at least 30 minutes before beginning travel.
- Warn the patient to avoid driving and other hazardous activities that require alertness until CNS effects of the drug are known.
- Advise patients that repeat doses may be necessary after 4 to 6 hours.

Evaluation
In patients receiving buclizine, appropriate evaluation statements may include:
- Patient demonstrates no signs of fluid volume deficit.
- Patient exhibits no signs of altered thought processes.
- Patient and family state an understanding of buclizine therapy.

---

bumetanide
(byoo met´ a nide)
Bumex, Burinex‡

- *Classification:* diuretic (loop diuretic)
- *Pregnancy Risk Category:* C

HOW SUPPLIED
Tablets: 0.5 mg, 1 mg, 2 mg
Injection: 0.25 mg/ml

ACTION
Mechanism: A loop diuretic that inhibits reabsorption of sodium and chloride at the proximal portion of the ascending loop of Henle.
Absorption: After oral administration, 85% to 95% of a dose is absorbed; food delays oral absorption; after I.M. administration, drug is completely absorbed.
Distribution: Approximately 92% to 96% protein-bound; it is unknown

whether bumetanide enters CSF or breast milk or crosses the placenta.
Metabolism: By the liver to at least five metabolites.
Excretion: In urine (80%) and in feces (10% to 20%). Half-life: Ranges from 1 to 1½ hours.
Onset, peak, duration: Diuresis begins a few minutes after I.V. administration and peaks in 15 to 30 minutes. Duration of effect is about 2 to 4 hours.

INDICATIONS & DOSAGE

Edema (congestive heart failure, hepatic and renal disease) –
Adults: 0.5 to 2 mg P.O. once daily. If diuretic response not adequate, a second or third dose may be given at 4- to 5-hour intervals. Maximum dosage is 10 mg/day. May be administered parenterally when P.O. not feasible. Usual initial dose is 0.5 to 1 mg I.V. or I.M. If response is not adequate, a second or third dose may be given at 2- to 3-hour intervals. Maximum dosage is 10 mg/day.
Children: 0.02 to 0.1 mg/kg P.O., I.M., or I.V. q 12 hours.

CONTRAINDICATIONS & PRECAUTIONS

Contraindicated in patients with hypersensitivity, anuria, hepatic coma, or electrolyte depletion, and patients with increasing BUN and creatinine levels or oliguria, despite its use as a diuretic in patients with renal impairment.

Use cautiously in patients allergic to sulfonamides, including furosemide, because cross-sensitivity may occur; in patients with hepatic cirrhosis and ascites because electrolyte alterations may precipitate hepatic encephalopathy; and in patients receiving cardiac glycosides (digoxin, digitoxin) because bumetanide-induced hypokalemia may predispose them to digitalis toxicity. Rapid I.V. administration increases hazard of ototoxicity.

ADVERSE REACTIONS

Common reactions are in italics; life-threatening reactions are in bold italics.
CNS: dizziness, headache.
CV: *volume depletion and dehydration, orthostatic hypotension,* ECG changes.
EENT: transient deafness.
GI: nausea.
Metabolic: *hypokalemia; hypochloremic alkalosis; asymptomatic hyperuricemia; fluid and electrolyte imbalances, including dilutional hyponatremia, hypocalcemia, hypomagnesemia;* hyperglycemia and impairment of glucose tolerance.
Skin: rash.
Other: muscle pain and tenderness.

INTERACTIONS

Aminoglycoside antibiotics: potentiated ototoxicity. Use together cautiously.
Probenecid, indomethacin, NSAIDs: inhibited diuretic response. Use cautiously.

EFFECTS ON DIAGNOSTIC TESTS

Electrolytes: altered results.
Liver and renal function tests: altered results.

NURSING CONSIDERATIONS

Besides those related universally to drug therapy (see "How to use this book"), consider the following specific recommendations:

Assessment

• Obtain a baseline assessment of urine output, vital signs, serum electrolytes, breath sounds, peripheral edema, and weight before initiating drug therapy.
• Be alert for adverse reactions and drug interactions throughout therapy.
• Evaluate the patient's and family's knowledge about drug therapy.

Nursing Diagnoses
• Fluid volume excess related to the patient's underlying condition as evidenced by edema.
• Altered urinary elimination related to bumetanide therapy (frequency, urgency).
• Knowledge deficit related to bumetanide therapy.

Planning and Implementation
Preparation and Administration
• ***I.V. use:*** Give drug by direct I.V. using a 21G or 23G needle over 1 to 2 minutes. If drug is ordered to be given by intermittent infusion give diluted drug through an intermittent infusion device or piggyback into an I.V. line containing a free-flowing, compatible solution. Infuse at ordered rate. Continuous infusion not needed.
• Give drug in a.m. to prevent nocturia. If second dose is necessary, give in the early afternoon.
• Be aware that intermittent dosage given on alternate days, or for 3 to 4 days with 1 to 2 days intervening, is recommended as the safest and most effective dosage schedule for control of edema.
Monitoring
• Monitor effectiveness by regularly checking urine output, weight, peripheral edema, and breath sounds.
• Monitor ECG for arrhythmias.
• Monitor serum electrolytes, CO_2, and BUN levels.
• Monitor vital signs: hypotension, dyspnea, tachycardia, and fever may indicate dehydration. Also monitor blood pressure and pulse rate during rapid diuresis for changes as drug is a potent loop diuretic.
• In the diabetic patient, monitor serum glucose.
• In the patient with gout, monitor serum uric acid.
• In the patient receiving digitalis, monitor for signs of digitalis toxicity.
• Monitor for signs of hypokalemia (muscle weakness and cramping).
• Monitor skin turgor and mucous membranes for signs of fluid volume depletion.
Supportive Care
• Hold drug and notify the doctor if hypersensitivity or adverse reactions occur. Be aware that oliguria or azotemia may require discontinuation of the drug.
• Keep accurate record of intake and output.
• Elevate the patient's legs to aid relief of peripheral edema.
• Encourage diet high in potassium and low in sodium.
• Provide frequent skin and mouth care to relieve dryness due to diuretic therapy.
• Answer the patient's call bells promptly; make sure bathroom or bedpan are easily accessible.
• Use safety precautions to avoid risk of falls due to hypotension.
• Notify doctor if drug-related hearing changes occur.
Patient Teaching
• Teach the patient to monitor fluid volume by daily weight and intake and output.
• Encourage the patient to avoid high-sodium foods and to choose high-potassium foods.
• Advise the patient to change positions slowly, especially when rising to a standing position, to avoid dizziness due to orthostatic hypotension, and to limit alcohol intake and strenuous exercise in warm weather.
• Advise the patient to take bumetanide early in the day to avoid sleep interruption due to nocturia.
• Teach the diabetic patient receiving bumetanide to monitor blood glucose.
• Teach the patient receiving bumetanide and digitalis to be aware of signs of digitalis toxicity and to store these drugs separately to avoid risk of dosage error.

Evaluation
In patients receiving bumetanide, appropriate evaluation statements may include:
- Patient is free of edema.
- Patient demonstrates adjustment of life-style to deal with altered patterns of urinary elimination.
- Patient and family state an understanding of bumetanide therapy.

bupivacaine hydrochloride
(byoo piv´ a kane)
Marcain‡, Marcaine, Sensorcaine

- *Classification:* amide-type local anesthetic (sodium-channel blockers)
- *Pregnancy Risk Category:* C

HOW SUPPLIED
Injection: 0.25%, 0.5%, 0.75%; also available with epinephrine 1:200,000

ACTION
Mechanism: Blocks depolarization by interfering with sodium-potassium exchange across the nerve cell membrane, preventing generation and conduction of the nerve impulse. When combined with epinephrine, action is prolonged because epinephrine causes local vasoconstriction, preventing diffusion of the drug into the bloodstream.
Absorption: Slowly absorbed into the systemic circulation. Caudal, epidural, or peripheral nerve block procedures provide peak systemic blood levels in about 45 minutes.
Distribution: More highly protein bound than any other local anesthetic (82% to 96%). It also has the lowest degree of placental transfer.
Metabolism: By the liver.
Excretion: In the urine, mostly as metabolites; 5% is excreted unchanged. Half life: 1.5 to 5.5 hours in adults, 8.1 hours in neonates.
Onset, peak, duration: When using 0.5% solutions for dental anesthesia, onset occurs in 2 to 10 minutes and lasts up to 7 hours. Using 0.5% solutions for epidural or peripheral nerve block, onset occurs in 4 to 17 minutes, with a duration of 3 to 7 hours.

INDICATIONS & DOSAGE
Dosages given are for drug without *epinephrine.*

Epidural:

Sol.	Vol. (ml)	Dose (mg)
0.25%	10 to 20	25 to 50
0.5%	10 to 20	50 to 100

Caudal:

Sol.	Vol. (ml)	Dose (mg)
0.25%	15 to 30	37.5 to 75
0.5%	15 to 30	75 to 150

Spinal:

Sol.	Vol. (ml)	Dose (mg)
0.75 (in dextrose 8.25%)	0.8 to 1.6	6 to 12

Peripheral nerve block:

Sol.	Vol. (ml)	Dose (mg)
0.25%	5	12.5
0.5%	5	25 (400 max.)

May repeat dose q 3 hours. Dosage and interval may be increased with epinephrine. Maximum 400 mg daily.

CONTRAINDICATIONS & PRECAUTIONS
Contraindicated in patients with hypersensitivity to this drug or other amide-type anesthetic agents. Also contraindicated in patients with inflammation or infection in puncture region, septicemia, severe hypertension, spinal deformities, and neurologic disorders.

Use cautiously in debilitated, elderly, acutely ill, or obstetric patients; and in those with severe shock, heart block, general drug allergies, and paracervical block.

Contraindications to epidural or spinal anesthesia include serious diseases of the CNS and spinal cord such as meningitis, tumors, cranial or spinal hemorrhage, poliomyelitis, syphilis, tuberculosis, or metastatic diseases of the spinal cord.

Local anesthetics should only be used by clinicians familiar with proper administration techniques. Individuals using these drugs should be familiar with the diagnosis and management of local anesthetic toxicity. Patients with mild-to-moderate cardiac disease, hyperthyroidism, or other endocrine abnormalities may be especially susceptible to the toxic effects of local anesthetics.

ADVERSE REACTIONS

Common reactions are in italics; life-threatening reactions are in bold italics.

Skin: dermatologic reactions.

Other: edema, status asthmaticus, ***anaphylaxis,*** anaphylactoid reactions.

The following systemic effects may result from high blood levels of the drug:

CNS: anxiety, nervousness, seizures followed by drowsiness, unconsciousness, tremors, twitches, shivering, *respiratory arrest.*

CV: myocardial depression, ***arrhythmias, cardiac arrest.***

EENT: blurred vision, tinnitus.

GI: nausea, vomiting.

INTERACTIONS

Chloroprocaine: may lessen bupivacaine's action. Don't use together.

Enflurane, halothane, isoflurane, and related drugs: cardiac arrhythmias when used with bupivacaine *with* epinephrine. Use with extreme caution.

MAO inhibitors, cyclic antidepressants: severe, sustained hypertension when used with bupivacaine *with* epinephrine. Use with extreme caution.

EFFECTS ON DIAGNOSTIC TESTS

None reported.

NURSING CONSIDERATIONS

Besides those related universally to drug therapy (see "How to use this book"), consider the following specific recommendations:

Assessment

- Obtain a baseline assessment of the patient's sensory status before therapy.
- Be alert for adverse reactions and drug interactions throughout therapy.
- Evaluate the patient's and family's knowledge about bupivacaine therapy.

Nursing Diagnoses

- Pain related to inadequate block.
- Decreased cardiac output related to adverse reaction to bupivacaine.
- Knowledge deficit related to bupivacaine therapy.

Planning and Implementation

Preparation and Administration

- Keep in mind that bupivacaine should not be used for I.V. regional anesthesia (Bier's anesthesia).
- Be aware that 0.75% solution is still available but should not to be used for obstetrical surgery. According to the FDA, lower concentrations are effective and much less hazardous.
- Remember that this drug should be administered only by persons who know how to recognize and manage adverse effects caused by epidural anesthetics.
- Use solutions with epinephrine cautiously in cardiovascular disorders and in body areas with limited blood supply (ears, nose, fingers, toes).
- ***Epidural use:*** Be aware that for epidural use, test doses are administered to verify needle or catheter placement. Initially, 2 to 3 ml is given to check for subarachnoid injection (which would cause extensive motor paralysis of the lower limbs and extensive sensory deficit). After about 5 minutes and in the absence of symptoms, a second, larger test dose of about 5 ml is given to check for intravascular injection (which would cause tinnitus, numbness around the lips, metallic taste, dysphoria, lethargy, or hypotension).

• Do not use solution with preservative for caudal or epidural block.
• Discard partially used vials without preservatives.
• Check solution for particles.

Monitoring

• Monitor effectiveness by evaluating pain relief. Continue to monitor sensory level every 15 minutes after completion of surgery or treatment until sympathetic innervation return.
• Monitor for evidence of anaphylaxis following administration of drug.
• Monitor for evidence of myocardial depression as well as respiratory depression, seizures, and other adverse reactions that may result from high blood levels of the drug.

Supportive Care

• Keep resuscitative equipment and drugs available.
• Consult with the doctor if pain relief is ineffective.
• Be aware that onset occurs in 4 to 17 minutes; duration is 3 to 6 hours.
• Notify the doctor immediately if the patient's CNS, cardiac or respiratory status deteriorates.
• Keep patient flat until sympathetic return has been established to prevent hypotension.

Patient Teaching

• Explain that the drug will cause a local loss of sensation providing pain relief in the selected body area, but unlike general anesthesia, will not cause unconsciousness.
• Describe the route of administration: epidural, caudal, spinal, or peripheral nerve block.

Evaluation

In the patient receiving bupivacaine, appropriate evaluation statements include:
• Effective sensory block achieved.
• Cardiac status within normal limits.
• Patient and family state an understanding of bupivacaine therapy.

buprenorphine hydrochloride

(byoo pre nor´ feen)
Buprenex, Temgesic Injection‡

• Controlled Substance Schedule V
• *Classification:* analgesic (narcotic agonist-antagonist, opioid partial agonist)
• *Pregnancy Risk Category:* C (D for prolonged use or use of high doses at term)

HOW SUPPLIED

Injection: 0.324 mg (equivalent to 0.3 mg base)/ml.

ACTION

Mechanism: An agonist-antagonist that binds with opiate receptors at many sites in the CNS (brain, brain stem, and spinal cord), altering both perception of and emotional response to pain through an unknown mechanism.
Absorption: Rapidly absorbed after I.M. administration.
Distribution: About 96% protein-bound. Drug enters CSF and crosses placenta.
Metabolism: Hepatic.
Excretion: In urine and feces. Half-life: About 2 to 3 hours.
Onset, peak, duration: Onset of action in 15 minutes; peak effect 1 hour after dosing. Duration of action is 6 hours.

INDICATIONS & DOSAGE

Moderate to severe pain–
Adults: 0.3 mg I.M. or slow I.V. q 6 hours, p.r.n. or around the clock. May administer up to 0.6 mg/dose if necessary.

CONTRAINDICATIONS & PRECAUTIONS

Contraindicated in patients with hypersensitivity to any semisynthetic opioid or thebaine derivative.

Use with extreme caution in patients with supraventricular arrhythmias; avoid or use with extreme caution in patients with head injury or increased intracranial pressure because drug obscures neurologic parameters; and during pregnancy and labor because drug readily crosses the placenta (premature infants are especially sensitive to the drug's respiratory and CNS depressant effects).

Use cautiously in patients with renal or hepatic dysfunction because drug accumulation or prolonged duration of action may occur; in patients with pulmonary disease (asthma, chronic obstructive pulmonary disease) because drug depresses respiration and suppresses cough reflex; in patients undergoing biliary tract surgery, because drug may cause biliary spasm; in patients with convulsive disorders, because drug may precipitate seizures; in elderly or debilitated patients, who are more sensitive to therapeutic and adverse drug effects; and in patients prone to addiction because of the high risk of addiction to this drug.

Buprenorphine has lower potential for abuse than do opioid agonists.

ADVERSE REACTIONS

Common reactions are in italics; life-threatening reactions are in bold italics.
CNS: *dizziness, sedation, headache,* confusion, nervousness, euphoria.
CV: hypotension.
EENT: *miosis.*
GI: *nausea,* vomiting, constipation.
Skin: pruritus, *sweating.*
Other: ***respiratory depression,*** hypoventilation.

INTERACTIONS

Alcohol, CNS depressants: additive effects. Use together cautiously.
Narcotic analgesics: avoid concomitant use. Possible decreased analgesic effect.

EFFECTS ON DIAGNOSTIC TESTS

None reported.

NURSING CONSIDERATIONS

Besides those related universally to drug therapy (see "How to use this book"), consider the following specific recommendations:

Assessment

- Obtain a baseline assessment of the patient's pain before therapy.
- Be alert for adverse reactions and drug interactions throughout therapy.
- Evaluate the patient's and family's knowledge about buprenorphine therapy.

Nursing Diagnoses

- Pain related to patient's underlying condition.
- Ineffective breathing pattern related to buprenorphine-induced respiratory depression.
- Knowledge deficit related to buprenorphine therapy.

Planning and Implementation

Preparation and Administration

- ***I.V. use:*** Give lower doses to elderly patients because of increased sensitivity to the drug and delayed clearance. Expect buprenorphine 0.3 mg to be equivalent to 10 mg morphine and 75 mg meperidine in analgesic potency. Burenorphine has longer duration of action than morphine or meperidine. Fixed dosage schedule helps to minimize breakthrough pain in chronic conditions.
- S.C. administration is not recommended.

Monitoring

- Monitor effectiveness by evaluating pain relief.
- Monitor respiratory status frequently for at least 1 hour after administration, noting any evidence of respiratory depression, such as decreased rate or depth of respiration.
- Regularly monitor blood pressure and heart rate.
- Monitor bowel function for constipation or ileus.

Supportive Care
• Notify the doctor and discuss increase of dosage or frequency if pain is not relieved.
• Hold dose, arouse patient to stimulate breathing, and notify the doctor if the patient's respiration rate falls below 8/minute.
• Keep narcotic antagonist (naloxone) and resuscitative equipment available. However, naloxone will not completely reverse the respiratory depression caused by buprenorphine overdose. Therefore, an overdose may necessitate mechanical ventilation. Larger than customary doses of naloxone (more than 0.4 mg) and doxapram may also be ordered.
• Because adverse CNS reactions are possible, institute safety precautions, such as supervising ambulation and keeping bed rails up.
• If not contraindicated, obtain an order for a stool softener and increase the patient's fluid and fiber intake to prevent or treat constipation, a possible adverse reaction to the drug.
• Anticipate that psychological and physical dependence may occur; withdrawal symptoms may appear up to 14 days after discontinuation of drug.
• Recognize that buprenorphine has narcotic antagonist properties and may precipitate abstinence syndrome in narcotic-dependent patients.

Patient Teaching
• Caution patient to change positions slowly and to avoid other activities that require alertness because drug may cause dizziness and drowsiness.
• Suggest measures, such as high-fiber diet and liberal fluid intake, to prevent constipation.
• Tell the patient or family to notify the doctor if patient's respiration rate decreases.

Evaluation

In patients receiving buprenorphine, appropriate evaluation statements may include:
• Patient reports relief of pain after administration of buprenorphine.
• Patient's respiratory status is within normal limits.
• Patient and family state an understanding of buprenorphine therapy.

bupropion hydrochloride
(byoo proe´ pee on)
Wellbutrin

• *Classification:* antidepressant (aminoketone)
• *Pregnancy Risk Category:* B

HOW SUPPLIED
Tablets: 75 mg, 100 mg

ACTION
Mechanism: Unknown. Bupropion is not a tricyclic antidepressant, does not inhibit monoamine oxidase (MAO), and is a weak inhibitor of norepinephrine, dopamine, and serotonin reuptake.
Absorption: Animal studies indicate that only 5% to 20% of the drug is bioavailable.
Distribution: At plasma concentrations up to 200 mcg/ml, the drug appears to be about 80% bound to plasma proteins.
Metabolism: Probably hepatic; several active metabolites have been identified. With prolonged use, the active metabolites are expected to accumulate in the plasma and their concentration may exceed that of the parent compound. Bupropion appears to induce its own metabolism.
Excretion: Primarily renal. Half-life: Between 8 to 24 hours.
Onset, peak, duration: Peak plasma levels are achieved within 2 hours; peak therapeutic effects may take several weeks.

INDICATIONS & DOSAGE

Treatment of depression–
Adults: initially, 100 mg P.O. b.i.d. If necessary, dosage is increased after 3 days to the usual dose of 100 mg P.O. t.i.d. If there is no response after several weeks of therapy, dosage may be increased to 150 mg t.i.d.

CONTRAINDICATIONS & PRECAUTIONS

Contraindicated in patients who are allergic to the drug, patients who have taken MAO inhibitors within the previous 14 days, and patients with a seizure disorder. (About 0.4% of patients treated at dosages up to 450 mg/day may experience seizures. If dosage increases to 600 mg/day, the incidence of seizures increases about 10-fold). Also contraindicated in patients with a history of bulimia or anorexia nervosa because studies have revealed a higher incidence of seizures in these patients.

ADVERSE REACTIONS

Common reactions are in italics; life-threatening reactions are in bold italics.
CNS: *headache,* akathisia, seizures, *agitation,* anxiety, *confusion,* decreased libido, delusions, euphoria, hostility, impaired sleep quality, insomnia, sedation, sensory disturbance, tremor.
CV: cardiac arrhythmias, hypertension, hypotension, palpitations, syncope, tachycardia.
GI: appetite increase, constipation, dyspepsia, nausea, vomiting, dry mouth.
GU: impotence, menstrual complaints, urinary frequency.
Skin: pruritus, rash, cutaneous temperature disturbance.
Other: arthritis, fever and chills, excessive sweating, auditory disturbance, gustatory disturbance, blurred vision.

INTERACTIONS

Levodopa, phenothiazines, MAO inhibitors, or tricyclic antidepressants; or recent and rapid withdrawal of benzodiazepines: increased risk of adverse reactions, including seizures.

EFFECTS ON DIAGNOSTIC TESTS

None reported.

NURSING CONSIDERATIONS

Besides those related universally to drug therapy (see "How to use this book"), consider the following specific recommendations:

Assessment
- Obtain a baseline assessment of depression before therapy.
- Be alert for adverse reactions and drug interactions throughout therapy.
- Evaluate the patient's and family's knowledge about bupropion therapy.

Nursing Diagnoses
- Ineffectve individual coping related to the patient's underlying condition.
- High risk for injury related to bupropion-induced adverse CNS reactions.
- Knowledge deficit related to bupropion therapy.

Planning and Implementation
Preparation and Administration
- Expect to give daily dosage in three divided doses to minimize the risk of seizures.

Monitoring
- Monitor effectiveness by encouraging the patient to discuss his feelings (ask broad, open-ended questions) and by evaluating his behavior.
- Monitor the patient for increased restlessness evidenced by agitation, insomnia, and anxiety, especially at start of therapy.

Supportive Care
- Institute safety precautions if patient shows severe restlessness and notify the doctor. Some patients require sedative/hypnotic agents; in about 2%, the drug must be discontinued.

• Be aware that this drug can cause manic episodes during the depressed phase of bipolar manic depression.
• Expect the doctor to consider implications of weight loss before providing this drug. Clinical trials revealed a 5 lb or greater weight loss in 28% of patients taking this drug.
Patient Teaching
• Notify the doctor if patient develops restlessness. Doctor may order a sedative-hypnotic agent or may discontinue the drug.
• Warn the patient to avoid driving and other hazardous activities that require alertness and good psychomotor coordination until CNS effects of the drug are known.
• Warn against combining drug with alcohol because this combination can result in seizures. Also warn patients not to take any OTC or other medications without first checking with their doctors.
• Advise the patient to take the drug regularly as scheduled. Emphasize that he should take each day's dosage in three divided doses to minimize the risk of seizures.
Evaluation
In patients receiving bupropion, appropriate evaluation statements may include:
• Patient behavior and communication indicate improvement of depression.
• Patient has not experienced injury from adverse CNS reactions.
• Patient and family state an understanding of bupropion therapy.

buspirone hydrochloride
(byoo spye´ rone)
BuSpar

• *Classification:* anxiolytic (azospirodecanedione)
• *Pregnancy Risk Category:* B

HOW SUPPLIED
Tablets: 5 mg, 10 mg

ACTION
Mechanism: An anxiolytic that may inhibit spontaneous firing of serotonin (5-HT) containing neurons and reduce 5-HT turnover in cortical, amygdaloid, and septohippocampal tissue. Drug is not a CNS depressant or anticonvulsant.
Absorption: Rapidly and completely absorbed after oral administration, but extensive first-pass metabolism limits absolute bioavailability to about 4%. Food slows absorption but increases the amount of unchanged drug in systemic circulation.
Distribution: 95% protein-bound; the drug does not displace other highly protein-bound medications, such as warfarin.
Metabolism: In the liver by hydroxylation and oxidation, resulting in at least one pharmacologically active metabolite–1, pyrimidinylpiperazine (1-PP).
Excretion: 29% to 63% is excreted in urine in 24 hours, primarily as metabolites; 18% to 38% is excreted in feces. Half-life: 2 to 4 hours.
Onset, peak, duration: Onset of therapeutic effect may require 1 to 2 weeks of daily therapy.

INDICATIONS & DOSAGE
Management of anxiety disorders; short-term relief of anxiety–
Adults: initially, 5 mg P.O. t.i.d. Dosage may be increased at 3-day intervals. Usual maintenance dosage is 20 to 30 mg daily in divided doses.

CONTRAINDICATIONS & PRECAUTIONS
Contraindicated in patients with hypersensitivity to the drug. Use cautiously in those with a history of drug abuse or dependence (because of potential misuse or abuse) and in those with impaired hepatic or renal

function because drug may cause impaired metabolism or excretion.

ADVERSE REACTIONS

Common reactions are in italics; life-threatening reactions are in bold italics.
CNS: *dizziness, drowsiness,* nervousness, insomnia, headache.
GI: nausea, dry mouth, diarrhea.
Other: fatigue.

INTERACTIONS

Alcohol, other CNS depressants: increased CNS depression. Avoid concomitant use.
MAO inhibitors: may elevate blood pressure.

EFFECTS ON DIAGNOSTIC TESTS

None reported.

NURSING CONSIDERATIONS

Besides those related universally to drug therapy (see "How to use this book"), consider the following specific recommendations:

Assessment

- Obtain a baseline assessment of the patient's underlying condition before drug therapy.
- Be alert for adverse reactions and drug interactions throughout therapy.
- Evaluate the patient's and family's knowledge about buspirone therapy.

Nursing Diagnoses

- Anxiety related to the patient's underlying condition.
- High risk for injury related to buspirone-induced CNS reaction.
- Knowledge deficit related to buspirone therapy.

Planning and Implementation

Preparation and Administration

- Signs of improvement are usually evident within 7 to 10 days; optimal results are achieved after 3 to 4 weeks of therapy.
- Dosage may be increased in 3-day intervals.

Monitoring

- Monitor for adverse reactions or drug interactions by frequently checking the patient's neuromuscular coordination and vital signs.
- Monitor effectiveness by frequently monitoring the patient's anxiety level.
- Be aware that although this drug is less sedating than other anxiolytics and does not produce any serious functional impairment, individual CNS effects may be unpredictable.
- Know that unlike the benzodiazepines, buspirone is not an effective anticonvulsant or skeletal muscle relaxant. Its use is limited to the treatment of anxiety.
- Monitor the patient's bowel patterns; drug may cause diarrhea.
- Monitor hydration status if patient develops diarrhea.
- Regularly monitor the effectiveness of alprazolam therapy by asking the patient about feelings of anxiety and by evaluating the patient's behavior.
- Know that this drug has shown no potential for abuse and has not been classified as a controlled substance. However, it is not recommended for use to relieve everyday stress.

Supportive Care

- Provide encouragement and support with other treatment measures, such as professional counseling.
- If drowsiness or dizziness occurs, institute safety measures, such as supervising patient activities. Reorient patient as needed and ensure a safe environment.
- Provide frequent sips of water or ice chips for dry mouth.
- Provide patient with additional fluids if he develops diarrhea.

Patient Teaching

- Warn the patient to avoid hazardous activities that require alertness and neuromuscular coordination until CNS effects of the drug are known.
- Recommend sugarless chewing gum, hard candy, or ice chips to relieve dry mouth.

• Tell the patient to take the drug with food.
• Before beginning buspirone therapy in patients already being treated with benzodiazepine, warn them that abrupt discontinuation of the benzodiazepine may cause a withdrawal reaction.

Evaluation

In patients receiving buspirone, appropriate evaluation statements may include:
• Patient states he is less anxious.
• Patient does not experience injury as a result of adverse CNS reactions.
• Patient and family state an understanding of buspirone therapy.

busulfan

(byoo sul′ fan)
Myleran

• *Classification:* antineoplastic (alkylating agent)
• *Pregnancy Risk Category:* D

HOW SUPPLIED

Tablets: 2 mg

ACTION

Mechanism: An alkylating agent that cross-links strands of cellular DNA and interferes with RNA transcription, causing an imbalance of growth that leads to cell death. Drug's predominant effects are against cells of the granulocytic series. Cell cycle–nonspecific.
Absorption: Although well absorbed from the GI tract, there is a 30-minute to 2-hour delay before drug appears in the blood.
Distribution: Rapidly cleared from the plasma. Distribution into the brain and CSF is unknown.
Metabolism: Extensively metabolized, probably in the liver.
Excretion: Excreted in the urine, mostly as metabolites.

INDICATIONS & DOSAGE

Chronic myelocytic (granulocytic) leukemia –
Adults: 4 to 8 mg P.O. daily up to 12 mg P.O. daily until WBC falls to 15,000/mm³; stop drug until WBC rises to 50,000/mm³, then resume treatment as before; or 4 to 8 mg P.O. daily until WBC falls to 10,000 to 20,000/mm³, then reduce daily dosage as needed to maintain WBC at this level (usually 2 mg daily).
Children: 0.06 to 0.12 mg/kg or 2.3 to 4.6 mg/m²/day P.O.; adjust dosage to maintain WBC at 20,000/mm³, but never less than 10,000/mm³.

CONTRAINDICATIONS & PRECAUTIONS

Contraindicated in patients with a history of resistance to therapy with busulfan. Use cautiously in men and women of childbearing age because it can impair fertility, in those with a history of gout from hyperuricemic effects of the drug, and in patients whose immune system is compromised because of potential for additive toxicity. The drug can cause further myelosuppression, increasing the patient's risk of infection.

ADVERSE REACTIONS

Common reactions are in italics; life-threatening reactions are in bold italics.
Blood: WBC falling after about 10 days and continuing to fall for 2 weeks after stopping drug; ***thrombocytopenia,*** leukopenia, anemia.
GI: nausea, vomiting, diarrhea, cheilosis, glossitis.
GU: amenorrhea, testicular atrophy, impotence.
Metabolic: Addison-like wasting syndrome, profound hyperuricemia due to increased cell lysis.
Skin: transient hyperpigmentation, anhidrosis.
Other: gynecomastia; alopecia; ***irreversible pulmonary fibrosis, commonly termed "busulfan lung."***

INTERACTIONS

None significant.

EFFECTS ON DIAGNOSTIC TESTS

Cytologic studies: interference with interpretation because of drug-induced cellular dysplasia.
Blood and urine uric acid: increased levels.

NURSING CONSIDERATIONS

Besides those related universally to drug therapy (see "How to use this book"), consider the following specific recommendations:

Assessment

- Obtain a baseline assessment of the patient's underlying condition; CBC, and differential, platelet, and uric acid levels before initiating therapy.
- Be alert for adverse reactions or drug interactions during therapy.
- Evaluate the patient's and family's knowledge about busulfan therapy.

Nursing Diagnoses

- High risk for infection related to the patient's busulfan-induced pancytopenia.
- Altered tissue perfusion (renal) related to hyperuricemia with resulting uric acid nephropathy.
- Knowledge deficit related to busulfan therapy.

Planning and Implementation

Preparation and Administration

- ***P.O. use:*** Give only by P.O. route and give at the same time each day.
- Remember that dosage is adjusted to weekly WBC counts and that severe leukocytopenia may temporarily halt busulfan therapy.
- Keep in mind that busulfan is often administered with allopurinol to prevent symptoms of gout.

Monitoring

- Monitor effectiveness by noting the results of follow-up diagnostic tests and overall physical status.
- Monitor WBC and platelet counts daily, then weekly. The drug should be temporarily discontinued when WBC count falls to 15,000/mm^3. It may be resumed when the WBC count rises to 50,000/mm^3.
- Monitor serum and urine uric acid levels frequently.
- Monitor for signs of bleeding and avoid all I.M. injections when the platelet count is below 100,000/mm^3.
- Monitor fluid and electrolyte balance and daily temperature, and watch for signs of infection (fever, sore throat, fatigue).

Supportive Care

- Use cautiously in patients recently given other myelosuppressive drugs or radiation, and in those with depressed neutophil or platelet count.
- Pulmonary fibrosis may occur as late as 4 to 6 months after treatment with busulfan.
- Increased appetite, sense of euphoria, decreased total leukocyte count, and reduction in the size of the spleen usually begins within 1 to 2 weeks.
- Give the patient extra fluids as needed. These are often required during busulfan therapy.
- Note the presence of persistent cough and progressive dyspnea with alveolar exudate, which may result from drug toxicity. Notify the doctor. Remember that therapeutic effects are often accompanied by toxicity.

Patient Teaching

- Instruct the patient to avoid taking any OTC product containing aspirin.
- Instruct the patient to use caution with shaving, using kitchen utensils; to take care to avoid bumping into objects; and to watch closely for signs of bleeding (easy bruising, nosebleeds, bleeding gums, melena).
- Instruct the patient to report any new, persistent cough or dyspnea.
- Instruct the patient to take daily temperatures and to report any signs of infection immediately.

Evaluation
In patients receiving busulfan, appropriate evaluation statements may include:
• Patient remains free of infection.
• Patient demonstrates adequate renal tissue perfusion and normal serum uric acid levels.
• Patient and family state an understanding of busulfan therapy.

butabarbital sodium
(byoo ta bar´ bi tal)
Barbased*, Butalan*, Buticaps, Butisol* **, Day-Barb†, Sarisol No. 2* **

• Controlled Substance Schedule III
• *Classification:* sedative-hypnotic (barbiturate)
• *Pregnancy Risk Category:* D

HOW SUPPLIED
Tablets: 15 mg, 30 mg, 50 mg, 100 mg
Capsules: 15 mg, 30 mg
Elixir: 30 mg/5 ml, 33.3 mg/5 ml

ACTION
Mechanism: Probably interferes with transmission of impulses from the thalamus to the cortex of the brain.
Absorption: Well absorbed after oral administration.
Distribution: Widely distributed. Crosses placenta and enters the CNS.
Metabolism: Metabolized extensively in the liver by oxidation.
Excretion: Inactive metabolites are excreted in urine. Only 1% to 2% of an oral dose is excreted in urine unchanged. Half-life: The terminal half-life ranges from 30 to 40 hours.
Onset, peak, duration: Peak concentrations occur in 3 to 4 hours; onset of action in 45 to 60 minutes; duration of action, 6 to 8 hours.

INDICATIONS & DOSAGE
Sedation–
Adults: 15 to 30 mg P.O. t.i.d. or q.i.d.
Children: 6 mg/kg P.O. divided t.i.d. Dosage range 7.5 to 30 mg P.O. t.i.d.
Preoperatively–
Adults: 50 to 100 mg P.O. 60 to 90 minutes before surgery.
Insomnia–
Adults: 50 to 100 mg P.O. h.s.

CONTRAINDICATIONS & PRECAUTIONS
Contraindicated in patients with hypersensitivity to barbiturates and in patients with bronchopneumonia, status asthmaticus, or other severe respiratory distress because of the potential for respiratory depression; in patients who are depressed or have suicidal ideation because the drug can worsen depression; in patients with uncontrolled acute or chronic pain because exacerbation of pain or paradoxic excitement can occur; in patients with porphyria because this drug can trigger symptoms of this disease; or in patients with a tartrazine sensitivity because butabarbital preparations contain tartrazine.

Use cautiously in patients who must perform hazardous tasks requiring mental alertness because the drug causes drowsiness. Prolonged use of high doses should be avoided because tolerance and physical or psychological dependence may occur.

Prenatal exposure to barbiturates is associated with an increased incidence of fetal abnormalaities, including brain tumors. Use of barbiturates in the third trimester may be associated with physical dependence in neonates.

Use cautiously in patients with renal or hepatic dysfunction because of the risk of drug accumulation.

ADVERSE REACTIONS
Common reactions are in italics; life-threatening reactions are in bold italics.

CNS: *drowsiness, lethargy, hangover,* paradoxical excitement in elderly patients.
GI: nausea, vomiting.
Skin: rash, urticaria.
Other: *Stevens-Johnson syndrome,* angioedema, exacerbation of porphyria.

INTERACTIONS

Alcohol or other CNS depressants, including narcotic analgesics: excessive CNS and respiratory depression. Use together cautiously.
Griseofulvin: decreased absorption of griseofulvin.
MAO inhibitors: inhibit the metabolism of barbiturates; may cause prolonged CNS depression. Reduce barbiturate dosage.
Oral anticoagulants, estrogens and oral contraceptives, doxycycline, corticosteroids: butabarbital may enhance the metabolism of these drugs. Monitor for decreased effect.
Rifampin: may decrease barbiturate levels. Monitor for decreased effect.

EFFECTS ON DIAGNOSTIC TESTS

Cyanocobalamin ^{57}Co: impaired absorption.
EEG: altered patterns (change in low voltage, fast activity). Changes persist for a time after discontinuation of therapy.
Phentolamine test: false-positive result.
Serum bilirubin: decreased concentrations in neonates, epileptic patients, and patients with congenital nonhemolytic unconjugated hyperbilirubinemia.
Sulfobromophthalein retention: increased.

NURSING CONSIDERATIONS

Besides those related universally to drug therapy (see "How to use this book"), consider the following specific recommendations:

Assessment
- Obtain a baseline assessment of sleeping patterns and CNS status before therapy.
- Be alert for adverse reactions and drug interactions throughout therapy.
- Evaluate the patient's and family's knowledge about butabarbital therapy.

Nursing Diagnoses
- Sleep pattern disturbance related to underlying patient problem.
- High risk for trauma related to adverse CNS reactions caused by butabarbital.
- Knowledge deficit related to butabarbital therapy.

Planning and Implementation

Preparation and Administration
- Before leaving the bedside, make sure the patient has swallowed the medication.
- Be aware that prolonged administration is not recommended; drug is not shown to be effective after 14 days. A drug-free interval of at least 1 week is advised after 14 days of therapy.

Monitoring
- Monitor effectiveness by regularlyevaluating patient's ability to sleep.
- Monitor CNS status for evidence of adverse reactions.
- Monitor for signs of barbiturate toxicity: coma, pupillary constriction, cyanosis, clammy skin, and hypotension. Overdose can be fatal.
- After drug discontinuation, be alert for withdrawal symptoms.

Supportive Care
- After administration, institute safety precautions: remove cigarettes; keep bed rails up, and supervise or assist ambulation.
- Withhold the drug if barbiturate toxicity is suspected.
- Do not discontinue the drug abruptly after prolonged high-dose therapy. The drug may cause dependence and severe withdrawal symptoms. Withdraw barbiturates gradually.

• Take precautions to prevent hoarding or self-overdosing, especially by patient who is depressed or suicidal or has a history of drug abuse.
• Keep in mind that butabarbital sodium elixer is sugar-free.

Patient Teaching

• Explain that morning "hangover" is common after hypnotic dose. Encourage the patient to report severe "hangover" or oversedation so the doctor can be consulted for change of dose or drug.
• Explain that because hypnotic drugs suppress rapid eye movement sleep, the patient may experience increased dreaming when the drug is discontinued.
• Instruct the patient to remain in bed after taking drug and to call for assistance to use the bathroom.
• Warn the patient that drug may cause physical dependence.
• Warn the patient to avoid hazardous activities that require mental alertness if adverse CNS reactions are present after awakening.
• Tell the patient to notify the nurse or doctor if sleep pattern disturbances persist despite therapy.
• Advise women who use oral contraceptives when taking this drug to discuss alternate birth control methods with their doctor. Explain that butabarbital may enhance contraceptive hormone metabolism and decrease its effect.

Evaluation

In patients receiving butabarbital, appropriate evaluation statements may include:

• Patient states drug was effective in inducing sleep.
• Patient's safety is maintained.
• Patient and family state an understanding of butabarbital therapy.

butoconazole nitrate

(byo toe koe´ na zole)
Femstat

• *Classification:* fungistat (imidazole derivative)
• *Pregnancy Risk Category:* C

HOW SUPPLIED

Vaginal cream: 2% supplied with applicators

ACTION

Mechanism: Controls or destroys fungus by disrupting cell membrane permeability and reducing osmotic resistance.
Absorption: Approximately 5.5% of the medication is absorbed through the vaginal walls.
Metabolism: Systemically absorbed drug appears to be metabolized, probably in the liver.
Excretion: Systemically absorbed drug appears to be excreted in the urine and feces. Half-life: Approximately 21 to 24 hours.
Onset, peak, duration: After vaginal administration, peak plasma levels of the drug and its metabolites are attained at 24 hours.

INDICATIONS & DOSAGE

Local treatment of vulvovaginal mycotic infections caused by Candida *species–*
Adults (nonpregnant): one applicatorful intravaginally at bedtime for 3 days.
Adults (pregnant): one applicatorful intravaginally at bedtime for 6 days. Use only during second and third trimester.

CONTRAINDICATIONS & PRECAUTIONS

Contraindicated in patients with hypersensitivity to the drug. Use cautiously in the first trimester of pregnancy.

ADVERSE REACTIONS

Common reactions are in italics; life-threatening reactions are in bold italics.
Skin: vulvar itching, soreness, and swelling; itching of the fingers.

INTERACTIONS

None significant.

EFFECTS ON DIAGNOSTIC TESTS

None reported.

NURSING CONSIDERATIONS

Besides those related universally to drug therapy (see "How to use this book"), consider the following specific recommendations:

Assessment

- Obtain a baseline assessment of vaginal drainage before therapy.
- Be alert for adverse reactions and drug interactions throughout therapy.
- Evaluate the patient's and family's knowledge about butoconazole nitrate therapy.

Nursing Diagnoses

- Impaired skin integrity related to patient's underlying condition.
- High risk for impaired skin integrity related to drug-induced adverse reaction.
- Knowledge deficit related to butoconazole nitrate therapy.

Planning and Implementation

Preparation and Administration

- Keep in mind that butoconazole may be used with oral contraceptive and antibiotic therapy.

Monitoring

- Monitor effectiveness by evaluating patient's vaginal discharge.
- Monitor symptom resolution. Effect of butoconazole is apparent after only 3 days of therapy as opposed to 7 days of miconazole cream therapy.

Supportive Care

- Confirm diagnosis of Candida vulvovaginal infection by smears or cultures.
- Withhold medication during first trimester of pregnancy.

Patient Teaching

- Teach patient how to apply. Tell patient not to use tampons during treatment.
- Inform patient that sexual partner should wear a condom during intercourse until treatment is complete. He should consult doctor if he experiences penile itching, redness or discomfort.
- Advise patient to do the following to prevent reinfection. Keep cool and dry, wear loose fitting cotton clothing, avoid feminine hygiene sprays, wash daily with unscented soap, dry thoroughly with clean towel, and maintain proper bowel hygiene by wiping from front to back.

Evaluation

In patients receiving butoconazole, appropriate evaluation statements may include:

- Patient no longer experiences vaginal discomfort or foul drainage.
- Patient did not experience itching.
- Patient and family state an understanding of butoconazole therapy.

butorphanol tartrate

(byoo tor´ fa nole)
Stadol

- *Classification:* analgesic, adjunct to anesthesia (opioid partial agonist, narcotic agonist-antagonist)
- *Pregnancy Risk Category:* B (D for prolonged use or use of high doses at term)

HOW SUPPLIED

Injection: 1 mg/ml, 2 mg/ml

*Liquid form contains alcohol. **May contain tartrazine.

ACTION

Mechanism: An agonist-antagonist that binds with opiate receptors at many sites in the CNS (brain, brain stem, and spinal cord), altering both perception of and emotional response to pain through an unknown mechanism.
Absorption: Well absorbed after I.M. administration.
Distribution: Rapidly crosses the placenta; neonatal serum concentrations are 0.4 to 1.4 times maternal concentrations.
Metabolism: Metabolized extensively in the liver, primarily by hydroxylation, to inactive metabolites.
Excretion: In inactive form, mainly by the kidneys. About 11% to 14% of a parenteral dose is excreted in feces. Half-life: About 2.5 hours.
Onset, peak, duration: Onset of analgesia is less than 10 minutes, with peak analgesic effect at 30 minutes to 1 hour. Duration of effect is 3 to 4 hours.

INDICATIONS & DOSAGE

Moderate to severe pain–
Adults: 1 to 4 mg I.M. q 3 to 4 hours, p.r.n. or around the clock; or 0.5 to 2 mg I.V. q 3 to 4 hours, p.r.n. or around the clock.

CONTRAINDICATIONS & PRECAUTIONS

Contraindicated in patients with hypersensitivity to the drug.

Administer with extreme caution to patients with supraventricular arrhythmias; avoid or use extreme caution in patients with head injury or increased intracranial pressure because neurologic parameters are obscured; and during pregnancy and labor because drug readily crosses placenta (premature infants are especially sensitive to respiratory and CNS depressant effects). Use cautiously in patients with renal or hepatic dysfunction, because drug accumulation or prolonged duration of action may occur; in patients with pulmonary disease (asthma, chronic obstructive pulmonary disease) because drug depresses respiration and suppresses cough reflex; in patients undergoing biliary tract surgery, because drug may cause biliary spasm; in patients with seizure disorders, because drug may precipitate seizures; in elderly or debilitated patients, who are more sensitive to drug's effects; and in patients prone to physical or psychological addiction because of the high risk of addiction to this drug.

Butorphanol has a lower potential for abuse than do narcotic agonists. It increases cardiac work, especially of the pulmonary circuit; therefore, use in patients with acute myocardial infarction or other cardiac abnormalities should be limited to those hypersensitive to other agents that might be used; for example, meperidine (cross-hypersensitivity to the morphine-allergic patient must be considered with butorphanol).

Use cautiously as a preoperative or preanesthetic drug in hypertensive patients because it may cause increases in systolic blood pressure.

ADVERSE REACTIONS

Common reactions are in italics; life-threatening reactions are in bold italics.
CNS: *sedation, headache, vertigo, floating sensation,* lethargy, confusion, nervousness, unusual dreams, agitation, euphoria, hallucinations, flushing.
CV: palpitations, fluctuation in blood pressure.
EENT: diplopia, blurred vision.
GI: *nausea,* vomiting, dry mouth, constipation.
Skin: rash, hives, *clamminess, excessive sweating.*
Other: ***respiratory depression.***

INTERACTIONS

Alcohol, CNS depressants: additive effects. Use together cautiously.
Narcotic analgesics: avoid concomitant use. Possible decreased analgesic effect.

EFFECTS ON DIAGNOSTIC TESTS

None reported.

NURSING CONSIDERATIONS

Besides those related universally to drug therapy (see "How to use this book"), consider the following specific recommendations:

Assessment

- Obtain a baseline assessment of the patient's pain before therapy.
- Be alert for adverse reactions and drug interactions throughout therapy.
- Evaluate the patient's and family's knowledge about butorphanol therapy.

Nursing Diagnoses

- Pain related to patient's underlying condition.
- High risk for trauma related to adverse CNS reactions induced by butorphanol.
- Knowledge deficit related to butorphanol therapy.

Planning and Implementation

Preparation and Administration

- ***I.V use:*** Do not administer rapid I.V. injection since this can can cause severe respiratory depression, hypotension, circulatory collapse, and cardiac arrest. Administer drug with patient in recumbent position to minimize hypotension and dizziness.
- S.C. route is not recommended.

Monitoring

- Monitor effectiveness after each dose by evaluating degree of pain relief.
- Monitor for adverse CNS reactions, such as vertigo, confusion, and floating sensation.
- Monitor respiratory status noting any evidence of respiratory depression, such as decreased rate or depth of respiration. Keep in mind that respiratory depression apparently does not increase with increased dosage.
- Regularly monitor blood pressure for fluctuations.
- Monitor bowel function for constipation.

Supportive Care

- Notify the doctor and discuss increase of dosage or frequency if pain persists.
- Keep narcotic antagonist (naloxone) and resuscitative equipment available.
- Because adverse CNS reactions are possible, institute safety precautions, such as supervising ambulation and keeping bed rails up.
- If not contraindicated, obtain an order for a stool softener and increase the patient's fluid and fiber intake to prevent or treat constipation, a possible reaction to therapy.
- Be aware that butorphanol can cause physical and psychological dependence. Abrupt withdrawal after chronic use produces intense withdrawal symptoms.
- Recognize that butorphanol has narcotic antagonist properties and may precipitate abstinence syndrome in narcotic-dependent patients.

Patient Teaching

- Warn patient to change positions slowly and to avoid activities that require alertness because drug may cause dizziness and drowsiness.
- Suggest high-fiber diet and liberal fluid intake to prevent constipation.
- Tell the patient or family caregiver to notify the nurse or doctor if respiration rate decreases.

Evaluation

In patients receiving butorphanol, appropriate evaluation statements may include:

- Patient reports relief of pain after administration of butorphanol.
- Adverse CNS reactions did not occur.
- Patient and family state an understanding of butorphanol therapy.

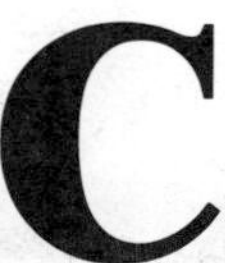

calcifediol

(kal si fe dye´ ole)
Calderol

• *Classification:* antihypocalcemic (vitamin analog)
• *Pregnancy Risk Category:* A

HOW SUPPLIED

Capsules: 20 mcg, 50 mcg

ACTION

Mechanism: A vitamin D analog (25-hydroxycholecalciferol) that stimulates calcium absorption from the GI tract and promotes bone resorption that releases calcium to blood.
Absorption: Readily absorbed from the small intestine.
Distribution: Widely distributed and highly protein-bound.
Metabolism: In the liver and kidney. It is activated to 1,25 dihydroxycholecalciferol.
Excretion: In urine and bile. Half-life: 16 days.
Onset, peak, and duration: Peak levels are seen within 4 hours of an oral dose.

INDICATIONS & DOSAGE

Treatment and management of metabolic bone disease associated with chronic renal failure–
Adults: initially, 300 to 350 mcg P.O. weekly, given on a daily or alternate-day schedule. Dosage may be increased at 4-week intervals. Optimal dosage must be carefully determined for each patient.

CONTRAINDICATIONS & PRECAUTIONS

Contraindicated in patients with hypercalcemia or sensitivity to vitamin D.

ADVERSE REACTIONS

Common reactions are in italics; life-threatening reactions are in bold italics.
Vitamin D intoxication associated with hypercalcemia:
CNS: headache, somnolence.
EENT: conjunctivitis, photosensitivity, rhinorrhea.
GI: nausea, vomiting, constipation, metallic taste, dry mouth, anorexia, diarrhea.
GU: polyuria.
Other: weakness, bone and muscle pain.

INTERACTIONS

Cholestyramine: may impair absorption of calcifediol.

EFFECTS ON DIAGNOSTIC TESTS

Cholesterol (Zlatkis-Zak reaction): falsely elevated.
Serum alkaline phosphatase: altered concentrations.
Serum and urine electrolytes (magnesium, phosphate, and calcium): altered results.

NURSING CONSIDERATIONS

Besides those related universally to drug therapy (see "How to use this book"), consider the following specific recommendations:
Assessment
• Obtain a baseline assessment of the patient's metabolic bone disease before initiating calcifediol therapy.
• Be alert for common adverse reac-

tions and drug interactions throughout therapy.
• Evaluate the patient's and family's knowledge about calcifediol therapy.

Nursing Diagnoses
• High risk for injury related to the patient's underlying bone condition.
• Altered protection related to potential for vitamin D intoxication caused by calcifediol therapy.
• Knowledge deficit related to calcifediol therapy.

Planning and Implementation
Preparation and Administration
• Be aware that optimal dosage is highly individualized.
Monitoring
• Monitor effectiveness by regularly checking the patient's serum calcium levels; serum calcium times serum phosphate should not exceed 70. During titration, serum calcium should be determined at least weekly.
• Monitor patient closely for vitamin D intoxication associated with hypercalcemia.
Supportive Care
• If hypercalcemia occurs, notify doctor because drug should be discontinued until serum calcium returns to normal.
• Ensure that patient is receiving adequate daily intake of calcium.
Patient Teaching
• Advise patient to adhere to diet and calcium supplementation and to avoid nonprescription drugs.
• Teach patient to report signs and symptoms of hypercalcemia.

Evaluation
In patients receiving calcifediol, appropriate evaluation statements may include:
• Patient exhibits improvement in serum calcium level amd his metabolic bone disease and as a result does not substain bone injury.
• Patient does not experience vitamin D intoxication because of calcifediol therapy.
• Patient and family express an understanding of calcifediol therapy.

calcitonin (human)
(kal si toe´ nin)
Cibacalcin

calcitonin (salmon)
Calcimar, Miacalcin

• *Classification:* hypocalcemic (polypeptide hormone)
• *Pregnancy Risk Category:* B

HOW SUPPLIED
Injection: salmon–100 IU/ml, 1-ml ampules; 200 IU/ml, 2-ml ampules; human–0.5 mg/vial

ACTION
Mechanism: A polypeptide hormone secreted by the parafollicular cells of the thyroid that decreases the number or function of osteoclasts. This decreases bone resorption (osteolysis).
Absorption: Because it is a polypeptide, calcitonin is destroyed in the GI tract. It must be administered parenterally.
Distribution: Endogenous calcitonin is found in breast milk; it is not known whether calcitonin (human) or calcitonin (salmon) enters the CNS or is found in milk.
Metabolism: Rapid metabolism occurs in the kidney, with additional metabolism in the blood and peripheral tissues.
Excretion: In urine as inactive metabolites. Half-life: About 1 hour.
Onset, peak, duration: Plasma concentrations of 0.1 to 0.4 mg/ml are achieved within 15 minutes of a 200 IU S.C. dose. The maximum effect is seen in 2 to 4 hours; duration of action may be 8 to 24 hours for S.C. or I.M. doses and 30 minutes to 12 hours for I.V. doses.

INDICATIONS & DOSAGE

Paget's disease of bone (osteitis deformans) –

Adults: initially, 100 IU of calcitonin (salmon) daily S.C. or I.M. Maintenance dosage is 50 to 100 IU daily or every other day. Alternatively, give calcitonin (human) 0.5 mg S.C. daily. If patient obtains sufficient improvement, dosage may be reduced to 0.25 mg. daily 2 or 3 times per week. Some patients may need as much as 1 mg daily.

Hypercalcemia –

Adults: 4 IU/kg of calcitonin (salmon) q 12 hours I.M.

Postmenopausal osteoporosis –

Adults: 100 of calcitonin (salmon) daily I.M. or S.C.

CONTRAINDICATIONS & PRECAUTIONS

Contraindicated in patients with hypersensitivity to the drug or its gelatin diluent.

ADVERSE REACTIONS

Common reactions are in italics; life-threatening reactions are in bold italics.

CNS: headaches.

GI: transient nausea with or without vomiting, diarrhea, anorexia.

GU: transient diuresis.

Metabolic: hyperglycemia.

Local: inflammation at injection site, skin rashes.

Other: *facial flushing;* hypocalcemia; swelling, tingling, and tenderness of hands; unusual taste sensation; ***anaphylaxis.***

INTERACTIONS

None significant.

EFFECTS ON DIAGNOSTIC TESTS

None reported.

NURSING CONSIDERATIONS

Besides those related universally to drug therapy (see "How to use this book"), consider the following specific recommendations:

Assessment

- Obtain a baseline assessment of the patient's serum calcium level before initiating calcitonin therapy.
- Be alert for common adverse reactions, especially facial flushing and anaphylaxis.
- Evaluate the patient's and family's knowledge about calcitonin therapy.

Nursing Diagnoses

- High risk for injury related to the patient's underlying bone condition.
- Altered protection related to potential for calcitonin-induced anaphylaxis.
- Knowledge deficit related to calcitonin therapy.

Planning and Implementation

Preparation and Administration

- Administer a skin test, as ordered, before beginning therapy.
- If possible, administer drug at bedtime to minimize nausea and vomiting.
- Use the freshly reconstituted solution within 2 hours.
- Be aware that the S.C. route is the preferred method of administration.

Monitoring

- Monitor effectiveness by regularly checking the patient's serum calcium levels. Be aware that serum alkaline phosphatase and 24-hour urine hydroxyproline levels should be determined periodically to evaluate drug effect.
- Monitor for signs of hypocalcemic tetany during therapy (muscle twitching, tetanic spasms, and seizures if hypocalcemia is severe), or watch for signs of hypercalcemic relapse: bone pain, renal calculi, polyuria, anorexia, nausea, vomiting, thirst, constipation, lethargy, bradycardia, muscle hypotonicity, pathologic fracture, psychosis, and coma.
- Be aware that periodic examinations of urine sediment are advisable.

Supportive Care
• Systemic allergic reactions are possible since calcitonin is a protein. Keep epinephrine handy when administering.
• Be aware that patients with good initial clinical response to calcitonin who suffer relapse should be evaluated for formation of antibodies response to the hormone protein.
• Keep parenteral calcium available during the first doses in case hypocalcemic tetany occurs.
Patient Teaching
• Teach the patient how to self-administer calcitonin until patient achieves proper technique.
• Tell the patient to handle missed doses as follows: With daily dosing, take as soon as possible; do not double up on doses. With every-other-day dosing, take as soon as possible, then restart the alternate days from this dose.
• Stress the importance of regular visits to the doctor to assess progress.
• If calcitonin is being taken to treat postmenopausal osteoporosis, remind patient to take adequate calcium and vitamin D supplements.
• Tell patients in whom calcitonin loses its hypocalcemic activity that further medication or increased dosages will be of no value.
• Facial flushing and warmth occur in 20% to 30% of all patients within minutes of injection and usually last about 1 hour. Reassure the patient that this is a transient effect.
Evaluation
In patients receiving calcitonin, appropriate evaluation statements may include:
• Patient's serum calcium levels are normal.
• Patient does not experience anaphylaxis.
• Patient and family state an understanding of calcitonin therapy.

calcitriol (1,25-dihydroxycholecalciferol)
(kal si trye´ ole)
Rocaltrol

• *Classification:* antihypocalcemic (vitamin analog)
• *Pregnancy Risk Category:* A (D if used in doses > RDA)

HOW SUPPLIED
Capsules: 0.25 mcg, 0.5 mcg

ACTION
Mechanism: A vitamin D analog that stimulates calcium absorption from the GI tract and promotes bone resorption that promotes the release of calcium to blood.
Absorption: Readily absorbed after oral administration if fat absorption is normal.
Distribution: Widely distributed and protein-bound.
Metabolism: In the liver and kidneys. No activation step is required.
Excretion: Primarily in the feces. Half-life: 3 to 8 hours.
Onset, peak, duration: The duration of activity is about 3 to 5 days. Peak serum concentrations are reached within 3 to 6 hours after dosing.

INDICATIONS & DOSAGE
Management of hypocalcemia in patients undergoing chronic dialysis–
Adults: initially, 0.25 mcg P.O. daily. Dosage may be increased by 0.25 mcg daily at 2- to 4-week intervals. Maintenance dosage is 0.25 mcg every other day up to 0.5 to 1.25 mcg daily.
Management of hypoparathyroidism and pseudohypoparathyroidism–
Adults and children over 1 year: initially, 0.25 mcg P.O. daily. Dosage may be increased at 2- to 4-week intervals. Maintenance dosage is 0.25 to 2 mcg daily.

CONTRAINDICATIONS & PRECAUTIONS

Contraindicated in patients with hypercalcemia or sensitivity to vitamin D. Use cautiously in patients taking digitalis, because dyshypercalcemia may precipitate cardiac arrhythmias.

ADVERSE REACTIONS

Common reactions are in italics; life-threatening reactions are in bold italics.
Vitamin D intoxication associated with hypercalcemia –
CNS: headache, somnolence.
EENT: conjunctivitis, photophobia, rhinorrhea.
GI: nausea, vomiting, constipation, metallic taste, dry mouth, anorexia.
GU: polyuria.
Other: weakness, bone and muscle pain.

INTERACTIONS

None significant.

EFFECTS ON DIAGNOSTIC TESTS

Cholesterol determinations (using the Zlatkis-Zak reaction): falsely elevated results.
Serum alkaline phosphatase: altered concentrations.
Serum and urine electrolytes (magnesium, phosphate, and calcium): altered results.

NURSING CONSIDERATIONS

Besides those related universally to drug therapy (see "How to use this book"), consider the following specific recommendations:

Assessment
- Obtain a baseline assessment of the patient's serum calcium level before initiating calcitriol therapy.
- Be alert for common adverse reactions and drug interactions throughout therapy.
- Evaluate the patient's and family's knowledge about calcitriol therapy.

Nursing Diagnoses
- High risk for injury related to the patient's underlying condition.
- Altered protection related to potential for calcitriol-induced vitamin D intoxication.
- Knowledge deficit related to calcitriol therapy.

Planning and Implementation

Preparation and Administration
- Protect drug from heat and light.

Monitoring
- Monitor effectiveness by regularly checking the patient's serum calcium levels; serum calcium times serum phosphate should not exceed 70. During titration, determine serum calcium twice weekly.
- Monitor patient for early signs of vitamin D toxicity.

Supportive Care
- Notify doctor if hypercalcemia occurs because drug should be discontinued, until serum calcium returns to normal.
- Ensure that patient is receiving adequate daily intake of calcium-1,000 mg.

Patient Teaching
- Instruct patient to adhere to diet and calcium supplementation and to avoid unapproved nonprescription drugs.
- Tell patient not to use magnesium-containing antacids while taking this drug.
- Instruct patient to report to doctor immediately any of the following symptoms: weakness, nausea, vomiting, dry mouth, constipation, muscle or bone pain, or metallic taste – early symptoms of vitamin D intoxication.
- Tell patient that although this drug is a vitamin, it must not be taken by anyone for whom it was not prescribed because of its potentially serious toxicities.

Evaluation

In patients receiving calcitriol, appropriate evaluation statements may include:

• Patient's serum calcium levels are normal.
• Patient does not experience vitamin D intoxication.
• Patient and family state an understanding of calcitriol therapy.

calcium salts

calcium carbonate
(kal′ see um kar′ boh nate)
Alka-Mints◇, Amitone◇, Cal Carb-HD◇, Cal-Plus◇, Chooz◇, Dicarbosil◇, Equilet◇, Mallamint◇, Rolaids Calcium Rich◇, Tums◇, Tums E-X Extra Strength◇, Tums Extra Strength◇

calcium chloride◇

calcium citrate◇

calcium glubionate◇

calcium gluceptate◇

calcium gluconate
Kalcinate◇

calcium lactate◇

calcium phosphate, dibasic◇

calcium phosphate, tribasic
Posture◇

• *Classification:* antacid, therapeutic agent for electrolyte imbalance, cardiotonic (calcium supplement)
• *Pregnancy Risk Category:* C

HOW SUPPLIED

calcium carbonate
Tablets◇: 650 mg, 667 mg, 750 mg, 1.25 g, 1.5 g (contains 400 mg calcium/g)
Tablets (chewable)◇: 350 mg, 420 mg, 500 mg, 625 mg, 750 mg, 850 mg, 1.25 g
Capsules: 1.512 g◇
Oral suspension: 1.25 g/5 ml (contains 400 mg of elemental calcium/g)◇
Chewy squares: 1.5 g◇
Powder packets: 6.5 g (2,400 mg calcium) per packet◇
calcium chloride
Injection: 10% solution in 10-ml ampules, vials, and syringes
calcium citrate
Tablets: 950 mg (contains 211 mg of elemental calcium/g)◇
calcium glubionate
Syrup: 1.8 g/5 ml (contains 64 mg of elemental calcium/g)
calcium gluceptate
Injection: 1.1 g/5 ml in 5-ml ampules or 50-ml vials
calcium gluconate
Tablets: 500 mg◇, 650 mg◇, 975 mg◇, 1 g◇ (contains 90 mg of elemental calcium/g)
Injection: 10% solution in 10-ml ampules and vials, 10-ml or 20-ml vials
calcium lactate
Tablets: 325 mg, 650 mg (contains 130 mg of elemental calcium/g)
calcium phosphate, dibasic
Tablets: 468 mg (contains 230 mg of elemental calcium/g)◇
calcium phosphate, tribasic
Tablets: 300 mg◇, 600 mg◇ (contains 400 mg of elemental calcium/g)

ACTION

Mechanism: Replaces and maintains calcium.
Absorption: The I.M. and I.V. calcium salts are absorbed directly into the bloodstream. I.V. injection gives an immediate blood level, which will decrease to previous levels in about 30 minutes to 2 hours. The oral dose is absorbed actively in the duodenum and proximal jejunum and, to a lesser extent, in the distal part of the small intestine. Calcium is absorbed only in the ionized form. Pregnancy and reduction of calcium intake may increase the efficiency of absorption.

Vitamin D in its active form is required for calcium absorption.
Distribution: Enters the extracellular fluid and is incorporated rapidly into skeletal tissue. Bone contains 99% of the total calcium; 1% is distributed equally between the intracellular and extracellular fluids. CSF concentrations are about 50% of serum calcium concentrations.
Metabolism: None significant.
Excretion: Mainly in the feces as unabsorbed calcium that was secreted via bile and pancreatic juice into the lumen of the GI tract. Most calcium entering the kidney is reabsorbed in the loop of Henle and the proximal and distal convoluted tubules. Only small amounts of calcium are excreted in the urine.

INDICATIONS & DOSAGE

Hypocalcemia, hypocalcemic tetany, hypocalcemia during exchange transfusions, cardiac resuscitation for inotropic effect when epinephrine has failed; magnesium intoxication; hypoparathyroidism–
Adults and children: initially, 500 mg to 1 g calcium salt I.V., with further dosage based on serum calcium determinations and specific calcium salt. See below for dosages with specific calcium salts.

Dosage with calcium chloride (1 g [10 ml] yields 13.5 mEq Ca^{++}):
Magnesium intoxication–
Adults and children: initially, 500 mg I.V., with further doses based on calcium and magnesium determinations.
Cardiac arrest–
0.5 to 1 g I.V., not to exceed 1 ml/minute; or 200 to 800 mg into the ventricular cavity.
Hypocalcemia–
500 mg to 1 g I.V. at intervals of 1 to 3 days, determined by serum calcium levels.
Calcium supplementation during total parenteral nutrition–
Adults: 10 to 15 mEq I.V. daily.
Children: 5 to 20 mEq I.V. daily.
Neonates: 0.5 to 3 mEq/kg I.V. daily.

Dosage with calcium gluconate (1 g [10 ml] yields 4.5 mEq Ca^{++}):
Hypocalcemia–
Adults: 500 mg to 1 g I.V., repeated q 1 to 3 days p.r.n. as determined by serum calcium levels. Further doses depend on serum calcium determinations.
Children: 100 to 150 mg/kg I.V. three to four times daily. Rate of infusion should not exceed 0.5 ml/minute.

Dosage with calcium gluceptate (1.1 g [5 ml] yields 4.5 mEq Ca^{++}) and calcium salts (18 mg [1 ml] yields 0.898 mEq Ca^{++}):
Hypocalcemia–
Adults: initially, 5 to 20 ml I.V., with further doses based on serum calcium determinations. If I.V. injection is impossible, 2 to 5 ml I.M. Average adult oral dose is 1 to 2 g elemental calcium P.O. daily, divided t.i.d. or q.i.d. Average oral dose for children is 45 to 65 mg/kg P.O. daily, divided t.i.d. or q.i.d.
During exchange transfusions–
Adults and children: 0.5 ml I.V. after each 100 ml blood exchanged.

CONTRAINDICATIONS & PRECAUTIONS

Use cautiously in patients with renal failure and hypercalcemia because calcium may accumulate and because patients with renal impairment or dehydration and electrolyte imbalance are predisposed to the milk-alkali syndrome. Use cautiously in patients with calcium loss secondary to decreased mobility (especially the elderly) and in patients with GI hemorrhage or obstruction.

ADVERSE REACTIONS

Common reactions are in italics; life-threatening reactions are in bold italics.

CNS: from I.V. use, tingling sensations, sense of oppression or heat waves; with rapid I.V. injection, syncope.
CV: mild fall in blood pressure; with rapid I.V. injection, vasodilation, *bradycardia,* ***cardiac arrhythmias, cardiac arrest.***
GI: with oral ingestion, irritation, hemorrhage, *constipation;*with I.V. administration, chalky taste; with oral calcium chloride, GI hemorrhage, nausea, vomiting, thirst, abdominal pain.
GU: hypercalcemia, hypophosphatemia, polyuria, renal calculi.
Skin: local reaction if calcium salts given I.M., burning, necrosis, tissue sloughing, cellulitis, soft tissue calcification.
Local: with S.C. injection, pain and irritation; *with I.V., vein irritation.*

INTERACTIONS

Cardiac glycosides: increased digitalis toxicity; administer calcium very cautiously (if at all) to digitalized patients.

EFFECTS ON DIAGNOSTIC TESTS

Blood and urine pH: possible increase.
Gastric acid secretion test: altered results by interference with penagastrin and histamine.
Serum calcium: increased concentrations (with high doses).
Serum gastrin: increased concentrations.
Serum phosphate: decreased concentrations (with excessive and prolonged use).

NURSING CONSIDERATIONS

Besides those related universally to drug therapy (see "How to use this book"), consider the following specific recommendations:

Assessment
- Obtain a baseline assessment of patient's serum calcium level before therapy.
- Be alert for adverse reactions or drug interactions throughout therapy.
- Evaluate the patient's and family's knowledge about calcium therapy.

Nursing Diagnoses
- Altered nutrition: Less than body requirements related to insufficient calcium.
- High risk for injury related to calcium-induced hypercalcemia.
- Knowledge deficit related to calcium therapy.

Planning and Implementation
Preparation and Administration
- Warm parenteral solution to body temperature before administering in nonemergencies.
- Crash carts usually contain both gluconate and chloride forms. Make sure doctor specifies form he wants administered.
- ***P.O. use:*** Give drug 1 to 1½ hours after meals if GI upset occurs.
- ***I.M. use:*** I.M. injection should be given in the gluteal region in adults; lateral thigh in infants; I.M. route is used only in emergencies when no I.V. route available. Patient should be recumbent for 15 minutes after administration.
- ***I.V. use (direct injection):*** Administer slowly through a small needle into a large vein or through an I.V. line containing a free-flowing, compatible solution at a rate not exceeding 1 ml/minute (1.5 mEq/minute) for calcium chloride, 1.5 to 5 ml/minute for calcium gluconate, and 2 ml/minute for calcium gluceptate. Do not use scalp veins in children.
- ***I.V. use (intermittent infusion):*** Infuse diluted solution through an I.V. line containing a compatible solution. Maximum rate of 200 mg/minute suggested for calcium gluceptate and calcium gluconate.

• ***I.V. use (continuous infusion):*** Infuse after addition of large volume of fluid at a maximum rate of 200 mg/minute for calcium gluceptate and calcium gluconate.
• Calcium chloride should be given I.V. only. When adding to parenteral solutions that contain other additives (especially phosphorus or phosphate), observe closely for precipitate. Use an in-line filter.
• During all I.V. administrations, the patient's ECG should be monitored. Discontinue the drug if patient complains of discomfort.
• Following all I.V. administrations patient should remain recumbent for 15 minutes.

Monitoring
• Monitor effectiveness by evaluating blood calcium level frequently.
• Monitor patient's vital signs and ECG with calcium therapy.
• Monitor patient for signs and symptoms of hypercalcemia, especially when large doses are given.
• Monitor I.V. site closely for extravasation as severe necrosis and tissue sloughing can occur. Be aware that calcium gluconate is less irritating to veins and tissues than calcium chloride.

Supportive Care
• Withhold drug and notify doctor if hypercalcemia occurs. Be prepared to provide emergency supportive care as needed until calcium level returns to normal.
• Stop drug immediately if extravasation occurs, and change I.V. site before continuing drug.
• Notify doctor if GI adverse reactions are present as hemorrhage may occur.

Patient Teaching
• Tell patient to take oral calcium 1 to 1½ hours after meals if GI upset occurs.
• Warn patient to avoid oxalic acid (found in rhubarb and spinach), phytic acid (in bran and whole cereals), and phosphorus (in milk and dairy products) because these substances may interfere with absorption of calcium.
• Teach patient the signs and symptoms of hypercalcemia and tell him to notify doctor if any occurs.
• Stress importance of follow-up care and regular blood samples to monitor calcium level.

Evaluation
In patients receiving calcium, appropriate evaluation statements may include:
• Patient's calcium level is normal.
• Patient does not develop hypercalcemia as a result of calcium therapy.
• Patient and family state an understanding of calcium therapy.

PHARMACOLOGIC CLASS

calcium channel blockers

bepridil hydrochloride
diltiazem
isradipine
nicardipine hydrochloride
nifedipine
nimodipine
verapamil hydrochloride

OVERVIEW

Calcium channel blockers (also called slow calcium channel blockers) were introduced in the United States in the early 1980s. The main physiologic action of calcium channel blockers is to inhibit calcium influx across the slow channels of myocardial and vascular smooth muscle cells. Calcium is especially important to these cells as well as specialized cardiac conduction cells. By inhibiting calcium influx into these cells, calcium channel blockers reduce intracellular calcium concentrations. This, in turn, dilates coronary arteries, peripheral arteries, and arterioles, and slows cardiac conduction.

When used to treat Prinzmetal's variant angina, calcium channel

COMPARING ORAL CALCIUM CHANNEL BLOCKERS

DRUG	ONSET OF ACTION	PEAK SERUM LEVEL	HALF-LIFE	THERAPEUTIC SERUM LEVEL
diltiazem	15 minutes	30 minutes	3 to 4 hours	50 to 200 ng/ml
nicardipine	20 minutes	1 hour	8.6 hours	28 to 50 ng/ml
nifedipine	5 to 30 minutes	30 minutes to 2 hours	2 to 5 hours	25 to 100 ng/ml
nimodipine	unknown	<1 hour	1 to 2 hours	unknown
verapamil	30 minutes (3 to 5 minutes after I.V. administration)	1 to 2.2 hours	6 to 12 hours	80 to 300 ng/ml

blockers inhibit coronary spasm, increasing oxygen delivery to the heart. Peripheral artery dilation leads to a decrease in total peripheral resistance; this reduces afterload, which, in turn, decreases myocardial oxygen consumption. Inhibition of calcium influx into the specialized cardiac conduction cells (specifically, those in the sinoatrial and atrioventricular nodes) slows conduction through the heart. This effect is most pronounced with verapamil.

Structurally dissimilar, diltiazem, nifedipine, and verapamil are thought to work at different receptor sites on the calcium channel. Consequently, their pharmacologic effects vary markedly in degree.

CLINICAL INDICATIONS AND ACTIONS

Angina

Calcium channel blockers are useful in managing Prinzmetal's variant angina, chronic stable angina, and unstable angina. In Prinzmetal's variant angina, they inhibit spontaneous and ergonovine-induced coronary spasm, thereby increasing coronary blood flow and maintaining myocardial oxygen delivery. By dilating peripheral arteries, these drugs decrease total peripheral resistance, reducing afterload and, in turn, myocardial oxygen consumption. In unstable and chronic stable angina, their effectiveness presumably stems from their ability to reduce afterload.

Arrhythmias

Of the calcium channel blockers, verapamil has the greatest effect on the AV node, slowing the ventricular rate in atrial fibrillation or flutter. Parenteral diltiazem has been used investigationally to treat supraventricular tachyarrhythmias.

Hypertension

Because they dilate systemic arteries, most calcium channel blockers are useful in treating mild to moderate hypertension.

Other actions

Calcium channel blockers (especially verapamil) may also prove to be effective as a hypertrophic cardiomyopathy therapy adjunct by improving left ventricular outflow as a result of negative inotropic effects and possibly improved diastolic function. They have been used to treat peripheral vascular disorders, and as adjunctive therapy in the treatment of esophageal spasm.

OVERVIEW OF ADVERSE REACTIONS

Adverse reactions vary in degree according to the specific drug used. Verapamil may cause adverse effects on the conduction system, including bradycardia, and various degrees of heart block, exacerbate heart failure, and cause hypotension after rapid I.V. administration. Prolonged oral verapamil therapy may cause constipation. Most adverse effects of nifedipine, such as hypotension (commonly accompanied by reflex tachycardia), peripheral edema, flushing, lightheadedness, and headache, result from its potent vasodilatory properties.

Diltiazem most commonly causes anorexia and nausea. It may also induce various degrees of heart block, bradycardia, congestive heart failure, and peripheral edema.

REPRESENTATIVE COMBINATIONS

None.

---

calcium polycarbophil

(kal´ see um pol ee kar´ boe fil)

Equalactin◇, FiberCon◇, Mitrolan◇

- *Classification:* bulk laxative, antidiarrheal (hydrophilic agent)
- *Pregnancy Risk Category:* C

HOW SUPPLIED

Tablets: 500 mg◇ (FiberCon◇)
Tablets (chewable): 500 mg◇ (Equalactin◇, Mitrolan◇)

ACTION

Mechanism: A bulk-forming laxative that absorbs water and expands to increase bulk and moisture content of the stool. The increased bulk encourages peristalsis and bowel movement. If administered with less water, drug acts as an antidiarrheal by absorbing free fecal water, thereby producing formed stools.
Absorption: None.
Distribution: None.
Metabolism: None.
Excretion: In feces.
Onset, peak, duration: Laxative effect is usually apparent within 12 to 24 hours, but full effect may not be seen for up to 3 days.

INDICATIONS & DOSAGE

Constipation (Equalactin and Mitrolan must be chewed before swallowing) –
Adults: 1 g P.O. q.i.d. as required. Maximum 6 g in 24-hour period.
Children 6 to 12 years: 500 mg P.O. t.i.d. as required. Maximum 3 g in 24-hour period.
Children 2 to 6 years: 500 mg P.O. b.i.d. as required. Maximum 1.5 g in 24-hour period.
Diarrhea associated with irritable bowel syndrome, as well as acute nonspecific diarrhea (Mitrolan must be chewed before swallowing) –
Adults: 1 g P.O. q.i.d. as required. Maximum 6 g in 24-hour period.
Children 6 to 12 years 500 mg P.O. t.i.d. as required. Maximum 3 g in 24-hour period.
Children 2 to 6 years: 500 mg P.O. b.i.d. as required. Maximum 1.5 g in 24-hour period.

CONTRAINDICATIONS & PRECAUTIONS

Contraindicated in patients with GI obstruction because the drug may exacerbate this condition.

ADVERSE REACTIONS

Common reactions are in italics; life-threatening reactions are in bold italics.
GI: abdominal fullness and increased flatus, intestinal obstruction.
Other: laxative dependence in long-term or excessive use.

INTERACTIONS
None significant.

EFFECTS ON DIAGNOSTIC TESTS
None reported.

NURSING CONSIDERATIONS
Besides those related universally to drug therapy (see "How to use this book"), consider the following specific recommendations:

Assessment

• Obtain a baseline assessment of history of bowel disorder, GI status, fluid intake, nutritional status, exercise habits, and normal pattern of elimination.
• Be alert for adverse reactions or drug interactions throughout therapy.
• Evaluate the patient's and family's knowledge about calcium polycarbophil therapy.

Nursing Diagnoses

• Constipation related to interruption of normal pattern of elimination characterized by infrequent or absent stools.
• Altered GI tissue perfusion related to drug-induced intestinal obstruction.
• Knowledge deficit related to calcium polycarbophil therapy.

Planning and Implementation

Preparation and Administration

• Give with a full glass of water when used for constipation.
• For severe diarrhea, the dose may be repeated every 30 minutes, but maximum daily dosage should not be exceeded.

Monitoring

• Monitor effectiveness by checking the frequency and characteristics of stools.
• Auscultate bowel sounds at least once a shift. Assess for pain, cramping, and abdominal distention.
• Monitor nutritional status and fluid intake.

Supportive Care

• Do not give to patients with signs of GI obstruction.
• Be aware that rectal bleeding or failure to respond may indicate need for surgery.
• Provide privacy for elimination.
• Unless contraindicated, encourage fluid intake up to 2500 ml a day.
• Consult with a dietitian to modify diet to increase fiber and bulk.

Patient Teaching

• Discourage excessive use of laxatives.
• Teach the patient about the relationship between fluid intake, dietary fiber, exercise, and constipation.
• Teach patient that dietary sources of fiber include bran and other cereals, fresh fruit, and vegetables.
• Advise patient to chew Equalactin or Mitrolan thoroughly and drink a full glass of water with each dose. However when used as an antidiarrheal, patient should not drink a glass of water afterward.

Evaluation

In patients receiving calcium polycarbophil, appropriate evaluation statements may include:
• Patient reports return of normal pattern of elimination.
• Patient remains free from intestinal obstruction.
• Patient and family state an understanding of calcium polycarbophil therapy.

---

capreomycin sulfate
(kap ree oh mye´ sin)
Capastat

• *Classification:* antitubular agent (polypeptide antibiotic)
• *Pregnancy Risk Category:* C

HOW SUPPLIED
Injection: 1 g/vial

ACTION

Mechanism: Bacteriostatic mechanism unknown.
Absorption: Not absorbed after oral administration; given by I.M. injection.
Excretion: Excreted primarily unchanged in urine by glomerular filtration. Half-life: 4 to 6 hours in adults, prolonged with elevated serum levels in renal impairment.
Onset, peak, duration: Peak serum concentrations in 1 to 2 hours; low serum concentrations occur 24 hours after I.M. injection.

INDICATIONS & DOSAGE

Adjunctive treatment in pulmonary tuberculosis–
Adults: 15 mg/kg/day up to 1 g I.M. daily injected deeply into large muscle mass for 60 to 120 days; then 1 g 2 to 3 times weekly for a period of 18 to 24 months. Maximum dosage should not exceed 20 mg/kg daily. Must be given in conjunction with another antitubercular drug.

CONTRAINDICATIONS & PRECAUTIONS

Contraindicated in patients with hypersensitivity to this drug. Use with great caution in patients taking other ototoxic or nephrotoxic drugs; in patients with tinnitus, vertigo, and high-frequency hearing loss, who are susceptible to ototoxicity; and in patients with decreased renal function. Use with caution in patients with allergies (particularly to drugs), and in those patients with hepatic disease, myasthenia gravis, or parkinsonism because this drug may exacerbate symptoms of these disorders.

ADVERSE REACTIONS

Common reactions are in italics; life-threatening reactions are in bold italics.
Blood: eosinophilia, leukocytosis, leukopenia.
CNS: headache, ***neuromuscular blockade.***
EENT: *ototoxicity* (tinnitus, vertigo, hearing loss).
GU: *nephrotoxicity* (elevated BUN and nonprotein nitrogen, casts, red blood cells, leukocytes; tubular necrosis; proteinuria; decreased creatinine clearance).
Metabolic: hypokalemia, alkalosis, hepatotoxicity.
Local: pain, induration, excessive bleeding and sterile abscesses at injection site.
Other: ***hypersensitivity,*** hepatotoxicity.

INTERACTIONS

None significant.

EFFECTS ON DIAGNOSTIC TESTS

BSP test: decreased excretion.
BUN and serum creatinine levels: elevated levels.
Urinalysis: increased WBC, RBC, casts, and protein.

NURSING CONSIDERATIONS

Besides those related universally to drug therapy (see "How to use this book"), consider the following specific recommendations:

Assessment
- Obtain a baseline assessment of infection before capreomycin therapy.
- Be alert for adverse reactions and drug interactions throughout therapy.
- Evaluate the patient's and family's knowledge about capreomycin therapy.

Nursing Diagnoses
- High risk for infection related to ineffectiveness of capreomycin to eradicate the infection.
- Sensory/perceptual alterations (auditory) related to capreomycin-induced ototoxicity.
- Knowledge deficit related to capreomycin.

Planning and Implementation
Preparation and Administration
• Obtain a specimen for culture and sensitivity tests before administering first dose.
• ***I.M. use:*** Administer deep into large muscle mass to minimize local reactions. As ordered, reconstitute I.M. dose with 0.5% lidocaine hydrochloride without epinephrine. Apply ice to injection site p.r.n. for pain.
• ***I.V. use:*** *Never administer drug I.V.* Intravenous use may cause neuromuscular blockade.
• Be aware that straw- or dark-colored solution does not indicate a loss of potency. Do not administer solutions that contain a precipitate.
• Expect to reduce dosage in patients with renal impairment.
Monitoring
• Monitor effectiveness by regularly assessing for improvement in infection and by evaluating results of periodic culture and sensitivity tests.
• Monitor patient's hearing before and every 1 to 2 weeks during therapy.
• Monitor renal function (output, specific gravity, urinalysis, BUN, and serum creatinine) before and during therapy.
Supportive Care
• Notify doctor if patient complains of tinnitus, vertigo, or hearing impairment, and if patient shows signs of decreasing renal function.
Patient Teaching
• Instruct a family member or friend how to administer an I.M. injection.
• Tell patient to promptly report tinnitus, vertigo, or any change in hearing to the doctor.
• Stress the importance of recommended laboratory tests to monitor for adverse reactions.
• Warn patient that injection may be painful and suggest applying ice to injection site p.r.n. for pain.
• Tell patient that a straw- or dark-colored solution may be used but that a solution that contains a precipitate should be discarded.

Evaluation
In patients receiving capreomycin, appropriate evaluation statements may include:
• Patient is free of infection.
• Patient's auditory function remains unchanged throughout capreomycin therapy.
• Patient and family state an understanding of capreomycin therapy.

captopril
(kap´ toe pril)
Capoten

• *Classification:* antihypertensive, adjunctive treatment of CHF (angiotensin-converting enzyme inhibitor)
• *Pregnancy Risk Category:* C (D in second and third trimester)

HOW SUPPLIED
Tablets: 12.5 mg, 25 mg, 50 mg, 100 mg

ACTION
Mechanism: By inhibiting angiotensin-converting enzyme (ACE), prevents pulmonary conversion of angiotensin I to angiotensin II.
Absorption: Absorbed through the GI tract; food may reduce absorption by up to 40%.
Distribution: Into most body tissues except the CNS; approximately 25% to 30% protein-bound.
Metabolism: About 50% is metabolized in the liver.
Excretion: Primarily in urine; small amounts are excreted in feces. Half-life: Less than 3 hours.
Onset, peak, duration: Antihypertensive effect begins in 15 minutes; peak blood levels occur at 1 hour. Maximum therapeutic effect may require

several weeks. Duration of effect is usually 2 to 6 hours; may be increased in patients with renal dysfunction.

INDICATIONS & DOSAGE

Hypertension–
Adults: 25 mg P.O. b.i.d. or t.i.d. initially. If blood pressure isn't satisfactorily controlled in 1 to 2 weeks, dosage may be increased to 50 mg t.i.d. If not satisfactorily controlled after another 1 to 2 weeks, a diuretic should be added to regimen. If further blood pressure reduction is necessary, dosage may be raised to as high as 150 mg t.i.d. while continuing the diuretic. Maximum dosage is 450 mg daily. Daily dose may also be administered b.i.d.
Congestive heart failure–
Adults: 6.25 to 12.5 mg P.O. t.i.d. initially. May be gradually increased to 50 mg t.i.d. Maximum dosage is 450 mg daily.

CONTRAINDICATIONS & PRECAUTIONS

Contraindicated in patients with hypersensitivity to captopril or other ACE inhibitors.

Use cautiously in patients with impaired renal function or collagen vascular disease and in patients taking drugs known to depress leukocytes or immune response; such patients are at increased risk of developing neutropenia, especially if they have impaired renal function.

ADVERSE REACTIONS

Common reactions are in italics; life-threatening reactions are in bold italics.
Blood: *leukopenia, agranulocytosis, pancytopenia.*
CNS: dizziness, fainting.
CV: *tachycardia, hypotension,* angina pectoris, CHF, pericarditis.
EENT: *loss of taste (dysgeusia).*
GI: anorexia.
GU: *proteinuria, nephrotic syndrome, membranous glomerulopathy,* ***renal failure*** (patients with preexisting renal disease or patients receiving high dosages), urinary frequency.
Metabolic: hyperkalemia.
Skin: *urticarial rash, maculopapular rash,* pruritus.
Other: fever, angioedema of face and extremities, transient increases in liver enzymes, persistent cough.

INTERACTIONS

Antacids: decreased captopril effect. Separate administration times.
Digitalis glycosides: may increase serum digoxin concentration by 15% to 30%.
NSAIDs: may reduce antihypertensive effect. Monitor blood pressure.
Potassium supplements: increased risk of hyperkalemia. Avoid these supplements unless hypokalemic blood levels are confirmed.

EFFECTS ON DIAGNOSTIC TESTS

Liver enzymes: transiently elevated levels.
Serum potassium: hyperkalemia.
Urinary acetone: false-positive results.

NURSING CONSIDERATIONS

Besides those related universally to drug therapy (see "How to use this book"), consider the following specific recommendations:

Assessment
- Obtain a baseline assessment of the patient's blood pressure before therapy.
- Be alert for adverse reactions and drug interactions throughout therapy.
- Evaluate the patient's and family's knowledge about captopril therapy.

Nursing Diagnoses
- High risk for injury related to the patient's underlying condition.
- Altered protection related to captopril-induced blood disorder or renal dysfunction.

• Knowledge deficit related to captopril therapy.

Planning and Implementation

Preparation and Administration

• ***P.O. use:*** Administer 1 hour before meals because food may reduce absorption.

• Antacids decrease captopril effect; therefore, separate administration times.

Monitoring

• Monitor effectiveness by regularly assessing the patient's blood pressure and pulse rate before administration.

• Carefully monitor elderly patients because they may be more sensitive to the drug's hypotensive effect.

• Monitor serum potassium level for hyperkalemia or hypokalemia.

• Monitor CBC, especially WBC and differential count, and observe for signs of infection every 2 weeks for the first 3 months of therapy.

• Monitor renal function (BUN and creatinine clearance levels, urinalysis). Drug may further impair renal function.

Supportive Care

• Notify the doctor if urinalysis reveals proteinuria, elevated BUN or creatinine levels, or a low creatinine clearance.

• Hold dose and notify the doctor if the patient develops fever, sore throat, or leukopenia, hypotension or tachycardia.

• Institute safety precautions if CNS reactions develop.

• Protect the patient from exposure to other patients with infection.

• Limit the patient's fluid intake if CHF or renal dysfunction occurs.

Patient Teaching

• Instruct the patient not to take antacids at the same time as captopril.

• Tell the patient that periodic blood tests (WBC with differential counts) will be required during therapy.

• Advise the patient to report any signs of infection (fever, sore throat).

• Tell the patient that captopril may cause dizziness or fainting, especially at start of therapy. Advise patient to avoid sudden postural changes and to sit down immediately if dizziness occurs.

• Explain the importance of taking this drug as prescribed, even when feeling well.

• Instruct the patient not to discontinue drug suddenly, but to call the doctor if unpleasant adverse reactions occur.

• Instruct the patient to check with the doctor or pharmacist before taking any OTC medications.

• Instruct the patient to take captopril 1 hour before meals.

Evaluation

In patients receiving captopril, appropriate evaluation statements may include:

• Patient's blood pressure is within normal limits.

• Patient's WBC and differential counts and renal function studies are normal.

• Patient and family state an understanding of captopril therapy.

carbachol (intraocular)

(kar´ ba kole)

Miostat

carbachol (topical)

Carbacel, Isopto Carbachol

• *Classification:* miotic (cholinergic agent)

• *Pregnancy Risk Category:* C

HOW SUPPLIED

Intraocular solution: 0.01%

Topical ophthalmic solution: 0.75%, 1.5%, 2.25%, 3%

ACTION

Mechanism: Acts on muscarinic acetylcholine receptors in the eye and causes contraction of the sphincter

muscles of the iris, resulting in miosis. Also produces ciliary spasm, deepening of the anterior chamber, and vasodilation of conjunctival vessels of the outflow tract.
Pharmacokinetics: Unknown.
Onset, peak, duration: Action begins within 10 to 20 minutes and peaks in less than 4 hours. Duration of effect is usually about 8 hours.

INDICATIONS & DOSAGE

Ocular surgery (to produce pupillary miosis) –
Adults: doctor gently instills 0.5 ml (intraocular form) into the anterior chamber for production of satisfactory miosis. It may be instilled before or after securing sutures.
Open-angle glaucoma –
Adults: instill 1 drop (topical form) into eye daily, b.i.d., t.i.d., or q.i.d.

CONTRAINDICATIONS & PRECAUTIONS

Contraindicated in patients with hypersensitivity to any components of the preparation or in patients in whom miosis is undesirable (acute iritis). Although systemic effects are uncommon with usual doses, use cautiously in patients with acute cardiac failure, bronchial asthma, peptic ulcer, hyperthyroidism, GI spasm, urinary tract obstruction, and Parkinson's disease, because drug may worsen these conditions.

ADVERSE REACTIONS

Common reactions are in italics; life-threatening reactions are in bold italics.
CNS: headache.
Eye: accommodative spasm, blurred vision, conjunctival vasodilation, eye and brow pain.
GI: abdominal cramps, diarrhea.
Other: sweating, flushing, asthma.

INTERACTIONS

Pilocarpine: additive effect.

EFFECTS ON DIAGNOSTIC TESTS

None significant.

NURSING CONSIDERATIONS

Besides those related universally to drug therapy (see "How to use this book"), consider the following specific recommendations:

Assessment
- Obtain a baseline assessment of the patient's vision, especially intraocular pressure.
- Be alert for adverse reactions and drug interactions throughout therapy.
- Evaluate the patient's and family's knowledge about carbachol therapy.

Nursing Diagnoses
- Sensory/perceptual alterations (visual) related to the patient's underlying condition.
- Pain related to carbachol-induced brow ache.
- Knowledge deficit related to carbachol therapy.

Planning and Implementation
Preparation and Administration
- Instill ointment or solution in lacrimal sac.
- Apply light finger pressure on lacrimal sac for 1 minute after drops are instilled.
- Patients with dark eyes (hazel or brown irises) may require stronger solution or more frequent instillation because the drug may be absorbed by the eye pigment.

Monitoring
- Monitor effectiveness by assessing the patient's visual status and intraocular pressure.
- Monitor the patient for drug-induced brow ache and other adverse reactions.
- Monitor for tolerance to the drug in long-term therapy, which may be restored by briefly substituting another miotic.

Supportive Care
- Notify the doctor immediately of changes in the patient's health status.

• Obtain an order for a mild analgesic if patient experiences brow aches.
• Keep parenteral atropine on hand to reverse toxicity.
Patient Teaching
• Tell the patient to take the medication regularly; long-term use may be necessary.
• Warn patient not to drive for 1 to 2 hours after administration, until effect on vision is determined.
• Reassure patient that blurred vision usually diminishes with prolonged use.
• Teach patient how to instill drops or solution, and advise him to wash his hands before and after administering the drug.
• Warn patient not to exceed the recommended dosage.
Evaluation
In the patient receiving carbachol, appropriate evaluation statements may include:
• Patient experiences a reduction in intraocular pressure.
• Patient does not experience browaches.
• Patient and family state an understanding of carbachol therapy.

carbamazepine
(kar ba maz´ e peen)
Apo-Carbamazepine†, Epitol, Mazepine†, Tegretol, Tegretol CR†, Teril‡

• *Classification:* anticonvulsant, analgesic (iminostilbene)
• *Pregnancy Risk Category:* C

HOW SUPPLIED
Tablets: 200 mg
Tablets (chewable): 100 mg
Oral suspension: 100 mg/5 ml

ACTION
Mechanism: Stabilizes neuronal membranes and limits seizure activity by either increasing efflux or decreasing influx of sodium ions across cell membranes in the motor cortex during generation of nerve impulses.
Absorption: Slowly absorbed from the GI tract.
Distribution: Widely distributed throughout the body; crosses the placenta, and accumulates in fetal tissue. The drug is approximately 75% protein-bound. Therapeutic serum levels are 3 to 14 mcg/ml; nystagmus can occur above 4 mcg/ml and ataxia, dizziness, and anorexia at or above 10 mcg/ml. Serum levels may be misleading because an unmeasured active metabolite also can cause toxicity.
Metabolism: By the liver to an active metabolite. It may also induce its own metabolism; over time, higher doses are needed to maintain plasma levels.
Excretion: In urine (70%) and feces (30%); carbamazepine levels in breast milk approach 60% of serum levels. Half-life: Initial half-life values range from 25 to 65 hours, with 12 to 17 hours on repeated doses.
Onset, peak, duration: Peak plasma concentrations occur at 2 to 8 hours.

INDICATIONS & DOSAGE
Generalized tonic-clonic and complex-partial seizures, mixed seizure patterns–
Adults and children over 12 years: initially, 200 mg P.O. b.i.d. May increase by 200 mg P.O. daily, in divided doses at 6- to 8-hour intervals. Adjust to minimum effective level when control achieved.
Children under 12 years: 10 to 20 mg/kg P.O. daily in two to four divided doses.
Trigeminal neuralgia–
Adults: initially, 100 mg P.O. b.i.d. with meals. Increase by 100 mg q 12 hours until pain is relieved. Don't exceed 1.2 g daily. Maintenance dose is 200 to 400 mg P.O. b.i.d.

CONTRAINDICATIONS & PRECAUTIONS

Contraindicated in patients with hypersensitivity to carbamazepine and tricyclic antidepressants and in patients with past or present bone marrow depression; MAO inhibitors or within 14 days of such use.

Use with caution in patients with cardiovascular, renal, or hepatic damage; increased intraocular pressure; or atypical absence seizures; and in elderly patients, in whom it may activate latent psychosis, agitation, or confusion.

ADVERSE REACTIONS

Common reactions are in italics; life-threatening reactions are in bold italics.

Blood: ***aplastic anemia, agranulocytosis,*** eosinophilia, leukocytosis, *thrombocytopenia.*

CNS: dizziness, *vertigo, drowsiness,* fatigue, *ataxia,* worsening of seizures.

CV: CHF, hypertension, hypotension, aggravation of coronary artery disease.

EENT: conjunctivitis, dry mouth and pharynx, blurred vision, diplopia, nystagmus.

GI: *nausea,* vomiting, abdominal pain, diarrhea, anorexia, *stomatitis,* glossitis.

GU: urinary frequency, urine retention, impotence, albuminuria, glycosuria, elevated BUN.

Hepatic: abnormal liver function tests, hepatitis.

Metabolic: water intoxication.

Skin: *rash,* urticaria, erythema multiforme, ***Stevens-Johnson syndrome.***

Other: diaphoresis, fever, chills, pulmonary hypersensitivity.

INTERACTIONS

Phenytoin, primidone, phenobarbital, nicotinic acid: may decrease carbamazepine levels. Monitor for decreased effect.

Phenytoin, warfarin, doxycycline, theophylline, haloperidol: carbamazepine may decrease blood levels of these drugs. Monitor for decreased effect.

Propoxyphene, troleandomycin, erythromycin, isoniazid, verapamil: may increase carbamazepine blood levels. Use cautiously.

EFFECTS ON DIAGNOSTIC TESTS

Liver enzymes: elevated levels.

Thyroid function tests: decreased values.

NURSING CONSIDERATIONS

Besides those related universally to drug therapy (see "How to use this book"), consider the following specific recommendations:

Assessment

- Obtain a baseline assessment of seizure activity before therapy.
- Be alert for adverse reactions and drug interactions throughout therapy.
- Evaluate the patient's and family's knowledge about carbamazepine therapy.

Nursing Diagnoses

- High risk for injury related to the underlying seizure disorder.
- Altered protection related to carbamazepine-induced blood disorders.
- Knowledge deficit related to carbamazepine therapy.

Planning and Implementation

Preparation and Administration

- Administer drug in divided doses, when possible, to maintain consistent blood levels.
- Administer with food to minimize GI distress.
- Increase dosage gradually, as ordered, to minimize adverse reactions.

Monitoring

- Monitor effectiveness by evaluating seizure activity.
- Monitor closely for therapeutic blood levels (3 to 9 mcg/ml). Ask patient when last dose of medication was taken to approximately evaluate blood levels.

• Obtain baseline determinations and periodically monitor urinalysis, BUN, liver function, CBC, platelet and reticulocyte counts, and serum iron levels.
• Monitor for mild-to-moderate dizziness and drowsiness at start of therapy. Effect usually disappears within 3 to 4 days.
• Monitor for signs of anorexia or subtle appetite changes, which may indicate excessive blood levels.
• Monitor for stomatitis (red, painful ulcerations in oral cavity) throughout therapy.
• Monitor for signs of anemia (pallor, fatigue), infection (fever, chills, drainage), or bleeding (easy bruising, spontaneous epistaxis).

Supportive Care

• Never discontinue the drug suddenly when treating seizures or status epilepticus.
• If anemia occurs, assist the patient with activities, schedule activities to allow frequent rest periods. Expect to administer additional agents to treat anemia.
• If the patient's WBC counts are low, institute infection control measures. Advise the patient to get adequate rest, maintain adequate hydration, and avoid exposure to colds and other infections.
• If the patient exhibits bleeding tendencies, institute bleeding precautions. Advise the patient to use an electric shaver and to avoid cuts and bruises.
• Advise meticulous oral hygiene for the patient with stomatitis; encourage a bland diet and obtain an order for a local anesthetic to ease mouth discomfort.
• Maintain seizure precautions.
• If CNS reactions occur, institute safety precautions.
• Be aware that carbamazepine may be used as an altermative to lithium in treatment of some affective disorders.
• Keep in mind that when carbamazepine is used for trigeminal neuralgia, an attempt should be made every 3 months to decrease dosage or discontinue the drug.

Patient Teaching

• Warn the patient to avoid hazardous activities that require alertness and good psychomotor coordination until CNS effects of the drug are known.
• Recommend periodic eye examinations during therapy.
• Tell the patient to notify the doctor immediately of fever, sore throat, mouth ulcers, easy bruising, or bleeding. Instruct the patient about appropriate protective measures.
• Tell the patient how to manage stomatitis.
• Instruct the patient to take the drug with food to minimize GI discomfort.
• Explain the importance of follow-up care, including periodic diagnostic studies.
• Reassure the patient that dizziness and drowsiness usually disappear after 3 to 4 days of therapy.

Evaluation

In patients receiving carbamazepine, appropriate evaluation statements may include:
• Patient remains free of seizure activity.
• Patient's CBC remains normal.
• Patient and family state an understanding of carbamazepine therapy.

carbenicillin indanyl sodium

(kar ben i sill´ in)
Geocillin, Geopen Oral†

• *Classification:* antibiotic (extended-spectrum penicillin)
• *Pregnancy Risk Category:* B

HOW SUPPLIED

Tablets: 382 mg

*Liquid form contains alcohol. **May contain tartrazine.

ACTION

Mechanism: Bactericidal by inhibiting cell wall synthesis during active multiplication. Bacteria resist carbenicillin by producing penicillinases—enzymes that hydrolyze its active form.
Absorption: Incompletely (30% to 90%) absorbed from GI tract.
Distribution: Widely distributed after oral administration, but concentrations are insufficient to treat systemic infections. Drug crosses the placenta and is 30% to 60% protein-bound.
Metabolism: Rapidly hydrolyzed in plasma to carbenicillin, which is metabolized partially.
Excretion: Drug and metabolites are excreted primarily (79% to 99%) in urine by renal tubular secretion and glomerular filtration; some are excreted in breast milk. In patients with severe renal failure, urine concentrations in renal parenchyma and urine levels of drug are insufficient for treating urinary tract infections. Half-life: In adults about 1 hour; with extensive renal impairment, 9½ to 23 hours.
Onset, peak, duration: Peak plasma concentrations occur at 30 minutes after oral dose; indanyl salt is completely hydrolyzed to carbenicillin in plasma within 90 minutes.

INDICATIONS & DOSAGE

Urinary tract infection and prostatitis caused by susceptible strains of gram-negative organisms—
Adults: 382 to 764 mg P.O. q.i.d.
Not recommended for children.

CONTRAINDICATIONS & PRECAUTIONS

Contraindicated in patients with hypersensitivity to any penicillin or cephalosporin. Use cautiously in patients with impaired renal function.

ADVERSE REACTIONS

Common reactions are in italics; life-threatening reactions are in bold italics.
Blood: leukopenia, neutropenia, eosinophilia, anemia, thrombocytopenia.
GI: *nausea,* vomiting, *diarrhea, flatulence, abdominal cramps, unpleasant taste.*
Other: *hypersensitivity (rash, chills, fever, urticaria, pruritus,* ***anaphylaxis****),* overgrowth of nonsusceptible organisms.

INTERACTIONS

None significant.

EFFECTS ON DIAGNOSTIC TESTS

Aminoglycoside serum levels: falsely decreased concentrations.
Coombs' tests: positive results.
Electrolytes: hypokalemia, hypernatremia.
HLA typing: inaccurate results.
Liver function tests: transient elevations.
Prothrombin times: prolonged.
RBC, WBC, platelet counts: transiently reduced.
Serum uric acid (copper sulfate method): increased values.
Urine glucose tests with copper sulfate (Benedict's reagent or Clinitest): false-positive results. Use glucose enzymatic methods (Clinistix or Tes-Tape).
Urine specific gravity: false elevations in dehydrated patients with low urine output.

NURSING CONSIDERATIONS

Besides those related universally to drug therapy (see "How to use this book"), consider the following specific recommendations:
Assessment
- Obtain a baseline assessment of infection before therapy.
- Be alert for adverse reactions or drug interactions during therapy.
- Evaluate the patient's and family's knowledge about carbenicillin.

Nursing Diagnoses
• High risk for injury related to ineffectiveness of carbenicillin to eradicate the infection.
• High risk for fluid volume deficit related to carbenicillin-induced adverse GI reactions.
• Knowledge deficit related to carbenicillin therapy.

Planning and Implementation

Preparation and Administration
• Obtain specimen for culture and sensitivity tests before first dose. Therapy may begin pending test results.
• Before first dose, ask the patient about previous allergic reactions to this drug or other penicillins. However, a negative history of penicillin allergy does not guarantee future safety.
• Give carbenicillin at least 1 hour before bacteriostatic antibiotics.
• Be aware that carbenicillin should only be used if patient's creatinine clearance is 10 ml/minute or more.
• ***P.O. use:*** Administer drug 1 to 2 hours before or 2 to 3 hours after meals because food may interfere with absorption.

Monitoring
• Monitor effectiveness by regularly assessing for improvement of infection.
• Monitor for bacterial or fungal superinfections during prolonged or high-dose therapy, especially in elderly, debilitated, or immunosuppressed patients.
• Monitor patient's hydration status if adverse GI reactions occur.

Supportive Care
• Obtain an order for an antiemetic or antidiarrheal agent as needed.

Patient Teaching
• Advise the patient who becomes allergic to carbenicillin to wear medical alert identification stating this information.
• Tell patient to call the doctor if he develops rash, fever, or chills. A rash is the most common allergic reaction.
• Advise patient to take the drug 1 to 2 hours before or 2 to 3 hours after meals as food may interfere with absorption.
• Tell patient to take drug exactly as prescribed, completing entire quantity even after he feels better.
• Warn patient never to use leftover carbenicillin for a new illness or to share it with others.

Evaluation

In patients receiving carbenicillin, appropriate evaluation statements may include:
• Patient is free of infection.
• Patient remains hydrated throughout carbenicillin therapy.
• Patient and family state an understanding of carbenicillin therapy.

PHARMACOLOGIC CLASS

carbonic anhydrase inhibitors

acetazolamide
dichlorphenamide
methazolamide

OVERVIEW

The carbonic anhydrase inhibitors were developed in the 1940s. They have been largely replaced by thiazides and are seldom used as diuretics because their propensity for causing metabolic acidosis makes patients refractory to their diuretic effects.

As their name implies, carbonic anhydrase inhibitors act by noncompetitive reversible inhibition of the enzyme carbonic anhydrase, which is responsible for formation of hydrogen and bicarbonate ions from carbon dioxide and water. This inhibition results in decreased hydrogen levels in the renal tubules, promoting excretion of bicarbonate, sodium, potassium, and water; because carbon dioxide is not eliminated as rapidly, systemic acidosis may occur.

CLINICAL INDICATIONS AND ACTIONS

Open-angle glaucoma and angle-closure glaucoma
Because carbonic anhydrase inhibitors reduce the formation of aqueous humor, lowering intraocular pressure, they are useful as adjunctive therapy in patients with glaucoma.
Epilepsy
Acetazolamide is used with other anticonvulsants in various types of epilepsy, particularly petit mal. It acts to inhibit seizures by an unknown mechanism; it may act by inducing metabolic acidosis or by increasing carbon dioxide tension within the CNS.
Diuresis
Acetazolamide, a carbonic anhydrase inhibitor, reversibly blocks the enzyme responsible for formation of hydrogen and bicarbonate ions from carbon dioxide and water. This decreases hydrogen concentration in the renal tubules, promoting excretion of bicarbonate, sodium, potassium, and water.
Mountain sickness
Acetazolamide shortens the period of high-altitude acclimatization; by inhibiting conversion of carbon dioxide to bicarbonate, it may increase carbon dioxide tension in tissues and decrease it in the lungs; the resultant etabolic acidosis may also increase oxygenation during hypoxia.

OVERVIEW OF ADVERSE REACTIONS

Many adverse reactions associated with carbonic anhydrase inhibitors are dose-related and respond to lowered dosage; each drug has a slightly different adverse reaction profile, and patients who cannot tolerate one of the drugs may be able to tolerate another. Serious adverse effects are infrequent, because drugs are primarily given for short-term use. Some of the more common adverse effects include generalized weakness, tiredness, or discomfort; nausea; vomiting; diarrhea; loss of appetite; metallic taste in the mouth; peripheral numbness or tingling in hands, fingers, toes, or tongue.

REPRESENTATIVE COMBINATIONS

None.

---

carboplatin

(kar´ boe pla tin)
Paraplatin

• *Classification:* antineoplastic (alklyating agent)
• *Pregnancy Risk Category:* D

HOW SUPPLIED

Injection: 50-mg, 150-mg, 450-mg vials

ACTION

Mechanism: A platinum coordination complex, carboplatin is a non-cell–cycle specific alkylating agent that produces cross-linking of strands of DNA.
Distribution: Carboplatin's volume of distribution is approximately equal to total body water; no significant protein binding of the drug occurs; however, the platinum from the drug becomes irreversibly bound to protein and is slowly eliminated from the body.
Metabolism: Hydrolyzed to form hydroxylated and aquated species.
Excretion: 65% of the drug is excreted by the kidneys within 12 hours, 71% within 24 hours. Half-life: Free platinum exhibits a half-life of 5 hours. Enterohepatic recirculation may occur.

INDICATIONS & DOSAGE

Palliative treatment of ovarian carcinoma –

Adults: 360 mg/m² I.V. on day 1 q 4 weeks; doses should not be repeated until platelet count exceeds 100,000/mm³ and neutrophil count exceeds 2,000/mm³. Subsequent doses are based on blood counts. Clinical trials have suggested the following dosage adjustments: if platelet count is above 100,000/mm³ and neutrophil count is above 2,000/mm³, dose administered should be 125% of the recommended starting dose. Dose should be reduced to 75% if platelet count falls below 50,000/mm³ or neutrophil count is below 500/mm³.

CONTRAINDICATIONS & PRECAUTIONS

Contraindicated in patients with a history of hypersensitivity to cisplatin, platinum-containing compounds, or mannitol. Avoid use in patients with severe bone marrow depression or bleeding. Transfusions may be necessary during treatment due to cumulative anemia. Bone marrow depression may be more severe in patients with creatinine clearance less than 60 ml/minute. Patients older than age 65 are at greater risk for neurotoxicity.

Use cautiously in patients with decreased renal function; use adjusted dose. Use extreme caution when preparing or administering carboplatin to avoid mutagenic, teratogenic, and carcinogenic risks. Use a biological containment cabinet, wear gloves and mask, and use syringes with Luer-Lok fittings to prevent leakage of drug solution. Also correctly dispose of needles, vials, and unused drug, and avoid contaminating work surfaces. Avoid inhalation of dust or vapors and contact with skin or mucous membranes.

ADVERSE REACTIONS

Common reactions are in italics; life-threatening reactions are in bold italics.

Blood: ***thrombocytopenia,*** *leukopenia, neutropenia, anemia.*

CNS: dizziness, confusion, peripheral neuropathy, ototoxicity, central neurotoxicity.

GI: constipation, diarrhea, *nausea, vomiting.*

Other: alopecia, hypersensitivity, hepatotoxicity, *increased BUN, AST, or alkaline phosphatase.*

INTERACTIONS

Bone marrow depressants (including radiotherapy): increased hematologic toxicity.

Nephrotoxic agents: added nephrotoxicity of carboplatin.

EFFECTS ON DIAGNOSTIC TESTS

Bilirubin, alkaline phosphatase, AST (SGOT), serum creatinine, and blood urea: elevated levels with high doses.

NURSING CONSIDERATIONS

Besides those related universally to drug therapy (see "How to use this book"), consider the following specific recommendations:

Assessment

- Obtain a baseline assessment of the extent of the patient's underlying condition and his alkaline phosphatase, serum electrolytes, creatinine, BUN, CBC and creatinine clearance levels before initiating therapy.
- Be alert for adverse reactions or drug interactions during therapy.
- Evaluate the patient's and family's knowledge about carboplatin therapy.

Nursing Diagnoses

- Altered nutrition related to nausea, vomiting, and resulting electrolyte imbalances.
- Altered urinary elimination related to nephrotoxic effects of carboplatin.
- Knowledge deficit related to carboplatin therapy.

Planning and Implementation

Preparation and Administration

• ***I.V. use:*** To avoid mutagenic, teratogenic, and carcinogenic risks, use extreme caution when preparing carboplatin; wear gloves and mask, use a biological containment cabinet, and prevent leakage of drug. Avoid inhalation of dust or vapors containing carboplatin when preparing I.V. solution. Immediately before use, reconstitute with dextrose 5% in water, 0.9% sodium choloride or sterile water for a concentration of 10 mg/ml. Solution will remain stable, at room temperature for up to 8 hours. Store unopened vials at room temperature, protected from light exposure. Do not use needles or administration sets containing aluminum as carboplatin may precipitate and lose potency. Infuse over 15 minutes or longer; direct injection and continuous infusion are not recommended.

• Patients with a creatinine clearance of 41 to 59 ml/minute should receive a starting dose of 250 mg/m^2 on day 1; creatinine clearance of 16 to 40 ml/minute, 200 mg/m^2. There is no recommended dose for when the creatinine clearance is below 15 ml/minute.

• Check ordered dose against laboratory results carefully. Only one increase in dosage is recommended. Subsequent doses should not exceed 125% of starting dose.

Monitoring

• Monitor effectiveness by noting results of follow-up diagnostic tests and overall physical status.

• Monitor serum electrolytes, creatinine, BUN, CBC, and creatinine clearance levels before the first initial infusion and before each course. Leukocyte and platelet nadirs usually occur by day 21; return to baseline values usually occurs by day 28.

• Monitor vital signs during infusion.

• Monitor for signs of nephrotoxicity, neurotoxicity, ototoxicity, and hepatotoxicity.

• Monitor the patient's skin color and any complaints that may be associated with anemia.

Supportive Care

• Determine if the patient has adverse reactions to mannitol or platinum compounds.

• Premedicate with antiemetics, as vomiting is a frequent side effect of carboplatin therapy.

• Have epinephrine, corticosteroids, and antihistamines available when administering this drug as anaphalaxis-type reactions may occur within 15 minutes of administration.

• Increased fluids may be necessary if creatinine clearance is adversly affected.

• Carboplatin therapy should be avoided in patients with severe bone marrow depression or bleeding. Patients with significant anemia may require transfusions.

• Mothers should discontinue breast-feeding during treatment with carboplatin.

• Intermittent audiometric testing may be necessary.

• Patients older than age 65 are at greater risk for neurotoxicity.

Patient Teaching

• Encourage patients to maintain an adequate fluid intake, especially those fluids containing high amounts of electrolytes.

• Warn the patient that nausea and vomiting can be expected.

• Instruct the patient to alert the doctor if rash, pruritus, redness, or increased warmth to the skin or severe dyspnea with bronchospasm occurs.

Evaluation

In patients receiving carboplatin, appropriate evaluation statements may include:

• Patient maintains adequate nutrition and electrolyte balance.

• Patient maintains adequate daily

urinary output and creatinine clearance greater than 15 ml/minute throughout treatment.
• Patient and family state an understanding of carboplatin therapy.

carboprost tromethamine
(kar´ boe prost)
Hemabate, Prostin/15 M

• *Classification:* oxytoric (prostaglandin)
• *Pregnancy Risk Category:* C

HOW SUPPLIED
Injection: 250 mcg/ml

ACTION
Mechanism: Produces strong, prompt contractions of uterine smooth muscle, possibly mediated by calcium and cyclic 3′, 5′-adenosine monophosphate. A prostaglandin.
Pharmacokinetics: Unknown.

INDICATIONS & DOSAGE
Abort pregnancy between 13th and 20th weeks of gestation–
Adults: initially, 250 mcg is administered deep I.M. Subsequent doses of 250 mcg should be administered at intervals of 1½ to 3½ hours, depending on uterine response. Increments in dosage may be increased to 500 mcg if contractility is inadequate after several 250-mcg doses. Total dosage should not exceed 12 mg.
Postpartum hemorrhage caused by uterine atony that has not responded to conventional management–
Adults: 250 mcg by deep I.M. injection. May administer repeat doses at 15- to 90-minute intervals. Maximum total dosage is 2 mg.

CONTRAINDICATIONS & PRECAUTIONS
Contraindicated when the fetus has reached the stage of viability and in patients with hypersensitivity to the drug, acute pelvic inflammatory disease, or active renal, cardiac, or hepatic disease, because of increased potential for adverse effects. Use cautiously in patients with asthma, epilepsy, diabetes, hypotension, or jaundice, because drug may exacerbate the symptoms or disorders; and in patients with compromised (scarred) uterus, because of drug's contractile effects on smooth muscle.

ADVERSE REACTIONS
Common reactions are in italics; life-threatening reactions are in bold italics.
GI: *vomiting, diarrhea,* nausea.
Other: *fever,* chills.

INTERACTIONS
None significant.

EFFECTS ON DIAGNOSTIC TESTS
None reported.

NURSING CONSIDERATIONS
Besides those related universally to drug therapy (see "How to use this book"), consider the following specific recommendations:
Assessment
• Obtain a baseline assessment of the patient's pregnancy status before therapy.
• Be alert for adverse reactions and drug interactions throughout therapy.
• Evaluate the patient's and family's knowledge about carboprost tromethamine therapy.
Nursing Diagnoses
• High risk for fluid volume deficit related to carboprost tromethamine-induced vomiting, diarrhea.
• High risk for altered body temperature related to possible carboprost-induced fever.
• Knowledge deficit related to carboprost tromethamine therapy.

Planning and Implementation
Preparation and Administration
• Keep in mind that unlike other prostaglandin abortifacients, carboprost tromethamine is administered by I.M. injection. Injectable form avoids risk of expelling vaginal suppositories, which may occur in the presence of profuse vaginal bleeding.
• Be aware that carboprost tromethamine should be administered only in a hospital setting by trained personnel.
Monitoring
• Monitor effectiveness by evaluating uterine contractions, expulsion of products of conception, or cessation of postpartum hemorrhage.
• Monitor for nausea or diarrhea after drug administration.
• Monitor body temperature after drug administration.
Supportive Care
• Maintain fluids to help prevent hyperthermia; replace fluids if nausea or diarrhea occurs. Ask doctor for medication to control symptoms.
• Consult with the doctor if uterine contractions are ineffective or if postpartum bleeding persists.
• Keep in mind that I.M. injection of this drug is technically less difficult and poses fewer potential risks than other prostaglandin abortifacients.
Patient Teaching
• Explain the importance of follow-up care to assess the patient's treatment.
• Tell the patient to report fever, nausea, vomiting, diarrhea or any other adverse reactions or feelings to the doctor.
Evaluation
In patients receiving carboprost tromethamine, appropriate evaluation statements may include:
• Adequate fluid volume is maintained.
• Body temperature is within normal limits.
• Patient and family state an understanding of carboprost tromethamine therapy.

carisoprodol
(kar eye soe proe´ dole)
Rela, Sodol, Soma, Soprodol, Soridol

• *Classification:* skeletal muscle relaxant (carbamate derivative)
• *Pregnancy Risk Category:* C

HOW SUPPLIED
Tablets: 350 mg

ACTION
Mechanism: Reduces transmission of impulses from the spinal cord to skeletal muscle.
Absorption: Rapidly absorbed from the GI tract.
Distribution: Widely distributed throughout the body.
Metabolism: Hepatic.
Excretion: In urine mainly as its metabolites; less than 1% of a dose is excreted unchanged. The drug may be removed by hemodialysis or peritoneal dialysis. Half-life: About 8 hours.
Onset, peak, duration: With usual therapeutic doses, onset of action occurs within 30 minutes and persists 4 to 6 hours.

INDICATIONS & DOSAGE
As an adjunct in acute, painful musculoskeletal conditions–
Adults and children over 12 years: 350 mg P.O. t.i.d. and h.s.

Not recommended for children under 12 years.

CONTRAINDICATIONS & PRECAUTIONS
Contraindicated in patients with acute intermittent porphyria because the drug may exacerbate the condition, and in those who have demonstrated allergic or idiosyncratic reac-

tions to the drug or its related compounds (meprobamate).

Use cautiously in patients with impaired renal or hepatic function; in patients with CNS depression because effects may be additive. Psychological dependence and abuse have been reported in those with a history of drug abuse or dependence. Patients allergic or sensitive to the dye tartrazine should avoid taking Rela tablets. Although tartrazine sensitivity is rare, it frequently occurs in patients sensitive to aspirin.

Avoid use in patients with head injury or coma.

ADVERSE REACTIONS

Common reactions are in italics; life-threatening reactions are in bold italics.

CNS: *drowsiness, dizziness,* vertigo, ataxia, tremor, agitation, irritability, headache, depressive reactions, insomnia.

CV: orthostatic hypotension, tachycardia, facial flushing.

GI: nausea, vomiting, hiccups, increased bowel activity, epigastric distress.

Skin: rash, *erythema multiforme,* pruritus.

Other: asthmatic episodes, fever, angioneurotic edema, ***anaphylaxis.***

INTERACTIONS

Alcohol, CNS depressants: increased CNS depression.

EFFECTS ON DIAGNOSTIC TESTS

None significant.

NURSING CONSIDERATIONS

Besides those related universally to drug therapy (see "How to use this book"), consider the following specific recommendations:

Assessment

- Obtain a baseline assessment of the patient's pain related to his underlying condition before drug therapy.
- Be alert for adverse reactions and drug interactions throughout therapy.
- Evaluate the patient's and family's knowledge about carisoprodol therapy.

Nursing Diagnoses

- Pain related to the patient's underlying condition.
- High risk for injury related to drug-induced drowsiness.
- Knowledge deficit related to carisoprodol therapy.

Planning and Implementation

Preparation and Administration

- Give with meals or milk to prevent GI distress.
- Amount of relief determines if amount of dosage can be reduced.

Monitoring

- Monitor effectiveness by regularly assessing the severity and frequency of muscle spasms.
- Monitor for adverse reactions by frequently checking vital signs for hypotension and tachycardia.
- Monitor for insomnia, headache, nausea, and abdominal cramps if drug is withdrawn.
- Monitor for idiosyncratic reactions, such as weakness, ataxia, visual and speech difficulties, fever, skin eruptions, and mental changes, or severe reactions, such as hypotension, bronchospasm, and anaphylactic shock.

Supportive Care

- Give the patient sugarless hard candy, ice chips, or sugarless gum to relieve dry mouth.
- Institute safety precautions if he develops blurred vision, confusion, or dizziness.
- Record the patient's degree of relief to determine whether dosage can be reduced.
- Do not withdraw the drug abruptly unless required by severe adverse reactions.
- Know that treatment of overdose is entirely supportive; do not induce emesis or use a respiratory stimulant in obtunded patients.

• Be prepared to withhold the drug and notify the doctor immediately if idiosyncratic or any reactions occur after the first to fourth dose.

Patient Teaching

• Warn the patient not to take the drug with alcohol or other depressants.

• Tell the patient to use ice chips, sugarless hard candy, or sugarless gum to relieve dry mouth.

• Warn the patient to avoid driving and other hazardous activities that require alertness until CNS effects of drug are known.

• Advise the patient not to suddenly stop taking the drug.

• Advise the patient to follow the doctor's recommendations regarding rest and physical therapy.

Evaluation

In patients receiving carisoprodol, appropriate evaluation statements may include:

• Patient reports pain has ceased.

• Patient does not experience injury as a result of drug-induced drowsiness.

• Patient and family state an understanding of carisoprodol therapy.

carmustine (BCNU)

(kar mus´ teen)

BiCNU

• *Classification:* antineoplastic (alklyating agent, nitrosourea)

• *Pregnancy Risk Category:* D

HOW SUPPLIED

Injection: 100-mg vial (lyophilized), with a 3-ml vial of absolute alcohol supplied as a diluent

ACTION

Mechanism: An alkylating agent that cross-links strands of cellular DNA and RNA; interferes with RNA transcription, causing an imbalance of growth that leads to cell death. Cell cycle–nonspecific.

Distribution: Rapidly cleared from the plasma. Because carmustine is lipid soluble and nonionized at physiological pH, it distributes rapidly into the CSF; also distributed in breast milk.

Metabolism: Extensively metabolized, probably in the liver. Some metabolites may be active.

Excretion: Approximately 60% to 70% of carmustine and its metabolites are excreted in urine within 96 hours, 6% to 10% are excreted as carbon dioxide by the lungs, and 1% are excreted in feces. Enterohepatic circulation and storage of the drug in adipose tissue can occur and may cause delayed hematologic toxicity.

INDICATIONS & DOSAGE

Brain, colon, and stomach cancer; Hodgkin's disease; non-Hodgkin's lymphomas; melanomas; multiple myeloma; and hepatoma –

Adults: 75 to 100 mg/m^2 I.V. by slow infusion daily for 2 days; repeat q 6 weeks if platelets are above 100,000/mm^3 and WBC is above 4,000/mm^3. Dosage is reduced 50% when WBC is less than 2,000/mm^3 and platelets are less than 25,000/mm^3.

Alternate therapy: 200 mg/m^2 I.V. slow infusion as a single dose, repeated q 6 to 8 weeks; or 40 mg/m^2 I.V. slow infusion for 5 consecutive days, repeated q 6 weeks.

CONTRAINDICATIONS & PRECAUTIONS

Contraindicated in patients with a history of hypersensitivity to the drug.

Drug should be withheld or dosage reduced in the presence of hepatic or renal insufficiency because drug accumulation may occur; in patients with compromised hematologic status because of the drug's adverse hematologic effects; and in patients with recent exposure to cytotoxic medications or radiation therapy.

ADVERSE REACTIONS

Common reactions are in italics; life-threatening reactions are in bold italics.

Blood: ***cumulative bone marrow depression,*** *delayed 4 to 6 weeks, lasting 1 to 2 weeks; leukopenia;* ***thrombocytopenia.***

CNS: ataxia, drowsiness.

GI: *nausea, which begins in 2 to 6 hours (can be severe); vomiting.*

GU: nephrotoxicity.

Hepatic: hepatotoxicity.

Metabolic: possible hyperuricemia in lymphoma patients when rapid cell lysis occurs.

Skin: facial flushing.

Local: *intense pain at infusion site from venous spasm.*

Other: ***pulmonary fibrosis.***

INTERACTIONS

Cimetidine: may increase carmustine's bone marrow toxicity. Avoid combination if possible.

EFFECTS ON DIAGNOSTIC TESTS

BUN, serum alkaline phosphatase, AST (SGOT), and bilirubin: increased concentrations.

NURSING CONSIDERATIONS

Besides those related universally to drug therapy (see "How to use this book"), consider the following specific recommendations:

Assessment

- Obtain a baseline assessment of the patient's underlying condition and CBC, platelets, uric acid, BUN, creatinine, alkaline phosphatase, bilirubin levels, and pulmonary function tests before initiating therapy.
- Be alert for adverse reactions or drug interactions during therapy.
- Evaluate the patient's and family's knowledge about carmustine therapy.

Nursing Diagnoses

- High risk for injury related to drug-induced bone marrow depression, hepatorenal toxicity, and pulmonary fibrosis.
- Pain related to venous spasm due to carmustine infusion.
- Knowledge deficit related to carmustine therapy.

Planning and Implementation

Preparation and Administration

- Preparation of parenteral form is associated with carcinogenic, mutagenic, and teratogenic risks for personnel. Follow institutional policy to reduce risks.
- ***I.V. use:*** To reconstitute, dissolve 100 mg carmustine in 3 ml absolute alcohol, provided by manufacturer. Dilute solution with 27 ml sterile water for injection. Resultant solution contains 3.3 mg carmustine/ml in 10% alcohol solution. Dilute in normal saline solution or dextrose 5% in water for I.V. infusion. Give at least 250 ml over 1 to 2 hours. Direct injection is contraindicated; continuous infusion is not used. Don't mix with other drugs during infusion. May store reconstituted solution in refrigerator for up to 24 hours; then discard, if not used. Do not use vial for multiple doses as there is no preservative in vial. May decompose at temperatures above 80° F (26.6° C). If powder liquefies or appears oily, it is a sign of decomposition and should be discarded.

Monitoring

- Monitor effectiveness by noting results of follow-up diagnostic tests and overall physical status.
- Monitor CBC and hepatic and renal functions throughout therapy.
- Monitor pulmonary function because toxicity increases in cummulative doses > 1,400 mg/m^2.
- Monitor serum uric acid levels.
- Monitor the patient for signs of bleeding (ecchymosis, petechiae, melena, hematuria).

• Monitor I.V. site for extravasation, pain, or burning.
• Monitor electrolytes if patient has experienced vomiting.
Supportive Care
• To reduce pain on infusion, dilute further or slow infusion rate.
• To reduce nausea, give antiemetic before administering carmustine.
• To prevent hyperuricemia with resulting uric acid nephropathy, allopurinol may be used along with increased hydration.
• Avoid contact with skin as carmustine leaves a brown stain. Wash off thoroughly with soap and water.
• Use anticoagulants and aspirin products cautiously in these patients.
• Do not give any I.M. injections if patient's platelet count falls below 100,000 mg/mm^3.
• Keep in mind that carmustine crosses blood-brain barriers and may be used to treat primary brain tumors.
Patient Teaching
• Warn patient to watch for signs of bleeding.
• Instruct patient to take daily temperature and report any signs of infection.
• Instruct patient to avoid the use of all OTC products containing aspirin.
• Tell the patient that he should not receive any immunizations during therapy and should avoid any contact with those newly exposed to the oral polio vaccine.
• Tell the patient not to take any OTC aspirin or aspirin products.
Evaluation
In patients receiving carmustine, appropriate evaluation statements may include:
• Injury to tissue is minimized and hepatic, renal, and pulmonary function remains effective.
• Pain is decreased during infusion of drug.
• Patient and family state an understanding of carmustine therapy.

carteolol
(kar´ tee oh lole)
Cartrol

• *Classification:* antihypertensive (beta-adrenergic blocking agent)
• *Pregnancy Risk Category:* C

HOW SUPPLIED
Tablets: 2.5 mg, 5 mg

ACTION
Mechanism: A nonselective beta-adrenergic blocking agent with intrinsic sympathomimetic activity (ISA). Its antihypertensive effects are probably caused by decreased sympathetic outflow from the brain and decreased cardiac output. No consistent effect on renin output.
Absorption: Rapid after oral administration; bioavailablity is about 85%.
Distribution: 20% to 30% bound to plasma proteins.
Metabolism: Only 30% to 50% of the drug is metabolized in the liver to 8-hydroxycarteolol, an active metabolite, and the inactive metabolite glucuronoside.
Excretion: Primarily renal. Half-life: About 6 hours.
Onset, peak, duration: Peak plasma levels occur in 1 to 3 hours.

INDICATIONS & DOSAGE
Hypertension–
Adults: initially, 2.5 mg P.O. as a single daily dose. Gradually increase dosage as required to 5 mg or 10 mg daily as a single dose.

CONTRAINDICATIONS & PRECAUTIONS
Contraindicated in patients with bronchial asthma because it may block bronchodilation by endogenous catecholamines or beta-receptor agonists; severe bradycardia and those with greater than first-degree heart

block, because it may further slow the heart rate; and cardiogenic shock or CHF, because it may worsen cardiac decompensation. Use cautiously in patients with CHF controlled by digitalis and diuretics because beta-adrenergic blocking agents do not block the inotropic effects of digitalis. Note that asymptomatic patients with a history of CHF may show signs of cardiac decompensation with beta blocker therapy.

Patients with unrecognized coronary artery disease may exhibit signs of angina pectoris upon withdrawal of the drug.

Beta blockade may mask tachycardia associated with hyperthyroidism, and the tachycardia and blood pressure changes associated with hypoglycemia, and may inhibit glycogenolysis. It may also attenuate insulin release. Drug should be withdrawn gradually in patients suspected of having thyrotoxicosis to avoid thyroid storm.

Withdrawal of beta blockers before surgery is controversial. Some clinicians advocate withdrawal to prevent any impairment of cardiac responsiveness to reflex stimuli and to prevent any decreased responsiveness to exogenous catecholamine administration. However, because the beta-blocking effects of carteolol may persist for weeks, discontinuing it before surgery may be impractical. The anesthesiologist should be informed that the patient is receiving a beta-blocking agent so that isoproterenol or dobutamine is readily available for the reversal of the drug's cardiac effects.

ADVERSE REACTIONS

Common reactions are in italics; life-threatening reactions are in bold italics.
CNS: weakness, lassitude, tiredness, fatigue, somnolescence.
CV: conduction disturbances.
Other: *muscle cramps, asthenia.*

INTERACTIONS

Calcium channel blocking agents: increased risk of hypotension, left ventricular failure, and AV conduction disturbances. I.V. calcium antagonists should be used with caution.
General anesthetics: increased hypotensive effects. Observe carefully for excessive hypotension or bradycardia, or orthostatic hypotension.
Insulin, oral hypoglycemic agents: hypoglycemic response may be altered by beta blockers. Dosage adjustments may be necessary.
Reserpine, catecholamine-depleting drugs: may have an additive effect when administered with a beta blocker.

EFFECTS ON DIAGNOSTIC TESTS

None reported.

NURSING CONSIDERATIONS

Besides those related universally to drug therapy (see "How to use this book"), consider the following specific recommendations:

Assessment

- Obtain a baseline assessment of patient's blood pressure before drug therapy.
- Be alert for adverse reactions and drug interactions throughout therapy.
- Evaluate the patient's and family's knowledge about cartelolol therapy.

Nursing Diagnoses

- High risk for injury related to ineffectiveness of carteolol to lower blood pressure.
- Pain related to carteolol-induced muscle cramps.
- Knowledge deficit related to carteolol.

Planning and Implementation

Preparation and Administration

- Be aware that patients with substantial renal failure should receive the usual dose of carteolol at longer intervals. If creatinine clearance is > 60 ml/minute, the drug is given at 24-hour intervals; if creatinine clearance is 20 to 60 ml/minute, at 48-hour intervals; if creatinine clearance is < 20 ml/minute, at 72-hour intervals.

• Don't discontinue abruptly in patients with suspected thyrotoxicosis; withdraw gradually to avoid thyroid storm.

• Be aware that withdrawal of beta blocker therapy before surgery is controversial.

Monitoring

• Monitor effectiveness by frequently monitoring patient's blood pressure.

• Monitor patients with a history of CHF for signs of cardiac decompensation.

• Monitor for signs of angina pectoris upon withdrawal of drug.

• Monitor ECG for conduction abnormalities.

• Monitor diabetic patient's blood glucose level closely as drug may inhibit glycogenolysis and mask the signs and symptoms of hypoglycemia (such as tachycardia and blood pressure changes). It may also attenuate insulin release.

• Monitor hyperthyroid patient closely for signs of thyroid storm other than tachycardia as drug may mask tachycardia associated with hyperthyroidism.

Supportive Care

• Be prepared to treat thyroid storm or hypoglycemia as this drug masks common signs of thyroid storm and hypoglycemia.

• Inform the anesthesiologist that the patient is receiving a beta blocking agent so that isoproterenol or dobutamine is made readily available for reversal of the cardiac effects of the drug.

• Institute safety measures if adverse CNS reactions occurs.

• Notify doctor if patient experiences muscle cramps.

• Be prepared to provide emergency treatment if conduction abnormalities occur.

• Assist patient with activities and provide frequent rest periods if patient experiences fatigue.

Patient Teaching

• Explain the importance of taking this drug as prescribed, even when feeling well. Tell patient not to discontinue drug suddenly, but to call the doctor if distressing reactions occur.

• Emphasize the importance of promptly reporting shortness of breath or difficulty breathing, unusually fast heartbeat, cough, or fatigue with exertion.

• Warn patient to avoid hazardous activities that require mental alertness if adverse CNS reactions occur.

Evaluation

In patients receiving carteolol, appropriate evaluation statements may include:

• Patient's blood pressure is within normal limits.

• Patient does not experience muscle cramps throughout carteolol therapy.

• Patient and family state an understanding of carteolol therapy.

cascara sagrada◇
(kas kar´ a)

cascara sagrada aromatic fluid extract*◇

cascara sagrada fluid extract*◇

• *Classification:* laxative (anthraquinone glycoside mixture)
• *Pregnancy Risk Category:* C

HOW SUPPLIED

Tablets: 150 mg◇, 325 mg◇
Aromatic fluid extract: 1 g/ml*◇
Fluidextract: 1 g/ml*◇

ACTION

Mechanism: A stimulant laxative that increases peristalsis by acting on the

smooth muscle of the intestine. Thought either to irritate the musculature or to stimulate the colonic intramural plexus. Also promotes fluid accumulation in the colon and small intestine.
Absorption: Minimal absorption in the small intestine.
Distribution: Found in bile, saliva, colonic mucosa, and breast milk.
Metabolism: Hydrolyzed by colonic flora enzymes to active, free anthraquinones, which are metabolized in the liver.
Excretion: In feces via biliary elimination; in urine; or in both.
Onset, peak, duration: Onset of action usually occurs in about 6 to 12 hours but may not occur for 3 or 4 days.

INDICATIONS & DOSAGE

Acute constipation; preparation for bowel or rectal examination–
Adults: 325 mg cascara sagrada tablets P.O. h.s.; or 1 ml fluid extract daily; or 5 ml aromatic fluid extract daily.
Children 2 to 12 years: ½ adult dose.
Children under 2 years: ¼ adult dose.

CONTRAINDICATIONS & PRECAUTIONS

Contraindicated in patients with fluid and electrolyte disturbances; appendicitis; nausea, vomiting, or abdominal pain; any abdominal condition necessitating immediate surgery; acute surgical delirium or fecal impaction; rectal bleeding; or intestinal obstruction, or perforation because the drug may exacerbate these conditions.

ADVERSE REACTIONS

Common reactions are in italics; life-threatening reactions are in bold italics.
GI: *nausea,* vomiting; diarrhea; loss of normal bowel function with excessive use; *abdominal cramps,* especially in severe constipation; malabsorption of nutrients; "cathartic colon" (syndrome resembling ulcerative colitis radiologically and pathologically) after chronic misuse; discoloration of rectal mucosa after long-term use.
Metabolic: hypokalemia, protein enteropathy, electrolyte imbalance in excessive use.
Other: laxative dependence in long-term or excessive use.

INTERACTIONS

None significant.

EFFECTS ON DIAGNOSTIC TESTS

None reported.

NURSING CONSIDERATIONS

Besides those related universally to drug therapy (see "How to use this book"), consider the following specific recommendations:

Assessment

- Obtain a baseline assessment of history of bowel disorder, GI status, fluid intake, nutritional status, exercise habits, and normal pattern of elimination.
- Be alert for adverse reactions or drug interactions throughout therapy.
- Evaluate the patient's and family's knowledge about cascara sagrada therapy.

Nursing Diagnoses

- Constipation related to interruption of normal pattern of elimination characterized by infrequent or absent stools.
- Pain related to cascara sagrada-induced abdominal cramps.
- Knowledge deficit related to cascara sagrada therapy.

Planning and Implementation

Preparation and Administration

- Check orders; read drug label carefully in order to give the correct form of the drug.

*Liquid form contains alcohol. **May contain tartrazine.

Monitoring
• Monitor effectiveness by checking the frequency and characteristics of stools.
• Auscultate bowel sounds at least once a shift. Assess for pain and cramping.
• Monitor nutritional status and fluid intake.
• Monitor serum electrolytes during prolonged use.
Supportive Care
• Note that onset of action is 6 to 12 hours.
• Be aware that aromatic cascara fluid extract is less active and less bitter than nonaromatic fluid extract and that liquid preparations are more reliable than solid dosage forms.
• Provide privacy for elimination.
• Unless contraindicated encourage fluid intake up to 2500 ml a day.
• Consult with a dietitian to modify diet to increase fiber and bulk.
Patient Teaching
• Discourage excessive use of laxatives.
• Teach the patient about the relationship between fluid intake, dietary fiber, exercise, and constipation.
• Teach patient that dietary sources of fiber include bran and other cereals, fresh fruit, and vegetables.
• Advise patient that cascara may turn alkaline urine red-pink and acidic urine yellow-brown.
• Warn patient that since cascara works by increasing intestinal peristalsis, abdominal cramping may occur.

Evaluation
In patients receiving cascara sagrada, appropriate evaluation statements may include:
• Patient reports return of normal pattern of elimination.
• Patient remians free from pain and abdominal cramping.
• Patient and family state an understanding of cascara sagrada therapy.

castor oil
(kas´ tor)
Alphamul◇, Emulsoil◇, Fleet Flavored Castor Oil◇, Kellogg's Castor Oil◇, Minims Castor Oil‡◇, Neoloid◇, Purge◇

• *Classification:* stimulant laxative (glyceride, *Ricinus communis* derivative)
• *Pregnancy Risk Category:* X

HOW SUPPLIED
Capsules: 0.62 ml oil◇
Oral liquid◇: 36.4% (Neoloid◇), 60% (Alphamul◇), 67% (Fleet◇), 95% (Purge◇, Emulsoil◇), 100% (Kellogg's◇, Minims◇).

ACTION
Mechanism: A stimulant laxative that increases peristalsis by direct effect on the smooth muscle of the intestine. Thought either to irritate the musculature or to stimulate the colonic intramural plexus. Also promotes fluid accumulation in the colon and small intestine.
Absorption: Unknown.
Distribution: Locally distributed, primarily in the small intestine.
Metabolism: Like other fatty acids, metabolized by intestinal enzymes into its active form, ricinoleic acid.
Excretion: In feces.
Onset, peak, duration: Action begins in 2 to 6 hours.

INDICATIONS & DOSAGE
Preparation for rectal or bowel examination, or surgery; acute constipation (rarely) –
Adults: 15 to 60 ml P.O.
Children over 2 years: 5 to 15 ml P.O.
Children under 2 years: 1.25 to 7.5 ml P.O.
Infants: up to 4 ml P.O. Increased dose produces no greater effect.

CONTRAINDICATIONS & PRECAUTIONS

Contraindicated in patients with fluid or electrolyte disturbances because it may worsen the imbalance; in patients with ulcerative bowel lesions, appendicitis, acute surgical abdomen, anal and rectal fissures, fecal impaction, intestinal obstruction, or intestinal perforation because excessive intestinal stimulation may exacerbate symptoms of these disorders; during pregnancy because it may induce labor; during menstruation; and in patients with hypersensitivity to castor beans. Use cautiously in patients with rectal bleeding.

ADVERSE REACTIONS

Common reactions are in italics; life-threatening reactions are in bold italics.

GI: *nausea;* vomiting; diarrhea; loss of normal bowel function with excessive use; *abdominal cramps,* especially in severe constipation; malabsorption of nutrients; "cathartic colon" (syndrome resembling ulcerative colitis radiologically and pathologically) in chronic misuse. May cause constipation after catharsis.

GU: pelvic congestion in menstruating women.

Metabolic: hypokalemia, protein-losing enteropathy, other electrolyte imbalance in excessive use.

Other: laxative dependence in long-term or excessive use.

INTERACTIONS

None significant.

EFFECTS ON DIAGNOSTIC TESTS

None reported.

NURSING CONSIDERATIONS

Besides those related universally to drug therapy (see "How to use this book"), consider the following specific recommendations:

Assessment

- Obtain a baseline assessment of history of bowel disorder, GI status, fluid intake, nutritional status, exercise habits, and normal pattern of elimination.
- Be alert for adverse reactions or drug interactions throughout therapy.
- Evaluate the patient's and family's knowledge about castor oil therapy.

Nursing Diagnoses

- Constipation related to interruption of normal pattern of elimination characterized by infrequent or absent stools.
- Pain related to castor oil-induced abdominal cramps.
- Knowledge deficit related to castor oil therapy.

Planning and Implementation

Preparation and Administration

- Check order; castor oil is available in two forms.
- Shake emulsion well. Store below 40° F (4.4° C).
- Give on an empty stomach for best results. Reschedule other P.O. drugs; increased intestinal motility caused by castor oil lessens absorption of concomitantly administered drugs.
- ***P.O. use:*** Give with juice or carbonated beverage to mask oily taste. Stir mixture and drink promptly.
- Schedule administration to avoid interference with scheduled activities or sleep. Be aware that castor oil produces complete evacuation after 3 hours.

Monitoring

- Monitor effectiveness by checking the frequency and characteristics of stools.
- Auscultate bowel sounds at least once a shift. Assess for pain and cramping.
- Monitor nutritional status and fluid intake.
- Monitor serum electrolytes during prolonged use. Castor oil affects the small intestine and may cause excessive loss of water and salt.

Supportive Care
• Generally used before diagnostic testing or therapy requiring thorough evacuation of the GI tract.
• Be aware that failure to respond to therapy may indicate an acute condition requiring surgery.
• Provide privacy for elimination.
• Unless contraindicated, encourage fluid intake up to 2500 ml a day.
• Consult with a dietitian to modify diet to increase fiber and bulk.
• Use for short-term treatment. Not recommended for routine use; useful for acute constipation not responsive to milder laxatives
Patient Teaching
• Discourage excessive use of laxatives.
• Teach the patient about the relationship between fluid intake, dietary fiber, exercise, and constipation.
• Teach patient that dietary sources of fiber include bran and other cereals, fresh fruit, and vegetables.
• Advise the patient that ice held in the mouth before taking the drug will help prevent tasting it. Inform the patient that castor oil emulsion is better tolerated but more expensive.
• Advise the patient that after castor oil has emptied the bowel he will not have a bowel movement for 1 to 2 days.
Evaluation
In patients receiving castor oil, appropriate evaluation statements may include:
• Patient reports return of normal pattern of elimination.
• Patient is pain free.
• Patient and family state an understanding of castor oil therapy.

cefaclor
(sef′ a klor)
Ceclor

• *Classification:* antibiotic (second-generation cephalosporin)
• *Pregnancy Risk Category:* B

HOW SUPPLIED
Capsules: 250 mg, 500 mg
Oral suspension: 125 mg/5 ml, 250 mg/5 ml

ACTION
Mechanism: A second-generation cephalosporin that inhibits cell wall synthesis during bacterial replication, promoting osmotic instability. Usually bactericidal.
Absorption: Well absorbed from the GI tract; food will delay but not prevent complete GI tract absorption.
Distribution: Distributed widely into most body tissues and fluids, with poor CSF penetration; crosses the placenta, and is 25% protein-bound.
Metabolism: Not metabolized.
Excretion: Primarily in urine by renal tubular secretion and glomerular filtration; small amounts are excreted in breast milk. Half-life: Elimination half-life is 30 minutes to 1 hour in patients with normal renal function; end-stage renal disease prolongs half-life to 3 to 5½ hours. Hemodialysis removes cefaclor.
Onset, peak, duration: Peak serum levels occur 30 to 60 minutes after oral dose.

INDICATIONS & DOSAGE
Treatment of infections of respiratory or urinary tracts, skin, and soft tissue; and otitis media due to Hemophilus influenzae, Streptococcus pneumoniae, S. pyogenes, Escherichia coli, Proteus mirabilis, Klebsiella *species, and staphylococci –*
Adults: 250 to 500 mg P.O. q 8 hours.

Total daily dose should not exceed 4 g.
Children: 20 mg/kg daily P.O. in divided doses q 8 hours. In more serious infections, 40 mg/kg daily are recommended, not to exceed 1 g per day.

CONTRAINDICATIONS & PRECAUTIONS

Contraindicated in patients with hypersensitivity to any cephalosporin. Use cautiously in patients with penicillin allergy, who usually are more susceptible to such reactions.

ADVERSE REACTIONS

Common reactions are in italics; life-threatening reactions are in bold italics.
Blood: transient leukopenia, lymphocytosis, anemia, eosinophilia.
CNS: dizziness, headache, somnolence.
GI: *nausea,* vomiting, *diarrhea,* anorexia, ***pseudomembranous colitis.***
GU: red and white cells in urine, vaginal moniliasis, vaginitis.
Skin: *maculopapular rash,* dermatitis.
Other: ***hypersensitivity,*** fever, cholestatic jaundice.

INTERACTIONS

Probenecid: may inhibit excretion and increase blood levels of cefaclor.

EFFECTS ON DIAGNOSTIC TESTS

Coombs' test: false-positive results.
Serum or urine creatinine: false elevations in tests using Jaffé's reaction.
Urine glucose tests with copper sulfate (Benedict's reagent or Clinitest): false-positive results; use glucose enzymatic tests (Clinistix or Tes-Tape) instead.

NURSING CONSIDERATIONS

Besides those related universally to drug therapy (see "How to use this book"), consider the following specific recommendations:

Assessment
- Obtain a baseline assessment of infection before therapy.
- Be alert for adverse reactions and drug interactions throughout therapy.
- Evaluate the patient's and family's knowledge about cefaclor therapy.

Nursing Diagnoses
- High risk for injury related to ineffectiveness of cefaclor to eradicate the infection.
- High risk for fluid volume deficit related to adverse GI reactions to cefaclor.
- Knowledge deficit related to cefaclor.

Planning and Implementation
Preparation and Administration
- Obtain specimen for culture and sensitivity tests before first dose. Therapy may begin pending test results.
- Ask patient about any reactions to previous cephalosporin or penicillin therapy before administering first dose.
- Be aware that total daily dose of cefaclor may be administered only twice daily instead of three times daily with similar therapeutic results.
- ***P.O. use:*** Store reconstituted suspension in refrigerator. Stable for 14 days if refrigerated. Keep tightly closed and shake well before using. Administer with food to prevent or minimize GI upset.

Monitoring
- Monitor effectiveness by regularly assessing for improvement of infection.
- Monitor for signs of an allergic or anaphylactic reaction.
- During prolonged or high-dose therapy, monitor for superinfection, especially in high-risk patients.
- Monitor hydration status if adverse GI reactions occur.

Supportive Care
- Obtain an order for an antiemetic or antidiarrheal agent as needed.
- Notify doctor if skin rash develops.

• When testing urine glucose, use only glucose enzymatic tests (Clinistix or Tes-Tape), because copper sulfate tests (Clinitest) may have false-positive results.

Patient Teaching

• Tell the patient to take medication exactly as prescribed, even after he feels better, and to take the entire amount prescribed.

• Tell the patient to take with food or milk to minimize GI discomfort.

• Inform the patient using oral suspension to shake it well before using. Tell the patient to store the mixture in a tightly closed container in refrigerator. Refrigerated suspension is stable for 14 days without significant loss of potency.

• Instruct patient to notify doctor if skin rash develops.

• Teach diabetic patients to test urine for glucose with a glucose enzymatic test such as Clinistix or Tes-Tape because copper sulfate tests (Clinitest) may yield false-positive results.

Evaluation

In patients receiving cefaclor, appropriate evaluation statements may include:

• Patient is free of infection.

• Patient maintains adequate hydration throughout cefaclor therapy.

• Patient and family state an understanding of cefaclor therapy.

cefadroxil monohydrate

(sef a drox´ ill)

Duricef, Ultracef

• *Classification:* (first-generation cehalosporin)

• *Pregnancy Risk Category:* B

HOW SUPPLIED

Tablets: 1 g

Capsules: 500 mg

Oral suspension: 125 mg/5 ml, 250 mg/5 ml, 500 mg/5 ml

ACTION

Mechanism: Inhibits cell wall synthesis during bacterial replication, promoting osmotic instability. Usually bactericidal.

Absorption: Rapid and complete from the GI tract after oral administration.

Distribution: Widely distributed into most body tissues and fluids, including the gallbladder, liver, kidneys, bone, bile, sputum, and pleural and synovial fluids. CSF penetration is poor. Cefadroxil crosses the placenta; it is 20% protein-bound.

Metabolism: Not metabolized.

Excretion: Primarily excreted unchanged in the urine via glomerular filtration and renal tubular secretion; small amounts may be excreted in breast milk. Half-life: About 1 to 2 hours in patients with normal renal function; 25 hours in end-stage renal disease.

Onset, peak, duration: Peak serum levels occur at 1 to 2 hours.

INDICATIONS & DOSAGE

Treatment of urinary tract infections caused by Escherichia coli, Proteus mirabilis, *and* Klebsiella *species; infections of skin and soft tissue; and streptococcal pharyngitis–*

Adults: 500 mg to 2 g P.O. per day, depending on the infection being treated. Usually given in once-daily or b.i.d. dosage.

Children: 30 mg/kg P.O. daily in 2 divided doses.

CONTRAINDICATIONS & PRECAUTIONS

Contraindicated in patients with hypersensitivity to any cephalosporin. Use cautiously in patients with penicillin allergy, who usually are more susceptible to such reactions.

ADVERSE REACTIONS

Common reactions are in italics; life-threatening reactions are in bold italics.

Blood: transient neutropenia, eosinophilia, leukopenia, anemia.
CNS: dizziness, headache, malaise, paresthesias.
GI: ***pseudomembranous colitis,*** nausea, anorexia, vomiting, *diarrhea,* glossitis, *dyspepsia,* abdominal cramps, anal pruritus, tenesmus, oral candidiasis (thrush).
GU: genital pruritus, moniliasis.
Skin: *maculopapular and erythematous rashes.*
Other: ***hypersensitivity,*** dyspnea.

INTERACTIONS

Probenecid: may inhibit excretion and increase blood levels of cefadroxil.

EFFECTS ON DIAGNOSTIC TESTS

Coombs' test: positive results in about 3% of patients.
Urine creatinine: falsely elevated levels in tests using Jaffé's reaction.
Urine glucose tests with copper sulfate (Benedict's reagent or Clinitest): false-positive results. Use glucose enzymatic test (Clinistix or Tes-Tape) instead.

NURSING CONSIDERATIONS

Besides those related universally to drug therapy (see "How to use this book"), consider the following specific recommendations:

Assessment
- Obtain a baseline assessment of infection before therapy.
- Be alert for adverse reactions or drug interactions during therapy.
- Evaluate the patient's and family's knowledge about cefadroxil.

Nursing Diagnoses
- High risk for injury related to ineffectiveness of cefadroxil to eradicate the infection.
- High risk for fluid volume deficit related to adverse GI reactions to cefadroxil.
- Knowledge deficit related to cefadroxil.

Planning and Implementation
Preparation and Administration
- Obtain specimen for culture and sensitivity tests before first dose. Therapy may begin pending test results.
- Before giving first dose, ask patient about any reaction to previous cephalosporin or penicillin therapy.
- Expect doctor to prescribe longer interval between doses to prevent accumulation of drug in patients with creatinine clearance below 50 ml/minute.
- ***P.O. use:*** Store reconstituted suspension in refrigerator. Keep container tightly closed and shake well before using. Administer the drug with food to prevent or minimize GI upset.

Monitoring
- Monitor effectiveness by regularly assessing for improvement of infection.
- Monitor for signs of an allergic or anaphylactic reaction.
- During prolonged or high-dose therapy, monitor for superinfection, especially in high-risk patients.
- Monitor hydration status if adverse GI reactions occur.

Supportive Care
- Obtain an order for an antiemetic or antidiarrheal agent as needed.
- Notify doctor if skin rash develops.
- When testing urine glucose, use only glucose enzymatic tests (Clinistix or Tes-Tape), because copper sulfate tests (Clinitest) may have false-positive results.

Patient Teaching
- Tell the patient to take medication exactly as prescribed, even after he feels better, and to take the entire amount prescribed.
- Tell the patient to take with food or milk to lessen GI discomfort.
- Inform the patient using oral suspension to shake it well before using. Tell the patient to store mixture in a tightly closed container in the refrigerator.

• Instruct patient to notify doctor if skin rash develops.
• Teach diabetic patients to test urine for glucose with a glucose enzymatic test such as Clinistix or Tes-Tape because copper sulfate tests (Clinitest) may yield false-positive results.

Evaluation

In patients receiving cefadroxil, appropriate evaluation statements may include:
• Patient is free of infection.
• Patient maintains adequate hydration throughout cefadroxil therapy.
• Patient and family state an understanding of cefadroxil therapy.

cefamandole nafate

(sef a man´ dole)
Mandol

• *Classification:* antibiotic (second-generation cephalosporin)
• *Pregnancy Risk Category:* B

HOW SUPPLIED

Injection: 500 mg, 1 g, 2 g, 10 g
Pharmacy bulk package: 10 g

ACTION

Mechanism: Inhibits cell wall synthesis during bacterial replication, promoting osmotic instability. Usually bactericidal.
Absorption: Not absorbed from the GI tract and must be given parenterally. Peak serum levels after an I.M. dose are lower than after I.V. infusion.
Distribution: Widely distributed into most body tissues and fluids, including the gallbladder, liver, kidney, bone, sputum, bile, and pleural and synovial fluids; CSF penetration is poor. Cefamandole crosses the placenta; it is 65% to 75% protein-bound.
Metabolism: Not metabolized.
Excretion: Primarily excreted in urine by renal tubular secretion and glomerular filtration; small amounts are excreted in breast milk. Half-life: about 30 minutes to 2 hours in patients with normal renal function; 12 to 18 hours in severe renal disease.
Onset, peak, duration: Peak serum levels occur 30 minutes to 2 hours after an I.M. dose.

INDICATIONS & DOSAGE

Treatment of serious infections of respiratory and genitourinary tracts, skin and soft-tissue infections, bone and joint infections, septicemia, and peritonitis due to Escherichia coli *and other coliform bacteria,* S. aureus *(penicillinase- and nonpenicillinase-producing),* S. epidermidis, *group A beta-hemolytic streptococci,* Klebsiella, Hemophilus influenzae, Proteus mirabilis, *and* Enterobacter–
Adults: 500 mg to 1 g q 4 to 8 hours. In life-threatening infections, up to 2 g q 4 hours may be needed.
Infants and children: 50 to 100 mg/kg daily in equally divided doses q 4 to 8 hours. May be increased to total daily dose of 150 mg/kg (not to exceed maximum adult dose) for severe infections.

Total daily dosage is same for I.M. or I.V. administration and depends on susceptibility of organism and severity of infection. In patients with impaired renal function, doses or frequency of administration must be modified according to degree of renal impairment, severity of infection, and susceptibility of organism.
Should be injected deep I.M. into a large muscle mass, such as gluteus or lateral aspect of thigh.

CONTRAINDICATIONS & PRECAUTIONS

Contraindicated in patients with hypersensitivity to any cephalosporin. Use cautiously in patients with penicillin allergy, who usually are more susceptible to such reactions; in patients with coagulopathy; and in severely debilitated and malnourished patients, who are at greater risk of bleeding complications.

ADVERSE REACTIONS

Common reactions are in italics; life-threatening reactions are in bold italics.
Blood: transient neutropenia, eosinophilia, hemolytic anemia, *hypoprothrombinemia,* bleeding.
CNS: headache, malaise, paresthesias, dizziness.
GI: ***pseudomembranous colitis,*** nausea, anorexia, vomiting, *diarrhea,* glossitis, dyspepsia, abdominal cramps, tenesmus, anal pruritus, oral candidiasis (thrush).
GU: genital pruritus and moniliasis.
Skin: *maculopapular and erythematous rashes, urticaria.*
Local: *at injection site—pain, induration, sterile abscesses,* temperature elevation, tissue sloughing; *phlebitis and thrombophlebitis with I.V. injection.*
Other: ***hypersensitivity,*** dyspnea.

INTERACTIONS

Ethyl alcohol: may cause a disulfiram-like reaction. Warn patients not to drink alcohol for several days after discontinuing cefamandole.
Oral anticoagulants, aspirin: increased risk of bleeding.
Probenecid: may inhibit excretion and increase blood levels of cefamandole.

EFFECTS ON DIAGNOSTIC TESTS

Coombs' test: positive results.
Liver function tests: elevated.
Prothrombin time: prolonged.
Serum or urine creatinine levels: false elevation in tests using Jaffe's reaction.
Urine glucose tests using copper sulfate (Benedict's reagent or Clinitest): false-positive results. Use glucose enzymatic tests (Clinistix or Tes-Tape) instead.

NURSING CONSIDERATIONS

Besides those related universally to drug therapy (see "How to use this book"), consider the following specific recommendations:

Assessment
- Obtain a baseline assessment of infection before therapy.
- Be alert for adverse reactions or drug interactions during therapy.
- Evaluate the patient's and family's knowledge about cefamandole.

Nursing Diagnoses
- High risk for injury related to ineffectiveness of cefamandole to eradicate the infection.
- High risk for fluid volume deficit related to adverse GI reactions to cefamandole.
- Knowledge deficit related to cefamandole.

Planning and Implementation

Preparation and Administration
- Obtain specimen for culture and sensitivity tests before first dose. Therapy may begin pending test results.
- Before giving first dose, ask patient about any reaction to previous cephalosporin or penicillin therapy.
- ***I.M. use:*** Administer deep into a large muscle mass, such as gluteus or lateral aspect of thigh. Reconstitute drug by following manufacturer's instructions.
- ***I.V. use:*** Reconstitute 1 g with 10 ml of sterile water for injection, dextrose 5%, or 0.9% sodium chloride for injection. Don't mix with I.V. infusions containing magnesium or calcium ions; they are chemically incompatible.
- After reconstitution, drug remains stable for 24 hours at room temperature or 96 hours under refrigeration.

Monitoring
- Monitor effectiveness by regularly assessing for improvement of infection.
- Monitor for signs of an allergic or anaphylactic reaction.

• During prolonged or high-dose therapy, monitor for superinfection, especially in high-risk patients.
• Monitor hydration status if adverse GI reactions occur.

Supportive Care
• Obtain an order for an antiemetic or antidiarrheal agent as needed.
• If bleeding occurs, be prepared to administer vitamin K as prescribed.
• When testing urine glucose, use only glucose enzymatic tests (Clinistix or Tes-Tape), because copper sulfate tests (Clinitest) may have false-positive results.

Patient Teaching
• Teach diabetic patients to test urine for glucose with a glucose enzymatic test such as Clinistrix or Tes-Tape because copper sulfate tests (Clinitest) may yield false-positive results.

Evaluation
In patients receiving cefamandole, appropriate evaluation statements may include:
• Patient is free of infection.
• Patient maintains adequate hydration throughout cefamandole therapy.
• Patient and family state an understanding of cefamandole therapy.

cefazolin sodium
(sef az´ oh linn)
Ancef, Kefzol

• *Classification:* antibiotic (first-generation cephalosporin)
• *Pregnancy Risk Category:* B

HOW SUPPLIED
Injection (parenteral): 250 mg, 500 mg, 1 g, 5 g, 10 g
Infusion: 500 mg/100 ml vial, 500-mg or 1-g Redi Vials, Faspaks, or ADD-Vantage vials

ACTION
Mechanism: Inhibits cell wall synthesis during bacterial replication, promoting osmotic instability. Usually bactericidal.
Absorption: Not well absorbed from the GI tract and must be given parenterally. Peak serum levels are lower after I.M. injection as compared to I.V. infusion.
Distribution: Widely distributed into most body tissues and fluids, including the gallbladder, liver, kidneys, bone, sputum, bile, and pleural and synovial fluids; CSF penetration is poor. Drug crosses the placenta; it is 74% to 86% protein-bound.
Metabolism: Not metabolized.
Excretion: Primarily excreted unchanged in urine by renal tubular secretion and glomerular filtration; small amounts are excreted in breast milk. Half-life: About 1 to 2 hours in patients with normal renal function; 12 to 50 hours in end-stage renal disease. Hemodialysis or peritoneal dialysis removes cefazolin.
Onset, peak, duration: Peak serum levels occur 1 to 2 hours after I.M. dose.

INDICATIONS & DOSAGE
Treatment of serious infections of respiratory and genitourinary tracts, skin and soft-tissue infections, bone and joint infections, septicemia, and endocarditis due to Escherichia coli, *Enterobacteriaceae, gonococci,* Hemophilus influenzae, Klebsiella, Proteus mirabilis, Staphylococcus aureus, Streptococcus pneumoniae, *and group A beta-hemolytic streptococci; and perioperative prophylaxis*—
Adults: 250 mg I.M. or I.V. q 8 hours to 1 g q 6 hours. Maximun 12 g/day in life-threatening situations.
Children over 1 month: 8 to 16 mg/kg I.M. or I.V. q 8 hours, or 6 to 12 mg/kg q 6 hours.

Total daily dosage is same for I.M. or I.V. administration and depends on susceptibility of organism and severity of infection. In patients with impaired renal function, doses or frequency of administration must be modified according to degree of renal impairment, severity of infection, and susceptibility of organism. Should be injected deep I.M. into a large muscle mass, such as gluteus or lateral aspect of thigh.

CONTRAINDICATIONS & PRECAUTIONS

Contraindicated in patients with hypersensitivity to any cephalosporin. Use cautiously in patients with penicillin allergy, who usually are more susceptible to such reactions.

ADVERSE REACTIONS

Common reactions are in italics; life-threatening reactions are in bold italics.
Blood: transient neutropenia, leukopenia, eosinophilia, anemia.
CNS: dizziness, headache, malaise, paresthesias.
GI: ***pseudomembranous colitis,*** nausea, anorexia, vomiting, *diarrhea,* glossitis, dyspepsia, abdominal cramps, anal pruritus, tenesmus, oral candidiasis (thrush).
GU: genital pruritus and moniliasis, vaginitis.
Skin: *maculopapular and erythematous rashes, urticaria.*
Local: *at injection site—pain, induration, sterile abscesses, tissue sloughing; phlebitis and thrombophlebitis with I.V. injection.*
Other: ***hypersensitivity,*** dyspnea.

INTERACTIONS

Probenecid: may inhibit excretion and increase blood levels of cefazolin.

EFFECTS ON DIAGNOSTIC TESTS

Coombs' test: positive results.
Liver function tests: elevated results.
Serum or urine creatinine: false elevations in tests using Jaffé's reaction.
Urine glucose tests with copper sulfate (Benedict's reagent or Clinitest): false-positive results. Use glucose enzymatic tests (Clinistix or Tes-Tape) instead.

NURSING CONSIDERATIONS

Besides those related universally to drug therapy (see "How to use this book"), consider the following specific recommendations:

Assessment
- Obtain a baseline assessment of infection before therapy.
- Be alert for adverse drug reactions or drug interactions during cefazolin therapy.
- Evaluate the patient's and family's knowledge about cefazolin.

Nursing Diagnoses
- High risk for injury related to ineffectiveness of cefazolin to eradicate the infection.
- High risk for fluid volume deficit related to adverse GI reactions to cefazolin.
- Knowledge deficit related to cefazolin.

Planning and Implementation

Preparation and Administration
- Obtain specimen for culture and sensitivity tests before first dose. Therapy may begin pending test results.
- Before giving first dose, ask about any reactions to previous cephalosporin or penicillin therapy.
- Be aware that doses greater than 4 g daily should be avoided in patients with severe renal impairment.
- ***I.M. use:*** Reconstitute with sterile water, bacteriostatic water, or 0.9% sodium chloride solution as follows: 2 ml to 250-mg vial; 2 ml to 500-mg vial; 2.5 ml to 1-g vial. Shake well until dissolved. Resultant concentration: 125 mg/ml, 225 mg/ml, 330 mg/ml, respectively. Administer deep into a large muscle mass, such as gluteus or lateral aspect of thigh.
- ***I.V. use:*** Reconstitute drug as for I.M. injection. For direct I.V. injection, further dilute drug with 10 ml of compatible solution; for intermit-

tent infusion, add reconstituted drug to 50 to 100 ml of compatible solution. Alternate injection sites if I.V. therapy lasts longer than 3 days. Use of small I.V. needles in the larger available veins may be preferable.
• After reconstitution, drug is stable for 24 hours at room temperature; for 96 hours under refrigeration.
Monitoring
• Monitor effectiveness by regularly assessing for improvement of infection.
• Monitor for signs of an allergic or anaphylactic reaction.
• During prolonged or high-dose therapy, monitor for superinfection, especially in high-risk patients.
• Monitor patient's hydration status if adverse GI reactions occur.
Supportive Care
• Obtain an order for an antiemetic or antidiarrheal agent as needed.
• When testing urine glucose, use only glucose enzymatic tests (Clinistix or Tes-Tape), because copper sulfate tests (Clinitest) may have false-positive results.
Patient Teaching
• Teach diabetic patients to test urine for glucose with a glucose enzymatic test such as Clinistix or Tes-Tape because copper sulfate tests (Clinitest) may yield false-positive results.
Evaluation
In patients receiving cefazolin, appropriate evaluation statements may include:
• Patient is free of infection.
• Patient maintains adequate hydration throughout cefazolin therapy.
• Patient and family state an understanding of cefazolin therapy.

cefixime
(sef ix´ eem)
Suprax

• *Classification:* antibiotic (third-generation cephalosporin)
• *Pregnancy Risk Category:* B

HOW SUPPLIED
Tablets: 200 mg, 400 mg
Oral suspension: 100 mg/5 ml (after reconstitution)

ACTION
Mechanism: Inhibits cell wall synthesis during bacterial replication, promoting osmotic instability. Usually bactericidal.
Absorption: About 30% to 50% of a dose is absorbed after oral administration. Food delays absorption but does not affect the total amount absorbed. Peak serum levels with oral suspension are 15% to 50% higher than with tablets.
Distribution: Distributes to sputum, bile, tonsils, maxillary sinus mucosa, middle ear discharge, and prostatic fluid; also distributes into amniotic fluid in low concentrations; crosses the placenta. Drug is about 65% bound to plasma proteins.
Metabolism: About 50% of the drug is metabolized.
Excretion: Primarily excreted in the urine. Half-life: 3 to 4 hours in patients with normal renal function; 11½ hours in patients with end-stage renal disease.
Onset, peak, duration: Peak serum levels occur 2 to 6 hours after an oral dose.

INDICATIONS & DOSAGE
Treatment of uncomplicated urinary tract infections caused by Escherichia coli *and* Proteus mirabilis; *otitis media caused by* Hemophilus influenzae *(beta-lactam positive and negative*

strains), Moraxella (Branhamella) catarrhalis, *and* Streptococcus pyogenes; *pharyngitis and tonsillitis caused by* S. pyogenes; *acute bronchitis and acute exacerbations of chronic bronchitis caused by* S. pneumoniae *and* H. influenzae *(beta-lactamase positive and negative strains)* –
Adults: 400 mg/day orally as a single 400-mg tablet or 200 mg q 12 hours.
Children: 8 mg/kg/day suspension orally as a single daily dose or 4 mg/kg orally q 12 hours.
Treat children over age 12 and those who weigh more than 50 kg with the recommended adult dose.

CONTRAINDICATIONS & PRECAUTIONS

Contraindicated in patients with allergy to cephalosporins. Use cautiously in patients with a history of hypersensitivity to penicillins, cephalosporins, or other drugs. Cross-hypersensitivity has been demonstrated in about 10% of patients with a penicillin allergy. Also administer cautiously to patients with a history of GI disease, particularly colitis. Pseudomembranous colitis has been reported in patients who have received cefixime. Symptoms can occur during or after therapy.

ADVERSE REACTIONS

Common reactions are in italics; life-threatening reactions are in bold italics.
Blood: thrombocytopenia, leukopenia, eosinophilia.
CNS: headaches, dizziness.
GI: *diarrhea,* loose stools, abdominal pain, nausea, vomiting, dyspepsia, flatulence, pseudomembranous colitis.
GU: genital pruritus, vaginitis, genital candidiasis.
Skin: pruritus, rash, urticaria.
Other: drug fever, ***hypersensitivity.***

INTERACTIONS

Probenecid: decreased elimination of cefixime. Clinical significance is not known.
Salicylates: may displace cefixime from protein binding sites, increasing serum levels of free cefixime. Clinical significance is not known.

EFFECTS ON DIAGNOSTIC TESTS

Coombs' test: false-positive results.
Urine glucose tests with copper sulfate (Benedict's reagent or Clinitest): false-positive results; use glucose enzymatic tests (Clinistix or Tes-Tape) instead.
Urine ketone tests (with nitroprusside): false-positive results with other cephalosporins.

NURSING CONSIDERATIONS

Besides those related universally to drug therapy (see "How to use this book"), consider the following specific recommendations:

Assessment
- Obtain a baseline assessment of infection before therapy.
- Be alert for adverse reactions or drug interactions during therapy.
- Evaluate the patient's and family's knowledge about cefixime.

Nursing Diagnoses
- High risk for injury related to ineffectiveness of cefixime to eradicate the infection.
- High risk for fluid volume deficit related to adverse GI reactions to cefixime.
- Knowledge deficit related to cefixime.

Planning and Implementation
Preparation and Administration
- Obtain specimen for culture and sensitivity tests before first dose. Therapy may begin pending test results.
- Before giving first dose, ask patient about any reaction to previous cephalosporin or penicillin therapy.
- Expect reduced dosage to avoid

drug accumulation if creatinine clearance is less than 60 ml/minute.
• ***P.O. use:*** To reconstitute, add required amount of water to powder in two portions. Shake well after each addition. Keep container tightly closed and shake it well before using. The reconstituted drug does not require refrigeration and is stable for 14 days.

Monitoring
• Monitor effectiveness by regularly assessing for improvement of infection.
• Monitor for signs of an allergic or anaphylactic reaction.
• During prolonged or high-dose therapy, monitor for superinfection, especially in high-risk patients.
• Monitor hydration status if adverse GI reactions occur.

Supportive Care
• Obtain an order for an antiemetic or antidiarrheal agent as needed.
• Notify doctor if skin rash develops.
• When testing urine glucose, use only glucose enzymatic tests (Clinistix or Tes-Tape), because copper sulfate tests (Clinitest) may have false-positive results.

Patient Teaching
• Tell the patient to take medication exactly as prescribed, even after he feels better, and to take the entire amount prescribed.
• Inform the patient using oral suspension to shake it well before using, and to store the mixture in a tightly closed container. Tell the patient suspension is stable for 14 days at room temperature without significant loss of potency.
• Instruct patient to notify doctor if skin rash develops.
• Teach diabetic patients to test urine for glucose with a glucose enzymatic test such as Clinistix or Tes-Tape because copper sulfate tests (Clinitest) may yield false-positive results.

Evaluation

In patients receiving cefixime, appropriate evaluation statements may include:
• Patient is free of infection.
• Patient maintains adequate hydration throughout cefixime therapy.
• Patient and family state an understanding of cefixime therapy.

cefmetazole sodium
(sef met´ a zole)
Zefazone

• *Classification:* antibiotic (second-generation cephalosporin)
• *Pregnancy Risk Category:* B

HOW SUPPLIED
Injection: 1 g, 2 g

ACTION
Mechanism: Inhibits cell wall synthesis during bacterial replication, promoting osmotic instability. Usually bactericidal.
Absorption: Not absorbed from the GI tract and must be given parenterally. Peak serum levels are lower after I.M. injection than after I.V. infusion.
Distribution: Widely distributed in most body tissues and fluids, including the gallbladder, liver, kidneys, bone, sputum, bile, and pleural and synovial fluids. CSF penetration is poor. Cefmetazole is 65% protein-bound.
Metabolism: About 15% of a dose is metabolized, probably in the liver.
Excretion: Primarily excreted in the urine by renal tubular secretion and glomerular filtration. Half-life: Approximately 1.5 hours in patients with normal renal function; patients with renal dysfunction require dosage adjustment.
Onset, peak, duration: Peak serum

levels occur 30 to 45 minutes after an I.M. dose.

INDICATIONS & DOSAGE

Lower respiratory tract infections caused by Streptococcus pneumoniae, Staphylococcus aureus *(penicillinase- and nonpenicillinase-producing strains),* Escherichia coli, *and* Hemophilus influenzae *(nonpenicillinase-producing strains) intra-abdominal infections caused by* E. coli*or* Bacteroides fragilis; *skin and skin-structure infections caused by* S. aureus *(penicillinase- and nonpenicillinase-producing strains),* Staphylococcus epidermidis, Streptococcus pyogenes, Streptococcus agalactiae, E. coli, Proteus mirabilis, Klebsiella pneumoniae, *and* B. fragilis–
Adults: 2 g I.V. q 6 to 12 hours for 5 to 14 days.
Urinary tract infections caused by E. coli–
Adults: 2 g I.V. q 12 hours.
Prophylaxis in patients undergoing vaginal hysterectomy–
Adults: 2 g I.V. 30 to 90 minutes before surgery as a single dose; or 1 g I.V. 30 to 90 minutes before surgery, repeated in 8 and 16 hours.
Prophylaxis in patients undergoing abdominal hysterectomy–
Adults: 1 g I.V. 30 to 90 minutes before surgery, repeated in 8 and 16 hours.
Prophylaxis in patients undergoing cesarean section–
Adults: 2 g I.V. as a single dose after clamping cord; or 1 g I.V. after clamping cord, repeated in 8 and 16 hours.
Prophylaxis in patients undergoing colorectal surgery–
Adults: 2 g I.V. as a single dose 30 to 90 minutes before surgery. Some clinicians follow with additional 2-g doses in 8 and 16 hours.
Prophylaxis in patients undergoing cholecystectomy (high risk)–
Adults: 1 g I.V. 30 to 90 minutes before surgery, repeated in 8 and 16 hours.

CONTRAINDICATIONS & PRECAUTIONS

Contraindicated in patients with hypersensitivity to any cephalosporin. Use cautiously in patients with penicillin allergy.

ADVERSE REACTIONS

Common reactions are in italics; life-threatening reactions are in bold italics.
CNS: headache.
CV: ***shock,*** hypotension.
EENT: epistaxis.
GI: nausea, vomiting, *diarrhea,* epigastric pain, ***pseudomembranous colitis.***
GU: vaginitis.
Respiratory: pleural effusion, dyspnea, respiratory distress.
Skin: rash, pruritus, generalized erythema.
Local: pain at injection site, phlebitis.
Other: fever, bacterial or fungal superinfection, ***hypersensitivity,*** altered color perception.

INTERACTIONS

Alcohol: disulfiram-like reaction. Alcohol should be avoided within 24 hours of administration.
Aminoglycosides: increased risk of nephrotoxicity.

EFFECTS ON DIAGNOSTIC TESTS

Coombs' test: positive results.
Liver function tests: elevated results.
Urine glucose tests with copper sulfate (Benedict's reagent or Clinitest): false-positive results; use glucose enzymatic tests (Clinistix or Tes-Tape) instead.

NURSING CONSIDERATIONS

Besides those related universally to drug therapy (see "How to use this

book"), consider the following specific recommendations:

Assessment

• Obtain baseline assessment of infection before therapy.
• Be alert for adverse reactions or drug interactions during therapy.
• Evaluate the patient's and family's knowledge about cefmetazole.

Nursing Diagnoses

• High risk for injury related to ineffectiveness of cefmetazole to eradicate the infection.
• High risk for fluid volume deficit related to adverse GI reactions to cefmetazole.
• Knowledge deficit related to cefmetazole.

Planning and Implementation

Preparation and Administration

• Obtain specimen for culture and sensitivity tests before first dose. Therapy may begin pending test results.
• Before giving first dose, ask patient about any reaction to previous cephalosporin or penicillin therapy.
• ***I.V. use:*** Reconstitute with bacteriostatic water for injection, sterile water for injection, or 0.9% sodium chloride for injection. After reconstitution, the drug may be further diluted to concentrations ranging from 1 to 20 mg/ml by adding it to 0.9% sodium chloride injection, 5% dextrose in water, or lactated Ringer's injection. Reconstituted or dilute solutions are stable for 24 hours at room temperature; for 1 week if refrigerated.

Monitoring

• Monitor effectiveness by regularly assessing for improvement of infection.
• Monitor for signs of an allergic or anaphylactic reaction.
• During prolonged or high-dose therapy, monitor for superinfection, especially in high-risk patients.
• Monitor hydration status if adverse GI reactions occur.
• Monitor prothrombin time because drug's chemical structure has been associated with bleeding disorders.

Supportive Care

• Obtain an order for an antiemetic or antidiarrheal agent as needed.
• If bleeding occurs, be prepared to administer vitamin K as prescribed.
• When testing urine glucose, use only glucose enzymatic tests (Clinistix or Tes-Tape), because copper sulfate tests (Clinitest) may have false-positive results.

Patient Teaching

• Teach diabetic patients to test urine for glucose with a glucose enzymatic test such as Clinistix or Tes-Tape because copper sulfate tests (Clinitest) may yield false-positive results.

Evaluation

In patients receiving cefmetazole, appropriate evaluation statements may include:
• Patient is free of infection.
• Patient maintains adequate hydration throughout cefmetazole therapy.
• Patient and family state an understanding of cefmetazole therapy.

cefonicid sodium

(se fon´ i sid)
Monocid

• *Classification:* antibiotic (second-generation cephalosporin)
• *Pregnancy Risk Category:* B

HOW SUPPLIED

Injection: 500 mg, 1 g
Infusion: 1 g/100 ml
Pharmacy bulk package: 10 g

ACTION

Mechanism: Inhibits cell wall synthesis during bacterial replication, promoting osmotic instability. Usually bactericidal.
Absorption: Not absorbed from the GI tract and must be given parenter-

ally. Peak serum levels are lower after I.M. injection than after I.V. infusion.
Distribution: Widely distributed into most body tissues and fluids, including the gallbladder, liver, kidneys, bone, sputum, bile, and pleural and synovial fluids; CSF penetration is poor. 90% to 98% protein-bound, and crosses the placenta.
Metabolism: Not metabolized.
Excretion: Primarily excreted in urine by renal tubular secretion and glomerular filtration; small amounts are excreted in breast milk. Half-life: About 3½ to 6 hours in patients with normal renal function; up to 100 hours in patients with severe renal disease.
Onset, peak, duration: Peak serum levels occur 1 to 2 hours after an I.M. dose.

INDICATIONS & DOSAGE

Treatment of serious infections of the lower respiratory and urinary tract; skin and skin structure infections; septicemia; and bone and joint infections. Susceptible microorganisms include Streptococcus pneumoniae, Klebsiella pneumoniae, Escherichia coli, Hemophilus influenzae, Proteus mirabilis, Staphyloccus aureus *and* epidermidis, *and* Streptococcus pyogenes–
Adults: usual dosage is 1 g I.V. or I.M. q 24 hours. In life-threatening infections, 2 g q 24 hours.

Total daily dosage is same for I.M. or I.V. administration and depends on susceptibility of organism and severity of infection. In patients with impaired renal function, doses or frequency of administration must be modified according to degree of renal impairment, severity of infection, and susceptibility of organism. Should be injected deep I.M. into a large muscle mass, such as gluteus or lateral aspect of thigh.

CONTRAINDICATIONS & PRECAUTIONS

Contraindicated in patients with hypersensitivity to any cephalosporin. Use cautiously in patients with penicillin allergy, who usually are more susceptible to such reactions.

ADVERSE REACTIONS

Common reactions are in italics; life-threatening reactions are in bold italics.
Blood: transient neutropenia, leukopenia, eosinophilia, anemia.
CNS: dizziness, headache, malaise, paresthesias.
GI: ***pseudomembranous colitis,*** nausea, anorexia, vomiting, diarrhea, glossitis, dyspepsia, abdominal cramps, anal pruritus, tenesmus, oral candidiasis (thrush).
GU: genital pruritus and moniliasis, vaginitis.
Skin: *maculopapular and erythematous rashes, urticaria.*
Local: *at injection site–pain, induration, sterile abscesses, tissue sloughing; phlebitis and thrombophlebitis with I.V. injection.*
Other: ***hypersensitivity,*** dyspnea.

INTERACTIONS

Probenecid: may inhibit excretion and increase blood levels of cefonicid.

EFFECTS ON DIAGNOSTIC TESTS

Serum or urine creatinine: false elevations in tests using Jaffé's reaction.
Urine glucose tests with copper sulfate (Benedict's reagent or Clinitest): false-positive results; use glucose enzymatic tests (Clinistix or Tes-Tape) instead.

NURSING CONSIDERATIONS

Besides those related universally to drug therapy (see "How to use this book"), consider the following specific recommendations:

Assessment
• Obtain a baseline assessment of infection before therapy.
• Be alert for adverse reactions or drug interactions during therapy.
• Evaluate the patient's and family's knowledge about cefonicid.

Nursing Diagnoses
• High risk for injury related to ineffectiveness of cefonicid to eradicate the infection.
• High risk for fluid volume deficit related to adverse GI reactions to cefonicid.
• Knowledge deficit related to cefonicid.

Planning and Implementation
Preparation and Administration
• Obtain specimen for culture and sensitivity tests before first dose. Therapy may begin pending test results.
• Before giving first dose, ask patient about any reaction to previous cephalosporin or penicillin therapy.
• ***I.M. use:*** Administer deep into a large muscle mass, such as gluteus or lateral aspect of thigh. Reconstitute drug following manufacturer's instructions. When administering 2-g I.M. doses once daily, one-half the dose should be administered in different large muscle masses.
• ***I.V. use:*** Reconstitute 500-mg vial with 2 ml of sterile water for injection (yields a concentration of 220 mg/ml) and 1-g vial with 2.5 ml of sterile water for injection (yields a concentration of 325 mg/ml). Shake well. Reconstitute piggyback vials with 50 to 100 ml of sterile water for injection, bacteriostatic water for injection, or 0.9% sodium chloride.
• After reconstitution, drug is stable for 24 hours at room temperature for 72 hours under refrigeration.

Monitoring
• Monitor effectiveness by regularly assessing for improvement of infection.
• Monitor for signs of an allergic or anaphylactic reaction.
• During prolonged or high-dose therapy, monitor for superinfection, especially in high-risk patients.
• Monitor hydration status if adverse GI reactions occur.

Supportive Care
• Obtain an order for an antiemetic or antidiarrheal agent as needed.

Patient Teaching
• Instruct the patient and family about cefonicid, including the dose, frequency, action, and adverse reactions.

Evaluation
In patients receiving cefonicid, appropriate evaluation statements may include:
• Patient is free of infection.
• Patient maintains adequate hydration throughout cefonicid therapy.
• Patient and family state an understanding of cefonicid therapy.

cefoperazone sodium
(sef oh per´ a zone)
Cefobid

• *Classification:* antibiotic (third-generation cephalosporin)
• *Pregnancy Risk Category:* B

HOW SUPPLIED
Infusion: 1 g, 2 g piggyback
Parenteral: 1 g, 2 g

ACTION
Mechanism: Inhibits cell wall synthesis during bacterial replication, promoting osmotic instability. Usually bactericidal.
Absorption: Not absorbed from the GI tract and must be given parenterally. Peak serum levels are lower after an I.M. dose than after an I.V. infusion.
Distribution: Widely distributed into most body tissues and fluids, includ-

†Available in Canada only. ‡Available in Australia only. ◊Available OTC.

ing the gallbladder, liver, kidneys, bone, sputum, bile, and pleural and synovial fluids; also crosses the placenta. CSF penetration is achieved in patients with inflamed meninges. Protein binding is dose-dependent and decreases as serum levels rise; average is 82% to 93%.
Metabolism: Not substantially metabolized.
Excretion: Primarily excreted in bile; some is excreted in urine by renal tubular secretion and glomerular filtration; small amounts are excreted in breast milk. Half-life: About 1½ to 2½ hours in patients with normal hepatorenal function; about 3½ to 7 hours in biliary obstruction or cirrhosis.
Onset, peak, duration: Peak serum levels occur 1 to 2 hours after I.M. dose.

INDICATIONS & DOSAGE

Treatment of serious infections of the respiratory tract; intra-abdominal, gynecologic, and skin infections; bacteremia, septicemia. Susceptible microorganisms include Streptococcus pneumoniae *and* pyogenes; Staphylococcus aureus *(penicillinase- and* nonpenicillinase-producing) *and* epidermidis; *enterococcus;* Escherichia coli; Klebsiella; Hemophilus influenzae; Enterobacter; Citrobacter; Proteus; *some* Pseudomonas, *including* P. aeruginosa; *and* Bacteroides fragilis–
Adults: Usual dosage is 1 to 2 g q 12 hours I.M. or I.V. In severe infections, or infections caused by less sensitive organisms, the total daily dosage or frequency may be increased up to 16 g/day in certain situations.

No dosage adjustment is usually necessary in patients with renal impairment. However, doses of 4 g/day should be given very cautiously in patients with hepatic disease. Should be injected deep I.M. into a large muscle mass, such as gluteus or lateral aspect of the thigh.

CONTRAINDICATIONS & PRECAUTIONS

Contraindicated in patients with hypersensitivity to any cephalosporin. Use with caution in patients with penicillin allergy, who usually are more susceptible to such reactions; in patients with coagulopathy; and in elderly, debilitated, or malnourished patients, who are at greater risk for bleeding complications.

ADVERSE REACTIONS

Common reactions are in italics; life-threatening reactions are in bold italics.
Blood: transient neutropenia, eosinophilia, hemolytic anemia, *hypoprothrombinemia, bleeding.*
CNS: headache, malaise, paresthesias, dizziness.
GI: ***pseudomembranous colitis,*** nausea, anorexia, vomiting, *diarrhea,* glossitis, dyspepsia, abdominal cramps, tenesmus, anal pruritus, oral candidiasis (thrush).
Hepatic: mildly elevated liver enzymes.
GU: genital pruritus and moniliasis.
Skin: *maculopapular and erythematous rashes, urticaria.*
Local: *at injection site–pain, induration, sterile abscesses, temperature elevation, tissue sloughing; phlebitis and thrombophlebitis with I.V. injection.*
Other: ***hypersensitivity,*** dyspnea.

INTERACTIONS

Ethyl alcohol: may cause a disulfiram-like reaction. Warn patients not to drink alcohol for several days after discontinuing cefoperazone.
Oral anticoagulants, aspirin: increased risk of bleeding.
Probenecid: may inhibit excretion and increase blood levels of cefoperazone.

EFFECTS ON DIAGNOSTIC TESTS

Coombs' test: positive results.
Liver function tests: elevated results.
Prothrombin time: prolonged.
Urine glucose tests with copper sulfate (Benedict's reagent or Clinitest): false-positive results; use glucose enzymatic tests (Clinistix or Tes-Tape) instead.

NURSING CONSIDERATIONS

Besides those related universally to drug therapy (see "How to use this book"), consider the following specific recommendations:

Assessment

• Obtain a baseline assessment of infection before therapy.
• Be alert for adverse reactions or drug interactions during therapy.
• Evaluate the patient's and family's knowledge about cefoperazone.

Nursing Diagnoses

• High risk for injury related to ineffectiveness of cefoperazone to eradicate the infection.
• High risk for fluid volume deficit related to adverse GI reactions to cefoperazone.
• Knowledge deficit related to cefoperazone.

Planning and Implementation

Preparation and Administration

• Obtain specimen for culture and sensitivity tests before first dose. Therapy may begin pending test results.
• Before giving first dose, ask patient about any reaction to previous cephalosporin or penicillin therapy.
• ***I.M. use:*** Reconstitute according to manufacturer's instructions. Administer deep into a large muscle mass, such as gluteus or lateral aspect of thigh.
• ***I.V. use:*** Reconstitute 1-g vial with 5 ml of compatible diluent. Shake vial vigorously until drug dissolves. Let vial stand to allow foam to dissipate before drawing up. After reconstitution, dilute further by adding 20 to 40 ml of compatible diluent for intermittent infusion and enough diluent to make a solution of 2 to 25 mg/ml for a continuous infusion.
• After reconstitution, drug is stable for 24 hours at room temperature; for 5 days under refrigeration.

Monitoring

• Monitor effectiveness by regularly assessing for improvement of infection.
• Monitor for signs of an allergic or anaphylactic reaction.
• During prolonged or high-dose therapy, monitor for superinfection, especially in high-risk patients.
• Monitor hydration status if adverse GI reactions occur.
• Monitor prothrombin time regularly as ordered because drug's chemical structure has been associated with bleeding disorders.

Supportive Care

• Obtain an order for an antiemetic or antidiarrheal agent as needed.
• When testing urine glucose, use only glucose enzymatic tests (Clinistix or Tes-Tape), because copper sulfate tests (Clinitest) may have false-positive results.
• If bleeding occurs, be prepared to administer vitamin K as prescribed.

Patient Teaching

• Teach diabetic patients to test urine for glucose with a glucose enzymatic test such as Clinistix or Tes-Tape because copper sulfate tests (Clinitest) may yield false-positive results.

Evaluation

In patients receiving cefoperazone, appropriate evaluation statements may include:
• Patient is free of infection.
• Patient maintains adequate hydration throughout cefoperazone therapy.
• Patient and family state an understanding of cefoperazone therapy.

ceforanide

(se for´ a nide)
Precef

- *Classification:* antibiotic (second-generation cephalosporin)
- *Pregnancy Risk Category:* B

HOW SUPPLIED

Injection: 500 mg, 1 g
Infusion: 500 mg, 1 g piggyback

ACTION

Mechanism: Inhibits cell wall synthesis during bacterial replication, promoting osmotic instability. Usually bactericidal.
Absorption: Poorly absorbed from the GI tract and must be given parenterally. Peak serum levels are lower after I.M. injection than after I.V. administration.
Distribution: Widely distributed into most body tissues and fluids, including the gallbladder, liver, kidneys, bone, skeletal muscle, uterus, jejunum, myocardium, and bile; CSF penetration is poor. It is unknown if ceforanide crosses the placenta. Ceforanide is about 80% protein-bound.
Metabolism: Not metabolized.
Excretion: Primarily excreted in urine by renal tubular excretion and glomerular filtration. Half-life: 2½ to 3½ hours in patients with normal renal function; 5½ to 25 hours in patients with end-stage renal disease.
Onset, peak, duration: Peak serum levels occur 1 hour after an I.M. dose.

INDICATIONS & DOSAGE

Treatment of serious infections of the lower respiratory and urinary tract, skin and skin structure infections, endocarditis, septicemia, and bone and joint infections. Susceptible microorganisms include Streptococcus pneumoniae *and* pyogenes, Klebsiella pneumoniae, Escherichia coli, Hemophilus influenzae, Proteus mirabilis, *and* Staphylococcus aureus *and* epidermidis–
Adults: 0.5 to 1 g I.V. or I.M. q 12 hours.
Children: 20 to 40 mg/kg/day in equally divided doses q 12 hours.
Prophylaxis of surgical infections–
Adults: 0.5 to 1 g I.M. or I.V. 1 hour prior to surgery.

Total daily dosage is same for I.M. or I.V. administration and depends on susceptibility of organism and severity of infection. In patients with impaired renal function, doses or frequency of administration must be modified according to degree of renal impairment, severity of infection, and susceptibility of organism. Should be injected deep I.M. into a large muscle mass, such as gluteus or lateral aspect of thigh.

CONTRAINDICATIONS & PRECAUTIONS

Contraindicated in patients with hypersensitivity to any cephalosporin. Use cautiously in patients with penicillin allergy, who usually are more susceptible to such reactions.

ADVERSE REACTIONS

Common reactions are in italics; life-threatening reactions are in bold italics.
Blood: transient neutropenia, leukopenia, eosinophilia, thrombocytopenia.
CNS: confusion, headache, lethargy.
GI: ***pseudomembranous colitis,*** nausea, anorexia, vomiting, diarrhea, glossitis, dyspepsia, abdominal cramps, oral candidiasis (thrush).
GU: genital pruritus and moniliasis, vaginitis.
Hepatic: transient elevation in liver enzymes.
Skin: *maculopapular and erythematous rashes, urticaria.*
Local: *at injection site–pain, induration, sterile abscesses, tissue slough-*

ing; phlebitis and thrombophlebitis with I.V. injection.
Other: ***hypersensitivity***, dyspnea.

INTERACTIONS

Aminoglycosides, diuretics: may increase the risk of nephrotoxicity. Use together cautiously.

EFFECTS ON DIAGNOSTIC TESTS

Coombs' test: positive results
Liver function tests: elevated results.
Serum or urine creatinine: false elevations in tests using Jaffé's reaction.
Urine glucose tests with copper sulfate (Benedict's reagent or Clinitest): false-positive results; use glucose enzymatic tests (Clinistix or Tes-Tape) instead.

NURSING CONSIDERATIONS

Besides those related universally to drug therapy (see "How to use this book"), consider the following specific recommendations:

Assessment

- Obtain a baseline assessment of infection before therapy.
- Be alert for adverse reactions and drug interactions throughout therapy.
- Evaluate the patient's and family's knowledge about ceforanide therapy.

Nursing Diagnoses

- High risk for injury related to ineffectiveness of ceforanide to eradicate the infection.
- High risk for fluid volume deficit related to adverse GI reactions to ceforanide.
- Knowledge deficit related to ceforanide.

Planning and Implementation

Preparation and Administration

- Obtain specimen for culture and sensitivity tests before first dose. Therapy may begin pending test results.
- Before giving first dose, ask patient about any reaction to previous cephalosporin or penicillin therapy.
- ***I.M. use:*** Reconstitute according to manufacturer's instructions. Administer deep into a large muscle mass, such as gluteus or lateral aspect of thigh.
- ***I.V. use:*** Dilute contents of 500-mg or 1-g vial or piggyback unit with 5 to 10 ml, respectively, of compatible solution; shake container immediately. Upon reconstitution, ceforanide solution may appear cloudy. Let it stand briefly to allow solution to deaerate and clarify.
- After reconstitution, drug is stable for 48 hours at room temperature, for 14 days under refrigeration, and for 90 days when frozen.

Monitoring

- Monitor effectiveness by regularly assessing for improvement of infection.
- Monitor for signs of an allergic or anaphylactic reaction.
- During prolonged or high-dose therapy, monitor for superinfection, especially in high-risk patients.
- Monitor hydration status if adverse GI reactions occur.

Supportive Care

- Obtain an order for an antiemetic or antidiarrheal agent as needed.

Patient Teaching

- Instruct the patient and family about ceforanide, including the dose, frequency, action, and adverse reactions.

Evaluation

In patients receiving ceforanide, appropriate evaluation statements may include:

- Patient is free of infection.
- Patient maintains adequate hydration throughout ceforanide therapy.
- Patient and family state an understanding of ceforanide therapy.

cefotaxime sodium

(sef oh taks´ eem)
Claforan

• *Classification:* antibiotic (third-generation cephalosporin)
• *Pregnancy Risk Category:* B

HOW SUPPLIED

Injection: 500 mg, 1 g, 2 g
Infusion: 1 g, 2 g
Pharmacy bulk package: 10-g vial

ACTION

Mechanism: Inhibits cell wall synthesis during bacterial replication, promoting osmotic instability. Usually bactericidal.
Absorption: Not absorbed from the GI tract and must be given parenterally. Peak serum levels are lower after I.M. injection as compared to I.V. administration.
Distribution: Widely distributed into most body tissues and fluids, including the gallbladder, liver, kidneys, bone, sputum, bile, pleural and synovial fluids. Unlike most other cephalosporins, CSF penetration is good; drug also crosses the placenta. It is 13% to 38% protein-bound.
Metabolism: Partially metabolized in the liver to an active metabolite, desacetylcefotaxime.
Excretion: Drug and its metabolite are excreted primarily in urine by renal tubular secretion; some may be excreted in breast milk; about 25% is excreted in urine as the active metabolite. Half-life: In normal adults, about 1 to 1½ hours for cefotaxime and about 1½ to 2 hours for desacetylcefotaxime; in severe renal impairment, 11½ hours for cefotaxime and 56 hours for the metabolite.
Onset, peak, duration: Peak levels occur 30 minutes after an I.M. injection.

INDICATIONS & DOSAGE

Treatment of serious infections of the lower respiratory and urinary tracts, CNS infections, gynecologic infections, bacteremia, septicemia, and skin infections. Among susceptible microorganisms are streptococci, including Streptococcus pneumoniae *and* pyogenes; Staphylococcus aureus *(penicillinase- and nonpenicillinase-producing) and* epidermidis; Escherichia coli; Klebsiella; Hemophilus influenzae; Enterobacter; Proteus; *and* Peptostreptococcus–
Adults: usual dose is 1 g I.V. or I.M. q 6 to 8 hours. Up to 12 g daily can be administered in life-threatening infections.

Total daily dosage is same for I.M. or I.V. administration and depends on susceptibility of organism and severity of infection. In patients with impaired renal function, doses or frequency of administration must be modified according to degree of renal impairment, severity of infection, and susceptibility of organism. Should be injected deep I.M. into a large muscle mass, such as gluteus or lateral aspect of thigh.
Children 1 month to 12 years: 50 to 180 mg/kg/day I.M. or I.V. in 4 to 6 divided doses.
Neonates to 1 week: 50 mg/kg I.V. q 12 hours.
Neonates 1 to 4 weeks: 50 mg/kg I.V. q 8 hours.

CONTRAINDICATIONS & PRECAUTIONS

Contraindicated in patients with hypersensitivity to any cephalosporin. Use cautiously in patients with penicillin allergy, who usually are more susceptible to such reactions.

ADVERSE REACTIONS

Common reactions are in italics; life-threatening reactions are in bold italics.
Blood: transient neutropenia, eosinophilia, hemolytic anemia.

CNS: headache, malaise, paresthesias, dizziness.
GI: ***pseudomembranous colitis,*** nausea, anorexia, vomiting, *diarrhea,* glossitis, dyspepsia, abdominal cramps, tenesmus, anal pruritus, oral candidiasis (thrush).
GU: genital pruritus and moniliasis.
Skin: *maculopapular and erythematous rashes, urticaria.*
Local: *at injection site—pain, induration, sterile abscesses, temperature elevation, tissue sloughing; phlebitis and thrombophlebitis with I.V. injection.*
Other: ***hypersensitivity,*** dyspnea, elevated temperature.

INTERACTIONS

Aminoglycosides: may increase the risk of nephrotoxicity. Use together cautiously.

EFFECTS ON DIAGNOSTIC TESTS

Coombs' test: positive results.
Liver function tests: elevated results.
Serum or urine creatinine: false elevations in tests using Jaffé's reaction.
Urine glucose tests with copper sulfate (Benedict's reagent or Clinitest): false-positive results; use glucose enzymatic tests (Clinistix or Tes-Tape) instead.

NURSING CONSIDERATIONS

Besides those related universally to drug therapy (see "How to use this book"), consider the following specific recommendations:

Assessment
- Obtain a baseline assessment of infection before therapy.
- Be alert for adverse reactions or drug interactions during therapy.
- Evaluate the patient's and family's knowledge about cefotaxime.

Nursing Diagnoses
- High risk for injury related to ineffectiveness of cefotaxime to eradicate the infection.
- High risk for fluid volume deficit related to adverse GI reactions to cefotaxime.
- Knowledge deficit related to cefotaxime.

Planning and Implementation
Preparation and Administration
- Obtain specimen for culture and sensitivity tests before first dose. Therapy may begin pending test results.
- Before giving first dose, ask patient about any reaction to previous cephalosporin or penicillin therapy.
- ***I.M. use:*** Reconstitute according to manufacturer's instructions. Administer deep into a large muscle mass, such as gluteus or lateral aspect of thigh.
- ***I.V. use:*** Reconstitute vial with 10 ml of sterile water for injection. Shake vial vigorously until drug dissolves. I.V. infusion bottles can be further diluted in 50 to 100 ml of dextrose 5% in water or 0.9% sodium chloride. Reconstituted drug can be diluted in 500 to 1,000 ml of compatible solution for continuous infusion.
- After reconstitution, drug remains stable for 24 hours at room temperature; for 10 days under refrigeration.

Monitoring
- Monitor effectiveness by regularly assessing for improvement of infection.
- Monitor for signs of an allergic or anaphylactic reaction.
- During prolonged or high-dose therapy, monitor for superinfection, especially in high-risk patients.
- Monitor hydration status if adverse GI reactions occur.

Supportive Care
- Obtain an order for an antiemetic or antidiarrheal agent as needed.
- When testing urine glucose, use only glucose enzymatic tests (Clinistix or Tes-Tape), because copper sulfate tests (Clinitest) may have false-positive results.

Patient Teaching
• Teach diabetic patients to test urine for glucose with a glucose enzymatic test such as Clinistix or Tes-Tape because copper sulfate tests (Clinitest) may yield false-positive results.

Evaluation
In patients receiving cefotaxime, appropriate evaluation statements may include:
• Patient is free of infection.
• Patient maintains adequate hydration throughout cefotaxime therapy.
• Patient and family state an understanding of cefotaxime therapy.

cefotetan disodium
(sef′ oh tee tan)
Cefotan

• *Classification:* antibiotic (second-generation cephalosporin)
• *Pregnancy Risk Category:* B

HOW SUPPLIED
Injection: 1 g, 2 g
Infusion: 1 g, 2 g piggyback

ACTION
Mechanism: Inhibits cell wall synthesis during bacterial replication, promoting osmotic instability. Usually bactericidal.
Absorption: Poorly absorbed from the GI tract and must be given parenterally. Peak serum levels are lower after I.M. injection than after I.V. administration.
Distribution: Widely distributed into most body tissues and fluids, including the gallbladder, liver, kidneys, bone, sputum, bile and pleural and synovial fluids; CSF penetration is poor. Biliary concentrations can be up to 20 times higher than serum concentrations in patients with good gallbladder function. Cefotetan crosses the placenta; it is 75% to 90% protein-bound.
Metabolism: Not metabolized.
Excretion: Primarily excreted in urine by glomerular filtration and some renal tubular secretion. Small amounts are excreted in breast milk. Half-life: About 3 to 9½ hours in patients with normal renal function.
Onset, peak, duration: Peak serum levels occur 1½ to 3 hours after I.M. dose.

INDICATIONS & DOSAGE
Treatment of serious infections of the urinary and lower respiratory tracts, and gynecologic, skin and skin structure, intra-abdominal, and bone and joint infections. Among susceptible microorganisms are streptococci, Staphylococcus aureus *(penicillinase- and nonpenicillinase-producing) and* epidermidis, Escherichia coli, Klebsiella, Enterobacter, Proteus, Hemophilus influenzae, Neisseria gonorrhoeae, *and* Bacteroides, *including* B. fragilis.
Adults: 1 to 2 g I.V. or I.M. q 12 hours for 5 to 10 days. Up to 6 g daily in life-threatening infections.

Total daily dosage is same for I.M. or I.V. administration and depends on susceptibility of organism and severity of infection. In patients with impaired renal function, doses or frequency of administration must be modified according to degree of renal impairment, severity of infection, and susceptibility of organism. Should be injected deep I.M. into a large muscle mass, such as gluteus or lateral aspect of thigh.

CONTRAINDICATIONS & PRECAUTIONS
Contraindicated in patients with hypersensitivity to any cephalosporin. Use with caution in patients with penicillin allergy, who usually are more susceptible to such reactions; in patients with coagulopathy; and in elderly, debilitated, or malnourished patients, who are at greater risk of bleeding complications.

ADVERSE REACTIONS

Common reactions are in italics; life-threatening reactions are in bold italics.
Blood: transient neutropenia, eosinophilia, hemolytic anemia, hypoprothrombinemia, bleeding.
CNS: headache, malaise, paresthesias, dizziness.
GI: ***pseudomembranous colitis,*** nausea, anorexia, vomiting, *diarrhea,* glossitis, dyspepsia, abdominal cramps, tenesmus, anal pruritus.
GU: genital pruritus and moniliasis.
Skin: *maculopapular and erythematous rashes, urticaria.*
Local: *at injection site–pain, induration, sterile abscesses, tissue sloughing; phlebitis and thrombophlebitis with I.V. injection.*
Other: ***hypersensitivity,*** dyspnea, elevated temperature.

INTERACTIONS

Aminoglycosides: may increase the risk of nephrotoxicity. Monitor renal function.
Ethyl alcohol: may cause a disulfiram-like reaction. Warn patients not to drink alcohol for several days after discontinuing cefotetan.
Oral anticoagulants, aspirin: increased risk of bleeding.

EFFECTS ON DIAGNOSTIC TESTS

Coombs' test: positive results.
Liver function tests: elevated results.
Prothrombin time: prolonged.
Serum or urine creatinine: false elevations in tests using Jaffé's reaction.
Urine glucose tests with copper sulfate (Benedict's reagent or Clinitest): false-positive results; use glucose enzymatic tests (Clinistix or Tes-Tape) instead.

NURSING CONSIDERATIONS

Besides those related universally to drug therapy (see "How to use this book"), consider the following specific recommendations:

Assessment
- Obtain a baseline assessment of infection before therapy.
- Be alert for adverse reactions and drug interactions throughout therapy.
- Evaluate the patient's and family's knowledge about cefotetan therapy.

Nursing Diagnoses
- High risk for injury related to ineffectiveness of cefotetan to eradicate the infection.
- High risk for fluid volume deficit related to adverse GI reactions to cefotetan.
- Knowledge deficit related to cefotetan.

Planning and Implementation
Preparation and Administration
- Obtain specimen for culture and sensitivity tests before first dose. Therapy may begin pending test results.
- Before giving first dose, ask patient about any reaction to previous cephalosporin or penicillin therapy.
- ***I.M. use:*** Reconstitute with sterile water or bacteriostatic water for injection, normal saline, or 0.5% or 1% lidocaine hydrochloride. Shake to dissolve and let solution stand until clear. Administer deep into a large muscle mass, such as gluteus or lateral aspect of thigh.
- ***I.V. use:*** Reconstitute with sterile water for injection. Then, may be mixed with 50 to 100 ml of dextrose 5% in water or 0.9% sodium chloride solution. After reconstitution, drug remains stable for 48 hours at room temperature; for 96 hours under refrigeration.

Monitoring
- Monitor effectiveness by regularly assessing for improvement of infection.
- Monitor for signs of an allergic or anaphylactic reaction.
- During prolonged or high-dose therapy, monitor for superinfection, especially in high-risk patients.

• Monitor hydration status if adverse GI reactions occur.

Supportive Care

• Obtain an order for an antiemetic or antidiarrheal agent as needed.

Patient Teaching

• Instruct the patient and family about cefotetan, including the dose, frequency, action, and adverse reactions.

Evaluation

In patients receiving cefotetan, appropriate evaluation statements may include:

• Patient is free of infection.
• Patient maintains adequate hydration throughout cefotetan therapy.
• Patient and family state an understanding of cefotetan therapy.

cefoxitin sodium

(se fox´ i tin)

Mefoxin

• *Classification:* antibiotic (second-generation cephalosporin)
• *Pregnancy Risk Category:* B

HOW SUPPLIED

Injection: 1 g, 2 g
Infusion: 1 g, 2 g in 50-ml or 100-ml container
Pharmacy bulk package: 10 g

ACTION

Mechanism: Inhibits cell wall synthesis during bacterial replication, promoting osmotic instability. Usually bactericidal.

Absorption: Not absorbed from the GI tract and must be given parenterally. Peak levels after I.M. injection are lower than after I.V. administration.

Distribution: Widely distributed into most body tissues and fluids, including the gallbladder, liver, kidneys, bone, sputum, bile, and pleural and synovial fluids; CSF penetration is poor. Cefoxitin crosses the placenta; it is 50% to 80% protein-bound.

Metabolism: About 2% is metabolized.

Excretion: Primarily excreted in urine by renal tubular secretion and glomerular filtration; small amounts are excreted in breast milk. Half-life: About 30 minutes to 1 hour in patients with normal renal function; 6½ to 21½ hours in patients with severe renal dysfunction.

Onset, peak, duration: Peak serum levels occur 20 to 30 minutes after an I.M. dose.

INDICATIONS & DOSAGE

Treatment of serious infection of respiratory and genitourinary tracts, skin and soft-tissue infections, bone and joint infections, bloodstream and intra-abdominal infections caused by Escherichia coli *and other coliform bacteria,* Staphylococcus aureus *(penicillinase- and nonpenicillinase-producing) and* epidermidis, *streptococci,* Klebsiella, Hemophilus influenzae, *and* Bacteroides, *including* B. fragilis–

Adults: 1 to 2 g q 6 to 8 hours for uncomplicated forms of infection. Up to 12 g daily in life-threatening infections.

Children: 80 to 160 mg/kg daily given in 4 to 6 equally divided doses.

Total daily dosage is same for I.M. or I.V. administration and depends on susceptibility of organism and severity of infection. In patients with impaired renal function, doses or frequency of administration must be modified according to degree of renal impairment, severity of infection, and susceptibility of organism. Should be injected deep I.M. into a large muscle mass, such as gluteus or lateral aspect of thigh.

CONTRAINDICATIONS & PRECAUTIONS

Contraindicated in patients with hypersensitivity to any cephalosporin. Use with caution in patients with penicillin allergy.

ADVERSE REACTIONS

Common reactions are in italics; life-threatening reactions are in bold italics.
Blood: transient neutropenia, eosinophilia, ***hemolytic anemia.***
CNS: headache, malaise, paresthesias, dizziness.
GI: ***pseudomembranous colitis,*** nausea, anorexia, vomiting, *diarrhea,* glossitis, dyspepsia, abdominal cramps, tenesmus, anal pruritus, oral candidiasis (thrush).
GU: genital pruritus and moniliasis.
Skin: *maculopapular and erythematous rashes, urticaria.*
Local: *at injection site–pain, induration, sterile abscesses, tissue sloughing; phlebitis and thrombophlebitis with I.V. injection.*
Other: ***hypersensitivity,*** dyspnea, elevated temperature.

INTERACTIONS

Nephrotoxic drugs: may increase the risk of nephrotoxicity. Monitor renal function.
Probenecid: may inhibit excretion and increase blood levels of cefoxitin. May be useful in treating some infections, such as gonorrhea.

EFFECTS ON DIAGNOSTIC TESTS

Coombs' test: positive results.
Liver function tests: elevated results.
Serum or urine creatinine: false elevations in tests using Jaffé's reaction.
Urine glucose tests with copper sulfate (Benedict's reagent or Clinitest): false-positive results; use glucose enzymatic tests (Clinistix or Tes-Tape) instead.

NURSING CONSIDERATIONS

Besides those related universally to drug therapy (see "How to use this book"), consider the following specific recommendations:

Assessment

- Obtain a baseline assessment of infection before therapy.
- Be alert for adverse reactions and drug interactions throughout therapy.
- Evaluate the patient's and family's knowledge about cefoxitin therapy.

Nursing Diagnoses

- High risk for injury related to ineffectiveness of cefoxitin to eradicate the infection.
- High risk for fluid volume deficit related to adverse GI reactions to cefoxitin.
- Knowledge deficit related to cefoxitin.

Planning and Implementation

Preparation and Administration

- Obtain specimen for culture and sensitivity tests before first dose. Therapy may begin pending test results.
- Before giving the first dose, ask patient about any reaction to previous cepalosporin or penicillin therapy.
- ***I.M. use:*** Reconstitute according to manufacturer's instructions. I.M. injection can be reconstituted with 0.5% or 1% lidocaine (without epinephrine) to minimize pain. Administer deep into a large muscle mass, such as gluteus or lateral aspect of thigh.
- ***I.V. use:*** Reconstitute 1-g vial with at least 10 ml of sterile water for injection, and 2-g vial with 10 to 20 ml. Solutions of dextrose 5% and 0.9% sodium chloride for injection can also be used. After reconstitution, drug remains stable for 24 hours at room temperature or 1 week under refrigeration.

Monitoring

- Monitor effectiveness by regularly assessing for improvement of infection.

• Monitor for signs of an allergic or anaphylactic reaction.
• During prolonged or high-dose therapy, monitor for superinfection, especially in high-risk patients.
• Monitor hydration status if adverse GI reactions occur.
Supportive Care
• Obtain an order for an antiemetic or antidiarrheal agent as needed.
• When testing urine glucose, use only glucose enzymatic tests (Clinistix or Tes-Tape), because copper sulfate tests (Clinitest) may have false-positive results.
Patient Teaching
• Teach diabetic patients to test urine for glucose with a glucose enzymatic test such as Clinistix or Tes-Tape because copper sulfate tests (Clinitest) may yield false-positive results.
• Warn patient that I.M. administration may cause pain at injection site.
Evaluation
In patients receiving cefoxitin, appropriate evaluation statements may include:
• Patient is free of infection.
• Patient maintains adequate hydration throughout cefoxitin therapy.
• Patient and family state an understanding of cefoxitin therapy.

ceftazidime
(sef′ tay zi deem)
Fortaz, Magnacef†, Tazicef, Tazidime

• *Classification:* antibiotic (third-generation cephalosporin)
• *Pregnancy Risk Category:* B

HOW SUPPLIED
Injection: 500 mg, 1 g, 2 g
Infusion: 1 g, 2 g in 100-ml vials and bags
Pharmacy bulk package: 6 g

ACTION
Mechanism: Inhibits cell wall synthesis during bacterial replication, promoting osmotic instability. Usually bactericidal.
Absorption: Not absorbed from the GI tract and must be given parenterally. Peak serum levels are lower after I.M. injection than after I.V. administration. The drug is absorbed from I.M. injection sites more slowly in women than in men; in women, higher serum levels are achieved after I.M. injection into the vastus lateralis as compared to the gluteus maximus.
Distribution: Widely distributed into most body tissues and fluids, including the gallbladder, liver, kidneys, bone, sputum, bile, and pleural and synovial fluids; unlike most other cephalosporins, CSF penetration is good; also it crosses the placenta, and is 5% to 24% protein-bound.
Metabolism: Not metabolized.
Excretion: Excreted primarily in urine by glomerular filtration; small amounts are excreted in breast milk. Half-life: About 1½ to 2 hours in patients with normal renal function; up to 35 hours in severe renal disease.
Onset, peak, duration: Peak serum levels occur 1 hour after an I.M. dose.

INDICATIONS & DOSAGE
Treatment of serious infections of the lower respiratory and urinary tracts, gynecologic infections, bacteremia, septicemia, intra-abdominal infections, CNS infections, and skin infections. Among susceptible microorganisms are streptococci, including Streptococcus pneumoniae *and* pyogenes; Staphylococcus aureus *(penicillinase- and nonpenicillinase-producing);*Escherichia coli; Klebsiella; Proteus; Enterobacter; Hemophilus influenzae; Pseudomonas; *and some strains of* Bacteroides–
Adults: 1 g I.V. or I.M. q 8 to 12

hours; up to 6 g daily in life-threatening infections.
Children 1 month to 12 years: 30 to 50 mg/kg I.V. q 8 hours.
Neonates 0 to 4 weeks: 30 mg/kg I.V. q 12 hours.

Total daily dosage is same for I.M. or I.V. administration and depends on susceptibility of organism and severity of infection. In patients with impaired renal function, doses or frequency of administration must be modified according to degree of renal impairment, severity of infection, and susceptibility of organism. Should be injected deep I.M. into a large muscle mass, such as gluteus or lateral aspect of thigh.

CONTRAINDICATIONS & PRECAUTIONS

Contraindicated in patients with hypersensitivity to any cephalosporin. Use cautiously in patients with penicillin allergy, who usually are more susceptible to such reactions.

ADVERSE REACTIONS

Common reactions are in italics; life-threatening reactions are in bold italics.
Blood: *eosinophilia; thrombocytosis,* leukopenia.
CNS: headache, dizziness.
GI: ***pseudomembranous enterocolitis,*** nausea, vomiting, diarrhea, dysgeusia, abdominal cramps.
GU: genital pruritus and moniliasis.
Hepatic: transient elevation in liver enzymes.
Skin: *maculopapular and erythematous rashes, urticaria.*
Local: *at injection site–pain, induration, sterile abscesses, tissue sloughing; phlebitis and thrombophlebitis with I.V. injection.*
Other: ***hypersensitivity,*** dyspnea, elevated temperature.

INTERACTIONS

Nephrotoxic drugs: increased risk of nephrotoxicity. Monitor renal function.
Sodium bicarbonate–containing solutions: make ceftazidime unstable. Don't mix together.

EFFECTS ON DIAGNOSTIC TESTS

Coombs' test: positive results.
Liver function tests: elevated results.
Serum or urine creatinine: false elevations in tests using Jaffé's reaction.
Urine glucose tests with copper sulfate (Benedict's reagent or Clinitest): false-positive results; use glucose enzymatic tests (Clinistix or Tes-Tape) instead.

NURSING CONSIDERATIONS

Besides those related universally to drug therapy (see "How to use this book"), consider the following specific recommendations:

Assessment
- Obtain a baseline assessment of infection before therapy.
- Be alert for adverse reactions and drug interactions throughout therapy.
- Evaluate the patient's and family's knowledge about ceftazidime therapy.

Nursing Diagnoses
- High risk for injury related to ineffectiveness of ceftazidime to eradicate the infection.
- High risk for fluid volume deficit related to adverse GI reactions to ceftazidime.
- Knowledge deficit related to ceftazidime.

Planning and Implementation
Preparation and Administration
- Obtain specimen for culture and sensitivity tests before first dose. Therapy may begin pending test results.
- Before giving first dose, ask patient about any reaction to previous cephalosporin or penicillin therapy.
- ***I.M. use:*** Reconstitute according to manufacturer's instructions; each

brand has specific instructions. Administer deep into a large muscle mass, such as gluteus or lateral aspect of thigh.
• *I.V. use:* Reconstitute according to manufacturer's instructions.
Monitoring
• Monitor effectiveness by regularly assessing for improvement of infection.
• Monitor for signs of an allergic or anaphylactic reaction.
• During prolonged or high-dose therapy, monitor for superinfection, especially in high-risk patients.
• Monitor hydration status if adverse GI reactions occur.
Supportive Care
• Obtain an order for an antiemetic or antidiarrheal agent as needed.
Patient Teaching
• Instruct the patient and family about ceftazidime, including the dose, frequency, action, and adverse reactions.

Evaluation
In patients receiving ceftazidime, appropriate evaluation statements may include:
• Patient is free of infection.
• Patient maintains adequate hydration throughout ceftazidime therapy.
• Patient and family state an understanding of ceftazidime therapy.

---

ceftizoxime sodium
(sef ti zox´ eem)
Cefizox

• *Classification:* antibiotic (third-generation cephalosporin)
• *Pregnancy Risk Category:* B

HOW SUPPLIED
Injection: 1 g, 2 g
Infusion: 1 g, 2 g in 100-mg vials, or 50 ml in D_5W

ACTION
Mechanism: Inhibits cell wall synthesis during bacterial replication, promoting osmotic instability. Usually bactericidal.
Absorption: Not absorbed from the GI tract and must be given parenterally. Peak serum levels are lower after I.M. injection than after I.V. administration.
Distribution: Widely distributed into most body tissues and fluids, including the gallbladder, liver, kidneys, bone, sputum, bile, and pleural and synovial fluids; good CSF penetration with adequate concentrations in inflamed meninges; also crosses the placenta. Ceftizoxime is 28% to 31% protein-bound.
Metabolism: Not metabolized.
Excretion: Primarily excreted in urine by renal tubular secretion and glomerular filtration; small amounts are excreted in breast milk. Half-life: About 1½ to 2 hours in patients with normal renal function; up to 30 hours in severe renal disease.
Onset, peak, duration: Peak serum levels occur at 30 minutes to 1½ hours after an I.M. dose.

INDICATIONS & DOSAGE
Treatment of serious infections of the lower respiratory and urinary tracts, gynecologic infections, bacteremia, septicemia, meningitis, intra-abdominal infections, bone and joint infections, and skin infections. Among susceptible microorganisms are streptococci, including Streptococcus pneumoniae *and* pyogenes; Staphylococcus aureus *(penicillinase- and nonpenicillinase-producing) and* epidermidis; Escherichia coli; Klebsiella; Hemophilus influenzae; Enterobacter; Proteus; *some* Pseudomonas; *and* Peptostreptococcus–
Adults: usual dosage is 1 to 2 g I.V. or I.M. q 8 to 12 hours. In life-threatening infections, up to 2 g q 4 hours.

Total daily dosage is same for I.M. or I.V. administration and depends on susceptibility of organism and severity of infection. In patients with impaired renal function, doses or frequency of administration must be modified according to degree of renal impairment, severity of infection, and susceptibility of organism. Should be injected deep I.M. into a large muscle mass, such as gluteus or lateral aspect of thigh.

CONTRAINDICATIONS & PRECAUTIONS

Contraindicated in patients with hypersensitivity to any cephalosporin. Use cautiously in patients with penicillin allergy, who usually are more susceptible to such reactions.

ADVERSE REACTIONS

Common reactions are in italics; life-threatening reactions are in bold italics.
Blood: transient neutropenia, eosinophilia, ***hemolytic anemia.***
CNS: headache, malaise, paresthesias, dizziness.
GI: ***pseudomembranous colitis,*** nausea, anorexia, vomiting, *diarrhea,* glossitis, dyspepsia, abdominal cramps, tenesmus, anal pruritus.
GU: genital pruritus and moniliasis.
Skin: *maculopapular and erythematous rashes, urticaria.*
Local: *at injection site—pain, induration, sterile abscesses, tissue sloughing; phlebitis and thrombophlebitis with I.V. injection.*
Other: ***hypersensitivity,*** dyspnea, elevated temperature.

INTERACTIONS

Nephrotoxic drugs (such as aminoglycosides): may increase the risk of nephrotoxicity. Monitor renal function.
Probenecid: may inhibit excretion and increase blood levels of ceftizoxime.

EFFECTS ON DIAGNOSTIC TESTS

Coombs' test: positive results.
Liver function tests: elevated results.
Serum or urine creatinine: false elevations in tests using Jaffé's reaction.
Urine glucose tests with copper sulfate (Benedict's reagent or Clinitest): false-positive results; use glucose enzymatic tests (Clinistix or Tes-Tape) instead.

NURSING CONSIDERATIONS

Besides those related universally to drug therapy (see "How to use this book"), consider the following specific recommendations:

Assessment

- Obtain a baseline assessment of infection before therapy.
- Be alert for adverse reactions and drug interactions throughout therapy.
- Evaluate the patient's and family's knowledge about ceftizoxime therapy.

Nursing Diagnoses

- High risk for injury related to ineffectiveness of ceftizoxime to eradicate the infection.
- High risk for fluid volume deficit related to adverse GI reactions to ceftizoxime.
- Knowledge deficit related to ceftizoxime.

Planning and Implementation

Preparation and Administration

- Obtain specimen for culture and sensitivity tests before first dose. Therapy may begin pending test results.
- Before giving first dose, ask patient about any reaction to previous cephalosporin or penicillin therapy.
- ***I.M. use:*** Reconstitute according to manufacturer's instructions. Administer deep into a large muscle mass, such as gluteus or lateral aspect of thigh.
- ***I.V. use:*** When reconstituting powder, add 10 ml of sterile water to the 1-g vial and 20 ml to the 2-g vial to yield a concentration of 95 mg/ml. Reconstitute piggyback vials with 50

to 100 ml of 0.9% sodium chloride or other suitable solution. Shake vial well.
• Solutions are stable for 24 hours at room temperature; for 96 hours if refrigerated. They may turn yellow to amber, but this color change doesn't affect potency. However, don't use solution that is cloudy or contains a precipitate.
Monitoring
• Monitor effectiveness by regularly assessing for improvement of infection.
• Monitor for signs of an allergic or anaphylactic reaction.
• During prolonged or high-dose therapy, monitor for superinfection, especially in high-risk patients.
• Monitor hydration status if adverse GI reactions occur.
Supportive Care
• Obtain an order for an antiemetic or antidiarrheal agent as needed.
Patient Teaching
• Instruct the patient and family about ceftizoxime, including the dose, frequency, action, and adverse reactions.
Evaluation
In patients receiving ceftizoxime, appropriate evaluation statements may include:
• Patient is free of infection.
• Patient maintains adequate hydration throughout ceftizoxime therapy.
• Patient and family state an understanding of ceftizoxime therapy.

ceftriaxone sodium
(sef try ax´ one)
Rocephin

• *Classification:* antibiotic (third-generation cephalosporin)
• *Pregnancy Risk Category:* B

HOW SUPPLIED
Injection: 250 mg, 500 mg, 1 g, 2 g
Infusion: 1 g, 2 g
Pharmacy bulk package: 10 g

ACTION
Mechanism: Inhibits cell wall synthesis during bacterial replication, promoting osmotic instability. Usually bactericidal.
Absorption: Not absorbed from the GI tract and must be given parenterally. Peak serum levels are higher after I.M. injection than after I.V. administration.
Distribution: Widely distributed into most body tissues and fluids, including the gallbladder, liver, kidneys, bone, sputum, bile, and pleural and synovial fluids; good CSF penetration; also crosses the placenta. Protein binding is dose-dependent and decreases as serum levels rise; average is 58% to 96%.
Metabolism: Partially metabolized.
Excretion: Primarily excreted in urine; some is excreted in bile by biliary mechanisms, and small amounts are excreted in breast milk. Half-life: Elimination half-life is 5½ to 11 hours in adults with normal renal function. Severe renal disease prolongs half-life only moderately.
Onset, peak, duration: Peak serum levels occur at 1½ to 4 hours after an I.M. dose.

INDICATIONS & DOSAGE
Treatment of serious infections of the CNS (meningitis), lower respiratory and urinary tracts, gynecologic infections, bacteremia, septicemia, intra-abdominal infections, and skin infections and Lyme disease. Susceptible microorganisms are streptococci, including Streptococcus pneumoniae *and* pyogenes; Staphylococcus aureus *(penicillinase- and nonpenicillinase-producing) and* epidermidis; Escherichia coli; Klebsiella; Hemophilus influenzae; Neisseria meningitidis;

Enterobacter; Proteus; Pseudomonas; Peptostreptococcus *and* Serratia marcescens–
Adults: 1 to 2 g I.M. or I.V. once daily or in equally divided doses twice daily. Total daily dose should not exceed 4 g.
Children: 50 to 75 mg/kg, given in divided doses q 12 hours.
Treatment of meningitis–
Adults and children: 100 mg/kg given in divided doses q 12 hours.
May give loading dose of 75 mg/kg.

Total daily dose is same for I.M. or I.V. administration and depends on susceptibility of organism and severity of infection. Should be injected deep I.M. into a large muscle mass, such as gluteus or lateral aspect of thigh.

CONTRAINDICATIONS & PRECAUTIONS

Contraindicated in patients with hypersensitivity to any cephalosporin. Use cautiously in patients with penicillin allergy, who usually are more susceptible to such reactions.

ADVERSE REACTIONS

Common reactions are in italics; life-threatening reactions are in bold italics.
Blood: *eosinophilia; thrombocytosis,* leukopenia.
CNS: headache, dizziness.
GI: ***pseudomembranous enterocolitis,*** nausea, vomiting, diarrhea, dysgeusia, abdominal cramps.
GU: genital pruritus and moniliasis.
Hepatic: transient elevation in liver enzymes.
Skin: *maculopapular and erythematous rashes, urticaria.*
Local: *at injection site–pain, induration, sterile abscesses, tissue sloughing; phlebitis and thrombophlebitis with I.V. injection.*
Other: ***hypersensitivity,*** dyspnea, elevated temperature.

INTERACTIONS

None significant.

EFFECTS ON DIAGNOSTIC TESTS

Coombs' test: positive results.
Liver function tests: elevated results.
Serum or urine creatinine: false elevations in tests using Jaffé's reaction.
Urine glucose tests with copper sulfate (Benedict's reagent or Clinitest): false-positive results; use glucose enzymatic tests (Clinistix or Tes-Tape) instead.

NURSING CONSIDERATIONS

Besides those related universally to drug therapy (see "How to use this book"), consider the following specific recommendations:

Assessment
- Obtain a baseline assessment of infection before therapy.
- Be alert for adverse reactions and drug interactions throughout therapy.
- Evaluate the patient's and family's knowledge about ceftriaxone therapy.

Nursing Diagnoses
- High risk for injury related to ineffectiveness of ceftriaxone to eradicate the infection.
- High risk for fluid volume deficit related to adverse GI reactions to ceftriaxone.
- Knowledge deficit related to ceftriaxone.

Planning and Implementation

Preparation and Administration
- Obtain specimen for culture and sensitivity tests before first dose. Therapy may begin pending test results.
- Before giving first dose, ask patient about any reaction to previous cephalosporin or penicillin therapy.
- ***I.M. use:*** Reconstitute according to manufacturer's instructions. Administer deep into a large muscle mass, such as gluteus or lateral aspect of thigh.
- ***I.V. use:*** Reconstitute with sterile water for injection, 0.9% sodium

chloride injection, dextrose 5% or 10% injection, or a combination of sodium chloride and dextrose injection and other compatible solutions. Reconstitute by adding 2.4 ml diluent to the 250-mg vial, 4.8 ml to the 500- mg vial, 9.6 ml to the 1-g vial, and 19.2 ml to the 2-g vial. All reconstituted solutions yield a concentration that averages 100 mg/ml. After reconstitution, dilute further for intermittent infusion to desired concentration. I.V. dilutions are stable for 24 hours at room temperature.

Monitoring

• Monitor effectiveness by regularly assessing for improvement of infection.
• Monitor for signs of an allergic or anaphylactic reaction.
• During prolonged or high-dose therapy, monitor for superinfection, especially in high-risk patients.
• Monitor hydration status if adverse GI reactions occur.

Supportive Care

• Obtain an order for an antiemetic or antidiarrheal agent as needed.

Patient Teaching

• Instruct the patient and family about ceftriaxone, including the dose, frequency, action, and adverse reactions.

Evaluation

In patients receiving ceftriaxone, appropriate evaluation statements may include:

• Patient is free of infection.
• Patient maintains adequate hydration throughout ceftriaxone therapy.
• Patient and family state an understanding of ceftriaxone therapy.

---

cefuroxime axetil

(se fyoor ox´ eem)

Ceftin

cefuroxime sodium

Kefurox, Zinacef

• *Classification:* antibiotic (second-generation cephalosporin)
• *Pregnancy Risk Category:* B

HOW SUPPLIED

axetil

Tablets: 125 mg, 250 mg, 500 mg

sodium

Injection: 750 mg, 1.5 g

Infusion: 750 mg, 1.5 g premixed, frozen solution

ACTION

Mechanism: Inhibits cell wall synthesis during bacterial replication, promoting osmotic instability. Usually bactericidal.

Absorption: Not well absorbed from the GI tract and must be given parenterally. Cefuroxime axetil is better absorbed orally; between 37% to 52% of an oral dose reaches the systemic circulation.

Distribution: Widely distributed into most body tissues and fluids, including the gallbladder, liver, kidneys, bone, sputum, bile, and pleural and synovial fluids; CSF penetration is greater than that of most cephalosporins, and drug achieves adequate therapeutic levels in inflamed meninges. Cefuroxime crosses the placenta; it is 33% to 50% protein-bound.

Metabolism: Not metabolized.

Excretion: Primarily excreted in urine by renal tubular secretion and glomerular filtration. Some is excreted in breast milk. Half-life: 1 to 2 hours in patients with normal renal function; 15 to 22 hours in end-stage renal disease.

Onset, peak, duration: Peak serum levels occur 15 to 60 minutes after an I.M. dose. Peak serum levels after oral administration occur in about 2 hours. Food appears to enhance absorption.

INDICATIONS & DOSAGE

Treatment of serious infections of the lower respiratory and urinary tract; skin and skin structure infections; septicemia, meningitis, and gonorrhea. Among susceptible organisms are Streptococcus pneumoniae *and* pyogenes, Hemophilus influenzae, Klebsiella, Staphylococcus aureus, Escherichia coli, Enterobacter, *and* Neisseria gonorrhoeae–

Adults: Usual dosage of cefuroxime sodium is 750 mg to 1.5 g I.M. or I.V. q 8 hours, usually for 5 to 10 days. For life-threatening infections and infections caused by less susceptible organisms, 1.5 g I.M. or I.V. q 6 hours; for bacterial meningitis, up to 3 g I.V. q 6 hours.

Alternatively, administer cefuroxime axetil 250 mg P.O. q 12 hours. For severe infections or less susceptible organisms, dosage may be increased to 500 mg P.O. q 12 hours.

Children and infants over 3 months: 50 to 100 mg/kg/day cefuroxime sodium I.M. or I.V. Higher doses are administered when treating meningitis. Alternatively, give cefuroxime axetil 125 mg P.O. q 12 hours.

Uncomplicated urinary tract infections –

Adults: 125 to 250 mg P.O. q 12 hours.

Otitis media –

Children under 2 years: 125 mg P.O. q 12 hours.

Children 2 years and over: 250 mg P.O. q 12 hours.

CONTRAINDICATIONS & PRECAUTIONS

Contraindicated in patients with hypersensitivity to any cephalosporin. Use cautiously in patients with penicillin allergy, who usually are more susceptible to such reactions.

ADVERSE REACTIONS

Common reactions are in italics; life-threatening reactions are in bold italics.

Blood: transient neutropenia, eosinophilia, ***hemolytic anemia,*** decrease in hemoglobin and hematocrit.

CNS: headache, malaise, paresthesias, dizziness.

GI: ***pseudomembranous colitis,*** nausea, anorexia, vomiting, *diarrhea,* glossitis, dyspepsia, abdominal cramps, tenesmus, anal pruritus.

GU: genital pruritus and moniliasis.

Skin: *maculopapular and erythematous rashes, urticaria.*

Local: *at injection site–pain, induration, sterile abscesses, temperature elevation, tissue sloughing; phlebitis and thrombophlebitis with I.V. injection.*

Other: ***hypersensitivity,*** dyspnea.

INTERACTIONS

Probenecid: may inhibit excretion and increase blood levels of cefuroxime.

EFFECTS ON DIAGNOSTIC TESTS

Coombs' test: positive results.

Liver function tests: elevated results.

Urine glucose tests with copper sulfate (Benedict's reagent or Clinitest): false-positive results; use glucose enzymatic tests (Clinistix or Tes-Tape) instead.

Serum or urine creatinine: false elevations in tests using Jaffé's reaction.

NURSING CONSIDERATIONS

Besides those related universally to drug therapy (see "How to use this book"), consider the following specific recommendations:

Assessment

- Obtain a baseline assessment of infection before therapy.
- Be alert for adverse reactions and drug interactions throughout therapy.
- Evaluate the patient's and family's knowledge about cefuroxime therapy.

Nursing Diagnoses

- High risk for injury related to ineffectiveness of cefuroxime to eradicate the infection.

• High risk for fluid volume deficit related to adverse GI reactions to cefuroxime.
• Knowledge deficit related to cefuroxime.

Planning and Implementation

Preparation and Administration

• Obtain specimen for culture and sensitivity tests before first dose. Therapy may begin pending test results.
• Before giving first dose, ask patient about any reaction to previous cephalosporin or penicillin therapy.
• Expect adjustments of dosage or frequency of administration in patients with impaired renal function.
• ***P.O. use:*** Administer with food because it enhances absorption. Tablets may be crushed for patients who cannot swallow them. However, drug has a bitter taste that is difficult to mask, even with food. Alternative therapy may be necessary.
• ***I.M. use:*** Reconstitute according to manufacturer's instructions. Administer deep into a large muscle mass, such as gluteus or lateral aspect of thigh.
• ***I.V. use:*** Reconstitute 750-mg vial with 9 ml of sterile water for injection, withdrawing 8 ml for 750-mg dose. For the 1.5 g vial, reconstitute with 16 ml of sterile water for injection, withdrawing the entire volume for a 1.5-g dose. For infusion, dilute 750 mg or 1.5 g in 50 to 100 ml of dextrose 5% in water for injection. Solution maintains potency for 24 hours at room temperature and for 7 days if refrigerated.

Monitoring

• Monitor effectiveness by regularly assessing for improvement of infection.
• Monitor for signs of an allergic or anaphylactic reaction.
• During prolonged or high-dose therapy, monitor for superinfection, especially in high-risk patients.
• Monitor hydration status if adverse GI reactions occur.

Supportive Care

• Obtain an order for an antiemetic or antidiarrheal agent as needed.

Patient Teaching

• Instruct patient to take oral cefuroxime with food to enhance absorption. Tell patient that the tablets may be crushed but drug has a bitter taste that is difficult to mask even with food.

Evaluation

In patients receiving cefuroxime, appropriate evaluation statements may include:
• Patient is free of infection.
• Patient maintains adequate hydration throughout cefuroxime therapy.
• Patient and family state an understanding of cefuroxime therapy.

cephalexin monohydrate
(sef a leks´ in)
Ceporex†‡, Keflet, Keflex, Keftab, Novolexin†

cephalexin hydrochloride
Keftab

• *Classification:* antibiotic (first-generation cephalosporin)
• *Pregnancy Risk Category:* B

HOW SUPPLIED

cephalexin monohydrate
Capsules: 500 mg, 1,250 mg
Oral suspension: 100 mg/5 ml, 125 mg/5 ml, 250 mg/5 ml
cephalexin hydrochloride
Tablets: 250 mg, 500 mg, 1 g

ACTION

Mechanism: Inhibits cell wall synthesis during bacterial replication, promoting osmotic instability. Usually bactericidal.
Absorption: Rapid and complete from the GI tract after oral adminis-

tration. Food delays but does not prevent complete absorption.
Distribution: Widely distributed into most body tissues and fluids, including the gallbladder, liver, kidneys, bone, sputum, bile, and pleural and synovial fluids.
Metabolism: Not metabolized.
Excretion: Primarily excreted unchanged in urine by glomerular filtration and renal tubular secretion; small amounts of drug may be excreted in breast milk. Half-life: About 30 minutes to 1 hour in patients with normal renal function; 7½ to 14 hours in severe renal impairment.
Onset, peak, duration: Peak serum levels occur within 1 hour.

INDICATIONS & DOSAGE

Treatment of infections of respiratory or genitourinary tract, skin and soft-tissue infections, bone and joint infections, and otitis media due to Escherichia coli *and other coliform bacteria, group A beta-hemolytic streptococci,* Hemophilus influenzae, Klebsiella, Proteus mirabilis, Streptococcus pneumoniae, *and staphylococci*–
Adults: 250 mg to 1 g P.O. q 6 hours.
Children: 6 to 12 mg/kg P.O. q 6 hours. Maximum 25 mg/kg q 6 hours.

CONTRAINDICATIONS & PRECAUTIONS

Contraindicated in patients with hypersensitivity to any cephalosporin. Use cautiously in patients with penicillin allergy, who usually are more susceptible to such reactions.

ADVERSE REACTIONS

Common reactions are in italics; life-threatening reactions are in bold italics.
Blood: transient neutropenia, eosinophilia, anemia.
CNS: dizziness, headache, malaise, paresthesias.
GI: ***pseudomembranous colitis,*** nausea, anorexia, vomiting, *diarrhea,* glossitis, dyspepsia, abdominal cramps, anal pruritus, tenesmus, oral candidiasis (thrush).
GU: genital pruritus and moniliasis, vaginitis.
Skin: *maculopapular and erythematous rashes, urticaria.*
Other: ***hypersensitivity,*** dyspnea.

INTERACTIONS

Probenecid: may increase blood levels of cephalosporins.

EFFECTS ON DIAGNOSTIC TESTS

Coombs' test: positive results (about 3%).
Liver function tests: elevated results.
Serum or urine creatinine: false elevations in tests using Jaffé's reaction.
Urine glucose tests with copper sulfate (Benedict's reagent or Clinitest): false-positive results; use glucose enzymatic tests (Clinistix or Tes-Tape) instead.

NURSING CONSIDERATIONS

Besides those related universally to drug therapy (see "How to use this book"), consider the following specific recommendations:

Assessment

- Obtain a baseline assessment of infection before therapy.
- Be alert for adverse reactions and drug interactions throughout therapy.
- Evaluate the patient's and family's knowledge about cephalexin therapy.

Nursing Diagnoses

- High risk for injury related to ineffectiveness of cephalexin to eradicate the infection.
- High risk for fluid volume deficit related to adverse GI reactions to cephalexin.
- Knowledge deficit related to cephalexin.

Planning and Implementation

Preparation and Administration

- Obtain specimen for culture and sensitivity tests before first dose.

Therapy may begin pending test results.
• Before giving first dose, ask patient about any reaction to previous cephalosporin or penicillin therapy.
• P.O. use: Administer the drug with food to prevent or minimize GI upset. To prepare oral suspension, add required amount of water to powder in two portions. Shake well after each addition. After mixing, store in refrigerator. Stable for 14 days without significant loss of potency. Keep container tightly closed and shake it well before using.

Monitoring
• Monitor effectiveness by regularly assessing for improvement of infection.
• Monitor for signs of an allergic or anaphylactic reaction, such as skin rash.
• During prolonged or high-dose therapy, monitor for superinfection, especially in high-risk patients.
• Monitor hydration status if adverse GI reactions occur.

Supportive Care
• Obtain an order for an antiemetic or antidiarrheal agent as needed.
• Notify doctor if skin rash develops.
• When testing urine glucose, use only glucose enzymatic tests (Clinistix or Tes-Tape), because copper sulfate tests (Clinitest) may have false-positive results.

Patient Teaching
• Tell the patient to take medication exactly as prescribed, even after he feels better, and to take the entire amount prescribed.
• Tell the patient to take with food or milk to minimize GI discomfort.
• Inform the patient using oral suspension to shake it well before using, and to store the mixture in a tightly closed container in the refrigerator. Tell the patient suspension is stable for 14 days without significant loss of potency.
• Instruct patient to notify doctor if skin rash develops.
• Teach diabetic patients to test urine for glucose with a glucose enzymatic test such as Clinistix or Tes-Tape because copper sulfate tests (Clinitest) may yield false-positive results.

Evaluation

In patients receiving cephalexin, appropriate evaluation statements may include:
• Patient is free of infection.
• Patient maintains adequate hydration throughout cephalexin therapy.
• Patient and family state an understanding of cephalexin therapy.

PHARMACOLOGIC CLASS

cephalosporins

First-generation cephalosporins
cefadroxil monohydrate
cefazolin sodium
cephalexin hydrochloride
cephalexin monohydrate
cephalothin sodium
cephapirin sodium
cephradine

Second-generation cephalosporins
cefaclor
cefamandole nafate
cefmetazole sodium
cefonicid sodium
ceforanide
cefotetan disodium
cefoxitin sodium
cefuroxime axetil
cefuroxime sodium

Third-generation cephalosporins
cefixime
cefoperazone sodium
cefotaxime sodium
ceftazidime
ceftizoxime sodium
ceftriaxone sodium

Oxa-beta lactam
moxalactam disodium

OVERVIEW

Cephalosporins are beta-lactam antibiotics first isolated in 1948 from the fungus *Cephalosporium acremonium.* Their mechanism of action is similar to that of penicillins, but their antibacterial spectra differ. Over the past 15 years, intensive research and development has resulted in the availability of many newer cephalosporins, which are now classified by generations. Generations are differentiated in terms of individual antimicrobial activity.

Cephalosporins are chemically and pharmacologically similar to penicillin and they act by inhibiting bacterial cell wall synthesis, causing rapid cell lysis.

Cephalosporins are bactericidal; they act against many gram-positive and gram-negative bacteria, and some anaerobic bacteria; they do not kill fungi or viruses.

First-generation cephalosporins act against many gram-positive cocci, including penicillinase-producing *Staphylococcus aureus* and *Staphylococcus epidermidis; Streptococcus pneumoniae,* group B streptococci, and group A beta-hemolytic streptococci; susceptible gram-negative organisms include *Klebsiella pneumoniae, Escherichia coli, Proteus mirabilis,* and *Shigella.*

Second-generation cephalosporins are effective against all organisms attacked by first-generation drugs and have additional activity against *Branhamella catarrhalis, Haemophilus influenzae, Enterobacter, Citrobacter, Providencia, Acinetobacter, Serratia,* and *Neisseria; Bacteroides fragilis* is susceptible to cefotetan and cefoxitin.

Third-generation cephalosporins are less active than first- and second-generation drugs against gram-positive bacteria, but more active against gram-negative organisms, including those resistant to first- and second-generation drugs; they have the greatest stability against beta-lactamases produced by gram-negative bacteria. Susceptible gram-negative organisms include *E. coli, Klebsiella, Enterobacter, Providencia, Acinetobacter, Serratia, Proteus, Morganella,* and *Neisseria;*some third-generation drugs are active against *Bacteroides fragilis* and *Pseudomonas.*

Oral absorption of cephalosporins varies widely; many must be given parenterally. Most are distributed widely into the body, the actual amount varying with individual drugs. CSF penetration by first- and second-generation drugs is minimal; third-generation drugs achieve much greater penetration. Cephalosporins cross the placenta. Degree of metabolism varies with individual drugs; some are not metabolized at all, and others are extensively metabolized.

Cephalosporins are excreted primarily in urine, chiefly by renal tubular effects; elimination half-life ranges from ½ to 10 hours in patients with normal renal function. Some drug is excreted in breast milk. Most cephalosporins can be removed by hemodialysis or peritoneal dialysis. Patients on dialysis may require dosage adjustment.

CLINICAL INDICATIONS AND ACTIONS

Infection caused by susceptible organisms

• *Parenteral cephalosporins:* Cephalosporins are used to treat serious infections of the lungs, skin, soft tissue, bones, joints, urinary tract, blood (septicemia), abdomen, and heart (endocarditis).

Third-generation cephalosporins (except moxalactam and cefoperazone) and the second-generation drug cefuroxime are used to treat CNS in-

COMPARING CEPHALOSPORINS

DRUG AND ROUTE	ELIMINATION HALF-LIFE (hours)		SODIUM (mEq/g)	CEREBROSPINAL FLUID PENETRATION
	NORMAL RENAL FUNCTION	END-STAGE RENAL DISEASE		
cefaclor oral	0.5 to 1	3 to 5.5	No data available	No
cefadroxil oral	1 to 2	20 to 25	No data available	No
cefamandole I.M., I.V.	0.5 to 2	12 to 18	3.3	No
cefazolin I.M., I.V.	1.2 to 2.2	12 to 50	2.0	No
cefixime oral	3-4	11.5	No data available	Unknown
cefmetazole I.V.	1.2	Unknown	49	Unknown
cefonicid I.M., I.V.	3.5 to 5.8	100	3.7	No
cefoperazone I.M., I.V.	1.5 to 2.5	3.4 to 7	1.5	Sometimes
ceforanide I.M., I.V.	2.5 to 3.5	5.5 to 25	No data available	No
cefotaxime I.M., I.V.	1 to 1.5	11.5 to 56	2.2	Yes
cefotetan I.M., I.V.	2.8 to 4.6	13 to 35	3.5	No
cefoxitin I.M., I.V.	0.5 to 1	6.5 to 21.5	2.3	No
ceftazidime I.M., I.V.	1.5 to 2	35	2.3	Yes
ceftizoxime I.M., I.V.	1.5 to 2	30	2.6	Yes
ceftriaxone I.M., I.V.	5.5 to 11	15.7	3.6	Yes
cefuroxime I.M., I.V.	1 to 2	15 to 22	2.4	Yes
cephalexin oral	0.5 to 1	7.5 to 14	No data available	No
cephalothin I.M., I.V.	0.5 to 1	19	2.8	No
cephaprin I.M., I.V.	0.5 to 1	1.0 to 1.5	2.4	No
cephradine oral, I.M., I.V.	0.5 to 2	8 to 15 hr	6	No
moxalactam I.M., I.V.	2 to 3.5	5 to 10	3.8	Yes

fections caused by susceptible strains of *N. meningitidis, H. influenzae,* and *S. pneumoniae;* meningitis caused by *E. coli* or *Klebsiella* can be treated by ceftriaxone, cefotaxime, or ceftizoxime.

First-generation, and some second-generation, cephalosporins also can be given prophylactically to reduce postoperative infection after surgical procedures classified as contaminated or potentially contaminated; third-generation drugs are not usually indicated.

Penicillinase-producing *N. gonorrhoeae* can be treated with cefoxitin, cefotaxime, ceftriaxone, ceftizoxime, or cefuroxime.

• *Oral cephalosporins:* Cephalosporins can be used to treat otitis media and infections of the respiratory tract, urinary tract, and skin and soft tissue; cefaclor is particularly effective against ampicillin-resistant middle ear infection caused by *H. influenzae.*

OVERVIEW OF ADVERSE REACTIONS

Many cephalosporins share a similar profile of adverse effects. Hypersensitivity reactions range from mild rashes, fever, and eosinophilia to fatal anaphylaxis, and are more common in patients with penicillin allergy. Hematologic reactions include positive direct and indirect antiglobulin (Coombs' test), thrombocytopenia or thrombocythemia, transient neutropenia, and reversible leukopenia. Adverse renal effects may occur with any cephalosporin; they are most common in older patients, those with decreased renal function, and those taking other nephrotoxic drugs. GI reactions include nausea, vomiting, diarrhea, abdominal pain, glossitis, dyspepsia, and tenesmus; minimal elevation of liver function test results occurs occasionally.

Local venous pain and irritation are common after I.M. injection; such reactions occur more often with higher doses and long-term therapy.

Disulfiram-type reactions occur when cefamandole, cefoperazone, moxalactam, cefonicid, or cefotetan are administered within 48 to 72 hours of alcohol ingestion.

Bacterial and fungal superinfection results from suppression of normal flora.

REPRESENTATIVE COMBINATIONS

None.

---

cephalothin sodium

(sef a´ loe thin)

Ceporacin†‡, Keflin

• *Classification:* antibiotic (first-generation cephalosporin)
• *Pregnancy Risk Category:* B

HOW SUPPLIED

Injection: 1 g, 2 g, 4 g
Infusion: 1 g/50 ml, 2 g/50 ml, 1 g/dl, 2 g/dl
Pharmacy bulk package: 10 g, 20 g

ACTION

Mechanism: Inhibits cell wall synthesis during bacterial replication, promoting osmotic instability. Usually bactericidal.
Absorption: Not absorbed from the GI tract and must be given parenterally. Peak serum levels are higher after I.M. injection than after I.V. administration.
Distribution: Widely distributed into most body tissues and fluids, including the gallbladder, liver, kidneys, bone, sputum, bile, and pleural and synovial fluids; CSF penetration is poor. Cephalothin crosses the placenta; it is 65% to 79% protein-bound.
Metabolism: Partially metabolized by the liver and kidneys.

Excretion: Primarily excreted in urine by renal tubular secretion and glomerular filtration; small amounts are excreted in breast milk. Half-life: 30 minutes to 1 hour in patients with normal renal function; 19 hours in severe renal disease.
Onset, peak, duration: Peak serum levels occur 30 minutes after an I.M. dose.

INDICATIONS & DOSAGE

Treatment of serious infections of respiratory, genitourinary, or gastrointestinal tract; skin and soft-tissue infections (including peritonitis); bone and joint infections; septicemia; and endocarditis due to Escherichia coli *and other coliform bacteria, Enterobacteriaceae, enterococci, gonococci, group A beta-hemolytic streptococci,* Hemophilus influenzae, Klebsiella, Proteus mirabilis, Salmonella, Staphylococcus aureus, Shigella, Streptococcus pneumoniae *and* viridans, *and staphylococci–*
Adults: 500 mg to 1 g I.M. or I.V. (or intraperitoneally) q 4 to 6 hours; in life-threatening infections, up to 2 g q 4 hours.
Children: 14 to 27 mg/kg I.V. q 4 hours, or 20 to 40 mg/kg q 6 hours; dose should be proportionately less in accordance with age, weight, and severity of infection.

Dosage schedule is determined by degree of renal impairment, severity of infection, and susceptibility of causative organism. Should be injected deep I.M. into a large muscle mass, such as gluteus or lateral aspect of thigh. I.V. route is preferable in severe or life-threatening infections.

CONTRAINDICATIONS & PRECAUTIONS

Contraindicated in patients with hypersensitivity to any cephalosporin. Use with caution in patients with penicillin allergy, who usually are more susceptible to such reactions.

ADVERSE REACTIONS

Common reactions are in italics; life-threatening reactions are in bold italics.
Blood: transient neutropenia, eosinophilia, ***hemolytic anemia.***
CNS: headache, malaise, paresthesias, dizziness.
GI: ***pseudomembranous colitis,*** nausea, anorexia, vomiting, *diarrhea,* glossitis, dyspepsia, abdominal cramps, tenesmus, anal pruritus, oral candidiasis (thrush).
GU: *nephrotoxicity,* genital pruritus and moniliasis.
Skin: *maculopapular and erythematous rashes, urticaria.*
Local: *at injection site–pain, induration, sterile abscesses, tissue sloughing; phlebitis and thrombophlebitis with I.V. injection.*
Other: ***hypersensitivity,*** dyspnea, fever.

INTERACTIONS

Aminoglycosides: increased risk of nephrotoxicity. Monitor renal function tests carefully.
Probenecid: may increase blood levels of cephalosporins. Use together cautiously.

EFFECTS ON DIAGNOSTIC TESTS

Coombs' test: positive results.
Liver function tests: elevated results.
Serum or urine creatinine: false elevations in tests using Jaffé's reaction.
Urine glucose tests with copper sulfate (Benedict's reagent or Clinitest): false-positive results; use glucose enzymatic tests (Clinistix or Tes-Tape) instead.

NURSING CONSIDERATIONS

Besides those related universally to drug therapy (see "How to use this book"), consider the following specific recommendations:
Assessment
• Obtain a baseline assessment of infection before therapy.

• Be alert for adverse reactions and drug interactions throughout therapy.
• Evaluate the patient's and family's knowledge about cephalothin therapy.

Nursing Diagnoses

• High risk for injury related to ineffectiveness of cephalothin to eradicate the infection.
• High risk for fluid volume deficit related to adverse GI reactions to cephalothin.
• Knowledge deficit related to cephalothin.

Planning and Implementation

Preparation and Administration

• Obtain specimen for culture and sensitivity tests before first dose. Therapy may begin pending test results.
• Before giving first dose, ask patient about any reaction to previous cephalosporin or penicillin therapy.
• ***I.M. use:*** Administer drug I.M. only when absolutely necessary because I.M. injection causes severe pain. Reconstitute each gram of the drug with 4 ml of sterile water for injection, to provide 500 mg in each 2.2 ml. If vial contents do not dissolve completely, add an additional 0.2 to 0.4 ml diluent, and warm contents slightly. Administer deep into a large muscle mass, such as gluteus or lateral aspect of thigh.
• ***I.V. use:*** Dilute contents of 4-g vial with at least 20 ml of sterile water for injection, dextrose 5% injection, or 0.9% sodium chloride injection and add to suitable I.V. solution according to patient's fluid and electrolyte status.

Monitoring

• Monitor effectiveness by regularly assessing for improvement of infection.
• Monitor I.V. site for vein irritation and phlebitis.
• Monitor for signs of an allergic or anaphylactic reaction.
• During prolonged or high-dose therapy, monitor for superinfection, especially in high-risk patients.
• Monitor hydration status if adverse GI reactions occur.

Supportive Care

• Obtain an order for an antiemetic or antidiarrheal agent as needed.
• Alternate infusion sites if I.V. therapy lasts longer than 3 days. Use of small I.V. needle in the larger available veins may be preferable. Addition of a small concentration of heparin (100 units) or hydrocortisone (10 to 25 mg) may reduce incidence of phlebitis.
• When testing urine glucose, use only glucose enzymatic tests (Clinistix or Tes-Tape), because copper sulfate tests (Clinitest) may have false-positive results.

Patient Teaching

• Warn patient I.M. injection will be painful.
• Teach diabetic patients to test urine for glucose with a glucose enzymatic test such as Clinistix or Tes-Tape because copper sulfate tests (Clinitest) may yield false-positive results.

Evaluation

In patients receiving cephalothin, appropriate evaluation statements may include:
• Patient is free of infection.
• Patient maintains adequate hydration throughout cephalothin therapy.
• Patient and family state an understanding of cephalothin therapy.

cephapirin sodium

(sef a pye´ rin)
Cefadyl

• *Classification:* antibiotic (first-generation cephalosporin)
• *Pregnancy Risk Category:* B

HOW SUPPLIED

Injection: 500-mg, 1-g, 2-g vials; 1-g, 2-g, 4-g piggyback vials; 20-g pharmacy bulk package

ACTION

Mechanism: Inhibits cell wall synthesis during bacterial replication, promoting osmotic instability. Usually bactericidal.
Absorption: Not absorbed from GI tract and must be given parenterally. Peak serum levels are higher after I.M. injection than after I.V. administration.
Distribution: Widely distributed into most body tissues and fluids, including the gallbladder, liver, kidneys, bone, sputum, bile, and pleural and synovial fluids; CSF penetration is poor. Cephapirin crosses the placenta.
Metabolism: Partially metabolized.
Excretion: Primarily excreted in urine by renal tubular secretion and glomerular filtration; small amounts are excreted in breast milk. Half-life: Elimination half-life is about 30 minutes to 1 hour in patients with normal renal function; 1 to 1½ hours in severe renal dysfunction.
Onset, peak, duration: Peak serum levels occur 30 minutes after an I.M. dose.

INDICATIONS & DOSAGE

Serious infections of respiratory, genitourinary, or gastrointestinal tract; skin and soft-tissue infections; bone and joint infections (including osteomyelitis); septicemia; endocarditis due to Streptococcus pneumoniae, Escherichia coli, *group A beta-hemolytic streptococci,* Hemophilus influenzae, Klebsiella, Proteus mirabilis, Staphylococcus aureus, *and* Streptococcus viridans–
Adults: 500 mg to 1 g I.V. or I.M. q 4 to 6 hours up to 12 g daily.
Children over 3 months: 10 to 20 mg/kg I.V. or I.M. q 6 hours; dose depends on age, weight, and severity of infection.

Should be injected deep I.M. into a large muscle mass, such as gluteus or lateral aspect of thigh. Depending on causative organism and severity of infection, patients with reduced renal function may be treated adequately with a lower dose (7.5 to 15 mg/kg q 12 hours). Patients with severely reduced renal function and who are to be dialyzed should receive same dose just before dialysis and q 12 hours thereafter.

CONTRAINDICATIONS & PRECAUTIONS

Contraindicated in patients with hypersensitivity to any cephalosporin. Use cautiously in patients with penicillin allergy, who usually are more susceptible to such reactions.

ADVERSE REACTIONS

Common reactions are in italics; life-threatening reactions are in bold italics.
Blood: transient neutropenia, eosinophilia, anemia.
CNS: dizziness, headache, malaise, paresthesias.
GI: ***pseudomembranous colitis,*** nausea, anorexia, vomiting, *diarrhea,* glossitis, dyspepsia, abdominal cramps, tenesmus, anal pruritus, oral candidiasis (thrush).
GU: genital pruritus and moniliasis, vaginitis.
Skin: *maculopapular and erythematous rashes, urticaria.*
Local: *at injection site–pain, induration, sterile abscesses, tissue sloughing; phlebitis and thrombophlebitis with I.V. injection.*
Other: ***hypersensitivity,*** dyspnea.

INTERACTIONS

Probenecid: may increase blood levels of cephalosporins. May be useful in treating some disorders.

EFFECTS ON DIAGNOSTIC TESTS

Coombs' test: positive results.
Liver function tests: elevated results.
Serum or urine creatinine: false elevations in tests using Jaffé's reaction.
Urine glucose tests with copper sulfate (Benedict's reagent or Clinitest): false-positive results; use glucose enzymatic tests (Clinistix or Tes-Tape) instead.

NURSING CONSIDERATIONS

Besides those related universally to drug therapy (see "How to use this book"), consider the following specific recommendations:

Assessment

- Obtain a baseline assessment of infection before therapy.
- Be alert for adverse reactions and drug interactions throughout therapy.
- Evaluate the patient's and family's knowledge about cephapirin therapy.

Nursing Diagnoses

- High risk for injury related to ineffectiveness of cephapirin to eradicate the infection.
- High risk for fluid volume deficit related to adverse GI reactions to cephapirin.
- Knowledge deficit related to cephapirin.

Planning and Implementation

Preparation and Administration

- Obtain specimen for culture and sensitivity tests before first dose. Therapy may begin pending test results.
- Before giving first dose, ask patient about any reaction to previous cephalosporin or penicillin therapy.
- Be aware that patients who are to be dialyzed should receive same dose just before dialysis and q 12 hours thereafter.
- ***I.M. use:*** Administer drug I.M. only when absolutely necessary because I.M. injection is painful. Reconstitute each gram of the drug with 2 ml of sterile water for injection or bacteriostatic water for injection, providing 500 mg in each 1.2 ml. Administer deep into a large muscle mass, such as gluteus or lateral aspect of thigh.
- ***I.V. use:*** Prepare I.V. infusion using dextrose injection, sodium chloride injection, or bacteriostatic water for injection as diluent: 20 ml yields 1 g per 10 ml; 50 ml yields 1 g per 25 ml; 100 ml yields 1 g per 50 ml. May use a Y-tubing when infusing drug I.V. During infusion stop other solution; check volume of cephapirin solution carefully so that calculated dose is infused. When Y-tubing is used, dilute 4-g vial with 40 ml of diluent.
- Reconstituted cephapirin is stable and compatible for 10 days under refrigeration and for 24 hours at room temperature.

Monitoring

- Monitor effectiveness by regularly assessing for improvement of infection.
- Monitor I.V. site for vein irritation and phlebitis.
- Monitor for signs of an allergic or anaphylactic reaction.
- Monitor hydration status if adverse GI reactions occur.

Supportive Care

- Obtain an order for an antiemetic or antidiarrheal agent as needed.
- Alternate infusion sites if I.V. therapy lasts longer than 3 days. Use of small I.V. needle in the larger available veins may be preferable.
- When testing urine glucose, use only glucose enzymatic tests (Clinistix or Tes-Tape), because copper sulfate tests (Clinitest) may have false-positive results.

Patient Teaching

- Warn patient I.M. injection may be painful.
- Teach diabetic patients to test urine for glucose with a glucose enzymatic test such as Clinistix or Tes-Tape because copper sulfate tests (Clinitest) may yield false-positive results.

Evaluation
In patients receiving cephapirin, appropriate evaluation statements may include:
• Patient is free of infection.
• Patient maintains adequate hydration throughout cephapirin therapy.
• Patient and family state an understanding of cephapirin therapy.

cephradine
(sef´ ra deen)
Anspor, Velosef**

• *Classification:* antibiotic (first-generation cephalosporin)
• *Pregnancy Risk Category:* B

HOW SUPPLIED
Capsules: 250 mg, 500 mg
Oral suspension: 125 mg/5 ml, 250 mg/5 ml
Injection: 250 mg, 500 mg, 1 g, 2 g, 4 g
Infusion: 2 g

ACTION
Mechanism: Inhibits cell wall synthesis during bacterial replication, promoting osmotic instability. Usually bactericidal.
Absorption: Well absorbed from the GI tract. Absorption rates may be faster with I.M. injection into the deltoid or vastus lateralis than into the gluteus maximus.
Distribution: Widely distributed into most body tissues and fluids, including the gallbladder, liver, kidneys, bone, sputum, bile, and pleural and synovial fluids; CSF penetration is poor. Cephradine crosses the placenta; it is 6% to 20% protein-bound.
Metabolism: Not metabolized.
Excretion: Primarily excreted in urine by renal tubular secretion and glomerular filtration; small amounts are excreted in breast milk. Half-life: About 30 minutes to 2 hours in normal renal function; 8 to 15 hours in end-stage renal disease.
Onset, peak, duration: Peak serum levels occur within 1 hour after an oral dose and between 1 and 2 hours after an I.M. dose.

INDICATIONS & DOSAGE
Serious infection of respiratory, genitourinary, or gastrointestinal tract; skin and soft-tissue infections; bone and joint infections; septicemia; endocarditis; and otitis media due to Escherichia coli *and other coliform bacteria, group A beta-hemolytic streptococci,* Hemophilus influenzae, Klebsiella, Proteus mirabilis, Staphylococcus aureus, Streptococcus pneumoniae *and* viridans, *and staphylococci–*
Adults: 500 mg to 1 g I.M. or I.V. 2 to 4 times daily; do not exceed 8 g daily. Or 250 to 500 mg P.O. q 6 hours. Severe or chronic infections may require larger and/or more frequent doses (up to 1 g P.O. q 6 hours).
Children over 1 year: 6 to 12 mg/kg P.O. q 6 hours. 12 to 25 mg/kg I.M. or I.V. q 6 hours.
Otitis media–19 to 25 mg/kg P.O. q 6 hours. Do not exceed 4 g daily.
All patients, regardless of age and weight: larger doses (up to 1 g q.i.d.) may be given for severe or chronic infections. Parenteral therapy may be followed by oral. Injections should be given deep I.M. into a large muscle mass, such as gluteus or lateral aspect of thigh.

CONTRAINDICATIONS & PRECAUTIONS
Contraindicated in patients with hypersensitivity to any cephalosporin. Use cautiously in patients with penicillin allergy, who usually are more susceptible to such reactions.

*Liquid form contains alcohol. **May contain tartrazine.

ADVERSE REACTIONS

Common reactions are in italics; life-threatening reactions are in bold italics.
Blood: transient neutropenia, eosinophilia.
CNS: dizziness, headache, malaise, paresthesias.
GI: ***pseudomembranous colitis,*** *nausea, anorexia,* vomiting, heartburn, glossitis, dyspepsia, abdominal cramping, *diarrhea,* tenesmus, anal pruritus, oral candidiasis (thrush).
GU: genital pruritus and moniliasis, vaginitis.
Skin: *maculopapular and erythematous rashes, urticaria.*
Local: *at injection site—pain, induration, sterile abscesses, tissue sloughing; phlebitis and thrombophlebitis with I.V. injection.*
Other: ***hypersensitivity,*** dyspnea.

INTERACTIONS

Probenecid: may increase blood levels of cephalosporins. May be useful in treating some disorders.

EFFECTS ON DIAGNOSTIC TESTS

Coombs' test: positive results.
Liver function tests: elevated results.
Serum or urine creatinine: false elevations in tests using Jaffé's reaction.
Urine glucose tests with copper sulfate (Benedict's reagent or Clinitest): false-positive results; use glucose enzymatic tests (Clinistix or Tes-Tape) instead.

NURSING CONSIDERATIONS

Besides those related universally to drug therapy (see "How to use this book"), consider the following specific recommendations:

Assessment
- Obtain a baseline assessment of infection before therapy.
- Be alert for adverse reactions and drug interactions throughout therapy.
- Evaluate the patient's and family's knowledge about cephradine therapy.

Nursing Diagnoses
- High risk for injury related to ineffectiveness of cephradine to eradicate the infection.
- High risk for fluid volume deficit related to adverse GI reactions to cephradine.
- Knowledge deficit related to cephradine.

Planning and Implementation
Preparation and Administration
- Obtain specimen for culture and sensitivity tests before first dose. Therapy may begin pending test results.
- Before giving first dose, ask patient about any reaction to previous cephalosporin or penicillin therapy.
- ***P.O. use:*** Administer drug with food or milk to minimize GI discomfort.
- ***I.M. use:*** Be aware that I.M. injection is painful. Reconstitute with sterile water for injection or with bacteriostatic water for injection as follows: 1.2 ml to 250-mg vial; 2 ml to 500-mg vial; 4 ml to 1-g vial. I.M. solutions must be used within 2 hours if kept at room temperature and within 24 hours if refrigerated. Solutions may vary in color from light straw to yellow without affecting potency.
- ***I.V. use:*** When available, use preparation specifically supplied for infusion. Follow specific product directions carefully when reconstituting.

Monitoring
- Monitor effectiveness by regularly assessing for improvement of infection.
- Monitor for signs of an allergic or anaphylactic reaction.
- During prolonged or high-dose therapy, monitor for superinfection, especially in high-risk patients.
- Monitor hydration status if adverse GI reactions occur.

Supportive Care
- Obtain an order for an antiemetic or antidiarrheal agent as needed.
- Alternate injection sites if I.V. ther-

apy lasts longer than 3 days. Use of small I.V. needle in the larger available veins may be preferable.
• When testing urine glucose, use only glucose enzymatic tests (Clinistix or Tes-Tape), because copper sulfate tests (Clinitest) may have false-positive results.
Patient Teaching
• Tell patient to take medication exactly as prescribed, even after he feels better.
• Instruct patient to take the oral dosage form with food or milk to lessen GI discomfort.
• Warn patient that I.M. injection will be painful.
• Teach diabetic patients to test urine for glucose with a glucose enzymatic test such as Clinistix or Tes-Tape because copper sulfate tests (Clinitest) may yield false-positive results.
Evaluation
In patients receiving cephradine, appropriate evaluation statements may include:
• Patient is free of infection.
• Patient maintains adequate hydration throughout cephradine therapy.
• Patient and family state an understanding of cephradine therapy.

chloral hydrate
(klor al hye´ drate)
Aquachloral Supprettes, Noctec, Novochlorhydrate†

• Controlled Substance Schedule IV
• *Classification:* sedative-hypnotic
• *Pregnancy Risk Category:* C

HOW SUPPLIED
Capsules: 250 mg, 500 mg
Syrup: 250 mg/5 ml, 500 mg/5 ml
Suppositories: 325 mg, 500 mg, 648 mg

ACTION
Mechanism: Unknown. Sedative effects may be caused by its primary metabolite, trichloroethanol.
Absorption: Well absorbed after oral and rectal administration.
Distribution: Chloral hydrate and its active metabolite trichloroethanol are distributed throughout the body tissue and fluids. Trichloroethanol is 35% to 41% protein-bound.
Metabolism: Rapidly and nearly completely metabolized in the liver and erythrocytes to the active metabolite trichloroethanol; is further metabolized in the liver and kidneys to trichloroacetic acid and other inactive metabolites.
Excretion: The inactive metabolites of chloral hydrate are excreted primarily in urine; minor amounts in bile. Half-life: Of trichloroethanol, 8 to 10 hours.
Onset, peak, duration: Sleep occurs 30 to 60 minutes after a 500-mg to 1-g dose.

INDICATIONS & DOSAGE
Sedation–
Adults: 250 mg P.O. or rectally t.i.d. after meals.
Children: 8 mg/kg P.O. t.i.d. Maximum dosage is 500 mg t.i.d.
Insomnia–
Adults: 500 mg to 1 g P.O. or rectally 15 to 30 minutes before bedtime.
Children: 50 mg/kg P.O. single dose. Maximum dosage is 1 g.
Premedication for EEG–
Children: 25 mg/kg P.O. single dose. Maximum dosage is 1 g.

CONTRAINDICATIONS & PRECAUTIONS
Contraindicated in patients with hypersensitivity to chloral derivatives; severe cardiac disease; and marked renal or hepatic failure because elimination of the drug will decrease.

Use cautiously in patients with depression, suicidal ideation, or history of drug abuse or addiction because the drug depresses CNS function; and in patients who need to perform hazardous tasks requiring mental alertness or physical coordination. Do not administer oral forms of chloral hydrate to patients with esophagitis, gastritis, or gastric or duodenal ulcers, because the drug is irritating to the GI tract. Rectal administration of chloral hydrate may exacerbate proctitis or ulcerative colitis.

ADVERSE REACTIONS

Common reactions are in italics; life-threatening reactions are in bold italics.
Blood: eosinophilia.
CNS: *hangover, drowsiness,* nightmares, dizziness, ataxia, paradoxical excitement.
GI: *nausea,* vomiting, diarrhea, flatulence.
Skin: hypersensitivity.

INTERACTIONS

Alcohol or other CNS depressants, including narcotic analgesics: excessive CNS depression or vasodilation reaction. Use together cautiously.
Furosemide I.V.: sweating, flushes, variable blood pressure, and uneasiness. Use together cautiously or use a different hypnotic drug.
Oral anticoagulants: increased risk of bleeding. Monitor patient closely.

EFFECTS ON DIAGNOSTIC TESTS

Phentolamine test: false-positive results.
Urine catecholamines: interference with fluorometric tests. Do not use drug for 48 hours before the test.
Urine 17-hydroxycorticosteroids (Reddy-Henkins-Thord test): interference.
Urine glucose with tests using copper sulfate, such as Benedict's reagent and Clinitest: false-positive results.

NURSING CONSIDERATIONS

Besides those related universally to drug therapy (see "How to use this book"), consider the following specific recommendations:

Assessment
- Obtain a baseline assessment of sleeping patterns and CNS status before therapy.
- Be alert for adverse reactions and drug interactions throughout therapy.
- Evaluate the patient's and family's knowledge about chloral hydrate therapy.

Nursing Diagnoses
- Sleep pattern disturbance related to underlying patient problem.
- High risk for trauma related to adverse CNS reactions caused by chloral hydrate.
- Knowledge deficit related to chloral hydrate therapy.

Planning and Implementation

Preparation and Administration
- ***P.O. use:*** Dilute syrup with adequate fluid (4 oz of water, fruit juice, or ginger ale) or administer with 8 oz of liquid to minimize unpleasant taste and stomach irritation. Keep in mind that aqueous solutions are incompatible with alkaline solutions. Administer after meals; store drug in dark container. Before leaving the bedside, make sure the patient has swallowed medication.
- Store rectal suppositories in refrigerator.

Monitoring
- Monitor effectiveness by evaluating the patient's ability to sleep after administration.
- Monitor for evidence of CNS or other adverse effects.

Supportive Care
- After administration, institute safety precautions: remove cigarettes; keep patient on bed rest, keep bed rails up, and supervise or assist ambulations.
- When interpreting test results, be aware that high dosage may raise

BUN level and may interfere with fluorometric tests for urine catecholamines and Reddy-Jenkins-Thorn test for urine 17-hydroxycorticosteroids. Do not administer drug for 48 hours before fluorometric test.
• Take precautions to prevent hoarding or self-overdosing by the patient who is depressed, suicidal, or drug-dependent or who has a history of drug abuse.

Patient Teaching

• Instruct the patient to remain in bed after taking the drug and to call for assistance to use the bathroom.
• Explain that drug may cause morning "hangover." Encourage the patient to report severe hangover or feelings of oversedation so the doctor can be consulted to adjust or change drug.
• Warn the patient to avoid hazardous activities that require mental alertness if CNS adverse reactions occur.
• Tell the patient to notify the nurse or doctor if sleep pattern disturbances persist.

Evaluation

In patients receiving chloral hydrate, appropriate evaluation statements include:
• Patient states drug was effective in inducing sleep.
• Patient's safety is maintained.
• Patient and family state an understanding of chloral hydrate therapy.

chlorambucil

(klor am´ byoo sil)
Leukeran

• *Classification:* antineoplastic (alkylating agent)
• *Pregnancy Risk Category:* D

HOW SUPPLIED

Tablets: 2 mg

ACTION

Mechanism: An alkylating agent that cross-links strands of cellular DNA and interferes with RNA transcription, causing an imbalance of growth that leads to cell death. Cell cycle–nonspecific.
Absorption: Rapidly and completely absorbed from the GI tract.
Distribution: Not well understood. However, the drug and its metabolites are highly bound to plasma and tissue proteins.
Metabolism: In the liver. The primary metabolite, phenylacetic acid mustard, also has cytotoxic activity.
Excretion: Metabolites of chlorambucil are excreted in urine. Half-life: Chlorambucil, 1½ hours; phenylacetic acid mustard, 2½ hours.
Onset, peak, duration: Peak serum levels of chlorambucil are seen within 1 hour of a dose; of phenylacetic acid mustard, within 2 to 4 hours.

INDICATIONS & DOSAGE

Chronic lymphocytic leukemia, diffuse lymphocytic lymphoma, nodular lymphocytic lymphoma, Hodgkin's disease, ovarian carcinoma, mycosis fungoides–
Adults: 0.1 to 0.2 mg/kg P.O. daily for 3 to 6 weeks, then adjust for maintenance (usually 2 mg daily).
Children: 0.1 to 0.2 mg/kg/day or 4.5 mg/m^2 P.O. daily as a single dose or in divided doses.

CONTRAINDICATIONS & PRECAUTIONS

Contraindicated in patients with a history of hypersensitivity to the drug or of resistance to previous therapy with the drug. Cross-sensitivity, which manifests as a rash, may occur between chlorambucil and other alkylating agents.

Dosage adjustments must be considered in patients with hematologic impairment because of the drug's hematologic toxicity.

Use cautiously in patients with a history of seizures, head trauma, or use of epileptogenic drugs. There is a small risk of chlorambucil-induced seizure.

Patients should not receive a full dose of chlorambucil if a full course of radiation therapy or other myelosuppressive drugs were administered within the preceding 4 weeks because of the potential for additive toxicity.

ADVERSE REACTIONS

Common reactions are in italics; life-threatening reactions are in bold italics.
Blood: leukopenia, delayed up to 3 weeks, lasting up to 10 days after last dose; ***thrombocytopenia;*** anemia; myelosuppression (usually moderate, gradual, and rapidly reversible).
CNS: seizures (with overdose).
GI: *nausea, vomiting.*
GU: *azoospermia, infertility.*
Metabolic: hyperuricemia, hepatotoxicity (rare).
Respiratory: interstitial pneumonitis or ***pulmonary fibrosis*** (rare).
Skin: ***exfoliative dermatitis,*** rash.
Other: allergic febrile reaction.

INTERACTIONS

None significant.

EFFECTS ON DIAGNOSTIC TESTS

Serum alkaline phosphatase, AST (SGOT), and blood and urine uric acid: increased concentrations.

NURSING CONSIDERATIONS

Besides those related universally to drug therapy (see "How to use this book"), consider the following specific recommendations:

Assessment

- Obtain a baseline assessment of the patient's underlying condition and CBC and uric acid levels before initiating therapy.
- Be alert for adverse reactions or drug interactions during therapy.
- Evaluate the patient's and familiy's knowledge about chlorambucil therapy.

Nursing Diagnoses

- Infection related to chlorambucil-induced neutropenia.
- Altered skin integrity related to resultant exfoliative dermatitis.
- Knowledge deficit related to chlorambucil therapy.

Planning and Implementation

Preparation and Administration

- ***P.O. use:*** Dose is individualized according to the response of the patient. Give the drug 1 hour before breakfast and at least 2 hours after the evening meal.

Monitoring

- Monitor effectiveness by noting the results of follow-up diagnostic tests and overall physical status.
- Monitor WBC, platelet, and uric acid levels.
- Monitor daily temperatures and watch for signs of infection (fever, sore throat, malaise).
- Monitor for skin reactions such as redness and exfoliation.

Supportive Care

- Place patient on neutropenic precautions if WBC falls below 2,000/mm³ or granulocytes fall below 1,000/mm³.
- Keep in mind that severe neutropenia is reversible up to cumulative dosage of 6.5 mg/kg in a single course.
- Allopurinol and increased fluids may be used to combat the nephrotoxic effects of increased uric acid levels.
- Do not give any I.M. injections when the patient's platelet count is $< 100{,}000/mm^3$.
- Remember that therapeutic effects are often accompanied by toxicity.

Patient Teaching

- Instruct the patient to take the drug 1 hour before breakfast and 2 hours after the evening meal.
- Instruct the patient to watch for signs of bleeding.

• Instruct the patient to take daily temperatures and report any signs of infection.
• Instruct the patient on how to keep diary of fluid intake and output—2,400 cc to 3,000 cc/day should be consumed.
• Instruct patient to refrain from taking any OTC drug containing aspirin.

Evaluation

In patients receiving chlorambucil, appropriate evaluation statements may include:
• Patient remains infection-free throughout drug treatment.
• Skin integrity is maintained, and patient did not experience exfoliation.
• Patient and family state an understanding of chlorambucil therapy.

chloramphenicol (systemic)

(klor am fen´ i kole)

Chloromycetin, Novochlorocap†

chloramphenicol palmitate

Chloromycetin Palmitate

chloramphenicol sodium succinate

Chloromycetin Sodium Succinate, Pentamycetin†

• *Classification:* antibiotic (dichloracetic acid derivative)
• *Pregnancy Risk Category:* C

HOW SUPPLIED

Capsules: 250 mg, 500 mg
Oral suspension: 150 mg/5 ml
Injection: 1-g, 10-g vials

ACTION

Mechanism: Inhibits bacterial protein synthesis by binding to the 50S subunit of the ribosome.
Absorption: After oral administration, well absorbed from GI tract. The palmitate salt is rapidly hydrolyzed in the stomach to free chloramphenicol. After I.V. administration, chloramphenicol sodium succinate produces variable plasma levels of free chloramphenicol; it is hydrolyzed by esterases in the liver, kidneys, and lungs. The rate and extent of hydrolysis is variable.
Distribution: Widely distributed into most body tissues and fluids, including CSF, liver, and kidneys; it readily crosses the placenta. About 50% to 60% of the drug binds to plasma protein.
Metabolism: Primarily by hepatic glucuronyl transferase to inactive metabolites. Premature and newborn infants lack these metabolic enzymes and may exhibit high and prolonged plasma levels of the drug.
Excretion: About 8% to 12% of dose is excreted unchanged by the kidneys, the remainder as inactive metabolites; some may be excreted in breast milk. Plasma chloramphenicol levels may be elevated in patients with renal impairment after I.V. administration because these patients show decreased excretion of the succinate ester. Half-life: Ranges from about 1½ to 4½ hours in adults with normal hepatic and renal function; plasma half-life of parent drug is prolonged in patients with hepatic dysfunction.
Onset, peak, duration: Peak serum concentrations occur in 1 to 3 hours. In patients receiving chloramphenicol palmitate, mean serum concentrations resemble those achieved by the base. Recommended therapeutic range is 10 to 20 mcg/ml for peak levels and 5 to 10 mcg/ml for trough levels.

INDICATIONS & DOSAGE

Haemophilus influenzae *meningitis, acute* Salmonella typhi *infection, and meningitis, bacteremia, or other severe infections caused by sensitive* Salmonella *species,* Rickettsia, *lym-*

phogranuloma, psittacosis, or various sensitive gram-negative organisms— **Adults and children:** 50 to 100 mg/kg P.O. or I.V. daily, divided q 6 hours. Maximum dosage is 100 mg/kg daily. **Premature infants and neonates 2 weeks or younger:** 25 mg/kg P.O. or I.V. daily, divided q 6 hours. I.V. route must be used to treat meningitis.

CONTRAINDICATIONS & PRECAUTIONS

Contraindicated in patients with minor infections (such as influenza, throat infections, and colds) or as prophylaxis against infection, because potential toxicity may outweigh therapeutic benefit; and in patients with hypersensitivity or history of toxic reaction to the drug.

Use cautiously in infants and in patients with renal or hepatic dysfunction, acute intermittent porphyria, or glucose-6-phosphate dehydrogenase (G6PD) deficiency because of potential for adverse hematopoietic effects (including gray syndrome).

ADVERSE REACTIONS

Common reactions are in italics; life-threatening reactions are in bold italics.
Blood: ***aplastic anemia,*** hypoplastic anemia,*granulocytopenia,* thrombocytopenia.
CNS: headache, mild depression, confusion, delirium, peripheral neuropathy with prolonged therapy.
EENT: optic neuritis (in patients with cystic fibrosis), glossitis, decreased visual acuity.
GI: nausea, vomiting, stomatitis, diarrhea, enterocolitis.
Other: infections by nonsusceptible organisms, hypersensitivity (fever, rash, urticaria, ***anaphylaxis***), jaundice, ***gray syndrome in premature and newborn infants*** *(abdominal distention, gray cyanosis, vasomotor collapse, respiratory distress, death within a few hours of onset of symptoms).*

INTERACTIONS

Acetaminophen: elevates chloramphenicol levels. Monitor for chloramphenicol toxicity.
Chlorpropamide, dicumarol, phenobarbital, phenytoin, tolbutamide: blood levels of these agents may be increased by chloramphenicol.
Penicillin: bactericidal activity reduced by chloramphenicol. Separate administration times.

EFFECTS ON DIAGNOSTIC TESTS

Bentiromide test for pancreatic function: false elevation of urinary para-aminobenzoic acid (PABA) levels.
CBC: decreased RBC, platelet, and WBC counts in the blood and possibly the bone marrow. Reversible bone marrow depression may become irreversible.
Lactic acid: increased lactate levels (lactic acidosis).
Urine glucose tests with copper sulfate (Clinitest): false-positive results.
Urine hemoglobin: increased.

NURSING CONSIDERATIONS

Besides those related universally to drug therapy (see "How to use this book"), consider the following specific recommendations:

Assessment

- Obtain a baseline assessment of infection before therapy.
- Be alert for adverse reactions and drug interactions throughout therapy.
- Evaluate the patient's and family's knowledge about chloramphenicol therapy.

Nursing Diagnoses

- High risk for injury related to ineffectiveness of chloramphenicol to eradicate the infection.
- Altered protection related to chloramphenicol-induced aplastic anemia.
- Knowledge deficit related to chloramphenicol.

Planning and Implementation

Preparation and Administration

• Expect to decrease the chloramphenicol dosage as prescribed in patients with serious hepatic dysfunction or renal failure, and in neonates to prevent bone marrow suppression, encephalitis, or gray syndrome.

• Obtain specimen for culture and sensitivity tests before first dose. Therapy may begin pending test results. Also obtain specimens for CBC, platelet count, serum iron, and reticulocyte count before administering first dose of chloramphenicol.

• ***I.V. use:*** Reconstitute 1-g vial of powder for injection with 10 ml sterile water for injection. Concentration will be 100 mg/ml. Give I.V. slowly over 1 minute. Reconstituted solution is stable for 30 days at room temperature, but refrigeration is recommended. Do not use cloudy solutions.

• If administering concomitantly with penicillin, give penicillin 1 hour or more before chloramphenicol to avoid reduction in penicillin's bactericidal activity.

Monitoring

• Monitor effectiveness by regularly assessing for improvement in the infection.

• Monitor hydration status if adverse GI reactions occur.

• Monitor CBC, platelet count, serum iron, and reticulocyte count every 2 days during therapy. Continue to monitor patient for signs and symptoms of aplastic anemia, such as anemia, infection, or bleeding, after chloramphenicol therapy has been discontinued.

• Monitor plasma concentrations. Therapeutic range is 5 to 25 mcg/ml.

Supportive Care

• Discontinue drug immediately if anemia, reticulocytopenia, leukopenia, or thrombocytopenia develops and prepare to treat patient's symptoms as indicated.

• If the patient's serum chloramphenicol concentration exceeds 25 mcg/ml, take bleeding precautions and infection-control measures because bone marrow suppression can occur.

• Obtain an order for an antiemetic or antidiarrheal agent as needed.

Patient Teaching

• Tell the patient to take medication for as long as prescribed, exactly as directed, and even after he feels better and to take entire amount prescribed.

• Stress the importance of having frequent blood tests done to monitor therapeutic effectiveness and potential for adverse drug reactions.

• Warn the patient about the unpleasant taste of oral chloramphenicol.

Evaluation

In patients receiving chloramphenicol, appropriate evaluation statements may include:

• Patient is free from infection.

• Patient's hematologic status remains unchanged with chloramphenicol therapy.

• Patient and family state an understanding of chloramphenicol therapy.

chloramphenicol (ophthalmic)

(klor am fen´ i kole)

AK-Chlor, Chloromycetin Ophthalmic, Chloroptic, Chloroptic S.O.P., Chlorsig‡, Fenicol†, Isopto Fenicol†, Ophthoclor Ophthalmic, Pentamycetin†

• *Classification:* antibiotic (dichloracetic acid derivative)

• *Pregnancy Risk Category:* C

HOW SUPPLIED

Ophthalmic ointment: 1%

Ophthalmic solution: 0.5%

ACTION

Mechanism: Inhibits protein synthesis in susceptible organisms by binding to the 50S ribosome. Bacteriostatic,

but may be bactericidal in high concentrations or against highly susceptible organisms.
Absorption: Limited evidence suggests that the drug may be absorbed into the aqueous humor after topical ophthalmic administration.

INDICATIONS & DOSAGE

Surface bacterial infection involving conjunctiva or cornea –
Adults and children: instill 1 drop of solution in eye q 1 to 4 hours until condition improves, or instill q.i.d., depending on severity of infection. Apply small amount of ointment to lower conjunctival sac at bedtime as supplement to drops. May use ointment alone by applying a small amount of ointment to lower conjunctival sac q 3 to 6 hours or more frequently, if necessary. Continue until condition improves.

CONTRAINDICATIONS & PRECAUTIONS

Contraindicated in patients with minor infections (such as influenza, throat infections, and colds) or as prophylaxis against infection because potential toxicity may outweigh therapeutic benefit; it is also contraindicated in patients with hypersensitivity or history of toxic reaction to the drug.

ADVERSE REACTIONS

Common reactions are in italics; life-threatening reactions are in bold italics.
Note: systemic adverse reactions have not been reported with short-term topical use.
Blood: ***bone marrow hypoplasia*** *with prolonged use,* ***aplastic anemia.***
Eye: optic atrophy in children, stinging or burning of eye after instillation, blurred vision (with ointment).
Other: overgrowth of nonsusceptible organisms; hypersensitivity, including itching and burning eye, dermatitis, angioedema.

INTERACTIONS

None significant.

EFFECTS ON DIAGNOSTIC TESTS

CBC: decreased platelet and WBC counts in the blood and possibly the bone marrow. Hemoglobinuria or lactic acidosis may also occur.
Urine glucose (copper sulfate [Clinitest]): false-positive results.
Urine para-aminobenzoic acid (PABA): falsely elevated levels during a bentiromide test for pancreatic function.

NURSING CONSIDERATIONS

Besides those related universally to drug therapy (see "How to use this book"), consider the following specific recommendations:

Assessment
- Obtain a baseline assessment of allergies before therapy.
- Be alert for adverse reactions or drug interactions during therapy.
- Evaluate the patient's and family's knowledge about chloramphenicol.

Nursing Diagnoses
- Altered protection related to ocular infection.
- Impaired gas exchange related to chloramphenicol-induced aplastic anemia.
- Knowledge deficit related to chloramphenicol therapy.

Planning and Implementation

Preparation and Administration
- Store in tightly closed, light-resistant container.
- Wash hands before and after administration.
- Cleanse eye area of excessive exudate before application.
- If chloramphenicol drops are given q1h and then tapered, follow order closely to ensure adequate anterior chamber levels.

Monitoring
- Monitor effectiveness by checking for microorganisms by culturing the eye exudate.

• Observe amount, color, and consistency of exudate.
• Monitor CBC and differential.

Supportive Care

• Apply warm moist compresses to aid removal of dried exudate.
• Start systemic therapy if more than superficial infection present.
• Notify the doctor if no improvement within 3 days; drug not for long-term use.
• One of the safest topical ocular antibiotics, especially for endophthalmitis.

Patient Teaching

• Teach the patient how to instill. Advise him to wash hands before and after administering ointment or solution. Warn him not to touch the tip of applicator to eye or surrounding tissue.
• Instruct the patient to apply light finger pressure to the lacrimal sac for 1 minute after drops are instilled.
• Stress the importance of compliance with recommended therapy.
• Instruct the patient to watch for signs of hypersensitivity (itching lids, swelling, or constant burning). Stop drug and notify the doctor immediately.
• Advise the patient not to share eye medications with family members. A family member who develops the same symptoms should contact the doctor.

Evaluation

In patients receiving chloramphenicol, appropriate evaluation statements may include:

• Patient remains free of signs and symptoms of infection.
• Patient exhibits no signs of chloramphenicol-induced aplastic anemia.
• Patient and family state an understanding of chloramphenicol therapy.

chloramphenicol (otic)

(klor am fen´ a kole)
Chloromycetin Otic, Sopamycetin†

• *Classification:* antibiotic (dichloracetic acid derivative)
• *Pregnancy Risk Category:* C

HOW SUPPLIED

Otic solution: 0.5%

ACTION

Mechanism: Inhibits or destroys bacteria present in the ear canal.
Pharmacokinetics: Unknown.

INDICATIONS & DOSAGE

External ear canal infection–
Adults and children: 2 to 3 drops into ear canal t.i.d. or q.i.d.

CONTRAINDICATIONS & PRECAUTIONS

Contraindicated in patients with minor infections (such as influenza, throat infections, and colds) or as prophylaxis against infection, because potential toxicity may outweigh therapeutic benefit; also contraindicated in patients with hypersensitivity or history of toxic reaction to the drug.

Use cautiously in infants and in patients with renal or hepatic dysfunction, acute intermittent porphyria, or glucose-6-phosphate dehydrogenase (G6PD) deficiency because of potential for adverse hematopoietic effects (including gray syndrome).

ADVERSE REACTIONS

Common reactions are in italics; life-threatening reactions are in bold italics.
Ear: itching or burning.
Local: pruritus, burning, urticaria, vesicular or maculopapular dermatitis.
Systemic: sore throat, angioedema.
Other: overgrowth of nonsusceptible organisms.

INTERACTIONS
None significant.

EFFECTS ON DIAGNOSTIC TESTS
Bentiromide test for pancreatic function: false elevations of urinary para-aminobenzoic acid (PABA) levels.
CBC: decreased RBC, WBC, and platelet counts in the blood and possibly in bone marrow.
Urine glucose tests with copper sulfate (Clinitest): false-positive results.

NURSING CONSIDERATIONS
Besides those related universally to drug therapy (see "How to use this book"), consider the following specific recommendations:

Assessment
- Obtain a baseline assessment of the patient's ear canal and tympanic membrane through otoscopic examination before therapy.
- Be alert for adverse reactions and drug interactions throughout therapy.
- Evaluate the patient's and family's knowledge about chloramphenicol therapy.

Nursing Diagnoses
- Sensory/perceptual alterations (auditory) related to the patient's underlying condition.
- High risk for infection related to overgrowth of nonsusceptible organisms.
- Knowledge deficit related to chloramphenicol therapy.

Planning and Implementation
Preparation and Administration
- Instill in ear canal; avoid touching ear with dropper.
- Screen patient history carefully for any reaction to the drug before administering.
- Avoid prolonged use.

Monitoring
- Monitor effectiveness by otoscopic examination of the ear canal.
- Monitor for superinfection: continued pain, inflammation, fever.
- Monitor for complaints of sore throat, an early sign of toxicity.

Supportive Care
- Culture any persistent ear drainage.
- Notify the doctor of signs of superinfection or severe side effects.

Patient Teaching
- Teach patient how to instill drops.
- Teach patient to report persistent pain, fever, and inflammation.

Evaluation
In patients receiving chloramphenicol, appropriate evaluation statements may include:
- Patient achieves relief of otic infection.
- Patient remains free of superinfection.
- Patient and family state an understanding of chloramphenicol therapy.

chloramphenicol (topical)
(klor am fen´ i kole)
Chloromycetin

- *Classification:* antibiotic (dichloracetic acid derivative)
- *Pregnancy Risk Category:* C

HOW SUPPLIED
Cream: 1%

ACTION
Mechanism: Binds to the 50S ribosomal subunit of susceptible bacteria and disrupts protein synthesis. May be bacteriostatic or bactericidal, depending upon concentration.
Pharmacokinetics: Unknown.

INDICATIONS & DOSAGE
Superficial skin infections caused by susceptible bacteria –
Adults and children: after thorough cleansing, apply t.i.d. or q.i.d.

CONTRAINDICATIONS & PRECAUTIONS

Contraindicated in patients with minor infections (such as influenza, throat infections, and colds) or as prophylaxis against infection, because potential toxicity may outweigh therapeutic benefit; and in patients with hypersensitivity or history of toxic reaction to the drug.

Use cautiously in infants and in patients with renal or hepatic dysfunction, acute intermittent porphyria, or glucose-6-phosphate dehydrogenase (G6PD) deficiency because of potential for adverse hematopoietic effects (including gray syndrome).

ADVERSE REACTIONS

Common reactions are in italics; life-threatening reactions are in bold italics.

Skin: possible contact sensitivity; itching, burning, urticaria, angioneurotic edema in patients hypersensitive to any of the components.

Other: ***blood dyscrasias*** (including ***bone marrow hypoplasia*** and ***aplastic anemia).***

INTERACTIONS

None significant.

EFFECTS ON DIAGNOSTIC TESTS

None reported.

NURSING CONSIDERATIONS

Besides those related universally to drug therapy (see "How to use this book"), consider the following specific recommendations:

Assessment

- Obtain a baseline assessment of skin infection before therapy.
- Be alert for adverse reactions and drug interactions throughout therapy.
- Evaluate the patient's and family's knowledge about chloramphenicol therapy.

Nursing Diagnoses

- Impaired skin integrity related to skin infection.
- Altered protection related to drug-induced adverse reactions.
- Knowledge deficit related to chloramphenicol therapy.

Planning and Implementation

Preparation and Administration

- ***Topical use:*** Cleanse area before application.

Monitoring

- Monitor effectiveness of drug by examining patient's skin.
- Monitor patient carefully. If condition worsens or does not improve, discontinue use and notify doctor.
- Monitor for adverse reactions or drug interactions by reviewing the patient's blood count; drug may cause aplastic anemia.
- Monitor vital signs.

Supportive Care

- Prolonged use may cause overgrowth of nonsusceptible organisms.
- Topical use of this drug should be supplemented by appropriate systemic medication for all but very superficial infections.
- Discontinue drug if signs of hypersensitivity develops and notify doctor.
- Provide relief from chills, fever, myalgias, and weakness if the patient becomes anemic.

Patient Teaching

- Teach patient to apply medication.
- Tell patient to continue using for full treatment period prescribed, even if condition has improved.
- Teach the patient protective measures: how to conserve energy, obtain adequate rest and eat balanced, nutritious meals.
- Promote personal and environmental cleanliness.

Evaluation

In patients receiving chloramphenicol, appropriate evaluation statements may include:

- Skin infection has resolved.
- The patient does not develop drug-induced aplastic anemia.
- Patient and family state an understanding of chloramphenicol therapy.

chlordiazepoxide

(klor dye az e pox´ ide)
Libritabs

chlordiazepoxide hydrochloride

Apo-Chlordiazepoxide†, Librium, Lipoxide, Medilium†, Mitran, Novopoxide†, Reposans, Sereen, Solium†

- Controlled Substance Schedule IV
- *Classification:* sedative-hypnotic (benzodiazepine)
- *Pregnancy Risk Category:* D

HOW SUPPLIED

chlordiazepoxide
Tablets: 5 mg, 10 mg, 25 mg
chlordiazepoxide hydrochloride
Capsules: 5 mg, 10 mg, 25 mg
Powder for injection: 100 mg/ampule

ACTION

Mechanism: Depresses the CNS at the limbic and subcortical levels of the brain.
Absorption: Well absorbed orally; I.M. administration results in erratic absorption.
Distribution: Enters CNS and crosses placenta; 80% to 90% protein-bound.
Metabolism: In the liver to active metabolites (demoxepam, desmethylchlordiazepoxide, desmethyldiazepam, and oxazepam) as well as inactive metabolites.
Excretion: Most metabolites of chlordiazepoxide are excreted in urine as glucuronide conjugates. Half-life: Chlordiazepoxide, 5 to 30 hours; demoxepam, 14 to 95 hours; desmethylchlordiazepoxide, 18 hours; desmethyldiazepam, 30 to 200 hours; and oxazepam, 3 to 21 hours.
Onset, peak, duration: After oral administration, action begins in 30 to 45 minutes and peaks in 1 to 3 hours. I.M. administration has onset of action in 15 to 30 minutes. After I.V. injection, onset occurs in 1 to 5 minutes.

INDICATIONS & DOSAGE

Mild to moderate anxiety and tension–
Adults: 5 to 10 mg P.O. t.i.d. or q.i.d.
Children over 6 years: 5 mg P.O. b.i.d. to q.i.d. Maximum dosage is 10 mg P.O. b.i.d. to t.i.d.
Severe anxiety and tension–
Adults: 20 to 25 mg P.O. t.i.d. or q.i.d.
Withdrawal symptoms of acute alcoholism–
Adults: 50 to 100 mg P.O., I.M., or I.V. Maximum dosage is 300 mg daily.
Preoperative apprehension and anxiety–
Adults: 5 to 10 mg P.O. t.i.d. or q.i.d. on day preceding surgery; or 50 to 100 mg I.M. 1 hour before surgery.

Note: Parenteral form not recommended in children under 12 years.

CONTRAINDICATIONS & PRECAUTIONS

Contraindicated in patients with hypersensitivity to the drug; acute narrow-angle glaucoma or untreated open-angle glaucoma because of possible anticholinergic effect; shock or coma because the drug's hypnotic or hypotensive effect may be prolonged or intensified; acute alcohol intoxication who have depressed vital signs because the drug will worsen CNS depression; and in infants younger than age 30 days in whom slow metabolism causes the drug to accumulate.

Use cautiously in patients with psychoses because drug is rarely beneficial in such patients and may induce paradoxical reactions; in patients with myasthenia gravis or Parkinson's disease because drug may exacerbate the disorder; in patients with impaired renal or hepatic function, which prolongs elimination of the drug; in elderly or debilitated patients, who are usually more sensitive to the drug's CNS effects; and in individuals prone to addiction or drug abuse.

ADVERSE REACTIONS

Common reactions are in italics; life-threatening reactions are in bold italics.
CNS: *drowsiness, lethargy, hangover,* fainting.
CV: transient hypotension.
GI: nausea, vomiting, abdominal discomfort.
Local: *pain at injection site.*

INTERACTIONS

Alcohol, other CNS depressants: increased CNS depression. Avoid concomitant use.
Cimetidine: increased sedation. Monitor carefully.

EFFECTS ON DIAGNOSTIC TESTS

EEG patterns: minor changes during and after therapy (low-voltage, fast activity).
Liver function tests: elevated results.
Pregnancy test: false-positive results, depending on method used.
Urine 17-ketosteroids (Zimmerman reaction), urine alkaloid determination (Frings thin-layer chromatography method), and urine glucose determinations (with Clinistix and Diastix, but not Tes-Tape): test interference.

NURSING CONSIDERATIONS

Besides those related universally to drug therapy (see "How to use this book"), consider the following specific recommendations:

Assessment
- Obtain a baseline assessment of the patient's anxiety level before drug therapy.
- Be alert for adverse reactions and drug interactions throughout therapy.
- Evaluate the patient's and family's knowledge about chlordiazepoxide therapy.

Nursing Diagnoses
- Anxiety related to the patient's underlying condition.
- High risk for injury related to chlordiazepoxide-induced CNS reactions.
- Knowledge deficit related to chlordiazepoxide therapy.

Planning and Implementation
Preparation and Administration
- Make sure the patient has swallowed the tablets before leaving the bedside.
- ***I.V use:*** Do not mix injectable form with any other parenteral drug. Use 5 ml of saline injection or sterile water or injection as diluent; do not give packaged diluent I.V. Give slowly over 1 minute.
- This drug may be given I.V., although package recommends I.M. use.
- Injectable form (as hydrochloride) comes in two ampules–diluent and powdered drug. Read directions carefully.
- ***I.M. use:*** Add 2 ml of diluent to powder and agitate gently until clear. Use immediately. I.M. form may be erratically absorbed.
- Store powder away from light and in the refrigerator; mix just before use; discard remainder.
- Dosage should be reduced in elderly or debilitated patients.

Monitoring
- Regularly monitor effectiveness by asking the patient about feelings of anxiety and by evaluating the patient's behavior.
- Monitor for adverse reactions by frequently checking his vital signs for hypotension.
- Monitor for possible abuse and addiction.
- If nausea and vomiting occur, evaluate the patient's hydration status.

Supportive Care
- Provide encouragement and support with other measures, such as professional counseling.

• If drowsiness, lethargy, or fainting occurs, institute safety measures, such as supervising patient activities. Reorient patient as needed and ensure a safe environment.
• Be aware that drug should not be prescribed regularly for everyday stress.
• Do not withdraw drug abruptly. Abuse or addiction is possible and withdrawal symptoms may occur.
Patient Teaching
• Warn the patient not to combine drug with alcohol or other CNS depressants and to avoid driving and other hazardous activities that require alertness and psychomotor coordination until adverse CNS effects of the drug are known.
• Caution the patient against giving medication to others.
• Warn the patient to take this drug only as directed and not discontinue it without the doctor's approval. Inform the patient of the drug's potential for dependence if taken longer than directed.
Evaluation
In patients receiving chlordiazepoxide, appropriate evaluation statements may include:
• Patient states he is less anxious.
• Patient does not experience injury as a result of adverse CNS reactions.
• Patient and family state an understanding of chlordiazepoxide therapy.

chloroprocaine hydrochloride
(klor oh proe´ kane)
Nesacaine, Nesacaine MPF

• *Classification:* local anesthetic
• *Pregnancy Risk Category:* C

HOW SUPPLIED
Nesacaine
Injection (for infiltration and regional anesthesia): 1%, 2%
Nesacaine MPF
Injection (preservative-free, for caudal and epidural anesthesia): 2%, 3%

ACTION
Mechanism: Blocks depolarization by interfering with sodium-potassium exchange across the nerve cell membrane, preventing generation and conduction of the nerve impulse.
Absorption: Slowly absorbed into the systemic circulation.
Metabolism: In the plasma, by pseudocholinesterase.
Excretion: Metabolites are excreted by the kidneys.
Onset, peak, duration: Shorter than procaine; 1% or 2% solutions without epinephrine exhibit an onset of 6 to 12 minutes and a duration of 30 minutes to 1 hour. Adding epinephrine 1:200,000 prolongs duration to 1 to 1½ hours.

INDICATIONS & DOSAGE
Infiltration and nerve block:
Adults: dosage limit is 11 mg/kg (14 mg/kg when used with epinephrine).

Sol.	Vol. (ml)	Dose (mg)
1%	3 to 20	30 to 200
2%	2 to 40	40 to 800

Caudal and epidural:

Sol.	Vol. (ml)	Dose (mg)
2% to 3%	15 to 25	300 to 750

May repeat with smaller doses q 40 to 50 minutes. Dose and interval may be increased with epinephrine. Maximum adult dosage is 800 mg, or 1 g when mixed with epinephrine.

CONTRAINDICATIONS & PRECAUTIONS
Contraindicated in patients hypersensitive to the drug or other ester-type anesthetics; in patients with myasthenia gravis; in patients with severe cardiac disease, including severe shock or impaired cardiac conduction. Use cautiously in patients with hepatic disease. Because they are me-

tabolized by plasma choliesterases, ester-type local anesthetics should be used with extreme caution, if at all, in patients with low plasma cholinesterase activity. Some clinicians suggest that ester-type local anesthetics should be avoided in patients receiving sulfonamides or aminosalicylic acid because these anesthetics are hydrolyzed to aminobenzoic acid derivatives which may antagonize their effects.

Contraindications to epidural or spinal anesthesia include serious diseases of the CNS and spinal cord, such as meningitis, tumors, cranial or spinal hemorrhage, poliomyelitis, syphilis, tuberculosis, or metastatic diseases of the spinal cord.

Local anesthetics should only be used by clinicians familiar with proper administration techniques. Individuals using these drugs should be familiar with the diagnosis and management of local anesthetic toxicity. Patients with mild-to-moderate cardiac disease, hyperthyroidism, or other endocrine abnormalities may be especially susceptible to the toxic effects of local anesthetics.

ADVERSE REACTIONS

Common reactions are in italics; life-threatening reactions are in bold italics.
Skin: dermatologic reactions.
Other: edema, status asthmaticus, ***anaphylaxis,*** anaphylactoid reactions.
The following systemic effects may result from high blood levels of the drug:
CNS: anxiety, nervousness, seizures followed by drowsiness, unconsciousness, tremors, twitches, shivering, ***respiratory arrest.***
CV: myocardial depression, ***arrhythmias, cardiac arrest.***
EENT: blurred vision, tinnitus.
GI: nausea, vomiting.

INTERACTIONS

None significant.

EFFECTS ON DIAGNOSTIC TESTS

None reported.

NURSING CONSIDERATIONS

Besides those related universally to drug therapy (see "How to use this book"), consider the following specific recommendations:

Assessment

- Obtain a baseline assessment of the patient's sensory status before therapy.
- Be alert for adverse reactions and drug interactions throughout therapy.
- Evaluate the patient's and family's knowledge about chloroprocaine hydrochloride therapy.

Nursing Diagnoses

- Pain related to inadequate block.
- Decreased cardiac output related to adverse reaction to chloroprocaine.
- Knowledge deficit related to chloroprocaine therapy.

Planning and Implementation

Preparation and Administration

- ***Epidural use:*** Be aware that for epidural use, test doses are administered to verify needle or catheter placement. Initially, 2 to 3 ml is given to check for subarachnoid injection (which would cause extensive motor paralysis of the lower limbs and extensive sensory deficit). After about 5 minutes and in the absence of symptoms, a second, larger test dose of about 5 ml is given to check for intravascular injection (which would cause tinnitus, numbness around the lips, metallic taste, dysphoria, lethargy, or hypotension). Repeat test dose if patient is moved in a way that might displace the epidural catheter. At least 5 minutes should elapse after each test dose before proceding further.
- Don't use discolored solution.
- Don't use solution with preservative for caudal or epidural block.
- Discard partially used vials without preservatives.
- Check solution for particles.

Monitoring
• Monitor effectiveness by evaluating pain relief. Continue to monitor sensory level every 15 minutes after completion of surgery or other treatment until sympathetic innervation return.
• Monitor for signs of anaphylaxis after administration of drug.
• Monitor for evidence of myocardial depression as well as respiratory depression, seizures, and other adverse reactions, which may result from high blood levels of the drug.
Supportive Care
• Keep resuscitative equipment and drugs available.
• Consult with the doctor if pain relief is ineffective.
• Be aware that duration of action is 30 minutes to 1 hour.
• Notify the doctor immediately if the patient's CNS, cardiac or respiratory status deteriorates.
• Keep patient flat until sympathetic return has been established in order to prevent hypotension.
Patient Teaching
• Explain that the drug will cause a local loss of sensation providing pain relief in the selected body area, but unlike general anesthesia, will not cause unconsciousness.
• Describe the route of administration: infiltration, epidural, caudal, spinal, or nerve block.
Evaluation
In patients receiving chloroprocaine, appropriate evaluation statements may include:
• Effective sensory block achieved.
• Cardiac status within normal limits.
• Patient and family state an understanding of chloroprocaine therapy.

chloroquine hydrochloride
(klor´ o kwin)
Aralen HCl, Chlorquin‡

chloroquine phosphate
Aralen Phosphate, Chlorquin‡

chloroquine sulphate
Nivaquine‡

• *Classification:* antimalarial, amebicide, anti-inflammatory agent (4-aminoquinoline)
• *Pregnancy Risk Category:* C

HOW SUPPLIED
hydrochloride
Injection: 50 mg/ml (40-mg/ml base)
phosphate
Tablets: 250 mg (150-mg base), 500 mg (300-mg base)
sulphate
Tablets: 200 mg (150-mg base)
Syrup: 68 mg (50-mg base)/5 ml

ACTION
Mechanism: As an antimalarial, may bind to and alter the properties of DNA in susceptible parasites. Mechanism of action of amebicide is unknown.
Absorption: Readily and almost completely after oral administration. Food may increase the extent of absorption, but apparently does not alter the absorption rate.
Distribution: 55% bound to plasma proteins. It concentrates in the liver, spleen, kidneys, heart, and brain and is strongly bound in melanin-containing cells.
Metabolism: About 30% of dose is metabolized by the liver to monodesethylchloroquine and bidesethylchloroquine.
Excretion: About 70% of dose is excreted unchanged in urine; unabsorbed drug is excreted in feces; some also excreted in breast milk. Small amounts may be present in urine for months after the drug is discontinued. Renal excretion is enhanced by urinary acidification.
Onset, peak, duration: Peak plasma concentrations occur at 1 to 2 hours.

INDICATIONS & DOSAGE

Suppressive prophylaxis and treatment of acute attacks of malaria due to Plasmodium vivax, P. malariae, P. ovale, *and susceptible strains of* P. falciparum–
Adults: initially, 600 mg (base) P.O., then 300 mg P.O. at 6, 24, and 48 hours. Or 160 to 200 mg (base) I.M. initially; repeat in 6 hours if needed. Switch to oral therapy as soon as possible.
Children: initially, 10 mg (base)/kg P.O., then 5 mg (base)/kg dose P.O. at 6, 24, and 48 hours (do not exceed adult dose). Or 5 mg (base)/kg I.M. initially; repeat in 6 hours if needed. Switch to oral therapy as soon as possible.
Malaria suppressive treatment–
Adults and children: 5 mg (base)/kg P.O. (not to exceed 300 mg) weekly on same day of the week (begin 2 weeks before entering endemic area and continue for 8 weeks after leaving). If treatment begins after exposure, double the initial dose (600 mg for adults, 10 mg/kg for children) in 2 divided doses P.O. 6 hours apart.
Extraintestinal amebiasis–
Adults: 160 to 200 mg chloroquine (hydrochloride) base I.M. daily for no more than 12 days. As soon as possible, substitute 1 g (600 mg base) chloroquine phosphate P.O. daily for 2 days; then 500 mg (300 mg base) daily for at least 2 to 3 weeks. Treatment is usually combined with an effective intestinal amebicide.
Children: 10 mg/kg of chloroquine (hydrochloride) base for 2 to 3 weeks. Maximum 300 mg daily.
Rheumatoid arthritis and lupus erythematosus–
250 mg chloroquine phosphate daily with evening meal.

CONTRAINDICATIONS & PRECAUTIONS

Contraindicated in patients who have experienced retinal or visual field changes or hypersensitivity reactions to 4-aminoquinoline compounds unless these compounds are the only ones to which the malarial strain is sensitive.

Use cautiously in patients with psoriasis, porphyria, or glucose-6-phosphate dehydrogenase (G6PD) deficiency because the drug may exacerbate these conditions. Because chloroquine concentrates in the liver and may cause adverse hepatic effects, it should be used cautiously in patients with hepatic disease or alcoholism and in those receiving other hepatotoxic drugs.

ADVERSE REACTIONS

Common reactions are in italics; life-threatening reactions are in bold italics.
Blood: ***agranulocytosis, aplastic anemia, hemolytic anemia,*** thrombocytopenia.
CNS: mild and transient headache, neuromyopathy, psychic stimulation, fatigue, irritability, nightmares, seizures, dizziness.
CV: hypotension, ECG changes.
EENT: *visual disturbances* (blurred vision; difficulty in focusing; reversible corneal changes; generally irreversible, sometimes progressive or delayed, retinal changes, such as narrowing of arterioles; macular lesions; pallor of optic disk; optic atrophy; patchy retinal pigmentation, often leading to blindness); ototoxicity (nerve deafness, vertigo, tinnitus).
GI: anorexia, abdominal cramps, diarrhea, nausea, vomiting, stomatitis.
Skin: pruritus, lichen planus-like eruptions, skin and mucosal pigmentary changes, pleomorphic skin eruptions.

INTERACTIONS

Magnesium and aluminum salts, kaolin: decreased GI absorption. Separate administration times.

EFFECTS ON DIAGNOSTIC TESTS

ECG: inversion or depression of the T wave; widening of the QRS complex.

WBC, RBC, platelet counts: decreased.

NURSING CONSIDERATIONS

Besides those related universally to drug therapy (see "How to use this book"), consider the following specific recommendations:

Assessment

• Obtain a baseline assessment of infection before therapy.

• Be alert for adverse reactions and drug interactions throughout therapy.

• Evaluate the patient's and family's knowledge about chloroquine therapy.

Nursing Diagnoses

• High risk for injury related to ineffective drug dosage.

• Sensory/perceptual alterations (visual or auditory) related to adverse reactions to chloroquine.

• Knowledge deficit related to chloroquine.

Planning and Implementation

Preparation and Administration

• Administer chloroquine at the same time of the same day each week.

• Missed doses should be given as soon as possible. To avoid doubling doses in regimens requiring more than one dose per day, administer the missed dose within 1 hour of scheduled time or omit the dose.

• ***P.O. use:*** Administer with milk or meals to minimize GI distress. Tablets may be crushed and mixed with food or chocolate syrup for patients with difficulty swallowing; however, the drug has a bitter taste and patients may find the mixture unpleasant. The crushed tablets may be placed inside empty gelatin capsules, which are easier to swallow.

• ***I.M. use:*** Substitute oral administration as soon as possible.

• Store drug in amber-colored containers to protect from light.

• Be aware that prophylactic antimalarial therapy should begin 2 weeks before exposure and should continue for 6 to 8 weeks after patient leaves the endemic area.

Monitoring

• Monitor effectiveness by regularly assessing for improvement of infection.

• Monitor the patient's weight for significant changes because dosage is calculated by patient's weight.

• Monitor patient for visual or auditory disturbances. Patient should have regular ophthalmologic and audiometric examinations before, during, and after therapy, especially if prolonged. Check patient periodically for ocular muscle weakness after prolonged use.

• Monitor CBC and liver function studies during prolonged therapy.

Supportive Care

• Notify doctor immediately if patient shows signs of severe blood disorder not attributable to disease under treatment. Discontinuation of drug may be required.

• Alert doctor to any significant weight changes in patient.

• Institute safety precautions if visual disturbances or adverse CNS reactions occur.

• Maintain seizure precautions throughout chloroquine therapy.

Patient Teaching

• To avoid exacerbated drug-induced dermatoses, warn the patient to avoid excessive exposure to sun.

• Review methods for reducing exposure to mosquitoes for the patient receiving this drug prophylactically.

• Warn the patient to avoid alcohol while taking this drug.

• Tell the patient to keep drug out of children's reach. Fatalities have followed accidental ingestion of as few as 3 or 4 tablets.

• Tell the patient to take drug with meals on the same day each week.

• Instruct patient how to take missed doses.

• Advise the patient to have regular ophthalmologic examinations and to report blurred vision, increased sensitivity to light, or muscle weakness as well as hearing changes.
• Advise the woman of childbearing age who is traveling to an endemic area to avoid pregnancy. Instruct her to continue contraceptive precautions for 2 months after the last dose of chloroquine.

Evaluation

In patients receiving chloroquine, appropriate evaluation statements may include:
• Patient is free of infection.
• Patient maintains normal visual and auditory function throughout chloroquine therapy.
• Patient and family state an understanding of chloroquine therapy.

chlorothiazide

(klor oh thye´ a zide)

Azide‡, Chlotride‡, Diachlor, Diuret‡, Diurigen, Diuril

chlorothiazide sodium

Diuril Sodium

• *Classification:* diuretic, antihypertensive (thiazide)
• *Pregnancy Risk Category:* D

HOW SUPPLIED

Tablets: 250 mg, 500 mg
Oral suspension: 250 mg/5 ml
Injection: 500-mg vial

ACTION

Mechanism: A thiazide diuretic that increases urine excretion of sodium and water by inhibiting sodium reabsorption in the cortical diluting site of the nephron.
Absorption: Incompletely and variably absorbed from the GI tract.
Distribution: Enters the extracellular space.
Metabolism: None.
Excretion: Unchanged in urine.

INDICATIONS & DOSAGE

Edema, hypertension–
Adults: 500 mg to 2 g P.O. or I.V. daily or in two divided doses.
Diuresis–
Children over 6 months: 20 mg/kg P.O. or I.V. daily in divided doses.
Children under 6 months: may require 30 mg/kg P.O. or I.V. daily in two divided doses.

CONTRAINDICATIONS & PRECAUTIONS

Contraindicated in patients with anuria and in those with sensitivity to the drug or to other sulfonamide derivatives. Use cautiously in patients with severe renal disease because it may decrease glomerular filtration rate and precipitate azotemia; in patients with impaired hepatic function or liver disease because electrolyte changes may precipitate coma; and in patients taking digoxin because hypokalemia may predispose them to digitalis toxicity.

ADVERSE REACTIONS

Common reactions are in italics; life-threatening reactions are in bold italics.
Blood: ***aplastic anemia, agranulocytosis,*** leukopenia, thrombocytopenia.
CV: *volume depletion and dehydration,* orthostatic hypotension.
GI: anorexia, nausea, pancreatitis.
Hepatic: hepatic encephalopathy.
Metabolic: *hypokalemia, asymptomatic hyperuricemia, hyperglycemia and impairment of glucose tolerance,* fluid and electrolyte imbalances including dilutional hyponatremia and hypochloremia, metabolic alkalosis, hypercalcemia, gout.
Skin: dermatitis, photosensitivity, rash.
Other: hypersensitivity such as pneumonitis and vasculitis.

INTERACTIONS

Cholestyramine, colestipol: intestinal absorption of thiazides decreased. Keep doses as separate as possible.
Diazoxide: increased antihypertensive, hyperglycemic, and hyperuricemic effects. Use together cautiously.
NSAIDs: decreased diuretic effectiveness. Avoid concomitant use.

EFFECTS ON DIAGNOSTIC TESTS

Serum electrolytes: altered levels.
Serum urate, glucose, cholesterol, and triglycerides: increased levels.
Parathyroid function tests: test interference. Drug should be discontinued before such tests.

NURSING CONSIDERATIONS

Besides those related universally to drug therapy (see "How to use this book"), consider the following specific recommendations:

Assessment

- Obtain a baseline assessment of blood pressure, serum electrolytes, urine output, weight, and peripheral edema before initiating drug therapy.
- Be alert for adverse reactions and drug interactions throughout therapy.
- Evaluate the patient's and family's knowledge about chlorothiazide therapy.

Nursing Diagnoses

- Fluid volume excess related to the patient's underlying condition as evidenced by edema.
- Altered urinary elimination related to chlorothiazide therapy.
- Knowledge deficit related to chlorothiazide therapy.

Planning and Implementation

Preparation and Administration

- ***P.O. use:*** If possible, give drug early in the day to prevent nocturia. Administer with food to enhance absorption.
- ***I.V. use:*** Reconstitute 500 mg with 18 ml of sterile water for injection. May store reconstituted solutions at room temperature up to 24 hours. Compatible with I.V. dextrose or sodium chloride solutions. Inject reconstituted drug directly into vein, through an I.V. line containing a free-flowing compatible solution, or through an intermittent infusion device. Also may be administered as an intermittent infusion; follow doctor's orders for administration.
- Parenteral solution should never be administered I.M. or S.C.

Monitoring

- Monitor effectiveness by regularly checking blood pressure, urine output, and weight.
- Monitor serum electrolytes, calcium, BUN, creatinine, glucose, and uric acid levels.
- Monitor CBC, differential, and platelet count.
- Monitor the patient receiving concomitant digitalis therapy for increased risk of digitalis toxicity.
- Monitor for signs of hypokalemia (for example, muscle weakness and cramps).
- Monitor the diabetic patient's insulin requirements because chlorothiazide has hyperglycemic effects.
- Monitor skin turgor and mucous membranes for signs of fluid volume deficit.
- Monitor elderly patients closely because they are especially susceptible to excessive diuresis.

Supportive Care

- Hold drug and notify the doctor if hypersensitivity reactions occur.
- Keep accurate records of intake and output, blood pressure, and weight.
- Provide frequent skin and mouth care to relieve dryness from diuretic therapy.
- Answer the patient's call bells promptly; make sure patient's bathroom or bedpan is easily accessible.
- Use safety precautions to minimize risk of falling due to hypotension.
- In the patient undergoing tests of parathyroid function, hold thiazide

and thiazidelike drugs before these tests are performed.
• Be aware that optimal antihypertensive effect may not occur for several days after beginning of therapy with chlorothiazide.
• Elevate the patient's legs to aid relief of peripheral edema.
• Administer potassium supplements as indicated and provide a high-potassium diet.
• Avoid I.V. infiltration; can be very painful.

Patient Teaching
• Teach the patient and family to identify and report signs of hypersensitivity reaction and hypokalemia.
• Teach the patient and family to monitor the patient's fluid volume by recording daily weight and intake and output.
• Inform the patient that optimal therapeutic response may not occur until several days after beginning chlorothiazide therapy.
• Teach the patient to avoid high-sodium and to choose high-potassium foods.
• Advise the patient to change positions slowly, especially when rising to standing position, to avoid dizziness and fainting due to orthostatic hypotension.
• Advise the patient to minimize risks of photosensitivity reaction by using a sunscreen when outdoors.
• Advise the diabetic patient that insulin dosage may require adjustment.
• Advise the patient who is taking digitalis that the drug's potassium-depleting effect may increase the risk of digitalis toxicity.
• Advise the patient to take chlorothiazide early in the day to avoid interruptions of sleep due to nocturia and to take with food to enhance absorption.

Evaluation
In patients receiving chlorothiazide, appropriate evaluation statements may include:
• Patient is free of edema.
• Patient demonstrates adjustment of life-style to deal with altered patterns of urinary elimination.
• Patient and family state an understanding of chlorothiazide therapy.

chlorotrianisene
(klor oh trye an´ i seen)
TACE**

• *Classification:* estrogen replacement, antineoplastic (estrogen)
• *Pregnancy Risk Category:* X

HOW SUPPLIED
Capsules: 12 mg, 25 mg

ACTION
Mechanism: Increases the synthesis of DNA, RNA, and protein in responsive tissues. Also reduces follicle-stimulating hormone and luteinizing hormone release from the pituitary.
Distribution: Stored in fat tissue, which may delay the onset of action as well as prolong the drug's effects. Estrogens are 50% to 80% bound to plasma proteins; they cross the placenta.
Metabolism: Probably hepatic.

INDICATIONS & DOSAGE
Prostatic cancer–
Men: 12 to 25 mg P.O. daily.
Atrophic vaginitis–
Women: 12 to 25 mg P.O. daily for 30 to 60 days.
Female hypogonadism–
Women: 12 to 25 mg P.O. for 21 days, followed by 1 dose of progesterone 100 mg I.M. or 5 days of oral progestogen given concurrently with last 5 days of chlorotrianisene (for example, medroxyprogesterone 5 to 10 mg).

Menopausal symptoms–
Women: 12 to 25 mg P.O. daily for 30 days or cyclic (3 weeks on, 1 week off).

CONTRAINDICATIONS & PRECAUTIONS

Contraindicated in patients with thrombophlebitis or thromboembolism, estrogen-responsive carcinoma (breast or genital tract cancer), or undiagnosed abnormal genital bleeding because the drug may aggravate these disorders; and during pregnancy and breast-feeding.

Use cautiously in patients with disorders that may be aggravated by fluid and electrolyte accumulation, such as asthma, seizure disorders, migraine, or cardiac, renal, or hepatic dysfunction. Carefully monitor female patients who have breast nodules, fibrocystic breast disease, or a family history of breast cancer. Because of the risk of thromboembolism, therapy with this drug should be discontinued at least 1 week before elective surgical procedures associated with an increased incidence of thromboembolism.

Chlorotrianisene capsules contain tartrazine, which may induce allergic reactions in aspirin-sensitive individuals.

ADVERSE REACTIONS

Common reactions are in italics; life-threatening reactions are in bold italics.
CNS: headache, dizziness, chorea, migraine, depression, libido changes.
CV: thrombophlebitis; ***thromboembolism;*** hypertension; edema; *increased risk of stroke,* ***pulmonary embolism, and myocardial infarction.***
EENT: worsening of myopia or astigmatism, intolerance to contact lenses.
GI: *nausea,* vomiting, abdominal cramps, bloating, diarrhea, constipation, anorexia, increased appetite, excessive thirst, weight changes, pancreatitis.
GU: in women–breakthrough bleeding, altered menstrual flow, dysmenorrhea, amenorrhea, cervical erosion or abnormal secretions, enlargement of uterine fibromas, vaginal candidiasis. In men–*gynecomastia, testicular atrophy, impotence.*
Hepatic: cholestatic jaundice.
Metabolic: hyperglycemia, hypercalcemia, folic acid deficiency.
Skin: melasma, urticaria, acne, seborrhea, oily skin, hirsutism or loss of hair.
Other: leg cramps, purpura, breast changes (tenderness, enlargement, secretion).

INTERACTIONS

None significant.

EFFECTS ON DIAGNOSTIC TESTS

Blood glucose: increased levels in diabetic patients necessitating dosage adjustment of insulin or oral hypoglycemic drugs.
Coagulation studies: potential to decrease the effects of warfarin-type anticoagulants.

NURSING CONSIDERATIONS

Besides those related universally to drug therapy (see "How to use this book"), consider the following specific recommendations:

Assessment
- Obtain a baseline assessment of the underlying condition before initiating therapy with chlorotrianisene.
- Be alert for adverse reactions and drug interactions throughout therapy.
- Evaluate the patient's and family's knowledge about chlorotrianisene therapy.

Nursing Diagnoses
- Sexual dysfunction related to the patient's hormonal deficiency.
- Altered cerebral, peripheral, pulmonary, or myocardial tissue perfusion related to potential for chlorotrianisene to cause thromboembolism.

• Knowledge deficit related to therapy with chlorotrianisene.

Plannning and Implementation

Preparation and Administration

• *P.O. use:* Administer oral preparations at mealtimes or bedtime (if only one daily dose is required) to minimize nausea.

Monitoring

• Monitor effectiveness by regularly assessing the underlying condition for signs of improvement.

• Monitor patient for thromboemboli formation by noting any changes in cerebral or cardiopulmonary function or peripheral circulation.

• Monitor the patient's blood glucose levels for alterations.

• Monitor patient for water retention; weigh daily.

Supportive Care

• Withhold drug and notify the doctor if a thromboembolic event is suspected; be prepared to provide supportive care as indicated.

• Alert the pathologist if a specimen is obtained during chlorotrianisene therapy.

• Be prepared to adjust diabetic patients' therapeutic regimen if blood glucose levels rise during therapy with chlorotrianisene.

• Institute safety measures if adverse CNS reactions occur.

• Obtain an order for an antiemetic, antidiarrheal, or laxative agent, as needed.

• Prepare patient for body changes that may occur, such as loss of hair.

• Limit patient's sodium intake if fluid retention occurs and it is not contraindicated.

Patient Teaching

• Warn the patient to report immediately abdominal pain; pain, numbness, or stiffness in legs or buttocks; pressure or pain in chest; shortness of breath; severe headaches; visual disturbances, such as blind spots, flashing lights, or blurriness; vaginal bleeding or discharge; breast lumps; swelling of hands or feet; yellow skin and sclera; dark urine; and light-colored stools.

• Tell male patients on long-term therapy about possible gynecomastia and impotence, which will disappear when therapy is terminated.

• Explain to patients on cyclic therapy for postmenopausal symptoms that, although withdrawal bleeding may occur in week off drug, fertility has not been restored; ovulation does not occur.

• Teach female patients how to perform routine breast self-examination.

• Inform the patient that nausea usually disappears with continued therapy, and can be relieved by taking medication at mealtimes or bedtime (if only one daily dose is required).

• Tell diabetic patients to report symptoms of hyperglycemia or glycosuria.

• Give the patient the package insert describing adverse reactions to chlorotrianisene, and also provide verbal explanation.

• Instruct patient to limit sodium intake if not contraindicated.

Evaluation

In patients receiving chlorotrianisene, appropriate evaluation statements may include:

• Patient exhibits improved health as a result of chlorotrianisene therapy.

• Patient does not experience a thromboembolic event during chlorotrianisene therapy.

• Patient and family state an understanding of chlorotrianisene therapy.

chlorphenesin carbamate

(klor fen´ e sin)

Maolate**

• *Classification:* skeletal muscle relaxant (carbamate derivative)

• *Pregnancy Risk Category:* C

HOW SUPPLIED

Tablets: 400 mg

ACTION

Mechanism: A centrally acting skeletal muscle relaxant that reduces transmission of impulses from the spinal cord to skeletal muscle.
Absorption: Rapidly and completely absorbed from the GI tract.
Distribution: Unknown.
Metabolism: Partially metabolized in the liver.
Excretion: Rapidly excreted in urine, mainly as the glucuronide metabolite and other metabolites. Half-life: 2.3 to 5.1 hours.
Onset, peak, duration: Peak effect occurs in 1 to 3 hours.

INDICATIONS & DOSAGE

As an adjunct in short-term, acute, painful musculoskeletal conditions–
Adults: initial dose is 800 mg P.O. t.i.d. Maintenance dose is 400 mg P.O. q.i.d. for maximum of 8 weeks.

CONTRAINDICATIONS & PRECAUTIONS

Contraindicated in patients with hypersensitivity to the drug. Use cautiously in patients with hepatic or renal impairment because the drug may accumulate in these patients upon chronic administration.

Patients allergic or sensitive to the dye tartrazine (FD&C Yellow No. 5) should not take chlorphenesin. Although tartrazine sensitivity is rare, it frequently occurs in patients sensitive to aspirin.

ADVERSE REACTIONS

Common reactions are in italics; life-threatening reactions are in bold italics.
Blood: thrombocytopenia, leukopenia, ***agranulocytosis.***
CNS: *drowsiness, dizziness,* confusion, headache, weakness. Dose-related adverse reactions include paradoxical stimulation, agitation, insomnia, nervousness, headache.
GI: *nausea, GI distress.*
Other: ***anaphylaxis.***

INTERACTIONS

Alcohol and CNS depressants: increased CNS depression.

EFFECTS ON DIAGNOSTIC TESTS

None reported.

NURSING CONSIDERATIONS

Besides those related universally to drug therapy (see "How to use this book"), consider the following specific recommendations:

Assessment
- Obtain a baseline assessment of the patient's pain related to his underlying condition before drug therpay.
- Be alert for adverse drug reactions and drug interactions throughout therapy.
- Evaluate the patient's and family's knowledge about chlorphenesin carbamate therapy.

Nursing Diagnoses
- Pain related to the patient's underlying condition.
- High risk for injury related to drug-induced drowsiness.
- Knowledge deficit related to chlorphenesin carbamate therapy.

Planning and Implementation

Preparation and Administration
- Give with meals or milk to prevent GI distress.
- Extent of relief determines if dosage (and drowsiness) can be reduced.

Monitoring
- Monitor effectiveness by regularly assessing the severity and frequency of muscle spasms.
- Monitor for adverse reactions by frequently checking the patient's CBC and platelet studies.
- Watch for abnormal bleeding and infections that may indicate blood dyscrasias.
- Monitor for drowsiness.

• Watch for sensivitity reactions, such as insomnia, nervousness, headache, and agitation.
• Know that safety of use for longer than 8 weeks has not been established.
Supportive Care
• Obtain an order for a mild analgesic if he develops a drug-induced headache.
• Institute safety precautions if he develops blurred vision, confusion, or dizziness.
• Be prepared to withhold dosage and notify the doctor at signs of adverse reactions.
• To reduce GI distress, give the drug with milk or meals.
Patient Teaching
• Advise the patient to report respiratory difficulties to the doctor.
• Warn the patient to avoid driving and other hazardous activities that require alertness until CNS effects of drug are known.
• Advise the patient to take the drug with food or milk to prevent GI distress.
Evaluation
In patients receiving chlorphenesin carbamate, appropriate evaluation statements may include:
• Patient reports pain has ceased.
• Patient does not experience injury as a result of drug-induced drowsiness.
• Patient and family state an understanding of chlorphenesin carbamate therapy.

chlorpheniramine maleate
(klor fen ir´ a meen)
Aller-Chlor*◇, Allergex‡, Chlo-Amine◇, Chlor-100◇, Chlorate◇, Chlor-Niramine◇, Chlor-Pro, Chlor-Pro 10, Chlorspan-12, Chlortab-4, Chlortab-8, Chlor-Trimeton*◇, Chlor-Trimeton Repetabs◇, Chlor-Tripolon†◇, Genallerate◇, Novopheniram‡◇, Pfeiffer's Allergy◇, Phenetron*, Piriton‡, Pyranistan◇, Telachlor, Teldrin◇, Trymegen◇

• *Classification:* Histamine 1-receptor antagonist, antihistamine (propylamine derivative)
• *Pregnancy Risk Category:* B

HOW SUPPLIED
Tablets: 4 mg◇
Tablets (chewable): 2 mg◇
Tablets (timed-release): 8 mg◇, 12 mg◇
Capsules (timed-release): 8 mg◇, 12 mg◇
Syrup: 2 mg/5 ml*◇
Injection: 10 mg/ml, 100 mg/ml

ACTION
Mechanism: Blocks the effects of histamine at H_1 receptors. Prevents but does not reverse histamine-mediated responses.
Absorption: Well absorbed from the GI tract; however, some drug is lost to first-pass hepatic metabolism. Food in the stomach delays absorption but does not affect bioavailability.
Distribution: Widely distributed; about 72% protein-bound.
Metabolism: Largely metabolized in GI mucosal cells and liver (first-pass effect).
Excretion: Drug and metabolites are excreted in urine. Half-life: 12 to 43 hours in adults and 10 to 13 hours in children.
Onset, peak, duration: Action begins within 30 minutes to 1 hour and peaks in 2 to 6 hours.

INDICATIONS & DOSAGE
Rhinitis, allergy symptoms–
Adults: 4 mg P.O. q 4 to 6 hours, not to exceed 24 mg/day; or (timed-release) 8 mg P.O. every 12 hours; or 5 to 40 mg I.M., I.V., or S.C. daily. Give I.V. injection over 1 minute.
Children 6 to 12 years: 2 mg P.O. q 4 to 6 hours, not to exceed 12 mg/day.

Alternatively, may give 8 mg (timed-release) at bedtime.
Children 2 to 6 years: 1 mg P.O. q 4 to 6 hours.

Note: Children under 12 years should use only as directed by a doctor.

CONTRAINDICATIONS & PRECAUTIONS

Contraindicated in patients with hypersensitivity to this medication or antihistamines with similar chemical structures, such as dexchlorpheniramine, brompheniramine, or triprolidine; during an acute asthmatic attack because it thickens bronchial secretions; in patients who have taken monoamine oxidase (MAO) inhibitors within the preceding 2 weeks; and during pregnancy (especially in the third trimester) or during breast-feeding. Antihistamines have caused seizures and other severe reactions, especially in premature infants.

Use cautiously in patients with narrow-angle glaucoma; pyloroduodenal obstruction or urinary bladder obstruction from prostatic hypertrophy or narrowing of the bladder neck because of their marked anticholinergic effects; cardiovascular disease, hypertension, or hyperthyroidism because of the risk of palpitations and tachycardia; and renal disease, diabetes, bronchial asthma, urinary retention, or stenosing peptic ulcers.

ADVERSE REACTIONS

Common reactions are in italics; life-threatening reactions are in bold italics.
CNS: *stimulation,* sedation, *drowsiness* (especially in elderly patients), excitability (in children).
CV: hypotension, palpitations.
GI: epigastric distress, *dry mouth.*
GU: urine retention.
Skin: rash, urticaria.
Other: thick bronchial secretions.
After parenteral administration: local stinging, burning sensation, pallor, weak pulse, transient hypotension.

INTERACTIONS

CNS depressants: increased sedation. Use together cautiously.
MAO inhibitors: increased anticholinergic effects. Don't use together.

EFFECTS ON DIAGNOSTIC TESTS

Diagnostic skin tests: test interference.

NURSING CONSIDERATIONS

Besides those related universally to drug therapy (see "How to use this book"), consider the following specific recommendations:

Assessment
• Obtain a baseline assessment of the patient's respiratory status before chlorpheniramine maleate therapy.
• Be alert for adverse reactions and drug interactions throughout therapy.
• Evaluate the patient's and family's knowledge about chlorpheniramine maleate therapy.

Nursing Diagnoses
• Ineffective airway clearance related to the patient's underlying condition.
• High risk for injury related to chlorpheniramine maleate-induced CNS adverse reactions.
• Knowledge deficit related to chlorpheniramine maleate therapy.

Planning and Implementation
Preparation and Administration
• ***P.O. use:*** Give with food or milk to reduce GI distress.
• ***I.V. use:*** Available in 1-ml ampules (concentration of 10 mg/ml). For intermittent infusion, dilute drug with 50 to 100 ml of a compatible solution (most solutions are compatible). Protect from light to prevent discoloration; discard if discolored. Store at room temperature or refrigerate. Only injectable forms without preservatives can be given I.V. Give slowly.

Monitoring
• Monitor effectiveness by frequently checking the patient's respiratory status and evaluating severity of allergy symptoms.
• Monitor the patient for adverse CNS reactions, especially drowsiness in elderly patients and excitability in children.
Supportive Care
• Notify the doctor if you notice tolerance. Doctor may substitute another antihistamine.
• If adverse CNS reactions develop in a hospitalized patient, institute safety measures, such as use of side rails to protect the patient from injury.
• Keep in mind that oral forms of chlorpheniramine maleate are available as a nonprescription item for self-medication by adults; use for children under 12 years of age is not recommended without a doctor's supervision.
• Remember that chlorpheniramine maleate causes less drowsiness than some other antihistamines.
Patient Teaching
• Suggest that patient drink coffee or tea to reduce drowsiness.
• Tell the patient to use sugarless gum, sour hard candy, or ice chips to relieve dry mouth.
• Warn patient to avoid drinking alcoholic beverages during therapy and to avoid hazardous activities that require alertness until CNS adverse effects are known.
• Warn patient to discontinue drug 4 days before allergy skin testing to preserve the accuracy of the tests.

Evaluation

In the patient receiving chlorpheniramine maleate, appropriate evaluation statements may include:
• Patient's allergic symptoms are relieved with chlorpheniramine maleate therapy.
• Patient did not develop chlorpheniramine maleate-induced CNS adverse reactions.
• Patient and family state an understanding of chlorpheniramine maleate therapy.

chlorpromazine hydrochloride
(klor proe´ ma zeen)
Chlorpromanyl†, Largactil†‡, Novo-Chlorpromazine†, Protran‡, Thorazine, Thor-Pram

• *Classification:* antipsychotic, antiemetic (phenothiazine)
• *Pregnancy Risk Category:* C

HOW SUPPLIED
Tablets: 10 mg, 25 mg, 50 mg, 100 mg, 200 mg
Capsules (sustained-release): 30 mg, 75 mg, 150 mg, 200 mg, 300 mg
Oral concentrate: 30 mg/ml, 100 mg/ml
Syrup: 10 mg/5ml
Injection: 25 mg/ml
Suppositories: 25 mg, 100 mg

ACTION
Mechanism: An aliphatic phenothiazine that blocks postsynaptic dopamine receptors in the brain. As an antiemetic, blocks dopamine receptors in the medullary chemoreceptor trigger zone.
Absorption: Rate and extent of absorption vary with route of administration. Oral tablet absorption is erratic and variable; absorption of oral concentrates and syrups is more predictable: I.M. drug is absorbed rapidly.
Distribution: Widely distributed into the body, including breast milk; concentration is usually higher in CNS than in plasma. Drug is 91% to 99% protein-bound.
Metabolism: Extensively by the liver and forms 10 to 12 metabolites; some are pharmacologically active.
Excretion: Most is excreted as metabolites in urine; some is excreted in

feces via the biliary tract. It may undergo enterohepatic circulation.
Onset, peak, duration: With onset ranging from 30 minutes to 1 hour; peak effects occur at 2 to 4 hours and duration of action is 4 to 6 hours. Sustained-release preparations have similar absorption, but action lasts for 10 to 12 hours. Suppositories act in 1 hour and last 3 to 4 hours. Steady-state serum level is achieved within 4 to 7 days.

INDICATIONS & DOSAGE

Intractable hiccups–
Adults: 25 to 50 mg P.O. or I.M. t.i.d. or q.i.d.
Mild alcohol withdrawal, acute intermittent porphyria, and tetanus–
Adults: 25 to 50 mg I.M. t.i.d. or q.i.d.
Psychosis–
Adults: initially, 30 to 75 mg P.O. daily in two to four divided doses. Increase dosage by 20 to 50 mg twice weekly until symptoms are controlled. Up to 800 mg daily may be required in some patients. Or give 25 to 50 mg I.M. q 1 to 4 hours p.r.n. Switch to oral therapy as soon as possible.
Children: 0.25 mg/kg P.O. q 4 to 6 hours; or 0.25 mg/kg I.M. q 6 to 8 hours; or 0.5 mg/kg rectally q 6 to 8 hours. Maximum I.M. dose is 40 mg in children under 5 years, and 75 mg in children 5 to 12 years.
Nausea and vomiting–
Adults: 10 to 25 mg P.O. or I.M. q 4 to 6 hours, p.r.n.; or 50 to 100 mg rectally q 6 to 8 hours, p.r.n.
Children: 0.25 mg/kg P.O. q 4 to 6 hours; or 0.25 mg/kg I.M. q 6 to 8 hours; or 0.5 mg/kg rectally q 6 to 8 hours.

CONTRAINDICATIONS & PRECAUTIONS

Contraindicated in patients with hypersensitivity to phenothiazines and related compounds, including allergic reactions involving hepatic function; blood dyscrasias and bone marrow depression because chlorpromazine may induce agranulocytosis; disorders accompanied by coma, brain damage, or CNS depression because of additive CNS depressant effects; in patients with circulatory collapse or cerebrovascular disease because of the potential for hypotensive or adverse cardiac effects; and for use with adrenergic-blocking agents or spinal or epidural anesthetics because of the drug's alpha-blocking potential.

Use cautiously in patients with cardiac disease (arrhythmias, CHF, angina pectoris, valvular disease, or heart block), encephalitis, Reye's syndrome, head injury, respiratory disease, epilepsy and other seizure disorders, glaucoma, prostatic hypertrophy, urine retention, hepatic or renal dysfunction, Parkinson's disease, pheochromocytoma, or hypocalcemia.

ADVERSE REACTIONS

Common reactions are in italics; life-threatening reactions are in bold italics.
Blood: transient leukopenia, ***agranulocytosis.***
CNS: *extrapyramidal reactions (moderate incidence), sedation (high incidence), tardive dyskinesia,* pseudoparkinsonism, EEG changes, dizziness.
CV: *orthostatic hypotension,* tachycardia, ECG changes.
EENT: ocular changes, *blurred vision.*
GI: *dry mouth, constipation.*
GU: *urine retention,* dark urine, menstrual irregularities, gynecomastia, inhibited ejaculation.
Hepatic: cholestatic jaundice, abnormal liver function tests.
Metabolic: hyperprolactinemia.
Skin: *mild photosensitivity,* dermal allergic reactions.
Local: *pain on I.M. injection,* sterile abscess.
Other: weight gain; increased appe-

tite; rarely, ***neuroleptic malignant syndrome*** (fever, tachycardia, tachypnea, profuse diaphoresis).
After abrupt withdrawal of long-term therapy: gastritis, nausea, vomiting, dizziness, tremors, feeling of warmth or cold, sweating, tachycardia, headache, insomnia.

INTERACTIONS

Alcohol, other CNS depressants: increased CNS depression. Avoid concomitant use.
Antacids: inhibit absorption of oral phenothiazines. Separate antacid and phenothiazine doses by at least 2 hours.
Anticholinergics (including antidepressant and antiparkinsonian agents): increased anticholinergic activity, aggravated parkinsonian symptoms. Use with caution.
Barbiturates, lithium: may decrease phenothiazine effect. Observe patient.
Centrally acting antihypertensive agents: decreased antihypertensive effect.
Lithium: possible decreased response to chlorpromazine. Observe patient.
Oral anticoagulants: decreased anticoagulant effect.
Propranolol: increased levels of both propranolol and chlorpromazine.

EFFECTS ON DIAGNOSTIC TESTS

ECG: quinidine-like effects.
Liver function tests: elevated results.
Urinary porphyrins, urobilinogen, amylase, and 5-HIAA: false-positive results because of darkening of urine by metabolites.
Urine pregnancy tests using human chorionic gonadotropin (HCG): false-positive results.

NURSING CONSIDERATIONS

Besides those related universally to drug therapy (see "How to use this book"), consider the following specific recommendations:

Assessment
- Obtain baseline assessment of patient's underlying condition.
- Be alert for adverse reactions and drug interactions throughout therapy.
- Evaluate the patient's and family's knowledge about chlorpromazine therapy.

Nursing Diagnoses
- Altered health maintenance related to patient's underlying condition.
- Impaired physical mobility related to extrapyramidal effects of adverse drug reactions.
- Knowledge deficit related to chlorpromazine therapy.

Planning and Implementation
Preparation and Administration
- Sustained-release preparations should not be crushed but rather swallowed whole.
- Because oral formulations may cause stomach upset, administer with food or milk.
- Dilute the concentrate in 2 to 4 oz of liquid, preferably water, carbonated drinks, fruit juice, tomato juice, milk, puddings, or applesauce.
- Shake the syrup before administration.
- Store suppositories in a cool place.
- Avoid skin contact with the injectable or liquid form because it may cause a rash.

Monitoring
- Regularly observe the patient and notice if symptoms have abated or diminished.
- Observe for adverse reactions, such as extrapyramidal or other CNS symptoms, cholinergic effects (blurred vision, dry mouth, constipation, urine retention), or allergic reactions.
- Monitor weekly bilirubin tests during the first month of therapy; regular blood tests (CBC and liver function), and ophthalmic tests during prolonged use.
- Observe the patient for orthostatic hypotension, especially after paren-

teral administration; monitor ECG for changes.
• Check and record blood pressure before and after I.M. administration.
• Monitor elderly patients carefully because they are more likely to develop adverse reactions, particularly tardive dyskinesia.

Supportive Care
• Hold dose and notify the doctor if the patient develops jaundice, symptoms of blood dyscrasia (fever, sore throat, infection, cellulitis, weakness), or severe adverse reactions.
• Keep the patient supine for 1 hour after I.M. administration. Then assist patient to get up slowly to avoid orthostatic hypotension.
• Do not discontinue drug abruptly unless required by severe adverse reactions.
• Assist the patient with ambulation and daily activities if extrapyramidal symptoms occur. Notify the doctor and expect dosage adjustment.
• Expect to treat acute dystonic reactions with I.V. diphenhydramine.
• Increase the patient's fluid and fiber intake–if not contraindicated–to prevent constipation. If necessary, request doctor's order for a laxative.
• Before administering chlorpromazine, ask the patient to void. If urine retention occurs, notify the doctor and prepare to perform catheterization.

Patient Teaching
• Tell the patient to avoid exposure to direct sunlight and to use a sunscreen when going outdoors to prevent photosensitivity reactions. (*Note:* Sunlamps and tanning beds may cause burning of the skin or skin discoloration.)
• Tell the patient to take the drug exactly as prescribed and not to take double doses to compensate for missed ones.
• Tell the patient not to stop taking the drug suddenly.
• Explain that many drug interactions are possible. Patient should seek medical approval before taking any OTC medication.
• Encourage the patient to report difficulty urinating, sore throat, dizziness, or fainting.
• Advise the patient to increase fluid and fiber in the diet, if appropriate.
• Tell the patient to avoid driving and other hazardous activities that require alertness until the effect of the drug is established. Excessive sedative effects tend to subside after several weeks.
• Explain which fluids are appropriate for diluting the concentrate and show the dropper technique for measuring dose. Warn patient to avoid spilling liquid preparation on skin because it may cause rash and irritation.
• Tell the patient to relieve dry mouth with sugarless hard candy, chewing gum, or ice chips.

Evaluation
In patients receiving chlorpromazine, appropriate evaluation statements may include:
• Patient is able to perform activities of daily living without assistance.
• Patient maintains physical mobility.
• Patient and family state an understanding of chlorpromazine therapy.

chlorpropamide
(klor proe´ pa mide)
Apo-Chlorpropamide†, Diabinese, Glucamide, Novo-propamide†

• *Classification:* antidiabetic, antidiuretic agent (sulfonylurea)
• *Pregnancy Risk Category:* D

HOW SUPPLIED
Tablets: 100 mg, 250 mg

ACTION
Mechanism: A sulfonylurea that lowers blood glucose by stimulating insulin release from the pancreatic beta

cells and reducing glucose output by the liver. An extrapancreatic effect increases peripheral sensitivity to insulin. Also exerts an antidiuretic effect in patients with pituitary-deficient diabetes insipidus.
Absorption: Readily absorbed from the GI tract.
Distribution: Not fully understood, but probably is similar to that of the other sulfonylureas; drug is highly protein-bound.
Metabolism: Approximately 80% is metabolized by the liver. Hypoglycemic activity of metabolites is unknown.
Excretion: In urine. The rate of excretion depends on urinary pH; it increases in alkaline urine and decreases in acidic urine. Half-life: 36 hours.
Onset, peak, duration: Onset of action within 1 hour, with a maximum decrease in serum glucose levels at 3 to 6 hours; duration of action is up to 60 hours.

INDICATIONS & DOSAGE

Adjunct to diet to lower blood glucose in patients with non-insulin-dependent diabetes mellitus (type II)—
Adults: 250 mg P.O. daily with breakfast or in divided doses if GI disturbances occur. First dosage increase may be made after 5 to 7 days because of extended duration of action, then dosage may be increased q 3 to 5 days by 50 to 125 mg, if needed, to maximum of 750 mg daily.
Adults over 65 years: initial dose should be in the range of 100 to 125 mg P.O. daily.
To change from insulin to oral therapy—
Adults: if insulin dosage is less than 40 units daily, insulin may be stopped and oral therapy started as above. If insulin dosage is 40 units or more daily, start oral therapy as above with insulin reduced 50%. Further insulin reductions should be made according to patient response.

CONTRAINDICATIONS & PRECAUTIONS

Contraindicated in patients with hypersensitivity to sulfonylureas or thiazides; burns, acidosis, diabetic coma, severe infection, ketosis, severe trauma, and major surgery because these conditions require treatment with insulin; and nonfunctioning beta cells. During periods of stress, insulin may be required temporarily.

Use cautiously in patients with impaired cardiac function because sodium and water retention may precipitate CHF; water retention because it may potentiate antidiuretic hormone; hepatic or renal insufficiency because it is metabolized in the liver and excreted in urine; and adrenal, pituitary, or thyroid dysfunction because of altered fluid and electrolyte balance.

ADVERSE REACTIONS

Common reactions are in italics; life-threatening reactions are in bold italics.
GI: nausea, heartburn, vomiting.
GU: tea-colored urine.
Metabolic: prolonged hypoglycemia, *dilutional hyponatremia.*
Skin: rash, pruritus, facial flushing.
Other: ***hypersensitivity.***

INTERACTIONS

Anabolic steroids, chloramphenicol, clofibrate, guanethidine, MAO inhibitors, oral anticoagulants, phenylbutazone, salicylates, sulfonamides: increased hypoglycemic activity. Monitor blood glucose level.
Beta blockers, clonidine: prolonged hypoglycemic effect and masked symptoms of hypoglycemia. Use together cautiously.
Corticosteroids, glucagon, rifampin, thiazide diuretics: decreased hypoglycemic response. Monitor blood glucose level.

EFFECTS ON DIAGNOSTIC TESTS

Cholesterol, alkaline phosphatase, bilirubin, urine phenyl ketone, porphyrins, and protein levels, and cephalin flocculation (thymol turbidity): altered results.

NURSING CONSIDERATIONS

Besides those related universally to drug therapy (see "How to use this book"), consider the following specific recommendations:

Assessment

- Obtain a baseline assessment of the patient's blood glucose level before initiating therapy.
- Be alert for common adverse reactions and drug interactions.
- Evaluate the patient's and family's knowledge about chlorpropamide therapy.

Nursing Diagnoses

- Altered nutrition: more than body requirements related to the patient's inability to release insulin to maintain normal blood glucose levels.
- High risk for injury related to chlorpropamide-induced hypoglycemia.
- Knowledge deficit related to chlorpropamide therapy.

Planning and Implementation

Preparation and Administration

- Consider that some patients taking drug may be controlled effectively on a once-daily regimen, whereas others show better response with divided dosing.
- ***P.O. use:*** Administer once-daily doses with breakfast; divided doses are usually given before the morning and evening meals.

Monitoring

- Monitor effectiveness by regularly checking patient's blood glucose levels. Monitor blood glucose levels more frequently if the patient is under stress, having difficulty controlling blood glucose levels, or is newly diagnosed.
- Monitor for signs and symptoms of both hyperglycemia and hypoglycemia; note time and circumstances of each reaction.
- Monitor the patient's hemoglobin A1C regularly as ordered.
- Monitor carefully for cardiovascular dysfunction because sulfonylureas have been associated with an increased risk of cardiovascular mortality as compared to diet or diet and insulin therapy.
- Monitor patient for signs of impending renal insufficiency, such as dysuria, anuria, and hematuria.
- Monitor elderly patients closely because they may be more sensitive to this drug's adverse reactions.

Supportive Care

- Notify the doctor if blood glucose levels remain elevated or frequent episodes of hypoglycemia occur.
- Treat a hypoglycemic reaction with an oral form of rapid-acting glucose if the patient is awake or with glucagon or I.V. glucose if the patient cannot be aroused. Follow up treatment with a complex carbohydrate snack when patient is awake, and determine cause of reaction.
- Be sure other treatment measures, such as diet and exercise programs, are being used appropriately.
- Discuss with the doctor how to deal with noncompliance.
- Patient transferring from insulin therapy to an oral antidiabetic requires blood glucose monitoring at least t.i.d. before meals. Patient may require hospitalization during transition.
- Report any signs of impending renal insufficiency to the doctor immediately.

Patient Teaching

- Emphasize to the patient the importance of following the prescribed diet, exercise, and medical regimens.
- Tell the patient to take the medication at the same time each day. If a dose is missed, it should be taken immediately, unless it's almost time to

take the next dose. Instruct the patient not to take double doses.
• Advise the patient to avoid alcohol while taking drug as chlorpropamide-alcohol flush can occur characterized by facial flushing, light-headedness, headache, and occasional breathlessness. Tell patient even very small amounts of alcohol can produce this reaction and remind him that many foods and nonprescription medications contain alcohol.
• Encourage the patient to wear a medical alert bracelet or necklace.
• Tell the patient to take drug with food; once-daily dosage should be taken with breakfast.
• Teach the patient how to monitor blood glucose levels as prescribed.
• Teach the patient how to recognize the signs and symptoms of hyperglycemia and hypoglycemia and what to do if they occur.
• Stress the importance of compliance and close follow-up with drug therapy. Make sure patient understands that therapy relieves symptoms but doesn't cure the disease.

Evaluation

In patients receiving chlorpropamide, appropriate evaluation statements may include:
• Patient's blood glucose level is normal.
• Patient recognizes hypoglycemia early and treats hypoglycemic episodes effectively before injury occurs.
• Patient and family express an understanding of chlorpropamide therapy.

---

chlorprothixene

(klor proe thix´ een)

Taractan**, Tarasan†

• *Classification:* antipsychotic (thioxanthene)
• *Pregnancy Risk Category:* C

HOW SUPPLIED

Tablets: 10 mg, 25 mg, 50 mg, 100 mg
Oral concentrate: 100 mg/5 ml (fruit)
Injection: 12.5 mg/ml

ACTION

Mechanism: A thioxanthene that blocks postsynaptic dopamine receptors in the brain.
Absorption: Both oral and I.M. absorption are rapid.
Distribution: Widespread; drug is 91% to 99% protein-bound.
Metabolism: Principally hepatic to chlorprothixine sulfoxide.
Excretion: Both parent drug and metabolite appear in urine and feces.
Onset, peak, duration: I.M. onset of action is 10 to 30 minutes. Peak effects occur at 1 to 3 hours. Duration of action is 6 hours.

INDICATIONS & DOSAGE

Psychotic disorders–
Adults: initially, 10 mg P.O. t.i.d. or q.i.d. Increase gradually to maximum of 600 mg daily.
Children over 6 years: 10 to 25 mg P.O. t.i.d. or q.i.d.
Agitation of severe neurosis, depression, schizophrenia–
Adults: 25 to 50 mg P.O. or I.M. t.i.d. or q.i.d. Increase as needed up to maximum of 600 mg.

CONTRAINDICATIONS & PRECAUTIONS

Contraindicated in patients with hypersensitivity to thioxanthenes, phenothiazines, and related compounds, including that evidenced by jaundice and other allergic symptoms; in patients with blood dyscrasias and bone marrow depression because of its potential for agranulocytosis; in patients with disorders accompanied by coma, brain damage, or CNS depression because of additive CNS depressant effects; and in patients with circulatory collapse or cerebrovascular disease because of potential arrhythmogenic effects.

Use cautiously in patients with cardiac disease (arrhythmias, CHF, angina pectoris, valvular disease, or heart block), encephalitis, Reye's syndrome, head injury, respiratory disease, epilepsy and other seizure disorders, glaucoma, prostatic hypertrophy, urine retention, hepatic or renal dysfunction, Parkinson's disease, pheochromocytoma, or hypocalcemia.

Oral preparations of chlorprothixene may contain tartrazine dye, which may cause allergic reaction in patients with aspirin allergy.

ADVERSE REACTIONS

Common reactions are in italics; life-threatening reactions are in bold italics.

Blood: transient leukopenia, ***agranulocytosis.***

CNS: extrapyramidal reactions (low incidence), tardive dyskinesia, *sedation,* pseudoparkinsonism, EEG changes, dizziness.

CV: *orthostatic hypotension,* tachycardia, ECG changes.

EENT: ocular changes, *blurred vision.*

GI: *dry mouth, constipation.*

GU: *urine retention,* dark urine, menstrual irregularities, gynecomastia, inhibited ejaculation.

Hepatic: cholestatic jaundice, abnormal liver function tests.

Metabolic: hyperprolactinemia.

Skin: *mild photosensitivity,* dermal allergic reactions.

Local: pain on I.M. injection, sterile abscess.

Other: weight gain; increased appetite; rarely, ***neuroleptic malignant syndrome*** (fever, tachycardia, tachypnea, profuse diaphoresis).

After abrupt withdrawal of long-term therapy: gastritis, nausea, vomiting, dizziness, tremors, feeling of warmth or cold, sweating, tachycardia, headache, insomnia.

INTERACTIONS

Alcohol, other CNS depressants: increased CNS depression. Avoid concomitant use.

Anticholinergics: potentiated central anticholinergic effects.

Centrally acting antihypertensives: decreased antihypertensive effect.

EFFECTS ON DIAGNOSTIC TESTS

ECG: quinidine-like effects.

Liver enzymes and protein-bound iodine: elevated results.

Urine porphyrins, urobilinogen, amylase, and 5-HIAA: false-positive results because of darkening of urine by metabolites.

Urine pregnancy tests using human chorionic gonadotropin: false-positive results.

NURSING CONSIDERATIONS

Besides those related universally to drug therapy (see "How to use this book"), consider the following specific recommendations:

Assessment

• Obtain a baseline assessment of the patient's underlying condition before drug therapy.

• Be alert for adverse reactions and drug interactions throughout therapy.

• Evaluate the patient's and family's knowledge about chlorprothixene therapy therapy.

Nursing Diagnoses

• Impaired thought processes related to the patient's underlying condition.

• Urine retention related to adverse drug reaction.

• Knowledge deficit related to chlorprothixene therapy.

Planning and Implementation

Preparation and Administration

• Protect medication from light. Slight yellowing of injection or concentrate is common and does not affect potency. Discard markedly discolored solutions.

• Dose of 100 mg is therapeutic

equivalent of 100 mg of chlorpromazine.
• *I.M. use:* Give injection deeply only in upper outer quadrant of buttocks. Massage slowly afterward to prevent sterile abscess.
• *P.O. use:* Dilute liquid concentrate with 60 ml tomato or fruit juice, carbonated beverages, coffee, tea, milk, water, or semisolid food just before giving.
• Store I.M. form in refrigerator.
• Avoid skin contact with the injectable or liquid form because it may cause a rash.

Monitoring
• Monitor effectiveness by regularly observing the patient's behavior and noting if psychotic symptoms have abated or diminished.
• Monitor for adverse reactions, especially extrapyramidal and anticholinergic effects (blurred vision, dry mouth, constipation, urine retention), and tardive dyskinesia, during prolonged therapy.
• Watch for orthostatic hypotension, especially parenteral administration.
• Monitor therapy by weekly bilirubin tests during the first month; periodic blood tests (CBC and liver function); and ophthalmic tests (long-term use).
• Monitor for neuroleptic malignant syndrome. This rare, potentially fatal reaction is not necessarily related to duration or type of neuroleptic therapy, but usually occurs in men (60% of affected patients).

Supportive Care
• Keep the patient supine for 1 hour after I.M. administration. Then assist patient to get up slowly to avoid orthostatic hypotension.
• Do not discontinue drug abruptly unless required by severe adverse reactions.
• Increase the patient's fluid and fiber intake–if not contraindicated–to prevent constipation. If necessary, request doctor's order for a laxative.
• Offer the patient sugarless gum, sour hard candy, ice chips, or have him rinse his mouth with mouthwash to relieve dryness.
• Treat acute dystonic reactions with I.V. diphenhydramine, as ordered.
• Hold dose if patient develops jaundice, symptoms of blood dyscrasias (fever, sore throat, infection, cellulitis, weakness), persistent (longer than a few hours) extrapyramidal reactions or any such reactions during pregnancy.
• Be prepared to give I.V. diphenhydramine for acute dystonic reactions.

Patient Teaching
• Tell the patient to avoid exposure to direct sunlight and to use a sunscreen when going outdoors to prevent photosensitivity reactions. (*Note:* Sunlamps and tanning beds may cause burning of the skin or skin discoloration.)
• Tell the patient not to stop taking the drug suddenly.
• Encourage the patient to report difficulty urinating, sore throat, dizziness, or fainting.
• Advise the patient to increase fluid and fiber in the diet, if appropriate.
• Tell the patient to avoid driving and other hazardous activities that require alertness until the effect of the drug is established. Excessive sedative effects tend to subside after several weeks.
• Explain which fluids are appropriate for diluting the concentrate and show the dropper technique for measuring dose. Warn the patient to avoid spilling liquid preparation on skin because it may cause rash and irritation.
• Tell the patient that sugarless hard candy, chewing gum, or ice chips can alleviate dry mouth.

Evaluation
In patients receiving chlorprothixene, appropriate evaluation statements may include:
• Patient demonstrates diminished psychotic behavior.

• Patient voids without difficulty.
• Patient and family state an understanding of chlorprothixene therapy.

---

chlortetracycline hydrochloride

(klor te tra sye´ kleen)
Aureomycin 3%◇

• *Classification:* antibiotic (tetracycline)
• *Pregnancy Risk Category:* D

HOW SUPPLIED

Ointment: 3% in 14.2-g, 30-g tubes◇

ACTION

Mechanism: Binds to the 30S ribosomal subunit of susceptible bacteria and disrupts protein synthesis. May be bacteriostatic or bactericidal, depending upon concentration.
Pharmacokinetics: Unknown.

INDICATIONS & DOSAGE

Superficial infections of the skin caused by susceptible bacteria –
Adults and children: rub into affected area b.i.d. or t.i.d.

CONTRAINDICATIONS & PRECAUTIONS

Contraindicated in patients with hypersensitivity to any of the tetracyclines and in pregnant patients in the second and third trimesters. Use with caution to avoid overgrowth of nonsusceptible organisms during long-term use.

ADVERSE REACTIONS

Common reactions are in italics; life-threatening reactions are in bold italics.
Skin: *dermatitis,* drying.

INTERACTIONS

None significant.

EFFECTS ON DIAGNOSTIC TESTS

None reported with topical or ophthalmic use.

NURSING CONSIDERATIONS

Besides those related universally to drug therapy (see "How to use this book"), consider the following specific recommendations:

Assessment
• Obtain a baseline assessment of skin infection before therapy.
• Be alert for adverse reactions and drug interactions throughout therapy.
• Evaluate the patient's and family's knowledge about chlortetracycline hydrochloride therapy.

Nursing Diagnoses
• Impaired skin integrity related to skin infection.
• High risk for infection related to chlortetracycline hydrochloride-induced dermatitis.
• Knowledge deficit related to chlortetracycline hydrochloride therapy.

Planning and Implementation
Preparation and Administration
• ***Cutaneous use:*** Rub into affected area as ordered. Cleanse area prior to application.
Monitoring
• Monitor effectiveness by regularly checking skin infection.
• Monitor carefully. If condition worsens or does not improve, discontinue use and notify doctor.
• Monitor the patient for adverse reactions or interactions by frequently assessing the patient's skin for infection
Supportive Care
• Drug has lanolin base. Don't use in persons allergic to wool.
• Prolonged use may result in overgrowth of nonsusceptible organisms.
• Be prepared to discontinue use, and notify doctor if condition worsens.
• Treated skin fluoresces under ultraviolet light.

Patient Teaching
- Teach patient to apply medication.
- Instruct patient to notify doctor if condition worsens.

Evaluation
In patients receiving chlortetracycline, appropriate evaluation statements may include:
- Patient states skin infection is resolving.
- Patient did not develop drug-induced dermatitis.
- Patient and family state an understanding of chlortetracycline therapy.

chlorthalidone
(klor thal′ i done)
Apo-Chlorthalidone†, Hygroton, Novothalidone†, Thalitone, Uridon†

- *Classification:* diuretic, antihypertensive (thiazidelike)
- *Pregnancy Risk Category:* D

HOW SUPPLIED
Tablets: 25 mg, 50 mg, 100 mg

ACTION
Mechanism: Although not a thiazide, chlorthalidone acts in a similar fashion. It increases urine excretion of sodium and water by inhibiting sodium reabsorption in the cortical diluting site of the nephron.
Absorption: From the GI tract; extent of absorption is unknown.
Distribution: 90% bound to erythrocytes.
Excretion: Between 30% and 60% of a given dose is excreted unchanged in urine. Half-life: 54 hours.

INDICATIONS & DOSAGE
Edema, hypertension–
Adults: 25 to 100 mg P.O. daily, or 100 mg 3 times weekly or on alternate days.
Children: 2 mg/kg P.O. 3 times weekly.

CONTRAINDICATIONS & PRECAUTIONS
Contraindicated in patients with anuria and in those with sensitivity to the drug or to other sulfonamide derivatives. Use cautiously in patients with severe renal disease because it may decrease glomerular filtration rate and precipitate azotemia; impaired hepatic function or liver disease because electrolyte changes may precipitate coma; and patients taking digoxin because hypokalemia may predispose them to digitalis toxicity.

ADVERSE REACTIONS
Common reactions are in italics; life-threatening reactions are in bold italics.
Blood: ***aplastic anemia, agranulocytosis,*** leukopenia, thrombocytopenia.
CV: *volume depletion and dehydration,* orthostatic hypotension.
GI: anorexia, nausea, pancreatitis.
GU: impotence.
Hepatic: hepatic encephalopathy.
Metabolic: *hypokalemia, asymptomatic hyperuricemia, hyperglycemia and impairment of glucose tolerance,* fluid and electrolyte imbalances including dilutional hyponatremia and hypochloremia, metabolic alkalosis, hypercalcemia, gout.
Skin: dermatitis, photosensitivity, rash.
Other: hypersensitivity, such as pneumonitis and vasculitis.

INTERACTIONS
Cholestyramine, colestipol: intestinal absorption of thiazides decreased. Keep doses as separate as possible.
Diazoxide: increased antihypertensive, hyperglycemic, and hyperuricemic effects. Use together cautiously.
NSAIDs: decreased diuretic effectiveness. Avoid concomitant use.

EFFECTS ON DIAGNOSTIC TESTS
Parathyroid function test: test inference. Drug should be discontinued before such tests.

Serum electrolytes: altered levels.
Serum urate, glucose, cholesterol, and triglycerides: increased levels.

NURSING CONSIDERATIONS

Besides those related universally to drug therapy (see "How to use this book"), consider the following specific recommendations:

Assessment

- Obtain a baseline assessment of blood pressure, serum electrolytes, urine output, weight, and peripheral edema before initiating chlorthalidone therapy.
- Be alert for adverse reactions and drug interactions throughout therapy.
- Evaluate the patient's and family's knowledge about chlorthalidone therapy.

Nursing Diagnoses

- Fluid volume excess related to the patient's underlying condition as evidenced by edema.
- Altered urinary elimination related to chlorthalidone therapy.
- Knowledge deficit related to chlorthalidone therapy.

Planning and Implementation

Preparation and Administration

- ***P.O. use:*** If possible, give drug early in the day to prevent nocturia.

Monitoring

- Monitor effectiveness by regularly checking blood pressure, urine output, and weight.
- Monitor serum electrolytes, calcium, BUN, creatinine, glucose, and uric acid levels.
- Monitor CBC, differential, and platelet count.
- For the patient receiving concomitant digitalis therapy, monitor for increased risk of digitalis toxicity.
- Monitor for signs of hypokalemia (for example, muscle weakness and cramps).
- Monitor the diabetic patient's insulin requirements because chlorothiazide has hyperglycemic effects.
- Monitor skin turgor and mucous membranes for signs of fluid volume deficit.
- Monitor elderly patients closely because they are especially susceptible to excessive diuresis.

Supportive Care

- Hold drug and notify the doctor if hypersensitivity reactions occur.
- Keep accurate records of intake and output, blood pressure, and weight.
- Provide frequent skin and mouth care to relieve dryness from diuretic therapy.
- Answer the patient's call bells promptly; make sure patient's bathroom or bedpan is easily accessible.
- Use safety precautions to minimize risk of falling due to hypotension.
- In the patient undergoing tests of parathyroid function, hold thiazide and thiazidelike drugs before these tests are performed.
- Be aware that optimal antihypertensive effect may occur several days after beginning of therapy with chlorthalidone.
- Elevate the patient's legs to aid relief of peripheral edema.
- Administer potassium supplements as indicated and provide a high-potassium diet.

Patient Teaching

- Teach the patient and family to identify and report signs of hypersensitivity reaction and hypokalemia.
- Teach the patient and family to monitor the patient's fluid volume by recording daily weight and intake and output.
- Inform the patient that optimal therapeutic response may not occur until several days after beginning chlorthalidone therapy.
- Teach the patient to avoid high-sodium foods and to choose high-potassium foods.
- Advise the patient to change positions slowly, especially when rising to standing position, to avoid dizziness and fainting due to orthostatic hypotension.

• Advise the patient to minimize risks of photosensitivity reaction by using a sunscreen when outdoors.
• Advise the diabetic patient that insulin dosage may require adjustment.
• Advise the patient who is taking digitalis that the drug's potassium-depleting effect may increase the risk of digitalis toxicity.
• Advise the patient to take drug early in the day to avoid interruptions of sleep due to nocturia.

Evaluation

In patients receiving chlorthalidone, appropriate evaluation statements may include:
• Patient is free of edema.
• Patient demonstrates adjustment of life-style to deal with altered patterns of urinary elimination.
• Patient and family state an understanding of chlorthalidone therapy.

cholestyramine

(koe less´ tir a meen)
Cholybar, Questran**

• *Classification:* antilipemic, bile acid sequestrant (anion exchange resin)
• *Pregnancy Risk Category:* C

HOW SUPPLIED

Bar: 4 g
Powder: 378-g cans, 9-g single-dose packets. Each scoop of powder or single-dose packet contains 4 g of cholestyramine resin.

ACTION

Mechanism: Combines with bile acid to form an insoluble compound that is excreted.
Absorption: Not absorbed.
Distribution: None.
Metabolism: None.
Excretion: Insoluble cholestyramine with bile acid complex is excreted in feces.
Onset, peak, duration: Cholesterol levels may begin to decrease 24 to 48 hours after the start of therapy and may continue to fall for up 12 months. In some patients, the initial decrease is followed by a return to baseline or higher cholesterol levels on continued therapy.

INDICATIONS & DOSAGE

Primary hyperlipidemia, pruritus, and diarrhea due to excess bile acid; as adjunctive therapy for the reduction of elevated serum cholesterol in patients with primary hypercholesterolemia; and to reduce the risks of atherosclerotic coronary artery disease and myocardial infarction–
Adults: 4 g before meals and h.s., not to exceed 32 g daily. Each scoop or packet of Questran contains 4 g cholestyramine. Also available as Cholybar, a chewable candy bar (raspberry or caramel flavored) containing 4 g cholestyramine.
Children: 240 mg/kg daily P.O. in three divided doses with beverage or food. Safe dosage not established for children under 6 years.

CONTRAINDICATIONS & PRECAUTIONS

Contraindicated in patients with complete biliary obstruction and in patients hypersensitive to any of its components. Cholestyramine powder contains tartrazine (FD&C Yellow No. 5), which may cause allergic reactions in susceptible individuals.

Use cautiously in patients with constipation because of the risk of fecal impaction; in patients with malabsorption, whose conditions may deteriorate from further decreased absorption of fats and fat-soluble vitamins E, A, D, and K; and in pregnant women, because impaired maternal absorption of vitamins and other nutrients is a potential threat to the fetus.

*Liquid form contains alcohol.
**May contain tartrazine.

ADVERSE REACTIONS

Common reactions are in italics; life-threatening reactions are in bold italics.

GI: *constipation,* fecal impaction, hemorrhoids, *abdominal discomfort,* flatulence, *nausea,* vomiting, steatorrhea.

Skin: *rashes,* irritation of skin, tongue, and perianal area.

Other: *vitamin A, D, and K deficiency from decreased absorption;* hyperchloremic acidosis with long-term use or very high dosage.

INTERACTIONS

Acetaminophen, coumarin anticoagulants, beta-adrenergic blocking agents, corticosteroids, digitalis glycosides, fat soluble vitamins (A,D,E and K), iron preparations, thiazide diuretics, thyroid hormone: absorption may be substantially decreased by cholestyramine. Separate administration times by at least 2 hours.

EFFECTS ON DIAGNOSTIC TESTS

Cholecystography using iopanoic acid: iopanoic acid is bound by cholestyramine.

Serum alkaline phosphatase, aspartate aminotransferase, chloride, phosphorus, potassium, calcium, and sodium: altered concentrations.

NURSING CONSIDERATIONS

Besides those related universally to drug therapy (see "How to use this book"), consider the following specific recommendations:

Assessment

- Obtain a baseline assessment of the patient's underlying condition before drug therapy.
- Be alert for adverse reactions and drug interactions throughout therapy.
- Evaluate the patient's and family's knowledge about cholestyramine therapy.

Nursing Diagnoses

- High risk for injury related to ineffectiveness of cholestyramine to lower blood lipid and cholesterol levels.
- Constipation related to adverse drug reactions.
- Knowledge deficit related to cholestyramine therapy.

Implementation

Preparation and Administration

- To mix powder, sprinkle on surface of preferred beverage or wet food. Let stand a few minutes, then stir to obtain uniform suspension. Mixing with carbonated beverages may result in excess foaming. Use large glass and mix slowly.
- Administer all other medications at least 1 hour before or 4 to 6 hours after cholestyramine to avoid blocking their absorption.
- Administer before meals and at bedtime.

Monitoring

- Monitor effectiveness by checking serum cholesterol and triglyceride levels every 4 weeks.
- Monitor the patient's bowel habits; drug may cause constipation.
- Monitor digitalis glycoside levels in patients receiving both medications concurrently. If cholestyramine therapy is discontinued, digitalis toxicity may result unless dosage is adjusted.
- Monitor for signs of vitamin deficiencies: A (visual disturbances, skin changes); D (alteration in calcium metabolism); and K (bleeding tendencies).

Supportive Care

- If severe constipation develops, decrease dosage, add a stool softener, or discontinue drug.

Patient Teaching

- Instruct the patient about all cardiac risk factors; advise patient about weight control, stop-smoking programs, and exercise.
- Teach the patient about proper dietary management. Recommend a diet low in saturated fats and high in fiber and vitamins A, D, and K.

• Tell the patient to take drug before meals and at bedtime.

Evaluation

In patients receiving cholestyramine, appropriate evaluation statements include:

• Patient's blood triglyceride and cholesterol levels are normal.
• Patient reports bowel habits are normal.
• Patient and family state an understanding of cholestyramine therapy.

choline magnesium trisalicylate (choline salicylate and magnesium salicylate)

(koe´ leen mag nee´ zhum trye sal´ i sye late)
Trilisate

choline salicylate

Antropan, Teejel†*

• *Classification:* non-narcotic analgesic, antipyretic, anti-inflammatory (salicylate)
• *Pregnancy Risk Category:* C

HOW SUPPLIED

Gel: 87 mg/g†*
Liquid: 870 mg/5 ml◇
Solution: 500 mg of salicylate/5 ml
Tablets: 500 mg, 750 mg, 1,000 mg of salicylate

ACTION

Mechanism: Produces analgesia by an ill-defined central effect; produces a peripheral anti-inflammatory effect by inhibiting prostaglandin synthesis. Relieves fever by acting on the hypothalamic heat-regulating center.
Absorption: Rapidly and completely absorbed from the GI tract.
Distribution: Protein binding depends on concentration and ranges from 75% to 90%, decreasing as serum concentration increases; severe toxic effects may occur at serum concentrations over 400 mcg/ml.
Metabolism: Hydrolyzed to salicylate in the liver.
Excretion: Metabolites are excreted in urine. Half-life: With the tablets, a steady-state condition is usually reached after 4 to 5 doses, half-life of elimination, on repeated administration of tablets, is 9 to 17 hours.
Onset, peak, duration: Peak therapeutic effect occurs in about 2 hours.

INDICATIONS & DOSAGE

Arthritis, mild–
Adults: 1 to 2 teaspoonfuls or tablets P.O. b.i.d. Total daily dosage can also be given at one time (usually h.s.)
Rheumatoid arthritis and osteoarthritis–
Adults: initially, 3 g P.O. daily either as a single dose h.s. or b.i.d. Dosage is adjusted according to patient response. Dosage range is 1 to 4.5 g daily.
Juvenile rheumatoid arthritis–
Children (12 to 37 kg): 50 mg/kg/day P.O. in divided doses.
Children (more than 37 kg): 2,250 mg P.O. given in divided doses.
Mild-to-moderate pain and fever
Adults: 2 to 3 g P.O. daily in divided doses.
Children: 2 g/m²/day in 4 to 6 divided doses or as shown below.
Children age 2 to 4: 217.5 mg q 4 hours, p.r.n.
Children age 4 to 6: 326.5 mg q 4 hours, p.r.n.
Children age 6 to 9: 435 mg q 4 hours, p.r.n.
Children age 9 to 11: 543.8 mg q 4 hours, p.r.n.
Children age 11 to 12: 652.5 mg q 4 hours, p.r.n.

CONTRAINDICATIONS & PRECAUTIONS

Contraindicated in patients with hypersensitivity to salicylates or other

NSAIDs and when GI ulcer or GI bleeding are present.

Use cautiously in patients with a history of GI disease and increased risk of GI bleeding because the drug may worsen these conditions; and in patients with decreased renal or hepatic function because of potential for drug accumulation (especially magnesium salicylate).

Patients with known "triad" symptoms (aspirin hypersensitivity, rhinitis/nasal polyps, and asthma) are at high risk of bronchospasm because of cross-sensitivity to NSAIDs. Salicylates may mask the signs and symptoms of acute infection (fever, myalgia, erythema); carefully evaluate patients with high risk (for example, those with diabetes).

ADVERSE REACTIONS

Common reactions are in italics; life-threatening reactions are in bold italics.
EENT: tinnitus and hearing loss.
GI: GI distress.
Skin: rash.
Other: ***hypersensitivity manifested by anaphylaxis (rare).***

INTERACTIONS

Alcohol, steroids, and other NSAIDs: enhanced risk of adverse GI effects.
Ammonium chloride (and other urine acidifiers): increased blood levels of salicylates. Monitor for salicylate toxicity.
Antacids in high doses (and other urine alkalinizers): decreased levels of salicylates. Monitor for decreased salicylate effect.
Corticosteroids: enhance salicylate elimination. Monitor for decreased salicylate effect.
Oral anticoagulants: increased risk of bleeding. Use together cautiously.

EFFECTS ON DIAGNOSTIC TESTS

Urinary glucose (Clinistix, Tes-Tape, Clinitest, and Benedict's solution): test interference.
Urine 5-HIAA: test interference.
Vanillymandelic acid (VMA): test interference.

NURSING CONSIDERATIONS

Besides those related universally to drug therapy (see "How to use this book"), consider the following specific recommendations:

Assessment
- Obtain a baseline assessment of pain level before therapy.
- Be alert for adverse reactions and drug interactions throughout therapy.
- Evaluate the patient's and family's knowledge about salicylate therapy.

Nursing Diagnoses
- Pain related to the patient's underlying condition.
- Sensory/perceptual alterations (auditory) related to adverse drug reactions.
- Knowledge deficit related to salicylate therapy.

Planning and Implementation

Preparation and Administration
- Keep in mind that each '500' tablet or teaspoonful equals salicylate content of 650 mg aspirin.
- Do not give this drug or other salicylates to children or teenagers with chicken pox or influenza-like illnesss because of epidemiologic association with Reye's syndrome.
- Give tablets with a full glass (8 oz.) of water or with food.
- Mix solution with fruit juice. Do not mix it with antacids.
- If GI distress occurs, give antacids 2 hours after meals and give choline magnesium trisalicylate before meals. This drug causes less GI distress than aspirin.

Monitoring
- Monitor effectiveness by regularly evaluating pain relief or reduction of fever.
- Monitor for toxicity, especially in febrile, dehydrated children.
- Monitor blood salicylate level. Therapeutic blood salicylate level in ar-

thritis is 10 to 30 mg/100 ml. Tinnitus may occur at plasma levels of 30 mg/100 ml and above, but does not reliably indicate toxicity, especially in very young patients and those older than age 60. With chronic therapy, mild toxicity may occur at plasma levels of 20 mg/100 ml.
• Obtain hemoglobin and prothrombin tests periodically in patients receiving prolonged treatment with large doses to monitor for increased tendency to bleed.
• Evaluate patient's hearing periodically and ask about tinnitus.

Supportive Care
• Notify the doctor if the patient develops salicylism (tinnitus, hearing), bleeding or GI distress.

Patient Teaching
• Tell the patient to take tablets with food or a full glass (8 oz) of water.
• Advise patient to mix drug solution with fruit juice but not with antacids.
• Instruct the patient to notify the doctor if tinnitus occurs or if or a family member notices any hearing loss.
• Explain the importance of periodically determining blood salicyclate levels in evaluating effectiveness and of measuring hemoglobin and prothrombin levels to evaluate risk of bleeding problems.

Evaluation
In patients receiving choline magnesium trisalicylate therapy appropriate evaluation statements may include:
• Patient states pain is relieved.
• Hearing is unchanged since initiation of therapy.
• Patient and family state an understanding of salicylate therapy.

PHARMACOLOGIC CLASS

cholinergics

acetylcholine chloride
bethanechol chloride
carbachol chloride

OVERVIEW

The basic components of cholinergic drugs were first synthesized in the 1860s; by the 1930s, physicians were using them and some of their synthetic analogues therapeutically.

These agents are used to simulate the actions of acetylcholine at postganglionic (muscarinic) neuroeffector sites. Acetylcholine is of little use clinically because of its susceptibility to acetylcholinesterase and butyrylcholinesterase and its relatively nonspecific action at both sympathetic and parasympathetic ganglia.

CLINICAL INDICATIONS AND ACTIONS

GI and urinary tract atony
Bethanechol is used to treat paralytic ileus, postoperative abdominal distention, and gastric atony or stasis. Bethanechol enhances gastric tone, contractions, and GI peristaltic activity, increasing gastric acid secretions. It also relieves gastric atony and retention after bilateral vagotomy for peptic ulcer. In some patients, bethanechol has proven effective in treating congenital megacolon. Bethanechol is used to treat postoperative or postpartum urinary retention and, in certain cases, neurogenic bladder; it increases ureteral peristalsis and induces contraction of the urinary bladder's detrusor muscle.

Glaucoma
Topical carbachol is used to treat glaucoma. In narrow-angle glaucoma, it causes the iris sphincter to contract; that allows aqueous humor to flow out through the trabecular space at Schlemm's canal. In open-angle glaucoma, physostigmine enhances trabecular network tone and alignment, permitting aqueous humor to flow through the Schlemm's canal, thereby reducing intraocular pressure.

Because of its short duration of action, acetylcholine is used only for perioperative miosis.

OVERVIEW OF ADVERSE REACTIONS

Cholinergics may cause dizziness, confusion, hallucinations, muscle weakness, nervousness, miosis, blurred vision, tearing, bronchospasm, bronchial constriction, nausea, vomiting, and belching. They may also precipitate asthma attacks in susceptible patients.

Clinical effects of overdose primarily involve muscarinic symptoms, such as nausea, vomiting, diarrhea, abdominal discomfort, involuntary defecation, urinary urgency, increased bronchial and salivary secretions, respiratory depression, skin flushing or heat sensation, and bradycardia; cardiac arrest has also occurred.

REPRESENTATIVE COMBINATIONS

Physostigmine salicylate with atropine: Atrophysine; with 1-hyoscyamine hydrobromide: Phyatromine-H; with pilocarpine and methylcellulose: Isopto P-ES, Miocel, Sol.

PHARMACOLOGIC CLASS

cholinesterase inhibitors

ambenonium chloride
demecarium bromide
edrophonium chloride
neostigmine bromide
neostigmine methylsulfate
physostigmine salicylate
physostigmine sulfate
pyridostigmine bromide
echothiophate iodide

OVERVIEW

The inhibition of cholinesterases has varied effects based on where the enzymes are inhibited, with the most significant effects occurring at sites of cholinergic neuroeffector transmission. Anticholinesterases are used both systemically and topically, and should be used under careful medical supervision as the therapeutic/toxic margin is quite small. Also, wide variations in response may occur even in the same patient; therefore, caution should be exercised because the first sign of adverse reactions may be subtle.

Some cholinesterase inhibitors are more selective for acetylcholinesterase and may enhance neuromuscular function with only a few autonomic side effects; however, some agents, like physostigmine, may cross the blood-brain barrier and cause central effects.

Echothiophate forms irreversible bonds at the site and is moderately selective. When neuromuscular transmission is enhanced by this agent, excessive effects on glands and smooth muscle can occur due to the presence of the enzyme in those sites. Because they are non-ionized, they readily penetrate the blood-brain barrier, causing central effects.

CLINICAL INDICATIONS AND ACTIONS

Muscle atony or paralysis; atropine or tricyclic antidepressant poisoning

Systemically, anticholinesterase agents are used to abolish muscle paralysis due to neuromuscular blocking agents, to improve muscle function in myasthenia gravis, to treat intestinal distention, and to restore GI tonicity postpartum and postoperatively. They also are used to treat atropine or tricyclic antidepressant poisoning.

Glaucoma and other ocular disorders

Topically, anticholinesterase agents are applied to the eye to treat wide-angle glaucoma, marginal corneal ulcers, accommodative convergent strabismus, accommodative esotropia, and to improve the function of extraocular muscles and eyelids in myasthenia gravis. They also may be used in the emergency treatment of acute congestive glaucoma. When alternated with mydriatics, reversibly acting anticholinesterases may be used to break adhesions between lens and iris.

OVERVIEW OF ADVERSE REACTIONS

Adverse systemic effects may result from systemic administration or systemic absorption following topical application. The most frequent of these include excessive salivation, sweating, lacrimation, bronchoconstriction, tracheobronchial secretion, marked miosis, blurred vision, nausea, vomiting, diarrhea, abdominal cramps, involuntary defecation, pallor, hypertension or hypotension, bradycardia, urinary frequency and urgency, and enuresis. Administration of atropine can antagonize these effects.

Topical application may result in stinging, lacrimation, ocular pain, browache, blurred vision, conjunctival and intraocular hyperemia, blepharospasm, transient rise in intraocular pressure, pigment cysts of the iris, anterior and posterior synechia, fibrinous iritis, cataracts (especially in elderly patients), and allergies. Atropine can antagonize these effects as well.

REPRESENTATIVE COMBINATIONS

None.

---

ciclopirox olamine

(sye kloe peer´ ox)
Loprox

• *Classification:* topical antifungal (N-hydroxypyridinone derivative)
• *Pregnancy Risk Category:* B

HOW SUPPLIED

Cream: 1%

ACTION

Mechanism: Blocks transmembrane transport of certain amino acids, ions, and other essential substrates, eventually resulting in decreased synthesis of cellular DNA, RNA and proteins.
Absorption: Rapid but minimal percutaneous absorption; only 1.3% of a dose appeared in the urine when applied under an occlusive dressing.
Distribution: Mostly local; drug concentrates in the stratum corneum, but inhibitory levels are found in dermis. About 98% bound to serum proteins.
Metabolism: Probably hepatic.
Excretion: After percutaneous absorption, ciclopirox and its metabolites are excreted rapidly in the urine. Half-life: About 2 hours.

INDICATIONS & DOSAGE

Treatment of tinea pedis, tinea cruris, tinea corporis, and tinea versicolor; cutaneous candidiasis–
Adults and children over 10 years: massage gently into the affected and surrounding areas b.i.d., in the morning and evening.

CONTRAINDICATIONS & PRECAUTIONS

Contraindicated in patients with hypersensitivity to the drug.

ADVERSE REACTIONS

Common reactions are in italics; life-threatening reactions are in bold italics.
Local: pruritus, burning.

INTERACTIONS

None reported.

EFFECTS ON DIAGNOSTIC TESTS

None reported.

NURSING CONSIDERATIONS

Besides those related universally to drug therapy (see "How to use this book"), consider the following specific recommendations:
Assessment
• Obtain a baseline assessment of infected area before therapy.

• Be alert for adverse reactions and drug interactions throughout therapy.
• Evaluate the patient's and family's knowledge about ciclopirox therapy.

Nursing Diagnoses

• Impaired skin integrity related to patient's underlying condition.
• Sensory/perceptual alterations, tactile related to ciclopirox-induced pruritis.
• Knowledge deficit related to ciclopirox therapy.

Planning and Implementation

Preparation and Administration

• ***Topical use:*** Massage gently into the affected and surrounding areas, in the morning and evening. Don't use occlusive dressings.

Monitoring

• Monitor effectiveness by checking the infected area.
• Monitor patient's condition; if there is no improvement after 4 weeks, stop using. Report to doctor.
• Check regularly for sensitivity or chemical irritation; if it occurs, discontinue treatment.
• Monitor for adverse reactions or interactions by frequently assessing the patient's skin.

Supportive Care

• Use the drug for the full treatment period even though symptoms may have improved (usually continued for 1 week after clearing). Notify doctor if there is no improvement after 4 weeks.
• Notify doctor if pruritus occurs.
• Keep in mind hypopigmentation from tinea versicolor will resolve gradually.

Patient Teaching

• Teach patient to apply medication.
• Teach the patient to take the drug for the full treatment even though the condition has improved.
• Tell the patient that a slight discoloration (hypopigmentation) from tinea versicolor will resolve gradually.

Evaluation

In patients receiving ciclopirox, appropriate evaluation statements may include:
• Patient's infection has resolved.
• Patient did not experience pruritis.
• Patient and family state an understanding of ciclopirox therapy.

cimetidine

(sye met´ i deen)

Doractin‡, Tagamet

• *Classification:* antiulcer agent (histamine$_2$-receptor antagonist
• *Pregnancy Risk Category:* B

HOW SUPPLIED

Tablets: 200 mg, 300 mg, 400 mg, 800 mg
Oral liquid: 300 mg/5 ml
Injection: 150 mg/ml, 200 mg/2 ml‡

ACTION

Mechanism: Competitively inhibits the action of histamine at H_2 receptor sites of the parietal cells, decreasing gastric acid secretion.
Absorption: Approximately 60% to 75% of oral dose is absorbed. Absorption rate (but not extent) may be affected by food.
Distribution: Well distributed to many body tissues. About 15% to 20% of drug is protein-bound. Cimetidine apparently crosses the placenta and is distributed in breast milk.
Metabolism: Approximately 30% to 40% of dose is metabolized in the liver.
Excretion: Primarily in urine (48% of oral dose, 75% of parenteral dose); 10% of oral dose is excreted in feces; some also in breast milk. Half-life: 2 hours in patients with normal renal function.
Onset, peak, duration: Onset and duration are dose-related; after oral administration of 300 mg, onset is less

than 1 hour and basal acid output is reduced by 90% for more than 4 hours. Some patients may have effects lasting as long as 8 hours. Higher doses taken at h.s. may suppress nocturnal acid secretion for 8 hours or more.

INDICATIONS & DOSAGE

Duodenal ulcer (short-term treatment)–
Adults and children over 16 years: 800 mg P.O. h.s. Alternatively, 400 mg P.O. b.i.d., or 300 mg P.O. q.i.d. (with meals and h.s.). Continue treatment for 4 to 6 weeks unless endoscopy shows healing. Maintenance therapy: 400 mg h.s. Parenteral: 300 mg diluted to 20 ml with 0.9% normal saline solution or other compatible I.V. solution by I.V. push over 1 to 2 minutes q 6 hours. Or 300 mg diluted in 50 ml dextrose 5% solution or other compatible I.V. solution by I.V. infusion over 15 to 20 minutes q 6 hours. Or 300 mg I.M. q 6 hours (no dilution necessary). To increase dose, give 300 mg doses more frequently to maximum daily dosage of 2,400 mg.
Duodenal ulcer prophylaxis–
Adults and children over 16 years: 400 mg P.O. h.s.
Active benign gastric ulcer–
Adults: 300 mg P.O. q.i.d. with meals and h.s. for up to 8 weeks.
Pathologic hypersecretory conditions (such as Zollinger-Ellison syndrome, systemic mastocytosis, and multiple endocrine adenomas)–
Adults and children over 16 years: 300 mg P.O. q.i.d. with meals and h.s.; adjust to individual needs. Maximum daily dosage is 2,400 mg.
Parenteral: 300 mg diluted to 20 ml with 0.9% normal saline solution or other compatible I.V. solutions by I.V. push over 1 to 2 minutes q 6 hours. Or 300 mg diluted in 50 ml dextrose 5% solution or other compatible I.V. solution by I.V. infusion over 15 to 20 minutes q 6 hours. To increase dosage, give 300-mg doses more frequently to maximum daily dosage of 2,400 mg.

CONTRAINDICATIONS & PRECAUTIONS

Contraindicated in patients with cimetidine allergy or cross-sensitivity to other H_2-receptor antagonists.

Use with caution when administering large parenteral doses to patients with asthma because the drug may exacerbate the symptoms of the disease; when administering to patients with cirrhosis, severely impaired hepatic function, and moderately to severely impaired renal function because drug accumulation may occur.

ADVERSE REACTIONS

Common reactions are in italics; life-threatening reactions are in bold italics.
Blood: ***agranulocytosis, neutropenia, thrombocytopenia, aplastic anemia (rare).***
CNS: mental confusion, dizziness, headaches, peripheral neuropathy.
CV: bradycardia.
GI: *mild and transient diarrhea.*
GU: transient elevations in serum creatinine.
Hepatic: jaundice (rare).
Skin: acne-like rash, urticaria.
Other: hypersensitivity, muscle pain, mild gynecomastia after use longer than 1 month.

INTERACTIONS

Antacids: interfere with absorption of cimetidine. Separate cimetidine and antacids by at least 1 hour if possible.

Cimetidine may inhibit hepatic microsomal enzyme metabolism of some drugs, like warfarin, phenytoin, some benzodiazepines, lidocaine, theophylline, and propranolol. Monitor serum levels of these drugs closely during cimetidine therapy.

EFFECTS ON DIAGNOSTIC TESTS

Gastric acid tests: antagonization of pentagastrin's effect.
Hemoccult and gastroccult tests: FD&C blue dye #2 in Tagamet tablets may impair interpretation. Draw sample of gastric content at least 15 minutes after tablet administration and follow test manufacturer's instructions closely.
Prolactin levels, serum alkaline phosphatase levels, and serum creatinine levels: increased levels.
Skin tests using allergen extracts: false-negative results.

NURSING CONSIDERATIONS

Besides those related universally to drug therapy (see "How to use this book"), consider the following specific recommendations:

Assessment

• Obtain a baseline assessment of the patient's GI pain before initiating cimetidine therapy.
• Be alert for common adverse reactions and drug interactions throughout therapy.
• Evaluate the patient's and family's knowledge about cimetidine therapy.

Nursing Diagnoses

• Pain related to the patient's underlying condition.
• Diarrhea related to cimetidine-induced adverse drug reactions.
• Knowledge deficit related to cimetidine therapy.

Planning and Implementation

Preparation and Administration

• ***P.O. use:*** Administering tablets with meals will ensure a more consistent therapeutic effect. After administration of the liquid via nasogastric tube, tube should be flushed to clear it and ensure drug's passage to stomach.
• ***I.M. use:*** This route of administration may be painful.
• ***I.V. use:*** I.V. solutions compatible for dilution with cimetidine are 0.9% sodium chloride solution, dextrose 5% and 10% (and combinations of these) in water solutions, lactated Ringer's solution, and 5% sodium bicarbonate injection. Do not dilute with sterile water for injection. Don't infuse I.V. drug too rapidly. It may cause bradycardia. When administering cimetidine as an I.V. infusion in 100 ml of diluent solution as it is sometimes ordered, do not infuse it so rapidly that circulatory overload is produced. Some authorities recommend that the drug in this much solution be infused over at least 30 minutes to minimize the risk of adverse cardiac reactions. I.V. cimetidine is often used in critically ill patients prophylactically to prevent GI bleeding.
• Hemodialysis reduces blood levels of cimetidine. Schedule cimetidine dose at end of hemodialysis treatment.

Monitoring

• Monitor effectiveness by regularly assessing for relief of or decrease in the patient's GI pain.
• Monitor the patient's stool for type, amount, and color.
• Frequently monitor I.V. site for signs of infiltration or phlebitis.
• Monitor for profound bradycardia and other cardiotoxic effects when giving drug rapidly by I.V.
• Evaluate hematologic studies for signs of abnormalities, such as thrombocytopenia and granulocytopenia.
• Monitor blood chemistry results for changes in creatinine and hepatic enzymes, which may reflect changes in the patient's renal or hepatic function.

Supportive Care

• If I.V. injection site becomes infiltrated or shows signs of phlebitis, discontinue I.V. and restart in another site. Notify the doctor and, if indicated, apply warm compress to site.
• Take seizure precautions if cimetidine accumulation occurs.
• Take safety precautions if the patient develops dizziness, confusion, or other mental status changes. For

example, keep bed in low position, keep side rails up, and supervise the patient's activity.
• If the patient develops diarrhea, notify the doctor and, if possible, obtain an order for an antidiarrheal. Also, if diarrhea is severe, encourage increased fluid intake.
• If the patient's stool becomes black and tarry, perform a test for occult blood and notify the doctor.
• Keep in mind that elderly or debilitated patients may be more susceptible to cimetidine-induced mental confusion.
• Remember that cimetidine is more effective for the treatment of duodenal ulcers than for the treatment of gastric ulcers.
• Remember that cimetidine may interfere with the results of several diagnostic tests. It antagonizes pentagastrin's effect during gastric acid secretion tests; may cause false-negative results in skin tests using allergen extracts; and increases prolactin, serum alkaline phosphatase, and serum creatinine levels. FD&C blue dye #2 used in Tagamet tablets may impair interpretation of tests for occult blood in gastric content aspirate. Be sure to wait at least 15 minutes after tablet administration before drawing the sample, and follow test manufacturer's instructions closely.

Patient Teaching

• Warn the patient to take drug as directed and to continue taking it even after pain subsides, to allow for adequate healing. Remind the patient not to take an antacid within 1 hour of taking drug.
• Remind the patient who is taking cimetidine once daily, to take it at bedtime for best results.
• Urge the patient to avoid smoking cigarettes, which may increase gastric acid secretion and worsen disease. Also tell the patient to avoid sources of GI irritation, such as alcohol, certain foods, and drugs containing aspirin.
• Instruct the patient to report immediately any signs of black, tarry stools; diarrhea; confusion; or rash.
• Advise the patient who is considering breast-feeding to consult with her doctor because drug is excreted in breast milk.

Evaluation

In patients receiving cimetidine, appropriate evaluation statements may include:
• Patient has experienced a decrease in or relief of GI pain.
• Patient has maintained normal bowel habits and has not experienced diarrhea.
• Patient and family state an understanding of cimetidine therapy.

cinoxacin

(sin ox´ a sin)
Cinobac

• *Classification:* urinary tract antiseptic (quinolone)
• *Pregnancy Risk Category:* B

HOW SUPPLIED

Capsules: 250 mg, 500 mg

ACTION

Mechanism: Inhibits microbial DNA synthesis.
Absorption: Well absorbed from the GI tract. Food decreases peak serum concentrations but not the extent of absorption.
Distribution: Concentrates in renal tissue; it is 60% to 80% protein-bound and has only fair prostatic penetration (30% to 60% of plasma levels).
Metabolism: Approximately 30% to 40% of cinoxacin dose is metabolized in the liver to inactive metabolites.
Excretion: Inactive metabolites and unchanged drug are excreted in the

urine. Half-life: 1 to 1½ hours in patients with normal renal function.
Onset, peak, duration: Peak plasma concentrations occur 1 to 2 hours after oral administration. Peak urine concentrations occur within 2 to 4 hours and usually exceed the minimum inhibitory concentration of susceptible organisms for 12 hours.

INDICATIONS & DOSAGE

Treatment of initial and recurrent urinary tract infections caused by susceptible strains of Escherichia coli, Klebsiella, Enterobacter, Proteus mirabilis, Proteus vulgaris, *and* Proteus morgani, Serratia, *and* Citrobacter–
Adults and children over 12 years: 1 g P.O. daily, in two to four divided doses for 7 to 14 days.

Not recommended for children under 12 years.

CONTRAINDICATIONS & PRECAUTIONS

Contraindicated in patients with hypersensitivity to the drug or to nalidixic acid. Use cautiously in patients with a history of hepatic or renal dysfunction, because drug accumulation may occur.

ADVERSE REACTIONS

Common reactions are in italics; life-threatening reactions are in bold italics.
CNS: *dizziness, headache,* drowsiness, insomnia, seizures.
EENT: photosensitivity, tinnitus.
GI: *nausea, vomiting, abdominal pain,* diarrhea.
Skin: rash, urticaria, pruritus, photosensitivity.

INTERACTIONS

Probenecid: may decrease urine levels of cinoxacin by inhibiting renal tubular secretion. Monitor for increased toxicity and reduced antibacterial effectiveness.

EFFECTS ON DIAGNOSTIC TESTS

Blood urea nitrogen: levels slightly increased.

NURSING CONSIDERATIONS

Besides those related universally to drug therapy (see "How to use this book"), consider the following specific recommendations:

Assessment
- Obtain a baseline assessment of infection before therapy.
- Be alert for adverse reactions and drug interactions throughout therapy.
- Evaluate the patient's and family's knowledge about cinoxacin therapy.

Nursing Diagnoses
- High risk for injury related to ineffectiveness of cinoxacin to eradicate the infection.
- High risk for fluid volume deficit related to adverse GI reactions caused by cinoxacin.
- Knowledge deficit related to cinoxacin.

Planning and Implementation

Preparation and Administration
- Obtain clean-catch urine specimen for culture and sensitivity tests before first dose. Therapy may begin pending test results.
- ***P.O. use:*** Administer drug with meals to minimize adverse GI reactions.

Monitoring
- Monitor effectiveness by regularly assessing for improvement in infection and by evaluating results of clean-catch urine specimens periodically as ordered.
- Monitor hydration status if adverse GI reactions occur.

Supportive Care
- Obtain an order for an antiemetic or antidiarrheal agent as needed.
- Impose safety precautions if the patient experiences adverse CNS reactions.
- Report adverse CNS reactions to the doctor immediately. They indicate

serious toxicity that usually requires discontinuation of drug.
• Take seizure precautions, such as padding bed rails, if needed. Notify the doctor if seizures occur.

Patient Teaching

• Because drug can cause dizziness or drowsiness, warn the patient to avoid driving and other hazardous tasks that require alertness until CNS effects of the drug are known.
• Instruct patient to notify the doctor if adverse CNS reactions occur because they may require discontinuation of the drug.
• Tell patient to take drug with meals to minimize adverse GI reactions.
• Remind patient to continue taking this drug, even when he feels better, and to take entire amount prescribed.

Evaluation

In patients receiving cinoxacin, appropriate evaluation statements may include:
• Patient is free of infection.
• Patient maintains adequate hydration throughout cinoxacin therapy.
• Patient and family state an understanding of cinoxacin therapy.

ciprofloxacin

(sip roe flox´ a sin)
Cipro, Cipro I.V., Ciproxin‡

• *Classification:* antibiotic (quinolone)
• *Pregnancy Risk Category:* C

HOW SUPPLIED

Tablets: 250 mg, 500 mg, 750 mg
Infusion (premixed): 200 mg in 100 ml 5% dextrose, 400 mg in 200 ml 5% dextrose
Vials: 200 mg (20 ml); 400 mg (40 ml)

ACTION

Mechanism: Exact mechanism unknown, but bactericidal effects may result from drug's ability to inhibit bacterial DNA gyrase and to prevent DNA replication in susceptible bacteria.
Absorption: About 70% is absorbed after oral administration. Food delays rate, but not extent, of absorption.
Distribution: 20% to 40% protein-bound. CSF levels are only about 10% of plasma levels.
Metabolism: Probably hepatic. Four metabolites have been identified; each has less antimicrobial activity than the parent compound.
Excretion: Primarily renal. Half-life: About 4 hours in adults with normal renal function.
Onset, peak, duration: Peak serum levels occur within 1 to 2 hours after oral administration.

INDICATIONS & DOSAGE

Mild to moderate urinary tract infections–
Adults: 250 mg P.O. or 200 mg I.V. q 12 hours.
Severe or complicated urinary tract infections; mild to moderate bone and joint infections; mild to moderate respiratory tract infections; mild to moderate skin and skin structure infections; infectious diarrhea–
Adults: 500 mg P.O. or 400 mg I.V. q 12 hours.
Severe or complicated bone or joint infections; severe respiratory tract infections; severe skin and skin structure infections–
Adults: 750 mg P.O. q 12 hours.

CONTRAINDICATIONS & PRECAUTIONS

Contraindicated in patients allergic to the drug or to other quinolone antibiotics, and in children because animal studies have shown that it can induce arthropathy in immature animals. Use cautiously in patients with suspected or known CNS disturbances, epilepsy, severe cerebral arterosclerosis, or other conditions that may induce seizures.

ADVERSE REACTIONS

Common reactions are in italics; life-threatening reactions are in bold italics.
CNS: headache, restlessness, tremor, light-headedness, confusion, hallucinations, *seizures.*
GI: *nausea, diarrhea,* vomiting, abdominal pain or discomfort, oral candidiasis.
GU: crystalluria.
Local: (with I.V. administration) thrombophlebitis, burning, pruritus, paresthesia, erythema, swelling.
Other: *rash,* eosinophilia.

INTERACTIONS

Antacids containing magnesium hydroxide or aluminum hydroxide: decreased ciprofloxacin absorption. Separate administration by at least 2 hours.
Probenecid: may elevate serum ciprofloxacin level.
Theophylline: increased plasma theophylline concentrations and prolonged theophylline half-life.

EFFECTS ON DIAGNOSTIC TESTS

None reported.

NURSING CONSIDERATIONS

Besides those related universally to drug therapy (see "How to use this book"), consider the following specific recommendations:

Assessment
- Obtain a baseline assessment of infection before therapy.
- Be alert for adverse reactions and drug interactions throughout therapy.
- Evaluate the patient's and family's knowledge about ciprofloxacin therapy.

Nursing Diagnoses
- High risk for injury related to ineffectiveness of ciprofloxacin to eradicate the infection.
- High risk for fluid volume deficit related to adverse GI reactions to ciprofloxacin.
- Knowledge deficit related to ciprofloxacin.

Planning and Implementation
Preparation and Administration
- Obtain specimen for culture and sensitivity tests before first dose. Therapy may begin pending test results.
- Dosage adjustments may be necessary in patients with renal dysfunction.
- ***P.O. use:*** Administer drug 2 hours after a meal. Food does not affect absorption but may delay peak serum levels. Administer antacids, if prescribed, at least 2 hours after administering drug.
- ***I.V. use:*** Vials (injection concentrate) must be diluted before use. Follow manufacturer's instructions for dilution. Infuse slowly (over 60 minutes) into a large vein.

Monitoring
- Monitor effectiveness by regularly assessing for improvement in infection.
- Monitor hydration status if adverse GI reactions occur.
- Periodically evaluate patient's and family's knowledge about ciprofloxacin.

Supportive Care
- Obtain an order for an antiemetic or antidiarrheal agent as needed.
- Impose safety precautions if the patient experiences adverse CNS reactions.
- Take seizure precautions, such as padding bed rails, if needed. Notify the doctor if seizures occur.
- Be aware that serious (even fatal) reactions have occurred in patients receiving I.V. theophylline and ciprofloxacin. If a patient must receive theophylline or aminophylline therapy with ciprofloxacin, closely monitor serum theophylline levels and expect dosage adjustments to be made accordingly.
- Because drug is excreted in breast milk, make sure patient has discon-

tinued breast-feeding during treatment.
• Have patient drink plenty of fluids to reduce the risk of crystalluria.
Patient Teaching
• May cause dizziness or light-headedness. Warn the patient to avoid driving or hazardous tasks that require alertness until CNS effects of the drug are known.
• Advise the patient to drink plenty of fluids to reduce the risk of crystalluria.
• Tell patient to take drug 2 hours after a meal and to take prescribed antacids at least 2 hours after taking the drug.
• Inform patients who are breast-feeding that drug is excreted in breast milk. Breast-feeding must be discontinued during drug therapy or a different drug used.
Evaluation
In patients receiving ciprofloxacin, appropriate evaluation statements may include:
• Patient is free of infection.
• Patient maintains adequate hydration throughout ciprofloxacin therapy.
• Patient and family state an understanding of ciprofloxacin therapy.

cisplatin (cis-platinum)
(sis´ pla tin)
Platamine‡, Platinol

• *Classification:* antineoplastic agent (alklyating agent)
• *Pregnancy Risk Category:* D

HOW SUPPLIED
Injection: 10-mg, 50-mg vials

ACTION
Mechanism: A platinum coordination complex that cross-links strands of cellular DNA and interferes with RNA transcription, causing an imbalance of growth that leads to cell death. Cell cycle–nonspecific.
Distribution: Widely distributed into tissues, with highest concentrations in the kidneys, liver, and prostate; can accumulate in body tissues and can be detected up to 6 months after the last dose; does not readily cross the blood-brain barrier. The drug is extensively and irreversibly bound to plasma proteins and tissue proteins.
Metabolism: No evidence of enzymatic metabolism; the drug probably undergoes spontaneous hydration, resulting in the release of free platinum.
Excretion: Primarily unchanged in urine. In patients with normal renal function. Half life: Initial elimination phase is 25 to 79 minutes; terminal phase is 58 to 78 hours. The terminal half-life of total cisplatin is up to 10 days.

INDICATIONS & DOSAGE
Adjunctive therapy in metastatic testicular cancer–
Adults: 20 mg/m² I.V. daily for 5 days. Repeat every 3 weeks for 3 cycles or longer.
Adjunctive therapy in metastatic ovarian cancer–
100 mg/m² I.V. Repeat every 4 weeks; or 50 mg/m² I.V. every 3 weeks with concurrent doxorubicin HCl therapy.
Treatment of advanced bladder cancer–
Adults: 50 to 70 mg/m² I.V. once every 3 to 4 weeks. Patients who have received other antineoplastics or radiation therapy should receive 50 mg/m² every 4 weeks.
Note: Prehydration and mannitol diuresis may reduce renal toxicity and ototoxicity significantly.

CONTRAINDICATIONS & PRECAUTIONS
Contraindicated in patients with a history of hypersensitivity to cisplatin or other platinum-containing com-

pounds; patients who have been previously exposed to these agents should undergo skin testing before cisplatin therapy because of potential for allergic reaction. Also contraindicated in patients with myelosuppression or hearing impairment because drug may worsen these conditions.

Use cautiously or adjust dosage in patients with impaired renal function because of the drug's nephrotoxic effects. Drug is usually not used in patients with a creatinine clearance below 50 ml/minute. Perform baseline audiometry before therapy begins. Cisplatin can impair fertility. Aspermia has been reported after cisplatin therapy.

ADVERSE REACTIONS

Common reactions are in italics; life-threatening reactions are in bold italics.

Blood: *mild myelosuppression in 25% to 30% of patients, leukopenia,* ***thrombocytopenia,*** anemia; nadirs in circulating platelets and leukocytes on days 18 to 23, with recovery by day 39.

CNS: peripheral neuritis, loss of taste, seizures.

EENT: *tinnitus, hearing loss.*

GI: *nausea, vomiting, beginning 1 to 4 hours after dose and lasting 24 hours;*diarrhea; metallic taste.

GU: *more prolonged and* ***severe renal toxicity*** with repeated courses of therapy.

Other: ***anaphylactoid reaction.***

INTERACTIONS

Aminoglycoside antibiotics: additive nephrotoxicity. Monitor renal function studies very carefully.

EFFECTS ON DIAGNOSTIC TESTS

BUN, serum creatinine, and serum uric acid: increased levels.

Creatinine clearance, serum calcium, magnesium, phosphate, and potassium: decreased levels indicating nephrotoxicity.

NURSING CONSIDERATIONS

Besides those related universally to drug therapy (see "How to use this book"), consider the following specific recommendations:

Assessment

- Obtain a baseline assessment of the patient's underlying condition and WBC, platelet, BUN, creatinine, and electrolyte levels before initiating therapy.
- Be alert for adverse reactions or drug interactions during therapy.
- Evaluate the patient's and family's knowledge about cisplatin therapy.

Nursing Diagnoses

- High risk for fluid volume deficit and renal tissue impairment related to physiologic renal needs.
- Sensory alteration (hearing) related to ototoxicty manifested by tinnitus and hearing loss.
- Knowledge deficit related to cisplatin therapy.

Planning and Implementation

Preparation and Administration

- Hydrate patient with 1 to 2 liters of I.V. normal saline solution before administering cisplatin. Maintain urine output of at least 100 ml/hour for 4 consecutive hours before and for 24 hours after infusion.
- Be aware that antiemetics are often started (up to 24 hours) before therapy.
- Expect that mannitol may be ordered to be given as 12.5 g I.V. bolus before starting cisplatin infusion. If ordered, a mannitol infusion may also follow cisplatin administration at a rate of up to 10 g/hour p.r.n. to maintain urine output during and for 6 to 24 hours after cisplatin infusion.
- ***I.V. use:*** Administer as an I.V. infusion in 2 liters normal saline solution with 37.5 g mannitol over 6 to 8 hours as recommended by the manufacturer. Reconstitute with sterile water for injection. Stable for 24 hours in normal saline solution at room temperature. Don't refrigerate.

Use a 0.45-mcg filter. Infusions are most stable in chloride-containing solutions. Keep in mind that preparation of parenteral form is associated with carcinogenic risks for personnel and that they must follow institutional policy to reduce these risks. Do not use needles or I.V. administration sets that contain aluminum as it will displace the platinum, causing precipitation and loss of potency. Add potassium chloride, as ordered, to I.V. fluids before and after cisplatin administration, to prevent deficiencies.
- Do not repeat dosage unless platelets are >100,000/mm³, WBC is >4,000/mm⁴, creatinine is <1.5 mg/dl, or BUN is <25 mg/dl.
- Be aware that investigational protocols may include administering cisplatin in 3% sodium chloride following intense prehydration with 0.9% sodium chloride.

Monitoring
- Monitor effectiveness by noting results of follow-up diagnostic tests and overall physical status.
- Monitor WBC, platelet, potassium, magnesium, BUN, and creatinine levels during therapy.
- Monitor efects of ototoxicity; have patient report tinnitus and hearing loss. Do audiometry prior to starting therapy.
- Monitor daily intake and output; report the first signs of oliguria.
- Monitor for facial edema, bronchospasm, tachydysrhythmias, and shock.
- Monitor for tremors, tetany, confusion, or other signs of hypomagnesemia or hypocalcemia. Do regular neurological examinations.

Supportive Care
- If ordered, administer metoclopramide. High-dose metoclopramide with dexamethasone and antihistamines has been effective in combating nausea and vomiting. Nausea and vomiting may be severe and last up to 24 hours after infusion has ended. Delayed-onset of up to 3 to 5 days has been reported.
- Remember that renal toxicity is cumulative. Function must return to normal before the next dose can be given. Also remember that cisplatin may be removed via hemodialysis for 3 hours after administration.
- If the patient has an anaphalactoid reaction, treat it immediately and notify the doctor. Anaphalactoid reactions usually respond to immediate treatment with epinephrine, corticosteroids, or antihistamines.

Patient Teaching
- Teach patient to record intake and output on a daily basis; and to report any edema or decrease in urine output.
- Teach patient to report any ringing in ears or hearing loss.
- Warn patient to watch for signs of infection and bleeding.
- Teach patient to take and record temperature daily.

Evaluation

In patients receiving cisplatin, appropriate evaluation statements may include:
- Patient's renal function was adequate; urinary output is maintained without collection of edema.
- Patient did not experience tinnitus nor hearing loss.
- Patient and family state an understanding of cisplatin therapy.

clemastine fumarate

(klem´ as teen)

Tavist*, Tavist-1

- *Classification:* antimuscarinic, GI antispasmodic (anticholinergic)
- *Pregnancy Risk Category:* C

HOW SUPPLIED

Tablets: 1.34 mg, 2.68 mg

Syrup: 0.67 mg/5 ml (equivalent to 0.5 mg base/5 ml)*

*Liquid form contains alcohol. **May contain tartrazine.

ACTION

Mechanism: Blocks the effects of histamine at H_1 receptors. Prevents but does not reverse histamine-mediated responses.
Absorption: Rapidly and completely absorbed from the GI tract.
Distribution: Drug enters breast milk, and probably enters CNS.
Metabolism: Extensively metabolized, probably in the liver.
Excretion: Drug and metabolites are excreted in urine.
Onset, peak, duration: Action begins in 15 to 30 minutes and peaks in 2 to 7 hours.

INDICATIONS & DOSAGE

Rhinitis, allergy symptoms–
Adults: 1.34 to 2.68 mg P.O. b.i.d. or t.i.d. Maximum recommended daily dosage is 8.04 mg.
Children 6 to 12 years: 0.67 mg P.O. b.i.d. Maximum dosage is 4.02 mg/day.
Allergic skin manifestation of urticaria and angioedema–
Adults: 2.68 mg P.O. up to t.i.d. maximum.
Children 6 to 12 years: 1.34 mg P.O. b.i.d. Maximum dosage is 4.02 mg/day.

Note: Children under 12 years should use only as directed by a doctor.

CONTRAINDICATIONS & PRECAUTIONS

Contraindicated in patients with hypersensitivity to this drug or other antihistamines with similar chemical structures (carbinoxamine and diphenhydramine); during an acute asthmatic attack because it thickens bronchial secretions; and in patients who have taken monoamine oxidase (MAO) inhibitors within the preceding 2 weeks; and during pregnancy (especially in the third trimester) or during breast-feeding. Antihistamines have caused seizures and other severe reactions, especially in premature infants.

Use cautiously in patients with narrow-angle glaucoma; in those with pyloroduodenal obstruction or urinary bladder obstruction from prostatic hypertrophy or narrowing of the bladder neck because of their marked anticholinergic effects; cardiovascular disease, hypertension, or hyperthyroidism because of the risk of palpitations and tachycardia; and renal disease, diabetes, bronchial asthma, urine retention, or stenosing peptic ulcers.

ADVERSE REACTIONS

Common reactions are in italics; life-threatening reactions are in bold italics.
Blood: ***hemolytic anemia,*** thrombocytopenia, ***agranulocytosis.***
CNS: (especially in elderly patients) *sedation, drowsiness.*
CV: hypotension, palpitations, tachycardia.
GI: epigastric distress, anorexia, nausea, vomiting, constipation, *dry mouth.*
GU: urine retention.
Skin: rash, urticaria.
Other: thick bronchial secretions.

INTERACTIONS

CNS depressants: increased sedation. Use together cautiously.
MAO inhibitors: increased anticholinergic effects. Don't use together.

EFFECTS ON DIAGNOSTIC TESTS

Diagnostic skin tests: test interference.

NURSING CONSIDERATIONS

Besides those related universally to drug therapy (see "How to use this book"), consider the following specific recommendations:

Assessment

• Obtain a baseline assessment of the patient's respiratory status before clemastine fumarate therapy.

• Be alert for adverse reactions and drug interactions throughout therapy.
• Evaluate the patient's and family's knowledge about clemastine fumarate therapy.

Nursing Diagnoses

• Ineffective airway clearance related to allergy symptoms.
• Hyperthermia related to potential clemastine fumarate-induced agranulocytosis.
• Knowledge deficit related to clemastine fumarate therapy.

Planning and Implementation

Preparation and Administration

• ***P.O. use:*** Reduce GI distress by giving with food or milk.

Monitoring

• Monitor effectiveness by frequently checking the patient's respiratory status and asking about the severity of allergy symptoms.
• Monitor blood counts during long-term therapy; watch for signs of blood dyscrasias.

Supportive Care

• Keep in mind that another antihistamine may be substituted if tolerance to this drug develops.
• Remember that clemastine fumarate is available as a nonprescription item for self-medication by adults; use in children under 12 years of age is not recommended without a doctor's supervision.
• Remember that clemastine fumarate causes less drowsiness than some other antihistamines.

Patient Teaching

• Suggest that the patient drink coffee or tea to reduce drowsiness.
• Tell the patient that sugarless gum, sour hard candy, or ice chips may relieve dry mouth.
• Warn patient to avoid alcoholic beverages during therapy and to avoid driving or other hazardous activities that require alertness until CNS adverse effects are known.
• Advise patient to stop taking clemastine fumarate 4 days before allergy skin testing to preserve the accuracy of the tests.

Evaluation

In patients receiving clemastine fumarate, appropriate evaluation statements may include:

• Patient's allergic symptoms are relieved with clemastine fumerate therapy.
• Patient does not experience significant CNS adverse effects.
• Patient and family state an understanding of clemastine fumarate therapy.

clidinium bromide

(kli di´ nee um)

Quarzan

• *Classification:* antimuscarinic, GI antispasmodic (anticholinergic)
• *Pregnancy Risk Category:* C

HOW SUPPLIED

Capsules: 2.5 mg, 5 mg

ACTION

Mechanism: A quartenary anticholinergic that competitively blocks the vagal effects of acetylcholine, decreasing GI motility and inhibiting gastric acid secretion.
Absorption: Only 10% to 25% of a dose is absorbed from the GI tract.
Distribution: As a quartenary ammonium compound, the drug is not expected to enter the CNS or aqueous humor of the eye.
Metabolism: Hepatic by enzymatic hydrolysis.
Excretion: In urine and feces.
Onset, peak, duration: Onset of action occurs within 1 hour, with duration of action about 3 hours.

INDICATIONS & DOSAGE

Adjunctive therapy for peptic ulcers—Dosage should be individualized according to severity of symptoms and occurrence of adverse reactions.
Elderly or debilitated patients: 2.5 to 5 mg P.O. t.i.d. or q.i.d. before meals and h.s.

CONTRAINDICATIONS & PRECAUTIONS

Contraindicated in patients with narrow-angle glaucoma because drug-induced cycloplegia and mydriasis may increase intraocular pressure; obstructive uropathy, obstructive GI tract disease, severe ulcerative colitis, myasthenia gravis, paralytic ileus, intestinal atony, or toxic megacolon because the drug may exacerbate these conditions; and hypersensitivity to anticholinergics.

Use cautiously in patients with autonomic neuropathy, hyperthyroidism, coronary artery disease, cardiac arrhythmias, CHF, or ulcerative colitis, because the drug may exacerbate symptoms of these disorders; hepatic or renal disease because toxic accumulation can occur; to patients over age 40 because the drug increases the glaucoma risk; hiatal hernia associated with reflux esophagitis because the drug may decrease lower esophageal sphincter tone; and in hot or humid environments because the drug may predispose the patient to heatstroke.

ADVERSE REACTIONS

Common reactions are in italics; life-threatening reactions are in bold italics.
CNS: headache, insomnia, drowsiness, dizziness, *confusion or excitement in elderly patients,* nervousness, weakness.
CV: *palpitations,* tachycardia.
EENT: *blurred vision,* mydriasis, increased ocular tension, cycloplegia, photophobia.
GI: *dry mouth,* dysphagia, heartburn, loss of taste, nausea, vomiting, *paralytic ileus, constipation.*
GU: *urinary hesitancy, urine retention,* impotence.
Skin: urticaria, decreased sweating or possible anhidrosis, other dermal manifestations.
Other: fever, allergic reactions.

Overdosage may cause curare-like symptoms.

INTERACTIONS

None significant.

EFFECTS ON DIAGNOSTIC TESTS

None reported.

NURSING CONSIDERATIONS

Besides those related universally to drug therapy (see "How to use this book"), consider the following specific recommendations:

Assessment

- Obtain a baseline assessment of the patient's underlying condition before drug therapy.
- Be alert for adverse reactions and drug interactions throughout therapy.
- Evaluate the patient's and family's knowledge about clidinium bromide therapy.

Nursing Diagnoses

- Altered health maintenance related to the patient's underlying condition.
- Constipation related to adverse drug reactions.
- Knowledge deficit related to clidinium bromide therapy.

Planning and Implementation

Preparation and Administration

- ***P.O. use:*** Give 30 minutes to 1 hour before meals and at mealtimes. Bedtime dose can be larger and should be given at least 2 hours after the last meal of the day.

Monitoring

- Monitor intake and output. Drug causes urine retention and urinary hesitancy; encourage the patient to void before receiving drug.
- Monitor closely for aspiration,

which may occur as a result of dysphagia.
• Monitor effectiveness by regularly assessing underlying condition.
• Monitor closely for urine retention in elderly men with benign prostatic hypertrophy.
Supportive Care
• Help the patient to get in and out of bed if he experiences dizziness or blurred vision.
• Provide gum or sugarless hard candy to relieve dry mouth.
• If constipation occurs, obtain an order for a laxative.
• Provide additional fluids to help prevent constipattion.
Patient Teaching
• Tell the patient to avoid driving and other hazardous activities that require alertness, if he is drowsy, dizzy, or has blurred vision.
• Encourage the patient to drink plenty of fluids to avoid constipation.
• Tell him to report any rash or skin eruptions.
• Tell the patient to take the drug 30 minutes to 1 hour before meals, and to take the bedtime dose at least 2 hours after the last meal of the day.
Evaluation
In patients receiving clidinium bromide, appropriate evaluation statements may include:
• Patient is able to perform activities of daily living without assistance.
• Patient does not develop constipation.
• Patient and family state an understanding of clidinium bromide therapy.

---

clindamycin hydrochloride
(klin da mye´ sin)
Cleocin HCl, Dalacin C†‡

clindamycin palmitate hydrochloride
Cleocin Pediatric, Dalacin C Palmitate†‡

clindamycin phosphate
Cleocin, Cleocin Phosphate, Dalacin C†‡, Dalacin C Phosphate

• *Classification:* antibiotic (lincomycin derivative)
• *Pregnancy Risk Category:* C

HOW SUPPLIED
Capsules: 75 mg, 150 mg
Oral solution: 75 mg/5 ml
Injection: 150 mg/ml

ACTION
Mechanism: Inhibits bacterial protein synthesis by binding to the 50S subunit of the ribosome.
Absorption: Absorbed rapidly and almost completely from the GI tract after oral administration, regardless of formulation. Clindamycin palmitate hydrochloride is hydrolyzed to free clindamycin before absorption. Phosphate salt is rapidly absorbed after I.M. injection, and is hydrolyzed in the plasma to free clindamycin after I.M. or I.V. administration.
Distribution: Widely distributed to most body tissues and fluids (except CSF); crosses the placenta. Approximately 93% is bound to plasma proteins.
Metabolism: Partially metabolized to inactive metabolites.
Excretion: About 10% of dose is excreted unchanged in urine, the remainder as inactive metabolites; some is excreted in breast milk. Half-life: 2½ to 3 hours in patients with normal renal function, 3½ to 5 hours in anephric patients, and 7 to 14 hours in patients with hepatic disease.
Onset, peak, duration: Peak concentrations of 1.9 to 3.9 mcg/ml occur in 45 to 60 minutes after oral administration. After I.M. injection, peak

concentrations occur in about 3 hours in adults and 1 hour in children.

INDICATIONS & DOSAGE

Infections caused by sensitive staphylococci, streptococci, pneumococci, Bacteroides, Fusobacterium, Clostridium perfringens, *and other sensitive aerobic and anaerobic organisms*– **Adults:** 150 to 450 mg P.O. q 6 hours; or 300 mg I.M. or I.V. q 6, 8, or 12 hours. Up to 2,700 mg I.M. or I.V. daily, divided q 6, 8, or 12 hours.

May be used for severe infections. **Children over 1 month:** 8 to 25 mg/kg P.O. daily, divided q 6 to 8 hours; or 15 to 40 mg/kg I.M. or I.V. daily, divided q 6 hours.

CONTRAINDICATIONS & PRECAUTIONS

Contraindicated in patients hypersensitive to the drug or to lincomycin, and those with a history of inflammatory bowel disease or antibiotic-induced colitis.

Use cautiously in patients with renal or hepatic dysfunction because it may exacerbate these conditions; with asthma or significant allergies; and in neonates with tartrazine sensitivity.

ADVERSE REACTIONS

Common reactions are in italics; life-threatening reactions are in bold italics.
Blood: transient leukopenia, eosinophilia, thrombocytopenia.
GI: *nausea,* vomiting, abdominal pain, *diarrhea,* ***pseudomembranous enterocolitis,*** esophagitis, flatulence, anorexia, ***bloody or tarry stools,*** *dysphagia.*
Hepatic: elevated AST (SGOT), alkaline phosphatase, bilirubin.
Skin: maculopapular rash, urticaria.
Local: *pain,* induration, *sterile abscess with I.M. injection;* thrombophlebitis, erythema, and pain after I.V. administration.
Other: unpleasant or bitter taste, ***anaphylaxis.***

INTERACTIONS

Erythromycin: antagonist that may block access of clindamycin to its site of action; don't use together.
Kaolin: decreased absorption of oral clindamycin.
Neuromuscular blocking agents: clindamycin may potentiate neuromuscular blockade.

EFFECTS ON DIAGNOSTIC TESTS

Liver function tests: abnormal results.

NURSING CONSIDERATIONS

Besides those related universally to drug therapy (see "How to use this book"), consider the following specific recommendations:

Assessment
- Obtain a baseline assessment of infection before therapy.
- Be alert for adverse reactions and drug interactions throughout therapy.
- Evaluate the patient's and family's knowledge about clindamycin therapy.

Nursing Diagnoses
- High risk for injury related to ineffectiveness of clindamycin to eradicate the infection.
- High risk for fluid volume deficit related to clindamycin-induced adverse GI reactions.
- Knowledge deficit related to clindamycin.

Planning and Implementation
Preparation and Administration
- Obtain specimen for culture and sensitivity tests before first dose. Therapy may begin pending test results.
- ***P.O. use:*** Administer capsule form with a full glass of water to prevent dysphagia. Don't refrigerate reconstituted oral solution because it will thicken. Drug is stable for 2 weeks at room temperature.
- ***I.M. use:*** Give deep I.M. Rotate

sites. Be aware that injection may be painful. Doses greater than 600 mg/injection are not recommended.
• ***I.V. use:*** Dilute each 300 mg in 50 ml solution and give no faster than 30 mg/minute.
Monitoring
• Monitor effectiveness by regularly assessing for improvement in the infection.
• Monitor renal, hepatic, and hematopoietic functions during prolonged therapy.
• Monitor hydration status if adverse GI reactions occur.
Supportive Care
• Obtain an order for an antiemetic or antidiarrheal agent as needed. Don't give diphenoxylate compound (Lomotil) to treat drug-induced diarrhea, because it may prolong and worsen diarrhea.
Patient Teaching
• Advise patient taking capsule form to take with a full glass of water to prevent dysphagia.
• Tell the patient to take medication for as long as prescribed, exactly as directed, and even after he feels better and to take entire amount prescribed.
• Instruct patient to keep drug at room temperature.
• Warn patient that I.M. injection may be painful.
• Instruct patient to report diarrhea and to avoid self-treatment.
• Tell patient receiving clindamycin I.V. to tell the nurse of discomfort at the infusion site.

Evaluation
In patients receiving clindamycin, appropriate evaluation statements may include:
• Patient is free from infection.
• Patient maintains adequate hydration throughout clindamycin therapy.
• Patient and family state an understanding of clindamycin therapy.

clindamycin phosphate
(klin da mye´ sin)
Cleocin T Gel, Lotion, Solution

• *Classification:* antibiotic (lincomycin derivative)
• *Pregnancy Risk Category:* B

HOW SUPPLIED
Gel: 1%
Lotion: 1%
Topical solution: 1%

ACTION
Mechanism: Suppresses growth of susceptible organisms in sebaceous glands.
Absorption: About 10% of a dose is absorbed into the stratum corneum.
Excretion: Less than 0.2% of a dose is found in the urine unchanged.
Onset, peak, duration: Very low serum levels are achieved after topical application, ranging from 0 to 3 ng/ml.

INDICATIONS & DOSAGE
Treatment of acne vulgaris, grades II and III–
Adults and adolescents: apply to skin b.i.d., morning and evening; solutions have been used once daily to q.i.d.

CONTRAINDICATIONS & PRECAUTIONS
Contraindicated in patients hypersensitive to the drug or to lincomycin.

Use cautiously in patients with renal or hepatic dysfunction. Also use cautiously in atopic patients because of potential for contact dermatitis.

ADVERSE REACTIONS
Common reactions are in italics; life-threatening reactions are in bold italics.
Skin: *dryness,* rash, redness, itching, swelling, irritation.

INTERACTIONS

Abrasive or medicated soaps or cleansers; acne preparations or any containing a peeling agent (benzoyl peroxide, salicylic acid, sulfur, resorcinol, tretinoin); alcohol-containing products (after-shave, perfumed toiletries, shaving creams or lotions, cosmetics); soaps or cosmetics with strong drying effect; isotretinoin; medicated cosmetics or "cover-ups": may cause cumulative drying or irritation, resulting in excessive skin irritation.

EFFECTS ON DIAGNOSTIC TESTS

None reported with topical use.

NURSING CONSIDERATIONS

Besides those related universally to drug therapy (see "How to use this book"), consider the following specific recommendations:

Assessment

- Obtain a baseline assessment of acne before therapy.
- Be alert for adverse reactions and drug interactions throughout therapy.
- Evaluate the patient's and family's knowledge about clindamycin therapy.

Nursing Diagnoses

- Impaired skin integrity related to acne blemishes.
- High risk for impaired skin integrity related to clindamycin-induced skin dryness.
- Knowledge deficit related to clindamycin therapy.

Planning and Implementation

Preparation and Administration

- ***Topical use:*** Apply to skin morning and evening. Use only as prescribed. Use dabbing motion rather than rolling action, when using an applicator-tip bottle.

Monitoring

- Monitor effectiveness by regularly examining acne blemishes.
- Monitor for adverse reactions by frequently assessing the patient's skin for dryness.

Supportive Care

- Keep in mind that clindamycin may be used concurrently with tretinoin and/or benzoyl peroxide as well as systemic antibiotics. Warn patient to notify doctor if skin becomes excessively dry.
- Be aware improvement is usually noticeable within 6 weeks; however, 8 to 12 weeks may be required for maximum benefit.

Patient Teaching

- Teach patient how to apply medication.
- Tell the patient that noticeable improvement may be seen within 6 weeks but may require 8 to 12 weeks for maximum benefit.
- Instruct patient to wash area with warm water and soap, and to rinse and pat dry before application; and allow 30 minutes after washing or shaving to apply. Warn patient to avoid too frequent washing of area. Tell patient to cover entire affected area, but to avoid contact with eyes, nose, mouth, and other mucous membranes.
- Warn patient not to smoke during application.

Evaluation

In patients receiving clindamycin, appropriate evaluation statements may include:

- Patient's acne has healed.
- Patient did not experience dryness.
- Patient and family state an understanding of clindamycin phosphate therapy.

---

clioquinol (iodochlorhydroxyquin)

(klye oh kwin´ ole

Torofor◇, Vioform◇

- *Classification:* antifungal (quinoline)
- *Pregnancy Risk Category:* C

HOW SUPPLIED

Cream: 3%
Ointment: 3%

ACTION

Mechanism: An 8-hydroxyquinoline derivative that has fungistatic and fungicidal activity.
Absorption: Variable; estimates range from 3% to 40%. Absorption is probably increased when an occlusive dressing is applied.

INDICATIONS & DOSAGE

Inflamed skin conditions, including eczema, athlete's foot, and other fungal infections; cutaneous or mucocutaneous mycotic infections caused by Candida *species* (monilia) –
Adults and children over 2 years: apply a thin layer b.i.d. or t.i.d., or as directed. Continue for 1 week after cessation of symptoms.

CONTRAINDICATIONS & PRECAUTIONS

Contraindicated in patients with hypersensitivity to iodine or iodine-containing preparations and in tuberculosis, vaccinia or varicella.

ADVERSE REACTIONS

Common reactions are in italics; life-threatening reactions are in bold italics.
CNS: neurotoxicity (with systemic absorption).
Metabolic: altered protein-bound iodine levels (with systemic absorption).
Skin: *possible burning, itching, acneiform eruptions,* allergic contact dermatitis.

INTERACTIONS

Systemic corticosteroids: possible increased absorption. Use together cautiously.

EFFECTS ON DIAGNOSTIC TESTS

None reported.

NURSING CONSIDERATIONS

Besides those related universally to drug therapy (see "How to use this book"), consider the following specific recommendations:

Assessment

• Obtain a baseline assessment of skin redness, dryness, and inflammation before therapy.

Nursing Diagnoses

• Impaired skin integrity related to patient's underlying condition.
• High risk for impaired skin integrity related to acneiform eruptions.
• Knowledge deficit related to clioquinol therapy.

Planning and Implementation

Preparation and Administration

• ***Topical use:*** Apply a thin layer on affected area. Continue for 1 week after cessation of symptoms.

Monitoring

• Monitor effectiveness by observing skin for erythema, swelling, and drainage.
• Monitor for adverse reactions or interactions by frequently assessing the patient's skin for burning, itching, contact dermatitis, and acneiform eruptions.
• Monitor for systemic absorption by checking for altered protein-bound iodine levels.
• Monitor for neurotoxicity with systemic absorption.

Supportive Care

• Note all adverse reactions and precautions of each component in the combination antifungals.
• Avoid use in diaper rash.
• Be aware, presence in urine may cause false-positive result for phenylketonuria (PKU) or inaccurate thyroid function tests. Discontinue at least 1 month before thyroid function tests.
• Notify doctor if adverse reactions occur.

Patient Teaching
• Teach patient to apply medication.
• Inform patient drug will stain fabric and hair.

Evaluation
In patients receiving clioquinol, appropriate evaluation statements may include:
• Superficial infection has resolved.
• Acneiform eruptions did not occur.
• Patient and family state an understanding of clioquinol therapy.

clobetasol propionate
(kloe bay´ ta sol)
Dermovate†, Temovate

• *Classification:* anti-inflammatory (adrenocorticoid)
• *Pregnancy Risk Category:* C

HOW SUPPLIED
Cream: 0.05%
Ointment: 0.05%

ACTION
Mechanism: Produces local anti-inflammatory, vasoconstrictor, and antipruritic actions. Diffuses across cell membranes to form complexes with specific cytoplasmic receptors, influencing cellular metabolism. Corticosteroids stabilize leukocyte lysosomal membranes, inhibit local actions and accumulation of macrophages, decrease local edema, and reduce the formation of scar tissue.
Absorption: Amount absorbed depends on amount applied and on nature of skin at the application site; it ranges from about 1% in areas with thick stratum corneum (on the palms, soles, elbows, and knees) to as high as 36% in thinner areas (face, eyelids, and genitals). Absorption increases in areas of skin damage, inflammation, or occlusion. Some systemic absorption of topical steroids may occur, especially through the oral mucosa.
Distribution: After topical application, distributed throughout the local skin. Any drug absorbed is rapidly removed from the blood and distributed into muscle, liver, skin, intestines, and kidneys.
Metabolism: After topical administration, metabolized primarily in the skin. The small amount absorbed into systemic circulation is metabolized primarily in the liver to inactive compounds.
Excretion: Inactive metabolites are excreted by the kidneys, primarily as glucuronides and sulfates, but also as unconjugated products. Small amounts of the metabolites are also excreted in feces.

INDICATIONS & DOSAGE
Inflammation of corticosteroid-responsive dermatoses–
Adults: apply a thin layer to affected skin areas b.i.d., once in the morning and once at night. Do not use more than 50 g of cream or ointment/week. Therapy should be limited to a maximum of 14 days.

CONTRAINDICATIONS & PRECAUTIONS
Contraindicated in patients with hypersensitivity to any component of the preparation and in patients with viral, fungal, or tubercular skin lesions. Use with extreme caution in patients with impaired circulation because the drug may increase the risk of skin ulceration.

ADVERSE REACTIONS
Common reactions are in italics; life-threatening reactions are in bold italics.
Skin: burning, itching, irritation, dryness, folliculitis, perioral dermatitis, allergic contact dermatitis, hypopigmentation, hypertrichosis, acneiform eruptions.

INTERACTIONS

None significant.

EFFECTS ON DIAGNOSTIC TESTS

None significant.

NURSING CONSIDERATIONS

Besides those related universally to drug therapy (see "How to use this book"), consider the following specific recommendations:

Assessment

• Obtain a baseline assessment of the patient's skin in the affected area before therapy.
• Be alert for adverse reactions and drug interactions throughout therapy.
• Evaluate the patient's and family's knowledge about clobetasol therapy.

Nursing Diagnoses

• Impaired skin integrity related to the patient's underlying condition.
• High risk for impaired skin integrity related to clobetasol-induced irritation.
• Knowledge deficit related to clobetasol therapy.

Planning and Implementation

Preparation and Administration

• ***Topical use:*** Wash skin gently before applying. Rub medication in gently, leaving a thin coat, to prevent skin damage. When treating hairy sites, part hair and apply directly to lesions.
• Occlusive dressings should not be used. Treated areas of skin should not be bandaged, covered, or wrapped.
• Do not refrigerate.

Monitoring

• Monitor effectiveness by regularly examining patient's skin.
• Monitor patient for signs of systemic absorption: skin irritation or ulceration, hypersensitivity, or infection. If they develop, stop drug and notify doctor. (If antifungals or antibiotics are being used with corticosteroids and infection does not respond immediately, corticosteroids should be discontinued until infection is controlled.)
• Monitor for adverse reactions and interactions by frequently inspecting the patient's skin for infection, striae and atrophy.

Supportive Care

• Be prepared to discontinue drug and notify doctor if infection, straie, or atrophy occur.

Patient Teaching

• Teach patient to apply medication.
• Instruct patient to avoid application near eyes or mucous membranes or in ear canal.
• Warn patient not to use for longer than 14 consecutive days because of the risk of systemic absorption and suppression of hypothalamic-pituitary-adrenal axis. Clobetasol is a potent fluoridated corticosteroid.
• Remind patient that diminished effectiveness can follow repeated application.

Evaluation

In patients receiving clobetasol, appropriate evaluation statements may include:

• Patient states his dermatosis has resolved.
• Patient does not develop skin irritation.
• Patient and family state an understanding of clobetasol therapy.

---

clocortolone pivalate

(kloe kor´ toe lone)
Cloderm

• *Classification:* anti-inflammatory (adrenocorticoid)
• *Pregnancy Risk Category:* C

HOW SUPPLIED

Cream: 0.1%

ACTION

Mechanism: Produces local anti-inflammatory, vasoconstrictor, and an-

*Liquid form contains alcohol. **May contain tartrazine.

tipruritic actions. Diffuses across cell membranes to form complexes with specific cytoplasmic receptors, influencing cellular metabolism. Corticosteroids stabilize leukocyte lysosomal membranes, inhibit local actions and accumulation of macrophages, decrease local edema, and reduce the formation of scar tissue.
Absorption: Amount absorbed depends on amount applied and on nature of skin at the application site; ranges from about 1% in areas with thick stratum corneum (on the palms, soles, elbows, and knees) to as high as 36% in thinner areas (face, eyelids, and genitals). Absorption increases in areas of skin damage, inflammation, or occlusion. Some systemic absorption of topical steroids may occur, especially through the oral mucosa.
Distribution: After topical application, distributed throughout the local skin. Any drug that is absorbed is removed rapidly removed from the blood and distributed into muscle, liver, skin, intestines, and kidneys.
Metabolism: After topical administration, metabolized primarily in the skin. The small amount that is absorbed into systemic circulation is metabolized primarily in the liver to inactive compounds.
Excretion: Inactive metabolites are excreted by the kidneys, primarily as glucuronides and sulfates, but also as unconjugated products. Small amounts of the metabolites are also excreted in feces.

INDICATIONS & DOSAGE

Inflammation of corticosteroid-responsive dermatoses, such as atopic dermatitis, contact dermatitis, seborrheic dermatitis–
Adults and children: apply cream sparingly to affected areas once daily to q.i.d. and rub in gently.

CONTRAINDICATIONS & PRECAUTIONS

Contraindicated in patients with hypersensitivity to any component of the preparation and in patients with viral, fungal, or tubercular skin lesions. Use with extreme caution in patients with impaired circulation because the drug may increase the risk of skin ulceration. Avoid use on the face or genital areas because increased absorption may result in striae.

ADVERSE REACTIONS

Common reactions are in italics; life-threatening reactions are in bold italics.
Skin: burning, itching, irritation, dryness, folliculitis, striae, acneiform eruptions, perioral dermatitis, hypertrichosis, hypopigmentation, allergic contact dermatitis. With occlusive dressings: *secondary infection, maceration, atrophy, striae, miliaria.*

INTERACTIONS

None significant.

EFFECTS ON DIAGNOSTIC TESTS

None reported.

NURSING CONSIDERATIONS

Besides those related universally to drug therapy (see "How to use this book"), consider the following specific recommendations:

Assessment

- Obtain a baseline assessment of patient's skin in the affected area before therapy.
- Be alert for adverse reactions and drug interactions throughout therapy.
- Evaluate the patient's and family's knowledge about clocortolone therapy.

Nursing Diagnoses

- Impaired skin integrity related to the patient's underlying condition.
- High risk for infection related to clocortolone-induced secondary infection.

• Knowledge deficit related to clocortolone therapy.

Planning and Implementation

Preparation and Administration

• ***Topical use:*** Wash skin gently, before applying. Rub medication in gently, leaving a thin coat, to prevent skin damage. When treating hairy sites, part hair and apply directly to lesion.

• To apply an occlusive dressing: Apply cream, then cover with a thin, pliable, nonflammable, plastic film, seal to adjacent normal skin with hypoallergenic tape. Minimize adverse reactions by using occlusive dressing intermittently. Don't leave in place longer than 16 hours each day. Occlusive dressings should not be used in presence of infections or weeping or exudative lesions.

For a patient with eczematous dermatitis who may develop irritation with adhesive material, hold dressing in place with gauze, elastic bandages, or stockinette.

Monitoring

• Monitor effectiveness by regularly examining patient's lesions.

• Observe for signs of systemic absorption: skin irritation or ulceration, hypersensitivity, or infection. If they develop, stop drug and notify doctor. (If antifungals or antibiotics are being used with corticosteroids and infection does not respond immediately, corticosteroids should be discontinued until infection is controlled.)

• Monitor the patient's temperature regularly, if fever develops, notify doctor and remove occlusive dressing.

• Monitor for adverse reactions and interactions by frequently inspecting the patient's skin for infection, striae and atrophy.

Supportive Care

• Change the patient's dressings as ordered. Be prepared to discontinue drug and notify doctor if infection, straie, or atrophy occue.

• Be aware that systemic absorption is especially likely with occlusive dressings, prolonged treatment, or extensive body surface treatment.

• When used on diaper area in young children, avoid the use of plastic pants and tight-fitting diapers.

• Expect treatment to continue for a few days after clearing of lesions to prevent recurrence.

Patient Teaching

• Teach patient to apply medication.

• Instruct patient to avoid application near eyes or mucous membranes.

• Inform patient of systemic and topical adverse reactions; if they occur, tell him to stop using the drug and notify doctor.

Evaluation

In patients receiving clocortolone, appropriate evaluation statements may include:

• Patient states his contact dermatitis is resolved.

• Patient does not develop a secondary infection.

• Patient and family state an understanding of clocortolone therapy.

clofazimine

(kloe fa´ zi meen)

Lamprene

• *Classification:* leprostatic (iminophenazine)

• *Pregnancy Risk Category:* C

HOW SUPPLIED

Capsules: 50 mg, 100 mg

ACTION

Mechanism: Inhibits mycobacterial growth by binding preferentially to mycobacterial DNA. Also has anti-inflammatory effects that suppress skin reactions of erythema nodosum leprosum.

Absorption: Variable (45% to 60%) after oral administration. Absorption

may be enhanced when taken with meals.
Distribution: Highly lipophilic; distributed widely into fatty tissues and is taken up by macrophages into the reticuloendothelial system. Little, if any, crosses the blood-brain barrier or enters the CNS.
Metabolism: Not completely defined; some evidence exists of enterohepatic cycling.
Excretion: Primarily in feces; some in sputum, sebum, and sweat and breast milk; very little in urine. Half-life: Up to 70 days.

INDICATIONS & DOSAGE

Treatment of dapsone-resistant leprosy (Hansen's disease) –
Adults: 100 mg P.O. daily in combination with other antileprotics for 3 years. Then, clofazimine *alone,* 100 mg daily.
Erythema nodosum leprosum –
Adults: 100 to 200 mg P.O. daily for up to 3 months. Taper dosage to 100 mg daily as soon as possible. Dosages above 200 mg daily are not recommended.

CONTRAINDICATIONS & PRECAUTIONS

Use cautiously in patients with abdominal pain or diarrhea; discontinue if patient becomes colicky or if pain and other symptoms worsen.

ADVERSE REACTIONS

Common reactions are in italics; life-threatening reactions are in bold italics.
EENT: conjunctival and corneal pigmentation.
GI: *epigastric pain, diarrhea, nausea, vomiting, GI intolerance, bowel obstruction, GI bleeding.*
Skin: *pink to brownish black pigmentation, ichthyosis and dryness,* rash, itching.
Other: ***splenic infarction,*** discolored body fluids and excrement.

INTERACTIONS

None significant.

EFFECTS ON DIAGNOSTIC TESTS

Bilirubin, AST (SGOT): elevated serum levels.
CBC: eosinophilia.
Glucose, sugar albumin: elevated blood levels.
Potassium level: hypokalemia.

NURSING CONSIDERATIONS

Besides those related universally to drug therapy (see "How to use this book"), consider the following specific recommendations:

Assessment

- Obtain a baseline assessment of patient's infection before therapy.
- Be alert for adverse reactions and drug interactions throughout therapy.
- Evaluate the patient's and family's knowledge about clofazimine therapy.

Nursing Diagnoses

- High risk for injury related to ineffectiveness of clofazimine to eradicate the infection.
- High risk for fluid volume deficit related to clofazimine-induced adverse GI reactions.
- Knowledge deficit related to clofazimine.

Planning and Implementation

Preparation and Administration

- Obtain a specimen for culture and sensitivity tests before administering the first dose.
- ***P.O. use:*** Administer the drug with meals.
- Be aware that doses that exceed 100 mg daily should be given for as short a period as possible and only under close medical supervision.

Monitoring

- Monitor effectiveness by regularly assessing for improvement in infection and by evaluating culture and sensitivity results.
- Monitor patient's hydration status if adverse GI reactions occur.

Supportive Care
• Notify doctor about colicky or burning abdominal pain or any adverse GI reaction, which may require discontinuing the drug.
• Apply skin oil or cream to ease skin dryness or ichthyosis.
Patient Teaching
• Advise patient to take the drug with meals.
• Warn patient that clofazimine may discolor skin, body fluids, and feces red to brownish black. Reassure patient that the unsightly skin discoloration is reversible but may not disappear until several months or years after drug treatment ends.
• Advise patient to apply skin oil or cream to reverse skin dryness or ichthyosis.
• Instruct patient to report adverse GI reactions because they may require dosage adjustment.

Evaluation
In patients receiving clofazimine, appropriate evaluation statements may include:
• Patient is free of infection.
• Patient maintains adequate hydration throughout clofazimine therapy.
• Patient and family state an understanding of clofazimine therapy.

clofibrate
(kloe fye´ brate)
Arterioflexin‡, Atromid-S, Claripex†, Novofibrate†

• *Classification:* antilipemic (fibric acid derivative)
• *Pregnancy Risk Category:* C

HOW SUPPLIED
Capsules: 500 mg

ACTION
Mechanism: Seems to inhibit biosynthesis of cholesterol at an early stage but the exact mechanism is unknown.
Absorption: Slowly but completely absorbed from the GI tract.
Distribution: Into extracellular space as the active form, clofibric acid, which is up to 98% protein-bound.
Metabolism: Hydrolyzed by serum enzymes to clofibric acid, which is metabolized by the liver.
Excretion: 20% excreted unchanged in urine; 70% is eliminated in urine as conjugated metabolite. Half-life: After a single dose, ranges from 6 to 25 hours; as long as 113 hours in patients with renal impairment and cirrhosis.
Onset, peak, duration: Peak plasma concentration occurs 2 to 6 hours after a single dose. Serum triglyceride levels decrease in 2 to 5 days, with peak clinical effect at 21 days.

INDICATIONS & DOSAGE
Hyperlipidemia and xanthoma tuberosum; Type III hyperlipidemia that does not respond adequately to diet—
Adults: 2 g P.O. daily in four divided doses. Some patients may respond to lower doses as assessed by serum lipid monitoring.

Should not be used in children.

CONTRAINDICATIONS & PRECAUTIONS
Contraindicated in patients with renal or hepatic dysfunction because drug accumulation increases the incidence of adverse reactions; in patients with primary biliary cirrhosis because their cholesterol levels may be raised not lowered; and in pregnant or lactating patients because fetal drug concentrations may exceed those in the mother and because it is believed that the fetus' immature liver may be unable to metabolize clofibrate.

Use cautiously in patients with a history of liver disease or peptic ulcer disease.

ADVERSE REACTIONS

Common reactions are in italics; life-threatening reactions are in bold italics.
Blood: leukopenia.
CNS: fatigue, weakness.
CV: arrhythmias.
GI: *nausea, diarrhea, vomiting,* stomatitis, *dyspepsia,* flatulence.
GU: impotence and decreased libido, acute renal failure.
Hepatic: gallstones, *transient and reversible elevations of liver function tests.*
Skin: rashes, urticaria, pruritus, dry skin and hair.
Other: myalgias and arthralgias, resembling a flu-like syndrome; *weight gain; polyphagia;*fever, decreased libido.

INTERACTIONS

Furosemide, sulfonylureas: clofibrate may potentiate the clinical effect of these agents. Monitor patient closely.
Lovastatin, simvastatin, and other cholesterol synthesis inhibitors: risk of myositis, rhabdomyolysis, and renal failute. Avoid concomitant use.
Oral anticoagulants: clofibrate may potentiate the anticoagulant effects of warfarin or dicoumarol. Decreased anticoagulant dosage is necessary.
Oral contraceptives, rifampin: may antagonize clofibrate's lipid-lowering effect. Monitor serum lipids.
Probenecid: increased clofibrate effect. Monitor for toxicity.

EFFECTS ON DIAGNOSTIC TESTS

Creatine phosphokinase, transaminase, amylase, ALT (SGPT), and AST (SGOT): increased serum levels.
Plasma beta-lipoprotein and plasma fibrinogen: decreased concentrations.

NURSING CONSIDERATIONS

Besides those related universally to drug therapy (see "How to use this book"), consider the following specific recommendations:

Assessment
- Obtain a baseline assessment of the patient's underlying condition before drug therapy.
- Be alert for adverse reactions and drug interactions throughout therapy.
- Evaluate the patient's and family's knowledge about clofibrate therapy.

Nursing Diagnoses
- High risk for injury related to the ineffectiveness of clofibrate to reduce blood lipid and cholesterol levels.
- Diarrhea related to adverse drug reaction.
- Knowledge deficit related to clofibrate therapy.

Planning and Implementation

Preparation and Administration
- If significant lipid lowering is not achieved within 3 months, drug should be discontinued.
- Clofibrate has been used investigationally to treat diabetes insipidus at doses of 1.5 to 2 g daily.
- Drug should not be used indiscriminately. May pose risk of gallstones, heart disease, and cancer.

Monitoring
- Monitor for adverse reactions or drug interactions to clofibrate therapy by frequently monitoring the patient's vital signs.
- Monitor intake and output.
- Monitor hydration status if diarrhea and vomiting occurs.
- Monitor serum cholesterol and triglycerides regularily to evaluate the effectiveness of drug therapy.
- Monitor renal and hepatic function, blood counts, and serum electrolyte and blood sugar levels.

Supportive Care
- Discontinue drug if liver function tests show steady rise.
- Provide fluids for the patient who has vomiting and diarrhea.

Patient Teaching
- Teach the patient about proper dietary management (restricting total fat and cholesterol intake), weight control, and exercise. Explain their

importance in controlling elevated serum lipids.
• Warn the patient to report flu-like symptoms immediately.

Evaluation
In patients receiving clofibrate, appropriate evaluation statements may include:
• Patient's blood triglyceride and cholesterol levels are normal.
• Patient does not develop diarrhea.
• Patient and family state an understanding of clofibrate therapy.

---

clomiphene citrate
(kloe´ mi feen)
Clomid

• *Classification:* ovulation stimulant (chlorotrianisene derivative)
• *Pregnancy Risk Category:* X

HOW SUPPLIED
Tablets: 50 mg

ACTION
Mechanism: Appears to stimulate release of pituitary gonadotropins, follicle-stimulating hormone (FSH), and luteinizing hormone (LSH). This results in maturation of the ovarian follicle, ovulation, and development of the corpus luteum.
Absorption: Readily absorbed from the GI tract.
Distribution: May undergo enterohepatic recirculation or may be stored in body fat.
Metabolism: By the liver.
Excretion: Drug is excreted principally in the feces via biliary elimination. Half life: Approximately 5 days.

INDICATIONS & DOSAGE
To induce ovulation–
Women: 50 to 100 mg P.O. daily for 5 days, starting any time; or 50 to 100 mg P.O. daily starting on day 5 of menstrual cycle (first day of menstrual flow is day 1). Repeat until conception occurs or until three courses of therapy are completed.

CONTRAINDICATIONS & PRECAUTIONS
Contraindicated in patients with liver disease or a history of liver dysfunction because of potential hepatotoxic effects; in patients with abnormal bleeding of undetermined origin; during pregnancy or suspected pregnancy because of its fetal effects; in those with fibroids or abnormal uterine bleeding; and in the presence of an ovarian cyst or in patients with polycystic ovary syndrome because drug may enlarge or promote cyst formation. Use cautiously in patients with visual disturbances, mental depression, or thrombophlebitis because drug may exacerbate these disorders.

ADVERSE REACTIONS
Common reactions are in italics; life-threatening reactions are in bold italics.
CNS: headache, restlessness, insomnia, dizziness, light-headedness, depression, fatigue, tension.
CV: hypertension.
EENT: blurred vision, diplopia, scotoma, photophobia (signs of impending visual toxicity).
GI: nausea, vomiting, bloating, distention, increased appetite, weight gain.
GU: urinary frequency and polyuria; ovarian enlargement and cyst formation, which regress spontaneously when drug is stopped.
Metabolic: hyperglycemia.
Skin: urticaria, rash, dermatitis.
Other: *hot flashes,* reversible alopecia, *breast discomfort.*

INTERACTIONS
None significant.

EFFECTS ON DIAGNOSTIC TESTS
FSH and LH: increased secretion.
Serum thyronine, thyroxine-binding

globulin, and sex hormone-binding globulin: increased levels.
Sulfobromophthalein: increased retention.

NURSING CONSIDERATIONS

Besides those related universally to drug therapy (see "How to use this book"), consider the following specific recommendations:

Assessment

- Obtain a baseline assessment of the patient's menstrual cycle before therapy.
- Be alert for adverse reactions and drug interactions throughout therapy.
- Evaluate the patient's and family's knowledge about clomiphene therapy.

Nursing Diagnoses

- Sexual dysfunction related to underlying condition.
- Fluid volume excess related to adverse reactions to the medication.
- Knowledge deficit related to clomiphene.

Planning and Implementation

Preparation and Administration

- Prepare administration instructions for the patient: Begin daily dosage on fifth day of menstrual flow for 5 consecutive days.
- Tell the patient to repeat the 5-day dosing until conception occurs or three courses of therapy are completed.
- Inform the patient about the risk of multiple births, which increases with higher doses.

Monitoring

- Monitor effectiveness by assessing menstrual cycle.
- Check the patient's visual acuity to determine signs of impending visual toxicity. Ophthalmoscopic examinations should be performed if treatment continues for more than 1 year.
- Test the patient's urine for hyperglycemia.
- Question the patient regarding restlessness, insomnia, fatigue, and tension to assess for adverse CNS effects.

Supportive Care

- Reassure patient that response (ovulation) generally occurs after the first course of therapy.
- Remind the patient that therapy may be repeated if pregnancy does not occur after the first course of treatment.
- Encourage the patient to call if she has any questions.

Patient Teaching

- Instruct the patient to report any visual disturbances to the doctor immediately.
- Teach the patient to take and chart basal body temperature to determine when ovulation occurs.
- Advise the patient to stop taking the drug immediately if abdominal symptoms or pain occur and to notify the doctor.
- Tell the patient to avoid hazardous tasks if dizziness or visual disturbances develop.

Evaluation

In patients receiving clomiphene, appropriate evaluation statements may include:

- Patient is ovaluating as shown by biphasic body temperature, postovulatory urinary levels of pregnanediol, estrogen excretion, and changes in endometrial tissues.
- Patient is free of fluid retention: within normal weight range, no evidence of bloating or dependent edema.
- Patient and family state an understanding of clomiphene therapy.

clomipramine hydrochloride

(kloe mi´ pra meen)
Anafranil

- *Classification:* antiobsessional agent (tricyclic antidepressant)

• *Pregnancy Risk Category:* C

HOW SUPPLIED

Capsules: 25 mg, 50 mg, 75 mg

ACTION

Mechanism: Mechanism is unknown; selectively inhibits reuptake of serotonin.
Absorption: Well absorbed from the GI tract, but extensive first-pass metabolism limits bioavailablity to about 50%.
Distribution: Well distributed into lipophilic tissues; volume of distribution is about 12 liters/kg; about 98% bound to plasma proteins.
Metabolism: Primarily hepatic. Several metabolites have been identified; desmethylclomipramine is the primary active metabolite.
Excretion: About 66% is excreted in the urine and the remainder in the feces. Half-life: Mean elimination half-life of the parent compound is about 36 hours; of desmethylclomipramine, from 4.4 to 233 days.

INDICATIONS & DOSAGE

Treatment of obsessive-compulsive disorder–
Adults: initially, 25 mg P.O. daily in divided doses with meals, gradually increasing to 100 mg daily during first 2 weeks. Maximum dosage, 250 mg/day in divided doses with meals. After titration, total daily dose may be given h.s.
Children and adolescents: initially, 25 mg P.O. daily, gradually increased to daily maximum of 3 mg/kg or 100 mg P.O., whichever is smaller; given in divided doses with meals during first 2 weeks. Maximum daily dosage is 3 mg/kg or 200 mg, whichever is smaller; may be given h.s. afer titration.

Maintenance dosage in children, adolescents, and adults is the lowest effective dose h.s. Periodic reassessment and adjustment are necessary.

CONTRAINDICATIONS & PRECAUTIONS

Contraindicated in patients with a history of hypersensitivity to clomipramine or other TCAs. Also contraindicated in combination with an MAO inhibitor, in patients who have received an MAO inhibitor within the previous 2 weeks, and during the acute recovery period after myocardial infarction.

Use cautiously in patients with a history of seizure disorders, brain damage of various causes, or who are using other seizure threshold–lowering drugs; in patients with narrow-angle glaucoma, increased intraocular pressure, cardiovascular disease, impaired hepatic function, or tumors of the adrenal medulla; in patients who are at risk for suicide, are hyperthyroid, or are receiving thyroid medication; and in those with urine retention or who are receiving electroshock therapy or electrocautery.

ADVERSE REACTIONS

Common reactions are in italics; life-threatening reactions are in bold italics.
CNS: *somnolence, tremor, dizziness,* headache, insomnia, *libido change, nervousness, myoclonus, increased appetite, fatigue.*
CV: postural hypotension, palpitations, tachycardia.
EENT: otitis media (children), *abnormal vision,* pharyngitis, rhinitis.
GI: *dry mouth, constipation, nausea, dyspepsia,* diarrhea, *anorexia,* abdominal pain, *nausea.*
GU: *micturition disorder,* urinary tract infection, dysmenorrhea, *ejaculation failure,* impotence.
Skin: *increased sweating,* rash, pruritus.
Other: myalgia.

INTERACTIONS

Barbiturates: decrease TCA blood levels. Monitor for decreased antidepressant effect.

Epinephrine, norepinephrine: increase hypertensive effect. Use with caution.
MAO inhibitors: hyperpyretic crisis, seizures, coma, death may result. Alcohol, barbiturates, other CNS depressants: exaggerated response.
Methylphenidate: increases TCA blood levels. Monitor for enhanced antidepressant effect.

EFFECTS ON DIAGNOSTIC TESTS
None reported.

NURSING CONSIDERATIONS
Besides those related universally to drug therapy (see "How to use this book"), consider the following specific recommendations:

Assessment
• Obtain a baseline assessment of depression before therapy.
• Be alert for adverse reactions and drug interactions throughout therapy.
• Evaluate the patient's and family's knowledge about clomipramine therapy.

Nursing Diagnoses
• Ineffective individual coping related to the patient's underlying condition.
• High risk for injury related to clomipramine-induced adverse reactions.
• Knowledge deficit related to clomipramine therapy.

Planning and Implementation
Preparation and Administration
• Total daily dose may be taken at bedtime after titration. During titration, the dose may be divided and given with meals to minimize GI effects.
Monitoring
• Monitor effectiveness by having the patient discuss his feelings (ask broad, open-ended questions) and by evaluating his behavior.
• Monitor bowel patterns for constipation and intake and output for urinary retention.
• Monitor for suicidal tendencies.
Supportive Care
• Institute safety precautions if adverse CNS reactions or abnormal vision occur.
• Do not withdraw drug abruptly.
• If not contraindicated, increase the patient's fluid and fiber intake to prevent constipation; if needed, obtain an order for a laxative or stool softener or a high-fiber diet.
Patient Teaching
• Tell the patient to relieve dry mouth with sugarless hard candy or gum. Explain that saliva substitutes may be necessary.
• Teach the patient how to manage constipation.
• Warn the patient to avoid driving and other hazardous activities that require alertness and good psychomotor coordination until CNS effects of the drug are known. Inform the patient that drug has strong sedative effects and may cause daytime sedation and dizziness.

Evaluation
In patients receiving clomipramine, appropriate evaluation statements may include:
• Patient's behavior and communication indicate improvement of depression.
• Patient does not experience injury from adverse CNS reactions.
• Patient and family state an understanding of clomipramine therapy.

clonazepam
(kloe na´ ze pam)
Klonopin, Rivotril

• Controlled Substance Schedule IV
• *Classification:* anticonvulsant (benzodiazepine)
• *Pregnancy Risk Category:* C

HOW SUPPLIED
Tablets: 0.5 mg, 1 mg, 2 mg
Drops: 2.5 mg/ml‡

Injection: 1 mg/ml‡

ACTION

Mechanism: A benzodiazepine that appears to act on the limbic system, thalamus, and hypothalamus to produce anticonvulsant effects.
Absorption: Well absorbed from the GI tract.
Distribution: Widely distributed throughout the body; it is approximately 47% protein-bound.
Metabolism: By the liver to several metabolites.
Excretion: In urine. Half-life: About 24 hours.
Onset, peak, duration: Action begins in 20 to 60 minutes and persists for 6 to 8 hours in infants and children and up to 12 hours in adults.

INDICATIONS & DOSAGE

Lennox-Gastaut syndrome and atypical absence seizures; akinetic and myoclonic seizures–
Adults: initial dosage should not exceed 1.5 mg P.O. daily in three divided doses. May be increased by 0.5 to 1 mg q 3 days until seizures are controlled. If given in unequal doses, the largest dose should be given h.s. Maximum recommended daily dosage is 20 mg.
Children up to 10 years or 30 kg: 0.01 to 0.03 mg/kg P.O. daily (not to exceed 0.05 mg/kg daily), divided q 8 hours. Increase dosage by 0.25 to 0.5 mg q third day to a maximum maintenance dosage of 0.1 to 0.2 mg/kg daily.
Status epilepticus (where parenteral form is available)–
Adults: 1 mg by slow I.V. infusion.
Children: 0.5 mg by slow I.V. infusion.

CONTRAINDICATIONS & PRECAUTIONS

Contraindicated in patients with hypersensitivity to clonazepam and other benzodiazepines and in patients with significant hepatic disease, chronic respiratory disease, and untreated open-angle glaucoma or narrow-angle glaucoma. Use with caution (and at lower doses) in patients with decreased renal function.

ADVERSE REACTIONS

Common reactions are in italics; life-threatening reactions are in bold italics.
Blood: leukopenia, thrombocytopenia, eosinophilia.
CNS: *drowsiness, ataxia, behavioral disturbances (especially in children),* slurred speech, tremor, confusion.
EENT: *increased salivation,* diplopia, nystagmus, abnormal eye movements.
GI: constipation, gastritis, change in appetite, nausea, abnormal thirst, sore gums.
GU: dysuria, enuresis, nocturia, urinary retention.
Skin: rash.
Other: ***respiratory depression.***

INTERACTIONS

Alcohol, CNS depressants: increased CNS depression. Monitor closely.

EFFECTS ON DIAGNOSTIC TESTS

Liver function tests: elevated values.

NURSING CONSIDERATIONS

Besides those related universally to drug therapy (see "How to use this book"), consider the following specific recommendations:

Assessment

- Obtain a baseline assessment of patient's seizure activities before therapy.
- Be alert for adverse reactions and drug interactions throughout therapy.
- Evaluate the patient's and family's knowledge about clonazepam therapy.

Nursing Diagnoses

- High risk for injury related to patient's underlying seizure disorder.
- Activity intolerance related to clonazepam-induced sedation.

• Knowledge deficit related to clonazepam therapy.

Planning and Implementation

Preparation and Administration

• ***P.O. use:*** Increase dosage gradually, as ordered.

• ***I.V. use:*** Administer by slow I.V. infusion.

Monitoring

• Monitor effectiveness by regularly evaluating seizure activity.

• Monitor for oversedation. Keep in mind that elderly patients are more sensitive to the drug's CNS effects.

• Monitor liver function tests and CBC periodically.

• After discontinuation of therapy, monitor for withdrawal symptoms, which may be similar to those of barbiturates.

Supportive Care

• Maintain seizure precautions.

• Institute safety precautions until sedative effects of the drug are known; assist the patient with daily activities as needed.

• Never withdraw drug suddenly. Call doctor at once if adverse reactions occur.

Patient Teaching

• Warn the patient to avoid hazardous activities that require alertness and good psychomotor coordination until CNS effects of the drug are known.

• Warn the patient not to discontinue the drug suddenly.

• Stress importance of follow-up care and periodic diagnostic tests.

• Tell the patient to notify the nurse or doctor if oversedation or other adverse reactions develop or questions arise about therapy.

• Instruct the parents to monitor child's school performance. Drug may interfere with children's attentiveness in school.

Evaluation

In patients receiving clonazepam, appropriate evaluation statements include:

• Patient is free of seizure activity.

• Patient's daily activity needs are met.

• Patient and family state an understanding of clonazepam therapy.

clonidine hydrochloride

(kloe´ ni deen)

Catapres, Catapres-TTS, Dixarit†‡

• *Classification:* antihypertensive (antiadrenergic agent)

• *Pregnancy Risk Category:* C

HOW SUPPLIED

Tablets: 0.025 mg†‡, 0.1 mg, 0.2 mg, 0.3 mg

Transdermal: TTS-1 (releases 0.1 mg/24 hours), TTS-2 (releases 0.2 mg/24 hours), TTS-3 (releases 0.3 mg/24 hours)

ACTION

Mechanism: Inhibits the central vasomotor centers, thereby decreasing sympathetic outflow.

Absorption: Well absorbed from the GI tract. Clonidine is absorbed well percutaneously after transdermal topical administration.

Distribution: Widely distributed.

Metabolism: In the liver, where nearly 50% is transformed to inactive metabolites.

Excretion: Approximately 65% of a given dose is excreted in urine; 20% in feces. Half-life: Variable; ranges from 6 to 20 hours in patients with normal renal function.

Onset, peak, duration: After oral administration, blood pressure begins to decline in 30 to 60 minutes, with maximal effect in 2 to 4 hours; transdermal therapeutic plasma levels are achieved 2 to 3 days after initial application. After oral administration, the antihypertensive effect lasts up to 8 hours; after transdermal application, for up to 7 days.

INDICATIONS & DOSAGE

Essential, renal, and malignant hypertension–
Adults: initially, 0.1 mg P.O. b.i.d. Then increase by 0.1 to 0.2 mg daily on a weekly basis. Usual dosage range is 0.2 to 0.8 mg daily in divided doses; infrequently, dosages as high as 2.4 mg daily. No dosing recommendations for children.

Or, apply transdermal patch to a hairless area of intact skin on the upper arm or torso, once every 7 days.

Prophylactic treatment of migraine; treatment of menopausal flushing–
Adults: 0.025 mg P.O. b.i.d. If there has been no remission after 2 weeks, increase dosage to 0.050 mg b.i.d.

To suppress abstinence symptoms during narcotics withdrawal–
Adults: 0.1 mg P.O. t.i.d.

CONTRAINDICATIONS & PRECAUTIONS

Contraindicated in patients with hypersensitivity to the drug. Use cautiously in patients with severe coronary insufficiency, diabetes mellitus, myocardial infarction, cerebrovascular disease, chronic renal failure, a history of depression, or those taking other antihypertensives.

ADVERSE REACTIONS

Common reactions are in italics; life-threatening reactions are in bold italics.
CNS: *drowsiness,* dizziness, fatigue, sedation, nervousness, headache, vivid dreams.
CV: orthostatic hypotension, bradycardia, ***severe rebound hypertension.***
EENT: *dry mouth.*
GI: *constipation.*
GU: urine retention, impotence.
Metabolic: transient glucose intolerance (after large doses).
Skin: *pruritus, dermatitis* (from transdermal patch).

INTERACTIONS

CNS depressants: enhanced CNS depression. Use together cautiously.
Propranolol and other beta blockers: paradoxic hypertensive response. Monitor carefully.
Tricyclic antidepressants and MAO inhibitors: may decrease antihypertensive effect. Use together cautiously.

EFFECTS ON DIAGNOSTIC TESTS

Coomb's test: weakly positive results.
Serum glucose: slightly increased blood or serum glucose.
Urinary vanillylmandelic acid and catecholamines: decreased levels.

NURSING CONSIDERATIONS

Besides those related universally to drug therapy (see "How to use this book"), consider the following specific recommendations:

Assessment
- Obtain a baseline assessment of patient's blood pressure before therapy.
- Be alert for adverse reactions and drug interactions throughout therapy.
- Evaluate the patient's and family's knowledge about clonidine therapy.

Nursing Diagnoses
- High risk for injury related to ineffectiveness of clonidine to lower blood pressure.
- Altered protection related to severe rebound hypertension caused by abrupt cessation of clonidine.
- Knowledge deficit related to clonidine therapy.

Planning and Implementation
Preparation and Administration
- Be prepared to adjust dose according to patient's blood pressure and tolerance.
- Be aware that drug dosage should be reduced gradually over 2 to 4 days. Abrupt discontinuation may cause severe hypertension.
- In patients receiving both clonidine and a beta blocker, the beta blocker should be gradually withdrawn as

prescribed before clonidine to minimize adverse reactions.
• Administer last dose of the day at bedtime.
• ***Transdermal use:*** To provide additional adherence of the patch, apply an adhesive "overlay." Place the patch at a different site each week.
• Be aware that antihypertensive effects of transdermal clonidine may take 2 to 3 days to become apparent. Oral antihypertensive therapy may have to be continued in the interim.

Monitoring
• Monitor effectiveness by regularly monitoring blood pressure and pulse rate.
• Monitor for tolerance evidenced by rising blood pressure readings.
• Be aware that periodic eye examinations are recommended.
• Monitor elderly patients closely because they are more sensitive to the hypotensive effects of the drug.
• Monitor closely for anticholinergic effects, such as constipation, dry mouth, and urine retention.
• Monitor patient receiving large doses for transient glucose intolerance.
• Monitor site of transdermal patch for dermatitis. Question patient about pruritus.

Supportive Care
• If a transdermal patch is used, remove before defibrillation to prevent arcing.
• Institute safety precautions if adverse CNS reactions occur.
• Have patient avoid sudden position changes to minimize orthostatic hypotension.
• Provide comfort and supportive measures to relieve anticholinergic reactions.
• Notify doctor immediately if severe hypertension occurs and be prepared to treat as a medical emergency.

Patient Teaching
• Explain the importance of taking this drug exactly as prescribed, even when feeling well.
• Stress importance of not discontinuing drug abruptly because this can cause severe rebound hypertension, but to call the doctor if unpleasant reactions occur.
• Warn patient that this drug can cause drowsiness but that this adverse effect will subside.
• Instruct patient to check with doctor or pharmacist before taking any OTC medications.
• Tell patient how to manage troublesome reactions, such as orthostatic hypotension and anticholinergic effects.
• Tell patient to take last dose immediately before retiring.
• Teach patient how to apply the transdermal patch. Tell patient patch usually adheres despite showering and other routine daily activities. However, an adhesive "overlay" is available to provide additional skin adherence if necessary. Instruct the patient to place the patch at a different site each week.
• Inform patient of the need for periodic eye examinations.

Evaluation
In patients receiving clonidine, appropriate evaluation statements may include:
• Patient's blood pressure is within normal limits.
• Patient states understanding of not abruptly stopping clonidine therapy to avoid severe rebound hypertension.
• Patient and family state an understanding of clonidine therapy.

clorazepate dipotassium
(klor az´ e pate)
Gen-Xene, Novoclopate†, Tranxene, Tranxene-SD, Tranxene-T-Tab

• Controlled Substance Schedule IV
• *Classification:* anxiolytic, anticonvulsant, sedative-hypnotic (benzodiazepine)
• *Pregnancy Risk Category:* C

HOW SUPPLIED

Tablets: 3.75 mg, 7.5 mg, 11.25 mg, 15 mg, 22.5 mg
Capsules: 3.75 mg, 7.5 mg, 15 mg

ACTION

Mechanism: Depresses the CNS at the limbic and subcortical levels of the brain. As an anticonvulsant, suppresses the spread of seizure activity produced by epileptogenic foci in the cortex, thalamus, and limbic structures.
Absorption: After oral administration, clorazepate is hydrolyzed in the stomach to desmethyldiazepam, which is absorbed completely and rapidly.
Distribution: Widely distributed; enters CNS and crosses placenta. Approximately 80% to 95% bound to plasma protein.
Metabolism: Desmethyldiazepam is metabolized in the liver to oxazepam.
Excretion: Inactive glucuronide metabolites are excreted in urine. Half-life: Desmethyldiazepam, 30 to 200 hours; oxazepam, 3 to 21 hours.
Onset, peak, duration: Peak serum levels occur at 1 to 2 hours.

INDICATIONS & DOSAGE

Acute alcohol withdrawal–
Adults: Day 1 – 30 mg P.O. initially, followed by 30 to 60 mg P.O. in divided doses; Day 2 – 45 to 90 mg P.O. in divided doses; Day 3 – 22.5 to 45 mg P.O. in divided doses; Day 4 – 15 to 30 mg P.O. in divided doses; gradually reduce daily dosage to 7.5 to 15 mg.
Anxiety–
Adults: 15 to 60 mg P.O. daily.
As an adjunct in epilepsy–
Adults and children over 12 years: Maximum recommended initial dosage is 7.5 mg P.O. t.i.d. Dosage increases should be no greater than 7.5 mg/week. Maximum daily dosage should not exceed 90 mg daily.
Children between 9 and 12 years: Maximum recommended initial dosage is 7.5 mg P.O. b.i.d. Dosage increases should be no greater than 7.5 mg/week. Maximum daily dosage should not exceed 60 mg/day.

CONTRAINDICATIONS & PRECAUTIONS

Contraindicated in patients with hypersensitivity to the drug; patients with acute narrow-angle glaucoma or untreated open-angle glaucoma because of the drug's possible anticholinergic effect; shock or coma because the drug's hypnotic or hypotensive effect may be prolonged or intensified; acute alcohol intoxication who have depressed vital signs because the drug will worsen CNS depression; and in infants younger than age 30 days, in whom slow metabolism of the drug causes it to accumulate.

Use cautiously in patients with psychoses, because the drug is rarely beneficial in such patients and may induce paradoxic reactions; in patients with myasthenia gravis or Parkinson's disease because it may exacerbate the disorder; in patients with impaired renal or hepatic function, which prolongs elimination of the drug; in elderly or debilitated patients, who are usually more sensitive to the drug's CNS effects; and in individuals prone to addiction or drug abuse.

ADVERSE REACTIONS

Common reactions are in italics; life-threatening reactions are in bold italics.
CNS: *drowsiness, lethargy, hangover,* fainting.
CV: transient hypotension.

GI: nausea, vomiting, abdominal discomfort.

INTERACTIONS

Alcohol, other CNS depressants: increased CNS depression. Avoid concomitant use.
Cimetidine: increased sedation. Monitor carefully.

EFFECTS ON DIAGNOSTIC TESTS

EEG patterns: minor changes (low-voltage, fast activity) during and after therapy.
Liver function tests: elevated results.

NURSING CONSIDERATIONS

Besides those related universally to drug therapy (see "How to use this book"), consider the following specific recommendations:

Assessment

- Obtain a baseline assessment of the patient's underlying condition before drug therapy.
- Be alert for adverse reactions and drug interactions throughout therapy.
- Evaluate the patient's and family's knowledge about clorazepate therapy.

Nursing Diagnoses

- Anxiety related to the patient's underlying condition.
- High risk for injury related to clorazepate-induced adverse reactions.
- Knowledge deficit related to clorazepate therapy.

Planning and Implementation

Preparation and Administration

- Expect to administer lower dosage in elderly or debilitated patients.

Monitoring

- Monitor for adverse reactions or drug interactions by frequently checking blood pressure for hypotension.
- Monitor effectiveness by regularly asking the patient about feelings of anxiety and by evaluating the patient's behavior.
- Monitor hydration status if patient develops nausea and vomiting.
- Know that the drug should not be perscribed regularly for everyday stress.

Supportive Care

- Provide encouragement and support with ancillary treatments, such as professional counseling and problem identification.
- If drowsiness or lethargy occurs, institute safety measures, such as supervising patient activities. Reorient patient as needed and ensure a safe environment.
- Provide frequent sips of water or ice chips for dry mouth.
- Provide patient with additional fluids if nausea and vomiting occur.
- Do not withdraw drug abruptly. Abuse or addiction is possible and withdrawal symptoms may occur.

Patient Teaching

- Warn the patient not to combine drug with alcohol or other CNS depressants, and to avoid driving and other hazardous activities that require alertness and psychomotor coordination until adverse CNS effects of the drug are known.
- Caution the patient against giving medication to others.
- Warn the patient to take this drug only as directed and not to discontinue taking it without the doctor's approval. Inform the patient of the drug's potential for dependence if taken longer than directed.
- Recommend sugarless chewing gum, hard candy, ice chips to relieve dry mouth.

Evaluation

In patients receiving clorazepate, appropriate evaluation statements may include:

- Patient states he is less anxious.
- Patient does not experience injury as a result of adverse CNS reactions.
- Patient and family state an understanding of clorazepate therapy.

clotrimazole

(kloe trim´ a zole)
Canesten†, Gyne-Lotrimin◇, Lotrimin (1% clotrimazole), Mycelex, Mycelex-G

- *Classification:* topical antifungal (imidazole derivative)
- *Pregnancy Risk Category:* B

HOW SUPPLIED

Lozenges: 1%
Cream: 1%
Topical lotion: 1%
Topical solution: 1%
Vaginal cream: 1%◇
Vaginal tablets: 100 mg◇, 500 mg

ACTION

Mechanism: Binds to phospholipids in the fungal cell wall and alters permeability.
Absorption: Limited with topical administration. After oral administration of a lozenge, dissolution occurs in 10 to 30 minutes and inhibitory concentrations of drug are present in the saliva for up to 3 hours. Only 3% to 10% of a dose is absorbed systemically with vaginal administration.
Distribution: With topical application, drug concentrates in the stratum corneum. With oral administration of lozenge, drug binds to and is slowly released from oral mucosa. Vaginal fluid levels of the drug are highly variable; adding lactic acid to the vaginal tablet preparation may enhance the aqueous solubility.
Onset, peak, duration: Serum levels corresponding to approximately 0.01 mg equivalents/1 ml were reached between 8 and 24 hours after application.

INDICATIONS & DOSAGE

Superficial fungal infections (tinea pedis, tinea cruris, tinea corporis, tinea versicolor, candidiasis)–
Adults and children: apply thinly and massage into affected and surrounding area, morning and evening, 2 to 8 weeks.
Candidal vulvovaginitis–
Adults: insert 1 applicatorful or 1 tablet intravaginally daily for 7 to 14 days at bedtime. Alternatively, insert two 100-mg tablets once daily for 3 consecutive days or one 500-mg tablet one time only at bedtime.
Oropharyngeal candidiasis–
Adults and children: dissolve lozenge in mouth five times daily for 14 consecutive days.

CONTRAINDICATIONS & PRECAUTIONS

Contraindicated in patients with hypersensitivity to the drug. Use cautiously in patients with hepatic impairment because abnormal liver function test results have been reported. Use intravaginally with caution during first trimester of pregnancy because of possible adverse fetal effects.

ADVERSE REACTIONS

Common reactions are in italics; life-threatening reactions are in bold italics.
GI: nausea and vomiting (with lozenges).
GU: (with vaginal use) *mild vaginal burning, irritation.*
Hepatic: elevated AST (SGOT) levels (from lozenges).
Skin: blistering, *erythema,* edema, pruritus, burning, stinging, peeling, urticaria, skin fissures, general irritation.

INTERACTIONS

None significant.

EFFECTS ON DIAGNOSTIC TESTS

Liver function tests: abnormal results (with lozenges).

NURSING CONSIDERATIONS

Besides those related universally to drug therapy (see "How to use this book"), consider the following specific recommendations:

Assessment

- Obtain a baseline assessment of the patient's skin in the affected area before therapy.
- Be alert for adverse reactions and drug interactions throughout therapy.
- Evaluate the patient's and family's knowledge about clotrimazole therapy.

Nursing Diagnoses

- Impaired skin integrity related to patient's underlying condition.
- High risk for impaired skin integrity related to clotrimazole-induced vaginal burning.
- Knowledge deficit related to clotrimazole therapy.

Planning and Implementation

Preparation and Administration

- ***Topical use:*** Apply thinly and massage into affected area. Clean area before applying.
- ***Intravaginal use:*** Insert the dose via applicator as ordered.
- ***Oral use:*** Lozenge must dissolve in mouth.

Monitoring

- Monitor effectiveness by regularly checking the affected area.
- Watch for and report irritation or sensitivity.
- Monitor for adverse reactions or interactions by reviewing the patient's AST (SGOT) levels during use of lozenges.
- Monitor hydration status if the patient develops nausea and vomiting with lozenge use.

Supportive Care

- Keep in mind that drug is not for ophthalmic use.
- Improvement usually occurs within a week; if no improvement in 4 weeks, diagnosis should be reviewed.
- Be prepared to discontinue the drug and notify the doctor if adverse reactions occur.
- Shortened dosage schedule may be used with tablets when compliance is a problem.
- Hypopigmentation from tinea versicolor will resolve gradually.

Patient Teaching

- Teach patient to apply medication.
- Emphasize the need to continue treatment for full course even if symptoms have improved.
- Warn patient not to use occlusive wrappings or dressings.
- Inform patient topical preparation may stain clothing.
- Inform the patient that slight discoloration (hypopigmentation) with tinea versicolor will disappear gradually.

Evaluation

In patients receiving clotrimazole, appropriate evaluation statements may include:

- Patient's underlying condition shows improvement.
- Patient does not develop drug-induced vaginal burning.
- Patient and family state an understanding of clotrimazole therapy.

---

cloxacillin sodium

(klox a sill´ in)

Alclox‡, Apo-Cloxi†, Austrastaph‡, Bactopen†, Cloxapen, Novocloxin†, Orbenin†, Orbenin Injection‡, Tegopen

- *Classification:* antibiotic (penicillinase-resistant penicillin)
- *Pregnancy Risk Category:* B

HOW SUPPLIED

Capsules: 250 mg, 500 mg
Oral solution: 125 mg/5 ml (after reconstitution)

Injection: 500 mg/vial‡

ACTION

Mechanism: Bactericidal against microorganisms by inhibiting cell wall synthesis during active multiplication. Bacteria resist penicillins by producing penicillinases–enzymes that convert penicillins to inactive penicilloic acid. Cloxacillin resists these enzymes.
Absorption: Rapidly but incompletely absorbed (37% to 60%) from the GI tract; it is relatively acid stable. Food may decrease both rate and extent of absorption.
Distribution: Widely distributed. CSF penetration is poor, but enhanced in patients with meningeal inflammation; also crosses the placenta and is 90% to 96% protein-bound.
Metabolism: Partially metabolized.
Excretion: Drug and metabolites excreted in urine by renal tubular secretion and glomerular filtration; also excreted in breast milk. Half-life: 30 minutes to 1 hour, extended minimally to 2½ hours in patients with renal impairment.
Onset, peak, duration: Peak plasma concentrations occur 30 minutes to 2 hours after an oral dose.

INDICATIONS & DOSAGE

Systemic infections caused by penicillinase-producing staphylococci–
Adults: 2 to 4 g P.O. daily, divided into doses given q 6 hours.
Children: 50 to 100 mg/kg P.O. daily, divided into doses given q 6 hours.

CONTRAINDICATIONS & PRECAUTIONS

Contraindicated in patients with hypersensitivity to any penicillin or cephalosporin. Use with caution in patients with renal impairment, because drug is excreted in urine; decreased dosage is required in moderate to severe renal failure.

ADVERSE REACTIONS

Common reactions are in italics; life-threatening reactions are in bold italics.
Blood: eosinophilia.
GI: *nausea,* vomiting, *epigastric distress, diarrhea.*
Other: ***hypersensitivity*** *(rash, urticaria, chills, fever, sneezing, wheezing,* ***anaphylaxis****),* intrahepatic cholestasis, overgrowth of nonsusceptible organisms.

INTERACTIONS

Probenecid: increases blood levels of cloxacillin and other penicillins. Probenecid may be used for this purpose.

EFFECTS ON DIAGNOSTIC TESTS

Aminoglycoside serum levels: falsely decreased concentrations.
Bence Jones protein (Bradshaw screening test): false results.
CBC: transient reductions in RBC, WBC, and platelet counts.
Liver function tests: transient elevations.
Urine and serum protein tests: false-positive or elevated results.

NURSING CONSIDERATIONS

Besides those related universally to drug therapy (see "How to use this book"), consider the following specific recommendations:
Assessment
- Obtain a baseline assessment of patient's infection before therapy.
- Be alert for adverse reactions and drug interactions throughout therapy.
- Evaluate the patient's and family's knowledge about cloxacillin therapy.

Nursing Diagnoses
- High risk for injury related to ineffectiveness of cloxacillin to eradicate the infection.
- High risk for fluid volume deficit related to cloxacillin-induced adverse GI reactions.
- Knowledge deficit related to cloxacillin therapy.

Planning and Implementation
Preparation and Administration
• Obtain specimen for culture and sensitivity tests before first dose. Therapy may begin pending test results.
• Before first dose, ask the patient about previous allergic reactions to this drug or other penicillins. However, a negative history of penicillin allergy does not guarantee future safety.
• Give cloxacillin at least 1 hour before bacteriostatic antibiotics.
• ***P.O. use:*** Administer drug 1 to 2 hours before meals or 2 to 3 hours after as food may interfere with absorption. Give each dose with a full glass of water, not fruit juice or carbonated beverage, because acid will inactivate the drug.
Monitoring
• Monitor the effectiveness of cloxacillin therapy by regularly assessing for improvement of infection.
• Monitor the patient's hydration status if adverse GI reactions occur.
• Monitor for bacterial and fungal superinfections during prolonged or high-dose therapy, especially in elderly, debilitated, or immunosuppressed patients.
Supportive Care
• Obtain an order for an antiemetic or antidiarrheal agent as needed.
• If the patient develops a rash, notify the doctor and expect to discontinue the drug.
Patient Teaching
• Advise the patient who becomes allergic to cloxacillin to wear medical alert identification stating this information.
• Tell the patient to call the doctor if rash, fever, or chills develop. A rash is the most common allergic reaction.
• Tell patient to take drug exactly as prescribed, and to complete entire quantity even if he feels better.
• Instruct patient to take the drug 1 to 2 hours before or 2 to 3 hours after meals because food may interfere with absorption. Tell patient to take cloxacillin with a full glass of water, not fruit juice or carbonated beverage, because acid will inactivate the drug.
• Warn patient never to use leftover cloxacillin for a new illness or to share it with others.
Evaluation
In patients receiving cloxacillin, appropriate evaluation statements may include:
• Patient is free of infection.
• Patient maintains adequate hydration throughout cloxacillin therapy.
• Patient and family state an understanding of cloxacillin therapy.

clozapine
(kloe´ za peen)
Clozaril

• *Classification:* antipsychotic (dibenzodiazepine)
• *Pregnancy Risk Category:* B

HOW SUPPLIED
Tablets: 25 mg, 100 mg

ACTION
Mechanism: Binds to dopamine receptors (both D-1 and D-2) within the limbic system of the CNS. It also may interfere with adrenergic, cholinergic, histaminergic, and serotoninergic receptors.
Absorption: Rapidly and completely absorbed after oral administration; however, hepatic first-pass effect limits bioavailability to 27% to 50%. Men have slightly lower plasma levels than women, and smoking appears to augment the first-pass effect. Food does not appear to interfere with bioavailability.
Distribution: Drug is about 95% bound to serum proteins.
Metabolism: Nearly complete; very

little unchanged drug appears in the urine.
Excretion: Approximately 50% of the drug appears in the urine and 30% in the feces, mostly as metabolites. Half-life: Elimination half-life appears proportional to dose and may range from 8 to 12 hours.
Onset, peak, duration: Peak levels occur about 1½ hours after oral administration.

INDICATIONS & DOSAGE

Treatment of schizophrenia in severely ill patients unresponsive to other therapies–
Adults: initially, 25 mg P.O. q.i.d. or b.i.d., titrated upward at 25 to 50 mg daily (if tolerated) to a daily dosage of 300 to 450 mg daily by the end of 2 weeks. Individual dosage is based on clinical response, patient tolerance, and adverse reactions. Subsequent dosage should not be increased more than once or twice weekly, and should not exceed 100 mg. Many patients respond to doses of 300 to 600 mg daily, but some may require as much as 900 mg daily. Do not exceed 900 mg/day.

CONTRAINDICATIONS & PRECAUTIONS

Contraindicated in patients with a history of clozapine-induced agranulocytosis or severe granulocytopenia and in patients with severe CNS depression or coma; in patients taking other drugs that suppress bone marrow function; and in those with myelosuppressive disorders.

Use cautiously in patients with prostatic hypertrophy or glaucoma because drug has potent anticholinergic effects.

Because clozapine therapy carries a significant risk of agranulocytosis (early trials estimate the incidence at 1.3%), patients should receive at least two trials of a standard antipsychotic drug before clozapine is used. Baseline WBC and differential counts are required before therapy; WBC counts must be monitored weekly and for at least 4 weeks after therapy is discontinued.

If WBC count drops below 3,500/mm³ or drops substantially from baseline, monitor patient closely for signs of infection. If WBC count is 3,000 to 3,500/mm³ and granulocyte count is above 1,500/mm³, perform twice weekly WBC and differential counts. If WBC count drops below 3,000/mm³ and granulocyte count drops below 1,500/mm³, therapy should be interrupted and the patient monitored for signs of infection. Therapy may be cautiously restarted if WBC count returns above 3,000/mm³ and granulocyte count returns above 1,500/mm³, but twice weekly monitoring of WBC and differential counts should continue until the WBC count exceeds 3,500/mm³.

If the WBC count drops below 2,000/mm³ and granulocyte count drops below 1,000/mm³, the patient may require protective isolation. If the patient develops an infection, prepare cultures and administer antibiotics as appropriate. Some clinicians may perform bone marrow aspiration to assess bone marrow function. Subsequent clozapine therapy is contraindicated.

ADVERSE REACTIONS

Common reactions are in italics; life-threatening reactions are in bold italics.
Blood: *leukopenia, granulocytopenia,* ***agranulocytosis.***
CNS: *drowsiness, sedation,* ***seizures,*** *dizziness,* syncope, vertigo, headache, tremor, disturbed sleep or nightmares, restlessness, hypokinesia or akinesia, agitation, rigidity, akathisia, confusion, fatigue, insomnia, hyperkinesia, weakness, lethargy, ataxia, slurred speech, depression, myoclonia, anxiety.

*Liquid form contains alcohol. **May contain tartrazine.

CV: *tachycardia, hypotension,* hypertension, chest pain, ECG changes.
GI: *constipation,* nausea, vomiting, *salivation, dry mouth.*
GU: urinary abnormalities, incontinence, abnormal ejaculation, urinary frequency or urgency, urine retention.
Other: fever, muscle pain or spasm, muscle weakness, weight gain, rash.

INTERACTIONS

Anticholinergics: may potentiate the anticholinergic effects of clozapine.
Antihypertensives: hypotensive effects may be potentiated by clozapine.
Bone marrow suppressant drugs: potentially increased bone marrow toxicity.
CNS-active drugs: possible additive effects. Use together cautiously.
Warfarin, digoxin, and other highly protein bound drugs: increased serum levels of these drugs may occur. Monitor closely for adverse reactions.

EFFECTS ON DIAGNOSTIC TESTS

CBC: depressed blood counts.

NURSING CONSIDERATIONS

Besides those related universally to drug therapy (see "How to use this book"), consider the following specific recommendations:

Assessment

- Obtain a baseline assessment of the patient's underlying condition before drug therapy.
- Be alert for adverse reactions and drug interactions throughout therapy.
- Evaluate the patient's and family's knowledge about clozapine therapy.

Nursing Diagnoses

- Altered thought processes related to the patient's underlying condition.
- High risk for injury related to adverse reactions.
- Knowledge deficit related to clozapine therapy.

Planning and Implementation

Preparation and Administration

- May be given with meals if patient develops GI distress.
- Store below 30° C (86° F) unless otherwise specified by manufacturer.
- Decrease initial dosage and increase titrated dose more slowly if the patient is malnourished or has hepatic, renal, or cardiovascular disease.

Monitoring

- Monitor for adverse reactions or drug interactions to therapy by frequently checking the patient's blood pressure, heart rate, and rhythm.
- Be alert for signs of agranulocytosis. Baseline WBC and differential counts must be monitored at least 4 weeks after clozapine therapy is discontinued.
- If possible, patients should receive at least two trials of a standard antipsychotic drug therapy before trial of clozapine therapy.
- Clozapine is available only through a special Clozapine Patient Management System that ensures weekly testing of WBC counts.
- Monitor the patient closely for signs of infection if WBC count drops below 3,500/mm^3 after initiating therpay or exhibits a substantial drop from baseline.
- Monitor the patient's WBC and differential counts twice weekly if the WBC count is 3,000 to 3,500/mm^3 and the granulocyte count is above 1,500/mm^3. These tests should be performed twice weekly until the WBC count exceeds 3,500/mm^3.
- Monitor for abnormal body movements; drug may cause seizures.
- If the drug is withdrawn, monitor for recurrence of psychotic symptoms.

Supportive Care

- Be prepared to interrupt therapy if the patient's WBC count drops below 3,000/mm^3 and granulocyte count is below 1,500/mm^3.

• Be prepared to cautiously restart therapy if WBC count returns above 3,000/mm³ and granulocyte count returns above 1,500/mm³.
• Be prepared to provide protective isolation for the patient if the WBC count drops below 2,000/mm³ and the granulocyte count drops below 1,000/mm³.
• If the patient develops infection, obtain cultures and administer antibiotics, as ordered. Also be prepared to assist with a bone marrow aspiration to assess bone marrow function.
• Monitor the patient for temperature above 100.4° F (38° C), especially in the first 3 weeks of therapy.
• Give the patient ice chips, sugarless candy, or gum to help relieve dry mouth.
• If the drug must be discontinued, expect to withdraw the drug gradually over a 1- to 2-week period. However, changes in the patient's condition (such as leukopenia) may require abrupt discontinuation.
• If therapy is reinstated after withdrawal, the usual guidelines for dosage buildup should be followed. However, reexposure of the patient to this drug may increase the severity of adverse reactions. If therapy was terminated because of WBC counts below 2,000/mm³ or granulocyte counts below 1,000/mm³, the drug should not be continued.

Patient Teaching

• Stress to the patient the importance of returning for WBC counts for 4 weeks after therapy is discontinued.
• Seizures may occur, especially in patients receiving high doses of the drug.
• Inform the patient that if his WBC and granulocyte counts drop to dangerous levels, the doctor may perform a bone marrow aspiration to ascess bone marrow function.
• Advise the patient to report flu-like symptoms, fever, lethargy, sore throat, malaise, or other signs of infection.
• Warn the patient about the risk of agranulocytosis.
• Tell the patient that the drug is available only through a special monitoring program that will require weekly blood tests for agranulocytosis.
• Inform the patient that he will receive only a 1-week supply of the drug from the program.
• Advise patients to check with their doctors before taking any OTC drugs or alcohol.
• Recommend ice chips, sugarless candy, or gum to help relieve dry mouth.
• Advise the patient to avoid hazardous activities that require alertness and good coordination, such as driving, swimming, and climbing, while taking this drug.

Evaluation

In patients receiving clozapine, appropriate evaluation statements may include:
• Patient demonstrates a reduction in psychotic symptoms.
• Patient does not experience any injuries.
• Patient and family state an understanding of clozapine therapy.

---

codeine phosphate

(koe´ deen)

Paveral†

codeine sulfate

• Controlled Substance Schedule II
• *Classification:* analgesic, antitussive (opioid)
• *Pregnancy Risk Category:* C (D for prolonged use or use of high doses at term)

HOW SUPPLIED

phosphate
Oral solution: 15 mg/5 ml, 10 mg/ml†
Injection: 30 mg/ml, 60 mg/ml
sulfate
Tablets: 15 mg, 30 mg, 60 mg
Soluble tablets: 15 mg, 30 mg, 60 mg

ACTION

Mechanism: Binds with opiate receptors at many sites in the CNS (brain, brain stem, and spinal cord), altering both perception of and emotional response to pain through an unknown mechanism. Supresses the cough reflex by direct action on the cough center in the medulla.
Absorption: Well absorbed after oral or parenteral administration. About two-thirds as potent orally as parenterally.
Distribution: Widely distributed throughout the body; crosses the placenta and enters breast milk.
Metabolism: Mainly in the liver, by demethylation, or conjugation with glucuronic acid.
Excretion: Mainly in the urine as norcodeine and free and conjugated morphine.
Onset, peak, duration: After oral or S.C. administration, action occurs in less than 30 minutes. Peak analgesic effect is seen at 30 minutes to 1 hour, and the duration of action is 4 to 6 hours.

INDICATIONS & DOSAGE

Mild to moderate pain–
Adults: 15 to 60 mg P.O. or 15 to 60 mg (phosphate) S.C. or I.M. q 4 hours, p.r.n. or around the clock.
Children: 3 mg/kg P.O. daily divided q 4 hours, p.r.n. or around the clock.
Nonproductive cough–
Adults: 10 to 20 mg P.O. q 4 to 6 hours. Maximum dosage is 120 mg/24 hours.
Children 6 to 12 years: 5 to 10 mg P.O. q 4 to 6 hours. Maximum dosage is 60 mg/24 hours.
Children 2 to 6 years: 2.5 to 5 mg P.O. q 4 to 6 hours. Do not exceed 30 mg in 24 hours.

CONTRAINDICATIONS & PRECAUTIONS

Contraindicated in patients with hypersensitivity to the drug or phenanthrene opioids (hydrocodone, hydromorphine, morphine, oxycodone, or oxymorphone).

Use with extreme caution in patients with supraventricular arrhythmias; avoid or use with extreme caution in patients with head injury or increased intracranial pressure because drug obscures signs of neurologic disproportion; and during pregnancy and labor because drug readily crosses placenta (premature infants are especially sensitive to respiratory and CNS depressant effects of opioids).

Use cautiously in patients with renal or hepatic dysfunction because drug accumulation or prolonged action may occur; in patients with pulmonary disease (asthma, COPD) because drug depresses respiration and suppresses cough reflex; in patients undergoing biliary tract surgery because drug may cause biliary spasm; in patients with seizure disorders because drug may precipitate seizures; in elderly or debilitated patients, who are more sensitive to drug effects; and in patients prone to physical or psychological addiction because of the high risk of addiction to this drug.

ADVERSE REACTIONS

Common reactions are in italics; life-threatening reactions are in bold italics.
CNS: *sedation, clouded sensorium, euphoria,* dizziness, seizures with large doses.
CV: *hypotension,* bradycardia.
GI: *nausea, vomiting, constipation, dry mouth,* ileus.
GU: *urine retention.*

†Available in Canada only. ‡Available in Australia only. ◊Available OTC.

Skin: pruritus, flushing.
Other: ***respiratory depression,*** physical dependence.

INTERACTIONS

Alcohol, CNS depressants: additive effects. Use together cautiously.

EFFECTS ON DIAGNOSTIC TESTS

Hepatobiliary imaging studies: test interference.
Plasma amylase and lipase: increased levels.

NURSING CONSIDERATIONS

Besides those related universally to drug therapy (see "How to use this book"), consider the following specific recommendations:

Assessment

- Obtain a baseline assessment of the patient's pain before therapy.
- Be alert for adverse reactions and drug interactions throughout therapy.
- Evaluate the patient's and family's knowledge about codeine therapy.

Nursing Diagnoses

- Pain related to patient's underlying condition.
- Constipation related to binding effect of codeine.
- Knowledge deficit related to codeine therapy.

Planning and Implementation

Preparation and Administration

- ***P.O. use:*** Expect to administer codeine with aspirin or acetaminophen together frequently as ordered to provide enhanced pain relief.
- ***I.V. use (phosphate):*** Do not administer by rapid infusion since this can cause life-threatening adverse reactions. To minimize hypotension, administer while patient is lying down.
- Do not administer discolored injection solution.
- For full analgesic effect, give before patient has intense pain.

Monitoring

- Monitor effectiveness after each dose by evaluating pain relief.
- Monitor respiratory and circulatory status.
- Monitor bowel and bladder function for constipation or ileus or urine retention.
- Be aware that use with general anesthetics, other narcotic analgesics, tranquilizers, sedatives, hypnotics, alcohol, tricyclic antidepressants, or MAO inhibitors, increases CNS depression. Codeine should be used with such drugs with extreme caution. Monitor patient response.
- Monitor cough type and frequency.

Supportive Care

- Notify the doctor and discuss increase of dosage or frequency if pain persists.
- Keep narcotic antagonist (naloxone) and resuscitative equipment available, if administering drug intravenously.
- If not contraindicated, obtain an order for a stool softener or other laxative and increase the patient's fluid and fiber intake to prevent or treat constipation.
- An antitussive; don't use when cough is a valuable diagnostic sign or beneficial (as after thoracic surgery).
- Recognize that the abuse potential is much less than that of morphine.

Patient Teaching

- Warn the ambulatory patient to avoid driving and other hazardous activities that require alertness.
- Suggest measures such as high-fiber diet and liberal fluid intake to prevent constipation.
- Encourage the patient to ask for medication before pain becomes severe.
- Inform the patient to promptly report constipation.

Evaluation

In patients receiving codeine, appropriate evaluation statements include:

- Patient reports relief of pain after administration of codeine.
- Patient reports normal bowel functioning.

• Patient and family state an understanding of codeine therapy.

colchicine

(kol´ chi seen)

Colchicine MR‡, Colgout‡, Colsalide, Novocolchicine†

• *Classification:* antigout (*Colchicum autumnale* alkaloid)
• *Pregnancy Risk Category:* D

HOW SUPPLIED

Tablets: 0.5 mg (1/120 grain), 0.6 mg (1/100 grain) as sugar-coated granules
Injection: 1 mg (1/60 g)/2 ml

ACTION

Mechanism: Interferes with microtubule function. In patients with gout, prevents the migration of polymorphonuclear lymphocytes into regions in which urate crystal deposits have formed. Drug also arrests dividing cells in metaphase by preventing normal function of mitotic spindle, which helps cells divide.
Absorption: Rapidly absorbed from the GI tract.
Distribution: Rapidly distributed into various tissues after reabsorption from the intestine. Concentrated in leukocytes and distributed into the kidneys, liver, spleen, and intestinal tract, but is absent in the heart, skeletal muscle, and brain.
Metabolism: Partially metabolized in the liver and also slowly metabolized in other tissues.
Excretion: Drug and metabolites are excreted in the bile. Parent drug may be reabsorbed in the intestine. Excretion is mainly in feces, with lesser amounts excreted in urine. Half life is about 60 hours in leukocytes.

INDICATIONS & DOSAGE

To prevent acute attacks of gout as prophylactic or maintenance therapy–
Adults: 0.5 or 0.6 mg P.O. daily; or 1 to 1.8 mg P.O. daily for more severe cases.
To prevent attacks of gout in patients undergoing surgery–
Adults: 0.5 to 0.6 mg P.O. t.i.d. 3 days before and 3 days after surgery.
To treat acute gout, acute gouty arthritis–
Adults: initially, 1 to 1.2 mg P.O., then 0.5 or 0.6 mg q hour, or 1 to 1.2 mg q 2 hours until pain is relieved or until nausea, vomiting, or diarrhea ensues. Or 2 mg I.V. followed by 0.5 mg q 6 hours if necessary. Total I.V. dosage over 24 hours (one course of treatment) not to exceed 4 mg.

Note: Give I.V. by slow I.V. push over 2 to 5 minutes. Avoid extravasation. Don't dilute colchicine injection with dextrose 5% injection or any other fluid that might change pH of colchicine solution. If lower concentration of colchicine injection is needed, dilute with normal saline solution or sterile water for injection and administer over 2 to 5 minutes by direct injection. Preferably, inject into the tubing of a free-flowing I.V. solution. However, if diluted solution becomes turbid, don't inject.
Familial Mediterranean fever suppression–
Adults: acute attack–P.O. 0.6 mg hourly for four doses, then q 2 hours for four doses on the first day. Then, give 1.2 mg P.O. q 12 hours for 2 days. Maintenance dosage is 0.5 to 0.6 mg P.O. b.i.d. to t.i.d.
Antiosteolytic treatment–
Adults: 0.6 mg t.i.d. Instruct patient in the proper methods of oral hygiene, including the use of a toothbrush, dental floss, and toothpicks.

CONTRAINDICATIONS & PRECAUTIONS

Contraindicated in patients with serious GI, renal, or cardiac disorders. Use cautiously in patients who may have early signs of these disorders because the drug may exacerbate these conditions; in patients with blood dyscrasia or hypersensitivity to colchicine; and in elderly or debilitated patients.

ADVERSE REACTIONS

Common reactions are in italics; life-threatening reactions are in bold italics.
Blood: ***aplastic anemia*** *and* ***agranulocytosis with prolonged use;*** nonthrombocytopenic purpura.
CNS: peripheral neuritis.
GI: *nausea, vomiting, abdominal pain, diarrhea.*
Skin: urticaria, dermatitis.
Local: severe local irritation if extravasation occurs.
Other: alopecia.

INTERACTIONS

Alcohol: may impair efficacy of colchicine prophylaxis.
Loop diuretics: may decrease efficacy of colchicine prophylaxis.
Phenylbutazone: may increase risk of leukopenia or thrombocytopenia.
Vitamin B_{12}: impaired absorption of vitamin B_{12}.

EFFECTS ON DIAGNOSTIC TESTS

Alkaline phosphatase, AST (SGOT), and ALT (SGPT): increased levels.
Serum carotene, cholesterol, and thrombocytes: decreased values.
Urine tests for RBC count or hemoglobin concentrations: false-positive results.

NURSING CONSIDERATIONS

Besides those related universally to drug therapy (see "How to use this book"), consider the following specific recommendations:

Assessment
- Obtain a baseline assessment of the patient's uric acid levels, joint pain, and stiffness before therapy.
- Be alert for adverse reactions and drug interactions throughout therapy.
- Evaluate the patient's and family's knowledge about colchicine therapy.

Nursing Diagnoses
- Pain (joint) related to patient's underlying condition.
- High risk for fluid volume deficit related to colchicine-induced adverse GI reactions.
- Knowledge deficit related to colchicine therapy.

Planning and Implementation
Preparation and Administration
- Store the drug in a tightly closed, light-resistant container, away from moisture and high temperatures.
- Review baseline laboratory study results, including CBC, which should precede therapy and be repeated periodically.
- Do not administer I.M. or S.C.; severe local irritation occurs.
- ***I.V. use:*** Give I.V. injection by slow I.V. push over 2 to 5 minutes or inject into tubing of a free-flowing I.V. with compatible I.V. fluid. Avoid extravasation. Change needle when making a direct I.V. injection. Don't dilute colchicine injection with dextrose 5% injection or any other fluid that might change pH of colchicine solution. If lower concentration of colchicine injection is needed, dilute with sterile water for injection or 0.9% sodium chloride solution. However, don't inject if diluted solution becomes turbid.
- As maintenance therapy, give with meals to reduce GI reactions.
- Expect to discontinue drug as soon as gout pain is relieved or at the first sign of GI symptoms.

Monitoring
- Monitor effectiveness by regularly assessing for relief of the patient's

discomfort and improved serum urate levels.
• Monitor intake and output and assess hydration status, particularly if adverse GI reactions occur.
• During prolonged use, monitor patient's CBC for evidence of aplastic anemia.
• Monitor I.V. injection site for signs of extravasation or phlebitis.
• Monitor serum uric acid test results.
Supportive Care
• Expect to discontinue drug as soon as gout pain is relieved or at the first sign of GI symptoms (anorexia, nausea, vomiting, or diarrhea) or weakness. First sign of acute overdosage may be GI symptoms, followed by vascular damage, muscle weakness, and ascending paralysis. Delirium and seizures may occur without loss of consciousness.
• If extravasation or phlebitis occurs during I.V. use, notify the doctor and apply heat or cold to relieve the discomfort.
• If the patient becomes noncompliant, discuss reasons why and suggest methods patient may use to help maintain compliance.
• To avoid cumulative toxicity, a course of I.V. colchicine should not be repeated for several weeks.
Patient Teaching
• Instruct the patient to keep colchicine readily available so it can be taken as soon as symptoms of an acute gout attack occur.
• Advise patient to report rash, sore throat, fever, unusual bleeding, bruising, fatigue, weakness, numbness, or tingling.
• Tell patient to discontinue colchicine as soon as gout pain is relieved or at the first sign of nausea, vomiting, stomach pain, or diarrhea. Advise patient to report persistent symptoms.
• Instruct the patient to avoid alcohol during colchicine therapy because alcohol may inhibit drug action.
• Inform the patient that colchicine has no effect on nongouty arthritis.
• Instruct patients with gout to avoid all medications containing aspirin as these may precipitate gout. Acetaminophen may be used for pain.
Evaluation
In patients receiving colchicine, appropriate evaluation statements may include:
• Patient expresses relief of discomfort from gout attacks.
• Patient does not develop a fluid volume deficit from adverse GI reactions.
• Patient and family state an understanding of colchicine therapy.

colestipol hydrochloride
(koe les´ ti pole)
Colestid

• *Classification:* antilipemic (anion exchange resin)
• *Pregnancy Risk Category:* C

HOW SUPPLIED
Granules: 500-g bottles, 5-g packets

ACTION
Mechanism: Combines with bile acid to form an insoluble compound that is excreted.
Absorption: Not absorbed.
Distribution: None.
Metabolism: None.
Excretion: In feces.
Onset, peak, duration: Cholesterol levels may decrease in 24 to 48 hours, with peak effect occurring at 1 month. In some patients, the initial decrease is followed by a return to baseline or higher cholesterol levels on continued therapy. Cholesterol levels return to baseline within 1 month after therapy stops.

INDICATIONS & DOSAGE

Primary hypercholesterolemia and xanthomas–
Adults: 15 to 30 g P.O. daily in two to four divided doses.

CONTRAINDICATIONS & PRECAUTIONS

Contraindicated in patients with complete biliary obstruction or atresia because bile is not secreted into the intestine; in patients with primary biliary cirrhosis because their cholesterol levels may be further increased; and in patients with hypersensitivity to the drug.

Use cautiously in patients with constipation because of the risk of fecal impaction; in patients with malabsorption because the condition may deteriorate from further decreased absorption of fats and fat-soluble vitamins E, A, D, and K; and in pregnant women because impaired maternal absorption of vitamins and other nutrients is a potential threat to the fetus.

ADVERSE REACTIONS

Common reactions are in italics; life-threatening reactions are in bold italics.
CNS: headache, dizziness.
GI: *constipation (common, may require decreasing the dosage),* fecal impaction, hemorrhoids, abdominal discomfort, flatulence, nausea, vomiting, steatorrhea.
Skin: rashes, irritation of skin, tongue, and perianal area.
Other: vitamin A, D, and K deficiency from decreased absorption; hyperchloremic acidosis with long-term use or very high dosage.

INTERACTIONS

Oral hypoglycemics: may antagonize response to colestipol. Monitor serum lipids.
Orally administered drugs: absorption may be decreased by colestipol. Separate administration times: other drugs should be taken at least 1 hour before or 4 hours after colestipol.

EFFECTS ON DIAGNOSTIC TESTS

Alkaline phosphatase, aspartate aminotransferase, chloride, phosphorus, potassium, and sodium: altered serum levels.

NURSING CONSIDERATIONS

Besides those related universally to drug therapy (see "How to use this book"), consider the following specific recommendations:

Assessment
- Obtain a baseline assessment of the patient's underlying condition before drug therapy.
- Be alert for adverse reactions and drug interactions throughout therapy.
- Evaluate the patient's and family's knowledge about colestipol therapy.

Nursing Diagnoses
- High risk for injury related to ineffectiveness of colestipol to reduce blood lipid and cholesterol levels.
- Constipation related to adverse drug reactions.
- Knowledge deficit related to colestipol therapy.

Planning and Implementation
Preparation and Administration
- To mix powder, sprinkle on surface of preferred beverage or wet food. Let stand a few minutes, then stir to obtain uniform suspension. Mixing with carbonated beverages may result in excess foaming. Use large glass and mix slowly.
- Administer all medications at least 1 hour before or 4 to 6 hours after colestipol to avoid blocking their absorption.
- Drug may bind with other drugs and cause decreased absorption.
- Administer this drug in at least 3 oz (90 ml) of juice, milk, or water. After drinking this preparation, patient should swirl a small additional amount of liquid in the same glass

and then drink it to ensure ingestion of the entire dose.

Monitoring

• Monitor for possible drug interactions if the patient is also receiving oral hypoglycemics or any orally administered drug.

• Monitor for signs of vitamin deficiencies: A (visual disturbances, skin changes); D (alteration in calcium metabolism); and K (bleeding tendencies).

• Monitor effectiveness by checking the patient's serum cholesterol and triglyceride levels every 4 weeks.

• Monitor levels of digitalis glycosides and other drugs to ensure appropriate dosage during and after therapy with colestipol.

• Monitor the patient's bowel patterns for constipation.

Supportive Care

• To enhance palatability, mix and refrigerate the next day's dose the previous evening.

• Digitalis dosage may need adjustment if digitalis glycoside toxicity follows discontinuation of colestipol.

• Lowering dosage, increasing dietary fiber, or adding a stool softener may relieve constipation.

Patient Teaching

• Teach the patient to take other drugs at least 1 hour before or 4 to 6 hours after colestipol to avoid blocking their absorption.

• Teach the patient about proper dietary management (restricting total fat and cholesterol intake), weight control, and exercise. Explain their importance in controlling elevated serum lipids.

• Teach the patient to take the drug with 3 oz of juice, milk, or water and then to add a small amount of liquid to the same glass, swirling and then drinking to ensure ingestion of the entire dose.

• To enhance palatability, advise the patient to make the next day's dose the previous evening and to refrigerate it.

• Teach the patient to increase dietary fiber or to take a stool softner if constipation develops.

Evaluation

In patients receiving colestipol, appropriate evaluation statements may include:

• Patient's blood triglyceride and cholesterol levels are normal.

• Patient does not develop constipation.

• Patient and family state an understanding of colestipol therapy.

PHARMACOLOGIC CLASS

corticosteroids (nasal and oral inhalation)

Nasal

beclomethasone dipropionate
dexamethasone sodium phosphate
flunisolide

Oral

triamcinolone acetonide

OVERVIEW

Topical administration via oral aerosol and nasal spray delivers adrenocorticoids to sites of inflammation in the nasal passages or the tracheobronchial tree. Because smaller doses are administered, less drug is absorbed systemically, with fewer systemic adverse effects.

Inhaled glucocorticoid is absorbed through the nasal mucosa or through the trachea, bronchi, and alveoli. The anti-inflammatory effects of the glucocorticoids depend upon the direct local action of the steroid. Glucocorticoids stimulate enzymes that decrease inflammation. These enzymes stimulate biochemical pathways that decrease the inflammatory response by stabilizing leukocyte lysosomal membranes, inhibiting macrophage accumulation in inflamed areas; reducing leukocyte adhesion to the capillary endothelium; reducing capillary wall permeability and edema formation.

CLINICAL INDICATIONS AND ACTIONS

Nasal inflammation

Nasal solutions are used to relieve symptoms of seasonal or perennial rhinitis when antihistamines and decongestants are ineffective; to treat inflammatory conditions of the nasal passages; and to prevent recurrence after surgical removal of nasal polyps.

Chronic bronchial asthma

Aerosols are used to treat chronic bronchial asthma not controlled by bronchodilators and other nonsteroidal medications.

OVERVIEW OF ADVERSE REACTIONS

• *Nasal:* local sensations of nasal burning and irritation in about 10% of patients; sneezing attacks immediately after the nasal application in about 10% of patients; and transient mild nosebleeds in 10% to 15% of patients, but it is unknown whether this is an effect of the nasal solution or of the dryness it induces in the nasal passages. Localized candidal infections of the nose or pharynx have occurred rarely.

• *Oral:* localized infections with *Candida albicans* or *Aspergillus niger,* which have occurred commonly in the mouth and pharynx and occasionally in the larynx. These infections may require treatment with appropriate antifungal therapy or discontinuation of treatment with the inhaled corticosteroid.

• *Systemic:* Systemic absorption may occur. This is more likely with large doses or with combined nasal and oral corticosteroid therapy.

Other: Hypersensitivity reactions are possible. Also, some patients may be intolerant of the fluorocarbon propellants in the preparations.

REPRESENTATIVE COMBINATIONS

None.

PHARMACOLOGIC CLASS

corticosteroids (ophthalmic)

dexamethasone
dexamethasone sodium phosphate
fluorometholone
medrysone
prednisolone acetate
prednisolone sodium phosphate

OVERVIEW

Topical ophthalmic steroids are effective for treating most external inflammatory conditions of the conjunctiva, sclera, cornea, and anterouveal tract. Ophthalmic corticosteroid preparations are available as sterile ointments, solutions, and suspensions. Solutions or suspensions, which cause minimal interference with vision and have minimal effect on corneal reepithelialization, usually are used during the day. Ointments provide longer contact with the eye and usually are used at night or to treat inflammatory conditions of the eyelid.

The anti-inflammatory effects of the corticosteroids depend on the direct local action of the steroid. Corticosteroids stimulate enzymes that decrease inflammation. These enzymes stimulate biochemical pathways that decrease the inflammatory response by stabilizing leukocyte lysosomal membranes, inhibiting macrophage accumulation in inflamed areas; reducing leukocyte adhesion to the capillary endothelium; reducing capillary wall permeability and edema formation.

CLINICAL INDICATIONS AND ACTIONS

Optic Inflammation

Ophthalmic corticosteroids provide symptomatic relief of allergic disorders involving the eyelid, conjunctiva, cornea, iris, or ciliary body. These disorders include nonpurulent blepharitis, nonpurulent phlyctenular keratoconjunctivitis, vernal conjunctivitis, acne rosacea, iritis, superficial punctate keratitis, cyclitis, contact dermatitis of the conjunctiva and eyelid, episcleritis, and uveitis.

Ophthalmic corticosteroids are used to treat corneal injuries from chemical, radiation, or thermal burns, or penetration by foreign bodies. In combination with anti-infective agents, they are effective in treating eye infections.

OVERVIEW OF ADVERSE REACTIONS

Topical ophthalmic corticosteroids may cause increased intraocular pressure. The magnitude of increase in intraocular pressure depends on the corticosteroid used, its concentration, and the frequency and duration of administration. A significant increase in intraocular pressure may develop after 1 to 6 weeks of therapy and is usually reversible within a few weeks after discontinuation. Prolonged use (usually longer than a year) may result in open-angle glaucoma, optic nerve damage, or defects in visual acuity and field of vision.

Patients with diabetes mellitus, preexisting glaucoma, or significant myopia are at much greater risk for increased intraocular pressure. In those patients susceptible to intraocular hypertension, a clinically significant increase in intraocular pressure occurs rarely with 1% medrysone; 0.1% fluorometholone is less likely to cause hypertension than 0.5% hydrocortisone or 0.1% prednisolone; and 0.5% hydrocortisone or 0.1% prednisolone is less likely to cause ocular hypertension than 0.1% dexamethasone.

Transient burning and stinging may occur after application. Rarely, mydriasis, ptosis, epithelial punctate keratitis, and possible corneal or scleral malacia may develop. Hypersensitivity has occurred rarely with topical corticosteroid therapy.

Prolonged use (more than 2 years) may result in posterior subcapsular cataracts that do not regress when the drugs are discontinued.

REPRESENTATIVE COMBINATIONS

Dexamethasone with neomycin sulfate: NeoDecadron Ocumeter Ophthalmic Solution, NeoDecadron Ophthalmic Ointment; with neomycin sulfate and polymixin B sulfate: Maxitrol Ophthalmic Suspension; with neomycin and polymixin B sulfate: Dexaridin Ophthalmic Suspension.

Hydrocortisone with neomycin sulfate: NeoCortef Ophthalmic Suspension; with neomycin sulfate and polymyxin B sulfate: Cortisporin.

Prednisolone acetate with neomycin sulfate: Neo-Delta-Cortef; with chloramphenicol: Chloroptic-P Ophthalmic Ointment; with sulfacetamide sodium: Cetapred Ophthalmic Ointment, Blephamide Liquifilm, Blephamide S.O.P., Metimyd Ophthalmic Ointment or Suspension, Pred-Forte, Predamide, Vasocidin; with phenylephrine: Predulose; with sulfacetamide and phenylephrine hydrochloride: Sulfapred; with atropine sulfate: Mydrapred.

Prednisolone sodium phosphate with neomycin sulfate: Neo-Hydeltrasol; with sodium sulfacetamide: Optimyd.

PHARMACOLOGIC CLASS

corticosteriods (systemic)

Glucocorticoids
betamethasone
betamethasone sodium phosphate
betamethasone sodium phosphate and betamethasone acetate
cortisone acetate
dexamethasone
dexamethasone acetate
dexamethasone sodium phosphate
hydrocortisone
hydrocortisone acetate
hydrocortisone cypionate
hydrocortisone sodium phosphate
hydrocortisone sodium succinate
methylprednisolone
methylprednisolone acetate
methylprednisolone sodium succinate
paramethasone acetate
prednisolone
prednisolone acetate
prednisolone sodium phosphate
prednisolone tebutate
prednisone
triamcinolone
triamcinolone acetonide
triamcinolone diacetate
triamcinolone hexacetonide

Mineralocorticoids
fludrocortisone acetate

OVERVIEW

Active adrenocortical extracts were first prepared in 1930; by 1942, chemists had isolated 28 steroids from the adrenal cortex. The corticosteroids are classified according to their activity into two groups: the glucocorticoids and the mineralocorticoids. The glucocorticoids regulate carbohydrate, lipid, and protein metabolism; inflammation; and the body's immune responses to diverse stimuli. The mineralocorticoids regulate electrolyte homeostasis. Many corticosteroids exert both kinds of activity.

The corticosteroids dramatically affect almost all body systems. They are thought to act by controlling the rate of protein synthesis. Because the maximum pharmacologic activity lags behind peak blood concentrations, corticosteroids' effects may result from modification of enzyme activity rather than from direct action by the drugs.

Mineralocorticoids act renally at the distal tubules to enhance the reabsorption of sodium ions (and thus water) from the tubular fluid into the plasma, and the urinary excretion of both potassium and hydrogen ions.

CLINICAL INDICATIONS AND ACTIONS

Inflammation
A major pharmacologic use of the glucocorticoids is treatment of inflammation. The anti-inflammatory effects depend on the direct local action of the steroids. Glucocorticoids decrease the inflammatory response by stabilizing leukocyte lysosomal membranes, which prevent the release of destructive acid hydrolases from leukocytes; inhibiting macrophage accumulation in inflamed areas; reducing leukocyte adhesion to the capillary endothelium; reducing capillary wall permeability and edema formation; decreasing complement components; antagonizing histamine activity and release of kinin from substrates; reducing fibroblast proliferation, collagen deposition, and subsequent scar tissue formation; and by other unknown mechanisms.

Immunosuppression
Another major pharmacologic use of the glucocorticoids is immunosuppression. The complete mechanisms of action are unknown, but glucocorticoids reduce activity and volume of the lymphatic system, producing lymphocytopenia, decreasing immunoglobulin and complement concentra-

tions, decreasing passage of immune complexes through basement membranes, and possibly depressing reactivity of tissue to antigen-antibody interaction.

Adrenal insufficiency

Combined mineralocorticoid and glucocorticoid therapy is used in treating adrenal insufficiency and in salt-losing forms of congenital adrenogenital syndrome.

Rheumatic and collagen diseases; other severe diseases: Glucocorticoids are used to treat rheumatic and collagen diseases (arthritis, polyarteritis nodosa, systemic lupus erythematosus); thyroiditis; severe dermatologic diseases, such as pemphigus, exfoliative dermatitis, lichen planus, and psoriasis; allergic reactions; ocular disorders (such as inflammations); respiratory diseases (asthma, sarcoidosis, lipid pneumonitis); hematologic diseases (autoimmune hemolytic anemia, idiopathic thrombocytopenia); neoplastic diseases (leukemias, lymphomas); and GI diseases (ulcerative colitis, regional enteritis, celiac disease). Other indications include myasthenia gravis, organ transplants, nephrotic syndrome, and septic shock.

OVERVIEW OF ADVERSE REACTIONS

Suppression of the hypothalamic-pituitary-adrenal (HPA) axis is the major effect of systemic therapy with corticosteroids. When administered in high doses or for prolonged therapy, the glucocorticoids suppress release of adrenocorticotropic hormone (ACTH) from the pituitary gland; subsequently, the adrenal cortex stops secreting endogenous corticosteroids. The degree and duration of HPA axis suppression produced by the drugs is highly variable among patients and depends on the dose, frequency and time of administration, and duration of therapy. Patients with a suppressed HPA axis resulting from exogenous glucocorticoid administration who abruptly discontinue therapy may experience severe withdrawal symptoms such as fever, myalgia, arthralgia, malaise, anorexia, nausea, desquamation of skin, orthostatic hypotension, dizziness, fainting, dyspnea, and hypoglycemia. Therefore, corticosteroid therapy should always be withdrawn gradually. Adrenal suppression may persist for as long as 12 months in patients who have received large doses for prolonged periods. Until complete recovery occurs, such patients subjected to stress may show signs and symptoms of adrenal insufficiency; they may require replacement therapy with both a glucocorticoid and a mineralocorticoid.

Cushingoid symptoms, the effects of excessive glucocorticoid therapy, may develop in patients receiving large doses of glucocorticoids over a period of several weeks or longer. These include moon face, central obesity, striae, hirsutism, acne, ecchymoses, hypertension, osteoporosis, muscle atrophy, sexual dysfunction, diabetes, cataracts, hyperlipidemia, peptic ulcer, increased susceptibility to infection, and fluid and electrolyte imbalance.

Other adverse reactions to normal or high dosages of corticosteroids may include CNS effects (euphoria, insomnia, psychotic behavior, pseudotumor cerebri, mental changes, nervousness, restlessness); cardiovascular effects (congestive heart failure, hypertension, edema); GI effects (peptic ulcer, irritation, increased appetite); metabolic effects (hypokalemia, sodium retention, fluid retention, weight gain, hyperglycemia, osteoporosis); dermatologic effects (delayed wound healing, acne, skin eruptions, muscle atrophy, striae); and immunosuppression (increased susceptibility to infection).

REPRESENTATIVE COMBINATIONS

Betamethasone sodium phosphate with betamethasone acetate: Celestone Soluspan.

Dexamethasone sodium phosphate with lidocaine hydrochloride: Decadron with Xylocaine.

Prednisolone sodium phosphate with prednisolone acetate: Dual-Pred, Soluject.

PHARMACOLOGIC CLASS

corticosteroids (topical)

alclometasone dipropionate
amcinonide
betamethasone benzoate
betamethasone dipropionate
betamethasone valerate
clobetasol propionate
clocortolone pivalate
desonide
desoximetasone
dexamethasone
dexamethasone sodium phosphate
diflorasone diacetate
fluocinolone acetonide
fluocinonide
flurandrenolide
fluticasone propionate
halcinonide
halobetasol propionate
hydrocortisone
hydrocortisone acetate
hydrocortisone butyrate
hydrocortisone valerate
methylprednisolone acetate
mometasone furoate
triamcinolone acetonide

OVERVIEW

Since topical hydrocortisone was introduced in the 1950s, numerous analogues have been developed to provide a wide range of potencies in creams, ointments, lotions, and gels.

The anti-inflammatory effects of topical glucocorticoids depend on the direct local action of the steroid. Although the exact mechanism of action is unclear, many researchers believe that glucocorticoids stimulate enzyme synthesis that decreases inflammation. These enzymes stimulate biochemical pathways that decrease the inflammatory response by stabilizing leukocyte lysosomal membranes, reducing leukocyte adhesion to the capillary endothelium; reducing capillary wall permeability and edema formation.

Topical corticosteroids are minimally absorbed systemically and cause fewer adverse effects than systemically administered corticosteroids. Fluorinated derivatives are absorbed to a greater extent than other topical steroids. The degree of absorption depends on the site of application, the amount applied, the relative potency, the presence of an occlusive dressing (may increase penetration by 10%), the condition of the skin, and the vehicle carrying the drug. Topical corticosteroids are used to relieve pruritus, inflammation, and other signs of corticosteroid-responsive dermatoses.

Among the several dosage forms available, ointments are preferred for dry, scaly areas; solutions, gels, aerosols, and lotions for hairy areas. Creams can be used for most areas except those in which additional dampness may cause maceration. Gels and lotions can be used for moist lesions; however, gels may contain alcohol, which can be drying and irritating to the skin. The topical preparations are classified by potency into six groups: group I is the most potent, group VI the least potent.

CLINICAL INDICATIONS AND ACTIONS

Inflammatory disorders of skin and mucous membranes

The topical adrenocorticoids relieve inflammatory and pruritic skin disorders, including localized neurodermatitis, psoriasis, atopic or seborrheic dermatitis, the inflammatory phase of

COMPARATIVE POTENCY OF TOPICAL CORTICOSTEROIDS

Topical corticosteroid preparations can be grouped according to relative anti-inflammatory activity. The following list arranges groups of topical corticosteroids in decreasing order of potency (based mainly on vasoconstrictor assay or clinical effectiveness in psoriasis). Preparations within each group are approximately equivalent.

GROUP	DRUG	CONCENTRATION (%)
I	betamethasone dipropionate (Diprolene)	0.05
	betamethasone dipropionate (Diprolene AF)	0.05
	clobetasol propionate (Temovate)	0.05
	diflorasone diacetate (Psorcon)	0.05
II	amcinonide (Cyclocort)	0.1
	betamethasone dipropionate ointment (Diprosone)	0.05
	desoximetasone (Topicort)	0.05, 0.25
	diflorasone diacetate (Florone, Maxiflor)	0.05
	fluocinonide (Lidex)	0.05
	fluocinonide gel	0.05
	halcinonide (Halog)	0.1
III	betamethasone benzoate gel	0.025
	betamethasone dipropionate cream (Diprosone)	0.05
	betamethasone valerate ointment (Valisone)	0.1
	diflorasone diacetate cream (Florone, Maxiflor)	0.05
	mometasone furoate (Elocon)	0.1
	triamcinolone acetonide cream (Artistocort)	0.5
IV	desoximetasone (Topicort LP)	0.05
	fluocinolone acetonide (Synalar-HP)	0.2
	fluocinolone acetonide ointment (Synalar)	0.025
	flurandrenolide (Cordran)	0.05
	triamcinolone acetonide ointment (Aristocort, Kenalog)	0.1
V	betamethasone benzoate cream	0.025
	betamethasone dipropionate lotion (Diprosone)	0.05
	betamethasone valerate cream or lotion (Valisone)	0.1
	fluocinolone acetonide cream (Synalar)	0.025
	flurandrenolide (Cordran)	0.05
	hydrocortisone butyrate (Locoid)	0.1
	hydrocortisone valerate (Westcort)	0.2
	triamcinolone acetonide cream or lotion (Kenalog)	0.1
VI	alclometasone dipropionate (Aclovate)	0.05
	desonide (Tridesilon)	0.05
	fluocinolone acetonide solution (Synalar)	0.01

xerosis, anogenital pruritus, discoid lupus erythematosus, lichen planus, granuloma annulare, and lupus erythematosus.

These drugs may also relieve irritant or allergic contact dermatitis; however, relief of acute dermatosis may require systemic adrenocorticoids.

Rectal disorders responsive to this class of drugs include ulcerative colitis, cryptitis, inflamed hemorrhoids, post-irradiation or factitial proctitis, and pruritus ani.

Oral lesions, such as nonherpetic oral inflammatory and ulcerative lesions and routine gingivitis, may respond to treatment with topical adrenocorticoids.

Nonprescription formulations of the topical corticosteroids are indicated for minor skin irritation such as itching; rashes due to eczema, dermatitis, insect bites, poison ivy, poison oak, or poison sumac; or dermatitis resulting from exposure to soaps, detergents, cosmetics, and jewelry.

OVERVIEW OF ADVERSE REACTIONS

Local effects include burning, itching, irritation, dryness, folliculitis, striae, miliaria, acne, perioral dermatitis, hypopigmentation, hypertrichosis, allergic contact dermatitis, secondary infection, and atrophy.

Systemic absorption may occur, leading to hypothalamic-pituitary-adrenal (HPA) axis suppression.

The risk of adverse reactions increases with the use of occlusive dressings or more potent steroids, in patients with liver disease, and in children (because of their greater ratio of skin surface to body weight).

Prolonged application around the eyes may lead to cataracts or glaucoma.

REPRESENTATIVE COMBINATIONS

Betamethasone with clotrimazole: Lotrisone.

Betamethasone diproprionate with clotrimazole: Lotrisone.

Dexamethasone with neomycin sulfate: NeoDecadron Cream; with neomycin sulfate and polymixin B sulfate: Dexacidin Ointment.

Fluocinolone acetonide with neomycin: Neo-Synalar.

Flurandrenolide with neomycin: Cordran-N.

Hydrocortisone with iodoquinol: Vytone; with iodochlorhydroxyquin: Racet, Vioform-hydrocortisone, AP, Caquin, Corque, Cortin, Lanvisone, Pedi-Cort-V, Viodo HC, Hysone; with pramoxine: Pramosone, FEP, Zone-A; with iodochlorhydroxyquin and pramoxine: Vipramosone, Dermarex, Stera-Foam, Vio-Hydrosone; with neomycin: Neo-Cortef, Neo-Cort-Dome; with neomycin and polymyxin B: Cortisporin Cream; with neomycin, bacitracin, and polymyxin B sulfate: Cortisporin Ointment; with neomycin sulfate and polymycin B sulfate: Cortisporin; with dibucaine: Corticaine; with pyrilamine maleate, pheniramine maleate, and chlorpheniramine: HC Derma-PAX Liquid; with benzocaine, oxyquinoline, ephedrine, menthol, ichthammol, and zinc oxide: Derma Medicone-HC Ointment; with chlorcyclizine: Mantadil Cream; with benzoyl peroxide and mineral oil: Vanoxide HC; with lidocaine and glycerin: Lida-Mantle-HC Cream; with sulfur and salicylic acid: Theracort Lotion; with sodium thiosulfate, salicylic acid, isopropyl alcohol, menthol, and camphor: Komed HC Lotion; with diperodone and zinc oxide: Allersone Ointment.

Methylprednisolone with neomycin: Neo-Medrol.

Prednisolone acetate with neomycin: Neo-Delta-Cortef.

Triamcinolone acetonide with nystatin: Mykacet, Mycogen II, Mycolog II, Myco-Triacet II, Mytrex F, N.G.T.; with neomycin, gramicidin, and nystatin: MycoTricet, Tri-Statin.

---

corticotropin (adrenocorticotropic hormone, ACTH)

(kor ti koe troe´ pin)

ACTH, Acthar, Acthar Gel (H.P.)†, ACTH Gel, Cortigel-40, Cortigel-80, Cortrophin Gel, Cortropic-Gel-40, Cortropic-Gel-80, H.P. Acthar Gel

- *Classification:* diagnostic aid,

replacement hormone, anti-inflammatory agent, and non-supportive thyroiditis treatment (anterior pituitary hormone)
• *Pregnancy Risk Category:* C

HOW SUPPLIED

Aqueous injection: 25 units/vial, 40 units/vial
Repository injection: 40 units/ml, 80 units/ml

ACTION

Mechanism: Stimulates the adrenal cortex to secrete corticosteroids.
Absorption: Rapidly absorbed after S.C. or I.M. administration; absorption occurs over 8 to 16 hours after I.M. administration of zinc or repository form.
Distribution: Exact distribution is unknown, but it is removed rapidly from plasma by many tissues.
Excretion: Probably excreted by the kidneys. Half-life: About 15 minutes.
Onset, peak, duration: Maximum stimulation occurs after infusing 1 to 6 units of corticotropin over 8 hours. Peak cortisol levels are achieved within 1 hour of I.M. or rapid I.V. administration of corticotropin. Peak 17-hydroxycorticosteroid levels are achieved within 7 to 24 hours with zinc and 3 to 12 hours with the repository form; duration of action is about 2 hours with zinc form and up to 3 days with the repository form.

INDICATIONS & DOSAGE

Diagnostic test of adrenocortical function–
Adults: up to 80 units I.M. or S.C. in divided doses; or a single dose of repository form; or 10 to 25 units (aqueous form) in 500 ml dextrose 5% in water I.V. over 8 hours, between blood samplings.

Individual dosages generally vary with adrenal glands' sensitivity to stimulation as well as with specific disease. Infants and younger children require larger doses per kilogram than do older children and adults.
For therapeutic use–
Adults: 40 units S.C. or I.M. in 4 divided doses (aqueous); 40 units q 12 to 24 hours (gel or repository form).

CONTRAINDICATIONS & PRECAUTIONS

Contraindicated in patients with hypersensitivity to corticotropin, primary adrenocortical insufficiency, or congenital adrenogenital syndrome (because corticotropin will be ineffective) and in any condition associated with adrenocortical hyperfunction (which may become exacerbated). Corticotropin also may exacerbate CHF or hypertension (because of sodium and fluid retention), ocular herpes simplex (because of the risk of corneal perforation), sensitivity to proteins of porcine origin (because corticotropin often is obtained from pigs), osteoporosis, and scleroderma.

Use cautiously in patients with acquired immune deficiency syndrome (AIDS) or a predisposition to AIDS because of an increased risk of uncontrollable infection or neoplasms; diabetes mellitus, which may become exacerbated; ulcerative colitis, diverticulitis, peptic ulcer, or gastritis because symptoms of disease progression may be masked or perforation may occur without warning; myasthenia gravis because it *may* cause muscle weakness; and systemic fungal or tuberculosis infection, which may become exacerbated.

Use in hypothyroidism and cirrhosis may result in an enhanced corticotropin effect. Use in gouty arthritis should be limited to a few days because rebound attacks may follow withdrawal after prolonged use. Corticotropin may aggravate existing emotional instability or psychotic tendencies.

ADVERSE REACTIONS

Common reactions are in italics; life-threatening reactions are in bold italics.

CNS: *seizures, dizziness,* papilledema, headache, *euphoria, insomnia,* mood swings, personality changes, depression, psychosis.
EENT: cataracts, glaucoma.
GI: peptic ulcer with perforation and hemorrhage, pancreatitis, abdominal distention, ulcerative esophagitis, nausea, vomiting.
GU: menstrual irregularities.
Metabolic: *sodium and fluid retention,* calcium and potassium loss, hypokalemic alkalosis, negative nitrogen balance.
Skin: *impaired wound healing,* thin fragile skin, petechiae, ecchymoses, facial erythema, increased sweating, acne, hyperpigmentation, allergic skin reactions, hirsutism.
Other: muscle weakness, steroid myopathy, loss of muscle mass, osteoporosis, vertebral compression fractures, cushingoid state, suppression of growth in children, *activation of latent diabetes mellitus,* progressive increase in antibodies, loss of ACTH stimulatory effect, and ***hypersensitivity.***

INTERACTIONS

None significant.

EFFECTS ON DIAGNOSTIC TESTS

Blood and urine glucose: altered levels.
CBC: altered leukocyte counts.
Plasma cortisol: falsely high concentrations with fluorometric analysis, not with radioimmunoassay or competitive protein-binding method.
Protein-bound iodine: altered levels.
Radioactive iodine (^{131}I) uptake and liothyronine (T_3) uptake: altered results.
Serum amylase: altered levels.
Sodium and potassium: altered levels.
Total protein: altered values.
Urine amino acid, serotonin, uric acid, calcium, and 17-ketosteroid: altered levels.

NURSING CONSIDERATIONS

Besides those related universally to drug therapy (see "How to use this book"), consider the following specific recommendations:

Assessment

- Obtain a baseline assessment of the patient's underlying condition before initiating corticotropin therapy.
- Be alert for common adverse reactions.
- Evaluate the patient's and family's knowledge about corticotropin.

Nursing Diagnoses

- Activity intolerance related to the patient's underlying condition.
- Fluid volume excess related to corticotropin-induced sodium and fluid retention.
- Knowledge deficit related to corticotropin therapy.

Planning and Implementation

Preparation and Administration

- Be aware that ACTH treatment should be preceded by verification of adrenal responsiveness and test for hypersensitivity and allergic reactions.
- Be aware that ACTH should be adjunctive not sole therapy.
- When possible ACTH dosage should be reduced to smallest effective dose to minimize induced adrenocortical insufficiency.
- Refrigerate reconstituted solution and use within 24 hours.
- ***I.M. use:*** If administering gel, warm it to room temperature, draw into large needle, and give slowly deep I.M. with 21G or 22G needle. Be aware injection is painful.
- ***I.V. use:*** When administering direct I.V., inject reconstituted drug directly into vein or through an I.V. line containing a free-flowing, compatible solution. When administering as a continuous infusion (not recommended

for intermittent infusion) infuse diluted solution, over 8 hours.

Monitoring

• Monitor patient for signs of improvement in underlying condition.

• Monitor patient for stress as unusual stress may require additional use of rapidly acting corticosteroids.

• Monitor neonates of corticotropin-treated mothers for signs of hypoadrenalism.

• Monitor weight changes, fluid exchange, and resting blood pressures until minimal effective dose is achieved.

• Monitor patient closely because drug may mask signs of chronic disease and decrease host resistance and ability to localize infection.

Supportive Care

• If stressful situations (trauma, surgery, severe illness) arise shortly after drug is stopped, notify doctor as corticotropin therapy will need to be reinstituted.

• Counteract edema by low-sodium, high-potassium intake; nitrogen loss by high-protein diet; and psychotic changes by reducing corticotropin dosage or administering sedatives as ordered.

Patient Teaching

• Stress importance of informing all members of the health care team about corticotropin use because unusual stress may require additional use of rapidly acting corticosteroids. If corticotropin was recently discontinued, therapy may have to be reinstituted.

• Tell patient to restrict sodium intake and consume a high-protein, high-potassium diet.

• Advise patient to have close follow-up care as drug may mask signs of chronic disease and decrease host resistance and ability to localize infection.

• Warn patient that injections, especially I.M. injections, are painful.

Evaluation

In patients receiving corticotropin, appropriate evaluation statements may include:

• Patient's tolerates normal activity level.

• Patient maintains normal fluid and electrolyte balance.

• Patient and family state an understanding of corticotropin therapy.

cortisone acetate

(kor´ ti sone)

Cortate‡, Cortone Acetate

• *Classification:* anti-inflammatory, replacement therapy (glucocorticoid, mineralocorticoid)

• *Pregnancy Risk Category:* D

HOW SUPPLIED

Tablets: 5 mg, 10 mg, 25 mg

Injection (suspension): 25 mg/ml, 50 mg/ml

ACTION

Mechanism: Decreases inflammation, mainly by stabilizing leukocyte lysosomal membranes. Also suppresses the immune response, stimulates bone marrow, and influences protein, fat, and carbohydrate metabolism.

Absorption: Rapidly absorbed after oral or I.M. administration.

Distribution: Rapidly distributed to muscle, liver, skin, intestines, and kidneys. Cortisone is extensively bound to plasma proteins (transcortin and albumin). Only the unbound portion is active. Cortisone is distributed into breast milk and through the placenta.

Metabolism: In the liver to the active metabolite hydrocortisone, which in turn is metabolized to inactive glucuronide and sulfate metabolites.

Excretion: The inactive metabolites and small amounts of unmetabolized drug are excreted by the kidneys. In-

significant amounts are also excreted in feces. Half-life: 8 to 12 hours.
Onset, peak, duration: Peak effects occur in about 1 to 2 hours after oral administration. The suspension for injection has a variable onset of 24 to 48 hours.

INDICATIONS & DOSAGE

Adrenal insufficiency, allergy, inflammation–
Adults: 25 to 300 mg P.O. or I.M. daily or on alternate days. Dosages highly individualized, depending on severity of disease.

CONTRAINDICATIONS & PRECAUTIONS

Contraindicated in patients with systemic fungal infections (except in adrenal insufficiency) or a hypersensitivity to ingredients of adrenocorticoid preparations. Patients who are receiving cortisone should not be given live virus vaccines because cortisone suppresses the immune response.

Use with extreme caution in patients with GI ulceration, renal disease, hypertension, osteoporosis, diabetes mellitus, thromboembolic disorders, seizures, myasthenia gravis, CHF, tuberculosis, hypoalbuminemia, hypothyroidism, cirrhosis of the liver, emotional instability, psychotic tendencies, hyperlipidemias, glaucoma, or cataracts because the drug may exacerbate these conditions.

Because adrenocorticoids increase the susceptibility to and mask symptoms of infection, cortisone should not be used (except in life-threatening situations) in patients with viral or bacterial infections not controlled by anti-infective agents.

ADVERSE REACTIONS

Common reactions are in italics; life-threatening reactions are in bold italics.

Most adverse reactions of corticosteroids are dose- or duration-dependent.
CNS: *euphoria, insomnia,* psychotic behavior, pseudotumor cerebri.
CV: ***CHF,*** hypertension, edema.
EENT: cataracts, glaucoma.
GI: *peptic ulcer,* GI irritation, increased appetite.
Metabolic: *possible hypokalemia, hyperglycemia and carbohydrate intolerance,* growth suppression in children.
Skin: delayed wound healing, acne, various skin eruptions.
Local: atrophy at I.M. injection sites.
Other: muscle weakness, pancreatitis, hirsutism, susceptibility to infections.
Acute adrenal insufficiency may follow increased stress (infection, surgery, or trauma) or abrupt withdrawal after long-term therapy.
Withdrawal symptoms: rebound inflammation, fatigue, weakness, arthralgia, fever, dizziness, lethargy, depression, fainting, orthostatic hypotension, dyspnea, anorexia, hypoglycemia. ***Sudden withdrawal may be fatal.***

INTERACTIONS

Barbiturates, phenytoin, rifampin: decreased corticosteroid effect. Corticosteroid dose may need to be increased.
Indomethacin, aspirin: increased risk of GI distress and bleeding. Give together cautiously.

EFFECTS ON DIAGNOSTIC TESTS

Diagnostic skin tests: suppresses reactions.
Glucose and cholesterol levels: may increase levels.
Nitroblue tetrazolium test for systemic bacterial infections: false-negative results.
Serum potassium, calcium, thyroxine, and triiodothyronine: decreased levels.
Thyroid function tests: decreases ^{131}I

uptake and protein-bound iodine concentrations in thyroid function tests. ***Urine glucose and calcium:*** increased levels.

NURSING CONSIDERATIONS

Besides those related universally to drug therapy (see "How to use this book"), consider the following specific recommendations:

Assessment

- Obtain a baseline assessment of the patient's condition before initiating drug therapy.
- Be alert for common adverse reactions and drug interactions throughout therapy.
- Evaluate the patient's and family's knowledge about cortisone therapy.

Nursing Diagnoses

- Fluid volume deficit related to the underlying condition.
- High risk for injury related to cortisone-induced adverse reactions.
- Knowledge deficit related to cortisone therapy.

Planning and Implementation

Preparation and Administration

- Gradually reduce drug dosage after long-term therapy. Never abruptly discontinue therapy as sudden withdrawal can be fatal.
- Always titrate to lowest effective dose as prescribed.
- Give a daily dosage in the morning for better results and less toxicity.
- Expect to increase dosage as prescribed during times of physiologic stress (surgery, trauma, or infection).
- ***P.O. use:*** Give with food when possible to avoid GI upset.
- ***I.M. use:*** Give injection deep into gluteal muscle. Rotate injection sites to prevent muscle atrophy. Be aware that I.M. route causes slow onset of action and should not be used in acute conditions when rapid effect is required. May be used on a twice-daily schedule matching diurnal variation.

Monitoring

- Monitor effectiveness by regularly assessing the patient for improvement of signs and symptoms of the underlying condition.
- Monitor for adverse reactions as drug can cause serious or life-threathening multisystem dysfunction.
- Monitor the patient's weight, blood pressure, blood glucose level, and serum electrolyte levels regularly.
- Monitor the patient for infection. Drug may mask or exacerbate infections.
- Monitor the patient's stress level. Stress (fever, trauma, surgery, or emotional problems) may increase adrenal insufficiency. Dose may have to be increased.
- Monitor patients receiving immunizations for decreased antibody response.
- Monitor the patient for signs of adrenal insufficiency, including hypoglycemia, areas of decreased skin pigmentation, hypotension, and symptoms of dehydration.

Supportive Care

- Notify the doctor if signs of adrenal insufficiency increase.
- Unless contraindicated, give the patient a low-sodium diet high in potassium and protein. Potassium supplement may be needed.

Patient Teaching

- Be sure that the patient understands the need to take the drug as prescribed. Tell patient if a dose is missed to take it as soon as the patient remembers. Warn the patient not to take two doses together.
- Warn the patient not to discontinue the drug abruptly or without the doctor's approval.
- Advise the patient to take oral form with meals to minimize GI adverse reactions.
- Tell the patient to carry a medical alert card indicating the need for supplemental adrenocorticoids during stress.

• Teach the patient to recognize signs of early adrenal insufficiency (fatigue, muscular weakness, joint pain, fever, anorexia, nausea, dyspnea, dizziness, and fainting) and to report them to the doctor promptly.
• Warn patients on long-term therapy about cushingoid symptoms, which may develop regardless of route of administration.
• Tell patient to eat a low-sodium diet that is high in potassium and protein unless contraindicated.

Evaluation

In patients receiving cortisone, appropriate evaluation statements may include:
• Fluid volume deficit shows improvement.
• Patient does not experience serious adverse reactions associated with cortisone.
• Patient and family state an understanding of cortisone therapy.

cosyntropin

(koe sin troe´ pin)

Cortrosyn

• *Classification:* diagnostic agent (anterior pituitary hormone)
• *Pregnancy Risk Category:* C

HOW SUPPLIED

Injection: 0.25 mg/vial

ACTION

Mechanism: By replacing the body's own tropic hormone, stimulates the adrenal cortex to secrete its entire spectrum of hormones.
Absorption: Inactivated by the proteolytic enzymes in the GI tract; rapidly absorbed after I.M. administration.
Distribution: Not fully understood, but the drug is removed rapidly from plasma by many tissues.
Excretion: Probably by the kidneys.
Onset, peak, duration: After rapid I.V. administration, plasma cortisol levels begin to rise within 5 minutes and double within 15 to 30 minutes. Peak levels occur within 1 hour after I.M. or rapid I.V. administration.

INDICATIONS & DOSAGE

Diagnostic test of adrenocortical function–
Adults and children: 0.25 to 1 mg I.M. or I.V. (unless label prohibits I.V. administration) between blood samplings.
Children under 2 years: 0.125 mg I.M. or I.V.

CONTRAINDICATIONS & PRECAUTIONS

Contraindicated in patients with hypersensitivity to the drug; however, it is less antigenic than corticotropin and less likely to produce allergic reactions. Use cautiously in patients with preexisting allergic disease or a history of allergic reactions to corticotropin, because hypersensitivity reactions are possible.

ADVERSE REACTIONS

Common reactions are in italics; life-threatening reactions are in bold italics.
Skin: pruritus.
Other: flushing, ***hypersensitivity.***

INTERACTIONS

None significant.

EFFECTS ON DIAGNOSTIC TESTS

Blood glucose: altered levels.

NURSING CONSIDERATIONS

Besides those related universally to drug therapy (see "How to use this book"), consider the following specific recommendations:

Assessment

• Obtain a baseline assessment of the patient's underlying condition before initiating cosyntropin test.
• Be alert for hypersensitivity.

• Evaluate the patient's and family's knowledge about cosyntropin test.

Nursing Diagnoses

• Altered protection related to cosyntropin-induced hypersensitivity.

• Knowledge deficit related to cosyntropin test.

Planning and Implementation

Preparation and Administration

• Check institutional protocol for guidelines used to administer drug.

Monitoring

• Monitor patient closely for hypersensitivity.

Supportive Care

• Notify doctor if hypersensitivity occurs, and be prepared to administer emergency care.

Patient Teaching

• Inform patient to notify a health professional promptly of pruritus or other signs of hypersensitivity.

• Explain how the cosyntropin test is performed.

Evaluation

In patients receiving cosyntropin, appropriate evaluation statements may include:

• Patient does not develop a hypersensitivity reaction.

• Patient and family state an understanding of cosyntropin test.

co-trimoxazole (sulfamethoxazole-trimethoprim)

(ko tri mox´ a zole)

Apo-Sulfatrim†, Apo-Sulfatrim DS†, Bactrim*, Bactrim DS, Bactrim I.V. Infusion, Cotrim, Cotrim D.S., Novotrimel†, Novotrimel DS†, Protrin†, Protrin DF†, Resprim‡, Roubac†, Roubac DS†, Septra*, Septra DS, Septra I.V. Infusion, Septrin‡, SMZ-TMP, Sulfamethoprim, Sulfamethoprim DS, Sulmeprim, Trib‡, Uroplus DS, Uroplus SS

• *Classification:* antibiotic (sulfonamide and folate antagonist)

• *Pregnancy Risk Category:* C (D if near term)

HOW SUPPLIED

Tablets: trimethoprim 80 mg and sulfamethoxazole 400 mg; trimethoprim 160 mg and sulfamethoxazole 800 mg

Oral suspension: trimethoprim 40 mg and sulfamethoxazole 200 mg/5 ml

Injection: trimethoprim 16 mg and sulfamethoxazole 80 mg/ml (5 ml/ampule)

ACTION

Mechanism: Sulfamethoxazole component inhibits formation of dihydrofolic acid from para-aminobenzoic acid (PABA). Trimethoprim component inhibits dihydrofolate reductase. Both decrease bacterial folic acid synthesis.

Absorption: Well absorbed from the GI tract after oral administration.

Distribution: Widely distributed into body tissues and fluids, including middle ear fluid, prostatic fluid, bile, aqueous humor, and CSF; also crosses the placenta. Protein binding is 44% for trimethoprim, 70% for sulfamethoxazole.

Metabolism: Metabolized by the liver.

Excretion: Primarily excreted in urine by glomerular filtration and renal tubular secretion; some is excreted in breast milk. Half-life: For trimethoprim, 8 to 11 hours in patients with normal renal function, extended to 26 hours in severe renal dysfunction; for sulfamethoxazole, normally 10 to 13 hours, extended to 30 to 40 hours in severe renal dysfunction.

INDICATIONS & DOSAGE

Urinary tract infections and shigellosis—

Adults: 160 mg trimethoprim/800 mg sulfamethoxazole (double strength tablet) P.O. q 12 hours for 10 to 14

days in urinary tract infections and for 5 days in shigellosis. For simple cystitis or acute urethral syndrome, may give one to three double strength tablets as a single dose. If indicated, give by I.V. infusion 8 to 10 mg/kg/day (based upon trimethoprim component) in two to four divided doses q 6, 8, or 12 hours for up to 14 days.
Children: 8 mg/kg trimethoprim/ 40 mg/kg sulfamethoxazole P.O. per 24 hours, in two divided doses q 12 hours (10 days for urinary tract infections; for 5 days in shigellosis).
Treatment of otitis media in patients with penicillin allergy or penicillin-resistant infections–
Children: 8 mg/kg trimethoprim/ 40 mg/kg sulfamethoxazole P.O. per 24 hours, in two divided doses q 12 hours for 10 days.
Pneumocystis carinii pneumonitis–
Adults and children: 20 mg/kg trimethoprim/100 mg/kg sulfamethoxazole P.O. per 24 hours, in equally divided doses q 6 hours for 14 days. If indicated, give by I.V. infusion 15 to 20 mg/kg/day (based upon trimethoprim component) in three or four divided doses q 6 to 8 hours for up to 14 days.
Chronic bronchitis–
Adults: 160 mg trimethoprim/800 mg sulfamethoxazole P.O. q 12 hours for 10 to 14 days. Not recommended for infants under 2 months old.
Prophylaxis of traveler's diarrhea–
Adults: 160 mg trimethoprim/800 mg sulfamethoxazole P.O. once daily, beginning on the first day of travel and continuing until 2 days after returning home.
Treatment of traveler's diarrhea–
Adults: 160 mg trimethoprim/800 mg sulfamethoxazole P.O. b.i.d. for 3 to 5 days. Some patients may require 2 days of therapy or less.
Treatment of urinary tract infections in males with prostatitis–
Adults: 160 mg trimethoprim/800 mg sulfamethoxazole P.O. b.i.d. for 3 to 6 months.
Prophylaxis of chronic urinary tract infections–
Adults: 40 mg trimethoprim/200 mg sulfamethoxazole (½ tablet) or 80 mg trimethoprim/400 mg sulfamethoxazole P.O. daily or three times a week for 3 to 6 months.

CONTRAINDICATIONS & PRECAUTIONS

Contraindicated in patients with hypersensitivity to sulfonamides (or any other drug containing sulfur, such as thiazides, furosemide, and oral sulfonylureas) and in patients with hypersensitivity to trimethoprim. Also contraindicated in patients with severe renal or hepatic dysfunction or porphyria; during pregnancy at term; and during lactation.

Use cautiously in patients with acquired immune deficiency syndrome (AIDS), because of the increased incidence of adverse reactions; and in patients with mild to moderate renal or hepatic impairment, urinary obstruction because of the hazard of drug accumulation, severe allergies, asthma, blood dyscrasias, and folate or glucose-6-phosphate dehydrogenase deficiency.

ADVERSE REACTIONS

Common reactions are in italics; life-threatening reactions are in bold italics.
Blood: ***agranulocytosis, aplastic anemia,*** megaloblastic anemia, thrombocytopenia, leukopenia, ***hemolytic anemia.***
CNS: headache, mental depression, seizures, hallucinations.
GI: *nausea, vomiting, diarrhea,* abdominal pain, anorexia, stomatitis.
GU: toxic nephrosis with oliguria and anuria, crystalluria, hematuria.
Hepatic: jaundice.

Skin: *erythema multiforme (Stevens-Johnson syndrome), generalized skin eruption, epidermal necrolysis, exfoliative dermatitis,* photosensitivity, urticaria, pruritus.
Other: ***hypersensitivity,*** *serum sickness, drug fever,* ***anaphylaxis.***

INTERACTIONS

Ammonium chloride, ascorbic acid: doses sufficient to acidify urine may cause precipitation of sulfonamide and crystalluria. Don't use together.
Oral anticoagulants: increased anticoagulant effect.
Oral antidiabetic agents: increased hypoglycemic effect.
Oral contraceptives: decreased contraceptive effectiveness and increased risk of breakthrough bleeding.

EFFECTS ON DIAGNOSTIC TESTS

CBC: decreased RBC, WBC, or platelet counts.
Liver function tests: false-positive results.
Urine glucose tests with copper sulfate (Benedict's reagent or Clinitest): false-positive results.

NURSING CONSIDERATIONS

Besides those related universally to drug therapy (see "How to use this book"), consider the following specific recommendations:

Assessment
- Obtain a baseline assessment of infection before therapy.
- Be alert for adverse reactions and drug interactions throughout therapy.
- Evaluate the patient's and family's knowledge about co-trimoxazole therapy.

Nursing Diagnoses
- High risk for injury related to ineffectiveness of co-trimoxazole to eradicate the infection.
- High risk for fluid volume deficit related to adverse GI reactions to co-trimoxazole.
- Knowledge deficit related to co-trimoxazole.

Planning and Implementation
Preparation and Administration
- Obtain specimen for culture and sensitivity tests before first dose. Therapy may begin pending test results.
- Note that the "DS" or "DP" product means "double strength."
- ***P.O. use:*** Administer with a full glass (8 oz or 240 ml) of water at least 1 hour before or 2 hours after meals for maximum absorption. Shake oral suspension thoroughly before administering.
- ***I.V. use:*** I.V. infusion must be diluted in dextrose 5% in water before administration. Don't mix with other drugs or solutions. Infuse slowly over 60 to 90 minutes; do not give by rapid infusion or bolus injection. Solution must be used within 2 hours of mixing. Do not refrigerate. Check solution carefully for precipitate before starting infusion. Do not use solution containing a precipitate.

Monitoring
- Monitor effectiveness of therapy by regularly assessing for improvement of infection.
- Monitor for adverse drug reactions, especially hypersensitivity reactions, rash, and fever, which occur more frequently in AIDS patients.
- Monitor intake and output. Urine output should be at least 1,500 ml/day to ensure proper hydration. Inadequate urine output can lead to crystalluria or tubular deposits of the drug.
- Monitor hydration status if adverse GI reactions occur.

Supportive Care
- Force fluid intake to 3,000 to 4,000 ml/day. (Patient's output should be at least 1,500 ml/day).
- Obtain an order for an antiemetic or antidiarrheal agent if needed.
- If I.V. administration is used,

change infusion site every 48 to 72 hours.

Patient Teaching

• Tell the patient to take medication exactly as prescribed, even if he feels better, and to take entire amount prescribed.

• Teach diabetic patients to test urine for glucose with a glucose enzymatic test such as Clinistix or Tes-Tape because copper sulfate tests (Clinitest) may yield false-positive results.

• Advise the patient to avoid exposure to direct sunlight because of risk of photosensitivity reaction.

• Tell the patient to take drug with a full glass of water and to drink at least 3,000 to 4,000 ml/day of water; explain that tablet may be crushed and swallowed with water.

Evaluation

In patients receiving co-trimoxazole, appropriate evaluation statements may include:

• Patient is free of infection.

• Patient maintains adequate hydration throughout co-trimoxazole therapy.

• Patient and family state an understanding of co-trimoxazole therapy.

cromolyn sodium (sodium cromoglycate) (systemic)

(kroe´ moe lin)

Gastrocrom, Intal**, Intal Inhaler, Intal Spincaps†, Nalcrom, Nasalcrom, Opticrom, Rynacrom†

• *Classification:* mast cell stabilizer, antiasthmatic (chromone derivative)

• *Pregnancy Risk Category:* B

HOW SUPPLIED

Capsules (for oral solution): 100 mg
Aerosol: 800 mcg/metered spray
Capsules (for inhalation): 20 mg
Nasal solution: 5.2 mg/metered spray (40 mg/ml)
Solution: 20 mg/2 ml for nebulization

ACTION

Mechanism: Inhibits the degranulation of sensitized mast cells that occurs after an exposure to specific antigens. It also inhibits release of histamine and slow-reacting substance of anaphylaxis (SRS-A).

Absorption: Only 0.5% to 2% of an oral dose is absorbed. After inhalation using capsules via an oral inhaler (Spinhaler), approximately 7.5% (range, 5% to 10%) of a dose reaches the lungs and is absorbed readily into the systemic circulation. The amount reaching the lungs depends on the patient's ability to use the inhaler correctly, the amount of bronchoconstriction, and the size or presence of mucous plugs. Degree of absorption depends on the method of administration: the most absorption occurs with the powder via the Spinhaler; next the aerosol via metered-dose inhaler; and the lowest with administration of the solution via power-operated nebulizer. Less than 7% of an intranasal dose is absorbed systemically.

Distribution: Does not cross most biological membranes because it is ionized and lipid-insoluble at the body's pH. Less than 0.1% of a dose crosses to the placenta; it is not known if the drug is distributed into breast milk.

Metabolism: Not significant.

Excretion: Unchanged in urine (50%) and bile (approximately 50%). Small amounts may be excreted in the feces or exhaled. Half life: Absorption half-life from the lung is 1 hour. A plasma concentration of 9 mcg/ml can be achieved 15 minutes after a 20-mg dose. Elimination half-life is 81 minutes.

INDICATIONS & DOSAGE

Adjunct in treatment of severe perennial bronchial asthma–
Adults and children over 5 years: contents of 20-mg capsule inhaled q.i.d. at regular intervals. Or administer 2 metered sprays using inhaler q.i.d. at regular intervals. Also available as an aqueous solution administered through a nebulizer.
Prevention and treatment of allergic rhinitis–
Adults and children over 5 years: 1 spray in each nostril t.i.d or q.i.d. May give up to 6 times daily.
Prevention of exercise-induced bronchospasm–
Adults and children over 5 years: contents of 20-mg capsule or 2 metered sprays inhaled no more than 1 hour before anticipated exercise.
Systemic mastocytosis–
Adults: 100 to 200 mg P.O. q.i.d.
Food allergy–
Adults: 200 mg P.O. q.i.d. 15 to 20 minutes before meals. Dosage may be doubled in 2 to 3 weeks if results are not satisfactory.
Children 2 to 13 years: 100 mg P.O. q.i.d. 15 to 20 minutes before meals. Dosage may be doubled in 2 to 3 weeks if results are not satisfactory. Do not exceed 40 mg/kg daily.
Children under 2 years: up to 20 mg/kg P.O. daily.
Inflammatory bowel disease–
Adults: 200 mg P.O. q.i.d. 15 to 20 minutes before meals.
Children 2 to 14 years: 100 mg P.O. q.i.d. 15 to 20 minutes before meals.

CONTRAINDICATIONS & PRECAUTIONS

Contraindicated in patients with a hypersensitivity to cromolyn or any ingredient (lactose) in these products. It should be not be used to treat acute asthma, especially status asthmaticus, because it is a prophylactic drug with no benefit in acute situations.

Cromolyn's safety in pregnancy has not been established; it should be used only when benefit clearly outweighs the risk to the fetus.

ADVERSE REACTIONS

Common reactions are in italics; life-threatening reactions are in bold italics.
CNS: dizziness, headache.
EENT: *irritation of the throat and trachea, cough,* ***bronchospasm following inhalation of dry powder;*** esophagitis; nasal congestion; pharyngeal irritation; wheezing.
GI: nausea.
GU: dysuria, urinary frequency.
Skin: rash, urticaria.
Other: joint swelling and pain, lacrimation, swollen parotid gland, angioedema, *eosinophilic pneumonia.*

INTERACTIONS

None significant.

EFFECTS ON DIAGNOSTIC TESTS

None reported.

NURSING CONSIDERATIONS

Besides those related universally to drug therapy (see "How to use this book"), consider the following specific recommendations:

Assessment
- Obtain a baseline assessment of respiratory status before therapy.
- Be alert for adverse reactions and drug interactions throughout therapy.
- Evaluate the patient's and family's knowledge about cromolyn therapy.

Nursing Diagnoses
- Ineffective breathing pattern related to underlying condition.
- High risk for impaired skin integrity due to adverse drug effects.
- Knowledge deficit related to cromolyn.

Planning and Implementation
Preparation and Administration
- Use only when acute episode has been controlled, airway is cleared, and patient is able to inhale.

• Be sure patients considered for cromolyn therapy have pulmonary function tests that show a significant bronchodilator-reversible component to their airway obstruction.
• Specific capsules are available for inhalation and for oral use. Make sure that inhalation capsules are not used for oral consumption. Store capsules for inhalation at room temperature in a tightly closed container, protected from moisture.
• ***P.O. use:*** Break capsule designated for oral use and dissolve in hot water. Further dilute with cold water as desired. Do not mix with fruit juice, milk, or food.
• ***Inhalation:*** Insert the inhalation capsule into the inhalation device as described in the manufacturer's directions. Have the patient exhale completely. Then place the mouthpiece between the patient's lips; have him inhale deeply and rapidly with a steady, even breath; remove the inhaler from the mouth, have the patient hold his breath for a few seconds, and then exhale. Repeat until all the powder has been inhaled.

Monitoring

• Monitor effectiveness by evaluating the patient's respiratory status and effort.
• Assess for recurrence of asthmatic symptoms as dosage is decreased.
• Monitor pulmonary function tests to demonstrate the bronchodilator-reversible component of the airway obstruction.
• Evaluate the patient for eosinophilic pneumonia.

Supportive Care

• Place the patient in a high semi-Fowler's position.
• Relieve esophagitis by use of antacids or a glass of milk.
• Notify the doctor if patient does not experience relief of symptoms after 15 to 30 minutes of receiving medication.

Patient Teaching

• Instruct the patient to avoid excessive handling of capsules for inhalation.
• Teach the patient proper use of the inhaler.
• Encourage the patient to notify the doctor if symptoms are not relieved by treatment.

Evaluation

In patients receiving cromolyn, appropriate evaluation statements may include:
• Patient will report an effective respiratory pattern as demonstrated by ease of respiratory effort and depth and regularity of respiratory rate.
• Patient will have an intact skin free of rash or vesicle formation.
• Patient and family state an understanding of cromolyn therapy.

cyclandelate

(sye klan´ de late)
Cyclan, Cyclospasmol

• *Classification:* antispasmodic, vasodilator (mandelic acid derivative)
• *Pregnancy Risk Category:* C

HOW SUPPLIED

Tablets: 200 mg, 400 mg
Capsules: 200 mg, 400 mg

ACTION

Mechanism: Directly relaxes smooth muscle by inhibiting phosphodiesterase, resulting in increased concentrations of cyclic adenosine monophosphate.
Absorption: Completely and rapidly absorbed from the GI tract.
Metabolism: Probably metabolized to mandelic acid by serum and hepatic enzymes.
Excretion: In urine. Half-life: Unknown.
Onset, peak, duration: Maximum effect of a single dose occurs in 1½

hours. Clinical improvement may require several weeks.

INDICATIONS & DOSAGE

Adjunct in intermittent claudication, arteriosclerosis obliterans, vasospasm and muscular ischemia associated with thrombophlebitis, nocturnal leg cramps, Raynaud's phenomenon, selected cases of ischemic cerebral vascular disease–

Adults: initially, 1.2 to 1.6 g P.O. daily, in divided doses before meals and at bedtime. For maintenance, decrease dosage by 200 mg/day to the lowest effective level. Maintenance dosage is usually 400 to 800 mg daily in two to four divided doses.

CONTRAINDICATIONS & PRECAUTIONS

Contraindicated in patients with hypersensitivity to the drug. Use with extreme caution in patients with severe obliterative coronary artery disease because the drug's vasodilating effects may compromise blood flow to diseased areas. Although prolonged bleeding time has not been reported clinically, it has occurred in animals treated with very high doses; keep this possibility in mind when giving drug to patients with active bleeding. Use cautiously in patients with glaucoma. Drug should not be used as a substitute for appropriate medical or surgical therapy for peripheral or cerebral vascular disease.

ADVERSE REACTIONS

Common reactions are in italics; life-threatening reactions are in bold italics.

CNS: *headache, tingling of the extremities, dizziness.*

CV: *mild flushing,* tachycardia.

GI: pyrosis, eructation, nausea, heartburn.

Other: *sweating.*

INTERACTIONS

None significant.

EFFECTS ON DIAGNOSTIC TESTS

None reported.

NURSING CONSIDERATIONS

Besides those related universally to drug therapy (see "How to use this book"), consider the following specific recommendations:

Assessment

- Obtain a baseline assessment of the patient's underlying condition before drug therapy.
- Be alert for adverse reactions and drug interactions throughout therapy.
- Evaluate the patient's and family's knowledge about cyclandelate therapy.

Nursing Diagnoses

- Impaired tissue integrity related to the patient's underlying condition.
- Pain related to adverse drug reactions.
- Knowledge deficit related to cyclandelate therapy.

Planning and Implementation

Preparation and Administration

- Give with food or antacids to minimize GI distress.
- Use with, not as a substitute for, appropriate medical or surgical treatment for peripheral or cerebrovascular disease.
- Short-term therapy is of little benefit.
- Adverse reactions usually disappear after several weeks of therapy.

Monitoring

- Monitor for adverse reactions or drug interactions by frequently monitoring the patient's vital signs.
- Monitor effectiveness by reduction of symptoms of the patient's underlying codition.

Supportive Care

- Give the patient food or antacids, if ordered, to lessen GI distress.
- Obtain an order for a mild analgesic for drug-induced headache.

Patient Teaching

- Instruct the patient to take a mild analgesic if headache occurs.
- Instruct the patient to expect long-

term treatment and to continue to take medication.

Evaluation

In patients receiving cyclandelate, appropriate evaluation statements may include:

- Patient demonstrates a reduction of symptoms of underlying condition.
- Patient's pain is relieved.
- Patient and family state an understanding of cyclandelate therapy.

cyclizine hydrochloride

(sye´ kli zeen)

Marezine◇

cyclizine lactate

Marezine, Marzine†

- *Classification:* antiemetic and antivertigo agent (piperazine derivative antihistamine)
- *Pregnancy Risk Category:* B

HOW SUPPLIED

hydrochloride

Tablets: 50 mg◇

lactate

Injection: 50 mg/ml

ACTION

Mechanism: An antihistamine that also blocks acetylcholine receptors; drug also has antispasmotic, local anesthetic, and CNS depressant effects. May affect neural pathways originating in the labyrinth to inhibit nausea and vomiting, but the exact mechanism of action is unknown.

Absorption: Not well characterized.

Metabolism: Probably in the liver. Norcyclizine is an inactive metabolite.

Onset, peak, duration: Onset of action is 30 minutes to 1 hour. Drug effect lasts 4 to 6 hours.

INDICATIONS & DOSAGE

Motion sickness (prevention and treatment) –

Adults: 50 mg P.O. (hydrochloride) one half hour before travel, then q 4 to 6 hours, p.r.n., to maximum of 200 mg daily; or 50 mg I.M. (lactate) q 4 to 6 hours, p.r.n.

Postoperative vomiting (prevention) –

Adults: 50 mg I.M. (lactate) preoperatively or 20 to 30 minutes before expected termination of surgery; then postoperatively 50 mg I.M. (lactate) q 4 to 6 hours, p.r.n.

Motion sickness and postoperative vomiting –

Children 6 to 12 years: 3 mg/kg (lactate) I.M. divided t.i.d., or 25 mg (hydrochloride) P.O. q 4 to 6 hours p.r.n. to a maximum of 75 mg daily.

CONTRAINDICATIONS & PRECAUTIONS

Contraindicated in patients with hypersensitivity to drug or other antiemetic antihistamines with a similar chemical structure, such as buclizine, meclizine, or dimenhydrinate.

Use cautiously in patients with narrow-angle glaucoma, asthma, prostatic hypertrophy (elderly men), or GU or GI obstruction because of its anticholinergic effects. Drug may mask signs of intestinal obstruction or brain tumor.

ADVERSE REACTIONS

Common reactions are in italics; life-threatening reactions are in bold italics.

CNS: *drowsiness,* dizziness, auditory and visual hallucinations.

CV: hypotension.

EENT: blurred vision, dry mouth.

GI: constipation.

GU: urine retention.

Other: may mask symptoms of ototoxicity, brain tumor, or intestinal obstruction.

INTERACTIONS

None significant.

EFFECTS ON DIAGNOSTIC TESTS

Diagnostic skin testing: test interference.

NURSING CONSIDERATIONS

Besides those related universally to drug therapy (see "How to use this book"), consider the following specific recommendations:

Assessment

- Obtain a baseline assessment of mental status and fluid balance before therapy.
- Be alert for adverse reactions and drug interactions throughout therapy.
- Evaluate the patient's and family's knowledge about cyclizine therapy.

Nursing Diagnoses

- High risk for fluid volume deficit related to nausea and vomiting induced by motion sickness.
- Sensory/perceptual alteration (visual or auditory) related to cyclizine-induced hallucinations.
- Knowledge deficit related to cyclizine therapy.

Planning and Implementation

Preparation and Administration

- Store in cool place. When stored at room temperature, injection may turn slightly yellow, but this color change does not indicate loss of potency.

Monitoring

- Monitor effectiveness by observing the patient for nausea and vomiting.
- Monitor blood pressure; hypotension may occur.
- Monitor for CNS adverse reactions (drowsiness, dizziness, hallucinations).
- Monitor fluid balance.

Supportive Care

- Be aware that drug is an antihistamine.
- Use safety precautions in patients with CNS adverse reactions.
- Encourage patient to maintain adequate fluid intake to prevent fluid volume deficit.

Patient Teaching

- Warn the patient against driving and other activities that require alertness until CNS adverse reactions are known.
- Instruct the patient to take cyclizine tablets at least 30 minutes before beginning travel.
- Advise patient that repeat doses may be necessary in 4 to 6 hours.

Evaluation

In patients receiving cyclizine, appropriate evaluation statements may include:

- Patient exhibits no signs of fluid deficit.
- Patient remains free from sensory/perceptual alterations.
- Patient and family state an understanding of cyclizine therapy.

cyclobenzaprine

(sye kloe ben´ za preen)

Flexeril

- *Classification:* skeletal muscle relaxant (tricyclic antidepressant)
- *Pregnancy Risk Category:* B

HOW SUPPLIED

Tablets: 10 mg

ACTION

Mechanism: A centrally acting skeletal muscle relaxant that reduces transmission of impulses from the spinal cord to skeletal muscle.

Absorption: Almost completely absorbed during first pass through GI tract.

Distribution: 93% plasma protein-bound.

Metabolism: During first pass through GI tract and liver, drug and metabolites undergo enterohepatic recycling.

Excretion: Primarily in urine as conjugated metabolites; also in feces via bile as unchanged drug.

Onset, peak, duration: Onset of action occurs within 1 hour, with peak concentrations in 3 to 8 hours. Duration of action is 12 to 24 hours.

INDICATIONS & DOSAGE

Short-term treatment of muscle spasm–
Adults: 10 mg P.O. t.i.d. for 7 days. Maximum dosage is 60 mg daily for 2 to 3 weeks.

CONTRAINDICATIONS & PRECAUTIONS

Contraindicated in patients with hyperthyroidism, CHF, arrhythmias, heart block, or conduction disorders because of its cardiovascular effects; in acute recovery stage after myocardial infarction; in patients with hypersensitivity to the drug; and in patients who have received monoamine oxidase (MAO) inhibitors within 14 days.

Use cautiously in patients with urinary retention, narrow-angle glaucoma, increased intraocular pressure, impaired hepatic or renal function, and those receiving anticholinergic drugs because of its adverse anticholinergic effects.

ADVERSE REACTIONS

Common reactions are in italics; life-threatening reactions are in bold italics.
CNS: *drowsiness,* euphoria, weakness, headache, insomnia, nightmares, paresthesias, dizziness, depression, visual disturbances, precipitation of seizures.
CV: tachycardia.
EENT: blurred vision, dry mouth.
GI: abdominal pain, dyspepsia, peculiar taste, constipation.
GU: urine retention.
Skin: rash, urticaria, pruritus.
Other: in high doses, watch for adverse reactions like those of other tricyclic drugs (e.g., amitriptyline, imipramine).

INTERACTIONS

None significant.

EFFECTS ON DIAGNOSTIC TESTS

None significant.

NURSING CONSIDERATIONS

Besides those related universally to drug therapy (see "How to use this book"), consider the following specific recommendations:

Assessment

- Obtain a baseline assessment of patient's muscle spasm before therapy.
- Be alert for adverse reactions and drug interactions throughout therapy.
- Evaluate the patient's and family's knowledge about cyclobenzaprine therapy.

Nursing Diagnoses

- Pain related to underlying condition.
- High risk for cyclobenzaprine-induced drowsiness.
- Knowledge deficit related to cyclobenzaprine therapy.

Planning and Implementation

Preparation and Administration

- Do not administer with other CNS depressants.

Monitoring

- Monitor effectiveness by regularly assessing the severity and frequency of muscle spasms.
- Monitor for adverse reactions by frequently checking the patient's vital signs for tachycardia.
- Monitor for drowsiness.
- Monitor closely for symptoms of overdose, such as cardiotoxicity, especially in patients receiving high doses.
- Monitor for visual and sleeping disturbances.
- Monitor for changes in bowel or bladder function, especially constipation or urine retention.

Supportive Care

- Notify the doctor immediately if symptoms of overdose occur; have

physostigmine readily available as an antidote.
• Be aware that withdrawal symptoms (nausea, headache, and malaise) may follow abrupt discontinuation after long-term use.
• Institute safety precautions until CNS adverse reactions are known.
• Maintain seizure precautions; drug may precipitate seizure activity.
• Provide sugarless hard candy, chewing gum, or ice chips to relieve dry mouth.

Patient Teaching
• Advise the patient to report urinary hesitancy or urine retention.
• If constipation is troublesome, advise patient to increase fluid intake and use a stool softener.
• Warn the patient to avoid driving and other hazardous activities that require alertness until CNS effects of drug are known. Drowsiness and dizziness usually subside after 2 weeks.
• Warn the patient to avoid alcohol and other CNS depressants during cyclobenzaprine therapy.
• Tell the patient that dry mouth may be relieved with sugarless hard candy, chewing gum, or ice chips.

Evaluation
In patients receiving cyclobenzaprine, appropriate evaluation statements may include:
• Patient reports pain and muscle spasms have ceased.
• Patient does not experience injury as a result of cyclobenzaprine-induced drowsiness.
• Patient and family state an understanding of cyclobenzaprine therapy.

cyclopentolate hydrochloride
(sye kloe pen´ toe late)
AK-Pentolate, Cyclogyl

• *Classification:* cycloplegic, mydriatic (anticholinergic agent)
• *Pregnancy Risk Category:* C

HOW SUPPLIED
Ophthalmic solution: 0.5%, 1%, 2%

ACTION
Mechanism: Blocks muscarinic acetylcholine receptors in the eye. Anticholinergic action leaves the pupil under unopposed adrenergic influence, causing it to dilate. A cycloplegic and mydriatic agent.
Pharmacokinetics: Unknown.
Onset, peak, duration: Peak mydriatic effect occurs within 30 to 60 minutes and cycloplegic effect within 25 to 75 minutes. Recovery from mydriasis usually occurs in about 24 hours; recovery from cycloplegia may occur in 6 to 24 hours.

INDICATIONS & DOSAGE
Diagnostic procedures requiring mydriasis and cycloplegia –
Adults: instill 1 drop of 1% solution in eye, followed by 1 more drop in 5 minutes. Use 2% solution in heavily pigmented irises.
Children: instill 1 drop of 0.5%, 1%, or 2% solution in each eye, followed in 5 minutes with 1 drop 0.5% or 1% solution, if necessary.

CONTRAINDICATIONS & PRECAUTIONS
Contraindicated in patients with narrow-angle glaucoma and in patients with hypersensitivity to any component of the preparation. Use cautiously in patients in whom increased intraocular pressure may occur; and in children because of increased risk of cardiovascular and CNS effects. Do not use solutions more concentrated than 0.5% in neonates.

ADVERSE REACTIONS
Common reactions are in italics; life-threatening reactions are in bold italics.
Eye: burning sensation on instillation, blurred vision, eye dryness, *pho-*

tophobia, ocular congestion, contact dermatitis, conjunctivitis.
Systemic: flushing, tachycardia, urine retention, dry skin, fever, ataxia, irritability, confusion, somnolence, hallucinations, seizures, behavioral disturbances in children.

INTERACTIONS

Carbachol, pilocarpine: may counteract mydriatic effect.
Long-acting cholinergic antiglaucoma agents: may inhibit miotic actions.

EFFECTS ON DIAGNOSTIC TESTS

None reported.

NURSING CONSIDERATIONS

Besides those related universally to drug therapy (see "How to use this book"), consider the following specific recommendations:

Assessment
- Obtain a baseline assessment of the patient's vision and pupil size.
- Be alert for adverse reactions and drug interactions throughout therapy.
- Evaluate the patient's and family's knowledge about cyclopentolate therapy.

Nursing Diagnoses
- Sensory/perceptual alterations (visual) related to the patient's underlying condition.
- High risk for poisoning related to the drug's systemic adrenergic effects.
- Knowledge deficit related to cyclopentolate therapy.

Planning and Implementation
Preparation and Administration
- Instill solution in lacrimal sac; remove excess solution around eyes with clean tissue or gauze and apply light finger pressure to lacrimal sac for 1 minute.

Monitoring
- Monitor effectiveness by assessing the patient's vision and pupil size.
- Monitor for systemic adrenergic effects, especially in children and elderly patients.

Supportive Care
- Notify the doctor immediately of any changes in the patient's health status.
- Keep physostigmine on hand to reverse systemic adrenergic effects.

Patient Teaching
- Teach patient how to instill the drops, and advise him to wash his hands before and after administering the drug.
- Warn the patient to expect transient mild burning when drug is instilled.
- Warn the patient to avoid driving and other hazardous activities until the temporary visual impairment caused by the drug wears off.
- Advise the patient that dark glasses will ease discomfort from photophobia.

Evaluation
In patients receiving cyclopentolate, appropriate evaluation statements include:
- Patient experiences therapeutic mydriasis.
- Patient remains free of systemic adrenergic effects.
- Patient and family state an understanding of cyclopentolate therapy.

cyclophosphamide

(sye kloe foss´ fa mide)
Cycoblastin‡, Cytoxan**, Cytoxan Lyophilized, Endoxan-Asta‡, Neosar, Procytox†

- *Classification:* antineoplastic (alkylating agent)
- *Pregnancy Risk Category:* D

HOW SUPPLIED

Tablets: 25 mg, 50 mg
Injection: 100-mg, 200-mg, 500-mg, 1-g, 2-g vials

ACTION

Mechanism: An alkylating agent that cross-links strands of cellular DNA

and interferes with RNA transcription, causing an imbalance of growth that leads to cell death. Cell-cycle–nonspecific.
Absorption: Almost completely absorbed from the GI tract when administered orally, at doses of 100 mg or less. Higher doses (300 mg) are approximately 75% absorbed.
Distribution: Throughout the body, although only minimal amounts have been found in saliva, sweat, and synovial fluid. CSF concentration is too low for treatment of meningeal leukemia. The active metabolites are approximately 50% bound to plasma proteins.
Metabolism: Metabolized to its active form by hepatic microsomal enzymes. The activity of these metabolites is terminated by metabolism to inactive forms.
Excretion: Drug and metabolites are eliminated primarily in urine, with 15% to 30% excreted as unchanged drug. Half-life: Ranges from 4 to 6½ hours.

INDICATIONS & DOSAGE

Breast, head, neck, lung, and ovarian cancer; Hodgkin's disease; chronic lymphocytic leukemia; chronic myelocytic leukemia; acute lymphoblastic leukemia; neuroblastoma; retinoblastoma; non-Hodgkin's lymphomas; multiple myeloma; mycosis fungoides; sarcomas–
Adults: initially, 40 to 50 mg/kg I.V. in divided doses over 2 to 5 days; then adjust for maintenance. Or 1 to 5 mg/kg P.O. daily, depending upon patient tolerance. Maintenance dosage is 1 to 5 mg/kg P.O. daily; or 10 to 15 mg/kg 0q 7 to 10 days I.V.; or 3 to 5 mg/kg I.V. twice weekly.
Children: 2 to 8 mg/kg daily or 60 to 250 mg/m² daily P.O. or I.V. for 6 days (dosage depends on susceptibility of neoplasm). Maintenance dosage 2 to 5 mg/kg or 50 to 150 mg/m² P.O. twice weekly.

CONTRAINDICATIONS & PRECAUTIONS

Use cautiously in young men and women of childbearing age because it may impair fertility; in pregnant women because it may be fetotoxic; in lactating women because of potential harm to the neonate; and in patients with myelosuppression or infections because of potentially severe immunosuppression.

ADVERSE REACTIONS

Common reactions are in italics; life-threatening reactions are in bold italics.
Blood: *leukopenia,* nadir between days 8 to 15, recovery in 17 to 28 days; thrombocytopenia; anemia.
CV: ***cardiotoxicity*** (with very high doses and in combination with doxorubicin).
GI: anorexia; *nausea and vomiting beginning within 6 hours, lasting 4 hours;* stomatitis; mucositis.
GU: gonadal suppression (may be irreversible), ***hemorrhagic cystitis,*** bladder fibrosis, nephrotoxicity.
Metabolic: hyperuricemia; syndrome of inappropriate antidiuretic hormone secretion (with high doses).
Other: *reversible alopecia in 50% of patients, especially with high doses;* secondary malignancies, ***pulmonary fibrosis (high doses).***

INTERACTIONS

Barbiturates: increased pharmacologic effect and enhanced cyclophosphamide toxicity due to induction of hepatic enzymes.
Cardiotoxic drugs: additive adverse cardiac effects.
Corticosteroids, chloramphenicol: reduced activity of cyclophosphamide. Use cautiously.
Succinylcholine: may cause apnea. Don't use together.

EFFECTS ON DIAGNOSTIC TESTS

Papanicolaou test: false-positive result.

Serum pseudocholinesterase: decreased concentrations.
Serum uric acid: increased concentrations.
Skin tests for* Candida, *mumps, tricophyton, and tuberculin: suppressed positive reaction.

NURSING CONSIDERATIONS

Besides those related universally to drug therapy (see "How to use this book"), consider the following specific recommendations:

Assessment

- Obtain a baseline assessment of the patient's underlying condition and CBC, platelet, and uric acid levels before therapy.
- Be alert for adverse reactions or drug interactions during therapy.
- Evaluate the patient's and family's knowledge about cyclophosphamide therapy.

Nursing Diagnoses

- High risk for infection related to immunosuppressive adverse reactions.
- Pain related to possible GU adverse reactions as evidenced by cystitis.
- Knowledge deficit related to cyclophosphamide therapy.

Planning and Implementation

Preparation and Administration

- Keep in mind that dosage modification may be required in severe leukopenia, thrombocytopenia, malignant cell infiltration of bone marrow, recent radiation or chemotherapy, or hepatic or renal disease.
- ***P.O. use:*** An oral solution of the drug can be made by dissolving cyclophosphamide in aromatic elixir. Oral solution should be given on an empty stomach, but may be given with meals when gastric disturbance is present. Always give the drug in the morning so it can be excreted from the kidneys before bedtime.
- ***I.M. use:*** Dissolve 100 mg cyclophosphamide in 5 ml sterile water for injection or bacteriostatic water for injection. Use a new site for each injection.
- ***I.V. use:*** Preparation of parenteral form is associated with carcinogenic, teratogenic, and mutagenic risks. Follow institutional policy to reduce risks. Lyophilized concentration is much easier to reconstitute. Request this form when preparing I.V. solution. Reconstituted solution is stable for up to 6 days refrigerated or 24 hours at room temperature. Always check reconstituted solution for precipitate. Filter solution if necessary.
- Drug can be given I.V. push into a running line or by infusion in 0.9% sodium chloride solution or dextrose 5% in water. High I.V. doses are associated with cardiotoxicity and syndrome of inappropriate antidiuretic hormone secretion.

Monitoring

- Monitor effectiveness by checking CBC, kidney and liver function, and uric acid levels.
- Monitor for the effects of cardiotoxicity, dyspnea, shortness of breath, presence of pulmonary crackles, or tachycardia.
- Monitor for cyclophosphamide toxicity if patient's corticosteroid therapy is altered or discontinued.
- Monitor serum glucose levels of insulin-dependent diabetics.
- Monitor for signs of hematuria or dysuria.
- Monitor for infection in patients with leukopenia

Supportive Care

- Keep in mind that apnea may be induced if cyclophosphamide is given in conjunction with succinylcholine.
- Encourage daily fluid intake of 3 liters or more. Also encourage frequent urination.
- If hemorrhagic cystitis occurs, stop treatment.
- Do not give any I.M. injections when the patient's platelet count is below 100,000/mm³.
- To prevent hyperuricemia with re-

sulting uric acid nephropathy, allopurinol and increased hydration may be used.
• Keep in mind that therapeutic effects are often accompanied by toxicity.
Patient Teaching
• Advise both male and female patients to practice contraception while taking this drug and for 4 months thereafter.
• Instruct patients to increase P.O. fluids to 3 liters each day.
• Instruct diabetic patients to perform daily glucometer analysis while receiving this drug.
• Have patients watch for signs of infection and to alert doctor to sore throat, fever, or fatigue.
• Instruct patients to notify doctor if dysuria or hematuria occurs.
• Warn the patient that alopecia is likely but is reversible.
• Advise women that this drug may cause a falsely positive Pap test.
Evaluation
In patients receiving cyclophosphamide, appropriate evaluation statements may include:
• Patient remained infection free during treatment.
• Patient demonstrated optimal intake and output without experiencing pain.
• Patient and family state an understanding of cyclophosphamide therapy.

cycloserine
(sye kloe ser´ een)
Seromycin

• *Classification:* antitubercular agent (isoxizolidone)
• *Pregnancy Risk Category:* C

HOW SUPPLIED
Capsules: 250 mg

ACTION
Mechanism: Inhibits cell wall biosynthesis by inhibiting the utilization of amino acids (bacteriostatic).
Absorption: About 80% of dose is absorbed from GI tract.
Distribution: Widely distributed into body tissues and fluids, including CSF; crosses the placenta and does not bind to plasma proteins.
Metabolism: May be metabolized partially.
Excretion: Primarily excreted in urine by glomerular filtration. Small amounts are excreted in feces and breast milk. Cycloserine is hemodialyzable. Half-life: 10 hours in adults.
Onset, peak, duration: Peak serum concentrations occur 3 to 4 hours after ingestion.

INDICATIONS & DOSAGE
Adjunctive treatment in pulmonary or extrapulmonary tuberculosis–
Adults: initially, 250 mg P.O. q 12 hours for 2 weeks; then, if blood levels are below 25 to 30 mcg/ml and there are no clinical signs of toxicity, dosage is increased to 250 mg P.O. q 8 hours for 2 weeks. If optimum blood levels are still not achieved, and there are no signs of clinical toxicity, then dosage is increased to 250 mg P.O. q 6 hours. Maximum dosage is 1 g/day. If CNS toxicity occurs, drug is discontinued for 1 week, then resumed at 250 mg daily for 2 weeks. If no serious toxic effects occur, dosage is increased by 250-mg increments q 10 days until blood level of 25 to 30 mcg/ml is obtained.

CONTRAINDICATIONS & PRECAUTIONS
Contraindicated in patients with hypersensitivity to cycloserine; mental depression, epilepsy, severe anxiety, or psychosis because drug may exacerbate symptoms of these disorders; severe renal impairment because of potential for drug accumulation; and

in frequent users of alcohol because of increased potential for seizures.

Use cautiously in patients taking isoniazid, ethionamide, or phenytoin.

ADVERSE REACTIONS

Common reactions are in italics; life-threatening reactions are in bold italics.
CNS: drowsiness, headache, tremor, dysarthria, vertigo, confusion, loss of memory, ***possible suicidal tendencies*** and other psychotic symptoms, nervousness, hallucinations, depression, hyperirritability, paresthesias, paresis, hyperreflexia.
Other: hypersensitivity (allergic dermatitis).

INTERACTIONS

Ethanol or ethionamide: increased risk of CNS toxicity (seizures).
Isoniazid: monitor for CNS toxicity (dizziness or drowsiness).

EFFECTS ON DIAGNOSTIC TESTS

Serum transaminase: elevated levels.

NURSING CONSIDERATIONS

Besides those related universally to drug therapy (see "How to use this book"), consider the following specific recommendations:

Assessment
- Obtain a baseline assessment of patient's infection before therapy.
- Be alert for adverse reactions and drug interactions throughout therapy.
- Evaluate the patient's and family's knowledge about cycloserine therapy.

Nursing Diagnoses
- High risk for infection related to ineffectiveness of cycloserine to eradicate the infection.
- Altered thought processes related to cycloserine-induced adverse CNS reactions.
- Knowledge deficit related to cycloserine.

Planning and Implementation

Preparation and Administration
- Obtain specimen for culture and sensitivity tests before therapy begins.
- ***P.O. use:*** Expect to adjust dose according to blood levels, clinical toxicity, or ineffectiveness.

Monitoring
- Monitor effectiveness by regularly assessing patient for improvement in infection and by evaluating culture and sensitivity results to detect possible drug resistance.
- Monitor for adverse CNS reactions.
- Monitor therapeutic blood levels regularly as prescribed. Toxic reactions may follow blood levels above 30 mcg/ml.

Supportive Care
- Institute safety precautions, including suicidal precautions, if CNS reactions occur.

Patient Teaching
- Instruct patient to take drug exactly as prescribed; warn against discontinuing drug without doctor's approval.
- Warn patient that ingestion of alcohol can cause serious neurologic effects and should be avoided. Provide supportive care as indicated.
- Stress the importance of having laboratory studies done as ordered to monitor drug effectiveness and toxicity.

Evaluation

In patients receiving cycloserine, appropriate evaluation statements may include:
- Patient is free of infection.
- Patient's thought processes remain unchanged throughout cycloserine therapy.
- Patient and family state an understanding of cycloserine therapy.

cyclosporine (cyclosporin)
(sye´ kloe spor een)
Sandimmun‡, Sandimmune

• *Classification:* immunosuppressant (polypeptide antibiotic)
• *Pregnancy Risk Category:* C

HOW SUPPLIED
Oral solution: 100 mg/ml
Injection: 50 mg/ml

ACTION
Mechanism: A polypeptide antibiotic that exhibits immunosuppressant activity. Blocks cell-mediated immunity by inhibiting the action of T lymphocytes; may also impair humoral immune responses.
Absorption: After oral administration, absorption varies widely among patients and in individuals. Conflicting evidence exists regarding the drug's activity against B cells.
Distribution: Widely distributed outside the blood volume. About 33% to 47% is found in plasma; 4% to 9%, in leukocytes; 5% to 12%, in granulocytes; and 41% to 58%, in erythrocytes. In plasma, approximately 90% is bound to proteins, primarily lipoproteins. Cyclosporine crosses the placenta; cord blood levels are about 60% those of maternal blood. Cyclosporine enters breast milk.
Metabolism: Extensively metabolized in the liver.
Excretion: Elimination is primarily in the feces (biliary excretion) with only 6% of the drug found in urine. Half-life: Biphasic; initial phase is 1.2 hours, and terminal elimination half-life is 19 to 27 hours.
Onset, peak, duration: Only 30% of an oral dose reaches systemic circulation; peak levels occur at 3 to 4 hours.

INDICATIONS & DOSAGE
Prophylaxis of organ rejection in kidney, liver, bone marrow, and heart transplants–
Adults and children: 15 mg/kg P.O. (oral solution) 4 to 12 hours before transplantation. Continue this daily dosage postoperatively for 1 to 2 weeks. Then, gradually reduce dosage by 5%/week to maintenance level of 5 to 10 mg/kg/day. Alternatively, administer I.V. concentrate 4 to 5 mg/kg 4 to 12 hours before transplantation. Postoperatively, repeat this dosage daily until patient can tolerate oral solution.

CONTRAINDICATIONS & PRECAUTIONS
Contraindicated in patients with hypersensitivity to the drug or to polyoxyethylated castor oil. Use cautiously in patients with renal or hepatic toxicity or hypertension because drug may exacerbate the signs and symptoms of these conditions.

ADVERSE REACTIONS
Common reactions are in italics; life-threatening reactions are in bold italics.
CNS: *tremor,* headache.
CV: hypertension.
GI: *gum hyperplasia,* nausea, vomiting, diarrhea, oral thrush.
GU: *nephrotoxicity.*
Hepatic: hepatotoxicity.
Skin: *hirsutism,* acne.
Other: sinusitis, flushing.

INTERACTIONS
Aminoglycosides, amphotericin B, co-trimoxazole, NSAIDs: increased risk of nephrotoxicity.
Azathioprine, corticosteroids, cyclophosphamide, verapamil: increased immunosuppression.
Carbamazepine, isoniazid, phenobarbital, phenytoin, rifampin: possible decreased immunosuppressant effect. May need to increase cyclosporine dosage.

Ketoconazole, amphotericin B, cimetidine, diltiazem, erythromycin, imipenem-cilastatin, metoclopramide, prednisolone: may increase blood levels of cyclosporine. Monitor for increased toxicity.

EFFECTS ON DIAGNOSTIC TESTS

BUN, and creatinine serum, and liver function tests: elevated results may signal nephrotoxicity or hepatotoxicity.
CBC and differential: altered results.
Serum lipid: increased levels.

NURSING CONSIDERATIONS

Besides those related universally to drug therapy (see "How to use this book"), consider the following specific recommendations:

Assessment

- Obtain a baseline assessment of the patient's immune status before therapy.
- Be alert for adverse reactions or drug interactions during therapy.
- Evaluate the patient's and family's knowledge about cyclosporine therapy.

Nursing Diagnoses

- Altered protection related to the threat of organ rejection.
- High risk for injury related to cyclosporine-induced nephrotoxicity.
- Knowledge deficit related to cyclosporine therapy.

Planning and Implementation

Preparation and Administration

- Always give cyclosporine concomitantly with adrenal corticosteroids.
- Dosage should be given once a day.
- Measure oral doses carefully in an oral syringe.
- ***P.O. use:*** To increase palatability, mix with whole milk, chocolate milk, or fruit juice. Use a glass container to minimize adherence to container walls.
- ***I.V. use:*** Cyclosporine I.V. concentrate is administered at one-third the oral dose.

Monitoring

- Monitor effectiveness by observing for signs of organ rejection.
- Monitor liver function tests for hepatotoxicity, which usually occurs during the first month after organ transplant.
- Monitor BUN and serum creatinine. Cyclosporine may cause nephrotoxicity, which develops 2 to 3 months after transplant.
- Monitor cyclosporine blood levels at regular intervals due to the erratic absorption of oral cyclosporine solution.
- Observe patient for tremors, which may indicate CNS adverse effects.

Supportive Care

- Report signs of nephrotoxicity to the doctor, a dosage reduction may be necessary.
- To prevent thrush, the patient should swish and swallow nystatin solution four times daily.
- Give cyclosporine with meals if the drug causes nausea.
- Obtain an order for an analgesic to relieve cyclosporine-induced headache.

Patient Teaching

- Advise the patient to take cyclosporine at the same time each day.
- Stress that cyclosporine therapy should not be discontinued without the doctor's approval.
- Instruct the patient to report even mild symptoms of infection (colds, fever, sore throat, malaise) immediately.
- Advise the patient to use a depilatory if hirsutism occurs.

Evaluation

In patients receiving cyclosporine, appropriate evaluation statements may include:

- Patient demonstrates no signs of organ rejection.
- Patient exhibits no signs and symptoms of nephrotoxicity.
- Patient and family state an understanding of cyclosporine therapy.

cyproheptadine hydrochloride

(si proe hep´ ta deen)
Periactin

• *Classification:* antihistamine, (histamine$_1$-receptor antagonist), antipruritic (piperidine derivative)
• *Pregnancy Risk Category:* B

HOW SUPPLIED

Tablets: 4 mg
Syrup: 2 mg/5 ml

ACTION

Mechanism: Blocks the effects of histamine at H_1-receptor sites on effector cells. Prevents but does not reverse histamine-mediated responses.
Absorption: Well absorbed from the GI tract.
Distribution: Unknown. Probably enters the CNS.
Metabolism: Almost completely metabolized in the liver.
Excretion: Metabolites are excreted primarily in urine; unchanged drug is not excreted in urine. Small amounts of unchanged cyproheptadine and metabolites are excreted in feces.
Onset, peak, duration: Peak action occurs in 6 to 9 hours.

INDICATIONS & DOSAGE

Allergy symptoms, pruritus–
Adults: 4 mg P.O. t.i.d. or q.i.d. Maximum dosage is 0.5 mg/kg daily.
Children 7 to 14 years: 4 mg P.O. b.i.d. or t.i.d. Maximum dosage is 16 mg daily.
Children 2 to 6 years: 2 mg P.O. b.i.d. or t.i.d. Maximum dosage is 12 mg daily.

Note: Children under 14 years should use only as directed by a doctor.

CONTRAINDICATIONS & PRECAUTIONS

Contraindicated in patients with hypersensitivity to this drug or other antihistamines with similar chemical structures, such as azatadine; in patients experiencing asthmatic attacks because cyproheptadine thickens bronchial secretions; and in patients who have taken monoamine oxidase (MAO) inhibitors within the preceding 2 weeks; and during pregnancy (especially in the third trimester) or during breast-feeding. Antihistamines have caused seizures and other severe reactions, especially in premature infants.

Use cautiously in patients with narrow-angle glaucoma; pyloroduodenal obstruction or urinary bladder obstruction from prostatic hyperthophy or narrowing of the bladder neck because of their marked anticholinergic effects; cardiovascular disease, hypertension, or hyperthyroidism because of the risk of palpitations and tachycardia; and in patients with renal disease, diabetes, bronchial asthma, urinary retention, or stenosing peptic ulcers.

ADVERSE REACTIONS

Common reactions are in italics; life-threatening reactions are in bold italics.
CNS: (especially in elderly patients) *drowsiness,* dizziness, headache, fatigue.
GI: nausea, vomiting, epigastric distress, *dry mouth.*
GU: urine retention.
Skin: rash.
Other: weight gain.

INTERACTIONS

CNS depressants: increased sedation. Use together cautiously.
MAO inhibitors: increased anticholinergic effects. Don't use together.

EFFECTS ON DIAGNOSTIC TESTS

Diagnostic skin tests: test interference.

NURSING CONSIDERATIONS

Besides those related universally to drug therapy (see "How to use this book"), consider the following specific recommendations:

Assessment

- Obtain a baseline assessment of the patient's symptoms and respiratory status before initiating cyproheptadine hydrochloride therapy.
- Be alert for adverse reactions and drug interactions throughout therapy.
- Evaluate the patient's and family's knowledge about cyproheptadine therapy.

Nursing Diagnoses

- Ineffective airway clearance related to the patient's underlying condition.
- High risk for injury to adverse CNS effects of cyproheptadine hydrochloride.
- Knowledge deficit related to cyproheptadine hydrochloride therapy.

Planning and Implementation

Preparation and Administration

- ***P.O. use:*** Administer with food or milk to reduce GI distress.

Monitoring

- Monitor effectiveness by evaluating severity of the patient's symptoms and frequently checking the patient's respiratory status.
- Monitor for CNS adverse reactions including drowsiness, especially in elderly patients.

Supportive Care

- If severe drowsiness occurs, institute safety measures, such as continuous use of side rails if the patient is hospitalized.
- Keep in mind that another antihistamine may be substituted if tolerance develops.
- Remember that cyproheptadine hydrochloride may be used experimentally to stimulate appetite and increase weight gain in children.

Patient Teaching

- Suggest to the patient that he drink coffee or tea to reduce drowsiness.
- Tell the patient that sugarless gum, sour hard candy, or ice chips may relieve dry mouth.
- Warn patient to avoid drinking alcoholic beverages during therapy and to avoid hazardous activities that require alertness until adverse CNS effects are known.
- Warn patient to discontinue cyproheptadine hydrochloride 4 days before allergy skin testing to preserve the accuracy of the tests.

Evaluation

In patients receiving cyproheptadine, appropriate evaluation statements may include:

- Patient's allergic symptoms are relieved with cyproheptadine hydrochloride therapy.
- Patient does not suffer any injuries related to cyproheptadine hydrochloride-induced CNS adverse reactions.
- Patient and family state an understanding of cyproheptadine hydrochloride therapy.

cytarabine (ara-C, cytosine arabinoside)

(sye tar´ a been)

Alexan‡, Cytosar-U

- *Classification:* antineoplastic (antimetabolite)
- *Pregnancy Risk Category:* D

HOW SUPPLIED

Injection: 40-mg‡, 100-mg, 500-mg vials

ACTION

Mechanism: A synthetic pyrimidine nucleoside that is converted to the nucleotide cytarabine triphosphate inside the cell. Inhibits DNA polymerase by competing with the naturally occuring substrate deoxycytidine tri-

phosphate, for the enzyme. Limited incorporation of the drug into DNA and RNA may also contribute to the cytotoxic effects of the drug. An antimetabolite.
Absorption: Usually given I.V. or intrathecally because drug is rapidly deactivated or poorly absorbed (less than 20%) from the GI tract.
Distribution: Rapidly distributes widely through the body. Approximately 13% of the drug is bound to plasma proteins. The drug penetrates the blood-brain barrier only slightly after a rapid I.V. dose; however, when the drug is administered by a continuous I.V. infusion, CSF levels achieve a concentration 40% to 60% of that of plasma levels.
Metabolism: Primarily metabolized in the liver but also in the kidneys, GI mucosa, and granulocytes.
Excretion: Drug and metabolites are excreted in urine. Less than 10% of a dose is excreted unchanged. Half-life: Biphasic, with an initial half-life of 8 minutes and a terminal half-life of 1 to 3 hours.

INDICATIONS & DOSAGE

Acute myelocytic and other acute leukemias–
Adults and children: 200 mg/m² daily by continuous I.V. infusion for 5 days.
Meningeal leukemias and meningeal neoplasms–
Adults and children: 10 to 30 mg/m² intrathecally once every 4 days.

CONTRAINDICATIONS & PRECAUTIONS

Contraindicated in patients with a history of hypersensitivity to the drug.

ADVERSE REACTIONS

Common reactions are in italics; life-threatening reactions are in bold italics.
Blood: WBC nadir 5 to 7 days after drug stopped; *leukopenia,* anemia, ***thrombocytopenia,*** reticulocytopenia; platelet nadir occurring on day 10; ***megaloblastosis.***
CNS: neurotoxicity with high doses.
EENT: *keratitis.*
GI: *nausea, vomiting,* diarrhea, dysphagia; reddened area at juncture of lips, followed by sore mouth, oral ulcers in 5 to 10 days; high dose given via rapid I.V. may cause projectile vomiting.
Hepatic: hepatotoxicity (usually mild and reversible).
Metabolic: hyperuricemia.
Skin: rash.
Other: flulike syndrome.

INTERACTIONS

None significant.

EFFECTS ON DIAGNOSTIC TESTS

Blood and urine uric acid: increased levels.
Serum alkaline phosphatase, AST (SGOT), and bilirubin: increased concentrations, which indicate drug-induced hepatotoxicity.

NURSING CONSIDERATIONS

Besides those related universally to drug therapy (see "How to use this book"), consider the following specific recommendations:
Assessment
- Obtain a baseline assessment of patient's overall physical status, CBC, serum uric acid, renal panel and hepatic profile before initiating therapy.
- Be alert for adverse reactions or drug interactions during therapy.
- Evaluate the patient's and family's knowledge about cytarabine therapy.

Nursing Diagnoses
- Altered protection related to cytarabine-induced myelosuppression and immunosuppression.
- Altered oral mucous membrane related to cytarabine-induced stomatitis.
- Knowledge deficit related to cytarabine therapy.

Planning and Implementation

Preparation and Administration

• Follow instititutional policy to reduce mutagenic, teratogenic, and carcinogenic risks.

• ***I.V. use:*** To reconstitute the 100-mg vial for I.V. administration, use 5 ml bacteriostatic water for injection (20 mg/ml) and for the 500-mg vial with 10 ml bacteriostatic water for injection (50 mg/ml). Drug may be further diluted with dextrose in water or normal saline for continuous I.V. infusion. Be aware that nausea and vomiting are more frequent when large doses are administered rapidly by I.V. push. These reactions are less frequent with infusion.

• Use preservative-free normal saline or Elliot's B solution for intrathecal use.

• Reconstituted solution is stable for 48 hours. Discard cloudy reconstituted solution.

• Keep in mind that dosage modification may be required in thrombocytopenia, leukopenia, renal or hepatic disease, and after chemotherapy or radiation therapy.

Monitoring

• Monitor effectiveness by noting results of follow-up diagnostic tests and patient's overall physical status.

• Monitor for signs of infection (cough, fever, sore throat) and bleeding (easy bruising, nosebleeds, bleeding gums). Monitor CBC.

• Monitor for signs of neurotoxicity in patients receiving high doses; may first appear as nystagmus, but can progress to ataxia and cerebellar dysfunction.

• Monitor hepatic function.

• Monitor intake and output and serum uric acid.

• Monitor for GI adverse reactions, such as stomatitis, nausea, vomiting, diarrhea.

• Monitor for skin reactions resulting from high-dose cytarabine. Reactions most commonly affect the palms, soles, and extensor surfaces.

Supportive Care

• If toxicity occurs, don't give next dose of cytarabine. Notify doctor, who may withhold drug for 24 hours if just one sign is present, or with multiple signs, may discontinue drug because high doses can cause permanent brain damage.

• To reduce nausea and vomiting, give antiemetics before administering.

• Avoid I.M. injections of any drugs in patients with thrombocytopenia to prevent bleeding.

• Administer excellent mouth care to help prevent stomatitis.

• Be aware that steroid eyedrops are often prescribed to prevent drug-induced keratitis.

• Prevent or minimize uric acid nephropathy by administering allopurinol and providing adequate hydration.

• Modify or discontinue therapy if polymorphonuclear granulocyte count is below 1,000/mm^3 or if platelet count is below 50,000/mm^3.

• To help prevent infection, maintain the patient's optimal health and protect him from undue exposure to environmental contagions. If signs of infection occur, notify doctor promptly; administer antibiotics, as ordered.

• Provide a safe environment to minimize risk of bleeding.

• If patient develops diarrhea, give meticulous skin care to avoid or treat perirectal abscess. Be alert for electrolyte imbalance, malabsorption, and pressure ulcers.

Patient Teaching

• Encourage the patient to drink at least 3 liters of fluids daily and to void as often as possible.

• Warn patients to watch for signs of infection (sore throat, fever, fatigue, and for signs of bleeding (easy bruising, nosebleeds, bleeding gums). Tell patient to take temperature daily and

to notify doctor promptly of fever, other signs of infection, or bleeding.
• Instruct patient about need for protective measures, including conservation of energy, maintenance of balanced diet, adequate rest, need for personal cleanliness and clean environment, and avoidance of exposure to persons with infections.
• Teach patient to avoid the use of all OTC products containing aspirin. Instruct patient about safety precautions to reduce risks of bleeding from falls, cuts, or other injuries.
• Instruct patient about the need for frequent oral hygiene.

Evaluation

In patients receiving cytarabine, appropriate evaluation statements may include:
• Patient does not demonstrate signs and symptoms of infection or bleeding.
• Oral lesions are absent.
• Patient and family state an understanding of cytarabine therapy.

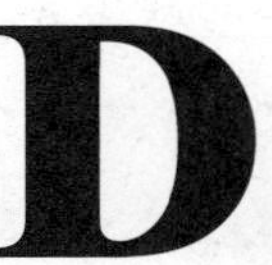

dacarbazine (DTIC)

(da kar´ ba zeen)
DTIC-Dome

- *Classification:* antineoplastic (alkylating agent)
- *Pregnancy Risk Category:* C

HOW SUPPLIED

Injection: 100-mg, 200-mg vials

ACTION

Mechanism: An alkylating agent that cross-links strands of cellular DNA and interferes with RNA transcription, causing an imbalance of growth that leads to cell death. Cell-cycle–nonspecific.
Absorption: Because of poor absorption from the GI tract, dacarbazine is not administered orally.
Distribution: Thought to localize in body tissues, especially the liver. The drug crosses the blood-brain barrier to a limited extent; minimally bound to plasma proteins.
Metabolism: Rapidly metabolized in the liver to several compounds, some of which may be active.
Excretion: Biphasic elimination. Approximately 30% to 45% of a dose is excreted in urine. Half-life: Initial phase half-life is 19 minutes; terminal phase is 5 hours in patients with normal renal and hepatic function.

INDICATIONS & DOSAGE

Metastatic malignant melanoma –
Adults: 2 to 4.5 mg/kg or 70 to 160 mg/m² I.V. daily for 10 days, then repeat q 4 weeks as tolerated; or 250 mg/m² I.V. daily for 5 days, repeated at 3-week intervals.
Hodgkin's disease –
Adults: 150 mg/m² I.V. daily (in combination with other agents) for 5 days, repeated q 4 weeks; or 375 mg/m² on the first day of a combination regimen, repeated q 15 days.

CONTRAINDICATIONS & PRECAUTIONS

Contraindicated in patients with a history of hypersensitivity to the drug.

ADVERSE REACTIONS

Common reactions are in italics; life-threatening reactions are in bold italics.
Blood: *leukopenia and thrombocytopenia,* nadir between 3 and 4 weeks.
GI: *severe nausea and vomiting begin within 1 to 3 hours in 90% of patients, last 1 to 12 hours; anorexia.*
Metabolic: increased liver enzymes, hepatotoxicity (rare).
Skin: phototoxicity.
Local: severe pain if I.V. infiltrates or if solution is too concentrated; tissue damage.
Other: *flu-like syndrome* (fever, malaise, myalgia beginning 7 days after treatment stopped and possibly lasting 7 to 21 days), alopecia, ***anaphylaxis.***

INTERACTIONS

None significant.

EFFECTS ON DIAGNOSTIC TESTS

BUN, serum ALT (SGPT), AST (SGOT), and alkaline phosphatase: transiently increased levels.

NURSING CONSIDERATIONS

Besides those related universally to drug therapy (see "How to use this

book"), consider the following specific recommendations:

Assessment

• Obtain a baseline assessment of the patient's underlying condition and CBC results and liver enzyme levels before initiating therapy.
• Be alert for adverse reactions and drug interactions throughout therapy.
• Evaluate the patient's and family's knowledge about dacarbazine therapy.

Nursing Diagnoses

• Altered nutrition: Less than body requirements, related to fasting prior to treatment and drug-induced adverse reactions.
• Altered protection related to flulike symptoms associated with dacarbazine therapy.
• Knowledge deficit related to dacarbazine therapy.

Planning and Implementation

Preparation and Administration

• Administer antiemetics as ordered before the start of drug therapy.
• ***I.V. use:*** Preparation of parenteral administration form is associated with carcinogenic, mutagenic, and teratogenic risks. Prepare in a biologic containment cabinet and wear gloves and mask.
• Give I.V. infusion in 50 to 100 ml dextrose 5% in water over 30 minutes. May dilute further or slow infusion to decrease pain at infusion site. Make sure drug does not infiltrate. If infusion infiltrates, stop immediately and apply ice to the area for 24 to 48 hours.
• Drug can be given by I.V. push over 1 minute, but a 30-minute infusion is preferred. During infusion, protect bag from direct sunlight to avoid possible drug breakdown. Protect dry vials from light as well. Discard refrigerated solution after 72 hours and room temperature solution after 8 hours. More dilute solutions are stable for 24 hours when stored at 2° to 8° C.

Monitoring

• Monitor effectiveness by noting results of follow-up diagnostic tests and overall physical status.
• Monitor CBC, platelets, and liver enzymes throughout therapy.
• Monitor electrolytes if nausea and vomiting cannot be controlled.
• Monitor fluid status when patient is fasting before the start of treatment.
• Monitor degree of flulike side effects and provide rest, antipyretics, and analgesia, as appropriate.
• Monitor for signs of bleeding.

Supportive Care

• Administer antiemetics as ordered. Keep in mind that nausea and vomiting may last up to 48 hours after treatment.
• Keep in mind that this drug is usually given with bleomycin, vinblastine, and doxorubicin when used for the treatment of Hodgkin's disease.
• Use anticoagulants and aspirin products with caution.
• Therapeutic side effects are often accompanied by toxicity.
• Do not give any I.M. injections when the platelet count is less than 100,000/mm³.
• Expect the doctor to discontinue drug if WBC count falls to 3,000/mm³ or platelets drop to 100,000/mm³.

Patient Teaching

• Advise the patient to avoid exposure to direct sunlight and sunlamps for the first 2 days after treatment.
• Warn the patient to watch for signs of infection and bleeding. Ask the patient to take his temperature daily. Tell the patient to notify the doctor if signs of infection or bleeding occur.
• Instruct the patient to avoid OTC drugs containing aspirin.
• Reassure the patient that nausea and vomiting usually cease after the first 2 days of therapy due to a buildup of tolerance to the drug.
• Explain all the possible adverse ef-

fects that may occur. Tell the patient how he can help prevent or alleviate their severity and when to notify the doctor. Be sure that the patient understands that this is a very toxic drug and that most patients experience some side effects.

Evaluation

In patients receiving dacarbazine, appropriate evaluation statements may include:

• Patient maintained adequate nutritional intake for healing and stabilization.

• Patient did not compromise protection when experiencing side effects to dacarbazine therapy.

• Patient and family state an understanding of dacarbazine therapy.

dactinomycin (actinomycin D)

(dak ti noe mye´ sin)

Cosmegen

• *Classification:* antineoplastic (antibiotic)

• *Pregnancy Risk Category:* C

HOW SUPPLIED

Injection: 500 mcg/vial

ACTION

Mechanism: An antineoplastic antibiotic that interferes with DNA-dependent RNA synthesis by intercalating guanine residues on DNA. Drug has some hypocalcemic and immunosuppressive activity; also is bacteriostatic against some gram-positive organisms, but toxicity precludes its use against infections.

Absorption: Because it is extremely irritating to tissues, drug must be administered intravenously.

Distribution: Rapidly distributed into tissues, with the highest levels in the bone marrow and nucleated cells, such as granulocytes and lymphocytes. Very little drug crosses the blood-brain barrier; probably crosses placenta.

Metabolism: Minimally metabolized in the liver.

Excretion: Dactinomycin and its metabolites are excreted in the urine and bile. Half-life: 36 hours.

INDICATIONS & DOSAGE

Dosage and indications may vary. Check patient's protocol with doctor.

Melanomas, sarcomas, trophoblastic tumors in women, testicular cancer–

Adults: 500 mcg I.V. daily for 5 days not to exceed 15 mg/kg or 400 to 600 mg/m^2 daily; wait 2 to 4 weeks and repeat. Or 2 mg I.V. single weekly dose for 3 weeks; wait for bone marrow recovery, then repeat in 3 to 4 weeks.

Wilms' tumor, rhabdomyosarcoma, Ewing's sarcoma–

Children: 15 mcg/kg I.V. daily for 5 days. Maximum dosage 500 mcg daily. Wait for bone marrow recovery.

CONTRAINDICATIONS & PRECAUTIONS

Contraindicated in patients who are infected with chickenpox or herpes zoster; in pregnant and breast-feeding women; and in infants younger than age 6 months because such treatment may lead to serious generalized disease and death.

Also contraindicated in patients with renal, hepatic, or bone marrow impairment and viral infections. Use cautiously in metastatic testicular tumors, in combination with chlorambucil and methotrexate therapy. Extreme bone marrow and GI toxicity can occur with this combined therapy.

Use cautiously in patients who have received cytotoxic drugs or radiation therapy within 6 weeks, or in patients with a history of gout, infection, or hematologic compromise because of increased potential for adverse effects.

ADVERSE REACTIONS

Common reactions are in italics; life-threatening reactions are in bold italics.
Blood: anemia, *leukopenia, thrombocytopenia,* ***pancytopenia.***
GI: *anorexia, nausea, vomiting,* abdominal pain, diarrhea, *stomatitis.*
Skin: *erythema;* desquamation; *hyperpigmentation of skin, especially in previously irradiated areas; acne-like eruptions (reversible).*
Local: phlebitis, severe damage to soft tissue.
Other: reversible alopecia, hepatotoxicity.

INTERACTIONS

None significant.

EFFECTS ON DIAGNOSTIC TESTS

Uric acid: increased concentrations in blood and urine.

NURSING CONSIDERATIONS

Besides those related universally to drug therapy (see "How to use this book"), consider the following specific recommendations:

Assessment
- Obtain a baseline assessment of patient's overall physical status, CBC, renal and hepatic function before initiating therapy.
- Be alert for adverse reactions and drug interactions throughout therapy.
- Evaluate the patient's and family's knowledge about dactinomycin therapy.

Nursing Diagnoses
- Impaired tissue integrity related to extravasation of dactinomycin.
- Altered protection related to dactinomycin-induced myelosuppression and immunosupression.
- Knowledge deficit related to dactinomycin therapy.

Planning and Implementation
Preparation and Administration
- Follow institutional policy when preparing and administering this drug to avoid mutagenic, teratogenic, and carcinogenic risks.
- Expect dosage and schedule modification in patients with leukopenia, thrombocytopenia, stomatitis, and diarrhea.
- Use only sterile water (without preservatives) as diluent for injection. Discard unused solutions since they do not contain a preservative.
- Keep in mind that dactinomycin is a vesicant. Administer through a running I.V. with good blood return.

Monitoring
- Monitor effectiveness by noting results of follow-up diagnostic tests and patient's overall physical status.
- Monitor for extravasation, which usually causes immediate pain. Extravasation can produce local tissue damage, cellulitis, phlebitis, necrosis, and possible muscle contracture.
- Monitor for signs of infection (cough, fever, sore throat) and bleeding (easy bruising, nosebleeds, bleeding gums).
- Monitor CBC daily and platelet counts frequently.
- Identify and monitor previously irradiated skin for radiation recall—a flare-up of skin irritation or even necrosis may appear.
- Monitor renal and hepatic functioning.
- Monitor for adverse GI reactions.

Supportive Care
- Avoid all I.M. injections when the platelet count is less than 100,000/ mm^3.
- Give antiemetics before administering to reduce nausea.
- Provide adequate hydration; alkalinizing urine or administering allopurinol may prevent or minimize uric acid nephropathy.
- To help prevent infection, maintain the patient's optimal health and pro-

tect him from undue exposure to environmental contagions. If signs of infection occur, notify doctor promptly; administer antibiotics, as ordered.
• Provide a safe environment to minimize risk of bleeding.
• If extravasation occurs, discontinue infusion and aspirate as much drug as possible. Minimize local reaction by immediately infiltrating the area with hydrocortisone sodium succinate injection (50 to 100 mg of hydrocortisone) or isotonic sodium thiosulfate injection (4.14% of the pentahydrate salt, 2.64% of the anhydrous salt, or a 4% solution prepared by diluting 4 ml of the 10% injection with 6 ml of sterile water for injection) or ascorbic acid injection (1 ml of 5% injection) and applying cold compresses.

Patient Teaching
• Warn patients to watch for signs of infection (sore throat, fever, fatigue) and for signs of bleeding (easy bruising, nosebleeds, bleeding gums). Tell patient to take temperature daily and to report fever, other signs of infection, or bleeding promptly.
• Instruct patient about need for protective measures, including conservation of energy, balanced diet, adequate rest, personal cleanliness, clean environment, and avoidance of exposure to persons with infections.
• Instruct patient about safety precautions to reduce risks of bleeding from falls, cuts, or other injuries.
• Instruct patient about the need for frequent oral hygiene.
• Inform patient that hair loss is possible but is usually reversible.
• Encourage the patient to drink at least 3 liters of fluids daily, unless contraindicated.

Evaluation
In patients receiving dactinomycin, appropriate evaluation statements may include:
• No local tissue damage is evidenced.
• Patient does not demonstrate signs and symptoms of infection or bleeding.
• Patient and family state an understanding of dactinomycin therapy.

danazol
(da´ na zole)
Cyclomen†, Danocrine

• *Classification:* antiestrogen, androgen (androgen)
• *Pregnancy Risk Category:* X

HOW SUPPLIED
Capsules: 50 mg, 100 mg, 200 mg

ACTION
Mechanism: A synthetic androgen that acts as a gonadotropin inhibitor; acts by direct enzyme inhibition of sex steroid synthesis and competitively blocks binding of sex hormones to their cytosol receptors. Suppresses the pituitary-ovarian axis; decreases the output of both follicle stimulating hormone and luteinizing hormone.
Absorption: The amount absorbed is not proportional to the administered doses; doubling the dose produces an increase of only 35% to 40% in drug absorption.
Metabolism: In 2-hydroxymethylethisterone.
Onset, peak, duration: Ovulation and cyclic bleeding return within about 60 to 90 days following discontinuation of therapy.

INDICATIONS & DOSAGE
Mild endometriosis–
Women: initially, 100 to 200 mg P.O. b.i.d. Subsequent dosage based upon patient response.

Moderate to severe endometriosis–
Women: 400 mg P.O. b.i.d. uninterrupted for 3 to 6 months; may continue for 9 months.
Fibrocystic breast disease–
Women: 100 to 400 mg P.O. daily in 2 divided doses uninterrupted for 2 to 6 months.
Prevention of hereditary angioedema–
Adults: 200 mg P.O. 2 to 3 times a day, continued until favorable response is achieved. Then dosage should be decreased by half at 1- to 3-month intervals.

CONTRAINDICATIONS & PRECAUTIONS

Contraindicated in patients with severe renal or cardiac disease because these conditions may be worsened by the fluid and electrolyte retention this drug may cause; hepatic disease because impaired elimination may cause toxic accumulation of the drug; undiagnosed abnormal genital bleeding because danazol can stimulate the growth of cancerous breast or prostate tissue in men; and in pregnant and breast-feeding patients because animal studies have shown that administration of androgens during pregnancy causes masculinization of the fetus.

Rule out breast cancer before beginning therapy for fibrocystic breast disease. Carefully evaluate breast nodules or masses that may appear or enlarge with danazol therapy.

Observe female patients carefully for signs of excessive virilization. If possible, discontinue therapy at the first sign of virilization because some adverse effects (deepening of the voice, clitoral enlargement) are not reversible.

ADVERSE REACTIONS

Common reactions are in italics; life-threatening reactions are in bold italics.
Androgenic: in women–acne, edema, *weight gain, hirsutism,* hoarseness, clitoral enlargement, *decrease in breast size,* changes in libido, male pattern baldness, *oiliness of skin or hair.*
Blood: thrombocytopenia.
CNS: dizziness, headache, sleep disorders, fatigue, tremor, irritability, excitation, lethargy, mental depression, chills, paresthesias.
CV: elevated blood pressure.
EENT: visual disturbances.
GI: gastric irritation, nausea, vomiting, diarrhea, constipation, change in appetite.
GU: hematuria.
Hepatic: reversible jaundice.
Hypoestrogenic: flushing; sweating; vaginitis, including itching, dryness, burning, and vaginal bleeding; nervousness, emotional lability, menstrual irregularities.
Other: muscle cramps or spasms.

INTERACTIONS

None significant.

EFFECTS ON DIAGNOSTIC TESTS

Glucose tolerance test: abnormal results.
Prothrombin time (especially in patients on anticoagulant therapy): prolonged.
Total serum thyroxine (T_4): decreased.
Triiodothyronine (T_3): increased.

NURSING CONSIDERATIONS

Besides those related universally to drug therapy (see "How to use this book"), consider the following specific recommendations:

Assessment

- Obtain a baseline assessment of the underlying condition being treated with danazol before therapy.
- Be alert for adverse reactions and drug interactions throughout therapy.
- Evaluate the patient's and family's knowledge about danazol therapy.

Nursing Diagnoses
• Pain related to implantation of endometrial tissue outside the uterine cavity.
• Body image disturbance related to adverse androgenic reactions associated with danazol.
• Knowledge deficit related to danazol therapy.

Planning and Implementation

Preparation and Administration
• Be aware that long-term therapy may be required.

Monitoring
• Monitor effectiveness by regularly assessing severity of pain and other signs and symptoms of the underlying condition.
• Monitor the patient's weight routinely for fluid retention.
• Monitor the female patient for virilization.

Supportive Care
• Report signs of virilization in women so the doctor can reevaluate treatment. Be aware that some androgenic effects, such as deepening of voice, may not be reversible.
• Give the patient a diet high in calories and protein unless contraindicated. Also implement salt restriction if edema occurs and expect to administer a diuretic concurrently, if needed.
• Prepare patient for altered body image as a result of potential androgenic adverse reaction.
• Administer other medications, such as mild analgesics for pain relief, as ordered.

Patient Teaching
• Explain to female patients that virilization may occur. Tell these patients to report androgenic effects immediately.
• Instruct patient to eat a diet high in calories and protein unless contraindicated and to restrict sodium intake if edema occurs.
• Advise patient who is taking drug for fibrocystic disease to examine breasts regularly. If breast nodule enlarges during treatment, tell patient to call doctor immediately.
• Instruct patient to wear cotton underwear only.
• Inform female patient that washing is recommended after intercourse to decrease the risk of vaginitis.

Evaluation
In patients receiving danazol, appropriate evaluation statements may include:
• Patient's underlying condition being treated with danazol shows improvement.
• Patient states acceptance of altered body image as a result of danazol therapy.
• Patient and family state an understanding of danazol therapy.

---

dantrolene sodium

(dan´ troe leen)
Dantrium, Dantrium I.V.

• *Classification:* skeletal muscle relaxant (hydantoin derivative)
• *Pregnancy Risk Category:* C

HOW SUPPLIED

Capsules: 25 mg, 50 mg, 100 mg
Injection: 20 mg/vial

ACTION

Mechanism: Acts directly on skeletal muscle to interfere with calcium movement.
Absorption: 35% of oral dose is absorbed through GI tract.
Distribution: Substantially plasma protein-bound, mainly to albumin.
Metabolism: In the liver to its less active 5-hydroxy derivatives, and to its amino derivative by reductive pathways.
Excretion: In urine as metabolites. Half-life: 7 to 9 hours.
Onset, peak, duration: Peak concentrations reached within 5 hours.

Therapeutic effect in patients with upper motor neuron disorders may take 1 week or more.

INDICATIONS & DOSAGE

Spasticity and sequelae secondary to severe chronic disorders (multiple sclerosis, cerebral palsy, spinal cord injury, stroke) –
Adults: 25 mg P.O. daily. Increase gradually in increments of 25 mg at 4- to 7-day intervals, up to 100 mg b.i.d. to q.i.d., to maximum of 400 mg daily.
Children: 1 mg/kg daily P.O. b.i.d. to q.i.d. Increase gradually as needed by 1 mg/kg daily to maximum of 100 mg q.i.d.
Management of malignant hyperthermia –
Adults and children: 1 mg/kg I.V. initially; may repeat dose up to cumulative dose of 10 mg/kg.
Prevention or attenuation of malignant hyperthermia in susceptible patients who require surgery–
Adults: 4 to 8 mg/kg P.O. daily given in three to four divided doses for 1 to 2 days before procedure. Administer final dose 3 to 4 hours before procedure.
Prevention of recurrence of malignant hyperthermia –
Adults: 4 to 8 mg/kg/day P.O. given in four divided doses for up to 3 days following hyperthermic crisis.

CONTRAINDICATIONS & PRECAUTIONS

Contraindicated in patients with active hepatic disease (hepatitis, cirrhosis), upper motor neuron disorders, and those in whom spasticity helps maintain upright posture and balance.

Use cautiously in patients with cardiac function impairment (may cause pleural effusion), pulmonary function impairment (especially chronic obstructive pulmonary disease), or preexisting hepatic disease. Also use cautiously in patients over age 35, especially women, and in patients receiving other drugs (especially estrogens) concomitantly, because of increased risk of hepatotoxicity.

There are no contraindications to the use of I.V. dantrolene in management of malignant hyperthermia crisis.

ADVERSE REACTIONS

Common reactions are in italics; life-threatening reactions are in bold italics.
CNS: *muscle weakness, drowsiness,* dizziness, light-headedness, malaise, headache, confusion, nervousness, insomnia, exacerbation of precipitation of seizures.
CV: tachycardia, blood pressure changes.
EENT: excessive tearing, visual disturbances.
GI: anorexia, constipation, cramping, dysphagia, metallic taste, *severe diarrhea.*
GU: urinary frequency, incontinence, nocturia, dysuria, crystalluria, difficulty achieving erection.
Hepatic: ***hepatitis.***
Skin: eczematous eruption, pruritus, urticaria, photosensitivity.
Other: abnormal hair growth, drooling, sweating, pleural effusion, myalgia, chills, fever.

INTERACTIONS

Alcohol, CNS depressants: increased CNS depression. Monitor for decreased alertness.
Verapamil (I.V.): may result in cardiovascular collapse. Stop drug before administering I.V. dantrolene.

EFFECTS ON DIAGNOSTIC TESTS

BUN: increased levels.
Liver function tests (ALT [SGPT], AST [SGOT], alkaline phosphatase, and lactic dehydrogenase): increased levels.
Total serum bilirubin: increased levels.

NURSING CONSIDERATIONS

Besides those related universally to drug therapy (see "How to use this book"), consider the following specific recommendations:

Assessment

- Obtain a baseline assessment of the patient's underlying condition before drug therapy.
- Be alert for adverse reactions and drug interactions throughout therapy.
- Evaluate the patient's and family's knowledge about dantrolene sodium therapy.

Nursing Diagnoses

- Hyperthermia related to the patient's underlying condition.
- High risk for injury related to drug-induced drowziness.
- Knowledge deficit related to dantrolene sodium therapy.

Planning and Implementation

Preparation and Administration

- ***P.O. use:*** Give with meals or milk to prevent GI distress.
- Prepare oral suspension for single dose by dissolving capsule contents in juice or other suitable liquid. For multiple doses, use acid vehicle, such as citric acid in USP syrup; refrigerate. Use within several days.
- ***I.V. use:*** Administer as soon as malignant hyperthermia reaction is recognized.
- Reconstitute each vial by adding 60 ml of sterile water for injection and shaking vial until clear. Don't use a diluent that contains a bacteriostatic agent.
- Protect contents from light and use within 6 hours.
- Be careful to avoid extravasation.

Monitoring

- Monitor liver function tests at the beginning of therapy.
- Watch for hepatitis (fever and jaundice), severe diarrhea, severe weakness, or sensivitity reactions (fever and skin eruptions).
- Monitor for adverse reactions and interactions by frequently checking vital signs for blood pressure changes and tachycardia.
- Monitor the patient's bowel pattern; drug may cause constipation or severe diarrhea.
- Monitor hydration status if the patient develops severe diarrhea.
- Monitor elimination pattern for urinary frequency.
- Monitor effectivenness by evaluating degree of hypothermia by monitoring vital signs, especially temperature.

Supportive Care

- Know that safety and efficacy for long-term use are not established; value may be determined by therapeutic trial. Do not give more than 45 days if no benefits are obtained.
- Extent of relief determines if dosage (and drowsiness) can be reduced.
- Be prepared to withhold dose and notify the doctor at first sign of hepatitis, severe diarrhea, severe weakness, or sensitivity reactions.
- If GI distress occurs, give the drug with meals or milk.
- Provide fluids if the patient develops severe diarrhea.
- Institute safety precautions if he develops muscle weakness, dizziness, light-headedness, or confusion.

Patient Teaching

- Warn patient to avoid driving and other hazardous activities that require alertness until CNS effects of the drug are known.
- Tell the patient to avoid combining the drug with alcohol or other depressants.
- Tell the patient to avoid photosensitivity reactions by using sunscreening agents and protective clothing when outdoors.
- Tell the patient to report abdominal discomfort or GI problems immediately.
- Tell him to follow his doctor's orders regarding rest and physical therapy.

Evaluation
In patients receiving dantrolene , appropriate evaluation statements may include:
- The patient does not develop hyperthermia.
- The patient does not experience injury related to drug-induced drowsiness.
- Patient and family state an understanding of dantrolene therapy.

dapsone
(dap´ sone)
Avlosulfon†, Dapsone 100‡

- *Classification:* antileprotic, antimalarial agent (sulfone)
- *Pregnancy Risk Category:* A

HOW SUPPLIED
Tablets: 25 mg, 100 mg

ACTION
Mechanism: Anti-infective action probably related to the inhibition of folic acid biosynthesis in susceptible organisms (bactericidal). Action in dermatitis herpetiformis is unknown.
Absorption: Completely, but rather slowly absorbed, from GI tract after oral administration.
Distribution: Widely distributed into most body tissues and fluids. It is 50% to 90% protein bound.
Metabolism: Undergoes acetylation by liver enzymes; rate varies and is genetically determined. Almost 50% of Blacks and Whites are slow acetylators; over 80% of Chinese, Japanese, and Eskimos are fast acetylators. Dosage adjustment may be required.
Excretion: Dapsone and metabolites are excreted primarily in urine; small amounts are excreted in feces and possibly in breast milk. Undergoes enterohepatic circulation. Orally administered charcoal may enhance excretion. Dapsone is dialyzable. Half-life: In adults, ranges between 10 and 50 hours (average, 28 hours).
Onset, peak, duration: Peak serum levels occur 2 to 8 hours after ingestion.

INDICATIONS & DOSAGE
All forms of leprosy (Hansen's disease)–
Adults: 100 mg P.O. daily for indefinite period, plus rifampin 600 mg daily for 6 months.
Children: 1.4 mg/kg P.O. daily.
Prophylaxis for leprosy patient's close contacts–
Adults: 50 mg P.O. daily.
Children age 6 to 12: 25 mg P.O. daily.
Children age 2 to 5: 25 mg P.O. three times weekly.
Infants age 6 to 23 months: 12 mg P.O. three times weekly.
Children under age 6 months: 6 mg P.O. three times weekly.
Dermatitis herpetiformis–
Adults: 50 mg. P.O. daily; may increase to 400 mg. daily.
Malaria suppression or prophylaxis due to chloroquine-resistant Plasmodium falciparum *when other agents aren't available–*
Adults: 100 mg. P.O. weekly; usually given with pyrimethimine 12.5 mg. P.O. weekly.
Children: 2 mg/kg P.O. weekly, with pyrimethamine 0.25 mg/kg weekly.

Continue prophylaxis during exposure and for 6 months after exposure.
Treatment of Pneumocystis carinii *pneumonia in patients with AIDS–*
Adults: 100 mg P.O. daily in conjunction with trimethoprim 20 mg/kg P.O. daily (usually divided q.i.d.).
Actinomycotic mycetoma–
Adults: 100 mg P.O. b.i.d. Treatment is usually continued for months after clinical symptoms abate.

CONTRAINDICATIONS & PRECAUTIONS

Contraindicated in patients with hypersensitivity to dapsone or its derivatives and in patients with severe anemia.

Use cautiously in patients with glucose-6-phosphate dehydrogenase (G6PD) deficiency, methemoglobin reductase deficiency, or hemoglobin M; in patients with predisposition to hemolysis induced by other drugs or conditions (certain infections or diabetic ketosis) because of potential adverse hematologic effects; and in patients taking probenecid because of decreased excretion and drug accumulation. Special care must be taken to recognize leprosy reactional states.

ADVERSE REACTIONS

Common reactions are in italics; life-threatening reactions are in bold italics.

Blood: ***aplastic anemia, agranulocytosis, hemolytic anemia;*** methemoglobinemia; possible leukopenia.
CNS: psychosis, headache, dizziness, lethargy, severe malaise, paresthesias.
EENT: tinnitus, allergic rhinitis.
GI: anorexia, abdominal pain, nausea, vomiting.
Hepatic: hepatitis, cholestatic jaundice.
Skin: allergic dermatitis (generalized or fixed maculopapular rash).

INTERACTIONS

Probenecid: elevates levels of dapsone. Use together with extreme caution.

EFFECTS ON DIAGNOSTIC TESTS

None reported.

NURSING CONSIDERATIONS

Besides those related universally to drug therapy (see "How to use this book"), consider the specific recommendations:

Assessment
- Obtain a baseline assessment of patient's infection before dapsone therapy.
- Be alert for adverse reactions and drug interactions throughout therapy.
- Evaluate the patient's and family's knowledge about dapsone therapy.

Nursing Diagnoses
- High risk for injury related to ineffectiveness of dapsone to eradicate the infection.
- High risk for impaired skin integrity related to dapsone-induced dermatologic reactions.
- Knowledge deficit related to dapsone.

Planning and Implementation

Preparation and Administration
- Obtain specimen for culture and sensitivity tests and CBC before administering the first dose of dapsone.

Monitoring
- Monitor effectiveness by regularly assessing for improvement of infection and evaluating culture and sensitivity test results as ordered.
- Monitor CBC closely as ordered (weekly for the first month, monthly for 6 months, and semiannually thereafter) because dapsone dosage should be reduced or temporarily discontinued if hemoglobin falls below 9 g/dl; if WBC count falls below 5,000/mm^3; and if RBC count falls below 2.5 million/mm^3 or remains low.
- Monitor patient for skin changes.

Supportive Care
- Withhold drug and notify doctor if generalized, diffuse dermatitis occurs.
- Expect to administer antihistamines for dapsone-induced allergic dermatitis.
- If erythema nodosum type of leprosy reaction occurs (malaise, fever, painful inflammatory induration in the skin and mucosa, iritis, and neuritis), notify the doctor. In severe cases, expect to withhold dapsone

and give glucocorticoids cautiously as prescribed.
• Institute safety precautions if adverse CNS reactions occur.

Patient Teaching
• Inform patient of the need for periodic laboratory studies.
• Teach patients to watch for and promptly report dermatologic changes to the doctor because such reactions may require discontinuation of the drug.
• Instruct a breast-feeding mother to report cyanosis in the infant because this indicates high sulfone level.
• Warn patient to avoid hazardous activities that require alertness if adverse CNS reactions occur.

Evaluation
In patients receiving dapsone, appropriate evaluation statements may include:
• Patient is free of infection.
• Patient maintains normal skin integrity throughout dapsone therapy.
• Patient and family state an understanding of dapsone therapy.

daunorubicin hydrochloride (DNR)
(daw noe roo´ bi sin)
Cerubidin‡, Cerubidine

• *Classification:* antineoplastic (antibiotic)
• *Pregnancy Risk Category:* D

HOW SUPPLIED
Injection: 20 mg/vial

ACTION
Mechanism: An antineoplastic antibiotic that interferes with DNA-dependent RNA synthesis by intercalating base pairs of DNA and causing an uncoiling of the helix, which interferes with the template function of DNA. May also block DNA polymerase. Also has some antibacterial and immunosuppressive activity. Drug is structurally related to doxorubicin.
Absorption: Because it is extremely irritating to tissues, drug must be given intravenously.
Distribution: Rapidly and widely distributed into tissues, with the highest concentrations found in the spleen, kidneys, liver, lungs, and heart. Does not cross the blood-brain barrier, but apparently crosses the placenta.
Metabolism: Extensively metabolized in the liver and other tissues. One metabolite, daunorubicinol, has cytotoxic activity; about 40% of a dose is converted to this metabolite within 30 minutes of administration.
Excretion: Primarily excreted in bile, with a small portion excreted in urine. Half-life: Biphasic, with an initial half-life of 45 minutes and a terminal half-life of 18½ hours. Average terminal half-life of daunorubicinol is about 27 hours.

INDICATIONS & DOSAGE
Dosage and indications may vary. Check patient's protocol with doctor.
Remission induction in acute nonlymphocytic leukemia (myelogenous, monocytic, erythroid) –
Adults: as a single agent, 60 mg/m^2 daily I.V. on days 1, 2, and 3 q 3 to 4 weeks; in combination, 45 mg/m^2 daily I.V. on days 1, 2, and 3 of the first course and on days 1 and 2 of subsequent courses with cytosine arabinoside infusions.
Note: Dose should be reduced if hepatic or renal function is impaired.

CONTRAINDICATIONS & PRECAUTIONS
Contraindicated in patients with severe myelosuppression, preexisting cardiac disease, severe infections, or hepatic or renal dysfunction because the drug may worsen these conditions; and in pregnant patients because of significant risk to the fetus.

ADVERSE REACTIONS

Common reactions are in italics; life-threatening reactions are in bold italics.
Blood: ***bone marrow suppression*** (lowest blood counts 10 to 14 days after administration).
CV: ***irreversible cardiomyopathy (dose-related),*** *ECG changes, arrhythmias,* pericarditis, myocarditis.
GI: *nausea, vomiting, stomatitis, esophagitis,* anorexia, diarrhea.
GU: nephrotoxicity, transient red urine.
Hepatic: hepatotoxicity.
Skin: rash, pigmentation of fingernails and toenails.
Local: *severe cellulitis or tissue sloughing if drug extravasates.*
Other: *generalized alopecia,* fever, chills.

INTERACTIONS

Heparin: don't mix. May form a precipitate.

EFFECTS ON DIAGNOSTIC TESTS

Serum alkaline phosphatase, AST (SGOT), and bilirubin: increased levels indicating drug-induced hepatotoxicity.
Uric acid: increased concentrations in blood and urine.

NURSING CONSIDERATIONS

Besides those related universally to drug therapy (see "How to use this book"), consider the following specific recommendations:

Assessment
- Obtain a baseline assessment of the patient's overall physical status, CBC, ECG, and renal and hepatic function before initiating therapy.
- Be alert for adverse reactions or drug interactions throughout therapy.
- Evaluate the patient's and family's knowledge about daunorubicin therapy.

Nursing Diagnoses
- Impaired tissue integrity related to extravasation of daunorubicin.
- Decreased cardiac output related to daunorubicin-induced cardiotoxicity.
- Knowledge deficit related to daunorubicin therapy.

Planning and Implementation

Preparation and Administration
- ***I.V. use:*** Follow institutional policy when preparing and administering this drug to avoid mutagenic, teratogenic, and carcinogenic risks.
- Expect to administer lower doses in renal, hepatic, or hematopoietic impairment.
- Stop drug immediately in patients with signs of CHF or cardiomyopathy. Prevent by limiting cumulative dose to 550 mg/m^2 (450 mg/m^2 when patient has been receiving radiation therapy that encompasses the heart, or any other cardiotoxic agent, such as cyclophosphamide.)
- Avoid extravasasation; inject into tubing of freely flowing I.V. solution.
- Do not administer I.M or S.C.
- Be aware that reconstituted solution is stable for 24 hours at room temperature or 48 hours refrigerated. Optimally, use within 8 hours of preparation.
- Since the reddish color of daunorubicin looks very similar to doxorubicin, be careful not to confuse the two drugs.

Monitoring
- Monitor effectiveness by noting results of follow-up diagnostic tests and patient's overall physical status.
- Monitor ECG during therapy; monitor for signs and symptoms of CHF.
- Monitor resting pulse rate; if high, may signal cardiac adverse reactions.
- Monitor CBC and hepatic function.
- Monitor for signs of extravasation, which usually causes an immediate burning sensation. Be aware that extravasation can produce severe local tissue necrosis, thrombophlebitis, cellulitis, or painful induration. Ulceration may require skin grafting.
- Monitor for nausea and vomiting,

which may be severe and last up to 48 hours.
• Identify and monitor previously irradiated skin for reactivated lesions. If present, reduce dosage as ordered.
• Monitor for signs of infection (cough, fever, sore throat) and bleeding (easy bruising, nosebleeds, bleeding gums).

Supportive Care

• Avoid all I.M. injections when the platelet count is less than 100,000/mm³.
• Give antiemetics to help control nausea and vomiting.
• Provide adequate hydration; alkalinizing urine or administering allopurinol may prevent or minimize uric acid nephropathy.
• To help prevent infection, maintain the patient's optimal health and protect him from undue exposure to environmental contagion. If signs of infection occur, notify doctor promptly; administer antibiotics, as ordered.
• Provide a safe environment to minimize risk of bleeding.
• If extravasation occurs, discontinue infusion and aspirate as much drug as possible. Minimize local reaction by immediately infiltrating the area with hydrocortisone sodium succinate injection (50 to 100 mg of hydrocortisone) or sodium bicarbonate (5 ml of 8.4% injection) and applying cold compresses.
• Report signs and symptoms of CHF promptly.

Patient Teaching

• Warn patients to watch for signs of infection (sore throat, fever, fatigue) and for signs of bleeding (easy bruising, nosebleeds, bleeding gums). Tell patient to take temperature daily and to report signs of infection or bleeding promptly.
• Inform the patient that hair loss is possible but is usually reversible.
• Warn patient that urine may appear red for 1 to 2 days and that it is a normal adverse reaction and not hematuria.
• Tell patient to report symptoms of CHF promptly to doctor.
• Instruct patient about need for protective measures, including conservation of energy, balanced diet, adequate rest, personal cleanliness, clean environment, and avoidance of exposure to persons with infections.
• Instruct patient about safety precautions to reduce risks of bleeding from falls, cuts, or other injuries.
• Instruct patient about the need for frequent oral hygiene.

Evaluation

In patients receiving daunorubicin, appropriate evaluation statements may include:
• No local tissue damage is evidenced.
• No decreased cardiac output is evidenced.
• Patient and family state an understanding of daunorubicin therapy.

deferoxamine mesylate

(de fer ox′ a meen)
Desferal

• *Classification:* heavy metal antagonist (chelating agent)
• *Pregnancy Risk Category:* C

HOW SUPPLIED

Powder for injection: 500 mg

ACTION

Mechanism: Chelates iron by binding ferric ions.
Absorption: Poorly absorbed after oral administration; however, oral absorption may occur in patients with acute iron toxicity.
Distribution: Widely distributed into the body after parenteral administration. Most of the chelating activity occurs in the plasma.

Metabolism: Small amounts of drug are metabolized by plasma enzymes.
Excretion: In urine as unchanged drug or as ferrioxamine, the deferoxamine-iron complex.

INDICATIONS & DOSAGE

Adjunctive treatment of acute iron intoxication–
Adults and children: 1 g I.M. or I.V. followed by 500 mg I.M. or I.V. for two doses, q 4 hours; then 500 mg I.M. or I.V. q 4 to 12 hours. Infusion rate shouldn't exceed 15 mg/kg hourly. Don't exceed 6 g in 24 hours.
Chronic iron overload resulting from multiple transfusions–
Adults and children: 500 mg to 1 g I.M. daily and 2 g slow I.V. infusion in separate solution along with each unit of blood transfused. Maximum dosage is 6 g daily. I.V. infusion rate shouldn't exceed 15 mg/kg hourly.
S.C.: 1 to 2 g via a subcutaneous infusion pump over 8 to 24 hours.

CONTRAINDICATIONS & PRECAUTIONS

Contraindicated in patients with severe renal failure or anuria, because the drug and ferrioxamine are excreted primarily by the kidneys (*except* for management of iron or aluminum intoxication in dialysis patients); and in pregnant women or in women who may become pregnant. Use cautiously in patients with pyelonephritis and in those with hearing or vision deficits, because drug may exacerbate these conditions.

ADVERSE REACTIONS

Common reactions are in italics; life-threatening reactions are in bold italics.
Local: pain and induration at injection site.
Other: *after rapid I.V. administration: erythema, urticaria, hypotension,* ***shock.***
With long-term use: sensitivity reaction (cutaneous wheal formation, pruritus, rash, ***anaphylaxis***), leg cramps, fever, tachycardia, dysuria, diarrhea, abdominal discomfort, blurred vision, cataracts.

INTERACTIONS

None significant.

EFFECTS ON DIAGNOSTIC TESTS

None reported.

NURSING CONSIDERATIONS

Besides those related universally to drug therapy (see "How to use this book"), consider the following specific recommendations:

Assessment
- Obtain a baseline assessment of allergies, serum iron levels, renal status, and urine output before therapy.
- Be alert for adverse reactions and drug interactions throughout therapy.
- Evaluate the patient's and family's knowledge about deferoxamine therapy.

Nursing Diagnoses
- High risk for injury related to acute iron intoxication.
- Ineffective airway clearance related to drug-induced anaphylaxis.
- Knowledge deficit related to deferoxamine therapy.

Planning and Implementation
Preparation and Administration
- For reconstitution, add 2 ml of sterile water for injection to each ampule. Make sure drug is completely dissolved.
- Reconstituted solution is good for 1 week at room temperature. Protect from light.
- ***I.M. use:*** Preferred method of administration is I.M. injection.
- ***I.V. use:*** Administer via I.V. route only when patient has cardiovascular collapse or shock. Dissolve drug as for I.M. use; dilute in 0.9% sodium chloride solution, dextrose 5% in water, or lactated Ringer's solution. Change to I.M. route as soon as possible.

Monitoring
• Monitor effectiveness by monitoring serum iron levels and decrease in signs of iron intoxication.
• Observe for signs of anaphylactic reaction immediately after injection.
• Check respiratory status and vital signs frequently until stable.
• Monitor intake and output carefully. Weigh patient daily to detect fluid volume deficit or retention.
• Monitor renal function studies and vision during long-term therapy.
• Observe injection site for local reaction.
Supportive Care
• Have epinephrine 1:1,000 available in case of anaphylaxis. Have airway, oxygen, and resuscitation equipment nearby.
• Do not give in severe renal disease or anuria.
• Use with caution in impaired renal function.
• Apply ice or cold compresses to injection site to alleviate local discomfort.
Patient Teaching
• Instruct patient to report respiratory difficulty or decrease in urine output immediately.
• Advise patient to notify doctor if blurred vision, leg cramps, abdominal discomfort, or rashes develop during deferoxamine therapy.
• Inform the patient that pain and induration may occur at the injection site.
• Warn patient that urine may be red.
• Recommend regular eye examinations during long-term therapy.
Evaluation
In patients receiving deferoxamine, appropriate evaluation statements may include:
• Patient is free from injury related to iron intoxication.
• Patient maintains patent and effective airway.
• Patient and family state an understanding of deferoxamine therapy.

demecarium bromide
(dem e kare´ ee um)
Humorsol

• *Classification:* miotic (cholinesterase inhibitor)
• *Pregnancy Risk Category:* X

HOW SUPPLIED
Ophthalmic solution: 0.125%, 0.25% (with benzalkonium chloride 1:5,000)

ACTION
Mechanism: Inhibits the enzymatic destruction of acetylcholine by inactivating cholinesterase. This leaves acetylcholine free to act on muscarinic receptors in the iridic sphincter and ciliary muscles, causing pupillary constriction and accommodation spasm.
Pharmacokinetics: Unknown.
Onset, peak, duration: Although a reversible inhibitor of cholinesterase, its duration of action is similar to that of irreversible cholinesterase inhibitors. Maximal decrease in intraocular pressure occurs in 24 hours and may persist for over a week.

INDICATIONS & DOSAGE
Angle-closure glaucoma after iridectomy, primary open-angle glaucoma –
Adults: instill 1 drop of 0.125% or 0.25% solution once or twice/day.
Treatment of accommodative esotropia (uncomplicated) –
Adults: instill 1 drop of 0.125% or 0.25% solution q.d for 2 to 3 weeks then reduce to 1 drop q 2 days for 3 to 4 weeks. After reevaluation, 1 drop once or twice/week to once q 2 days as determined by patient's condition. Reevaluate q 4 to 12 weeks, adjusting dose as needed. Discontinue after 4 months if dose required is 1 drop q 2 days.

Diagnostic use–
Adults: 1 drop q.d. for 2 weeks then 1 drop q 2 days for 2 to 3 weeks.

CONTRAINDICATIONS & PRECAUTIONS

Contraindicated in patients with active uveal inflammation, narrow-angle glaucoma, secondary glaucoma resulting from iridocyclitis, ocular hypertension, vasomotor instability, bronchial instability, bronchial asthma, spastic GI conditions, peptic ulcer, severe bradycardia, hypotension, recent MI, seizure disorder, Parkinson's disease, or history of retinal detachment, because the drug may aggravate the signs or symptoms of these disorders.

Use cautiously in patients with myasthenia gravis who are also receiving systemic anticholinesterase therapy and in patients exposed to organophosphate insecticides.

ADVERSE REACTIONS

Common reactions are in italics; life-threatening reactions are in bold italics.
CNS: browache, unusual fatigue or weakness, headache.
CV: slow or irregular heartbeat.
Eye: eye pain, retinal detachment, iris cysts, conjunctival thickening, lens opacities, paradoxic increase in intraocular pressure, *lacrimation,* obstruction of nasolacrimal canals, burning, redness, stinging, irritation, twitching of eyelids, *blurred vision,* visual disturbances.
GI: nausea, vomiting, diarrhea, stomach cramps or pain.
GU: loss of bladder control.

INTERACTIONS

Anticholinergics, antimyasthenics, other cholinesterase inhibitors: potential for additive toxicity.
Carbamate or organophosphate-type insecticides: increased risk of systemic effects through respiratory tract or skin. Protective measures advised.
Cocaine: increased risk of cocaine toxicity; anticholinesterase effects may last weeks or months.
Edrophonium: worsening of patient's condition.
Local anesthetics, ophthalmic tetracaine: increased risk of systemic toxicity, prolonged ocular anesthetic effect.
Ophthalmic adrenocorticoids: increased intraocular pressure, decreased effectiveness of antiglaucoma agent.
Ophthalmic belladonna alkaloids, cyclopentolate: may antagonize miotic effects.
Succinylcholine: enhanced neuromuscular blockade, possible cardiovascular collapse, prolonged respiratory depression or apnea; effects may occur for several weeks or months after demecarium is discontinued.

EFFECTS ON DIAGNOSTIC TESTS

None reported.

NURSING CONSIDERATIONS

Besides those related universally to drug therapy (see "How to use this book"), consider the following specific recommendations:

Assessment

- Obtain a baseline assessment of the patient's vision, especially ocular pressure.
- Be alert for adverse reactions and drug interactions throughout therapy.
- Evaluate the patient's and family's knowledge about demecarium therapy.

Nursing Diagnoses

- Sensory/perceptual alterations (visual) related to the patient's underlying condition.
- Sensory/perceptual alterations (visual) related to demecarium-induced adverse reactions affecting the eye.
- Knowledge deficit related to demecarium bromide therapy.

Planning and Implementation
Preparation and Administration
• Instill drops in lacrimal sac; remove excess solution around eyes with clean tissue.
• May be administered concurrently with phenylephrine (to reduce incidence of iris cyst formation) or epinephrine (additive therapeutic effect).
Monitoring
• Monitor effectiveness by assessing the patient's visual status and intraocular pressure.
• Monitor for systemic cholinergic effects: toxicity is cumulative and may not appear for weeks or months after start of therapy.
• Monitor for tolerance to the drug in long-term therapy; effectiveness may be restored by briefly substituting another miotic.
Supportive Care
• Notify the doctor immediately if changes in the patient's health status occur.
• Obtain an order for a mild analgesic if the patient experiences head or brow aches.
• Keep atropine sulfate (I.M. or I.V.) on hand to reverse systemic cholenergic effects.
Patient Teaching
• Teach the patient how to instill the drops, and advise him to wash his hands before and after administering the drug.
• Advise the patient to carry a medical alert card during therapy because the drug has many potential interactions.
• Warn the patient not to exceed the recommended dosage. If a dose is missed, he should not double dose.
• Advise the patient to continue with regular medical supervision during therapy.
Evaluation
In patients receiving demecarium, appropriate evaluation statements may include:
• Patient experiences a reduction in introcular pressure.
• Patient does not experience demecarium-induced visual alterations.
• Patient and family state an understanding of demecarium bromide therapy

demeclocycline hydrocholoride
(de me kloe sye´ kleen)
Declomycin, Ledermycin‡

• *Classification:* antibiotic (tetracycline)
• *Pregnancy Risk Category:* D

HOW SUPPLIED
Tablets: 150 mg, 300 mg
Capsules: 150 mg

ACTION
Mechanism: Exerts bacteriostatic effect by binding to the 30S ribosomal subunit of microorganisms, thus inhibiting protein synthesis.
Absorption: 60% to 80% is absorbed from the GI tract after oral administration. Food or milk reduces absorption by 50%; antacids chelate with tetracyclines and further reduce absorption. Drug has greatest affinity of all tetracyclines for calcium ions.
Distribution: Widely distributed into body tissues and fluids, including synovial, pleural, prostatic, and seminal fluids; bronchial secretions; saliva; and aqueous humor; CSF penetration is poor. Demeclocycline crosses the placenta; it is 36% to 91% protein-bound.
Metabolism: Not metabolized.
Excretion: Primarily excreted unchanged in urine by glomerular filtration; some drug may be excreted in breast milk. Half-life: 10 to 17 hours in adults with normal renal function.
Onset, peak, duration: Peak serum levels occur at 3 to 4 hours after oral administration.

INDICATIONS & DOSAGE

Infections caused by susceptible gram-negative and gram-positive organisms, trachoma, rickettsiae–
Adults: 150 mg P.O. q 6 hours or 300 mg P.O. q 12 hours.
Children over 8 years: 6 to 12 mg/kg P.O. daily, divided q 6 to 12 hours.
Gonorrhea–
Adults: 600 mg P.O. initially, then 300 mg P.O. q 12 hours for 4 days (total 3 g).
Uncomplicated urethral, endocervical, or rectal infection caused by Chlamydia trachomatis–
Adults: 300 mg P.O. q.i.d. for at least 7 days.
Syndrome of inappropriate antidiuretic hormone (a hyposmolar state)–
Adults: 600 to 1,200 mg P.O. daily in divided doses.

CONTRAINDICATIONS & PRECAUTIONS

Contraindicated in patients with hypersensitivity to any tetracycline; during the second half of pregnancy because it may cause maternal fatty infiltration of the liver and may cause permanent discoloration or hypoplasia of tooth enamel or impaired skeletal growth in the fetus; and in children under age 8 because it may cause permanent discoloration of teeth, enamel defects, and retardation of bone growth.

Use with caution in patients with decreased renal function, because it may elevate BUN levels and exacerbate renal dysfunction, and in patients likely to be exposed to direct sunlight or ultraviolet light because of the risk of photosensitivity reactions.

ADVERSE REACTIONS

Common reactions are in italics; life-threatening reactions are in bold italics.
Blood: neutropenia, eosinophilia, thrombocytopenia, **hemolytic anemia.**
CNS: pseudotumor cerebri.
CV: pericarditis.
EENT: dysphagia, glossitis.
GI: anorexia, *nausea, vomiting, diarrhea,* enterocolitis, anogenital inflammation.
Metabolic: *increased BUN,* diabetes insipidus syndrome (polyuria, polydipsia, weakness).
Skin: *maculopapular and erythematous rashes, photosensitivity, increased pigmentation, urticaria.*
Other: ***hypersensitivity.***

INTERACTIONS

Antacids (including sodium bicarbonate) and laxatives containing aluminum, magnesium, or calcium; food, milk, or other dairy products: decrease antibiotic absorption. Give antibiotic 1 hour before or 2 hours after any of the above.
Ferrous sulfate and other iron products, zinc: decrease antibiotic absorption. Give demeclocycline 3 hours after or 2 hours before iron administration.
Methoxyflurane: may cause nephrotoxicity with tetracyclines. Monitor carefully.
Oral contraceptives: decreased contraceptive effectiveness and increased risk of breakthrough bleeding.

EFFECTS ON DIAGNOSTIC TESTS

BUN: elevated levels in patients with decreased renal function.
Urinary catecholamines: false elevations in fluorometric tests.
Urine glucose tests using glucose enzymatic method (Clinistix or Tes-Tape): false-negative results.

NURSING CONSIDERATIONS

Besides those related universally to drug therapy (see "How to use this book"), consider the following specific recommendations:
Assessment
• Obtain a baseline assessment of infection before therapy.

• Be alert for adverse reactions and drug interactions throughout therapy.
• Evaluate the patient's and family's knowledge about demeclocycline therapy.

Nursing Diagnoses

• High risk for infection related to ineffectiveness of demeclocycline to eradicate the infection.
• High risk for fluid volume deficit related to adverse GI reactions to demeclocycline therapy.
• Knowledge deficit related to demeclocycline.

Planning and Implementation

Preparation and Administration

• Obtain specimen for culture and sensitivity tests before first dose. Therapy may begin pending test results.
• Check expiration date. Outdated or deteriorated demeclocycline has been associated with reversible nephrotoxicity (Fanconi's syndrome).
• Do not expose drug to light or heat; store in tight container.
• Be aware that use of demeclocycline during last half of pregnancy and in children under age 8 may cause permanent discoloration of teeth, enamel defects, and retardation of bone growth, so always question order for demeclocycline for these patients before administering first dose.
• ***P.O. use:*** Do not administer with milk or other dairy products, food, antacids, or iron products because they reduce effectiveness. Administer with a full glass of water on an empty stomach, at least 1 hour before meals or 2 hours afterward. Give at least 1 hour before bedtime to prevent esophagitis.

Monitoring

• Monitor effectiveness by regularly assessing for improvement of infection.
• Monitor hydration status if adverse GI reactions occur.
• During prolonged or high-dose therapy, monitor for superinfection, especially in high-risk patients.

Supportive Care

• If the patient develops a superinfection, or new infection, notify the doctor. Prepare to discontinue demeclocycline and substitute another antibiotic. If the patient develops oral thrush, provide good mouth care.
• If the patient develops diarrhea, nausea, or vomiting, request an antiemetic or antidiarrheal agent, if needed. Expect to substitute to a different antibiotic as prescribed.
• When testing urine glucose, remember that glucose enzymatic methods (Clinistix or Tes-Tape) may cause false-negative results.

Patient Teaching

• Advise the patient to avoid direct exposure to sunlight and ultraviolet light and to use a sunscreen with a sun protection factor of 15 or higher to help prevent photosensitivity reactions. Remind the patient that photosensitivity persists for some time after discontinuation of drug.
• Tell the patient to take the drug with a full glass of water (to facilitate passage to the stomach), 1 hour before or 2 hours after meals for maximum absorption, and not less than 1 hour before bedtime (to prevent irritation from esophageal reflux).
• Tell the patient not to take the drug with food, milk or other dairy products, antacids, or iron compounds because these may interfere with absorption.
• Emphasize importance of completing prescribed regimen exactly as ordered and keeping follow-up appointments.
• Tell the patient to check expiration dates and discard any outdated demeclocycline because it may become toxic.
• Teach the patient to recognize and report signs of superinfection (furry overgrowth on tongue, vaginal itch or

discharge, foul-smelling stool). Stress good oral hygiene.
• Instruct diabetic patients to avoid using Clinistix or Tes-Tape to test urine for glucose because it may yield a false-negative reading.
• Advise patient taking an oral contraceptive to use an alternative means of contraception during demeclocycline therapy and for 1 week after it is discontinued.

Evaluation
In patients receiving demeclocycline, appropriate evaluation statements may include:
• Patient is free of infection.
• Patient remains adequately hydrated throughout demeclocycline therapy.
• Patient and family state an understanding of demeclocycline therapy.

desipramine hydrochloride
(dess ip´ ra meen)
Norpramin**, Pertofran‡, Pertofrane

• *Classification:* antidepressant, antianxiety agent (tricyclic dibenzazepine)
• *Pregnancy Risk Category:* C

HOW SUPPLIED
Tablets: 10 mg, 25 mg, 50 mg, 75 mg, 100 mg, 150 mg
Capsules: 25 mg, 50 mg

ACTION
Mechanism: Increases the amount of norepinephrine or serotonin, or both, in the CNS by blocking their reuptake by the presynaptic neurons.
Absorption: Absorbed rapidly after oral administration.
Distribution: Widely distributed; enters CNS and is found in breast milk. Drug is 90% protein-bound.
Metabolism: By the liver; a significant first-pass effect may explain variability of serum concentrations in different patients taking the same dosage.
Excretion: Primarily in urine. Half-life: Estimates range from 7 to more than 60 hours.
Onset, peak, duration: Peak effect occurs in 4 to 6 hours; steady state, within 2 to 11 days, with full therapeutic effect in 4 or more weeks. Proposed therapeutic plasma levels (parent drug and metabolite) range from 125 to 300 ng/ml.

INDICATIONS & DOSAGE
Treatment of depression–
Adults: 75 to 150 mg P.O. daily in divided doses, increasing to maximum of 300 mg daily. Alternatively, the entire dosage can be given at bedtime.
Elderly and adolescents: 25 to 50 mg P.O. daily, increasing gradually to maximum of 100 mg daily.

CONTRAINDICATIONS & PRECAUTIONS
Contraindicated in patients with hypersensitivity to tricyclic antidepressants, trazodone, and related compounds; in the acute recovery phase of myocardial infarction because of potential arrhythmogenic effects and ECG changes; in patients in coma or severe respiratory depression because of added CNS depressant effects; and during or within 14 days of therapy with monoamine oxidase (MAO) inhibitors.

Use cautiously in patients with other cardiac disease (arrhythmias, CHF, angina pectoris, valvular disease, or heart block); respiratory disorders; seizure disorders; bipolar disease, glaucoma, hyperthyroidism, or patients taking thyroid replacement; Type I and Type II diabetes; prostatic hypertrophy, paralytic ileus, or urine retention; hepatic or renal dysfunction; or Parkinson's disease; and in those undergoing electroconvulsive therapy or those undergoing surgery using general anesthesia.

If product contains tartrazine, drug may precipitate asthma in patients with aspirin allergy.

ADVERSE REACTIONS

Common reactions are in italics; life-threatening reactions are in bold italics.
CNS: *drowsiness, dizziness,* excitation, tremors, weakness, confusion, headache, nervousness.
CV: *orthostatic hypotension, tachycardia, ECG changes,* hypertension.
EENT: *blurred vision,* tinnitus, mydriasis.
GI: *dry mouth, constipation,* nausea, vomiting, anorexia, paralytic ileus.
GU: *urine retention.*
Skin: rash, urticaria.
Other: *sweating,* allergy.
After abrupt withdrawal of long-term therapy: nausea, headache, malaise. (Does not indicate addiction.)

INTERACTIONS

Barbiturates: decrease TCA blood levels. Monitor for decreased antidepressant effect.
Cimetidine: may increase desipramine serum levels. Monitor for increased adverse reactions.
Epinephrine, norepinephrine: increase hypertensive effect. Use with caution.
MAO inhibitors: may cause severe excitation, hyperpyrexia, or seizures, usually with high dose. Use together cautiously.
Methylphenidate: increases TCA blood levels. Monitor for enhanced antidepressant effect.

EFFECTS ON DIAGNOSTIC TESTS

CBC: decreased WBC count.
ECG: elongation of Q-T and PR intervals; flattened T waves.
Liver function tests: elevated results.
Serum glucose: decreased or increased levels.

NURSING CONSIDERATIONS

Besides those related universally to drug therapy (see "How to use this book"), consider the following specific recommendations:

Assessment
- Obtain a baseline assessment of depression before therapy.
- Be alert for adverse reactions and drug interactions throughout therapy.
- Evaluate the patient's and family's knowledge about desipramine therapy.

Nursing Diagnoses
- Ineffective individual coping related to the patient's underlying condition.
- High risk for injury related to desipramine-induced adverse reactions.
- Knowledge deficit related to desipramine therapy.

Planning and Implementation

Preparation and Administration
- Whenever possible, patient should take full dose at bedtime.
- Expect reduced dosage in elderly or debilitated patients and adolescents.

Monitoring
- Monitor effectiveness by having the patient discuss his feelings (ask broad, open-ended questions) and by evaluating his behavior.
- Monitor blood pressure (supine and standing) for changes, heart rate for tachycardia, and ECG for changes.
- Monitor bowel patterns for constipation, and check for urine retention.
- Monitor for suicidal tendencies.

Supportive Care
- Institute safety precautions if adverse CNS reactions, orthostatic hypotension, or blurred vision occur. Keep in mind that orthostatic hypotension with this drug is less severe than with other tricyclic antidepressants.
- Do not withdraw drug abruptly.
- If psychotic signs increase, notify doctor and expect dosage to be reduced.
- If not contraindicated, increase the patient's fluid and fiber intake to pre-

vent constipation; if needed, obtain an order for a laxative.
• Expect this drug to be ordered more frequently for cardiac patients because it produces less tachycardia and other anticholinergic effects than with other tricyclics.
Patient Teaching
• Tell the patient to relieve dry mouth with sugarless hard candy or gum, but explain that saliva substitutes may be necessary.
• Teach the patient to increase fluids to lessen constipation. Suggest stool softener or high-fiber diet, if needed.
• Warn the patient to avoid driving and other hazardous activities that require alertness and good psychomotor coordination until CNS effects of the drug are known. Tell the patient that drowsiness and dizziness usually subside after first few weeks. Warn against combining drug with alcohol or other CNS depressants.
• Tell the patient that treatment must continue for 2 weeks or more before noticeable effect and for at least 4 weeks for full effect.
• Encourage the patient to continue to take medication until it achieves full therapeutic effect.
• Advise the patient not to take any other drugs (prescription or OTC) without first consulting the doctor.
Evaluation
In patients receiving desipramine, appropriate evaluation statements may include:
• Patient behavior and communication indicate improvement of depression.
• Patient has not experienced injury from desipramine-induced adverse reactions.
• Patient and family state an understanding of desipramine therapy.

deslanoside (desacetyl-lanatoside C)
(des lan´ oh side)
Cedilanid†, Cedilanid-D

• *Classification:* antiarrhythmic, inotropic (digitalis glycoside)
• *Pregnancy Risk Category:* C

HOW SUPPLIED
Injection: 0.2 mg/ml

ACTION
Mechanism: Inhibits sodium-potassium–activated adenosine triphosphatase (Na/K ATPase). Intracellular sodium accumulation leads to calcium accumulation within the myocardial cell. Increased calcium availability strengthens myocardial contraction. Digitalis glycosides also act on the CNS to increase vagal tone and slow heart rate.
Absorption: Inconsistently and incompletely absorbed from the GI tract; usually given I.V.
Distribution: Widespread in body tissues; highest concentrations occur in the heart, kidneys, intestine, stomach, liver, and skeletal muscle; lowest concentrations in the plasma and the brain. Deslanoside crosses both the blood-brain barrier and the placenta; consequently, fetal and maternal serum drug levels are presumably similar. About 25% of drug is bound to plasma proteins.
Metabolism: Minimal metabolism.
Excretion: Unchanged in the urine. Half-life: About 33 hours.
Onset, peak, duration: After I.V. administration, effects occur in about 10 minutes; peak effects occur in about 20 minutes.

INDICATIONS & DOSAGE
CHF, paroxysmal supraventricular tachycardia, atrial fibrillation and flutter–

Adults: loading dose is 1.2 to 1.6 mg I.M. or slow I.V. in two divided doses over 24 hours; for maintenance, use another glycoside. Not recommended for children.

CONTRAINDICATIONS & PRECAUTIONS

Contraindicated in patients with ventricular fibrillation because it may cause ventricular asystole; in patients with digitalis toxicity because of potential for additive toxicity; and in patients with hypersensitivity to the drug.

Use with extreme caution, if at all, in patients with idiopathic hypertrophic subaortic stenosis because the drug may increase obstruction of left ventricular outflow; in patients with incomplete atrioventricular (AV) block who do not have an artificial pacemaker (especially those with Stokes-Adams syndrome) because the drug may induce advanced or complete AV block; in patients with hypersensitive carotid sinus syndrome because the drug increases vagal tone (carotid sinus massage has induced ventricular fibrillation in patients receiving digitalis glycosides); in patients with Wolff-Parkinson-White syndrome because the drug may increase conduction through accessory pathways; in patients with sinus node disease (for example, sick sinus syndrome), because the drug may worsen sinus bradycardia or SA block; and in patients with acute glomerulonephritis and CHF because the drug may accumulate rapidly to toxic levels.

Use with caution in patients with severe pulmonary disease, hypoxia, myxedema, acute myocardial infarction, severe heart failure, acute myocarditis, or an otherwise damaged myocardium because of the increased risk of drug-induced arrhythmias in these patients; with chronic constrictive pericarditis because such patients may respond unfavorably to the drug; in patients with frequent premature ventricular contractions or ventricular tachycardia (especially if these arrhythmias are not caused by heart failure) because the drug may induce additional arrhythmias; low cardiac output states caused by valvular stenosis, chronic pericarditis, or chronic cor pulmonale because the drug may decrease heart rate and subsequently further reduce cardiac output; conditions that increase cardiac sensitivity to digitalis glycosides, including hypokalemia, chronic pulmonary disease, and acute hypoxemia; and, hypertension, because I.V. administration may transiently increase blood pressure.

ADVERSE REACTIONS

Common reactions are in italics; life-threatening reactions are in bold italics.

The following are signs of toxicity that may occur with all digitalis glycosides:

CNS: *fatigue, generalized muscle weakness, agitation,* hallucinations, headache, malaise, dizziness, vertigo, stupor, paresthesias.

CV: ***increased severity of CHF,*** *arrhythmias (most commonly conduction disturbances with or without AV block, premature ventricular contractions, and supraventricular arrhythmias),* hypotension.

Toxic effects on heart may be life-threatening and require immediate attention.

EENT: *yellow-green halos around visual images, blurred vision,* light flashes, photophobia, diplopia.

GI: *anorexia, nausea,* vomiting, diarrhea.

INTERACTIONS

Amphotericin B, carbenicillin, ticarcillin, corticosteroids, and diuretics (including loop diuretics, chlorthalidone, metolazone, and thiazides): hypokalemia, predisposing patient to

digitalis toxicity. Monitor serum potassium.
Parenteral calcium, thiazides: hypercalcemia and hypomagnesemia, predisposing patient to digitalis toxicity. Monitor serum calcium and serum magnesium.

EFFECTS ON DIAGNOSTIC TESTS

None reported.

NURSING CONSIDERATIONS

Besides those related universally to drug therapy (see "How to use this book"), consider the following specific recommendations:

Assessment

- Obtain a baseline assessment of the patient's heart rate and rhythm or degree of CHF present before deslanoside therapy.
- Be alert for adverse reactions and drug interactions throughout therapy.
- Evaluate the patient's and family's knowledge about deslanoside therapy.

Nursing Diagnoses

- Decreased cardiac output related to ineffectiveness of deslanoside.
- High risk for injury related to toxicity caused by deslanoside.
- Knowledge deficit related to deslanoside.

Planning and Implementation

Preparation and Administration

- Obtain baseline data (heart rate and rhythm, blood pressure, and electrolyte levels) before giving first dose.
- Ask patient about recent use of digitalis glycosides (within the previous 2 to 3 weeks) before administering a loading dose.
- Always divide loading dose over first 24 hours unless clinical situation indicates otherwise.
- Be aware that drug is used only for rapid digitilization, not maintenance therapy. Maintenance therapy with an oral digitalis glycoside is usually initiated within 12 to 24 hours.
- ***I.V. use:*** Infuse drug slowly over at least 5 minutes.

Monitoring

- Monitor effectiveness by taking an apical-radial pulse for a full minute before each dose, evaluating continuous ECG readings, and regularly assessing patient's cardiopulmonary status for signs of improvement.
- Monitor serum calcium, potassium, and magnesium levels.
- Monitor closely for deslanoside toxicity.

Supportive Care

- Withhold drug and notify doctor if excessive slowing of the pulse rate (60 beats/minute or less) occurs as this may be a sign of deslanoside toxicity.
- Notify doctor if significant changes, such as a sudden increase or decrease in heart rate, pulse deficit, irregular beats, and particularly regularization of a previously irregular rhythm, occurs. Check blood pressure and obtain 12-lead ECG with these changes.
- Institute safety precautions if CNS reactions occur.
- Obtain an order for an antiemetic or antidiarrheal agent if GI reactions occur.

Patient Teaching

- Encourage patient to eat potassium-rich foods.
- Tell the patient that maintenance therapy will be necessary with an oral digitalis glycoside and instruct him on the prescribed agent accordingly.

Evaluation

In patients receiving deslanoside, appropriate evaluation statements may include:

- Patient's cardiopulmonary function has returned to patient's baseline status.
- Patient does not experience deslanoside toxicity throughout therapy.
- Patient and family state an understanding of deslanoside therapy.

desmopressin acetate

(des moe press´ in)
DDAVP, Minirin‡, Stimate

• *Classification:* antidiuretic, hemostatic agent (posterior pituitary hormone)
• *Pregnancy Risk Category:* B

HOW SUPPLIED

Nasal solution: 0.1 mg/ml
Injection: 4 mcg/ml

ACTION

Mechanism: Increases the permeability of the renal tubular epithelium to adenosine monophosphate and water; the epithelium promotes reabsorption of water and produces a concentrated urine (antidiuretic hormone effect); also increases factor VIII activity by releasing endogenous factor VIII from plasma storage sites.
Absorption: After intranasal administration, 10% to 20% of the dose is absorbed through nasal mucosa. Desmopressin is destroyed in the GI tract.
Excretion: Plasma levels decline in two phases. Half-life: Of the fast phase, about 8 minutes; the slow phase, 75½ minutes.
Onset, peak, duration: Antidiuretic action occurs within 1 hour and peaks in 1 to 5 hours. After I.V. infusion, plasma factor VIII activity increases within 15 to 30 minutes and peaks between 1½ and 3 hours. Duration of action after intranasal administration is 8 to 20 hours; after I.V. administration, it is 12 to 24 hours for mild hemophilia and approximately 3 hours for von Willebrand's disease.

INDICATIONS & DOSAGE

Nonnephrogenic diabetes insipidus, temporary polyuria and polydipsia associated with pituitary trauma –
Adults: 0.1 to 0.4 ml intranasally daily in 1 to 3 doses. Adjust morning and evening doses separately for adequate diurnal rhythm of water turnover. Alternatively, may administer injectable form in dosage of 0.5 to 1 ml I.V. or S.C. daily, usually in two divided doses.
Children 3 months to 12 years: 0.05 to 0.3 ml intranasally daily in 1 or 2 doses.
Treatment of hemophilia A and von Willebrand's disease –
Adults and children: 0.3 mcg/kg diluted in normal saline and infused I.V. slowly over 15 to 30 minutes. May repeat dose if necessary as indicated by laboratory response and the patient's clinical condition.
Primary nocturnal enuresis –
Children 5 years and over: initially, 20 mcg intranasally h.s. Adjust dose according to response. Maximum recommended dose is 40 mcg daily.

CONTRAINDICATIONS & PRECAUTIONS

Contraindicated in patients with hypersensitivity to the drug. Use cautiously in patients with allergic rhinitis, nasal congestion, or upper respiratory infection because these states may interfere with the drug's absorption. Large doses may produce a slight rise in blood pressure when used in patients with coronary artery disease or hypertension.

ADVERSE REACTIONS

Common reactions are in italics; life-threatening reactions are in bold italics.
CNS: headache.
CV: slight rise in blood pressure at high dosage.
EENT: nasal congestion, rhinitis.
GI: nausea.
GU: vulval pain.
Other: flushing.

INTERACTIONS

None significant.

EFFECTS ON DIAGNOSTIC TESTS

None reported.

NURSING CONSIDERATIONS

Besides those related universally to drug therapy (see "How to use this book"), consider the following specific recommendations:

Assessment

• Obtain a baseline assessment of the patient's underlying condition before initiating desmopressin therapy.
• Be alert for adverse reactions throughout therapy.
• Evaluate the patient's and family's knowledge about desmopressin therapy.

Nursing Diagnoses

• Fluid volume deficit related to the patient's underlying condition.
• Pain related to desmopressin-induced headache.
• Knowledge deficit related to desmopressin therapy.

Planning and Implementation

Preparation and Administration

• Check expiration date before administering.
• ***Intranasal route use:*** Administer desmopressin through a flexible catheter called a rhinyle. Draw up the correct dosage into the catheter, and insert one end into the patient's nose. The patient blows on the other end to deposit drug into nasal cavity.
• When desmopressin is used to treat diabetes insipidus, dosage or frequency of administration may be adjusted according to the patient's fluid output; adjust morning and evening doses separately for adequate diurnal rhythm of water turnover.
• For treating nocturnal enuresis, the recommended method of administration is one-half of the calculated dose in each nostril.
• Do not administer a desmopressin injection to treat hemophilia with factor VIII levels of 0% to 5% or to treat severe cases of von Willebrand's disease.

Monitoring

• Monitor effectiveness by regularly checking the patient's intake and output, serum and urine osmolality, and urine specific gravity for treatment of diabetes insipidus or relief of symptoms of other disorders.
• Monitor for early signs of water intoxication—drowsiness, listlessness, headache, confusion, anuria, and weight gain—to prevent seizures, coma, and death.
• Monitor the patient's weight daily and observe for edema.
• Monitor carefully for hypertension during high-dose treatment.

Supportive Care

• Adjust the patient's fluid intake to reduce risk of water intoxication and of sodium depletion, especially in young or elderly patients.
• Overdose may cause oxytoxic or vasopressor activity. Withhold drug as prescribed until effects subside. Furosemide may be used if fluid retention is excessive.
• Be aware that intranasal use can cause changes in the nasal mucosa resulting in erratic, unreliable absorption. Report any patient's worsening condition to doctor, who may prescribe injectable DDAVP.
• Administer a mild analgesic for drug-induced headache, if not contraindicated.
• Offer patient ice chips or frequent sips of water if nausea occurs. If nausea persists or becomes severe, obtain an order for an antiemetic.

Patient Teaching

• Some patients may have difficulty measuring and inhaling drug into nostrils. Teach them correct administration technique, then evaluate their proficiency at drug administration and accurate measurement on return visits.
• Warn the patient not to increase or decrease dosage unless instructed by doctor.
• Review fluid intake measurement

and methods for measuring fluid output with patient.
• Tell the patient to contact doctor if signs of water intoxication (drowsiness, listlessness, headache, or shortness of breath) develop.
• Advise the patient to wear medical alert identification.
• Instruct the patient to clear nasal passages before administering drug.
• Teach patients using S.C. desmopressin to rotate injection sites to prevent tissue damage.
• Nasal congestion, allergic rhinitis, or upper respiratory infections may impair drug absorption. Advise the patient to report such conditions to the doctor because they may require dosage adjustment.
• Tell patient to store drug away from heat and direct light. Do not store in bathroom, where heat and moisture can cause drug to deteriorate.

Evaluation

In patients receiving desmopressin, appropriate evaluation statements may include:
• Patient achieves normal fluid and electrolyte balance.
• Headache is relieved with mild analgesic.
• Patient and family state an understanding of desmopressin therapy.

desonide

(dess´ oh nide)
DesOwen, Tridesilon

• *Classification:* topical anti-inflammatory (adrenocorticoid)
• *Pregnancy Risk Category:* C

HOW SUPPLIED

Cream: 0.05%
Ointment: 0.05%

ACTION

Mechanism: Produces local anti-inflammatory, vasoconstrictor, and antipruritic actions. Drug diffuses across cell membranes to form complexes with specific cytoplasmic receptors, influencing cellular metabolism. Corticosteroids stabilize leukocyte lysosomal membranes, inhibit local actions and accumulation of macrophages, decrease local edema, and reduce the formation of scar tissue.
Absorption: Amount absorbed depends on the amount applied and on the nature of the skin at the application site. It ranges from about 1% in areas with thick stratum corneum (on the palms, soles, elbows, and knees) to as high as 36% in thinner areas (face, eyelids, and genitals). Absorption increases in areas of skin damage, inflammation, or occlusion. Some systemic absorption of topical steroids may occur, especially through the oral mucosa.
Distribution: After topical application, distributed throughout the local skin layer. Any drug that is absorbed is removed rapidly from the blood and distributed into muscle, liver, skin, intestines, and kidneys.
Metabolism: After topical administration, metabolized primarily in the skin. The small amount absorbed into systemic circulation is metabolized primarily in the liver to inactive compounds.
Excretion: Inactive metabolites are excreted by the kidneys, primarily as glucuronides and sulfates, but also as unconjugated products. Small amounts of the metabolites are also excreted in feces.

INDICATIONS & DOSAGE

Adjunctive therapy for inflammation in acute and chronic corticosteroid-responsive dermatoses–
Adults and children: clean area; apply cream or lotion sparingly b.i.d. to q.i.d.

CONTRAINDICATIONS & PRECAUTIONS

Contraindicated in patients who are hypersensitive to any component of the preparation and in patients with viral, fungal, or tubercular skin lesions. Use with extreme caution in patients with impaired circulation, because the drug may increase the risk of skin ulceration.

ADVERSE REACTIONS

Common reactions are in italics; life-threatening reactions are in bold italics.

Skin: burning, itching, irritation, dryness, folliculitis, perioral dermatitis, allergic contact dermatitis, hypertrichosis, hypopigmentation, acneiform eruptions. With occlusive dressings: *maceration of skin, secondary infection, atrophy, striae, miliaria.*

INTERACTIONS

None significant.

EFFECTS ON DIAGNOSTIC TESTS

None reported.

NURSING CONSIDERATIONS

Besides those related universally to drug therapy (see "How to use this book"), consider the following specific recommendations:

Assessment

- Obtain a baseline assessment of patient's skin in the affected area before therapy.
- Be alert for adverse reactions and drug interactions throughout therapy.
- Evaluate the patient's and family's knowledge about desonide therapy.

Nursing Diagnoses

- Impaired skin integrity related to the patient's underlying condition.
- High risk for impaired skin integrity related to desonide-induced skin macerations.
- Knowledge deficit related to desonide therapy.

Planning and Implementation

Preparation and Administration

- ***Topical use:*** Wash skin gently before applying. Rub medication in gently to prevent skin damage, leaving a thin coat. When treating hairy sites, part hair and apply directly to lesion.
- To apply an occlusive dressing: Apply cream or ointment, then cover with a thin, pliable, nonflammable plastic film; seal to adjacent normal skin with hypoallergenic tape. Minimize adverse reactions by using occlusive dressing intermittently. Don't leave in place longer than 16 hours each day. Occlusive dressings should not be used in presence of infection or with weeping or exudative lesions.
- For patient with eczematous dermatitis who may develop irritation with adhesive material, hold dressings in place with gauze, elastic bandages, stockings, or stockinette.

Monitoring

- Monitor effectiveness by checking patient's skin regularly in the affected area.
- Observe patient for signs of systemic absorption: skin irritation or ulceration, hypersensitivity, or infection. If these develop, stop drug and notify doctor. (If antifungals or antibiotics are being used with corticosteroids and infection does not respond immediately, corticosteroids should be discontinued until infection is controlled.)
- Check patient's temperature regularly; if fever develops, remove occlusive dressing and notify doctor.
- Monitor for adverse reactions and interactions by frequently inspecting his skin for infection, striae, and atrophy.

Supportive Care

- Change the patient's dressings as ordered and be prepared to discontinue drug and notify doctor if infection, striae, or atrophy occur.
- Use cautiously in patients with viral skin diseases, such as varicella, vacci-

nia, or herpes simplex; fungal infections; or bacterial skin infections.
• Systemic absorption is especially likely with occlusive dressings, prolonged treatment, or extensive body-surface treatment.
• When used on diaper area in young children, avoid the use of plastic pants or tight-fitting diapers.
• Notify doctor if adverse reactions occur.
• Expect treatment to continue for a few days after clearing of lesions to prevent recurrence.

Patient Teaching
• Teach patient how to apply medication.
• Instruct patient to avoid application near eyes, mucous membranes, or in ear canal.
• Inform patient of adverse reactions and instruct him to notify doctor if they occur.

Evaluation
In patients receiving desonide, appropriate evaluation statements may include:
• Patient states his dermatoses is resolving.
• Patient did not develop drug-induced impaired skin integrity.
• Patient and family state an understanding of desonide therapy.

desoximetasone
(des ox i met´ a sone)
Topicort

• *Classification:* topical anti-inflammatory (adrenocorticoid)
• *Pregnancy Risk Category:* C

HOW SUPPLIED
Cream: 0.05%, 0.25%
Gel: 0.05%
Ointment: 0.25%

ACTION
Mechanism: Produces local anti-inflammatory, vasoconstrictor, and antipruritic actions. Drug diffuses across cell membranes to form complexes with specific cytoplasmic receptors, influencing cellular metabolism. Corticosteroids stabilize leukocyte lysosomal membranes, inhibit local actions and accumulation of macrophages, decrease local edema, and reduce the formation of scar tissue.
Absorption: Amount absorbed depends on the amount applied and on the nature of the skin at the application site. It ranges from about 1% in areas with thick stratum corneum (on the palms, soles, elbows, and knees) to as high as 36% in thinnest areas (face, eyelids, and genitals). Absorption increases in areas of skin damage, inflammation, or occlusion. Some systemic absorption of topical steroids may occur, especially through the oral mucosa.
Distribution: After topical application, distributed throughout the local skin layer. Absorbed drug is removed rapidly from the blood and distributed into muscle, liver, skin, intestines, and kidneys.
Metabolism: After topical administration, metabolized primarily in the skin. The small amount that is absorbed into systemic circulation is metabolized primarily in the liver to inactive compounds.
Excretion: Inactive metabolites are excreted by the kidneys, primarily as glucuronides and sulfates, but also as unconjugated products. Small amounts of the metabolites are also excreted in feces.

INDICATIONS & DOSAGE
Inflammation of corticosteroid-responsive dermatoses—
Adults and children: clean area; apply cream, gel, or ointment sparingly once daily to b.i.d.

CONTRAINDICATIONS & PRECAUTIONS

Contraindicated in patients who are hypersensitive to any component of the preparation and in patients with viral, fungal, or tubercular skin lesions. Use with extreme caution in patients with impaired circulation, because the drug may increase the risk of skin ulceration. Avoid using on the face and genital areas because increased absorption may result in striae.

ADVERSE REACTIONS

Common reactions are in italics; life-threatening reactions are in bold italics.
Skin: burning, itching, irritation, dryness, folliculitis, hypertrichosis, acneiform eruptions, perioral dermatitis, hypopigmentation, allergic contact dermatitis. With occlusive dressings: *maceration of skin, secondary infection, atrophy, striae, miliaria.*

INTERACTIONS

None significant.

EFFECTS ON DIAGNOSTIC TESTS

None reported.

NURSING CONSIDERATIONS

Besides those related universally to drug therapy (see "How to use this book"), consider the following specific recommendations:

Assessment

- Obtain a baseline assessment of patient's skin in the affected area before therapy.
- Be alert for adverse reactions and drug interactions throughout therapy.
- Evaluate the patient's and family's knowledge about desoximetasone therapy.

Nursing Diagnoses

- Impaired skin integrity related to the patient's underlying condition.
- High risk for impaired skin integrity related to desoximetasone-induced skin maceration.
- Knowledge deficit related to desoximetasone therapy.

Planning and Implementation

Preparation and Administration

- ***Topical use:*** Wash skin gently before applying. Rub medication in gently to prevent damage to skin, leaving a thin coat. When treating hairy sites, part hair and apply directly to lesions.
- To apply an occlusive dressing: Apply cream, then cover with a thin, pliable, nonflammable plastic film; seal to adjacent normal skin with hypoallergenic tape. To minimize adverse reactions, use occlusive dressing intermittently. Don't leave in place longer than 16 hours each day. Occlusive dressing should not be used in presence of infection or with weeping or exudative lesions.
- For patient with eczematous dermatitis who may develop irritation with adhesive material, hold dressings in place with gauze, elastic bandages, stockings, or stockinette.
- Store in tightly sealed containers.

Monitoring

- Monitor effectiveness by regularly examining the affected area of the skin.
- Observe patient for signs of systemic absorption: skin irritation or ulceration, hypersensitivity, or infection. If these develop, stop drug and notify doctor. (If antifungals or antibiotics are being used with corticosteroids and infection does not respond immediately, corticosteroids should be stopped until infection is controlled.)
- Check patient's temperature; if fever occurs, notify doctor and remove occlusive dressing.
- Monitor for adverse reactions and interactions by observing for secondary infection.

Supportive Care

- Change dressing as ordered. Inspect skin for infection, striae, and atrophy.

Discontinue drug and notify doctor if these occur.
- Use cautiously in patients with viral skin diseases such as varicella, vaccinia, or herpes simplex; fungal infections; or bacterial skin infections.
- When used on diaper area in young children, avoid the use of plastic pants or tight-fitting diapers.
- Systemic absorption is especially likely with occlusive dressings, prolonged treatment, or extensive body-surface treatment.
- Expect treatment to continue for a few days after clearing of lesions to prevent recurrence.
- Notify doctor if adverse drug reactions occur.

Patient Teaching
- Teach patient how to apply medication.
- Inform patient that gel contains alcohol and may cause burning or irritation in open lesions.

Evaluation

In patients receiving desoximetasone, appropriate evaluation statements may include:
- Patient states his dermatoses has healed.
- Patient did not develop skin maceration.
- Patient and family state an understanding of desoximetasone therapy.

---

dexamethasone (ophthalmic)
(dex a meth´ a sone)
Maxidex Ophthalmic Suspension

dexamethasone sodium phosphate
Decadron Phosphate Ophthalmic, Maxidex Ophthalmic

- *Classification:* anti-inflammatory, immunosuppressant (glucocorticoid)
- *Pregnancy Risk Category:* C

HOW SUPPLIED
dexamethasone
Ophthalmic suspension: 0.01%
dexamethasone sodium phosphate
Ophthalmic ointment: 0.05%
Ophthalmic solution: 0.1%

ACTION
Mechanism: A corticosteroid that decreases the inflammatory response. Exact mechanism unknown; drug inhibits edema formation, prevents fibrin deposition, and blocks infiltration of phagocytes and leukocytes at the site of inflammation.
Absorption: After ophthalmic administration, dexamethasone is absorbed through the aqueous humor. Because only low doses are administered, little if any systemic absorption occurs.
Distribution: Throughout the local tissue layers.
Metabolism: Primarily metabolized locally. The small amount that is absorbed into systemic circulation is metabolized primarily in the liver to inactive compounds.

INDICATIONS & DOSAGE
Uveitis; iridocyclitis; inflammatory conditions of eyelids, conjunctiva, cornea, anterior segment of globe; corneal injury from chemical or thermal burns, or penetration of foreign bodies; allergic conjunctivitis–
Adults and children: instill 1 to 2 drops of 0.01% suspension or 0.1% solution into conjunctival sac. In severe disease, drops may be used hourly, tapering to discontinuation as condition improves. In mild conditions, drops may be used up to four to six times daily or ointment applied q.i.d. As condition improves, taper dosage to b.i.d. then once daily. Treatment may extend from a few days to several weeks.

CONTRAINDICATIONS & PRECAUTIONS

Contraindicated in patients who are hypersensitive to any component of the preparation; in patients with fungal infections of the eye; and in patients with acute, untreated purulent bacterial, viral, or fungal ocular infections. Use cautiously in patients with corneal abrasions. If a bacterial infection does not respond promptly to appropriate anti-infective therapy, discontinue therapy.

ADVERSE REACTIONS

Common reactions are in italics; life-threatening reactions are in bold italics.

Eye: increased intraocular pressure; thinning of cornea, interference with corneal wound healing, increased susceptibility to viral or fungal corneal infection, corneal ulceration; with excessive or long-term use, glaucoma exacerbations, cataracts, defects in visual acuity and visual field, optic nerve damage; mild blurred vision; burning, stinging, or redness of eyes; watery eyes.

Other: systemic effects and adrenal suppression with excessive or long-term use.

INTERACTIONS

None significant.

EFFECTS ON DIAGNOSTIC TESTS

None reported.

NURSING CONSIDERATIONS

Besides those related universally to drug therapy (see "How to use this book"), consider the following specific recommendations:

Assessment

- Obtain a baseline assessment of the patient's allergies and report of culture of the eye before therapy.
- Be alert for adverse reactions or drug interactions throughout therapy.
- Evaluate the patient's and family's knowledge about ophthalmic dexamethasone therapy.

Nursing Diagnoses

- Altered protection related to ocular inflammatory process.
- High risk for infection related to dexamethasone-induced viral or fungal infections.
- Knowledge deficit related to ophthalmic dexamethasone therapy.

Planning and Implementation

Preparation and Administration

- Read label carefully; give the correct form of the drug.
- Shake the suspension well before using.
- Wash hands before and after administration.
- May use eye pad with ointment.

Monitoring

- Monitor effectiveness by checking the eye for decreasing signs of inflammation.
- Monitor the patient for changes in visual acuity or visual field.
- Intraocular pressure should be measured every 2 to 4 weeks for the first 2 months of ophthalmic corticosteroid therapy and then, if no increase in intraocular pressure has occurred, every 1 to 2 months thereafter. Dexamethasone is more likely than other ophthalmic products to increase intraocular pressure in susceptible patients.

Supportive Care

- Use safety precautions if vision is impaired. Assist with activities.
- Dexamethasone has greater anti-inflammatory effect than dexamethasone sodium phosphate.
- Do not give in acute superficial herpes simplex (dendritic keratitis), vaccinia, varicella, or other fungal or viral diseases of cornea and conjunctiva; ocular tuberculosis, or any acute, purulent, untreated infection of the eye.
- Use with caution in corneal abrasions, since these may be infected (especially with herpes); in glaucoma

(any form) because of the possibility of increasing intraocular pressure (glaucoma medications may need to be increased to compensate).
• Viral and fungal infections of the cornea may be exacerbated by the application of steroids.
• Not for long-term use.
Patient Teaching
• Teach the patient to instill. Advise him to wash hands before and after administration. Warn him not to touch dropper tip to eye or surrounding tissues.
• Instruct the patient to apply light finger pressure to the lacrimal sac for 1 minute after instilling the drops. Caution him to avoid scratching or rubbing the eye area.
• Warn the patient to notify the doctor immediately and stop using the drug if visual acuity changes or visual field diminishes.
• Advise the patient not to use leftover medications for a new eye inflammation.
• Instruct the patient not to share eye medication with family members. If a family member develops the same symptoms, contact the doctor.
Evaluation
In patients receiving ophthalmic dexamethasone, appropriate evaluation statements may include:
• Patient demonstrates decrease or absence of inflammation.
• Patient remains free from signs and symptoms of viral or fungal infection.
• Patient and family state an understanding of ophthalmic dexamethasone therapy.

---

dexamethasone (systemic)
(dex a meth´ a sone)
Decadron, Deronil, Dexasone†, Dexone, Hexadrol, Mymethasone

dexamethasone acetate
Dalalone D.P., Dalalone L.A., Decadron L.A., Decaject-L.A., Decameth L.A., Dexacen LA, Dexasone-LA, Dexone LA, Dexon LA, Solurex-LA

dexamethasone sodium phosphate
Ak-Dex, Dalalone, Decadrol, Decadron Phosphate, Decaject, Decameth, Dex, Dexacen, Dexasone, Dexon, Dexone, Hexadrol Phosphate, Solurex

• *Classification:* anti-inflammatory agent (glucocorticoid)
• *Pregnancy Risk Category:* C

HOW SUPPLIED
dexamethasone
Tablets: 0.25 mg, 0.5 mg, 0.75 mg, 1 mg, 1.5 mg, 2 mg, 4 mg, 6 mg
Oral solution: 0.5 mg/5 ml, 0.5 mg/0.5 ml
Elixir: 0.5 mg/5 ml
dexamethasone acetate
Injection: 8 mg/ml, 16 mg/ml suspension
dexamethasone sodium phosphate
Injection: 4 mg/ml, 10 mg/ml, 20 mg/ml, 24 mg/ml

ACTION
Mechanism: Decreases inflammation, mainly by stabilizing leukocyte lysosomal membranes. Also suppresses the immune response, stimulates bone marrow, and influences protein, fat, and carbohydrate metabolism.
Absorption: Readily absorbed after oral administration.
Distribution: Rapidly removed from the blood and distributed to muscle, liver, skin, intestines, and kidneys; weakly bound to plasma proteins (transcortin and albumin). Only the unbound portion is active. Adrenocorticoids are distributed into breast milk and through the placenta.

Metabolism: In the liver to inactive glucuronide and sulfate metabolites.
Excretion: The inactive metabolites and small amounts of unmetabolized drug are excreted by the kidneys. Insignificant amounts are also excreted in feces. Half-life: 36 to 54 hours.
Onset, peak, duration: After oral administration, peak effects occur in about 1 to 2 hours. The suspension for injection has a variable onset and duration of action (ranging from 2 days to 3 weeks), depending on site of injection (intra-articular space, muscle, or the blood supply to the muscle).

INDICATIONS & DOSAGE

Cerebral edema –
Adults: initially, 10 mg (phosphate) I.V., then 4 to 6 mg I.M. q 6 hours for 2 to 4 days, then tapered over 5 to 7 days.
Children: initially, 0.5 to 1.5 mg/kg I.V. daily; then 0.2 to 0.5 mg/kg I.V. daily in divided doses q 6 hours.
Inflammatory conditions, allergic reactions, neoplasias –
Adults: 0.25 to 4 mg P.O. b.i.d., t.i.d., or q.i.d.; or 4 to 16 mg (acetate) I.M. into joint or soft tissue q 1 to 3 weeks; or 0.8 to 1.6 mg (acetate) into lesions q 1 to 3 weeks.
Shock –
Adults: 1 to 6 mg/kg (phosphate) I.V. single dosage; or 40 mg I.V. q 2 to 6 hours, p.r.n.
Dexamethasone suppression test –
Adults: 0.5 mg P.O. q 6 hours for 48 hours.

CONTRAINDICATIONS & PRECAUTIONS

Contraindicated in patients who are hypersensitive to ingredients of adrenocorticoid preparations and in those with systemic fungal infections (except in adrenal insufficiency). Patients who are receiving dexamethasone should not be given live virus vaccines because dexamethasone suppresses the immune response.

Use with extreme caution in patients with GI ulceration, renal disease, hypertension, osteoporosis, diabetes mellitus, thromboembolytic disorders, seizures, myasthenia gravis, CHF, tuberculosis, hypoalbuminemia, hypothyroidism, cirrhosis of the liver, emotional instability, psychotic tendencies, hyperlipidemias, glaucoma, or cataracts because the drug may exacerbate these conditions.

Because adrenocorticoids increase susceptibility to and mask symptoms of infection, do not use (except in life-threatening situations) in patients with viral or bacterial infections not controlled by anti-infective agents.

ADVERSE REACTIONS

Common reactions are in italics; life-threatening reactions are in bold italics.

Most adverse reactions of corticosteroids are dose- or duration-dependent.
CNS: *euphoria, insomnia,* psychotic behavior, pseudotumor cerebri.
CV: ***CHF,*** hypertension, edema.
EENT: cataracts, glaucoma.
GI: *peptic ulcer,* GI irritation, increased appetite.
Metabolic: *possible hypokalemia, hyperglycemia and carbohydrate intolerance,* growth suppression in children.
Skin: delayed wound healing, acne, various skin eruptions.
Local: atrophy at I.M. injection sites.
Other: muscle weakness, pancreatitis, hirsutism, susceptibility to infections.
Acute adrenal insufficiency may follow increased stress (infection, surgery, or trauma) or abrupt withdrawal after long-term therapy.
Withdrawal symptoms: rebound inflammation, fatigue, weakness, arthralgia, fever, dizziness, lethargy, depression, fainting, orthostatic hypotension, dyspnea, anorexia, hypogly-

cemia. ***Sudden withdrawal may be fatal.***

INTERACTIONS

Barbiturates, phenytoin, rifampin: decreased corticosteroid effect. Corticosteroid dose may need to be increased.
Indomethacin, aspirin: increased risk of GI distress and bleeding. Give together cautiously.

EFFECTS ON DIAGNOSTIC TESTS

Diagnostic skin tests: suppressed reactions.
Glucose and cholesterol levels: increased levels.
Nitroblue tetrazolium test for systemic bacterial infections: false-negative results.
Serum potassium, calcium, thyroxine, and triiodothyronine: decreased levels.
Thyroid function tests: decreases ^{131}I uptake and protein-bound iodine concentrations.
Urine glucose and calcium levels: increased levels.

NURSING CONSIDERATIONS

Besides those related universally to drug therapy (see "How to use this book"), consider the following specific recommendations:

Assessment
- Obtain a baseline assessment of the underlying condition before initiating drug therapy.
- Be alert for common adverse reactions and drug interactions throughout therapy.
- Evaluate the patient's and family's knowledge about dexamethasone therapy.

Nursing Diagnoses
- Impaired tissue integrity related to the underlying condition.
- High risk for injury related to dexamethasone-induced adverse reactions.
- Knowledge deficit related to dexamethasone therapy.

Planning and Implementation

Preparation and Administration
- Do not use for alternate-day therapy.
- Gradually reduce drug dosage after long-term therapy. Never abruptly discontinue therapy as sudden withdrawal can be fatal.
- Always titrate to lowest effective dose as prescribed.
- Give a daily dosage in the morning for better results and less toxicity.
- Expect to increase dosage as prescribed during times of physiological stress (surgery, trauma, or infection).
- ***P.O. use:*** Give with food when possible to avoid GI upset.
- ***I.M. use:*** Give injection deep into gluteal muscle. Rotate injection sites to prevent muscle atrophy. Avoid S.C. injection, because atrophy and sterile abscesses may occur.
- ***I.V. use:*** When administering as direct injection, inject undiluted over at least 1 minute. When administering as an intermittent or continuous infusion, dilute solution according to manufacturer's instructions and give over the prescribed duration. If used for continuous infusion, change solution every 24 hours.

Monitoring
- Monitor effectiveness by regularly assessing for improvement of signs and symptoms of the underlying condition.
- Monitor for signs of peptic ulcer, hypokalemia, and hyperglycemia because dexamethasone can cause serious or even life-threatening multisystem dysfunction.
- Monitor the patient's weight, blood pressure, blood glucose level, and serum electrolyte levels regularly.
- Monitor the patient for infection. Drug may mask or exacerbate infections.
- Monitor the patient's stress level. Stress (fever, trauma, surgery, or emo-

tional problems) may increase adrenal insufficiency. Dose may have to be increased.
• Monitor the patient's mental status for depression or psychotic episodes, especially in high-dose therapy.
• Monitor the patient's skin for petechiae.
• Monitor growth in infants and children on long-term therapy.
• Monitor patients receiving immunizations for decreased antibody response.
• Monitor the patient for early signs of adrenal insufficiency or cushingoid symptoms.

Supportive Care
• Unless contraindicated, give the patient a low-sodium diet high in potassium and protein. Potassium supplement may be needed.
• Be aware that diabetic patients may have increased insulin requirements.

Patient Teaching
• Be sure that the patient understands the need to take the drug as prescribed. Tell the patient if a dose is inadvertently missed, to take it as soon as the patient remembers. However, the patient should not take two doses together.
• Warn the patient not to discontinue the drug abruptly or without the doctor's approval.
• Advise the patient to take oral form with meals to minimize GI adverse reactions.
• Inform the patient of the possible therapeutic and adverse effects of the drug, so that he may report complications to the doctor as soon as possible.
• Tell the patient to carry a medical alert card indicating the need for supplemental adrenocorticoids during stress.
• Teach the patient to recognize signs of early adrenal insufficiency (fatigue, muscular weakness, joint pain, fever, anorexia, nausea, dyspnea, dizziness, and fainting) and to notify the doctor promptly if they occur.
• Warn patients on long-term therapy about cushingoid symptoms, which may develop regardless of route of administration.
• Warn patient about easy bruising.
• Tell patient to eat a low-sodium diet that is high in potassium and protein unless contraindicated.

Evaluation
In patients receiving dexamethasone, appropriate evaluation statements may include:
• Patient's condition being treated with dexamethasone therapy shows improvement.
• Patient does not experience serious adverse reactions associated with dexamethasone.
• Patient and family state an understanding of dexamethasone therapy.

dexamethasone (topical)
(dex a meth´ a sone)
Aeroseb-Dex, Decaderm, Decaspray

dexamethasone sodium phosphate
Decadron Phosphate

• *Classification:* anti-inflammatory agent (glucocorticoid)
• *Pregnancy Risk Category:* C

HOW SUPPLIED
dexamethasone
Aerosol: 0.01%, 0.04%
Gel: 0.1%
dexamethasone sodium phosphate
Cream: 0.1%

ACTION
Mechanism: Produces local anti-inflammatory, vasoconstrictor, and antipruritic actions. Drug diffuses across cell membranes to form complexes with specific cytoplasmic receptors, influencing cellular metabo-

lism. Corticosteroids stabilize leukocyte lysosomal membranes, inhibit local actions and accumulation of macrophages, decrease local edema, and reduce the formation of scar tissue.
Absorption: Once absorbed through the skin, topical corticosteroids are handled through pharmacokinetic pathways similar to systemically administered corticosteroids.
Distribution: Bound to plasma proteins in varying degrees.
Metabolism: Primarily in the liver.
Excretion: By the kidneys. Some topical corticosteroids and their metabolites are also excreted into the bile.

INDICATIONS & DOSAGE

Inflammation of corticosteroid-responsive dermatoses–
Adults and children: clean area; apply cream, gel, or aerosol sparingly b.i.d. to q.i.d.

Aerosol use on scalp–shake can well and apply to dry scalp after shampooing. Hold can upright. Slide applicator tube under hair so that it touches scalp. Spray while moving tube to all affected areas, keeping tube under hair and in contact with scalp throughout spraying, which should take about 2 seconds. Inadequately covered areas may be spot sprayed. Slide applicator tube through hair to touch scalp, press and immediately release spray button. Don't massage medication into scalp or spray forehead or eyes.

CONTRAINDICATIONS & PRECAUTIONS

Contraindicated in patients who are hypersensitive to any component of the preparation and in patients with viral, fungal, or tubercular skin lesions. Use with extreme caution in patients with impaired circulation, because the drug may increase the risk of skin ulceration.

ADVERSE REACTIONS

Common reactions are in italics; life-threatening reactions are in bold italics.
Skin: burning, itching, irritation, dryness, folliculitis, hypertrichosis, acneiform eruptions, perioral dermatitis, hypopigmentation, allergic contact dermatitis. With occlusive dressings: *maceration of skin, secondary infection, atrophy, striae, miliaria.*

INTERACTIONS

None significant.

EFFECTS ON DIAGNOSTIC TESTS

None reported.

NURSING CONSIDERATIONS

Besides those related universally to drug therapy (see "How to use this book"), consider the following specific recommendations:

Assessment
- Obtain a baseline assessment of patient's skin in the affected area before therapy.
- Be alert for adverse reactions and drug interactions throughout therapy.
- Evaluate the patient's and family's knowledge about dexamethasone therapy.

Nursing Diagnoses
- Impaired skin integrity related to the patient's underlying condition.
- High risk for infection related to dexamethasone-induced secondary infection.
- Knowledge deficit related to topical dexamethasone therapy.

Planning and Implementation
Preparation and Administration
- ***Topical use:*** Wash skin gently before applying. Rub medication in gently to prevent damage to skin, leaving a thin coat. When treating hairy sites, part hair and apply directly to lesions.
- For patient with eczematous dermatitis who may develop irritation with adhesive material, hold dressing in

place with gauze, elastic bandages, stockings, or stockinette.
• Occlusive dressing should not be used in presence of infection or weeping or exudative lesions.
Monitoring
• Monitor effectiveness by examining patient's skin in the affected area.
• Observe for signs of systemic absorption–skin irritation, or ulceration, hypersensitivity, or infection. If these occur, discontinue drug and notify doctor. (If antifungals or antibiotics are being used with corticosteroids and infection does not respond immediately, corticosteroids should be stopped until infection is controlled.)
• Check patient's temperature; if fever develops, notify doctor and remove dressing.
• Monitor for adverse reactions or interactions by frequently inspecting the patient's skin for infection, striae, and atrophy.
Supportive Care
• Change the patient's dressings as ordered by the doctor and be prepared to discontinue drug and notify doctor if infection, striae, or atrophy occur.
• Use cautiously in patients with viral skin diseases, such as varicella, vaccinia, or herpes simplex; fungal infections; or bacterial skin infections.
• When used on diaper area in young children, avoid the use of plastic pants or tight-fitting diapers.
• Systemic absorption is especially likely with occlusive dressings, prolonged treatment, or extensive body-surface treatment.
• Expect treatment to continue for a few days after clearing of lesions to prevent recurrence.
Patient Teaching
• Teach patient how to apply medication.
• Instruct patient to avoid application near eyes, mucous membranes, or in ear canal.
• Inform patient that aerosol preparation contains alcohol and may produce irritation or burning in open lesions. When using about the face, cover patient's eyes and warn against inhalation of the spray. To avoid freezing tissues, do not spray longer than 3 seconds or closer than 6″ (15 cm).
• Inform patient about adverse reactions; if they occur, tell patient to notify doctor and stop drug.
Evaluation
In patients receiving topical dexamethasone, appropriate evaluation statements may include:
• Patient states his dermatoses is healing.
• Patient does not develop secondary infection.
• Patient and family state an understanding of topical dexamethasone therapy.

dexamethasone sodium phosphate
(dex a meth´ a sone)
Decadron Phosphate Turbinaire

• *Classification:* anti-inflammatory agent (glucocorticoid)
• *Pregnancy Risk Category:* C

HOW SUPPLIED
Nasal aerosol: 84 mcg/metered spray, 170 doses/canister

ACTION
Mechanism: Produces local anti-inflammatory, vasoconstrictor, and antipruritic actions. Diffuses across cell membranes to form complexes with specific cytoplasmic receptors, influencing cellular metabolism. Corticosteroids stabilize leukocyte lysosomal membranes, inhibit local actions and accumulation of macrophages, decrease local edema, and reduce the formation of scar tissue.

Absorption: Drug is absorbed from the nasal mucosa. Systemic effects may occur after prolonged use.
Distribution: Rapidly removed from the blood and distributed to muscle, liver, skin, intestines, and kidneys; weakly bound to plasma proteins (transcortin and albumin). Only the unbound protein is active. Adrenocorticoids are distributed into breast milk and through the placenta.
Metabolism: In the liver to inactive glucuronide and sulfate metabolites.
Excretion: The inactive metabolites and small amounts of unmetabolized drug are excreted by the kidneys; insignificant amounts are also excreted in feces. Half-life: 36 to 54 hours.

INDICATIONS & DOSAGE

Allergic or inflammatory conditions, nasal polyps–
Adults: 2 sprays in each nostril b.i.d. or t.i.d. Maximum 12 sprays daily.
Children 6 to 12 years: 1 or 2 sprays in each nostril b.i.d. Maximum 8 sprays daily.

Each spray delivers 0.1 mg dexamethasone sodium phosphate equal to 0.084 mg dexamethasone.

CONTRAINDICATIONS & PRECAUTIONS

Contraindicated in patients with acute status asthmaticus, hypersensitivity to any component of the preparation, or nasal infections. Use with caution in patients receiving systemic corticosteroids, because of increased risk of hypothalamic-pituitary-adrenal axis suppression; when substituting inhalant for oral systemic administration, because withdrawal symptoms may occur; and in patients with healing nasal septal ulcers, oral or nasal surgery, or trauma.

Prolonged use may produce posterior subcapsular cataracts or glaucoma with possible damage to the optic nerves, and may enhance secondary ocular infections from fungi or viruses.

ADVERSE REACTIONS

Common reactions are in italics; life-threatening reactions are in bold italics.
EENT: nasal irritation, dryness, rebound nasal congestion.
Other: hypersensitivity, systemic effects with prolonged use (pituitary-adrenal suppression, sodium retention, ***congestive heart failure,*** hypertension, hypokalemia, headaches, convulsions, peptic ulcer, ecchymoses, petechiae, masking of infection).

INTERACTIONS

None significant.

EFFECTS ON DIAGNOSTIC TESTS

None reported.

NURSING CONSIDERATIONS

Besides those related universally to drug therapy (see "How to use this book"), consider the following specific recommendations:

Assessment
- Obtain a baseline assessment of the patient's breathing pattern and degree of nasal congestion, and vital signs.
- Be alert for adverse reactions and drug interactions throughout therapy.
- Evaluate the patient's and family's knowledge about dexamethasone sodium phosphate therapy.

Nursing Diagnoses
- Ineffective airway clearance related to the patient's underlying condition.
- Impaired tissue integrity related to nasal irritation and dryness.
- Knowledge deficit related to dexamethasone sodium phosphate therapy.

Planning and Implementation
Preparation and Administration
- ***Inhalation:*** Shake container and invert. Patient should first clear nasal passages, then tilt head back. Insert nozzle into nostril, holding other nostril closed. Deliver spray while pa-

tient inspires. Shake container again and repeat in other nostril.

• Do not break, incinerate or store container in extreme heat (contents under pressure).

Monitoring

• Monitor effectiveness by assessing the patient's breathing pattern and degree of nasal congestion.

• Monitor BP, and fluid and electrolytes (especially serum potassium) for drug-induced fluid or sodium retention, hypertension, or hypokalemia.

• Frequently ask the patient about nasal irritation.

Supportive Care

• Notify the doctor immediately of any changes in the patient's health status including nasal irritation. The drug may have to be discontinued.

Patient Teaching

• Teach the patient how to use the spray and warn him that the medicine should be used by one person only.

• Teach the patient good nasal and oral hygiene.

• Warn mothers to avoid breast-feeding because systemic absorption may occur.

• Tell the patient that the drug is not for prolonged use; dosage should be reduced gradually as congestion improves.

• Advise the patient to report any unusual symptoms, and to continue with regular medical supervision.

Evaluation

In patients receiving dexamethasone sodium phosphate, appropriate evaluation statements may include:

• Patient achieves relief from nasal congestion.

• Nasal irritation has not occurred.

• Patient and family state an understanding of dexamethasone sodium phosphate therapy.

dexchlorpheniramine maleate

(dex klor fen eer´ a meen)

Dexchlor, Poladex TD, Polaramine*, Polaramine Repetabs, Polargen

• *Classification:* antihistamine (H_1-receptor antagonist), antipruritic (propylamine derivative)

• *Pregnancy Risk Category:* B

HOW SUPPLIED

Tablets: 2 mg

Tablets (timed-release): 4 mg, 6 mg

Syrup: 2 mg/5 ml*

ACTION

Mechanism: Competes with histamine for H_1-receptor sites on effector cells. Prevents but does not reverse histamine-mediated responses.

Absorption: Well absorbed from the GI tract.

Distribution: 70% protein-bound.

Metabolism: Hepatic.

Excretion: Drug and metabolites are excreted in urine. Half-life: Plasma half-life ranges from 20 to 24 hours.

Onset, peak, duration: Action begins within 30 minutes to 1 hour.

INDICATIONS & DOSAGE

Rhinitis, allergy symptoms, contact dermatitis, pruritus–

Adults: 2 mg P.O. q 4 to 6 hours, not to exceed 12 mg/day; or (timed-release) 4 to 6 mg b.i.d. or t.i.d.

Children 6 to 12 years: 1 mg P.O. q 4 to 6 hours, not to exceed 6 mg/day; or 4 mg (timed-release tablet) at bedtime.

Children 2 to 6 years: 0.5 mg P.O. q 4 to 6 hours, not to exceed 3 mg/day.

Note: Children under 6 years should use only as directed by a doctor. Do not use timed-release tablets for children younger than 6 years.

CONTRAINDICATIONS & PRECAUTIONS

Contraindicated in patients with hypersensitivity to this drug or other antihistamines with similar chemical structures (brompheniramine, chlorpheniramine, and triprolidine); during an acute asthmatic attack because dexchlorpheniramine thickens bronchial secretions; in patients who have taken monoamine oxidase (MAO) inhibitors within the preceding 2 weeks because these drugs prolong and intensify the effects of antihistamines; and during pregnancy (especially in the third trimester) or during breast-feeding. Antihistamines have caused seizures and other severe reactions have occurred, especially in premature infants.

Use cautiously in patients with narrow-angle glaucoma; in those with pyloroduodenal obstruction or urinary bladder obstruction from prostatic hypertrophy or narrowing of the bladder neck because of their marked anticholinergic effects; cardiovascular disease, hypertension, or hyperthyroidism because of the risk of palpitations and tachycardia; and renal disease, diabetes, bronchial asthma, urine retention, or stenosing peptic ulcers.

ADVERSE REACTIONS

Common reactions are in italics; life-threatening reactions are in bold italics.

CNS: (especially in elderly patients) *drowsiness,* dizziness, *stimulation.*

GI: nausea, *dry mouth.*

GU: polyuria, dysuria, urine retention.

INTERACTIONS

CNS depressants: increased sedation. Use together cautiously.

MAO inhibitors: increased anticholinergic effects. Don't use together.

EFFECTS ON DIAGNOSTIC TESTS

Diagnostic skin tests: test interference.

NURSING CONSIDERATIONS

Besides those related universally to drug therapy (see "How to use this book"), consider the following specific recommendations:

Assessment

- Obtain a baseline assessment of the patient's respiratory status and symptoms before beginning dexchlorpheniramine therapy.
- Be alert for adverse reactions or drug interactions during therapy.
- Evaluate the patient's and family's knowledge about dexchlorpheniramine therapy.

Nursing Diagnoses

- Ineffective airway clearance related to the patient's underlying condition.
- High risk for injury related to dexchlorpheniramine-induced CNS adverse reactions.
- Knowledge deficit related to dexchlorpheniramine maleate therapy.

Planning and Implementation

Preparation and Administration

- ***P.O. use:*** Store syrup between 15° C and 30° C (59° and 80° F) in a tightly closed container unless otherwise specified. Protect from freezing. Store tablets below 25° C (72° F) in a light-resistant, tight container unless otherwise specified.

Monitoring

- Monitor effectiveness by frequently evaluating severity of patient's symptoms and the patient's respiratory status, if the drug is given for rhinitis; and patient's comfort level and relief of allergic symptoms.
- Monitor for adverse CNS reactions, including drowsiness and stimulation.

Supportive Care

- Keep in mind that another antihistamine may be substituted if tolerance develops.

Patient Teaching
• Suggest to the patient that he drink coffee or tea to reduce drowsiness.
• Tell the patient that sugarless gum, sour hard candy, or ice chips may relieve dry mouth.
• Warn patient to avoid drinking alcoholic beverages during therapy and to avoid hazardous activities that require alertness until CNS effects are known. However, this drug causes less drowsiness than some other antihistamines.
• Warn patient to discontinue dexchlorpheniramine maleate 4 days before allergy skin testing to preserve the accuracy of the tests.
• Tell the patient that this drug is available as an OTC item for self-medication by adults; but use in children under age 6 is not recommended without a doctor's supervision.

Evaluation
In patients receiving dexchlorpheniramine maleate, appropriate evaluation statements may include:
• Patient's allergic symptoms are relieved with dexchlorpheniramine maleate.
• Injury did not occur; patient did not experience CNS adverse reactions.
• Patient and family state an understanding of dexchlorpheniramine maleate therapy.

dextroamphetamine sulfate

(dex troe am fet´ a meen)
Dexedrine* **, Ferndex, Oxydess II, Robese, Spancap #1

• Controlled Substance Schedule II
• *Classification:* CNS stimulant, short-term adjunctive anorexigenic, sympathomimetic amine (amphetamine)
• *Pregnancy Risk Category:* C

HOW SUPPLIED
Tablets: 5 mg, 10 mg
Capsules (sustained-release): 5 mg, 10 mg, 15 mg
Elixir: 5 mg/5 ml

ACTION
Mechanism: Promotes nerve impulse transmission by releasing stored norepinephrine from nerve terminals in the brain. In children with hyperkinesia, amphetamines have a paradoxical calming effect.
Absorption: Rapidly absorbed from the GI tract.
Distribution: Widely distributed throughout the body.
Excretion: In urine.
Onset, peak, duration: Peak serum concentrations occur 2 to 4 hours after oral administration; long-acting capsules are absorbed more slowly and have a longer duration of action.

INDICATIONS & DOSAGE
Narcolepsy–
Adults: 5 to 60 mg P.O. daily in divided doses.
Children over 12 years: 10 mg P.O. daily, with 10-mg increments weekly, p.r.n.
Children 6 to 12 years: 5 mg P.O. daily, with 5-mg increments weekly, p.r.n.
Short-term adjunct in exogenous obesity–
Adults: single 10- to 15-mg long-acting capsule, up to 30 mg daily; or in divided doses, 5 to 10 mg half hour before meals.
Attention deficit disorders with hyperactivity (ADDH)–
Children 6 years and older: 5 mg P.O. once daily or b.i.d., with 5-mg increments weekly, p.r.n.
Children 3 to 5 years: 2.5 mg P.O. daily, with 2.5-mg increments weekly, p.r.n.

*Liquid form contains alcohol. **May contain tartrazine.

CONTRAINDICATIONS & PRECAUTIONS

Contraindicated in patients with hypersensitivity or idiosyncratic reaction to amphetamines; in patients with hyperthyroidism, angina pectoris, glaucoma, any degree of hypertension, or other severe cardiovascular disease; and in patients with a history of substance abuse; also contraindicated for concomitant use with monoamine oxidase (MAO) inhibitors or within 14 days of discontinuing MAO inhibitors.

Use cautiously in patients with diabetes mellitus; in elderly, debilitated, or hyperexcitable patients; and in children with Gilles de la Tourette's syndrome. Amphetamine-induced CNS stimulation superimposed on CNS depression can cause seizures. Some formulations (Dexedrine) contain tartrazine, which may induce allergic reactions in hypersensitive individuals.

ADVERSE REACTIONS

Common reactions are in italics; life-threatening reactions are in bold italics.

CNS: *restlessness,* tremor, *hyperactivity, talkativeness, insomnia,* irritability, dizziness, headache, chills, overstimulation, dysphoria.
CV: *tachycardia, palpitations,* hypertension, hypotension.
GI: nausea, vomiting, cramps, dry mouth, diarrhea, constipation, metallic taste, anorexia, weight loss.
Skin: urticaria.
Other: impotence, altered libido.

INTERACTIONS

Ammonium chloride, ascorbic acid: observe for decreased amphetamine effects.
Antacids, sodium bicarbonate, acetazolamide: increased renal reabsorption. Monitor for enhanced amphetamine effects.
MAO inhibitors: severe hypertension; possible hypertensive crisis. Don't use together.
Phenothiazines, haloperidol: observe for decreased amphetamine effects.

EFFECTS ON DIAGNOSTIC TESTS

Plasma corticosteroids: elevated levels.
Urinary steroid determinations: test interference.

NURSING CONSIDERATIONS

Besides those related universally to drug therapy (see "How to use this book"), consider the following specific recommendations:

Assessment
- Obtain a baseline assessment of the patient's CNS status, behavior, or weight, depending on underlying disorder.
- Be alert for common adverse reactions and drug interactions during therapy.
- Evaluate the patient's and family's knowledge about dextroamphetamine therapy.

Nursing Diagnoses
- Ineffective individual coping related to patient's underlying disorder.
- Sleep pattern disturbance related to dextroamphetamine sulfate-induced insomnia.
- Knowledge deficit related to dextroamphetamine sulfate therapy.

Planning and Implementation
Preparation and Administration
- Administer drug at least 6 hours before bedtime to avoid interference with sleep.
- When used for obesity, administer drug 30 minutes to 1 hour before meals.
- Avoid prolonged administration because psychological dependence or habituation may occur, especially in patients with a history of drug addiction. After prolonged use, reduce dosage gradually to prevent acute rebound depression.

Monitoring
• Monitor effectiveness regularly by observing the patient's CNS status and behavior or assessing the patient's weight.
• Monitor vital signs for evidence of tachycardia or blood pressure changes; question the patient regularly about palpitations.
• Monitor sleeping pattern, and observe for signs of excessive stimulation.
• Monitor blood glucose levels in diabetic patients because drug may alter daily insulin needs.
• Monitor dietary intake, when used for obesity.
Supportive Care
• Provide frequent rest periods and assistance with activities as needed; fatigue may result as drug effects wear off.
• Institute safety precautions by making environment safe and providing supervision of patient's activities.
• When used for obesity, make sure the patient is also on a weight-reduction program. Do calorie counts, if necessary. Be aware that this drug is not recommended for first-line treatment of obesity and use as an anorexigenic agent is prohibited in some states.
• Be aware that this drug should not be used to overcome fatigue. Use as an analeptic is usually discouraged, since CNS stimulation superimposed on CNS depression can lead to neuronal instability and seizures.
Patient Teaching
• Warn the patient to avoid activities that require alertness or good psychomotor coordination until CNS effects of the drug are known.
• Tell the patient to avoid beverages containing caffeine, which increase the stimulant effects of amphetamines and related amines.
• Have the patient report severe insomnia and other signs of excessive stimulation.
• Tell the patient to weigh himself weekly in the same clothes at the same time of day to evaluate effectiveness in obesity therapy.
• Tell the diabetic patient to monitor blood glucose levels closely.
• Teach the patient how to take the drug to minimize insomnia and enhance effectiveness.
• Tell the patient that, when tolerance to anorexigenic effect develops, dosage should not be increased, but drug discontinued. Patient should call the doctor to report decreased effectiveness of drug. Warn the patient against stopping drug abruptly.

Evaluation
In patients receiving dextroamphetamine, appropriate evaluation statements may include:
• Patient demonstrates clinical improvement and related improved coping ability.
• Patient is able to sleep without difficulty.
• Patient and family state an understanding of dextroamphetamine therapy.

dextromethorphan hydrobromide

(dex troe meth or´ fan)
Balminil D.M.◇, Benylin DM◇, Broncho-Grippol-DM†, Congespirin for Children◇, Cremacoat 1◇, Delsym◇, DM Cough*◇, Hold◇, Koffex†, Mediquell◇, Neo-DM†, Pediacare 1◇, Pertussin 8 Hour Cough Formula◇, Robidex†, Sedatuss†, St. Joseph for Children◇, Sucrets Cough Control Formula◇.
More commonly available in combination products such as Contac Cough and Sore Throat Formula◇, Contact Cough Formula◇, Contac Jr. Children's Cold Medicine◇, Contac Nighttime Cold Medicine◇, Contac Severe Cold Formula Caplets◇, Novahistine DMX Liquid, Phenergan

*Liquid form contains alcohol. **May contain tartrazine.

with Dextromethorphan*, Robitussin-DM*◇, Rondec-DM*◇, Triaminicol Multi-Symptom Cold◇, Trind-DM Liquid*◇, Tussi-Organidin-DM Liquid*

• *Classification:* nonnarcotic antitussive (levorphanol derivative)
• *Pregnancy Risk Category:* C

HOW SUPPLIED

Chewable pieces: 15 mg◇
Liquid (sustained-action): 30 mg/5 ml◇
Lozenges: 5 mg◇
Syrup: 5 mg/5 ml*◇, 7.5 mg/5 ml*◇, 10 mg/5 ml*◇, 15 mg/5 ml*◇

ACTION

Mechanism: A chemical analogue of levorphanol, an opiate analgesic. No analgesic activity and shows little potential for abuse. Suppresses the cough reflex by direct action on the cough center in the medulla.
Absorption: Readily absorbed from the GI tract.
Metabolism: Extensively metabolized by the liver.
Excretion: Minimally excreted unchanged; metabolites are excreted primarily in urine, about 7% to 10% is excreted in feces. Half-life: Approximately 11 hours.
Onset, peak, duration: Action begins within 15 to 30 minutes. Antitussive effect persists for 5 to 6 hours.

INDICATIONS & DOSAGE

Nonproductive cough–
Adults: 10 to 20 mg P.O. q 4 hours, or 30 mg q 6 to 8 hours. Or the controlled-release liquid twice daily (60 mg b.i.d.). Maximum 120 mg daily.
Children 6 to 12 years: 5 to 10 mg P.O. q 4 hours, or 15 mg q 6 to 8 hours. Or the controlled-release liquid twice daily (30 mg b.i.d.). Maximum 60 mg daily.
Children 2 to 6 years: 2.5 to 5 mg P.O. q 4 hours, or 7.5 mg q 6 to 8 hours. Maximum 30 mg daily.

CONTRAINDICATIONS & PRECAUTIONS

Contraindicated in patients with hypersensitivity to this drug; and in patients who have taken MAO inhibitors within the preceding 2 weeks.

Use cautiously in patients with asthma and other respiratory conditions in which thick secretions are present because this drug may impair mobilization of secretions.

ADVERSE REACTIONS

Common reactions are in italics; life-threatening reactions are in bold italics.
CNS: drowsiness, dizziness.
GI: nausea.

INTERACTIONS

MAO inhibitors: hypotension, coma, hyperpyrexia, and death have occurred. Do not use together.

EFFECTS ON DIAGNOSTIC TESTS

None reported.

NURSING CONSIDERATIONS

Besides those related universally to drug therapy (see "How to use this book"), consider the following specific recommendations:

Assessment
• Obtain a baseline assessment of the patient's cough before initiating therapy.
• Be alert for common adverse reactions and drug interactions throughout therapy.
• Evaluate the patient's and family's knowledge about dextromethorphan therapy.

Nursing Diagnoses
• Ineffective airway clearance related to the patient's underlying condition producing cough.
• High risk for injury related to dextromethorphan-induced CNS reactions.

• Knowledge deficit related to dextromethorphan therapy.

Planning and Implementation

Preparation and Administration

• Do not administer an antitussive, such as dextromethorphan, to a patient if the effect of the drug may mask an underlying condition.

• Administer dextromethorphan exactly as directed.

Monitoring

• Monitor effectiveness by regularly evaluating relief of the patient's cough.

• Monitor hydration status; record intake and output.

• Monitor for dizziness and drowsiness. Keep in mind that this drug produces little or no CNS depression.

Supportive Care

• Notify the doctor if cough is unrelieved with dextromethorphan.

• Encourage the patient to take 2,000 to 3,000 ml of liquids daily.

• Perform percussion and chest vibration during dextromethorphan therapy.

• Institute safety precautions if CNS adverse reactions occur.

• Obtain an order for an antiemetic if nausea persists or becomes severe.

Patient Teaching

• Instruct the patient to follow the directions on the medication bottle exactly; explain the importance of not taking more of the drug than directed.

• Tell the patient to call the doctor if cough persists more than 7 days.

• Suggest sugarless throat lozenges to decrease throat irritation and resulting cough.

• Advise the patient to use a humidifier to filter out dust, smoke, and air pollutants.

Evaluation

In patients receiving dextromethorphan, appropriate evaluation statements may include:

• Patient's cough is relieved.

• Patient does not experience injury as a result of dextromethorphan-induced CNS reactions.

• Patient and family state an understanding of dextromethorphan therapy.

dextrothyroxine sodium (d-thyroxine sodium)

(dex troe thye rox´ een)

Choloxin**

• *Classification:* antilipemic (thyroid hormone)

• *Pregnancy Risk Category:* C

HOW SUPPLIED

Tablets: 1 mg, 2 mg, 4 mg, 6 mg

ACTION

Mechanism: The dextro isomer of the thyroid hormone thyroxine that accelerates hepatic catabolism of cholesterol and increases bile secretion to lower cholesterol levels.

Absorption: About 25% absorbed from the GI tract.

Distribution: Almost completely protein-bound.

Metabolism: Some drug is deiodinated in peripheral tissues; a small amount is metabolized by the liver.

Excretion: In urine and feces. Half-life: Plasma half-life is 18 hours.

Onset, peak, duration: Serum lipids return to pretreatment levels 6 weeks to 3 months after discontinuing therapy.

INDICATIONS & DOSAGE

Hyperlipidemia in euthyroid patients, especially when cholesterol and triglyceride levels are elevated–

Adults: initial dose 1 to 2 mg P.O. daily, increased by 1 to 2 mg daily at monthly intervals to a total of 4 to 8 mg daily.

Children: initial dose 0.05 mg/kg P.O. daily, increased by 0.05 mg/kg daily

*Liquid form contains alcohol.

**May contain tartrazine.

at monthly intervals to a total of 4 mg daily.

CONTRAINDICATIONS & PRECAUTIONS

Contraindicated in patients with heart disease or a history of hypertension or rheumatic heart disease because drug increases myocardial oxygen demand and such patients are at increased risk of angina or myocardial infarction; in patients with advanced liver or kidney disease or a history of iodism because the drug may exacerbate these conditions; and in pregnant or lactating women because thyroid hormones cross the placenta and enter breast milk.

Dextrothyroxine 2-mg and 6-mg tablets contain tartrazine dye (FD&C Yellow No. 5), which may cause allergic reactions in some patients, usually those who are sensitive to aspirin.

ADVERSE REACTIONS

Common reactions are in italics; life-threatening reactions are in bold italics.
CV: palpitations, angina pectoris, arrhythmias, ischemic myocardial changes on ECG, ***myocardial infarction.***
EENT: visual disturbances, ptosis.
GI: nausea, vomiting, diarrhea, constipation, decreased appetite.
Metabolic: *insomnia, weight loss, sweating,* flushing, hyperthermia, hair loss, menstrual irregularities.

INTERACTIONS

Digitalis glycosides: dextrothyroxine may enhance clinical effect. Use together cautiously.
Oral anticoagulants: dextrothyroxine may potentiate the anticoagulant effect of warfarin or dicumarol.
Sympathomimetics: dextrothyroxine may precipitate arrhythmias or coronary insufficiency in patients with cardiac disease.

EFFECTS ON DIAGNOSTIC TESTS

Radioactive iodine uptake: decreased.
Thyroxine (T_4), alkaline phosphatase, aspartate aminotransferase, and bilirubin: altered serum levels.
Urine and blood glucose: altered levels.

NURSING CONSIDERATIONS

Besides those related universally to drug therapy (see "How to use this book"), consider the following specific recommendations:

Assessment
- Obtain a baseline assessment of the patient's underlying condition before drug therapy.
- Be alert for adverse reactions and drug interactions throughout therapy.
- Evaluate the patient's and family's knowledge about dextrothyroxine therapy.

Nursing Diagnoses
- High risk for injury related to the patient's elevated blood lipid and cholesterol levels.
- Constipation related to adverse drug reaction.
- Knowledge deficit related to dextrothyroxine therapy.

Planning and Implementation

Preparation and Administration
- Drug should be given with food to minimize GI distress.

Monitoring
- Monitor the patient's vital signs.
- Monitor for signs of hypothyroidism, such as nervousness, insomnia, and weight loss.
- Monitor the patient's bowel habits; drug may cause diarrhea.

Supportive Care
- Administer the drug with food to minimize GI distress.
- Discontinue drug 2 weeks before surgery if anticoagulant therapy is being considered to avoid possible potentiation of anticoagulant effect.
- Diabetic patient may require more insulin, diet therapy, or oral hypoglycemics.

• Discontinue the drug or decrease the dosage as ordered if signs of hypothyroidism occur.

Patient Teaching

• Teach the patient proper dietary management (restricting total fat and cholesterol intake), weight control, and exercise. Explain their importance in controlling elevated serum lipids.

• Teach the patient to take the drug with food to reduce possible GI distress.

Evaluation

In patients receiving dextrothyroxine, appropriate evaluation statements may include:

• Patient's serum lipoprotein and total cholesterol levels are within normal limits.

• Patient does not develop diarrhea.

• Patient and family state an understanding of dextrothyroxine therapy.

dezocine

(dez´ oh seen)

Dalgan

• *Classification:* analgesic (opiate agonist-antagonist)

• *Pregnancy Risk Category:* C

HOW SUPPLIED

Injection: 5 mg/ml, 10 mg/ml, 15 mg/ml

ACTION

Mechanism: A synthetic opioid agonist-antagonist that produces postoperative analgesia qualitatively similar to morphine.

Absorption: Rapidly and completely absorbed after I.M. administration.

Distribution: The average volume of distribution is 10.1 liters/kg and is increased by hepatic disease. The degree of serum protein binding is not known.

Metabolism: Probably hepatic. A glucuronide conjugate has been identified.

Excretion: Approximately 66% of a dose appears in the urine: about 1% is unchanged drug; the remainder is the metabolite. Half-life: About 2.4 hours; prolonged in hepatic disease.

Onset, peak, duration: Peak levels appear 10 to 90 minutes after I.M. administration, and peak analgesic effects appear to follow blood levels by 20 to 60 minutes.

INDICATIONS & DOSAGE

Management of moderate to severe pain–

Adults: 5 to 20 mg I.M. q 3 to 6 hours or 2.5 to 10 mg I.V. q 2 to 4 hours. Maximum recommended single I.M. dose is 20 mg, with a maximum daily dosage of 120 mg. Maximum dosage for I.V. use has not been determined.

Dosage in renal and hepatic failure: Limited studies suggest that the drug should be used with caution and in lower doses. The half-life increases hepatic failure. The primary means of drug elimination is renal excretion of the metabolite.

CONTRAINDICATIONS & PRECAUTIONS

Contraindicated in patients hypersensitive to the drug.

Dezocine produces a dose-dependent respiratory depression similar to that of morphine, usually peaking within 15 minutes of administration. The drug should be used only in clinical settings where adequate respiratory support and an opiate antagonist (naloxone [Narcan]) is available. Use of dezocine is not recommended in patients who are opioid-dependent because it may precipitate a withdrawal syndrome. In animal studies, dezocine had greater antagonist activity than pentazocine but less than nalorphine.

Use with extreme caution in patients with head injury because dezocine can obscure clinical signs in such patients. Related drugs have been associated with respiratory-depressant effects and elevations of CSF pressure (caused by cerebral vasodilation as a response to elevated CO_2 levels). Use with caution and in lower doses in patients with chronic respiratory disease. Use cautiously in patients undergoing biliary surgery. Related drugs have caused significant increases in pressure within the common bile duct. Plasma concentrations higher than 45 ng/ml are associated with an increased incidence of adverse effects.

Note that the injection contains sulfite preservatives, which may cause allergic reactions in certain hypersensitive patients.

ADVERSE REACTIONS

Common reactions are in italics; life-threatening reactions are in bold italics.

Blood: low hemoglobin.

CNS: *sedation, dizziness, vertigo,* anxiety, mood disorders, sleep disturbances, headache, slurred speech.

CV: edema, hypotension, irregular heartbeat, hypertension, chest pain.

GI: *nausea, vomiting,* dry mouth, constipation, diarrhea, abdominal distress.

Skin: rash, pruritus, *local irritation at the injection site.*

Other: sweating, chills, flushing, pallor, thrombophlebitis.

INTERACTIONS

Alcohol or other CNS depressants: may increase the risk of CNS depression.

Opiates: patients receiving chronic opioid therapy (opioid-dependent patients) may experience withdrawal symptoms after receiving dezocine. May increase the risk of CNS depression.

EFFECTS ON DIAGNOSTIC TESTS

Alkaline phosphatase and AST (SGOT): increased levels in $<1\%$ of patients.

NURSING CONSIDERATIONS

Besides those related universally to drug therapy (see "How to use this book"), consider the following specific recommendations:

Assessment

- Obtain a baseline assessment of the patient's pain before therapy.
- Be alert for adverse reactions and drug interactions throughout therapy.
- Evaluate the patient's and family's knowledge about dezocine therapy.

Nursing Diagnoses

- Pain related to patient's underlying condition.
- Ineffective breathing pattern related to dezocine-induced respiratory depression.
- Knowledge deficit related to dezocine therapy.

Planning and Implementation

Preparation and Administration

- ***I.V. use:*** Be aware that I.V. dosage has not been determined.
- ***I.M. use:*** Maximum recommended single I.M. dose is 20 mg; a maximum daily I.M. dosage is 120 mg.

Monitoring

- Monitor effectiveness by evaluating pain relief.
- Monitor respiratory status throughout dezocine therapy noting any evidence of respiratory depression, such as decreased rate or depth of respiration. Dezocine produces a dose-dependent respiratory depression similar to that of morphine, usually peaking within 15 minutes of administration.
- Keep in mind that plasma concentrations higher than 45 ng/ml are associated with an increased incidence of adverse reactions.

Supportive Care
• Notify the doctor and discuss increase of dosage or frequency if pain is not relieved.
• Hold dose and notify the doctor if the patient's respirations are below 12 breaths/minute.
• Keep narcotic antagonist (naloxone) and resuscitative equipment available.
• Because adverse CNS reactions are possible, institute safety precautions: supervise ambulation and keep bed rails up.
• Be aware that the injection contains sulfite preservatives, which may cause allergic reactions in hypersensitive patients.
Patient Teaching
• Warn the ambulatory patient to move about cautiously because the drug may cause dizziness.
• Tell the patient or family to notify the doctor if respiratory rate decreases.
Evaluation
In patients receiving dezocine, appropriate evaluation statements may include:
• Patient reports relief of pain after administration of dezocine.
• Respiratory rate and pattern are within normal limits after administration of dezocine.
• Patient and family state an understanding of dezocine therapy.

diazepam
(dye az´ e pam)
Apo-Diazepam†, Diazemuls†, Diazepam Intensol, E-Pam†, Meval†, Novodipam†, Q-Pam, Rival†, Valium, Valrelease, Vasepam, Vivol†, Zetran

• Controlled Substance Schedule IV
• *Classification:* anxiolytic, skeletal muscle relaxant, amnesic agent, anticonvulsant, sedative-hypnotic (benzodiazepine)
• *Pregnancy Risk Category:* D

HOW SUPPLIED
Tablets: 2 mg, 5 mg, 10 mg
Capsules (extended-release): 15 mg
Oral solution: 5 mg/5 ml, 5 mg/ml
Injection: 5 mg/ml
Sterile emulsion for injection: 5 mg/ml†

ACTION
Mechanism: Depresses the CNS at the limbic and subcortical levels of the brain. As an anticonvulsant, suppresses the spread of seizure activity produced by epileptogenic foci in the cortex, thalamus, and limbic structures.
Absorption: Well absorbed through the GI tract. I.M. administration results in erratic absorption of the drug.
Distribution: Widely distributed throughout the body. Approximately 85% to 95% of an administered dose is bound to plasma protein.
Metabolism: In the liver to the active metabolites desmethyldiazepam, 3-hydroxydiazepam, and oxazepam.
Excretion: Most metabolites of diazepam are excreted in urine, with only small amounts excreted in feces. Half-life: Diazepam, 20 to 50 hours; desmethyldiazepam, 30 to 200 hours; 3-hydroxydiazepam, 5 to 20 hours; oxazepam, 3 to 21 hours.
Onset, peak, duration: Onset of action occurs within 30 minutes to 1 hour, with peak action in 1 to 2 hours. After I.M. administration, onset of action usually occurs in 15 to 30 minutes; after I.V. administration, onset occurs 1 to 5 minutes after injection. Duration of effect is 3 hours; may be prolonged up to 90 hours in elderly patients and those with hepatic or renal dysfunction.

INDICATIONS & DOSAGE

Tension, anxiety, adjunct in seizure disorders or skeletal muscle spasm–
Adults: 2 to 10 mg P.O. t.i.d. or q.i.d. Or, 15 to 30 mg of extended-release capsule once daily.
Children over 6 months: 1 to 2.5 mg P.O. t.i.d. or q.i.d.
Tension, anxiety, muscle spasm, endoscopic procedures, seizures–
Adults: 5 to 10 mg I.V. initially, up to 30 mg in 1 hour or possibly more for cardioversion or status epilepticus, depending on response.
Children 5 years and older: 1 mg I.V. or I.M. slowly q 2 to 5 minutes to maximum of 10 mg. Repeat q 2 to 4 hours.
Children 30 days to 5 years: 0.2 to 0.5 mg I.V. or I.M. slowly q 2 to 5 minutes to maximum of 5 mg. Repeat q 2 to 4 hours.
Tetanic muscle spasms–
Children over 5 years: 5 to 10 mg I.M. or I.V. q 3 to 4 hours, p.r.n.
Infants over 30 days: 1 to 2 mg I.M. or I.V. q 3 to 4 hours, p.r.n.
Status epilepticus–
Adults: 5 to 20 mg slow I.V. push 2 to 5 mg/minute; may repeat q 5 to 10 minutes up to maximum total dose of 60 mg. Use 2 to 5 mg in elderly or debilitated patients. May repeat therapy in 20 to 30 minutes with caution if seizures recur.
Children: 0.1 to 0.3 mg/kg slow I.V. push (1 mg/minute over 3 minutes). May repeat q 15 minutes for 2 doses. Maximum single dose in children under 5 years is 5 mg; in children over 5 years, 10 mg.

CONTRAINDICATIONS & PRECAUTIONS

Contraindicated in patients with hypersensitivity to the drug; acute narrow-angle glaucoma or untreated open-angle glaucoma because of the drug's possible anticholinergic effect; shock or coma because the drug's hypnotic or hypotensive effect may be prolonged or intensified; acute alcohol intoxication who have depressed vital signs because the drug will worsen CNS depression; and in infants younger than age 30 days in whom slow metabolism of the drug causes it to accumulate.

Use cautiously in patients with psychoses because the drug is rarely beneficial in such patients and may induce paradoxic reactions; myasthenia gravis or Parkinson's disease because it may exacerbate the disorder; impaired renal or hepatic function, which prolongs elimination of the drug; in elderly or debilitated patients, who are usually more sensitive to the drug's CNS effects; and in individuals prone to addiction or drug abuse. Abrupt withdrawal of diazepam may precipitate seizures in patients with seizure disorders. Use of I.V. diazepam in patients with petit mal or Lennox-Gastaut syndrome may precipitate tonic status epilepticus.

ADVERSE REACTIONS

Common reactions are in italics; life-threatening reactions are in bold italics.
CNS: *drowsiness, lethargy, hangover, ataxia,* fainting, slurred speech, tremor.
CV: transient hypotension, bradycardia, ***cardiovascular collapse.***
EENT: diplopia, blurred vision, nystagmus.
GI: nausea, vomiting, abdominal discomfort.
Skin: rash, urticaria.
Local: desquamation, *pain, phlebitis at injection site.*
Other: respiratory depression.

INTERACTIONS

Alcohol, other CNS depressants: increased CNS depression. Avoid concomitant use.
Cimetidine: increased sedation. Monitor carefully.

Phenobarbital: increased effects of both drugs. Use together cautiously.

EFFECTS ON DIAGNOSTIC TESTS

EEG: minor changes (usually low-voltage, fast activity) during and after therapy.
Liver function tests: elevated results.

NURSING CONSIDERATIONS

Besides those related universally to drug therapy (see "How to use this book"), consider the following specific recommendations:

Assessment

- Obtain a baseline assessment of the patient's underlying condition before drug therapy.
- Be alert for adverse reactions and drug interactions throughout therapy.
- Evaluate the patient's and family's knowledge about diazepam therapy.

Nursing Diagnoses

- Anxiety related to the patient's underlying condition.
- Altered tissue perfusion (cardiopulmonary) related to adverse drug reactions.
- Knowledge deficit related to diazepam therapy.

Planning and Implementation

Preparation and Administration

- ***I.V. use:*** Give slowly at a rate not exceeding 5 mg/minute. When injecting I.V., best to administer directly into the vein. If this is not possible, inject slowly through the infusion tubing as close as possible to the vein insertion site.
- I.V. route is more reliable; I.M. administration is not recommended because absorption is variable and injection is painful (because the solution is highly alkaline).
- Dosage should be reduced in elderly and debilitated patients because they may be more susceptible to the adverse CNS effects.
- Avoid extravasation. Do not inject into small veins.
- Know that this is the drug of choice (I.V. form) for status epilepticus.
- Continuous infusions of 1 to 10 mg hourly have been used to prevent seizure recurrence.
- Do not store diazepam in plastic syringes.
- Do not mix injectable form with other drugs because diazepam is incompatable with most drugs.
- There is considerable controvery about the use of diluted diazepam solutions for continuous I.V. infusions because of the low aqueous solubility. Under certain conditions, it may be compatible with sodium chloride 0.9% or Ringer's lactate injection, but the solution may not be stable. Consult hospital pharmacy for further information.

Monitoring

- Monitor effectiveness regularly by asking the patient about feelings of anxiety and by evaluating the patient's behavior.
- Monitor the patient for adverse reactions by frequently monitoring vital signs for hypotension and bradycardia.
- Monitor the patient daily for possible phlebitis at the injection site.
- Monitor CBC and hepatic function during long-term use.
- Monitor respirations every 5 to 15 minutes and before each repeated I.V. dose.
- Monitor for seizures, which may recur within 20 to 30 minutes of initial control, because of redistribution of the drug.
- Monitor hydration status if patient develops nausea and vomiting.

Supportive Care

- If drowsiness, light-headedness, ataxia, or fainting occurs, institute safety measures, such as supervising patient activities. Reorient patient as needed and ensure a safe environment.
- Be aware that drug should not be prescribed for everyday stress.

• Do not withdraw drug abruptly. Abuse or addiction is possible and withdrawal symptoms may occur.
• Have emergency resuscitative equipment and oxygen at the bedside. Note that naloxone does not reverse the respiratory depression produced by diazepam.
• Provide additional fluids if the patient develops nausea and vomiting.

Patient Teaching

• Warn the patient not to combine drug with alcohol or other CNS depressants and to avoid driving and other hazardous activities that require alertness and psychomotor coordination until adverse CNS effects of the drug are known.
• Caution the patient against giving medication to others.
• Warn the patient to take this drug only as directed and not to discontinue it without the doctor's approval. Inform the patient of the drug's potential for causing dependence if taken longer than directed.
• Recommend frequent ophthalmic examinations during therapy and tell patient to report any visual changes.

Evaluation

In patients receiving diazepam, appropriate evaluation statements may include:
• The patient states he is less anxious.
• The patient does not develop respiratory depression.
• Patient and family state an understanding of diazepam therapy.

diazoxide (oral)

(dye az ox´ ide)
Proglycem

• *Classification:* antihypertensive, antihypoglycemic (peripheral vasodilator)
• *Pregnancy Risk Category:* C

HOW SUPPLIED

Capsules: 50 mg
Oral suspension: 50 mg/ml in 30-ml bottle

ACTION

Mechanism: Raises serum glucose levels by inhibiting the release of insulin from the pancreas and decreasing peripheral utilization of glucose.
Absorption: Over 98% of a dose is absorbed from the GI tract.
Distribution: Highest concentrations are found in the kidneys; lower concentrations in the liver and adrenal glands. About 90% bound to plasma proteins.
Metabolism: Probably in the liver; over 98% of a dose is excreted as metabolites.
Excretion: In urine; unabsorbed drug is found in feces. Half life: Plasma half-life is 2.8 to 8.3 hours
Onset, peak, duration: After administration of oral solution, hyperglycemic effect begins within an hour and generally lasts no more than 8 hours in the presence of normal renal function.

INDICATIONS & DOSAGE

Management of hypoglycemia from a variety of conditions resulting in hyperinsulinism–
Adults and children: 3 to 8 mg/kg P.O. daily, in three equally divided doses q 8 hours.
Infants and newborns: 8 to 15 mg/kg P.O. daily, in two or three equally divided doses q 8 to 12 hours.

CONTRAINDICATIONS & PRECAUTIONS

Contraindicated in patients with hypersensitivity to the drug or to other thiazide derivatives. I.V. diazoxide is contraindicated in patients with coarctation of the aorta or an atrioventricular shunt; oral diazoxide is contraindicated in patients with functional hypoglycemia.

Use cautiously in patients who may be harmed by sodium and water retention and in patients with impaired cerebral, cardiac, or renal function, because the drug may reduce blood pressure abruptly, resulting in decreased perfusion.

ADVERSE REACTIONS

Common reactions are in italics; life-threatening reactions are in bold italics.
Blood: *leukopenia,* ***thrombocytopenia.***
CV: ***cardiac arrhythmias.***
EENT: diplopia.
GI: nausea, vomiting, anorexia, taste alteration.
Metabolic: sodium and fluid retention, ketoacidosis and hyperosmolar nonketotic syndrome, hyperuricemia.
Other: *severe hypertrichosis (hair growth) in 25% of adults and higher percentage of children.*

INTERACTIONS

Alpha-adrenergic blocking agents: antagonize inhibition of insulin release by diazoxide.
Anticoagulants: increased anticoagulant effect. Adjust dosage of anticoagulant.
Antigout agents: increased serum uric acid. Adjust dosage of antigout agent.
Antihypertensive agents, peripheral vasodilators: additive hypotensive effects.
Beta-adrenergic blocking agents: increased hypotensive effect.
Hydantoin anticonvulsants: decreased anticonvulsant effects and decreased hyperglycemic effect of diazoxide. Don't use together.
Thiazide diuretics: may potentiate hyperglycemic, hyperuricemic, and hypotensive effects. Monitor appropriate laboratory values.

EFFECTS ON DIAGNOSTIC TESTS

Glucagon: false-negative insulin response.
Hemoglobin and hematocrit: decreased with prolonged use.

NURSING CONSIDERATIONS

Besides those related universally to drug therapy (see "How to use this book"), consider the following specific recommendations:

Assessment
- Obtain a baseline assessment of urine and serum glucose before therapy.

Nursing Diagnoses
- Altered nutrition: Less than body requirements, related to decreased glucose available due to underlying condition.
- High risk for fluid volume excess related to adverse effects of drug.
- Knowledge deficit related to oral diazoxide.

Planning and Implementation

Preparation and Administration
- Note the administration of concurrent medications that may interfere with metabolism of diazoxide.
- Discontinue medication if not effective after 2 to 3 weeks of therapy.

Monitoring
- Monitor effectiveness by testing urine and serum glucose levels.
- Evaluate the patient for signs of hypoglycemia.

Supportive Care
- Report any abnormalities in serum or urine glucose to the doctor.
- Expect discontinuation of therapy if the drug is not effective within 2 or 3 weeks.

Patient Teaching
- Teach the patient how to monitor serum glucose levels.
- Explain the importance of following dietary restrictions for successful therapy.
- Tell the patient to report any adverse reactions, including excessive thirst, fruity breath, or urinary frequency.
- Reassure patient that hair growth on the arms and forehead is a com-

mon adverse reaction to the medication and will subside once treatment is completed.

Evaluation

In patients receiving oral diazoxide, appropriate evaluation statements may include:

- Patient reports normal serum and urine glucose levels.
- Patient is free of dependent edema.
- Patient and family state an understanding of oral diazoxide therapy.

diazoxide (parenteral)

(dye az ox´ ide)

Hyperstat

- *Classification:* antihypertensive, antihypoglycemic (peripheral vasodilator)
- *Pregnancy Risk Category:* C

HOW SUPPLIED

Injection: 300 mg/20 ml

ACTION

Mechanism: Directly relaxes arteriolar smooth muscle.

Absorption: For maximal antihypertensive effect, diazoxide is administered I.V.

Distribution: Distributed throughout the body; highest concentration is found in kidneys, liver, and adrenal glands; crosses the placenta and blood-brain barrier. Drug is approximately 90% protein-bound.

Metabolism: Partially metabolized in the liver.

Excretion: Drug and metabolites are excreted slowly by the kidneys. Half-life: About 28 hours.

Onset, peak, duration: After I.V. administration, blood pressure should decrease promptly, with maximum decrease in less than 5 minutes. Duration of antihypertensive effect varies widely, ranging from 30 minutes to 72 hours (average 3 to 12 hours) after I.V. administration; may be prolonged in patients with renal dysfunction.

INDICATIONS & DOSAGE

Hypertensive crisis–

Adults and children: 1 to 3 mg/kg I.V. bolus (up to a maximum of 150 mg) q 5 to 15 minutes until adequate response is seen. Repeat at intervals q 4 to 24 hours p.r.n.

CONTRAINDICATIONS & PRECAUTIONS

Contraindicated in patients with hypersensitivity to the drug or to other thiazide derivatives. I.V. diazoxide is contraindicated in patients with coarctation of the aorta or an atrioventricular shunt; oral diazoxide is contraindicated in patients with functional hypoglycemia.

Use cautiously in patients who may be harmed by sodium and water retention and in patients with impaired cerebral, cardiac, or renal function because the drug may reduce blood pressure abruptly, resulting in decreased perfusion.

ADVERSE REACTIONS

Common reactions are in italics; life-threatening reactions are in bold italics.

CNS: *headaches,* dizziness, lightheadedness, euphoria.

CV: *sodium and water retention, orthostatic hypotension,* sweating, flushing, warmth, angina, myocardial ischemia, arrhythmias, ECG changes.

GI: *nausea, vomiting,* abdominal discomfort.

Metabolic: *hyperglycemia,* hyperuricemia.

Local: inflammation and pain from extravasation.

INTERACTIONS

Hydralazine: may cause severe hypotension. Use together cautiously.

Thiazide diuretics: may increase the

effects of diazoxide. Use together cautiously.

EFFECTS ON DIAGNOSTIC TESTS

Glucagon: false-negative insulin response.
Hemoglobin and hematocrit: decreased with prolonged use.

NURSING CONSIDERATIONS

Besides those related universally to drug therapy (see "How to use this book"), consider the following specific recommendations:

Assessment

- Obtain a baseline assessment of the patient's blood pressure before beginning therapy.
- Be alert for adverse reactions and drug interactions throughout therapy.
- Evaluate the patient's and family's knowledge about diazoxide therapy.

Nursing Diagnoses

- Altered tissue perfusion (renal, cerebral, cardiopulmonary, and peripheral) related to the patient's underlying condition.
- Fluid volume excess related to diazoxide-induced adverse reactions.
- Knowledge deficit related to diazoxide therapy.

Planning and Implementation

Preparation and Administration

- ***I.V. use:*** Infusion of diazoxide is as effective as a bolus in some patients. Take care to avoid extravasation. Keep the patient supine or in Trendenlenberg's position during and for 1 hour after infusion. Protect I.V. solutions from light. Darkened solutions of diazoxide are subpotent and should not be used.

Monitoring

- Continuously monitor the patient's blood pressure and ECG during diazoxide therapy.
- Monitor the patient's intake and output carefully. If fluid or sodium retention develops, doctor may want to order diuretics.
- Weigh patient daily and notify the doctor of any weight increase.
- Monitor the patient's uric acid levels frequently.
- Monitor blood glucose daily if the patient has diabetes. Drug may alter requirements for insulin, diet, or oral hypoglycemic drugs in previously controlled diabetics.
- Stay alert for signs of severe hyperglycemia or hyperosmolar nonketotic coma. Insulin may be needed.

Supportive Care

- Notify the doctor immediately if severe hypotension develops and keep norepinephrine available.
- Report uric acid abnormalities to the doctor.
- Administer insulin to diabetics as needed.
- Check the patient's standing blood pressure for hypotension before discontinuing close monitoring for this reaction.

Patient Teaching

- Advise patient to minimize risk of dizziness or fainting by rising slowly and avoiding sudden position changes. Instruct the patient to remain supine for up to 1 hour after injection.

Evaluation

In patients receiving diazoxide, appropriate evaluation statements may include:

- Blood pressure is controlled within normal limits for this patient.
- Patient did not retain fluid or sodium.
- Patient and family state an understanding of diazoxide therapy.

diclofenac sodium

(dye kloe´ fen ak)
Voltaren, Voltaren SR†

- *Classification:* antiarthritic (nonsteroidal anti-inflammatory agent)

- *Pregnancy Risk Category:* B

HOW SUPPLIED

Tablets (enteric-coated): 25 mg, 50 mg, 75 mg
Tablets (slow-release): 100 mg†
Suppositories: 50 mg†, 100 mg†

ACTION

Mechanism: Produces anti-inflammatory, analgesic, and antipyretic effects, possibly through inhibition of prostaglandin synthesis.
Absorption: Rapidly and almost completely absorbed after oral, rectal, or I.M. administration.
Distribution: Highly (nearly 100%) protein-bound.
Metabolism: Undergoes first-pass metabolism, with 60% of unchanged drug reaching systemic circulation. The principal and only active metabolite, 4′-hydroxydiclofenac, has approximately 3% the activity of the parent compound. The mean terminal half-life is approximately 1.2 to 1.8 hours after an oral dose.
Excretion: About 40% to 60% of diclofenac is excreted in the urine; the remainder in the bile. The 4′-hydroxy metabolite accounts for 20% to 30% of the dose excreted in the urine; the other metabolites account for 10% to 20%; 5% to 10% is excreted unchanged in the urine. More than 90% is excreted within 72 hours. Moderate renal impairment does not alter the elimination rate of unchanged diclofenac but may reduce the elimination rate of the metabolites. Half-life: Terminal elimination half-life is 1 to 2 hours.
Onset, peak, duration: Peak plasma concentrations occur in 10 to 30 minutes. After oral, rectal, or I.M. administration, absorption is delayed by food, with peak plasma concentrations occurring in 2½ to 12 hours; however, bioavailability is unchanged.

INDICATIONS AND DOSAGE

Ankylosing spondylitis–
Adults: 25 mg P.O. q.i.d. and h.s.
Osteoarthritis–
Adults: 50 mg P.O. b.i.d. or t.i.d., or 75 mg P.O. b.i.d.
Rheumatoid arthritis–
Adults: 75 to 100 mg P.O. b.i.d., or 50 to 100 mg P.R. (where available) h.s. as a substitute for the last oral dose of the day. Do not exceed 150 mg daily.

CONTRAINDICATIONS & PRECAUTIONS

Contraindicated in patients with hypersensitivity to it and those in whom diclofenac, aspirin, or other NSAIDs induce asthma, urticaria, or other allergic reactions. Allergic reactions, including anaphylaxis, have been reported. Diclofenac should not be used in patients with hepatic porphyria because it may exacerbate this condition.

Serious GI toxicity, including ulceration and hemorrhage, can occur at any time in patients on chronic NSAID therapy. Peptic ulceration and GI bleeding have been reported. Monitor for ulceration and bleeding in all patients who receive prolonged treatment with diclofenac sodium, even those without previous GI symptoms. Maintain therapy with lowest effective dosage.

Periodically monitor serum transaminase levels (particularly ALT [SGPT]) and other indicators of liver function because mild-to-moderate hepatic dysfunction has been reported during therapy with diclofenac.

Use cautiously in patients with impaired renal function because this drug is eliminated by the kidneys. Fluid retention and edema have occurred in some patients.

ADVERSE REACTIONS

Common reactions are in italics; life-threatening reactions are in bold italics.
CNS: anxiety, depression, drowsiness, insomnia, irritability, *headache.*
CV: *CHF,* hypertension.
EENT: *tinnitus,* laryngeal edema, swelling of the lips and tongue.
GI: *abdominal pain or cramps, constipation, diarrhea, indigestion, nausea,* abdominal distention, flatulence, peptic ulceration, GI bleeding, melena, bloody diarrhea, appetite change, colitis.
GU: azotemia, proteinuria, acute renal failure, oliguria, interstitial nephritis, papillary necrosis, nephrotic syndrome, *fluid retention.*
Hepatic: elevated hepatic enzymes, jaundice, hepatitis, hepatotoxicity.
Respiratory: asthma.
Skin: rash, pruritus, urticaria, eczema, dermatitis, alopecia, photosensitivity, bullous eruption, ***Stevens-Johnson syndrome (rare),*** allergic purpura.
Other: ***anaphylaxis,*** anaphylactoid reactions, angioedema.

INTERACTIONS

Anticoagulants (including warfarin): possible increased incidence of bleeding. Monitor patient closely.
Aspirin: concomitant use not recommended by manufacturer.
Cyclosporine, digoxin, lithium, methotrexate: diclofenac may reduce renal clearance of these drugs, and increase risk of toxicity. Monitor patient closely.
Diuretics: diclofenac may decrease the effectiveness of diuretics.
Insulin, oral hypoglycemic agents: diclofenac may alter requirements for hypoglycemic agents. Monitor patient closely.
Potassium-sparing diuretics: diclofenac may enhance potassium retention resulting in increased serum potassium levels.

EFFECTS ON DIAGNOSTIC TESTS

Platelet aggregation time: prolonged. No effect on bleeding time, plasma thrombin clotting time, plasma fibrinogen, or Factors V and VII to XII.

NURSING CONSIDERATIONS

Besides those related universally to drug therapy (see "How to use this book"), consider the following specific recommendations:

Assessment
- Obtain a baseline assessment of patient's pain before therapy.
- Be alert for adverse reactions and drug interactions throughout therapy.
- Evaluate the patient's and family's knowledge about diclofenac therapy.

Nursing Diagnoses
- Pain related to the patient's underlying condition.
- Constipation related to diclofenac sodium-induced GI reactions.
- Knowledge deficit related to diclofenac therapy.

Planning and Implementation

Preparation and Administration

P.O. use: Administer each dose with milk or with meals to minimize GI distress.

Monitoring
- Regularly monitor the patient for relief of pain.
- Monitor carefully for peptic ulceration and GI bleeding because these problems have occurred despite the absence of symptoms.
- Monitor for signs of hepatoxicity: nausea, fatigue, lethargy, pruritus, jaundice, right upper quadrant tenderness, and flu-like symptoms.
- Measure serum transaminase, especially ALT (SGPT), periodically, in patients undergoing long-term therapy. The first serum transaminase measurement should be made no later than 8 weeks after beginning therapy. Keep in mind that elevations of liver tests can occur during therapy.

Supportive Care
• Notify the doctor immediately if the patient develops signs of GI bleeding or hepatotoxicity.
• Encourage intake of high-fiber foods for the patient with constipation.
Patient Teaching
• Teach the patient the signs and symptoms of GI bleeding and of hepatotoxicity. Tell him to notify the doctor immediately if any of these signs occur.
• Tell the patient to take the drug with milk or with meals to minimize GI distress.
• Tell the patient not to crush, break, or chew the enteric-coated tablets.
Evaluation
In patients receiving diclofenac, appropriate evaluation statements may include:
• Pain is relieved by diclofenac sodium therapy.
• Constipation did not occur.
• Patient and family state an understanding of diclofenac therapy.

dicloxacillin sodium
(dye klox a sill′ in)
Dycill, Dynapen, Pathocil

• *Classification:* antibiotic (penicillinase-resistant penicillin)
• *Pregnancy Risk Category:* B

HOW SUPPLIED
Capsules: 125 mg, 250 mg, 500 mg
Oral suspension: 62.5 mg/5 ml (after reconstitution)

ACTION
Mechanism: Bactericidal against microorganisms by inhibiting cell wall synthesis during active multiplication. Bacteria resist penicillins by producing penicillinases—enzymes that convert penicillins to inactive penicilloic acid. Dicloxacillin resists these enzymes.
Absorption: Absorbed rapidly but incompletely (35% to 76%) from the GI tract; it is relatively acid stable. Food may decrease both rate and extent of absorption.
Distribution: Widely distributed into bone, bile, and pleural and synovial fluids. CSF penetration is poor but is enhanced by meningeal inflammation. Dicloxacillin crosses the placenta; it is 95% to 99% protein-bound.
Metabolism: Metabolized only partially.
Excretion: Metabolites are excreted in urine by renal tubular secretion and glomerular filtration; they are also excreted in breast milk. Half-life: 30 minutes to 1 hour in adults, extended minimally to 2½ hours in patients with renal impairment.
Onset, peak, duration: Peak plasma levels occur 30 minutes to 2 hours after oral dose.

INDICATIONS & DOSAGE
Systemic infections caused by penicillinase-producing staphylococci—
Adults: 1 to 2 g daily P.O., divided into doses given q 6 hours.
Children: 25 to 50 mg/kg P.O. daily, divided into doses given q 6 hours.

CONTRAINDICATIONS & PRECAUTIONS
Contraindicated in patients with hypersensitivity to any penicillin or cephalosporin. Use cautiously in patients with renal impairment because drug is excreted in urine; decreased dosage is required in moderate to severe renal failure.

ADVERSE REACTIONS
Common reactions are in italics; life-threatening reactions are in bold italics.
Blood: eosinophilia.

CNS: neuromuscular irritability, seizures.
GI: *nausea,* vomiting, *epigastric distress,* flatulence, *diarrhea.*
Other: *hypersensitivity (pruritus, urticaria, rash,* ***anaphylaxis****),* overgrowth of nonsusceptible organisms.

INTERACTIONS

Probenecid: increases blood levels of dicloxacillin and other penicillins. Probenecid may be used for this purpose.

EFFECTS ON DIAGNOSTIC TESTS

Aminoglycoside serum levels: falsely decreased concentrations.
Bence Jones protein (Bradshaw screening test): false-positive results.
CBC: transient reductions in RBC, WBC, and platelet counts.
Liver function tests: transient elevations may indicate drug-induced cholestasis or hepatitis.
Urine and serum proteins: false-positive results.

NURSING CONSIDERATIONS

Besides those related universally to drug therapy (see "How to use this book"), consider the following specific recommendations:

Assessment
- Obtain a baseline assessment of patient's infection before therapy.

Nursing Diagnoses
- High risk for injury related to ineffectiveness of dicloxacillin to eradicate the infection.
- High risk for fluid volume deficit related to dicloxacillin-induced adverse GI reactions.
- Knowledge deficit related to dicloxacillin therapy.

Planning and Implementation
Preparation and Administration
- Obtain specimen for culture and sensitivity tests before first dose. Therapy may begin pending test results.
- Before first dose, ask the patient about previous allergic reactions to this drug or other penicillins. However, a negative history of penicillin allergy does not guarantee future safety.
- Give dicloxacillin at least 1 hour before bacteriostatic antibiotics.
- ***P.O. use:*** Administer drug 1 to 2 hours before or 2 to 3 hours after meals because food may interfere with absorption.

Monitoring
- Monitor effectiveness by regularly assessing for improvement of infection.
- Monitor hydration status if adverse GI reactions occur.
- Monitor for bacterial and fungal superinfections during prolonged or high-dose therapy, especially in elderly, debilitated, or immunosuppressed patients.
- Regularly monitor renal, hepatic, and hematopoietic function periodically as ordered during prolonged therapy.

Supportive Care
- Obtain an order for an antiemetic or antidiarrheal agent as needed.
- If the patient develops a rash, notify the doctor and expect to discontinue the drug.

Patient Teaching
- Advise the patient who becomes allergic to dicloxacillin to wear medical alert identification stating this information.
- Tell the patient to call the doctor if rash, fever, or chills develop. A rash is the most common allergic reaction.
- Tell patient to take drug exactly as prescribed, and to take entire quantity even if he feels better.
- Instruct patient to take the drug 1 to 2 hours before or 2 to 3 hours after meals because food may interfere with absorption.
- Warn patient never to use leftover dicloxacillin for a new illness or to share it with others.

Evaluation
In patients receiving dicloxacillin, appropriate evaluation statements may include:
• Patient is free of infection.
• Patient maintains adequate hydration throughout dicloxacillin therapy.
• Patient and family state an understanding of dicloxacillin therapy.

dicumarol (bishydroxycoumarin)
(dye koo´ ma role)

• *Classification:* oral anticoagulant (coumarin derivative)
• *Pregnancy Risk Category:* D

HOW SUPPLIED
Tablets: 25 mg, 50 mg

ACTION
Mechanism: Inhibits vitamin K-dependent activation of clotting factors II, VII, IX, and X, which are formed in the liver.
Absorption: Slowly and incompletely absorbed from the GI tract, causing erratic bioavailability.
Distribution: Highly bound to plasma proteins, primarily albumin; it crosses the placenta.
Metabolism: Hydroxylated by the liver to inactive metabolites.
Excretion: Metabolites are reabsorbed from bile and excreted in urine and breast milk. Unabsorbed drug is excreted in feces. Half-life: 1 to 2 days; half-life is dose-dependent.
Onset, peak, duration: Therapeutic effect is relatively more dependent on clotting factor depletion (factor X half-life is 40 hours), and prothrombin time (PT) will not peak for 1 to 3 days. Duration of action more closely reflects drug's half-life, ranging from 2 to 10 days.

INDICATIONS & DOSAGE
Treatment of pulmonary emboli; prevention and treatment of deep vein thrombosis, myocardial infarction, rheumatic heart disease with heart valve damage, atrial arrhythmias—
Adults: 200 to 300 mg P.O. on first day, 25 to 200 mg P.O. daily thereafter, based on prothrombin times.

CONTRAINDICATIONS & PRECAUTIONS
Contraindicated in patients with hemophilia, thrombocytopenic purpura, leukemia with pronounced bleeding tendency, open wounds or ulcers, impaired hepatic or renal function, severe hypertension (diastolic pressure over 110 mm Hg), acute nephritis, or subacute bacterial endocarditis because of the potential for excessive bleeding.

Use with extreme caution (avoid when possible) in psychiatric patients and debilitated or cachectic patients; also use cautiously during menses or when any drainage tube is being used, and in any patient in whom slight bleeding is dangerous.

ADVERSE REACTIONS
Common reactions are in italics; life-threatening reactions are in bold italics.
Blood: ***hemorrhage with excessive dosage,*** leukopenia, ***agranulocytosis.***
GI: anorexia, nausea, vomiting, cramps, *diarrhea,* mouth ulcers.
GU: hematuria.
Skin: dermatitis, urticaria, alopecia, *rash.*
Other: *fever.*

INTERACTIONS
Acetaminophen: increased bleeding possible with chronic (greater than 2 weeks) therapy with acetaminophen. Monitor very carefully.
Allopurinol, amiodarone, chloramphenicol, clofibrate, diflunisal, thyroid drugs, heparin, anabolic steroids, cimetidine, disulfiram, gluca-

gon, inhalation anesthetics, metronidazole, quinidine, influenza vaccine, sulindac, sulfinpyrazone, sulfonamides, tricyclic antidepressants: increased prothrombin time. Monitor patient carefully for bleeding. Consider anticoagulant dosage reduction.
Barbiturates: inhibition of hypoprothrombinemic effect of anticoagulants. If barbiturates are withdrawn, reduce anticoagulant dosage; inhibition may last weeks after barbiturate is withdrawn, but fatal hemorrhage can occur when inhibiting effect disappears.
Cholestyramine: decreased response when administered too close together. Administer 6 hours after oral anticoagulants.
Ethacrynic acid, indomethacin, mefenamic acid, oxyphenbutazone, phenylbutazone, salicylates: increased prothrombin time; ulcerogenic effects. Don't use together.
Glutethimide, chloral hydrate, sulfinpyrazone, triclofos sodium: increased or decreased prothrombin time. Avoid use if possible, or monitor patient carefully.
Griseofulvin, haloperidol, ethchlorvynol, carbamazepine, rifampin: decreased prothrombin time with reduced anticoagulant effect. Monitor patient carefully.

EFFECTS ON DIAGNOSTIC TESTS

PT and partial thromboplastin time: prolonged.
Serum theophylline (Schack and Waxler ultraviolet method): falsely decreased levels.

NURSING CONSIDERATIONS

Besides those related universally to drug therapy (see "How to use this book"), consider the following specific recommendations:

Assessment

- Obtain a baseline assessment of prothrombin time before therapy.
- Be alert for adverse reactions or drug interactions during therapy.
- Evaluate the patient's and family's knowledge about dicumarol therapy.

Nursing Diagnoses

- Altered tissue perfusion (renal, cerebral, cardiopulmonary, gastrointestional, peripheral) related to the patient's underlying condition.
- High risk for fluid volume deficit related to adverse effects of dicumarol therapy
- Knowledge deficit related to dicumarol therapy.

Planning and Implementation

Preparation and Administration

- ***P.O. use:*** Dose given depends on PT. The treatment goal is usually to maintain the PT at 1½ to 2 times normal. PT values may vary depending on individual laboratory procedures. The dose should be given at the same time daily. Because onset of action is delayed, heparin sodium is often given during the first few days of treatment. Don't draw blood for PT when heparin is being given simultaneously, or within 5 hours of intermittent I.V. heparin administration. However, blood for PT may be drawn anytime during continuous heparin infusion.

Monitoring

- Monitor effectiveness by regularly checking the patient's PT.
- Check the patient regularly for bleeding gums, bruises on arms or legs, petechiae, nosebleeds, melena, tarry stools, hematuria, hematemesis. Notify the doctor immediately if any of these symptoms occur.
- Monitor the patient for fever and skin rash, which may signal a severe adverse reaction. Stop the drug and notify the doctor immediately.

Supportive Care

- Remember that the clotting status may be affected by the addition or withdrawal of other drugs.
- Keep in mind that the duration of action of dicumarol is 2 to 5 days.

Patient Teaching
• Tell the patient to carry a card that identifies him as a potential bleeder due to anticoagulant therapy.
• Teach the patient to avoid OTC products containing aspirin, other salicylates, or drugs that may interact with dicumarol.
• Advise the patient to notify doctor if menses is heavier than usual.
• Tell the patient to use an electric shaver to avoid scratches and a soft toothbrush to brush the teeth.
• Teach the patient that dicumarol may turn alkaline urine orange-red.

Evaluation

In patients receiving dicumarol, appropriate evaluation statements may include:
• PT reflects the goal of dicumarol therapy.
• Patient has not experienced any hemorrhagic episodes related to the adverse effects of dicumarol therapy.
• Patient and family state an understanding of dicumarol therapy.

dicyclomine hydrochloride

(dye sye´ kloe meen)

Antispas, Bemote, Bentyl, Bentylol†, Byclomine, Dibent, Di-Cyclonex, Dilomine, Di-Spaz, Formulex†, Lomine†, Merbentyl‡, Neoquess Injection, Or-Tyl, Spasmoban†, Spasmoject, Viscerol†

• *Classification:* antimuscarinic, GI antispasmodic (anticholinergic)
• *Pregnancy Risk Category:* B

HOW SUPPLIED

Tablets: 10 mg‡, 20 mg
Capsules: 10 mg, 20 mg
Syrup: 5 mg/5 ml‡, 10 mg/5 ml
Injection: 10 mg/ml

ACTION

Mechanism: Exerts a nonspecific, direct spasmolytic action on smooth muscle. Also possesses local anesthetic properties that may be partly responsible for spasmolysis.
Absorption: About 67% of an oral dose is absorbed from the GI tract; well absorbed after I.M. injection.
Excretion: After oral administration, 50% of a dose is excreted in urine and 50% in feces. Half-life: Approximately 1.8 hours.

INDICATIONS & DOSAGE

Adjunctive therapy for peptic ulcers and other functional GI disorders–
Adults: 10 to 20 mg P.O. t.i.d. or q.i.d.; 20 mg I.M. q 4 to 6 hours.

Always adjust dosage according to patient's needs and response.

CONTRAINDICATIONS & PRECAUTIONS

Contraindicated in patients with obstructive uropathy, obstructive GI tract disease, severe ulcerative colitis, myasthenia gravis, paralytic ileus, intestinal atony, or toxic megacolon because the drug may exacerbate these conditions; and in patients with hypersensitivity to anticholinergics; also contraindicated in infants under age 6 months.

Use cautiously in patients with narrow-angle glaucoma because drug-induced cycloplegia and mydriasis may increase intraocular pressure; autonomic neuropathy, hyperthyroidism, coronary artery disease, cardiac arrhythmias, CHF, or ulcerative colitis, because the drug may exacerbate the symptoms associated with these disorders; in patients with hepatic or renal disease because toxic accumulation can occur; hiatal hernia associated with reflux esophagitis because the drug may decrease lower esophageal sphincter tone; in patients over age 40 because the drug increases the glaucoma risk; in hot or humid environments because the drug may predispose the patient to heatstroke.

ADVERSE REACTIONS

Common reactions are in italics; life-threatening reactions are in bold italics.
CNS: *headache,* insomnia, drowsiness, *dizziness.*
CV: *palpitations,* tachycardia.
GI: nausea, *constipation,* vomiting, *paralytic ileus.*
GU: *urinary hesitancy, urine retention, impotence.*
Skin: urticaria, decreased sweating or possible anhidrosis, other dermal manifestations.
Other: fever, allergic reactions.

Overdosage may cause curare-like symptoms.

INTERACTIONS

None significant.

EFFECTS ON DIAGNOSTIC TESTS

None reported.

NURSING CONSIDERATIONS

Besides those related universally to drug therapy (see "How to use this book"), consider the following specific recommendations:

Assessment

- Obtain a baseline assessment of the patient's underlying condition before drug therapy.
- Be alert for adverse reactions and drug interactions during dicyclomine therapy.
- Evaluate the patient's and family's knowledge about dicyclomine therapy.

Nursing Diagnoses

- Pain related to the patient's underlying condition.
- Urinary retention related to adverse drug reactions.
- Knowledge deficit related to dicyclomine therapy.

Planning and Implementation

Preparation and Administration

- Never give this drug I.V. or S.C.
- ***P.O. use:*** Give this drug 30 minutes to 1 hour before meals and at bedtime. Bedtime dose can be larger and should be given at least 2 hours after the last meal of the day.

Monitoring

- Monitor for adverse reactions or drug interactions by frequently checking the patient's vital signs.
- Monitor effectiveness by regularly assessing underlying condition.
- Monitor intake and output.

Supportive Care

- A synthetic tertiary derivative that may have fewer atropine-like adverse reactions.
- Help the patient to get in and out of bed if he has dizziness or blurred vision.
- Provide gum or sugarless hard candy to relieve dry mouth.
- If constipation occurs, obtain an order for a laxative.
- Provide additional fluids to help prevent constipation.
- Encourage the patient to void before taking this medication.

Patient Teaching

- Instruct the patient to avoid driving and other hazardous activities that require alertness if he is drowsy, dizzy, or has blurred vision.
- Encourage the patient to drink plenty of fluids to avoid constipation.
- Tell him to report any rash or skin eruptions.

Evaluation

In patients receiving dicyclomine, appropriate evaluation statements may include:

- Patient is able to perform activities of daily living without pain.
- Patient does not develop urine retention.
- Patient and family state an understanding of dicyclomine therapy.

dienestrol (dienoestrol)

(dye en ess´ trole)
DV, Ortho Dienestrol

- *Classification:* topical estrogen

• *Pregnancy Risk Category:* X

HOW SUPPLIED
Vaginal cream: 0.01%

ACTION
Mechanism: Increases the synthesis of DNA, RNA, and protein in responsive tissues. Also reduces follicle stimulating hormone and luteinizing hormone release from the pituitary.
Absorption: Although applied topically for a local effect, some of the drug is absorbed systemically.
Distribution: Absorbed drug is 50% to 80% bound to plasma proteins; like other estrogens, it probably crosses the placenta.

INDICATIONS & DOSAGE
Atrophic vaginitis and kraurosis vulvae–
Postmenopausal women: 1 to 2 intravaginal applications of vaginal cream daily for 1 to 2 weeks (as directed), then half that dose for the same period. A maintenance dosage of 1 applicatorful one to three times a week may be ordered.

CONTRAINDICATIONS & PRECAUTIONS
Contraindicated in patients with estrogen-responsive carcinoma (breast or genital tract cancer) or undiagnosed abnormal genital bleeding because it may worsen these conditions; in pregnant patients because it may be fetotoxic; and in breast-feeding women because it may adversely affect the infant.

Carefully monitor patients who have breast nodules, fibrocystic breast disease, or a family history of breast cancer. Because of the risk of thromboembolism, therapy with this drug should be discontinued at least 1 week before elective surgical procedures associated with an increased incidence of thromboembolism.

ADVERSE REACTIONS
Common reactions are in italics; life-threatening reactions are in bold italics.
GU: vaginal discharge; with excessive use, uterine bleeding.
Local: increased discomfort, burning sensation. Systemic effects possible.
Other: breast tenderness.

INTERACTIONS
None significant.

EFFECTS ON DIAGNOSTIC TESTS
Antithrombin III: decreased concentration.
Free triiodothyronine resin uptake: decreased.
Glucose tolerance: impaired.
Pregnanediol excretion: decreased.
Serum folate and pyridoxine: decreased concentrations.
Sulfobromophthalein retention, prothrombin time and clotting Factors VII to X, and norepinephrine-induced platelet aggregability: increased levels.
Thyroid-binding globulin: increased concentration.
Total thyroid concentration (measured by protein-bound iodine or total thyroxine): increased levels.
Triglyceride, glucose, and phospholipid: increased levels.

NURSING CONSIDERATIONS
Besides those related universally to drug therapy (see "How to use this book"), consider the following specific recommendations:
Assessment
• Obtain a baseline assessment of the patient's atrophic vaginitis and kraurosis vulvae condition before initiating therapy with dienestrol.
• Be alert for local or GU adverse reactions or drug interactions.
• Evaluate the patient's and family's knowledge about dienestrol therapy.
Nursing Diagnoses
• Impaired tissue integrity related to the underlying condition.

• Pain related to local discomfort or burning sensation caused by dienestrol therapy.
• Knowledge deficit related to therapy with dienestrol.

Planning and Implementation

Preparation and Administration

• ***Vaginal use:*** Wash vaginal area with soap and water before application. Have patient remain recumbent for 30 minutes after administration to prevent loss of drug. Supply sanitary pad for patient to wear to prevent staining clothing. Apply drug at bedtime to increase effectiveness.

Monitoring

• Monitor effectiveness by regularly assessing the patient for improvement.
• Monitor patient's level of local discomfort.
• Monitor patient closely for possible systemic reactions.

Supportive Care

• Be aware that withdrawal bleeding may occur if drug is suddenly stopped.

Patient Teaching

• Instruct patient how to insert suppositories or cream and to remain recumbent for 30 minutes after administration.
• Advise patient to administer the drug at bedtime to increase effectiveness.
• Warn patient not to exceed the prescribed dose.
• Tell patient not to wear tampon while receiving vaginal therapy but to protect clothing with a sanitary pad.
• Warn the patient that local discomfort or burning sensation may occur with drug use.
• Teach female patients how to perform routine breast self-examination.
• Give the patient the package insert describing adverse reactions to dienestrol, and also provide verbal explanation.

Evaluation

In patients receiving dienestrol, appropriate evaluation statements may include:
• Patient maintains normal tissue integrity in vaginal area as a result of dienestrol therapy.
• Patient does not experience increased local discomfort or burning sensation during dienestrol therapy.
• Patient and family state an understanding of dienestrol therapy.

diethylstilbestrol (stilboestrol)

(dye eth il stil bess´ trole)
DES

diethylstilbestrol diphosphate

Honvol†

• *Classification:* estrogen replacement, antineoplastic (estrogen)
• *Pregnancy Risk Category:* X

HOW SUPPLIED

diethylstilbestrol
Tablets: 1 mg, 2.5 mg, 5 mg
Tablets (enteric-coated): 1 mg, 5 mg
diethylstilbestrol diphosphate
Tablets: 83 mg†
Injection: 50 mg/ml

ACTION

Mechanism: Increases the synthesis of DNA, RNA, and protein in responsive tissues. Also reduces follicle stimulating hormone and luteinizing hormone release from the pituitary.
Absorption: Well absorbed from the GI tract when administered orally.
Distribution: Like other estrogen derivatives, drug is 50% to 80% bound to plasma proteins. Crosses the placenta.
Metabolism: Hepatic conjugation with glucuronic acid.
Excretion: In both urine and feces, primarily as the glucuronide conjugate.

INDICATIONS & DOSAGE

Hypogonadism, castration, primary ovarian failure–
Women: 0.2 to 0.5 mg P.O. daily.
Menopausal symptoms–
Women: 0.1 to 2 mg P.O. daily in cycles of 3 weeks on and 1 week off.
Postcoital contraception ("morning-after pill")–
Women: 25 mg P.O. b.i.d. for 5 days, starting within 72 hours after coitus.
Postpartum breast engorgement–
Women: 5 mg P.O. daily or t.i.d. up to total dose of 30 mg.
Prostatic cancer–
Men: initially, 1 to 3 mg P.O. daily; may be reduced to 1 mg P.O. daily, or 5 mg I.M. twice weekly initially, followed by up to 4 mg I.M. twice weekly. Or 50 to 200 mg (diphosphate) P.O. t.i.d.; or 0.25 to 1 g I.V. daily for 5 days, then once or twice weekly.
Breast cancer–
Men and postmenopausal women: 15 mg P.O. daily.

CONTRAINDICATIONS & PRECAUTIONS

Contraindicated in patients with thrombophlebitis, thromboembolism or history of thromboembolism associated with estrogen use, estrogen-responsive carcinoma (breast or genital tract cancer), or undiagnosed abnormal genital bleeding; and in pregnant and breast-feeding women.

Use cautiously in patients with disorders that may be aggravated by fluid and electrolyte accumulation, such as asthma, seizure disorders, migraine, or cardiac, renal, or hepatic dysfunction. Carefully monitor female patients who have breast nodules, fibrocystic breast disease, or a family history of breast cancer. Because of the risk of thromboembolism, therapy with this drug should be discontinued at least 1 week before elective surgical procedures associated with an increased incidence of thromboembolism.

ADVERSE REACTIONS

Common reactions are in italics; life-threatening reactions are in bold italics.
CNS: headache, dizziness, chorea, depression, lethargy.
CV: *thrombophlebitis; thromboembolism;* hypertension; edema; ***increased risk of stroke, pulmonary embolism, and myocardial infarction.***
EENT: worsening of myopia or astigmatism, intolerance to contact lenses.
GI: *nausea,* vomiting, abdominal cramps, bloating, diarrhea, constipation, anorexia, increased appetite, excessive thirst, weight changes, pancreatitis.
GU: in women–breakthrough bleeding, altered menstrual flow, dysmenorrhea, amenorrhea, cervical erosion, altered cervical secretions, enlargement of uterine fibromas, vaginal candidiasis, loss of libido. In men–gynecomastia, testicular atrophy, impotence.
Hepatic: cholestatic jaundice.
Metabolic: hyperglycemia, hypercalcemia, folic acid deficiency.
Skin: melasma, urticaria, acne, seborrhea, oily skin, hirsutism or loss of hair.
Other: leg cramps, breast tenderness or enlargement.

INTERACTIONS

None significant.

EFFECTS ON DIAGNOSTIC TESTS

Antithrombin III: decreased concentrations.
Blood glucose: increased levels, necessitating dosage adjustment of insulin or oral hypoglycemic drugs.
Free triiodothyronine resin: decreased uptake.
Glucose tolerance: impaired.
Serum folate and pyridoxine and pregnanediol excretion: decreased.
Sulfobromophthalein, prothrombin

and clotting Factors VII to X, and norepinephrine-induced platelet aggregability: increased.
Thyroid-binding globulin: increased concentration.
Total thyroid concentrations (measured by protein-bound iodine or total thyroxine): increased.
Triglyceride, glucose, and phospholipid: increased levels.

NURSING CONSIDERATIONS

Besides those related universally to drug therapy (see "How to use this book"), consider the following specific recommendations:

Assessment

- Obtain a baseline assessment of the patient's underlying condition before initiating therapy with diethylstibestrol.
- Be alert for common adverse reactions and drug interactions during therapy.
- Evaluate the patient's and family's knowledge about diethylstilbestrol therapy.

Nursing Diagnoses

- Sexual dysfunction related to the patient's underlying condition.
- Altered tissue perfusion (cerebral, peripheral, pulmonary, or myocardial) related to potential for diethylstilbestrol to cause thromboembolism.
- Knowledge deficit related to therapy with diethylstilbestrol.

Planning and Implementation

Preparation and Administration

- ***P.O. use:*** Be aware that only the 25- mg tablet is approved by FDA as the "morning-after pill." To be effective, it must be taken within 72 hours after coitus.
- ***I.M. use:*** When administering I.M., rotate injection sites to prevent muscle atrophy.
- ***I.V. use:*** Not recommended to be given by direct I.V. or by continuous infusion. When giving as an intermittent infusion, inject diluted drug into an I.V. line containing a free-flowing compatible solution, and infuse at 1 to 2 ml/minute for 10 to 15 minutes. Adjust rate so that remaining solution infuses within 1 hour. Infuse drug slowly; rapid infusion can cause perineal or vaginal burning.

Monitoring

- Monitor effectiveness by regularly assessing underlying condition for signs of improvement.
- Monitor for thromboemboli formation by noting any changes in cerebral or cardiopulmonary function or peripheral circulation.
- Monitor blood glucose levels for alterations.
- Monitor hydration status if administering the 25-mg tablet P.O. as nausea and vomiting are common with this large dose.
- Monitor female patients for pregnancy, which requires discontinuation of drug.

Supportive Care

- Withhold drug and notify the doctor if a thromboembolic event is suspected; be prepared to provide supportive care as indicated.
- Alert the pathologist if a specimen is obtained during estrogen therapy.
- Be prepared to adjust diabetic patients' therapeutic regimen if blood glucose levels rise during therapy with diethylstilbestrol.
- Institute safety measures if CNS adverse reactions occur.
- Obtain an order for an antiemetic, antidiarrheal, or laxative agent, as needed.
- Prepare patient for body changes that may occur, such as loss of hair.

Patient Teaching

- Warn the patient to report immediately abdominal pain; pain, numbness, or stiffness in legs or buttocks; pressure or pain in chest; shortness of breath; severe headaches; visual disturbances, such as blind spots, flashing lights, or blurriness; vaginal bleeding or discharge; breast lumps;

swelling of hands or feet; yellow skin and sclera; dark urine; and light-colored stools.
• Explain to patients on cyclic therapy for postmenopausal symptoms that, although withdrawal bleeding may occur in week off drug, fertility has not been restored; ovulation does not occur.
• Teach female patients how to perform routine breast self-examination.
• Teach the patient that medical supervision is essential during therapy. Use of this drug is associated with increased risk of endometrial cancer and possible increased risk of breast cancer. Also be aware that an increased number of cardiovascular deaths has been reported in men taking the 5-mg tablet daily for prostate cancer over a long period.
• Tell diabetic patients to report symptoms of hyperglycemia or glycosuria.
• Tell patients who become pregnant during therapy with diethylstilbestrol to stop taking the drug immediately because it may adversely affect the fetus.
• Give the patient the package insert describing adverse reactions to diethylstilbestrol, and also provide verbal explanation.

Evaluation

In patients receiving diethylstilbestrol, appropriate evaluation statements may include:
• Patient exhibits improved health as a result of diethylstilbestrol therapy.
• Patient does not experience a thromboembolic event during diethylstilbestrol therapy.
• Patient and family state an understanding of diethylstilbestrol therapy.

difenoxin hydrochloride

(dye fen ox´ in)
Lyspafen‡, Motofen

• *Classification:* antidiarrheal (opioid agonist)
• *Pregnancy Risk Category:* C

HOW SUPPLIED

Tablets: 0.5 mg (with atropine sulphate, 0.025 mg)‡, 1 mg (with atropine sulfate, 0.025 mg)

ACTION

Mechanism: Difenoxin is an opiate chemically related to meperidine; it is the active metabolite of diphenoxylate. Atropine has been added to the compound to discourage abuse. Drug exerts a direct effect on the intestinal smooth muscle to slow motility.
Absorption: Rapidly absorbed after oral administration.
Metabolism: Metabolized to an inactive hydroxylated metabolite and conjugates.
Excretion: In urine and feces, as parent drug and metabolites. Over 90% of the drug is excreted within 24 hours of a single dose. Half life: 12 to 14 hours.
Onset, peak, duration: Peak levels occur about 1 hour after a dose.

INDICATIONS AND DOSAGE

Adjunct in acute nonspecific diarrhea, and acute exacerbations of chronic functional diarrhea –
Adults: initially, 2 mg P.O., then 1 mg P.O. after each loose bowel movement. Total dosage should not exceed 8 mg daily. Not recommended for use longer than 2 days.

CONTRAINDICATIONS & PRECAUTIONS

Contraindicated in patients allergic to difenoxin or atropine, in children under age 2, and in patients with diarrhea from pseudomembranous colitis associated with antibiotic administration; in patients with jaundice or diarrhea from organisms that may penetrate the intestinal mucosa (including toxigenic *Escherichia coli, Salmonella,* or *Shigella*). Difenoxin is the principal metabolite of diphenoxylate (Lomotil) and is chemically related to meperidine. Use cautiously in patients with a history of drug abuse or in those currently receiving drugs with a high abuse potential.

Atropine has been added to the medication to prevent abuse. The small amount of atropine in the medication is unlikely to cause clinical problems, but patients may experience dry mouth, tachycardia, urine retention, and flushing. The atropine may exacerbate preexisting glaucoma.

ADVERSE REACTIONS

Common reactions are in italics; life-threatening reactions are in bold italics.
CNS: dizziness and light-headedness, drowsiness, headache, fatigue, nervousness, insomnia, confusion.
EENT: burning eyes, blurred vision.
GI: nausea, vomiting, dry mouth, epigastric distress, constipation.

INTERACTIONS

Alcohol, CNS depressants, tranquilizers, narcotics, barbiturates: enhanced CNS depression. Closely monitor patients.
MAO inhibitors: potential hypertensive crisis. Avoid concomitant use.

EFFECTS ON DIAGNOSTIC TESTS

None reported.

NURSING CONSIDERATIONS

Besides those related universally to drug therapy (see "How to use this book"), consider the following specific recommendations:

Assessment

- Obtain a baseline assessment of history of bowel disorders, GI status, allergies, and frequency of loose stools before therapy.
- Be alert for adverse reactions or drug interactions during therapy.
- Evaluate the patient's and family's knowledge about difenoxin .

Nursing Diagnoses

- Diarrhea related interruption in normal pattern of elimination characterized by frequent loose stools.
- Altered thought processes related to drug-induced adverse CNS reactions.
- Knowledge deficit related to difenoxin therapy.

Planning and Implementation

Preparation and Administration

- Read label carefully; check dosage and strength.
- ***P.O. use:*** Give 2 mg initially, then 1 mg after each loose stool.

Monitoring

- Monitor effectiveness by checking the frequency and characteristics of stools.
- Auscultate bowel sounds at least once a shift. Assess for pain and cramping.
- Monitor closely for fluid and electrolyte balance. Difenoxin-induced decreases in peristalsis may result in fluid retention in the colon, with subsequent dehydration and possibly difenoxin intoxication.
- Weigh patient daily until diarrhea is controlled to detect fluid loss or retention.
- Check skin in perianal area to detect and prevent breakdown.
- Monitor mental and neurologic status. Be alert for development of adverse CNS reactions (confusion, dizziness, light-headedness, drowsiness).
- Monitor for adverse reactions due to atropine.
- Observe for changes in respiratory status, which may indicate difenoxin toxicity.

Supportive Care

- Encourage patient to drink fluids to prevent fluid loss.

• Provide good skin care especially in the perianal area; use soothing powders and lotions.
• Use safety precautions for those patient's with CNS adverse reactions. If patient is confused, reorient to person, time, and place.
• Patients who overdose with difenoxin should be observed for at least 48 hours. Respiratory depression may occur up to 30 hours after ingestion. Gastric lavage, establishment of patent airway, and mechanically assisted ventilation are advised. Naloxone will reverse the respiratory depression. Because difenoxin has longer duration of action than naloxone, repeated injections of naloxone will be necessary.

Patient Teaching
• Advise the patient to adhere to dosing schedule. Overdose with difenoxin may result in respiratory depression and coma.
• Encourage proper storage to keep drug out of children's reach.
• Warn patients that they may experience dry mouth, tachycardia, urine retention, and flushing due to the atropine added to the drug.
• Advise patients to avoid hazardous activities that may require mental alertness until the CNS effects of the drug are known.

Evaluation
In patients receiving difenoxin, appropriate evaluation statements may include:
• Patient reports decrease or absence of loose stools.
• Patient exhibits no signs of CNS adverse reactions.
• Patient and family state an understanding of difenoxin therapy.

diflorasone diacetate
(dye flor´ a sone)
Florone, Flutone, Maxiflor, psorcon

• *Classification:* topical anti-inflammatory (adrenocorticoid)
• *Pregnancy Risk Category:* C

HOW SUPPLIED
Cream: 0.05%
Ointment: 0.05%

ACTION
Mechanism: Produces local anti-inflammatory, vasoconstrictor, and antipruritic actions. Drug diffuses across cell membranes to form complexes with specific cytoplasmic receptors, influencing cellular metabolism. Corticosteroids stabilize leukocyte lysosomal membranes, inhibit local actions and accumulation of macrophages, decrease local edema, and reduce the formation of scar tissue.
Absorption: Amount absorbed depends on the amount applied and on the nature of the skin at the application site. It ranges from about 1% in areas with thick stratum corneum (on the palms, soles, elbows, and knees) to as high as 36% in thinnest areas (face, eyelids, and genitals). Absorption increases in areas of skin damage, inflammation, or occlusion. Some systemic absorption of topical steroids may occur, especially through the oral mucosa.
Distribution: After topical application, distributed throughout the local skin. If absorbed into the circulation, drug is rapidly removed from the blood and distributed into muscle, liver, skin, intestines, and kidneys.
Metabolism: After topical administration, metabolized primarily in the skin. The small amount absorbed into systemic circulation is metabolized primarily in the liver to inactive compounds.

Excretion: Inactive metabolites are excreted by the kidneys, primarily as glucuronides and sulfates, but also as unconjugated products. Small amounts of the metabolites are also excreted in feces.

INDICATIONS & DOSAGE

Inflammation of corticosteroid-responsive dermatoses–
Adults and children: clean area; apply ointment daily to t.i.d.; apply cream b.i.d. to q.i.d. Apply sparingly in a thin film.

CONTRAINDICATIONS & PRECAUTIONS

Contraindicated in patients who are hypersensitive to any component of the preparation and in those with viral, fungal, or tubercular skin lesions. Use with extreme caution in patients with impaired circulation, because its use may increase the risk of skin ulceration. Avoid using on the face and genital areas because increased absorption may result in striae.

ADVERSE REACTIONS

Common reactions are in italics; life-threatening reactions are in bold italics.
Skin: burning, itching, irritation, dryness, folliculitis, perioral dermatitis, hypertrichosis, hypopigmentation, acneiform eruptions. With occlusive dressings: *maceration, secondary infection, atrophy, striae, miliaria.*

INTERACTIONS

None significant.

EFFECTS ON DIAGNOSTIC TESTS

None reported.

NURSING CONSIDERATIONS

Besides those related universally to drug therapy (see "How to use this book"), consider the following specific recommendations:

Assessment

- Obtain a baseline assessment of skin in the affected area before therapy.
- Be alert for adverse reactions and drug interactions throughout therapy.
- Evaluate the patient's and family's knowledge about diflorasone therapy.

Nursing Diagnoses

- Impaired skin integrity related to the patient's underlying condition.
- High risk for infection related to drug-induced adverse reactions.
- Knowledge deficit related to diflorasone therapy.

Planning and Implementation

Preparation and Administration

- ***Topical use:*** Wash skin gently before applying. Rub medication in gently to prevent damage to skin, leaving a thin coat.
- To apply an occlusive dressing: Apply cream or ointment, then cover with a thin, pliable, nonflammable plastic film; seal to adjacent normal skin with hypoallergenic tape. Minimize adverse reactions by using occlusive dressing intermittently. Don't leave in place longer than 16 hours each day. Occlusive dressings should not be used in presence of infection or with weeping or exudative lesions.
- For patient with dermatitis who may develop irritation with adhesive material, hold dressing in place with gauze, elastic bandages, stockings, or stockinettes.
- Diflorasone is often effective with once-daily application.

Monitoring

- Monitor effectiveness by regularly checking patient's skin.
- Observe patient for signs of systemic absorption: skin irritation or ulceration, hypersensitivity, or infection; if these occur, stop drug and notify doctor. (If antifungals or antibiotics are being used concomitantly, corticosteroids should be stopped until infection is controlled.)
- Monitor for adverse reactions and

interactions by frequently inspecting the patient's skin for infection, striae, and atrophy.
• Monitor patient's temperature; if fever develops, notify doctor and remove occlusive dressing.
Supportive Care
• Be prepared to discontinue drug and notify doctor if secondary infection, striae, or atrophy occur.
• Change patient's dressings as ordered.
• Remember that occlusive dressing should not be used with psorcon.
• When used on diaper area in young children, avoid the use of plastic pants or tight-fitting diapers.
• Systemic absorption is especially likely with occlusive dressings, prolonged treatment, or extensive body surface treatment.
• Use cautiously in patients with viral skin diseases, such as varicella, vaccinia, or herpes simplex; fungal infections; or bacterial skin infections.
• Use very cautiously in young children. A high-potency corticosteroid.
Patient Teaching
• Teach patient how to apply medication.
• Instruct patient to avoid application near eyes, mucous membranes, or in ear canal.
• Inform patient about adverse reactions such as secondary infection; if theyoccur, tell patient to stop drug and notify doctor.
Evaluation
In patients receiving diflorasone, appropriate evaluation statements may include:
• Patient states his dermatoses has healed.
• Patient does not develop secondary infection.
• Patient and family state an understanding of diflorasone therapy.

diflunisal
(dye floo´ ni sal)
Dolobid

• *Classification:* nonnarcotic, nonsteroidal analgesic, antipyretic (salicylic acid derivative)
• *Pregnancy Risk Category:* C

HOW SUPPLIED
Tablets: 250 mg, 500 mg

ACTION
Mechanism: Probably related to inhibition of prostaglandin synthesis.
Absorption: Is rapidly and completely absorbed via the GI tract. Peak plasma concentrations occur in 2 to 3 hours. Analgesia is achieved within 1 hour and peaks within 2 to 3 hours.
Distribution: Highly protein-bound.
Metabolism: Hepatic. Diflunisal is not metabolized to salicylic acid.
Excretion: In urine. Half-life: 8 to 12 hours.
Onset, peak, duration: Peak plasma concentrations occur in 2 to 3 hours. Analgesia is achieved within 1 hour and peaks within 2 to 3 hours.

INDICATIONS & DOSAGE
Mild to moderate pain and osteoarthritis–
Adults: 500 to 1,000 mg P.O. daily in two divided doses, usually q 12 hours. Maximum dosage 1,500 mg daily.
Adults over 65: Start with one-half the usual adult dose.

CONTRAINDICATIONS & PRECAUTIONS
Contraindicated in patients with hypersensitivity to the drug or other NSAIDs, and in patients in whom aspirin or other salicylates provoke asthma, urticaria, and rhinitis. Patients with known "triad" symptoms (aspirin hypersensitivity, rhinitis/na-

sal polyps, and asthma) are at high risk of bronchospasm.

Serious GI toxicity, particularly ulceration or hemorrhage, can occur at any time in patients on chronic NSAID therapy. Diflunisal should be administered cautiously to patients with active GI bleeding or history of peptic ulcer disease because the drug may exacerbate these conditions; and to patients with renal impairment or compromised cardiac function because peripheral edema has been seen in some patients. Diflunisal may mask the signs and symptoms of acute infection (fever, myalgia, erythema); carefully evaluate patients with high risk (such as those with diabetes).

ADVERSE REACTIONS

Common reactions are in italics; life-threatening reactions are in bold italics.

CNS: *dizziness,* somnolence, insomnia, *headache,* fatigue.
EENT: *tinnitus, visual disturbances (rare).*
GI: *nausea, dyspepsia, gastrointestinal pain, diarrhea,* vomiting, constipation, flatulence.
Skin: *rash,* pruritus, sweating, dry mucous membranes, stomatitis.

INTERACTIONS

Aspirin, antacids: decreased diflunisal blood levels. Monitor for possible decreased therapeutic effect.
Oral anticoagulants, thrombolytic agents: diflunisal may enhance pharmacologic effects of these agents. Use together cautiously.
Sulindac: diflunisal decreases blood levels of sulindac's active metabolite. Monitor for decreased pharmacologic effect.

EFFECTS ON DIAGNOSTIC TESTS

Bleeding time: prolonged.
BUN, serum creatinine and potassium: increased levels.
Serum transaminase, alkaline phosphatase, and lactic dehydrogenase: increased levels.
Serum uric acid: decreased.

NURSING CONSIDERATIONS

Besides those related universally to drug therapy (see "How to use this book"), consider the following specific recommendations:

Assessment

- Obtain a baseline assessment of pain before therapy.
- Be alert for adverse reactions and drug interactions throughout therapy.
- Evaluate the patient's and family's knowledge about diflunisal therapy.

Nursing Diagnoses

- Pain related to the patient's underlying condition.
- High risk for injury related to adverse reactions.
- Knowledge deficit related to diflunisal therapy.

Planning and Implementation

Preparation and Administration

- Administer drug with water, milk, or meals.
- Avoid use in children and teenagers with viral illnesses and flu because of possible association with Reye's syndrome.

Monitoring

- Monitor effectiveness by regularly evaluating pain relief.
- Monitor platelet function. Drug is similar to aspirin but is metabolized differently and has less effect on platelet function.

Supportive Care

- Notify the doctor if dizziness, headache, tinnitus, or GI disturbances occurs.
- If patient experiences dizziness, take safety precautions, such as using side rails and assisting the patient when out of bed.

Patient Teaching

- Advise patient to take the drug with water, milk, or meals.
- Because of possible interactions with drugs, such as those containing

aspirin, warn the patient to check with the doctor or pharmacist before taking any OTC medications.

Evaluation

In patients receiving diflunisal, appropriate evaluation statements may include:

- Patient states that pain is relieved.
- Patient exhibits no evidence of injury from adverse reactions.
- Patient and family state an understanding of diflunisal therapy.

digitoxin

(di ji tox´ in)

Crystodigin

- *Classification:* antiarrhythmic, inotropic agent (digitalis glycoside)
- *Pregnancy Risk Category:* C

HOW SUPPLIED

Tablets: 0.05 mg, 0.1 mg, 0.15 mg, 0.2 mg

ACTION

Mechanism: A cardiac glycoside that inhibits sodium-potassium activated adenosine triphosphatase (Na/K ATPase). Intracellular sodium accumulation leads to calcium accumulation within the myocardial cell. Increased calcium availability strengthens myocardial contraction. Cardiac glycosides also act on the CNS to increase vagal tone and slow heart rate.

Absorption: Rapidly and completely absorbed from the GI tract.

Distribution: Widely distributed in body tissues; highest concentrations appear in the heart, kidneys, intestine, stomach, liver, and skeletal muscle; lowest concentrations appear in the plasma and brain. Little of the drug crosses the blood-brain barrier. About 97% is bound to plasma proteins. Usual therapeutic steady-state serum levels range from 20 to 35 ng/ml.

Metabolism: Extensively metablized in the liver to active metabolites (one of which is digoxin) and inactive metabolites. Dosage reduction may be necessary in patients with hepatic impairment.

Excretion: After it is metabolized and enters the enterohepatic recirculation, digitoxin is eventually excreted in urine. Half-life: Ranges from 5 to 14 days.

Onset, peak, duration: After oral administration, therapeutic effects appear in 1 to 2 hours, with peak effects occurring in 8 to 12 hours. Drug effects can persist for 3 to 5 weeks.

INDICATIONS & DOSAGE

CHF, paroxysmal supraventricular tachycardia, atrial fibrillation and flutter–

Adults: loading dose is 1.2 to 1.6 mg P.O. in divided doses over 24 hours; average maintenance dosage is 0.15 mg daily (range: 0.05 to 0.3 mg daily).

Children 2 to 12 years: loading dose is 0.03 mg/kg or 0.75 mg/m² P.O. in divided doses over 24 hours; maintenance dosage is one-tenth of loading dose or 0.003 mg/kg or 0.075 mg/m² daily. Monitor closely for toxicity.

Children 1 to 2 years: loading dose is 0.04 mg/kg P.O. over 24 hours in divided doses; maintenance dosage is 0.004 mg/kg daily. Monitor closely for toxicity.

Children 2 weeks to 1 year: loading dose is 0.045 mg/kg P.O. in divided doses over 24 hours; maintenance dosage is 0.0045 mg/kg daily. Monitor closely for toxicity.

Premature infants, neonates, severely ill older infants: loading dose is 0.022 mg/kg P.O. in divided doses over 24 hours; maintenance dosage is 0.0022 mg/kg daily. Monitor closely for toxicity.

CONTRAINDICATIONS & PRECAUTIONS

Contraindicated in patients with ventricular fibrillation because the drug may induce arrhythmias; in patients with digitoxin toxicity; and in patients with hypersensitivity to the drug.

Use with extreme caution, if at all, in patients with idiopathic hypertrophic subaortic stenosis because the drug may cause increased obstruction of left ventricular outflow; incomplete atrioventricular (AV) block who do not have an artificial pacemaker (especially those with Stokes-Adams syndrome) because the drug may induce advanced or complete AV block; hypersensitive carotid sinus syndrome because the drug increases vagal tone (carotid sinus massage has induced ventricular fibrillation in patients receiving cardiac glycosides); Wolff-Parkinson-White syndrome because the drug may cause fatal ventricular arrhythmias; in patients with sinus node disease (such as sick sinus syndrome), because the drug may worsen sinus bradycardia or SA block; severe pulmonary disease, hypoxia, myxedema, acute myocardial infarction, severe heart failure, acute myocarditis, or an otherwise damaged myocardium because the drug increases the risk of arrhythmias in these patients; chronic constrictive pericarditis because such patients may respond unfavorably to the drug; frequent premature ventricular contractions or ventricular tachycardia (especially if these arrhythmias do not result from heart failure) because the drug may induce arrhythmias; with low cardiac output states caused by valvular stenosis, chronic pericarditis, or chronic cor pulmonale because the drug may decrease heart rate, which, in turn, may reduce cardiac output; and conditions that increase cardiac sensitivity to digitalis, including hypokalemia, chronic pulmonary disease, and acute hypoxemia.

ADVERSE REACTIONS

Common reactions are in italics; life-threatening reactions are in bold italics. *The following are signs of toxicity that may occur with all cardiac glycosides:*

CNS: *fatigue, generalized muscle weakness, agitation, hallucinations,* headache, malaise, dizziness, vertigo, stupor, paresthesias.

CV: ***increased severity of CHF,*** *arrhythmias (most commonly conduction disturbances with or without AV block, premature ventricular contractions, and supraventricular arrhythmias),* hypotension.

Toxic effects on heart may be life-threatening and require immediate attention.

EENT: *yellow-green halos around visual images, blurred vision,* light flashes, photophobia, diplopia.

GI: *anorexia, nausea,* vomiting, diarrhea.

INTERACTIONS

Amphotericin B, carbenicillin, ticarcillin, corticosteroids, and diuretics (including loop diuretics, chlorthalidone, metolazone, and thiazides): hypokalemia, predisposing patient to digitalis toxicity. Monitor serum potassium.

Antacids, kaolin-pectin: decreased absorption of oral digitoxin. Schedule doses as far as possible from oral digitoxin administration.

Cholestyramine, colestipol, metoclopramide: decreased absorption of oral digitoxin. Monitor for decreased effect and low blood levels. Dosage may have to be increased.

Cimetidine: decreased digitoxin metabolism. Monitor for digitoxin toxicity.

Parenteral calcium, thiazides: hypercalcemia and hypomagnesemia, predisposing patient to digitalis toxicity.

Monitor serum calcium and serum magnesium.
Phenylbutazone, phenobarbital, phenytoin, rifampin: faster metabolism and shorter duration of digitoxin. Observe for underdigitalization.
Quinidine, verapamil: Possible increased serum digitoxin levels. Monitor patient closely.

EFFECTS ON DIAGNOSTIC TESTS

Urine 17-ketogenic steroid (Zimmerman reaction): falsely elevated levels.

NURSING CONSIDERATIONS

Besides those related universally to drug therapy (see "How to use this book"), consider the following specific recommendations:

Assessment

- Obtain a baseline assessment of the patient's heart rate and rhythm or degree of CHF present before digitoxin therapy.
- Be alert for adverse reactions and drug interactions throughout therapy.
- Evaluate the patient's and family's knowledge about digitoxin therapy.

Nursing Diagnoses

- Decreased cardiac output related to ineffectiveness of digitoxin.
- High risk for injury related to digitalis toxicity caused by digitoxin.
- Knowledge deficit related to digitoxin therapy.

Planning and Implementation

Preparation and Administration

- Obtain baseline data (heart rate and rhythm, blood pressure, and electrolyte levels) before giving first dose.
- Ask patient about recent use of digitalis glycosides (within the previous 2 to 3 weeks) before administering a loading dose.
- Always divide loading dose over first 24 hours unless clinical situation indicates otherwise.
- Before giving each dose, take apical-radial pulse for a full minute.

Monitoring

- Monitor effectiveness by taking an apical-radial pulse for a full minute before each dose, evaluating ECG when ordered, and regularly assessing patient's cardiopulmonary status for signs of improvement.
- Monitor serum calcium, potassium, and magnesium levels.
- Monitor serum digitoxin levels. Obtain blood for digitoxin levels 8 hours after last oral dose. Therapeutic blood levels of digitoxin range from 25 to 35 ng/ml.
- Regularly monitor for digitalis toxicity.

Supportive Care

- Withhold drug and notify doctor if excessive slowing of the pulse rate (60 beats/minute or less) occurs as this may be a sign of digitalis toxicity. Also notify doctor of any significant changes, such as a sudden increase or decrease in rate, pulse deficit, irregular beats, and particularly regularization of a previously irregular rhythm. Check blood pressure and obtain 12-lead ECG with these changes.
- Obtain a serum digitoxin level as ordered if digitalis toxicity is suspected. Be prepared to treat digitoxin toxicity by withholding drug and administering agents that bind the drug in the intestine (for example, colestipol and cholestyramine). Arrhythmias may be treated with phenytoin I.V. Potentially life-threatening toxicity may be treated by specific antigen-binding fragments (digoxin immune FAB).
- Institute safety precautions if CNS reactions occur.
- Obtain an order for an antiemetic or antidiarrheal agent if GI reactions occur.

Patient Teaching

- Teach the patient and family how to take a pulse before each dose.
- Stress the importance of notifying the doctor if digitalis toxicity is sus-

pected because of visual disturbances, change in mental status, irregular pulse, or GI dysfunction.
• Encourage patient to eat potassium-rich foods.
• Tell the patient that regular follow-up and periodic laboratory tests will be needed to evaluate the effectiveness of the drug.

Evaluation
In patients receiving digitoxin, appropriate evaluation statements may include:
• Patient's cardiopulmonary function has returned to patient's baseline status.
• Patient does not experience digitalis toxicity during digitoxin therapy.
• Patient and family state an understanding of digitoxin therapy.

---

digoxin
(di jox´ in)
Lanoxicaps, Lanoxin*, Novodigoxin†

• *Classification:* antiarrhythmic, inotropic agent (digitalis glycoside)
• *Pregnancy Risk Category:* C

HOW SUPPLIED
Tablets: 0.125 mg, 0.25 mg, 0.5 mg
Capsules: 0.05 mg, 0.1 mg, 0.2 mg
Elixir: 0.05 mg/ml
Injection: 0.05 mg/ml†, 0.1 mg/ml (pediatric), 0.25 mg/ml

ACTION
Mechanism: Promotes movement of calcium from extracellular to intracellular cytoplasm and inhibits sodium-potassium–activated adenosine triphosphatase. These actions strengthen myocardial contraction.
Absorption: With tablet or elixir administration, 60% to 85% of dose is absorbed. With capsule form, bioavailability is greater; about 90% to 100% of a dose is absorbed. With I.M. administration, absorption can be erratic; about 80% of dose is absorbed.
Distribution: Widely distributed in body tissues; highest concentrations occur in the heart, kidneys, intestine, stomach, liver, and skeletal muscle; lowest concentrations are in the plasma and brain. Digoxin crosses both the blood-brain barrier and the placenta; fetal and maternal digoxin levels are equivalent at birth. About 20% to 30% of drug is bound to plasma proteins. Usual therapeutic range for steady-state serum levels is 0.5 to 2 ng/ml. In treatment of atrial tachyarrhythmias, higher serum levels (such as 2 to 4 ng/ml) may be needed. Because of drug's long half-life, achievement of steady-state levels may take 7 days or longer, depending on patient's renal function. Toxic symptoms may appear within the usual therapeutic range; however, these are more frequent and serious with levels above 2.5 ng/ml.
Metabolism: In most patients, a small amount of digoxin apparently is metabolized in the liver and gut by bacteria. This metabolism varies and may be substantial in some patients. Drug undergoes some enterohepatic recirculation (also variable). Metabolites have minimal cardiac activity.
Excretion: Most of dose is excreted by the kidneys as unchanged drug. Some patients excrete a substantial amount of metabolized or reduced drug. In patients with renal failure, biliary excretion is a more important excretion route. Half life: In healthy patients, terminal half-life is 30 to 40 hours; in those lacking functioning kidneys, half-life increases to at least 4 days.

Promotes movement of calcium from extracellular to intracellular cytoplasm and inhibits sodium-potassium activated adenosine triphosphatase. These actions strengthen myocardial contraction.
Onset, peak, and duration: With oral

administration, onset of action occurs in 30 minutes to 2 hours, with peak effects in 6 to 8 hours. With I.M. administration, onset of action occurs in 30 minutes, with peak effects in 4 to 6 hours. With I.V. administration, onset of action occurs in 5 to 30 minutes, peak effects in 1 to 5 hours, and duration is for 6 to 8 days.

INDICATIONS & DOSAGE

CHF, paroxysmal supraventricular tachycardia, atrial fibrillation and flutter–

Adults: loading dose is 0.5 to 1 mg I.V. or P.O. in divided doses over 24 hours; maintenance dosage is 0.125 to 0.5 mg I.V. or P.O. daily (average 0.25 mg). Larger doses are often needed for treatment of arrhythmias, depending on patient response. Smaller loading and maintenance doses should be given in patients with impaired renal function.

Adults over 65 years: 0.125 mg P.O. daily as maintenance dose. Frail or underweight elderly patients may require only 0.0625 mg daily or 0.125 mg every other day.

Children over 2 years: loading dose is 0.02 to 0.04 mg/kg P.O. divided q 8 hours over 24 hours; I.V. loading dose is 0.015 to 0.035 mg/kg; maintenance dosage is 0.012 mg/kg P.O. daily divided q 12 hours.

Children 1 month to 2 years: loading dose is 0.035 to 0.06 mg/kg P.O. in three divided doses over 24 hours; I.V. loading dose is 0.03 to 0.05 mg/kg; maintenance dosage is 0.01 to 0.02 mg/kg P.O. daily divided q 12 hours.

Neonates under 1 month: loading dose is 0.035 mg/kg P.O. divided q 8 hours over 24 hours; I.V. loading dose is 0.02 to 0.03 mg/kg; maintenance dosage is 0.01 mg/kg P.O. daily divided q 12 hours.

Premature infants: loading dose is 0.025 mg/kg I.V. in three divided doses over 24 hours; maintenance dosage is 0.01 mg/kg I.V. daily divided q 12 hours.

CONTRAINDICATIONS & PRECAUTIONS

Contraindicated in patients with ventricular fibrillation because the drug may induce arrhythmias; in patients with digoxin toxicity; and in patients with hypersensitivity to the drug.

Use with extreme caution, if at all, in patients with idiopathic hypertrophic subaortic stenosis because the drug may cause increased obstruction of left ventricular outflow; incomplete atrioventricular (AV) block who do not have an artificial pacemaker (especially those with Stokes-Adams syndrome) because the drug may induce advanced or complete AV block; hypersensitive carotid sinus syndrome, because the drug increases vagal tone (carotid sinus massage has induced ventricular fibrillation in patients receiving cardiac glycosides); Wolff-Parkinson-White syndrome because the drug may cause fatal ventricular arrhythmias; sinus node disease (such as sick sinus syndrome) because the drug may worsen sinus bradycardia or SA block; in patients with severe pulmonary disease, hypoxia, myxedema, acute myocardial infarction, severe heart failure, acute myocarditis, or an otherwise damaged myocardium because the drug increases the risk of arrhythmias; chronic constrictive pericarditis because such patients may respond unfavorably to the drug; frequent premature ventricular contractions or ventricular tachycardia (especially if these arrhythmias do not result from heart failure) because the drug may induce arrhythmias; low cardiac output states caused by valvular stenosis, chronic pericarditis, or chronic cor pulmonale because the drug may decrease heart rate, which, in turn, may reduce cardiac output; and conditions that increase cardiac sensitivity to digitalis, including hypokalemia, chronic pulmonary disease, and acute hypoxemia.

I.V. digoxin should be used with caution in patients with hypertension, because I.V. administration may increase blood pressure transiently.

ADVERSE REACTIONS

Common reactions are in italics; life-threatening reactions are in bold italics. *The following are signs of toxicity that may occur with all cardiac glycosides:*

CNS: *fatigue, generalized muscle weakness, agitation, hallucinations,* headache, malaise, dizziness, vertigo, stupor, paresthesias.

CV: ***increased severity of CHF,*** *arrhythmias (most commonly conduction disturbances with or without AV block, premature ventricular contractions, and supraventricular arrhythmias),* hypotension.

Toxic effects on heart may be life-threatening and require immediate attention.

EENT: *yellow-green halos around visual images, blurred vision,* light flashes, photophobia, diplopia.

GI: *anorexia, nausea,* vomiting, diarrhea.

INTERACTIONS

Amiloride: inhibits and increases digoxin excretion. Monitor for altered digoxin effect.

Amphotericin B, carbenicillin, ticarcillin, corticosteroids, and diuretics (including loop diuretics, chlorthalidone, metolazone, and thiazides): hypokalemia, predisposing patient to digitalis toxicity. Monitor serum potassium.

Antacids, kaolin-pectin: decreased absorption of oral digoxin. Schedule doses as far as possible from oral digoxin administration.

Anticholinergics: may increase digoxin absorption of oral tablets. Monitor blood levels and observe for toxicity.

Cholestyramine, colestipol, metoclopramide: decreased absorption of oral digoxin. Monitor for decreased effect and low blood levels. Dosage may have to be increased.

Parenteral calcium, thiazides: hypercalcemia and hypomagnesemia, predisposing patient to digitalis toxicity. Monitor serum calcium and serum magnesium.

Quinidine, diltiazem, amiodarone, nifedipine, verapamil: increased digoxin blood levels. Monitor for toxicity.

EFFECTS ON DIAGNOSTIC TESTS

None reported.

NURSING CONSIDERATIONS

Besides those related universally to drug therapy (see "How to use this book"), consider the following specific recommendations:

Assessment

- Obtain a baseline assessment of the patient's heart rate and rhythm or degree of CHF present before digoxin therapy.
- Be alert for adverse drug reactions or drug interactions throughout digoxin therapy.
- Evaluate the patient's and family's knowledge about digoxin therapy.

Nursing Diagnoses

- Decreased cardiac output related to ineffectiveness of digoxin.
- High risk for injury related to digitalis toxicity caused by digoxin.
- Knowledge deficit related to digoxin therapy.

Planning and Implementation

Preparation and Administration

- Obtain baseline data (heart rate and rhythm, blood pressure, and electrolyte levels) before giving first dose.
- Ask patient about recent use of digitalis glycosides (within the previous 2 to 3 weeks) before administering a loading dose.

• Withhold drug for 1 to 2 days before elective electrocardioversion as prescribed. Expect dosage adjustment after cardioversion.
• Always divide loading dose over first 24 hours unless clinical situation indicates otherwise.
• Be aware that when changing from oral tablets or elixir to parenteral therapy or to liquid-filled capsules, the dosage is reduced by 20% to 25%. When changing from liquid-filled capsules to parenteral therapy, dosage is about equivalent because liquid-filled capsules are readily absorbed.
• Be aware that, in obese patients, dosage should be based on ideal body weight.
• Before giving each dose, take apical-radial pulse for a full minute.
• ***I.V. use:*** Infuse drug slowly over at least 5 minutes.

Monitoring

• Monitor effectiveness by taking an apical-radial pulse for a full minute before each dose, evaluating ECG when ordered, and regularly assessing patient's cardiopulmonary status for signs of improvement.
• Monitor serum calcium, potassium, and magnesium levels.
• Monitor serum digoxin levels. Obtain blood for digoxin levels 8 hours after last oral dose. Therapeutic blood levels of digoxin range from 0.5 to 2 ng/ml.
• Regularly monitor for digitalis toxicity.

Supportive Care

• Withhold drug and notify doctor if excessive slowing of the pulse rate (60 beats/minute or less) occurs as this may be a sign of digitalis toxicity. Obtain a serum digoxin level and be prepared to treat digitalis toxicity if confirmed by withholding the drug and administering agents that bind the drug in the intestine (for example, colestipol and cholestyramine). Arrrhythmias may be treated with phenytoin I.V. Potentially life-threathening toxicity may be treated by specific antigen-binding fragments (digoxin immune FAB).
• Notify doctor if significant changes, such as a sudden increase or decrease in heart rate, pulse deficit, irregular beats, and particularly regularization of a previously irregular rhythm, occurs. Check blood pressure and obtain 12-lead ECG with these changes.
• Do not administer calcium salts to patients receiving digoxin; calcium affects cardiac contractility and excitability and may lead to serious arrhythmias.
• Institute safety precautions if CNS reactions occur.
• Obtain an order for an antiemetic or antidiarrheal agent if GI reactions occur. Also obtain a digoxin blood level to determine if symptoms are a result of toxicity. If so, expect to withhold dose.

Patient Teaching

• Teach the patient and family how to take a pulse before each dose.
• Stress the importance of notifying the doctor if digitalis toxicity is suspected because of visual disturbances, change in mental status, irregular pulse, or GI dysfunction.
• Encourage patient to eat potassium-rich foods.
• Tell the patient that regular follow-up and periodic laboratory tests will be needed to evaluate the effectiveness of the drug.

Evaluation

In patients receiving digoxin, appropriate evaluation statements may include:
• Patient's cardiopulmonary function has returned to patient's baseline status.
• Patient does not experience digitalis toxicity throughout digoxin therapy.
• Patient and family state an understanding of digoxin therapy.

digoxin immune FAB (ovine)

(di jox´ in)
Digibind

• *Classification:* digitalis antidote (antibody fragment)
• *Pregnancy Risk Category:* C

HOW SUPPLIED

Injection: 40-mg vial

ACTION

Mechanism: An antibody fragment derived from horse serum that binds molecules of digoxin and digitoxin rendering them inactive.
Absorption: The binding between FAB fragments and glycoside molecules appears to occur rapidly; data are limited.
Distribution: After I.V. administration, it appears to distribute rapidly throughout extracellular space, into both plasma and interstitial fluid. It is not known if digoxin immune FAB crosses the placental barrier or is distributed into breast milk.
Excretion: In urine via glomerular filtration. Half-life: 15 to 20 hours.
Onset, peak, duration: Peak serum concentrations occur at the completion of I.V. infusion.

INDICATIONS & DOSAGE

Treatment of potentially life-threatening digoxin or digitoxin intoxication–
Adults and children: administered I.V. over 30 minutes or as a bolus if cardiac arrest is imminent. The dosage varies according to the amount of digoxin or digitoxin to be neutralized. Each vial binds about 0.6 mg digoxin or digitoxin. Average dosage is 10 vials (400 mg). However, if the toxicity resulted from acute digoxin ingestion, and neither a serum digoxin level nor an estimated ingestion amount is known, 20 vials (800 mg) should be administered. See package insert for complete, specific dosage instructions.

CONTRAINDICATIONS & PRECAUTIONS

There are no known contraindications. No systemic allergic reactions have been reported; however, patients sensitive to or intolerant of sheep or other products of ovine origin may be intolerant of digoxin immune FAB. In these high-risk patients, skin testing is recommended. Use cautiously in patients with low cardiac output and CHF because the condition may worsen from the subsequent decrease in effective inotropic concentrations of digoxin. A causal relationship has not been established.

Ventricular tachycardia may develop in patients with preexisting atrial fibrillation because of the reversal of the glycoside effects on the AV node.

Renal impairment may delay elimination of FAB-digoxin complex.

ADVERSE REACTIONS

Common reactions are in italics; life-threatening reactions are in bold italics.
CV: CHF, rapid ventricular rate (both caused by reversal of the cardiac glycoside's therapeutic effects).
Metabolic: hypokalemia.
Other: ***hypersensitivity.***

INTERACTIONS

None reported.

EFFECTS ON DIAGNOSTIC TESTS

Digitalis glycosides: altered determinations by radioimmunoassay (falsely increased or decreased, depending on separation method).
Serum potassium: rapidly decreased levels.

NURSING CONSIDERATIONS

Besides those related universally to drug therapy (see "How to use this

book"), consider the following specific recommendations:

Assessment

• Obtain a baseline assessment of serum digoxin or digitoxin levels, allergies, and cardiopulmonary status before therapy.

• Be alert for adverse reactions and drug interactions throughout therapy.

• Evaluate the patient's and family's knowledge about digoxin immune FAB therapy.

Nursing Diagnoses

• High risk for injury related to life-threatening digoxin or digitoxin intoxication.

• Decreased cardiac output related to drug-induced CHF.

• Knowledge deficit related to digoxin immune FAB therapy.

Planning and Implementation

Preparation and Administration

• Refrigerate powder for reconstitution. Reconstituted product should be used immediately, but it may be stored for up to 4 hours in the refrigerator.

• ***I.V. use:*** Infuse drug through a 0.22 membrane filter. Give by bolus injection if cardiac arrest seems imminent.

Monitoring

• Monitor effectiveness by observing for decreased signs and symptoms of digitalis toxicity; in most patients, they disappear within a few hours.

• Monitor vital signs, ECG, and serum potassium levels during and after administration.

• Monitor for signs of CHF: auscultate lungs; observe for dyspnea and jugular vein distention; observe skin color and turgor; check peripheral pulses and for the presence of edema; monitor intake and output, urine specific gravity and daily weight.

• Monitor mental status, including orientation and level of consciousness.

• Observe for signs of hypersensitivity, serum sickness, or febrile reaction.

• Check serum digoxin level; digoxin immune FAB may interfere with digoxin immunoassay measurements, so standard serum digoxin levels may be misleading until the drug is cleared from the body (about 2 days). Total serum digoxin levels may rise after administration of this drug, but this reflects FAB-bound (inactive) digoxin.

Supportive Care

• Use with caution in patients allergic to ovine proteins. Digoxin immune FAB is derived from digoxin-specific antibody fragments obtained from immunized sheep. Skin testing is recommended in high-risk patients.

• This antidote should only be used for life-threatening overdose in patients in shock or cardiac arrest; with ventricular arrhythmias, such as ventricular tachycardia or fibrillation; with progressive bradycardia, such as severe sinus bradycardia; or with second- or third-degree AV block not responsive to atropine.

• Administer oxygen as ordered. Keep resuscitation equipment nearby.

• Elevate head of bed to alleviate orthopnea.

• Cover patient lightly; keep patient warm but avoid overheating.

• Relieve anxiety and pain; offer emotional support and reassurance.

Patient Teaching

• Instruct the patient to report respiratory difficulty, chest pain, or dizziness immediately.

• Advise patient to avoid straining at stool to prevent bradycardia and decreased cardiac output.

• Encourage proper storage of medication to avoid accidental poisoning.

Evaluation

In patients receiving digoxin immune FAB, appropriate evaluation statements may include:

• Patient remains free from injury related to digitalis intoxication.

• Patient's cardiac output remains adequate.
• Patient and family state an understanding of digoxin immune FAB therapy.

---

dihydroergotamine mesylate
(dye hye droe er got´ a meen)
D.H.E. 45, Dihydergot‡

• *Classification:* vasoconstrictor (ergot alkaloid)
• *Pregnancy Risk Category:* X

HOW SUPPLIED
Injection: 1 mg/ml

ACTION
Mechanism: A semisynthetic ergot alkaloid that inhibits the effects of epinephrine, norepinephrine, and other sympathomimetic amines. Also has antiserotonin effects.
Absorption: Incompletely and irregularly absorbed from the GI tract.
Distribution: Drug is 90% plasma protein-bound.
Metabolism: In the liver; undergoes extensive first-pass metabolism.
Excretion: 10% of a dose is excreted in urine within 72 hours as metabolites; the rest in feces by biliary elimination.
Onset, peak, duration: Onset of action is probably dependent on how promptly after onset of headache the drug is given. After I.M. injection, the onset of action occurs within 15 to 30 minutes, and after I.V. injection, within a few minutes. Duration of action persists 3 to 4 hours after I.M. injection.

INDICATIONS & DOSAGE
Vascular or migraine headache–
Adults: 1 mg I.M. or I.V. May repeat q 1 to 2 hours, p.r.n., up to total of 3 mg per attack. Maximum weekly dosage is 6 mg.

CONTRAINDICATIONS & PRECAUTIONS
Contraindicated in patients with peripheral vascular disease, coronary artery disease, hypertension, or sepsis because of the cardiovascular effects of the drug; impaired hepatic or renal function because of the potential for accumulation and toxicity; hypersensitivity to the drug; and during pregnancy.

ADVERSE REACTIONS
Common reactions are in italics; life-threatening reactions are in bold italics.
CV: numbness and tingling in fingers and toes, transient tachycardia or bradycardia, precordial distress and pain, increased arterial pressure.
GI: nausea, vomiting.
Skin: itching.
Other: weakness in legs, muscle pains in extremities, localized edema.

INTERACTIONS
Propranolol and other beta blockers: blocked natural pathway for vasodilation in patients receiving ergot alkaloids and thus could result in excessive vasoconstriction. Watch closely if drugs are used together.

EFFECTS ON DIAGNOSTIC TESTS
None reported.

NURSING CONSIDERATIONS
Besides those related universally to drug therapy (see "How to use this book"), consider the following recommendations:
Assessment
• Obtain a baseline assessment of the patient's pain before drug therapy.
• Be alert for adverse reactions and drug interactions during therapy.
• Evaluate the patient's and family's knowledge about dihydroergotamine mesylate therapy.
Nursing Diagnoses
• Pain related to the patient's underlying condition.

• Sensory/perceptual alteration (tactile) related to adverse drug reactions.
• Knowledge deficit related to dihydroergotamine mesylate therapy.

Planning and Implementation

Preparation and Administration
• Avoid prolonged administration; don't exceed recommended dosage.
• Know that the drug is most effective when used at first sign of migraine or soon after onset.
• ***I.V. use:*** Continuous and intermittent infusions are not recommended. Directly inject the solution into the vein over 3 minutes. Protect ampules from heat and light. Discard if solution is discolored.
• For short-term use only.

Monitoring
• Monitor for adverse reactions or drug interactions by frequently asking the patient about any numbness and tingling or loss of sensation in the extremities, fingers, and toes. Severe vasoconstriction may result in tissue damage.
• Monitor the patient's vital signs.
• Monitor hydration status if he develops nausea and vomiting.
• Monitor for ergotamine rebound, or an increase in frequency and duration of headache, which may occur when the drug is discontinued.

Supportive Care
• Be prepared to adjust the dose, as ordered, to determine the most effective minimal dose.
• Provide fluids if he develops nausea and vomiting.
• Obtain an order for a mild antipruretic if he develops itching.
• Help the patient to evaluate his underlying causes of stress.
• Provide a quiet, low-light environment to help the patient relax.

Patient Teaching
• Tell the patient to use a mild antipruritic to relieve itching.
• Tell the patient to take the drug at the first sign of a migraine or soon after the onset.
• Tell the patient to report any feeling of coldness in his extremities or tingling of fingers and toes from vasoconstriction.

Evaluation

In patients receiving dihydroergotamine mesylate, appropriate evaluation statements may include:
• Patient's pain is relieved.
• Patient does not develop numbness and tingling.
• Patient and family state an understanding of dihydroergotamine mesylate therapy.

dihydrotachysterol

(dye hye droe tak iss´ ter ole)
AT-10‡, DHT*, Hytakerol

• *Classification:* antihypocalcemic (vitamin D analog)
• *Pregnancy Risk Category:* A (D if used in doses > RDA)

HOW SUPPLIED

Tablets: 0.125 mg, 0.2 mg, 0.4 mg
Capsules: 0.125 mg
Oral solution: 0.2 mg/5 ml, 0.2 mg/ml* (Intensol*), 0.25 mg/ml (in sesame oil)

ACTION

Mechanism: A vitamin D analog that stimulates calcium absorption from the GI tract and promotes bone resorption that releases calcium to blood.
Absorption: Readily absorbed from the small intestine if fat absorption is normal.
Distribution: Widely distributed; it is largely protein-bound.
Metabolism: In the liver.
Excretion: Dihydrotachysterol is excreted in urine and bile.
Onset, peak, duration: Increases in serum calcium can be seen within

several hours of an oral dose; maximal effect is seen within about 2 weeks of starting daily administration. Duration of action is up to 9 weeks.

INDICATIONS & DOSAGE

Familial hypophosphatemia –
Adults and children: 0.5 to 2 mg P.O. daily. Maintenance dosage is 0.3 to 1.5 mg daily.
Hypocalcemia associated with hypoparathyroidism and pseudohypoparathyroidism–
Adults: initially, 0.8 to 2.4 mg P.O. daily for several days. Maintenance dosage is 0.2 to 2 mg daily, as required for normal serum calcium. Average dose is 0.6 mg daily.
Children: initially, 1 to 5 mg P.O. for several days. Maintenance dosage is 0.2 to 1 mg daily, as required for normal serum calcium.
Renal osteodystrophy in chronic uremia –
Adults: 0.1 to 0.6 mg P.O. daily.
Prophylaxis of hypocalcemic tetany following thyroid surgery–
Adults: 0.25 mg P.O. daily (with calcium supplements).

CONTRAINDICATIONS & PRECAUTIONS

Contraindicated in patients with hypercalcemia or sensitivity to vitamin D.

ADVERSE REACTIONS

Common reactions are in italics; life-threatening reactions are in bold italics.
Vitamin D intoxication associated with hypercalcemia:
CNS: headache, somnolence.
EENT: conjunctivitis, photophobia, rhinorrhea.
GI: nausea, vomiting, constipation, metallic taste, dry mouth, anorexia, diarrhea.
GU: polyuria.
Other: weakness, bone and muscle pain.

INTERACTIONS

Thiazide diuretics: possible hypercalcemia in hypoparathyroid patients. Avoid concomitant use.

EFFECTS ON DIAGNOSTIC TESTS

Cholesterol: altered levels.
Serum alkaline phosphatase: altered concentrations.
Serum and urine electrolytes (magnesium, phosphate, and calcium): altered results.

NURSING CONSIDERATIONS

Besides those related universally to drug therapy (see "How to use this book"), consider the following specific recommendations:

Assessment

- Obtain a baseline assessment of the patient's underlying condition and serum and urine calcium levels before initiating dihydrotachysterol therapy.
- Be alert for common adverse reactions and drug interactions throughout therapy.
- Evaluate the patient's and family's knowledge about dihydrotachysterol therapy.

Nursing Diagnoses

- Altered nutrition: Less than body requirements related to patient's deceased ability to absorb calcium from the GI tract.
- Altered protection related to potential for vitamin D intoxication caused by dihydrotachysterol therapy.
- Knowledge deficit related to dihydrotachysterol therapy.

Planning and Implementation

Preparation and Administration

- Be aware that optimal dosage is highly individualized.
- Store in tightly closed, light-resistant container. Don't refrigerate.

Monitoring

- Monitor effectiveness by regularly checking the patient's serum and urine calcium levels.
- Monitor for hypercalcemia (early

signs include thirst, headache, vertigo, tinnitus, and anorexia).
• Monitor closely for vitamin D intoxication associated with hypercalcemia.
Supportive Care
• If hypercalcemia occurs, notify doctor.
• Ensure that patient is receiving adequate daily intake of calcium. Expect to administer 10 to 15 g oral calcium lactate or gluconate daily.
Patient Teaching
• Advise patient to adhere to diet and calcium supplementation and to avoid nonprescription drugs.
• Teach patient to report signs and symptoms of hypercalcemia.
• Inform patient how to store drug correctly.
Evaluation
In patients receiving dihydrotachysterol, appropriate evaluation statements may include:
• Patient serum calcium levels are within normal range, and patient exhibits improvement in his underlying condition.
• Patient does not experience vitamin D intoxication because of dihydrotachysterol therapy.
• Patient and family state an understanding of dihydrotachysterol therapy.

dihydroxyaluminum sodium carbonate

(dye hye drox´ i a loo´ mi num)
Rolaids◇

• *Classification:* antacid (aluminum salt)
• *Pregnancy Risk Category:* C

HOW SUPPLIED

Tablets: 334 mg◇

ACTION

Mechanism: An antacid that reacts with gastric hydrochloric acid to form aluminum chloride, carbon dioxide, and water. Reduces total acid load in the GI tract and elevates gastric pH to reduce pepsin activity.
Absorption: About 17% to 30% of the aluminum chloride formed is absorbed.
Metabolism: None.
Excretion: Most excreted in feces; absorbed aluminum chloride is excreted by the kidneys. Some aluminum may be excreted in breast milk.

INDICATIONS & DOSAGE

Antacid–
Adults: chew 1 to 2 tablets (334 to 668 mg), p.r.n.

CONTRAINDICATIONS & PRECAUTIONS

Contraindicated in patients with renal failure, hypophosphatemia, appendicitis, undiagnosed rectal or GI bleeding, constipation, fecal impaction, chronic diarrhea, or intestinal obstruction because drug may exacerbate the symptoms associated with these conditions.

Use cautiously in patients with restricted sodium intake or CHF because of high sodium content (53 mg sodium/tablet); hemorrhoids because the drug may exacerbate this condition; and decreased GI motility, such as elderly patients and those receiving such drugs as anticholinergics or antidiarrheals, because these patients may be predisposed to intestinal obstruction.

ADVERSE REACTIONS

Common reactions are in italics; life-threatening reactions are in bold italics.
GI: anorexia, *constipation,* intestinal obstruction.

INTERACTIONS

Allopurinol, antibiotics (including quinolones and tetracyclines), corticosteroids, diflunisal, digoxin, iron, isoniazid, penicillamine, phenothiazines, ranitidine: decreased pharmacologic effect because absorption may be impaired. Separate administration times.

EFFECTS ON DIAGNOSTIC TESTS

Imaging tests using radiopaque media: test interference.
Serum gastrin levels: increased levels.

NURSING CONSIDERATIONS

Besides those related universally to drug therapy (see "How to use this book"), consider the following specific recommendations:

Assessment
- Obtain a baseline assessment of the patient's pain or discomfort before beginning therapy.
- Be alert for adverse reactions and drug interactions during therapy.
- Evaluate the patient's and family's knowledge about dihydroxyaluminum sodium carbonate therapy.

Nursing Diagnoses
- Pain related to gastric hyperacidity.
- Constipation related to dihydroxyaluminum sodium carbonate-induced adverse reactions.
- Knowledge deficit related to dihydroxyaluminum sodium carbonate therapy.

Planning and Implementation
Preparation and Administration
- ***P.O. use:*** Do not give other oral medications within 1 to 2 hours of antacid administration. May cause enteric-coated drugs to be released prematurely in stomach. Tablets should be chewed completely before swallowing and followed by a glass of water.

Monitoring
- Monitor by regularly assessing reduction or relief of the patient's pain.
- Carefully monitor long-term, high-dose use in patients on restricted sodium intake.
- Monitor the patient's bowel pattern. Watch for development of constipation, especially in the elderly patient.
- Monitor patient for water retention because this drug has a high sodium content. Periodically monitor serum sodium level if patient shows signs of water retention.

Supportive Care
- If the patient develops constipation, notify the doctor and obtain an order for a laxative or stool softener and monitor its effectiveness. Also, if not contraindicated, encourage the patient to eat a high-fiber diet and to drink 8 to 13 8-oz glasses (2 to 3 liters) of water per day to help prevent constipation. Alternate this drug with magnesium-containing antacids (if the patient does not have renal disease).
- Encourage the patient to discuss any emotional factors or dietary habits that may be contributing to the his GI problems.

Patient Teaching
- Tell the patient receiving the tablet form of the drug to chew the tablets completely before swallowing and, after swallowing, to drink a glass of milk or water, if possible.
- As indicated, instruct the patient to restrict sodium intake and drink plenty of fluids
- Warn the patient not to take this drug indiscriminately.
- Teach the patient how to prevent constipation during therapy.
- Explain the importance of taking this medication as prescribed and not taking other medications at the same time.

Evaluation
In patients receiving dihydroxyaluminum sodium carbonate, appropriate evaluation statements may include:
- Patient's pain subsides or is relieved.

• Patient experiences no constipation and maintains normal bowel function during therapy.
• Patient and family state an understanding of dihydroxyaluminum sodium carbonate therapy.

diltiazem hydrochloride

(dil tye´ a zem)
Cardizem, Cardizem SR

• *Classification:* antianginal (calcium channel blocker)
• *Pregnancy Risk Category:* C

HOW SUPPLIED

Tablets: 30 mg, 60 mg, 90 mg, 120 mg
Capsules (sustained-release): 60 mg, 90 mg, 120 mg

ACTION

Mechanism: Inhibits calcium ion influx across cardiac and smooth muscle cells, decreasing myocardial contractility and oxygen demand, and dilates coronary arteries and peripheral arterioles.
Absorption: Approximately 80% of a dose of diltiazem is absorbed rapidly from the GI tract. However, only about 40% of the drug enters systemic circulation because of a significant first-pass effect in the liver.
Distribution: About 70% to 85% of circulating diltiazem is bound to plasma proteins.
Metabolism: Hepatic.
Excretion: About 35% of the drug is excreted in the urine and about 65% in the bile as unchanged drug and inactive and active metabolites. Half-life: 3 to 9 hours, possibly longer in elderly patients; however, renal dysfunction does not appear to affect half-life.
Onset, peak, duration: Peak serum levels occur in about 2 to 3 hours.

INDICATIONS & DOSAGE

Management of vasospastic (also called Prinzmetal's or variant) angina and classic chronic stable angina pectoris–
Adults: 30 mg P.O. t.i.d. or q.i.d. before meals and at bedtime. Dosage may be gradually increased to a maximum of 360 mg/day, in divided doses.
Hypertension–
Adults: 60 mg P.O. b.i.d. (sustained-release capsule). Titrate dosage to effect. Maximum recommended dosage is 360 mg/day.

CONTRAINDICATIONS & PRECAUTIONS

Contraindicated in patients with severe hypotension (systolic blood pressure below 90 mm Hg), because of the drug's hypotensive effect; in patients with second- or third-degree atrioventricular (AV) block or sick sinus syndrome (unless a functioning artificial ventricular pacemaker is in place) because of the drug's effect on the cardiac conduction system; and in patients with hypersensitivity to the drug.

Use with caution in patients with CHF; impaired ventricular function or conduction abnormalities because the drug may worsen this condition; beta blocker or digoxin therapy because this may result in excessive bradycardia or conduction abnormalities; impaired liver or kidney function; and in elderly patients because plasma half-life may be prolonged.

ADVERSE REACTIONS

Common reactions are in italics; life-threatening reactions are in bold italics.
CNS: *headache, fatigue, drowsiness,* dizziness, nervousness, depression, insomnia, confusion.
CV: *edema, arrhythmias,* flushing, bradycardia, hypotension, conduction abnormalities, CHF.
GI: *nausea,* vomiting, diarrhea.

GU: nocturia, polyuria.
Hepatic: transient elevation of liver enzymes.
Skin: *rash,* pruritus.
Other: photosensitivity.

INTERACTIONS

Cimetidine: may inhibit diltiazem metabolism. Monitor for toxicity.
Digoxin: diltiazem may increase serum levels of digoxin. Monitor for toxicity.
Propranolol (and other beta blockers): may prolong cardiac conduction time. Use together cautiously.

EFFECTS ON DIAGNOSTIC TESTS

None reported.

NURSING CONSIDERATIONS

Besides those related universally to drug therapy (see "How to use this book"), consider the following specific recommendations:

Assessment

- Obtain a baseline assessment of the patient's anginal state before diltiazem therapy.
- Be alert for adverse reactions and drug interactions throughout therapy.
- Evaluate the patient's and family's knowledge about diltiazem therapy.

Nursing Diagnoses

- Pain related to ineffectiveness of diltiazem therapy.
- Altered protection related to diltiazem-induced arrhythmia.
- Knowledge deficit related to diltiazem therapy.

Planning and Implementation

Preparation and Administration

- Monitor blood pressure during initiation of therapy and dosage adjustment.
- ***P.O. use:*** Administer tablets before meals and at bedtime.

Monitoring

- Monitor effectiveness by regularly evaluating the severity and frequency of the patient's anginal pain.
- Monitor patient's blood pressure regularly.
- Monitor patient's ECG and heart rate and rhythm regularly.

Supportive Care

- Consult the doctor if the patient does not experience pain relief.
- If nitrate therapy is prescribed during titration of diltiazem dosage, be sure patient continues nitrate therapy. Be aware that sublingual nitroglycerin, especially, may be taken concomitantly as needed when anginal symptoms are acute.
- If systolic pressure is less than 90 mm Hg, or heart rate is less than 60 beats/minute, withhold dose and notify doctor.
- Have emergency drugs readily available to treat any arrhythmia that may occur.
- Maintain safety precautions if dizziness occurs; assist the patient with daily activities to minimize energy expenditure.
- Restrict the patient's fluid and sodium intake to minimize edema.
- Obtain an order for an antiemetic or antidiarrheal agent as needed.

Patient Teaching

- Stress importance of taking the drug exactly as prescribed even when feeling well.
- Instruct patient taking tablet form to take drug before meals and at bedtime (if ordered q.i.d.).
- Stress the importance of compliance with concomitant nitrate therapy during titration of diltiazem dosage. Tell him sublinguinal nitroglycerin, especially, may be taken concomitantly as needed when anginal symptoms are acute.
- Tell the patient to schedule activities to allow adequate rest.
- Encourage the patient to restrict fluid and sodium intake to minimize edema.
- Advise patient to minimize exposure to direct sunlight and to take

precautions when in the sun because of diltiazem-induced photosensitivity.

Evaluation

In patients receiving diltiazem, appropriate evaluation statements may include:

• Patient states anginal pain relief occurs with diltiazem therapy.

• Patient's ECG and heart rate and rhythm are unchanged with diltiazem therapy.

• Patient and family state an understanding of diltiazem therapy.

dimenhydrinate

(dye men hye´ dri nate)

Andrumin‡, Apo-Dimenhydrinate†, Calm X◇, Dimentabs, Dinate, Dommanate, Dramamine◇*, Dramamine Chewable◇**, Dramamine Liquid◇*, Dramanate, Dramilin, Dramocen, Dramoject, Dymenate, Gravol†, Hydrate, Marmine◇, Motion-Aid, Nauseatol†, Novodimenate†, PMS-Dimenhydrinate†, Reidamine, Tega-Vert◇, Travamine†, Travs‡, Triptone Caplets◇, Wehamine

• *Classification:* antihistamine (H_1-receptor antagonist) antiemetic and antivertigo agent (ethanolamine derivative)

• *Pregnancy Risk Category:* B

HOW SUPPLIED

Tablets: 50 mg◇
Tablets (chewable): 50 mg◇
Capsules: 50 mg◇
Oral liquid: 12.5 mg/4 ml*◇, 15.62 mg/5 ml
Injection: 50 mg/ml

ACTION

Mechanism: An antihistamine that also blocks acetylcholine receptors; drug also has antispasmodic, local anesthetic, and CNS depressant effects. May affect neural pathways originating in the labyrinth to inhibit nausea and vomiting, but the exact mechanism of action is unknown.

Absorption: Well absorbed after oral or parenteral administration.

Distribution: Widely distributed; crosses the placenta.

Metabolism: Probably in the liver.

Excretion: Probably in urine.

Onset, peak, duration: Action begins within 15 to 30 minutes after oral administration, 30 minutes after I.M. absorption, and almost immediately after I.V. administration.

INDICATIONS & DOSAGE

Nausea, vomiting, dizziness of motion sickness (treatment and prevention)—

Adults: 50 mg P.O. q 4 hours, or 100 mg q 4 hours if drowsiness is not objectionable; or 50 mg I.M., p.r.n.; or 50 mg I.V. diluted in 10 ml sodium chloride solution, injected over 2 minutes.

Children: 5 mg/kg P.O. or I.M., divided q.i.d. Maximum dosage is 300 mg daily. Don't use in children under 2 years.

CONTRAINDICATIONS & PRECAUTIONS

Contraindicated in patients with hypersensitivity to this drug or to other antiemetic antihistamines with a similar chemical structure, such as diphenhydramine; and in those sensitive to theophylline, because dimenhydrinate is the 8-chlorotheophylline salt of diphenhydramine.

Use cautiously in patients with narrow-angle glaucoma, asthma, prostatic hypertrophy, or GU or GI obstruction, because of the drug's anticholinergic effects; and in patients with seizure disorders. Drug may mask signs of brain tumor or intestinal obstruction.

ADVERSE REACTIONS

Common reactions are in italics; life-threatening reactions are in bold italics.

CNS: *drowsiness,* headache, incoordination, dizziness.
CV: palpitations, hypotension.
EENT: blurred vision, tinnitus, dry mouth and respiratory passages.
Other: may mask symptoms of ototoxicity, brain tumor, or intestinal obstruction.

INTERACTIONS

None significant.

EFFECTS ON DIAGNOSTIC TESTS

Caffeine and other xanthines: altered results.
Diagnostic skin tests: test interference.

NURSING CONSIDERATIONS

Besides those related universally to drug therapy, (see "How to use this book"), consider the following specific recommendations:

Assessment

- Obtain a baseline assessment of cardiovascular status, blood pressure, and fluid balance before therapy.
- Be alert for adverse reactions or drug interactions during therapy.
- Evaluate the patient's and family's knowledge about dimenhydrinate.

Nursing Diagnoses

- High risk for fluid volume deficit related to nausea and vomiting induced by motion sickness.
- Pain related to dimenhydrinate-induced headache.
- Knowledge deficit related to dimenhydrinate therapy.

Planning and Implementation

Preparation and Administration

- Check order carefully; drug is available in multiple forms.
- ***I.V. use:*** Not for direct I.V. injection; undiluted solution is irritating to veins and may cause sclerosis.
- ***I.M. use:*** Be sure to aspirate syringe before injecting drug to avoid inadvertent I.V. administration.
- Do not mix parenteral preparations with other drugs; incompatible with many solutions.

Monitoring

- Monitor effectiveness by observing the patient for nausea and vomiting.
- Check blood pressure and pulse; may cause hypotension and palpitations.
- Observe for CNS adverse reactions (dizziness, incoordination, drowsiness).
- Monitor fluid balance.

Supportive Care

- Use cautiously in seizures, narrow-angle glaucoma, or enlargement of the prostate. Be aware that dimenhydrinate may mask ototoxicity of aminoglycoside antibiotics.
- Be aware that dimenhydrinate is an antihistamine.
- Encourage patient to maintain adequate fluid intake.
- Obtain order for medication to relieve drug-induced headache.
- Use safety precautions for patients who develop CNS adverse reactions.

Patient Teaching

- Warn patient to avoid driving and other hazardous activities that require alertness until CNS adverse reactions are known.
- Advise patient to take tablets at least 30 minutes before beginning traveling.

Evaluation

In patients receiving dimenhydrinate, appropriate evaluation statements may include:

- Patient exhibits no signs of fluid deficit.
- Patient remains free from drug-induced headache.
- Patient and family state an understanding of dimenhydrinate therapy.

dimercaprol

(dye mer kap′ role)
BAL in Oil

• *Classification:* heavy metal antagonist (chelating agent)
• *Pregnancy Risk Category:* D

HOW SUPPLIED

Injection: 100 mg/ml

ACTION

Mechanism: A chelating agent that forms complexes with heavy metals.
Absorption: Slowly absorbed through the skin after topical application. Well absorbed from I.M. injection sites.
Distribution: Distributed to all tissues, mainly the intracellular space, with highest concentrations in the liver and kidneys.
Metabolism: Rapidly metabolized to inactive products.
Excretion: Most dimercaprol-metal complexes and inactive metabolites are excreted in urine and feces.
Onset, peak, duration: After I.M. injection, peak serum levels occur in 30 minutes to 1 hour.

INDICATIONS & DOSAGE

Severe arsenic or gold poisoning–
Adults and children: 3 mg/kg deep I.M. q 4 hours for 2 days, then q.i.d. on third day, then b.i.d. for 10 days.
Mild arsenic or gold poisoning–
Adults and children: 2.5 mg/kg deep I.M. q.i.d. for 2 days, then b.i.d. on third day, then once daily for 10 days.
Mercury poisoning–
Adults and children: 5 mg/kg deep I.M. initially, then 2.5 mg/kg daily or b.i.d. for 10 days.
Acute lead encephalopathy or lead level more than 100 mcg/ml–
Adults and children: 4 mg/kg deep I.M. injection, then q 4 hours with edetate calcium disodium (12.5 mg/kg I.M.). Use separate sites. Maximum dosage is 5 mg/kg per dose.

CONTRAINDICATIONS & PRECAUTIONS

Contraindicated in patients with iron, cadmium, selenium, or uranium poisoning, because the complexes formed are more toxic than the free metals; and in patients with impaired hepatic function except those with postarsenical jaundice.

Use cautiously in patients with impaired renal function because toxic levels may result; and in patients with hypertension because drug may worsen the hypertension.

ADVERSE REACTIONS

Common reactions are in italics; life-threatening reactions are in bold italics.
CNS: pain or tightness in throat, chest, or hands; headache; paresthesias; muscle pain or weakness.
CV: *transient increase in blood pressure, returns to normal in 2 hours; tachycardia.*
EENT: blepharospasm, conjunctivitis, lacrimation, rhinorrhea, excessive salivation.
GI: *halitosis; nausea; vomiting; burning sensation in lips, mouth, and throat; abdominal pain.*
GU: *dysuria;* renal damage if alkaline urine not maintained.
Metabolic: decreased iodine uptake.
Local: sterile abscess, pain at injection site.
Other: *fever (especially in children),* sweating, pain in teeth.

INTERACTIONS

^{131}I uptake thyroid tests: decreased; don't schedule patient for this test during course of dimercaprol therapy.
Iron: forms toxic metal complex; concurrent therapy contraindicated. Wait 24 hours after last dimercaprol dose.

EFFECTS ON DIAGNOSTIC TESTS

Thyroid uptake of ^{131}I: decreased values.

NURSING CONSIDERATIONS

Besides those related universally to drug therapy (see "How to use this book"), consider the following specific recommendations:

Assessment

• Obtain a baseline assessment of circumstances surrounding situation, substance reportedly ingested, allergies, blood pressure, hepatic and renal function before therapy.
• Be alert for adverse reactions and drug interactions throughout therapy.
• Evaluate the patient's and family's knowledge about dimercaprol therapy.

Nursing Diagnoses

• High risk for injury related to ingestion of poisonous substance.
• High risk for fluid volume deficit related to drug induced nausea and vomiting.
• Knowledge deficit related to dimercaprol therapy.

Planning and Implementation

Preparation and Administration

• Solution with slight sediment is usable.
• ***I.M. use:*** Give by deep I.M. injection only. Do not give I.V.
• Aspirate syringe before injection to avoid inadvertent I.V. administration.
• Massage the injection site after administration.
• Avoid contact with skin to prevent skin reaction.

Monitoring

• Monitor effectiveness by monitoring serum level of substance ingested and for improvement in patient's condition.
• Monitor blood pressure for transient hypertension.
• Monitor renal and liver function studies.
• Monitor fluid and electrolyte balance; check urine output, urine pH, and daily weight.
• Observe injection site for local reaction.

Supportive Care

• Do not give in hepatic dysfunction (except post-arsenical jaundice), or in acute renal insufficiency.
• Should not be used in pregnancy except to treat life-threatening poisoning.
• Do not use for iron, cadmium, or selenium toxicity. Complex formed is highly toxic, even fatal.
• Ephedrine or antihistamine may prevent or relieve mild adverse reactions.
• Dimercaprol is ineffective in arsine gas poisoning.
• Keep patient well hydrated; if patient is alert, encourage fluid intake.
• Treat drug-induced fever with antipyretics.
• Apply ice or cold compresses to injection site to alleviate local discomfort.
• Obtain order for pain medication to alleviate drug-induced pain, burning, and discomfort.
• Provide mouth care after emesis is complete.

Patient Teaching

• Warn the patient that the drug has an unpleasant garliclike odor.
• Advise the patient that the drug may cause pain at the injection site.
• Instruct the patient to report changes in urine output, fever, pain, nausea or vomiting immediately.
• Encourage proper storage of medication and hazardous materials to prevent accidental poisoning.

Evaluation

In patients receiving dimercaprol, appropriate evaluation statements may include:

• Patient remains free from injury related to ingestion of poisonous substance.
• Patient exhibits no signs of fluid volume deficit.
• Patient and family state an understanding of dimercaprol therapy.

dinoprostone

(dye noe prost´ one)
Prostin E_2

• *Classification:* oxytocic (prostaglandin)
• *Pregnancy Risk Category:* ?????

HOW SUPPLIED

Vaginal suppositories: 20 mg

ACTION

Mechanism: A prostaglandin that produces strong, prompt contractions of uterine smooth muscle, possibly mediated by calcium and cyclic 3′,5′-adenosine monophosphate.
Absorption: Following vaginal insertion, dinoprostone is diffused slowly into the maternal blood. Some local absorption into the uterus through the cervix or local vascular and lymphatic channels, but this accounts for only a small portion of the dose.
Distribution: Widely distributed in the mother.
Metabolism: In the lungs, liver, kidneys, spleen, and other maternal tissues to at least nine inactive metabolites.
Excretion: Primarily in urine, with small amounts in feces.
Onset, peak, duration: Contractions appear within 10 minutes of dosing, with a peak effect in 17 hours. There is no correlation of activity with plasma concentrations.

INDICATIONS & DOSAGE

Abort second trimester pregnancy, evacuate uterus in cases of missed abortion, intrauterine fetal deaths up to 28 weeks of gestation, or benign hydatidiform mole–
Adults: insert 20-mg suppository high into posterior vaginal fornix. Repeat q 3 to 5 hours until abortion is complete.

CONTRAINDICATIONS & PRECAUTIONS

Contraindicated in patients sensitive to the drug; in patients with acute pelvic inflammatory disease, because drug may worsen fever and associated symptoms; in pregnant women when membranes have ruptured; and in patients with history of pelvic surgery, uterine fibroid disease, or cervical stenosis, because of risk of retention of placenta and hemorrhage. Use cautiously in patients with epilepsy, diabetes, and hypotension or hypertension, because drug may exacerbate symptoms of these disorders.

ADVERSE REACTIONS

Common reactions are in italics; life-threatening reactions are in bold italics.
CNS: headache, *dizziness.*
CV: hypotension (in large doses).
GI: *nausea, vomiting, diarrhea.*
GU: vaginal pain, vaginitis.
Other: *fever, shivering, chills, joint inflammation, nocturnal leg cramps,* ***bronchospasm.***

INTERACTIONS

Alcohol (I.V. infusions of 500 ml of 10% over 1 hour): inhibited uterine activity.

EFFECTS ON DIAGNOSTIC TESTS

None reported.

NURSING CONSIDERATIONS

Besides those related universally to drug therapy (see "How to use this book"), consider the following specific recommendations:
Assessment
• Obtain a baseline assessment of the patient's pregnancy status before therapy.
• Be alert for adverse reactions and drug interactions throughout therapy.
• Evaluate the patient's and family's knowledge about dinoprostone therapy.

Nursing Diagnoses
- High risk for fluid volume deficit related to possible dinoprostone-induced vomiting, diarrhea.
- High risk for altered body temperature related to possible dinoprostone-induced fever.
- Knowledge deficit related to dinoprostone therapy.

Planning and Implementation
Preparation and Administration
- Administer only when critical care facilities are readily available.
- Just before use, warm dinoprostone suppositories in their wrapping to room temperature.
- Store suppositories in freezer at temperature of − 4° F (− 20° C).

Monitoring
- Monitor effectiveness by evaluating uterine contractions, and expulsion of products of conception. Keep in mind that abortion should be complete within 30 hours.
- Monitor for nausea and diarrhea after drug administration.
- Monitor the patient's body temperature after drug administration.
- Check vaginal discharge daily.

Supportive Care
- Be aware that dinoprostone-induced fever is self-limiting and transient and occurs in approximately 50% of patients. Treat with water or alcohol sponging and increased fluid intake rather than with aspirin.
- Replace fluids if nausea or diarrhea occurs. Keep in mind that the patient may be pretreated with an antiemetic and an antidiarrheal agent.
- Know that dinoprostone is being investigated as an agent that promotes cervical inducibility (cervical "ripening") before induction of labor with oxytocin.

Patient Teaching
- Explain the importance of follow-up care to assess treatment.
- Tell the patient to report suspected fever, nausea, vomiting, diarrhea or any other adverse reactions or feelings to the doctor.
- Instruct the patient to remain supine for 10 minutes after administration.

Evaluation
In patients receiving dinoprostone, appropriate evaluation statements may include:
- Adequate fluid volume is maintained.
- Body temperature is within normal limits.
- Patient and family state an understanding of dinoprostone therapy.

diphenhydramine hydrochloride
(dye fen hye´ dra meen)
Allerdryl†◇, AllerMax◇, Beldin*◇, Belix◇, Bena-D, Bena-D 50◇, Benadryl*◇, Benadryl Complete Allergy◇, Benahist 10, Benahist 50, Ben-Allergen-50, Benaphen◇, Benoject-10, Benoject-50, Benylin Cough*◇, Benylin Dietetic†, Benylin Expectorant†, Benylin Pediatric†, Bydramine Cough◇, Compoz Diahist◇, Dihydrex, Diphenacen-50, Diphenadryl◇, Diphen Cough*◇, Diphenhist◇, Dormarex 2◇, Fenylhist◇, Fynex◇, Hydramine*, Hydramyn, Hydril◇, Hyrexin-50, Insomnal†, Nervine Nighttime Sleep-Aid◇, Noradryl, Nordryl, Nytol with DPH◇, Sleep-Eze 3◇, Sominex◇, Sominex Liquid◇, Tusstat*◇, Twilite◇, Valdrene*◇, Wehdryl

- *Classification:* antihistamine (H_1-receptor antagonist) antiemetic and antivertigo agent, antitussive, sedative-hypnotic, topical anesthetic, antidyskinetic (anticholinergic agent) (ethanolamine derivative)
- *Pregnancy Risk Category:* B

HOW SUPPLIED

Tablets: 25 mg◇, 50 mg◇
Capsules: 25 mg◇, 50 mg◇
Elixir: 12.5 mg/5 ml (14% alcohol)*◇
Syrup: 12.5 mg/5 ml◇, 13.3 mg/5 ml (5% alcohol)◇
Injection: 10 mg/ml, 50 mg/ml

ACTION

Mechanism: Competes with histamine for H_1-receptor sites on effector cells. Prevents but does not reverse histamine-mediated responses, particularly histamine's effects on the smooth muscle of the bronchial tubes, GI tract, uterus, and blood vessels. Structurally related to local anesthetics, diphenhydramine provides local anesthesia by preventing initiation and transmission of nerve impulses. Also suppresses the cough reflex by a direct effect in the medulla of the brain.
Absorption: Well absorbed from the GI tract; however substantial portions of drug are lost to first-pass metabolism.
Distribution: Widely distributed throughout the body, including the CNS; drug crosses the placenta and is excreted in breast milk; approximately 82% protein-bound.
Metabolism: About 50% to 60% of an oral dose of diphenhydramine is metabolized by the liver before reaching the systemic circulation (first-pass effect); virtually all available drug is metabolized by the liver within 24 to 48 hours.
Excretion: Drug and metabolites are excreted primarily in urine. Half-life: Plasma elimination half-life is about 3½ hours.
Onset, peak, duration: Action begins within 15 to 30 minutes and peaks in 1 to 4 hours.

INDICATIONS & DOSAGE

Rhinitis, allergy symptoms, nighttime sedation, motion sickness, antiparkinsonism–
Adults: 25 to 50 mg P.O. t.i.d. or q.i.d.; or 10 to 50 mg deep I.M. or I.V. Maximum dosage is 400 mg daily.
Children under 12 years: 5 mg/kg daily P.O., deep I.M., or I.V. divided q.i.d. Maximum dosage is 300 mg daily.
Sedation–
Adults: 25 to 50 mg P.O., or deep I.M., p.r.n.
As a nighttime sleep aid–
Adults: 50 mg P.O. at bedtime.
Nonproductive cough–
Adults: 25 mg P.O. q 4 hours (not to exceed 100 mg daily).
Children 6 to 12 years: 12.5 mg P.O. q 4 hours (not to exceed 50 mg daily).
Children 2 to 6 years: 6.25 mg P.O. q 4 hours (not to exceed 25 mg daily).

Note: Children under 12 years should use only as directed by a doctor.

CONTRAINDICATIONS & PRECAUTIONS

Contraindicated in patients with hypersensitivity to this drug or antihistamines with similar chemical structures (carbinoxamine and clemastine); during an acute asthma attack because diphenhydramine thickens bronchial secretions; and in patients who have taken monoamine oxidase (MAO) inhibitors within the past 2 weeks; and during pregnancy, especially in the third trimester, or during breast-feeding. Antihistamines have caused convulsions and other severe reactions, especially in premature infants (see Interactions).

Use cautiously in patients with narrow-angle glaucoma; in those with pyloroduodenal obstruction or urinary bladder obstruction from prostatic hypertrophy or narrowing of the bladder neck because of their marked anticholinergic effects; cardiovascular disease, hypertension, or hyperthyroidism because of the risk of palpitations and tachycardia; and renal disease, diabetes, bronchial asthma, urinary retention, or stenosing peptic ulcers.

Benadryl 25 contains bisulfites, which can cause severe reactions in individuals allergic to these chemicals.

ADVERSE REACTIONS

Common reactions are in italics; life-threatening reactions are in bold italics.
CNS: (especially in elderly patients) *drowsiness,* confusion, insomnia, headache, vertigo.
CV: palpitations.
EENT: diplopia, nasal stuffiness.
GI: *nausea,* vomiting, diarrhea, *dry mouth,* constipation.
GU: dysuria, urine retention.
Skin: urticaria, photosensitivity.

INTERACTIONS

CNS depressants: increased sedation. Use together cautiously.
MAO inhibitors: increased anticholinergic effects. Don't use together.

EFFECTS ON DIAGNOSTIC TESTS

Diagnostic skin tests: test interference.

NURSING CONSIDERATIONS

Besides those related universally to drug therapy (see "How to use this book"), consider the following specific recommendations:

Assessment
- Obtain a baseline assessment of the patient's underlying condition before therapy.
- Be alert for adverse reactions or drug interactions during therapy.
- Evaluate the patient's and family's knowledge about diphenhydramine therapy.

Nursing Diagnoses
- Ineffective airway clearance related to the patient's underlying condition.
- High risk for injury related to diphenhydramine-induced drowsiness.
- Knowledge deficit related to diphenhydramine therapy.

Planning and Implementation

Preparation and Administration
- ***P.O. use:*** Administer with food or milk, if oral forms cause GI distress. Administer 30 minutes before travel, if medication is being used for motion sickness.
- ***I.M. use:*** Administer I.M. injection deep into a large muscle. Alternate injection sites to prevent irritation.

Monitoring
- Monitor effectiveness by regularly assessing for relief of symptoms.
- Monitor patient for CNS adverse reactions, such as drowsiness.
- Monitor elderly patients carefully because they are especially vulnerable to reactions, such as drowsiness, confusion, insomnia, headaches, and vertigo.
- Monitor lung sounds and characteristics of bronchial secretions.
- Monitor patient's intake and output for possible urine retention.

Supportive Care
- Ensure adequate fluid intake to decrease the viscosity of the secretions in patients with bronchial secretions.
- Take safety precautions with all patients, particularly during ambulation. Diphenhydramine is one of the most sedating antihistamines and is often used as a hypnotic.
- Keep in mind that if tolerance develops, another antihistamine may be substituted.

Patient Teaching
- Explain that drug interactions are likely to occur with simultaneous use of CNS depressants. The patient should seek medical approval before taking any OTC medication.
- Warn the patient to avoid alcoholic beverages during therapy.
- Warn the patient to avoid driving and other hazardous activities that require alertness until the CNS ef-

fects of the drug are established. The patient who experiences excessive sedation may be better able to tolerate terfenadine or astemizole, which are less likely to cause drowsiness.

• Tell the patient that coffee or tea may reduce drowsiness and that dry mouth may be relieved with sugarless gum, hard candy, or ice chips.

• Encourage the patient to notify the doctor if dysuria or urine retention occurs and if allergy symptoms persist.

• Tell the patient not to take the medication for 4 days before allergy skin tests. Diphenhydramine must be discontinued 4 days before testing to preserve the accuracy of the tests.

Evaluation

In patients receiving diphenhydramine, appropriate evaluation statements may include:

• Patient's allergic symptoms are relieved with diphenhydramine hydrochloride.

• Patient does not experience injury as a result of diphenhydramine-induced drowsiness.

• Patient and family state an understanding of diphenhydramine therapy.

diphenoxylate hydrochloride

(dye fen ox´ i late)

Diphenatol, Lofene, Logen, Lomanate, Lomotil*, Lonox, Lo-Trol, Low-Quel, Nor-Mil

• Controlled Substance Schedule V
• *Classification:* antidiarrheal (opiate)
• *Pregnancy Risk Category:* C

HOW SUPPLIED

Tablets: 2.5 mg (with atropine sulfate, 0.025 mg)
Liquid: 2.5 mg/5 ml (with atropine sulfate, 0.025 mg/5 ml)*

ACTION

Mechanism: An opiate chemically related to meperidine. Atropine has been added to the compound to discourage abuse. Drug increases smooth muscle tone in the GI tract, inhibits motility and propulsion, and diminishes secretions.
Absorption: About 90% of an oral dose is absorbed.
Distribution: Found in breast milk.
Metabolism: Extensively metabolized by the liver to the active metabolite difenoxin.
Excretion: Mainly in feces via the biliary tract, with lesser amounts excreted in urine. Half-life: The elimination half-life of diphenoxylic acid is approximately 12 to 14 hours.
Onset, peak, duration: Action begins in 45 minutes to 1 hour.

INDICATIONS & DOSAGE

Acute, nonspecific diarrhea –
Adults: initially, 5 mg P.O. q.i.d., then adjust dosage.
Children 2 to 12 years: 0.3 to 0.4 mg/kg P.O. daily in 4 divided doses, using liquid form only. For maintenance, initial dose may be reduced by as much as 75%.

Don't use in children under 2 years.

CONTRAINDICATIONS & PRECAUTIONS

Contraindicated in patients with hypersensitivity to this drug, atropine, or meperidine; in patients with obstructive jaundice because of potential for hepatic coma; in patients with diarrhea caused by pseudomembranous colitis because of potential for toxic megacolon. Use cautiously in patients with diarrhea caused by poisoning or by infection by *Shigella, Salmonella,* and some strains of *Escherichia coli* because expulsion of intestinal contents may be protective.

Use with extreme caution in patients with impaired hepatic function, cirrhosis, advanced hepatorenal disease, or abnormal liver function test results because the drug may precipitate hepatic coma. The atropine component may exacerbate preexisting glaucoma.

ADVERSE REACTIONS

Common reactions are in italics; life-threatening reactions are in bold italics.
CNS: *sedation, dizziness,* headache, drowsiness, lethargy, restlessness, depression, euphoria.
CV: tachycardia.
EENT: mydriasis.
GI: *dry mouth,* nausea, vomiting, abdominal discomfort or distention, *paralytic ileus,* anorexia, fluid retention in bowel (may mask depletion of extracellular fluid and electrolytes, especially in young children treated for acute gastroenteritis).
GU: urine retention.
Skin: pruritus, giant urticaria, rash.
Other: possibly physical dependence in long-term use, angioedema, respiratory depression.

INTERACTIONS

None significant.

EFFECTS ON DIAGNOSTIC TESTS

Phenolsulfonphthalein excretion test: decreased excretion.
Serum amylase: increased levels.

NURSING CONSIDERATIONS

Besides those related universally to drug therapy (see "How to use this book"), consider the following specific recommendations:

Assessment
- Obtain a baseline assessment of history of bowel disorders, GI status, and frequency of loose stool before therapy.
- Be alert for adverse reactions or drug interactions during therapy.
- Evaluate the patient's and family's knowledge about diphenoxylate therapy.

Nursing Diagnoses
- Diarrhea related to interruption of normal elimination pattern characterized by frequent loose stools.
- Altered thought processes related to drug-induced CNS adverse reactions.
- Knowledge deficit related to diphenoxylate therapy.

Planning and Implementation

Preparation and Administration
- Read label carefully; note dosage and strength.
- ***P.O. use:*** Available in liquid and tablet form.
- Dose of 2.5 mg is as effective as 5 ml camphorated tincture of opium.

Monitoring
- Monitor effectiveness by checking the frequency and characteristics of stool.
- Auscultate bowel sounds at least once a shift. Assess for pain and cramping.
- Monitor closely for fluid and electrolyte balance.
- Weigh patient daily until diarrhea is controlled to detect fluid loss or retention.
- Check skin in perianal area to prevent and detect breakdown.
- Assess neurological and mental status to detect CNS adverse reactions (sedation, dizziness, lethargy, restlessness).

Supportive Care
- Provide good skin care, especially to the perianal area; apply soothing lotions and powder.
- Consult with dietitian to modify diet to help control diarrhea.
- Use safety precautions in those patients with CNS adverse reactions.
- Correct fluid and electrolyte disturbances before starting the drug. Make sure patient is well hydrated; dehydration, especially in young children, may increase risk of delayed toxicity.
- Do not give to patients with acute diarrhea resulting from poison until

*Liquid form contains alcohol. **May contain tartrazine.

toxic material is eliminated from the GI tract; acute diarrhea caused by organisms that penetrate the intestinal mucosa; diarrhea resulting from antibiotic-induced pseudomembraneous enterocolitis; and in jaundiced patients. Diphenoxylate is not indicated in the treatment of antibiotic-induced diarrhea.

• Use cautiously in children; in patients with hepatic disease, narcotic dependence, and pregnant women. Use cautiously in acute ulcerative colitis. Stop therapy immediately if abdominal distention or other signs of toxic megacolon develop.

• Be aware that risk of physical dependence increases with high dosage and long-term use. Atropine sulfate is included to discourage abuse.

• Consider change in therapy if no improvement within 48 hours.

Patient Teaching

• Advise the patient that diphenoxylate should not be used to treat acute diarrhea for longer than 2 days and that they should seek medical attention if diarrhea continues.

• Warn the patient not to exceed the recommended dosage.

• Encourage proper storage to keep the drug out of children's reach.

Evaluation

In patients receiving diphenoxylate, appropriate evaluation statements may include:

• Patient reports decrease or absence of loose stools.

• Patient remains free from signs and symptoms of CNS adverse reactions.

• Patient and family state an understanding of diphenoxylate therapy.

diphtheria and tetanus toxoids, adsorbed

(dif theer´ ee a and *tet´ nus)*

• *Classification:* diphtheria and tetanus prophylaxis (triod)

• *Pregnancy Risk Category:* C

HOW SUPPLIED

Available in pediatric (DT) and adult (Td) strengths

Injection (for pediatric use): diphtheria toxoid 6.6 Lf units and tetanus toxoid 5 Lf units per 0.5 ml; diphtheria toxoid 10 Lf units and tetanus toxoid 5 Lf units per 0.5 ml; diphtheria toxoid 12.5 Lf units and tetanus toxoid 5 Lf units per 0.5 ml; diphtheria toxoid 15 Lf units and tetanus toxoid 10 Lf units per 0.5 ml

Injection (for adult use): diphtheria toxoid 1.5 Lf units and tetanus toxoid 5 Lf units per 0.5 ml; diphtheria toxoid 2 Lf units and tetanus toxoid 5 Lf units per 0.5 ml; diphtheria toxoid 2 Lf units and tetanus toxoid 10 Lf units per 0.5 ml

ACTION

Mechanism: Promotes immunity to diphtheria and tetanus by inducing production of antitoxins.

Pharmacokinetics: Unknown.

INDICATIONS & DOSAGE

Primary immunization–

Adults and children over 7 years: use adult strength; 0.5 ml I.M. 4 to 6 weeks apart for two doses and a third dose 1 year later. Booster is 0.5 ml I.M. q 10 years.

Children 1 to 6 years: use pediatric strength; 0.5 ml I.M. at least 4 weeks apart for two doses. Give booster dosage 6 to 12 months after the second injection. If the final immunizing dose is given after the 7th birthday, use the adult strength.

Infants 6 weeks to 1 year: use pediatric strength; 0.5 ml I.M. at least 4 weeks apart for three doses. Give booster dose 6 to 12 months after third injection.

CONTRAINDICATIONS & PRECAUTIONS

Contraindicated in patients with a history of systemic or anaphylactic reactions to the use of this product.

Some clinicians recommend deferring (if possible) elective immunization under the following conditions: poliomyelitis outbreaks, acute respiratory or other active infection, or febrile illness. Patients receiving immunosuppressive agents (corticosteroids, antimetabolites, alkylating agents, or radiation therapy), immunosuppressed patients, or patients who have recently received an injection of immune globulin may not respond optimally.

ADVERSE REACTIONS

Common reactions are in italics; life-threatening reactions are in bold italics.

Systemic: chills, fever, malaise, ***anaphylaxis.***

Local: stinging, edema, erythema, pain, induration.

INTERACTIONS

None significant.

EFFECTS ON DIAGNOSTIC TESTS

None reported.

NURSING CONSIDERATIONS

Besides those related universally to drug therapy (see "How to use this book"), consider the following specific recommendations:

Assessment

- Obtain a baseline assessment of the patient's allergies, immunization history and reaction to immunization before therapy.
- Be alert for adverse reactions or drug interactions during therapy.
- Evaluate the patient's and family's knowledge about diphtheria and tetanus toxoids, adsorbed.

Nursing Diagnoses

- Altered protection related to lack of immunity to diphtheria and tetanus.
- Ineffective breathing pattern related to possible toxoid-induced anaphylaxis.
- Knowledge deficit related to diphtheria and tetanus toxoids.

Planning and Implementation

Preparation and Administration

- Verify strength (pediatric or adult) of toxoids used.
- ***I.M. use:*** Give in site not recently used for vaccines or toxoids.

Monitoring

- Monitor effectiveness by checking patient's antibody titers for diphteria and tetanus.
- Check vital signs.
- Observe injection site for local adverse reactions (edema, erythema, induration).

Supportive Care

- Do not administer toxoid to patients undergoing immunosuppressive, radiation, or corticosteroid therapy.
- Defer administration in respiratory illness, polio outbreaks, or acute illness except in emergency. Use single antigen during polio risks.
- Use only when diphtheria, tetanus, and pertussis combination is contraindicated in children under 6 years, due to pertussis component.
- Keep epinephrine 1:1000 available to treat possible anaphylaxis.
- Apply ice or cold compresses to injection site to alleviate local reaction.

Patient Teaching

- Instruct the patient or parent to report difficulty breathing, fever, and chills immediately.
- Inform the patient or parent about probable expected local reactions to the toxoid.
- Advise the patient or parent that the toxoid must be administered in multiple doses 4 to 6 weeks apart, followed by a booster 1 year later in children; and every 10 years for adults.

Evaluation
In patients receiving diphteria and tetanus toxoids, appropriate evaluation statements may include:
• Patient exhibits immunity to diphtheria and tetanus.
• Patient demonstrates no signs of anaphylaxis.
• Patient and family state an understanding of diphtheria and tetanus toxoid, adsorbed.

diphtheria and tetanus toxoids and pertussis vaccine (DPT)

(dif theer´ ee a, tet´ nus, and *per tuss´ iss)*
Tri-Immunol

• *Classification:* diphtheria, tetanus, and pertussis prophylaxis (toixoid and vaccine)
• *Pregnancy Risk Category:* D

HOW SUPPLIED

Injection: 12.5 Lf units inactivated diphtheria, 5 Lf units inactivated tetanus, and 4 protective units pertussis per 0.5 ml, in 7.5-ml vials

ACTION

Mechanism: Promotes active immunity to diphtheria, tetanus, and pertussis by inducing production of antitoxins and antibodies.
Pharmacokinetics: Unknown.
Onset, peak, duration: Immunity against diptheria and tetanus persists at least 10 years in persons who complete the initial four dose primary immunization series; less than 50% of these persons have adequate immunity against pertussis after 10 years.

INDICATIONS & DOSAGE

Primary immunization–
Children 6 weeks to 6 years: 0.5 ml I.M. 2 months apart for three doses and a fourth dose 1 year later. Booster is 0.5 ml I.M. when starting school.

Not advised for adults or children over 6 years.

CONTRAINDICATIONS & PRECAUTIONS

Do not use in adults or children age 7 and over (use diphtheria and tetanus toxoids). Defer immunization during acute illness or if the patient has a history of seizures after use of this product.

Children with a history of neurologic disorders (including seizures) should not receive the pertussis component.

A history of any of the following effects from a previous administration of pertussis vaccine precludes further use of this component (use diphtheria and tetanus toxoids instead): fever greater than 103° F (39.4° C), focal neurologic signs, screaming episodes, shock, collapse, somnolence, or encephalopathy. Also contraindicated in patients with hypersensitivity to thimerosal, which is a component of this vaccine.

ADVERSE REACTIONS

Common reactions are in italics; life-threatening reactions are in bold italics.
Systemic: slight fever, chills, malaise, ***seizures, encephalopathy, anaphylaxis,*** anorexia, vomiting.
Local: *soreness, redness,* expected nodule remaining several weeks.
Other: ***sudden infant death syndrome.***

INTERACTIONS

Immunosuppressive therapy: may reduce response to DPT vaccine. Avoid if possible.

EFFECTS ON DIAGNOSTIC TESTS

None reported.

NURSING CONSIDERATIONS

Besides those related universally to drug therapy (see "How to use this book"), consider the following specific recommendations:

Assessment

- Obtain a baseline assessment of the patient's allergies, immunization history, and reaction to immunization before therapy.
- Be alert for adverse reactions or drug interactions during therapy.
- Evaluate the patient's and family's knowledge about diphtheria and tetanus toxoids and pertussis vaccine.

Nursing Diagnoses

- Altered protection due to lack of immunity to diphtheria, tetanus, and pertussis.
- High risk for injury related to DPT-induced seizure.
- Knowledge deficit related to DPT vaccine.

Planning and Implementation

Preparation and Administration

- Shake before using and refrigerate.
- ***I.M. use:*** Administer DPT by deep I.M. injection only, preferably in thigh or deltoid muscle. Do not give S.C.

Monitoring

- Monitor effectiveness by checking the patient's antibody titer to diphtheria, tetanus, and pertussis.
- Observe the patient for signs of anaphylaxis immediately after injection.
- Check vital signs.
- Observe injection site for expected nodule and redness.

Supportive Care

- Do not administer DPT to patients receiving corticosteroid or immunosuppressive therapy. DPT is also contraindicated in patients with an acute febrile illness or a history of seizure disorder.
- Do not administer the pertussis component to children with preexisting neurological disorders or who reacted to previous DPT injection with neurologic signs. Give diphtheria and tetanus toxoids instead.
- Keep epinephrine 1:1000 available in case of anaphylaxis.
- Institute seizure precautions. Place an airway or tongue blade nearby.
- DPT is not to be used for active infection.
- Apply ice or cold compress to expected nodule at injection site.
- Obtain order for antipyretic to alleviate DPT-induced fever.

Patient Teaching

- Instruct parent to report respiratory difficulty and seizure immediately.
- Advise the parent that slight fever, malaise, and a local reaction at the injection site are common and expected reactions to DPT vaccination.
- Inform the parent that multiple doses of DPT are necessary including a booster when the child starts school.

Evaluation

In patients receiving DPT vaccination, appropriate evaluation statements may include:

- Patient demonstrates active immunity to diphtheria, tetanus, and pertussis.
- Patient is seizure free.
- Patient and family state an understanding of diphtheria and tetanus toxoids and pertussis vaccine.

dipivefrin

(dye pi´ ve frin)

Propine

- *Classification:* antiglaucoma agent (sympathomimetic)
- *Pregnancy Risk Category:* B

HOW SUPPLIED

Ophthalmic solution: 0.1%

ACTION

Mechanism: In the eye, dipivefrin is converted to epinephrine. The liber-

*Liquid form contains alcohol.

**May contain tartrazine.

ated epinephrine appears to decrease aqueous production and increase aqueous outflow.
Absorption: In animal studies, about 10% of a dose is absorbed into ocular fluids and tissues, mainly as epinephrine within about 10 minutes.
Distribution: Highest concentrations are found in the conjunctiva, iris, aqueous humor, and cornea. Degree of systemic availability of the drug is not known.
Metabolism: Rapidly and almost completely metabolized to epinephrine by esterases present in the cornea, conjunctiva, and aqueous humor. Epinephrine is subsequently metabolized by monoamine oxidase (MAO) and catechol O-methyl transferase (COMT) within the eye. Small amounts of epinephrine that reach the systemic circulation are metabolized by these enzymes in the liver and other tissues.
Excretion: Most of the metabolites are excreted in the urine; small amounts are excreted in the feces. Half life: In the cornea is about 1.8 hours; in the aqueous humor, about 0.9 hours; and in the ciliary body, about 3.1 hours.
Onset, peak, duration: Action begins in about 30 minutes, with peak effect in 1 hour.

INDICATIONS & DOSAGE

To reduce intraocular pressure in chronic open-angle glaucoma –
Adults: for initial glaucoma therapy, 1 drop in eye q 12 hours.

CONTRAINDICATIONS & PRECAUTIONS

Contraindicated in patients with hypersensitivity to any component of the preparation and in narrow-angle glaucoma. Use with caution in aphakic patients, because macular edema may occur.

ADVERSE REACTIONS

Common reactions are in italics; life-threatening reactions are in bold italics.
CV: tachycardia, hypertension.
Eye: burning, stinging.

INTERACTIONS

Digitalis glycosides, inhalational hydrocarbon anesthetics, tricyclic antidepressants: increased risk of cardiac side effects if significant systemic absorption occurs.
Ophthalmic beta blockers: monitor for potential adverse effects.
Systemic sympathomimetics: possible additive effects if significant systemic absorption occurs.

EFFECTS ON DIAGNOSTIC TESTS

None reported.

NURSING CONSIDERATIONS

Besides those related universally to drug therapy, (see "How to use this book"), consider the following specific recommendations:

Assessment

- Obtain a baseline assessment of the patient's visual status, ocular pressure, and vital signs.
- Be alert for adverse reactions and drug interactions throughout therapy.
- Evaluate the patient's and family's knowledge about dipivefrin therapy.

Nursing Diagnoses

- Sensory/perceptual alterations (visual) related to the patient's underlying condition.
- Decreased cardiac output related to cardiovascular adverse effects.
- Knowledge deficit related to dipivefrin therapy.

Planning and Implementation

Preparation and Administration

- Instill in lacrimal sac; remove excess solution from around eyes with clean tissue or gauze.

Monitoring

- Monitor effectiveness by assessing the patient's visual status and intraocular pressure.

• Monitor blood pressure and apical rate for drug-induced tachycardia and hypertension; obtain ECG as indicated.

Supportive Care

• Notify the doctor immediately of any changes in the patient's health status occur.

Patient Teaching

• Teach patient how to instill the solution and advise him to wash his hands before and after administering the drug.

• Encourage the patient to continue regular medical supervision during therapy, especially if he has underlying cardiac disease.

Evaluation

In patients receiving dipivefrin, appropriate evaluation statements may include:

• Patient experiences therapeutic reduction in introcular pressure.

• Patient remains free of systemic cardiac effects.

• Patient and family state an understanding of dipivefrin therapy.

dipyridamole

(dye peer id´ a mole)

Apo-Dipyridamole†, Persantin 100‡, Persantine**

• *Classification:* coronary vasodilator, platelet aggregation inhibitor (pyrimidine analogue)

• *Pregnancy Risk Category:* C

HOW SUPPLIED

Tablets: 25 mg, 50 mg, 75 mg

Injection: 10 mg/2 ml†

ACTION

Mechanism: Inhibits platelet adhesion and the action of the enzymes adenosine deaminase and phosphodiesterase.

Absorption: Variable and slow after oral administration. Bioavailability ranges from 27% to 59%.

Distribution: Animal studies indicate wide distribution in body tissues; small amounts cross the placenta. Protein binding ranges from 91% to 97%.

Metabolism: Hepatic.

Excretion: Via biliary excretion of glucuronide conjugates. Some dipyridamole and conjugates may undergo enterohepatic circulation and fecal excretion; a small amount is excreted in urine. Half-life: Estimates vary from 1 to 12 hours.

Onset, peak, duration: Serum concentrations of dipyridamole peak 2 to 2½ hours after oral administration.

INDICATIONS & DOSAGE

Inhibition of platelet adhesion in prosthetic heart valves, in combination with warfarin or aspirin–

Adults: 75 to 100 mg P.O. q.i.d.

Transient ischemic attack–

Adults: 400 to 800 mg P.O. daily in divided doses.

As an alternative to exercise in the evaluation of coronary artery disease during thallium myocardial perfusion imaging–

Adults: 0.57 mg/kg as an I.V. infusion at a constant rate over 4 minutes (0.142 mg/kg/minute). Do not give more than 60 mg.

Acute coronary insufficiency‡ –

Adults: 10 mg I.V.

CONTRAINDICATIONS & PRECAUTIONS

Drug is ineffective in acute angina; it should not be substituted for other appropriate treatments, such as nitroglycerin. Contraindicated in patients with hypersensitivity to the drug. Use cautiously in patients with hypotension and in patients taking anticoagulants.

ADVERSE REACTIONS

Common reactions are in italics; life-threatening reactions are in bold italics.
CNS: *headache, dizziness,* weakness.
CV: flushing, fainting, *hypotension; chest pain, ECG abnormalities, blood pressure lability, hypertension* (with I.V. infusion).
GI: *nausea,* vomiting, diarrhea.
Local: irritation (with undiluted injection).
Skin: rash.

INTERACTIONS

None significant.

EFFECTS ON DIAGNOSTIC TESTS

Bleeding time: prolonged.

NURSING CONSIDERATIONS

Besides those related universally to drug therapy (see "How to use this book"), consider the following specific recommendations:

Assessment

- Obtain a baseline assessment of the patient's underlying condition before drug therapy.
- Be alert for adverse reactions and drug interactions throughout therapy.
- Evaluate the patient's and family's knowledge about dipyridamole therapy.

Nursing Diagnoses

- Altered tissue perfusion (cardiopulmonary) related to the patient's underlying condition.
- Pain related to adverse drug reactions.
- Knowledge deficit related to dipyridamole therapy.

Implementation

Preparation and Administration

- ***I.V. use:*** Dilute in 0.455 or 0.9% sodium chloride injection or dextrose 5% in water in at least a 1:2 ratio for a total volume of 20 to 50 ml when given as a diagnostic agent. Inject thallium-201 within 5 minutes after completion of the 4-minute dipyridamole injection.
- Drug should not be used alone for the prophylaxis of thromboembolism in postoperative prosthetic valve patients; it should be used with oral anticoagulants. Its value as part of an antithrombotic regimen is controversial and may not be significantly better than aspirin alone.
- Administer 1 hour before meals.

Monitoring

- Monitor the patient's blood pressure, heart rate and rhythm especially with I.V. administration.
- Monitor the patient for drug-induced headache.
- Watch for signs of bleeding and prolonged bleeding times, especially in patients receiving high-dose and long-term therapy.

Supportive Care

- Obtain an order for a mild analgesic if the patient develops a headache.
- If the patient develops GI distress, give doses with meals instead of 1 hour before.

Patient Teaching

- Tell the patient to take the drug 1 hour before meals or with meals if GI distress occurs.
- Tell the patient to have his blood pressure checked frequently.
- Tell the patient he may take a mild analgesic if he develops a headache.
- Tell him to notify the doctor if he develops chest pain.

Evaluation

In patients receiving dipyridamole, appropriate evaluation statements may include:

- Patient maintains tissue perfusion and cellular oxygenation.
- Patient does not develop a headache.
- Patient and family state an understanding of dipyridamole therapy.

---

disopyramide

(dye soe peer´ a mide)
Rythmodan†

disopyramide phosphate

Napamide, Norpace, Norpace CR, Rythmodan LA†

• *Classification:* antiarrhythmic (pyridine derivative)
• *Pregnancy Risk Category:* C

HOW SUPPLIED

disopyramide
Capsules: 100 mg†, 150 mg†
disopyramide phosphate
Tablets (sustained-release): 250 mg†
Capsules: 100 mg, 150 mg
Capsules (controlled-release): 100 mg, 150 mg
Injection: 10 mg/ml†

ACTION

Mechanism: A class Ia antiarrhythmic that depresses phase O. It prolongs the action potential. All class I drugs have membrane stabilizing effects.
Absorption: Rapidly and well absorbed from the GI tract; about 60% to 80% of the drug reaches systemic circulation.
Distribution: Well distributed throughout extracellular fluid but not extensively bound to tissues. Plasma protein binding varies, depending on drug concentration levels, but ranges from about 50% to 65%. Usual therapeutic serum level ranges from 2 to 4 mcg/ml, but some patients may require up to 7 mcg/ml. Levels above 9 mcg/ml generally are considered toxic.
Metabolism: In the liver to one major metabolite that has little antiarrhythmic activity but greater anticholinergic activity than the parent compound.
Excretion: About 90% of an orally administered dose is excreted in the urine as unchanged drug and metabolites; 40% to 60% is excreted as unchanged drug. Half-life: Usually about 7 hours; longer in patients with renal or hepatic insufficiency.
Onset, peak, duration: Onset of action usually occurs in 30 minutes; peak blood levels occur approximately 2 hours after administration of regular capsules, 5 hours after extended-release capsules. Duration of effect is usually 6 to 7 hours.

INDICATIONS & DOSAGE

Premature ventricular contractions (unifocal, multifocal, or coupled); ventricular tachycardia not severe enough to require electrocardioversion; to convert atrial fibrillation or flutter to normal sinus rhythm–
Adults: usual maintenance dosage 150 to 200 mg P.O. q 6 hours; for patients who weigh less than 50 kg or those with renal, hepatic, or cardiac impairment–100 mg P.O. q 6 hours. May give sustained-release capsule q 12 hours.

Recommended dosages in advanced renal insufficency: creatinine clearance 15 to 40 ml/minute–100 mg q 10 hours; creatinine clearance 5 to 15 ml/minute–100 mg q 20 hours; creatinine clearance 1 to 5 ml/minute–100 mg q 30 hours.
Children 12 to 18 years: 6 to 15 mg/kg P.O. daily.
Children 4 to 12 years: 10 to 15 mg/kg P.O. daily.
Children 1 to 4 years: 10 to 20 mg/kg P.O. daily.
Children less than 1 year: 10 to 30 mg/kg P.O. daily.

All children's dosages should be divided into equal amounts and given q 6 hours.

CONTRAINDICATIONS & PRECAUTIONS

Contraindicated in patients with second- or third-degree heart block (unless a pacemaker is in place), because of the drug's effects on atrioventricular (AV) conduction; myasthenia gravis because the drug's anticholinergic effect may precipitate a myasthenic crisis; untreated glaucoma or urinary retention (particularly from prostatic hypertrophy) because of the drug's anticholinergic effect (however, disopyramide may be used with caution in such patients if they are treated appropriately and monitored carefully); uncompensated CHF and cardiogenic shock because of the drug's negative inotropic effect; and hypersensitivity to the drug.

Use with caution in patients with sick sinus syndrome, Wolff-Parkinson-White syndrome, or bundle branch block because of the drug's unpredictable effects on AV conduction; and in patients with renal or hepatic insufficiency because decreased drug elimination may cause toxicity.

ADVERSE REACTIONS

Common reactions are in italics; life-threatening reactions are in bold italics.
CNS: dizziness, agitation, depression, fatigue, muscle weakness, syncope.
CV: *hypotension, **CHF**, heart block, edema, weight gain, arrhythmias.*
EENT: *blurred vision, dry eyes, dry nose.*
GI: nausea, vomiting, anorexia, bloating, abdominal pain, *constipation, dry mouth.*
GU: urine retention and urinary hesitancy.
Hepatic: cholestatic jaundice.
Metabolic: hypoglycemia.
Skin: rash in 1% to 3% of patients.

INTERACTIONS

Antiarrhythmics: possible additive or antagonized antiarrhythmic effects.
Phenytoin: increases disopyramide's metabolism. Monitor for decreased antiarrhythmic effect.

EFFECTS ON DIAGNOSTIC TESTS

Blood glucose: decreased concentrations.

NURSING CONSIDERATIONS

Besides those related universally to drug therapy (see "How to use this book"), consider the following specific recommendations:

Assessment
- Obtain a baseline assessment of the patient's heart rate and rhythm before disopyramide.
- Be alert for adverse reactions and drug interactions throughout therapy.
- Evaluate the patient's and family's knowledge about disopyramide therapy.

Nursing Diagnoses
- Decreased cardiac output related to ineffectiveness of disopyramide.
- Altered protection related to disopyramide-induced proarrthymias.
- Knowledge deficit related to disopyramide.

Planning and Implementation

Preparation and Administration
- Expect to decrease dosage in patients with renal impairment.
- Correct any underlying electrolyte abnormalities before use as ordered.
- Check apical pulse before administering drug. Notify doctor if pulse rate is slower than 60 beats/minute or faster than 120 beats/minute prior to administration.
- ***P.O. use:*** Be aware that sustained-release capsules should not be used for rapid control of ventricular arrhythmias. If patient is unable to take capsule or tablet form, ask pharmacist to prepare a suspension from 100-mg capsules using cherry syrup. Protect suspension from light and store in amber glass bottles.

Monitoring
- Monitor effectiveness by regularly assessing ECG pattern and apical heart rate.
- Monitor the patient's serum electrolyte levels.
- Monitor patient for anticholinergic effects.
- Monitor hydration status if adverse GI disturbances occur.

Supportive Care
• Discontinue if heart block develops, if QRS complex widens by more than 25%, or if Q-T interval lengthens by more than 25% above baseline and notify the doctor.
• If recurrence of arrhythmia occurs, obtain a rhythm strip and notify the doctor.
• Relieve discomfort of dry mouth by chewing gum or hard candy.
• Manage constipation with proper diet or bulk laxatives.
• Institute safety precautions if adverse CNS reactions occur.
Patient Teaching
• When transferring patient from immediate-release to sustained-release capsules, advise him to begin a sustained-release capsule 6 hours after the last immediate-release capsule was taken.
• Stress importance of taking the drug exactly as prescribed. Patient may have to set an alarm clock for night doses.
• Teach patient how to minimize troublesome anticholinergic effects, such as constipation or dry mouth.
• Warn patient to avoid hazardous activities that require mental alertness until CNS effects of drug are known.
Evaluation
In patients receiving disopyramide, appropriate evaluation statements may include:
• Patient's ECG reveals arrhythmia has been corrected.
• Patient does not develop a new arrhythmia as a result of disopyramide therapy.
• Patient and family state an understanding of disopyramide therapy.

disulfiram
(dye sul´ fi ram)
Antabuse, Cronetal, Ro-Sulfiram-500

• *Classification:* alcohol abuse deterrent (aldehyde dehydrogenase inhibitor)
• *Pregnancy Risk Category:* X

HOW SUPPLIED
Tablet: 250 mg, 500 mg

ACTION
Mechanism: Competes with nicotinamide adenine dinucleotide (NAD) for aldehyde reductase and irreversibly inhibits the enzyme. Blocks oxidation of alcohol at the acetaldehyde stage. Excess acetaldehyde produces a highly unpleasant reaction in the presence of even small amounts of alcohol.
Absorption: Completely absorbed after oral administration, but 3 to 12 hours may be required before effects occur. Toxic reactions to alcohol may occur up to 2 weeks after the last dose of disulfiram.
Distribution: Highly lipid-soluble and is initially localized in adipose tissue.
Metabolism: Mostly oxidized in the liver and excreted in urine as free drug and metabolites (for example, diethyldithiocarbamate, diethylamine, and carbon disulfide.)
Excretion: 5% to 20% is unabsorbed and is eliminated in feces. A small amount is eliminated through the lungs, but most is excreted in the urine. Up to 20% of a dose remains in the body after 6 days. Several days may be required for total elimination of the drug.

INDICATIONS & DOSAGE
Adjunct in management of chronic alcoholism–
Adults: maximum of 500 mg P.O. q morning for 1 to 2 weeks. Can be taken in evening if drowsiness occurs. Maintenance: 125 to 500 mg P.O. daily (average dose 250 mg) until permanent self-control is established. Treatment may continue for months or years.

CONTRAINDICATIONS & PRECAUTIONS

Contraindicated in patients with severe myocardial disease or coronary occlusion because of the potential for adverse cardiac effects; psychosis; hypersensitivity to disulfiram or to other thiuram derivatives; chronic intoxication; and in pregnant women.

Use cautiously in patients with a history of rubber contact dermatitis or hypersensitivity to thiuram derivatives; and in patients with diabetes mellitus, chronic or acute nephritis, hepatitis, cirrhosis or insufficiency, seizure disorders, cerebral damage, abnormal ECG results, or drug dependence. Patients who have received metronidazole, paraldehyde, alcohol, or alcohol-containing preparations (such as vitamin tonics and cough syrups) may experience a disulfiram reaction.

ADVERSE REACTIONS

Common reactions are in italics; life-threatening reactions are in bold italics.
CNS: drowsiness, headache, fatigue, delirium, depression, neuritis.
EENT: optic neuritis.
GI: metallic or garliclike aftertaste.
GU: impotence.
Skin: acneiform or allergic dermatitis.
Other: peripheral neuritis; polyneuritis; disulfiram reaction, which may include flushing, throbbing headache, dyspnea, nausea, copious vomiting, sweating, thirst, chest pain, palpitations, hyperventilation, hypotension, syncope, anxiety, weakness, blurred vision, confusion. *In severe reactions, **respiratory depression, cardiovascular collapse, arrhythmias, myocardial infarction, acute CHF, seizures, unconsciousness, and even death can occur.***

INTERACTIONS

Alfentanil: prolonged duration of effect.
Anticoagulants: increased anticoagulant effect. Adjust dosage of anticoagulant.
Ascorbic acid: may interfere with disulfiram-alcohol interaction.
Bacampicillin: use with caution, because its metabolism produces low concentrations of alcohol and acetaldehyde.
CNS depressants: increased CNS depression.
Isoniazid (INH): ataxia or marked change in behavior. Don't use together.
Metronidazole: psychotic reaction. Do not use together.
Midazolam: increased plasma levels of midazolam.
Paraldehyde: toxic levels of the acetaldehyde. Don't use together.
Tricyclic antidepressants, especially amitriptylene: transient delirium.

EFFECTS ON DIAGNOSTIC TESTS

Radioactive iodine (^{131}I) uptake of protein-bound iodine: decreased levels (rarely).
Serum cholesterol: elevated levels.
Urinary vanillmandelic acid excretion: decreased.
Urinalysis: increased homovanillic acid concentrations.

NURSING CONSIDERATIONS

Besides those related universally to drug therapy (see "How to use this book"), consider the following specific recommendations:

Assessment
- Obtain a baseline assessment of alcohol consumption behaviors before therapy.
- Be alert for adverse reactions and drug interactions throughout therapy.
- Evaluate the patient's and family's knowledge about disulfiram therapy.

Nursing Diagnoses
- High risk for toxicity related to underlying condition.
- Pain related to disulfiram-induced headache.

• Knowledge deficit related to disulfiram.

Planning and Implementation

Preparation and Administration

• Administer only after patient has abstained from alcohol for at least 12 hours and when the patient can be closely supervised by medical and nursing personnel.

• Check that patient has given permission for administration of the drug. Ensure that patient understands the consequences of disulfiram therapy.

• Administer the drug only to patients who are cooperative, well-motivated and receiving supportive psychiatric care.

• Check to be sure that a complete physical examination and laboratory studies, including CBC, SMA-12, and transaminase are performed before therapy begins.

• Anticipate maximum dose for 1 to 2 weeks.

• ***P.O. use:*** Administration is usually a daytime dose although it may be given at night is drowsiness occurs. Establish lowered maintenance dose until permanent self-control is practiced. Keep in mind that treatment may continue for months or years.

Monitoring

• Monitor effectiveness by assessing the patient's abstinence from alcohol.

• Observe the patient with alcohol levels of 5 to 10 mg/100 ml for mild reaction to the medication.

• Obtain serum alcohol levels on a weekly basis.

Supportive Care

• Obtain a complete patient physical examination and laboratory studies regularly during therapy.

• Notify the doctor of signs of severe disulfiram reaction: respiratory depression, cardiovascular collapse, arrhythmias, or seizures.

Patient Teaching

• Explain the expected interaction of disulfiram with alcohol.

• Tell the patient to avoid all sources of alcohol including cough syrups, external liniments, shaving lotion, and back-rub preparations.

• Encourage the patient to wear a bracelet or carry a card identifying him as a disulfiram user.

• Reassure the patient the disulfiram-induced reactions subside after about 2 weeks of therapy.

• Encourage the patient to seek emotional support when needed.

• Warn the patient's family to *never* give the patient disulfiram without his knowledge as it may result in a severe reaction if alcohol is then ingested.

Evaluation

In patients receiving disulfiram, appropriate evaluation statements may include:

• Patient will be free of symptoms of disulfiram-induced reaction.

• Patient reports freedom from headache related to adverse effects of medication.

• Patient and family state an understanding of disulfiram therapy.

PHARMACOLOGIC CLASS

diuretics, loop

bumetanide
ethacrynate sodium
ethacrynic acid
furosemide

OVERVIEW

Loop diuretics are sometimes referred to as high-ceiling diuretics because they produce a peak diuresis greater than that produced by other agents. Loop diuretics are particularly useful in edema associated with compromised renal function.

Loop diuretics inhibit sodium and chloride reabsorption in the ascending loop of Henle, thus increasing renal excretion of sodium, chloride, and water; like thiazide diuretics, loop diuretics increase excretion of

COMPARING LOOP DIURETICS

DRUG AND ROUTE	ONSET	PEAK	DURATION	USUAL DOSAGE
bumetanide				
I.V.	≤5 min	15 to 45 min	4 to 6 hr	0.5 to 1 mg ≤ t.i.d
P.O.	30 to 60 min	1 to 2 hr	4 to 6 hr	0.5 to 2 mg/day
ethacrynic acid				
I.V.	≤5 min	¼ to ½ hr	2 hr	50 mg/day
P.O.	≤30 min	2 hr	6 to 8 hr	50 to 100 mg/day
furosemide				
I.V.	≤5 min	⅓ to 1 hr	2 hr	20 to 40 mg q 2 hr, p.r.n.
P.O.	30 to 60 min	1 to 2 hr	6 to 8 hr	20 to 80 mg ≤b.i.d.

potassium. Loop diuretics produce greater maximum diuresis and electrolyte loss than thiazide diuretics.

Furosemide and bumetanide, but not ethacrynic acid, have some renal vasodilatory effect, which may temporarily increase glomerular filtration rate (GFR), and peripheral vasodilatory effect, which may decrease peripheral vascular resistance.

CLINICAL INDICATIONS AND ACTIONS

Edema

Loop diuretics effectively relieve edema associated with congestive heart failure (CHF). They may be useful in patients refractory to other diuretics; because furosemide and bumetanide may increase GFR, they are useful in patients with renal impairment. I.V. loop diuretics are used adjunctively in acute pulmonary edema to decrease peripheral vascular resistance. Loop diuretics also are used to treat edema associated with hepatic cirrhosis and nephrotic syndrome.

Hypertension

Loop diuretics are used in patients with mild to moderate hypertension, although thiazides are the initial diuretics of choice in most patients. Loop diuretics are preferred in patients with CHF or renal impairment; used I.V., they are a helpful adjunct in managing hypertensive crises.

OVERVIEW OF ADVERSE REACTIONS

The most common adverse effects associated with therapeutic doses of loop diuretics are metabolic and electrolyte disturbances, particularly potassium depletion, which may require replacement by other diuretic therapy. Loop diuretics may also cause hypochloremic alkalosis, hyperglycemia, hyperuricemia, and hypomagnesemia. Rapid parenteral administration of loop diuretics may cause hearing loss (including deafness) and tinnitus. Toxic doses produce profound diuresis, leading to hypovolemia and cardiovascular collapse.

REPRESENTATIVE COMBINATIONS
None.

PHARMACOLOGIC CLASS

diuretics, osmotic
mannitol
urea

OVERVIEW
Osmotic diuretics are used to reduce intraocular and intracranial pressure. Most clinicians prefer mannitol because it is relatively less toxic and more stable in solution. Mannitol, but not urea, is approved for prevention and, adjunctively, for treatment of acute renal failure or oliguria.

Osmotic diuretics elevate osmotic pressure of the glomerular filtrate, thereby hindering tubular reabsorption of solutes and water and promoting renal excretion of water, sodium, potassium, chloride, calcium, phosphorus, magnesium, and uric acid. Osmotic diuretics also elevate osmotic pressure in blood and promote the shift of intracellular water into the blood.

CLINICAL INDICATIONS AND ACTIONS
Acute renal failure or oliguria
Mannitol is used to prevent and treat the oliguric phase of acute renal failure. It enhances renal blood flow by its osmotic diuretic effect and by vasodilating effects.

Reduction of intracranial pressure
Osmotic diuretics reduce intracranial pressure and control cerebral edema caused by trauma or disease and during surgery by drawing water from cells (including those in the brain and CSF) into the blood. A rebound effect may occur 12 hours after the administration of urea.

Reduction of intraocular pressure
Osmotic diuretics are used to reduce intraocular pressure when it cannot be reduced by other means; these drugs are especially useful in acute angle-closure glaucoma, in absolute or secondary glaucoma, and before surgery. Their osmotic effect draws fluid from the anterior chamber of the eye, reducing intraocular pressure. Urea, unlike mannitol, penetrates the eye and may cause a rebound increase in intraocular pressure if plasma urea levels fall below that in the vitreous humor. Because urea penetrates the eye, it should not be used when irritation is present.

Drug intoxication
Mannitol is used alone or with other diuretics to enhance urinary excretion of toxins, including aspirin, some barbiturates, bromides, imipramine, and lithium. Besides promoting diuresis, mannitol maintains renal blood flow.

OVERVIEW OF ADVERSE REACTIONS
The most severe adverse effects associated with mannitol are fluid and electrolyte imbalance. Circulatory overload may follow administration of mannitol to patients with inadequate urine output. The most common adverse reactions associated with urea are headache, nausea, and vomiting; a rebound increase in intraocular pressure also may occur.

REPRESENTATIVE COMBINATIONS
None.

PHARMACOLOGIC CLASS

diuretics, potassium-sparing
amiloride hydrochloride
spironolactone
triamterene

OVERVIEW
Potassium-sparing diuretics are less potent than many others; in particular, amiloride and triamterene have little clinical effect when used alone. However, because they protect against

*Liquid form contains alcohol.

**May contain tartrazine.

potassium loss, they are used with other more potent diuretic agents. Spironolactone, an aldosterone antagonist, is particularly useful in patients with edema and hypertension associated with hyperaldosteronism.

Amiloride and triamterene act directly on the distal renal tubules, inhibiting sodium reabsorption and potassium excretion, thereby reducing the potassium loss associated with other diuretic therapy. Spironolactone competitively inhibits aldosterone at the distal renal tubules, also promoting sodium excretion and potassium retention.

CLINICAL INDICATIONS AND ACTIONS

Edema

All potassium-sparing diuretics are used to manage edema associated with hepatic cirrhosis, nephrotic syndrome, and congestive heart failure.

Hypertension

Amiloride and spironolactone are used to treat mild and moderate hypertension; the exact mechanism is unknown. Spironolactone may block the effect of aldosterone on arteriolar smooth muscle.

Diagnosis of primary hyperaldosteronism

Because spironolactone inhibits aldosterone, correction of hypokalemia and hypertension is presumptive evidence of primary hyperaldosteronism.

OVERVIEW OF ADVERSE REACTIONS

Hyperkalemia is the most important adverse reaction; it occurs with all drugs in this class and may lead to cardiac arrhythmias. Other adverse reactions include nausea, vomiting, headache, weakness, fatigue, bowel disturbances, cough, and dyspnea.

Potassium-sparing diuretics are contraindicated in patients with serum potassium levels above 5.5 mEq/liter, in those receiving other potassium-sparing diuretics or potassium supplements, and in patients with anuria, acute or chronic renal insufficiency, diabetic nephropathy, or known hypersensitivity to the drug. They should be used cautiously in patients with severe hepatic insufficiency because electrolyte imbalance may precipitate hepatic encephalopathy, and in patients with diabetes, who are at increased risk of hyperkalemia.

REPRESENTATIVE COMBINATIONS

Amiloride with hydrochlorothiazide: Moduretic.

Spironolactone with hydrochlorothiazide: Aldactazide, Spiranazide.

Triamterene with hydrochlorothiazide: Dyazide, Maxzide.

PHARMACOLOGIC CLASS

diuretics, thiazide

bendroflumethiazide
benzthiazide
chlorothiazide
hydrochlorothiazide
hydroflumethiazide
methyclothiazide
polythiazide
trichlormethiazide

diuretics, thiazidelike

chlorthalidone
indapamide
metolazone
quinethazone

OVERVIEW

Thiazide diuretics were discovered and synthesized as an outgrowth of studies on carbonic anhydrase inhibitors. Until the 1950s, organic mercurials were the only effective diuretics available; though potent, they were also toxic. Introduction of the thiazides in 1957 proved a major advance because these were the first potent – and safe – diuretics.

Thiazide diuretics interfere with

COMPARING THIAZIDES

Under most conditions, thiazide diuretics differ mainly in duration of action.

DRUG	EQUIVALENT DOSE	ONSET	PEAK	DURATION
bendroflumethiazide	5 mg	Within 2 hr	4 hr	6 to 12 hr
benzthiazide	50 mg	Within 2 hr	4 to 6 hr	6 to 12 hr
chlorothiazide	500 mg	Within 2 hr	4 hr	6 to 12 hr
cyclothiazide	2 mg	Within 6 hr	7 to 12 hr	18 to 24 hr
hydrochlorothiazide	50 mg	Within 2 hr	4 to 6 hr	6 to 12 hr
hydroflumethiazide	50 mg	Within 2 hr	4 hr	6 to 12 hr
methyclothiazide	5 mg	Within 2 hr	4 to 6 hr	24 hr
polythiazide	2 mg	Within 2 hr	6 hr	24 to 48 hr
trichlormethiazide	2 mg	Within 2 hr	6 hr	24 hr

sodium transport thereby increasing renal excretion of sodium, chloride, water, potassium, and calcium.

The exact mechanism of thiazides' antihypertensive effect is unknown; however, it is thought to be partially caused by direct arteriolar dilatation.

In diabetes insipidus, thiazides cause a paradoxical decrease in urine volume and increase in renal concentration of urine, possibly because of sodium depletion and decreased plasma volume, which leads to an increase in renal water and sodium reabsorption.

CLINICAL INDICATIONS AND ACTIONS

Edema

Thiazide diuretics are used to treat edema associated with right-sided heart failure, mild to moderate left-sided heart failure, and nephrotic syndrome and, with spironolactone, to treat edema and ascites secondary to hepatic cirrhosis.

Efficacy and toxicity profiles of thiazide and thiazide-like diuretics are equivalent at comparable dosages; the single exception is metolazone, which may be more effective in patients with impaired renal function. Usually, thiazide diuretics are less effective than loop diuretics in patients with renal insufficiency.

Hypertension

Thiazide diuretics are commonly used for initial management of all degrees of hypertension. Used alone, they reduce mean blood pressure by only 10 to 15 mm Hg; in mild hypertension, thiazide diuresis alone will usually reduce blood pressure to desired levels. However, in moderate to severe hypertension that does not respond to thiazides alone, combination therapy with another antihypertensive agent is necessary.

Diabetes insipidus

In diabetes insipidus, thiazides cause a paradoxical decrease in urine volume; urine becomes more concentrated, possibly because of sodium depletion and decreased plasma volume. Thiazides are particularly effective in nephrogenic diabetes insipidus.

*Liquid form contains alcohol. **May contain tartrazine.

OVERVIEW OF ADVERSE REACTIONS
Therapeutic doses of thiazide diuretics cause electrolyte and metabolic disturbances, the most common being potassium depletion; patients may require dietary supplementation. Other abnormalities include hypochloremic alkalosis, hyponatremia, hypercalcemia, hyperuricemia, elevated cholesterol levels, and hyperglycemia. Overdose of thiazides may produce lethargy that can progress to coma within a few hours.

REPRESENTATIVE COMBINATIONS
Bendroflumethiazide with nadolol: Corzide; with potassium chloride: Naturetin W/K; with rauwolfia serpentina: Rauzide; with raudixin and potassium chloride: Rautrax; with rauwolfia serpentina and potassium chloride: Rautrax-N; with raudixin and potassium chloride: Rautrax-N, modified; with reserpine: Exna-R.

Chlorthalidone with reserpine: Regroton.

Chlorothiazide with methyldopa: Aldochlor; with reserpine: Diupres.

Hydrochlorothiazide with deserpidine: Oreticyl; with guanethidine monosulfate: Esimil; with hydralazine: Apresazide, Apresoline-Esidrix, Hydralazide; with methyldopa: Aldoril; with propranolol: Inderide; with reserpine: Hydropine, Hydropres, Hydroserp, Hydroserpine, Hydrotensin, Mallopress, Serpasil-Esidrex, Thia-Serp; with hydralazine and reserpine: Harbolin, Ser-Ap-Es, Serapine, Serpahyde, Thia-Serpa-Zine, Unipres; with spironolactone: Aldactazide; with timolol maleate: Timolide; with triamterene: Dyazide, Maxzide; with amiloride: Moduretic.

Hydroflumethiazide with reserpine: Salutensin.

Methyclothiazide with cryptenamine: Diutensin; with reserpine: Diutensin-R; with deserpidine: Enduronyl; with pargyline: Eutron.

Polythiazide with prazosin: Minizide; with reserpine: Renese-R.

Quinethazone with reserpine: Hydromox R.

Trichlormethiazide with reserpine: Metatensin, Naquival.

---

dobutamine hydrochloride
(doe byoo´ ta meen)
Dobutrex

- *Classification:* inotropic agent (adrenergic beta, agonist)
- *Pregnancy Risk Category:* C

HOW SUPPLIED
Injection: 12.5 mg/ml in 20-ml vials (parenteral)

ACTION
Mechanism: Directly stimulates $beta_1$ receptors of the heart to increase myocardial contractility and stroke volume, resulting in increased cardiac output.
Absorption: Drug is administered I.V. because it is rapidly metabolized in the GI tract after oral administration.
Distribution: Unknown if drug enters breast milk or crosses the placenta.
Metabolism: By the liver to inactive metabolites.
Excretion: Mainly in urine, with minor amounts in feces, as its metabolites and conjugates. Half-life: About 2 minutes.
Onset, peak, duration: After I.V. administration, onset of action occurs within 2 minutes, with peak concentrations achieved within 10 minutes of starting an infusion. Effects persist a few minutes after I.V. is discontinued.

INDICATIONS & DOSAGE
Refractory heart failure and as adjunct in cardiac surgery—
Adults: 2.5 to 10 mcg/kg/minute as an I.V. infusion. Rarely, infusion

rates up to 40 mcg/kg/minute may be needed.

CONTRAINDICATIONS & PRECAUTIONS

Contraindicated in patients with idiopathic hypertrophic subaortic stenosis or hypersensitivity to the drug or its ingredients. Use with extreme caution after myocardial infarction (may intensify or extend myocardial ischemia). Dobutamine increases atrioventricular (AV) conduction; therefore, patients with atrial fibrillation should have therapeutic levels of a cardiac glycoside before administration of dobutamine.

Drug contains sodium bisulfite and may trigger allergic reaction in patients with sulfite sensitivity.

ADVERSE REACTIONS

Common reactions are in italics; life-threatening reactions are in bold italics.
CNS: headache.
CV: *increased heart rate, hypertension,* ***premature ventricular contractions,*** angina, nonspecific chest pain.
GI: nausea, vomiting.
Other: shortness of breath.

INTERACTIONS

Beta blockers: may antagonize dobutamine effects. Do not use together.
General anesthetics: greater incidence of ventricular arrhythmias.

EFFECTS ON DIAGNOSTIC TESTS

None reported.

NURSING CONSIDERATIONS

Besides those related universally to drug therapy (see "How to use this book"), consider the following specific recommendations:

Assessment

- Obtain a baseline assessment of the patient's underlying condition before drug therapy.
- Be alert for adverse reactions and drug interactions during dobutamine therapy.
- Evaluate the patient's and family's knowledge about dobutamine therapy.

Nursing Diagnoses

- Decreased cardiac output related to the patient's underlying condition.
- Ineffective breathing pattern related to adverse drug reactions.
- Knowledge deficit related to dobutamine hydrochloride therapy.

Planning and Implementation

Preparation and Administration

- Know that this drug is a chemical modification of isoproterenol.
- Drug is often used with nitroprusside for additive effects.
- Drug is incompatable with alkaline solutions, such as sodium bicarbonate injection.
- ***I.V. use:*** Direct and intermittent infusion not used; administer continuous infusion through a central venous line, using an infusion pump for precise titration.
- Long infusions (up to 72 hours) produce no more adverse effects than shorter infusions.
- Oxidation of drug may discolor admixtures containing dobutamine. This not does indicate a significant loss of potency.
- Solutions remain stable for 24 hours.
- Know that this drug is a unique agent that increases contractility of the heart without inducing marked tachycardia, except at high doses.

Monitoring

- Continuously monitor for adverse reactions or drug interactions by monitoring ECG, blood pressure, pulmonary wedge pressure, and cardiac output continuously.
- Monitor for hypovolemia, which should be corrected with plasma expanders before initiating therapy with dobutamine.
- Monitor for drug-induced headache.
- Monitor patient's respirations; drug may cause dyspnea.

• Monitor patient's hydration status by monitoring intake and output if the patient develops nausea and vomiting.

Supportive Care

• Provide fluids if the patient develops nausea and vomiting.

• Provide respiratory support if the patient develops dyspnea.

Patient Teaching

• Teach the patient to report shortness of breath and a drug-induced headache.

Evaluation

In patients receiving dobutamine, appropriate evaluation statements may include:

• Patient's cardiac output remains adaquate.

• Patient does not develop dyspnea.

• Patient and family state an understanding of dobutamine therapy.

docusate calcium (dioctyl calcium sulfosuccinate)

(dok´ yoo sate)

Pro-Cal-Sof◇, Surfak◇

docusate potassium (dioctyl potassium sulfosuccinate)

Dialose◇, Diocto-K◇, Kasof◇

docusate sodium (dioctyl sodium sulfosuccinate)

Afko-Lube◇, Colace◇, Coloxyl‡, Coloxyl Enema Concentrate‡, Diocto◇, Dioeze◇, Diosuccin◇, Dio-Sul◇, Disonate◇, Di-Sosul◇, DOK-250◇, DOK Liquid◇, Doss 300◇, Doxinate◇, D-S-S◇, Duosol◇, Genasoft◇, Laxinate 100◇, Modane Soft◇, Pro-Sof◇, Pro-Sof 250◇, Pro-Sof Liquid Concentrate◇, Regulax SS◇, Regutol◇, Stulex◇

• *Classification:* emollient laxative (surfactant)

• *Pregnancy Risk Category:* C

HOW SUPPLIED

calcium

Capsules: 50 mg◇, 240 mg◇

potassium

Capsules: 100 mg◇, 240 mg◇

sodium

Tablets: 50 mg◇, 100 mg◇

Capsules◇: 50 mg, 60 mg, 100 mg, 240 mg, 250 mg, 300 mg

Oral liquid: 50 mg/ml◇

Syrup: 50 mg/15 ml◇, 60 mg/15 ml◇

Enema concentrate: 18 g/100 ml (must be diluted)‡

ACTION

Mechanism: A stool softener that reduces surface tension of interfacing liquid contents of the bowel. This detergent activity promotes incorporation of additional liquid into the stool, forming a softer mass.

Absorption: Minimally absorbed in the duodenum and jejunum.

Distribution: Primarily distributed locally, in the gut.

Metabolism: None.

Excretion: In feces.

Onset, peak, duration: Drug acts in 1 to 3 days.

INDICATIONS & DOSAGE

Stool softener–

Adults and older children: 50 to 300 mg (docusate sodium) P.O. daily or 50 to 300 mg (docusate calcium and docusate potassium) P.O. daily until bowel movements are normal. Alternatively, give enema (where available). Dilute 1:24 with sterile water before administration, and give 100 to 150 ml (retention enema), 300 to 500 ml (evacuation enema), or 0.5 to 1.5 liters (flushing enema).

Children 6 to 12 years: 40 to 120 mg (docusate sodium) P.O. daily.

Children 3 to 6 years: 20 to 60 mg (docusate sodium) P.O. daily.

Children under 3 years: 10 to 40 mg (docusate sodium) P.O. daily.

Higher dosages are for initial therapy. Adjust dosage to individual response. Usual dosage in children and adults with minimal needs: 50 to 150 mg (docusate calcium) P.O. daily.

CONTRAINDICATIONS & PRECAUTIONS

Contraindicated in patients receiving mineral oil because they may increase absorption to dangerous levels.

ADVERSE REACTIONS

Common reactions are in italics; life-threatening reactions are in bold italics.
EENT: throat irritation.
GI: bitter taste, mild abdominal cramping, diarrhea.
Other: laxative dependence in long-term or excessive use.

INTERACTIONS

Mineral oil: may increase mineral oil absorption and cause lipoid pneumonia. Don't administer together.

EFFECTS ON DIAGNOSTIC TESTS

None reported.

NURSING CONSIDERATIONS

Besides those related universally to drug therapy (see "How to use this book"), consider the following specific recommendations:

Assessment
- Obtain a baseline assessment of history of bowel disorder, GI status, fluid intake, nutritional status, exercise habits, and normal pattern of elimination.
- Be alert for adverse reactions or drug interactions during therapy.
- Evaluate the patient's and family's knowledge about docusate.

Nursing Diagnoses
- Constipation related to interruption of normal pattern of elimination characterized by infrequent or absent stools.
- Diarrhea related to prolonged or excessive use of docusate.
- Knowledge deficit related to docusate therapy.

Planning and Implementation

Preparation and Administration
- Store at 59° to 86° F (15° to 30° C). Protect liquid from light.
- ***P.O. use:*** Give liquid in milk, fruit juice or infant formula to mask bitter taste.
- Minimum effective dose is 300 mg daily. A lower dosage may not produce satisfactory results.

Monitoring
- Monitor effectiveness by checking the frequency and characteristics of stools.
- Auscultate bowel sounds at least once a shift. Assess for pain and cramping.
- Monitor nutritional status and fluid intake.

Supportive Care
- Be aware that docusate prevents but does not treat constipation.
- Laxative of choice for patients who should not strain during defecation, such as those recovering from myocardial infarction or rectal surgery; in disease of the rectum and anus that makes passage of firm, hard stool difficult; or in postpartum constipation.
- Acts within 24 to 48 hours to produce firm, semisolid stool.
- Discontinue if abdominal cramping occurs; docusate does not stimulate intestinal peristaltic movements.
- Provide privacy for elimination.
- Unless contraindicated, encourage fluid intake up to 2500 ml a day.
- Consult with a dietitian to modify diet to increase fiber and bulk.

Patient Teaching
- Discourage excessive use of laxatives by patient. Instruct the patient not to use for more than 1 week without doctor's knowledge.
- Teach the patient about the relationship between fluid intake, dietary fiber, exercise, and constipation.
- Teach patient that dietary sources of

fiber include bran and other cereals, fresh fruit, and vegetables.

Evaluation

In patients receiving docusate, appropriate evaluation statements may include:

- Patient reports return of normal pattern of elimination.
- Patient remains free from diarrhea.
- Patient and family state an understanding of docusate therapy.

dopamine hydrochloride

(doe´ pa meen)

Intropin, Revimine†‡

- *Classification:* inotropic agent, vasopressor (adrenergic)
- *Pregnancy Risk Category:* C

HOW SUPPLIED

Injection: 40 mg/ml, 80 mg/ml, 160 mg/ml parenteral concentrate for injection for I.V. infusion; 0.8 mg/ml (200 or 400 mg) in dextrose 5%; 1.6 mg/ml (400 or 800 mg) in dextrose 5%, 3.2 mg/ml (800 mg) in dextrose 5% parenteral injection for I.V. infusion.

ACTION

Mechanism: Stimulates dopaminergic, beta-adrenergic, and alpha-adrenergic receptors of the sympathetic nervous system.

Absorption: Rapidly metabolized in the GI tract after oral administration.

Distribution: Unknown if drug enters breast milk or crosses the placenta. Does not enter the CNS.

Metabolism: To inactive compounds in the liver, kidneys, and plasma by monoamine oxidase and catechol-O-methyltransferase. About 25% is metabolized to norepinephrine within adrenergic nerve terminals.

Excretion: In urine, mainly as its metabolites. Half-life: About 2 minutes.

Onset, peak, duration: Onset of action after starting an I.V. infusion is 5 minutes and persists for less than 10 minutes.

INDICATIONS & DOSAGE

To treat shock and correct hemodynamic imbalances; to improve perfusion to vital organs; to increase cardiac output; to correct hypotension; to treat acute renal failure—

Adults: 2 to 5 mcg/kg/minute I.V. infusion, up to 50 mcg/kg/minute. Titrate the dosage to the desired hemodynamic and/or renal response.

CONTRAINDICATIONS & PRECAUTIONS

Contraindicated in patients with pheochromocytoma and in those with uncorrected tachyarrhythmias or ventricular fibrillation because of potential for severe cardiovascular effects.

Commercially available dopamine solutions containing sulfites should be used cautiously in patients with asthma and other patients with hypersensitivity to them; also use cautiously in patients with ischemic heart disease. Monitor patients with a history of occlusive vascular disease for decreased circulation to extremities.

ADVERSE REACTIONS

Common reactions are in italics; life-threatening reactions are in bold italics.

CNS: headache.

CV: ectopic beats, tachycardia, anginal pain, palpitations, *hypotension.* Less frequently, bradycardia, widening of QRS complex, conduction disturbances, vasoconstriction.

GI: nausea, vomiting.

Local: necrosis and tissue sloughing with extravasation.

Other: piloerection, dyspnea.

INTERACTIONS

Beta blockers: may antagonize dopamine's effects.

Ergot alkaloids: extreme elevations in blood pressure. Don't use together.
MAO inhibitors: may cause hypertensive crisis. Avoid if possible.
Phenytoin: may lower blood pressure of dopamine-stabilized patients. Monitor carefully.

EFFECTS ON DIAGNOSTIC TESTS

Serum glucose: elevation in levels (usually within normal limits).

NURSING CONSIDERATIONS

Besides those related universally to drug therapy (see "How to use this book"), consider the following specific recommendations:

Assessment

- Obtain a baseline assessment of the patient's underlying condition before initiating dopamine therapy.
- Be alert for common adverse reactions.
- Evaluate the patient's and family's knowledge about dopamine therapy.

Nursing Diagnoses

- Altered tissue perfusion (cerebral, cardiopulmonary, and renal) related to patient's underlying condition.
- Impaired tissue integrity related to adverse drug reactions.
- Knowledge deficit related to dopamine therapy.

Planning and Implementation

Preparation and Administration

- Use large vein, as in the antecubital fossa, to minimize risk of extravasation.
- ***I.V. use:*** Don't mix with alkaline solutions. Use dextrose 5% in water (D_5W), 0.9% sodium chloride solution, or combination of D_5W and 0.9% sodium chloride solution. Mix just before use.
- Dopamine solutions deteriorate after 24 hours. Discard at that time or earlier if solution is discolored.
- Do not mix other drugs in I.V. container with dopamine.
- Do not give alkaline drugs (for example, sodium bicarbonate, phenytoin sodium) through I.V. line containing dopamine.
- Use a continuous infusion pump to regulate flow rate.
- Be aware that dopamine is not a substitute for blood or fluid volume deficit. Volume deficit should be corrected before vasopressors, such as dopamine, are administered.
- Be aware that the patient's response depends on dosage and pharmacologic effect. Dosage of 0.5 to 2 mcg/kg/minute predominantly stimulates dopamine receptors and produces vasodilation. Dosage of 2 to 10 mcg/kg/minute stimulates beta-adrenergic receptors. Higher dosage also stimulates alpha-adrenergic receptors. Most patients are satisfactorily maintained on less than 20 mcg/kg/minute.

Monitoring

- During infusion, monitor effectiveness by frequently checking blood pressure, cardiac output, pulse rate, urine output, and color and temperature of extremities.
- Monitor for adverse reactions by carefully observing the I.V. site for signs of extravasation.
- Monitor ECG for arrhythmias.
- Monitor hydration status if nausea and vomiting occur.
- Monitor for drug interactions if patient is receiving beta blockers, ergot alkaloids, MAO inhibitors, or phenytoin.
- Frequently monitor urine output if doses exceed 50 mcg/kg/minute.

Supportive Care

- Titrate infusion rate according to assessment findings, using doctor's guidelines.
- If the patient develops a disproportionate rise in the diastolic pressure (a marked decrease in pulse pressure), decrease infusion rate and observe carefully for further evidence of predominant vasoconstrictor activity, unless such an effect is desired.
- If urine flow decreases without hypotension, consider reducing dose.

• Be aware that acidosis decreases effectiveness of dopamine.
• If extravasation occurs, stop infusion immediately and call the doctor for instructions; doctor may order infiltration of the area with 5 to 10 mg phentolamine and 10 to 15 ml 0.9% sodium chloride solution to counteract this effect.
• Adverse reactions may require dosage adjustment or discontinuation of the drug.

Patient Teaching
• Emphasize the importance of reporting discomfort at I.V. site immediately.
• Tell the patient that this drug will help to correct hypotension.

Evaluation
In patients receiving dopamine, appropriate evaluation statements may include:
• Cerebral, cardiopulmonary, and renal tissue perfusion remains adequate.
• Tissue integrity is maintained at the I.V. site and extravasation does not occur.
• Patient and family state an understanding of dopamine therapy.

doxapram hydrochloride
(dox´ a pram)
Dopram

• *Classification:* CNS and respiratory stimulant (analeptic)
• *Pregnancy Risk Category:* C

HOW SUPPLIED
Injection: 20 mg/ml (benzyl alcohol 0.9%)

ACTION
Mechanism: Acts either directly on the central respiratory centers in the medulla or indirectly on the chemoreceptors.
Distribution: Widely distributed; drug enters the CNS.
Metabolism: Drug is 99% metabolized by the liver.
Excretion: Metabolites are excreted in urine. Half-life: Plasma ranges from about 2½ to 4 hours.
Onset, peak, duration: After I.V. administration, action begins within 20 to 40 seconds; peak effect occurs in 1 to 2 minutes. Pharmacologic action persists for 5 to 12 minutes.

INDICATIONS & DOSAGE
Postanesthesia respiratory stimulation, drug-induced CNS depression, and chronic pulmonary disease associated with acute hypercapnia –
Adults: 0.5 to 1 mg/kg of body weight (up to 2 mg/kg in CNS depression), I.V. injection or infusion. Maximum dosage is 4 mg/kg, up to 3 g/day. Infusion rate is 1 to 3 mg/minute (initial: 5 mg/minute for postanesthesia).
Chronic obstructive pulmonary disease –
Adults: infusion, 1 to 2 mg/minute. Maximum is 3 mg/minute for a maximum duration of 2 hours.

CONTRAINDICATIONS & PRECAUTIONS
Contraindicated in patients with head trauma and epilepsy or other seizure disorders because of the risk of drug-induced convulsions; with acute bronchial asthma, pulmonary embolism, pneumothorax, pulmonary fibrosis, airway obstruction, severe dyspnea and respiratory failure from muscle paresis because of risk of hypoxia and subsequent arrhythmias; and in patients with coronary artery disease, severe hypertension, frank uncompensated heart failure, or cerebrovascular accident, because of drug's vasopressor effects.

Use cautiously in patients with a history of severe tachycardia or cardiac arrhythmia, because of the risk of hypoxia and subsequent arrhythmia; and in patients with increased cerebrospinal fluid pressure or cerebral edema, pheochromocytoma, or hyperthyroidism, because of drug's vasopressor effects.

ADVERSE REACTIONS

Common reactions are in italics; life-threatening reactions are in bold italics.
CNS: ***seizures,*** *headache,* dizziness, apprehension, disorientation, pupillary dilation, bilateral Babinski's signs, flushing, sweating, paresthesias.
CV: *chest pain and tightness, variations in heart rate, hypertension,* lowered T waves.
GI: nausea, vomiting, diarrhea.
GU: urine retention, or stimulation of the bladder with incontinence.
Other: sneezing, coughing, laryngospasm, ***bronchospasm,*** hiccups, rebound hypoventilation, pruritus.

INTERACTIONS

MAO inhibitors, sympathomimetics: potentiate adverse cardiovascular effects. Use together cautiously.

EFFECTS ON DIAGNOSTIC TESTS

BUN: increased levels.
CBC: decreased RBC and WBC counts.
ECG: T-wave depression.
Hemoglobin and hematocrit: reduced levels.
Urinalysis: albuminuria.

NURSING CONSIDERATIONS

Besides those related universally to drug therapy (see "How to use this book"), consider the following specific recommendations:

Assessment
- Obtain a baseline assessment of arterial blood gases, heart rate and rhythm, and deep tendon reflexes before therapy.
- Be alert for adverse reactions and drug interactions throughout therapy.
- Evaluate the patient's and family's knowledge about doxapram therapy.

Nursing Diagnoses
- Ineffective breathing pattern related to anesthesia-induced respiratory depression.
- High risk for injury related to doxapram-induced seizure.
- Knowledge deficit related to doxapram therapy.

Planning and Implementation

Preparation and Administration
- Establish adequate airway before administering drug.
- ***I.V. use:*** Administer slowly; rapid administration may cause hemolysis.
- Do not combine with alkaline solutions such as thiopental sodium; doxapram is acidic.

Monitoring
- Monitor effectiveness by observing the patient for decrease in CNS and respiratory depression.
- Monitor blood pressure, heart rate, rhythm, deep tendon reflexes, and arterial blood gases every 30 minutes after administering doxapram.
- Observe for signs of overdosage: hypertension, tachycardia, arrhythmias, skeletal muscle hyperactivity, or dyspnea.
- Monitor infusion rate and I.V. patency carefully to prevent extravasation-induced thrombophlebitis and local skin irritation.

Supportive Care
- Be aware that use as an analeptic is strongly discouraged.
- Keep airway patent, position patient on side to prevent aspiration of vomitus. Have suction equipment nearby.
- Discontinue drug if patient shows signs of increased arterial carbon dioxide or oxygen tension, or if mechanical ventilation is started. Give I.V. injection of anticonvulsant.
- Use only in surgical or emergency room situations.
- Use seizure precautions.

Patient Teaching
- Instruct patient to report chest pain or tightness, headache, or palpitations immediately.

Evaluation
In patients receiving doxapram hydrochloride, appropriate evaluation statements may include:
- Patient exhibits no signs of respiratory difficulty related to anesthesia.
- Patient remains free from injury related to drug-induced seizure.
- Patient and family state an understanding of doxapram hydrochloride therapy.

---

doxazosin mesylate
(dox ay′ zoe sin)
Cardura

- *Classification:* antihypertensive (alpha-adrenergic blocking agent)
- *Pregnancy Risk Category:* B

HOW SUPPLIED
Tablets: 1 mg, 2 mg, 4 mg, 8 mg

ACTION
Mechanism: An alpha-adrenergic blocking agent that acts on the peripheral vasculature to produce vasodilation.
Absorption: Readily absorbed from the GI tract after oral administration. The effect of food on the bioavailability has not been determined.
Distribution: 98% protein-bound. Distributed to breast milk in concentrations about 20 times greater than maternal plasma.
Metabolism: Bioavailability is approximately 65% reflecting first-pass metabolism of doxazosin by the liver. Drug extensively metabolized in the liver.
Excretion: 63% is excreted in bile and feces (4.8% as unchanged drug); 9% is excreted in urine. Half-life: Plasma elimination is biphasic with a terminal elimination half-life of about 22 hours.
Onset, peak, duration: Peak plasma levels occur about 2 to 3 hours after an oral dose.

INDICATIONS & DOSAGE
Essential hypertension–
Adults: initiate dosage at 1 mg P.O. daily and determine effect on standing and supine blood pressure at 2 to 6 hours and 24 hours after dosing. If necessary, increase dose to 2 mg daily. To minimize adverse reactions, titrate dosage slowly (usually increased dosage only q 2 weeks). Dose may be increased to a daily dose of 4 mg, then 8 mg if necessary. Maximum daily dosage is 16 mg, but dosage that exceeds 4 mg daily is associated with a greater incidence of adverse reactions.

CONTRAINDICATIONS & PRECAUTIONS
Contraindicated in patients with hypersensitivity to quinazolines. Use with caution in patients with impaired hepatic function or those receiving drugs known to influence hepatic metabolism. Concurrent use with other antihypertensives may result in marked hypotension, especially postural hypotension, and syncope with sudden loss of consciousness, particularly with the first few doses; use with caution.

ADVERSE REACTIONS
Common reactions are in italics; life-threatening reactions are in bold italics.
CNS: dizziness, vertigo, headache, somnolence, drowsiness, fatigue, malaise, syncope, paresthesia.
CV: *orthostatic hypotension,* hypotension, edema, palpitations, arrhythmias, tachycardia, peripheral ischemia.
Skin: rash, pruritus.
Other: arthralgia, myalgia, muscle weakness, rhinitis.

INTERACTIONS
None reported.

EFFECTS ON DIAGNOSTIC TESTS

WBC and neutrophil counts: may be decreased.

NURSING CONSIDERATIONS

Besides those related universally to drug therapy (see "How to use this book"), consider the following specific recommendations:

Assessment

• Obtain a baseline assessment of the patient's blood pressure before beginning therapy.

• Be alert for adverse reactions and drug interactions throughout therapy.

• Evaluate the patient's and family's knowledge about doxazosin therapy.

Nursing Diagnoses

• Altered tissue perfusion (renal, cerebral, cardiopulmonary and peripheral) related to the patient's underlying condition.

• Decreased cardiac output related to doxazosin mesylate-induced adverse reactions.

• Knowledge deficit related to doxazosin mesylate therapy.

Planning and Implementation

Preparation and Administration

• ***P.O. use:*** Dosage increases must be titrated gradually, with adjustments every 2 weeks. The 2-, 4- and 8-mg tablets are not indicated for initial therapy.

Monitoring

• Monitor effectiveness by regularly checking the patient's blood pressure, pulse and ECG.

• Monitor for marked orthostatic hypotension, which may be accompanied by dizziness and syncope. Keep in mind that patients taking doxazosin mesylate are susceptible to "first dose" effect similar to that produced by other alpha-adrenergic blocking agents. Orthostatic hypotension is most common after the first dose but can also occur when therapy is interrupted for a few days and during periods of dosage adjustment.

Supportive Care

• Place the patient in a recumbent position and treat supportively if syncope occurs. A transient hypotensive response is not considered a contraindication to continued therapy.

Patient Teaching

• Warn the patient to avoid driving and other hazardous activities or situations because drug may cause dizziness or fainting.

• Warn the patient that the drug may cause drowsiness. Tell the patient to avoid driving and other hazardous activities that require alertness until the adverse CNS effects of the drug are known.

• Teach the patient how to take his own blood pressure. Tell the patient to notify the doctor if there is a significant change in blood pressure measurement.

• Stress the importance of regular follow-up visits for evaluation of the drug therapy.

Evaluation

In patients receiving doxazosin, appropriate evaluation statements may include:

• Blood pressure is controlled within normal limits for this patient.

• Patient did not experience decreased cardiac output.

• Patient and family state an understanding of doxazosin therapy.

doxepin hydrochloride

(dox´ e pin)

Adapin**, Deptran‡, Sinequan, Triadapin†

• *Classification:* tricyclic antidepressant
• *Pregnancy Risk Category:* C

HOW SUPPLIED

Tablets: 10 mg, 25 mg, 50 mg, 75 mg, 100 mg, 150 mg
Capsules: 10 mg‡, 25 mg‡
Oral concentrate: 10 mg/ml

ACTION

Mechanism: Increases the amount of norepinephrine or serotonin, or both, in the CNS by blocking their reuptake by the presynaptic neurons.
Absorption: Rapidly absorbed after oral administration.
Distribution: Widely distributed; enters the CNS and is found in breast milk. Drug is 90% protein-bound.
Metabolism: By the liver to the active metabolite desmethyldoxepin. A significant first-pass effect may explain variability of serum concentrations in different patients taking the same dosage.
Excretion: Most is excreted in urine. Half-life: 6 to 8 hours.
Onset, peak, duration: Peak effect occurs in 2 to 4 hours; steady state is achieved within 7 days. Therapeutic concentrations (parent drug and metabolite) are thought to range from 150 to 250 ng/ml.

INDICATIONS & DOSAGE

Treatment of depression–
Adults: initially, 50 to 75 mg P.O. daily in divided doses, to maximum of 300 mg daily. Alternatively, entire dosage may be given at bedtime.

CONTRAINDICATIONS & PRECAUTIONS

Contraindicated in patients with hypersensitivity to tricyclic antidepressants, trazodone, and related compounds; in the acute recovery phase of myocardial infarction (MI) because of its potential arrhythmogenic effects and ECG changes; in patients in coma or severe respiratory depression because of additive CNS depression; during or within 14 days of therapy with monoamine oxidase inhibitors; and in breast-feeding women because of the hazard of respiratory depression in the infant.

Use cautiously in patients with other cardiac disease (arrhythmias, CHF, angina pectoris, valvular disease, or heart block); respiratory disorders; alcoholism, seizure disorders; scheduled electroconvulsive therapy; bipolar disease; glaucoma; hyperthyroidism, or in those taking thyroid replacement; Type I and Type II diabetes; prostatic hypertrophy, paralytic ileus, or urine retention; hepatic or renal dysfunction; or Parkinson's disease; and in those undergoing surgery with general anesthesia.

ADVERSE REACTIONS

Common reactions are in italics; life-threatening reactions are in bold italics.
CNS: *drowsiness, dizziness,* excitation, tremors, weakness, confusion, headache, nervousness.
CV: *orthostatic hypotension, tachycardia, ECG changes,* hypertension.
EENT: *blurred vision,* tinnitus, glossitis, mydriasis.
GI: *dry mouth, constipation,* nausea, vomiting, anorexia, paralytic ileus.
GU: *urine retention.*
Skin: rash, urticaria.
Other: *sweating,* allergy.
After abrupt withdrawal of long-term therapy: nausea, headache, malaise. (Does not indicate addiction.)

INTERACTIONS

Barbiturates: decrease TCA blood levels. Monitor for decreased antidepressant effect.
Cimetidine: may increase doxepin serum levels. Monitor for increased adverse reactions.
MAO inhibitors: may cause severe excitation, hyperpyrexia, or seizures, usually with high dose. Use together cautiously.
Methylphenidate: increases TCA blood levels. Monitor for enhanced antidepressant effect.

EFFECTS ON DIAGNOSTIC TESTS

CBC: decreased WBC counts.
ECG: elongated Q-T and PR intervals; flattened T-waves.
Liver function tests: elevated results.

Serum glucose: increased or decreased levels.

NURSING CONSIDERATIONS

Besides those related universally to drug therapy (see "How to use this book"), consider the following specific recommendations:

Assessment

- Obtain a baseline assessment of depression before therapy.
- Be alert for adverse reactions and drug interactions throughout therapy.
- Evaluate the patient's and family's knowledge about doxepin therapy.

Nursing Diagnoses

- Ineffectve individual coping related to the patient's underlying condition.
- High risk for injury related to doxepin-induced CNS and CV adverse reactions.
- Knowledge deficit related to doxepin therapy.

Planning and Implementation

Preparation and Administration

- Whenever possible, patient should take full dose at bedtime.
- Expect reduced dosage in elderly patients even though this drug is well-tolerated by the elderly, debilitated patients, adolescents and those receiving other medications (especially anticholinergics).
- ***P.O. use:*** Dilute oral concentrate with 120 ml water, milk, or juice (orange, grapefruit, tomato, prune, or pineapple). The drug is incompatible with carbonated beverages.

Monitoring

- Monitor effectiveness by encouraging the patient to discuss his feelings (ask broad, open-ended questions) and by evaluating his behavior.
- Monitor blood pressure (supine and standing) and ECG for changes and heart rate for tachycardia.
- Watch for signs of oversedation, especially in the elderly patient.
- Monitor bowel patterns for constipation and check for urine retention.
- Note mood changes and monitor for suicidal tendencies.

Supportive Care

- Institute safety precautions if adverse CNS and CV reactions occur.
- If psychotic signs increase, notify doctor and expect dosage to be reduced.
- If not contraindicated, increase the patient's fluid and fiber intake to prevent constipation; if needed, obtain an order for a stool softener or laxative.

Patient Teaching

- Tell the patient to relieve dry mouth with sugarless hard candy or gum but explain that saliva substitutes may be necessary.
- Teach the patient to increase fluid intake to minimize constipation. Suggest stool softener or high-fiber diet, if needed.
- Warn the patient to avoid driving and other hazardous activities that require alertness and good psychomotor coordination until CNS effects of the drug are known. Tell the patient that drowsiness and dizziness usually subside after first few weeks. Inform the patient that drug has strong sedative effects. Warn against combining it with alcohol or other CNS depressants.
- Tell the patient therapy must continue for 2 weeks or more before noticeable effect, and for at least 4 weeks for full effect. Encourage the patient to continue to take medication until it achieves its full therapeutic effect.
- Advise the patient not to take any other drugs (prescription or OTC) without first consulting the doctor.
- Warn the patient about the possibility of morning orthostatic hypotension. Instruct the patient to rise slowly and to sit for several minutes before standing up.

Evaluation
In the patient receiving doxepin, appropriate evaluation statements include:
- Patient behavior and communication indicate improvement of depression.
- Patient has not experienced injury from adverse CNS reactions.
- Patient and family state an understanding of doxepin therapy.

doxorubicin hydrochloride

(dox oh roo´ bi sin)
Adriamycin‡, Adriamycin PFS, Adriamycin RDF

- *Classification:* antineoplastic (antibiotic)
- *Pregnancy Risk Category:* D

HOW SUPPLIED

Injection (preservative-free): 2 mg/ml
Powder for injection: 10-mg, 20-mg, 50-mg vials.

ACTION

Mechanism: An antineoplastic antibiotic that interferes with DNA-dependent RNA synthesis by intercalating base pairs of DNA and causing an uncoiling of the helix, which interferes with the template function of DNA. Also has antibacterial activity, but toxicity precludes its usefulness against infections. Chemically related to daunorubicin.
Absorption: Unstable in gastric acid and extremely irritating to tissues. Animal studies reveal that GI absorption is poor. Drug must be administered intravenously.
Distribution: Widely distributed into body tissues, with the highest concentrations found in the liver, heart, lungs, and kidneys. Drug is present in these tissues within 30 seconds of administration. Drug does not cross the blood-brain barrier. Concentrates in breast milk; limited evidence suggests that it crosses the placenta.
Metabolism: Rapidly and extensively metabolized in the liver and other tissues to several metabolites. Doxorubinol, also known as adriamycinol, is pharmacologically active. There is a significant first-pass effect of the liver on the drug; most of the drug is metabolized before the entire dose is administered.
Excretion: Primarily excreted in the feces; 50% appears as parent drug, and 23% is doxorubinol. Only 4% to 5% is eliminated in urine after 5 days, mostly as unchanged drug; however, it may be of sufficient quantity to turn the urine red. Half-life: Plasma elimination is triphasic, with the initial half-life of about 30 minutes for the parent compound and 3.3 hours for metabolites representing the distribution of the drug into the tissues. A second phase has a half-life of 16½ hours for doxorubicin and 31.7 hours for metabolites, reflecting tissue binding of drug. The final elimination phase takes about 7 days.

INDICATIONS & DOSAGE

Dosage and indications may vary. Check patient's protocol with doctor.
Bladder, breast, cervical, head, neck, liver, lung, ovarian, prostatic, stomach, testicular, and thyroid cancer; Hodgkin's disease; acute lymphoblastic and myeloblastic leukemia; Wilms' tumor; neuroblastomas; lymphomas; sarcomas–
Adults: 60 to 75 mg/m² I.V. as single dose q 3 weeks; or 30 mg/m² I.V. in single daily dose, days 1 to 3 of 4-week cycle. Alternatively, 20 mg/m² I.V. once weekly or 30 mg/m² I.V. on 3 successive days, repeated every 4 weeks. Maximum cumulative dose 550 mg/m².

CONTRAINDICATIONS & PRECAUTIONS

Contraindicated in patients with hepatic dysfunction, depressed bone marrow function, or impaired cardiac function and in patients who have previously received lifetime cumulative doses of doxorubicin or daunorubicin because of increased potential for cardiac or hematopoietic toxicity.

ADVERSE REACTIONS

Common reactions are in italics; life-threatening reactions are in bold italics.

Blood: *leukopenia,* ***especially agranulocytosis,*** *during days 10 to 15, with recovery by day 21;* ***thrombocytopenia.***

CV: ***cardiac depression,*** *seen in such ECG changes as sinus tachycardia, T wave flattening, ST segment depression, voltage reduction; arrhythmias in 11% of patients;* ***irreversible cardiomyopathy*** *(sometimes with pulmonary edema) with mortality of 30% to 75%.*

GI: *nausea, vomiting,* diarrhea, *stomatitis,* esophagitis.

GU: enhancement of cyclophosphamide-induced bladder injury, transient red urine.

Skin: *hyperpigmentation of skin, especially in previously irradiated areas.*

Local: *severe cellulitis or tissue sloughing if drug extravasates.*

Other: hyperpigmentation of nails and dermal creases, *complete alopecia within 3 to 4 weeks;* hair may regrow 2 to 5 months after drug is stopped.

INTERACTIONS

Heparin: don't mix together. May form a precipitate.

Streptozocin: increased and prolonged blood levels. Dosage may have to be adjusted.

EFFECTS ON DIAGNOSTIC TESTS

Blood and urine: increased uric acid concentrations.

NURSING CONSIDERATIONS

Besides those related universally to drug therapy (see "How to use this book"), consider the following specific recommendations:

Assessment

- Obtain a baseline assessment of the patient's overall physical status, CBC, ECG, and renal and hepatic function before initiating therapy.
- Be alert for common adverse reactions and drug interactions during therapy.
- Evaluate the patient's and family's knowledge about doxorubicin therapy.

Nursing Diagnoses

- Impaired tissue integrity related to extravasation of doxorubicin.
- Decreased cardiac output related to doxorubicin-induced cardiotoxicity.
- Knowledge deficit related to doxorubicin therapy.

Planning and Implementation

Preparation and Administration

- Use extreme caution to avoid confusing doxorubicin with daunorubicin (which is a similar reddish color).
- Follow institutional policy during preparation and administration to minimize carcinogenic, mutagenic, and teratogenic risks for personnel.
- Never give I.M. or S.C.
- Be aware that refrigerated, reconstituted solution is stable for 48 hours; at room temperature, it's stable for 24 hours.
- Dosage modification may be required in patients with myelosuppression or impaired cardiac or hepatic function.
- Be aware that the alternative dosage schedule (once-weekly dosing), has been found to lower the incidence of cardiomyopathy.
- Decrease dosage, as ordered, if serum bilirubin level is increased: 50% dosage when bilirubin is 1.2 to

3 mg/100 ml; 25% dosage when bilirubin is greater than 3 mg/100 ml.
• Avoid extravasation; inject slowly by I.V. push into tubing of freely flowing infusion. Don't place I.V. line over joints or in extremities with poor venous or lymphatic drainage.
• Stop drug or slow rate of infusion if tachycardia develops.
• Stop drug immediately in signs of CHF. Prevent by limiting cumulative dose to 550 mg/m^2 (450 mg/m^2 when patient has been receiving radiation therapy that encompasses the heart, or any other cardiotoxic agent, such as cyclophosphamide.)
• If vein streaking occurs, slow administration rate. However, if welts occur, stop administration and report to doctor.

Monitoring

• Monitor effectiveness by noting results of follow-up diagnostic tests and patient's overall physical status.
• Monitor ECG during and following therapy; monitor for early signs and symptoms of CHF.
• Monitor for GI adverse reactions. Keep in mind that esophagitis is very common in patients who have also received radiation therapy.
• Monitor CBC and hepatic functioning.
• Monitor cardiac function studies for evidence of cardiomyopathy.
• Monitor the patient for signs of infection (fever, sore throat, or fatigue).
• Monitor the patient for signs of bleeding (epistaxis, petechiae, melena, or hematuria).
• Monitor for signs of extravasation, which can produce local tissue necrosis, vesication, thrombophlebitis, lymphangitis, cellulitis, painful induration, and result in limited mobility of adjacent joints.

Supportive Care

• Provide frequent mouth care, using a soft toothbrush and mild mouthwash to avoid trauma to oral mucosa.
• If extravasation occurs, discontinue I.V. immediately and apply ice to area for 24 to 48 hours. Some clinicians will infiltrate the area with a parenteral corticosteroid.
• Premedicate the patient with an antiemetic to decrease nausea and vomiting.
• Avoid all I.M. injections when the platelet count is less than 100,000/mm^3.
• Provide adequate hydration; alkalinizing urine or administering allopurinol may prevent or minimize uric acid nephropathy.
• To help prevent infection, maintain the patient's optimal health and protect him from undue exposure to environmental contagions. If signs of infection occur, notify doctor promptly; administer antibiotics, as ordered.
• Provide a safe environment to minimize risk of bleeding.
• Report signs and symptoms of cardiac adverse reactions. If cumulative dose exceeds 550 mg/m^2 body surface area, 30% of patients develop cardiac adverse reactions, which begin 2 weeks to 6 months after stopping drug.

Patient Teaching

• Advise the patient that hyperpigmentation of skin and nails may occur, especially in previously irradiated areas.
• Warn the patient that alopecia will occur, but it is usually reversible.
• Warn patients to watch for signs of infection (sore throat, fever, fatigue) and for signs of bleeding (easy bruising, nosebleeds, bleeding gums). Tell patient to take temperature daily and to report signs of infection or bleeding promptly.
• Tell patient to report symptoms of CHF promptly to doctor.
• Instruct patient about need for protective measures, including conservation of energy, balanced diet, adequate rest, personal cleanliness, clean

environment, and avoidance of exposure to persons with infections.
• Instruct patient about safety precautions to reduce risks of bleeding from falls, cuts, or other injuries.
• Instruct patient about the need for frequent oral hygiene.
• Warn the patient that urine will be orange to red for 1 to 2 days. Explain that this is not blood, but it is caused by the appearance of the drug in the urine.

Evaluation

In patients receiving doxorubicin, appropriate evaluation statements may include:
• No local tissue damage is evidenced.
• No decreased cardiac output is evidenced.
• Patient and family state an understanding of doxorubicin therapy.

doxycycline

(dox i sye´ kleen)

Doxylin‡, Vibramycin

doxycycline hyclate

Doxy-100, Doxy-200, Doxy-Caps, Doxychel, Doxy-Lemmon, Doxy-Tabs, Vibramycin, Vibra-Tabs

doxycycline hydrochloride

Cyclidox‡, Doryx‡, Vibramycin‡, Vibramycin IV‡, Vibra-Tabs 50‡

• *Classification:* antibiotic (tetracycline)
• *Pregnancy Risk Category:* D

HOW SUPPLIED

doxycycline
Tablets: 50 mg‡, 100 mg‡
Oral suspension: 25 mg/5 ml
Syrup: 50 mg/5 ml
doxycycline hyclate
Tablets: 50 mg, 100 mg
Capsules: 50 mg, 100 mg
Capsules (coated pellets): 100 mg
Injection: 100 mg, 200 mg
doxycycline hydrochloride
Tablets: 50 mg‡, 100 mg‡
Capsules: 50 mg‡, 100 mg‡, 250 mg‡
Injection: 100 mg‡

ACTION

Mechanism: Exerts bacteriostatic effect by binding to the 30S ribosomal subunit of microorganisms, thus inhibiting protein synthesis.
Absorption: 90% to 100% absorbed after oral administration. Doxycycline has the least affinity for calcium of all tetracyclines; its absorption is insignificantly altered by milk or other dairy products.
Distribution: Widely distributed into body tissues and fluids, including synovial, pleural, prostatic, and seminal fluids; bronchial secretions; saliva; and aqueous humor. CSF penetration is poor. Doxycycline readily crosses the placenta; it is 25% to 93% protein-bound.
Metabolism: Insignificantly metabolized; some hepatic degradation occurs.
Excretion: Primarily excreted unchanged in urine by glomerular filtration; some drug may be excreted in breast milk and some in the feces. Half-life: 22 to 24 hours after multiple dosing in adults with normal renal function; 20 to 30 hours in patients with severe renal impairment.
Onset, peak, duration: Peak serum levels occur at 1½ to 4 hours after an oral dose.

INDICATIONS & DOSAGE

Infections caused by sensitive gram-negative and gram-positive organisms, trachoma, rickettsiae, Mycoplasma, Chlamydia, *and Lyme disease –*
Adults: 100 mg P.O. q 12 hours on first day, then 100 mg P.O. daily; or 200 mg I.V. on first day in one or two infusions, then 100 to 200 mg I.V. daily.
Children over 8 years (under 45 kg):

4.4 mg/kg P.O. or I.V. daily, divided q 12 hours first day, then 2.2 to 4.4 mg/kg daily. For children over 45 kg, dosage is same as adults.

Give I.V. infusion slowly (minimum 1 hour). Infusion must be completed within 12 hours (within 6 hours in lactated Ringer's solution or dextrose 5% in lactated Ringer's solution).

Gonorrhea in patients allergic to penicillin–
Adults: 200 mg P.O. initially, followed by 100 mg P.O. at bedtime, and 100 mg P.O. b.i.d. for 3 days; or 300 mg P.O. initially and repeat dose in 1 hour.

Primary or secondary syphilis in patients allergic to penicillin–
Adults: 300 mg P.O. daily in divided doses for 10 days.

Uncomplicated urethral, endocervical, or rectal infections caused by Chlamydia trachomatis *or* Ureaplasma urealyticum–
Adults: 100 mg P.O. b.i.d. for at least 7 days.

To prevent "traveler's diarrhea" commonly caused by enterotoxigenic Escherichia coli–
Adults: 100 mg P.O. daily.

CONTRAINDICATIONS & PRECAUTIONS

Contraindicated in patients with hypersensitivity to any tetracycline; during the second half of pregnancy; and in children under age 8 because of the risk of permanent discoloration of teeth, enamel defects, and retardation of bone growth.

Use with caution in patients with impaired renal function, as serum half-life is prolonged; and in patients likely to be exposed to direct sunlight or ultraviolet light because of the risk of photosensitivity reactions.

ADVERSE REACTIONS

Common reactions are in italics; life-threatening reactions are in bold italics.
Blood: neutropenia, eosinophilia.
CNS: intracranial hypertension.
CV: pericarditis.
EENT: sore throat, glossitis, dysphagia.
GI: anorexia, *epigastric distress, nausea,* vomiting, *diarrhea,* enterocolitis, anogenital inflammation.
Skin: *maculopapular and erythematous rashes, photosensitivity, increased pigmentation, urticaria.*
Local: thrombophlebitis.
Other: hypersensitivity.

INTERACTIONS

Antacids (including sodium bicarbonate) and laxatives containing aluminum, magnesium, or calcium: decrease antibiotic absorption. Give antibiotic 1 hour before or 2 hours after any of the above.
Ferrous sulfate and other iron products, zinc: decrease antibiotic absorption. Give doxycycline 3 hours after or 2 hours before iron administration.
Oral contraceptives: decreased contraceptive effectiveness and increased risk of breakthrough bleeding.
Phenobarbital, carbamazepine, alcohol: decrease antibiotic effect. Avoid if possible.

EFFECTS ON DIAGNOSTIC TESTS

Urine catecholamines (fluorometric tests): false elevations.
Urine glucose using copper sulfate method (Clinitest): false-negative results with parenteral dosage.
Urine glucose tests using glucose enzymatic method (Clinistix or Tes-Tape): false-negative results.

NURSING CONSIDERATIONS

Besides those related universally to drug therapy (see "How to use this book"), consider the following specific recommendations:

Assessment
- Obtain a baseline assessment of infection before therapy.

• Be alert for adverse reactions and drug interactions throughout therapy.
• Evaluate the patient's and family's knowledge about doxycycline therapy.

Nursing Diagnoses

• High risk for infection related to ineffectiveness of doxycycline to eradicate the infection.
• High risk for fluid volume deficit related to adverse GI reactions to doxycycline therapy.
• Knowledge deficit related to doxycycline.

Planning and Implementation

Preparation and Administration

• Obtain specimen for culture and sensitivity tests before first dose. Therapy may begin pending test results.
• Check expiration date. Outdated or deteriorated tetracyclines have been associated with reversible nephrotoxicity (Fanconi's syndrome).
• Be aware that use of doxycycline during the last half of pregnancy and in children under age 8 may cause permanent discoloration of teeth, enamel defects, and retardation of bone growth. Question an order for doxycycline in these patients before administering the first dose.
• Do not expose drug to light or heat.
• ***P.O. use:*** Administer with milk or food if GI adverse reactions develop. However, do not administer with antacids. Do not administer drug within 1 hour of bedtime because of increased incidence of dysphagia.
• ***I.V. use:*** Reconstitute powder for injection with sterile water for injection. Use 10 ml in 100-mg vial and 20 ml in 200-mg vial. Dilute solution to 100 to 1,000 ml for I.V. infusion. Do not infuse solutions more concentrated than 1 mg/ml. Reconstituted solution is stable for 72 hours refrigerated. Protect from sunlight during infusion.

Monitoring

• Monitor effectiveness by regularly assessing for improvement of infection.
• During prolonged or high-dose therapy, monitor for superinfection, especially in high-risk patients.
• Monitor hydration status if adverse GI reactions occur.
• Monitor I.V. site for phlebitis.

Supportive Care

• If the patient develops a superinfection or new infection, notify the doctor and expect to discontinue doxycycline and substitute another antibiotic. If the patient develops oral thrush, provide good mouth care.
• If the patient develops diarrhea, nausea, or vomiting, request an antiemetic or antidiarrheal agent, if needed. Expect to substitute parenteral doxycycline or a different antibiotic, as prescribed.
• Because drug may alter results of urine glucose tests, monitor diabetic patients with blood glucose techniques.
• Rotate I.V. therapy sites to minimize irritation.

Patient Teaching

• Tell the patient to take oral doxycycline with milk or food but not with antacids if adverse GI reactions develop and not less than 1 hour before bedtime (to prevent irritation from esophageal reflux).
• Emphasize importance of completing prescribed regimen exactly as ordered and keeping follow-up appointments.
• Inform diabetic patients that drug may interfere with urine glucose test results. Teach patient to monitor glucose level with blood glucose tests.
• Tell the patient to check expiration dates and discard any outdated doxycycline because it may become toxic.
• Teach the patient to recognize and report signs of superinfection (furry overgrowth on tongue, vaginal itch or

discharge, foul-smelling stool). Stress good oral hygiene.
• Advise patient taking an oral contraceptive to use an alternative means of contraception during doxycycline therapy and for 1 week after therapy is discontinued.

Evaluation

In patients receiving doxycycline, appropriate evaluation statements may include:
• Patient is free of infection.
• Patient remains adequately hydrated during doxycycline therapy.
• Patient and family state an understanding of doxycycline therapy.

dronabinol (tetrahydrocannabinol)

(droe nab´ i nol)
Marinol

• Controlled Substance Schedule II
• *Classification:* antiemetic (cannabiniod)
• *Pregnancy Risk Category:* B

HOW SUPPLIED

Capsules: 2.5 mg, 5 mg, 10 mg

ACTION

Mechanism: The principal psychoactive ingredient of marijuana; mechanism of antiemetic action is unknown.
Absorption: About 10% to 20% of dose is absorbed.
Distribution: Rapidly distributed into many tissue sites; drug enters the CNS. Drug is 97% to 99% protein-bound.
Metabolism: Extensively metabolized in the liver. Not known if metabolites are active.
Excretion: Primarily in feces, via the biliary tract. Drug effect may persist for several days after treatment ends; duration varies considerably among patients. Half-life: Terminal plasma half-life for the 11-OH-delta-9-THc is approximately 15 to 18 hours.
Onset, peak, duration: Action begins in 30 to 60 minutes, with peak action in 1 to 3 hours.

INDICATIONS & DOSAGE

Treatment of nausea and vomiting associated with cancer chemotherapy—
Adults: 5 mg/m² P.O. 1 to 3 hours before administration of chemotherapy. Then give same dose q 2 to 4 hours after chemotherapy is administered for a total of four to six doses per day. Dosage may be increased in increments of 2.5 mg/m² to a maximum of 15 mg/m² per dose.

CONTRAINDICATIONS & PRECAUTIONS

Contraindicated in patients with nausea and vomiting not secondary to cancer chemotherapy or not refractory to conventional antiemetics; and in patients with hypersensitivity to sesame oil or dronabinol.

Use cautiously in elderly patients and patients with hypertension, cardiac disease, or psychiatric illness because of possible CNS and cardiovascular adverse effects. Drug may exacerbate underlying psychiatric illness.

ADVERSE REACTIONS

Common reactions are in italics; life-threatening reactions are in bold italics.
CNS: *dizziness, ataxia,* depersonalization, disorientation, hallucinations, headache, irritability, memory lapse, muddled thinking, paranoia, perceptual difficulties, weakness, paresthesias.
CV: tachycardia, orthostatic hypotension.
Other: *dry mouth,* visual distortions.

INTERACTIONS

Alcohol, CNS depressants, sedatives, psychotomimetic substances: additive effects. Don't use together.

EFFECTS ON DIAGNOSTIC TESTS

None reported.

NURSING CONSIDERATIONS

Besides those related universally to drug therapy (see "How to use this book"), consider the following specific recommendations:

Assessment

- Obtain a baseline assessment of allergies, mental status, and blood pressure before therapy.
- Be alert for adverse reactions or drug interactions during therapy.
- Evaluate the patient's and family's knowledge about dronabinol therapy.

Nursing Diagnoses

- High risk for fluid volume deficit related to nausea and vomiting induced by chemotherapy.
- Altered thought processes related to dronabinol-induced CNS adverse reactions.
- Knowledge deficit related to dronabinol therapy.

Planning and Implementation

Preparation and Administration

- Give 1 to 3 hours prior to beginning chemotherapy and again 2 to 4 hours after chemotherapy is administered.

Monitoring

- Monitor effectiveness by monitoring the patient for nausea and vomiting.
- Observe for changes in mental status, mood, and behavior.
- Monitor fluid balance.
- Check for orthostatic hypotension.
- Continue to observe for adverse reactions until it is certain that patient is no longer experiencing effects of the drug. There are many variations in persistent effects among individual patients.

Supportive Care

- Be aware that drug effects may persist for days after treatment ends. CNS effects are intensified at higher doses.
- Dronabinol is the principal active substance in *Cannabis sativa* (marijuana). High potential exists for physical and psychological dependence and abuse.
- Use safety precautions; patients should be supervised during and after treatment.
- If patient is alert, encourage adequate fluid intake to prevent fluid volume deficit.

Patient Teaching

- Warn patient to avoid hazardous activities that require alertness until the CNS effects of the drug are known.
- To prevent panic and anxiety, tell the patient that this drug may induce unusual changes in mood and behavioral effects.
- Emphasize to the family that patient should be under the supervision of a responsible person during and immediately after treatment.
- Advise patient to change positions slowly to prevent orthostatic hypotension.

Evaluation

In patients receiving dronabinol, appropriate evaluation statements may include:

- Patient exhibits no signs of fluid volume deficit.
- Patient demonstrates no signs of altered thought processes.
- Patient and family state an understanding of dronabinol therapy.

droperidol

(droe per´ i dole)

Droleptan‡, Inapsine

- *Classification:* tranquilizer (butyrophenone derivative)
- *Pregnancy Risk Category:* C

HOW SUPPLIED

Tablets: 10 mg‡
Oral solution: 1 mg/ml‡
Injection: 2.5 mg/ml, 5 mg/ml‡

*Liquid form contains alcohol. **May contain tartrazine.

ACTION

Mechanism: Blocks postsynaptic dopamine receptors in the CNS. Acts on subcortical levels of the CNS to produce sedation.
Absorption: Well absorbed after I.M. injection.
Distribution: Crosses the blood-brain barrier and is distributed in the CSF; also crosses the placenta.
Metabolism: By the liver to p-fluorophenylacetic acid and p-hydroxypiperidine.
Excretion: Drug and its metabolites are excreted in urine and feces.
Onset, peak, duration: Sedation begins in 3 to 10 minutes, peaks at 30 minutes, and lasts for 2 to 4 hours; some alteration of consciousness may persist for 12 hours.

INDICATIONS & DOSAGE

Premedication–
Adults: 2.5 to 10 mg (1 to 4 ml) I.M. 30 to 60 minutes preoperatively.
Children 2 to 12 years: 1 to 1.5 mg (0.4 to 0.6 ml)/20 to 25 lb body weight I.M.
As an induction agent–
Adults: 2.5 mg (1 ml)/20 to 25 lb body weight I.V. with analgesic and/or general anesthetic.
Children 2 to 12 years: 1 to 1.5 mg (0.4 to 0.6 ml)/20 to 25 lb I.V. Dosage should be titrated.
Elderly and debilitated patients: initial dose should be decreased.
Maintenance dosage in general anesthesia–
Adults: 1.25 to 2.5 mg (0.5 to 1 ml) I.V.
To suppress nystagmus, nausea, vomiting, and vertigo associated with an acute attack of Meniere's disease–
Adults: 5 mg I.M. as a single dose.
Management of severe agitation of psychotic disorders‡ –
Adults: 10 to 25 mg P.O. daily in divided doses.

CONTRAINDICATIONS & PRECAUTIONS

Contraindicated in patients with hypersensitivity or intolerance to the drug. Use cautiously in patients with hypotension and other cardiovascular disease because of its vasodilatory effects; with hepatic or renal disease, in whom drug clearance may be impaired; and in those taking other CNS depressants, including alcohol, opiates, and sedatives because droperidol may potentiate the effects of these drugs.

ADVERSE REACTIONS

Common reactions are in italics; life-threatening reactions are in bold italics.
Blood: ***agranulocytosis.***
CNS: extrapyramidal reactions (dystonia, akathisia), upward rotation of eyes and oculogyric crises, extended neck, flexed arms, fine tremor of limbs, dizziness, chills or shivering, facial sweating, restlessness, decreased seizure threshold.
CV: *hypotension,* tachycardia.
Respiratory: ***laryngospasm, bronchospasm.***

INTERACTIONS

None significant.

EFFECTS ON DIAGNOSTIC TESTS

EEG: temporarily altered pattern.
Pulmonary artery pressure: decreased.

NURSING CONSIDERATIONS

Besides those related universally to drug therapy (see "How to use this book"), consider the following specific recommendations:
Assessment
- Obtain a baseline assessment of the patient's vital signs and overall physical status before therapy.
- Be alert for adverse reactions and drug interactions throughout therapy.
- Evaluate the patient's and family's knowledge about droperidol therapy.

Nursing Diagnoses
• High risk for injury related to droperidol-induced sedation.
• Decreased cardiac output related to droperidol-induced hypotension.
• Knowledge deficit related to droperidol therapy.

Planning and Implementation
Preparation and Administration
• ***I.V. use:*** Give I.V. injection slowly. When giving a narcotic analgesic with droperidol, reduce narcotic dosage by one quarter to one third for up to 12 hours or until patient becomes fully alert.
Monitoring
• Monitor effectiveness by evaluating degree of sedation.
• Frequently monitor vital signs, especially hypotension.
• Watch for extrapyramidal reactions. Keep in mind that droperidol, a butyrophenone compound, related to haloperiodol, has greater tendency to cause extrapyramidal reactions than other antipsychotics.
Supportive Care
• Notify the doctor immediately if vital signs change, if extrapyramidal reactions occur, or if any other adverse reaction develops.
• Be aware that droperidol has been used as an I.V. antiemetic in cancer chemotherapy.
• Keep I.V. fluids and vasopressors available for treatment of hypotension.
• Keep resuscitative equipment available during I.V. administration.
• Move and position the patient slowly during anesthesia to avoid orthostatic hypotension.
• Do not place patient in Trendelenburg's position (that is, shock position); severe hypotension and deeper anesthesia may result, causing respiratory arrest.
• Implement safety measures to protect the sedated patient, such as raising bedrails.
Patient Teaching
• Explain that this drug causes marked sedation. Advise the patient not to ambulate without assistance if drug is administered preoperatively.
• If appropriate, tell the patient what to expect during induction of anesthesia and during recovery from general anesthesia. As needed, clarify any other information provided by the anesthesiologist.

Evaluation
In patients receiving droperidol, appropriate evaluation statements may include:
• Sedation is achieved.
• Blood pressure is within normal limits.
• Patient and family state an understanding of droperidol therapy.

dyphylline
(dye´ fi lin)
Brophylline, Dilin, Dilor*, Dyflex, Dylline*, Emfabid, Lufyllin*, Protophylline†

• *Classification:* bronchodilator (xanthine derivative)
• *Pregnancy Risk Category:* C

HOW SUPPLIED
Tablets: 200 mg, 400 mg
Elixir: 100 mg/15 ml, 160 mg/15 ml*
Injection: 250 mg/ml

ACTION
Mechanism: A structural analog of theophylline; unlike other xanthine derivatives, dyphylline does not release free theophylline. Inhibits phosphodiesterase, the enzyme that degrades cyclic 3',5' adenosine monophosphate (cyclic AMP). Increased cyclic AMP levels alter intracellular calcium movement, which results in relaxation of smooth muscle of the bronchial tree, bronchodilation, and increased pulmonary blood flow.

Absorption: Approximately 75% of an oral dose is absorbed rapidly through the gastric mucosa.
Distribution: Rapidly and widely distributed in body fluids and tissues.
Excretion: About 88% of the drug is excreted unchanged in urine. Half-life: Approximately 2 hours; prolonged in patients with decreased renal function.
Onset, peak, duration: Peak concentration in 1 hour after oral administration.

INDICATIONS & DOSAGE

For relief of acute and chronic bronchial asthma and reversible bronchospasm associated with chronic bronchitis and emphysema –
Adults: 15 mg/kg P.O. q 6 hours. I.M. route is rarely used, but patients may receive 250 to 500 mg I.M. injected slowly at 6-hour intervals.
Dosage should be decreased in renal insufficiency.

CONTRAINDICATIONS & PRECAUTIONS

Contraindicated in patients with hypersensitivity to xanthines. Use cautiously in patients with compromised cardiac or circulatory function, diabetes, glaucoma, hypertension, hyperthyroidism, peptic ulcer, or gastroesophageal reflux because drug may worsen these symptoms or conditions.

ADVERSE REACTIONS

Common reactions are in italics; life-threatening reactions are in bold italics.
CNS: *restlessness, dizziness,* headache, *insomnia,* light-headedness, ***seizures,*** muscle twitching.
CV: *palpitations, sinus tachycardia,* extrasystoles, flushing, marked hypotension, increase in respiratory rate.
GI: *nausea, vomiting, anorexia,* bitter aftertaste, dyspepsia, heavy feeling in stomach.
Skin: urticaria.

INTERACTIONS

Barbiturates, phenytoin, rifampin: enhanced metabolism and decreased theophylline blood levels. Monitor for decreased theophylline effect.
Beta-adrenergic blockers: antagonism. Propanolol and nadolol, especially, may cause bronchospasm in sensitive patients. Use together cautiously.
Influenza virus vaccine, oral contraceptives, troleandomycin, erythromycin, cimetidine: decreased hepatic clearance of theophylline; elevated theophylline levels. Monitor for signs of toxicity.

EFFECTS ON DIAGNOSTIC TESTS

None reported.

NURSING CONSIDERATIONS

Besides those related universally to drug therapy (see "How to use this book"), consider the following specific recommendations:

Assessment

- Obtain a baseline assessment of the patient's cardiopulonary status by taking vital signs, evaluating ECG results and auscultating the heart and lungs.
- Be alert for any adverse reactions or drug interactions throughout therapy.
- Evaluate the patient and family's knowledge about dyphylline therapy.

Nursing Diagnoses

- Ineffective airway clearance related to patient's underlying condition.
- Sleep pattern disturbance related to CNS adverse effects of dyphylline.
- Knowledge deficit related to use of dyphylline.

Planning and Implementation

Preparation and Adminstration

- ***P.O. use:*** Gastric irritation may be relieved by taking oral drugs after meals; there is no evidence that antacids reduce this adverse reaction. May produce less gastric discomfort than theophylline.
- ***I.M. use:*** Discard injectable dyphyl-

line if precipitate is present. Protect from light.
• Remember that dyphylline is metabolized faster than theophylline so dosage intervals may have to be decreased to ensure continual therapeutic effect. Higher daily dosages may be needed.
• Do not administer I.V.

Monitoring
• Monitor effectiveness by regularly auscultating lungs, taking respiratory rate and pulse rate and noting results of laboratory studies such as arterial blood gases. Also measure intake and output. Expected clinical effects include improvement in quality of pulse and respirations.
• Monitor for dizziness especially in elderly patients. Dizziness is a common adverse reaction at the start of therapy.
• Evaluate the patient for insomnia and restlessness after therapy begins.

Supportive Care
• Notify the doctor if patient experiences dizziness or significant changes in sleep patterns.

Patient Teaching
• Provide instructions for home care and dosage schedule.
• Warn the patient, especially if elderly, that dizziness, a common adverse reaction, may occur at the start of therapy.
• Tell the patient to check with his the doctor or pharmacist before taking any other medications, as OTC remedies may contain ephedrine, which if combined with theophylline salts may cause excessive CNS stimulation.

Evaluation

In patients receiving dyphylline, appropriate evaluation statements may include:
• Patient exhibits improved respiratory status.
• Patient maintains a sleeping pattern that allows for adequate rest.
• Patient and family state an understanding of dyphylline therapy.

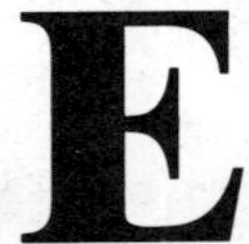

echothiophate iodide (ecothiopate iodide)
Phospholine Iodide
(ek oh thye´ oh fate)

• *Classification:* miotic (cholinesterase inhibitor)
• *Pregnancy Risk Category:* C

HOW SUPPLIED

Ophthalmic powder for solution: for reconstitution to make 0.03%, 0.06%, 0.125%, and 0.25% solutions

ACTION

Mechanism: A long-acting miotic that inhibits the enzymatic destruction of acetylcholine by inactivating cholinesterase. This leaves acetylcholine free to act on muscarinic receptors on the iridic sphincter and ciliary muscles, causing pupillary constriction and accommodation spasm. Contraction of the ciliary muscle widens the trabecular meshwork, facilitating the outflow of aqueous humor, and decreases intraocular pressure.
Pharmacokinetics: Unknown.
Onset, peak, duration: Onset occurs within 10 to 30 minutes; maximal effects are usually evident within 30 minutes. Decreases in intraocular pressure are evident within 4 to 8 hours and are maximal within 24 hours. The duration of effect can be several days up to 4 weeks.

INDICATIONS & DOSAGE

Primary open-angle glaucoma, conditions obstructing aqueous outflow–
Adults and children: instill 1 drop of 0.03% to 0.125% solution into conjunctival sac daily. Maximum 1 drop b.i.d. Use lowest possible dosage to continuously control intraocular pressure.
Diagnosis of accommodative esotropia–
Adults: instill 1 drop of 0.125% solution daily at h.s. for 2 to 3 weeks.
Accommodative esotropia (treatment)–
Adults: instill 1 drop of 0.03% to 0.125% solution q.d. or q.o.d. at h.s.

CONTRAINDICATIONS & PRECAUTIONS

Contraindicated in patients with hypersensitivity to cholinesterase inhibitors, active uveal inflammation or inflammatory diseases of the iris or ciliary body, narrow-angle or angle-closure glaucoma (most cases), seizures disorders, vasomotor instability, parkinsonism, hypersensitivity to iodides, bronchial asthma, spastic GI conditions, urinary tract obstruction, peptic ulcer, severe bradycardia or hypotension, vascular hypertension, MI, or a history of retinal detachment because the drug can worsen these symptoms or disorders.

Use cautiously in patients routinely exposed to organophosphate insecticides because of potential for additive toxicity; it may cause nausea, vomiting, and diarrhea, progressing to muscle weakness and respiratory difficulty. Also use cautiously in patients with myasthenia gravis who are receiving anticholinesterase therapy.

ADVERSE REACTIONS

Common reactions are in italics; life-threatening reactions are in bold italics.
CNS: fatigue, muscle weakness, paresthesias, headache.

CV: bradycardia, hypotension.
Eye: ciliary or accommodative spasm, ciliary or conjunctival injection, nonreversible cataract formation (time- and dose-related), reversible iris cysts, pupillary block, blurred or dimmed vision, eye or brow pain, lid twitching, hyperemia, photophobia, lens opacities, lacrimation, retinal detachment.
GI: diarrhea, nausea, vomiting, abdominal pain, intestinal cramps, salivation.
GU: frequent urination.
Other: flushing, sweating, bronchial constriction.

INTERACTIONS

Anticholinergics, ophthalmic belladonna alkaloids (such as atropine), cyclopentolate: antagonized miotic effects.
Cocaine: increased risk of cocaine toxicity.
Local anesthetics, ophthalmic tetracaine: increased rate of systemic toxicity; prolonged ocular anesthesia.
Ophthalmic adrenocorticoids: increased intraocular pressure and decreased antiglaucoma effect.
Other cholinesterase inhibitors, edrophonium, organophosphorus insecticides (parathion, malathion): may have an additive effect that could cause systemic effects. Warn patient exposed to insecticides of this danger.
Succinylcholine: respiratory and cardiovascular collapse. Don't use together.
Systemic anticholinesterase for myasthenia gravis, pilocarpine: effects may be additive. Monitor patient for signs of toxicity.

EFFECTS ON DIAGNOSTIC TESTS

Plasma cholinesterase activity: decreased levels.

NURSING CONSIDERATIONS

Besides those related universally to drug therapy (see "How to use this book"), consider the following specific recommendations:

Assessment

- Obtain a baseline assessment of the patient's vision, especially ocular pressure, before therapy.
- Be alert for adverse reactions and drug interactions throughout therapy.
- Evaluate the patient's and family's knowledge about echothiophate therapy.

Nursing Diagnoses

- Sensory/perceptual alterations (visual) related to the patient's underlying condition.
- High risk for poisoning related to the drug's systemic cholinergic effects.
- Knowledge deficit related to echothiophate therapy.

Planning and Implementation

Preparation and Administration

- Reconstitute powder carefully, using only the diluent provided.
- Instill solution in lacrimal sac and apply light finger pressure for 1 minute after instillation.
- Reconstituted solution should be discarded after 1 month if kept at room temperature; 6 months, if refrigerated.

Monitoring

- Monitor effectiveness by assessing the patient's visual status and intraocular pressure.
- Monitor for systemic cholinergic effects. Toxicity is cumulative and may not appear for weeks or months after start of therapy.
- Monitor blood pressure and pulse for drug-induced hypotension and bradycardia.

Supportive Care

- Notify the doctor immediately of any changes in the patient's health status.
- Obtain an order for a mild analge-

sic if the patient experiences headaches or brow aches.
• Keep atropine sulfate (S.C., I.M., or I.V.) on hand to reverse systemic cholinergic effects.
• Stop drug at least 2 weeks before any surgery if succinylcholine is to be used operatively.
Patient Teaching
• Teach the patient how to instill the drops, and advise him to wash his hands before and after administering the drug.
• Advise the patient to carry a medical alert card during therapy because the drug has many potential interactions.
• Warn the patient not to exceed the recommended dosage.
• Advise the patient to continue with regular medical supervision during therapy.
• Tell the patient to instill the drug at bedtime because it causes transient blurring of vision. Reassure him that blurred or dimmed vision usually improves after 5 to 10 days of therapy.
Evaluation
In patients receiving echothiophate, appropriate evaluation statements may include:
• Patient experiences a reduction in intraocular pressure.
• Patient does not experience systemic cholinergic effects.
• Patient and family state an understanding of echothiophate therapy.

econazole nitrate
(e kone´ a zole)
Ecostatin, Spectazole

• *Classification:* antifungal (imidazole derivative)
• *Pregnancy Risk Category:* C

HOW SUPPLIED
Cream: 1%

ACTION
Mechanism: Alters fungal cell wall permeability.
Absorption: Minimal but rapid percutaneous absorption. Less than 1% of a dose reaches the systemic circulation.
Distribution: 7.6% to 9.6% of a dose is present in the stratum corneum after topical application.
Excretion: Mostly in urine; some in feces.

INDICATIONS & DOSAGE
Treatment of tinea pedis, tinea cruris, and tinea corporis; cutaneous candidiasis–
Adults and children: apply sufficient quantity to cover affected areas b.i.d., in the morning and evening for at least 2 weeks.
Tinea versicolor–
Adults and children: apply once daily.

CONTRAINDICATIONS & PRECAUTIONS
Contraindicated in patients with hypersensitivity to the drug and during the first trimester of pregnancy. Use in second and third trimesters only if essential to patient's welfare.

ADVERSE REACTIONS
Common reactions are in italics; life-threatening reactions are in bold italics.
Local: burning, itching, stinging, erythema.

INTERACTIONS
Topical corticosteroids: may inhibit antifungal effect.

EFFECTS ON DIAGNOSTIC TESTS
None reported.

NURSING CONSIDERATIONS
Besides those related universally to drug therapy (see "How to use this book"), consider the following specific recommendations:

Assessment
• Obtain a baseline assessment of the patient's skin in the affected area before therapy.
• Be alert for adverse reactions and drug interactions throughout therapy.
• Evaluate the patient's and family's knowledge about econazole therapy.
Nursing Diagnoses
• Body image disturbance related to patient's underlying condition.
• High risk for impaired skin integrity related to econazole-induced erythema.
• Knowledge deficit related to econazole therapy.
Planning and Implementation
Preparation and Administration
• ***Topical use:*** Clean affected area before application. Apply sufficient quantity to cover area.
Monitoring
• Monitor effectiveness by regularly checking the skin of the affected area.
• If condition persists or worsens or if irritation occurs, discontinue use and report to doctor.
• Monitor for adverse reactions or drug interactions by frequently assessing patient's skin for erythema.
Supportive Care
• Keep in mind that hypopigmentation of tinea versicolor will resolve gradually.
Patient Teaching
• Teach patient to apply medication.
• Inform patient to use medication for entire treatment period, even though symptoms may have improved. Notify doctor if no improvement after 2 weeks or 4 weeks, depending on diagnosis.
• Instruct patient not to use occlusive dressings.
• Tell patient medication may stain clothing.
Evaluation
In patients receiving econazole, appropriate evaluation statements may include:
• Patient's body image is improved.
• Patient does not develop drug-induced erythema.
• Patient and family state an understanding of econazole therapy.

edetate calcium disodium
(ed´ e tate)
Calcium Disodium Versenate, Calcium EDTA

• *Classification:* heavy metal antagonist (chelating agent)
• *Pregnancy Risk Category:* C

HOW SUPPLIED
Injection: 200 mg/ml

ACTION
Mechanism: A chelating agent that forms stable, soluble complexes with metals, particularly lead.
Absorption: Well absorbed after I.M. or S.C. injection.
Distribution: Primarily in extracellular fluid.
Metabolism: None.
Excretion: Rapidly excreted in urine. After I.V. administration, 50% of drug is excreted in urine unchanged or as a metal chelate in 1 hour; 95% of drug is excreted in 24 hours.
Onset, peak, duration: After I.V. administration, chelated lead appears in urine within 1 hour; peak excretion of lead occurs in 24 to 48 hours.

INDICATIONS & DOSAGE
Lead poisoning (blood levels greater than 50 mcg/dl)–
Adults and children: 1 g/m² in dextrose 5% in water or normal saline solution I.V. over 1 to 2 hours daily for 3 to 5 days.
Acute lead encephalopathy or lead levels above 100 mcg/dl–
Adults and children: 1.5 g/m² I.V. daily for 3 to 5 days, usually in conjunction with dimercaprol. A second

course may be administered at least 4 days later, but preferably 2 to 3 weeks should elapse between courses.

CONTRAINDICATIONS & PRECAUTIONS

Contraindicated in patients with severe renal disease and anuria because of drug's possible nephrotoxic effects. Avoid rapid I.V. infusion in patients with lead encephalopathy because drug may increase intracranial pressure to lethal levels. Use cautiously in patients with renal insufficiency or dehydration, who are at increased risk of renal failure because of drug's potential for nephrotoxicity.

ADVERSE REACTIONS

Common reactions are in italics; life-threatening reactions are in bold italics.
CNS: headache, paresthesias, numbness.
CV: cardiac arrhythmias, hypotension.
GI: anorexia, nausea, vomiting.
GU: *proteinuria, hematuria;* ***nephrotoxicity with renal tubular necrosis leading to fatal nephrosis.***
Other: arthralgia, myalgia, hypercalcemia.

4 to 8 hours after infusion: sudden fever and chills, fatigue, excessive thirst, sneezing, nasal congestion.

INTERACTIONS

None significant.

EFFECTS ON DIAGNOSTIC TESTS

None reported.

NURSING CONSIDERATIONS

Besides those related universally to drug therapy (see "How to use this book"), consider the following specific recommendations:

Assessment
- Obtain a baseline assessment of the patient's serum lead level and renal status before therapy.
- Be alert for adverse reactions and drug interactions throughout therapy.
- Evaluate the patient's and family's knowledge about edetate calcium disodium therapy.

Nursing Diagnoses
- High risk for injury related to lead poisoning.
- Altered renal tissue perfusion related to drug-induced fatal nephrosis.
- Knowledge deficit related to edetate calcium disodium therapy.

Planning and Implementation
Preparation and Administration
- Read label carefully; do not confuse this drug with edetate disodium, which is used to treat hypercalcemia.
- ***I.V. use:*** Infuse slowly, diluted into an established I.V. line. I.V. use contraindicated in lead encephalopathy; may increase intracranial pressure. Use I.M. route instead.
- ***I.M. use:*** Add procaine hydrochloride to I.M. solutions to minimize pain. I.M. route preferred method of administration, especially in children.
- Administer with dimercaprol to avoid toxicity.

Monitoring
- Monitor effectiveness by checking serum lead levels and observing for decreasing signs and symptoms of lead poisoning.
- Monitor intake and output, urinalysis, blood pressure, BUN level, and ECG daily.
- Monitor for signs of increased intracranial pressure in lead encephalopathy.
- Observe injection site for local reaction.

Supportive Care
- Force fluid to facilitate excretion of lead in all patients except those with lead encephalopathy.
- Obtain order for medication to relieve headache, nausea, and vomiting.
- Apply ice or cold compresses to injection site to ease local reaction.

Patient Teaching
• Warn patient that fever, chills, thirst, and nasal congestion may occur 4 to 8 hours after administration.
• Advise patient to get up from lying or sitting position slowly to avoid dizziness.
• Encourage patient and family to identify and remove source of lead in home.

Evaluation
In patients receiving edetate calcium disodium, appropriate evaluation statements may include:
• Patient does not demonstrate signs of injury related to lead poisoning.
• Patient does not exhibit signs of altered renal tissue perfusion.
• Patient and family state an understanding of edetate calcium disodium therapy.

edetate disodium
(ed´ e tate)
Disodium EDTA, Disotate, Endrate

• *Classification:* antihypercalcemic (chelating agent)
• *Pregnancy Risk Category:* C

HOW SUPPLIED
Injection: 150 mg/ml

ACTION
Mechanism: A chelating agent that binds with metals and ions, such as calcium, to form a stable, soluble complex.
Absorption: Poorly absorbed from the GI tract.
Distribution: Widely distributed throughout the rest of the body but does not enter the CSF in significant amounts.
Metabolism: None.
Excretion: After I.V. administration, excreted rapidly in urine; 95% of the dose is excreted within 24 hours.

INDICATIONS & DOSAGE
Hypercalcemic crisis–
Adults: 50 mg/kg by slow I.V. infusion added to 500 ml of dextrose 5% in water or normal saline solution. Maximum dosage is 3 g/day.
Children: 40 to 70 mg/kg by slow I.V. infusion, diluted to a maximum concentration of 30 mg/ml in dextrose 5% in water or normal saline solution. Maximum dosage is 70 mg/kg/day.

CONTRAINDICATIONS & PRECAUTIONS
Contraindicated in patients with severe renal failure or anuria; in patients with suspected or known hypocalcemia, active or healed tuberculosis, or severe heart, renal, or coronary artery disease; in elderly patients with generalized arteriosclerosis; and in those with a history of seizures because drug may exacerbate the signs and symptoms of these conditions. Do not use to treat lead poisoning; edetate calcium disodium should be used instead.

Use cautiously in patients with renal impairment; in patients with incipient CHF because its effect on calcium concentration depresses cardiac function and because large sodium and fluid loads are delivered during therapy; in those with hypokalemia or hypomagnesemia because drug may lower total body stores via increased renal excretion; and in patients with diabetes.

ADVERSE REACTIONS
Common reactions are in italics; life-threatening reactions are in bold italics.
CNS: circumoral paresthesias, numbness, headache, malaise, fatigue, muscle pain or weakness.
CV: hypertension, thrombophlebitis, orthostatic hypotension.
GI: nausea, vomiting, diarrhea, anorexia, abdominal cramps.
GU: in excessive doses– ***nephrotoxic-***

ity with urgency, nocturia, dysuria, polyuria, proteinuria, renal insufficiency and failure, tubular necrosis.
Metabolic: *severe hypocalcemia,* decreased magnesium.
Local: pain at site of infusion, erythema, dermatitis.

INTERACTIONS

None significant.

EFFECTS ON DIAGNOSTIC TESTS

Alkaline phosphatase: decreased levels related to drug-induced hypomagnesemia.
Blood glucose: lower concentration in diabetic patients.
Serum calcium: lower concentrations when measured by oxalate or other precipitation methods and by colorimetry.

NURSING CONSIDERATIONS

Besides those related universally to drug therapy (see "How to use this book"), consider the following specific recommendations:

Assessment
- Obtain a baseline assessment of urine output, blood pressure, serum calcium level, and renal function before therapy.
- Be alert for adverse reactions and drug interactions throughout therapy.
- Evaluate the patient's and family's knowledge about edetate disodium therapy.

Nursing Diagnoses
- High risk for injury related to hypercalcemic crisis.
- Pain related to drug-induced headache and muscle pain.
- Knowledge deficit related to edetate disodium therapy.

Planning and Implementation
Preparation and Administration
- Read label carefully; do not confuse with edetate calcium disodium which is used for lead toxicity.
- ***I.V. use:*** Drug must be diluted before administration. Avoid rapid I.V. infusion; profound hypocalcemia may occur, leading to tetany, seizures, cardiac arrhythmias, and respiratory arrest.
- Not recommended for direct or intermittent injection.
- Avoid extravasation of I.V.

Monitoring
- Monitor effectiveness by checking the patient's serum calcium level.
- Frequently monitor ECG and renal function studies.
- Obtain serum calcium level after each dose. Be alert for signs of severe hypocalcemia (tetany, seizure).
- Monitor blood pressure and respiratory status closely.
- Frequently check I.V. site and patency.
- Observe for generalized systemic reaction 4 to 8 hours after drug administration: fever, chills, back pain, emesis, muscle cramps, and urinary urgency.

Supportive Care
- Keep I.V. calcium and resuscitation equipment available.
- Record I.V. site used and try to avoid repeated use of the same site, which increases the likelihood of thrombophlebitis.
- Keep patient in bed for 15 minutes after administration to avoid orthostatic hypotension.
- Obtain an order for an analgesic to relieve drug-induced headache and muscle pain.
- Treatment for generalized systemic reaction is supportive.
- Be aware that edetate disodium is not currently the drug of choice for treatment of hypercalcemia; other treatments are safer and more effective. Edetate disodium therapy has also been inappropriately recommended for treatment of arteriosclerosis and related disorders. There is no scientific evidence that the drug is safe or effective for these indications.

Patient Teaching
• Instruct patient to report respiratory difficulty, dizziness, and muscle cramping immediately.
• Advise the patient to move from sitting or lying position slowly to avoid dizziness.
• Reassure patient that generalized systemic reaction usually subsides within 12 hours.

Evaluation

In patients receiving edetate disodium, appropriate evaluation statements may include:
• Patient remains free of injury related to hypercalcemic crisis.
• Patient remains free of drug-induced headache and muscle pain.
• Patient and family state an understanding of edetate disodium therapy.

edrophonium chloride

(ed roe foe´ nee um)
Enlon, Reversol, Tensilon

• *Classification:* anticholinergic agonist, diagnostic agent (cholinesterase inhibitor)
• *Pregnancy Risk Category:* C

HOW SUPPLIED

Injection: 10 mg/ml in 1-ml ampules or 10-ml vials

ACTION

Mechanism: Inhibits the destruction of acetylcholine released from the parasympathetic and somatic efferent nerves. Acetylcholine accumulates, promoting increased stimulation of the receptor. Drug has a very short duration of action.
Absorption: Not applicable as drug is given I.V.
Distribution: May cross the placenta; little else is known. As a quaternary ammonium compound, drug is not expected to enter the CNS.
Metabolism: Exact metabolic fate is unknown; drug is not hydrolyzed by cholinesterases.
Excretion: Exact excretion mode is unknown.
Onset, peak, duration: After I.V. administration, action begins in 30 to 60 seconds and lasts from 5 to 10 minutes. Although not usually administered I.M., onset begins in 2 to 10 minutes and lasts 5 to 30 minutes.

INDICATIONS & DOSAGE

As a curare antagonist (to reverse neuromuscular blocking action)–
Adults: 10 mg I.V. given over 30 to 45 seconds. Dose may be repeated as necessary to 40 mg maximum dosage. Larger dosages may potentiate rather than antagonize effect of curare.
Diagnostic aid in myasthenia gravis (Tensilon test)–
Adults: 1 to 2 mg I.V. within 15 to 30 seconds, then 8 mg if no response (increase in muscular strength).
Children over 34 kg: 2 mg I.V. If no response within 45 seconds, give 1 mg q 45 seconds to maximum of 10 mg.
Children up to 34 kg: 1 mg I.V. If no response within 45 seconds, give 1 mg q 45 seconds to maximum of 5 mg.
Infants: 0.5 mg I.V.
To differentiate myasthenic crisis from cholinergic crisis–
Adults: 1 mg I.V. If no response in 1 minute, repeat dose once. Increased muscular strength confirms myasthenic crisis; no increase or exaggerated weakness confirms cholinergic crisis.
Paroxysmal supraventricular tachycardia–
Adults: 5 to 10 mg I.V. given over 1 minute or less.
Children: 2 mg I.V. Administer slowly.

CONTRAINDICATIONS & PRECAUTIONS

Contraindicated in patients with mechanical obstruction of the GI or urinary tract because of its stimulatory effect on smooth muscle and in patients with bradycardia, hyperthyroidism, or hypotension because it may exacerbate these conditions.

Use cautiously in patients with cardiac disease because of stimulating effects on cardiovascular system; in patients with peptic ulcer disease because it may increase gastric acid secretion; and in patients with bronchial asthma because it may precipitate asthma attacks.

ADVERSE REACTIONS

Common reactions are in italics; life-threatening reactions are in bold italics.

CNS: seizures, weakness, dysphagia, respiratory paralysis, sweating.
CV: hypotension, bradycardia, AV block.
EENT: excessive lacrimation, diplopia, miosis.
GI: nausea, vomiting, *diarrhea, abdominal cramps,* excessive salivation.
GU: urinary frequency.
Other: increased bronchial secretions, ***bronchospasm,*** muscle cramps, muscle fasciculation.

INTERACTIONS

Digitalis glycosides: may increase the heart's sensitivity to edrophonium. Use together cautiously.
Procainamide, quinidine: may reverse cholinergic effects. Observe for lack of drug effect.

EFFECTS ON DIAGNOSTIC TESTS

None reported.

NURSING CONSIDERATIONS

Besides those related universally to drug therapy (see "How to use this book"), consider the following specific recommendations:

Assessment

- Obtain a baseline assessment of the patient's underlying condition before drug therapy.
- Be alert for adverse reactions and drug interactions throughout therapy.
- Evaluate the patient and family's knowledge about edrophonium therapy.

Nursing Diagnoses

- Altered health maintenance related to underlying condition.
- Urine retention related to adverse drug reactions.
- Knowledge deficit related to edrophonium therapy.

Planning and Implementation

Preparation and Administration

- Discontinue all other cholinergic drugs before giving this drug.
- Be prepared to administer atropine if adverse reactions ocur. Give atropine 0.5 mg subcutaneoulsy or slow I.V. push, as ordered.
- Drug may not be effective if used to treat muscle relaxation induced by decamethonium bromide and succinylcholine chloride.
- This drug has the most rapid onset but shortest duration; therefore, do not use to treat myasthenia gravis.
- Use a tuberculin syringe with an I.V. needle for easier parenteral administration.
- Administer to children by I.M. route because of difficulty with I.V. route. For children under 34 kg, inject 2 mg I.M.; children over 34 kg, 5 mg I.M. Some reactions may occur as with the I.V. test, but these appear after 2- to 10-minute delay.
- ***I.V. use:*** Continuous I.V. infusions have been used to control atrial tachycardia or supraventricular tachycardia associated with Wolf-Parkinson-White syndrome that is unresponsive to digitalis glycosides.

Monitoring

- Monitor effectiveness by evaluating the reduction of symptoms of the underlying condition.
- Monitor for adverse reactions and drug interactions by frequently checking the patient's vital signs, especially respirations.

• Observe the patient's muscle strength closely when giving drug to differentiate myasthenia gravis from cholinergic crisis.

Supportive Care

• Provide respiratory support if adverse reactions occur.

Patient Teaching

• Teach the patient to notify the doctor of adverse reactions, such as diarrhea, abdominal cramps, or increased bronchial secretions.

Evaluation

In patients receiving edrophonium therapy, appropriate evaluation statements may include:

• Patient demonstrates no further symptoms of underlying condition.

• Patient's elimination pattern is unaffected by drug therapy.

• Patient and family state an understanding of edrophonium therapy.

enalaprilat

(e nal´ a pril at)

Vasotec I.V.

enalapril maleate

Amprace‡, Renitec‡, Vasotec

• *Classification:* antihypertensive (angiotensin-converting enzyme inhibitor)

• *Pregnancy Risk Category:* C (D in second and third trimester)

HOW SUPPLIED

Tablets: 2.5 mg, 5 mg, 10 mg, 20 mg
Injection: 1.25 mg/ml in 2-ml vials

ACTION

Mechanism: By inhibiting angiotensin-converting enzyme, prevents pulmonary conversion of angiotensin I to angiotensin II.

Absorption: Approximately 60% of an oral dose is absorbed; absorption is not affected by food.

Distribution: Full distribution pattern of enalapril is unknown; drug does not appear to cross the blood-brain barrier.

Metabolism: Enalapril is inactive; drug is hydrolyzed in the plasma to the active metabolite enalaprilat.

Excretion: About 94% of a dose of enalapril is excreted in urine and feces as enalaprilat and enalapril. Half-life: Of enalapril, about 1.3 hours; of enalaprilat, 11 hours.

Onset, peak, duration: After oral administration, blood pressure decreases within 1 hour, with peak antihypertensive effect at 4 to 6 hours. Duration of effect is about 24 hours. After I.V. administration, onset is about 15 minutes, and duration is about 6 hours.

INDICATIONS & DOSAGE

Treatment of hypertension–

Adults: initially, 5 mg P.O. once daily, then adjust according to response. Usual dosage range is 10 to 40 mg daily as a single dose or two divided doses. Alternatively, give by I.V. infusion 1.25 mg q 6 hours over 5 minutes.

To convert from I.V. therapy to oral therapy–

Adults: initially, 5 mg P.O. once a day. Adjust dosage to response.

To convert from oral therapy to I.V. therapy–

Adults: 1.25 mg I.V. over 5 minutes q 6 hours. Higher doses have not demonstrated greater efficacy.

Adjunctive treatment of heart failure (with diuretics and digitalis)–

Adults: initially, 2.5 mg P.O. b.i.d. Adjust dosage based on clinical or hemodynamic response. Usual range is 5 to 20 mg daily in two divided doses; maximum dosage is 40 mg/day.

CONTRAINDICATIONS & PRECAUTIONS

Contraindicated in patients with hypersensitivity to the drug. Use cautiously in patients with collagen vascular disease or immune disease and in patients taking drugs that may depress immune function or cause decreased WBC count; such patients are at increased risk of developing enalapril-induced neutropenia, especially if they also have renal impairment. Also use cautiously in patients with renal dysfunction because the drug may worsen this condition.

ADVERSE REACTIONS

Common reactions are in italics; life-threatening reactions are in bold italics.
Blood: neutropenia, ***agranulocytosis.***
CNS: *headache, dizziness, fatigue,* insomnia.
CV: *hypotension.*
GI: diarrhea, nausea.
GU: decreased renal function (patients with bilateral renal artery stenosis or CHF).
Skin: rash.
Other: persistent cough, ***angioedema.***

INTERACTIONS

Lithium: lithium toxicity can occur. Monitor lithium levels.
NSAIDs: may reduce antihypertensive effect. Monitor blood pressure.
Potassium supplements: increased risk of hyperkalemia. Avoid these supplements unless hypokalemic blood levels are confirmed.

EFFECTS ON DIAGNOSTIC TESTS

BUN and serum creatinine: elevated levels.
Hemoglobin and hematocrit: slightly decreased levels.
Liver enzymes and bilirubin: elevated levels.

NURSING CONSIDERATIONS

Besides those related universally to drug therapy (see "How to use this book"), consider the following specific recommendations:

Assessment
- Obtain a baseline assessment of the patient's blood pressure before beginning therapy.
- Be alert for adverse reactions and drug interactions throughout therapy.
- Evaluate the patient's and family's knowledge about enalapril therapy.

Nursing Diagnoses
- Altered tissue perfusion (renal, cerebral, cardiopulmonary, and peripheral) related to the patient's underlying condition.
- Decreased cardiac output related to enalapril-induced adverse reactions.
- Knowledge deficit related to enalapril therapy.

Planning and Implementation
Preparation and Administration
- ***I.V. use:*** Not recommended for intermittent or continuous use. May be administered by direct injection as provided or diluted with up to 50 ml of a compatible diluent. Infuse slowly over at least 5 minutes. A response to I.V. enalaprilat is usually seen in 15 minutes, but peak effects may not be seen for up to 4 hours.
- Keep in mind that elderly patients may need lower doses because of impaired drug clearance.

Monitoring
- Monitor effectiveness by regularly checking the patient's blood pressure.
- Monitor the patient closely for hypotension, especially during use to treat heart failure. Keep in mind that hypotension frequently occurs after the initial dose. Observe the patient after the initial dose for at least 2 hours and then for at least 1 hour after blood pressure has stabilized.
- Monitor WBC count and liver and kidney function.
- Observe the patient for facial swelling and difficulty breathing, which may indicate angioedema. Angioedema may occur at any time but especially after the initial dose.
- Monitor potassium intake and

serum potassium. Drug can cause hyperkalemia.
• Observe the patient for signs of infection, such as sore throat, fever, and malaise.

Supportive Care
• Discontinue diuretics 2 to 3 days before beginning enalapril therapy to reduce the risk of hypotension. Then, if this drug does not control blood pressure, diuretic therapy may be added.
• Keep in mind that many patients taking enalapril get therapeutic results by taking the drug once a day. This occurs because enalapril, although similar to captopril, another angiotension-converting enzyme inhibitor, has a longer duration of action.
• If angioedema of the face, extremities, lips, tongue, glottis, or larynx occurs, notify the doctor and discontinue treatment immediately. Institute appropriate therapy–epinephrine solution 1:1000 (0.3 to 0.5 ml) S.C.–and take measures to ensure a patent airway.

Patient Teaching
• Explain the importance of taking this drug as prescribed, even when feeling well. Also tell the patient not to discontinue the drug suddenly if unpleasant adverse reactions occur.
• Tell the patient to check with the doctor or pharmacist before taking OTC medications.
• Advise the patient to report any light-headedness, which is most likely to occur during the first few days of therapy; any signs of infection; or any signs or symptoms of angioedema: swelling of the face, eyes, lips, or tongue or difficulty breathing.
• Teach the patient and family caregiver how to take blood pressure measurements. Tell them to notify the doctor of any significant change in blood pressure measurement.

Evaluation
In patients receiving enalapril, appropriate evaluation statements may include:
• Patient's blood pressure remains within normal limits.
• Patient does not experience any signs of decreased cardiac output.
• Patient and family state an understanding of enalapril therapy.

epinephrine bitartrate (ophthalmic)
(ep i nef′ rin)
Epitrate, Mytrate

epinephrine hydrochloride
Epifrin, Glaucon

epinephryl borate
(ep i nef′ rill)
Epinal, Eppy/N

• *Classification:* antiglaucoma agent (adrenergic)
• *Pregnancy Risk Category:* C

HOW SUPPLIED
epinephrine bitartrate
Ophthalmic solution: 2%
epinephrine hydrochloride
Ophthalmic solution: 0.1%, 0.25%, 0.5%, 1%, 2%
epinephryl borate
Ophthalmic solution: 0.5%, 1%, 2%

ACTION
Mechanism: An adrenergic that dilates the pupil by contracting the dilator muscle. Activates ophthalmic $alpha_2$- or $beta_2$-adrenergic receptors.
Absorption: Little systemic absorption.
Distribution: Animal studies show that application to the eye can result in highest drug levels in the pituitary gland.
Metabolism: Occurs primarily in adrenergic nerve endings; circulating

drug is metabolized by catechol-O-methyltransferase and MAO.
Excretion: Metabolites are excreted by the kidneys.
Onset, peak, duration: Reductions in intraocular pressure are measurable within 1 hour, peak in 4 to 8 hours, and may persist for 12 to 24 hours or more.

INDICATIONS & DOSAGE

Open-angle glaucoma –
Adults: instill 1 to 2 drops of 1% or 2% bitartrate solution in eye with frequency determined by tonometric readings (once q 2 to 4 days up to q.i.d.), or instill 1 drop of 0.5%, 1%, or 2% hydrochloride solution (or 0.5% or 1% epinephryl borate solution) in eye b.i.d.
During surgery–
Adults: instill 1 or more drops of 0.1% solution up to three times.

CONTRAINDICATIONS & PRECAUTIONS

Contraindicated in patients with narrow-angle glaucoma because the drug may worsen the condition and in patients with sensitivity to the drug.

Administer with extreme caution to patients with hypertension or hyperthyroidism and to elderly patients; diabetic patients; those with cardiovascular diseases, history of sensitivity to sympathomimetics, Parkinson's disease (temporary increase in tremor or rigidity), bronchial asthma, or psychoneurotic disorders; and patients receiving inhalational anesthetics because of the potential for cardiac arrhythmias. Use cautiously in patients with sulfite hypersensitivity; some epinephrine preparations contain sulfites.

ADVERSE REACTIONS

Common reactions are in italics; life-threatening reactions are in bold italics.
Eye: corneal or conjunctival pigmentation or corneal edema in long-term use; follicular hypertrophy; chemosis; conjunctivitis; iritis; hyperemic conjunctiva; maculopapular rash; severe stinging, burning, and tearing upon instillation; browache.
Systemic: palpitations, tachycardia.

INTERACTIONS

Cyclopropane or halogenated hydrocarbons: arrhythmias, tachycardia. Use together cautiously, if at all.
Digitalis glycosides: increased risk of cardiac arrhythmias.
Local or systemic sympathomimetics: additive toxic effects.
MAO inhibiters: exaggerated adrenergic effects. Adjust dose of epinephrine carefully.
Pilocarpine: additive effect in lowering intraocular pressure.
Tricyclic antidepressants, antihistamines (diphenhydramine, dexchlorpheniramine): potentiated cardiac effects of epinephrine.

EFFECTS ON DIAGNOSTIC TESTS

Blood glucose and serum lactic acid: possibly increased levels.
BUN: increased levels.
Urine catecholamines: test interference.

NURSING CONSIDERATIONS

Besides those related universally to drug therapy (see "How to use this book"), consider the following specific recommendations:

Assessment
- Obtain a baseline assessment of the patient's vision, ocular pressure, and pupil size before therapy.
- Be alert for adverse reactions and drug interactions throughout therapy.
- Evaluate the patient's and family's knowledge about epinephrine therapy.

Nursing Diagnoses
- Sensory/perceptual alterations (visual) related to the patient's underlying condition.

• High risk for poisoning (systemic adrenergic effects).
• Knowledge deficit related to epinephrine therapy.

Planning and Implementation

Preparation and Administration

• Epinephrine salts are not interchangeable: don't substitute one if another is ordered.
• Examine solution; do not use if darkened.
• Instill in lacrimal sac; remove excess solution around eyes with clean tissue or gauze and apply light finger pressure to lacrimal sac for 1 minute.

Monitoring

• Monitor effectiveness by assessing the patient's visual status, intraocular pressure, and pupil size.
• Monitor for systemic adrenergic effects, especially if the patient is receiving other sympathomimetic drugs.
• Monitor apical rate for drug-induced tachycardia or arrhythmia; obtain ECG as indicated.

Supportive Care

• Notify the doctor immediately if changes in the patient's health status occur.
• Obtain an order for a mild analgesic if the patient experiences brow ache.

Patient Teaching

• Teach the patient how to instill the solution, and advise him to wash his hands before and after administering the drug.
• Warn the patient that the drug may stain soft contact lenses.
• Advise the patient to continue with regular medical supervision during therapy.

Evaluation

In patients receiving epinephrine, appropriate evaluation statements may include:

• Patient experiences therapeutic mydriasis and reduction in intraocular pressure.
• Patient remains free of systemic adrenergic effects.
• Patient and family state an understanding of epinephrine therapy.

epinephrine

(ep i nef′ rin)

Adrenalin◇, Bronkaid Mist◇, Bronkaid Mistometer†, Dysne-Inhal†, Primatene Mist Solution◇

epinephrine bitartrate

AsthmaHaler◇, Broniten Mist◇, Bronkaid Mist Suspension◇, Medihaler-Epi◇, Primatene Mist Suspension◇

epinephrine hydrochloride

Adrenalin Chloride◇, Epi-Pen, Epi-Pen Jr., Sus-Phrine

• *Classification:* bronchodilator, vasopressor, cardiac stimulant, local anesthetic (adjunct), topical antihemorrhagic (adrenergic)
• *Pregnancy Risk Category:* C

HOW SUPPLIED

Aerosol inhaler: 160 mcg◇, 200 mcg◇, 250 mcg/metered spray◇
Nebulizer inhaler: 1% (1:100)†◇, 1.25%†◇, 2.25%†◇
Injection: 0.01 mg/ml (1:100,000), 0.1 mg/ml (1:10,000), 0.5 mg/ml (1:2,000), 1 mg/ml (1:1,000) parenteral; 5 mg/ml (1:200) parenteral suspension

ACTION

Mechanism: A naturally occurring catecholamine that is secreted by the adrenal medulla. It stimulates alpha- and beta-adrenergic receptors within the sympathetic nervous system.
Absorption: Well absorbed after S.C. or I.M. injection.
Distribution: Distributed widely; crosses placenta and enters breast milk but does not enter CNS.

Metabolism: Metabolized at sympathetic nerve endings, liver, and other tissues to inactive metabolites by monoamine oxidase (MAO) and catechol-O-methyltransferase. Action is also terminated by uptake into nerve terminals.
Excretion: In urine, mainly as metabolites and conjugates.
Onset, peak, duration: Epinephrine has a rapid onset of action and short duration of action. Bronchodilation occurs within 5 to 10 minutes and peaks in 20 minutes after S.C. injection; onset after oral inhalation is within 1 minute.

INDICATIONS & DOSAGE

Bronchospasm, hypersensitivity reactions, anaphylaxis–
Adults: 0.1 to 0.5 ml of 1:1,000 S.C. or I.M. Repeat q 10 to 15 minutes, p.r.n. Or 0.1 to 0.25 ml 1:1,000 I.V.
Children: 0.01 ml (10 mcg) of 1:1,000/kg S.C. Repeat q 20 minutes to 4 hours, p.r.n.; 0.005 ml/kg of 1:200 (Sus-Phrine). Repeat q 8 to 12 hours, p.r.n.
Hemostasis–
Adults: 1:50,000 to 1:1,000, applied topically.
Acute asthmatic attacks (inhalation)–
Adults and children: 1 or 2 inhalations of 1:100 or 2.25% racemic, every 1 to 5 minutes until relief is obtained; 0.2 mg/dose usual content.
To prolong local anesthetic effect–
Adults and children: 0.2 to 0.4 ml of 1:1,000 intraspinal; 1:500,000 to 1:50,000 local mixed with local anesthetic.
To restore cardiac rhythm in cardiac arrest–
Adults: 0.5 to 1 mg I.V. or into endotracheal tube. May be given intracardiac if no I.V. route or intratracheal route available. Some clinicians advocate higher dose (up to 5 mg), especially in patients who don't respond to usual I.V dose. Following initial I.V. administration, may be infused I.V. at a rate of 1 to 4 mcg/minute.
Children: 10 mcg/kg I.V. or 5 to 10 mcg (0.05 to 0.1 ml of 1:10,000)/kg intracardiac.

Note: 1 mg = 1 ml of 1:1,000 or 10 ml of 1:10,000.

CONTRAINDICATIONS & PRECAUTIONS

Contraindicated in patients with shock (except anaphylactic shock), organic heart disease, cardiac dilatation, and arrhythmias because it increases myocardial oxygen demand; organic brain damage or cerebral arteriosclerosis because of potential adverse CNS effects; in patients with narrow-angle glaucoma because the drug may worsen the condition; and sensitivity to the drug. Contraindicated in conjunction with local anesthetics in fingers, toes, ears, nose, or genitalia because vasoconstriction in these extremities may induce tissue necrosis.

Use with extreme caution in patients with hypertension or hyperthyroidism; in elderly patients, diabetic patients, and those with cardiovascular diseases, history of sensitivity to sympathomimetics, Parkinson's disease (temporary increase in tremor or rigidity), bronchial asthma, or psychoneurotic disorders; and in patients receiving inhalational anesthetics because of the potential for cardiac arrhythmias. Use cautiously in patients with sulfite hypersensitivity; some epinephrine preparations contain sulfites. Epinephrine may delay the second stage of labor in pregnant women because the drug inhibits spontaneous or oxytocin-induced uterine contractions. It may also cause anoxia in the fetus. However, some evidence suggests that epinephrine can be safely added to lidocaine to prolong epidural anesthesia.

ADVERSE REACTIONS

Common reactions are in italics; life-threatening reactions are in bold italics.
CNS: *nervousness,* tremor, euphoria, anxiety, coldness of extremities, vertigo, *headache,* sweating, disorientation, agitation. In patients with Parkinson's disease, the drug increases rigidity and tremor.
CV: *palpitations;* widened pulse pressure; hypertension; *tachycardia;* ***ventricular fibrillation; CVA;*** anginal pain; ECG changes, including a decrease in the T wave amplitude.
Metabolic: *hyperglycemia,* glycosuria.
Other: pulmonary edema, dyspnea, *pallor.*

INTERACTIONS

Alpha-adrenergic blocking agents: hypotension due to unopposed beta-adrenergic effects.
Beta blockers, such as propranolol: vasoconstriction and reflex bradycardia. Monitor patient carefully.
Digitalis glycosides, general anesthetics (halogenated hydrocarbons): increased risk of ventricular arrhythmias.
Doxapram, mazindol, methylphenidate: enhanced CNS stimulation or pressor effects.
Ergot alkaloids: enhanced vasoconstrictor activity.
Guanadrel, guanethidine: enhanced pressor effects of epinephrine.
Levodopa: enhanced risk of cardiac arrhythmias.
MAO inhibitors: increased risk of hypertensive crisis.
Tricyclic antidepressants, antihistamines, thyroid hormones: when given with sympathomimetics, may cause severe adverse cardiac effects. Avoid giving together.

EFFECTS ON DIAGNOSTIC TESTS

Blood glucose and serum lactic acid: increased levels.
BUN: increased levels.
Urine catecholamines: test interference.

NURSING CONSIDERATIONS

Besides those related universally to drug therapy (see "How to use this book"), consider the following specific recommendations:

Assessment

- Obtain a baseline assessment of the patient's cardiopulmonary status by assessing the patient's vital signs, evaluating ECG results, and auscultating heart and lung sounds before therapy.
- Be alert for adverse reactions and drug interactions throughout therapy.
- Evaluate the patient and family's knowledge about epinephrine therapy.

Nursing Diagnoses

- Ineffective airway clearance related to patient's underlying condition.
- Decreased cardiac output related to epinphrine-induced CV adverse effects.
- Knowledge deficit related to epinephrine therapy.

Planning and Implementation

Preparation and Administration

- ***I.V. use:*** Epinephrine should not be mixed with an alkaline solution. Use dextrose 5% in water (D_5W), 0.9% sodium chloride solution, or a combination of D_5W and 0.9% sodium chloride solution. Mix the solution just before using it. Don't mix with other drugs, and don't use discolored solutions. Discard the solution after 24 hours as epinephrine solutions deteriorate after that time. Discard earlier if the solution is discolored or contains precipitates. Store solution in a light-resistant container and do not remove it before use.
- ***S.C. use:*** Massage the injection site to counteract possible vasoconstriction. Avoid repeated injections at the same site. Repeated local injections can cause local vasoconstriction and necrosis at the site.
- ***Inhalant use:*** Always wait 2 min-

utes between inhalations, if bronchodilator is administered via inhalant and more than 1 inhalation is ordered. Always administer the bronchodilator first and wait 5 minutes before administering the other, if more than one type of inhalant is ordered. Remember that the patient should not receive more than 12 bronchodilator inhalations in 24 hours.

• Giving the medication on time is extremely important.

• Administer the medication around the clock for greatest effectiveness.

• Keep in mind that epinephrine is rapidly destroyed by oxidizing agents, such as iodine, chromates, nitrates, and salts of easily reducible metal (such as iron).

Monitoring

• Monitor effectiveness by regularly checking the patient's vital signs and ECG pattern (if applicable) and auscultating the lungs and heart. Note widened pulse pressure, elevated blood pressure, tachycardia, ventricular fibrillation, ECG changes, dyspnea, and crackles in lung fields.

• Monitor for distended neck veins, peripheral edema, and sudden weight gain, which suggest fluid retention.

• Monitor blood glucose levels regularly because drug may cause hyperglycemia.

• Monitor patients with Parkinson's disease for increased rigidity and tremor.

Supportive Care

• Hold dose and notify the doctor if CV symptoms, such as palpitations, hypertension, tachycardia, or anginal pain, occur. Also report signs and symptoms of pulmonary edema. In the event of sharp blood pressure rise, rapid acting vasodilators, such as nitrites or alpha-adrenergic blocking agents, can be given to counteract the marked pressor effect of large doses of epinephrine.

• Notify the doctor if the patient's pulse increases by 20% or more when epinephrine is administered.

Patient Teaching

• Tell the patient to always take the medication exactly as prescribed and to take it around the clock.

• Instruct the patient to perform oral inhalation correctly as follows: Clear nasal passages and throat. Breathe out, expelling as much air from the lungs as possible. Place the mouthpiece well into the mouth as the dose from the inhaler is released, and inhale deeply. Hold breath for several seconds, remove the mouthpiece, and exhale slowly.

• Explain that if more than one inhalation is ordered, he should wait at least 2 minutes before repeating the procedure for a second dose.

• Explain why it is necessary to use the bronchodilator first if other inhalants, such as a steroid inhaler, are prescribed. (This allows the bronchodilator to open air passages for maximum effectiveness.) Tell the patient to allow 5 minutes between the inhalant treatments.

• Warn the patient to avoid accidentally spraying the inhalant into the eyes, which may cause temporary blurring of vision.

• Tell the patient to reduce the intake of foods containing caffeine, such as coffee, colas, and chocolates, when taking a bronchodilator.

• Instruct the patient to contact the doctor immediately if he experiences a fluttering of the heart, rapid beating of the heart, shortness of breath, or chest pain.

• Warn elderly patients that dizziness may occur at start of the therapy, and they should take precautions to avoid injury from falls.

• Tell the patient not to self-medicate with any OTC drugs without medical approval while taking this drug.

• Warn the patient against increasing the dosage or frequency of administration. Advise the patient to notify

the doctor if the prescribed dosage does not relieve symptoms.
• Show the patient how to check the pulse. Instruct him to check the pulse before and after using a bronchodilator and to call the doctor if pulse rate increases more than 20 to 30 beats/minute.
• The patient who has an acute hypersensitivity reaction may require instruction for self-injection of epinephrine at home.

Evaluation
In patients receiving epinephrine, appropriate evaluation statements may include:
• Patient's respiratory signs and symptoms are relieved by epinephrine.
• Patient does not experience serious adverse reactions during therapy.
• Patient and family state an understanding of epinephrine therapy.

epoetin alfa (erythropoietin)
(eh poh´ ee tin)
Epogen, Procrit

• *Classification:* antianemic agent (glycoprotein)
• *Pregnancy Risk Category:* C

HOW SUPPLIED
Injection: 2,000 units/ml, 3,000 units/ml, 4,000 units/ml, 6,000 units/ml

ACTION
Mechanism: A glycoprotein produced by recombinant DNA technology that has all of the properties of the naturally occuring hormone, erythropoietin, which is produced by the kidneys. Influences the rate of red blood cell production by bone marrow by acting on erythyroid tissues to stimulate the mitotic activity of erythroid progenitor cells and early precursor cells. It functions as a growth factor and as a differentiating factor, increasing the production or erythrocytes (red blood cells).
Absorption: Epoetin alfa may be given S.C. or I.V. After S.C. administration, peak serum levels occur within 5 to 24 hours.
Excretion: Half-life: Approximately 4 to 13 hours in patients with chronic renal failure; may be about 20% shorter in normal patients.

INDICATIONS & DOSAGE
Anemia due to reduced production of endogenous erythropoietin, end-stage renal disease–
Adults: dosage is individualized. Starting dose is 50 to 100 units/kg I.V. three times weekly. (Nondialysis patients with chronic renal failure may receive the drug by S.C. injection or I.V.) Reduce dosage when target hematocrit is reached or if the hematocrit rises more than 4 points in any 2-week period. Increase dosage if hematocrit does not increase by 5 to 6 points after 8 weeks of therapy. Maintenance dose is usually 25 units/kg three times weekly.
Adjunctive treatment of HIV-infected patients with anemia secondary to zidovudine therapy–
Adults: 100 units/kg I.V. or S.C. three times weekly for 8 weeks or until target hemoglobin is reached.

CONTRAINDICATIONS & PRECAUTIONS
Contraindicated in patients hypersensitive to mammalian cell-derived products or to human albumin. Also contraindicated in patients with uncontrolled hypertension.

ADVERSE REACTIONS
Common reactions are in italics; life-threatening reactions are in bold italics.
Blood: iron deficiency, elevated platelet count.
CNS: headache, ***seizures.***
CV: hypertension.
GI: nausea, vomiting, diarrhea.

Skin: rash.
Other: increased clotting of arteriovenous grafts.

INTERACTIONS

None reported.

EFFECTS ON DIAGNOSTIC TESTS

BUN, uric acid, creatinine, phosphorus, and potassium levels: moderately increased levels.

NURSING CONSIDERATIONS

Besides those related universally to drug therapy (see "How to use this book"), consider the following specific recommendations:

Assessment

- Obtain a baseline assessment of the patient's blood count and blood pressure before therapy.
- Be alert for adverse reactions and drug interactions throughout therapy.
- Evaluate the patient's and family's knowledge about epoetin alfa therapy.

Nursing Diagnoses

- Altered protection related to reduced production of endogenous erythropoietin.
- High risk for injury related to epoetin-alfa–induced seizure.
- Knowledge deficit related to epoetin alfa therapy.

Planning and Implementation

Preparation and Administration

- ***I.V. use:*** Administer by direct IV injection; not recommended for continuous or intermittent infusion.
- Reduce dosage in patients who exhibit a rapid rise in hematocrit (more than 4 points in any 2-week period) because of the risk of hypertension.
- Adjust dosage on individual basis according to patient's response in HIV infection. Dosage recommendations are for patients with endogenous erythropoietin levels of 500 units/liter or less and cumulative zidovudine doses of 4.2 g/week or less.

Monitoring

- Monitor effectiveness by checking erythropoietin levels.
- Monitor complete blood count and clotting times. Hematocrit may rise and cause excessive clotting.
- Monitor hematocrit for rapid rise, which can cause loss of control of blood pressure. Dosage should be adjusted to allow for no more than a 4 point rise within any 2-week period. The drug may have to be temporarily withheld until blood pressure is controlled.
- Monitor blood pressure regularly. Up to 80% of patients with chronic renal failure have hypertension. Blood pressure may rise, especially when the hematocrit is increasing in the early part of epoetin alfa therapy.
- Observe the patient for pain or discomfort in long bones and pelvis, chills, and diaphoresis about 2 hours after injection.

Supportive Care

- Use seizure precautions. Have an airway or padded tongue blade nearby.
- Obtain order for medication to alleviate bone pain induced by epoetin alfa.
- Provide comfort measures to relieve chills and diaphoresis. Include good skin care, additional clothing or blankets, and environmental control.
- Dietary restrictions and drug therapy may be necessary to control hypertension.
- Dialysis patients may require additional anticoagulation to prevent clotting during epoetin alfa treatment.
- Do not give to patients with uncontrolled hypertension.
- Epoetin alfa has been used to correct the hemostatic defect associated with uremia.
- Additional clinical trials are investigating epoetin alfa for the treatment of anemia of AIDS patients receiving zidovudine, of cancer patients undergoing chemotherapy, and of patients

with rheumatoid arthritis. It is also being investigated for facilitating autologous transfusion by helping to produce more units of blood before surgery.

Patient Teaching

• Inform the patient that blood specimens will be drawn weekly for blood counts and, depending on the results, dosage adjustments may be necessary.
• Reassure patient that bone pain, chills, and diaphoresis are temporary and will eventually subside.
• Arrange for dietitian to teach patient about low-salt diet.
• Advise patient to avoid hazardous activities, such as driving or operating heavy machinery, during the initiation of therapy. There may be a relationship between rapidly rising hematocrit levels and seizures.

Evaluation

In patients receiving epoetin alfa, appropriate evaluation statements may include:

• Patient's endogenous erythropoietin remains within normal range.
• Patient is seizure free.
• Patient and family state an understanding of epoetin alfa therapy.

ergonovine maleate (ergometrine maleate)

(er goe noe´ veen)
Ergotrate Maleate

• *Classification:* oxytocic (ergot alkaloid)

HOW SUPPLIED

Tablets: 0.2 mg
Injection: 0.2 mg/ml

ACTION

Mechanism: Increases motor activity of the uterus by direct stimulation. Prolonged uterine contraction helps control hemorrhage.

Absorption: Rapidly absorbed after oral and I.M. administration.
Metabolism: In the liver.
Excretion: Primarily renal, although nonrenal elimination in feces has been suggested.
Onset, peak, duration: Onset of action is immediate for I.V., 2 to 5 minutes for I.M., and 6 to 15 minutes for oral doses. Duration of contractions is 3 hours for oral and I.M. doses and 45 minutes for I.V. doses. Some rhythmic contractions may persist for up to 3 hours after an I.V. dose.

INDICATIONS & DOSAGE

Prevent or treat postpartum and postabortion hemorrhage from uterine atony or subinvolution–
Adults: 0.2 mg I.M. q 2 to 4 hours, maximum of 5 doses; or 0.2 mg I.V. (only for severe uterine bleeding or other life-threatening emergency) over 1 minute while blood pressure and uterine contractions are monitored. I.V. dose may be diluted to 5 ml with normal saline injection. After initial I.M. or I.V. dose, may give 0.2 to 0.4 mg P.O. q 6 to 12 hours for 2 to 7 days. Decrease dosage if severe uterine cramping occurs.

CONTRAINDICATIONS & PRECAUTIONS

Contraindicated in patients with sensitivity to ergot preparations; in threatened spontaneous abortion, induction of labor, or before delivery of placenta because captivation of placenta may occur; and in patients with a history of allergic or idiosyncratic reactions to the drug. Because of the potential for adverse CV effects, use cautiously in patients with hypertension, toxemia, sepsis, occlusive vascular disease, and hepatic, renal, and cardiac disease.

ADVERSE REACTIONS

Common reactions are in italics; life-threatening reactions are in bold italics.
CNS: dizziness, headache.
CV: ***hypertension,*** chest pain.
EENT: tinnitus.
GI: nausea, vomiting.
GU: uterine cramping.
Other: sweating, dyspnea, ***hypersensitivity.***

INTERACTIONS

Regional anesthetics, dopamine, I.V. oxytocin: excessive vasoconstriction. Use together cautiously.

EFFECTS ON DIAGNOSTIC TESTS

Serum prolactin: possibly decreased levels.

NURSING CONSIDERATIONS

Besides those related universally to drug therapy (see "How to use this book"), consider the following specific recommendations:

Assessment

• Obtain a baseline assessment of the patient's hemodynamic status and condition of uterine musculature before therapy.
• Be alert for adverse reactions and drug interactions throughout therapy.
• Evaluate the patient's and family's knowledge about ergonovine therapy.

Nursing Diagnoses

• Fluid volume deficit related to postpartum hemorrhage.
• Pain related to ergonovine-induced uterine cramping.
• Knowledge deficit related to ergonovine therapy.

Planning and Implementation

Preparation and Administration

• Administer only under conditions of meticulous observation. Uterine hyperstimulation during labor may lead to uterine tetany, which may impair placental blood flow and cause amniotic fluid embolism.
• ***I.V. use:*** Avoid rapid injection because of severe CV effects. Store I.V. solutions below 46.4° F (8° C).
• Keep in mind that I.V. ergonovine is used to diagnose coronary artery spasm (Prinzmetal's angina).
Daily stock may be kept at cool room temperature for 60 days.
• Have drug available for immediate use if it is to be given postpartum.
• Store in tightly closed, light-resistant container. Discard if discolored.

Monitoring

• Monitor effectiveness by evaluating blood pressure, pulse rate, contractions, uterine tone, and character and amount of bleeding after administration of the drug.
• Be aware that contractions begin 5 to 15 minutes after P.O. administration; immediately after I.V. injection. May continue 3 hours or more after P.O. or I.M. injection; 45 minutes after I.V. injection.

Supportive Care

• Report sudden changes in vital signs, frequent periods of uterine relaxation, and character and amount of vaginal bleeding.
• Maintain or restore adequate blood volume.
• Keep in mind that, if hypertension occurs, it may respond to chlorpromazine or hydralazine.
• Administer analgesics as ordered. Assist patient with relaxation techniques.
• Keep patient warm.
• Be aware that hypocalcemia may decrease patient response. If patient is not also taking digitalis, cautious administration of calcium gluconate I.V. may produce desired oxytocic action.

Patient Teaching

• Explain that this drug stimulates uterine musculature, controlling postpartum bleeding and atonia.
• Tell the patient to report pain, dizziness or other adverse reactions to the drug.

Evaluation
In patients receiving ergonovine, appropriate evaluation statements may include:
• Patient's vital signs are stable and she experiences, reduction in amount of or absence of uterine bleeding, as well as effective uterine contractions.
• Patient is free of pain.
• Patient and family state an understanding of ergonovine therapy.

ergotamine tartrate
(er got´ a meen)
Ergomar, Ergostat, Gynergen†, Medihaler-Ergotamine

• *Classification:* vasoconstrictor (ergot alkaloid)
• *Pregnancy Risk Category:* X

HOW SUPPLIED
Tablets (sublingual): 2 mg
Aerosal inhaler: 360 mcg/metered spray
Suppositories: 2 mg

ACTION
Mechanism: An ergot alkaloid that inhibits the effects of epinephrine, norepinephrine, and other sympathomimetic amines. Also has antiserotonin effects.
Absorption: Rapidly absorbed after inhalation and variably absorbed after oral administration. Caffeine may increase rate and extent of absorption. Drug undergoes first-pass metabolism after oral administration; this is avoided by administering drug rectally.
Distribution: Widely distributed; crosses placenta and enters the CNS.
Metabolism: Extensively metabolized in the liver.
Excretion: 4% of a dose is excreted in urine within 96 hours; remainder of a dose presumed to be excreted in feces. Ergotamine is dialyzable. Half-life: Terminal elimination half-life is about 21 hours.
Onset, peak, duration: Peak concentrations are reached within 30 minutes to 3 hours. Onset of action depends on how promptly drug is given after onset of headache.

INDICATIONS & DOSAGE
Vascular or migraine headache–
Adults: initially, 2 mg S.L., then 1 to 2 mg S.L. q ½ hour, to maximum of 6 mg daily and 10 mg weekly. Alternatively, use aerosol inhaler: 1 spray (360 mcg) initially, repeated every 5 minutes p.r.n. to a maximum of 6 sprays (2.16 mg) per 24 hours or 15 sprays (5.4 mg) per week.

Patient may also use rectal suppositories. Initially, 2 mg rectally at the onset of the attack, repeated in 1 hour p.r.n. Maximum dose is 2 suppositories per attack or 5 suppositories per week.

CONTRAINDICATIONS & PRECAUTIONS
Contraindicated in patients with sepsis or peripheral vascular disease, because of adverse vascular effects; in patients with impaired renal or hepatic function because of the potential for accumulation and toxicity; and in patients with malnutrition, severe pruritus, severe hypertension, or hypersensitivity to drug or ergot alkaloids; also contraindicated in women who are or who may become pregnant.

ADVERSE REACTIONS
Common reactions are in italics; life-threatening reactions are in bold italics.
CV: numbness and tingling in fingers and toes, transient tachycardia or bradycardia, precordial distress and pain, increased arterial pressure, angina pectoris.
GI: nausea, vomiting, diarrhea, abdominal cramps.
Skin: itching.

Other: weakness in legs, muscle pains in extremities, localized edema.

INTERACTIONS

Propranolol and other beta blockers: blocked natural pathway for vasodilation in patients receiving ergot alkaloids and thus could result in excessive vasoconstriction. Watch closely if drugs are used together.

EFFECTS ON DIAGNOSTIC TESTS

None reported.

NURSING CONSIDERATIONS

Besides those related universally to drug therapy (see "How to use this book"), consider the following specific recommendations:

Assessment

- Obtain a baseline assessment of the patient's pain before therapy.
- Be alert for adverse reactions and drug interactions throughout therapy.
- Evaluate the patient's and family's knowledge about ergotamine therapy.

Nursing Diagnoses

- Pain related to the patient's underlying condition.
- Fluid volume deficit related to adverse drug reactions.
- Knowledge deficit related to ergotamine therapy.

Planning and Implementation

Preparation and Administration

- Avoid prolonged administration; do not exceed recommended dosage.
- Store in light-resistant containers.
- Sublingual tablets are preferred for use during early stage of attack because of its rapid absorption.

Monitoring

- Monitor for drug interactions or adverse reactions by frequently checking the patient's vital signs for transient tachycardia or bradycardia.
- Monitor hydration status if nausea, vomiting, and diarrhea occur.
- Monitor skin for possible loss of skin integrity resulting from severe vasoconstriction.

Supportive Care

- Provide additional fluids if patient develops nausea, vomiting, and diarrhea.
- Obtain an order for a mild antipruritic if patient develops itching.
- Provide a quiet, low-light environment to help the patient relax.
- Help the patient to evaluate underlying causes of physical or emotional stress, which may precipitate attacks.
- Know that cold may increase the occurrence of adverse effects.
- Obtain an accurate dietary history from the patient to identify if a relationship exists between certain foods and onset of headache.
- Do not stop the drug abruptly. Be prepared to gradually discontinue the drug to avoid ergotamine rebound, which may increase frequency and duration of headache.

Patient Teaching

- Instruct the patient how to use the inhaler properly.
- Tell the patient to use a mild antipruretic if he develops itching.
- Warn the patient not to increase dosage without first consulting the doctor.
- Tell the patient not to stop taking the drug abruptly.
- Tell the patient to avoid prolonged exposure to cold to avoid a possible increase in adverse reactions.
- Tell the patient that the drug is most effective during the prodromal stage of the headache or as soon as possible after onset.
- Instruct the patient on long-term therapy to check for and report feeling of coldness in extremities or tingling of fingers and toes due to vasoconstriction.
- Tell the patient to report chest pain to the doctor.

Evaluation

In patients receiving ergotamine tartrate, appropriate evaluation statements may include:

- Patient's pain is relieved.

• Patient's fluid and electrolyte balance is maintained.
• Patient and family state an understanding of ergotamine therapy.

erythrityl tetranitrate
(e ri´ thri till)
Cardilate

• *Classification:* antianginal, vasodilator (nitrate)
• *Pregnancy Risk Category:* C

HOW SUPPLIED
Tablets (chewable): 10 mg
Tablets (oral, sublingual, buccal): 5 mg, 10 mg

ACTION
Mechanism: A vasodilator that reduces cardiac oxygen demand by decreasing left ventricular end-diastolic pressure (preload) and, to a lesser extent, systemic vascular resistance (afterload). Increases blood flow through the collateral coronary vessels.
Absorption: Readily absorbed when administered orally, sublingually, and intrabuccally.
Distribution: Probably similar to that of nitroglycerin and other nitrates.
Metabolism: Drug is metabolized in the liver and serum similarly to other nitrates. Metabolites are unknown.
Excretion: In urine. Half-life: About 40 minutes.
Onset, peak, duration: Onset of action occurs within 5 to 10 minutes after administration of sublingual, intrabuccal, and chewable tablets; within 30 minutes with other oral forms. Duration of effect for sublingual, intrabuccal, and chewable tablets is 30 minutes to 3 hours; for other oral forms, 1 to 1½ hours to maximal effect, lasting up to 6 hours.

INDICATIONS & DOSAGE
Prophylaxis and long-term management of frequent or recurrent anginal pain, reduced exercise tolerance associated with angina pectoris–
Adults: 5 mg orally, sublingually, or buccally t.i.d., increasing in 2 to 3 days if needed.

CONTRAINDICATIONS & PRECAUTIONS
Contraindicated in patients with head trauma or cerebral hemorrhage, because it may increase intracranial pressure, or in patients with a history of hypersensitivity or idiosyncratic reaction to nitrates; and in patients with severe anemia, because nitrate ions readily oxidize hemoglobin to methemoglobin.

Use cautioulsy in patients with increased intracranial pressure because the drug dilates meningeal vessels; open- or closed-angle glaucoma, although intraocular pressure is increased only briefly and aqueous humor drainage from the eye is unimpeded; diuretic-induced fluid depletion or low systolic blood pressure (below 90 mm Hg) because of the drug's hypotensive effect; and in the initial days after acute MI, because the drug may cause excessive hypotension and tachycardia.

ADVERSE REACTIONS
Common reactions are in italics; life-threatening reactions are in bold italics.
CNS: *headache, sometimes with throbbing; dizziness;* weakness.
CV: *orthostatic hypotension, tachycardia, flushing, palpitations,* fainting.
GI: nausea, vomiting.
Skin: cutaneous vasodilation.
Local: sublingual burning.
Other: hypersensitivity.

INTERACTIONS
None significant.

*Liquid form contains alcohol.

**May contain tartrazine.

EFFECTS ON DIAGNOSTIC TESTS

Serum cholesterol (Zlatkis-Zak color reaction): falsely decreased value.

NURSING CONSIDERATIONS

Besides those related universally to drug therapy (see "How to use this book"), consider the following specific recommendations:

Assessment

• Obtain a baseline assessment of the patient's anginal state before therapy.
• Be alert for adverse reactions and drug interactions throughout therapy.
• Evaluate the patient's and family's knowledge about erythrityl therapy.

Nursing Diagnoses

• Pain related to ineffectiveness of erythrityl therapy.
• High risk for injury related to erythrityl-induced dizziness or orthostatic hypotension.
• Knowledge deficit related to erythrityl therapy.

Planning and Implementation

Preparation and Administration

• ***S.L. use:*** Administer at first sign of attack. Have patient wet the tablet with saliva, place it under his tongue until completely absorbed, and sit down and rest. Dose may be repeated every 10 to 15 minutes for a maximum of three doses.
• ***P.O. use:*** Administer oral tablet on empty stomach, either 30 minutes before or 1 to 2 hours after meals, and have patient swallow oral tablets whole.
• Provide additional dose at bedtime if nocturnal angina occurs or before anticipated stress as ordered.
• Do not discontinue drug abruptly as coronary vasospasm may occur.
• Store drug in cool place, in a tightly closed container, away from light.
• Remove cotton from container because it absorbs drug.

Monitoring

• Monitor effectiveness by regularly evaluating the severity and frequency of the patient's anginal pain.
• Monitor patient's heart rate and rhythm regularly.
• Monitor blood pressure and intensity and duration of response to drug.

Supportive Care

• Consult the doctor if the patient does not experience pain relief.
• Obtain an order for a mild analgesic if headache occurs. Be aware that dosage may need to be reduced temporarily but tolerance usually develops.
• To minimize orthostatic hypotension, have patient change to upright position slowly, go up and down stairs carefully, and lie down at the first sign of dizziness.
• To ensure freshness of tablets, replace supply every 3 months.
• Maintain safety precautions if dizziness occurs; assist the patient with daily activities to minimize energy expenditure.
• Obtain an order for an antiemetic agent as needed.

Patient Teaching

• Teach patient how to take drug form prescribed. Stress importance of taking the drug exactly as prescribed and to keep it easily accessible at all times.
• Tell patient to take additional dose before anticipated stress or at bedtime if angina is nocturnal.
• Teach patient to take sublingual tablet at first sign of attack and to sit down and rest. Dose may be repeated every 10 to 15 minutes for a maximum of three doses. If no relief, patient should call doctor or go to hospital emergency room. If patient complains of tingling sensation with drug placed sublingually, tell him he may try holding tablet in buccal pouch.
• Warn patient that discontinuing the

drug abruptly may cause coronary vasospasm.
• Tell the patient to schedule activities to allow adequate rest.
• Reassure patient that if headache occurs it is usually temporary and to take a mild analgesic until tolerance occurs. However, if headache is severe tell patient to notify doctor as dosage may need to be reduced temporarily until tolerance occurs.
• Advise patient to avoid alcoholic beverages; may produce increased hypotension.
• Tell patient how to minimize effects of orthostatic hypotension.
• Instruct patient to store drug in cool place, in a tightly closed container, away from light. To ensure freshness, tell patient to replace supply every 3 months. Also tell him to remove cotton from container since it absorbs drug.

Evaluation
In patients receiving erythrityl, appropriate evaluation statements may include:
• Patient states anginal pain relief occurs with erythrityl therapy.
• Patient does not experience injury as a result of dizziness or orthostatic hypotension caused by erythrityl therapy.
• Patient and family state an understanding of erythrityl therapy.

---

erythromycin base (systemic)
(er ith roe mye´ sin)
Apo-Erythro base†, EMU-V‡, E-Mycin, Eryc, Eryc Sprinkle, Ery-Tab, Erythromid†, Ilotycin, Novorythro†, PCE Dispersatabs, Robimycin

erythromycin estolate
Ilosone, Novorythro†

erythromycin ethylsuccinate
Apo-Erythro-ES†, E.E.S., E-Mycin E, EryPed, Erythrocin, Pediamycin, Wyamycin E

erythromycin gluceptate
Ilotycin

erythromycin lactobionate
Erythrocin

erythromycin stearate
Apo-Erythro-S†, Erypar, Erythrocin, Novorythro†, Wyamycin S

• *Classification:* antibiotic (erythromycin)
• *Pregnancy Risk Category:* B

HOW SUPPLIED
base
Tablets (enteric-coated): 250 mg, 330 mg, 500 mg
Pellets (enteric-coated): 250 mg
Oral suspension: 125 mg/5 ml, 200 mg/5 ml, 400 mg/5 ml
estolate
Tablets: 250 mg, 500 mg
Tablets (chewable): 125 mg, 250 mg
Capsules: 125 mg, 250 mg
Oral suspension: 125 mg/5 ml, 250 mg/5 ml
Drops: 100 mg/ml
ethylsuccinate
Tablets (chewable): 200 mg, 400 mg
gluceptate
Injection: 250-mg, 500-mg, 1-g vials
lactobionate
Injection: 500-mg, 1-g vials
stearate
Tablets (film-coated): 250 mg, 500 mg

ACTION
Mechanism: Inhibits bacterial protein synthesis by binding to the 50S subunit of the ribosome.
Absorption: Most erythromycin salts are absorbed in the duodenum. Because erythromycin base is acid-sensitive, it must be buffered or have enteric coating to prevent destruction

by gastric acid. Acid salts and esters (estolate, ethylsuccinate, and stearate) are not affected by gastric acidity and therefore are well absorbed; they are unaffected or possibly even enhanced by presence of food. Base and stearate preparations should be given on empty stomach. Gluceptate and lactobionate salts are given I.V., and result in higher peak levels of free erythromycin.
Distribution: Widely distributed to most body tissues and fluids except CSF, where it appears only in low concentrations; also crosses the placenta. About 80% of erythromycin base and 96% of erythromycin estolate are protein-bound.
Metabolism: Partially metabolized in the liver to inactive metabolites.
Excretion: Mainly excreted unchanged in bile; small amounts (less than 5%) are excreted in urine; some in breast milk. Half-life: About 1½ hours in patients with normal renal function. Peritoneal hemodialysis does not remove drug.
Onset, peak, duration: Peak levels usually occur 1 to 4 hours after an oral dose; peak levels are higher when the drug is given in divided doses (q.i.d.) as compared to a single dose.

INDICATIONS & DOSAGE

Acute pelvic inflammatory disease caused by Neisseria gonorrhoeae–
Women: 500 mg I.V. (erythromycin gluceptate, lactobionate) q 6 hours for 3 days, then 250 mg (erythromycin base, estolate, stearate) or 400 mg (erythromycin ethylsuccinate) P.O. q 6 hours for 7 days.
Endocarditis prophylaxis for dental procedures in patients allergic to penicillin–
Adults: 1 g (erythromycin base, estolate, stearate) P.O. 1 hour before procedure, then 500 mg P.O. 6 hours later.
Intestinal amebiasis–
Adults: 250 mg (erythromycin base, estolate, stearate) P.O. q 6 hours for 10 to 14 days.
Children: 30 to 50 mg/kg (erythromycin base, estolate, stearate) P.O. daily, divided q 6 hours for 10 to 14 days.
Mild-to-moderately severe respiratory tract, skin, and soft tissue infections caused by sensitive group A beta-hemolytic streptococci, Diplococcus pneumoniae, Mycoplasma pneumoniae, Corynebacterium diphtheriae, Bordetella pertussis, Listeria monocytogenes–
Adults: 250 to 500 mg (erythromycin base, estolate, stearate) P.O. q 6 hours; or 400 to 800 mg (erythromycin ethylsuccinate) P.O. q 6 hours; or 15 to 20 mg/kg I.V. daily, as continuous infusion or divided q 6 hours.
Children: 30 mg/kg to 50 mg/kg (oral erythromycin salts) P.O. daily, divided q 6 hours; or 15 to 20 mg/kg I.V. daily, divided q 4 to 6 hours.
Syphilis–
Adults: 500 mg (erythromycin base, estolate, stearate) P.O. q.i.d. for 15 days.
Legionnaire's disease–
Adults: 500 mg to 1 g I.V. or P.O. q 6 hours for 21 days.
Uncomplicated urethral, endocervical, or rectal infections where tetracyclines are contraindicated–
Adults: 500 mg P.O. q.i.d. for at least 7 days.
Urogenital Chlamydia trachomatis *infections during pregnancy–*
Adults: 500 mg P.O. q.i.d. for at least 7 days or 250 mg P.O. q.i.d. for at least 14 days.
Conjunctivitis caused by Chlamydia trachomatis *in newborns–*
Newborns: 50 mg/kg P.O. daily in four divided doses for at least 2 weeks.
Pneumonia of infancy due to Chlamydia trachomatis–
Infants: 50 mg/kg/day in four divided doses for at least 3 weeks.

CONTRAINDICATIONS & PRECAUTIONS

Contraindicated in patients with hypersensitivity to drug. Erythromycin estolate is contraindicated in patients with hepatic disease because drug may be hepatotoxic.

Use other erythromycin forms cautiously in patients with preexisting hepatic disease because drug may exacerbate hepatic dysfunction.

ADVERSE REACTIONS

Common reactions are in italics; life-threatening reactions are in bold italics.
EENT: hearing loss with high I.V. doses.
GI: *abdominal pain and cramping, nausea, vomiting, diarrhea.*
Hepatic: cholestatic jaundice (with erythromycin estolate).
Skin: urticaria, rashes.
Local: *venous irritation, thrombophlebitis following I.V. injection.*
Other: overgrowth of nonsusceptible bacteria or fungi; ***anaphylaxis;*** fever.

INTERACTIONS

Clindamycin, lincomycin: may be antagonistic. Don't use together.
Oral anticoagulants: increased anticoagulant effects.
Theophylline: decreased erythromycin blood level and increased theophylline toxicity. Use together cautiously.

EFFECTS ON DIAGNOSTIC TESTS

Fluorometric tests of urinary catecholamines: interference.
Liver function tests: abnormal results.

NURSING CONSIDERATIONS

Besides those related universally to drug therapy (see "How to use this book"), consider the following specific recommendations:

Assessment

- Obtain a baseline assessment of patient's infection before therapy.
- Be alert for adverse reactions and drug interactions throughout therapy.
- Evaluate the patient's and family's knowledge about erythromycin therapy.

Nursing Diagnoses

- High risk for injury related to ineffectiveness of erythromycin to eradicate the infection.
- High risk for fluid volume deficit related to erythromycin-induced adverse GI reactions.
- Knowledge deficit related to erythromycin therapy.

Planning and Implementation

Preparation and Administration

- Obtain specimen for culture and sensitivity tests before first dose. Therapy may begin pending test results.
- ***P.O. use:*** For best absorption, administer with a full glass of water 1 hour before or 2 hours after meals. Coated tablets may be taken with meals. Do not administer erythromycin stearate with meals or food, or any oral form with fruit juice. Make sure patient does not swallow chewable erythromycin tablets whole. When administering suspension, be sure to note the concentration.
- ***I.V. use:*** Reconstitute according to manufacturer's instructions and dilute each 250 mg in at least 100 ml 0.9% sodium chloride solution. Infuse over 60 minutes.
- Do not administer erythromycin lactobionate with other drugs because of chemical instability.
- Do not administer erythromycin by I.M. injection; it is painful and may cause abscess or local tissue necrosis.

Monitoring

- Monitor effectiveness by regularly assessing for improvement in the infection.
- Monitor hydration status if adverse GI reactions occur.
- Monitor hepatic function for evidence of hepatotoxicity.
- Monitor serum theophylline levels

during concomitant use with theophylline.
• Monitor prothrombin time and observe for signs of bleeding during concomitant use with warfarin.

Supportive Care
• Obtain an order for an antiemetic or antidiarrheal agent as needed and ask doctor about coated forms of erythromycin, which are associated with lower incidence of GI distress.
• If adverse reactions occur (especially the signs and symptoms of cholestatic hepatitis), expect to discontinue the drug and substitute another antibiotic.

Patient Teaching
• Tell the patient to take medication for as long as prescribed, exactly as directed, and even after he feels better and to take entire amount prescribed.
• For best absorption, instruct the patient to take oral form with full glass of water 1 hour before or 2 hours after meals, but never with fruit juice. (However, enteric-coated tablets may be taken with meals.) Instruct the patient taking chewable tablets not to swallow them whole.
• Inform the patient on long-term erythromycin therapy of the importance of having routine liver function studies as prescribed.
• Instruct the patient receiving I.V. erythromycin lactobionate to notify the nurse of any hearing changes.

Evaluation

In patients receiving erythromycin, appropriate evaluation statements may include:
• Patient is free from infection.
• Patient maintains adequate hydration throughout erythromycin therapy.
• Patient and family state an understanding of erythromycin therapy.

erythromycin (topical)

(er ith roe mye´ sin)
Akne-mycin, A/T/S, Erycette, EryDerm, EryGel, Ery-Sol†, ETS†, Sans-Acne†, T-Stat†, Staticin

• *Classification:* topical antibiotic
• *Pregnancy Risk Category:* B

HOW SUPPLIED

Ointment: 2%
Topical gel: 2%
Pledgets: 2%
Topical solution: 2%*

ACTION

Mechanism: Binds to the 50S ribosomal subunit of susceptible bacteria and disrupts protein synthesis. Bacteriostatic or bactericidal, depending on concentration.
Pharmacokinetics: Unknown.

INDICATIONS & DOSAGE

Superficial skin infections due to susceptible organisms, acne vulgaris–
Adults and children: clean affected area; apply b.i.d.

CONTRAINDICATIONS & PRECAUTIONS

Contraindicated in patients with hypersensitivity to drug. Topical use of the drug can result in an overgrowth of nonsusceptible organisms, especially fungi. Drug is for external use only; do not use near the eyes, ears, nose, mouth, or other mucous membranes. Skin dryness may result because some of the topical preparations may contain alcohol.

ADVERSE REACTIONS

Common reactions are in italics; life-threatening reactions are in bold italics.
Skin: sensitivity reactions, erythema, *burning, dryness, pruritus.*

INTERACTIONS

None significant.

EFFECTS ON DIAGNOSTIC TESTS

None reported.

NURSING CONSIDERATIONS

Besides those related universally to drug therapy (see "How to use this book"), consider the following specific recommendations:

Assessment

- Obtain a baseline assessment of the patient's skin infections before therapy.
- Be alert for adverse reactions and drug interactions throughout therapy.
- Evaluate the patient's and family's knowledge about erythromycin therapy.

Nursing Diagnoses

- Impaired skin integrity related to acne blemishes.
- High risk for impaired skin integrity related to erythromycin-induced skin dryness.
- Knowledge deficit related to topical erythromycin therapy.

Planning and Implementation

Preparation and Administration

- ***Topical use:*** Wash, rinse, and dry affected area, then apply.

Monitoring

- Monitor effectiveness by regularly checking the skin in affected area.
- Monitor carefully. If no improvement or condition worsens, stop using and notify doctor.
- Monitor for adverse reactions and drug interactions by frequently evaluating the patient's skin for dryness.

Supportive Care

- Be prepared to discontinue the drug and notify doctor if adverse reactions occur.
- Keep in mind that prolonged use may cause overgrowth of nonsusceptible organisms.
- Avoid use near eyes, nose, mouth, or other mucous membranes.

Patient Teaching

- Teach patient how to apply medication and to avoid using the drug near his eyes, nose, mouth, or other mucous membranes.

Evaluation

In patients receiving erythromycin, appropriate evaluation statements may include:

- Patient states his skin infection has been resolved.
- Patient does not develop drug-induced erythema and dryness.
- Patient and family state an understanding of topical erythromycin therapy.

erythromycin (ophthalmic)

(er ith roe mye´ sin)

Ilotycin Ophthalmic

- *Classification:* antibiotic (erythromycin)
- *Pregnancy Risk Category:* C

HOW SUPPLIED

Ophthalmic ointment: 5 mg/g

ACTION

Mechanism: Inhibits protein synthesis by binding to the 50S ribosome in susceptible bacteria. Bacteriostatic, but may be bactericidal in high concentrations or against highly susceptible organisms.

Absorption: After topical ophthalmic administration, antibacterial concentrations of the drug are probably not reached within the aqueous humor or deep layers of the cornea. Unknown if drug is absorbed from mucous membranes.

INDICATIONS & DOSAGE

Acute and chronic conjunctivitis, trachoma, other eye infections–

Adults and children: apply 0.5% ointment 1 or more times daily, depending upon severity of infection.

Prophylaxis of ophthalmia neonatorum–
Neonates: a ribbon of ointment approximately 0.5 to 1 cm long placed in the lower conjunctival sacs shortly after birth.

CONTRAINDICATIONS & PRECAUTIONS

Contraindicated in patients with hypersensitivty to erythromycin. Because of the risk of development of bacterial resistance and overgrowth of other organisms, use cautiously. Ophthalmic ointments can temporarily obscure the patient's vision, possibly increasing the risk of injury from falling.

ADVERSE REACTIONS

Common reactions are in italics; life-threatening reactions are in bold italics.
Eye: slowed corneal wound healing, blurred vision.
Other: overgrowth of nonsusceptible organisms with long-term use; hypersensitivity, including itching and burning eyes, urticaria, dermatitis, angioedema.

INTERACTIONS

None significant.

EFFECTS ON DIAGNOSTIC TESTS

None reported.

NURSING CONSIDERATIONS

Besides those related universally to drug therapy (see "How to use this book"), consider the following specific recommendations:

Assessment
- Obtain a baseline assessment of allergies before therapy.
- Be alert for adverse reactions or drug interactions throughout therapy.
- Evaluate the patient's and family's knowledge about ophthalmic erythromycin.

Nursing Diagnoses
- Altered protection related to ocular infection.
- Sensory/perceptual alterations (visual) related to erythromycin-induced blurred vision.
- Knowledge deficit related to ophthalmic erythromycin therapy.

Planning and Implementation

Preparation and Administration
- Store at room temperature in tightly sealed, light-resistant container.
- Wash hands before and after administration.
- Cleanse eye area of excessive exudate before application.
- For prophylaxis of ophthalmia neonatorum, apply ointment no later than 1 hour after birth.

Monitoring
- Monitor effectiveness by checking for the presence of microorganisms by culture test of the eye.
- Observe amount, color, and consistency of exudate.
- Check patient's vision.

Supportive Care
- Apply warm, moist compress to aid removal of dried exudate before administration.
- Use safety precautions if vision is impaired. Assist with activities.
- Use only when sensitivity studies show effectiveness; drug has limited antibacterial spectrum.
- Do not use in infection of unknown etiology.

Patient Teaching
- Teach the patient how to apply ointment. Advise him to wash hands before and after administration of ointment and warn patient not to touch tip of applicator to eye or surrounding tissue.
- Instruct patient to apply light finger pressure on lacrimal sac for 1 minute after administration. Caution patient not to scratch or rub eyes.
- Warn the patient that ointment may cause blurred vision.

• Instruct the patient to watch for signs of sensitivity (itching lids, swelling, constant burning). If signs develop, stop drug and inform doctor immediately.
• Warn patient to avoid sharing washcloths and towels with family members during infection.
• Advise the patient not to share eye medication with family members. If a family member develops the same symptoms, instruct him to contact the doctor.

Evaluation
In patients receiving erythromycin, appropriate evaluation statements may include:
• Patient remains free from signs and symptoms of infection.
• Patient reports decrease or absence in visual blurring.
• Patient and family state an understanding of ophthalmic erythromycin therapy.

esmolol hydrochloride
(ess´ moe lol)
Brevibloc

• *Classification:* antiarrhythmic ($beta_1$-adrenergic blocking agent)
• *Pregnancy Risk Category:* C

HOW SUPPLIED
Injection: 10 mg/ml in 10-ml vials; 250 mg/ml in 10-ml ampules

ACTION
Mechanism: A class II antiarrhythmic that is an ultrashort-acting beta-adrenergic blocking agent. Decreases heart rate, myocardial contractility, and blood pressure.
Absorption: Immediate after I.V. infusion.
Distribution: Rapidly distributed throughout the plasma and is 35% protein-bound.
Metabolism: Hydrolyzed rapidly by plasma esterases.
Excretion: By the kidneys as metabolites. Half-life: Distribution half-life is about 2 minutes. Elimination half-life is about 9 minutes.
Onset, peak, duration: Onset and peak drug effects are variable and depend upon loading dose; patients are titrated to maximal drug effect. Duration of action is short, lasting only 5 to 10 minutes after infusion is discontinued.

INDICATIONS & DOSAGE
Supraventricular tachycardia –
Adults: loading dose is 500 mcg/kg/minute by I.V. infusion over 1 minute, followed by a 4-minute maintenance infusion of 50 mcg/kg/minute. If adequate response does not occur within 5 minutes, repeat the loading dose. followed by a maintenance infusion of 100 mcg/kg/minute for 4 minutes. Maximum maintenance infusion is 200 mcg/kg/minute.

CONTRAINDICATIONS & PRECAUTIONS
Contraindicated in patients hypersensitive to the drug; patients with cardiac failure, cardiogenic shock, second- or third-degree atrioventricular block, or sinus bradycardia (less than 45 beats/minute) because the drug may worsen cardiac depression. Esmolol is not for long-term use when transfer to another agent is anticipated.

Use with caution in atopic patients, and in patients with bronchial asthma, emphysema, or bronchitis because it may precipitate bronchospasm; in patients with diabetes, because it may mask tachycardia associated with hypoglycemia.

ADVERSE REACTIONS
Common reactions are in italics; life-threatening reactions are in bold italics.

CNS: dizziness, somnolence, headache, agitation, fatigue.
CV: *hypotension* (sometimes with diaphoresis).
GI: *nausea,* vomiting.
Local: inflammation and induration at infusion site.
Other: ***bronchospasm.***

INTERACTIONS

Digoxin: esmolol may increase serum digoxin levels by 10% to 20%.
Morphine: may increase esmolol blood levels. Titrate esmolol carefully.
Reserpine (and other catecholamine-depleting drugs): may cause additive bradycardia and hypotension. Titrate esmolol carefully.
Succinylcholine: esmolol may prolong neuromuscular blockade.

EFFECTS ON DIAGNOSTIC TESTS

None reported.

NURSING CONSIDERATIONS

Besides those related universally to drug therapy (see "How to use this book"), consider the following specific recommendations:

Assessment

- Obtain a baseline assessment of the patient's heart rate and rhythm before therapy.
- Be alert for adverse reactions and drug interactions throughout therapy.
- Evaluate the patient's and family's knowledge about esmolol therapy.

Nursing Diagnoses

- Decreased cardiac output related to ineffectiveness of esmolol therapy.
- Altered tissue perfusion (cerebral) related to esmolol-induced hypotension.
- Knowledge deficit related to esmolol therapy.

Planning and Implementation

Preparation and Administration

- Be aware that esmolol is recommended only for short-term use, no longer than 48 hours.
- ***I.V. use:*** Before infusion, reconstitute 2 ampules with 20 ml of diluent to yield a concentration of 10 mg/ml. Administer loading dose of 500 mcg/kg over 1 minute, followed by a 4-minute maintenance infusion of 50 mcg/kg/minute using a controlled infusion device. Drug should never be administered as direct I.V. push.
- Be aware that esmolol solutions are incompatible with diazepam, furosemide, sodium bicarbonate, and thiopental sodium.
- Be aware that when patient's heart rate becomes stable, esmolol will be replaced by alternative (longer-acting) antiarrhythmics, such as propranolol, digoxin, or verapamil. As the replacement drug is started, the esmolol infusion should be gradually reduced over 1 hour.

Monitoring

- Monitor effectiveness by evaluating continuous ECG recordings as well as blood pressure and heart rate. Up to 50% of all patients treated with esmolol develop hypotension. Monitor closely, especially if patient's pretreatment blood pressure was low.
- Monitor patient for thrombophlebitis at I.V. site regularly.

Supportive Care

- Notify the doctor if hypotension occurs. Hypotension can usually be reversed within 30 minutes by decreasing the dose, or if necessary, by stopping the infusion.
- Change I.V. site if a local reaction develops at the infusion site. Avoid butterfly needles.
- Institute safety precautions if adverse CNS reactions occur.

Patient Teaching

- Inform patient of the need for continuous ECG, blood pressure, and heart rate monitoring to assess effectiveness of drug and detect adverse reactions.

Evaluation

In patients receiving esmolol, appropriate evaluation statements may include:

• Patient's ECG reveals arrhythmia has been corrected.
• Patient's blood pressure remains normal throughout esmolol therapy.
• Patient and family state an understanding of esmolol therapy.

estazolam

(es tay´ zoe lam)
ProSom

• Controlled Substance Schedule IV
• *Classification:* hypnotic (benzodiazepine)
• *Pregnancy Risk Category:* X

HOW SUPPLIED

Tablets: 1 mg, 2 mg

ACTION

Mechanism: Acts on the limbic system and thalamus of the CNS by binding to specific benzodiazepine receptors.
Absorption: Tablets are well absorbed.
Distribution: About 93% protein bound.
Metabolism: Extensively metabolized; metabolites are excreted primarily in the urine.
Excretion: Less than 5% of a 2-mg dose is excreted unchanged in the urine; only 4% of the dose appears in the feces. Half-life: Elimination half-life varies from 10 to 24 hours.
Onset, peak, duration: Peak plasma concentrations occur within 2 hours after dosing (range 30 minutes to 6 hours).

INDICATIONS & DOSAGE

Adjunctive treatment of insomnia –
Adults: 1 mg P.O. h.s. Some patients may require 2 mg.
Elderly patients: 1 mg P.O. h.s. Use higher doses with extreme care. Frail elderly or debilitated patients may take 0.5 mg, but this low dose may be only marginally effective.

CONTRAINDICATIONS & PRECAUTIONS

Contraindicated in patients with a history of hypersensitivity to benzodiazepines and during pregnancy because of the risk of fetal damage. Use with caution in elderly and debilitated patients and in those with hepatic impairment, compromised respiratory function, depression, impaired renal function, or sleep apnea.

ADVERSE REACTIONS

Common reactions are in italics; life-threatening reactions are in bold italics.
CNS: fatigue, dizziness, *daytime drowsiness,* headache.

INTERACTIONS

Alcohol, CNS depressants including antihistamines, opiate analgesics, and other benzodiazepines: increased CNS depression. Avoid concomitant use.
Cimetidine, oral contraceptives, disulfiram, isoniazid: may impair the metabolism and clearance of benzodiazepines and prolong their plasma half-life. Monitor for increased CNS depression.
Rifampin, cigarette smoking: may increase metabolism and clearance and decrease plasma half-life. Monitor for decreased effectiveness.
Theophylline: pharmacologic antagonism. Monitor for decreased effectiveness.

EFFECTS ON DIAGNOSTIC TESTS

AST (SGOT): increased levels.

NURSING CONSIDERATIONS

Besides those related universally to drug therapy (see "How to use this book"), consider the following specific recommendations:

Assessment
• Obtain a baseline assessment of sleeping patterns and CNS status before therapy.
• Be alert for adverse reactions and drug interactions throughout therapy.
• Evaluate the patient's and family's knowledge about estazolam therapy.
Nursing Diagnoses
• Sleep pattern disturbance related to underlying patient problem.
• High risk for trauma related to adverse CNS reactions caused by estazolam.
• Knowledge deficit related to estazolam therapy.
Planning and Implementation
Preparation and Administration
• Before leaving the bedside, make sure the patient has swallowed the medication.
Monitoring
• Monitor effectiveness regularly by evaluating the patient's ability to sleep.
• Monitor CNS status for evidence of adverse reactions.
• After drug discontinuation, be alert for possible withdrawal symptoms.
Supportive Care
• After administration, institute safety precautions: remove cigarettes; keep bed rails up, and supervise or assist ambulation.
• Do not discontinue the drug abruptly after prolonged use (possibly after 6 weeks of continuous therapy) because withdrawal symptoms may occur.
• Take precautions to prevent hoarding or self-overdosing, especially by patients who are depressed, suicidal, or have a history of drug abuse.
Patient Teaching
• Encourage the patient to report severe drowsiness or dizziness so the doctor can be consulted for change of dose or drug.
• Instruct the patient to remain in bed after taking drug and to call for assistance to use the bathroom.
• Warn the patient about dizziness and drowsiness. Tell the patient to avoid hazardous activities that require mental alertness until the adverse CNS effects are known.
• Tell the patient not to increase dosage but to inform the doctor that the drug is no longer effective. Also advise patient to notify the doctor if adverse reactions develop.
• Warn the patient that additive depressant effects can occur if alcohol is consumed on the day after use of the drug.
Evaluation
In patients receiving estazolam, appropriate evaluation statements may include:
• Patient states drug was effective in inducing sleep.
• Patient's safety is maintained.
• Patient and family state an understanding of estazolam therapy.

esterified estrogens
(es ter´ i fied ess´ troe jenz)
Estratab, Estromed†, Menest, Neo-Estrone†

• *Classification:* estrogen replacement, antineoplastic (estrogen)
• *Pregnancy Risk Category:* X

HOW SUPPLIED
Tablets: 0.3 mg, 0.625 mg, 1.25 mg, 2.5 mg

ACTION
Mechanism: Increases the synthesis of DNA, RNA, and protein in responsive tissues. Also reduces release of follicle-stimulating hormone and luteinizing hormone from the pituitary.
Distribution: Approximately 50% to 80% plasma protein-bound, particularly the estradiol-binding globulin. Distribution occurs throughout the

body with highest concentrations appearing in fat.
Metabolism: Primarily in the liver, where they are conjugated with sulfate and glucuronide.
Excretion: Through the kidneys, in the form of sulfate or glucuronide conjugates.

INDICATIONS & DOSAGE

Inoperable prostatic cancer–
Men: 1.25 to 2.5 mg P.O. t.i.d.
Breast cancer–
Men and postmenopausal women: 10 mg P.O. t.i.d. for 3 or more months.
Hypogonadism, castration, primary ovarian failure–
Women: 2.5 mg P.O. daily to t.i.d. in cycles of 3 weeks on, 1 week off.
Menopausal symptoms–
Women: average 0.3 to 3.75 mg P.O. daily in cycles of 3 weeks on, 1 week off.

CONTRAINDICATIONS & PRECAUTIONS

Contraindicated in patients with thrombophlebitis or thromboembolism because of drug's association with thromboembolic disorders; estrogen-responsive carcinoma (breast or genital tract cancer); undiagnosed abnormal genital bleeding; during pregnancy because drug may be fetotoxic; and in breast-feeding women because drug may adversely affect the infant.

Use cautiously in patients with disorders that may be aggravated by fluid and electrolyte accumulation, such as asthma, seizure disorders, migraine, or cardiac, renal, or hepatic dysfunction. Carefully monitor female patients who have breast nodules, fibrocystic breast disease, or a family history of breast cancer. Because of the risk of thromboembolism, therapy with esterified estrogens should be discontinued at least 1 week before elective surgical procedures associated with an increased incidence of thromboembolism.

ADVERSE REACTIONS

Common reactions are in italics; life-threatening reactions are in bold italics.
CNS: headache, dizziness, chorea, depression, libido changes, lethargy.
CV: thrombophlebitis; ***thromboembolism;*** hypertension; edema; ***increased risk of stroke, pulmonary embolism, and myocardial infarction.***
EENT: worsening of myopia or astigmatism, intolerance to contact lenses.
GI: *nausea,* vomiting, abdominal cramps, bloating, diarrhea, constipation, anorexia, increased appetite, weight changes, pancreatitis.
GU: in women–breakthrough bleeding, altered menstrual flow, dysmenorrhea, amenorrhea, cervical erosion, altered cervical secretions, enlargement of uterine fibromas, vaginal candidiasis. In men–gynecomastia, testicular atrophy, impotence.
Hepatic: cholestatic jaundice.
Metabolic: hyperglycemia, hypercalcemia, folic acid deficiency.
Skin: melasma, rash, acne, hirsutism or hair loss, seborrhea, oily skin.
Other: breast changes (tenderness, enlargement, secretion).

INTERACTIONS

None significant.

EFFECTS ON DIAGNOSTIC TESTS

Free triiodothyronine resin: decreased uptake.
Glucose tolerance: impaired.
Pregnanediol excretion: decreased.
Serum folate, pyridoxine, and antithrombin III: decreased concentrations.
Sulfobromophthalein retention, prothrombin time and clotting Factors VII to X, and norepinephrine-induced platelet aggregability: increased.
Thyroid-binding globulin: increased concentration.

Total thyroid concentrations (measured by protein-bound iodine or total thyroxine): increased.
Triglyceride, glucose, and phospholipid: increased levels.

NURSING CONSIDERATIONS

Besides those related universally to drug therapy (see "How to use this book"), consider the following specific recommendations:

Assessment

- Obtain a baseline assessment of the patient's underlying condition before initiating therapy with esterified estrogens.
- Be alert for adverse reactions and drug interactions throughout therapy.
- Evaluate the patient's and family's knowledge about esterified estrogen therapy.

Nursing Diagnoses

- Altered protection related to the patient's underlying condition.
- Altered (cerebral, peripheral, pulmonary, or myocardial) tissue perfusion related to high risk for esterified estrogens to cause thromboembolism.
- Knowledge deficit related to therapy with esterified estrogens.

Planning and Implementation

Preparation and Administration

- ***P.O. use:*** Administer oral preparations at mealtimes or bedtime (if only one daily dose is required) to minimize nausea.

Monitoring

- Monitor effectiveness by regularly assessing the patient's underlying condition for signs of improvement.
- Monitor patient for thromboemboli formation by noting any changes in cerebral or cardiopulmonary function or peripheral circulation.
- Monitor the patient's blood glucose levels for alterations.

Supportive Care

- Withhold drug and notify the doctor if a thromboembolic event is suspected; be prepared to provide supportive care as indicated.
- Alert the pathologist if a specimen is obtained during estrogen therapy.
- Be prepared to adjust diabetic patients' therapeutic regimen if blood glucose levels rise during therapy with esterified estrogens.
- Institute safety measures if adverse CNS reactions occur.
- Obtain an order for an antiemetic, antidiarrheal, or laxative agent, as needed.
- Prepare patient for body changes that may occur, such as loss of hair.

Patient Teaching

- Warn the patient to report immediately abdominal pain; pain, numbness, or stiffness in legs or buttocks; pressure or pain in chest; shortness of breath; severe headaches; visual disturbances, such as blind spots, flashing lights, or blurriness; vaginal bleeding or discharge; breast lumps; swelling of hands or feet; yellow skin and sclera; dark urine; and light-colored stools.
- Explain to patients on cyclic therapy for postmenopausal symptoms that, although withdrawal bleeding may occur in week off drug, fertility has not been restored; ovulation does not occur.
- Teach female patients how to perform routine breast self-examination.
- Teach the patient that medical supervision is essential during prolonged therapy with esterified estrogens.
- Inform the patient that nausea may be relieved by taking medication at mealtimes or bedtime (if only one daily dose is required).
- Tell diabetic patients to report symptoms of hyperglycemia or glycosuria.
- Tell patients who become pregnant during therapy with esterified estrogens to stop taking the drug immediately because it may adversely affect the fetus.
- Give the patient the package insert describing adverse reactions to ester-

ified estrogens, and also provide verbal explanation.

Evaluation

In patients receiving esterified estrogens, appropriate evaluation statements may include:

• Patient exhibits improved health as a result of therapy with esterified estrogens.

• Patient does not experience a thromboembolic event during therapy with esterified estrogens.

• Patient and family state an understanding of therapy with esterified estrogens.

estradiol (oestradiol)

(ess tra dye´ ole)

Estrace**, Estrace Vaginal Cream, Estraderm

estradiol cypionate

depGynogen, Depo-Estradiol, Dura-Estrin, E-Cypionate, Estro-Cyp, Estrofem, Estroject-L.A., Estronol-LA

estradiol valerate (oestradiol valerate)

Delestrogen, Dioval, Duragen 10, Duragen 20, Duragen 40, Estradiol L.A., Estraval, Estraval P.A., Estra-L 20, Estra-L 40, Feminate, Femogex, Gynogen L.A., L.A.E., Menaval, Primogyn Depot‡, Ru-Est-Span 20, Ru-Est-Span 40, Valergen 10, Valergen 20, Valergen 40

• *Classification:* estrogen replacement, antineoplastic (estrogen)

• *Pregnancy Risk Category:* X

HOW SUPPLIED

estradiol

Tablets (micronized): 1 mg, 2 mg**

Transdermal: 4 mg/10 cm² (delivers 0.05 mg/24 hours); 8 mg/20 cm² (delivers 0.1 mg/24 hours)

Vaginal cream (in nonliquefying base): 0.1 mg/g

estradiol cypionate

Injection (in oil): 1 mg/ml, 5 mg/ml

estradiol valerate

Injection (in oil): 10 mg/ml, 20 mg/ml, 40 mg/ml

ACTION

Mechanism: Increases the synthesis of DNA, RNA, and protein in responsive tissues. Also reduces release of follicle-stimulating hormone and luteinizing hormone from the pituitary.

Absorption: After I.M. administration, absorption begins rapidly and continues for days. The cypionate and valerate esters administered in oil have prolonged durations of action because of slow absorption.

Topically applied estradiol is absorbed readily into the systemic circulation.

Distribution: Estradiol and the other natural estrogens are approximately 50% to 80% plasma protein-bound, particularly the estradiol-binding globulin. Distribution occurs throughout the body, with highest concentrations in fat.

Metabolism: Primarily in the liver, where they are conjugated with sulfate and glucuronide. Because of the rapid rate of metabolism, nonesterified forms of estrogen, including estradiol, must usually be administered daily.

Excretion: Primarily through the kidneys in the form of sulfate and/or glucuronide conjugates.

INDICATIONS & DOSAGE

Menopausal symptoms, hypogonadism, castration, primary ovarian failure–

Women: 1 to 2 mg P.O. daily, in cycles of 21 days on and 7 days off, or cycles of 5 days on and 2 days off; or 0.2 to 1 mg I.M. weekly.

Kraurosis vulvae–

Women: 1 to 1.5 mg I.M. once or more per week.

Atrophic vaginitis–
Women: 2 to 4 g intravaginal applications of cream daily for 1 to 2 weeks. When vaginal mucosa is restored, begin maintenance dosage of 1 g one to three times weekly.
Menopausal symptoms–
Women: 1 to 5 mg (cypionate) I.M. q 3 to 4 weeks. Or 5 to 20 mg (valerate) I.M., repeated once after 2 to 3 weeks.
Postpartum breast engorgement–
Women: 10 to 25 mg (valerate) I.M. at end of first stage of labor.
Inoperable breast cancer–
Women: 10 mg P.O. (oral estradiol) t.i.d. for 3 months.
Treatment of moderate to severe symptoms of menopause, female hypogonadism, female castration, primary ovarian failure, and atrophic conditions caused by deficient endogenous estrogen production–
Women: place one Estraderm transdermal patch on trunk of the body twice weekly. Administer on an intermittent cyclic schedule (3 weeks of therapy followed by discontinuation for 1 week).
Inoperable prostatic cancer–
Men: 30 mg (valerate) I.M. q 1 to 2 weeks. Or, 1 to 2 mg (oral estradiol) t.i.d.

CONTRAINDICATIONS & PRECAUTIONS

Contraindicated in patients with thrombophlebitis or thromboembolism, estrogen-responsive carcinoma (breast or genital tract cancer), or undiagnosed abnormal genital bleeding; and in pregnant or breast-feeding women.

Use cautiously in patients with disorders that may be aggravated by fluid and electrolyte accumulation, such as asthma, seizure disorders, migraine, or cardiac, renal, or hepatic dysfunction. Carefully monitor female patients who have breast nodules, fibrocystic breast disease, or a family history of breast cancer. Because of the risk of thromboembolism, therapy with this drug should be discontinued at least 1 week before elective surgical procedures associated with an increased incidence of thromboembolism.

The 2-mg tablet of Estrace contains tartrazine dye, which may cause hypersensitivity reactions (bronchial asthma, anaphylaxis) in rare individuals. These individuals are commonly also sensitive to aspirin and have nasal polyps.

ADVERSE REACTIONS

Common reactions are in italics; life-threatening reactions are in bold italics.
CNS: headache, dizziness, chorea, depression, libido changes, lethargy.
CV: thrombophlebitis, ***thromboembolism,*** hypertension, edema.
EENT: worsening of myopia or astigmatism, intolerance to contact lenses.
GI: *nausea,* vomiting, abdominal cramps, bloating, diarrhea, constipation, anorexia, increased appetite, weight changes, pancreatitis.
GU: in women–breakthrough bleeding, altered menstrual flow, dysmenorrhea, amenorrhea, cervical erosion, altered cervical secretions, enlargement of uterine fibromas, vaginal candidiasis. In men–gynecomastia, testicular atrophy, impotence.
Hepatic: cholestatic jaundice.
Metabolic: hyperglycemia, hypercalcemia, folic acid deficiency.
Skin: melasma, urticaria, acne, seborrhea, oily skin, hirsutism or hair loss.
Other: breast changes (tenderness, enlargement, secretion), leg cramps.

INTERACTIONS

None significant.

EFFECTS ON DIAGNOSTIC TESTS

Free triiodothyronine resin: decreased uptake.
Glucose tolerance: impaired.
Pregnanediol excretion: decreased.

Serum folate, pyridoxine, and antithrombin III: decreased concentrations.
Sulfobromophthalein retention, prothrombin time, clotting Factors VII to X, and norepinephrine-induced platelet aggregability: increased.
Thyroid-binding globulin: increased concentration.
Total thyroid concentrations (measured by protein-bound iodine or total thyroxine): increased.
Triglyceride, glucose, and phospholipid: increased levels.

NURSING CONSIDERATIONS

Besides those related universally to drug therapy (see "How to use this book"), consider the following specific recommendations:

Assessment

• Obtain a baseline assessment of the patient's underlying condition before therapy.
• Be alert for adverse reactions and drug interactions throughout therapy.
• Evaluate the patient's and family's knowledge about estradiol therapy.

Nursing Diagnoses

• Sexual dysfunction related to the patient's underlying hormonal deficiency.
• Altered (cerebral, peripheral, pulmonary, or myocardial) tissue perfusion related to high risk for estradiol to cause thromboembolism.
• Knowledge deficit related to estradiol therapy.

Planning and Implementation

Preparation and Administration

• Ask patient about allergies, especially to foods or plants, before administering drug.
• ***P.O. use:*** Administer oral preparations at mealtimes or bedtime (if only one daily dose is required) to minimize nausea.
• ***I.M. use:*** Before injection, make sure drug is well dispersed in solution by rolling vial between palms. Inject deep I.M. into large muscle. Rotate injection sites to prevent muscle atrophy.
• Never administer drug I.V.
• ***Transdermal use:*** Be aware that women who are currently taking oral estrogen can begin Estraderm transdermal patch therapy 1 week after withdrawal of oral therapy or sooner if symptoms appear before the end of the week. Patch should be applied to the trunk of the body.

Monitoring

• Monitor effectiveness by regularly assessing the patient's underlying condition for signs of improvement.
• Monitor patient for thromboemboli formation by noting any changes in cerebral or cardiopulmonary function or peripheral circulation.
• Monitor the patient's blood glucose levels for alterations.

Supportive Care

• Withhold drug and notify the doctor if a thromboembolic event is suspected; be prepared to provide supportive care as indicated.
• Alert the pathologist if a specimen is obtained during estrogen therapy.
• Be prepared to adjust diabetic patients' therapeutic regimen if blood glucose levels rise during therapy with estradiol.
• Institute safety measures if adverse CNS reactions occur.
• Obtain an order for an antiemetic, antidiarrheal, or laxative agent, as needed.
• Prepare patient for body changes that may occur, such as loss of hair.

Patient Teaching

• Instruct patient how to administer vaginal cream or transdermal patch if prescribed.
• Warn the patient to report immediately abdominal pain; pain, numbness, or stiffness in legs or buttocks; pressure or pain in chest; shortness of breath; severe headaches; visual disturbances, such as blind spots, flashing lights, or blurriness; vaginal bleeding or discharge; breast lumps;

swelling of hands or feet; yellow skin and sclera; dark urine; and light-colored stools.

• Explain to patients on cyclic therapy for postmenopausal symptoms that, although withdrawal bleeding may occur in week off drug, fertility has not been restored; ovulation does not occur.

• Teach female patients how to perform routine breast self-examination.

• Teach the patient that medical supervision is essential during prolonged therapy with estradiol. Be aware that risk of endometrial cancer is increased in postmenopausal women who take estrogens for more than 1 year.

• Tell diabetic patients to report symptoms of hyperglycemia or glycosuria.

• Give the patient the package insert describing adverse reactions to estradiol, and also provide verbal explanation.

Evaluation

In patients receiving estradiol, appropriate evaluation statements may include:

• Patient hormonal deficiency improves as a result of estradiol therapy.

• Patient does not experience a thromboembolic event during estradiol therapy.

• Patient and family state an understanding of estradiol therapy.

estramustine phosphate sodium

(ess tra muss´ teen)

Emcyt, Estracyst‡

• *Classification:* antineoplastic (estrogen, aklylating agent)

• *Pregnancy Risk Category:* D

HOW SUPPLIED

Capsules: 140 mg

ACTION

Mechanism: A combination of estrogen and an alkylating agent; acts by its ability to bind selectively to a protein present in the human prostate.

Absorption: After oral administration, about 75% of a dose is absorbed across the GI tract.

Distribution: Widely distributed into body tissues.

Metabolism: Extensively metabolized in the liver.

Excretion: Drug and metabolites are eliminated primarily in feces, with a small amount excreted in urine. Half-life: Terminal phase of plasma elimination has a half-life of 20 hours.

INDICATIONS & DOSAGE

Palliative treatment of metastatic or progressive cancer of the prostate–

Adults: 10 to 16 mg/kg P.O. in three to four divided doses. Usual dosage is 14 mg/kg daily. Therapy should continue for up to 3 months and, if successful, be maintained as long as the patient responds.

CONTRAINDICATIONS & PRECAUTIONS

Contraindicated in patients with a history of hypersensitivity to the drug or to estradiol or mechlorethamine; cross-sensitivity may occur; in patients with peptic ulcers, severe liver disease, cardiac disease, or impaired bone marrow function because it may worsen these conditions.

Use cautiously in patients with thromboembolic disorders, cerebrovascular disorders, or coronary artery disease because of the drug's cardiovascular toxicity.

ADVERSE REACTIONS

Common reactions are in italics; life-threatening reactions are in bold italics.

Blood: leukopenia, thrombocytopenia.

CV: ***myocardial infarction, CVA,*** *edema,* ***pulmonary emboli,*** thrombophlebitis, CHF, hypertension.

GI: *nausea, vomiting,* diarrhea.
Skin: rash, pruritus.
Other: *painful gynecomastia and breast tenderness,* thinning of hair, hyperglycemia, fluid retention.

INTERACTIONS

Calcium-rich foods (milk and dairy products): impaired absorption of estramustine.

EFFECTS ON DIAGNOSTIC TESTS

Glucose tolerance: decreased.
Metyrapone test: reduced response.
Platelet aggregability (norepinephrine-induced): increased.

NURSING CONSIDERATIONS

Besides those related universally to drug therapy (see "How to use this book"), consider the following specific recommendations:

Assessment

- Obtain a baseline assessment of CBC, ECG, glucose and glucose tolerance testing, chest X-ray, serum calcium, and weight before therapy.
- Be alert for adverse reactions or drug interactions throughout therapy.
- Evaluate the patient's and family's knowledge about estramustine therapy.

Nursing Diagnoses

- High risk for fluid volume deficit related to drug-induced nausea and vomiting.
- High risk for injury related to drug-induced adverse cardiac reactions.
- Knowledge deficit related to estramustine therapy.

Planning and Implementation

Preparation and Administration

- ***P.O. use:*** Each 140-mg capsule contains 12.5 mg sodium.
- Store capsules in refrigerator.
- Capsules should be taken with water or juice 1 hour before or 2 hours after meals.

Monitoring

- Monitor effectiveness by noting the results of follow-up diagnostic tests and overall physical status.
- Monitor effectiveness by obtaining glucose tolerance tests and daily glucose monitoring.
- Monitor CBC, calcium, and ECG periodically during therapy.
- Monitor daily weights and report any gains.
- Monitor blood pressure daily and watch for hypertension.
- Monitor the patient's hydration status if the patient develops nausea, vomiting, and diarrhea.
- Monitor for increased peripheral edema because estramustine may exaggerate preexisting peripheral edema or CHF.

Supportive Care

- Be prepared to withhold drug if serum calcium levels rise.
- Provide the patient with fluids if he develops nausea, vomiting, and diarrhea.
- Know that estramustine is a combination of estradiol and nitrogen mustard. It is effective in patients refractory to estrogen therapy alone.

Patient Teaching

- Encourage increased fluid intake to lessen the effects of hypercalcemia.
- Encourage patient to use contraceptives; drug is known to be teratogenic and mutagenic.
- Tell the patient that he may continue therapy as long as he is responding favorably.
- Tell the patient that breast tenderness to painful gynocomastia is common.
- Have patient or family member monitor patient's blood pressure daily.

Evaluation

In patients receiving estramustine, appropriate evaluation statements may include:

- Patient's fluid volume remains within established limits.

• Patient does not develop drug-induced adverse cardiac reactions.
• Patient and family state an understanding of estramustine therapy.

PHARMACOLOGIC CLASS

estrogens

chlorotrianisene
dienestrol
diethylstilbestrol
diethylstilbestrol diphosphate
esterified estrogens
estradiol
estradiol cypionate
estradiol valerate
estrogen and progestin
estrogenic substances, conjugated
estrone
estropipate
ethinyl estradiol
polyestradiol phosphate
quinestrol

OVERVIEW

Estrogens were first discovered in the urine of humans and animals in 1930. Since that time, numerous synthetic modifications of the naturally occurring estrogen molecules and completely synthetic estrogenic compounds have been developed.

Conjugated estrogens and estrogenic substances are normally obtained from the urine of pregnant mares. Other estrogens are manufactured synthetically. Of the six naturally occurring estrogens in humans, three (estradiol, estrone, and estriol) are present in significant quantities. The estrogens promote the development and maintenance of the female reproductive system and secondary sexual characteristics.

Estrogens inhibit the release of pituitary gonadotropins and also have various metabolic effects, including retention of fluid and electrolytes, retention and deposition in bone of calcium and phosphorus, and mild anabolic activity. Estrogens and estrogenic substances administered as drugs have effects related to endogenous estrogen's mechanism of action. They can mimic the action of endogenous estrogen when used as replacement therapy or produce such useful effects as inhibiting ovulation or inhibiting growth of certain hormone-sensitive cancers.

Use of estrogens is not without risk. Long-term use is associated with an increased incidence of endometrial cancer, gall bladder disease, and thromboembolic disease. Elevations in blood pressure often occur as well.

CLINICAL INDICATIONS AND ACTIONS

Moderate to severe vasomotor symptoms of menopause
Endogenous estrogens are markedly reduced in concentration after menopause. This commonly results in vasomotor symptoms, such as hot flashes and dizziness. Chlorotrianisene, diethylstilbestrol, estradiol cypionate, and ethinyl estradiol serve to mimic the action of endogenous estrogens in preventing these symptoms.

Atrophic vaginitis/kraurosis vulvae
Chlorotrianisene and diethylstilbestrol stimulate development, cornification, and secretory activity in vaginal tissues.

Carcinoma of the breast
Conjugated estrogens, diethylstilbestrol, esterified estrogens, estradiol, and ethinyl estradiol inhibit the growth of hormone-sensitive cancers in certain carefully selected male and post-menopausal female patients.

Carcinoma of the prostate
Chlorotrianisene, conjugated estrogens, diethylstilbestrol, esterified estrogens, estradiol, estradiol valerate, estrone, and ethinyl estradiol inhibit growth of hormone-sensitive cancer tissue in males with advanced disease.

Prophylaxis of postmenopausal osteoporosis
Conjugated estrogens serve to replace or augment the activity of endogenous estrogen in causing calcium and phosphate retention and preventing bone decalcification.
Contraception
Estrogens are also used in combination with progestins for ovulation control to prevent conception.

OVERVIEW OF ADVERSE REACTIONS
Acute reactions: changes in menstrual bleeding patterns (spotting, prolongation or absence of bleeding), abdominal cramps, swollen feet or ankles, bloated sensation (fluid and electrolyte retention), breast swelling and tenderness, weight gain, nausea, loss of appetite, headache, photosensitivity, loss of libido.

With chronic administration: increased blood pressure (sometimes into the hypertensive range), thromboembolic disease, cholestatic jaundice, benign hepatomas, endometrial carcinoma (rare). Risk of thromboembolic disease increases markedly with cigarette smoking, especially in women older than age 35.

REPRESENTATIVE COMBINATIONS
Ethynodiol diacetate with ethinyl estradiol: Demulen; with mestranol: Ovulen.

Estradiol with testosterone: Testrolix; with testosterone and chlorobutanol: Depo-Testadiol.

Estradiol cypionate with testosterone: D-Diol, Dep-Tesestro, Dep-Testradiol, Duo-Cyp, Duo-Ionate, Duracrine, Estran-C, Menoject, T.E. Ionate.

Estradiol valerate with testosterone enanthate: Bi-Nate, Deladumone, Delatestadiol, Duoval-P.A., Estran E.V., Estra-Testrin, Teev, Tesogen, Testanate, Valertest.

Estrogenic substances (conjugated) with meprobamate: Milprem, PMB 200, PMB 400; with methyltestosterone: Menotab-M, Premarin with Methyltestosterone.

Estrone with hydrocortisone acetate: Estro-V HC; with estradiol: Tri-Orapin; with estradiol and vitamin B_{12}: Ovest, Ovulin; with estriol and estradiol: Estro Plus, Hormonin; with potassium estrone sulfate: Dura-Keelin, Estro-Plus, Gynlin, Mer-Estrone, Sodestrin, Spanestrin; with testosterone: Andesterone, Anestro, Di-Hormone, Di-Met, Diorapin, Di-Steroid, Estratest; with testosterone and vitamins: Android-G, Geratic Forte, Geriamic, Geritag; with testosterone, vitamins and minerals: Geramine.

---

estrogens, conjugated (estrogenic substances, conjugated; oestrogens, conjugated)
OESTROGENS CONJUGATES)
(ess´ troe jenz)
C.E.S.†, Conjugated Estrogens C.S.D.†, Premarin, Premarin Intravenous, Progens

• *Classification:* estrogen replacement, antineoplastic, antiosteoporotic (estrogen)
• *Pregnancy Risk Category:* X

HOW SUPPLIED
Tablets: 0.3 mg, 0.625 mg, 0.9 mg, 1.25 mg, 2.5 mg
Injection: 25 mg/5 ml
Vaginal cream: 0.625 mg/g

ACTION
Mechanism: Increases the synthesis of DNA, RNA, and protein in responsive tissues. Also reduces release of follicle-stimulating hormone and luteinizing hormone from the pituitary.
Absorption: Not well characterized.

After I.M. administration, absorption begins rapidly and continues for days.
Distribution: Conjugated estrogens are approximately 50% to 80% plasma protein-bound, particularly the estradiol-binding globulin. Distribution occurs throughout the body, with highest concentrations in fat.
Metabolism: Primarily in the liver, where they are conjugated with sulfate and glucuronide. Because of the rapid rate of metabolism, nonesterified forms of estrogen, including estradiol, must usually be administered daily.
Excretion: Primarily through the kidneys, in the form of sulfate or glucuronide conjugates, or both.

INDICATIONS & DOSAGE

Abnormal uterine bleeding (hormonal imbalance) –
Women: 25 mg I.V. or I.M. Repeat in 6 to 12 hours.
Breast cancer (at least 5 years after menopause) –
Women: 10 mg P.O. t.i.d. for 3 months or more.
Castration, primary ovarian failure, and osteoporosis –
Women: 1.25 mg P.O. daily in cycles of 3 weeks on, 1 week off.
Hypogonadism –
Women: 2.5 mg P.O. b.i.d. or t.i.d. for 20 consecutive days each month.
Menopausal symptoms –
Women: 0.3 to 1.25 mg P.O. daily in cycles of 3 weeks on, 1 week off.
Postpartum breast engorgement –
Women: 3.75 mg P.O. q 4 hours for five doses or 1.25 mg q 4 hours for 5 days.
Treatment of atrophic vaginitis, kraurosis vulvae associated with menopause –
Women: 2 to 4 g intravaginally on a cyclical basis (3 weeks on, 1 week off).
Inoperable prostatic cancer –
Men: 1.25 to 2.5 mg P.O. t.i.d.

CONTRAINDICATIONS & PRECAUTIONS

Contraindicated in patients with thrombophlebitis or thromboembolism because of the potential for increased clotting abnormalities; estrogen-responsive carcinoma (breast or genital tract cancer) because drug may stimulate tumor growth; undiagnosed abnormal genital bleeding; in pregnant women because drug may be fetotoxic; and in breast-feeding women because drug may have adverse effects upon the infant.

Use cautiously in patients with disorders that may be aggravated by fluid and electrolyte accumulation, such as asthma, seizure disorders, migraine, or cardiac, renal, or hepatic dysfunction. Carefully monitor female patients who have breast nodules, fibrocystic breast disease, or a family history of breast cancer. Because of the risk of thromboembolism, therapy with this drug should be discontinued at least 1 week before elective surgical procedures associated with an increased incidence of thromboembolism.

ADVERSE REACTIONS

Common reactions are in italics; life-threatening reactions are in bold italics.
CNS: headache, dizziness, chorea, depression, libido changes, lethargy.
CV: thrombophlebitis; ***thromboembolism;*** hypertension; edema; ***increased risk of stroke, pulmonary embolism, and myocardial infarction.***
EENT: worsening of myopia or astigmatism, intolerance to contact lenses.
GI: *nausea,* vomiting, abdominal cramps, bloating, diarrhea, constipation, anorexia, increased appetite, weight changes, pancreatitis.
GU: in women–breakthrough bleeding, altered menstrual flow, dysmenorrhea, amenorrhea, cervical erosion, altered cervical secretions, enlargement of uterine fibromas, vaginal

candidiasis. In men–gynecomastia, testicular atrophy, impotence.
Hepatic: cholestatic jaundice.
Metabolic: hyperglycemia, hypercalcemia, folic acid deficiency.
Skin: melasma, urticaria, acne, seborrhea, oily skin, flushing (when given rapidly I.V.), hirsutism or loss of hair.
Other: breast changes (tenderness, enlargement, secretion), leg cramps.

INTERACTIONS

None significant.

EFFECTS ON DIAGNOSTIC TESTS

Free triiodothyronine resin: decreased uptake.
Glucose tolerance: impaired.
Pregnanediol excretion: decreased.
Serum folate, pyridoxine, and antithrombin III: decreased concentrations.
Sulfobromophthalein retention, prothrombin time, clotting Factors VII to X, and norepinephrine-induced platelet aggregability: increased.
Thyroid-binding globulin: increased concentration.
Total thyroid concentrations (measured by protein-bound iodine or total thyroxine): increased.
Triglyceride, glucose, and phospholipid: increased levels.

NURSING CONSIDERATIONS

Besides those related universally to drug therapy (see "How to use this book"), consider the following specific recommendations:

Assessment

- Obtain a baseline assessment of the patient's underlying condition before initiating therapy with conjugated estrogens.
- Be alert for adverse reactions and drug interactions throughout therapy.
- Evaluate the patient's and family's knowledge about therapy with conjugated estrogens.

Nursing Diagnoses

- Sexual dysfunction related to hormonal imbalance.
- Altered (cerebral, peripheral, pulmonary, or myocardial) tissue perfusion related to high risk for conjugated estrogens to cause thromboembolism.
- Knowledge deficit related to therapy with conjugated estrogens.

Planning and Implementation

Preparation and Administration

- Refrigerate parenteral solution before reconstituting. Agitate gently after adding diluent.
- Be aware that I.M. or I.V. use is preferred for rapid treatment of dysfunctional uterine bleeding or reduction of surgical bleeding.
- ***P.O. use:*** Administer oral preparations at mealtimes or bedtime (if only one daily dose is required) to minimize nausea.
- ***I.M. use:*** Be aware that this route is usually only used to treat abnormal uterine bleeding caused by hormonal imbalance.
- ***I.V. use:*** Inject reconstituted drug directly into a vein over 1 to 5 minutes or into an established I.V. line containing free-flowing compatible solution; inject just distal to the infusion needle. Do not administer by intermittent or continuous infusion.

Monitoring

- Monitor effectiveness by regularly assessing the patient's underlying condition for signs of improvement.
- Monitor patient for thromboemboli formation by noting any changes in cerebral or cardiopulmonary function or peripheral circulation.
- Monitor the patient's blood glucose, calcium, and folic acid levels for alterations.

Supportive Care

- Withhold drug and notify the doctor if a thromboembolic event is suspected; be prepared to provide supportive care as indicated.

• Alert the pathologist if a specimen is obtained during estrogen therapy.
• Be prepared to adjust diabetic patients' therapeutic regimen if blood glucose levels rise during therapy with conjugated estrogens.
• Institute safety measures if adverse CNS reactions occur.
• Obtain an order for an antiemetic, antidiarrheal, or laxative agent, as needed.
• Prepare patient for possible body changes, such as loss of hair.

Patient Teaching

• Warn the patient to report immediately abdominal pain; pain, numbness, or stiffness in legs or buttocks; pressure or pain in chest; shortness of breath; severe headaches; visual disturbances, such as blind spots, flashing lights, or blurriness; vaginal bleeding or discharge; breast lumps; swelling of hands or feet; yellow skin and sclera; dark urine; and light-colored stools.
• Tell male patients on long-term therapy about possible gynecomastia and impotence, which will disappear when therapy is terminated.
• Explain to patients on cyclic therapy for postmenopausal symptoms that, although withdrawal bleeding may occur in week off drug, fertility has not been restored; ovulation does not occur.
• Teach female patients how to perform routine breast self-examination.
• Teach the patient that medical supervision is essential during prolonged therapy with conjugated estrogens.
• Inform the patient that nausea, when present, usually disappears with continued therapy. Nausea can be relieved by taking medication at mealtimes or bedtime (if only one daily dose is required).
• Tell diabetic patients to report symptoms of hyperglycemia or glycosuria.
• Tell patients who are planning to breast-feed not to take conjugated estrogens.
• Tell patients who become pregnant during therapy with conjugated estrogens to stop taking the drug immediately because it may adversely affect the fetus.
• Give the patient the package insert describing adverse reactions to conjugated estrogens, and also provide verbal explanation.

Evaluation

In patients receiving conjugated estrogens, appropriate evaluation statements may include:
• Patient states that sexual dysfunction improves.
• Patient does not experience a thromboembolic event during therapy with conjugated estrogens.
• Patient and family state an understanding of therapy with conjugated estrogens.

estrone (oestrone)

(ess´ trone)

Estrone "5", Estrone Aqueous, Estronol, Kestrone, Theelin Aqueous

• *Classification:* estrogen replacement (estrogen)
• *Pregnancy Risk Category:* X

HOW SUPPLIED

Injection (aqueous suspension): 2 mg/ml, 5 mg/ml

ACTION

Mechanism: Increases the synthesis of DNA, RNA, and protein in responsive tissues. Also reduces release of follicle-stimulating hormone and luteinizing hormone from the pituitary.

Absorption: After I.M. administration, absorption begins rapidly and continues for days. The cypionate and valerate esters administered in

oil have prolonged durations of action because of their slow absorption.
Distribution: Approximately 50% to 80% plasma protein-bound, particularly the estradiol-binding globulin. Distribution occurs throughout the body, with highest concentrations in fat.
Metabolism: Primarily metabolized in the liver, where they are conjugated with sulfate and glucuronide. Because of the rapid rate of metabolism, drug must usually be administered daily.
Excretion: Primarily through the kidneys in the form of sulfate and/or glucuronide conjugates.

INDICATIONS & DOSAGE

Atrophic vaginitis and menopausal symptoms–
Women: 0.1 to 0.5 mg I.M. two or three times weekly.
Female hypogonadism and primary ovarian failure–
Women: 0.1 to 1 mg I.M. weekly in single or divided doses.
Inoperable prostatic cancer–
Men: 2 to 4 mg I.M. 2 to 3 times weekly.

CONTRAINDICATIONS & PRECAUTIONS

Contraindicated in patients with thrombophlebitis or thromboembolism because of drug's association with thromboembolic disorders; estrogen-responsive carcinoma (breast or genital tract cancer); undiagnosed abnormal genital bleeding; and in pregnant and breast-feeding women.

Use cautiously in patients with disorders that may be aggravated by fluid and electrolyte accumulation, such as asthma, seizure disorders, migraine, or cardiac, renal, or hepatic dysfunction. Carefully monitor female patients who have breast nodules, fibrocystic breast disease, or a family history of breast cancer. Because of the risk of thromboembolism, therapy with this drug should be discontinued at least 1 week before elective surgical procedures associated with an increased incidence of thromboembolism.

ADVERSE REACTIONS

Common reactions are in italics; life-threatening reactions are in bold italics.
CNS: headache, dizziness, chorea, depression, libido changes, lethargy.
CV: thrombophlebitis, ***thromboembolism,*** hypertension, edema.
EENT: worsening of myopia or astigmatism, intolerance to contact lenses.
GI: *nausea,* vomiting, abdominal cramps, bloating, diarrhea, constipation, anorexia, increased appetite, weight changes, pancreatitis.
GU: in women–breakthrough bleeding, altered menstrual flow, dysmenorrhea, amenorrhea, cervical erosion, altered cervical secretions, enlargement of uterine fibromas, vaginal candidiasis. In men–gynecomastia, testicular atrophy, impotence.
Hepatic: cholestatic jaundice.
Metabolic: hyperglycemia, hypercalcemia, folic acid deficiency.
Skin: melasma, urticaria, acne, seborrhea, oily skin, hirsutism or hair loss.
Other: breast changes (tenderness, enlargement, secretion), leg cramps.

INTERACTIONS

None significant.

EFFECTS ON DIAGNOSTIC TESTS

Free triiodothyronine resin: decreased uptake.
Glucose tolerance: impaired.
Pregnanediol excretion: decreased.
Serum folate, pyridoxine, and antithrombin III: decreased concentrations.
Sulfobromophthalein retention, prothrombin time, clotting Factors VII to X, and norepinephrine-induced platelet aggregability: increased.
Thyroid-binding globulin: increased concentration.

Total thyroid concentrations (measured by protein-bound iodine or total thyroxine): increased.
Triglyceride, glucose, and phospholipid: increased levels.

NURSING CONSIDERATIONS

Besides those related universally to drug therapy (see "How to use this book"), consider the following specific recommendations:

Assessment

- Obtain a baseline assessment of the patient's underlying condition before therapy.
- Be alert for adverse reactions and drug interactions throughout therapy.
- Evaluate the patient's and family's knowledge about estrone therapy.

Nursing Diagnoses

- Impaired tissue integrity related to vaginitis.
- Altered (cerebral, peripheral, pulmonary, or myocardial) tissue perfusion related to high risk for estrone to cause thromboembolism.
- Knowledge deficit related to estrone therapy.

Planning and Implementation

Preparation and Administration

- ***I.M. use:*** Rotate injection sites to prevent muscle atrophy.

Monitoring

- Monitor effectiveness by regularly assessing the patient's underlying condition for signs of improvement.
- Monitor for thromboemboli formation by noting any changes in cerebral or cardiopulmonary function or peripheral circulation.
- Monitor the patient's blood glucose levels for alterations.

Supportive Care

- Withhold drug and notify the doctor if a thromboembolic event is suspected; be prepared to provide supportive care as indicated.
- Alert the pathologist if a specimen is obtained during estrone therapy.
- Be prepared to adjust diabetic patients' therapeutic regimen if blood glucose levels rise during therapy with estrone.
- Institute safety measures if adverse CNS reactions occur.
- Obtain an order for an antiemetic, antidiarrheal, or laxative agent, as needed.
- Prepare patient for possible body changes, such as loss of hair.

Patient Teaching

- Warn the patient to report immediately abdominal pain; pain, numbness, or stiffness in legs or buttocks; pressure or pain in chest; shortness of breath; severe headaches; visual disturbances, such as blind spots, flashing lights, or blurriness; vaginal bleeding or discharge; breast lumps; swelling of hands or feet; yellow skin and sclera; dark urine; and light-colored stools.
- Explain to patients on cyclic therapy for postmenopausal symptoms that, although withdrawal bleeding may occur in week off drug, fertility has not been restored; ovulation does not occur.
- Teach female patients how to perform routine breast self-examination.
- Teach the patient that medical supervision is essential during prolonged therapy with estrone. Be aware that use of estrogens is associated with increased risk of endometrial cancer and possible increased risk of breast cancer.
- Tell diabetic patients to report symptoms of hyperglycemia or glycosuria.
- Give the patient the package insert describing adverse reactions to estrone, and also provide verbal explanation.

Evaluation

In patients receiving estrone, appropriate evaluation statements may include:

- Patient's vaginal symptoms improve as a result of estrone therapy.
- Patient does not experience a

thromboembolic event during estrone therapy.
• Patient and family state an understanding of estrone therapy.

estropipate (piperazine estrone sulfate)
(ess´ troe pih pate)
Ogen

• *Classification:* estrogen replacement (estrone conjugate)
• *Pregnancy Risk Category:* X

HOW SUPPLIED
Tablets: 0.625 mg, 1.25 mg, 2.5 mg, 5 mg
Vaginal cream: 1.5 mg estropipate/g

ACTION
Mechanism: Increases synthesis of DNA, RNA, and protein in responsive tissues. Also reduces release of follicle-stimulating hormone and luteinizing hormone from the pituitary.
Distribution: Approximately 50% to 80% plasma protein-bound, particularly the estradiol-binding globulin. Distribution occurs throughout the body, with highest concentrations in fat.
Metabolism: Primarily in the liver, where it is conjugated with sulfate and glucuronide. Because of the rapid rate of metabolism, drug must usually be administered daily.
Excretion: Primarily through the kidneys in the form of sulfate and glucuronide conjugates, or both.

INDICATIONS & DOSAGE
Atrophic vaginitis, kraurosis vulvae, or moderate to severe vasomotor symptoms associated with menopause–
Women: 0.625 to 5 mg P.O. daily. Dosage is usually given on a cyclical, short-term basis.
Primary ovarian failure, female castration, or female hypogonadism–
Women: administer on a cyclical basis–1.25 to 7.5 mg P.O. daily for the first 3 weeks, followed by a rest period of 8 to 10 days. If bleeding does not occur by the end of the rest period, repeat cycle.
Atrophic vaginitis or kraurosis vulvae–
Women: 2 to 4 g of vaginal cream daily. Administration should be cyclic and short term (3 weeks on and 1 week off).

CONTRAINDICATIONS & PRECAUTIONS
Contraindicated in patients with thrombophlebitis or thromboembolism because of drug's association with thromboembolic disorders; estrogen-responsive carcinoma (breast or genital tract cancer); undiagnosed abnormal genital bleeding; and during pregnancy or breast-feeding.

Use cautiously in patients with disorders that may be aggravated by fluid and electrolyte accumulation, such as asthma, seizure disorders, migraine, or cardiac, renal, or hepatic dysfunction. Carefully monitor female patients who have breast nodules, fibrocystic breast disease, or a family history of breast cancer. Because of the risk of thromboembolism, therapy with this drug should be discontinued at least 1 week before elective surgical procedures associated with an increased incidence of thromboembolism.

ADVERSE REACTIONS
Common reactions are in italics; life-threatening reactions are in bold italics.
CNS: depression, headache, dizziness, migraine, changes in libido.
CV: edema, thrombophlebitis, ***thromboembolism.***
GI: *nausea,* vomiting, abdominal cramps, *bloating,* cholestatic jaundice.

GU: increased size of uterine fibromyomata, vaginal candidiasis, cystitis-like syndrome, dysmenorrhea, amenorrhea, *breakthrough bleeding, premenstrual-like syndrome.*
Skin: hemorrhagic eruption, erythema nodosum, erythema multiforme, hirsutism, chloasma, hair loss.
Other: breast engorgement or enlargement, *weight changes,* aggravation of porphyria.

INTERACTIONS

None significant.

EFFECTS ON DIAGNOSTIC TESTS

Free triiodothyronine resin: decreased uptake.
Glucose tolerance: impaired.
Pregnanediol excretion: decreased.
Serum folate, pyridoxine, and antithrombin III: decreased concentrations.
Sulfobromophthalein retention, prothrombin time, clotting Factors VII to X, and norepinephrine-induced platelet aggregability: increased.
Thyroid-binding globulin: increased concentration.
Total thyroid concentrations (measured by protein-bound iodine or total thyroxine): increased.
Triglyceride, glucose, and phospholipid: increased levels.

NURSING CONSIDERATIONS

Besides those related universally to drug therapy (see "How to use this book"), consider the following specific recommendations:

Assessment

- Obtain a baseline assessment of the patient's underlying condition before therapy.
- Be alert for adverse reactions and drug interactions throughout therapy.
- Evaluate the patient's and family's knowledge about estropipate therapy.

Nursing Diagnoses

- Impaired tissue integrity related to the patient's underlying condition.
- Fluid volume excess related to estropipate-induced edema.
- Knowledge deficit related to estropipate therapy.

Planning and Implementation

Preparation and Administration

- Be aware that dosage is usually given on a cyclical, short-term basis.

Monitoring

- Monitor effectiveness by regularly assessing the patient's underlying condition for signs of improvement.
- Monitor patient for fluid retention; weigh daily.

Supportive Care

- Institute safety measures if CNS adverse reactions occur.
- Obtain an order for an antiemetic agent, as needed.
- Prepare patient for body changes that may occur, such as loss of hair.
- Limit sodium intake if not contraindicated.

Patient Teaching

- Warn the patient to report immediately abdominal pain; pain, numbness, or stiffness in legs or buttocks; pressure or pain in chest; shortness of breath; severe headaches; visual disturbances, such as blind spots, flashing lights, or blurriness; vaginal bleeding or discharge; breast lumps; swelling of hands or feet; yellow skin and sclera; dark urine; and light-colored stools.
- Explain to patients treated for hypogonadism that the duration of therapy necessary to produce withdrawal bleeding depends on individual's endometrial response to the drug. If satisfactory withdrawal bleeding does not occur, an oral progestin may have to be added to the regimen. Explain that despite the return of withdrawal bleeding, pregnancy is not possible because patient is not ovulating.
- Teach female patients how to perform routine breast self-examination.
- Give the patient the package insert describing adverse reactions to estro-

pipate, and also provide verbal explanation.
• Instruct patient to weigh herself daily and to report any sudden weight gain. Also tell her to limit sodium intake if appropriate and not contraindicated.

Evaluation

In patients receiving estropipate, appropriate evaluation statements may include:
• Patient exhibits improved health as a result of estropipate therapy.
• Patient does not develop edema.
• Patient and family state an understanding of estropipate therapy.

ethacrynate sodium
(eth a kri´ nate)
Edecrin Sodium

ethacrynic acid
Edecril‡, Edecrin

• *Classification:* diuretic (loop diuretic)
• *Pregnancy Risk Category:* D

HOW SUPPLIED
Tablets: 25 mg, 50 mg
Injection: 50 mg (with 62.5 mg of mannitol and 0.1 mg of thimerosal)

ACTION
Mechanism: A loop diuretic that inhibits reabsorption of sodium and chloride at the proximal portion of the ascending loop of Henle.
Absorption: Rapidly absorbed from the GI tract.
Distribution: In animal studies, ethacrynic acid was found to accumulate in the liver; it does not enter CSF, and its distribution into breast milk or the placenta is unknown.
Metabolism: In animals, metabolized by the liver to a potentially active metabolite.
Excretion: According to animal studies, 30% to 65% of ethacrynate sodium is excreted in urine and 35% to 40% is excreted in bile, as the metabolite.
Onset, peak, duration: After oral administration, diuresis occurs in 5 minutes and peaks in 15 to 30 minutes. Duration of action is 6 to 8 hours after oral administration and about 2 hours after I.V. administration.

INDICATIONS & DOSAGE
Acute pulmonary edema –
Adults: 50 to 100 mg of ethacrynate sodium I.V. slowly over several minutes.
Edema –
Adults: 50 to 200 mg P.O. daily. Refractory cases may require up to 200 mg b.i.d.
Children: initial dose is 25 mg P.O., cautiously, increased in 25-mg increments daily until desired effect is achieved.

CONTRAINDICATIONS & PRECAUTIONS
Contraindicated in patients with hypersensitivity to the drug and with anuria, hypotension, dehydration with low serum sodium levels, or metabolic alkalosis with hypokalemia because the drug may exacerbate these conditions. Use cautiously in patients with hearing impairment or cirrhosis, especially those with a history of electrolyte imbalance or hepatic encephalopathy; diabetes because drug may alter carbohydrate metabolism; and increasing azotemia or oliguria and in patients receiving cardiac glycosides (digoxin, digitoxin) because ethacrynic acid–induced hypokalemia may predispose them to digitalis toxicity.

ADVERSE REACTIONS
Common reactions are in italics; life-threatening reactions are in bold italics.
Blood: ***agranulocytosis,*** neutropenia, thrombocytopenia.

CV: *volume depletion and dehydration,* orthostatic hypotension.
EENT: transient deafness with too-rapid I.V. injection.
GI: abdominal discomfort and pain, diarrhea.
Metabolic: *hypokalemia; hypochloremic alkalosis; asymptomatic hyperuricemia; fluid and electrolyte imbalances including dilutional hyponatremia, hypocalcemia, hypomagnesemia;* hyperglycemia and impairment of glucose tolerance.
Skin: dermatitis.

INTERACTIONS

Aminoglycoside antibiotics: potentiated ototoxic adverse reactions of both ethacrynic acid and aminoglycosides. Use together cautiously.
Warfarin: potentiated anticoagulant effect. Use together cautiously.

EFFECTS ON DIAGNOSTIC TESTS

Electrolytes: altered results.
Liver and renal function tests: altered results.

NURSING CONSIDERATIONS

Besides those related universally to drug therapy (see "How to use this book"), consider the following specific recommendations:

Assessment

- Obtain a baseline assessment of urine output, vital signs, serum electrolytes, breath sounds, peripheral edema, and weight before therapy.
- Be alert for adverse reactions and drug interactions throughout therapy.
- Evaluate the patient's and family's knowledge about ethacrynate therapy.

Nursing Diagnoses

- Fluid volume excess related to the patient's underlying condition as evidenced by edema.
- Altered urinary elimination related to diuretic therapy.
- Knowledge deficit related to ethacrynate therapy.

Planning and Implementation

Preparation and Administration

- ***P.O. use:*** Give in morning to prevent nocturia.
- ***I.V. use:*** Reconstitute vacuum vial with 50 ml of dextrose 5% injection or sodium chloride injection. Discard unused solution after 24 hours. Don't use cloudy or opalescent solutions. Administer slowly through tubing of running infusion over several minutes.

Monitoring

- Monitor effectiveness by regularly checking urine output, weight, peripheral edema, and breath sounds.
- Monitor serum electrolytes and BUN levels.
- Monitor vital signs: hypotension, dyspnea, tachycardia, and fever may indicate dehydration.
- In the diabetic patient, monitor serum glucose.
- In the patient with gout, monitor serum uric acid.
- In the patient receiving digitalis, monitor for signs of digitalis toxicity.
- Monitor for signs of hypokalemia (muscle weakness and cramping).
- Monitor skin turgor and mucous membranes for signs of fluid volume depletion.
- Monitor elderly patients closely because they are especially susceptible to excessive diuresis.
- Monitor I.V. site for thrombophlebitis.

Supportive Care

- Hold drug and notify the doctor if hypersensitivity or adverse reactions occur.
- Keep accurate record of intake and output.
- Elevate the patient's legs to aid relief of peripheral edema.
- Encourage low-sodium/high-potassium diet.
- Provide frequent skin and mouth care to relieve dryness due to diuretic therapy.
- Answer the patient's call bells

promptly; make sure patient's bathroom or bedpan are easily accessible.
• Use safety precautions to avoid risk of falls due to hypotension.
Patient Teaching
• Teach the patient and family to identify and report signs of hypersensitivity or fluid and electrolyte disturbances.
• Teach the diabetic patient to monitor blood glucose.
• Teach the patient receiving ethacrynic and digitalis to be aware of signs of digitalis toxicity and to store these drugs separately to avoid risk of dosage error.
• Teach the patient to monitor fluid volume by daily weight and intake and output.
• Encourage the patient to avoid foods high in sodium and to choose foods high in potassium.
• Advise the patient to change positions slowly, especially when rising to a standing position, to avoid dizziness due to orthostatic hypotension, and to limit alcohol intake and strenuous exercise in warm weather.
• Advise the patient to take drug early in the day to avoid interruption of sleep by nocturia.
Evaluation
In patients receiving ethacrynate or ethacrynic acid, appropriate evaluation statements may include:
• Patient is free of edema.
• Patient demonstrates adjustment of life-style to deal with altered patterns of urinary elimination.
• Patient and family state an understanding of ethacrynate or ethacrynic acid therapy.

ethambutol hydrochloride
(e tham´ byoo tole)
Etibi†, Myambutol

• *Classification:* antitubercular agent
• *Pregnancy Risk Category:* B

HOW SUPPLIED
Tablets: 100 mg, 400 mg

ACTION
Mechanism: Interferes with the synthesis of RNA, thus inhibiting protein metabolism (bacteriostatic).
Absorption: About 75% to 80% of dose is absorbed rapidly from the GI tract; absorption is not affected by food.
Distribution: Widely distributed into body tissues and fluids, especially into lungs, RBCs, saliva, and kidneys; lesser amounts distribute into brain, ascitic and pleural fluids, and CSF. Ethambutol is 8% to 22% protein-bound.
Metabolism: Partially metabolized by hepatic process.
Excretion: After 24 hours, about 50% of a dose appears in the urine as unchanged drug and 8% to 15% as metabolites; 20% to 25% is excreted in feces as unchanged drug; small amounts may be excreted in breast milk. The drug can be removed by peritoneal dialysis and to a lesser extent by hemodialysis. Half-life: About 3½ hours in adults; prolonged in decreased renal or hepatic function.
Onset, peak, duration: Peak serum levels occur 2 to 4 hours after ingestion.

INDICATIONS & DOSAGE
Adjunctive treatment in pulmonary tuberculosis—
Adults and children over 13 years: initial treatment for patients who have not received previous antitubercular therapy is 15 mg/kg P.O. daily single dose.
Re-treatment: 25 mg/kg P.O. daily single dose for 60 days with at least one other antitubercular drug; then decrease to 15 mg/kg P.O. daily single dose.

CONTRAINDICATIONS & PRECAUTIONS

Contraindicated in patients with hypersensitivity to ethambutol.

Use cautiously in patients with preexisting visual disturbances, in whom ethambutol-induced visual changes are difficult to identify; monthly vision tests are mandatory at high dosage levels. Also cautiously in patients with gout and in those with decreased renal or hepatic function.

ADVERSE REACTIONS

Common reactions are in italics; life-threatening reactions are in bold italics.

CNS: headache, dizziness, mental confusion, possible hallucinations, peripheral neuritis (numbness and tingling of extremities).

EENT: optic neuritis (vision loss and loss of color discrimination, especially red and green).

GI: anorexia, nausea, vomiting, abdominal pain.

Metabolic: *elevated uric acid.*

Other: ***anaphylactoid reactions,*** fever, malaise, bloody sputum.

INTERACTIONS

None significant.

EFFECTS ON DIAGNOSTIC TESTS

Liver function tests: elevated results.
Serum urate: elevated levels.

NURSING CONSIDERATIONS

Besides those related universally to drug therapy (see "How to use this book"), consider the following specific recommendations:

Assessment

- Obtain a baseline assessment of patient's infection before therapy.
- Be alert for adverse reactions and drug interactions throughout therapy.
- Evaluate the patient's and family's knowledge about ethambutol therapy.

Nursing Diagnoses

- High risk for injury related to ineffectiveness of ethambutol to eradicate the infection.
- Altered health maintenance related to ethambutol-induced gout caused by elevated uric acid levels.
- Knowledge deficit related to ethambutol therapy.

Planning and Implementation

Preparation and Administration

- Obtain specimen for culture and sensitivity tests before the first dose of ethambutol.
- Perform visual acuity and color discrimination tests before administering the first dose of ethambutol if possible.
- Expect to reduce dosage in patients with impaired renal function.

Monitoring

- Monitor effectiveness by regularly assessing for improvement in infection and by evaluating culture and sensitivity test results.
- Monitor serum uric acid levels and patient for symptoms of gout.
- Regularly monitor patient's visual acuity and color discrimination during ethambutol therapy.

Supportive Care

- Institute safety precautions if visual disturbances or adverse CNS reactions occur.
- Obtain an order for an antiemetic or antidiarrheal agent as needed.
- Notify doctor if gout occurs.

Patient Teaching

- Emphasize the need for periodic laboratory tests to monitor serum uric acid level and drug effectiveness.
- Teach patient the signs of gout and tell him to report them to doctor.
- Caution patient not to perform hazardous activities if visual disturbances or adverse GI reactions occur.

Evaluation

In patients receiving ethambutol, appropriate evaluation statements may include:

- Patient is free of infection.

• Patient's uric acid levels remain normal throughout therapy.
• Patient and family state an understanding of ethambutol therapy.

ethchlorvynol

(eth klor vi´ nole)
Placidyl**

• Controlled Substance Schedule IV
• *Classification:* sedative-hypnotic (chlorinated acetylenic carbinol)
• *Pregnancy Risk Category:* C

HOW SUPPLIED

Capsules: 200 mg, 500 mg, 750 mg**

ACTION

Mechanism: Depresses the CNS by an unknown mechanism.
Absorption: Completely and rapidly absorbed after oral administration.
Distribution: Throughout the body, including the CNS, with extensive storage in fatty tissue.
Metabolism: Primarily in the liver with significant metabolism also in the kidneys. In overdose, the metabolic pathways can be saturated.
Excretion: Inactive metabolites of the drug are excreted in urine. Half-life: 10 to 20 hours.
Onset, peak, duration: Peak serum concentrations occur within 2 hours. Action begins in 15 minutes to 1 hour. The duration of sleep is about 5 hours.

INDICATIONS & DOSAGE

Sedation–
Adults: 100 to 200 mg P.O. b.i.d. or t.i.d.
Insomnia–
Adults: 500 mg to 1 g P.O. h.s. May repeat 100 to 200 mg if awakened in early morning.

CONTRAINDICATIONS & PRECAUTIONS

Contraindicated in patients with hypersensitivity to the drug; in patients with porphyria; and in patients with persistent pain and insomnia unless the insomnia persists after the pain is controlled, because the drug increases sensitivity to pain. The 750-mg dosage form is contraindicated in individuals allergic to aspirin, because it contains tartrazine and because significant cross-reactivity has been demonstrated.

Because drug depresses the CNS, use cautiously in patients who are depressed or have suicidal tendencies and in those with a history of drug abuse or addiction. Also use cautiously in patients with hepatic or renal dysfunction because decreased elimination of the drug may lead to accumulation and toxicity and in patients who have shown unpredictable or paradoxic reactions to barbiturates or chloral hydrate because drug may cause a similar reaction.

ADVERSE REACTIONS

Common reactions are in italics; life-threatening reactions are in bold italics.
Blood: thrombocytopenia.
CNS: facial numbness, drowsiness, fatigue, nightmares, dizziness, *residual sedation,* muscular weakness, syncope, ataxia.
CV: hypotension.
EENT: unpleasant aftertaste, blurred vision.
GI: distress, nausea, vomiting.
Skin: rashes, urticaria.

INTERACTIONS

Alcohol or other CNS depressants, including narcotic analgesics, tricyclic antidepressants, and MAO inhibitors: excessive CNS depression. Use together cautiously.
Oral anticoagulants: ethchlorvynol may enhance the metabolism of cou-

marin derivatives, decreasing their effectiveness. Monitor closely.

EFFECTS ON DIAGNOSTIC TESTS

Phentolamine test: false-positive results.

NURSING CONSIDERATIONS

Besides those related universally to drug therapy (see "How to use this book"), consider the following specific recommendations:

Assessment

- Obtain a baseline assessment of sleeping patterns and CNS status before therapy.
- Be alert for adverse reactions and drug interactions throughout therapy.
- Evaluate the patient's and family's knowledge about ethchlorvynol therapy.

Nursing Diagnoses

- Sleep pattern disturbance related to underlying patient problem.
- High risk for trauma related to adverse CNS reactions caused by ethchlorvynol.
- Knowledge deficit related to ethchlorvynol therapy.

Planning and Implementation

Preparation and Administration

- Before leaving the bedside, make sure the patient has swallowed the medication.
- Give with milk or food to minimize transient dizziness or ataxia caused by rapid absorption.
- Slight darkening of liquid from exposure to air and light doesn't affect safety or potency, but store in tight, light-resistant container to avoid possible deterioration.

Monitoring

- Regularly monitor effectiveness by evaluating the patient's ability to sleep after administration.
- Monitor the patient's CNS status for evidence of adverse reactions.
- Monitor for signs of toxicity, such as poor muscle coordination, confusion, hypothermia, speech or vision disturbances, tremors, and weakness.
- After drug discontinuation, be alert for withdrawal symptoms.

Supportive Care

- After administration, institute safety precautions, such as: remove cigarettes; keep bed rails up, and supervise or assist ambulation.
- Keep in mind that the 750-mg strength capsule contains tartrazine dye. May cause allergic reactions in susceptible patients.
- Do not discontinue the drug abruptly. The drug may cause dependence and severe withdrawal symptoms. Withdraw gradually.
- Take precautions to prevent hoarding or self-overdosing, especially by a patient who is depressed, suicidal, or has a history of drug abuse. Overdosage is difficult to treat and has a high mortality.
- Be aware that the drug is effective for only short-term use; treatment period should not exceed 1 week.

Patient Teaching

- Encourage the patient to report severe dizziness or daytime drowsiness so the doctor can be consulted for change of dose or drug.
- Instruct the patient to remain in bed after taking drug and to call for assistance to use the bathroom.
- Warn the patient that drug may cause physical dependence.
- Warn the patient to avoid hazardous activities that require mental alertness until CNS effects are known.
- Tell the patient to notify the nurse or doctor if sleep pattern disturbances continue despite therapy.

Evaluation

In patients receiving ethchlorvynol, appropriate evaluation statements mayinclude:

- Patient states drug was effective in inducing sleep.
- Patient's safety is maintained.

• Patient and family state an understanding of ethchlorvynol therapy.

ethinyl estradiol (ethinyloestradiol)

(eth´ in il ess tra dye´ ole)
Estinyl**, Feminone

• *Classification:* estrogen replacement, antineoplastic (estrogen)
• *Pregnancy Risk Category:* X

HOW SUPPLIED

Tablets: 0.02 mg, 0.05 mg, and 0.5 mg

ACTION

Mechanism: Increases the synthesis of DNA, RNA, and protein in responsive tissues. Also reduces release of follicle-stimulating hormone and luteinizing hormone from the pituitary.
Absorption: Absolute bioavailability about 40%.
Distribution: About 98% bound to plasma protein (mostly albumin). Distribution occurs throughout the body, with highest concentrations in fat.
Metabolism: Mostly hepatic; ethinyl estradiol undergoes extensive enterohepatic recycling, where the drug is excreted in bile, and bacteria in the GI tract hydrolyze the glucuronide and sulfate conjugates. Free ethinyl estradiol is reabsorbed.
Excretion: Primarily through the kidneys in the form of sulfate and/or glucuronide conjugates. Half life: 5 to 20 hours.

INDICATIONS & DOSAGE

Breast cancer (at least 5 years after menopause)–
Women: 1 mg P.O. t.i.d.
Hypogonadism–
Women: 0.05 mg P.O. daily to t.i.d. for 2 weeks a month, followed by 2 weeks progesterone therapy; continue for 3 to 6 monthly dosing cycles, followed by 2 months off.
Menopausal symptoms–
Women: 0.02 to 0.05 mg P.O. daily for cycles of 3 weeks on, 1 week off.
Postpartum breast engorgement–
Women: 0.5 to 1 mg P.O. daily for 3 days, then taper over 7 days to 0.1 mg and discontinue.
Inoperable prostatic cancer–
Men: 0.15 to 2 mg P.O. daily.

CONTRAINDICATIONS & PRECAUTIONS

Contraindicated in patients with thrombophlebitis or thromboembolism because of its association with thromboembolic disorders; in patients with estrogen-responsive carcinoma (breast or genital tract cancer) because the drug may induce tumor growth; in patients with undiagnosed abnormal genital bleeding; in pregnant women because drug may be fetotoxic; and in breast-feeding women because of the potential for adverse effects on the infant.

Use cautiously in patients with disorders that may be aggravated by fluid and electrolyte accumulation, such as asthma, seizure disorders, migraine, or cardiac, renal, or hepatic dysfunction. Carefully monitor female patients who have breast nodules, fibrocystic breast disease, or a family history of breast cancer. Because of the risk of thromboembolism, therapy with this drug should be discontinued at least 1 week before elective surgical procedures associated with an increased incidence of thromboembolism.

ADVERSE REACTIONS

Common reactions are in italics; life-threatening reactions are in bold italics.
CNS: headache, dizziness, chorea, depression, libido changes, lethargy.
CV: thrombophlebitis, ***thromboembolism,*** hypertension, edema.

EENT: worsening of myopia or astigmatism, intolerance to contact lenses.
GI: *nausea,* vomiting, abdominal cramps, bloating, diarrhea, constipation, anorexia, increased appetite, weight changes.
GU: in women–*breakthrough bleeding, altered menstrual flow,* dysmenorrhea, amenorrhea, cervical erosion, altered cervical secretions, enlargement of uterine fibromas, vaginal candidiasis. In men–gynecomastia, testicular atrophy, impotence.
Hepatic: cholestatic jaundice.
Metabolic: hyperglycemia, hypercalcemia, folic acid deficiency.
Skin: melasma, urticaria, acne, seborrhea, oily skin, hirsutism or hair loss.
Other: breast changes (tenderness, enlargement, secretion), leg cramps.

INTERACTIONS

None significant.

EFFECTS ON DIAGNOSTIC TESTS

Free triiodothyronine resin: decreased uptake.
Glucose tolerance: impaired.
Pregnanediol excretion: decreased.
Serum folate, pyridoxine, and antithrombin III: decreased concentrations.
Sulfobromophthalein retention, prothrombin time, clotting Factors VII to X, and norepinephrine-induced platelet aggregability: increased.
Thyroid-binding globulin: increased concentration.
Total thyroid concentrations (measured by protein-bound iodine or total thyroxine): increased.
Triglyceride, glucose, and phospholipid: increased levels.

NURSING CONSIDERATIONS

Besides those related universally to drug therapy (see "How to use this book"), consider the following specific recommendations:

Assessment
- Obtain a baseline assessment of the patient's underlying condition before therapy.
- Be alert for adverse reactions and drug interactions throughout therapy.
- Evaluate the patient's and family's knowledge about ethinyl estradiol therapy.

Nursing Diagnoses
- Sexual dysfunction related to the patient's underlying condition.
- Altered (cerebral, peripheral, pulmonary, or myocardial) tissue perfusion related to high risk for ethinyl estradiol to cause thromboembolism.
- Knowledge deficit related to ethinyl estradiol therapy.

Planning and Implementation
Preparation and Administration
- ***P.O. use:*** Administer at mealtimes or bedtime (if only one daily dose is required) to minimize nausea.

Monitoring
- Monitor effectiveness by regularly assessing the patient's underlying condition for signs of improvement.
- Monitor for thromboemboli formation by noting any changes in cerebral or cardiopulmonary function or peripheral circulation.
- Monitor the patient's blood glucose levels for alterations.

Supportive Care
- Withhold drug and notify the doctor if a thromboembolic event is suspected; be prepared to provide supportive care as indicated.
- Alert the pathologist if a specimen is obtained during estrogen therapy.
- Be prepared to adjust diabetic patients' therapeutic regimen if blood glucose levels rise during therapy with ethinyl estradiol.
- Institute safety measures if CNS adverse reactions occur.
- Obtain an order for an antiemetic, antidiarrheal, or laxative agent, as needed.
- Prepare patient for possible body changes, such as loss of hair.

Patient Teaching

• Warn the patient to report immediately abdominal pain; pain, numbness, or stiffness in legs or buttocks; pressure or pain in chest; shortness of breath; severe headaches; visual disturbances, such as blind spots, flashing lights, or blurriness; vaginal bleeding or discharge; breast lumps; swelling of hands or feet; yellow skin and sclera; dark urine; and light-colored stools.

• Explain to patients on cyclic therapy for postmenopausal symptoms that, although withdrawal bleeding may occur in week off drug, fertility has not been restored; ovulation does not occur.

• Teach female patients how to perform routine breast self-examination.

• Teach the patient that medical supervision is essential during prolonged therapy with ethinyl estradiol because use of estrogens are associated with increased risk of endometrial cancer and possible increased risk of breast cancer.

• Inform the patient that nausea, when present, may be relieved by taking medication at mealtimes or bedtime (if only one daily dose is required).

• Tell diabetic patients to report symptoms of hyperglycemia or glycosuria.

• Give the patient the package insert describing adverse reactions to ethinyl estradiol, and also provide verbal explanation.

Evaluation

In patients receiving ethinyl estradiol, appropriate evaluation statements may include:

• Patient's sexual dysfunction improves; patient exhibits improved health as a result of ethinyl estradiol therapy.

• Patient does not experience a thromboembolic event during ethinyl estradiol therapy.

• Patient and family state an understanding of ethinyl estradiol therapy.

---

ethinyl estradiol and ethynodiol diacetate

(eth´ in il ess tra dye´ ole and *e thye noe dye´ ole)*

monophasic: Demulen 1/35, Demulen 1/50

ethinyl estradiol and levonorgestrel

(lee´ voe nor jess trel)

monophasic: Levlen, Nordette
triphasic: Tri-Levlen, Triphasil

ethinyl estradiol and norethindrone

(nor eth in´ drone)

monophasic: Brevicon, Genora 0.5/35, Genora 1/35, Modicon, N.E.E. 1/35, Nelova 0.5/35 E, Nelova 1/35 E, Norcept-E 1/35, Norethin 1/35 E, Norinyl 1 + 35, Ortho-Novum 1/35, Ovcon-35, Ovcon-50
biphasic: Nelova 10/11, Ortho Novum 10/11
triphasic: Ortho Novum 7/7/7, Tri-Norinyl

ethinyl estradiol and norethindrone acetate

monophasic: Loestrin 21 1/20, Loestrin 21 1.5/30, Norlestrin 21 1/50, Norlestrin 21 2.5/50

ethinyl estradiol and norgestrel

(nor jess´ trel)

monophasic: Lo/Ovral, Ovral

ethinyl estradiol, norethindrone acetate, and ferrous fumarate

monophasic: Loestrin Fe 1/20, Loestrin Fe 1.5/30, Norlestrin Fe 1/50, Norlestrin Fe 2.5/50

mestranol and norethindrone

(mes´ tra nole)

monophasic: Genora 1/50, Nelova 1/50 M, Norethin 1/50 M, Norinyl 1 + 50, Ortho-Novum 1/50

• *Classification:* hormonal contraceptive (estrogen with progestin)
• *Pregnancy Risk Category:* X

HOW SUPPLIED

Monophasic oral contraceptives

ethinyl estradiol and ethynodiol diacetate

Tablets: ethinyl estradiol 35 mcg and ethynodiol diacetate 1 mg (Demulen 1/35); ethinyl estradiol 50 mcg and ethynodiol diacetate 1 mg (Demulen 1/50)

ethinyl estradiol and levonorgestrel

Tablets: ethinyl estradiol 30 mcg and levonorgestrel 0.15 mg (Levlen, Nordette)

ethinyl estradiol and norethindrone

Tablets: ethinyl estradiol 35 mcg and norethindrone 0.4 mg (Ovcon-35); ethinyl estradiol 35 mcg and norethindrone 0.5 mg (Brevicon, Genora 0.5/35, Modicon, Nelova 0.5/35E); ethinyl estradiol 35 mcg and norethindrone 1 mg (Genora 1/35, N.E.E 1/35, Nelova 1/35 E, Norcept-E 1/35, Norethin 1/35 E, Norinyl 1 + 35, Ortho-Novum 1/35), ethinyl estradiol 50 mcg and norethindrone 1 mg (Ovcon-50)

ethinyl estradiol and norethindrone acetate

Tablets: ethinyl estradiol 20 mcg and norethindrone acetate 1 mg (Loestrin 21 1/20); ethinyl estradiol 30 mcg and norethindrone acetate 1.5 mg (Loestrin 21 1.5/30); ethinyl estradiol 50 mcg and norethindrone acetate 1 mg (Norlestrin 21 1/50); ethinyl estradiol 50 mcg and norethindrone acetate 2.5 mg (Norlestrin 21 2.5/50)

ethinyl estradiol and norgestrel

Tablets: ethinyl estradiol 30 mcg and norgestrel 0.3 mg (Lo/Ovral); ethinyl estradiol 50 mcg and norgestrel 0.5 mg (Ovral)

ethinyl estradiol, norethindrone acetate, and ferrous fumarate

Tablets: ethinyl estradiol 20 mcg, norethindrone acetate 1 mg, and ferrous fumarate 75 mg (Loestrin Fe 1/20); ethinyl estradiol 30 mcg, norethindrone acetate 1.5 mg, and ferrous fumarate 75 mg (Loestrin Fe 1.5/30); ethinyl estradiol 50 mcg, norethindrone acetate 1 mg, and ferrous fumarate 75 mg (Norlestrin Fe 1/50); ethinyl estradiol 50 mcg, norethindrone acetate 2.5 mg, and ferrous fumarate 75 mg (Norlestrin Fe 2.5/50)

mestranol and norethindrone

Tablets: mestranol 50 mcg and norethindrone 1 mg Genora 1/50, Nelova 1/50 M, Norethin 1/50 M, Norinyl 1 + 50, Ortho-Novum 1/50)

Biphasic oral contraceptives

ethinyl estradiol and norethindrone

Tablets: ethinyl estradiol 35 mcg and norethindrone 0.5 mg during phase 1 [10 days]; ethinyl estradiol 35 mcg and norethindrone 1 mg during phase 2 [11 days] (Nelova 10/11, Ortho Novum 10/11)

Triphasic oral contraceptives

ethinyl estradiol and levonorgestrel

Tablets: (Tri-Levlen, Triphasil) ethinyl estradiol 35 mcg and levonorgesntrel 0.05 mg during phase 1 [6 days]; ethinyl estradiol 35 mcg and levonorgestrel 0.075 mg during phase 2 [5 days]; ethinyl estradiol 35 mcg and levonorgestrel 0.125 mg during phase 3 [10 days]

ethinyl estradiol and norethindrone

Tablets: (Tri-Norinyl) ethinyl estradiol 35 mcg and norethindrone 0.5 mg during phase 1 [7 days]; ethinyl estradiol 35 mcg and norethindrone 1 mg during phase 2 [9 days]; ethinyl estradiol 35 mcg and norethindrone 0.5 mg during phase 3 [5 days]; (Ortho Novum 7/7/7) ethinyl estradiol 35 mcg and norethindrone 0.5 mg during phase 1 [7 days]; ethinyl estradiol 35 mcg and norethindrone

0.75 mg during phase 2 [7 days]; ethinyl estradiol 35 mcg and norethindrone 1 mg during phase 3 [7 days]

ACTION

Mechanism: Oral contraceptives inhibit ovulation through a negative feedback mechanism directed at the hypothalamus. They may also prevent transport of the ovum through the fallopian tubes.

Estrogen suppresses secretion of follicle-stimulating hormone, blocking follicular development and ovulation.

Progestin suppresses luteinizing hormone secretion so ovulation can't occur even if the follicle develops. Progestin thickens cervical mucus, which interferes with sperm migration, and also causes endometrial changes that prevent implantation of the fertilized ovum.

Absorption: Most drugs are well absorbed from the GI tract; levonorgestrel is completely absorbed. Absolute bioavailability is about 40% for ethinyl estradiol and 65% for norethindrone.

Distribution: Widely distributed and extensively bound to plasma proteins. Ethinyl estradiol is about 98% bound to plasma protein (mostly albumin). Levonorgestrel is about 93% to 95% bound, and norethindrone is about 80% bound, to both albumin and sex hormone binding globulin. Oral contraceptives distribute into bile; small amounts enter breast milk.

Metabolism: Mostly hepatic; ethinyl estradiol undergoes extensive enterohepatic recycling, where the drug is excreted in bile, and bacteria in the GI tract hydrolyze the glucuronide and sulfate conjugates. Free ethinyl estradiol is reabsorbed.

Excretion: In both urine and feces. Half-life: 11 to 45 hours for levonorgestrel, 5 to 14 hours for norethindrone, and 6 to 20 hours for ethinyl estradiol.

INDICATIONS & DOSAGE

Contraception–

Women: 1 tablet P.O. daily, beginning on day 5 of menstrual cycle (first day of menstrual flow is day 1). With 20- and 21-tablet packages, new dosing cycle begins 7 days after last tablet taken. With 28-tablet packages, dosage is 1 tablet daily without interruption; extra tablets are placebos or contain iron. If only 1 or 2 doses are missed, dosage may continue on schedule. If 3 or more doses are missed, remaining tablets in monthly package must be discarded and another contraceptive method substituted. If next menstrual period doesn't begin on schedule, rule out pregnancy before starting new dosing cycle. If menstrual period begins, start new dosing cycle 7 days after last tablet was taken. If all doses have been taken on schedule and 1 menstrual period is missed, continue dosing cycle. If 2 consecutive menstrual periods are missed, pregnancy test is required before new dosing cycle is started.

Biphasic oral contraceptives–
1 color tablet P.O. daily for 10 days, then next color tablet for 11 days.

Triphasic oral contraceptives–
1 tablet P.O. daily in the sequence specified by the brand.

Endometriosis–

Women: Enovid 5 mg or 10 mg–1 tablet P.O. daily for 2 weeks starting on day 5 of menstrual cycle. Continue without interruption for 6 to 9 months, increasing dose by 5 to 10 mg q 2 weeks, up to 20 mg daily. Up to 40 mg daily may be needed if breakthrough bleeding occurs.

CONTRAINDICATIONS & PRECAUTIONS

Contraindicated in patients with thromboembolic disorders, cerebrovascular or coronary artery disease, or myocardial infarction because of drug's association with thromboembolic disease; known or suspected cancer of the breast or reproductive organs or with benign or malignant liver tumors because of drug's association with tumorigenesis; undiagnosed abnormal vaginal bleeding; in women known or believed to be pregnant or breast-feeding; in adolescents with incomplete epiphyseal closure; in women smokers over age 35; and in all women over age 40.

Use cautiously in patients with systemic lupus erythematosus, hypertension, mental depression, migraine, epilepsy, asthma, diabetes mellitus, amenorrhea, scanty or irregular periods, fibrocystic breast disease, family history (mother, grandmother, sister) of breast or genital tract cancer, or renal or gallbladder disease. Development or worsening of any of these conditions should be reported. Prolonged therapy may be inadvisable in women who plan to become pregnant.

ADVERSE REACTIONS

Common reactions are in italics; life-threatening reactions are in bold italics.
CNS: *headache, dizziness,* depression, libido changes, lethargy, migraine.
CV: ***thromboembolism,*** hypertension, edema.
EENT: worsening of myopia or astigmatism, intolerance to contact lenses.
GI: *nausea,* vomiting, abdominal cramps, bloating, diarrhea, constipation, anorexia, changes in appetite, weight gain, *bowel ischemia,* pancreatitis.
GU: *breakthrough bleeding, granulomatous colitis,* dysmenorrhea, amenorrhea, cervical erosion or abnormal secretions, enlargement of uterine fibromas, vaginal candidiasis.
Hepatic: gallbladder disease, cholestatic jaundice, liver tumors.
Metabolic: hyperglycemia, hypercalcemia, folic acid deficiency.
Skin: rash, acne, seborrhea, oily skin, erythema multiforme, hyperpigmentation.
Other: *breast tenderness,* enlargement, secretion.

Adverse reactions may be more serious, frequent, and rapid in onset with high-dose than with low-dose combinations.

INTERACTIONS

Barbiturates, anticonvulsants, rifampin, ampicillin, phenylbutazone, tetracycline: may diminish contraceptive effectiveness. Use supplemental form of contraception.

EFFECTS ON DIAGNOSTIC TESTS

Antithrombin III, metyrapone, pregnanediol excretion, free triiodothyronine resin uptake, glucose tolerance, zinc, vitamin B_{12}, and urine 17-hydroxycorticosteroids: decreased results.
Sulfobromophthalein retention, prothrombin time, clotting Factors VII to X, plasminogen, norepinephrine-induced platelet aggregation, fibrinogen, thyroid-binding globulin, serum bilirubin AST (SGOT), ALT (SGPT), protein-bound iodine, triglycerides, phospholipids, transcortin and corticosteroids, transferrin, prolactin, renin, and vitamin A: elevated results.

NURSING CONSIDERATIONS

Besides those related universally to drug therapy (see "How to use this book"), consider the following specific recommendations:

Assessment

- Obtain a baseline assessment of the patient's pregnancy status before therapy.
- Be alert for adverse reactions and drug interactions throughout therapy.
- Evaluate the patient's and family's knowledge about oral contraceptive therapy.

Nursing Diagnoses

- Pain related to drug-induced headache.
- Altered (cerebral, pulmonary, or pe-

ripheral) tissue perfusion related to drug-induced thromboembolism.
• Knowledge deficit related to oral conceptive therapy.

Planning and Implementation

Preparation and Administration
• Ensure that the patient has been properly instructed about the prescribed oral conceptive drug before patient administers first dose.
• Check to be sure a negative pregnancy test has been obtained before drug is initiated.

Monitoring
• Monitor effectiveness by regularly assessing that pregnancy has not occurred; have pregnancy test performed if menstruation does not occur when expected.
• Monitor the patient's blood glucose, calcium, and folic acid levels regularly.
• Monitor the patient's mental status for CNS changes, such as depression.
• Regularly monitor blood pressure and weight.
• Regularly monitor the patient for breakthrough bleeding or abnormal vaginal secretions.

Supportive Care
• Alert the doctor immediately if a thromboembolic event is suspected and be prepared to provide supportive care as indicated.
• Evaluate laboratory study findings carefully. Anticipate increase in serum bilirubin, alkaline phosphatase, AST (SGOT), ALT (SGPT), and protein-bound iodine levels and decreases in glucose tolerance and urine excretion of 17-hydroxycorticosteroids.
• Take the patient's blood pressure and administer a mild analgesic, as ordered. Notify the doctor if headache is severe or if it is not relieved with a mild analgesic.

Patient Teaching
• Instruct patient how to take the prescribed oral contraceptive drug.
• Warn the patient that headache, nausea, dizziness, breast tenderness, spotting, and breakthrough bleeding are common at first. These should diminish after three to six dosing cycles (months). However, breakthrough bleeding in patients taking high-dose estrogen-progestin combinations for menstrual disorders may necessitate dosage adjustment.
• Advise the patient to use an additional method of birth control for the first week of administration in the initial cycle.
• Tell the patient to take tablets at the same time each day for efficacy of medication; nighttime dosing may reduce incidence of nausea and headaches.
• If one menstrual period is missed and tablets have been taken on schedule, tell the patient to continue taking them. If two consecutive menstrual periods are missed, tell the patient to stop drug and have a pregnancy test performed. Progestins may cause birth defects if taken early in pregnancy.
• Teach the patient to keep tablets in original container and to take them in correct (color-coded) sequence.
• Suggest that the patient take the drug with or immediately after food to reduce nausea.
• Stress importance of annual Papanicolaou tests and gynecologic examinations while taking an oral contraceptive drug.
• Warn the patient of possible delay in achieving pregnancy when drug is discontinued.
• Advise the patient of increased risks associated with simultaneous use of cigarettes and oral contraceptives.
• Instruct the patient to weigh herself at least twice a week and to report any sudden weight gain or edema to the doctor.
• Warn the patient to avoid exposure to ultraviolet light or prolonged exposure to sunlight; chloasma seems to

be aggravated by sunlight. With anticipated exposure (as in summer), taking pill at bedtime will reduce daytime levels of circulating hormone.

• Many doctors recommend that women not become pregnant within 2 months after stopping oral contraceptive therapy. Advise the patient to check with her doctor about how soon pregnancy may be safely attempted after oral contraceptive therapy is stopped.

• Inform the patient that oral contraceptives decrease viscosity of the cervical mucus and increase susceptibility to vaginal infections. Good hygienic practices are essential.

• Instruct the patient to ask her doctor for another form of contraception if she is receiving ampicillin, anticonvulsants, phenylbutazone, rifampin, or tetracycline because intermittent bleeding and unwanted pregnancy might result from effect of drug interactions.

• Instruct the patient as follows regarding missed doses. *Monophasic or biphasic cycles* for 20-, 21-, or 24-day dosing schedule: if one regular dose is missed, take tablet as soon as possible; if remembered on the next day, take 2 tablets, then continue regular dosing schedule. If two consecutive doses are missed, take 2 tablets a day for next 2 days, then resume regular dosing schedule. If 3 consecutive days are missed, discontinue drug and substitute other contraceptive method until period begins or pregnancy is ruled out. Then start new cycle of tablets. For 28-day dosing schedule, follow instructions for 21-day dosing schedule; if 1 of the last 7 tablets is missed, be sure to take first tablet of next month's cycle on regularly scheduled day.

– *Triphasic cycle:* If one dose is missed, take dose as soon as possible; if remembered on the next day, take 2 tablets, then continue regular dosing schedule while using additional method of contraception for remainder of cycle. If two consecutive doses are missed, take 2 tablets/day for next 2 days, then continue regular schedule while using additional contraceptive method for remainder of cycle. If three consecutive doses are missed, discontinue drug and use other contraceptive method until period begins or pregnancy is ruled out. Then start new cycle of tablets. For 28-day dosing schedule, follow instructions for 21-day dosing schedule; if 1 of the last 7 tablets was missed, be sure to take first tablet of next month's cycle on regularly scheduled day.

Evaluation

In patients receiving oral contraceptives, appropriate evaluation statements may include:

• Patient's headache is mild and relieved with mild analgesic.

• Patient does not experience a thromboembolic event during oral contraceptive therapy.

• Patient and family state an understanding of oral contraceptive therapy.

ethosuximide

(eth oh sux´ i mide)

Zarontin

• *Classification:* anticonvulsant (succinimide derivative)

• *Pregnancy Risk Category:* C

HOW SUPPLIED

Capsules: 250 mg

Syrup: 250 mg/5 ml

ACTION

Mechanism: Increases seizure threshold. Reduces the paroxysmal spike-and-wave pattern of absence seizures by depressing nerve transmission in the motor cortex.

Absorption: Completely absorbed from the GI tract.
Distribution: Widely distributed throughout the body; protein binding is minimal. After long-term therapy, CSF levels are similar to those in plasma.
Metabolism: Extensively metabolized in the liver to several inactive metabolites.
Excretion: About 25% of a dose is excreted in urine unchanged; the rest appears as metabolites. Small amounts of drug and metabolites are excreted in bile and feces. Half-life: 40 to 50 hours in adults; 30 hours in children.
Onset, peak, duration: Peak levels are seen about 3 hours after an oral dose. Therapeutic plasma levels are 40 to 100 mcg/ml.

INDICATIONS & DOSAGE

Absence seizure–
Adults and children over 6 years: initially, 250 mg P.O. b.i.d. May increase by 250 mg q 4 to 7 days up to 1.5 g daily.
Children 3 to 6 years: 250 mg P.O. daily or 125 mg P.O. b.i.d. May increase by 250 mg q 4 to 7 days up to 1.5 g daily.

CONTRAINDICATIONS & PRECAUTIONS

Contraindicated in patients with hypersensitivity to succinimides. Use with extreme caution in patients with hepatic or renal disease and in those taking other CNS depressants or anticonvulsants. Ethosuximide may increase the incidence of generalized tonic-clonic seizures if used alone to treat patient with mixed seizures; abrupt withdrawal may precipitate absence seizures. Anticonvulsants have been associated with an increased incidence of birth defects.

ADVERSE REACTIONS

Common reactions are in italics; life-threatening reactions are in bold italics.
Blood: leukopenia, eosinophilia, ***agranulocytosis,*** pancytopenia, ***aplastic anemia.***
CNS: *drowsiness,* headache, *fatigue, dizziness,* ataxia, irritability, hiccups, *euphoria, lethargy.*
EENT: myopia.
GI: *nausea, vomiting,* diarrhea, gum hypertrophy, weight loss, cramps, tongue swelling, *anorexia, epigastric and abdominal pain.*
GU: vaginal bleeding.
Skin: urticaria, pruritic and erythematous rashes, hirsutism.

INTERACTIONS

None significant.

EFFECTS ON DIAGNOSTIC TESTS

Coombs' test: false-positive results.
Liver enzymes: elevated levels.
Renal function tests: abnormal results.

NURSING CONSIDERATIONS

Besides those related universally to drug therapy (see "How to use this book"), consider the following specific recommendations:

Assessment
- Obtain a baseline assessment of patient's seizure activity before therapy.
- Be alert for adverse reactions and drug interactions throughout therapy.
- Evaluate the patient's and family's knowledge of ethosuximide therapy.

Nursing Diagnoses
- Altered thought processes related to patient's underlying absence seizure disorder.
- Altered protection related to ethosuximide-induced blood disorders.
- Knowledge deficit related to ethosuximide therapy.

Planning and Implementation

Preparation and Administration

• Administer drug with food to minimize GI distress.

Monitoring

• Monitor effectiveness by regularly assessing seizure activity. However, keep in mind that this drug may increase frequency of generalized tonic-clonic seizures when used alone in patients who have mixed types of seizures.

• Monitor CBC every 3 to 6 months and monitor continuously for dermatologic reactions, joint pain, unexplained fever, or unusual bruising or bleeding (which may signal hematologic or other severe adverse reactions).

• Monitor serum blood levels; therapeutic levels range between 40 and 80 mcg/ml.

Supportive Care

• Never withdraw drug suddenly. Abrupt withdrawal may precipitate absence seizures.

• Institute safety precautions if the patient develops adverse CNS reactions.

• If blood disorders occur, provide supportive measures, such as assisting the anemic patient with activities and providing frequent rest periods, and implementing measures to protect the patient with agranulocytosis from infection.

• Be aware that ethosuximide is currently the drug of choice for treating absence seizures.

Patient Teaching

• Tell the patient to take drug with food or milk to prevent GI distress and to avoid use with alcoholic beverages.

• Advise the patient to avoid hazardous tasks that require alertness until CNS effects of the drug are known.

• Warn the patient not to discontinue drug abruptly; this may cause seizures.

• Encourage the patient to wear medical alert identification indicating seizure disorder and ethosuximide use.

• Tell the patient to report the following reactions to the doctor: skin rash, mouth ulcers, joint pain, fever, sore throat, or unusual bleeding or bruising.

Evaluation

In patients receiving ethosuximide, appropriate evaluation statements may include:

• Patient is free of seizures.

• Patient's CBC is normal.

• Patient and family state an understanding of ethosuximide therapy.

etidronate disodium

(e ti droe´ nate)

Didronel

• *Classification:* antihypercalcemic (pyrophosphate analog)

• *Pregnancy Risk Category:* B

HOW SUPPLIED

Tablets: 200 mg, 400 mg

ACTION

Mechanism: Decreases bone resorption by decreasing the number of osteoclasts. Also decreases mineral release and matrix or collagen breakdown in bone by binding to hydroxyaptite crystals.

Absorption: Variable after an oral dose and decreased in the presence of food. May also be dose-related; only 1% to 1.5% of a 5-mg/kg dose is absorbed, whereas 6% to 10% of a 20-mg/kg dose is absorbed.

Distribution: Approximately half of the dose is distributed to bone. No drug distributes to soft tissue.

Metabolism: Not metabolized.

Excretion: About 50% of the drug is excreted within 24 hours in urine. Half-life of the dose after binding to bone exceeds 90 days. Plasma half-life is about 6 hours.

INDICATIONS & DOSAGE

Symptomatic Paget's disease–
Adults: 5 mg/kg P.O. daily as a single dose 2 hours before a meal with water or juice. Patient should not eat for 2 hours after dose. May give up to 10 mg/kg daily in severe cases. Maximum dosage is 20 mg/kg daily.
Heterotopic ossification in spinal cord injuries–
Adults: 20 mg/kg P.O. daily for 2 weeks, then 10 mg/kg daily for 10 weeks. Total treatment period is 12 weeks.
Heterotopic ossification after total hip replacement–
Adults: 20 mg/kg daily P.O. for 1 month before total hip replacement and for 3 months afterward.

CONTRAINDICATIONS & PRECAUTIONS

No known contraindications. Use cautiously in patients with restricted calcium and vitamin D intake. Because of potential for intestinal irritation, use cautiously in patients with enterocolitis. Closely monitor patients with impaired renal function because the drug may accumulate.

ADVERSE REACTIONS

Common reactions are in italics; life-threatening reactions are in bold italics.
GI: (seen most frequently at 20 mg/kg daily) diarrhea, increased frequency of bowel movements, nausea.
Other: increased or recurrent bone pain at pagetic sites, pain at previously asymptomatic sites, increased risk of fracture, *elevated serum phosphate.*

INTERACTIONS

None significant.

EFFECTS ON DIAGNOSTIC TESTS

Serum phosphate: elevated levels.

NURSING CONSIDERATIONS

Besides those related universally to drug therapy (see "How to use this book"), consider the following specific recommendations:

Assessment

- Obtain a baseline assessment of the patient's underlying condition, including bone pain and loss of function, before therapy.
- Be alert for adverse reactions and drug intereactions throughout therapy.
- Evaluate the patient's and family's knowledge about etidronate therapy.

Nursing Diagnoses

- High risk for injury related to the patient's underlying bone condition.
- Diarrhea related to etidronate-induced adverse GI reactions.
- Knowledge deficit related to etidronate therapy.

Planning and Implementation

Preparation and Administration

- Be aware that therapy should not last more than 6 months. After 3 months, therapy may be resumed as prescribed if needed. Also be aware that drug should not be given longer than 3 months at doses above 10 mg/kg daily.
- ***P.O. use:*** Don't give drug with food, milk, or antacids; may reduce absorption.

Monitoring

- Monitor effectiveness by regularly checking serum alkaline phosphatase and urinary hydroxyproline excretion (both lowered if therapy effective).
- Monitor hydration status if patient develops diarrhea.
- Monitor renal function before and during therapy as ordered.

Supportive Care

- Notify doctor if elevated serum phosphate occurs, especially in patients receiving higher doses. Be aware that serum phosphate usually returns to normal 2 to 4 weeks after drug is discontinued.

• Obtain an order for an antidiarrheal agent as needed.

Patient Teaching

• Tell patient that improvement may not occur for up to 3 months but may continue for months after drug is stopped.

• Stress importance of good nutrition, especially diet high in calcium and vitamin D.

• Inform patient that taking drug with food, milk, or antacids may reduce absorption.

Evaluation

In patients receiving etidronate, appropriate evaluation statements may include:

• Patient exhibits improvement of underlying condition.

• Patient does not experience diarrhea with use of etidronate.

• Patient and family state an understanding of etidronate therapy.

etoposide (VP-16)

(e toe poe´ side)

VePesid

• *Classification:* antineoplastic (podophyllotoxin)

• *Pregnancy Risk Category:* D

HOW SUPPLIED

Capsules: 50 mg

Injection: 100-mg/5-ml multiple-dose vials

ACTION

Mechanism: A semisynthetic derivative of podophyllotoxin that arrests cell mitosis. Probably acts by directly damaging DNA. A cell-cycle–dependent agent that induces arrest in G-2 phase and kills cells in G-2 or S-phase.

Absorption: Moderately absorbed across the GI tract after oral administration. The bioavailability averages 50% (range: 25% to 75%).

Distribution: Widely distributed into body tissues; in animals, the highest concentrations are found in the liver, kidney, and small intestine. The drug crosses the blood-brain barrier to a limited and variable extent; higher levels are found in brain tumor tissue than normal brain tissue; approximately 94% bound to serum albumin.

Metabolism: Only a small portion of a dose is metabolized in the liver.

Excretion: Primarily excreted in the urine as unchanged drug. A smaller portion of a dose is excreted in the feces. Half-life: Biphasic; initial half-life is about 30 minutes to 2 hours and terminal elimination half-life is about 5½ to 11 hours.

INDICATIONS & DOSAGE

Small-cell carcinoma of the lung, acute nonlymphocytic leukemia, lymphosarcoma, Hodgkin's disease, testicular carcinoma –

Adults: 45 to 75 mg/m² daily I.V. or P.O. for 3 to 5 days repeated q 3 to 5 weeks; or 200 to 250 mg/m² I.V. or P.O. weekly; or 125 to 140 mg/m² daily I.V. or P.O. three times a week q 5 weeks.

CONTRAINDICATIONS & PRECAUTIONS

Contraindicated in patients with a history of hypersensitivity to the drug.

ADVERSE REACTIONS

Common reactions are in italics; life-threatening reactions are in bold italics.

Blood: ***myelosuppression*** *(dose-limiting),* ***leukopenia, thrombocytopenia.***

CV: hypotension from rapid infusion.

GI: nausea and vomiting.

Local: infrequent phlebitis.

Other: occasional headache and fever, *reversible alopecia,* ***anaphylaxis*** (rare).

INTERACTIONS

Warfarin: etoposide may further increase prothrombin time.

EFFECTS ON DIAGNOSTIC TESTS

None reported.

NURSING CONSIDERATIONS

Besides those related universally to drug therapy (see "How to use this book"), consider the following specific recommendations:

Assessment

- Obtain a baseline assessment of the patient's underlying condition before therapy.
- Be alert for adverse reactions or drug interactions throughout therapy.
- Evaluate the patient's and family's knowledge about etoposide therapy.

Nursing Diagnoses

- High risk for impaired skin integrity related to drug-induced adverse reactions.
- Altered protection related to adverse reactions.
- Knowledge deficit related to etoposide therapy.

Planning and Implementation

Preparation and Administration

- Avoid all I.M. injections when platelet count is below 100,000/mm^3.
- ***I.V. use:*** Exercise caution when preparing and administering this drug to avoid mutagenic, teratogenic, and carcinogenic risks. Use a biological containment cabinet, wear gloves and mask, and avoid contaminating work surfaces.
- Reconstitute with sterile water for injection or sterile saline to make a 0.2 or 0.4 mg/ml solution. Higher concentrations may crystallize.
- Reconstituted 0.2 mg/ml solution is stable for 96 hours at room temperature in plastic or glass, protected from light; solutions diluted to 0.4 mg/ml are stable for 48 hours under the same conditions.
- Give drug slowly over 30 minutes to prevent severe hypotension.
- Do not administer via membrane-type in-line filters because the diluent may dissolve the filter.
- Intrapleural and intrathecal administration of the drug is contraindicated.

Monitoring

- Obtain baseline blood pressure, CBC, and platelet count before initiating therapy.
- Monitor effectiveness by noting the results of follow-up diagnostic tests and overall physical status; by regularly checking tumor size and rate of growth through appropriate studies.
- Monitor for signs of bleeding (hematuria, ecchymosis, petechiae, epistaxis, melena).
- Monitor for signs of infection (temperature elevation, sore throat, malaise).
- Monitor CBC.
- Monitor vital signs frequently during I.V. infusion of this drug. Blood pressure needs to be taken before infusion and at 30-minute intervals during infusion. If systolic blood pressure falls below 90 mm Hg, discontinue infusion and notify doctor.
- Monitor the I.V. site for possible extravasation.

Supportive Care

- Be prepared to stop the infusion and notify the doctor immediately if the patient's systolic blood pressure falls below 90 mm Hg.
- Know that etoposide has produced complete remissions in small-cell lung cancer and testicular cancer.
- Anticoagulants and aspirin products should be used with extreme caution.
- Be prepared to administer epinephrine, corticosteroids, or antihistamines for anaphalactoid reactions, which usually respond to immediate treatment.
- Suggest that the patient obtain a wig or a hairpiece if hair loss is a problem.

Patient Teaching
- Warn patients to watch for signs of infection (sore throat, fever, fatigue), and for signs of bleeding (easy bruising, nosebleeds, bleeding gums). Tell him to take his temperature daily.
- Teach patient to avoid the use of all OTC products containing aspirin.
- Reassure the patient that hair loss is possible but reversible.
- Tell the patient to report discomfort, pain, or burning at the injection site.

Evaluation
In patients receiving etoposide, appropriate evaluation statements may include:
- Patient does not develop impaired skin integrity related to adverse reactions.
- Patient's immune system response improves.
- Patient and family state an understanding of etoposide therapy.

etretinate
(e tret′ i nate)
Tegison

- *Classification:* antipsoriatic (retinoid)
- *Pregnancy Risk Category:* X

HOW SUPPLIED
Capsules: 10 mg, 25 mg

ACTION
Mechanism: Unknown. Drug is related to retinoic acid and retinol.
Absorption: Absorption from the GI tract is increased by whole milk or a high-lipid diet.
Distribution: More than 99% of drug is bound to plasma lipoproteins, whereas its active metabolite, the all-trans acid form, is predominantly bound to albumin.
Metabolism: Extensively metabolized with first-pass metabolism to acid form, which is active. Subsequent metabolism results in breakdown products and conjugates that are ultimately excreted.
Excretion: In bile and urine. Half-life: Terminal half-life after 6 months of therapy is approximately 120 days.

INDICATIONS & DOSAGE
Treatment of severe recalcitrant psoriasis, including the erythrodermic and generalized pustular types in patients unresponsive to standard therapy (topical tar plus UVB light, psoralens plus UVA light, systemic corticosteroids, and methotrexate) –
Adults: initially, 0.75 to 1 mg/kg P.O. daily in divided doses. Don't exceed maximum initial dose of 1.5 mg/kg daily. After initial response, begin maintenance dosage of 0.5 to 0.75 mg/kg daily (usually after 8 to 16 weeks).

CONTRAINDICATIONS & PRECAUTIONS
Contraindicated in women who are pregnant or intend to become pregnant and in women who may not reliably use effective means of birth control during treatment. Drug has caused teratogenic effects in humans, but the blood levels for these effects is not known. Measurable blood levels of the drug have been detected in patients over 2 years after treatment was discontinued. Also contraindicated in patients with hypersensitivity to the drug. Drug has been associated with corneal erosion, abrasion, irregularity and with punctate staining. Because there have been a number of cases of decreased night vision, often with sudden onset, warn patients against driving at night. Patients experiencing visual difficulties should be immediately assessed by an ophthalmologist.

ADVERSE REACTIONS
Common reactions are in italics; life-threatening reactions are in bold italics.

Blood: ***blood dyscrasia,*** anemia, altered prothrombin time.
CNS: *benign intracranial hypertension (pseudotumor cerebri), fatigue, headache,* dizziness, lethargy.
CV: thrombosis, edema.
EENT: dry eyes, *eye pain; sore tongue; chapped lips; corneal erosion, abrasion, irregularity; punctate staining; decreased night vision.*
GI: *appetite change, nausea, dry mouth, abdominal pain, changes in appetite.*
GU: *white blood cells in urine,* proteinuria, hematuria.
Hepatic: *hepatitis, elevated liver enzymes.*
Metabolic: *hypokalemia or hyperkalemia, hyperlipidemia.*
Skin: *peeling, itching, dryness.*
Other: *bone pain,* dyspnea, photosensitivity.

INTERACTIONS

Alcohol: increased risk of hypertriglyceridemia.
Hepatotoxic medications (including methotrexate): increased risk of hepatotoxicity.
Milk, high-fat diet: increases etretinate's absorption.
Tetracyclines: increased risk of pseudotumor cerebri.
Vitamin A: additive toxic effects. Avoid concomitant use.

EFFECTS ON DIAGNOSTIC TESTS

Serum triglycerides, serum cholesterol, AST (SGOT), ALT (SGPT), lactate dehydrogenase: increased levels.
Serum high-density lipoproteins: decreased levels.

NURSING CONSIDERATIONS

Besides those related universally to drug therapy (see "How to use this book"), consider the following specific recommendations:

Assessment

- Obtain a baseline assessment of the patient's integumentary status before therapy.
- Be alert for adverse reactions and drug interactions throughout therapy.
- Evaluate the patient's and family's knowledge about etretinate therapy.

Nursing Diagnoses

- Impaired skin intergrity related to underlying condition.
- Altered nutrition: Less than body requirements, related to adverse reactions to etretinate.
- Knowledge deficit related to etretinate therapy.

Planning and Implementation

Preparation and Administration

- Administer the drug with milk or fatty foods to enhance absorption.
- Rule out pregnancy by performing a pregnancy test within 2 weeks of beginning therapy. Therapy may begin on the second or third day of the next normal menstrual period.

Monitoring

- Monitor effectiveness by evaluating the patient's skin for severity and number of lesions associated with the underlying condition.
- Assess pain related to the underlying condition.
- Monitor liver function tests at 1- to 2-week intervals for the first 2 months of therapy and then at intervals of 1 to 3 months.
- Review blood lipids every 1 to 2 weeks during treatment.
- Assess for signs of CNS involvement (dizziness, lethargy, changes in sensation).
- Monitor blood glucose daily if the patient has diabetes.

Supportive Care

- Provide sugarless gum or hard candy or ice chips to help relieve dry mouth.
- Administer antihistamines if ordered to control pruritus related to underlying condition.

• Adjust hypoglycemic medications of diabetic patients as ordered.

Patient Teaching

• Tell women of childbearing age to use effective contraception for 1 month before therapy begins, during therapy, and for an indefinite time after treatment is discontinued. Explain that the exact period of time after therapy in which pregnancy must be avoided is not known.

• Instruct the patient to report immediately the development of headache or visual disturbances.

• Advise the patient to avoid taking vitamin A supplements, which can cause additive adverse reactions.

• Instruct the patient to take a missed dose as soon as possible, unless it is nearly time for the next dose; if so, he should omit the missed dose and resume the usual schedule.

• Inform the patient that dry skin and drying of the eyes are common adverse reactions to etretinate. Tell him that eye dryness may cause discomfort if he is wearing contact lenses.

• Tell the patient to take drug with milk or fatty foods to enhance absorption.

• Advise the patient to avoid exposure to excess bright light and to use a sunscreen.

• Teach the diabetic patient to monitor blood glucose daily.

• Tell the patient to notify the doctor of decreased night vision.

Evaluation

In patients receiving etretinate, appropriate evaluation statements may include:

• Patient reports decrease of skin lesions and associated discomfort.

• Patient does not experience any gastric symptoms and can eat and drink a regular diet.

• Patient and family state an understanding of etretinate therapy.

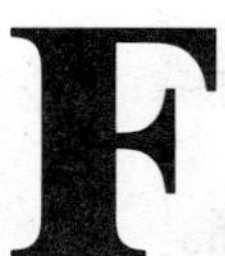

Factor IX complex

Konyne-HT, Profilnine Heat-Treated, Proplex T

• *Classification:* systemic hemostatic (blood derivative)
• *Pregnancy Risk Category:* C

HOW SUPPLIED

Injection: vials, with diluents. Units specified on label.

ACTION

Mechanism: Directly replaces deficient clotting factor.
Absorption: Must be administered intravenously; drug is destroyed in the GI tract.
Distribution: Equilibration within extravascular space takes 4 to 6 hours.
Metabolism: Rapidly cleared by plasma.
Excretion: Half-life: Approximately 24 hours.

INDICATIONS & DOSAGE

Factor IX deficiency (hemophilia B or Christmas disease), anticoagulant overdosage–
Adults and children: units required equal 0.8 to 1 × body weight in kg × percentage of desired increase of factor IX level, by slow I.V. infusion or I.V. push. Dosage is highly individualized, depending on degree of deficiency, level of factor IX desired, weight of patient, and severity of bleeding.

CONTRAINDICATIONS & PRECAUTIONS

Contraindicated in hepatic disease, intravascular coagulation, or fibrinolysis. Administer factor IX complex cautiously to neonates and infants susceptible to hepatitis, which factor IX complex may transmit; presently available heat-treated products reduce this risk. Only Proplex T may be used to treat factor VII deficiency.

ADVERSE REACTIONS

Common reactions are in italics; life-threatening reactions are in bold italics.
CNS: headache.
CV: *thromboembolic reactions,* possible ***intravascular hemolysis*** in patients with blood type A, B, or AB.
Other: *transient fever, chills, flushing, tingling,* hypersensitivity.

INTERACTIONS

None significant.

EFFECTS ON DIAGNOSTIC TESTS

None reported.

NURSING CONSIDERATIONS

Besides those related universally to drug therapy (see "How to use this book"), consider the following specific recommendations:
Assessment
• Obtain a baseline assessment of vital signs and coagulation studies before therapy.
• Be alert for adverse reactions and drug interactions throughout therapy.
• Evaluate the patient's and family's knowledge about factor IX complex therapy.
Nursing Diagnoses
• Fluid volume deficit related to the patient's underlying condition.
• High risk for altered body temperature related to adverse effects of factor IX complex.

• Knowledge deficit related to factor IX complex therapy.

Planning and Implementation

Preparation and Administration

• ***Direct injection:*** Available in kit that includes concentrate, diluent (10 to 30 ml, depending on manufacturer), and filter needle. Number of international units of factor per vial appears on label. Refrigerate but do not freeze. After warming concentrate and diluent to room temperature, reconstitute using aseptic technique. Follow manufacturer's directions. Administer within 3 hours. Do not refrigerate after reconstitution. Specific dose depends on the patient and the type of bleeding episode. Using a 21G or 23G winged infusion set, inject slowly (do not exceed 3 ml/minute). Slow injection minimizes the risk of thrombosis. If facial flushing or tingling occurs during infusion, stop momentarily and resume at a slower rate.

• ***Intermittent infusion:*** not recommended.

• ***Continuous infusion:*** not recommended.

Monitoring

• Monitor effectiveness by carefully checking vital signs and coagulation assays.

• Monitor the patient for alterations in temperature, chills, headache, pulse and blood pressure changes, tingling, and urticaria.

Supportive Care

• Remember that the international committee on thrombosis and hemostasis recommends adding 5 units of heparin per milliliter of diluent when treating factor IX deficient patients. This practice isn't recommended for patients with factor VIII inhibitors.

Patient Teaching

• Educate the patient about acquired immunodeficiency syndrome, and encourage immunization against hepatitis B in HBsAg-negative patients. Explain that the risk of infection with human immunodeficiency virus is low in patients receiving heat-treated factor IX concentrate from screened donors.

Evaluation

In patients receiving factor IX, appropriate evaluation statements may include:

• Patient has normal fluid volume and hemostasis has occurred.

• Patient has vital signs within normal limits and experienced no alteration in temperature.

• Patient and family state an understanding of factor IX complex therapy.

---

famotidine

(fa moe´ ti deen)

Pepcid, Pepcidin‡

• *Classification:* antiulcer agent (histamine$_2$-receptor antagonist)

• *Pregnancy Risk Category:* B

HOW SUPPLIED

Tablets: 20 mg, 40 mg

Powder for oral suspension: 40 mg/5 ml after reconstituting

Injection: 10 mg/ml

ACTION

Mechanism: Competitively inhibits the action of histamine at H_2 receptor sites of the parietal cells, decreasing gastric acid secretion.

Absorption: When administered orally, approximately 40% to 45% of dose is absorbed.

Distribution: Widely distributed to many body tissues.

Metabolism: About 30% to 35% of an administered dose is metabolized by the liver (minimal first-pass metabolism).

Excretion: Most excreted unchanged in urine. Half-life: 2½ to 4 hours in patients with normal renal function.

Onset, peak, duration: Onset of action occurs in 1 hour, with peak action in 1 to 3 hours. After parenteral administration, peak action occurs in 30 minutes. Duration of effect is dose-related. Following a single 40-mg oral dose at h.s., 24-hour gastric acid secretion is inhibited by about 70%, while 95% of nocturnal and 32% of daytime secretion is blocked.

INDICATIONS & DOSAGE

Duodenal ulcer–
Adults: For acute therapy, 40 mg P.O. once daily h.s. For maintenance therapy, 20 mg P.O. once daily h.s.
Pathologic hypersecretory conditions (such as Zollinger-Ellison syndrome)–
Adults: 20 mg P.O. q 6 hours. As much as 160 mg q 6 hours may be administered.
Hospitalized patients with intractable ulcers or hypersecretory conditions, or patients who cannot take oral medication–
Adults: 20 mg I.V. q 12 hours.

CONTRAINDICATIONS & PRECAUTIONS

Contraindicated in patients with famotidine allergy. Use cautiously in patients with severely impaired hepatic function because inadequate hepatic metabolism may cause accumulation of the drug and toxic effects. Dosage increase may be necessary in patients with creatinine clearance less than 10 ml/minute.

ADVERSE REACTIONS

Common reactions are in italics; life-threatening reactions are in bold italics.
Blood: thrombocytopenia (rare).
CNS: *headache,* dizziness, hallucinations.
GI: diarrhea, constipation, nausea, flatulence.
GU: increased BUN and creatinine.
Skin: acne, pruritus, rash.
Local: transient irritation at I.V. site.

INTERACTIONS

None significant.

EFFECTS ON DIAGNOSTIC TESTS

Gastric acid secretion tests: antagonism of pentagastrin.
Hepatic enzymes: elevated levels.
Skin tests using allergen extracts: false-negative results.

NURSING CONSIDERATIONS

Besides those related universally to drug therapy (see "How to use this book"), consider the following specific recommendations:

Assessment
- Obtain a baseline assessment of the patient's GI pain before initiating famotidine therapy.
- Be alert for adverse reactions and drug interactions throughout therapy.
- Evaluate the patient's and family's knowledge about famotidine therapy.

Nursing Diagnoses
- Pain related to the patient's underlying condition.
- High risk for injury related to famotidine-induced CNS adverse reactions.
- Knowledge deficit related to famotidine therapy.

Planning and Implementation
Preparation and Administration
- Be sure that gastric cancer has been ruled out before administering famotidine.
- ***P.O. use:*** Give this drug at bedtime. Give with a snack if the patient desires. Expect some patients to have this drug prescribed to be taken 20 mg twice daily instead of 40 mg at bedtime. This alternate dosing schedule is effective, but at least one dose should be taken at bedtime.
- Store reconstituted suspension below 85° F (30° C). Discard after 30 days.
- ***I.V. use:*** To prepare I.V. direct injection, dilute 2 ml (20 mg) famotidine

with compatible I.V. solution to a total volume of either 5 or 10 ml, and inject slowly (over at least 2 minutes). Compatible solutions include sterile water for injection, 0.9% sodium chloride injection, 5% or 10% dextrose injection, 5% sodium bicarbonate injection, or latated Ringer's injection.

Alternatively, famotidine may be given by I.V. infusion. Dilute 20 mg (2 ml) famotidine in 100 ml of compatible solution and infuse over 15 to 30 minutes. Solution is stable for 48 hours at room temperature after dilution.

- Store I.V. injection in refrigerator at 35.6° to 46.4° F (2° to 8° C).

Monitoring

- Monitor effectiveness by regularly observing potential for relief of GI pain.
- Evaluate hematologic studies for signs of abnormalities, such as thrombocytopenia.
- Frequently monitor I.V. site for signs of infiltration or phlebitis.

Supportive Care

- If I.V. injection site becomes infiltrated or shows signs of phlebitis, discontinue I.V. and restart in another site. Notify the doctor and, if indicated, apply warm compress to site.
- Take safety precautions if the patient develops dizziness, confusion, or other mental status changes. For example, keep bed in low position, keep side rails up, and supervise the patient's activity.
- If the patient develops diarrhea, notify the doctor and obtain an order for an antidiarrheal. Also encourage the patient to increase fluid intake.

Patient Teaching

- Tell the patient that he may take antacids concomitantly with this drug as long as the doctor is aware that he is taking them. Explain that the doctor often permits patients to take antacids concomitantly with this drug at the beginning of therapy when pain is severe.
- Remind the patient that, if he's taking famotidine once daily, he should take it at bedtime for best results.
- Advise the patient not to take the drug for longer than 8 weeks unless the doctor specifically orders it.
- Tell the patient that he may take famotidine with a snack if he desires.
- Urge the patient to avoid smoking cigarettes, which may increase gastric acid secretion and worsen disease. Also instruct the patient to avoid sources of GI irritation, such as alcohol, certain foods, and drugs containing aspirin.
- Instruct the patient to report immediately headache or any signs of diarrhea, confusion, or rash.

Evaluation

In patients receiving famotidine, appropriate evaluation statements may include:

- Patient has decrease in or relief of GI pain.
- Patient injury did not occur; no CNS adverse reactions were experienced.
- Patient and family state an understanding of famotidine therapy.

fat emulsions

Intralipid 10%, Intralipid 20%, Liposyn 10%, Liposyn 20%, Liposyn II 10%, Liposyn II 20%, Soyacal 10%, Soyacal 20%, Travamulsion 10%, Travamulsion 20%

- *Classification:* nutritional agent (lipid)
- *Pregnancy Risk Category:* B for Soyacal 10%; C for all others

HOW SUPPLIED

Injection: 50 ml (10%, 20%), 100 ml (10%, 20%), 200 ml (10%, 20%), 250 ml (10%, 20%), 500 ml (10%, 20%).

ACTION

Mechanism: Acts as a source of calories. Each ml of a 10% solution provides about 1.1 calories; each ml of a 20% solution provides about 2 calories. Provides neutral triglycerides predominantly as saturated fatty acids. Most contain soybean or safflower oil, glycerin, water, and fatty acids (linoleic, oleic, palmitic, linolenic, and stearic), and egg yolk phospholipids, which act as emulsifiers.
Absorption: Administered as an I.V. infusion.
Distribution: Throughout the plasma compartment.
Metabolism: Metabolized and used as an energy source, causing increased heat production, decreased respiratory quotient, and increased oxygen consumption.
Excretion: The infused fat particles are cleared from the bloodstream in a manner similar to chylomicrons.

INDICATIONS & DOSAGE

Intralipid:
Source of calories adjunctive to total parenteral nutrition–
Adults: 1 ml/minute I.V. for 15 to 30 minutes (10% emulsion); 0.5 ml/minute I.V. for 15 to 30 minutes (20% emulsion). If no adverse reactions, increase rate to deliver 500 ml over 4 to 8 hours. Total daily dosage should not exceed 2.5 g/kg.
Children: 0.1 ml/minute for 10 to 15 minutes (10% emulsion); 0.05 ml/minute I.V. for 10 to 15 minutes (20% emulsion). If no adverse reactions, increase rate to deliver 1 g/kg over 4 hours. Daily dosage should not exceed 4 g/kg. Equals 60% of daily caloric intake. Protein-carbohydrate total parenteral nutrition should supply remaining 40%.
Fatty acid deficiency–
Adults and children: 8% to 10% of total caloric intake I.V.

Liposyn:
Prevention of fatty acid deficiency–
Adults: 500 ml (10% emulsion) I.V. twice weekly. Infuse initially at a rate of 1 ml/minute for 30 minutes. Rate may be increased but should not exceed 500 ml over 4 to 6 hours.
Children: 5 to 10 ml/kg (10% emulsion) I.V. daily. Infuse initially at a rate of 0.1 ml/minute for 30 minutes. Rate may be increased but should not exceed 100 ml/hour.

CONTRAINDICATIONS & PRECAUTIONS

Contraindicated in patients with impaired fat metabolism, such as pathologic hyperlipidemia, lipoid nephrosis, and in those with acute pancreatitis if accompanied by hyperlipidemia. Because I.V. fat emulsions contain egg yolk phospholipids, they should not be administered to patients with severe egg allergies.

Use cautiously in patients with severe liver damage, pulmonary disease, anemia, or blood coagulation disorders; and when danger of fat embolism exists. All patients must have their capacity to eliminate I.V. fat emulsions monitored to ensure clearance of the lipemia between daily infusions. Discontinue use if abnormal parameters result.

ADVERSE REACTIONS

Common reactions are in italics; life-threatening reactions are in bold italics.
Early reactions of fat overload:
Blood: hyperlipemia, hypercoagulability, thrombocytopenia in neonates (rare).
CNS: headache, sleepiness, dizziness.
EENT: pressure over eyes.
GI: nausea, vomiting.
Skin: flushing, diaphoresis.
Local: irritation at infusion site.
Other: fever, dyspnea, chest and back pains, cyanosis, ***allergic reactions,*** deposition of I.V. fat.

Delayed reactions:
Blood: thrombocytopenia, leukopenia, leukocytosis.
CNS: focal seizures.
CV: ***shock.***
Hepatic: transient increased liver function test results, hepatomegaly.
Other: fever, splenomegaly, ***fat accumulation in lungs.***

INTERACTIONS
None significant.

EFFECTS ON DIAGNOSTIC TESTS
Hemoglobin: abnormally high mean corpuscular hemoglobin concentration in blood samples drawn during or shortly after fat emulsion infusion.
Liver function tests: transient abnormalities.
Serum bilirubin: altered results (especially in infants).

NURSING CONSIDERATIONS
Besides those related universally to drug therapy (see "How to use this book"), consider the following specific recommendations:

Assessment
- Obtain a baseline assessment of the patient's underlying condition before therapy.
- Be alert for adverse reactions and drug interactions throughout therapy.
- Evaluate the patient's and family's knowledge about fat emulsion therapy.

Nursing Diagnoses
- Altered nutrition: Less than body requirements related to the patient's underlying condition.
- Pain related to fat emulsion-induced headache, pressure over eyes and chest, and back discomfort related to adverse drug reaction.
- Knowledge deficit related to fat emulsion therapy.

Planning and Implementation
Preparation and Administration
- Do not use if solution separates or becomes oily.
- Refrigeration is not necessary.
- ***I.V. use:*** Do not use an in-line filter when administering this drug because the fat particles are larger than the 0.22-micron cellulose filter. Avoid rapid infusion and use an infusion pump to regulate rate.
- Keep in mind that fat emulsion may be mixed with amino acid solution, dextrose, electrolytes, and vitamins in the same I.V. container. Check with the pharmacist for acceptable proportions and compatibility information.
- Keep in mind that Intralipid, Travamulsion, and Liposyn differ mainly in their fatty acid components.

Monitoring
- Monitor effectiveness by assessing patient's overall condition, especially noting nutritional status.
- Monitor the patient closely for adverse reactions, especially during the first half hour of infusion.
- Monitor serum lipid levels closely throughout fat emulsion therapy. Lipemia must clear between dosing.
- Monitor hepatic function carefully in long-term use.
- Carefully monitor platelet count in neonates, and triglycerides and free fatty acids in premature infants receiving fat emulsion because they are susceptible to I.V. fat overload.
- Check the injection site frequently for signs of inflammation and infection.

Supportive Care
- Change all I.V. tubing before each infusion. Lipids support bacterial growth.
- Report signs of inflammation or infection at the infusion site promptly.
- Notify the doctor before giving an infusion if lipemia has not cleared as evidenced by serum lipid level after the last infusion.

Patient Teaching
- Tell the patient to notify the nurse or doctor of any burning, stinging,

redness, or swelling at the infusion site.

• Explain the early and delayed reactions to fat overload, and tell the patient to report these symptoms if they occur.

Evaluation

In patients receiving fat emulsions, appropriate evaluation statements may include:

• Patient's nutritional status is improving.

• Patient did not experience discomfort from fat emulsion-induced adverse reactions.

• Patient and family state an understanding of fat emulsion therapy.

fenfluramine hydrochloride

(fen flure´ a meen)

Ponderal†, Ponderal Pacaps†, Ponderax‡, Ponderax Pacaps‡, Pondimin, Pondimin Extentabs

• Controlled Substance Schedule IV
• *Classification:* short-term adjunctive anorexigenic agent, indirect-acting sympathomimetic amine (amphetamine congener)
• *Pregnancy Risk Category:* C

HOW SUPPLIED

Tablets: 20 mg, 40 mg
Capsules (sustained-release): 60 mg†‡

ACTION

Mechanism: An anorexigenic agent that probably acts by stimulating the ventromedial nucleus of the hypothalamus. May also affect serotonin metabolism.

Absorption: Well absorbed after oral administration.

Distribution: Widely distributed throughout the body, including the CNS.

Metabolism: Hepatic.

Excretion: Most drug and metabolites are excreted in urine; rate of elimination is pH-dependent. Half-life: About 20 hours; may decrease to 11 hours with acidic urine.

Onset, peak, duration: Maximal anorexia occurs 2 to 4 hours after ingestion.

INDICATIONS & DOSAGE

Short-term adjunct in exogenous obesity–

Adults: initially, 20 mg P.O. t.i.d. before meals. Maximum dosage is 40 mg t.i.d. Adjust dosage according to patient's response.

CONTRAINDICATIONS & PRECAUTIONS

Contraindicated in patients with hypersensitivity or idiosyncratic reaction to sympathomimetic amines; in depressed or alcoholic patients; symptomatic cardiovascular disease; and a history of substance abuse: for use with monoamine oxidase (MAO) inhibitors or within 14 days of such use.

Use cautiously in patients with hypertension, diabetes mellitus, or a history of depressive disorder. Habituation or psychological dependence may occur with prolonged use.

Use cautiously in patients undergoing general anesthesia; fatal cardiac arrest has been reported. Therefore, when possible, discontinue drug for 1 week before surgery; if surgery cannot be postponed, full cardiac monitoring and resuscitative equipment must be available.

Do not use for intermittent courses of therapy in weight control.

ADVERSE REACTIONS

Common reactions are in italics; life-threatening reactions are in bold italics.

CNS: *drowsiness,* dizziness, incoordination, headache, euphoria or depression, anxiety, *insomnia,* weakness, fatigue, agitation.

CV: *palpitations,* hypotension, hypertension, chest pain.
EENT: eye irritation, blurred vision.
GI: *diarrhea, dry mouth,* nausea, vomiting, abdominal pain, constipation.
GU: dysuria, increased urinary frequency, impotence.
Skin: rashes, urticaria, burning sensation.
Other: sweating, chills, fever, increased libido.

INTERACTIONS

Alcohol, CNS depressants: enhanced CNS depression.
Centrally acting antihypertensives: decreased antihypertensive effect.
MAO inhibitors: severe hypertension; possible hypertensive crisis. Don't use together.

EFFECTS ON DIAGNOSTIC TESTS

None reported.

NURSING CONSIDERATIONS

Besides those related universally to drug therapy (see "How to use this book"), consider the following specific recommendations:

Assessment

- Obtain a baseline assessment of the patient's weight and dietary intake.
- Be alert for adverse reactions and drug interactions throughout therapy.
- Evaluate the patient's and family's knowledge about fenfluramine hydrochloride therapy.

Nursing Diagnoses

- Altered nutrition: More than body requirements related to obesity.
- High risk for injury related to CNS adverse reactions to drug therapy.
- Knowledge deficit related to fenfluramine hydrochloride therapy.

Planning and Implementation

Preparation and Administration

- Avoid prolonged administration. Tolerance or dependence may occur.

Monitoring

- Monitor effectiveness regularly by assessing the patient's weight and monitoring dietary intake.
- Closely monitor blood pressure; regularly question the patient about palpitations or chest pain.
- Monitor blood glucose. Because of possible hypoglycemia, patients with diabetes may have altered insulin or sulfonylurea requirements.
- Monitor for signs of excessive sedation, depression, or excessive stimulation. Keep in mind that this drug differs pharmacologically from amphetamines in that it produces CNS depression more often than stimulation.

Supportive Care

- If CNS disturbances occur, institute precautions, such as providing a safe environment and supervising activities.
- Make sure the patient is also on a weight-reduction program. Do calorie counts, if necessary.
- Be aware that this drug has proven effective for autistic children.

Patient Teaching

- Warn the patient to avoid hazardous activities that require alertness or good psychomotor coordination until CNS effects of the drug are known.
- Have the patient report signs of excessive drowsiness, dizziness, or stimulation.
- Tell patient to weigh himself weekly in the same clothes at the same time of day to evaluate effectiveness of drug therapy.
- Tell the diabetic patient to monitor blood glucose levels closely.
- Warn the patient not to stop taking the drug abruptly because this may precipitate an acute depressive reaction.

Evaluation

In patients receiving fenfluramine hydrochloride, appropriate evaluation statements may include:

- Patient demonstrates safe, targeted weight loss.

• Patient's safety is maintained. CNS adverse reactions did not occur.
• Patient and family state an understanding of fenfluramine hydrochloride therapy.

fenoprofen calcium

(fen oh proe´ fen)
Nalfon

• *Classification:* nonnarcotic analgesic, antipyretic (nonsteroidal anti-inflammatory agent)
• *Pregnancy Risk Category:* B (D in 3rd trimester)

HOW SUPPLIED

Tablets: 600 mg
Capsules: 200 mg, 300 mg, 600 mg

ACTION

Mechanism: Produces anti-inflammatory, analgesic, and antipyretic effects, possibly through inhibition of prostaglandin synthesis.
Absorption: Rapidly and completely absorbed from the GI tract.
Distribution: 99% protein-bound.
Metabolism: Hepatic.
Excretion: Mainly in urine; a small amount in feces. Half-life: 2½ to 3 hours.
Onset, peak, duration: The onset of analgesic activity occurs within 15 to 30 minutes, with peak plasma levels in 2 hours. The duration of action is approximately 4 to 6 hours.

INDICATIONS & DOSAGE

Rheumatoid arthritis and osteoarthritis–
Adults: 300 to 600 mg P.O. q.i.d. Maximum dosage is 3.2 g daily.
Mild to moderate pain–
Adults: 200 mg P.O. q 4 to 6 hours, p.r.n.

CONTRAINDICATIONS & PRECAUTIONS

Contraindicated in patients with hypersensitivity to the drug; in patients in whom aspirin or other NSAIDs induce symptoms of asthma, urticaria, or rhinitis; and in patients with renal impairment because it may induce renal failure. Patients with known "triad" symptoms (aspirin hypersensitivity, rhinitis/nasal polyps, and asthma) are at high risk for bronchospasm).

Because serious GI toxicity, including ulceration or hemorrhage, can occur at any time in patients on chronic NSAID therapy, use cautiously in patients with a history of GI disease and in patients with impaired cardiac function and bleeding abnormalities.

NSAIDs may mask the signs and symptoms of acute infection (fever, myalgia, erythema); carefully evaluate patients with high risk (such as those with diabetes).

ADVERSE REACTIONS

Common reactions are in italics; life-threatening reactions are in bold italics.
Blood: prolonged bleeding time, anemia.
CNS: *headache, drowsiness, dizziness.*
CV: peripheral edema.
GI: *epigastric distress, nausea, vomiting, occult blood loss, peptic ulceration,* constipation, anorexia.
GU: reversible renal failure.
Hepatic: elevated enzymes.
Skin: *pruritus,* rash, urticaria.

INTERACTIONS

Aspirin: decreases fenoprofen half-life.
Oral anticoagulants, sulfonylureas: fenoprofen enhances pharmacologic effects of these drugs. Use together cautiously.

EFFECTS ON DIAGNOSTIC TESTS

Bleeding time: prolonged.
BUN, serum creatinine, potassium, alkaline phosphatase, lactic dehydrogenase, and transaminase: increased concentrations.

NURSING CONSIDERATIONS

Besides those related universally to drug therapy (see "How to use this book"), consider the following specific recommendations:

Assessment
- Obtain a baseline assessment of pain before therapy.
- Be alert for adverse reactions and drug interactions throughout therapy.
- Evaluate the patient's and family's knowledge about fenoprofen therapy.

Nursing Diagnoses
- Pain related to the patient's underlying condition.
- High risk for injury related to CNS adverse reactions to fenoprofen therapy.
- Knowledge deficit related to fenoprofen therapy.

Planning and Implementation
Preparation and Administration
- Give each dose of the drug 30 minutes before or 2 hours after meals. If GI adverse reactions occur, give with milk or meals.

Monitoring
- Regularly evaluate the patient's pain relief.
- Check renal, hepatic, and auditory function periodically during prolonged therapy. Discontinue drug if abnormalities occur.
- Monitor for signs of serious GI toxicity, such as GI bleeding. Keep in mind that concomitant use with aspirin, alcohol, or steroids may increase the risk of GI reactions.

Supportive Care
- Keep in mind that prothrombin time may be prolonged in patients receiving coumarin-type anticoagulants. Fenoprofen decreases platelet aggregation and may prolong bleeding time.
- If CNS adverse reactions, such as dizziness or drowsiness, occur, impose safety precautions; for example, use side rails to protect the patient from injury.

Patient Teaching
- Tell the patient who is receiving the drug for arthritis that the full therapeutic effect of the drug may be delayed for 2 to 4 weeks.
- Teach the patient and family the signs and symptoms of GI bleeding and tell them to report the occurrence of any of these signs to the doctor immediately.

Evaluation
In patients receiving fenoprofen, appropriate evaluation statements may include:
- Patient states that pain was relieved by fenoprofen.
- No adverse CNS reactions and no injury occurred.
- Patient and family state an understanding of fenoprofen therapy.

---

fentanyl citrate
(fen´ ta nil)
Sublimaze

fentanyl transdermal system
Duragesic-25, Duragesic-50, Duragesic-75, Duragesic-100

- Controlled Substance Schedule II
- *Classification:* analgesic, anesthetic (opioid agonist)
- *Pregnancy Risk Category:* B (D for prolonged use or use of high doses at term)

HOW SUPPLIED

Injection: 50 mcg/ml
Transdermal system: patches designed to release 25, 50, 75, or 100 mcg of fentanyl/hour.

ACTION

Mechanism: Binds with opiate receptors at many sites in the CNS (brain, brain stem, and spinal cord), altering both perception of and emotional response to pain through an unknown mechanism.
Absorption: For acute analgesic effects, fentanyl is usually administered I.V. The drug is absorbed through the skin when administered by transdermal system.
Distribution: Redistribution has been suggested as the main cause of the brief analgesic effect of parenterally administered fentanyl. With transdermal administration, drug accumulates in the layers of skin adjacent to the transdermal system.
Metabolism: Hepatic.
Excretion: In the urine as metabolites and unchanged drug. Half-life: Terminal elimination half-life is 3 to 12 hours after I.V. administration; about 17 hours after transdermal administration.
Onset, peak, duration: Rapid onset after I.V. administration; peak levels occur within 5 to 15 minutes, with peak analgesia within 30 minutes. Duration of action is 1 to 2 hours. When given by transdermal system, serum fentanyl levels rise for the first 12 to 24 hours after application and remain relatively constant for up to 3 days.

INDICATIONS & DOSAGE

Adjunct to general anesthetic–
Adults: 0.05 to 0.1 mg I.V. repeated q 2 to 3 minutes, p.r.n. Dose should be reduced in elderly and high-risk patients.
Postoperatively–
Adults: 0.05 to 0.1 mg I.M. q 1 to 2 hours p.r.n.
Preoperatively–
Adults: 0.05 to 0.1 mg I.M. 30 to 60 minutes before surgery.
Children 2 to 12 years: 1.7 to 3.3 mcg/kg I.M.
Management of chronic pain–
Adults: Apply one transdermal system to a portion of the upper torso on an area of skin that is not irritated and has not been irradiated. Initiate therapy with the 25-mcg/hr system; adjust dosage as needed and tolerated. Each system may be worn for 72 hours.

CONTRAINDICATIONS & PRECAUTIONS

Contraindicated in patients with hypersensitivity to the drug.

Use with extreme caution in patients with supraventricular arrhythmias or bradycardia. Avoid or use with extreme caution in patients with head injury or increased intracranial pressure because drug obscures neurologic parameters. Avoid during pregnancy and labor because drug readily crosses the placenta (premature infants are especially sensitive to respiratory and CNS depressant effects of fentanyl).

Use cautiously in patients with renal or hepatic dysfunction because drug accumulation or prolonged duration of action may occur; in patients with pulmonary disease (asthma, chronic obstructive pulmonary disease) because drug depresses respiration and suppresses cough reflex; in patients undergoing biliary tract surgery because drug may cause biliary spasm; in patients with seizure disorders because drug may precipitate seizures; in elderly or debilitated patients, who are more sensitive to drug's effects; and in patients prone to physical or psychological addiction because of the high abuse potential for this drug.

Muscle rigidity that may be associated with reduced pulmonary compliance or apnea, laryngospasm, and bronchoconstriction may occur and may be treated with assisted ventilation or I.V. neuromuscular blocking drugs.

The manufacturer states that use of fentanyl is not recommended in patients who have received monoamine oxidase (MAO) inhibitors within the preceding 14 days.

ADVERSE REACTIONS

Common reactions are in italics; life-threatening reactions are in bold italics.

CNS: *sedation, somnolence, clouded sensorium, euphoria,* dizziness, seizures with large doses.

CV: *hypotension,* bradycardia.

GI: nausea, vomiting, *constipation,* ileus.

GU: *urine retention.*

Local: reaction at application site (erythema, papules, edema, itching).

Other: ***respiratory depression,*** muscle rigidity, physical dependence.

INTERACTIONS

Alcohol, CNS depressants: additive effects. Use together cautiously.

EFFECTS ON DIAGNOSTIC TESTS

Plasma amylase and lipase: increased levels.

NURSING CONSIDERATIONS

Besides those related universally to drug therapy (see "How to use this book"), consider the following specific recommendations:

Assessment

• Obtain a baseline assessment of the patient's pain before therapy.

• Be alert for adverse reactions and drug interactions throughout therapy.

• Evaluate the patient's and family's knowledge about fentanyl therapy.

Nursing Diagnoses

• Pain related to patient's underlying condition.

• Ineffective breathing pattern related to fentanyl-induced respiratory depression.

• Knowledge deficit related to fentanyl therapy.

Planning and Implementation

Preparation and Administration

• Reduce fentanyl citrate dose by one-fourth to one-third, as ordered, if used with other narcotic analgesics, general anesthetics, tranquilizers, alcohol, sedatives, hypnotics, tricyclic antidepressants, or MAO inhibitors because such use may cause respiratory depression, hypotension, profound sedation, and coma. Also give above drugs in reduced dosages.

• ***I.V. use:*** Only staff trained in administration of I.V. anesthetics and managing their potential adverse reactions should administer I.V. fentanyl.

• ***Epidural use:*** Be aware that epidural injection or infusion has been used for postoperative analgesia, chronic pain management, or postpartum pain control.

• ***Transdermal use:*** Remove transdermal system from package only immediately before applying. Hold in place for 10 to 20 seconds, and be sure the edges of the system are in contact with the patient's skin. Refer to dosage equivalent charts as needed to calculate the fentanyl transdermal dose based on the daily morphine intake. An approximation: For every 90 mg of oral morphine or 15 mg of I.M. morphine per 24 hours, 25 mcg/hour of transdermal fentanyl is required. Make gradual dosage adjustments in patients using the transdermal system. Reaching steady-state levels of a new dose may take up to 6 days; patients should delay adjusting dose until after at least two applications. Some patients will require alternate means of opiate administration when the dose exceeds 300 mcg/hour.

If another transdermal system is needed after 72 hours, it should be applied to a new site. When reducing opiate therapy or substituting a different analgesic, gradually withdraw the drug in patients using the transdermal system. Because the serum level of fentanyl declines gradually after removal, give half of the equianalgesic dose of the new analgesic 12 to 18 hours after removal.

Monitoring

• Monitor effectiveness by evaluating pain relief. Because serum fentanyl concentration rises during the first 24 hours after application of the transdermal system, do not expect to evaluate the analgesic effect for the first day.

• Monitor respirations of neonates exposed to drug during labor.

• Monitor for muscle rigidity, leading to problems with ventilation, which may occur with high doses. Note that these problems may occur during emergence from anesthesia. This effect can be reversed by administration of neuromuscular blocking agents.

• Monitor for evidence of respiratory depression, such as decreased rate or depth of respirations.

• Monitor circulatory status carefully.

• Monitor bladder function in postoperative patients.

• Closely monitor patients who discontinue using the transdermal system because of adverse reaction, for at least 12 hours after removal. Serum levels of fentanyl decline gradually after transdermal use and may take as long as 17 hours to decline by 50%.

Supportive Care

• Notify the doctor if pain is not relieved.

• Notify the doctor if the patient's respirations are below 12/minute.

• Realize that when I.V. fentanyl is used in high doses, respiratory depression may persist for several hours after the patient awakens, making ventilatory support necessary.

• Keep narcotic antagonist (naloxone) and resuscitative equipment available when giving drug I.V.

• **Treatment of overdose:** For hypoventilation or apnea, give oxygen and positive pressure ventilation via bag and mask or endotracheal tube to maintain a patent airway and ventilation. To reverse respiratory depression, as ordered, administer naloxone in divided doses. Continue supportive therapy until the drug is metabolized

• Be aware that fentanyl is often used with droperidol (Innovar) to produce neuroleptanalgesia.

• For better analgesic effect, give fentanyl before patient has intense pain. Remember that transdermal fentanyl is not recommended for postoperative pain.

• Be sure the patient using the transdermal system has adequate supplemental analgesic to prevent breakthrough pain.

Patient Teaching

• When used postoperatively, encourage turning, coughing, and deep breathing to avoid atelectasis.

• Tell the patient or family to notify the doctor if respiration rate decreases.

• Teach the proper application of the transdermal system. Clip hair at the application site. Do not use a razor because shaving may irritate the skin. Wash area with clear water if necessary, but do not use soaps, oils, lotions, alcohol, or any other substance that may irritate the skin or interfere with the adhesive. Be sure area is completely dry before applying.

• Teach patient to dispose of the transdermal system by folding the system so the adhesive side adheres to itself and then flushing the system down the toilet.

Evaluation

In patients receiving fentanyl, appropriate evaluation statements include:

• Patient reports relief of pain after administration of fentanyl.

• Respiratory status is within normal limits.

• Patient and family state an understanding of fentanyl therapy.

fentanyl citrate with droperidol

(fen′ ta nil/droe per′ i dol)
Innovar

• Controlled Substance Schedule II
• *Classification* analgesic, anesthetic (opioid agonist)
• *Pregnancy Risk Category:* C

HOW SUPPLIED

Injection: 0.5 mg fentanyl and 2.5 mg droperidol per ml

ACTION

Mechanism: Acts as a CNS depressant to produce a general calming effect, reduced motor activity, and analgesia.
Absorption: Rapidly absorbed from I.M. injection sites.
Distribution: Distribution time is 1.7 minutes, redistribution is 13 minutes. The volume of distribution for fentanyl citrate is 4 L/kg.
Metabolism: In the liver.
Excretion: Metabolites are excreted in urine and feces. Half-life: Terminal elimination half-life is 219 minutes.
Onset, peak, duration: The onset of action of fentanyl citrate is almost immediate when given I.V. Usual duration of action of the analgesic effect is 30 to 60 minutes after a single I.V. dose of up to 100 mg. After I.M. administration, onset of action is from 7 to 8 minutes; duration of action is 1 to 2 hours.

INDICATIONS & DOSAGE

Dosages vary depending on application; use of other agents; and patient's age, body weight, and clinical status.

Anesthesia–
Adults:
Premedication–0.5 to 2 ml I.M. 45 to 60 minutes before surgery.
Adjunct to general anesthesia–Induction: 1 ml/20 to 25 lb body weight by slow I.V. to produce neuroleptanalgesia.

Maintenance: not indicated as sole agent for maintenance of surgical anesthesia. Used in combination with other agents. To prevent excessive accumulation of the relatively long-acting droperidol component, fentanyl alone should be used in increments of 0.025 to 0.05 mg (0.5 to 1 ml) for maintenance of analgesia. However, during prolonged surgery, additional 0.5- to 1-ml amounts of Innovar may be given with caution.
Diagnostic procedures–0.5 to 2 ml I.M. 45 to 60 minutes before procedure. In prolonged procedure, give 0.5 to 1 ml I.V. with caution and without a general anesthetic.
Adjunct in regional anesthesia–1 to 2 ml I.M. or slow I.V.
Children:
Premedication–0.25 ml/20 lb body weight I.M. 45 to 60 minutes before surgery.
Adjunct to general anesthesia–0.5 ml/20 lb body weight I.V. (total combined dose for induction and maintenance). Following induction with Innovar, fentanyl alone in a dose of ¼ to ⅓ of adult dosage should be used to avoid accumulation of droperidol. However, during prolonged surgery, additional amounts of Innovar may be administered with caution. Safety of use in children under 2 years has not been established.

CONTRAINDICATIONS & PRECAUTIONS

Contraindicated in patients with hypersensitivity to the drug.

Use with extreme caution in patients with supraventricular arrhythmias or bradycardia; avoid or use with extreme caution in patients with head injury or increased intracranial pressure because drug obscures neurologic parameters; and during pregnancy and labor because drug readily crosses the placenta (premature infants are especially sensitive to respiratory and CNS depressant effects of fentanyl). Use cautiously in patients with renal or hepatic dysfunction because drug accumulation or prolonged duration of action may occur; in patients with pulmonary disease (asthma, chronic obstructive pulmonary disease) because drug depresses respiration and suppresses cough reflex; in patients undergoing biliary tract surgery because drug may cause biliary spasm; in patients with seizure disorders because drug may precipitate seizures; in elderly or debilitated patients, who are more sensitive to drug's effects; and in patients prone to physical or psychological addiction because of the high abuse potential for this drug.

Muscle rigidity that may be associated with reduced pulmonary compliance or apnea, laryngospasm, and bronchoconstriction may occur and may be treated with assisted ventilation or I.V. neuromuscular blocking drugs.

The manufacturer states that use of fentanyl is not recommended in patients who have received monoamine oxidase (MAO) inhibitors within the preceding 14 days.

ADVERSE REACTIONS

Common reactions are in italics; life-threatening reactions are in bold itallics.

CNS: emergence delirium and hallucinations, postoperative drowsiness.
CV: vasodilation, *hypotension,* decreased pulmonary arterial pressure, bradycardia, tachycardia.
EENT: blurred vision, ***laryngospasms.***
GI: *nausea, vomiting.*
Respiratory: ***respiratory depression, apnea,*** or ***arrest.***
Other: drug dependence, muscle rigidity, chills, *shivering,* diaphoresis.

INTERACTIONS

CNS depressants (such as barbiturates, tranquilizers, narcotics, and general anesthetics): additive or potentiating effect. Dosage should be reduced.
MAO inhibitors: severe and unpredictable potentiation of Innovar. Do not use together or within 2 weeks of MAO inhibitor therapy.

EFFECTS ON DIAGNOSTIC TESTS

Plasma amylase and lipase: increased levels.

NURSING CONSIDERATIONS

Besides those related universally to drug therapy (see "How to use this book"), consider the following specific recommendations:

Assessment

• Obtain a baseline assessment of the patient's vital signs, CNS status, and overall physical status before therapy.
• Be alert for adverse reactions and drug interactions throughout therapy.
• Evaluate the patient's and family's knowledge about fentanyl citrate with droperidol therapy.

Nursing Diagnoses

• High risk for injury related to adverse CNS reactions induced by fentanyl citrate with droperidol.
• Ineffective breathing pattern related to fentanyl citrate with droperidol-induced respiratory depression.
• Knowledge deficit related to fentanyl citrate with droperidol therapy.

Planning and Implementation

Preparation and Administration

• ***I.V. use:*** Keep in mind that only staff specially trained in giving I.V. anesthetics and managing potential adverse reactions should administer this drug.

Monitoring
• Monitor effectiveness by evaluating effects of CNS depression.
• Frequently monitor patient's vital signs. Be aware that hypotension is a common adverse reaction. However, if blood pressure drops, also consider hypovolemia as a possible cause. Use appropriate parenteral fluids to help restore blood pressure.
• Monitor respiratory status frequently. Be aware that respiratory depression, rigidity of respiratory muscles, and respiratory arrest can occur.
Supportive Care
• Notify the doctor immediately of any changes in CNS, respiratory, or cardiovascular status.
• Maintain a patent airway.
• Have resuscitative equipment and a narcotic antagonist available.
• Keep in mind that after use of high doses, respiratory depression may persist for several hours after the patient awakens, making ventilatory assistance necessary.
• Move and position the patient slowly during anesthesia to avoid orthostatic hypotension.
• Implement safety measures to protect the unconscious patient.
• Be aware that postoperative EEG pattern may return to normal slowly.
• If narcotic analgesics are required postoperatively, use initially in reduced doses, as low as ¼ to ⅓ those usually recommended.
• Keep in mind that when fentanyl citrate with droperidol is given for anesthesia induction, fentanyl should be used for maintenance analgesia during procedure.
• Be aware that premedication with this drug has sometimes been associated with patient agitation and refusal of surgery. Administration of diazepam may prevent this reaction.
Patient Teaching
• Explain that this drug is used to induce a calming effect, reduce motor activity, and provide analgesia during surgery.
• Tell the patient what to expect during induction of general anesthesia and during recovery afterward. As needed, clarify any other information provided by the anesthesiologist, including possible risks.
Evaluation
In patients receiving fentanyl citrate with droperidol, appropriate evaluation statements include:
• Effective CNS depression is achieved; patient safety maintained.
• Patent airway and adequate ventilatory status are maintained.
• Patient and family state an understanding of fentanyl citrate with droperidol.

fibrinolysin and desoxyribonuclease
(fye bri nol´ ih sin/des ock see rye bo nu´ klee aze)
Elase

• *Classification:* topical debriding agent (proteolytic enzyme)
• *Pregnancy Risk Category:* C

HOW SUPPLIED
Dry powder: 25 units fibrinolysin and 15,000 units deoxyribonuclease in 30-ml vial
Ointment: 30 units fibrinolysin and 20,000 units deoxyribonuclease in 30-g tube

ACTION
Mechanism: Desoxyribonuclease attacks DNA, and fibrinolysin attacks fibrin of blood clots and fibrinous exudates. Enzymatic action produces clean surfaces and promotes healing.
Absorption: Limited with topical use.

INDICATIONS & DOSAGE
Debridement of inflammatory and infected lesions (surgical wounds, ulcer-

ative lesions, second- and third-degree burns, circumcision, episiotomy, cervicitis, vaginitis, abscesses, fistulas, and sinus tracts) –
Intravaginally–
Adults and children: 5 ml ointment may be inserted using applicator supplied, once daily h.s. for vaginitis or cervicitis for 5 days or until tube is empty.
Topical use–
Adults and children: apply ointment at intervals as long as enzyme action is desired.
Irrigating agent for infected wounds, empyema cavities, abscesses, otorhinolaryngologic wounds, subcutaneous hematomas–
Adults and children: dilution for irrigation depends on extent and severity of wound.

CONTRAINDICATIONS & PRECAUTIONS

Contraindicated in patients with hypersensitivity to bovine products or mercury compounds.

ADVERSE REACTIONS

Common reactions are in italics; life-threatening reactions are in bold italics.
Local: hyperemia with high doses, allergic reactions.

INTERACTIONS

None significant.

EFFECTS ON DIAGNOSTIC TESTS

None reported.

NURSING CONSIDERATIONS

Besides those related universally to drug therapy (see "How to use this book"), consider the following specific recommendations:

Assessment
- Obtain a baseline assessment of the patient's inflammatory or infected lesions before therapy.
- Be alert for adverse reactions and drug interactions throughout therapy.
- Evaluate the patient's and family's knowledge about fibrinolysin and desoxyribonuclease therapy.

Nursing Diagnoses
- Impaired tissue integrity related to inflammatory or infected lesion.
- High risk for impaired skin integrity related to possible allergic reaction to drug therapy.
- Knowledge deficit related to fibrinolysin and desoxyribonuclease therapy.

Planning and Implementation
Preparation and Administration
- Keep in mind that dense, dry eschar must be removed surgically before enzymatic debridement. Enzyme must be in constant contact with substrate. Accumulated necrotic debris must be removed periodically and the enzyme replenished at least once daily.
- Clean wound with water, normal saline solution, or peroxide and dry gently; cover with thin layer of fibrinolysin and desoxyribonuclease. Cover with nonadhesive dressing.
- To use solution as wet to dry dressing: Mix 1 vial of fibrinolysin and desoxyribonuclease powder with 10 to 50 ml saline solution; saturate strips of fine gauze with solution. Pack ulcerated area with medicated gauze. Allow gauze to remain in contact with ulcerated lesion for about 6 to 8 hours. Remove dried gauze and repeat 3 to 4 times daily.
- To use solution as irrigating agent: Drain cavity and replace fibrinolysin and desoxyribonuclease every 6 to 10 hours to reduce amount of by-product accumulation and to minimize loss of enzyme activity. Although parenteral use is contraindicated, this drug is used as an irrigating agent in certain specific conditions.
- Prepare solution just before use. Discard after 24 hours.

Monitoring
• Monitor effectiveness by evaluating the healing of lesions.
• Monitor for signs of an allergic reaction.
Supportive Care
• Report indications of allergic reaction or signs of poor healing.
• Change dressing at least once and preferably two to three times daily. Flush away necrotic debris and reapply ointment. Frequency of application may be more important than the amount of drug used.
Patient Teaching
• Inform the patient that this medication is used to promote healing.
• Describe the dressing, irrigation and application procedure. Tell the patient how often to expect it.
• Tell the patient to report signs of allergic reaction.
Evaluation
In patients receiving fibrinolysin and desoxyribonuclease, appropriate evaluation statements include:
• Forms a healthy, clean lesion surface.
• No allergic reactions occur.
• Patient and family state an understanding of fibrinolysin and desoxyribonuclease therapy.

filgrastim (granulocyte colony stimulating factor; G-CSF)
(fil grass´ tim)
Neupogen

• *Classification:* colony stimulating factor (biological response modifier)
• *Pregnancy Risk Category:* C

HOW SUPPLIED
Injection: 300 mcg/ml

ACTION
Mechanism: A glycoprotein produced by recombinant DNA technology that stimulates proliferation and differentiation of hematopoietic cells. Filgrastim is specific for neutrophils.
Absorption: Rapidly absorbed after S.C. administration.
Excretion: The elimination half-life, in both normal subjects and cancer patients, was approximately 3½ hours.
Onset, peak, duration: Peak levels occur in 4 to 5 hours after S.C. administration.

INDICATIONS & DOSAGE
To decrease the incidence of infection in patients with nonmyeloid malignancies receiving myelosuppressive antineoplastic agents–
Adults and children: 5 mcg/kg/day I.V. or S.C. as a single dose. Doses may be increased in increments of 5 mcg/kg for each chemotherapy cycle depending on the duration and severity of the nadir of the absolute neutrophil count (ANC).

CONTRAINDICATIONS & PRECAUTIONS
Do not use in patients with malignancies with myeloid characteristics because filgrastim may act as a growth factor for any tumor.

ADVERSE REACTIONS
Common reactions are in italics; life-threatening reactions are in bold italics.
Blood: ***thrombocytopenia.***
GU: hematuria, proteinuria.
Skin: alopecia, exacerbation of preexisting conditions (such as psoriasis).
Other: *skeletal pain,* fever, splenomegaly, osteoporosis.

INTERACTIONS
Chemotherapeutic agents: rapidly dividing myeloid cells are potentially sensitive to cytotoxic agents. Do not use filgrastim concomitantly with chemotherapy.

EFFECTS ON DIAGNOSTIC TESTS

Blood pressure: transient decreases.
CBC: increased WBC counts (100,000/mm³ or more); transiently increased neutrophils.
Serum creatinine and aminotransferase: increased levels.
Uric acid, lactate dehydrogenase, and alkaline phosphatase levels: reversible elevations.

NURSING CONSIDERATIONS

Besides those related universally to drug therapy (see "How to use this book"), consider the following specific recommendations:

Assessment

- Obtain a baseline assessment of the patient's allergies, CBC count with differential, and platelet count before therapy.
- Be alert for adverse reactions and drug interactions throughout therapy.
- Evaluate the patient's and family's knowledge about filgrastim therapy.

Nursing Diagnoses

- High risk for infection related to myelosuppression induced by antineoplastic agents.
- Pain (skeletal) induced by filgrastim therapy.
- Knowledge deficit related to filgrastim therapy.

Planning and Implementation

Preparation and Administration

- Store in the refrigerator at 36° to 46° F (2° to 8° C). Do not freeze. The drug may be stored at room temperature for a maximum of 6 hours; discard any vial that has been at room temperature for more than 6 hours.
- Avoid shaking.
- Do not reenter a vial once a dose is withdrawn. Vials are intended for single use only and contain no preservatives.
- ***I.V. use:*** Give filgrastim daily for up to 2 weeks until the ANC has returned to 10,000 mm³ after the expected chemotherapy-induced neutrophil nadir.
- May also be administered by S.C. injection.

Monitoring

- Monitor effectiveness by reviewing the neutrophil count. Note that a transiently increased neutrophil count is common 1 to 2 days after the start of therapy.
- Monitor CBC and platelet count twice weekly during therapy.
- Monitor urine, stool, secretions, and emesis fluid for occult blood. Observe for bruising.
- Observe for hypersensitivity reaction.

Supportive Care

- Obtain order for medication to relieve drug-induced skeletal pain. Use comfort measures, such as positioning and padding; provide assistance with activities and ambulation.
- Be aware that patients receiving filgrastim have the potential for receiving higher doses of chemotherapy, which may increase the risk of chemotherapy-induced toxicity.
- Do not give the drug within 24 hours of cytotoxic chemotherapy.
- Do not give to patients hypersensitive to proteins derived from *Escherichia coli.* Although the drug is a growth factor for neutrophils only, the potential exists for stimulation of myeloid tumor growth.

Patient Teaching

- Teach patients to self-administer drug and to correctly dispose of used needles, syringes, and drug containers.
- Go over "Information for patients" section of material included with the product information. Ensure that patient understands all information.
- Advise the patient that hair loss may follow filgrastim therapy.
- Instruct the patient to notify the doctor if hematuria or bruising occurs.

Evaluation
In patients receiving filgrastim, appropriate evaluation statements may include:
• Patient remains free from signs and symptoms of infection.
• Patient reports decrease or absence in skeletal pain.
• Patient and family state an understanding of filgrastim therapy.

flecainide acetate
(fle kay′ nide)
Tambocor

• *Classification:* ventricular antiarrhythmic (benzamide derivative)
• *Pregnancy Risk Category:* C

HOW SUPPLIED
Tablets: 100 mg
Injection: 10 mg/ml‡

ACTION
Mechanism: A class Ic antiarrhythmic that depresses phase O. Unlike class Ia and Ib agents, however, it does not prolong or shorten the action potential. All class I drugs have membrane stabilizing effects.
Absorption: Rapidly and almost completely absorbed from the GI tract; bioavailability of tablets is 85% to 90%. Absorption is not affected by food or antacids.
Distribution: Well distributed throughout the body. Only about 40% binds to plasma proteins. Trough serum levels ranging from 0.2 to 1 mcg/ml provide the greatest therapeutic benefit. Trough serum levels higher than 0.7 mcg/ml have been associated with increased adverse effects.
Metabolism: Hepatic conversion to inactive metabolites.
Excretion: About 30% of an orally administered dose escapes metabolism and is excreted in the urine unchanged. Half-life: About 20 hours; may be prolonged in patients with CHF or renal disease.
Onset, peak, duration: Peak plasma levels usually occur within 2 to 3 hours. After multiple oral doses, steady-state levels are reached in 3 to 5 days.

INDICATIONS & DOSAGE
Treatment of life-threatening ventricular arrhythmias, such as sustained ventricular tachycardia –
Adults: 100 mg P.O. q 12 hours. May be increased in increments of 50 mg b.i.d. q 4 days until efficacy is achieved. Maximum dosage is 400 mg daily for most patients.

Initial dosage for patients with CHF is 50 mg q 12 hours.

Where available, flecainide may be given by I.V. injection–
Adults: 2 mg/kg I.V. push over not less than 10 minutes; or the dose may be diluted with dextrose 5% in water and administered as an infusion. Do not use any other solutions for infusion.

CONTRAINDICATIONS & PRECAUTIONS
Contraindicated in patients with hypersensitivity to this drug; in patients with significant conduction delay, including second- or third-degree heart block, sick sinus syndrome, and right bundle-branch block with bifascicular block (unless an artificial pacemaker is in place) because it may further depress cardiac conduction; and in patients with cardiogenic shock because of its mild negative inotropic and arrhythmogenic effects.

Use only in patients with life-threatening arrhythmias. Data from the Cardiac Arrhythmia Suppression Trial (CAST) showed that the drug may increase the risk of sudden death in patients who have had a myocardial infarction and who have asymptomatic nonsustained ventricular tachycardia.

Use with caution in patients with preexisting left ventricular dysfunction because it may worsen cardiac function; atrial flutter because it may accelerate the ventricular rate; preexisting sinus node dysfunction because it may cause marked effects on the sinus node; in patients with permanent artificial pacemakers or temporary pacing electrodes because the drug may increase pacing thresholds and may suppress ventricular escape rhythms; preexisting left ventricular dysfunction or sustained ventricular tachycardia because the drug may cause proarrhythmic effects; and renal or hepatic dysfunction because these conditions can cause increased drug levels and subsequent toxicity.

ADVERSE REACTIONS

Common reactions are in italics; life-threatening reactions are in bold italics.

CNS: *dizziness, headache,* fatigue, tremor.
CV: ***new or worsened arrhythmias,*** chest pain, *CHF,* ***cardiac arrest.***
EENT: *blurred vision and other visual disturbances.*
GI: nausea, constipation, abdominal pain.
Other: *dyspnea,* edema, skin rash.

INTERACTIONS

Amiodarone, cimetidine, digoxin, propranolol: altered pharmacokinetics. Monitor for toxicity.
Digitalis glycosides: flecainide may increase plasma digoxin levels by 15% to 25%.
Propranolol, beta-adrenergic blocking agents: both flecainide and propranolol plasma levels increase by 20% to 30%.
Urine acidifying and alkalinizing agents: extremes of urine pH may substantially alter excretion of flecainide.

EFFECTS ON DIAGNOSTIC TESTS

None reported.

NURSING CONSIDERATIONS

Besides those related universally to drug therapy (see "How to use this book"), consider the following specific recommendations:

Assessment

- Obtain a baseline assessment of the patient's heart rate and rhythm before flecainide therapy.
- Be alert for adverse reactions and drug interactions throughout therapy.
- Evaluate the patient's and family's knowledge about flecainide therapy.

Nursing Diagnoses

- Decreased cardiac output related to ineffectiveness of flecainide therapy.
- Altered sensory/perceptual alterations (visual) related to flecainide-induced visual disturbances.
- Knowledge deficit related to flecainide therapy.

Planning and Implementation

Preparation and Administration

- Determine pacing threshold 1 week before and after initiating therapy in patients with pacemakers as flecainide can alter endocardial pacing thresholds.
- Correct hypokalemia or hyperkalemia before this drug is given because both may alter the effect of flecainide.
- ***P.O. use:*** Expect to increase dosage in increments of 50 mg b.i.d. every 4 days until efficacy is achieved or a maximum dosage of 400 mg daily is reached.
- ***I.V. use:*** When administering flecainide by I.V. push, give over at least 10 minutes. When administering as an I.V. infusion, mix only with dextrose 5% in water.
- Expect to administer I.V. lidocaine while awaiting full therapeutic effect of flecainide.

Monitoring

- Monitor effectiveness by continuous ECG monitoring initially; long-term

oral administration requires regular ECG readings to monitor rhythm.
• Monitor the patient's vital signs, weight, and breath and heart sounds for evidence of CHF.
• Monitor therapeutic blood levels of flecainide. Normal levels range from 0.2 to 1 mcg/ml. Incidence of adverse reactions increases when trough blood levels exceed 1 mcg/ml.
• Monitor serum potassium levels regularly.
• Monitor patient for visual disturbances.

Supportive Care
• If ECG disturbances occur, withhold the drug, obtain a rhythm strip, and notify the doctor immediately.
• Keep emergency equipment nearby.
• Be aware that full therapeutic effects may take 3 to 5 days.
• Institute measures to minimize CHF, such as fluid and sodium restriction, as needed.
• Maintain seizure precautions.
• Institute safety precautions if adverse CNS reactions or visual disturbances occur.

Patient Teaching
• Stress importance of taking the drug exactly as prescribed.
• Warn the patient against hazardous activities that require alertness or good vision if adverse CNS or visual reactions occur.
• Emphasize the importance of close follow-up care that includes frequent ECGs and blood tests.
• Tell the patient to limit fluid and sodium intake to minimize CHF or fluid retention and to weigh himself daily. Emphasize that a sudden weight gain of 3 to 5 lb (1.4 to 2.3 kg) in 1 week should be reported to the doctor promptly.

Evaluation

In patients receiving flecainide, appropriate evaluation statements may include:
• Patient's ECG reveals arrhythmia has been corrected.
• Patient states vision is unaffected by flecainide therapy.
• Patient and family state an understanding of flecainide therapy.

floxuridine

(flox yoor´ i deen)
FUDR

• *Classification:* antineoplastic (antimetabolite)
• *Pregnancy Risk Category:* D

HOW SUPPLIED

Injection: 500-mg vials (50 mg/ml in 10-ml vials or 100 mg/ml in 5-ml vials)

ACTION

Mechanism: Drug is anabolized to 5-fluoro-2'-deoxyuridine-5'-phosphate (FUDR-MP), which inhibits DNA synthesis by blocking the enzyme thymidylate synthetase. Some may be catabolized to fluorouracil, which intereferes with both DNA and RNA synthesis. An antimetabolite.
Absorption: Administered intra-arterially.
Distribution: Crosses the blood-brain barrier to a limited extent.
Metabolism: Metabolized to fluorouracil in the liver after intra-arterial infusions and rapid I.V. injections.
Excretion: Approximately 60% of a dose is excreted through the lungs as carbon dioxide. A small amount is excreted by the kidneys as unchanged drug and metabolites.

INDICATIONS & DOSAGE

Brain, breast, head, neck, liver, gallbladder, and bile duct cancer–
Adults: 0.1 to 0.6 mg/kg daily by intraarterial infusion (use pump for continuous, uniform rate); or 0.4 to 0.6 mg/kg daily into hepatic artery.

CONTRAINDICATIONS & PRECAUTIONS

Contraindicated in patients with poor nutritional status, depressed bone marrow function, or serious infections, because they are at high risk for serious drug-related toxicity.

ADVERSE REACTIONS

Common reactions are in italics; life-threatening reactions are in bold italics.

Blood: ***leukopenia,*** *anemia,* thrombocytopenia.
CNS: cerebellar ataxia, vertigo, nystagmus, seizures, depression, hemiplegia, hiccups, lethargy.
EENT: blurred vision.
GI: *stomatitis, cramps, nausea, vomiting, diarrhea, bleeding, enteritis.*
Hepatic: cholangitis, jaundice, elevated liver enzymes.
Skin: *erythema,* dermatitis, pruritus, rash.

INTERACTIONS

None significant.

EFFECTS ON DIAGNOSTIC TESTS

Serum ALT (SGPT), alkaline phosphatase, AST (SGOT), bilirubin, and LDH: increased concentrations indicate drug-induced hepatotoxicity.

NURSING CONSIDERATIONS

Besides those related universally to drug therapy (see "How to use this book"), consider the following specific recommendations:

Assessment

- Obtain a baseline assessment of patient's overall physical status, CBC, renal panel, and hepatic profile before initiating therapy.
- Be alert for adverse reactions and drug interactions throughout therapy.
- Evaluate the patient's and family's knowledge of floxuridine therapy.

Nursing Diagnoses

- Altered protection related to floxuridine-induced myelosuppression and immunosuppression.
- Altered oral mucous membrane related to floxuridine-induced stomatitis.
- Knowledge deficit related to floxuridine therapy.

Planning and Implementation

Preparation and Administration

- Expect dosage modification in patients with poor nutritional state, bone marrow depression, or serious infection.
- Follow institutional policy to reduce mutagenic, teratogenic, and carcinogenic risks.
- Reconstitute this drug with sterile water for injection then further dilute with dextrose 5% in water or normal saline solution for infusion. Discard refrigerated solution after 2 weeks.
- Keep in mind that floxuridine is often administered via hepatic arterial infusion in treating hepatic metastasis.
- To maintain continuous intra-arterial infusion, administer by infusion pump.

Monitoring

- Monitor effectiveness by noting results of follow-up diagnostic tests and patient's overall physical status. Keep in mind that therapeutic effects may be delayed 1 to 6 weeks.
- Monitor for signs of infection (cough, fever, sore throat) and bleeding (easy bruising, nosebleeds, bleeding gums). Monitor CBC.
- Monitor intake and output and renal and hepatic function.
- Monitor for severe GI or skin adverse reactions; these require stopping the drug.
- Monitor arterial perfusion area. Check line for bleeding, blockage, displacement, or leakage.

Supportive Care

- Provide excellent mouth care to help prevent stomatitis.

• Remember that antiemetics may be given preceding or during infusion of this drug to decrease severe nausea, and vomiting. Use of antacid eases but probably won't prevent GI distress.
• Discontinue drug if WBC count is less than 3,500/mm³ or if platelets are less than 100,000/mm³.
• Avoid I.M. injections of any drugs in patients with thrombocytopenia to prevent bleeding.
• To prevent infection, maintain the patient's optimal health and protect him from undue exposure to environmental contagions. If signs of infection occur, notify doctor promptly; administer antibiotics, as ordered.
• Provide a safe environment to minimize risk of bleeding.

Patient Teaching

• Make sure patient knows theraputic effects may be delayed from 1 to 6 weeks.
• Warn patients to watch for signs of infection (sore throat, fever, fatigue), and for signs of bleeding (easy bruising, nosebleeds, bleeding gums). Tell patient to take temperature daily and to notify the doctor promptly if signs of infection or bleeding occur.
• Instruct patient about need for protective measures, including conservation of energy, balanced diet, adequate rest, personal cleanliness, clean environment, and avoidance of exposure to persons with infections.
• Teach patient to avoid the use of all OTC products containing aspirin. Instruct patient about safety precautions to reduce risks of bleeding from falls, cuts, or other injuries.
• Instruct patient about the need for frequent oral hygiene.

Evaluation

In patients receiving floxuridine, appropriate evaluation statements may include:

• Patient does not demonstrate signs and symptoms of infection or bleeding.
• Oral lesions are absent.
• Patient and family state an understanding of floxuridine therapy.

fluconazole

(floo koe´ na zole)
Diflucan

• *Classification:* antifungal (bis-triazole derivative)
• *Pregnancy Risk Category:* C

HOW SUPPLIED

Tablets: 50 mg, 100 mg, 200 mg
Injection: 200 mg/100 ml, 400 mg/200 ml

ACTION

Mechanism: Inhibits fungal cytochrome P-450, an enzyme responsible for fungal sterol synthesis. This results in weakening of fungal cell walls.
Absorption: After oral administration, absorption is rapid and complete; the oral and I.V. dose is the same.
Distribution: Well distributed to various sites, including CNS, saliva, sputum, blister fluid, urine, normal skin, nails, and blister skin; CNS concentrations approach 50% to 90% of that of serum. Fluconazole is 12% protein-bound.
Metabolism: Partially metabolized (less than 20% of a dose).
Excretion: Primarily excreted via the kidneys; over 80% of dose is excreted unchanged in the urine. The excretion rate diminishes as renal function decreases. Half-life: Approximately 30 hours (range 20 to 50 hours) after oral administration.
Onset, peak, duration: Peak plasma concentration after an oral dose occurs in 1 to 2 hours.

INDICATIONS & DOSAGE

Oropharyngeal candidiasis–
Adults: 200 mg P.O. or I.V. on the first day, followed by 100 mg once daily. Therapy should continue for 2 weeks.
Esophageal candidiasis–
Adults: 200 mg P.O. or I.V. on the first day, followed by 100 mg once daily. Higher doses (up to 400 mg daily) have been used, depending upon the patient's condition and tolerance of treatment. Patients should receive the drug for at least 3 weeks and for 2 weeks after symptoms resolve.
Systemic candidiasis–
Adults: 400 mg P.O. or I.V. on the first day, followed by 200 mg once daily. Treatment should continue for at least 4 weeks or for 2 weeks after symptoms resolve.
Cryptococcal meningitis–
Adults: 400 mg P.O. or I.V. on the first day, followed by 200 mg once daily. Higher doses (up to 400 mg daily) may be used. Treatment should continue for 10 to 12 weeks after cultures of the cerebrospinal fluid are negative.
Suppression of relapse of cryptococcal meningitis in patients with AIDS–
Adults: 200 mg P.O. or I.V. daily.

CONTRAINDICATIONS & PRECAUTIONS

Contraindicated in patients with hypersensitivity to the drug.

ADVERSE REACTIONS

Common reactions are in italics; life-threatening reactions are in bold italics.
CNS: headache.
GI: *nausea,* vomiting, abdominal pain, diarrhea.
Skin: rash, ***Stevens-Johnson syndrome (rare).***
Other: hepatotoxicity (rare), elevated liver enzymes.

INTERACTIONS

Cyclosporine, phenytoin, oral antidiabetic agents (tolbutamide, glyburide, glipizide): may cause increased plasma concentrations of these drugs.
Isoniazid, phenytoin, rifampin, valproic acid, oral sulfonylureas: increased incidence of abnormally elevated hepatic transaminases.
Rifampin: enhanced metabolism of fluconazole.
Warfarin: increased prothrombin time.

EFFECTS ON DIAGNOSTIC TESTS

Liver function tests: increased serum levels.

NURSING CONSIDERATIONS

Besides those related universally to drug therapy (see "How to use this book"), consider the following specific recommendations:

Assessment
- Obtain a baseline assessment of fungal infection, including appropriate specimens to identify fungi, before therapy.
- Be alert for adverse reactions and drug interactions throughout therapy.
- Evaluate the patient's and family's knowledge about fluconazole therapy.

Nursing Diagnoses
- High risk for injury related to ineffectiveness of fluconazole in eradicating the infection.
- High risk for fluid volume deficit related to fluconazole induced nausea.
- Knowledge deficit related to fluconazole.

Planning and Implementation
Preparation and Administration
- Be aware that because drug is excreted unchanged by the kidneys, dosage should be reduced in patients with renal failure. If creatinine clearance is 21 to 50 ml/minute, expect dosage to be reduced 50%; if 11 to 20 ml/minute, expect it to be reduced by 75%. Patients receiving regular

hemodialysis treatment will receive the usual dose after each dialysis session.

• ***I.V. use:*** I.V. fluconazole may be administered by continuous infusion at a rate not to exceed 200 mg/hour. Use an infusion pump. Do not connect in series with other infusions to prevent air embolism. Do not add any other drugs to the solution. Protective wrapping of I.V. fluconazole should not be removed until just before use to help ensure sterility. The plastic container may show some opacity from moisture absorbed during sterilization. This is normal, will not affect the drug, and will diminish over time.

Monitoring

• Monitor effectiveness by regularly assessing for improvement of infection.

• The incidence of adverse reactions appears to be greater in HIV-infected patients.

• Monitor patient's hydration status if adverse GI reactions occur.

• Monitor regularly for elevation of liver enzymes.

Supportive Care

• Obtain an order for an antiemetic to manage persistent or severe nausea or diarrhea.

• Obtain an order for an analgesic for fluconazole-induced headache.

Patient Teaching

• Urge the patient to adhere to regimen and to return as instructed for follow-up.

Evaluation

In patients receiving fluconazole, appropriate evaluation statements may include:

• Patient's infection is alleviated.

• Patient maintains adequate hydration throughout fluconazole therapy.

• Patient and family state an understanding of fluconazole therapy.

flucytosine (5-FC)

(floo sye´ toe seen)

Ancobon

• *Classification:* antifungal (fluorinated pyrimidine)

• *Pregnancy Risk Category:* C

HOW SUPPLIED

Capsules: 250 mg, 500 mg

ACTION

Mechanism: Penetrates fungal cells, where fungal enzymes converted it to fluorouracil, a known metabolic antagonist. Causes defective protein synthesis.

Absorption: About 75% to 90% of an oral dose of flucytosine is absorbed. Food decreases the rate, but not extent of absorption.

Distribution: Widely distributed into the liver, kidneys, spleen, heart, bronchial secretions, joints, peritoneal fluid, and aqueous humor; CSF levels vary from 60% to 100% of serum levels. Drug is 2% to 4% bound to plasma proteins.

Metabolism: Only small amounts are metabolized.

Excretion: About 75% to 95% of a dose is excreted unchanged in urine; less than 10% is excreted unchanged in feces. Half-life: 2½ to 6 hours with normal renal function; as long as 1,160 hours with creatinine clearance below 2 ml/min.

Onset, peak, duration: Peak serum concentrations occur at 2 to 6 hours after a dose.

INDICATIONS & DOSAGE

For severe fungal infections caused by susceptible strains of Candida *(including septicemia, endocarditis, urinary tract and pulmonary infections) and* Cryptococcus *(meningitis, pulmonary infection, and possible urinary tract infections)–*

Adults and children weighing more than 50 kg: 50 to 150 mg/kg daily q 6 hours P.O.
Adults and children weighing less than 50 kg: 1.5 to 4.5 g/m²/day in four divided doses P.O.

Severe infections, such as meningitis, may require doses up to 250 mg/kg.

CONTRAINDICATIONS & PRECAUTIONS

Contraindicated in patients with hypersensitivity to the drug. Use with caution in patients with bone marrow depression (regardless of origin), as it may exacerbate this condition; and in patients with impaired renal function, to prevent toxic drug accumulation. In patients with impaired renal function, serum concentrations should be determined to maintain therapeutic range (25 to 120 mcg/ml).

ADVERSE REACTIONS

Common reactions are in italics; life-threatening reactions are in bold italics.
Blood: anemia, ***leukopenia, bone marrow suppression, thrombocytopenia.***
CNS: dizziness, drowsiness, confusion, headache, vertigo.
GI: *nausea, vomiting, diarrhea,* abdominal bloating.
Hepatic: elevated AST (SGOT), ALT (SGPT).
Metabolic: elevated serum alkaline phosphatase, BUN, serum creatinine.
Skin: occasional rash.

INTERACTIONS

None significant.

EFFECTS ON DIAGNOSTIC TESTS

Alkaline phosphatase, AST (SGOT), ALT (SGPT): increased levels.
BUN and serum creatinine: increased levels.
RBC, WBC, and platelet counts: may be decreased.
Serum creatinine (iminohydrolase enzymatic assay): falsely elevated values.

NURSING CONSIDERATIONS

Besides those related universally to drug therapy (see "How to use this book"), consider the following specific recommendations:

Assessment
- Obtain a baseline assessment of fungal infection, including appropriate specimens to establish sensitivity to flucytosine, before therapy.
- Be alert for adverse reactions and drug interactions throughout therapy.
- Evaluate the patient's and family's knowledge about flucytosine therapy.

Nursing Diagnoses
- High risk for injury related to ineffectiveness of flucytosine in eradicating the fungal infection.
- Altered protection related to flucytosine-induced hematologic adverse reactions.
- Knowledge deficit related to flucytosine.

Planning and Implementation

Preparation and Administration
- Hematologic, renal and liver function studies should precede flucytosine therapy. Check to be sure these tests were done before administering first dose.
- ***P.O. use:*** Administer capsules over a 15-minute period to minimize adverse GI reactions.
- Expect to administer concurrently with amphotericin B for synergistic effects.

Monitoring
- Monitor effectiveness by regularly assessing for improvement of infection.
- Monitor susceptibility tests weekly to detect drug resistance.
- If possible, monitor blood level assays of the drug regularly to maintain flucytosine at therapeutic level (25 to 120 mcg/ml). Higher blood levels may be toxic.
- Monitor patient's hematologic,

renal, and liver function studies at frequent intervals throughout therapy.
• Monitor patient for infection or bleeding if hematologic studies are abnormal.
• Monitor patient's intake and output.
Supportive Care
• Institute infection control and bleeding precautions as indicated by patient's hematologic status.
• Obtain an order for an antiemetic or antidiarrheal agent as needed.
• Institute safety precautions if adverse CNS reactions occur.
Patient Teaching
• Inform patient that adequate therapeutic response may take weeks or months.
• Tell patient to take capsules over a 15-minute period to minimize adverse GI reactions.
• Teach patient precautions to control infection and bleeding.
• Warn patient to avoid hazardous activities requiring mental alertness if adverse CNS reactions occur.
• Stress importance of compliance with drug therapy, recommended laboratory studies, and close follow-up care.

Evaluation

In patients receiving flucytosine, appropriate evaluation statements may include:
• Patient's infection is alleviated.
• Patient's hematologic status remains normal throughout flucytosine therapy.
• Patient and family state an understanding of flucytosine therapy.

fludrocortisone acetate
(floo droe kor´ ti sone)
Florinef

• *Classification:* mineralocorticoid replacement (mineralocorticoid, glucocorticoid)
• *Pregnancy Risk Category:* C

HOW SUPPLIED
Tablets: 0.1 mg

ACTION
Mechanism: Increases sodium reabsorption, and potassium and hydrogen secretion at the nephron's distal convoluted tubule.
Absorption: Readily absorbed from the GI tract.
Distribution: Rapidly removed from the blood and distributed to muscle, liver, skin, intestines, and kidneys. It is extensively bound to plasma proteins (transcortin and albumin). Only the unbound portion is active. Adrenocorticoids are distributed into breast milk and through the placenta.
Metabolism: In the liver to inactive glucuronide and sulfate metabolites.
Excretion: The inactive metabolites and small amounts of unmetabolized drug are excreted by the kidneys. Insignificant amounts are also excreted in feces. Half-life: About 30 minutes; biological half-life is 18 to 36 hours.
Onset, peak, duration: Peak concentration is reached in about 1½ hours.

INDICATIONS & DOSAGE
Adrenal insufficiency (partial replacement), adrenogenital syndrome—
Adults: 0.1 to 0.2 mg P.O. daily.

CONTRAINDICATIONS & PRECAUTIONS
Contraindicated in patients with hypersensitivity to the drug. Use with extreme caution in patients with hypertension, CHF, or cardiac disease. Discontinue if a significant increase in weight or blood pressure, edema, or cardiac enlargement occurs.

Drug use should be accompanied by adequate glucocorticoid therapy in adrenal insufficiency or the salt-losing form of adrenogenital syndrome.

Patients with Addison's disease are more sensitive to the drug's action and may develop exaggerated adverse reactions. Stop treatment in the event of a significant increase in weight or blood pressure, or the development of edema or cardiac enlargement.

Sodium retention and potassium loss are accelerated by a high-sodium intake. If edema develops, restriction of dietary sodium and administration of potassium supplements may be necessary.

ADVERSE REACTIONS

Common reactions are in italics; life-threatening reactions are in bold italics.

CV: *sodium and water retention,* hypertension, cardiac hypertrophy, edema.

Metabolic: hypokalemia.

INTERACTIONS

None significant.

EFFECTS ON DIAGNOSTIC TESTS

Serum potassium: decreased levels.

Serum sodium: increased levels.

NURSING CONSIDERATIONS

Besides those related universally to drug therapy (see "How to use this book"), consider the following specific recommendations:

Assessment

- Obtain a baseline assessment of the patient's adrenal insufficiency or adrenogenital syndrome before initiating drug therapy.
- Be alert for adverse reactions and drug interactions throughout therapy.
- Evaluate the patient's and family's knowledge about fludrocortisone therapy.

Nursing Diagnoses

- Fluid volume deficit related to the patient's underlying condition.
- Fluid volume excess related to high risk of sodium and water retention.
- Knowledge deficit related to fludrocortisone therapy.

Planning and Implementation

Preparation and Administration

- Expect to use fludrocortisone with cortisone or hydrocortisone in patients with adrenal insufficiency.

Monitoring

- Monitor effectiveness by regularly assessing for signs of improving mineralocortical function.
- Monitor the patient's blood pressure and serum electrolyte levels regularly.
- Monitor the patient's weight daily and observe for evidence of fluid retention.
- Know that glucose tolerance tests should be performed only if necessary in addisonian patients because they tend to develop severe hypoglycemia within 3 hours of the test.

Supportive Care

- Report any significant patient weight gain, edema, hypertension, or severe headaches to the doctor.
- Unless contraindicated, give the patient a low-sodium diet high in potassium and protein. Potassium supplement may be needed.

Patient Teaching

- Teach the patient to recognize signs of fluid and electrolyte imbalance: muscle weakness, paresthesia, numbness, fatigue, anorexia, nausea, altered mental status, increased urination, altered heart rhythm, severe or continuing headaches, unusual weight gain, or swelling of the feet and to report any such symptoms to the doctor.
- Tell the patient to take missed doses as soon as possible, unless it is almost time for the next dose, and not to double doses.
- Inform patient of the long-term need for the drug and stress the importance of compliance.
- Tell patient to eat a low-sodium diet that is high in potassium and protein unless contraindicated.

Evaluation
In patients receiving fludrocortisone, appropriate evaluation statements may include:
• Patient's dosage regimen relieves fluid volume deficit and other signs and symptoms of mineralocorticoid insufficiency.
• Patient does not develop sodium and water retention.
• Patient and family state an understanding of fludrocortisone therapy.

flunisolide
(floo niss´ oh lide)
Nasalide, Rhinalar Nasal Mist‡

• *Classification:* anti-inflammatory agent (glucocorticoid)
• *Pregnancy Risk Category:* C

HOW SUPPLIED
Nasal inhalant: 25 mcg/metered spray, 200 doses/bottle
Nasal solution: 0.25 mg/ml in pump spray bottle

ACTION
Mechanism: Produces local anti-inflammatory, vasoconstrictor, and antipruritic actions. Diffuses across cell membranes to form complexes with specific cytoplasmic receptors, influencing cellular metabolism. Corticosteroids stabilize leukocyte lysosomal membranes, inhibit local actions and accumulation of macrophages, decrease local edema, and reduce the formation of scar tissue.
Absorption: Approximately 50% of a nasally inhaled dose is absorbed systemically.
Distribution: Distribution after intranasal administration has not been described.
Metabolism: Flunisolide and its 6-beta-hydroxy metabolite are eventually conjugated in the liver, by glucuronic acid or surface sulfate, to inactive metabolites.
Excretion: Excretion of inhaled flunisolide has not been described, however, after systemic administration, metabolites are excreted in approximately equal portions in feces and urine. Half-life: Averages about 2 hours.
Onset, peak, duration: Peak plasma concentrations occur within 10 to 30 minutes. Onset of action usually occurs in a few days but may take as long as 4 weeks in some patients.

INDICATIONS & DOSAGE
Relief of symptoms of seasonal or perennial rhinitis–
Adults: Starting dose is 2 sprays (50 mcg) in each nostril b.i.d. Total daily dosage is 200 mcg. If necessary, dose may be increased to 2 sprays in each nostril t.i.d. Maximum total daily dosage is 8 sprays in each nostril (400 mcg daily).
Children 6 to 14 years: Starting dose is 1 spray (25 mcg) in each nostril t.i.d. or 2 sprays (50 mcg) in each nostril b.i.d. Total daily dosage is 150 to 200 mcg. Maximum total daily dosage is 4 sprays in each nostril (200 mcg daily).

Not recommended for children under age 6.

CONTRAINDICATIONS & PRECAUTIONS
Contraindicated in patients with acute status asthmaticus; tuberculosis or viral, fungal, or bacterial respiratory infections; and hypersensitivity to any component of the preparation.

Use cautiously in patients receiving systemic corticosteroids because of increased risk of hypothalamic-pituitary-adrenal axis suppression; when substituting inhalant for oral systemic administration (because withdrawal symptoms may occur); and in patients with healing nasal septal ulcers, and those who have had recent oral or nasal surgery, or trauma.

ADVERSE REACTIONS

Common reactions are in italics; life-threatening reactions are in bold italics.

CNS: headache.

EENT: *mild, transient nasal burning and stinging,* nasal congestion, sneezing, epistaxis, watery eyes.

GI: nausea, vomiting.

Other: development of nasopharyngeal fungal infections.

INTERACTIONS

None reported.

EFFECTS ON DIAGNOSTIC TESTS

None reported.

NURSING CONSIDERATIONS

Besides those related universally to drug therapy (see "How to use this book"), consider the following specific recommendations:

Assessment

- Obtain a baseline assessment of the patient's breathing pattern and degree of nasal congestion.
- Be alert for adverse reactions and drug interactions throughout therapy.
- Evaluate the patient's and family's knowledge about flunisolide therapy.

Nursing Diagnosis

- Ineffective breathing pattern related to the patient's underlying condition.
- Pain related to flunisolide-induced nasal burning and stinging.
- Knowledge deficit related to flunisolide therapy.

Planning and Implementation

Preparation and Administration

- ***Nasal inhalation:*** Patient should first clear nasal passages, then tilt head slightly forward. Prime inhaler, and insert tip into nostril (pointing away from septum) while holding other nostril closed. Deliver spray while patient inspires. Repeat in other nostril.

Monitoring

- Monitor effectiveness by assessing the patient's breathing pattern and degree of nasal congestion.
- Monitor compliance. Flunisolide is not effective for acute exacerbations because its effects are not immediate. Most patients achieve a benefit in a few days, but some may need to continue the drug for 2 to 3 weeks before achieving maximum benefit.
- Observe for signs of fungal infection. Obtain culture as necessary.

Supportive Care

- Notify the doctor if relief is not obtained, if signs of infection appear, or if nasal stinging or burning on application is severe.

Patient Teaching

- Teach the patient how to use the spray, and tell him it should be used by one person only.
- Teach the patient good nasal and oral hygiene.
- Warn the patient that he may experience a mild transient nasal burning or stinging when the spray is administered.
- Advise the patient to discontinue use and notify the doctor if symptoms do not improve after 3 weeks or if irritation persists.
- Advise the patient to use the drug regularly as prescribed, and tell him effectiveness depends on regular use.

Evaluation

In patients receiving flunisolide, appropriate evaluation statements may include:

- Patient obtains relief from nasal congestion.
- Nasal stinging or burning is mild and well tolerated by the patient.
- Patient and family state an understanding of flunisolide therapy.

flunisolide

(floo niss´ oh lide)
AeroBid Inhaler

• *Classification:* anti-inflammatory agent, antiasthmatic (glucocorticoid)
• *Pregnancy Risk Category:* C

HOW SUPPLIED

Oral inhalant: 250 mcg/metered spray, 50 doses/inhaler

ACTION

Mechanism: Produces local anti-inflammatory, vasoconstrictor, and antipruritic actions. Diffuses across cell membranes to form complexes with specific cytoplasmic receptors, influencing cellular metabolism. Corticosteroids stabilize leukocyte lysosomal membranes, inhibit local actions and accumulation of macrophages, decrease local edema, and reduce the formation of scar tissue.
Absorption: After oral inhalation, about 70% of the dose is absorbed from the lungs and GI tract. Only about 20% of an orally inhaled dose of flunisolide reaches systemic circulation unmetabolized because of extensive metabolism in the liver.
Distribution: After oral inhalation, 10% to 25% of the drug is distributed to the lungs; the remainder is deposited in the mouth and swallowed; No evidence of tissue storage of flunisolide or its metabolites. Absorbed drug is 50% bound to plasma proteins.
Metabolism: Rapidly metabolizes in the liver or GI tract to various metabolites, one of which has glucocorticoid activity. Flunisolide and its 6-beta-hydroxy metabolite are eventually conjugated in the liver, by glucuronic acid or surface sulfate, to inactive metabolites.
Excretion: Excretion of the inhaled form has not been described; Half-life: Biological half-life averages about 2 hours.
Onset, peak, duration: Onset of action usually occurs in a few days but may take as long as 4 weeks.

INDICATIONS & DOSAGE

Steroid-dependent asthma –
Adults and children over 6 years: 2 oral inhalations (500 mcg) b.i.d. Don't exceed 4 inhalations b.i.d.

CONTRAINDICATIONS & PRECAUTIONS

Contraindicated in patients with acute status asthmaticus; in patients with tuberculosis or viral, fungal, or bacterial respiratory infections; and in patients who are hypersensitive to any component of the preparation.

Use cautiously in patients receiving systemic corticosteroids because of increased risk of hypothalamic-pituitary-adrenal axis suppression; when substituting inhalant for oral systemic administration (because withdrawal symptoms may occur); and in patients with healing nasal septal ulcers, oral or nasal surgery, or trauma.

ADVERSE REACTIONS

Common reactions are in italics; life-threatening reactions are in bold italics.
CNS: headache.
EENT: watery eyes, throat irritation, hoarseness.
GI: nausea, vomiting, dry mouth.
Other: development of oropharyngeal fungal infections.

INTERACTIONS

None significant.

EFFECTS ON DIAGNOSTIC TESTS

None reported.

NURSING CONSIDERATIONS

Besides those related universally to drug therapy (see "How to use this

book"), consider the following specific recommendations:

Assessment

• Obtain a baseline assessment of the patient's asthmatic condition before initiating drug therapy.
• Assess patient for oral fungal infections with drug therapy.
• Be alert for adverse reactions or drug interactions throughout therapy.
• Evaluate the patient's and family's knowledge about flunisolide.

Nursing Diagnoses

• Ineffective airway clearance related to the patient's underlying condition.
• Altered oral mucous membranes related to drug-induced fungal infections.
• Knowledge deficit related to flunisolide therapy.

Planning and Implementation

Preparation and Administration

• Never administer the drug to relieve an emergency asthmatic attack because onset of action takes too long.
• Be aware that oral glucocorticoid therapy should be tapered slowly.
• Expect to administer systemic corticosteroids during times of stress (trauma, surgery, infection) to prevent adrenal insufficiency in previously steroid-dependent patients.
• Always administer prescribed bronchodilators several minutes before flunisolide.
• ***Oral inhalation:*** Have patient rest 1 minute between puffs and hold breath for a few seconds after each puff to enhance drug action.

Monitoring

• Monitor effectiveness by regularly assessing the patient's respiratory status for improvement.
• Monitor the patient's oral mucous membranes for early signs of a fungal infection.

Supportive Care

• Notify the doctor if decreased response is noted after administration of drug.
• Have patient drink a glass of water following inhalations to help prevent oral fungal infections.
• Keep inhaler clean and unobstructed by washing it with warm water and drying it thoroughly after each use.

Patient Teaching

• Teach patient how to administer the drug and care for the inhaler device.
• Be sure that the patient understands the need to take the drug as prescribed. Tell the patient not to take two doses at once if he inadvertently misses one.
• Stress the importance of never using the drug to alleviate an acute asthmatic attack because drug takes too long to work.
• Warn the patient not to discontinue the drug abruptly or without the doctor's approval and not to exceed the recommended dose.
• Instruct the patient to contact the doctor if he notices a decreased response or if symptoms don't improve within 3 weeks of initiating therapy.
• Tell patient to drink a glass of water after inhalations to help prevent oral fungal infections.
• Tell the patient to carry a medical identification card indicating the need for supplemental adrenocorticoids during stress.

Evaluation

In the patient receiving flunisolide, appropriate evaluation statements may include:

• Patient's lungs are clear and breathing pattern and skin color are normal.
• Patient does not exhibit an oral fungal infection during flunisolide therapy.
• Patient and family state an understanding of flunisolide therapy.

fluocinolone acetonide

(floo oh sin´ oh lone)
Fluocet, Fluonid, Flurosyn, Synalar, Synemol

- *Classification:* topical anti-inflammatory (adrenocorticoid)
- *Pregnancy Risk Category:* C

HOW SUPPLIED

Cream: 0.01%, 0.025%, 0.2%
Ointment: 0.025%
Topical solution: 0.01%

ACTION

Mechanism: Produces local anti-inflammatory, vasoconstrictor, and antipruritic actions. Drug diffuses across cell membranes to form complexes with specific cytoplasmic receptors, influencing cellular metabolism. Corticosteroids stabilize leukocyte lysosomal membranes, inhibit local actions and accumulation of macrophages, decrease local edema, and reduce the formation of scar tissue.
Absorption: Amount absorbed depends on the amount applied and on the nature of the skin at the application site. It is lowest in areas with thick stratum corneum (palms, soles, elbows, and knees) and higher in thinner areas (face, eyelids, and genitalia). Absorption increases in areas of skin damage, inflammation, or occlusion. Some systemic absorption of topical steroids may occur, especially through the oral mucosa.
Distribution: After topical application, distributed throughout the local skin. If absorbed, it is rapidly removed from the blood and distributed into muscle, liver, skin, intestines, and kidneys.
Metabolism: After topical application, metabolized primarily in the skin. The small amount that is absorbed into systemic circulation is metabolized primarily in the liver to inactive compounds.
Excretion: Inactive metabolites are excreted by the kidneys, primarily as glucuronides and sulfates, but also as unconjugated products. Small amounts of the metabolites are also excreted in feces.

INDICATIONS & DOSAGE

Inflammation of corticosteroid-responsive dermatoses–
Adults and children over 2 years: Clean area; apply cream, ointment, or solution sparingly b.i.d. to q.i.d. Treat multiple or extensive lesions sequentially, applying preparation to only small areas at any one time.

CONTRAINDICATIONS & PRECAUTIONS

Contraindicated in patients who are hypersensitive to any component of the preparation and in patients with viral, fungal, or tubercular skin lesions. Use with extreme caution in patients with impaired circulation because the drug may increase the risk of skin ulceration.

Avoid using on the face or genital areas because increased absorption may result in striae.

ADVERSE REACTIONS

Common reactions are in italics; life-threatening reactions are in bold italics.
Skin: burning, itching, irritation, dryness, folliculitis, hypertrichosis, hypopigmentation, acneiform eruptions, perioral dermatitis, allergic contact dermatitis. With occlusive dressings: *maceration of skin, secondary infection, atrophy, striae, miliaria.*

INTERACTIONS

None significant.

EFFECTS ON DIAGNOSTIC TESTS

None significant.

NURSING CONSIDERATIONS

Besides those related universally to drug therapy (see "How to use this book"), consider the following specific recommendations:

Assessment

• Obtain a baseline assessment of the patient's skin condition before initiating drug therapy.

• Be alert for adverse reactions and drug interactions throughout therapy.

• Evaluate the patient's and family's knowledge about fluocinolone therapy.

Nursing Diagnoses

• Impaired skin integrity related to the patient's underlying condition

• High risk for infection related to drug-induced adverse reaction.

• Knowledge deficit related to fluocinolone therapy.

Planning and Implementation

Preparation and Administration

• Read order and drug labels carefully.

• Wear gloves when administering drug.

• Before applying, gently wash the patient's skin. Apply a thin layer of medication and rub in gently.

• When treating hairy sites, part hair and apply directly to lesion.

• To apply an occlusive dressing (only if ordered by doctor), apply cream heavily, then cover with a thin, pliable, nonflammable plastic film; seal to adjacent normal skin with hypoallergenic tape.

• To prevent recurrence, treatment should continue for a few days after lesions have cleared.

Monitoring

• Monitor effectiveness by regularly assessing skin for extent and severity of inflammation.

• Monitor for hypersensitivity reaction to fluocinolone.

• Monitor for evidence of secondary infection.

• Monitor for adverse reactions and drug interactions by frequently assessing the patient's skin for burning, itching, and dryness.

• Monitor patient who must use occlusive dressings for maceration of the skin and secondary infection.

Supportive Care

• To minimize adverse reactions, use occlusive dressings intermittently. Don't use occlusive dressings in the presence of infection or on weeping or exudative lesions, and don't leave dressings in place longer than 16 hours each day.

• For patients with eczematous dermatitis, who may develop irritation with adhesive material, hold dressing in place with gauze, elastic bandage, or stockings.

• Notify the doctor and remove occlusive dressing if fever develops.

• Withhold the drug and notify the doctor if hypersensitivity reaction or infection occurs.

• Have the patient's fingernails cut short to minimize skin trauma from scratching.

• Apply cool, moist compresses to involved areas to relieve itching and burning.

• Use hypoallergenic tape, gauze, stockings, or elastic bandage to secure occlusive dressings.

Patient Teaching

• Instruct the patient to clean involved area before applying fluocinolone in a thin layer to cover the entire surface.

• Teach the patient how to apply an occlusive dressing.

• Teach the patient and family how to recognize signs of a hypersensitivity reaction or an infection. Advise them to discontinue the drug and notify the doctor immediately if either of these occur.

• Instruct the patient to complete the entire treatment regimen as prescribed, even if the lesions appear to have healed.

• Tell the patient and family not to

share the fluocinolone prescription with others.

Evaluation

In patients receiving fluocinolone, appropriate evaluation statements include:

- Patient maintains skin integrity.
- Patient does not develop secondary infection.
- Patient and family state an understanding of fluocinolone therapy.

fluocinonide

(floo oh sin´ oh nide)

Lidemol†, Lidex, Lidex-E, Topsyn

- *Classification:* topical anti-inflammatory (adrenocorticoid)
- *Pregnancy Risk Category:* C

HOW SUPPLIED

Cream: 0.05%
Gel: 0.05%
Ointment: 0.05%
Topical solution: 0.05%

ACTION

Mechanism: Diffuses across cell membranes and complexes with specific cytoplasmic receptors.

Absorption: Amount absorbed depends on the amount applied and on the nature of the skin at the application site. It is lowest in areas with thick stratum corneum (palms, soles, elbows, and knees) and higher in thinner areas (face, eyelids, and genitalia). Absorption increases in areas of skin damage, inflammation, or occlusion. Some systemic absorption of topical steroids may occur, especially through the oral mucosa.

Distribution: After topical application, distributed throughout the local skin. If absorbed, it is rapidly removed from the blood and distributed into muscle, liver, skin, intestines, and kidneys.

Metabolism: After topical application, metabolized primarily in the skin. The small amount absorbed into systemic circulation is metabolized primarily in the liver to inactive compounds.

Excretion: Inactive metabolites are excreted by the kidneys, primarily as glucuronides and sulfates, but also as unconjugated products. Small amounts of the metabolites are also excreted in feces.

INDICATIONS & DOSAGE

Inflammation of corticosteroid-responsive dermatoses—

Adults and children: Clean area; apply cream, ointment, solution, or gel sparingly t.i.d. or q.i.d.

CONTRAINDICATIONS & PRECAUTIONS

Contraindicated in patients who are hypersensitive to any component of the preparation and in patients with viral, fungal, or tubercular skin lesions. Use with extreme caution in patients with impaired circulation because the drug may increase the risk of skin ulceration. Avoid using on the face or genital areas because increased absorption may result in striae.

ADVERSE REACTIONS

Common reactions are in italics; life-threatening reactions are in bold italics.

Skin: burning, itching, irritation, dryness, folliculitis, hypertrichosis, hypopigmentation, acneiform eruptions, perioral dermatitis, allergic contact dermatitis. With occlusive dressings: *maceration of skin, secondary infection, atrophy, striae, miliaria.*

INTERACTIONS

None significant.

EFFECTS ON DIAGNOSTIC TESTS

None reported.

NURSING CONSIDERATIONS

Besides those related universally to drug therapy (see "How to use this book"), consider the following specific recommendations:

Assessment

• Obtain a baseline assessment of the patient's skin integrity before fluocinonide therapy.
• Be alert for adverse reactions and drug interactions throughout therapy.
• Evaluate the patient's and family's knowledge about fluocinonide therapy.

Nursing Diagnoses

• Impaired skin integrity related to the patient's underlying condition.
• High risk for infection related to drug-induced adverse reaction.
• Knowledge deficit related to fluocinonide therapy.

Planning and Implementation

Preparation and Administration

• Read order and drug labels carefully.
• Wear gloves when administering drug.
• Before applying, gently wash the patient's skin. Apply a thin layer of medication and rub in gently.
• When treating hairy sites, part hair and apply directly to lesion.
• To apply an occlusive dressing (only if ordered by doctor), apply cream heavily, then cover with a thin, pliable, nonflammable plastic film; seal to adjacent normal skin with hypoallergenic tape.
• To prevent recurrence, treatment should continue for a few days after lesions have cleared.

Monitoring

• Monitor effectiveness by regularly assessing skin for extent and severity of inflammation.
• Monitor for hypersensitivity reaction to fluocinonide.
• Monitor for evidence of secondary infection.
• Monitor for adverse reactions and drug interactions by frequently assessing the patient's skin for burning, itching, and dryness.
• Monitor patient who must use occlusive dressings for maceration of the skin and secondary infection.

Supportive Care

• To minimize adverse reactions, use occlusive dressings intermittently. Don't use occlusive dressings in the presence of infection or on weeping or exudative lesions, and don't leave dressings in place longer than 16 hours each day.
• For patients with eczematous dermatitis, who may develop irritation with adhesive material, hold dressing in place with gauze, elastic bandage, or stockings.
• Notify the doctor and remove occlusive dressing if fever develops.
• Withhold the drug and notify the doctor if hypersensitivity reaction or infection occurs.
• Have the patient's fingernails cut short to minimize skin trauma from scratching.
• Apply cool, moist compresses to involved areas to relieve itching and burning.
• Use hypoallergenic tape, gauze, stockings, or elastic bandage to secure occlusive dressings.
• Be prepared to discontinue the drug if burning or stinging persists and dermatitis has not improved.

Patient Teaching

• Instruct the patient to clean involved area before applying fluocinonide in a thin layer to cover the entire surface.
• Teach the patient how to apply an occlusive dressing.
• Teach the patient and family how to recognize signs of a hypersensitivity reaction or an infection. Advise them to discontinue the drug and notify the doctor immediately if either of these occurs.
• Instruct the patient to complete the entire treatment regimen as pre-

scribed, even if the lesions appear to have healed.
• Tell the patient and family not to share the fluocinonide prescription with others.

Evaluation

In the patient receiving fluocinonide, appropriate evaluation statements include:
• Patient maintains skin integrity.
• Patient does not develop secondary infection.
• Patient and family state an understanding of fluocinonide therapy.

fluorometholone

(flure oh meth´ oh lone)
FML Liquifilm Ophthalmic, FML S.O.P.

• *Classification:* ophthalmic anti-inflammatory agent (corticosteroid)
• *Pregnancy Risk Category:* C

HOW SUPPLIED

Ophthalmic ointment: 0.1%
Ophthalmic suspension: 0.1%, 0.25%

ACTION

Mechanism: A corticosteroid that decreases the inflammatory response. Exact mechanism unknown; drug inhibits edema formation, prevents fibrin deposition, and blocks infiltration of phagocytes and leukocytes at the site of inflammation.
Absorption: After ophthalmic administration, fluorometholone is absorbed mainly into the aqueous humor. Slight systemic absorption typically occurs.
Distribution: Throughout the local tissue layers.

INDICATIONS & DOSAGE

Inflammatory and allergic conditions of cornea, conjunctiva, sclera, anterior uvea –
Adults and children: instill 1 to 2 drops in conjunctival sac b.i.d. to q.i.d. May use q hour during first 1 to 2 days if needed. Alternatively, apply thin strip of ointment to conjunctiva q 4 hours, decreasing to one to three times a day as inflammation subsides.

CONTRAINDICATIONS & PRECAUTIONS

Contraindicated in patients who are hypersensitive to any component of the preparation; in patients with fungal infections of the eye; and in patients with acute, untreated purulent bacterial, viral, or fungal ocular infections. If a bacterial infection does not respond promptly to appropriate anti-infective therapy, fluorometholone should be discontinued and another therapy applied.

ADVERSE REACTIONS

Common reactions are in italics; life-threatening reactions are in bold italics.
Eye: increased intraocular pressure, thinning of cornea, interference with corneal wound healing, corneal ulceration, increased susceptibility to viral or fungal corneal infections; with excessive or long-term use, glaucoma exacerbations, cataracts, decreased visual acuity, diminished visual field, optic nerve damage.
Other: systemic effects and adrenal suppression in excessive or long-term use.

INTERACTIONS

None significant.

EFFECTS ON DIAGNOSTIC TESTS

None reported.

NURSING CONSIDERATIONS

Besides those related universally to drug therapy (see "How to use this book"), consider the following specific recommendations:

Assessment

• Obtain a baseline assessment of the patient's allergies and culture of the eye before therapy.
• Be alert for adverse reactions and drug interactions throughout therapy.
• Evaluate the patient's and family's knowledge about fluorometholone therapy.

Nursing Diagnoses

• Altered protection related to ocular inflammatory process.
• High risk for injury related to fluorometholone-induced corneal ulceration.
• Knowledge deficit related to fluorometholone therapy.

Planning and Implementation

Preparation and Administration

• Store in a tightly covered, light-resistant container.
• Wash hands before and after administration.
• Shake well before using.

Monitoring

• Monitor effectiveness by observing for signs of decreased eye inflammation.
• Intraocular pressure should be measured every 2 to 4 weeks for the first 2 months of ophthalmic corticosteroid therapy; then, if no increase in intraocular pressure has occurred, every 1 to 2 months thereafter.
• Monitor for changes in visual acuity and visual field.
• Observe for hypersensitivity.

Supportive Care

• Use safety precautions if vision is impaired. Assist with activities.
• Do not give to patients with vaccinia, varicella, acute superficial herpes simplex (dendritic keratitis), or other fungal or viral eye diseases; ocular tuberculosis; or any other acute, purulent, untreated eye infection.
• Use with caution in corneal abrasions because these may be contaminated (especially with herpes).
• Not for long-term use.
• Less likely to cause increased intraocular pressure with long-term use than other ophthalmic anti-inflammatory drugs (except medrysone).

Patient Teaching

• Teach the patient how to instill. Advise him to wash hands before and after administration. Warn him not to touch applicator tip to eye or surrounding tissues.
• Instruct the patient to apply light finger pressure to the lacrimal sac for 1 minute after instilling drops. Caution him to avoid scratching or rubbing the eye area.
• Instruct the patient to notify the doctor immediately if changes occur in visual acuity or visual field.
• Advise the patient not to use leftover eye medication for a new eye inflammation and not to share eye medications with family members. A family member who develops the same symptoms should contact the doctor.

Evaluation

In patients receiving fluorometholone, appropriate evaluation statements may include:

• Patient demonstrates decrease in or absence of eye inflammation.
• Patient's cornea remains free from ulceration.
• Patient and family state an understanding of fluorometholone therapy.

fluorouracil (5-fluorouracil, 5-FU)

(flure oh yoor´ a sill)

Adrucil, Efudex, Fluoroplex

• *Classification:* antineoplastic (antimetabolite)
• *Pregnancy Risk Category:* D

HOW SUPPLIED

Injection: 50 mg/ml
Cream: 1%, 5%
Topical solution: 1%, 2%, 5%

ACTION

Mechanism: A pyrimidine antagonist that inhibits DNA synthesis by several mechanisms. The drug is converted to the deoxyribonucleotide, which blocks thymidylate synthesis. It may also be incorporated into RNA, resulting in fraudulent RNA. By blocking uracil phosphatase, the drug may inhibit utilization of preformed uracil.
Absorption: Poorly absorbed after oral or topical administration.
Distribution: Distributes into all areas of body water and tissues, including tumors, bone marrow, liver, and intestinal mucosa; also crosses the blood-brain barrier. After I.V. administration, no drug is found in plasma after 3 hours.
Metabolism: A small amount is converted in the tissues to the active metabolite, with a majority of the drug degraded in the liver.
Excretion: Metabolites are primarily excreted through the lungs as carbon dioxide. About 15% of a dose is excreted in urine as unchanged drug within 6 hours; most of this excretion occurs in the first hour. Half-life: About 16 minutes.

INDICATIONS & DOSAGE

Colon, rectal, breast, ovarian, cervical, bladder, liver, and pancreatic cancer–
Adults: 12.5 mg/kg I.V. daily for 3 to 5 days q 4 weeks; or 15 mg/kg weekly for 6 weeks. (Dosages recommended based on lean body weight.) Maximum single recommended dose is 800 mg, although higher single doses (up to 1.5 g) have been used. The injectable form has been given orally but is not recommended.
Multiple actinic (solar) keratoses; superficial basal cell carcinoma–
Adults: Apply cream or topical solution b.i.d.

CONTRAINDICATIONS & PRECAUTIONS

Contraindicated in patients with poor nutritional status, depressed bone marrow function, recent major surgery, or serious infections because of the increased potential for toxicity; and in pregnant patients because the drug may be fetotoxic.

ADVERSE REACTIONS

Common reactions are in italics; life-threatening reactions are in bold italics.
Blood: ***leukopenia,*** thrombocytopenia, anemia; WBC nadir 9 to 14 days after first dose; platelet nadir in 7 to 14 days.
CNS: acute cerebellar syndrome.
GI: *stomatitis, GI ulcer may precede leukopenia, nausea, vomiting in 30% to 50% of patients; diarrhea.*
Skin: (I.V. use) *dermatitis,* hyperpigmentation (especially in blacks), nail changes, pigmented palmar creases.
Local: *erythema, pain, burning, scaling, pruritus;* (topical use) contact dermatitis, *hyperpigmentation,* soreness, suppuration, swelling.
Other: *reversible alopecia in 5% to 20% of patients, weakness, malaise.*

INTERACTIONS

None significant.

EFFECTS ON DIAGNOSTIC TESTS

Plasma albumin: decreased concentration because of drug-induced protein malabsorption.

NURSING CONSIDERATIONS

Besides those related universally to drug therapy (see "How to use this book"), consider the following specific recommendations:
Assessment
• Obtain a baseline assessment of patient's overall physical status, CBC, renal panel and hepatic profile before initiating therapy.

• Be alert for adverse reactions and drug interactions throughout therapy.
• Evaluate the patient's and family's knowledge about fluorouracil therapy.

Nursing Diagnoses

• Altered protection related to fluorouracil-induced myelosuppression and immunosuppression.
• Altered oral mucous membrane related to fluorouracil-induced stomatitis.
• Knowledge deficit related to fluorouracil therapy.

Planning and Implementation

Preparation and Administration

• ***I.V. use:*** Follow institutional policy to reduce carcinogenic, mutagenic, and teratogenic risks associated with preparation of parenteral form of drug.
• Read order and drug label carefully before administering fluorouracil. It is sometimes ordered as 5-fluorouracil or 5-FU. The numeral 5 is part of the drug name; don't confuse it with dosage units.
• Don't refrigerate fluorouracil or use cloudy solution. If crystals form, redissolve by warming.
• Solution is more stable in plastic I.V. bags than in glass bottles. Use plastic I.V. containers for administering continuous infusions.
• Be aware that fluorouracil is sometimes administered via hepatic arterial infusion in treatment of hepatic metastases.
• Keep in mind that slowing the infusion rate from 2 to 8 hours lessens potential toxicity.
• Be aware that for injection, the drug requires no further dilution. For infusion, dilute with dextrose 5% in water or 0.9% sodium chloride in an appropriate volume based on the patient's condition.
• ***Topical application:*** Apply topical drug while using plastic gloves. Wash hands immediately after handling medication.
• Avoid occlusive dressings because they increase the risk of inflammatory reactions in adjacent normal skin.
• Apply with caution near eyes, nose, and mouth.
• Expect to use 1% concentration on the face. Higher concentrations are used for thicker-skinned areas or resistant lesions.
• Expect to use 5% strength for superficial basal cell carcinoma confirmed by biopsy.

Monitoring

• Expect toxic effects with therapeutic doses; monitor for severity. Be aware that toxicity may be delayed for 1 to 3 weeks.
• Monitor effectiveness by noting results of follow-up diagnostic tests and patient's overall physical status.
• Monitor WBC and platelet counts daily. Drug should be discontinued when WBC count is below 3,500/mm^3 and platelet count is below 100,000/mm^3.
• Monitor for signs of infection (cough, fever, sore throat) and bleeding (easy bruising, nosebleeds, bleeding gums).
• Monitor intake and output and renal and hepatic function.
• Watch for signs of stomatitis or diarrhea (signs of toxicity).
• Monitor for adverse skin reactions.

Supportive Care

• Premedicate the patient with an antiemetic to decrease nausea and vomiting.
• Notify the doctor if severe diarrhea or other toxic reactions occur. Stop drug if severe diarrhea occurs.
• Provide frequent mouth care with a soft toothbrush and mild mouthwash to prevent trauma to oral mucosa.
• Use a topical oral anesthetic to soothe lesions if stomatitis occurs.
• Be aware that drug does not reach therapeutic concentrations in CSF.
• To prevent bleeding, avoid I.M. injections in patients with thrombocytopenia.

• To help prevent infection, maintain the patient's optimal health and protect him from undue exposure to environmental contagions. If signs of infection occur, notify doctor promptly; administer antibiotics, as ordered.
• Provide a safe environment to minimize risk of bleeding.
• Keep in mind that ingestion and systemic absorption of topical drug may cause leukopenia, thrombocytopenia, stomatitis, diarrhea, or GI ulcerations, bleeding, and hemorrhage; application of topical drug to large ulcerated areas may cause systemic toxicity.

Patient Teaching
• Teach the patient and family how to identify and report signs of infection and bleeding.
• Instruct patient about need for protective measures, including conservation of energy, balanced diet, eating frequent small meals, adequate rest, personal cleanliness, clean environment, and avoidance of exposure to persons with infections.
• Warn the patient that alopecia may occur but is reversible.
• Encourage good and frequent oral hygiene to prevent superinfection of denuded areas. Tell the patient to use a soft-bristled toothbrush and nonalcoholic mouthwash. If oral lesions are present, tell the patient to avoid drinking alcohol, smoking, and eating extremely hot or spicy foods. If lesions are painful, tell the patient to consult with the doctor about using a topical oral anesthetic.
• Warn patient to avoid exposure to strong sunlight or ultraviolet light because it will intensify the skin reaction. Encourage use of sunscreens. Explain that dermatologic effects are reversible when drug is discontinued.
• Warn patients receiving topical fluorouracil that treated area may be unsightly during therapy and for several weeks after therapy. Complete healing may take 1 or 2 months.
• Instruct the patient and family members to wear gloves when applying the topical preparation and to avoid occlusive dressings.
• Tell the patient to apply topical drug with caution on areas near eyes, nose, and mouth.
• Instruct the patient and family to wash hands thoroughly after handling fluorouracil cream or solution.

Evaluation
In patients receiving fluorouracil, appropriate evaluation statements may include:
• Patient does not demonstrate signs and symptoms of infection or bleeding.
• Oral lesions are absent or, if present, complications are avoided or minimized.
• Patient and family state an understanding of fluorouracil therapy.

fluoxetine hydrochloride
(floo ox´ e teen)
Prozac

• *Classification:* antidepressant (serotonin uptake inhibitor)
• *Pregnancy Risk Category:* B

HOW SUPPLIED
Pulvules: 20 mg.

ACTION
Mechanism: Inhibits the CNS neuronal uptake of serotonin.
Absorption: Well absorbed after oral administration; absorption is not altered by food.
Distribution: Apparently highly protein-bound (about 95%).
Metabolism: Primarily metabolized in the liver to active metabolites.
Excretion: Drug is excreted by the kidneys. Half-life: Elimination half-life is 2 to 3 days. Norfluoxetine (the

primary active metabolite) has an elimination half-life of 7 to 9 days.
Onset, peak, duration: Peak levels are seen within 8 hours of oral administration. Onset of therapeutic activity may take several weeks.

INDICATIONS & DOSAGE

Short-term management of depressive illness–
Adults: Initially, 20 mg P.O. in the morning; dosage increased according to patient response. May be given b.i.d. in the morning and at noon. Maximum dosage is 80 mg/day.

CONTRAINDICATIONS & PRECAUTIONS

Because patients taking fluoxetine may experience anxiety, nervousness, and insomnia, administering it early in the day may avoid sleep disturbance. Monitor changes in weight during therapy because significant weight loss may occur, especially in underweight patients.

ADVERSE REACTIONS

Common reactions are in italics; life-threatening reactions are in bold italics.
CNS: *nervousness, anxiety, insomnia, headache, drowsiness, tremor, dizziness,* abnormal dreams.
CV: palpitations, flushing, bradycardia, arrhythmias.
EENT: flu-like syndrome, nasal congestion, upper respiratory infection, pharyngitis, cough, sinusitis, visual disturbances, tinnitus, respiratory distress.
GI: *nausea, diarrhea, dry mouth, anorexia, dyspepsia,* constipation, abdominal pain, vomiting, taste change, flatulence, increased appetite.
GU: sexual dysfunction, urine retention.
Other: muscle pain, *weight loss, rash, pruritus, urticaria, asthenia,* edema, lymphadenopathy.

INTERACTIONS

Diazepam: half-life may be prolonged. Drugs highly bound to plasma proteins (warfarin, digitoxin) can displace drug and cause toxic effects.
Tryptophan: agitation, GI distress, and restlessness.

EFFECTS ON DIAGNOSTIC TESTS

None reported.

NURSING CONSIDERATIONS

Besides those related universally to drug therapy (see "How to use this book"), consider the following specific recommendations:

Assessment
- Obtain a baseline assessment of depression before therapy.
- Be alert for adverse reactions and drug interactions throughout therapy.
- Evaluate the patient's and family's knowledge about fluoxetine therapy.

Nursing Diagnoses
- Ineffective individual coping related to the patient's underlying condition.
- Sleep pattern disturbance related to fluoxetine-induced insomnia and drowsiness.
- Knowledge deficit related to fluoxetine therapy.

Planning and Implementation
Preparation and Administration
- Do not give the patient this drug in the afternoon to prevent sleep pattern disturbances because this drug commonly causes nervousness and drowsiness.
- Expect lower dosages or less frequent dosing for elderly patients, debilitated patients, and patients with impaired renal or hepatic function.

Monitoring
- Monitor effectiveness by having the patient discuss his feelings (ask broad, open-ended questions) and by evaluating his behavior.
- Record mood changes and monitor for suicidal tendencies.

• Monitor bowel patterns for diarrhea and check for urine retention

Supportive Care

• Institute safety precautions if adverse CNS reactions occur.

Patient Teaching

• Tell the patient that clinical effects of dosage changes may not be evident for weeks and that full antidepressant effect may take 4 weeks or more of treatment.

• Because this drug can cause nervousness and insomnia, tell the patient to avoid taking it in the afternoon.

• Tell the patient to relieve dry mouth with sugarless hard candy or gum, but explain that saliva substitutes may be necessary.

• Warn the patient to avoid driving and other hazardous activities that require alertness and good psychomotor coordination until CNS effects of the drug are known. Explain that this drug may cause drowsiness and dizziness. Warn against combining it with alcohol or other CNS depressants.

Evaluation

In patients receiving fluoxetine, appropriate evaluation statements include:

• Patient behavior and communication indicate improvement of depression.

• Insomnia and drowsiness from adverse CNS reactions has not occurred.

• Patient and family state an understanding of fluoxetine therapy.

fluoxymesterone

(floo ox i mes´ te rone)

Android F, Halotestin**, Ora-Testryl

• Controlled Substance Schedule III

• *Classification:* androgen replacement, antineoplastic (androgen)

• *Pregnancy Risk Category:* X

HOW SUPPLIED

Tablets: 2 mg, 5 mg, 10 mg

ACTION

Mechanism: An androgen that stimulates cytosol steroid receptors in tissues to effect protein synthesis. Stimulates target tissues to develop normally in androgen-deficient men. Approximately five times as potent as methyltestosterone.

Pharmacokinetics: Unknown.

INDICATIONS & DOSAGE

Hypogonadism and impotence caused by testicular deficiency–

Adults: 2 to 10 mg P.O. daily.

Palliation of breast cancer in women–

Adults: 15 to 30 mg P.O. daily in divided doses. All dosages should be individualized and reduced to minimum when effect is noted.

Postpartum breast engorgement–

Adults: 2.5 mg P.O. followed by 5 to 10 mg daily for 5 days.

CONTRAINDICATIONS & PRECAUTIONS

Contraindicated in patients with severe renal or cardiac disease (fluid and sodium retention caused by fluoxymesterone may aggravate renal and cardiac disease); in patients with hepatic disease because impaired elimination of the drug may cause this accumulation; undiagnosed abnormal genital bleeding because drug can stimulate the growth of cancerous breast or prostate tissue; in male patients with prostate or breast cancer or benign prostatic hypertrophy with obstruction; in pregnant or breast-feeding women because animal studies have shown that administration of androgens during pregnancy causes masculinization of the fetus; and in patients with hypersensitivity to the drug.

The brands Halotestin and Ora-Testryl contain the dye tartrazine. Rare individuals, particularly those who are known to be sensitive to aspirin and who have nasal polyps, may suffer severe hypersensitivity reactions (for example, anaphylaxis) after ingesting tartrazine.

ADVERSE REACTIONS

Common reactions are in italics; life-threatening reactions are in bold italics.

Androgenic: in women–*acne, edema, oily skin, weight gain, hirsutism, hoarseness,* clitoral enlargement, change in libido. In men–prepubertal: premature epiphyseal closure, acne, priapism, growth of body and facial hair, phallic enlargement; postpubertal: testicular atrophy, oligospermia, decreased ejaculatory volume, impotence, gynecomastia, epididymitis.

CV: edema.

GI: gastroenteritis, nausea, vomiting, constipation, change in appetite, diarrhea.

GU: bladder irritability.

Hepatic: reversible jaundice.

Hypoestrogenic: in women–flushing; sweating; vaginitis with itching, drying, burning, or bleeding; menstrual irregularities; emotional lability.

Other: hypercalcemia.

INTERACTIONS

None significant.

EFFECTS ON DIAGNOSTIC TESTS

Glucose tolerance test: abnormal results.

Liver function tests: abnormal results.

Prothrombin time (especially during anticoagulant therapy): prolonged.

Serum sodium, potassium, calcium, phosphate, and cholesterol: increased levels.

Thyroid function tests: (protein-bound iodine, radioactive iodine uptake, thyroid-binding capacity); decreased results.

NURSING CONSIDERATIONS

Besides those related universally to drug therapy (see "How to use this book"), consider the following specific recommendations:

Assessment

• Obtain a baseline assessment of the patient's underlying condition before initiating therapy.

• Be alert for adverse reactions and drug interactions throughout therapy.

• Evaluate the patient's and family's knowledge about fluoxymesterone therapy.

Nursing Diagnoses

• Sexual dysfunction related to hormonal dysfunction.

• Body image disturbance related to adverse androgenic reactions associated with fluoxymesterone.

• Knowledge deficit related to fluoxymesterone therapy.

Planning and Implementation

Preparation and Administration

P.O. use: Administer with food or meals if GI upset occurs.

• Be aware that when used in breast cancer, subjective effects may not be seen for about 1 month and objective effects not for 3 months.

Monitoring

• Monitor effectiveness by regularly assessing the patient's condition for signs of improvement.

• Monitor the patient for hypercalcemia and obtain calcium levels regularly. Hypercalcemia is particularly likely to occur in patients with metastatic breast cancer and may indicate bone metastases.

• Monitor female patients for signs of virilization and menstrual irregularities.

• Monitor the patient for symptoms of jaundice, which may be reversed by dosage adjustment. Periodic liver function tests should be performed.

• Monitor the patient on concomitant anticoagulant therapy for ecchymotic areas, petechiae, or abnormal bleeding. Monitor prothrombin time.
• Monitor the patient's weight routinely for fluid retention.
• Monitor for signs of hypoglycemia in patients with diabetes. Check blood glucose levels frequently as dosage of antidiabetic drug may need to be adjusted.

Supportive Care

• Report signs of virilization or menstrual irregularities to the doctor.
• Give the patient a diet high in calories and protein unless contraindicated. Give small, frequent feedings. Also implement salt restriction if edema occurs; expect to administer a diuretic concurrently, if needed.
• Carefully evaluate results of laboratory studies. Many laboratory results may be altered during therapy and for 2 to 3 weeks after therapy ends.
• Obtain an order for an antiemetic, antidiarrheal, or laxative, as indicated.
• Prepare patient for altered body image if androgenic adverse reactions occur.

Patient Teaching

• Tell the patient to take drug with food or meals if GI upset occurs.
• Tell female patients to report menstrual irregularities; therapy should be discontinued pending etiologic determination.
• Explain to female patients that virilization may occur, especially to patients on drug for palliation of breast cancer, because of dosage required. Tell these patients to report such effects immediately as effects may be irreversible.
• Tell patient to eat a diet high in calories and protein and low in sodium if not contraindicated and to eat small frequent meals.
• Warn the diabetic patient about the potential for hypoglycemia and instruct him how to manage symptoms and to notify doctor if it occurs.

Evaluation

In patients receiving fluoxymesterone, appropriate evaluation statements may include:
• Patient's underlying condition exhibits improvement.
• Patient states acceptance of body image changes caused by fluoxymesterone therapy.
• Patient and family state an understanding of fluoxymesterone therapy.

fluphenazine decanoate

(floo fen´ a zeen)
Modecate Decanoate†‡, Prolixin Decanoate

fluphenazine enanthate

Moditen Enanthate†, Prolixin Enanthate

fluphenazine hydrochloride

Anatensol‡*, Apo-Fluphenazine†, Moditen HCl†, Moditen HCl-HP†, Permitil* **, Prolixin* **

• *Classification:* antipsychotic (piperazine phenothiazine)
• *Pregnancy Risk Category:* C

HOW SUPPLIED

decanoate
Depot injection: 25 mg/ml
enanthate
Depot injection: 25 mg/ml
hydrochloride
Tablets: 1 mg, 2.5 mg, 5 mg, 10 mg
Oral concentrate: 5 mg/ml (contains 14% alcohol)
Elixir: 2.5 mg/5 ml (with 14% alcohol)
I.M. injection: 2.5 mg/ml

ACTION

Mechanism: Blocks postsynaptic dopamine receptors in the brain.
Absorption: Rate and extent of ab-

sorption vary with route of administration; oral tablet absorption is erratic and variable. Absorption of enanthate and decanoate esters from I.M. injection sites is slow.
Distribution: Widely distributed into the body, including breast milk. CNS concentrations are usually higher than those in plasma. Drug is 91% to 99% protein-bound.
Metabolism: Extensively metabolized by the liver, but no active metabolites are formed.
Excretion: Most of drug is excreted in urine via the kidneys; some is excreted in feces via the biliary tract.
Onset, peak, duration: After oral administration, peak serum levels are seen in about 1 hour. After I.M. injection, peak serum levels occur within 1 hour for hydrochloride; 24 to 72 hours for decanoate or enanthate. Duration of action of these depot forms averages 2 weeks.

INDICATIONS & DOSAGE

Psychotic disorders–
Adults: initially, 0.5 to 10 mg (fluphenazine hydrochloride) P.O. daily in divided doses q 6 to 8 hours; may increase cautiously to 20 mg. Higher doses (50 to 100 mg) have been given. Maintenance dosage is 1 to 5 mg P.O. daily. I.M. doses are ⅓ to ½ oral doses. Lower dosages for geriatric patients (1 to 2.5 mg daily).
Children: 0.25 to 3.5 mg fluphenazine hydrochloride P.O. daily in divided doses q 4 to 6 hours; or ⅓ to ½ of oral dose I.M.; maximum dosage is 10 mg daily.
Adults and children over 12 years: 12.5 to 25 mg of long-acting esters (fluphenazine decanoate and enanthate) I.M. or S.C. q 1 to 6 weeks. Maintenance dosage is 25 to 100 mg, p.r.n.

CONTRAINDICATIONS & PRECAUTIONS

Contraindicated in patients with hypersensitivity to phenothiazines and related compounds, including allergic reactions involving hepatic function; blood dyscrasias and bone marrow depression because of possible agranulocytosis; disorders accompanied by coma, brain damage, or CNS depression because of additive CNS depression; in patients with circulatory collapse or cerebrovascular disease because of its hypotensive effect; and for use with adrenergic-blocking agents or spinal or epidural anesthetics because of potential hypotension and alpha blockade.

Use cautiously in patients with cardiac disease (arrhythmias, CHF, angina pectoris, valvular disease, or heart block), encephalitis, Reye's syndrome, head injury, respiratory disease, epilepsy and other seizure disorders, glaucoma, prostatic hypertrophy, urinary retention, hepatic or renal dysfunction, Parkinson's disease, pheochromocytoma, or hypocalcemia. Some oral preparations of fluphenazine contain tartrazine; use of such products may cause allergic reaction in patients with aspirin allergy.

ADVERSE REACTIONS

Common reactions are in italics; life-threatening reactions are in bold italics.
Blood: transient leukopenia, ***agranulocytosis.***
CNS: *extrapyramidal reactions (high incidence), tardive dyskinesia,* sedation (low incidence), pseudoparkinsonism, EEG changes, dizziness.
CV: *orthostatic hypotension,* tachycardia, ECG changes.
EENT: ocular changes, *blurred vision.*
GI: *dry mouth, constipation.*
GU: *urine retention,* dark urine, menstrual irregularities, gynecomastia, inhibited ejaculation.

Hepatic: cholestatic jaundice, abnormal liver function tests.
Metabolic: hyperprolactinemia.
Skin: *mild photosensitivity,* dermal allergic reactions.
Other: weight gain; increased appetite; rarely, ***neuroleptic malignant syndrome*** (fever, tachycardia, tachypnea, profuse diaphoresis).
After abrupt withdrawal of long-term therapy: gastritis, nausea, vomiting, dizziness, tremors, feeling of warmth or cold, sweating, tachycardia, headache, insomnia.

INTERACTIONS

Alcohol, other CNS depressants: increased CNS depression. Avoid concomitant use.
Antacids: inhibit absorption of oral phenothiazines. Separate antacid and phenothiazine doses by at least 2 hours.
Barbiturates, lithium: may decrease phenothiazine effect. Observe patient.
Centrally acting antihypertensives: decreased antihypertensive effect.

EFFECTS ON DIAGNOSTIC TESTS

ECG: quinidine-like effects.
Liver enzymes and protein-bound iodine: elevated results.
Urine porphyrins, urobilinogen, amylase, and 5-HIAA: false-positive results because of darkening of urine by metabolites.
Urine pregnancy test results using human chorionic gonadotropin: false-positive results.

NURSING CONSIDERATIONS

Besides those related universally to drug therapy (see "How to use this book"), consider the following specific recommendations:

Assessment
- Obtain a baseline assessment of the patient's mental status, including symptoms, before drug therapy.
- Be alert for adverse reactions and drug interactions throughout therapy.
- Evaluate the patient's and family's knowledge about fluphenazine therapy.

Nursing Diagnoses
- Impaired thought processes related to the patient's underlying condition.
- Sensory/perceptual (visual) alterations related to adverse drug reactions.
- Knowledge deficit related to fluphenazine therapy.

Planning and Implementation
Preparation and Administration
- Protect medication from light. Slight yellowing of injection or concentrate is common and does not affect potency. Discard markedly discolored solutions.
- Dose of 2 mg is therapeutic equivalent of 100 mg of chlorpromazine.
- ***P.O. use:*** Dilute liquid concentrate with 60 ml tomato or fruit juice, carbonated beverages, coffee, tea, milk, water, or semisolid food just before giving.
- Avoid skin contact with the injectable or liquid form because it may cause a rash.
- Decanoate and enanthate may be given subcutaneously.
- Note that Prolixin Concentrate and Permitil Concentrate are 10 times more concentrated than Prolixin Elixir (5 mg/ml vs. 0.5 mg/ml).
- ***I.M. use:*** For long-acting oil preparations (decanoate and enanthate), use a dry needle of at least 21 G. Allow 24 to 96 hours for onset of action.

Monitoring
- Monitor effectiveness by regularly observing the patient's behavior and noting if psychotic symptoms have abated or diminished.
- Monitor for adverse reactions, especially extrapyramidal and anticholinergic effects (blurred vision, dry mouth, constipation, urine retention),

and tardive dyskinesia, during prolonged therapy.
• Watch for orthostatic hypotension, especially after parenteral administration.
• Monitor therapy by weekly bilirubin tests during the first month; periodic blood tests (CBC and liver function); and ophthalmic tests (long-term use).
• Monitor for neuroleptic malignant syndrome. This rare, potentially fatal reaction is not necessarily related to duration or type of neuroleptic therapy, but usually occurs in men (60% of affected patients).

Supportive Care
• Keep the patient supine for 1 hour after I.M. administration. Then assist patient to get up slowly to avoid orthostatic hypotension.
• Do not discontinue drug abruptly unless required by severe adverse reactions.
• Increase the patient's fluid and fiber intake if not contraindicated–to prevent constipation. If necessary, request doctor's order for a laxative.
• Give the patient sugarless gum, sour hard candy, ice chips, or a mouthwash rinse to relieve dryness.
• Be prepared to give I.V. diphenhydramine, as ordered, to treat acute dystonic reactions.
• Hold the dose if patient develops signs of jaundice, symptoms of blood dyscrasias (fever, sore throat, infection, cellulitis, weakness), persistent (longer than a few hours) extrapyramidal reactions, or any such reactions during pregnancy.

Patient Teaching
• Tell the patient to avoid exposure to direct sunlight and to use a sunscreen when going outdoors to prevent photosensitivity reactions. (**Note:** Sunlamps and tanning beds may cause burning of the skin or skin discoloration.)
• Tell the patient not to stop taking the drug suddenly.
• Encourage the patient to report difficulty urinating, sore throat, dizziness, or fainting.
• Advise the patient to increase fluid and fiber in the diet, if appropriate.
• Tell the patient to avoid driving and other hazardous activities that require alertness until the effect of the drug is established. Excessive sedative effects tend to subside after several weeks.
• Explain which fluids are appropriate for diluting the concentrate and show the dropper technique for measuring dose. Warn the patient to avoid spilling liquid on skin because it may cause a rash and irritation.
• Tell the patient to relieve dry mouth with sugarless hard candy or chewing gum or ice chips.

Evaluation

In patients receiving fluphenazine, appropriate evaluation statements may include:
• Patient demonstrates a decrease in psychotic behavior.
• Patient does not experience blurred vision.
• Patient voids without difficulty.
• Patient and family state an understanding of fluphenazine therapy.

flurandrenolide

(flure an dren´ oh lide)

Cordran, Cordran SP, Cordran Tape, Drenison†, Drenison 1/4†, Drenison Tape†

• *Classification:* topical anti-inflammatory (adrenocorticoid)
• *Pregnancy Risk Category:* C

HOW SUPPLIED

Cream: 0.025%, 0.05%
Lotion: 0.05%
Ointment: 0.025%, 0.05%
Tape: 4 mcg/cm^2

ACTION

Mechanism: Diffuses across cell membranes and complexes with specific cytoplasmic receptors.
Absorption: Amount absorbed depends on the amount applied and on the nature of the skin at the application site. Absorption is lowest in areas with thick stratum corneum (palms, soles, elbows, and knees) and higher in thinner areas (face, eyelids, and genitalia). Absorption increases in areas of skin damage, inflammation, or occlusion. Some systemic absorption of topical steroids may occur, especially through the oral mucosa.
Distribution: After topical application, distributed throughout the local skin. If absorbed into the circulation, it is rapidly removed from the blood and distributed into muscle, liver, skin, intestines, and kidneys.
Metabolism: After topical administration, metabolized primarily in the skin. The small amount that is absorbed into systemic circulation is metabolized primarily in the liver to inactive compounds.
Excretion: Inactive metabolites are excreted by the kidneys, primarily as glucuronides and sulfates, but also as unconjugated products. Small amounts of the metabolites are also excreted in feces.

INDICATIONS & DOSAGE

Inflammation of corticosteroid-responsive dermatoses–
Adults and children: clean area; apply cream, lotion, or ointment sparingly b.i.d. or t.i.d. Apply tape q 12 to 24 hours. Before applying tape, cleanse skin carefully, removing scales, crust, and dried exudates. Allow skin to dry for 1 hour before applying new tape. Shave or clip hair to allow good contact with skin and comfortable removal. If tape ends loosen prematurely, trim off and replace with fresh tape. Lowest incidence of adverse reactions if tape is replaced q 12 hours, but may be left in place for 24 hours if well tolerated and adheres satisfactorily.
Drenison 1/4 – for maintenance therapy of widespread or chronic lesions.

CONTRAINDICATIONS & PRECAUTIONS

Contraindicated in patients who are hypersensitive to any component of the preparation and in patients with viral, fungal, or tubercular skin lesions. Use with extreme caution in patients with impaired circulation because it may increase the risk of skin ulceration. Avoid using on the face or genital areas because increased absorption may result in striae.

ADVERSE REACTIONS

Common reactions are in italics; life-threatening reactions are in bold italics.
Skin: burning, itching, irritation, dryness, folliculitis, hypertrichosis, hypopigmentation, acneiform eruptions, allergic contact dermatitis. With occlusive dressings: *maceration of skin, secondary infection, atrophy, striae, miliaria.* With tape: purpura, stripping of epidermis, furunculosis.

INTERACTIONS

None significant.

EFFECTS ON DIAGNOSTIC TESTS

None significant.

NURSING CONSIDERATIONS

Besides those related universally to drug therapy (see "How to use this book"), consider the following specific recommendations:
Assessment
- Obtain a baseline assessment of patient's skin integrity before flurandrenolide therapy.
- Be alert for adverse reactions and drug interactions throughout therapy.
- Evaluate the patient's and family's

knowledge about flurandrenolide therapy.

Nursing Diagnoses

• Impaired skin integrity related to the patient's underlying condition.
• High risk for infection related to drug-induced adverse reaction.
• Knowledge deficit related to flurandrenolide therapy.

Planning and Implementation

Preparation and Administration

• Read order and drug labels carefully.
• Wear gloves when administering drug.
• Before applying, gently wash the patient's skin. Apply a thin layer of medication and rub in gently.
• When treating hairy sites, part hair and apply directly to lesion.
• To apply an occlusive dressing (only if ordered by doctor), apply cream heavily, then cover with a thin, pliable, nonflammable plastic film; seal to adjacent normal skin with hypoallergenic tape.
• To prevent recurrence, treatment should continue for a few days after lesions have cleared.

Monitoring

• Monitor effectiveness by regularly assessing skin for extent and severity of inflammation.
• Monitor for hypersensitivity reaction to flurandrenolide.
• Monitor for evidence of secondary infection.
• Monitor for adverse drug reaction and drug interactions by frequently assessing the patient's skin for burning, itching, and dryness.
• Monitor patient who must use occlusive dressings for maceration of the skin and secondary infection.

Supportive Care

• To minimize adverse reactions, use occlusive dressings intermittently. Don't use occlusive dressings in the presence of infection or on weeping or exudative lesions, and don't leave in place longer than 16 hours each day.
• For patients with eczematous dermatitis, who may develop irritation with adhesive material, hold dressing in place with gauze, elastic bandage, or stockings.
• Notify the doctor and remove occlusive dressing if fever develops.
• Withhold the drug and notify the doctor if hypersensitivity reaction or infection occurs.
• Have the patient's fingernails cut short to minimize skin trauma from scratching.
• Apply cool, moist compresses to involved areas to relieve itching and burning.
• Use hypoallergenic tape, gauze, stockings, or elastic bandage to secure occlusive dressings.
• Be prepared to stop the drug and notify the doctor if patient develops signs of systemic absorption, skin irritation or ulceration, hypersensitivity, or infection. (If antifungals or antibiotics are being used with corticosteroids and infection does not respond immediately, corticosteroids should be stopped until infection is controlled.)

Patient Teaching

• Instruct the patient to clean involved area before applying flurandrenolide in a thin layer to cover the entire surface.
• Teach the patient how to apply an occlusive dressing.
• Teach the patient and family how to recognize signs of a hypersensitivity reaction or an infection. Advise them to discontinue the drug and notify the doctor immediately if either of these occur.
• Instruct the patient to complete the entire treatment regimen as prescribed, even if the lesions appear to have healed.
• Tell the patient and family not to share the flurandrenolide prescription with others.

Evaluation
In patients receiving flurandrenolide, appropriate evaluation statements include:
• Patient maintains skin integrity.
• Patient does not develop secondary infection.
• Patient and family state an understanding of flurandrenolide therapy.

flurazepam hydrochloride
(flure az´ e pam)
Apo-Flurazepam†, Dalmane, Durapam, Novoflupam†, Sam-Pam†

• Controlled Substance Schedule IV
• *Classification:* sedative-hypnotic (benzodiazepine)
• *Pregnancy Risk Category:* D

HOW SUPPLIED
Capsules: 15 mg, 30 mg

ACTION
Mechanism: Acts on the limbic system, thalamus, and hypothalamus of the CNS to produce hypnotic effects.
Absorption: When administered orally, rapidly absorbed through the GI tract.
Distribution: Widely distributed throughout the body. Approximately 97% of an administered dose is bound to plasma protein.
Metabolism: Hepatic conversion to the active metabolite desalkylflurazepam.
Excretion: Desalkylflurazepam is excreted in urine. Half-life: 50 to 100 hours.
Onset, peak, duration: Onset of action within 20 minutes; peak action in 1 to 2 hours; duration of action, 7 to 10 hours. The drug has a substantial carry-over effect, becoming more effective after 2 or more days of therapy because of the accumulation of an active metabolite.

INDICATIONS & DOSAGE
Insomnia –
Adults: 15 to 30 mg P.O. h.s. May repeat dose once.
Adults over 65 years: 15 mg P.O. h.s.

CONTRAINDICATIONS & PRECAUTIONS
Contraindicated in patients with hypersensitivity to the drug; acute narrow-angle glaucoma or untreated open-angle glaucoma because of the drug's possible anticholinergic effect; shock or coma because the drug's hypnotic or hypotensive effect may be prolonged or intensified; and acute alcohol intoxication who have depressed vital signs because the drug will worsen CNS depression.

Use cautiously in psychotic patients because the drug is rarely beneficial in such patients and may induce paradoxical reactions; in patients with myasthenia gravis or Parkinson's disease because it may exacerbate the disorder; in patients with impaired renal or hepatic function, which prolongs elimination of the drug; in elderly or debilitated patients, who are usually more sensitive to the drug's CNS effects; and in persons prone to addiction or drug abuse.

ADVERSE REACTIONS
Common reactions are in italics; life-threatening reactions are in bold italics.
Blood: leukopenia, granulocytopenia.
CNS: *daytime sedation, dizziness, drowsiness, disturbed coordination,* lethargy, confusion, *headache.*
GI: nausea, vomiting, heartburn.
Metabolic: elevated liver enzymes.

INTERACTIONS
Alcohol or other CNS depressants, including narcotic analgesics: excessive CNS depression. Use together cautiously.
Cimetidine: increased sedation. Monitor carefully.

EFFECTS ON DIAGNOSTIC TESTS

EEG: Minor changes in patterns, (usually low-voltage, fast activity).
Liver function tests: elevated results.

NURSING CONSIDERATIONS

Besides those related universally to drug therapy (see "How to use this book"), consider the following specific recommendations:

Assessment

- Obtain a baseline assessment of sleeping patterns and CNS status before therapy.
- Be alert for adverse reactions and drug interactions throughout therapy.
- Evaluate the patient's and family's knowledge about flurazepam therapy.

Nursing Diagnoses

- Sleep pattern disturbance related to underlying patient problem.
- High risk for trauma related to adverse CNS reactions caused by flurazepam.
- Knowledge deficit related to flurazepam therapy.

Planning and Implementation

Preparation and Administration

- Before leaving the bedside, make sure the patient has swallowed capsule.

Monitoring

- Regularly monitor effectiveness by evaluating the patient's ability to sleep. Be aware that drug is more effective on second, third, and fourth nights of use.
- Monitor for CNS and other adverse reactions. Remember that elderly patients are more sensitive to the drug's CNS effects.
- Monitor for evidence of dependency during prolonged use.

Supportive Care

- After administration, institute safety precautions: remove cigarettes; keep bed rails up, and supervise or assist ambulation.
- Take precautions to prevent hoarding or self-overdosing, especially by patient who is depressed, suicidal, or drug-dependent or who has a history of drug abuse.

Patient Teaching

- Explain that drug is more effective on second, third, and fourth nights of use because active metabolite accumulates. Encourage the patient to continue drug if it doesn't work the first night.
- Instruct the patient to remain in bed after taking drug and to call for assistance to use bathroom.
- Warn the patient to avoid driving and other hazardous activities that require mental alertness if adverse CNS reactions are present after awakening.
- Tell the patient that prolonged use may cause dependency; encourage the patient to induce sleep with nonpharmacologic measures.
- Tell the patient to notify the nurse or doctor if sleep pattern disturbances persist.

Evaluation

In patients receiving flurazepam, appropriate evaluation statements may include:

- Patient states drug was effective in inducing sleep.
- Patient's safety is maintained.
- Patient and family state an understanding of flurazepam therapy.

flurbiprofen (systemic)

(flure bi´ proe fen)
Ansaid

- *Classification:* ophthalmic anti-inflammatory agent, antimitotic (nonsteroidal anti-inflammatory drug)
- *Pregnancy Risk Category:* B

HOW SUPPLIED

Tablets: 50 mg, 100 mg

*Liquid form contains alcohol.

**May contain tartrazine.

ACTION

Mechanism: An anti-inflammatory agent that interferes with prostaglandin synthesis.
Absorption: Well absorbed after oral administration. Administering with food alters the rate, but not extent, of absorption.
Distribution: Highly bound (>99%) to plasma proteins.
Metabolism: Primarily in the liver. The major metabolite shows little anti-inflammatory activity.
Excretion: Primarily in the urine. Half-life: Average elimination half-life is 6½ hours.
Onset, peak, duration: Peak levels occur in about 1½ hours.

INDICATIONS & DOSAGE

Rheumatoid arthritis and osteoarthritis–
Adults: 200 to 300 mg P.O. daily, divided b.i.d. to q.i.d.

CONTRAINDICATIONS & PRECAUTIONS

Contraindicated in patients with a history of an allergic response (including asthma or urticaria) to aspirin or NSAIDs. Serious GI toxicity, including ulceration and hemorrhage, can occur at any time in patients receiving chronic NSAID therapy.

ADVERSE REACTIONS

Common reactions are in italics; life-threatening reactions are in bold italics.
CNS: *headache,* anxiety, insomnia, increased reflexes, tremors, amnesia, asthenia, drowsiness, malaise, depression, dizziness.
CV: *edema.*
EENT: rhinitis, tinnitus, visual changes.
GI: *dyspepsia, diarrhea, abdominal pain, nausea,* constipation, *GI bleeding,* flatulence, vomiting.
GU: *symptoms suggesting urinary tract infection.*
Hepatic: elevated liver enzymes.
Skin: rash.
Other: weight changes.

INTERACTIONS

Aspirin: decreased flurbiprofen levels. Concomitant use is not recommended.
Diuretics: possible decreased diuretic effect. Monitor patient closely.
Oral anticoagulants: increased bleeding tendencies. Monitor patient closely.

EFFECTS ON DIAGNOSTIC TESTS

None reported.

NURSING CONSIDERATIONS

Besides those related universally to drug therapy (see "How to use this book"), consider the following specific recommendations:

Assessment
- Obtain a baseline assessment of pain before therapy.
- Be alert for adverse reactions and drug interactions throughout therapy.
- Evaluate the patient's and family's knowledge about flurbiprofen therapy.

Nursing Diagnoses
- Pain related to the patient's underlying condition.
- Diarrhea related to adverse GI reactions to flurbiprofen therapy.
- Knowledge deficit related to flurbiprofen therapy.

Planning and Implementation

Preparation and Administration
- Give this drug with food, milk, or an antacid if GI upset occurs.
- Give lower doses to elderly or debilitated patients with impaired renal or hepatic function, as ordered, because of increased possibility of renal impairment.

Monitoring
- Regularly evaluate for pain relief.
- Monitor the patient for signs of serious GI toxicity, such as GI bleeding. Notify the doctor if these signs occur.

• Monitor liver function studies, hematocrit levels, and results of eye examinations if the patient is receiving long-term therapy with this drug.
• Monitor renal function in elderly or debilitated patients with impaired hepatic or renal function.
• Monitor the frequency and character of stools and record the number of stools in patients experiencing diarrhea as an adverse reaction.

Supportive Care

• Administer antidiarrheal therapy, as ordered, if patient experiences diarrhea.

Patient Teaching

• Tell the patient to take the drug with food, milk, or an antacid if GI upset occurs.
• Advise the patient to call the doctor immediately if edema, black stools, skin rash, itching, or visual disturbances occur.
• Advise the patient to avoid hazardous activities that require mental alertness until the CNS effects of the drug are known.
• Encourage the patient to have periodic eye examinations during long-term therapy. Also explain the importance of periodic liver function studies and hematocrit determiniations to these patients.

Evaluation

In patients receiving flurbiprofen, appropriate evaluation statements may include:

• Patient states pain is relieved by flurbiprofen.
• Diarrhea did not occur.
• Patient and family state an understanding of flurbiprofen therapy.

flurbiprofen sodium (ophthalmic)

(flure bi´ proe fen)

Ocufen

• *Classification:* anti-inflammatory agent (nonsteroidal anti-inflammatory agent, phenylalkanoic acid derivative)
• *Pregnancy Risk Category:* C

HOW SUPPLIED

Ophthalmic solution: 0.03%

ACTION

Mechanism: Blocks the production of prostaglandins in the aqueous humor of the eye, which may cause postoperative miosis; prostaglandins are released as a result of trauma. Drug is not effective if miosis is already present.

Absorption: Following topical administration to the eye, drug is found in aqueous humor; peak levels do not increase as dose increases.

Distribution: Rapidly distributes throughout ocular tissues and fluids. Little is found in the contralateral eye.

Metabolism: After ophthalmic administration, flurbiprofen is absorbed systemically and is metabolized primarily in the liver, where it is converted mainly to inactive glucuronide and sulfate compounds.

Excretion: Inactive metabolites are excreted by the kidneys, primarily as glucuronides and sulfates. Half-life: About 1½ hours.

Onset, peak, duration: Peak levels in aqueous humor are found within 30 minutes to 1 hour of instillation.

INDICATIONS & DOSAGE

Inhibition of intraoperative miosis–
Adults: Instill 1 drop approximately every ½ hour, beginning 2 hours before surgery. Give a total of 4 drops.

CONTRAINDICATIONS & PRECAUTIONS

Contraindicated in patients who are hypersensitive to any component of the preparation. Ophthalmic flurbiprofen is contraindicated in patients with active epithelial herpes simplex keratitis and should be used with extreme caution in patients with a history of this disorder, because it *may worsen* this condition and may delay wound healing. It should be used with caution in patients who may be affected adversely by a prolonged bleeding time because flurbiprofen can inhibit platelet aggregation.

Because of a potential for cross-sensitivity between flurbiprofen and aspirin or other NSAIDs, flurbiprofen should be used with particular caution in patients in whom aspirin or other NSAIDs may trigger asthma, rhinitis, or urticaria.

ADVERSE REACTIONS

Common reactions are in italics; life-threatening reactions are in bold italics.

Eye: transient burning and stinging upon instillation, ocular irritation.

INTERACTIONS

Acetylcholine, carbachol: may be rendered ineffective.

Epinephrine or other antiglaucoma agents: reduced ability to lower intraocular pressure.

EFFECTS ON DIAGNOSTIC TESTS

None reported.

NURSING CONSIDERATIONS

Besides those related universally to drug therapy (see "How to use this book"), consider the following specific recommendations:

Assessment

- Obtain a baseline assessment of the patient's allergies (especially to aspirin and other NSAIDs) and clotting time before therapy.
- Be alert for adverse reactions and drug interactions throughout therapy.
- Evaluate the patient's and family's knowledge about ophthalmic flurbiprofen therapy.

Nursing Diagnoses

- Altered protection related to ocular inflammatory process.
- Pain related to ophthalmic flurbiprofen-induced burning and stinging on instillation.
- Knowledge deficit related to ophthalmic flurbiprofen therapy.

Planning and Implementation

Preparation and Administration

- Wash hands before and after administration.
- Give preoperatively only unless otherwise ordered.

Monitoring

- Monitor effectiveness by checking the eye for decreasing signs of inflammation.
- Observe for bleeding.
- Check prothrombin time and partial thromboplastin time.
- Monitor for signs of hypersensitivity.

Supportive Care

- Do not give in epithelial herpes simplex keratitis.
- Use with caution in patients allergic to aspirin and other NSAIDs; and in patients with bleeding tendencies or who are receiving medications that may prolong clotting time.

Patient Teaching

- Warn the patient that the eyedrops may burn or sting on instillation. Reassure him that these sensations will subside.

Evaluation

In patients receiving ophthalmic flurbiprofen, appropriate evaluation statements may include:

- Patient demonstrates decrease in or absence of eye inflammation.
- Patient reports decrease in or absence of pain on instillation.
- Patient and family state an understanding of ophthalmic flurbiprofen therapy.

flutamide

(floo´ ta mide)
Eulexin

• *Classification:* antineoplastic (nonsteroidal antiandrogen)
• *Pregnancy Risk Category:* D

HOW SUPPLIED

Capsules: 125 mg

ACTION

Mechanism: Inhibits androgen uptake or prevents binding of androgens in nucleus of cells within target tissues.
Absorption: Rapid and complete absorption occurs after oral administration.
Distribution: Studies in animals show that the drug concentrates in the prostate. The drug and its active metabolite is about 95% protein-bound.
Metabolism: Rapid, with at least six metabolites identified. Over 97% of the drug is metabolized within 1 hour of administration. The alpha-hydroxy form of the drug is biologically active and forms rapidly.
Excretion: Over 95% in the urine. Half-life: About 6 hours for the active metabolite.
Onset, peak, duration: Peak levels of the active alpha-hydroxy metabolite appear within 2 hours of administration.

INDICATIONS & DOSAGE

Treatment of metastatic prostatic carcinoma (stage D_2) in combination with luteinizing hormone-releasing hormone analogs such as leuprolide acetate–
Adults: 250 mg P.O. q. 8 hours.

CONTRAINDICATIONS & PRECAUTIONS

Contraindicated in patients allergic to the drug. Periodic liver tests should be performed in patients receiving prolonged therapy with flutamide. Animal studies indicate harmful fetal effects.

ADVERSE REACTIONS

Common reactions are in italics; life-threatening reactions are in bold italics.
CNS: *loss of libido.*
CV: edema, hypertension.
GI: *diarrhea, nausea, vomiting.*
GU: *impotence.*
Metabolic: gynecomastia, elevated of hepatic enzymes, hepatitis.
Skin: rash, photosensitivity.
Other: *hot flashes.*

INTERACTIONS

None reported.

EFFECTS ON DIAGNOSTIC TESTS

Plasma testosterone and estradiol: elevated levels.

NURSING CONSIDERATIONS

Besides those related universally to drug therapy (see "How to use this book"), consider the following specific recommendations:

Assessment
• Obtain a baseline assessment of the patient's underlying condition before initiating therapy.
• Be alert for adverse reactions and drug interactions throughout therapy.
• Evaluate the patient's and family's knowledge about flutamide therapy.

Nursing Diagnoses
• High risk for fluid volume deficit related to adverse drug reactions.
• Sexual dysfunction related to drug-induced impotence.
• Knowledge deficit related to flutamide therapy.

Planning and Implementation
Preparation and Administration
• ***P.O. use:*** Administered in combination with luteinizing hormone releasing hormone–antagonist (such as leuprolide acetate).

• Generally taken in three divided doses daily.

Monitoring

• Monitor effectiveness by noting the results of follow-up diagnostic tests and overall physical status; by periodically evaluating liver function studies.

• Monitor hydration status if nausea, vomiting, and diarrhea occur.

• Monitor the patient's vital signs for hypertension.

• Monitor the patient for edema.

Supportive Care

• Know that leuprolide suppresses testosterone production, while flutamide inhibits testosterone action at the cellular level. Together they can impair growth of androgen-responsive tumors.

• Provide the patient with fluids if he develops nausea, vomiting, and diarrhea.

• Encourage the patient to discuss his feeling and concerns about sexual dysfunction.

• Encourage the patient to seek professional evaluation and therapy for sexual dysfunction.

Patient Teaching

• Warn patient not to interrupt or discontinue drug therapy without consulting the doctor.

• Inform the patient that flutamide must be taken continuously with the agent used for medical castration (such as leuprolide acetate) to allow the full benefits of therapy.

Evaluation

In patient's receiving flutamide, appropriate evaluation statements may include:

• Patient does not experience fluid volume deficit.

• Sexual dysfunction is supported by patient and significant other.

• Patient and family state an understanding of flutamide therapy.

---

furosemide (frusemide)

(fur oh´ se mide)

Apo-Furosemide†, Furomide M.D., Furoside†, Lasix*, Lasix Special†, Myrosemide*, Novosemide†, Urex‡, Urex-M‡, Uritol†

• *Classification:* diuretic, antihypertensive (loop diuretic)

• *Pregnancy Risk Category:* C

HOW SUPPLIED

Tablets: 20 mg, 40 mg, 80 mg, 500 mg†

Oral solution: 8 mg/ml, 10 mg/ml, 50 mg/ml

Injection: 10 mg/ml

ACTION

Mechanism: A loop diuretic that inhibits reabsorption of sodium and chloride at the proximal portion of the ascending loop of Henle.

Absorption: About 60% of a given dose is absorbed from the GI tract after oral administration. Food delays oral absorption but does not alter diuretic response. Well absorbed after I.M. injection.

Distribution: About 95% plasma protein-bound. It crosses the placenta and distributes into breast milk.

Metabolism: Minimally metabolized by the liver.

Excretion: About 50% to 80% of a dose is excreted in urine. Half-life: Plasma half-life is about 30 minutes.

Onset, peak, duration: Diuresis begins in 30 minutes to 1 hour; peak diuresis occurs 1 to 2 hours after oral administration. Diuresis follows I.V. administration within 5 minutes and peaks in 20 minutes to 1 hour. Duration of action is 6 to 8 hours after oral administration and about 2 hours after I.V. administration.

INDICATIONS & DOSAGE

Acute pulmonary edema–
Adults: 40 mg I.V. injected slowly; then 40 mg I.V. in 1 to 1½ hours if needed.
Edema–
Adults: 20 to 80 mg P.O. daily in a.m., second dose can be given in 6 to 8 hours; carefully titrated up to 600 mg daily if needed; or 20 to 40 mg I.M. or I.V. Increase by 20 mg q 2 hours until desired response is achieved. I.V. dose should be given slowly over 1 to 2 minutes.
Hypertension–
Adults: 40 mg P.O. b.i.d. Adjust dose according to response.
Infants and children: 2 mg/kg P.O. daily; dose increased by 1 to 2 mg/kg in 6 to 8 hours if needed; carefully titrated up to 6 mg/kg daily if needed.
Hypertensive crisis, acute renal failure–
Adults: 100 to 200 mg I.V. over 1 to 2 minutes.
Chronic renal failure–
Adults: initially, 80 mg P.O. daily. Increase by 80 to 120 mg daily until desired response is achieved.

CONTRAINDICATIONS & PRECAUTIONS

Contraindicated in patients with hypersensitivity, anuria, hepatic coma, or electrolyte depletion and in the presence of rising BUN and serum creatinine levels or oliguria, even though it is used to produce diuresis in patients with renal impairment, because rapid fluid and electrolyte changes can exacerbate these conditions.

Use cautiously in patients hypersensitive to sulfonamides; in patients with hepatic cirrhosis and ascites because changes in electrolyte balance may precipitate hepatic encephalopathy; and in patients receiving digitalis glycosides because furosemide-induced hypokalemia may predispose them to digitalis toxicity. Rapid I.V. administration of furosemide increases risk of ototoxicity.

ADVERSE REACTIONS

Common reactions are in italics; life-threatening reactions are in bold italics.
Blood: ***agranulocytosis,*** leukopenia, thrombocytopenia.
CV: *volume depletion and dehydration,* orthostatic hypotension.
EENT: transient deafness with too rapid I.V. injection.
GI: abdominal discomfort and pain, diarrhea (with oral solution).
Metabolic: *hypokalemia; hypochloremic alkalosis; asymptomatic hyperuricemia, fluid and electrolyte imbalances including dilutional hyponatremia, hypocalcemia, hypomagnesemia;* hyperglycemia and impairment of glucose tolerance.
Skin: dermatitis.

INTERACTIONS

Aminoglycoside antibiotics: potentiated ototoxicity. Use together cautiously.
Chloral hydrate: sweating, flushing with I.V. furosemide.
Clofibrate: enhanced furosemide effects. Use cautiously.
Indomethacin: inhibited diuretic response. Use cautiously.

EFFECTS ON DIAGNOSTIC TESTS

Electrolytes: altered results.
Liver and renal function tests: altered results.

NURSING CONSIDERATIONS

Besides those related universally to drug therapy (see "How to use this book"), consider the following specific recommendations:
Assessment
• Obtain a baseline assessment of urine output, vital signs, serum electrolytes, breath sounds, peripheral

edema, and weight before initiating therapy.
• Be alert for adverse reactions and drug interactions throughout therapy.
• Evaluate the patient's and family's knowledge about furosemide therapy.

Nursing Diagnoses

• Fluid volume excess related to the patient's underlying condition as evidenced by edema.
• Altered urinary elimination related to diuretic therapy (frequency, urgency).
• Knowledge deficit related to furosemide therapy.

Planning and Implementation

Preparation and Administration

• Check injectable preparation for discoloration (yellow); discard if present.
• Avoid parenteral route of administration in infants and children if possible.
• ***I.V. use:*** Check patency of I.V. line and site before administration of I.V. furosemide. When giving by direct I.V., to avoid transient hearing impairment administer over 1 to 2 minutes directly into a vein or through tubing of a free-flowing compatible solution. When giving as intermittent infusion, infuse diluted drug at appropriate rate, but not to exceed 4 mg/minute. Continuous infusion of drug not recommended.
• ***P.O. use:*** Store tablets in light-resistant container to avoid discoloration. Store oral furosemide solution in refrigerator to ensure drug stability.
• Give P.O. or I.M. preparations early in the morning to avoid nocturia. Give second doses in early afternoon.

Monitoring

• Monitor effectiveness by regularly checking urine output, weight, peripheral edema, and breath sounds.
• Monitor ECG for arrhythmias.
• Monitor serum electrolytes and BUN levels.
• Monitor vital signs: hypotension, dyspnea, tachycardia, and fever may indicate dehydration.
• In the diabetic patient, monitor serum glucose.
• In the patient with gout, monitor serum uric acid.
• Monitor the patient receiving digitalis for signs of digitalis toxicity.
• Monitor for signs of hypokalemia (muscle weakness and cramping).
• Monitor skin turgor and mucous membranes for signs of fluid volume depletion.

Supportive Care

• Hold drug and notify the doctor if hypersensitivity or adverse reactions occur.
• Keep accurate record of intake and output.
• Weigh the patient daily.
• Elevate the patient's legs to aid relief of peripheral edema.
• Encourage low-sodium/high-potassium diet.
• Provide frequent skin and mouth care to relieve dryness due to diuretic therapy.
• Answer the patient's call bells promptly; make sure patient's bathroom or bedpan are easily accessible.
• Use safety precautions to avoid risk of falls due to hypotension.
• Use written communication for the patient who experiences drug-related deafness.

Patient Teaching

• Teach the patient and family to identify and report signs of hypersensitivity or furosemide toxicity (ringing ears, severe abdominal pain, sore throat, or fever).
• Teach the diabetic patient receiving furosemide to monitor blood glucose.
• Teach the patient receiving furosemide and digitalis to be aware of signs of digitalis toxicity and to store these drugs separately to avoid risk of dosage error.
• Teach the patient to monitor fluid volume by daily weight and intake and output.

• Encourage the patient to avoid foods high in sodium and to choose foods high in potassium.
• Advise the patient to change positions slowly, especially when rising to a standing position, to avoid dizziness due to orthostatic hypotension and to limit alcohol intake and strenuous exercise in warm weather.
• Advise the patient to take drug early in the day to avoid interruption of sleep by nocturia.

Evaluation

In the patient receiving furosemide, appropriate evaluation statements may include:
• Patient is free of edema.
• Patient demonstrates adjustment of life-style to deal with altered patterns of urinary elimination.
• Patient and family state an understanding of furosemide therapy.

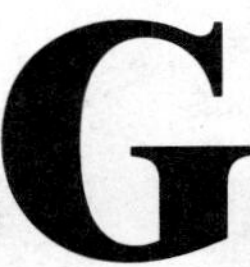

gallamine triethiodide

(gal´ a meen)
Flaxedil

• *Classification:* skeletal muscle relaxant (nondepolarizing neuromuscular blocking agent)
• *Pregnancy Risk Category:* C

HOW SUPPLIED

Injection: 20 mg/ml

ACTION

Mechanism: Prevents acetylcholine from binding to the receptors on the muscle end plate, thus blocking depolarization. Nondepolarizing agent.
Distribution: After I.V. administration, distributed in the extracellular fluid and rapidly reaches its site of action. Termination of pharmacologic activity depends on drug redistribution. It is substantially bound to serum albumin; the extent of binding is pH dependent. Drug crosses the placenta.
Metabolism: Not metabolized.
Excretion: Unchanged in urine.
Onset, peak, duration: After I.V. administration, muscle relaxation occurs rapidly and reaches a maximum in about 3 minutes. The duration is related to total dosage, anesthetic used, and depth of anesthesia. After usual doses, the duration of action averages 15 to 20 minutes.

INDICATIONS & DOSAGE

Adjunct to anesthesia to induce skeletal muscle relaxation; facilitate intubation, reduction of fractures and dislocations; lessen muscle contractions in pharmacologically or electrically induced seizures; assist with mechanical ventilation–
Dosage depends on anesthetic used, individual needs, and response. Dosages are representative and must be adjusted.
Adults and children over 1 month: initially, 1 mg/kg I.V. to maximum of 100 mg, regardless of patient's weight; then 0.5 mg to 1 mg/kg q 30 to 40 minutes.
Children under 1 month but over 5 kg (11 lb): initially, 0.25 to 0.75 mg/kg I.V., then may give additional doses of 0.1 to 0.5 mg/kg q 30 to 40 minutes.

CONTRAINDICATIONS & PRECAUTIONS

Contraindicated in patients with myasthenia gravis because of potential for prolonged neuromuscular blockade; impaired renal function because of decreased elimination of drug and potential for accumulation and toxicity; shock or hypersensitivity to gallamine or iodides, in whom tachycardia may be hazardous. Use cautiously in elderly or debilitated patients; in those with cardiac, hepatic, or pulmonary impairment, respiratory depression, myasthenic syndrome of lung cancer, dehydration, thyroid disorders, collagen diseases, porphyria, familial periodic paralysis, or electrolyte disturbances; and in those undergoing cesarean section. Commercially available formulations containing sulfites should be used cautiously in patients with sensitivity to sulfites.

Neonates are particularly sensitive to the effects of the drug and respond to usual doses with prolonged neuromuscular blockade.

The drug may increase blood pressure. Hyperthermia may increase the duration and intensity of drug's effects; hypothermia may decrease its duration and intensity.

Use cautiously at reduced dose in pregnant women receiving magnesium sulfate.

ADVERSE REACTIONS

Common reactions are in italics; life-threatening reactions are in bold italics.

CV: tachycardia.

Other: ***respiratory paralysis, dose-related prolonged apnea,*** residual muscle weakness, increased oropharyngeal secretions, allergic or idiosyncratic hypersensitivity reactions.

INTERACTIONS

Aminoglycoside antibiotics (amikacin, gentamicin, kanamycin, neomycin, streptomycin); polymyxin antibiotics (polymyxin B sulfate, colistin); clindamycin; quinidine; general anesthetics (such as halothane, enflurane, isoflurane): potentiated neuromuscular blockade, leading to increased skeletal muscle relaxation and possible respiratory paralysis. Use cautiously during surgical and postoperative periods.

Narcotic analgesics, I.V. diazepam: potentiated neuromuscular blockade, leading to increased skeletal muscle relaxation and possible respiratory paralysis. Use with extreme caution, and reduce dose of gallamine.

EFFECTS ON DIAGNOSTIC TESTS

None reported.

NURSING CONSIDERATIONS

Besides those related universally to drug therapy (see "How to use this book"), consider the following specific recommendations:

Assessment

- Obtain a baseline assessment of skeletal muscle function and respiratory pattern before drug therapy.
- Be alert for adverse reactions and drug interactions throughout therapy.
- Evaluate the patient's and family's knowledge about gallamine triethiodide therapy.

Nursing Diagnoses

- Ineffective breathing pattern related to the patient's underlying condition.
- Impaired verbal communication related to drug-induced paralysis.
- Knowledge deficit related to gallamine triethiodide therapy.

Planning and Implementation

Preparation and Administration

- Gallamine should be administered only by personnel experienced in airway management.
- Have emergency respiratory support equipment (endotracheal equipment, ventilator, oxygen, atropine, edrophonium, epinephrine, and neostigmine) on hand before administration.
- Protect drug from light or excessive heat; use only fresh solution.
- Do not mix with meperidine hydrochloride or barbiturate solutions (precipitate will form).
- Usually administered with a cholinergic blocker (such as atropine or glycopyrrolate).
- If succinylcholine is used, allow effects to subside before giving pancuronium.
- ***I.V. use:*** Continuous and intermittent infusion are not recommended.
- Determine if the patient has iodide allergy before administration.
- Know that this drug may be preferred in patients who have bradycardia.

Monitoring

- Monitor effectiveness by regularly checking relaxation state of the patient's skeletal muscles; close observation of the patient is mandatory.
- Closely monitor baseline electrolyte determinations (electrolyte imbalance can potentiate neuromuscular effects) and vital signs (watch respiration and heart rate).
- Measure intake and output (renal

dysfunction may prolong duration of action, since the drug is unchanged before excretion).
• Monitor respirations and respiratory status closely until patient recovers fully from neuromuscular blockade, as evidenced by tests of muscle strength (hand grip, head lift, and ability to cough).
• Monitor for drug interactions and adverse reactions by frequently checking the patient's vital signs every 15 minutes for tachycardia.

Supportive Care

• Maintain adequate ventilation through respiratory support equipment throughout drug therapy and provide pulmonary care as indicated.
• Once spontaneous recovery starts, pancuronium-induced neuromuscular blockade may be reversed with an anticholinesterase agent (such as neostigmine or edrophonium).
• Provide emotional support for the intubated patient who is awake.
• Administer pain medication on regular basis (as condition dictates) because the patient will be unable to communicate that pain is present.
• Anticipate the patient's needs and try to meet them. Explain everything thoroughly before performing any procedure. Use nonverbal communication especially eye contact.
• Protect the patient from injury when moving him in bed.
• Provide meticulous eye care since blink reflex will be absent.

Patient Teaching

• Reassure the patient that necessary pain management will be provided regularly.
• Inform the patient that drug-induced paralysis will inhibit his ability to communicate but that he will receive continuous monitoring and care.
• Reassure the patient that as soon as the need for neuromuscular blockade is no longer necessary, the drug-induced paralysis will be reversed.

Evaluation

In patients receiving gallamine triethiodide, appropriate evaluation statements may include:
• Patient maintains adequate ventilation.
• Patient's basic needs are anticipated and met.
• Patient and family state an understanding of gallamine triethiodide therapy.

gallium nitrate

(gal´ ee um)
Ganite

• *Classification:* skeletal muscle relaxant (nondepolarizing neuromuscular blocking agent)
• *Pregnancy Risk Category:* C

HOW SUPPLIED

Injection: 25 mg/ml

ACTION

Mechanism: Precise mechanism unknown; the drug has no cytotoxic effects in animals. It appears to reduce hypercalcemia by inhibiting the resorption of bone and reducing bone turnover in patients with increased bone turnover.
Metabolism: Not metabolized.
Excretion: By the kidneys.
Onset, peak, duration: In most patients, apparent steady-state is achieved in 24 to 48 hours.

INDICATIONS & DOSAGE

Treatment of symptomatic, unresponsive hypercalcemia caused by cancer—
Adults: 200 mg/m² I.V. daily for 5 consecutive days or until serum calcium is normal. Administer as a constant infusion over 24 hours. Lower doses (100 mg/m²) may be given to patients with mild hypercalcemia.

CONTRAINDICATIONS & PRECAUTIONS

Contraindicated in patients hypersensitive to the drug and in those with severe renal impairment.

ADVERSE REACTIONS

Common reactions are in italics; life-threatening reactions are in bold italics.
Blood: anemia, leukopenia.
CNS: lethargy, confusion.
CV: tachycardia, lower extremity edema, decreased mean systolic and diastolic blood pressures.
GI: nausea and vomiting, diarrhea, constipation.
GU: ***acute renal failure,*** *increased BUN and creatinine levels.*
Respiratory: dyspnea, crackles and rhonchi, pulmonary infiltrates, pleural effusion.
Metabolic: *hypophosphatemia, hypocalcemia, decreased serum bicarbonate.*
Other: visual or hearing impairment, acute optic neuritis.

INTERACTIONS

Nephrotoxic drugs, such as aminoglycosides or amphotericin B: increased risk of nephrotoxicity. Avoid concomitant use.

EFFECTS ON DIAGNOSTIC TESTS

Serum calcium: will be decreased.
Serum creatinine, BUN: may be elevated.

NURSING CONSIDERATIONS

Besides those related universally to drug therapy (see "How to use this book"), consider the following specific recommendations:

Assessment

- Obtain a baseline assessment of serum calcium levels before therapy.
- Be alert for adverse reactions and drug interactions throughout therapy.
- Evaluate the patient's and family's knowledge about gallium nitrate therapy.

Nursing Diagnoses

- Pain related to the underlying disease.
- Diarrhea related to adverse effects of the drug.
- Knowledge deficit related to gallium nitrate.

Planning and Implementation

Preparation and Administration

- Keep in mind that this drug is administered only as an I.V. infusion. Direct injection is not recommended.
- Be sure to hydrate the patient either with oral fluids or I.V. saline before using the drug and during the infusion. Avoid over hydration, especially in patients with decreased overhydration. It is important to establish a urine flow rate (2 liters per day) before treatment. Diuretic therapy is not recommended before the correction of hypovolemia.
- After reconstitution the drug is stable for at least 48 hours at 59° to 86° F, or for 7 days if refrigerated.
- ***I.V. use:*** Dilute the daily dose in 1 liter of 0.9% sodium chloride or 5% dextrose in water and infuse over 24 hours. Discard the unused portion as the medication does not contain preservatives. Rapid infusion of doses greater than 200 mg/m^2 may increase risk of nephrotoxicity, or cause nausea and vomiting, and substantially increase the risk of renal insufficiency.

Monitoring

- Monitor effectiveness by evaluating the patient's serum calcium and phosphorous levels twice weekly.
- Assess the patient's intake and output to determine an adequate hydration level.
- Monitor renal function (serum creatinine and BUN) closely.
- Assess the patient for signs of hypocalcemia throughout therapy.
- Assess the patient for pain relating to the underlying condition.
- Evaluate the patient's neurological status to evaluate CNS involvement.

Supportive Care
• Expect to discontinue gallium nitrate if concurrent nephrotoxic drugs are needed. Continue to hydrate the patient for several days following administration of the nephrotoxic drug.
• Expect to discontinue the drug if hypocalcemia occurs or if serum creatinine level rises above 2.5 mg/dl.
• Treat overdose with vigorous hydration, sometimes with diuretics, for 2 to 3 days. Short-term therapy with I.V. calcium may be needed.
• Administer oral phosphorous supplements if transient hypophosphatemia is common.
Patient Teaching
• Advise the patient to report hearing or vision problems.
• Instruct the patient in the need for adequate fluid intake.
• Teach the patient and family to measure intake and output.
Evaluation
In patients receiving gallium nitrate, appropriate evaluation statements may include:
• Patient denies bone pain related to underlying condition.
• Patient reports normal bowel movements.
• Patient and family state an understanding of gallium nitrate therapy.

---

ganciclovir
(gan sye´ kloe vir)
Cytovene

• *Classification:* antiviral (synthetic nucleoside)
• *Pregnancy Risk Category:* C

HOW SUPPLIED
Injection: 500 mg/vial

ACTION
Mechanism: Inhibits viral DNA synthesis of the cytomegalovirus (CMV).
Absorption: Ganciclovir is administered I.V. because less than 7% is absorbed after oral administration.
Distribution: The drug is only 2% to 3% protein-bound. It preferentially concentrates within CMV-infected cells because of the action of cellular kinases that convert it to ganciclovir triphosphate.
Metabolism: Most (79%) of the drug is excreted unchanged.
Excretion: Primarily through the kidneys by glomerular filtration and some renal tubular secretion. Half-life: About 3 hours in patients with normal renal function; as long as 30 hours in severe renal failure.
Onset, peak, duration: Peak serum levels occur after the completion of an I.V. infusion. Limited studies show that most patients respond to treatment within 7 to 8 days of therapy.

INDICATIONS & DOSAGE
CMV retinitis treatment of immunocompromised individuals, including patients with acquired immunodeficiency syndrome (AIDS)–
Adults: induction treatment: initially, 5 mg/kg I.V. q 12 hours for 14 to 21 days (normal renal function); maintenance treatment: 5 mg/kg I.V. once daily, for 7 days each week, or 6 mg/kg once daily, for 5 days each week.

CONTRAINDICATIONS & PRECAUTIONS
Contraindicated in patients who are hypersensitive to ganciclovir or acyclovir.

About 40% of the patients who receive the drug experience some form of hematologic toxicity, including granulocytopenia or thrombocytopenia. Granulocytopenia usually occurs during the first week, but may occur anytime during therapy. Patients with drug-induced immunosuppression seem more likely to develop thrombocytopenia than patients with AIDS. Cell counts usually recover within 3 to 7 days after discontinuing the drug.

In animal studies, the drug has shown carcinogenic and mutagenic activity and has also caused aspermatogenesis. It should be used only to treat immunocompromised patients with CMV retinitis.

ADVERSE REACTIONS

Common reactions are in italics; life-threatening reactions are in bold italics.

Blood: *granulocytopenia, thrombocytopenia.*
CNS: altered dreams, confusion, ataxia, dizziness, headache.
CV: arrhythmias, hypotension, hypertension.
GI: nausea, vomiting, diarrhea, anorexia.
GU: hematuria.
Local: injection site inflammation, pain, phlebitis.
Other: retinal detachment in CMV retinitis patients.

INTERACTIONS

Cytotoxic agents: additive toxic effects, especially hematologic effects and stomatitis.
Imipenem/cilastatin: reports of seizure activity with concomitant use.
Probenecid: increased ganciclovir blood levels.
Zidovudine: increased incidence of granulocytopenia with concurrent use.

EFFECTS ON DIAGNOSTIC TESTS

None reported.

NURSING CONSIDERATIONS

Besides those related universally to drug therapy (see "How to use this book"), consider the following specific recommendations:

Assessment

- Obtain a baseline assessment of infection before therapy.
- Be alert for adverse reactions and drug interactions throughout therapy.
- Evaluate the patient's and family's knowledge about ganciclovir therapy.

Nursing Diagnoses

- High risk for injury related to ineffectiveness of ganciclovir to eradicate the infection.
- Altered protection related to ganciclovir induced blood disorders.
- Knowledge deficit related to ganciclovir.

Planning and Implementation

Preparation and Administration

- Be aware that patient must be adequately hydrated throughout drug administration, and that dosage should be reduced in patients with renal dysfunction.
- ***I.V. use:*** Reconstitute by adding 10 ml of sterile water without perservatives to one 500 mg vial to produce a solution of 50 mg/ml. Shake vial until solution is clear to ensure complete dissolution of particles. Infuse over at least 1 hour, using infusion pump; faster infusions increase toxicity. Do not administer as an I.V. bolus. Do not refrigerate drug.

Monitoring

- Monitor effectiveness by regularly assessing for improvement in the infection.
- Monitor neutrophil and platelet counts every 2 days during twice-daily ganciclovir dosing and at least weekly thereafter.
- Monitor hydration status if adverse GI reactions occur with oral administration of the drug.

Supportive Care

- Institute infection control or bleeding precautions if hematologic studies become abnormal.
- Obtain an order for an antiemetic or antidiarrheal agent as needed.
- Keep patient adequately hydrated throughout ganciclovir therapy.
- Institute safety precautions if adverse CNS reactions occur.

Patient Teaching
• Encourage patient to drink adequate amounts of fluid throughout ganciclovir therapy.
• Advise patient to tell the nurse promptly of pain or discomfort at the site of I.V. injection.

Evaluation
In patients receiving ganciclovir, appropriate evaluation statements may include:
• Patient's infection remains controlled.
• Patient maintains adequate hydration throughout ganciclovir therapy.
• Patient and family state an understanding of ganciclovir therapy.

gemfibrozil
(jem fi´ broe zil)
Lopid

• *Classification:* antilipemic (fibric acid derivative)
• *Pregnancy Risk Category:* B

HOW SUPPLIED
Tablets: 600 mg
Capsules: 300 mg

ACTION
Mechanism: Inhibits peripheral lipolysis and also reduces triglyceride synthesis in the liver.
Absorption: Well absorbed from the GI tract.
Distribution: 95% protein-bound.
Metabolism: Hepatic.
Excretion: Mainly in urine; some in feces. Half-life: After a single dose, half-life is 1½ hours; after multiple doses, half-life decreases to about 1¼ hours.
Onset, peak, duration: Peak plasma concentrations occur 1 to 2 hours after an oral dose. Plasma levels of very low-density lipoprotein (VLDL) decrease in 2 to 5 days; peak clinical effect occurs in 4 weeks. Further decreases in plasma VLDL levels occur over several months.

INDICATIONS & DOSAGE
Treatment of type IV hyperlipidemia (hypertriglyceridemia) and severe hypercholesterolemia unresponsive to diet and other drugs–
Adults: 1,200 mg P.O. administered in two divided doses. Usual dosage range is 900 to 1,500 mg daily. If no beneficial effect is seen after 3 months of therapy, drug should be discontinued.

CONTRAINDICATIONS & PRECAUTIONS
Contraindicated in patients with hypersensitivity to the drug; gallbladder disease because it may increase cholesterol excretion through the bile and cause cholelithiasis; and hepatic dysfunction (including primary biliary cirrhosis) or severe renal dysfunction. Drug may cause paradoxic increase in serum cholesterol levels in patients with primary biliary cirrhosis. Hepatic or severe renal disease may increase drug's adverse reactions.

ADVERSE REACTIONS
Common reactions are in italics; life-threatening reactions are in bold italics.
Blood: anemia, leukopenia.
CNS: blurred vision, headache, dizziness.
GI: *abdominal and epigastric pain, diarrhea, nausea,* vomiting, flatulence.
Hepatic: bile duct obstruction, elevated enzymes.
Skin: rash, dermatitis, pruritus.
Other: painful extremities.

INTERACTIONS
Oral anticoagulants: gemfibrozil may enhance the clinical effects of oral anticoagulants. Monitor patient closely.

EFFECTS ON DIAGNOSTIC TESTS

CBC: decreased leukocyte counts.
Creatine phosphokinase, ALT (SGOT), AST (SGPT), alkaline phosphatase, and LDH: elevated serum levels.
Serum potassium, hematocrit, hemoglobin: decreased.

NURSING CONSIDERATIONS

Besides those related universally to drug therapy (see "How to use this book"), consider the following specific recommendations:

Assessment
- Obtain a baseline assessment of the patient's underlying condition before drug therapy.
- Be alert for adverse reactions and drug interactions throughout therapy.
- Evaluate the patient's and family's knowledge about gemfibrozil therapy.

Nursing Diagnoses
- High risk for injury related to elevated blood lipids and cholesterol levels.
- Sensory/perceptual alteration (visual) related to adverse drug reactions.
- Knowledge deficit related to gemfibrozil therapy.

Planning and Implementation
Preparation and Administration
- Drug should be given 30 minutes before breakfast and dinner.
- Drug should not be used indiscriminately. May pose risk of gallstones, heart disease, and cancer.
- If significant lipid lowering is not achieved within 3 months, drug should be discontinued.
- Gemfibrozil is pharmacologically related to clofibrate.

Monitoring
- Monitor for adverse reactions or drug interactions to gemfibrozil therapy by monitoring the patient's vital signs.
- Monitor hydration status if diarrhea and vomiting occurs.
- Monitor serum cholesterol and triglycerides regularly to evaluate the effectiveness of therapy.
- Monitor CBC and liver function tests periodically during the first 12 months of therapy.
- Observe patient's bowel movements for evidence of steatorrhea or other signs of bile-duct obstruction.
- Monitor the patient's intake and output.

Supportive Care
- Assist the patient who experiences dizziness or blurred vision with getting in and out of bed.
- Provide fluids to the patient who has vomiting and diarrhea.
- Because of possible dizziness and blurred vision, patient should avoid driving or other hazardous activities until CNS effects of the drug are known.

Patient Teaching
- Teach the patient about proper dietary management (restricting total fat and cholesterol intake), weight control, and exercise. Explain their importance in controlling elevated serum lipids.
- Tell the patient to avoid hazardous activities until CNS effects of the drug are known.

Evaluation
In patients receiving gemfibrozil, appropriate evaluation statements may include:
- Patient's blood triglyceride and cholesterol levels are normal.
- Patient does not develop dizziness and blurred vision.
- Patient and family state an understanding of gemfibrozil therapy.

gentamicin (ophthalmic)

(jen ta mye´ sin)
Gentacidin

gentamicin sulfate
Garamycin Ophthalmic, Genoptic

• *Classification:* antibiotic (aminoglycoside)
• *Pregnancy Risk Category:* C

HOW SUPPLIED
gentamicin
Ophthalmic ointment: 3 mg/g
gentamicin sulfate
Ophthalmic ointment: 3 mg/g
Ophthalmic solution: 3 mg/ml

ACTION
Mechanism: An aminoglycoside antibiotic that inhibits protein synthesis by irreversibly binding to the 30S ribosome in susceptible bacteria. Usually bactericidal.
Absorption: After topical ophthalmic administration of ointment or solution, animal studies show that the drug is absorbed into the aqueous humor. Absorption is greater if the cornea is abraded.

INDICATIONS & DOSAGE
External ocular infections (conjunctivitis, keratoconjunctivitis, corneal ulcers, blepharitis, blepharoconjunctivitis, meibomianitis, and dacryocystitis) caused by susceptible organisms, especially Pseudomonas aeruginosa, Proteus, Klebsiella pneumoniae, Escherichia coli, *and other gram-negative organisms–*
Adults and children: instill 1 to 2 drops in eye q 4 hours. In severe infections, may use up to 2 drops q 1 hour. Apply ointment to lower conjunctival sac b.i.d. or t.i.d.

CONTRAINDICATIONS & PRECAUTIONS
Contraindicated in patients with hypersensitivity to gentamicin or any other aminoglycoside.

ADVERSE REACTIONS
Common reactions are in italics; life-threatening reactions are in bold italics.
Note: systemic absorption from excessive use may cause systemic toxicities.
Eye: *burning, stinging or blurred vision* (with ointment), *transient irritation* (from solution).
Other: hypersensitivity, overgrowth of nonsusceptible organisms with long-term use.

INTERACTIONS
None significant.

EFFECTS ON DIAGNOSTIC TESTS
None reported.

NURSING CONSIDERATIONS
Besides those related universally to drug therapy (see "How to use this book"), consider the following specific recommendations:
Assessment
• Obtain a baseline assessment of allergies before therapy.
• Be alert for adverse reactions and drug interactions throughout therapy.
• Evaluate the patient's and family's knowledge about gentamicin therapy.
Nursing Diagnoses
• Altered protection related to ocular infection.
• High risk for infection related to gentamicin-induced overgrowth of nonsusceptible organisms.
• Knowledge deficit related to gentamicin therapy.
Planning and Implementation
Preparation and Administration
• Obtain culture before giving drug.
• Wash hands before and after administration.
• Cleanse eye area of excessive exudate before administration.
• Do not inject solution into conjunctiva or anterior chamber of the eye.

Monitoring
- Monitor effectiveness by checking for the presence of microorganisms by culturing the eye.
- Monitor serum gentamicin carefully if ophthalmic gentamicin is given concomitantly with systemic gentamicin.
- Observe amount, color, and consistency of exudate.
- Check patient's vision.

Supportive Care
- Apply warm moist compresses to aid removal of dried exudate.
- Do not give in aminoglycoside hypersensitivity. Use with caution in impaired renal function.

Patient Teaching
- Teach the patient how to instill. Advise him to wash hands before and after administration and not to touch the tip of the applicator to eye or surrounding tissue.
- Advise the patient to apply light finger pressure to lacrimal sac for 1 minute after drops are administered. Instruct him to avoid scratching or rubbing eyes.
- Warn the patient to watch for signs of hypersensitivity (itching lids, swelling, constant burning). Stop the drug and notify the doctor if they occur.
- Stress importance of following recommended therapy. *Pseudomonas* infections can cause complete vision loss within 24 hours if not controlled.
- Warn the patient not to share washcloths and towels with family members during infection.
- Instruct the patient not to share eye medication with family members. A family member who develops the same symptoms, should contact the doctor.

Evaluation

In patients receiving gentamicin, appropriate evaluation statements may include:
- Patient remains free from signs and symptoms of infection.
- Patient demonstrates no signs of infection by nonsusceptible organisms.
- Patient and family state an understanding of gentamicin therapy.

gentamicin sulfate (systemic)

(jen ta mye´ sin)

Cidomycin†‡, Garamycin, Gentafair, Jenamicin

- *Classification:* antibiotic (aminoglycoside)
- *Pregnancy Risk Category:* C

HOW SUPPLIED

Injection: 40 mg/ml (adult), 10 mg/ml (pediatric), 2 mg/ml (intrathecal)
Injection, for I.V. infusion: 0.6 mg/ml, 0.8 mg/ml, 0.9 mg/ml, 1 mg/ml, 1.2 mg/ml, 1.4 mg/ml, 1.6 mg/ml, 2 mg/ml.

ACTION

Mechanism: Inhibits protein synthesis by binding directly to the 30S ribosomal subunit in susceptible bacteria. Generally bactericidal.
Absorption: Poorly absorbed after oral administration and is given parenterally. Peak plasma levels are similar after I.M. or I.V. administration.
Distribution: Widely distributed after parenteral administration; intraocular penetration is poor; CSF penetration is low even in patients with inflamed meninges. Intraventricular administration produces high concentration throughout the CNS. Protein binding is minimal. Gentamicin crosses the placenta.
Metabolism: Not metabolized.
Excretion: Primarily excreted in urine by glomerular filtration; small amounts may be excreted in bile and breast milk. Half-life: 2 to 3 hours in adults; 24 to 60 hours in severe renal disease.
Onset, peak, duration: Following I.M. administration, peak serum con-

*Liquid form contains alcohol. **May contain tartrazine.

centrations occur at 30 to 90 minutes; peak levels occur immediately after completion of an I.V. infusion.

INDICATIONS & DOSAGE

Serious infections caused by sensitive Pseudomonas aeruginosa, Escherichia coli, Proteus, Klebsiella, Serratia, Enterobacter, Citrobacter, Staphylococcus–

Adults with normal renal function: 3 mg/kg daily in divided doses q 8 hours I.M. or I.V. infusion (in 50 to 200 ml of normal saline solution or dextrose 5% in water infused over 30 minutes to 2 hours). May be given by direct I.V. push if necessary. For life-threatening infections, patient may receive up to 5 mg/kg daily in 3 to 4 divided doses.

Children with normal renal function: 2 to 2.5 mg/kg I.M. or I.V. infusion q 8 hours.

Infants and neonates over 1 week with normal renal function: 2.5 mg/kg q 8 hours I.M. or I.V. infusion.

Neonates under 1 week: 2.5 mg/kg I.V. q 12 hours. For I.V. infusion, dilute in normal saline solution or dextrose 5% in water and infuse over 30 minutes to 2 hours.

Meningitis–

Adults: systemic therapy as above; may also use 4 to 8 mg intrathecally daily.

Children: systemic therapy as above; may also use 1 to 2 mg intrathecally daily.

Endocarditis prophylaxis for GI or GU procedure or surgery–

Adults: 1.5 mg/kg I.M. or I.V. 30 to 60 minutes before procedure or surgery and q 8 hours after, for 2 doses. Given with aqueous penicillin G or ampicillin.

Children: 2.5 mg/kg I.M. or I.V. 30 to 60 minutes before procedure or surgery and q 8 hours after, for 2 doses. Given with aqueous penicillin G or ampicillin.

Patients with impaired renal function: initial dose is same as for those with normal renal function. Subsequent doses and frequency determined by renal function studies and serum concentrations of gentamicin.

Posthemodialysis to maintain therapeutic blood levels–

Adults: 1 to 1.7 mg/kg I.M. or I.V. infusion after each dialysis.

Children: 2 mg/kg I.M. or I.V. infusion after each dialysis.

CONTRAINDICATIONS & PRECAUTIONS

Contraindicated in patients with hypersensitivity to gentamicin or any aminoglycoside.

Use cautiously in patients with decreased renal function because of potential for decreased drug clearance; tinnitus, vertigo, or high-frequency hearing loss, who are susceptible to ototoxicity; dehydration because of increased risk of ototoxicity and nephrotoxicity; myasthenia gravis, parkinsonism, or hypocalcemia because it may aggravate muscle weakness; in neonates and other infants; and in elderly patients because of decreased renal clearance.

ADVERSE REACTIONS

Common reactions are in italics; life-threatening reactions are in bold italics.

CNS: headache, lethargy, ***neuromuscular blockade.***

EENT: *ototoxicity (tinnitus, vertigo, hearing loss).*

GU: *nephrotoxicity (cells or casts in the urine; oliguria; proteinuria; decreased creatinine clearance; increased BUN, nonprotein nitrogen, and serum creatinine levels).*

Other: ***hypersensitivity, hepatic necrosis.***

INTERACTIONS

Cephalothin: increases nephrotoxicity. Use together cautiously.

Dimenhydrinate: may mask symptoms of ototoxicity. Use with caution.

General anesthetics, neuromuscular blocking agents: may potentiate neuromuscular blockade.
I.V. loop diuretics (e.g. furosemide): increase ototoxicity. Use cautiously.
Other aminoglycosides, methoxyflurane: increase ototoxicity and nephrotoxicity. Use together cautiously.
Parenteral penicillins (e.g. carbenicillin and ticarcillin): gentamicin inactivation in vitro. Don't combine in I.V.

EFFECTS ON DIAGNOSTIC TESTS

BUN, nonprotein nitrogen, or serum creatinine: elevated levels and increased urinary excretion of casts.

NURSING CONSIDERATIONS

Besides those related universally to drug therapy (see "How to use this book"), consider the following specific recommendations:

Assessment

- Obtain a baseline assessment of patient's infection before gentamicin therapy.
- Be alert for adverse reactions and drug interactions throughout therapy.
- Evaluate the patient's and family's knowledge about gentamicin therapy.

Nursing Diagnoses

- High risk for injury related to dosage regimen inadequate to alleviate infection.
- Sensory/perceptual alterations (auditory) related to ototoxicity induced by gentamicin.
- Knowledge deficit related to gentamicin.

Planning and Implementation

Preparation and Administration

- Obtain specimen for culture and sensitivity tests before first dose. Therapy may begin pending test results.
- Ensure that the patient is well hydrated before therapy (unless contraindicated) to decrease the risk of nephrotoxicity.
- Weigh the patient and obtain baseline renal function studies before therapy begins.
- Always consult manufacturer's directions for reconstitution, dilution, and storage. Check expiration dates. Solutions should always be clear, colorless to pale yellow (darkening usually indicates deterioration), and free of particles; do not give solutions containing precipitates or other particles.
- Administer gentamicin and an extended-spectrum penicillin or cephalosporin at least 2 hours apart to prevent a decrease in the drug level and half-life in a patient with normal renal function.
- Expect to reduce the dosage as prescribed for an elderly patient, or one with renal impairment, or one who is receiving hemodialysis. Don't administer the drug before dialysis treatment.
- After loading dose, all doses should be based on renal studies and serum levels of the drug.
- ***I.M. use:*** Administer I.M. dose deep into large muscle mass (gluteal or midlateral thigh); rotate injection sites to minimize tissue injury; do not inject more than 2 g of drug per injection site. Apply ice to injection site for pain.
- ***I.V. use:*** Refrigerate prepared I.V. aminoglycoside solution until use; infuse I.V. drug continuously or intermittently over 30 to 60 minutes for adults; 1 to 2 hours for infants. Too rapid I.V. administration may cause neuromuscular blockade. At end of infusion, flush line with 0.9% sodium chloride solution in water or dextrose 5% solution. Adequate dilution of I.V. solution and rotation of injection site every 48 hours help minimize local irritation.

  Do not administer through heparinized I.V. line. If administering intermittent dose through heparin lock, flush with 0.9% sodium chloride solution before and after infusing gentamicin to separate gentamicin and the heparin used to keep the lock patent.

Monitoring

• Monitor effectiveness by regularly assessing for improvement in infection process.
• Monitor serum gentamicin level. Draw blood for peak gentamicin level 1 hour after I.M. injection and 30 minutes to 1 hour after infusion ends; for trough levels, draw levels, draw blood just before the next dose. Do not collect blood in a heparinized tube because heparin is incompatible with aminoglycosides. Acceptable peak levels are 4 to 12 mcg/dl. Peak blood levels above 12 mcg/dl and trough levels above 2 mcg/dl may be associated with higher incidence of toxicity.
• Monitor renal function, including intake and output, serum creatinine and BUN levels, weight, urinalysis and specific gravity.
• Monitor the patient's hearing and for signs of vestibular toxicity (dizziness, vertigo, nystagmus).

Supportive Care

• Notify the doctor of increased serum creatinine or BUN levels, decreased intake and output, increased weight gain, increased casts in urine, and decreased specific gravity.
• Encourage the patient to maintain fluid intake of at least 2,000 ml/day (unless contraindicated).
• If you suspect ototoxicity, notify the doctor and prepare the patient for audiometric testing. Expect to discontinue gentamicin and substitute another antibiotic. If the patient has signs of vestibular toxicity (dizziness), impose safety precautions, such as supervising ambulation.
• Notify the doctor if patient's serum gentamicin peak or trough levels fall outside the recommended range.
• Usual duration of therapy is 7 to 10 days. If no response in 3 to 5 days, drug may be discontinued and new specimens obtained for culture and sensitivity.
• After drawing a blood specimen for determining serum gentamicin level, immediately place it on ice for transport to the laboratory to prevent false changes of the gentamicin level.

Patient Teaching

• Instruct the patient to notify the doctor immediately if hearing changes occur.
• Instruct the patient to notify the doctor if the infection does not improve or if it worsens.
• Stress the importance of blood tests to monitor gentamicin level and renal function, to determine the effectiveness of therapy, or detect any increased risk of adverse reactions.
• Instruct female patients to notify the doctor of suspected or confirmed pregnancy during therapy.
• Emphasize the need to drink 2,000 ml of fluid each day, not including coffee, tea, or other caffeinated beverages.

Evaluation

In patients receiving gentamicin, appropriate evaluation statements may include:

• Patient is free of infection.
• Patient maintains normal auditory function throughout therapy.
• Patient and family state an understanding of gentamicin therapy.

gentamicin sulfate (topical)

(jen ta mye´ sin)
Garamycin

• *Classification:* antibiotic (aminoglycoside)
• *Pregnancy Risk Category:* C

HOW SUPPLIED

Cream: 0.1%
Ointment: 0.1%

ACTION

Mechanism: Binds to the 30S ribosomal subunit of susceptible bacteria and disrupts protein synthesis. Usually bactericidal.
Absorption: Not usually absorbed, unless applied to denuded skin or areas that have lost their keratin layer, such as ulcers, wounds, or burns.
Distribution: Absorbed drug is widely distributed; intraocular penetration is poor; CSF penetration is low even in patients with inflamed meninges. Protein binding is minimal. Gentamicin crosses the placenta.
Metabolism: Not metabolized.
Excretion: Absorbed drug is primarily excreted in urine by glomerular filtration; small amounts may be excreted in bile and breast milk. Half-life: 2 to 3 hours in adults; 24 to 60 hours in severe renal disease.

INDICATIONS & DOSAGE

Primary and secondary bacterial infections, superficial burns, skin ulcers, infected insect bites and stings, infected lacerations and abrasions, wounds from minor surgery–
Adults and children over 1 year: rub in small amount gently t.i.d. or q.i.d., with or without gauze dressing.

CONTRAINDICATIONS & PRECAUTIONS

Contraindicated in patients with hypersensitivity to gentamicin or any other aminoglycoside.

Use cautiously in patients with decreased renal function because of potential for decreased drug clearance; tinnitus, vertigo, or high-frequency hearing loss, who are susceptible to ototoxicity; dehydration because of increased risk of ototoxicity and nephrotoxicity; myasthenia gravis, parkinsonism, or hypocalcemia because it may aggravate muscle weakness; in neonates and other infants; and in elderly patients because of decreased renal clearance.

ADVERSE REACTIONS

Common reactions are in italics; life-threatening reactions are in bold italics.
Skin: *minor skin irritation;* possible photosensitivity; allergic contact dermatitis.

INTERACTIONS

Patients hypersensitive to neomycin may exhibit cross-sensitivity.

EFFECTS ON DIAGNOSTIC TESTS

None reported for topical use.

NURSING CONSIDERATIONS

Besides those related universally to drug therapy (see "How to use this book"), consider the following specific recommendations:

Assessment
- Obtain a baseline assessment of wound before therapy.
- Be alert for adverse reactions and drug interactions throughout therapy.
- Evaluate the patient's and family's knowledge about gentamicin therapy.

Nursing Diagnoses
- Impaired skin integrity related to patient's underlying condition.
- High risk for impaired skin integrity related to gentamicin-induced dermatitis.
- Knowledge deficit related to gentamicin therapy.

Planning and Implementation

Preparation and Administration
- ***Topical use:*** Clean affected area before applying. Rub a small amount into affected area. Remove crusts before application of gentamicin in impetigo contagiosa.
- Store in cool place.

Monitoring
- Monitor effectiveness by regularly evaluating wounds.
- Monitor patient's progress. If condition worsens, stop using and report to doctor.

• Monitor for adverse reactions or drug interactions by frequently assessing the patient's skin for contact dermatitis.

Supportive Care

• Notify doctor if adverse reactions occur.

• Avoid use on large skin lesions or over a wide area because of possible systemic toxic effects.

• Be aware that gentamicin should be used in selected patients. Widespread use may lead to resistant organisms.

• Prolonged use may result in overgrowth of nonsusceptible organisms.

• Keep in mind that gentamicin may treat bacterial infections that have not responded to other antibacterial agents.

Patient Teaching

• Teach patient how to apply medication.

Evaluation

In patients receiving gentamicin, appropriate evaluation statements may include:

• Patient states wounds have healed.

• Patient did not develop drug-induced dermatitis.

• Patient and family state an understanding of gentamicin therapy.

glipizide

(glip´ i zide)

Glucotrol, Minidiab‡

• *Classification:* antidiabetic (sulfonylurea)

• *Pregnancy Risk Category:* C

HOW SUPPLIED

Tablets: 5 mg, 10 mg

ACTION

Mechanism: A sulfonylurea that lowers blood glucose by stimulating insulin release from the pancreatic beta cells and reducing glucose output by the liver. An extrapancreatic effect increases peripheral sensitivity to insulin.

Absorption: Rapidly and completely absorbed from the GI tract.

Distribution: Probably distributed within the extracellular fluid; approximately 92% to 99% protein-bound.

Metabolism: Almost completely metabolized by the liver to inactive metabolites.

Excretion: Primarily in urine; small amounts in feces. Renal clearance of unchanged glipizide increases with increasing urinary pH. Half-life: 2 to 4 hours.

Onset, peak, duration: Onset of action within 1½ hours, with maximum hypoglycemic effects within 2 to 3 hours; duration of action, 10 to 24 hours.

INDICATIONS & DOSAGE

Adjunct to diet to lower the blood glucose in patients with non-insulin-dependent diabetes mellitus (type II)–

Adults: initially, 5 mg P.O. daily given before breakfast. Elderly patients or those with liver disease may be started on 2.5 mg. Usual maintenance dosage is 10 to 15 mg. Maximum recommended daily dosage is 40 mg.

To replace insulin therapy–

Adults: if insulin dosage is more than 20 units daily, patient may be started at usual dosage in addition to 50% of the insulin. If insulin dosage is less than 20 units, insulin may be discontinued.

CONTRAINDICATIONS & PRECAUTIONS

Contraindicated in patients with hypersensitivity to sulfonylureas or thiazides; in those with nonfunctioning beta cells; in those with impaired adrenal, pituitary, or thyroid function; in patients with burns, acidosis, diabetic coma, severe infection, ketosis, or severe trauma or in those requiring major surgery because such conditions of severe physiologic stress require insulin for adequate control of serum glucose levels.

Use cautiously in patients with hepatic or renal insufficiency because of the important roles of the liver in metabolism and the kidneys in elimination.

ADVERSE REACTIONS

Common reactions are in italics; life-threatening reactions are in bold italics.

CNS: dizziness.
GI: nausea, vomiting, constipation.
Hepatic: *cholestatic jaundice.*
Metabolic: *hypoglycemia.*
Skin: rash, pruritus, facial flushing.

INTERACTIONS

Anabolic steroids, chloramphenicol, clofibrate, guanethidine, MAO inhibitors, oral anticoagulants, phenylbutazone, salicylates, sulfonamides: increased hypoglycemic activity. Monitor blood glucose level.

Beta blockers, clonidine: prolonged hypoglycemic effect and masked symptoms of hypoglycemia. Use together cautiously.

Corticosteroids, glucagon, rifampin, thiazide diuretics: decreased hypoglycemic response. Monitor blood glucose level.

EFFECTS ON DIAGNOSTIC TESTS

Cholesterol, alkaline phosphatase, AST (SGOT), lactic dehydrogenase, and BUN: altered levels.

NURSING CONSIDERATIONS

Besides those related universally to drug therapy (see "How to use this book"), consider the following specific recommendations:

Assessment

- Obtain a baseline assessment of the patient's blood glucose level before initiating therapy.
- Be alert for adverse reactions and drug interactions throughout therapy.
- Evaluate the patient's and family's knowledge about glipizide therapy.

Nursing Diagnoses

- Altered nutrition: More than body requirements related to the patient's inability to produce sufficient insulin to maintain normal blood glucose levels.
- High risk for injury related to glipizide-induced hypoglycemia.
- Knowledge deficit related to glipizide therapy.

Planning and Implementation

Preparation and Administration

- Consider that some patients taking glipizide may be controlled effectively on a once-daily regimen, whereas others show better response with divided dosing.
- ***P.O. use:*** Administer approximately 30 minutes before meals.

Monitoring

- Monitor effectiveness by regularly checking patient's blood glucose levels. Monitor blood glucose levels more frequently if the patient is under stress, having difficulty controlling blood glucose levels, or is newly diagnosed.
- Monitor for signs and symptoms of both hyperglycemia and hypoglycemia; note time and circumstances of each reaction.
- Be aware that glipizide is a second-generation sulfonylurea that appears to cause fewer adverse reactions than first-generation drugs.
- Monitor the patient's hemoglobin A_1C regularly as ordered.
- Monitor the patient carefully for cardiovascular dysfunction because sulfonylureas have been associated with an increased risk of cardiovascular mortality as compared to diet or diet and insulin therapy.
- Monitor elderly patients closely for adverse reactions because they may be more sensitive to this drug's adverse reactions.

Supportive Care
• Notify the doctor if blood glucose levels remain elevated or frequent episodes of hypoglycemia occur.
• Treat a hypoglycemic reaction with an oral form of rapid-acting glucose if the patient is awake or with glucagon or I.V. glucose if the patient cannot be aroused. Follow up treatment with a complex carbohydrate snack when patient is awake, and determine cause of reaction.
• Be sure ancillary treatment measures, such as diet and exercise programs, are being used appropriately.
• Discuss with the doctor how to deal with noncompliance.
• Patient transferring from insulin therapy to an oral antidiabetic requires blood glucose monitoring at least t.i.d. before meals. Patient may require hospitalization during transition.
Patient Teaching
• Emphasize the importance of following the prescribed diet, exercise, and medical regimens.
• Tell the patient to take the medication at the same time each day. If a dose is missed, it should be taken immediately, unless it's almost time to take the next dose. Instruct the patient not to take double doses.
• Advise the patient to avoid alcohol while taking glipizide. Remind him that many foods and nonprescription medications contain alcohol.
• Encourage the patient to wear a medical alert bracelet or necklace.
• Tell the patient to take drug 30 minutes before meals.
• Teach the patient how to monitor blood glucose levels as prescribed.
• Teach the patient how to recognize the signs and symptoms of hyperglycemia and hypoglycemia and what to do if they occur.
• Stress the importance of compliance and close follow-up with glipizide therapy.

Evaluation
In patients receiving glipizide, appropriate evaluation statements may include:
• Patient's blood glucose level is normal.
• Patient recognizes hypoglycemia early and treats hypoglycemic episodes effectively before injury occurs.
• Patient and family express an understanding of glipizide therapy.

glucagon
(gloo´ ka gon)

• *Classification:* antihypoglycemic agent, diagnostic agent
• *Pregnancy Risk Category:* B

HOW SUPPLIED
Powder for injection: 1 mg (1 unit)/vial, 10 mg (10 units)/vial

ACTION
Mechanism: Raises blood glucose level by promoting depolymerization of hepatic glycogen to glucose.
Absorption: Glucagon is destroyed in the GI tract; therefore, it must be given parenterally. Drug is rapidly absorbed after S.C. or I.M. injection.
Metabolism: Degraded extensively by the liver, in the kidneys and plasma, and at its tissue receptor sites in plasma membranes.
Excretion: By the kidneys. Half-life: About 3 to 10 minutes.
Onset, peak, duration: After I.V. administration, hyperglycemic activity peaks within 30 minutes; relaxation of the GI smooth muscle occurs within 1 minute; after I.M. administration, relaxation of the GI smooth muscle occurs within 10 minutes. Administration to comatose hypoglycemic patients (with normal liver glycogen stores) usually produces a return to consciousness within 20 minutes. Duration after I.M. administration is

up to 32 minutes; after I.V. administration, up to 25 minutes.

INDICATIONS & DOSAGE

Coma of insulin-shock therapy–
Adults: 0.5 to 1 mg S.C., I.M., or I.V. 1 hour after coma develops; may repeat within 25 minutes, if necessary. In very deep coma, also give glucose 10% to 50% I.V. for faster response. When patient responds, give additional carbohydrate immediately.
Severe insulin-induced hypoglycemia during diabetic therapy–
Adults and children: 0.5 to 1 mg S.C., I.M., or I.V.; may repeat q 20 minutes for 2 doses, if necessary. If coma persists, give glucose 10% to 50% I.V.
Diagnostic aid for radiologic examination–
Adults: 0.25 to 2 mg I.V. or I.M. before initiation of radiologic procedure.

CONTRAINDICATIONS & PRECAUTIONS

Contraindicated in patients with hypersensitivity to the drug, often a result of its protein nature. Use cautiously in patients with a history of insulinoma because, although it initially raises blood glucose levels in patients with insulinoma, its insulin-releasing effect subsequently may cause hypoglycemia. Also use with caution in patients with pheochromocytoma because the drug stimulates release of catecholamines.

ADVERSE REACTIONS

Common reactions are in italics; life-threatening reactions are in bold italics.
GI: nausea, vomiting.
Other: hypersensitivity.

INTERACTIONS

Phenytoin: inhibited glucagon-induced insulin release. Use cautiously.

EFFECTS ON DIAGNOSTIC TESTS

Serum potassium: decreased levels.

NURSING CONSIDERATIONS

Besides those related universally to drug therapy (see "How to use this book"), consider the following specific recommendations:

Assessment

- Obtain a baseline assessment of the patient's blood glucose level before initiating glucagon therapy.
- Be alert for adverse reactions and drug interactions throughout therapy.
- Evaluate the patient's and family's knowledge about glucagon therapy.

Nursing Diagnoses

- High risk for injury related to the patient's severe hypolycemia.
- High risk for fluid volume deficit related to glucagon-induced vomiting.
- Knowledge deficit related to glucagon therapy.

Planning and Implementation

Preparation and Administration

- Repeat dose within 25 minutes, as needed.
- ***I.V. use:*** Use dextrose solution for I.V. drip infusion, as glucagon is compatible to it; drug forms a precipitate in chloride solutions. Give directly into vein or into I.V. tubing of a free-flowing compatible solution over 2 to 5 minutes. Interrupt primary infusion during glucagon injection if you're using the same I.V. line.

Monitoring

- Monitor effectiveness by checking patient's blood glucose level after administration and noting patient's response.
- Monitor patient for hypersensitivity reaction after administration.

Supportive Care

- Notify the doctor that patient's hypoglycemic episode required glucagon use. Be prepared to provide emergency intervention if patient does not respond to glucagon administration.
- Be aware that unstable hypoglycemic diabetics may not respond to glucagon. Give dextrose I.V. instead.
- It is vital to arouse the patient from coma as quickly as possible and to

give additional carbohydrates orally to prevent secondary hypoglycemic reactions.
• Identify the cause of the hypoglycemic episode and determine if the patient is able to recognize early warning signs (may be blunted in patients with chronic diabetes or masked by other drug therapies).
• If the patient experiences nausea and vomiting from glucagon administration and cannot retain some form of sugar for 1 hour, notify the doctor.
Patient Teaching
• Teach the family how to mix and inject the medication properly, using an appropriate-sized syringe and injecting at a 90° angle.
• Recommend that the patient use medication within 3 months after mixing and store the mixed solution in refrigerator. Patient should store unmixed medication at room temperature and not in the bathroom, which often becomes hot and humid.
• Instruct family how to recognize hypoglycemia. Urge them to call a doctor immediately in emergencies.
• Tell the family to expect a response usually within 20 minutes after injection and that injection may be repeated if no response occurs. Tell the family to seek medical assistance if second injection is needed.
Evaluation
In patients receiving glucagon, appropriate evaluation statements may include:
• Patient's blood glucose level returns to normal.
• Patient does not experience fluid volume deficit.
• Patient and family state an understanding of glucagon therapy and demonstrate appropriate administration techniques.

glutethimide
(gloo teth´ i mide)
Doriden, Doriglute

• Controlled Substance Schedule III
• *Classification:* sedative-hypnotic (piperidinedione)
• *Pregnancy Risk Category:* C

HOW SUPPLIED
Tablets: 250 mg, 500 mg
Capsules: 500 mg

ACTION
Mechanism: Unknown. A CNS depressant.
Absorption: Erratically absorbed after oral administration.
Distribution: Widely distributed throughout the body and concentrates in fat. Slightly more than 50% of the drug is protein-bound.
Metabolism: Hepatic conversion to inactive metabolites.
Excretion: Inactive metabolites are excreted primarily in urine, with minor excretion in feces. Less than 2% of the drug is excreted unchanged. Half-life: 10 to 12 hours.
Onset, peak, duration: Peak serum levels may occur at any point from 1 to 6 hours. Action may begin in 30 minutes. Duration of action is 4 to 8 hours.

INDICATIONS & DOSAGE
Insomnia –
Adults: 250 to 500 mg P.O. h.s. May be repeated, but not less than 4 hours before intended awakening. Total daily dosage should not exceed 1 g.

CONTRAINDICATIONS & PRECAUTIONS
Contraindicated in patients with hypersensitivity to the drug and in those with porphyria, severe renal failure, or uncontrolled pain.
Use cautiously in patients with

conditions that may be worsened by the drug's anticholinergic effects: prostatic hypertrophy, bladder-neck obstruction, narrow-angle glaucoma, or stenosing peptic ulcer.

Because this drug depresses the CNS, avoid use in depressed patients or those with suicidal tendencies and in patients with a history of drug abuse or addiction. The abuse potential, persistence of side effects, and potential lethality of glutethimide overdose mandates the use of other agents in these patients.

ADVERSE REACTIONS

Common reactions are in italics; life-threatening reactions are in bold italics.
CNS: *residual sedation, dizziness, ataxia,* paradoxical excitation, headache, vertigo.
EENT: dry mouth, blurred vision.
GI: irritation, nausea.
GU: bladder atony.
Skin: rash, urticaria.

INTERACTIONS

Alcohol or other CNS depressants, including narcotic analgesics: excessive CNS depression. Use together cautiously.
Oral anticoagulants: glutethimide enhances the metabolism of coumarin derivitives. Monitor for decreased effect.

EFFECTS ON DIAGNOSTIC TESTS

Phentolamine test: false-positive results.
Urine 17-hydroxycorticosteroids (Glenn-Nelson technique): test interference.

NURSING CONSIDERATIONS

Besides those related universally to drug therapy (see "How to use this book"), consider the following specific recommendations:

Assessment
• Obtain a baseline assessment of sleeping patterns and CNS status before therapy.
• Be alert for adverse reactions and drug interactions throughout therapy.
• Evaluate the patient's and family's knowledge about gluthethimide therapy.

Nursing Diagnoses
• Sleep pattern disturbance related to underlying patient problem.
• High risk for trauma related to adverse CNS reactions caused by gluthethimide.
• Knowledge deficit related to gluthethimide therapy.

Planning and Implementation
Preparation and Administration
• Before leaving the bedside, make sure the patient has swallowed the medication.
Monitoring
• Regularly monitor the effectiveness of gluthethimide by evaluating the patient's ability to sleep after administration.
• Monitor the patient after initiating therapy for evidence of CNS and other adverse reactions.
• Monitor prothrombin times carefully when patient on glutethimide starts or ends anticoagulant therapy. Anticoagulant dose may need to be adjusted.
Supportive Care
• After administration, institute safety precautions: remove cigarettes; keep bed rails up, and supervise or assist ambulation.
• Do not discontinue the drug abruptly since this may produce nausea, vomiting, nervousness, tremors, chills, fever, nightmares, insomnia, tachycardia, delirium, numbness of extremities, hallucinations, dysphagia, and seizures. Withdraw gradually.
• Take precautions to prevent hoarding or self-overdosing, especially by the patient who is depressed or suicidal or has a history of drug abuse.

• Be aware that drug is intended for short-term use only.

Patient Teaching

• Encourage the patient to report severe dizziness, or feeling oversedated so the doctor can be consulted for change of dose or drug.

• Explain that hypnotic drugs suppress rapid eye movement sleep. When drug is discontinued, the patient may experience increased dreaming.

• Instruct the patient to remain in bed after taking drug and to call for assistance to use the bathroom.

• Warn the patient to avoid hazardous activities that require mental alertness if adverse CNS reactions are present after awakening.

• Tell the patient to notify the nurse or doctor if sleep pattern disturbances continue despite therapy.

Evaluation

In patients receiving glutethimide, appropriate evaluation statements may include:

• Patient states drug was effective in inducing sleep.

• Patient's safety is maintained.

• Patient and family state an understanding of glutethimide therapy.

glyburide

(glye´ byoor ide)

DiaBeta**, Euglucon†, Micronase

• *Classification:* antidiabetic agent (sulfonylurea)

• *Pregnancy Risk Category:* B

HOW SUPPLIED

Tablets: 1.25 mg, 2.5 mg, 5 mg

ACTION

Mechanism: A sulfonylurea that lowers blood glucose by stimulating insulin release from the pancreatic beta cells and reducing glucose output by the liver. An extrapancreatic effect increases peripheral sensitivity to insulin.

Absorption: Almost completely absorbed from the GI tract.

Distribution: Not fully understood; is 99% protein-bound.

Metabolism: Completely metabolized by the liver to inactive metabolites.

Excretion: As metabolites in urine and feces in equal proportions. Half-life: 10 hours.

Onset, peak, duration: Onset of action within 2 hours; hypoglycemic effects peak in 3 to 4 hours; duration of action is 24 hours.

INDICATIONS & DOSAGE

Adjunct to diet to lower the blood glucose in patients with non-insulin-dependent diabetes mellitus (type II)–

Adults: initially, 2.5 to 5 mg P.O. daily administered with breakfast. Patients who are more sensitive to hypoglycemic drugs should be started at 1.25 mg daily. Usual maintenance dosage is 1.25 to 20 mg daily, given either as a single dose or in divided doses.

To replace insulin therapy–

Adults: if insulin dosage is more than 40 units daily, patient may be started on 5 mg glyburide daily in addition to 50% of the insulin dosage.

CONTRAINDICATIONS & PRECAUTIONS

Contraindicated in patients with hypersensitivity to sulfonylureas or thiazides; nonfunctioning pancreatic beta cells and patients with burns, acidosis, diabetic coma, severe infection, ketosis, or severe trauma or in patients requiring major surgery because such conditions of severe physiologic stress require insulin for adequate control of blood glucose.

Use cautiously in patients with hepatic or renal insufficiency because of the important roles of the liver in metabolism and the kidneys in elimination; and in patients with impaired adrenal, pituitary, or thyroid function.

ADVERSE REACTIONS

Common reactions are in italics; life-threatening reactions are in bold italics.
GI: nausea, epigastric fullness, heartburn.
Hepatic: *cholestatic jaundice.*
Metabolic: *hypoglycemia.*
Skin: rash, pruritus, facial flushing.

INTERACTIONS

Anabolic steroids, chloramphenicol, clofibrate, guanethidine, MAO inhibitors, oral anticoagulants, phenylbutazone, salicylates, sulfonamides: increased hypoglycemic activity. Monitor blood glucose level.
Beta blockers, clonidine: prolonged hypoglycemic effect and masked symptoms of hypoglycemia. Use together cautiously.
Corticosteroids, glucagon, rifampin, thiazide diuretics: decreased hypoglycemic response. Monitor blood glucose level.

EFFECTS ON DIAGNOSTIC TESTS

Cholesterol, alkaline phosphatase, and BUN: altered levels.

NURSING CONSIDERATIONS

Besides those related universally to drug therapy (see "How to use this book"), consider the following specific recommendations:

Assessment
- Obtain a baseline assessment of the patient's blood glucose level before initiating therapy.
- Be alert for adverse reactions and drug interactions throughout therapy.
- Evaluate the patient's and family's knowledge about glyburide therapy.

Nursing Diagnoses
- Altered nutrition: More than body requirements related to the patient's inability to produce sufficient insulin to maintain normal blood glucose levels.
- High risk for injury related to glyburide-induced hypoglycemia.
- Knowledge deficit related to glyburide therapy.

Planning and Implementation

Preparation and Administration
- Consider that some patients taking glyburide may be controlled effectively on a once-daily regimen, whereas others show better response with divided dosing.
- Remember that in elderly, debilitated, or malnourished patients or those with renal or liver dysfunction, glyburide therapy should start with 1.25 mg once a day.
- ***P.O. use:*** Administer once-daily doses with breakfast. Be aware that to improve control in patients receiving 10 mg/day or more, divided doses are usually given before the morning and evening meals.

Monitoring
- Monitor effectiveness by regularly checking patient's blood glucose levels. Monitor blood glucose levels more frequently if the patient is under stress, having difficulty controlling blood glucose levels, or is newly diagnosed.
- Monitor for signs and symptoms of both hyperglycemia and hypoglycemia; note time and circumstances of each reaction.
- Be aware that glyburide is a second-generation sulfonylurea that appears to cause fewer adverse reactions than first-generation drugs.
- Monitor the patient's hemoglobin A_1C regularly as ordered.
- When substituting glyburide for chlorpropamide, monitor the patient closely during the first week because of the prolonged retention of chlorpropamide in the body.
- Monitor the patient carefully for cardiovascular dysfunction, because sulfonylureas have been associated with an increased risk of cardiovascular mortality as compared to diet or diet and insulin therapy.

Supportive Care
- Notify the doctor if blood glucose levels remain elevated or frequent episodes of hypoglycemia occur.
- Treat a hypoglycemic reaction with an oral form of rapid-acting glucose if the patient is awake or with glucagon or I.V. glucose if the patient cannot be aroused. Follow up treatment with a complex carbohydrate snack when patient is awake, and determine cause of reaction.
- Be sure ancillary treatment measures, such as diet and exercise programs, are being used appropriately.
- Discuss with the doctor how to approach noncompliance issues.
- Patient transferring from insulin therapy to an oral antidiabetic requires blood glucose monitoring at least t.i.d. before meals. Patient may require hospitalization during transition.

Patient Teaching
- Emphasize to the patient the importance of following the prescribed diet, exercise, and medical regimens.
- Tell the patient to take the medication at the same time each day. If a dose is missed, it should be taken immediately, unless it's almost time to take the next dose. Instruct the patient not to take double doses.
- Advise the patient to avoid alcohol while taking glyburide. Remind him that many foods and nonprescription medications contain alcohol.
- Encourage the patient to wear a medical alert bracelet or necklace.
- Tell the patient to take drug with food; once-daily dosage should be taken with breakfast.
- Teach the patient how to monitor blood glucose levels as prescribed.
- Teach the patient how to recognize the signs and symptoms of hyperglycemia and hypoglycemia and what to do if they occur.
- Stress the importance of compliance and close follow-up with glyburide therapy.

Evaluation

In patients receiving glyburide, appropriate evaluation statements may include:
- Patient's blood glucose level is normal.
- Patient recognizes hypoglycemia early and treats hypoglycemic episodes effectively before injury occurs.
- Patient and family express an understanding of glyburide therapy.

glycerin
(gli´ ser in)

Fleet Babylax◇, Sani-Supp◇

- *Classification:* osmotic laxative, ophthalmic osmotic agent, lubricant, adjunct in glaucoma (trihydric alcohol)
- *Pregnancy Risk Category:* C

HOW SUPPLIED
Enema (pediatric): 4 ml/applicator◇
Suppositories: adult, children, and infant sizes◇

ACTION
Mechanism: A hyperosmolar laxative that draws water from the tissues into the feces and thus stimulates evacuation.
Absorption: Poorly absorbed.
Distribution: When administered by suppository, glycerin is distributed locally.
Metabolism: None.
Excretion: In the feces.
Onset, peak, duration: After rectal administration, laxative effect occurs in 15 to 30 minutes.

INDICATIONS & DOSAGE
Constipation–
Adults and children over 6 years: 3 g as a rectal suppository; or 5 to 15 ml as an enema.
Children under 6 years: 1 to 1.5 g as

a rectal suppository; or 2 to 5 ml as an enema.

CONTRAINDICATIONS & PRECAUTIONS

Contraindicated in patients with glycerin hypersensitivity. Glycerin suppositories are contraindicated in patients who are recovering from rectal surgery.

Orally administered glycerin should be used cautiously in patients with cardiac, renal, or hepatic disease, because it may cause a fluid shift precipitating pulmonary edema or CHF; in elderly and dehydrated patients because it may cause seizures and disorientation; and in diabetic patients because it may lead to diabetic ketoacidosis and coma.

ADVERSE REACTIONS

Common reactions are in italics; life-threatening reactions are in bold italics.
GI: *cramping pain,* rectal discomfort, hyperemia of rectal mucosa.

INTERACTIONS

None significant.

EFFECTS ON DIAGNOSTIC TESTS

None reported.

NURSING CONSIDERATIONS

Besides those related universally to drug therapy (see "How to use this book"), consider the following specific recommendations:

Assessment
- Obtain a baseline assessment of history of bowel disorder, GI status, fluid intake, nutritional status, exercise habits, and normal pattern of elimination.
- Be alert for adverse reactions and drug interactions throughout therapy.
- Evaluate the patient's and family's knowledge about glycerin therapy.

Nursing Diagnoses
- Constipation related to interruption of normal pattern of elimination characterized by infrequent or absent stools.
- Pain related to glycerin-induced abdominal cramping.
- Knowledge deficit related to glycerin therapy.

Planning and Implementation
Preparation and Administration
- Must be retained for at least 15 minutes; usually acts within 1 hour.
- Entire suppository need not melt to be effective.

Monitoring
- Monitor effectiveness by checking the frequency and characteristics of stools.
- Auscultate bowel sounds at least once a shift. Assess for pain and cramping.
- Monitor nutritional status and fluid intake.

Supportive Care
- A hyperosmolar laxative used mainly to reestablish proper toilet habits in laxative-dependent patients.
- Provide privacy for elimination.
- Unless contraindicated, encourage fluid intake up to 2,500 ml a day.
- Consult with a dietitian to modify diet to increase fiber and bulk.

Patient Teaching
- Discourage excessive use of laxatives by patient to prevent dependence.
- Teach the patient about the relationship between fluid intake, dietary fiber, exercise, and constipation.
- Teach patient that dietary sources of fiber include bran and other cereals, fresh fruit, and vegetables.
- Warn patient that abdominal cramping may occur but will subside when the bowel is emptied.

Evaluation
In patients receiving glycerin, appropriate evaluation statements may include:
- Patient reports return of normal pattern of elimination.
- Patient remains free from abdominal cramping.

• Patient and family state an understanding of glycerin therapy.

glycerin, anhydrous

(gli´ ser in)
Ophthalgan

• *Classification:* adjunctive agent in diagnosing glaucoma (ophthalmic osmotic vehicle)
• *Pregnancy Risk Category:* C

HOW SUPPLIED

Ophthalmic solution: 7.5-ml containers

ACTION

Mechanism: Topical application to the eye removes excess fluid from the cornea, decreasing edema and improving visualization.
Pharmacokinetics: Unknown.

INDICATIONS & DOSAGE

Corneal edema before ophthalmoscopy or gonioscopy in acute glaucoma and bullous keratitis–
Adults and children: instill 1 to 2 drops glycerin solution after instilling a local anesthetic.

CONTRAINDICATIONS & PRECAUTIONS

Contraindicated in patients with glycerin hypersensitivity.

Use orally administered glycerin cautiously in patients with cardiac, renal, or hepatic disease, because it may cause a fluid shift precipitating pulmonary edema or congestive heart failure; in elderly and dehydrated patients because it may cause seizures and disorientation; and in diabetic patients because it may lead to diabetic ketoacidosis and coma.

ADVERSE REACTIONS

Common reactions are in italics; life-threatening reactions are in bold italics.
Eye: *pain* if instilled without topical anesthetic.

INTERACTIONS

None significant.

EFFECTS ON DIAGNOSTIC TESTS

None reported.

NURSING CONSIDERATIONS

Besides those related universally to drug therapy (see "How to use this book"), consider the following recommendations.

Assessment
• Obtain a baseline assessment of the patient's visual status and ocular appearance.
• Be alert for adverse reactions and drug interactions throughout therapy.
• Evaluate the patient's and family's knowledge about anhydrous glycerin therapy.

Nursing Diagnoses
• Sensory/perceptual alterations (visual) related to the patient's underlying condition.
• Pain related to unanesthetized instillation.
• Knowledge deficit related to anhydrous glycerin therapy.

Planning and Implementation
Preparation and Administration
• Store solution in tightly closed container.
• A topical anesthetic such as tetracaine or proparacaine must be used before instilling to prevent discomfort.
• Avoid touching the dropper to the eye, surrounding tissue or tear-film, as glycerin will readily absorb moisture.

Monitoring
• Monitor effectiveness by assessing the patient's visual status and degree of corneal edema.

Patient Teaching
• Tell the patient how the drug will be administered and elicit his cooperation.

• Warn the patient not to touch or rub his eye after it has been anesthetized, as he may inadvertently injure or abrade it.

Evaluation

In patients receiving anhydrous glycerin, appropriate evaluation statements may include:

• Patient experiences a therapeutic reduction in corneal edema.

• Patient remains free of drug-induced ocular pain.

• Patient and family state an understanding of anhydrous glycerin therapy.

glycopyrrolate

(glue koe pye´ roe late)

Robinul, Robinul Forte

• *Classification:* antimuscarinic, GI antispasmodic (anticholinergic)

• *Pregnancy Risk Category:* B

HOW SUPPLIED

Tablets: 1 mg, 2 mg

Injection: 0.2 mg/ml

ACTION

Mechanism: A quaternary anticholinergic that blocks the cholinergic (muscarinic) actions of acetylcholine on autonomic effectors innervated by postganglionic cholinergic nerves.

Absorption: Poorly absorbed from the GI tract (10% to 25%) after oral administration. Glycopyrrolate is rapidly absorbed when given I.M. or S.C.

Distribution: Does not cross the blood-brain barrier or enter the eye.

Excretion: Primarily renal. Half-life: 1.7 hours.

Onset, peak, duration: When given I.M., serum concentrations peak in 30 to 45 minutes. Action begins in 1 minute after I.V. and 15 to 30 minutes after I.M. or S.C. administrtion. Duration of effect is up to 7 hours when given parenterally and up to 12 hours when given orally.

INDICATIONS & DOSAGE

To reverse neuromuscular blockade–

Adults: 0.2 mg I.V. for each 1 mg neostigmine or 5 mg of pyridostigmine. May be given I.V. without dilution or may be added to dextrose injection and given by infusion.

Preoperatively to diminish secretions and block cardiac vagal reflexes–

Adults: 0.002 mg/lb of body weight I.M. 30 to 60 minutes before anesthesia.

Adjunctive therapy in peptic ulcers and other GI disorders–

Adults: 1 to 2 mg P.O. t.i.d. or 0.1 mg I.M. t.i.d. or q.i.d. Dosage must be individualized. Maximum P.O. dose is 8 mg/day.

CONTRAINDICATIONS & PRECAUTIONS

Contraindicated in patients with narrow-angle glaucoma because drug-induced cycloplegia and mydriasis may increase intraocular pressure; obstructive uropathy because the drug may exacerbate urinary retention; and myasthenia gravis, paralytic ileus, intestinal atony, or toxic megacolon because the drug may worsen these conditions.

Use cautiously in patients with hyperthyroidism, ulcerative colitis, coronary artery disease, CHF, cardiac arrhythmias, or hypertension because it may exacerbate these conditions; hiatal hernia associated with reflux esophagitis because the drug may decrease lower esophageal sphincter tone, thus worsening the condition; in patients over age 40 because it increases the glaucoma risk; and in hot or humid environments because it may predispose the patient to heatstroke.

ADVERSE REACTIONS

Common reactions are in italics; life-threatening reactions are in bold italics.
CNS: disorientation, irritability, incoherence, weakness, nervousness, drowsiness, dizziness, headache.
CV: palpitations, tachycardia, paradoxical bradycardia.
EENT: *dilated pupils, blurred vision,* photophobia, increased intraocular pressure, difficulty swallowing.
GI: *constipation, dry mouth,* nausea, vomiting, epigastric distress.
GU: *urinary hesitancy, urine retention,* impotence.
Skin: urticaria, decreased sweating or anhidrosis, other dermal manifestations.
Local: burning at injection site.
Other: bronchial plugging, fever.

INTERACTIONS

None significant.

EFFECTS ON DIAGNOSTIC TESTS

None reported.

NURSING CONSIDERATIONS

Besides those related universally to drug therapy (see "How to use this book"), consider the following specific recommendations:

Assessment
- Obtain a baseline assessment of the patient's underlying condition before drug therapy.
- Be alert for adverse drug reactions and drug interactions throughout glycopyrrolate therapy.
- Evaluate the patient's and family's knowledge about glycopyrrolate therapy.

Nursing Diagnoses
- Altered health maintenance related to the patient's underlying condition.
- Sensory/perceptual alteration (visual) related to adverse drug reaction.
- Knowledge deficit related to glycopyrrolate therapy.

Planning and Implementation

Preparation and Administration
- ***I.V. use:*** Do not mix with I.V. solutions containing sodium bicarbonate or alkaline solutions with a pH > 6.
- Administer 30 minutes to 1 hour before meals.
- Administer smaller doses to elderly patients.
- Check all dosages carefully. Even a slight overdose could lead to toxicity.

Monitoring
- Monitor for adverse reactions or drug interactions especially in debilitated or elderly patients by checking vital signs carefully for tachycardia or paradoxical bradycardia.
- Monitor intake and output carefully.
- Evaluate the patient's visual ability and ask about blurred vision.
- Monitor the patient's bowel pattern; drug may cause constipation.

Supportive Care
- Assist the patient to get in and out of bed if he experiences blurred vision. Institute safety precautions.
- Give the patient gum or hard sugarless candy to help relieve dry mouth.
- If constipation occurs, obtain an order for a laxative.

Patient Teaching
- Tell the patient to report any signs of urinary hesitancy or retention.
- Warn the patient to avoid activities that require alertness until CNS effects of the drug are known.

Evaluation

In patients receiving glycopyrrolate, appropriate evaluation statements may include:
- Patient is able to perform activities of daily living without assistance.
- Patient does not experience any blurred vision.
- Patient and family state an understanding of glycopyrrolate therapy.

gonadorelin acetate

(goe nad oh rell′ in)
Lutrepulse

- *Classification:* fertility agent (gonadotropin releasing hormone [GNrH])
- *Pregnancy Risk Category:* B

HOW SUPPLIED

Injection: 0.8-mg/10-ml, 3.2-mg/10-ml vials; supplied as a kit with I.V. supplies and ambulatory infusion pump

ACTION

Mechanism: Mimics the action of gonadotropin releasing hormone, which results in the synthesis and release of luteinizing hormone (LH) from the anterior pituitary. LH subsequently acts upon the reproductive organs to regulate hormone synthesis.
Absorption: Because the drug is a polypeptide, it is destroyed in the GI tract after oral administration. Gonadorelin must be administered I.V. using a pump designed to deliver the drug in a pulsatile fashion to mimic the endogenous hormone.
Distribution: The drug has a low plasma volume of distribution (10 to 15 liters) and a high rate of clearance from plasma.
Metabolism: Rapidly metabolized. Several biologically inactive peptide fragments have been identified.
Excretion: Primarily in urine. Half-life: Initial phase, 2 to 10 minutes; terminal phase, 10 to 40 minutes.

INDICATIONS & DOSAGE

Induction of ovulation in women with primary hypothalamic amenorrhea –
Women: 5 mcg I.V. q 90 minutes for 21 days. If no response follows three treatment intervals, dosage may be increased.

CONTRAINDICATIONS & PRECAUTIONS

Contraindicated in patients hypersensitive to the drug, with conditions that could be complicated by pregnancy (such as a pituitary prolactinoma), who are anovulatory from any cause other than a hypothalamic disorder, and with ovarian cysts.

ADVERSE REACTIONS

Common reactions are in italics; life-threatening reactions are in bold italics.
GU: ovarian hyperstimulation.
Local: hematoma, infection, inflammation, mild phlebitis.
Other: multiple pregnancy.

INTERACTIONS

None reported.

EFFECTS ON DIAGNOSTIC TESTS

None reported.

NURSING CONSIDERATIONS

Besides those related universally to drug therapy (see "How to use this book"), consider the following specific recommendations:
Assessment
- Obtain a baseline assessment of the patient's primary hypothalamic amenorrhea before initiating therapy with gonadorelin.
- Be alert for adverse reactions and drug interactions throughout therapy.
- Evaluate the patient's and family's knowledge about gonadorelin therapy.

Nursing Diagnoses
- Sexual dysfunctional related to the patient's underlying condition.
- High risk for infection related to need for maintaining an I.V. site for extended period.
- Knowledge deficit related to therapy with gonadorelin.

Planning and Implementation
Preparation and Administration
- ***I.V. use:*** To mimic the naturally occurring hormone, gonadorelin acetate must be administered in a pulsatile

fashion with the available ambulatory infusion pump. The pulse period is set at 1 minute (drug is infused over 1 minute) and pulse interval is set at 90 minutes. To administer 2.5 mcg/pulse, reconstitute the 0.8-mg vial with 8 ml of supplied diluent, and set the pump to deliver 25 microliters/pulse. To administer 5 mcg/pulse, use the same dosage strength and dilution but set the pump to deliver 50 microliters/pulse. Some patients may require higher doses. To administer 10 mcg/pulse, reconstitute the 3.2-mg vial with 8 ml of supplied diluent, and set the pump to deliver 25 microliters/pulse. To administer 20 mcg/pulse, use the same dosage strength and dilution but set the pump to deliver 50 microliters/pulse.

Monitoring

- Monitor effectiveness by ensuring that patient has regular pelvic examinations, midluteal phase serum progesterone determinations and pelvic ultrasound on days 7 and 14 after establishment of a baseline scan. (Be aware that some clinicians prefer shorter intervals between scans).
- Monitor patient closely for anaphylaxis, which has been reported with similiar drugs.
- Closely monitor the patient response; this is critical to ensure adequate ovarian stimulation without hyperstimulation (sudden ovarian enlargement, ascites, or pleural effusion).
- Monitor for abdominal pain and discomfort, which may indicate ovarian enlargement.
- Monitor I.V. site at each visit.

Supportive Care

- Be aware that cannula and I.V. site should be changed every 48 hours.

Patient Teaching

- Instruct patient how to recognize the signs and symptoms of hypersensitivity reactions (hives, wheezing, difficulty breathing) and encourage her to report these as soon as possible.
- Warn the patient to report immediately symptoms of ovarian hyperstimulation syndrome: abdominal distention and pain, dyspnea, and vaginal bleeding.
- Inform patient that multiple births are possible. (Incidence is about 12%).
- Stress importance of adhering to the close monitoring schedule required by therapy.
- Teach patient about proper aseptic technique and care of the I.V. site. Cannula and I.V. site should be changed every 48 hours. Provide written instructions.

Evaluation

In patients receiving gonadorelin acetate, appropriate evaluation statements include:

- Patient ovulates during gonadorelin acetate therapy.
- Infection at the I.V. site did not develop.
- Patient and family state an understanding of gonadorelin acetate therapy.

gonadorelin hydrochloride (luteinizing hormone-releasing hormone, LHRH; gonadotropin releasing hormone, GnRH)

(goe nad oh rell′ in)

Factrel

- *Classification:* diagnostic agent (luteinizing hormone releasing hormone)
- *Pregnancy Risk Category:* B

HOW SUPPLIED

Injection: 100 mcg, 500 mcg

ACTION

Mechanism: A synthetic luteinizing hormone that releases LHRH.

Absorption: Because the drug is a polypeptide, it is destroyed in the GI tract after oral administration.

Excretion: Primarily renal as metabolites. Half-life: About 10 minutes.
Onset, peak, duration: Gonadorelin has a duration of action of 3 to 5 hours.

INDICATIONS & DOSAGE

Evaluation of the functional capacity and response of gonadotropic hormones–
Adults: 100 mcg S.C. or I.V. In women for whom the phase of the menstrual cycle can be established, perform the test between day 1 and day 7.

CONTRAINDICATIONS & PRECAUTIONS

Contraindicated in patients who have demonstrated hypersensitivity to it.

ADVERSE REACTIONS

Common reactions are in italics; life-threatening reactions are in bold italics.
CNS: headache, flushing, light-headedness.
GI: *nausea, abdominal discomfort.*
Local: swelling, occasionally with pain and pruritus when administered S.C.; skin rash after chronic S.C. administration.

INTERACTIONS

Digoxin, oral contraceptives: may depress gonadotropin levels. Monitor results carefully.
Levodopa, spironolactone: may elevate gonadotropin levels. Monitor results carefully.

EFFECTS ON DIAGNOSTIC TESTS

Luteinizing hormone: increased levels.

NURSING CONSIDERATIONS

Besides those related universally to drug therapy (see "How to use this book"), consider the following specific recommendations:

Assessment
- Evaluate the patient's and family's knowledge about the gonadorelin hydrochloride test.
- Be alert for adverse reactions and drug interactions throughout therapy.
- Evaluate the patient's knowledge about gonadorelin hydrochloride therapy.

Nursing Diagnoses
- Sexual dysfunction related to the patient's underlying condition.
- Pain related to gonadorelin hydrochloride-induced headache and abdominal discomfort.
- Knowledge deficit related to the gonadorelin hydrochloride test.

Planning and Implementation
Preparation and Administration
- For specific test methodology and interpretation of test results, refer to the manufacturer's full product information. Ask pharmacist for a copy.
- ***I.V. use:*** Reconstitute vial with 1 ml of accompanying sterile diluent. Prepare solution immediately before use. Inject drug directly into vein over 3 to 5 minutes. Alternatively, inject into an I.V. line containing a free-flowing compatible solution.
- After reconstitution, store at room temperature and use within 1 day. Discard unused reconstituted solution and diluent.

Monitoring
- Monitor the patient for a hypersensitivity reaction throughout the test.

Supportive Care
- Keep epinephrine readily available in case of hypersensitivity.

Patient Teaching
- Inform patient about test procedure. Tell the patient that, as a single injection, this drug can aid in evaluating the functional capacity and response of the gonadotropins of the anterior pituitary.
- Instruct patient how to recognize the signs and symptoms of hypersensitivity reactions (hives, wheezing, dif-

ficulty breathing) and encourage her to report these immediately.

Evaluation

In patients receiving the gonadorelin hydrochloride test, appropriate evaluation statements may include:

- Gonadorelin hydrochloride test aided evaluation of the functional capacity and response of gonadotropic hormones.
- Pain did not occur.
- Patient and family state an understanding of the gonadorelin hydrochloride test.

gonadotropin, chorionic (HCG)

(goe nad´ oh troe pin)

Antuitrin, A.P.L., Chorex, Follutein, Pregnyl, Profasi HP

- *Classification:* gonadotropin (ovulation stimulant; spermatogenesis stimulant)
- *Pregnancy Risk Category:* C

HOW SUPPLIED

Injection: 200 units/ml, 500 units/ml, 1,000 units/ml, 2,000 units/ml (after reconstitution)

ACTION

Mechanism: Serves as a substitute for luteinizing hormone to stimulate ovulation of a human menopausal gonadotropin–prepared follicle; promotes secretion of gonadal steroid hormones by stimulating production of androgen by the interstitial cells of the testes (Leydig's cells).

Absorption: Because the drug is a polypeptide, it is destroyed in the GI tract after oral administration. Usually administered I.M.

Distribution: Found primarily in the testes in men and ovaries in women; small amounts may also be distributed into the proximal tubules of the renal cortex.

Excretion: In the urine. Half-life: Initial phase, 11 hours; terminal phase, 23 hours.

Onset, peak, duration: Serum-HCG levels increase within 2 hours of administration; drug levels peak within 6 hours, persist for about 36 hours, begin to decline at 48 hours, and are nearly undetectable at 72 hours.

INDICATIONS & DOSAGE

Anovulation and infertility–

Women: 10,000 units I.M. 1 day after last dose of menotropins.

Hypogonadism–

Men: 500 to 1,000 units I.M. three times weekly for 3 weeks, then twice weekly for 3 weeks; or 4,000 units I.M. three times weekly for 6 to 9 months, then 2,000 units three times weekly for 3 more months.

Nonobstructive cryptorchidism–

Boys 4 to 9 years: 5,000 units I.M. every other day for four doses.

CONTRAINDICATIONS & PRECAUTIONS

Contraindicated in patients with precocious puberty or androgen-responsive cancer (prostatic, testicular, male breast) because it stimulates androgen production, and in patients with hypersensitivity to HCG.

HCG should be used only by clinicians experienced in treating infertility disorders. Use cautiously in patients with asthma, seizure disorders, migraines, or cardiac or renal diseases because it may exacerbate these conditions.

ADVERSE REACTIONS

Common reactions are in italics; life-threatening reactions are in bold italics.

CNS: headache, fatigue, irritability, restlessness, depression.

GU: early puberty (growth of testes, penis, pubic and axillary hair; voice change; down on upper lip; growth of body hair).

Local: *pain at injection site.*

Other: gynecomastia, edema.

INTERACTIONS

None significant.

EFFECTS ON DIAGNOSTIC TESTS

None reported.

NURSING CONSIDERATIONS

Besides those related universally to drug therapy (see "How to use this book"), consider the following specific recommendations:

Assessment

- Obtain a baseline assessment of the patient's underlying condition before initiating therapy with HCG.
- Be alert for adverse reactions and drug interactions throughout therapy.
- Evaluate the patient's and family's knowledge about HCG therapy.

Nursing Diagnoses

- Sexual dysfunction related to the patient's underlying condition.
- Pain related to HCG administration.
- Knowledge deficit related to therapy with HCG.

Planning and Implementation

Preparation and Administration

- ***I.M. use:*** Rotate injection sites to prevent muscle atrophy.

Monitoring

- Monitor effectiveness by ensuring that patient has regular pelvic examinations, midluteal phase serum progesterone determinations, and pelvic ultrasound as ordered.
- Regularly inspect boys' genitalia for signs of early puberty.
- Monitor patient for ectopic pregnancy, which is usually evident between week 8 to 12 of gestation.
- Be aware that drug is usually used only after failure of clomiphene in anovulatory patients.
- Limit sodium intake if not contraindicated to limit fluid retention.

Patient Teaching

- Warn patient about possibility of pain at injection site.
- Warn patient that multiple births are possible when used with menotropins to induce ovulation.
- Encourage daily intercourse from day before HCG is given until ovulation occurs when used in infertility.
- Tell patient to limit sodium intake if not contraindicated.

Evaluation

In patients receiving HCG, appropriate evaluation statements include:

- Patient's underlying condition is improved or corrected.
- Patient experiences only minimal pain at injection site of HCG.
- Patient and family state an understanding of HCG therapy.

---

goserelin acetate

(goe´ se rel in)

Zoladex

- *Classification:* luteinizing hormone releasing hormone (synthetic decapeptide)
- *Pregnancy Risk Category:* X

HOW SUPPLIED

Implants: 3.6 mg

ACTION

Mechanism: A luteinizing hormone-releasing hormone (LHRH) analog that acts on the pituitary to decrease the release of follicle-stimulating hormone and luteinizing hormone. In men, the result is dramatically lowered serum levels of testosterone.

Absorption: Slowly absorbed from implant site; absorption during the first 8 days is slower than during the remainder of the 28-day dosing cycle.

Excretion: Half-life: Elimination half-life is about 4.2 hours in patients with normal renal function. Substantial renal impairment prolongs half-life, but this does not appear to increase the incidence of adverse effects.

Onset, peak, duration: Drug levels peak in 12 to 15 days after implantation.

INDICATIONS & DOSAGE

Palliative treatment of advanced carcinoma of the prostate–
Adults: 1 implant S.C. q 28 days into the upper abdominal wall.

CONTRAINDICATIONS & PRECAUTIONS

Contraindicated during pregnancy. Initially, LHRH analogs such as goserelin may cause a worsening of the symptoms of prostatic cancer because the drug initially increases testosterone serum levels. A few patients may experience increased bone pain. Rarely, disease exacerbation (spinal cord compression or ureteral obstruction) has occurred.

ADVERSE REACTIONS

Common reactions are in italics; life-threatening reactions are in bold italics.
Blood: anemia.
CNS: lethargy, pain (worsened in the first 30 days), dizziness, insomnia, anxiety, depression, headache, chills, fever.
CV: edema, CHF, arrhythmias, CVA, hypertension, myocardial infarction, peripheral vascular disorder, chest pain.
EENT: upper respiratory infection.
GI: nausea, vomiting, diarrhea, constipation, ulcer.
GU: *decreased erections, lower urinary tract symptoms,* renal insufficiency, urinary obstruction, urinary tract infection.
Skin: rash, sweating.
Other: *hot flashes, sexual dysfunction,* gout, hyperglycemia, weight increase, breast swelling and tenderness.

INTERACTIONS

None reported.

EFFECTS ON DIAGNOSTIC TESTS

None reported.

NURSING CONSIDERATIONS

Besides those related universally to drug therapy (see "How to use this book"), consider the following specific recommendations:

Assessment

- Obtain a baseline assessment of patient's underlying condition before initiating therapy.
- Be alert for adverse reactions and drug interactions throughout therapy.
- Evaluate the patient's and family's knowledge about goserelin therapy.

Nursing Diagnoses

- Anxiety related to drug-induced adverse reactions.
- Sexual dysfunction related to drug-induced impotence.
- Knowledge deficit related to goserelin therapy.

Planning and Implementation

Preparation and Administration

- Goserelin is supplied as implants contained in sterile syringes.
- Do not remove drug from packaging until ready to use.
- The upper abdominal area should be cleaned with alcohol; a local anesthetic may also be administered to reduce pain.
- The skin is stretched with one hand while the barrel of the syringe is grasped with the other. The needle is inserted into the subcutaneous fat and not aspirated. The direction of the needle must parallel with the abdominal wall. The needle is then be inserted until the hub touches the patient's skin and then withdrawn 1 cm to create a space for the drug. The plunger is then depressed to deliver the drug.
- Store drug at room temperature, but not exceeding 77° F.
- The drug should be administered under the supervision of a doctor.
- It should be delivered into the patient every 28 days.

Monitoring
• Monitor effectiveness by obtaining a CBC, renal and hepatic function tests periodically and by noting results of follow-up diagnostic tests and overall physical status.
• Monitor for bone pain, spinal cord compression and pain, and ureteral obstruction. These may be side effects of drug therapy.
• Monitor the patient for worsening symptoms of prostatic cancer. This is a transient result of increased testosterone and will abate.
• Assess the patient's anxiety level.
• Monitor the patient's elimination patttern—drug may cause urinary obstruction and infection.
• Monitor the patient's weight and assess for potential weight gain.
Supportive Care
• After implantation, the area requires a bandage after the needle is withdrawn.
• Be prepared to schedule patient for ultrasound to locate the goserelin implants if there is a need to remove them.
• Encourage the patient to seek alternate coping methods to deal with anxiety.
• Encourage the patient to express his fears and concerns about sexual dysfunction.
• Encourage the pateint to seek professional evaluation and therapy for sexual dysfunction.
Patient Teaching
• Advise the patient to keep his 28-day schedule for receiving a new implant of the drug.
• Tell the patient that the common side effects of hot flashes, decreased erections, and sexual dysfunction are due to lower testosterone levels.
• Suggest that individual and family counseling be started to help with the adjustment to impotence.
• Teach the patient ways to deal with anxiety such as relaxation techniques and imagery.

Evaluation
In patients receiving goserelin, appropriate evaluation statements may include:
• Patient does not develop drug-induced anxiety.
• Sexual dysfunction is supported by patient and significant other.
• Patient and family state an understanding of goserelin therapy.

griseofulvin microsize
(gri see oh ful´ vin)
Fulcin‡, Fulvicin-U/F, Grifulvin V, Grisactin, Grisovin‡, Grisovin 500‡, Grisovin-FP

griseofulvin ultramicrosize
Fulvicin P/G, Grisactin Ultra, Griseostatin‡, Gris-PEG

• *Classification:* antifungal (penicillin antibiotic)
• *Pregnancy Risk Category:* C

HOW SUPPLIED
microsize
Tablets: 125 mg, 250 mg, 500 mg
Capsules: 125 mg, 250 mg
Oral suspension: 125 mg/5ml
ultramicrosize
Tablets: 125 mg, 165 mg, 250 mg, 330 mg

ACTION
Mechanism: Arrests fungal cell division in metaphase by disrupting its mitotic spindle structure. May also cause the production of defective DNA in dividing fungal cells.
Absorption: Primarily absorbed in the duodenum. Ultramicrosize preparations are absorbed almost completely; microsize absorption ranges from 25% to 70% and may be increased by giving with a high-fat meal.
Distribution: Concentrates in skin, hair, nails, fat, liver, and skeletal

muscle; drug is tightly bound to new keratin.
Metabolism: Oxidatively demethylated and conjugated with glucuronic acid to inactive metabolites in the liver.
Excretion: About 50% of griseofulvin and its metabolites is excreted in urine and 33% in feces within 5 days. Less than 1% of a dose appears unchanged in urine; also excreted in sweat. Half-life: 9 to 24 hours.
Onset, peak, duration: Peak serum levels occur 4 to 8 hours after dosing.

INDICATIONS & DOSAGE
Ringworm infections of skin, hair, nails (tinea corporis, tinea pedis, tinea capitis) when caused by Trichophyton, Microsporum, *or* Epidermophyton–
Adults: 500 mg (microsize) P.O. daily in single or divided doses. Severe infections may require up to 1 g daily. Alternatively, may give 330 to 375 mg ultramicrosize in single or divided doses.
Tinea pedis and tinea unguium–
Adults: 0.75 to 1 g (microsize) P.O. daily. Alternatively, may give 660 to 750 mg ultramicrosize P.O. daily.
Children: 11 mg/kg/day (microsize) P.O. Alternatively, may give 7.3 mg/kg/day of the ultramicrosize.

CONTRAINDICATIONS & PRECAUTIONS
Contraindicated in patients with hypersensitivity to the drug; in patients with hepatocellular failure, and in patients with porphyria because it interferes with porphyrin metabolism. Use with caution in patients with penicillin hypersensitivity because both drugs are produced by *Penicillium.* Drug should be reserved for mycotic disease unresponsive to other topical treatment.

ADVERSE REACTIONS
Common reactions are in italics; life-threatening reactions are in bold italics.
Blood: leukopenia, ***granulocytopenia*** (requires discontinuation of drug).
CNS: *headaches* (in early stages of treatment), transient decrease in hearing, fatigue with large doses, occasional mental confusion, impaired performance of routine activities, psychotic symptoms, dizziness, insomnia.
GI: nausea, vomiting, excessive thirst, flatulence, diarrhea.
Metabolic: porphyria.
Skin: rash, urticaria, photosensitivity (may aggravate lupus erythematosus).
Other: estrogen-like effects in children, oral thrush.

INTERACTIONS
Alcohol: may cause tachycardia, diaphoresis, and flushing. Avoid alcohol.
Barbiturates: decreased griseofulvin blood levels due to decreased absorption or increased metabolism. Avoid using together or administer griseofulvin t.i.d.
Coumarin anticoagulants: decreased effectiveness. Monitor prothrombin times when used concurrently.
Oral contraceptives: decreased effectiveness. Suggest alternate methods of contraception.

EFFECTS ON DIAGNOSTIC TESTS
CBC: decreased granulocyte counts.
Renal function: proteinuria.

NURSING CONSIDERATIONS
Besides those related universally to drug therapy (see "How to use this book"), consider the following specific recommendations:
Assessment
- Obtain a baseline assessment of patient's fungal infection including appropriate specimens for identification of fungi before therapy.
- Be alert for adverse reactions and drug interactions throughout therapy.

• Evaluate the patient's and family's knowledge about griseofulvin therapy.

Nursing Diagnoses

• High risk for injury related to ineffectiveness of griseofulvin to eradicate the fungus infection.

• Altered protection related to griseofulvin induced granulocytopenia.

• Knowledge deficit related to griseofulvin.

Planning and Implementation

Preparation and Administration

• ***P.O. use:*** Administer the drug after a high-fat meal to minimize GI distress and increase absorption.

• Be aware that because griseofulvin ultramicrosize is dispersed in polyethylene glycol, it is absorbed more rapidly and completely than microsize preparations and is therefore effective at one half to two thirds the usual griseofulvin dose.

• Be aware that effective treatment of tinea pedis may require concomitant use of a topical agent.

Monitoring

• Monitor effectiveness by regularly assessing for improvement of infection and for laboratory confirmation of complete eradication of the organism.

• Monitor CBC regularly, especially noting granulocytopenia or leukopenia.

• Monitor patient's hydration status if adverse GI reactions occur.

Supportive Care

• Notify doctor immediately of granulocytopenia, which requires discontinuation of drug.

• Institute safety precautions if adverse CNS reactions occur.

• Obtain an order for an antiemetic or antidiarrheal agent as needed.

Patient Teaching

• Tell patient that prolonged treatment may be needed to control infection and prevent relapse, even if symptoms abate in first few days of therapy.

• Stress importance of compliance with drug therapy, recommended laboratory studies, and close follow up care.

• Instruct patient to keep skin clean and dry and to maintain good hygiene.

• Warn patient to avoid exposure to intense sunlight.

• Instruct patient to take the drug after a high-fat meal to minimize GI distress and increase absorption.

• Inform patient with tinea pedis that a topical treatment may also be required.

• Advise patient to avoid alcoholic beverages.

• Warn patient to avoid hazardous activities that require alertness if adverse CNS reactions occur.

Evaluation

In patients receiving griseofulvin, appropriate evaluation statements may include:

• Patient's infection is alleviated.

• Patient's CBC remains within normal limits throughout griseofulvin therapy.

• Patient and family state an understanding of griseofulvin therapy.

guaifenesin (glyceryl guaiacolate)

(gwye fen´ e sin)

Anti-Tuss*◇, Balminil Expectorant†, Baytussin◇, Breonesin◇, Colrex Expectorant*◇, Cremacoat 2◇, Gee-Gee◇, GG-CEN*◇, Glyate*◇, Glycotuss◇, Glytuss◇, Guiatuss*◇, Halotussin◇, Humibid L.A.◇, Hytuss◇, Hytuss-2X◇, Malotuss◇, Naldecon Senior EX◇, Neo-Spec†, Nortussin◇, Resyl†◇, Robafen◇, Robitussin*◇, S-T Expectorant◇

• *Classification:* expectorant (propanediol derivative)

• *Pregnancy Risk Category:* C

*Liquid form contains alcohol.

**May contain tartrazine.

HOW SUPPLIED

Tablets: 100 mg◇, 200 mg◇
Capsules: 200 mg◇
Syrup: 67 mg/5 ml*◇, 100 mg/5 ml*◇

ACTION

Mechanism: Increases production of respiratory tract fluids to help liquefy and reduce the viscosity of thick, enacious secretions.
Pharmacokinetics: Unknown.

INDICATIONS & DOSAGE

As expectorant–
Adults: 100 to 400 mg P.O. q 4 hours. Maximum 2,400 mg daily.
Children 6 to 12 years: 100 to 200 mg P.O. q 4 hours. Maximum 600 mg daily.
Children 2 to 5 years: 50 to 100 mg P.O. q 4 hours. Maximum 300 mg daily.

CONTRAINDICATIONS & PRECAUTIONS

Contraindicated in patients with hypersensitivity to this drug.

ADVERSE REACTIONS

Common reactions are in italics; life-threatening reactions are in bold italics.
CNS: drowsiness.
GI: vomiting and nausea occur with large doses.

INTERACTIONS

Heparin: increased risk of bleeding. Use together cautiously.

EFFECTS ON DIAGNOSTIC TESTS

None significant.

NURSING CONSIDERATIONS

Besides those related universally to drug therapy (see "How to use this book"), consider the following specific recommendations:

Assessment

- Obtain a baseline assessment of the patient's cough and sputum production before initiating therapy.
- Be alert for adverse reactions and drug interactions throughout therapy.
- Evaluate the patient's and family's knowledge about guaifenesin.

Nursing Diagnoses

- Ineffective airway clearance related to the patient's underlying condition.
- Fluid volume deficit related to guaifenesin-induced nausea and vomiting.
- Knowledge deficit related to guaifenesin therapy.

Planning and Implementation

Preparation and Administration

- Administer drug with a glass of water to help loosen mucus in lungs.

Monitoring

- Monitor effectiveness by regularly evaluating the patient's cough and sputum production.
- Monitor hydration status; record intake and output.
- Monitor for drowsiness.
- Monitor for bleeding if used concurrently with heparin.

Supportive Care

- Provide the patient with the necessary tissues and waste receptacles for disposing of expectorated respiratory secretions.
- Provide for good oral hygiene for the patient receiving an expectorant.
- Encourage fluid intake to at least 3,000 ml/day if not contraindicated to help liquefy and reduce the viscosity of thick, tenacious secretions.
- Be aware that guaifenesin may interfere with certain laboratory tests for 5-hydroxyindoleacetic acid and vanillylmandelic acid.
- Encourage deep-breathing exercises.
- Obtain an order for an antiemetic as needed.
- Institute safety precautions if drowsiness occurs.

Patient Teaching

- Instruct the patient to follow the directions on the medication label exactly. Explain the importance of not taking more of the drug than directed.
- Explain that the patient should

monitor the type and frequency of his sputum and cough and notify his doctor if the medication has not improved his condition within 10 days. This drug should not be used for prolonged periods unless the patient is under direct medical supervision.

• Tell the patient to increase fluid intake to at least 8 full (8-oz) glasses of fluid per 24 hours.

• Encourage the patient to do deep-breathing exercises. The patient should sit properly in a straight chair, take several deep breaths, and then attempt to cough.

• Tell the patient to avoid sources of respiratory irritants, such as fumes, smoke, and dust.

• Explain that this drug may cause drowsiness or dizziness; therefore, warn patient to avoid driving or other hazardous activities that require alertness until CNS adverse reactions are known.

Evaluation

In patients receiving guaifenesin, appropriate evaluation statements may include:

• Patient's lungs are clear and respiratory secretions and cough are decreased.

• Patient maintains adequate hydration.

• Patient and family state an understanding of guaifenesin therapy.

guanabenz acetate

(gwahn´ a benz)

Wytensin

• *Classification:* anithypertensive (antiadrenergic agent)

• *Pregnancy Risk Category:* C

HOW SUPPLIED

Tablets: 4 mg, 8 mg

ACTION

Mechanism: Inhibits the central vasomotor centers, thereby decreasing sympathetic outflow.

Absorption: After oral administration, 70% to 80% of guanabenz is absorbed from the GI tract.

Distribution: Widely distributed in the body; about 90% protein-bound.

Metabolism: Extensively metabolized in the liver; several metabolites are formed.

Excretion: Primarily in urine; unabsorbed drug is excreted in feces. Half-life: About 6 hours.

Onset, peak, duration: Antihypertensive effect occurs within 60 minutes, peaking at 2 to 4 hours. Duration of antihypertensive effect varies from 6 to 12 hours.

INDICATIONS & DOSAGE

Treatment of hypertension–

Adults: initially, 4 mg P.O. b.i.d. Dosage may be increased in increments of 4 to 8 mg/day q 1 to 2 weeks. Maximum dosage is 32 mg b.i.d. To ensure adequate overnight blood pressure control, give last dose h.s.

CONTRAINDICATIONS & PRECAUTIONS

Contraindicated in patients with hypersensitivity to the drug. Use cautiously in patients with vascular insufficiency, severe coronary insufficiency, recent myocardial infarction, cerebrovascular disease, or severe hepatic or renal failure.

ADVERSE REACTIONS

Common reactions are in italics; life-threatening reactions are in bold italics.

CNS: *drowsiness, sedation, dizziness, weakness,* headache, ataxia, depression.

CV: ***severe rebound hypertension.***

EENT: *dry mouth.*

GU: sexual dysfunction.

INTERACTIONS

CNS depressants: may cause increased sedation. Use together cautiously.
Tricyclic antidepressants, MAO inhibitors: may decrease antihypertensive effect.

EFFECTS ON DIAGNOSTIC TESTS

Liver enzyme levels: nonprogressive elevations.
Plasma norepinephrine, dopamine, beta-hydroxylase, and plasma renin activity: decreased (with chronic use).
Serum cholesterol and total triglyceride: slightly reduced levels, but it does not alter high-density lipoprotein fraction.

NURSING CONSIDERATIONS

Besides those related universally to drug therapy (see "How to use this book"), consider the following specific recommendations:

Assessment
- Obtain a baseline assessment of the patient's blood pressure before beginning therapy.
- Be alert for adverse reactions and drug interactions throughout therapy.
- Evaluate the patient's and family's knowledge about guanabenz therapy.

Nursing Diagnoses
- Altered tissue perfusion (renal, cerebral, cardiopulmonary, peripheral) related to the patient's underlying condition.
- High risk for injury related to guanabenz-induced adverse reactions.
- Knowledge deficit related to guanabenz therapy.

Planning and Implementation

Preparation and Administration
- Give last dose of day just before sleep to help ensure adequate blood pressure control.

Monitoring
- Monitor effectiveness by regularly monitoring the patient's blood pressure and ECG results.
- Monitor for hypotension, especially in elderly patients who are often more sensitive to drug's hypotensive effects.

Supportive Care
- Don't discontinue guanabenz therapy abruptly. Rebound hypertension may occur.
- Keep in mind that this drug may be used alone or in combination with a thiazide diuretic.

Patient Teaching
- Advise the patient to avoid driving and other hazardous activities until the CNS effects of the drug are known.
- Warn the patient that drug may diminish tolerance to alcohol or other CNS depressants.
- Explain the importance of taking the drug as prescribed, even when feeling well.
- Tell the patient not to suddenly discontinue using the drug even if unpleasant adverse reactions occur, but to report such effect to the doctor. Warn patient that rebound hypertension can occur if the drug is suddenly withdrawn.
- Instruct the patient to check with the doctor or pharmacist before taking OTC medications.
- Advise the patient to relieve dry mouth with sugarless gum or ice chips.
- Teach the patient or a family caregiver how to take blood pressure measurements. Tell them to notify the doctor of any significant change in blood pressure measurement.

Evaluation

In patients receiving guanabenz, appropriate evaluation statements may include:
- Blood pressure is controlled within normal limits for this patient.
- Patient has not experienced adverse CNS reactions.
- Patient and family state an understanding of guanabenz therapy.

guanadrel sulfate

(gwahn´ a drel)
Hylorel

• *Classification:* antihypertensive (adrenergic neuron blocking agent)
• *Pregnancy Risk Category:* B

HOW SUPPLIED

Tablets: 10 mg, 25 mg

ACTION

Mechanism: Acts peripherally, inhibiting norepinephrine release and depleting norepinephrine stores in adrenergic nerve endings.
Absorption: Rapidly and almost completely absorbed from the GI tract.
Distribution: Widely disributed in the body; about 20% protein-bound; does not enter the CNS.
Metabolism: Approximately 40% to 50% of a given dose is metabolized by the liver.
Excretion: Guanadrel and its metabolites are eliminated primarily in urine. Half-life: Varies widely; average about 10 hours.
Onset, peak, duration: Antihypertensive effect usually occurs at 30 minutes to 2 hours; peak effect occurs at 4 to 6 hours. Antihypertensive activity persists for 4 to 14 hours.

INDICATIONS & DOSAGE

Treatment of hypertension—
Adults: initially, 5 mg P.O. b.i.d. Dosage can be adjusted until blood pressure is controlled. Most patients require doses of 20 to 75 mg/day, usually given b.i.d.; however, tolerance to hypotensive effect may necessitate upward titration of dosage to 100 to 400 mg daily, given in three to four divided doses.

CONTRAINDICATIONS & PRECAUTIONS

Contraindicated in patients with hypersensitivity to the drug; in patients with known or suspected pheochromocytoma because guanadrel may increase sensitivity to circulating catecholamines; and in patients with CHF because the drug may interfere with normal sympathetic compensation.

Use cautiously in patients with bronchial asthma, peptic ulcer disease, or regional vascular disease because the drug may worsen these conditions.

ADVERSE REACTIONS

Common reactions are in italics; life-threatening reactions are in bold italics.
CNS: *fatigue, dizziness,* drowsiness, faintness.
CV: *orthostatic hypotension,* edema.
GI: diarrhea.
Other: impotence, ejaculation disturbances.

INTERACTIONS

MAO inhibitors, ephedrine, norepinephrine, methylphenidate, tricyclic antidepressants, amphetamines, phenothiazines: may inhibit the antihypertensive effect of guanadrel. Adjust dose accordingly.

EFFECTS ON DIAGNOSTIC TESTS

None reported.

NURSING CONSIDERATIONS

Besides those related universally to drug therapy (see "How to use this book"), consider the following specific recommendations:

Assessment

• Obtain a baseline assessment of the patient's lying and standing blood pressure and his pulse before beginning therapy.
• Be alert for adverse reactions and drug interactions throughout therapy.

• Evaluate the patient's and family's knowledge about guanadrel therapy.

Nursing Diagnoses

• Altered tissue perfusion (renal, cerebral, cardiopulmonary, peripheral) related to the patient's underlying condition.

• High risk for injury related to guanadrel-induced hypotension and CNS adverse reactions.

• Knowledge deficit related to guanadrel therapy.

Planning and Implementation

Preparation and Administration

• Do not give guanadrel concurrently or within 1 week of therapy with an MAO inhibitor.

• Remember that this drug should be discontinued 48 to 72 hours before surgery to minimize the risk of vascular collapse during anesthesia.

Monitoring

• Monitor the effectiveness of therapy by frequently checking the patient's blood pressure, pulse rate, and ECG.

• Monitor patient's supine and standing blood pressure, especially during periods of dosage adjustment. Patient response varies widely and dosage must be individualized. Also keep in mind that elderly patients are often more sensitive to drug's hypotensive effects.

• Institute safety measures until CNS and hypotensive effects of the drug are known. Keep bed side rails and assist the patient from a sitting or lying position to a standing position, as appropriate.

Supportive Care

• Administer this medication with a diuretic, if ordered. A diuretic is sometimes administered concurrently with this drug to decrease fluid retention.

Patient Teaching

• Explain the importance of taking this drug as prescribed, even when feeling well.

• Tell the patient not to discontinue the drug suddenly, even if unpleasant adverse reactions occur, but to call the doctor.

• Instruct the patient to check with the doctor or pharmacist before taking OTC medications, such as cough, cold, or allergy medications.

• Tell the patient to avoid strenuous exercise, and warn that hot showers may cause a hypotensive reaction.

• Teach the patient to minimize orthostatic hypotension by rising slowly from a supine position and by avoiding sudden position changes.

• Teach the patient and the family caregiver how to take blood pressure measurements. Stress the importance of checking patient's blood pressure at least once weekly during antihypertensive drug therapy.

• Tell the patient to report significant changes in blood pressure to the doctor.

• Tell the patient to avoid driving and other activities that require alertness until the CNS effects of the drug are known. Explain that this drug can cause fatigue and drowsiness.

Evaluation

In patients receiving guanadrel, appropriate evaluation statements may include:

• Blood pressure is within normal limits for this patient.

• Hypotension and CNS adverse reactions did not occur.

• Patient and family state an understanding of guanadrel therapy.

guanethidine sulfate

(gwahn eth´ i deen)

Apo-Guanethidine†, Ismelin

• *Classification:* antihypertensive (adrenergic neuron blocking agent)

• *Pregnancy Risk Category:* C

HOW SUPPLIED

Tablets: 10 mg, 25 mg

ACTION

Mechanism: Acts peripherally, inhibiting norepinephrine release and depleting norepinephrine stores in adrenergic nerve endings.
Absorption: Incompletely absorbed from the GI tract.
Distribution: Widley distributed throughout the body; it is not protein-bound but demonstrates extensive tissue binding.
Metabolism: Undergoes partial hepatic metabolism to pharmacologically less-active metabolites.
Excretion: Guanethidine and metabolites are excreted primarily in urine; small amounts are excreted in feces. Half-life: Elimination half-life after chronic administration is biphasic: initial half-life is 1½ days followed by a terminal elimination of 4 to 8 days.
Onset, peak, duration: Maximal effects appear 1 to 3 weeks after therapy begins.

INDICATIONS & DOSAGE

For moderate to severe hypertension; usually used in combination with other antihypertensives–
Adults: initially, 10 mg P.O. daily. Increase by 10 mg at weekly to monthly intervals, p.r.n. Usual dose is 25 to 50 mg daily. Some patients may require up to 300 mg.
Children: initially, 200 mcg/kg P.O. daily. Increase gradually q 1 to 3 weeks to maximum of 8 times initial dose.

CONTRAINDICATIONS & PRECAUTIONS

Contraindicated in patients with hypersensitivity to the drug; in patients with overt CHF not caused by hypertension, because the drug may interfere with normal sympathetic compensation; and in patients with pheochromocytoma because the drug may increase sensitivity to circulating catecholamines.

Use cautiously in patients with recent myocardial infarction, severe cardiac disease, cerebrovascular disease, peptic ulcer disease, impaired renal function, or bronchial asthma because the drug may precipitate or worsen these conditions.

ADVERSE REACTIONS

Common reactions are in italics; life-threatening reactions are in bold italics.
CNS: *dizziness, weakness, syncope.*
CV: *orthostatic hypotension, bradycardia,* CHF, arrhythmias.
EENT: *nasal stuffiness.*
GI: *diarrhea.*
Other: *edema, weight gain, inhibition of ejaculation.*

INTERACTIONS

Levodopa, alcohol: may increase hypotensive effect of guanethidine. Use together cautiously.
MAO inhibitors, ephedrine, norepinephrine, methylphenidate, tricyclic antidepressants, amphetamines, phenothiazines: may inhibit the antihypertensive effect of guanethidine. Adjust dose accordingly.

EFFECTS ON DIAGNOSTIC TESTS

None reported.

NURSING CONSIDERATIONS

Besides those related universally to drug therapy (see "How to use this book"), consider the following specific recommendations:

Assessment

- Obtain a baseline assessment of the patient's blood pressure before beginning therapy.
- Be alert for adverse reactions and drug interactions throughout therapy.
- Evaluate the patient's and family's knowledge about guanethidine sulfate therapy.

Nursing Diagnoses

- Altered tissue perfusion (renal, cerebral, cardiopulmonary, peripheral) related to the patient's underlying condition.

- High risk for injury related to orthostatic hypotension and guanethidine sulfate CNS adverse reactions.
- Knowledge deficit related to guanethidine sulfate therapy.

Planning and Implementation

Preparation and Administration

- Keep in mind that this drug should be discontinued 2 to 3 weeks before elective surgery to reduce the possibility of vascular collapse and cardiac arrest during anesthesia.
- ***P.O. use:*** If the patient has difficulty swallowing, crush the tablet and allow the patient to take the drug with the fluid of his choice.

Monitoring

- Monitor effectiveness by regularly checking the patient's blood pressure, pulse, and ECG.
- Monitor the patient's blood pressure in both the supine and standing positions during the initial dosage adjustment period to check for orthostatic hypotension. Keep in mind that elderly patients may be more sensitive to hypotensive effects.
- Monitor for CNS adverse reactions such as dizziness and weakness.
- Monitor the patient's weight regularly and observe for edema.

Supportive Care

- Keep in mind that the full antihypertensive effect of this drug may not appear for 2 to 3 weeks.
- If the patient experiences dizziness, weakness, or orthostatic hypotension, institute safety precautions: such as continuous use of side rails.
- Keep in mind that if the patient develops diarrhea, the doctor may prescribe atropine or paregoric.

Patient Teaching

- Explain the importance of taking this drug as prescribed even when feeling well.
- Tell the patient not to discontinue the drug suddenly but to call the doctor if unpleasant adverse reactions occur.
- Instruct the patient to check with the doctor or pharmacist before taking OTC drugs, such as cold or allergy remedies.
- Tell the patient to avoid strenuous exercise, and warn him that hot showers or a hot environment may cause hypotensive effects.
- Teach the patient how to follow a low-sodium diet, and explain that it can help decrease hypertension.
- Teach the patient or family caregiver to take blood pressure measurements. Tell them to notify the doctor of any significant changes.

Evaluation

In patients receiving guanethidine sulfate, appropriate evaluation statements may include:

- Blood pressure is controlled within normal limits for this patient.
- Orthostatic hypotension and CNS adverse reactions did not occur.
- Patient and family state an understanding of guanethidine sulfate therapy.

guanfacine hydrochloride

(gwahn´ fa seen)

Tenex

- *Classification:* antihypertensive (centrally acting antiadrenergic)
- *Pregnancy Risk Category:* B

HOW SUPPLIED

Tablets: 1 mg

ACTION

Mechanism: Inhibits the central vasomotor center, thereby decreasing sympathetic outflow.
Absorption: Well and completely absorbed after oral administration and is approximately 80% bioavailable.
Distribution: Approximately 70% protein-bound.
Metabolism: Hepatic.
Excretion: About 50% is eliminated in urine as unchanged drug, the re-

mainder as metabolites. Half-life: With normal renal function, the average half-life is about 17 hours (range 10 to 30 hours); 13 to 14 hours in younger patients. Older patients tend to have half-lives at the upper end of the range. Steady-state blood levels were obtained within 4 days in most subjects.
Onset, peak, duration: Peak plasma concentrations occur in 1 to 4 hours; average is about 2½ hours.

INDICATIONS & DOSAGE

Treatment of mild to moderate hypertension–
Adults: initially, 0.5 to 1 mg P.O. daily, h.s. Average dose is 1 to 3 mg daily.

CONTRAINDICATIONS & PRECAUTIONS

Contraindicated in patients with hypersensitivity to the drug.

Use cautiously in patients with cerebrovascular disease, coronary insufficiency, recent myocardial infarction (which may be aggravated by reduced blood pressure); chronic hepatic function impairment, or a history of mental depression.

ADVERSE REACTIONS

Common reactions are in italics; life-threatening reactions are in bold italics.
CNS: *drowsiness, dizziness,* fatigue, headache, insomnia.
CV: bradycardia, orthostatic hypotension, ***rebound hypertension.***
EENT: dry mouth.
GI: *constipation,* diarrhea, nausea.
Skin: dermatitis, pruritus.

INTERACTIONS

None significant.

EFFECTS ON DIAGNOSTIC TESTS

Plasma growth hormone: increased levels (after a single dose).
Urinary catecholamine: altered concentrations.
Urine vanillylmandelic acid (VMA): decreased excretion during therapy; possible increase on abrupt withdrawal.

NURSING CONSIDERATIONS

Besides those related universally to drug therapy (see "How to use this book"), consider the following specific recommendations:

Assessment

- Obtain a baseline assessment ofthe patient's blood pressure before beginning therapy.
- Be alert for adverse reactions and drug interactions throughout therapy.
- Evaluate the patient's and family's knowledge about guanfacine hydrochloride therapy.

Nursing Diagnoses

- Altered tissue perfusion (renal, cerebral, cardiopulmonary and peripheral) related to the patient's underlying condition.
- High risk for injury related to guanfacine-induced adverse reactions.
- Knowledge deficit related to guanfacine therapy.

Planning and Implementation

Preparation and Administration

- Keep in mind that guanfacine appears to be as effective as methyldopa and clonidine; a long half-life permits once-daily dosing.
- Remember that this drug may be given alone or with a diuretic.
- Give daily dose at bedtime to minimize daytime drowsiness.

Monitoring

- Monitor effectiveness by regularly checking the patient's blood pressure, pulse and ECG.
- Monitor patient's blood pressure in the supine and the standing position, during the initial dosage adjustment period to check for orthostatic hypotension.
- Monitor for CNS effects including dizziness and drowsiness and other adverse reactions.

Supportive Care
• If the patient experiences dizziness, drowsiness or orthostatic hypotension, institute safety precautions such as continuous use of side rails.
Patient Teaching
• Explain the importance of taking this drug as prescribed even when feeling well.
• Tell the patient not to discontinue the drug suddenly but to call the doctor if unpleasant adverse reactions occur.
• Instruct the patient to check with the doctor or pharmacist before taking OTC drugs such as cold or allergy remedies.
• Advise the patient to avoid activities that require alertness until response to the drug is established because this drug causes drowiness.
• Teach the patient and family caregiver how to take blood pressure measurements. Tell them to notify the doctor of a significant change in blood pressure.

Evaluation

In patients receiving guanfacine, appropriate evaluation statements may include:
• Blood pressure is controlled within normal limits for this patient.
• CNS adverse reactions did not occur.
• Patient and family state an understanding of guanfacine therapy.

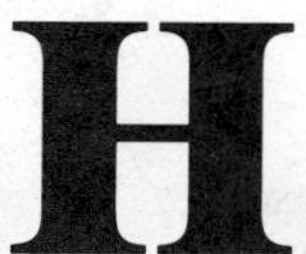

Haemophilus b conjugate vaccines (*Hemophilus* b conjugate vaccines)
(hem off′ il us)

Haemophilus b conjugate vaccine, diphtheria CRM_{197} protein conjugate
HibTITER

Haemophilus b conjugate vaccine, diphtheria toxoid conjugate
ProHIBiT

Haemophilus b conjugate vaccine, meningococcal protein conjugate
PedvaxHIB

• *Classification:* bacterial vaccine

HOW SUPPLIED

conjugate vaccine, diphtheria CRM_{197} protein conjugate
Injection: 10 mcg purified *Haemophilus* b saccharide and approximately 25 mcg CRM_{197} protein per 0.5 ml
conjugate vaccine, diphtheria toxoid conjugate
Injection: 25 mcg of *Haemophilus influenzae* type b (Hib) capsular polysaccharide and 18 mcg of diphtheria toxoid protein per 0.5 ml
conjugate vaccine, meningococcal protein conjugate
Powder for injection: 15 mcg *Haemophilus* b PRP, 250 mcg *Neisseria meningitidis* OMPC per dose

ACTION

Mechanism: Promotes active immunity to Hib.
Distribution: Limited data indicate that antibodies to *H. influenzae* type b can be detected in fetal blood and in breast milk after administration of the vaccine to pregnant and breast-feeding women.
Excretion: The vaccine polysaccharide has been detected in urine for up to 11 days after administration to children.
Onset, peak, duration: After I.M. or S.C. administration, increases in *H. influenzae* type b capsular antibody levels in serum are detectable in about 2 weeks and peak within 3 weeks.

INDICATIONS & DOSAGE

Immunization against Hib infection–
Children 15 months to 5 years: 0.5 ml I.M.

CONTRAINDICATIONS & PRECAUTIONS

Contraindicated in children with any febrile illness or active infection and in those with hypersensitivity to thimerosal, a component of some of the commercially available preparations (check package insert). Also contraindicated in children who are immunosuppressed or who are receiving immunosuppressive therapy.

ADVERSE REACTIONS

Common reactions are in italics; life-threatening reactions are in bold italics.
Systemic: fever, ***anaphylaxis.***
Local: *erythema and pain at injection site.*

INTERACTIONS

Immunosuppressive agents: may suppress antibody response to Hib vaccine.

EFFECTS ON DIAGNOSTIC TESTS

None reported.

NURSING CONSIDERATIONS

Besides those related universally to drug therapy (see "How to use this book"), consider the following specific recommendations:

Assessment

• Obtain a baseline assessment of allergies, immunization history, and reaction to immunization before therapy.
• Be alert for adverse reactions and drug interactions throughout therapy.
• Evaluate the patient's and family's knowledge about *Haemophilus* b conjugate vaccines therapy.

Nursing Diagnoses

• Altered protection related to lack of immunity to Hib infection.
• Ineffective breathing pattern related to vaccine-induced anaphylaxis.
• Knowledge deficit related to *Haemophilus* b conjugate vaccine.

Planning and Implementation

Preparation and Administration

• ***I.M. use:*** Do not administer intradermally or I.V.
• Inject in the anterolateral aspect of the upper thigh in small children. Injection may be made into the deltoid of larger children if sufficient muscle mass is present.
• This vaccine and diphtheria and tetanus toxoids and pertussis vaccine (DTP) can be given simultaneously, but should be administered in different sites.

Monitoring

• Monitor effectiveness by checking the patient's antibody titers to Hib infection.
• Observe patient for signs of anaphylaxis immediately after injection.
• Check vital signs.
• Observe injection site for local reaction to vaccine.

Supportive Care

• Do not administer vaccine during immunosuppressive therapy or during acute or febrile illness.
• Keep epinephrine 1:1,000 available in case of anaphylaxis. Have oxygen and resuscitation equipment nearby.
• Obtain order for antipyretic medication to alleviate vaccine-induced fever.
• Apply ice or cold compress to injection site to alleviate erythema and pain.
• Be aware that Hib is an important cause of meningitis in infants and preschool children.
• The conjugate vaccine is formed when Hib is chemically bound to other protein antigens. It produces a stronger immune response in most patients.
• This vaccine protects only against Hib infection; it will not protect against other microorganisms that cause meningitis.
• The vaccine is not routinely given to adults or children over age 5 unless they are at risk for infection (including patients with chronic conditions, such as functional asplenia, Hodgkin's disease, or sickle cell anemia, or those who have undergone splenectomy).

Patient Teaching

• Instruct parent to report respiratory difficulty or other signs of anaphylactic reaction immediately.
• Inform parents that slight fever, redness, and soreness at the injection site may occur.
• Advise the parent that children vaccinated with nonconjugated vaccine (no longer available in the United States) need not be routinely revaccinated if the primary immunization occurred at age 24 months. However, if the first vaccination occurred between ages 18 and 23 months, the child should be revaccinated with

conjugate vaccine, provided at least 2 months has elapsed.

Evaluation

In patients receiving *Haemophilus* b conjugate vaccine, appropriate evaluation statements may include:

• Patient exhibits active immunity to Hib infection.

• Patient demonstrates no signs and symptoms of anaphylaxis.

• Patient and family state an understanding of *Haemophilus* b conjugate vaccine.

halazepam

(hal az´ e pam)

Paxipam

• Controlled Substance Schedule IV

• *Classification:* anxiolytic (benzodiazepine)

• *Pregnancy Risk Category:* D

HOW SUPPLIED

Tablets: 20 mg, 40 mg

ACTION

Mechanism: Depresses the CNS at the limbic and subcortical levels of the brain.

Absorption: Well absorbed when administered orally.

Distribution: Widely distributed throughout the body. Drug is approximately 85% to 95% protein-bound.

Metabolism: In the liver to the active metabolite desmethyldiazepam.

Excretion: The metabolites are excreted in urine as glucuronide conjugates. Half-life: Halazepam, 14 hours; desmethyldiazepam, 30 to 200 hours.

Onset, peak, duration: Peak levels occur in 1 to 3 hours.

INDICATIONS & DOSAGE

Relief of anxiety and tension–

Adults: Usual dose is 20 to 40 mg P.O. t.i.d. or q.i.d. Optimal daily dosage is generally 80 to 160 mg. Daily dosages up to 600 mg have been given. In elderly or debilitated patients, initial dosage is 20 mg once or twice daily.

CONTRAINDICATIONS & PRECAUTIONS

Contraindicated in patients with hypersensitivity to the drug; in patients with acute narrow-angle glaucoma or untreated open-angle glaucoma because of the drug's possible anticholinergic effect; in shock or coma because the drug's hypnotic or hypotensive effect may be prolonged or intensified; and in patients with acute alcohol intoxication who have depressed vital signs because the drug will worsen CNS depression.

Use cautiously in patients with psychoses, because the drug is rarely beneficial in such patients and may induce paradoxical reactions; in patients with myasthenia gravis or Parkinson's disease because it may exacerbate these disorders; in patients with impaired renal or hepatic function, which prolongs elimination of the drug; in elderly or debilitated patients, who are usually more sensitive to the drug's CNS effects; and in individuals prone to addiction or drug abuse.

ADVERSE REACTIONS

Common reactions are in italics; life-threatening reactions are in bold italics.

CNS: *drowsiness, lethargy, hangover,* fainting.

CV: transient hypotension.

EENT: dry mouth.

GI: nausea and vomiting, discomfort.

INTERACTIONS

Alcohol, other CNS depressants: increased CNS depression. Avoid concomitant use.

Cimetidine: possible increased sedation. Monitor carefully.

EFFECTS ON DIAGNOSTIC TESTS

EEG: changes (low-voltage, fast activity) during and after therapy.
Liver function tests: elevated results.

NURSING CONSIDERATIONS

Besides those related universally to drug therapy (see "How to use this book"), consider the following specific recommendations:

Assessment

- Obtain a baseline assessment of the patient's anxiety before therapy.
- Be alert for adverse reactions and drug interactions throughout therapy.
- Evaluate the patient's and family's knowledge about halazepam therapy.

Nursing Diagnoses

- Anxiety related to the patient's underlying condition.
- High risk for injury related to drug-induced CNS reactions.
- Knowledge deficit related to halazepam therapy.

Planning and Implementation

Preparation and Administration

- Dosage should be reduced in elderly or debilitated patients who may be more susceptible to CNS reactions from the drug.
- Know that drug should not be prescribed for everyday stress.
- Halazepam is not recommended for long-term use (> 4 months).

Monitoring

- Monitor for adverse reactions or drug interactions by frequently checking the patient's vital signs for hypotension.
- Regularly monitor effectiveness by asking the patient about feelings of anxiety and by observing the patient's behavior.
- Monitor the patient for adverse reactions by monitoring the degree of dry mouth.
- Monitor for drug interactions by observing for excessive sedation due to potentiation by other CNS drugs.
- Monitor hydration status if patient develops nausea and vomiting.

Supportive Care

- Provide frequent sips of water or ice chips for dry mouth.
- If patient experiences drowsiness, light-headedness, lethargy, or fainting, institute safety measures, such as supervising patient activities. Reorient patient as needed and ensure a safe environment.
- Be aware that drug should not be prescribed for everyday stress.
- Do not withdraw drug abruptly. Abuse or addiction is possible and withdrawal symptoms may occur. Provide additional fluids if patient develops nausea and vomiting.

Patient Teaching

- Suggest sugarless hard candy, ice chips, or gum to relieve dry mouth.
- Warn the patient not to combine drug with alcohol or other CNS depressants and to avoid driving and other hazardous activities that require alertness and psychomotor coordination until adverse CNS effects of the drug are known.
- Warn the patient against giving medication to others.
- Warn the patient to take this drug only as directed and not to discontinue taking it without the doctor's approval. Inform the patient of the drug's potential for dependence if taken longer than directed.

Evaluation

In patients receiving halazepam, appropriate evaluation statements may include:

- Patient states he is less anxious.
- Patient does not experience injury as a result of adverse CNS reactions.
- Patient and family state an understanding of halazepam therapy.

halcinonide

(hal sin´ oh nide)
Halciderm, Halog

- *Classification:* topical anti-inflammatory (adrenocorticoid)
- *Pregnancy Risk Category:* C

HOW SUPPLIED

Cream: 0.025%, 0.1%
Ointment: 0.1%
Topical solution: 0.1%

ACTION

Mechanism: Diffuses across cell membranes and complexes with specific cytoplasmic receptors.
Absorption: The amount of drug absorbed depends on the amount applied and on the nature of the skin at the application site. It is lowest in areas with thick stratum corneum (on the palms, soles, elbows, and knees) and higher in thinner areas (face, eyelids, and genitals). Absorption increases in areas of skin damage, inflammation, or occlusion. Some systemic absorption of topical steroids may occur, especially through the oral mucosa.
Distribution: After topical application, distributed throughout the local skin. If absorbed into the circulation, it is rapidly removed from the blood and distributed into muscle, liver, skin, intestines, and kidneys.
Metabolism: After topical administration, metabolized primarily in the skin. The small amount absorbed into systemic circulation is metabolized primarily in the liver to inactive compounds.
Excretion: Inactive metabolites are excreted by the kidneys, primarily as glucuronides and sulfates, but also as unconjugated products. Small amounts of the metabolites are also excreted in feces.

INDICATIONS & DOSAGE

Inflammation of acute and chronic corticosteroid-responsive dermatoses–
Adults and children: clean area; apply cream, ointment, or solution sparingly b.i.d. or t.i.d.

CONTRAINDICATIONS & PRECAUTIONS

Contraindicated in patients who are hypersensitive to any component of the preparation and in patients with viral, fungal, or tubercular skin lesions. Use with extreme caution in patients with impaired circulation because the drug may increase the risk of skin ulceration. Avoid using on the face or genital areas because increased absorption may result in striae.

ADVERSE REACTIONS

Common reactions are in italics; life-threatening reactions are in bold italics.
Skin: burning, itching, irritation, dryness, folliculitis, hypertrichosis, hypopigmentation, acneiform eruptions, allergic contact dermatitis. With occlusive dressings: *maceration of skin, secondary infection, atrophy, striae, miliaria.*

INTERACTIONS

None significant.

EFFECTS ON DIAGNOSTIC TESTS

None reported.

NURSING CONSIDERATIONS

Besides those related universally to drug therapy (see "How to use this book"), consider the following specific recommendations:
Assessment
- Obtain a baseline assessment of patient's skin integrity before halcinonide therapy.
- Be alert for adverse reactions and drug interactions throughout therapy.

• Evaluate the patient's and family's knowledge about halcinonide therapy.

Nursing Diagnoses

• Impaired skin integrity related to the patient's underlying condition.
• High risk for infection related to drug-induced adverse reaction.
• Knowledge deficit related to halcinonide therapy.

Planning and Implementation

Preparation and Administration

• Read order and drug labels carefully.
• Wear gloves when administering drug.
• ***Topical use:*** Before applying, gently wash the patient's skin. Apply a thin layer of medication and rub in gently.
• When treating hairy sites, part hair and apply directly to lesion.
• To apply an occlusive dressing (only if ordered by doctor), apply cream heavily, then cover with a thin, pliable, nonflammable plastic film; seal to adjacent normal skin with hypoallergenic tape.
• To prevent recurrence, treatment should continue for a few days after clearing of lesions.

Monitoring

• Monitor effectiveness by regularly assessing skin for extent and severity of inflammation.
• Monitor for hypersensitivity reaction to halcinonide.
• Monitor for signs of secondary infection.
• Frequently assess the patient's skin for burning, itching, and dryness.
• Monitor patient who must use occlusive dressings for maceration of the skin and secondary infection.

Supportive Care

• To minimize adverse reactions, use occlusive dressing intermittently. Don't use occlusive dressings in the presence of infection or on weeping or exudative lesions, and don't leave in place longer than 16 hours each day.
• For patients with eczematous dermatitis who may develop irritation with adhesive material, hold dressing in place with gauze, elastic bandage, or stockings.
• Notify the doctor and remove occlusive dressing if fever develops.
• Withhold the drug and notify the doctor if hypersensitivity reaction or infection occurs.
• Have the patient's fingernails cut short to minimize skin trauma from scratching.
• Apply cool, moist compresses to involved areas to relieve itching and burning.

Patient Teaching

• Instruct the patient to cleanse involved area before applying halcinonide in a thin layer to cover the entire surface.
• Teach the patient how to apply an occlusive dressing.
• Teach the patient and family how to recognize signs of a hypersensitivity reaction or infection. Advise them to discontinue the drug and notify the doctor immediately if these occur.
• Instruct the patient to complete the entire treatment regimen as prescribed, even if the lesions appear to have healed.
• Tell the patient and family not to share the halcinonide prescription with others.

Evaluation

In patients receiving halcinonide, appropriate evaluation statements may include:

• Patient's skin maintains integrity.
• Patient does not develop secondary infection.
• Patient and family state an understanding of halcinonide therapy.

---

haloperidol

(ha loe per´ i dole)

Apo-Haloperidol†, Haldol**, Halperon, Novoperidol†, Peridol†, Serenace‡

haloperidol decanoate
Haldol Decanoate, Haldol LA†

haloperidol lactate
Haldol

- *Classification:* antipsychotic (butyrophenone)
- *Pregnancy Risk Category:* C

HOW SUPPLIED
haloperidol
Tablets: 0.5 mg, 1 mg, 2 mg, 5 mg, 10 mg, 20 mg
haloperidol decanoate
Injection: 50 mg/ml
haloperidol lactate
Oral concentrate: 2 mg/ml
Injection: 5 mg/ml

ACTION
Mechanism: A butyrophenone that blocks postsynaptic dopamine receptors in the brain.
Absorption: Rate and extent of absorption vary with route of administration: oral tablet absorption yields 60% to 70% bioavailability. I.M. dose is 70% absorbed within 30 minutes.
Distribution: Widely distributed into the body, with high concentrations in adipose tissue. Drug is 91% to 99% protein-bound.
Metabolism: Extensively metabolized by the liver; there may be only one active metabolite that is less active than the parent drug.
Excretion: About 40% of a given dose is excreted in urine within 5 days; about 15% is excreted in feces via the biliary tract. Half-life: About 3 weeks.
Onset, peak, duration: Peak plasma levels after oral administration occur at 2 to 6 hours; after I.M. administration, 30 to 45 minutes; and after long-acting I.M. (decanoate) administration, 4 to 11 days.

INDICATIONS & DOSAGE
Psychotic disorders–
Adults: dosage varies for each patient. Initial range is 0.5 to 5 mg P.O. b.i.d. or t.i.d.; or 2 to 5 mg I.M. q 4 to 8 hours, increasing rapidly if necessary for prompt control. Maximum dosage is 100 mg P.O. daily. Doses over 100 mg have been used for patients with severely resistant conditions.
Chronic psychotic patients who require prolonged therapy–
Adults: 50 to 100 mg I.M. haloperidol decanoate q 4 weeks.
Control of tics, vocal utterances in Gilles de la Tourette's syndrome–
Adults: 0.5 to 5 mg P.O. b.i.d. or t.i.d., increasing p.r.n.

CONTRAINDICATIONS & PRECAUTIONS
Contraindicated in patients with hypersensitivity to haloperidol, phenothiazines, and related compounds, including that expressed by jaundice because haloperidol may impair liver function; blood dyscrasias and bone marrow depression because *agranulocytosis* can occur; disorders accompanied by coma, brain damage, or CNS depression because of additive CNS depression; and in circulatory collapse or cerebrovascular disease because of the drug's hypotensive and arrhythmogenic effects.

Use cautiously in patients with cardiac disease (arrhythmias, CHF, angina pectoris, valvular disease, or heart block), encephalitis, Reye's syndrome, head injury, respiratory disease, seizure disorders, glaucoma, prostatic hypertrophy, urinary retention, hepatic or renal dysfunction, Parkinson's disease, pheochromocytoma, or hypocalcemia.

ADVERSE REACTIONS
Common reactions are in italics; life-threatening reactions are in bold italics.

Blood: transient leukopenia and leukocytosis.
CNS: *high incidence of severe extrapyramidal reactions, tardive dyskinesia,* low incidence of sedation.
CV: low incidence of cardiovascular effects with therapeutic dosages.
EENT: *blurred vision, dry mouth.*
GU: urine retention, menstrual irregularities, gynecomastia.
Skin: rash.
Other: rarely, ***neuroleptic malignant syndrome*** (fever, tachycardia, tachypnea, profuse diaphoresis).

INTERACTIONS

Alcohol, other CNS depressants: increased CNS depression. Avoid concomitant use.
Lithium: lethargy and confusion with high doses. Observe patient.
Methyldopa: possible symptoms of dementia. Observe patient.

EFFECTS ON DIAGNOSTIC TESTS

ECG: quinidine-like effects.

NURSING CONSIDERATIONS

Besides those related universally to drug therapy (see "How to use this book"), consider the following specific recommendations:

Assessment

- Obtain a baseline assessment of the patient's mental status, including psychotic symptoms, before therapy.
- Be alert for adverse reactions and drug interactions throughout therapy.
- Evaluate the patient's and family's knowledge about haloperidol therapy.

Nursing Diagnoses

- Impaired thought processes related to the patient's underlying condition.
- Impaired physical mobility related to high risk for extrapyramidal effects.
- Knowledge deficit related to haloperidol therapy.

Planning and Implementation

Preparation and Administration

- When changing from tablets to decanoate injection, patient should receive 10 to 15 times the oral dose once a month (maximum 100 mg).
- Don't administer the decanoate form I.V.
- Protect medication from light. Slight yellowing of injection or concentrate is common and does not affect potency. Discard markedly discolored solutions.
- Dose of 2 mg is therapeutic equivalent of 100 mg of chlorpromazine.
- Elderly patients usually require lower initial dosage and more gradual dosage titration.

Monitoring

- Monitor effectiveness by regularly observing the patient's behavior and noting changes in psychotic symptoms.
- Monitor for extrapyramidal and anticholinergic effects (blurred vision, dry mouth, constipation, urine retention) and tardive dyskinesia during prolonged therapy.
- Monitor for drug interactions if the patient is also receiving alcohol or other CNS depressants, lithium, or methyldopa.

Supportive Care

- Do not withdraw drug abruptly unless required by severe adverse reactions.
- Assist the patient with ambulation and daily activities if extrapyramidal symptoms occur. Notify doctor of symptoms and expect to implement change of drug or dosage.
- Expect to treat dystonic reactions with I.V. diphenhydramine.
- Institute safety precautions if the patient develops blurred vision.

Patient Teaching

- Tell the patient to take drug exactly as prescribed and not to double doses to compensate for missed ones.
- Warn the patient to avoid alcohol and other CNS depressants during

haloperidol therapy because their combined use causes excessive CNS depression.

- Advise the patient to avoid driving and other hazardous activities that require alertness or normal vision until full effect of the drug is known.
- Recommend sugarless hard candy, chewing gum, or ice chips to relieve dry mouth.

Evaluation

In patients receiving haloperidol, appropriate evaluation statements may include:

- Patient demonstrates decreased psychotic behavior.
- Patient maintains physical mobility.
- Patient and family state an understanding of haloperidol therapy.

haloprogin

(ha loe proe´ jin)

Halotex

- *Classification:* topical antifungal
- *Pregnancy Risk Category:* B

HOW SUPPLIED

Cream: 1%
Topical solution: 1%

ACTION

Mechanism: Unknown. Drug has fungistatic and fungicidal activity.
Pharmacokinetics: Unknown.

INDICATIONS & DOSAGE

Superficial fungal infections (tinea pedis, tinea cruris, tinea corporis, tinea manuum, and tinea versicolor) –
Adults and children: apply liberally b.i.d. for 2 to 3 weeks.

CONTRAINDICATIONS & PRECAUTIONS

Contraindicated in patients with hypersensitivity to the drug.

ADVERSE REACTIONS

Common reactions are in italics; life-threatening reactions are in bold italics.
Skin: burning sensation, irritation, vesicle formation, increased maceration, *pruritus or exacerbation of preexisting lesions.*

INTERACTIONS

None significant.

EFFECTS ON DIAGNOSTIC TESTS

None reported.

NURSING CONSIDERATIONS

Besides those related universally to drug therapy (see "How to use this book"), consider the following specific recommendations:

Assessment

- Obtain a baseline assessment of skin color or drainage before therapy.
- Be alert for adverse reactions and drug interactions throughout therapy.
- Evaluate the patient's and family's knowledge about haloprogin therapy.

Nursing Diagnoses

- Impaired skin integrity related to patient's underlying condition.
- High risk for impaired skin integrity related to haloprogin-induced exacerbation of lesions.
- Knowledge deficit related to haloprogin therapy.

Planning and Implementation

Preparation and Administration

- ***Topical use:*** Cleanse area before application. Apply liberally.

Monitoring

- Monitor effectiveness by regularly checking affected area for erythema or drainage.
- Monitor for pruritus or exacerbation of preexisting lesions. Notify doctor if these occur.

Supportive Care

- Remember, diagnosis should be reconsidered if no improvement is seen in 4 weeks.
- Avoid contact of drug with the eyes.

Patient Teaching
• Teach patient how to apply medication.
• Tell patient to notify doctor if increased irritation occurs.
• Instruct patient to continue using for full treatment period prescribed, even if condition has improved.

Evaluation
In patients receiving haloprogin therapy, appropriate evaluation statements may include:
• Infection has resolved.
• Lesions did not occur.
• Patient and family state an understanding of haloprogin therapy.

heparin calcium
(hep´ a rin)
Calcilean†, Calciparine, Caprin‡, Uniparin-Ca‡

heparin sodium
Hepalean†, Heparin Lock Flush Solution (Tubex), Hep Lock, Liquaemin Sodium, Uniparin‡

• *Classification:* anticoagulant (blood derivative)
• *Pregnancy Risk Category:* C

HOW SUPPLIED
Products are derived from bovine lung or porcine intestinal mucosa.
heparin calcium
Ampule: 12,500 units/0.5 ml; 20,000 units/0.8 ml
Syringe: 5,000 units/0.2 ml
heparin sodium
Carpuject: 5,000 units/ml
Disposable syringes: 1,000 units/ml, 2,500 units/ml, 5,000 units/ml, 7,500 units/ml, 10,000 units/ml, 20,000 units/ml, 40,000 units/ml
Premixed I.V. solutions: 1,000 units in 500 ml normal saline solution; 2,000 units in 1,000 ml normal saline solution; 12,500 units in 250 ml 0.45% saline solution; 25,000 units in 250 ml 0.45% saline solution; 25,000 units in 500 ml 0.45% saline solution; 10,000 units in 100 ml 5% dextrose in water (D_5W); 12,500 units in 250 ml D_5W; 25,000 units in 250 ml D_5W; 25,000 units in 500 ml D_5W
Unit-dose ampules: 1,000 units/ml, 5,000 units/ml, 10,000 units/ml
Vials: 1,000 units/ml, 2,500 units/ml, 5,000 units/ml, 7,500 units/ml, 10,000 units/ml, 15,000 units/ml, 20,000 units/ml, 40,000 units/ml
heparin sodium flush
Disposable syringes: 10 units/ml, 100 units/ml
Vials: 10 units/ml, 100 units/ml

ACTION
Mechanism: Accelerates formation of an antithrombin III–thrombin complex. It inactivates thrombin and prevents conversion of fibrinogen to fibrin.
Absorption: Not absorbed from the GI tract; must be given parenterally. Absorption after deep S.C. administration is highly variable; preliminary studies indicate that the extent and rate of absorption of heparin calcium is lower.
Distribution: Extensively bound to lipoprotein, globulins, and fibrinogen; it does not cross the placenta.
Metabolism: Though metabolism is not completely described, heparin is thought to be removed by the reticuloendothelial system, with some metabolism occurring in the liver.
Excretion: Little is known; a small fraction is excreted in urine as unchanged drug. Drug is not excreted into breast milk. Half-life: Plasma half-life is between 1 and 2 hours.
Onset, peak, duration: After I.V. use, onset of action is almost immediate; after S.C. injection, onset of action occurs in 20 minutes to 1 hour.

INDICATIONS & DOSAGE

Treatment of deep vein thrombosis, myocardial infarction–
Adults: initially, 5,000 to 7,500 units I.V. push, then adjust dose according to PTT results and give dose I.V. q 4 hours (usually 4,000 to 5,000 units); or 5,000 to 7,500 units I.V. bolus, then 1,000 units/hour by I.V. infusion pump. Wait 8 hours following bolus dose, and adjust hourly rate according to PTT.
Treatment of pulmonary embolism–
Adults: initially, 7,500 to 10,000 units I.V. push, then adjust dose according to PTT results and give dose I.V. q 4 hours (usually 4,000 to 5,000 units); or 7,500 to 10,000 units I.V. bolus, then 1,000 units hourly by I.V. infusion pump. Wait 8 hours following bolus dose, and adjust hourly rate according to PTT.
Prophylaxis of embolism–
Adults: 5,000 units S.C. q 12 hours.
Open heart surgery–
Adults: (total body perfusion) 150 to 300 units/kg continuous I.V infusion.
Treatment of pulmonary emboli; prevention and treatment of deep vein thrombosis–
Children: initially, 50 units/kg I.V. drip. Maintenance dose is 100 units/kg I.V. drip q 4 hours. Constant infusion: 20,000 units/m^2 daily. Dosages adjusted according to PTT.
As an I.V. flush to maintain patency of I.V. indwelling catheters–
10 to 100 units as an I.V. flush. Not intended for therapeutic use.

Heparin dosing is highly individualized, depending upon disease state, age, renal and hepatic status.

CONTRAINDICATIONS AND PRECAUTIONS

Conditionally contraindicated in patients with active bleeding; blood dyscrasias; or bleeding tendencies, such as hemophilia, thrombocytopenia, or hepatic disease with hypoprothrombinemia; suspected intracranial hemorrhage; suppurative thrombophlebitis; inaccessible ulcerative lesions (especially of GI tract); open ulcerative wounds; extensive denudation of skin; ascorbic acid deficiency and other conditions causing increased capillary permeability; subacute bacterial endocarditis; shock; advanced renal disease; threatened abortion; or severe hypertension; during or after brain, eye, or spinal cord surgery; and during continuous tube drainage of stomach or small intestine. Although the use of heparin is clearly hazardous in these conditions, a decision to use it depends on the comparative risk of failure to treat the coexisting thromboembolic disorder.

Use cautiously during menses; in patients with mild hepatic or renal disease, or alcoholism; in patients in occupations with the risk of physical injury; immediately postpartum; and in patients with history of allergies, asthma, or GI ulcers.

ADVERSE REACTIONS

Common reactions are in italics; life-threatening reactions are in bold italics.
Blood: ***hemorrhage with excessive dosage,*** *overly prolonged clotting time, thrombocytopenia.*
Local: irritation, mild pain.
Other: ***"white clot" syndrome,*** hypersensitivity including chills, fever, pruritus, rhinitis, burning of feet, conjunctivitis, lacrimation, arthralgia, urticaria.

INTERACTIONS

Anticoagulants, oral: additive anticoagulation. Monitor prothrombin time and partial thromboplastin time.
Salicylates: increased anticoagulant effect. Don't use together.

EFFECTS ON DIAGNOSTIC TESTS

Partial thromboplastin time: prolonged.
AST (SGOT), ALT (SGPT), serum thyroxine levels: false elevations.

NURSING CONSIDERATIONS

Besides those related universally to drug therapy (see "How to use this book"), consider the following specific recommendations:

Assessment

• Obtain a baseline assessment of blood pressure, serum electrolytes, APTT, PT, hematocrit, and platelet count before heparin therapy.

• Be alert for adverse reactions and drug interactions throughout therapy.

• Evaluate the patient's and family's knowledge about heparin therapy.

Nursing Diagnoses

• Altered tissue perfusion (renal, cerebral, cardiopulmonary, GI, peripheral) related to the patient's underlying condition.

• High risk for fluid volume deficit related to adverse effects of heparin therapy.

• Knowledge deficit related to heparin therapy.

Planning and Implementation

Preparation and Administration

• ***I.V. use:*** Direct injection: Give diluted or undiluted drug through intermittent infusion device or into I.V. tubing containing a free-flowing compatible solution.

• Intermittent infusion: Give drug diluted or undiluted in 50 to 100 ml of 0.9% sodium chloride solution. Using an infusion pump, administer through a peripheral or central venous line over prescribed duration. Draw blood 30 minutes before next scheduled dose to avoid a falsely prolonged partial thromboplastin time (PTT).

• Continuous infusion: Using an infusion pump, give diluted solution over 24 hours. Blood for PTT can be drawn anytime after 8 hours of initiation of continuous I.V. heparin therapy. Do not draw blood from the infusion tubing or the vein used for infusion. Always draw blood from the other arm.

• I.V. heparin should be given on time; try not to skip a dose or "catch up" with an I.V. containing heparin.

• Do not piggyback other drugs into an infusion line while a heparin infusion is running; many drugs, including antibiotics, inactivate heparin. Never mix any drug with heparin in a syringe when bolus therapy is used. Remember that concentrated heparin solutions (greater than 100 units/ml) can irritate blood vessels.

• ***S.C. injection:*** Give the low-dose injection sequentially between iliac crests in lower abdomen deep into subcutaneous fat. Inject drug slowly subcutaneously into fat pad. Leave needle in place for 10 seconds after injection; then withdraw needle. Alternate site every 12 hours right for a.m., left for p.m. Don't massage the injection site. Check the site for bleeding. I.M. injection is not recommended.

• ***I.M. use:*** Try to avoid excessive I.M. injections to prevent or minimize hematomas. If possible, do not give I.M. injections.

Monitoring

• Monitor effectiveness by regularly checking PTT or APTT (activated partial thromboplastin time).

• Monitor platelet counts regularly. Notify the doctor of any thrombocytopenia. Arterial thrombosis known as "white clot" syndrome may be associated with thrombocytopenia caused by heparin.

• Check the patient for bleeding gums, bruises on arms or legs, petechiae, nosebleeds, melena, tarry stools, hematuria, and hematemesis.

Supportive Care

• Check continuous and intermittent heparin infusions regularly to ensure proper infusion rate. Use an infusion pump for maximum safety.

• Place a notice above the patient's bed to remind team members to apply pressure dressings after taking blood.

• Be aware that abrupt withdrawal may cause increased coagulability. Heparin therapy is usually followed by oral anticoagulant prophylaxis.
Patient Teaching
• Tell the patient to report signs of bleeding, such as bleeding gums, bruises on arms or legs, petechiae, nosebleeds, melena, tarry stools, hematuria, and hematemesis, immediately.
• Tell the patient to avoid OTC medications containing aspirin, other salicylates, or drugs that may interact with heparin.
Evaluation
In patients receiving heparin, appropriate evaluation statements may include:
• Patient's PTT or APTT are reflective of the goal of the heparin therapy.
• Patient has not experienced a hemorrhagic fluid volume deficit related to heparin therapy.
• Patient and family state an understanding of heparin therapy.

hepatitis B immune globulin, human
(hep ah ty´ tiss)
H-BIG, Hep-B-Gammagee, HyperHep

• *Classification:* hepatitis B prophylaxis (immune serum)
• *Pregnancy Risk Category:* C

HOW SUPPLIED
Injection: 1-ml, 4-ml, 5-ml vials

ACTION
Mechanism: Provides passive immunity to hepatitis B.
Absorption: Slowly absorbed after I.M. injection.
Distribution: Probably does not cross the placenta or distribute into breast milk.
Excretion: Half-life: The serum half-life for antibodies to HB_sAg is reportedly 21 days.
Onset, peak, duration: Antibodies to hepatitis B surface antigen (HB_sAg) appear in serum within 1 to 6 days, peak within 3 to 11 days, and persist for about 2 to 6 months.

INDICATIONS & DOSAGE
Hepatitis B exposure—
Adults and children: 0.06 ml/kg I.M. within 7 days after exposure. Repeat 28 days after exposure.
Neonates born to women who test positive for hepatitis B surface antigen (HB_sAg): 0.5 ml within 12 hours of birth. Repeat dose at ages 3 months and 6 months.

CONTRAINDICATIONS & PRECAUTIONS
Contraindicated in patients with hypersensitivity to thimerosal, a component of this immune serum.

ADVERSE REACTIONS
Common reactions are in italics; life-threatening reactions are in bold italics.
Systemic: ***anaphylaxis.***

INTERACTIONS
Other vaccines: Hepatitis B immune globulin may interfere with response to live virus vaccines. Defer administration for 3 months.

EFFECTS ON DIAGNOSTIC TESTS
None reported.

NURSING CONSIDERATIONS
Besides those related universally to drug therapy (see "How to use this book"), consider the following specific recommendations:
Assessment
• Obtain a baseline assessment of the patient's allergies and reaction to immunization before therapy.
• Be alert for adverse reactions and drug interactions throughout therapy.
• Evaluate the patient's and family's

knowledge about hepatitis B immune globulin therapy.

Nursing Diagnoses

• Altered protection related to lack of immunity to hepatitis B.
• Ineffective breathing pattern related to immunization-induced anaphylaxis.
• Knowledge deficit related to hepatitis B immune globulin.

Planning and Implementation

Preparation and Administration

• ***I.M. use:*** Give in anterolateral aspect of thigh or deltoid areas in adults. Give in anterolateral aspect of thigh in neonates and children under 3 years.

Monitoring

• Monitor effectiveness by checking the patient's antibody titers.
• Observe the patient for signs of anaphylaxis immediately after injection.
• Check vital signs.

Supportive Care

• Keep epinephrine 1:1000 available in case of anaphylaxis. Have oxygen and resuscitation equipment nearby.
• Health care personnel should receive immunization if exposed to hepatitis B (needle stick, direct contact).

Patient Teaching

• Instruct the patient to report respiratory difficulty immediately.
• Advise the patient that immunization should take place no longer than 7 days after exposure with a booster 28 days after exposure.

Evaluation

In patients receiving hepatitis B immune globulin, appropriate evaluation statements may include:

• Patient exhibits passive immunity to hepatitis B.
• Patient demonstrates no signs of anaphylaxis.
• Patient and family state an understanding of hepatitis B immune globulin.

hepatitis B vaccine, recombinant

(hep ah ty´ tiss)

Engerix-B, Recombivax HB

• *Classification:* hepatitis B prophylaxis (vaccine)
• *Pregnancy Risk Category:* C

HOW SUPPLIED

recombinant form

Injection: 5 mcg HB_sAg/0.5 ml (Recombivax HB, pediatric injection); 10 mcg HB_sAg/0.5 ml (Engerix-B, pediatric injection); 10 mcg HB_sAg/ml (Recombivax HB); 20 mcg HB_sAg/ml (Engerix-B); 40 mcg HB_sAg/ml (Recombivax HB Dialysis Formulation)

ACTION

Mechanism: Promotes active immunity to hepatitis B.

Onset, peak, duration: After I.M. administration, antibody to HB_sAg appears in serum within about 2 weeks, peaks after 6 months and persists for at least 3 years.

INDICATIONS & DOSAGE

Immunization against infection from all known subtypes of hepatitis B; primary preexposure prophylaxis against hepatitis B; or postexposure prophylaxis (when given with hepatitis B immune globulin)–

Recombinant form (Engerix-B)

Adults and children over 10 years: initially, give 20 mcg (1-ml adult formulation) I.M., followed by a second dose of 20 mcg I.M. 30 days later. Give a third dose of 20 mcg I.M. 6 months after the initial dose.

Neonates and children up to 10 years: initially, give 10 mcg (0.5-ml pediatric formulation) I.M., followed by a second dose of 10 mcg I.M. 30 days later. Give a third dose of

10 mcg I.M. 6 months after the initial dose.
Adults undergoing dialysis or receiving immunosuppressant therapy: initially, give 40 mcg I.M. (divided into two 20-mcg doses and administered at different sites). Follow with a second dose of 40 mcg I.M. in 30 days, and a final dose of 40 mcg I.M. 6 months after the initial dose.

Note: Certain populations (neonates born to infected mothers, persons recently exposed to the virus, and travelers to high-risk areas) may receive the vaccine on an abbreviated schedule, with the initial dose followed by a second dose in 1 month, and the third dose after 2 months. For prolonged maintenance of protective antibody titers, a booster dose is recommended 12 months after the initial dose.

Recombinant form (Recombivax HB)
Adults: initially, give 10 mcg (1-ml adult formulation) I.M., followed by a second dose of 10 mcg I.M. 30 days later. Give a third dose of 10 mcg I.M. 6 months after the initial dose.
Children 11 to 19 years: initially, give 5 mcg (0.5-ml pediatric formulation) I.M., followed by a second dose of 5 mcg I.M. 30 days later. Give a third dose of 5 mcg I.M. 6 months after the initial dose.
Neonates (born to HB_sAg-negative mothers) and children to 11 years: initially, give 2.5 mcg (0.25-ml pediatric formulation) I.M., followed by a second dose of 2.5 mcg I.M. 30 days later. Give a third dose of 2.5 mcg I.M. 6 months after the initial dose.
Neonates born to HB_sAg-positive mothers: initially, give 5 mcg (0.5-ml pediatric formulation) I.M., followed by a second dose of 5 mcg I.M. 30 days later. Give a third dose of 5 mcg I.M. 6 months after the initial dose.
Adults undergoing dialysis or receiving immunosuppressant therapy: initially, give 40 mcg I.M. (use dialysis formulation, which contains 40 mcg/ml). Follow with a second dose of 40 mcg I.M. in 30 days, and give a final dose of 40 mcg I.M. 6 months after the initial dose.

CONTRAINDICATIONS & PRECAUTIONS

Contraindicated in patients with hypersensitivity to thimerosal, a component of the vaccine. (Some clinicians will use the vaccine cautiously in these persons.) Use cautiously in patients with any serious, active infection; in patients with compromised cardiac or pulmonary status; and in those for whom a febrile or systemic reaction could pose a serious risk.

ADVERSE REACTIONS

Common reactions are in italics; life-threatening reactions are in bold italics.
Systemic: slight fever, transient malaise, headache, dizziness, nausea, vomiting, flu-like symptoms, myalgia.
Local: discomfort at injection site, local inflammation.

INTERACTIONS

None reported.

EFFECTS ON DIAGNOSTIC TESTS

None reported.

NURSING CONSIDERATIONS

Besides those related universally to drug therapy (see "How to use this book"), consider the following specific recommendations:
Assessment
- Obtain a baseline assessment of allergies, immunization history, and reaction to immunization before therapy.
- Be alert for adverse reactions and drug interactions throughout therapy.
- Evaluate the patient's and family's knowledge about hepatitis B vaccine.

Nursing Diagnoses
• Altered protection related to lack of immunity to hepatitis.
• Hyperthermia related to vaccine-induced fever.
• Knowledge deficit related to hepatitis B vaccine immunization.

Planning and Implementation
Preparation and Administration
• Thoroughly agitate vial just before administration to restore suspension.
• Store both open and unopened vials in the refrigerator. Do not freeze.
• ***I.M. use:*** The Centers for Disease Control reports that response to hepatitis B vaccine is significantly better when administered intramuscularly in the arm rather than the buttock.
• ***S.C. use:*** The vaccine may be administered S.C. but only to persons, such as hemophiliacs, who are at risk of hemorrhage.

Monitoring
• Monitor effectiveness by checking the patient's antibody titers to hepatitis.
• Observe injection site for local reaction.
• Monitor patient's temperature for vaccine-induced fever.
• Observe for signs of anaphylactic reaction to the vaccine.

Supportive Care
• Recombivax HB and Engerix-B are manufactured by recombinant DNA technology. Human plasma is *not* used.
• Use cautiously in patients with any serious, active infections; compromised cardiac or pulmonary status; and in those for whom a febrile or systemic reaction could pose a serious risk.
• Hepatitis B vaccine has *not* been associated with an increased incidence of AIDS.
• Although anaphylaxis has not been reported, epinephrine should always be available when administering the drug to counteract any possible reaction.
• Obtain an order for antipyretic medication to alleviate vaccine-induced fever.
• Apply ice or cold compresses to injection site to relieve local redness and pain.

Patient Teaching
• Inform the patient that a slight fever, headache, and malaise may occur after vaccination.
• Instruct the patient to use ice or cold compresses for local reaction to the vaccine.
• Advise the patient that the following people are at increased risk of infection and should be considered for the vaccine: certain health care personnel (especially those working with dialysis patients, in blood banks, and in emergency medicine); selected patients and patient contacts; certain endemic populations (Alaskan Eskimos, Indochinese and Haitian refugees); certain military personnel; morticians and embalmers; sexually active male homosexuals; prostitutes; prisoners; and users of illicit injectable drugs.

Evaluation
In patients receiving hepatitis B vaccine, appropriate evaluation statements may include:
• Patient exhibits active immunity to hepatitis B.
• Patient's temperature remains within normal range.
• Patient and family state an understanding of hepatitis B vaccine.

PHARMACOLOGIC CLASS

histamine$_2$-receptor antagonists
cimetidine
famotidine
nizatidine
ranitidine

OVERVIEW
The introduction of histamine$_2$ (H_2)-receptor antagonists has revolution-

ized the treatment of peptic ulcer disease. These drugs structurally resemble histamine and competitively inhibit histamine's action on gastric H_2-receptors. Cimetidine, approved for clinical use in 1977, is the prototype of this class.

All H_2-receptor antagonists inhibit histamine's action at H_2-receptors in gastric parietal cells, reducing gastric acid output and concentration regardless of the stimulatory agent (histamine, food, insulin, caffeine) or basal conditions.

CLINICAL INDICATIONS AND ACTIONS

Duodenal ulcer
All four H_2-receptor antagonists are used to treat acute duodenal ulcer and to prevent ulcer recurrence.

Gastric ulcer
Cimetidine, famotidine, nizatidine, and ranitidine are indicated for acute gastric ulcer. However, the benefits of long-term therapy (greater than 8 weeks) with these drugs remain unproven.

Hypersecretory states
All four H_2-receptor antagonists are used to treat hypersecretory states such as Zollinger-Ellison syndrome. Because patients with these conditions require much higher doses than patients with peptic ulcer disease, they may experience more pronounced adverse effects.

Reflux esophagitis
H_2-receptor antagonists are used to provide short-term relief from gastroesophageal reflux in patients who don't respond to conventional therapy (life-style changes, antacids, diet modification). They act by raising the stomach pH. Some clinicians prefer to combine the H_2-receptor antagonist with metoclopramide, but further study is necessary to confirm effectiveness of the combination.

Stress ulcer prophylaxis
H_2-receptor antagonists are used to prevent stress ulcers in critically ill patients, particularly those in intensive care units. However, this remains an unlabeled (FDA unapproved) indication; some physicians prefer intensive antacid therapy for such patients.

Other uses
H_2-receptor antagonists have been used for a number of other unlabeled indications, including short-bowel syndrome and prophylaxis for allergic reactions to I.V. contrast medium.

OVERVIEW OF ADVERSE REACTIONS

H_2-receptor antagonists rarely cause adverse reactions. However, mild transient diarrhea, neutropenia, dizziness, fatigue, cardiac arrhythmias, and gynecomastia have been reported.

Cimetidine may inhibit hepatic enzymes, thereby impairing the metabolism of certain drugs. Ranitidine may also produce this effect, but to a lesser extent. Famotidine has not been shown to inhibit hepatic enzymes or drug clearance.

REPRESENTATIVE COMBINATIONS

None.

---

homatropine hydrobromide

(hoe ma´ troe peen)
Homatrine, Homatropine, Isopto Homatropine

- *Classification:* cycloplegic, mydriatic (anticholinergic agent)
- *Pregnancy Risk Category:* C

HOW SUPPLIED

Ophthalmic solution: 2%, 5%

ACTION

Mechanism: A mydriatic and cycloplegic agent that blocks muscarinic

*Liquid form contains alcohol.

**May contain tartrazine.

cholinergic receptors in the eye. Anticholinergic action leaves the pupil under unopposed adrenergic influence, causing it to dilate.
Pharmacokinetics: Unknown.
Onset, peak, duration: Peak effect is reached in 40 minutes to 1 hour. Recovery from cycloplegic and mydriatic effects usually occurs within 1 to 3 days.

INDICATIONS & DOSAGE

Cycloplegic refraction–
Adults and children: instill 1 to 2 drops of 2% or 5% solution in eye; repeat in 5 to 10 minutes if needed, for two or three doses.
Uveitis–
Adults and children: instill 1 to 2 drops of 2% or 5% solution in eye up to q 3 to 4 hours.

CONTRAINDICATIONS & PRECAUTIONS

Contraindicated in patients with narrow-angle glaucoma or hypersensitivity to belladonna alkaloids (such as atropine) or any other component of the medication. Use cautiously in patients with hypertension, cardiac disease, or increased intraocular pressure.

ADVERSE REACTIONS

Common reactions are in italics; life-threatening reactions are in bold italics.
Eye: irritation, *blurred vision, photophobia.*
Systemic: flushing, dry skin and mouth, fever, tachycardia, ataxia, irritability, confusion, somnolence.

INTERACTIONS

None significant.

EFFECTS ON DIAGNOSTIC TESTS

None significant.

NURSING CONSIDERATIONS

Besides those related universally to drug therapy (see "How to use this book"), consider the following specific recommendations:

Assessment
- Obtain a baseline assessment of the patient's vision and pupil size.
- Be alert for adverse reactions and drug interactions throughout therapy.
- Evaluate the patient's and family's knowledge about homatropine therapy.

Nursing Diagnoses
- Sensory/perceptual alterations (visual) related to the patient's underlying condition.
- High risk for poisoning related to the drug's systemic adrenergic effects.
- Knowledge deficit related to homatropine therapy.

Planning and Implementaton
Preparation and Administration
- Check the patient's history before administering: patients hypersensitive to atropine will also be hypersensitive to homatropine.
- Instill in lacrimal sac; remove excess solution from around eyes with a clean tissue or gauze and apply light finger pressure to the lacrimal sac for 1 minute.

Monitoring
- Monitor effectiveness by assessing the patient's visual status and pupil size.
- Monitor for systemic adrenergic effects.

Supportive Care
- Notify the doctor immediately of any changes in the patient's health status.

Patient Teaching
- Teach the patient how to instill the solution, and advise him to wash his hands before and after administering the drug.
- Tell the patient that dark glasses should be worn to ease any discomfort from photophobia.
- Advise the patient that gum or hard candy can be used to relieve dry mouth.

Evaluation
In patients receiving homatropine, appropriate evaluation statements may include:
• Patient experiences therapeutic mydriasis.
• Patient remains free of systemic adrenergic effects.
• Patient and family state an understanding of homatropine therapy.

hydralazine hydrochloride
(hye dral´ a zeen)
Alazine, Apresoline**, Novo-Hylazin†, Supres‡

• *Classification:* antihypertensive (peripheral vasodilator)
• *Pregnancy Risk Category:* C

HOW SUPPLIED
Tablets: 10 mg, 25 mg, 50 mg, 100 mg
Injection: 20 mg/ml

ACTION
Mechanism: Directly relaxes arteriolar smooth muscle.
Absorption: Rapidly absorbed from the GI tract after oral administration. Food enhances absorption. Little is known about the pharmacokinetics of injectable hydralazine.
Distribution: Widely distributed throughout the body; approximately 88% to 90% protein-bound.
Metabolism: Extensively metabolized in the GI mucosa and the liver.
Excretion: Most of a given dose is excreted in urine, primarily as metabolites; about 10% of an oral dose is excreted in feces. Half-life: Varies from 3 to 7 hours.
Onset, peak, duration: Peak plasma levels occur in 1 to 2 hours. Antihypertensive effect occurs 20 to 30 minutes after oral dose, 5 to 20 minutes after I.V. administration, and 10 to 30 minutes after I.M. administration. Antihypertensive effect persists 2 to 4 hours after an oral dose and 2 to 6 hours after I.V. or I.M. administration.

INDICATIONS & DOSAGE
Essential hypertension (oral, alone or in combination with other antihypertensives); to reduce afterload in severe CHF (with nitrates); and severe essential hypertension (parenteral to lower blood pressure quickly) –
Adults: initially, 10 mg P.O. q.i.d.; gradually increased to 50 mg q.i.d. Maximum recommended dosage is 200 mg daily, but some patients may require 300 to 400 mg daily. Can be given b.i.d. for CHF.
I.V. – 10 to 20 mg given slowly and repeated as necessary, generally q 4 to 6 hours. Switch to oral antihypertensives as soon as possible.
I.M. – 20 to 40 mg repeated as necessary, generally q 4 to 6 hours. Switch to oral antihypertensives as soon as possible.
Children: initially, 0.75 mg/kg P.O. daily in four divided doses (25 mg/m² daily). May increase gradually to 10 times this dosage, if necessary.
I.V. – give slowly 1.7 to 3.5 mg/kg daily or 50 to 100 mg/m² daily in four to six divided doses.
I.M. – 1.7 to 3.5 mg/kg daily or 50 to 100 mg/m² daily in four to six divided doses.

CONTRAINDICATIONS & PRECAUTIONS
Contraindicated in patients with hypersensitivity to the drug and in patients with mitral valve rheumatic heart disease or coronary artery disease. Use cautiously in patients with a history of stroke or severe renal damage because these conditions may be exacerbated by hypotension.

ADVERSE REACTIONS
Common reactions are in italics; life-threatening reactions are in bold italics.
Blood: neutropenia, leukopenia.

CNS: peripheral neuritis, *headache*, dizziness.
CV: orthostatic hypotension, *tachycardia,* ***arrhythmias,*** *angina, palpitations, sodium retention.*
GI: *nausea, vomiting, diarrhea, anorexia.*
Skin: rash.
Other: *lupus erythematosus-like syndrome (especially with high doses), weight gain.*

INTERACTIONS

Diazoxide: may cause severe hypotension. Use together cautiously.

EFFECTS ON DIAGNOSTIC TESTS

ANA: positive titer.
CBC: decreased RBC and WBC.
Hemoglobin: decreased.
Lupus erythematosus (LE) cell preparation: positive result.

NURSING CONSIDERATIONS

Besides those related universally to drug therapy (see "How to use this book"), consider the following specific recommendations:

Assessment

- Obtain a baseline assessment of the patient's blood pressure before beginning therapy.
- Be alert for adverse reactions and drug interactions throughout therapy.
- Evaluate the patient's and family's knowledge about hydralazine therapy.

Nursing Diagnoses

- Altered tissue perfusion (renal, cerebral, cardiopulmonary, and peripheral) related to the patient's underlying condition.
- Pain related to hydralazine-induced headache.
- Knowledge deficit related to hydralazine therapy.

Planning and Implementation

Preparation and Administration

- Check to be sure that CBC, LE cell preparation, and ANA titer determinations were performed before therapy.
- Compliance with the drug therapy may be improved if the drug is administered b.i.d. Check with the doctor to see if this is possible for the patient.
- ***P.O. use:*** Give the drug with meals to increase absorption.
- ***I.V. use:*** For direct injection, inject undiluted drug directly into the vein or as close to I.V. insertion site as possible. Give at a rate of 10 mg/minute.

Monitoring

- Monitor effectiveness by frequently monitoring the patient's blood pressure, pulse, and ECG.
- Monitor the patient's body weight frequently. Some clinicians combine hydralazine therapy with diuretics and beta-adrenergic blocking agents to decrease sodium retention and tachycardia and to prevent anginal attacks.
- Watch the patient closely for signs of lupus-like syndrome (sore throat, fever, muscle and joint aches, skin rash).
- Periodically ask if patient is experiencing headache.
- Monitor for orthostatic hypotension by taking the patient's blood pressure in the supine and the standing positions. Keep in mind that elderly patients are often more sensitive to the drug's hypotensive effects.
- Monitor results of CBC, LE cell preparation, and ANA titer determinations throughout therapy.

Supportive Care

- Notify the doctor immediately if lupus-like syndrome develops.

Patient Teaching

- Explain the importance of taking this drug as prescribed even when feeling well.
- Tell the patient not to discontinue the drug suddenly but to call the doctor if unpleasant adverse reactions occur.
- Instruct the patient to check with the doctor or pharmacist before tak-

ing OTC drugs, such as cold or allergy remedies.
• Inform the patient that orthostatic hypotension can be minimized by rising slowly and avoiding sudden position changes.
• Teach the patient and a family caregiver to take blood pressure measurements. Tell them to notify the doctor of any significant change.

Evaluation

In patients receiving hydralazine, appropriate evaluation statements may include:
• Patient's blood pressure is controlled within normal limits for this patient.
• Headache did not occur.
• Patient and family state an understanding of hydralazine therapy.

hydrochlorothiazide

(hye droe klor oh thye´ a zide)

Apo-Hydro†, Dichlotride‡, Diuchlor H†, Esidrix, HydroDIURIL, Mictrin, Natrimax†, Novohydrazide†, Oretic, Thiuretic, Urozide†

• *Classification:* diuretic, antihypertensive (thiazide)
• *Pregnancy Risk Category:* D

HOW SUPPLIED

Tablets: 25 mg, 50 mg, 100 mg
Oral solution: 10 mg/ml, 100 mg/ml

ACTION

Mechanism: A thiazide diuretic that increases urine excretion of sodium and water by inhibiting sodium reabsorption in the cortical diluting site of the nephron.
Absorption: Variety absorbed from the GI tract depending on different formulations of this drug.
Distribution: Enters the extracellular space.
Excretion: Unchanged in urine, usually within 24 hours.

INDICATIONS & DOSAGE

Edema –
Adults: initially, 25 to 100 mg P.O. daily or intermittently for maintenance dosage.
Children over 6 months: 2.2 mg/kg P.O. daily divided b.i.d.
Children under 6 months: up to 3.3 mg/kg P.O. daily divided b.i.d.
Hypertension –
Adults: 25 to 100 mg P.O. daily or divided dosage. Daily dosage increased or decreased according to blood pressure.

CONTRAINDICATIONS & PRECAUTIONS

Contraindicated in patients with hypersensitivity to the drug or to sulfonamide derivatives. Use cautiously in patients with severe renal disease because reduced glomerular filtration rate may cause azotemia and in patients with impaired hepatic function or liver disease because electrolyte alterations may precipitate hepatic coma. Hydrochlorothiazide-induced hypokalemia may predispose patients taking digoxin to digitalis toxicity.

ADVERSE REACTIONS

Common reactions are in italics; life-threatening reactions are in bold italics.
Blood: ***aplastic anemia, agranulocytosis,*** leukopenia, thrombocytopenia.
CV: *volume depletion and dehydration,* orthostatic hypotension.
GI: anorexia, nausea, pancreatitis.
Hepatic: hepatic encephalopathy.
Metabolic: *hypokalemia, asymptomatic hyperuricemia, hyperglycemia and impairment of glucose tolerance,* fluid and electrolyte imbalances including dilutional hyponatremia and hypochloremia, metabolic alkalosis, hypercalcemia, gout.
Skin: dermatitis, photosensitivity, rash.
Other: hypersensitivity, such as pneumonitis and vasculitis.

*Liquid form contains alcohol. **May contain tartrazine.

INTERACTIONS

Cholestyramine, colestipol: intestinal absorption of thiazides decreased. Keep doses as separate as possible.
Diazoxide: increased antihypertensive, hyperglycemic, and hyperuricemic effects. Use together cautiously.
NSAIDs: decreased diuretic effectiveness. Avoid concomitant use.

EFFECTS ON DIAGNOSTIC TESTS

Blood glucose levels: hyperglycemia.
Parathyroid function tests: test interference. Drug should be discontinued before such tests.
Serum electrolytes: altered levels.
Serum urate, cholesterol, and triglycerides: altered levels.

NURSING CONSIDERATIONS

Besides those related universally to drug therapy (see "How to use this book"), consider the following specific recommendations:

Assessment

- Obtain a baseline assessment of blood pressure, serum electrolytes, urine output, weight, and peripheral edema before initiating hydrochlorothiazide therapy.
- Be alert for adverse reactions and drug interactions throughout therapy.
- Evaluate the patient's and family's knowledge about hydrochlorothiazide therapy.

Nursing Diagnoses

- Fluid volume excess related to ineffectiveness of hydrochlorothiazide to relieve edema.
- Altered urinary elimination related to hydrochlorothiazide therapy.
- Knowledge deficit related to hydrochlorothiazide therapy.

Planning and Implementation

Preparation and Administration

- ***P.O. use:*** If possible, give drug early in the day to prevent nocturia.

Monitoring

- Monitor effectiveness by regularly checking blood pressure, urine output, and weight.
- Monitor serum electrolytes, BUN, creatinine, glucose, and uric acid levels.
- Monitor CBC, differential, and platelet count.
- Monitor the patient receiving concomitant digitalis therapy for increased risk of digitalis toxicity.
- Monitor for signs of hypokalemia (for example, muscle weakness and cramps).
- Monitor the diabetic patient's insulin requirements because hydrochlorothiazide has hyperglycemic effects.
- Monitor skin turgor and mucous membranes for signs of fluid volume deficit.

Supportive Care

- Hold drug and notify the doctor if hypersensitivity reactions occur.
- Keep accurate records of intake and output, blood pressure, and weight.
- Provide frequent skin and mouth care to relieve dryness from diuretic therapy.
- Answer the patient's call bells promptly; make sure patient's bathroom or bedpan is easily accessible.
- Use safety precautions to minimize risk of falling due to hypotension.
- In the patient undergoing tests of parathyroid function, hold thiazide and thiazide-like drugs before these tests are performed.
- Be aware that optimal antihypertensive effect may not occur for several days after beginning of therapy with hydrochlorothiazide.
- Elevate the patient's legs to aid relief of peripheral edema.
- Administer potassium supplements as indicated.

Patient Teaching

- Teach the patient and family to identify and report signs of hypersensitivity reaction and hypokalemia.
- Teach the patient and family to monitor the patient's fluid volume by recording daily weight and intake and output.
- Inform the patient that optimal

therapeutic response may not occur until several days after beginning hydrochlorothiazide therapy.
• Teach the patient to avoid high-sodium foods and to choose high-potassium foods.
• Advise the patient to change positions slowly, especially when rising to standing position, to avoid dizziness and fainting due to orthostatic hypotension.
• Advise the patient to minimize risks of photosensitivity reaction by using a sunscreen when outdoors.
• Advise the diabetic patient that insulin dosage may require adjustment.
• Advise the patient who is taking digitalis that the drug's potassium-depleting effect may increase the risk of digitalis toxicity.
• Advise the patient to take hydrochlorothiazide early in the day to avoid interruptions of sleep due to nocturia.

Evaluation
In patients receiving hydrochlorothiazide, appropriate evaluation statements may include:
• Patient is free of edema.
• Patient demonstrates adjustment of life-style to deal with altered patterns of urinary elimination.
• Patient and family state an understanding of hydrochlorothiazide therapy.

hydrocortisone (systemic)
(hye droe kor´ ti sone)
Cortef, Cortenema, Hycort†, Hydrocortone

hydrocortisone acetate
Biosone, Cortifoam, Cortamed, Hydrocortone Acetate

hydrocortisone cypionate
Cortef

hydrocortisone sodium phosphate
Hydrocortone Phosphate

hydrocortisone sodium succinate
A-HydroCort, Solu-Cortef

• *Classification:* adrenocorticoid replacement (glucocorticoid, mineralocorticoid)
• *Pregnancy Risk Category:* C

HOW SUPPLIED
hydrocortisone
Tablets: 5 mg, 10 mg, 20 mg
Injection: 25 mg/ml, 50 mg/ml suspension
Enema: 100 mg/60 ml
hydrocortisone acetate
Injection: 25 mg/ml, 50 mg/ml suspension
Enema: 10% aerosol foam (provides 90 mg/application)
hydrocortisone cypionate
Oral suspension: 10 mg/5 ml
hydrocortisone sodium phosphate
Injection: 50 mg/ml solution
hydrocortisone sodium succinate
Injection: 100 mg, 250 mg, 500 mg, 1,000 mg/vial

ACTION
Mechanism: Decreases inflammation, mainly by stabilizing leukocyte lysosomal membranes. Also suppresses the immune response, stimulates bone marrow, and influences protein, fat, and carbohydrate metabolism.
Absorption: Readily absorbed after oral or I.M. administration.
Distribution: Rapidly removed from the blood and distributed to muscle, liver, skin, intestines, and kidneys. Bound extensively to plasma proteins (transcortin and albumin); only the unbound portion is active. Adrenocorticoids are distributed into breast milk and cross the placenta.
Metabolism: In the liver to inactive glucuronide and sulfate metabolites.

Excretion: The inactive metabolites and small amounts of unmetabolized drug are excreted by the kidneys. Insignificant amounts are excreted in feces. Half-life: 8 to 12 hours.
Onset, peak, duration: After oral and I.V. administration, peak effects occur in about 1 to 2 hours. The acetate suspension for injection has a variable absorption over 24 to 48 hours, depending on site of injection (intra-articular space, muscle, or the blood supply to the muscle).

INDICATIONS & DOSAGE

Severe inflammation, adrenal insufficiency–
Adults: 5 to 30 mg P.O. b.i.d., t.i.d., or q.i.d. (as much as 80 mg P.O. q.i.d. may be given in acute situations); or initially, 100 to 250 mg (succinate) I.M. or I.V., then 50 to 100 mg I.M., as indicated; or 15 to 240 mg (phosphate) I.M. or I.V. q 12 hours; or 5 to 75 mg (acetate) into joints and soft tissue. Dosage varies with size of joint. Often local anesthetics are injected with dose.
Shock–
Adults: 500 mg to 2 g (succinate) q 2 to 6 hours.
Children: 0.16 to 1 mg/kg (phosphate or succinate) I.M. or I.V., b.i.d. or t.i.d.
Adjunctive treatment of ulcerative colitis and proctitis–
Adults: 1 enema (100 mg) nightly for 21 days.

CONTRAINDICATIONS & PRECAUTIONS

Contraindicated in patients with systemic fungal infections (except in adrenal insufficiency) and in those with a hypersensitivity to ingredients of adrenocorticoid preparations. Patients who are receiving hydrocortisone should not be given live virus vaccines because hydrocortisone suppresses the immune response.

Use with extreme caution in patients with GI ulceration, renal disease, hypertension, osteoporosis, diabetes mellitus, thromboembolic disorders, seizures, myasthenia gravis, CHF, tuberculosis, hypoalbuminemia, hypothyroidism, cirrhosis of the liver, emotional instability, psychotic tendencies, hyperlipidemias, glaucoma, or cataracts because the drug may exacerbate these conditions.

Because adrenocorticoids increase the susceptibility to and mask symptoms of infection, hydrocortisone should not be used (except in life-threatening situations) in patients with viral or bacterial infections not controlled by anti-infective agents.

ADVERSE REACTIONS

Common reactions are in italics; life-threatening reactions are in bold italics. Most adverse reactions of corticosteroids are dose- or duration-dependent.
CNS: *euphoria, insomnia,* psychotic behavior, pseudotumor cerebri.
CV: ***CHF,*** hypertension, edema.
EENT: cataracts, glaucoma.
GI: *peptic ulcer,* GI irritation, increased appetite.
Metabolic: *possible hypokalemia, hyperglycemia and carbohydrate intolerance,* growth suppression in children.
Skin: delayed wound healing, acne, various skin eruptions.
Other: muscle weakness, pancreatitis, hirsutism, susceptibility to infections. Acute adrenal insufficiency may occur with increased stress (infection, surgery, or trauma) or abrupt withdrawal after long-term therapy.
Withdrawal symptoms: rebound inflammation, fatigue, weakness, arthralgia, fever, dizziness, lethargy, depression, fainting, orthostatic hypotension, dyspnea, anorexia, hypoglycemia. ***Sudden withdrawal may be fatal.***

INTERACTIONS

Barbiturates, phenytoin, rifampin: decreased corticosteroid effect. Corticosteroid dose may need to be increased.

Indomethacin, aspirin: increased risk of GI distress and bleeding. Give together cautiously.

EFFECTS ON DIAGNOSTIC TESTS

Diagnostic skin tests: suppressed reactions.

Glucose and cholesterol: increased levels.

Nitroblue tetrazolium tests for systemic bacterial infections: false-negative results.

Serum potassium, calcium, thyroxine, and triiodothyronine: decreased levels.

Thyroid function tests(^{131}I uptake and protein-bound iodine): decreased concentrations.

Urine glucose and calcium: increased levels.

NURSING CONSIDERATIONS

Besides those related universally to drug therapy (see "How to use this book"), consider the following specific recommendations:

Assessment

- Obtain a baseline assessment of the patient's underlying condition before initiating drug therapy.
- Be alert for adverse reactions and drug interactions throughout therapy.
- Evaluate the patient's and family's knowledge about hydrocortisone therapy.

Nursing Diagnoses

- Fluid volume deficit related to volume depletion from adrenal insufficiency.
- High risk for injury related to hydrocortisone-induced adverse reactions.
- Knowledge deficit related to hydrocortisone therapy.

Planning and Implementation

Preparation and Administration

- Do not confuse Solu-Cortef (hydrocortisone sodium succinate) with Solu-Medrol (methylprednisolone sodium succinate).
- Do not use injectable forms for alternate-day therapy.
- Gradually reduce drug dosage after long-term therapy. Never abruptly discontinue therapy as sudden withdrawal can be fatal.
- Always titrate to lowest effective dose as prescribed.
- Give a daily dosage in the morning for better results and less toxicity.
- Expect to increase dosage as prescribed during times of physiological stress (surgery, trauma, or infection).
- ***P.O. use:*** Give with food when possible to avoid GI upset.
- ***I.M. use:*** Give injection deep into gluteal muscle. Rotate injection sites to prevent muscle atrophy. Avoid S.C. injection because atrophy and sterile abscesses may occur.
- ***I.V. use:*** Do not use the acetate form for I.V. use. When administering as direct injection, inject directly into vein or into an I.V. line containing a free-flowing compatible solution over 30 seconds to several minutes. When administering as an intermittent or continuous infusion, dilute solution according to manufacturer's instructions and give over the prescribed duration. If used for continuous infusion change solution every 24 hours.
- ***Rectal use:*** Be aware that enema may produce same systemic effects as other forms of hydrocortisone. If enema therapy must exceed 21 days, discontinue gradually by reducing administration to every other night for 2 or 3 weeks.

Monitoring

- Monitor effectiveness by regularly assessing for improvement of signs and symptoms of the underlying condition.
- Monitor for adverse reactions be-

cause drug can cause serious or even life-threatening multisystem dysfunction.
• Monitor the patient's weight, blood pressure, blood glucose level, and serum electrolyte levels regularly.
• Monitor the patient for infection. Drug may mask or exacerbate infections.
• Monitor the patient's stress level. Stress (fever, trauma, surgery, or emotional problems) may increase adrenal insufficiency. Higher dose may be needed.
• Monitor the patient's mental status for depression or psychotic episodes, especially in high-dose therapy.
• Monitor the patient's skin for petechiae.
• Monitor growth in infants and children on long-term therapy.
• Monitor patients receiving immunizations for decreased antibody response.
• Monitor the patient for early signs of adrenal insufficiency or cushingoid symptoms.

Supportive Care

• Unless contraindicated, give the patient a low-sodium diet high in potassium and protein. Potassium supplement may be needed.

Patient Teaching

• Be sure that the patient understands the need to take the drug as prescribed. Tell the patient that if a dose is missed inadvertently, to take it immediately. Advise the patient not to take two doses together.
• Warn the patient not to discontinue the drug abruptly or without the doctor's approval.
• Advise the patient to take oral form with meals to minimize GI adverse reactions.
• Warn the patient about easy bruising.
• Inform the patient of the possible therapeutic and adverse effects of the drug, so that he may report complications to the doctor as soon as possible.
• Tell the patient to carry a medical alert card indicating the need for supplemental adrenocorticoids during stress.
• Teach the patient to recognize signs of early adrenal insufficiency (fatigue, muscular weakness, joint pain, fever, anorexia, nausea, dyspnea, dizziness, and fainting) and to notify the doctor promptly if they occur.
• Warn patients on long-term therapy about cushingoid symptoms, which may develop regardless of route of administration.
• Tell patient to eat a low-sodium diet that is high in potassium and protein if not contraindicated.

Evaluation

In patients receiving hydrocortisone, appropriate evaluation statements may include:
• Patient's condition being treated with hydrocortisone therapy shows improvement.
• Patient does not experience serious adverse reactions associated with hydrocortisone.
• Patient and family state an understanding of hydrocortisone therapy.

hydrocortisone (topical)

(hye droe kor´ ti sone)

Acticort, Aeroseb-HC, Carmol HC, Cetacort, Cort-Dome, Cortef◇, Cortinal, Cortizone 5◇, Cortril, Cremesone, Delacort, DermiCort◇, Dermolate◇, Durel-Cort, Ecosone, HC Cream, HI-Cor-2.5, Hycortole, Hydrocortex, Hytone, Ivocort, Maso-Cort, Microcort, Orabase HCA, Penecort, Proctocort, Rhus Tox HC, Rocort, Squibb-HC‡, Unicort

hydrocortisone acetate

Cortaid◇, Cortamed†, Cortef, Corticreme†, Cortifoam, Dermacort‡, Dermacort Ointment‡, Epifoam,

Hydrocortisone Acetate, MyCort Lotion, Proctofoam-HC

hydrocortisone valerate
Westcort Cream

- *Classification:* topical anti-inflammatory (adrenocorticoid)
- *Pregnancy Risk Category:* C

HOW SUPPLIED

hydrocortisone
Aerosol: 0.5%
Cream: 0.25%◇, 0.5%◇, 1%, 2.5%
Gel: 1%
Lotion: 0.125%, 0.25%, 0.5%◇, 1%, 2%, 2.5%
Ointment: 0.5%◇, 1%, 2.5%
Topical solution: 1%
hydrocortisone acetate
Cream: 0.5%◇
Lotion: 0.5%◇
Ointment: 0.5%◇, 1%
Rectal foam: 90 mg/application
hydrocortisone valerate
Ointment: 0.2%
Cream: 0.2%

ACTION

Mechanism: Diffuses across cell membranes and complexes with specific cytoplasmic receptors.
Absorption: Amount absorbed depends on the amount applied and on the nature of the skin at the application site. It is lowest in areas with thick stratum corneum (on the palms, soles, elbows, and knees) and highest in thinner areas (face, eyelids, and genitals). Absorption increases in areas of skin damage, inflammation, or occlusion. Some systemic absorption may occur, especially through the oral mucosa.
Distribution: After topical application, distributed throughout the local skin. If absorbed, it is rapidly removed from the blood and distributed into muscle, liver, skin, intestines, and kidneys.
Metabolism: After topical administration, metabolized primarily in the skin. The small amount absorbed into systemic circulation is metabolized primarily in the liver to inactive compounds.
Excretion: Inactive metabolites are excreted by the kidneys, primarily as glucuronides and sulfates, but also as unconjugated products. Small amounts of the metabolites are also excreted in feces.

INDICATIONS & DOSAGE

Inflammation of corticosteroid-responsive dermatoses; adjunctive topical management of seborrheic dermatitis of scalp; may be safely used on face, groin, armpits, and under breasts–
Adults and children: clean area; apply cream, gel, lotion, ointment, topical solution, or aerosol sparingly daily to q.i.d.
Aerosol–shake can well. Direct spray onto affected area from a distance of 6″ (15 cm). Apply for only 3 seconds (to avoid freezing tissues). Apply to dry scalp after shampooing; no need to massage or rub medication into scalp after spraying. Apply daily until acute phase is controlled, then reduce dosage to 1 to 3 times a week as needed to maintain control.
Rectal form–shake can well. One applicatorful daily to b.i.d. for 2 to 3 weeks, then every other day as necessary.

CONTRAINDICATIONS & PRECAUTIONS

Contraindicated in patients who are hypersensitive to any component of the preparation and in patients with viral, fungal, or tubercular skin lesions. Use with extreme caution in patients with impaired circulation because it may increase the risk of skin ulceration.

ADVERSE REACTIONS

Common reactions are in italics; life-threatening reactions are in bold italics.
Skin: burning, itching, irritation, dryness, folliculitis, hypertrichosis, hypopigmentation, acneiform eruptions, allergic contact dermatitis. With occlusive dressings: *maceration of skin, secondary infection, atrophy, striae, miliaria.*

INTERACTIONS

None significant.

EFFECTS ON DIAGNOSTIC TESTS

None reported.

NURSING CONSIDERATIONS

Besides those related universally to drug therapy (see "How to use this book"), consider the following specific recommendations:

Assessment

- Obtain a baseline assessment of patient's skin integrity before topical hydrocortisone therapy.
- Be alert for adverse reactions and drug interactions throughout therapy.
- Evaluate the patient's and family's knowledge about topical hydrocortisone therapy.

Nursing Diagnoses

- Impaired skin integrity related to the patient's underlying condition.
- High risk for infection related to drug-induced adverse reaction.
- Knowledge deficit related to topical hydrocortisone therapy.

Planning and Implementation

Preparation and Administration

- Read order and drug labels carefully.
- Wear gloves when administering drug.
- Before applying, gently wash the patient's skin. Apply a thin layer of medication and rub in gently.
- When treating hairy sites, part hair and apply directly to lesion.
- To apply an occlusive dressing (only if ordered by doctor), apply cream heavily, then cover with a thin, pliable, nonflammable plastic film; seal to adjacent normal skin with hypoallergenic tape.
- Know that aerosol preparation contains alcohol and may produce irritation or burning when used on open lesions. When using on the face, cover the patient's eyes and warn against inhalation of the spray. To avoid freezing tissues, do not spray longer than 3 seconds or closer than 6" (15 cm).
- To prevent recurrence, treatment should continue for a few days after clearing of lesions.

Monitoring

- Monitor effectiveness by regularly assessing skin for extent and severity of inflammation.
- Monitor for hypersensitivity reaction to hydrocortisone.
- Monitor for evidence of secondary infection.
- Frequently assess the patient's skin for burning, itching, and dryness.
- Monitor patients with occlusive dressings for maceration of the skin and secondary infection.

Supportive Care

- To minimize adverse reactions, use occlusive dressing intermittently. Don't use occlusive dressings in the presence of infection or on weeping or exudative lesions. Do not leave in place longer than 16 hours each day.
- For patients with eczematous dermatitis who may develop irritation with adhesive material, hold dressing in place with gauze, elastic bandage, or stockings.
- Notify the doctor and remove occlusive dressing if fever develops.
- Withhold the drug and notify the doctor if hypersensitivity reaction or infection occurs.
- Have the patient's fingernails cut short to minimize skin trauma from scratching.
- Apply cool, moist compresses to in-

volved areas to relieve itching and burning.

Patient Teaching

• Instruct the patient to cleanse involved area before applying hydrocortisone in a thin layer to cover the entire surface.

• Teach the patient how to apply an occlusive dressing.

• Teach the patient and family how to recognize signs of a hypersensitivity reaction or infection. Advise them to discontinue the drug and notify the doctor immediately if they occur.

• Instruct the patient to complete the entire treatment regimen as prescribed, even if the lesions appear to have healed.

• Tell the patient and family not to share the hydrocortisone prescription with others and not to administer topical hydrocortisone to children under age 2 without a doctor's order.

Evaluation

In patients receiving topical hydrocortisone, appropriate evaluation statements may include:

• Patient's skin maintains integrity.

• Patient does not develop secondary infection.

• Patient and family state an understanding of topical hydrocortisone therapy.

hydromorphone hydrochloride

(hye droe mor´ fone)

Dilaudid, Dilaudid HP

• Controlled Substance Schedule II

• *Classification:* analgesic antitussive (opioid)

• *Pregnancy Risk Category:* B (D for prolonged use or use of high doses at term)

HOW SUPPLIED

Tablets: 1 mg, 2 mg, 3 mg, 4 mg

Injection: 1 mg/ml, 2 mg/ml, 3 mg/ml, 4 mg/ml, 10 mg/ml

Suppositories: 3 mg

ACTION

Mechanism: Binds with opiate receptors at many sites in the CNS (brain, brain stem, and spinal cord), altering both perception of and emotional response to pain through an unknown mechanism. Suppresses the cough reflex by direct action on the cough center in the medulla.

Absorption: Well absorbed after oral, rectal, or parenteral administration.

Distribution: Unknown.

Metabolism: Primarily in the liver, where it undergoes conjugation with glucuronic acid.

Excretion: Primarily in the urine as the glucuronide conjugate. Half-life: 2 to 3 hours.

Onset, peak, duration: Onset of action occurs in 15 to 30 minutes, with peak effect at 30 minutes to 1 hour after dosing. Duration of action is 4 to 5 hours.

INDICATIONS & DOSAGE

Moderate to severe pain—

Adults: 1 to 6 mg P.O. q 4 to 6 hours, p.r.n. or around the clock; or 2 to 4 mg I.M., S.C., or I.V. q 4 to 6 hours, p.r.n., or q 6 to 8 hours around the clock (I.V. dose should be given over 3 to 5 minutes); or 3 mg rectal suppository h.s., p.r.n., or q 6 to 8 hours around the clock.

Cough—

Adults: 1 mg P.O. q 3 to 4 hours p.r.n.

Children 6 to 12 years: 0.5 mg P.O. q 3 to 4 hours p.r.n.

CONTRAINDICATIONS & PRECAUTIONS

Contraindicated in patients with hypersensitivity to the drug or other phenanthrene opioids (codeine, hydrocodone, morphine, oxymorphone, or oxycodone).

Use with extreme caution in patients with supraventricular arrhythmias; avoid or use with extreme caution in patients with head injury or increased intracranial pressure because drug obscures neurologic parameters; avoid or use with extreme caution during pregnancy and labor because drug readily crosses the placenta (premature infants are especially sensitive to respiratory and CNS depressant effects).

Use cautiously in patients with renal or hepatic dysfunction because drug accumulation or prolonged duration of action may occur; in patients with asthma or COPD because drug depresses respiration and suppresses cough reflex; in patients with seizure disorders because drug may precipitate seizures; in patients undergoing biliary tract surgery, because drug may cause biliary spasm; or in elderly or debilitated patients, who are more sensitive to both therapeutic and adverse drug effects; and in patients prone to physical or psychological addiction, because of the high risk of addiction to this drug.

ADVERSE REACTIONS

Common reactions are in italics; life-threatening reactions are in bold italics.

CNS: *sedation, somnolence, clouded sensorium,* dizziness, *euphoria,* seizures with large doses.

CV: *hypotension,* bradycardia.

GI: *nausea, vomiting, constipation,* ileus.

GU: *urine retention.*

Local: induration with repeated S.C. injections.

Other: ***respiratory depression,*** physical dependence.

INTERACTIONS

Alcohol, CNS depressants: additive effects. Use together cautiously.

EFFECTS ON DIAGNOSTIC TESTS

Hepatobiliary imaging studies: test interference.

Plasma amylase and lipase: increased levels.

NURSING CONSIDERATIONS

Besides those related universally to drug therapy (see "How to use this book"), consider the following specific recommendations:

Assessment

- Obtain a baseline assessment of the patient's pain before therapy.
- Be alert for adverse reactions and drug interactions throughout therapy.
- Evaluate the patient's and family's knowledge about hydromorphone therapy.

Nursing Diagnoses

- Pain related to patient's underlying condition.
- Ineffective breathing pattern related to hydromorphone-induced respiratory depression.
- Knowledge deficit related to hydromorphone therapy.

Planning and Implementation

Preparation and Administration

- ***I.V. use:*** Give drug slowly and with patient lying down to minimize hypotensive effect. Be aware that repeated doses prolong duration of effects because of drug accumulation.
- Check access site before giving drug by I.V. push; local tissue irritation can occur with infiltration. Give concentrate (10 mg/ml) only in patients tolerant of opiate agonists who are receiving high doses.
- ***S.C. use:*** Rotate injection sites to avoid induration.
- ***P.O. use:*** Be aware that the oral dosage form is particularly convenient for patients with chronic pain because of availability of tablets in 1-, 2-, 3-, and 4-mg strengths. This enables these patients to titrate their own dose.
- Consider that Dilaudid HP, a highly concentrated form (10 mg/ml), may be administered in smaller volumes, preventing the discomfort associated with large-volume I.M. or S.C. injections.
- Expect to administer reduced dose of hydromorphone, as ordered, when

using with general anesthetics, other narcotic analgesics, tranquilizers, sedatives, hypnotics, alcohol, tricyclic antidepressants, or MAO inhibitors, because continued use increases CNS depression. Use together with extreme caution, and monitor patient response.

Monitoring

• Monitor effectiveness after each dose by evaluating pain relief.

• Monitor for signs of respiratory depression, such as decreased rate and depth of respirations.

• Also monitor circulatory status and bowel function.

Supportive Care

• Notify the doctor and discuss increase of dosage or frequency if pain persists.

• If respiratory rate drops below 8 breaths/minute, after I.V. administration, arouse the patient to stimulate breathing, and notify the doctor. Also notify the doctor if significant hypotension occurs.

• Keep narcotic antagonist (naloxone) and resuscitative equipment available.

• **Treatment of overdose:** Maintain patent airway and provide respiratory support. Give 0.4 mg of naloxone by I.V. push, as needed, to reverse respiratory depression. Administer I.V. fluids and vasopressors to maintain blood pressure.

• Because adverse CNS reactions are possible, institute safety precautions, such as supervising ambulation and keeping bed rails up.

• Be aware that hydromorphone may worsen or mask gallbladder pain.

• Recognize that habituation and psychological dependence can develop with long-term use.

• For better analgesic effect, give before patient has intense pain.

Patient Teaching

• Warn the ambulatory patient to avoid hazardous activities that require alertness.

• When used postoperatively, encourage turning, coughing, and deep breathing and use of the incentive spirometer to avoid atelectasis.

• Suggest measures such as high-fiber diet and liberal fluid intake to prevent constipation during maintenance therapy.

• Encourage the patient to ask for medication before pain becomes severe.

• Tell the patient or family caregiver to notify the nurse or doctor if patient's respiratory rate decreases.

Evaluation

In patients receiving hydromorphone, appropriate evaluation statements include:

• Patient reports relief of pain after administration of hydromorphone.

• Patient maintains normal respiratory rate and pattern after administration of hydromorphone.

• Patient and family state an understanding of hydromorphone therapy.

hydroxychloroquine sulfate

(hye drox ee klor´ oh kwin)

Plaquenil

• *Classification:* antimalarial, anti-inflammatory agent (4-aminoquinoline)

• *Pregnancy Risk Category:* C

HOW SUPPLIED

Tablets: 200 mg (150-mg base)

ACTION

Mechanism: As an antimalarial, hydroxychloroquine may bind to and alter the properties of DNA in susceptible parasites. Mechanism of antinflammatory action is unknown, but the drug inhibits the synthesis of prostaglandins in mammalian cells.

Absorption: Absorbed readily and almost completely from the GI tract; absorption may be enhanced by food.

Distribution: Widely distributed and

probably crosses the placenta; concentrates in the liver, spleen, kidneys, heart, and brain and is strongly bound in erythrocytes and melanin-containing cells of the skin and eyes.
Metabolism: Metabolized by the liver to desethylchloroquine and desethyl hydroxychloroquine.
Excretion: Most of dose is excreted unchanged in urine. The drug and its metabolites are excreted slowly in urine; unabsorbed drug is excreted in feces. The drug is excreted in breast milk.
Onset, peak, duration: Peak plasma concentration occurs at 1 to 2 hours. Small amounts may be present in urine for months after the drug is discontinued.

INDICATIONS & DOSAGE

Suppressive prophylaxis of attacks of malaria due to Plasmodium vivax, P. malariae, P. ovale, *and susceptible strains of* P. falciparum–
Adults and children: for suppression: 5 mg (base)/kg body weight P.O. (not to exceed 310 mg) weekly on same day of the week (begin 2 weeks prior to entering and continue for 8 weeks after leaving endemic area). If not started prior to exposure, double initial dose (620 mg for adults, 10 mg/kg for children) in 2 divided doses P.O. 6 hours apart.
Treatment of acute malarial attacks–
Adults and children over 15 years: initially, 800 mg (sulfate) P.O., then 400 mg after 6 to 8 hours, then 400 mg daily for 2 days (total 2 g sulfate salt).
Children 11 to 15 years: 600 mg (sulfate) P.O. stat, then 200 mg 8 hours later, then 200 mg 24 hours later (total 1 g sulfate salt).
Children 6 to 10 years: 400 mg (sulfate) P.O. stat, then 2 doses of 200 mg at 8-hour intervals (total 800 mg sulfate salt).
Children 2 to 5 years: 400 mg (sulfate) P.O. stat, then 200 mg 8 hours later (total 600 mg sulfate salt).
Children under 1 year: 100 mg (sulfate) P.O. stat; then 3 doses of 100 mg 6 to 9 hours apart (total 400 mg sulfate salt).
Lupus erythematosus (chronic discoid and systemic)–
Adults: 400 mg P.O. daily or b.i.d., continued for several weeks or months, depending on response. Prolonged maintenance dosage–200 to 400 mg P.O. daily.
Rheumatoid arthritis–
Adults: initially, 400 to 600 mg P.O. daily. When good response occurs (usually in 4 to 12 weeks), cut dosage in half.

CONTRAINDICATIONS & PRECAUTIONS

Contraindicated in patients who have experienced retinal or visual field changes or hypersensitivity reactions to 4-aminoquinoline compounds, unless these compounds are the only agents to which the malarial strain is sensitive.

Use cautiously in patients with psoriasis, porphyria, or G6PD deficiency because the drug may exacerbate these conditions; and hepatic disease, alcoholism, and in those receiving other hepatotoxic drugs because hydroxychloroquine concentrates in the liver and may cause adverse hepatic effects.

ADVERSE REACTIONS

Common reactions are in italics; life-threatening reactions are in bold italics.
Blood: ***agranulocytosis, leukopenia,*** thrombocytopenia, ***hemolysis in patients with G6PD deficiency, aplastic anemia.***
CNS: irritability, nightmares, ataxia, seizures, psychic stimulation, toxic psychosis, vertigo, tinnitus, nystagmus, lassitude, fatigue, dizziness, hypoactive deep tendon reflexes, skeletal muscle weakness.

EENT: visual disturbances (blurred vision; difficulty in focusing; reversible corneal changes; generally irreversible, sometimes progressive or delayed, retinal changes, e.g., narrowing of arterioles; macular lesions; pallor of optic disk; optic atrophy; visual field defects; patchy retinal pigmentation, often leading to blindness), ototoxicity (irreversible nerve deafness, tinnitus, labyrinthitis).
GI: anorexia, abdominal cramps, diarrhea, nausea, vomiting.
Skin: pruritus, lichen planus-like eruptions, skin and mucosal pigmentary changes, pleomorphic skin eruptions.
Other: weight loss, alopecia, bleaching of hair.

INTERACTIONS

Magnesium and aluminum salts, kaolin: decreased GI absorption. Separate administration times.

EFFECTS ON DIAGNOSTIC TESTS

CBC: decreased WBC, RBC, or platelet counts.
ECG: inverted or depressed T wave; widened QRS complex.

NURSING CONSIDERATIONS

Besides those related universally to drug therapy (see "How to use this book"), consider the following specific recommendations:

Assessment
- Obtain a baseline assessment of infection before therapy.
- Be alert for adverse reactions and drug interactions throughout therapy.
- Evaluate the patient's and family's knowledge about hydroxychloroquine therapy.

Nursing Diagnoses
- High risk for injury related to ineffectiveness of hydroxychloroquine.
- Sensory/perceptual alterations (visual and auditory) related to adverse reactions associated with hydroxychloroquine.
- Knowledge deficit related to hydroxychloroquine.

Planning and Implementation
Preparation and Administration
- ***P.O. use:*** Drug should be administered immediately before or after meals on same day of each week.

Monitoring
- Monitor effectiveness by regularly assessing for improvement of infection.
- Monitor for toxic symptoms, especially in children. Watch for headache, drowsiness, visual disturbances, cardiovascular collapse, and seizures, which may be followed by respiratory and cardiac arrest.
- Monitor for visual or auditory disturbances with ophthalmologic and audiometric examinations before, during, and after therapy, especially if prolonged. Check periodically for ocular muscle weakness after prolonged use.
- Monitor CBC and liver function studies during prolonged therapy.

Supportive Care
- Notify doctor immediately of severe blood disorder not attributable to disease under treatment. Blood reaction may require discontinuation of drug.
- Institute safety precautions if visual or other adverse CNS reactions occur.
- Obtain an order for an antiemetic or antidiarrheal agent if adverse GI reactions occur.

Patient Teaching
- Review methods for reducing exposure to mosquitoes for the patient receiving this drug prophylactically.
- Warn patient to avoid hazardous activities requiring alertness if adverse CNS or visual disturbances occur.
- Tell patient to take drug immediately before or after meals on the same day each week.
- Advise the patient to have baseline and periodic ophthalmologic examinations, and to promptly report blurred vision, increased sensitivity

to light or muscle weakness as well as any hearing changes.

Evaluation

In patients receiving hydroxychloroquine, appropriate evaluation statements may include:

• Patient is free of infection.

• Patient maintains normal visual and auditory function throughout therapy.

• Patient and family state an understanding of hydroxychloroquine therapy.

---

hydroxyprogesterone caproate

(hye drox ee proe jess´ ter one)

Delalutin†, Duralutin, Gesterol L.A., Hy-Gesterone, Hylutin, Hyprogest, Hyproval P.A., Hyroxon, Pro-Depo, Prodrox

• *Classification:* progestin, antineoplastic (progestin)

• *Pregnancy Risk Category:* X

HOW SUPPLIED

Injection: 125 mg/ml, 250 mg/ml

ACTION

Mechanism: Suppresses ovulation, possibly by inhibiting pituitary gonadotropin secretion. Also forms a thick cervical mucus.

Absorption: Slowly absorbed after I.M. injection.

Metabolism: Primarily hepatic; not well characterized.

Excretion: Primarily renal; not well characterized.

Onset, peak, duration: Duration of action is 9 to 17 days.

INDICATIONS & DOSAGE

Menstrual disorders–

Women: 125 to 375 mg I.M. q 4 weeks. Stop after 4 cycles.

Uterine cancer–

Women: 1 to 5 g I.M. weekly.

CONTRAINDICATIONS & PRECAUTIONS

Contraindicated in patients with hypersensitivity to progestins; history of thromboembolic disorders because of its potential for causing thromboembolic disorders; severe hepatic disease because impaired hepatic metabolism may cause the drug to accumulate; breast or genital cancer because it may induce tumor growth; undiagnosed abnormal vaginal bleeding (origin should be determined); and in pregnant or breast-feeding women.

Use cautiously in patients with existing conditions that might be aggravated by fluid and electrolyte retention, such as cardiac or renal disease, seizure disorders, or migraine; and in diabetic patients (because decreased glucose tolerance may occur) or patients with a history of mental depression.

ADVERSE REACTIONS

Common reactions are in italics; life-threatening reactions are in bold italics.

CNS: dizziness, migraine headache, lethargy, depression.

CV: hypertension, thrombophlebitis, ***pulmonary embolism,*** *edema.*

GI: nausea, vomiting, abdominal cramps.

GU: breakthrough bleeding, dysmenorrhea, amenorrhea, cervical erosion, or abnormal secretions, uterine fibromas, vaginal candidiasis.

Hepatic: cholestatic jaundice.

Metabolic: hyperglycemia.

Skin: melasma, rash.

Local: irritation and pain at injection site.

Other: breast tenderness, enlargement, or secretion; decreased libido.

INTERACTIONS

Rifampin: decreased progestogen effects. Monitor for diminished therapeutic response.

EFFECTS ON DIAGNOSTIC TESTS

Glucose tolerance test: decreased in a small percentage of patients.
Metyrapone test: altered results.
Pregnanediol: decreased excretion.
Thyroid or liver function tests: abnormal results.

NURSING CONSIDERATIONS

Besides those related universally to drug therapy (see "How to use this book"), consider the following specific recommendations:

Assessment

- Obtain a baseline assessment of the patient's underlying condition before initiating therapy with hydroxyprogesterone.
- Be alert for adverse reactions and drug interactions throughout therapy.
- Evaluate the patient's and family's knowledge about hydroxyprogesterone therapy.

Nursing Diagnoses

- Sexual dysfunction related to the patient's underlying condition.
- Fluid volume excess related to hydroxyprogesterone-induced edema.
- Knowledge deficit related to therapy with hydroxyprogesterone.

Planning and Implementation

Preparation and Administration

- FDA regulations require that, before receiving first dose, patients read package insert explaining possible progestin adverse reactions. Provide verbal explanation as well.
- ***I.M. use:*** Give oil solutions (sesame oil and castor oil) deep I.M. in gluteal muscle. Rotate injection sites to prevent muscle atrophy. Be aware that effects last 7 to 14 days.

Monitoring

- Monitor effectiveness by regularly assessing the patient's underlying condition for signs of improvement.
- Monitor patient for edema; weigh daily.

Supportive Care

- Withhold drug and notify the doctor if a pulmonary embolism is suspected; be prepared to provide supportive care as indicated.
- Institute safety measures if adverse CNS reactions occur.
- Obtain an order for an antiemetic agent, as needed.
- Notify doctor if hyperglycemia occurs, especially in a diabetic client as therapy may need to be adjusted.
- Limit patient's sodium intake if not contraindicated.

Patient Teaching

- Instruct patients to report any unusual symptoms immediately and to discontinue the drug and call the doctor if visual disturbances or migraine occurs.
- Check patient's understanding of the package insert information.
- Tell diabetic patients to report symptoms of hyperglycemia or glycosuria.
- Tell patients who become pregnant during therapy with hydroxyprogesterone to stop taking the drug immediately because it may adversely affect the fetus.
- Warn patient that edema and weight gain are likely. Advise them to restrict sodium intake.
- Instruct patients how to perform a monthly breast self-examination.
- Inform patient that normal menstrual cycles may not resume for 2 to 3 months after drug is stopped.

Evaluation

In patients receiving hydroxyprogesterone, appropriate evaluation statements may include:

- Patient exhibits improved health as a result of hydroxyprogesterone therapy.
- Patient does not exhibit fluid excess.
- Patient verbalizes an understanding of hydroxyprogesterone therapy.

hydroxyurea

(hye drox ee yoor ee´ a)
Hydrea**

- *Classification:* antineoplastic (antimetabolite)
- *Pregnancy Risk Category:* D

HOW SUPPLIED

Capsules: 500 mg

ACTION

Mechanism: Inhibits DNA synthesis by inhibiting the incorporation of thymidine onto DNA. Drug also inhibits urease and may block the production of ammonia and thus the increase in urinary pH in patients with urea-producing bacteria in the urinary tract. Drug may be useful in the treatment of sickle cell disease because it increases the production of fetal hemoglobin.
Absorption: Readily absorbed from the GI tract.
Distribution: Readily crosses the blood-brain barrier. Peak CSF levels are seen 3 hours after an oral dose.
Metabolism: About 50% is metabolized in the liver.
Excretion: About 50% of the drug is excreted unchanged in the urine; the rest is excreted in expired air as carbon dioxide or in the urine as urea.
Onset, peak, duration: Peak serum levels occur 2 hours after a dose. Because it is cleared rapidly, higher peak levels may be seen after a large, single dose rather than divided doses.

INDICATIONS & DOSAGE

Melanoma; resistant chronic myelocytic leukemia; recurrent, metastatic, or inoperable ovarian cancer–
Adults: 80 mg/kg P.O. as single dose q 3 days; or 20 to 30 mg/kg P.O. daily.

CONTRAINDICATIONS & PRECAUTIONS

Contraindicated in patients with a leukocyte count below 2,500/mm^3; in those with a platelet count below 100,000/mm^3; and in severely anemic patients because of the drug's hematologic toxicity. Also contraindicated in pregnant patients because it may be fetotoxic.

Use with extreme caution in patients with impaired renal function; they are susceptible to the development of visual and auditory hallucinations and pronounced hematologic toxicity. Hydroxyurea can impair fertility. Reversible germ cell toxicity has followed treatment with hydroxyurea.

ADVERSE REACTIONS

Common reactions are in italics; life-threatening reactions are in bold italics.
Blood: ***leukopenia,*** thrombocytopenia, anemia, ***megaloblastosis; dose-limiting and dose-related bone marrow suppression,*** with rapid recovery.
CNS: drowsiness, hallucinations.
GI: *anorexia, nausea, vomiting, diarrhea,* stomatitis.
GU: increased BUN and serum creatinine levels.
Metabolic: hyperuricemia.
Skin: rash, pruritus.

INTERACTIONS

None significant.

EFFECTS ON DIAGNOSTIC TESTS

BUN, serum creatinine, and serum uric acid: elevated levels.

NURSING CONSIDERATIONS

Besides those related universally to drug therapy (see "How to use this book"), consider the following specific recommendations:
Assessment
- Obtain a baseline assessment of patient's overall physical status, CBC,

serum uric acid, BUN, and serum creatinine before initiating therapy.
- Be alert for adverse reactions and drug interactions throughout therapy.
- Evaluate the patient's and family's knowledge about hydroxyurea therapy.

Nursing Diagnoses
- Altered protection related to hydroxyurea-induced myelosuppression and immunosuppression.
- Altered oral mucous membrane related to hydroxyurea-induced stomatitis.
- Knowledge deficit related to hydroxyurea therapy.

Planning and Implementation

Preparation and Administration
- If patient can't swallow capsule, it may be opened into water and taken immediately.
- Keep in mind that dosage modification may be required following other chemotherapy or radiation therapy.

Monitoring
- Monitor effectiveness by noting results of follow-up diagnostic tests and patient's overall physical status.
- Monitor for signs of infection (cough, fever, sore throat) and bleeding (easy bruising, nosebleeds, bleeding gums). Monitor CBC.
- Monitor intake and output.
- Routinely monitor BUN, uric acid, and serum creatinine levels.
- Monitor for skin reaction. Keep in mind that this drug may exaccerbate postirradiation erythema.
- Monitor for GI adverse reactions, such as nausea, vomiting, diarrhea, and stomatitis.

Supportive Care
- Keep patient well hydrated.
- Keep in mind that this drug crosses the blood-brain barrier.
- Do not give I.M. injections when platelet count is less than 100,000/mm^3.
- Be aware that auditory and visual hallucinations and blood toxicity increase when decreased renal function exists.
- Discontinue therapy if WBC is less than 3,500/mm^3 or if platelet count is less than 100,000/mm^3.
- Administer excellent mouth care to help prevent stomatitis.
- To help prevent infection, maintain the patient's optimal health and protect him from undue exposure to environmental contagions. If signs of infection occur, notify doctor promptly; administer antibiotics, as ordered.
- Provide a safe environment to minimize risk of bleeding.

Patient Teaching
- Warn patients to watch for signs of infection (sore throat, fever, fatigue), and for signs of bleeding (easy bruising, nosebleeds, bleeding gums). Tell patient to take temperature daily and to promptly report signs of infection or bleeding.
- Instruct patient about need for protective measures, including conservation of energy, balanced diet, adequate rest, personal cleanliness, clean environment, and avoidance of exposure to persons with infections.
- Teach patient to avoid the use of all OTC products containing aspirin. Instruct patient about safety precautions to reduce risk of bleeding from falls, cuts, or other injuries.
- Instruct patient about the need for frequent oral hygiene.
- Encourage the patient to drink at least 3 liters of fluids daily to increase urine output and facilitate excretion of uric acid.
- Tell the patient to call immediately if vomiting occurs shortly after taking a dose.

Evaluation

In patients receiving hydroxyurea, appropriate evaluation statements may include:
- Patient does not demonstrate signs and symptoms of infection or bleeding.

• Oral lesions are absent.
• Patient and family state an understanding of hydroxyurea therapy.

hydroxyzine hydrochloride (hydroxyzine embonate)

(hye drox´ i zeen)

Anxanil, Apo-Hydroxyzine†, Atarax*, Atozine, Durrax, E-Vista, Hydroxacen, Hyzine-50, Multipax†, Novohydroxyzin†, Quiess, Vistacon, Vistaject, Vistaquel, Vistaril, Vistazine

hydroxyzine pamoate

Hy-Pam, Vamate, Vistaril

• *Classification:* anxiolytic, sedative, antipruritic, antiemetic, antispasmodic (antihistamine)
• *Pregnancy Risk Category:* C

HOW SUPPLIED

hydrochloride
Tablets: 10 mg, 25 mg, 50 mg, 100 mg
Capsules: 10 mg†‡, 25 mg†‡, 50 mg†‡
Syrup: 10 mg/5 ml
Injection: 25 mg/ml, 50 mg/ml
pamoate
Capsules: 25 mg, 50 mg, 100 mg
Oral suspension: 25 mg/5 ml

ACTION

Mechanism: Depresses the CNS at the limbic and subcortical levels of the brain.
Absorption: Rapidly and completely absorbed after oral administration.
Distribution: Not well understood.
Metabolism: Almost completely metabolized in the liver.
Excretion: Metabolites are excreted primarily in urine; small amounts of drug and metabolites are found in feces. Half-life: 3 hours. Sedative effects can last for 4 to 6 hours, and antihistamine effects can persist for up to 4 days.
Onset, peak, duration: Peak serum levels occur within 2 to 4 hours. Sedation and other clinical effects are usually noticed in 15 to 30 minutes.

INDICATIONS & DOSAGE

Anxiety and tension–
Adults: 25 to 100 mg P.O. t.i.d. or q.i.d.
Anxiety, tension, hyperkinesia–
Children 6 years and over: 50 to 100 mg P.O. daily in divided doses.
Children under 6 years: 50 mg P.O. daily in divided doses.
Preoperative and postoperative adjunctive therapy–
Adults: 25 to 100 mg I.M. q 4 to 6 hours.
Children: 1.1 mg/kg I.M. q 4 to 6 hours.
Rashes, pruritus–
Adults: 25 mg P.O. t..i.d. or q.i.d.
Children 6 years and over: 50 to 100 mg P.O. daily in divided doses.
Children under 6 years: 50 mg P.O. daily in divided doses.

CONTRAINDICATIONS & PRECAUTIONS

Contraindicated in patients with hypersensitivity to the drug. Use cautiously in patients with open-angle glaucoma, urinary retention, or any other condition where anticholinergic effects would be detrimental.

ADVERSE REACTIONS

Common reactions are in italics; life-threatening reactions are in bold italics.
CNS: *drowsiness,* involuntary motor activity.
GI: *dry mouth.*
Local: marked discomfort at site of I.M. injection.

INTERACTIONS

Alcohol, other CNS depressants: increased CNS depression. Avoid concomitant use.

EFFECTS ON DIAGNOSTIC TESTS

Skin allergen tests: false-negative tests by inhibiting cutaneous response to histamine.
Urine 17-hydroxycorticosteroid: falsely elevated levels.

NURSING CONSIDERATIONS

Besides those related universally to drug therapy (see "How to use this book"), consider the following specific recommendations:

Assessment
- Obtain a baseline assessment of the patient's anxiety level before therapy.
- Be alert for adverse reactions and drug interactions throughout therapy.
- Evaluate the patient's and family's knowledge about hydroxyzine therapy.

Nursing Diagnoses
- Anxiety related to patient's underlying condition.
- Altered oral mucous membrane related to hydroxyzine-induced dry mouth.
- Knowledge deficit related to hydroxyzine therapy.

Planning and Implementation

Preparation and Administration
- Parenteral form (hydrochloride) for I.M. use only (Z-track injection is preferred). Never administer I.V.
- ***I.M. use:*** Aspirate injection carefully to prevent inadvertent intravascular injection. Inject deep into a large muscle.
- Dosage should be reduced in elderly or debilitated patients.

Monitoring
- Regularly monitor effectiveness by asking the patient about feelings of anxiety and by observing his behavior.
- Monitor frequently for degree of dry mouth.
- Monitor for excessive sedation due to potentiation with other CNS drugs.

Supportive Care
- If drowsiness or involuntary motor activity occurs, institute safety precautions, such as supervising ambulation.
- Provide frequent sips of water or ice chips for dry mouth.
- Encourage and support ancillary treatments such as professional counseling and problem identification.

Patient Teaching
- Warn the patient to avoid driving and other hazardous activities that require alertness and good psychomotor coordination until CNS effects of the drug are known.
- Warn the patient not to combine drug with alcohol or other CNS depressants.
- Alert the patient to expect some marked discomfort at the injection site.
- Suggest sugarless hard candy, ice chips, or gum to relieve dry mouth.

Evaluation

In the patient receiving hydroxyzine, appropriate evaluation statements include:
- Patient states he is less anxious.
- Patient states that use of sugarless candy, ice chips, or gum relieves the discomfort of dry mouth.
- Patient and family state an understanding of hydroxyzine therapy.

*Liquid form contains alcohol.

**May contain tartrazine.

IJK

ibuprofen

(eye byoo proe´ fen)

Aches-N-Pain◇, Advil◇, Amersol†, Apo-Ibuprofen†, Brufen‡, Cap-Profen◇, Genpril◇, Haltran◇, Ibuprin◇, Inflam‡, Medipren Caplets◇, Medipren Tablets◇, Midol-200◇, Motrin, Motrin IB◇, Novoprofen†, Nuprin◇, Pamprin-IB◇, Rafen‡, Rufen, Trendar◇

- *Classification:* nonnarcotic analgesic, antipyretic (nonsteroidal anti-inflammatory agent)
- *Pregnancy Risk Category:* B (D in 3rd trimester)

HOW SUPPLIED

Tablets: 200 mg◇, 300 mg, 400 mg, 600 mg, 800 mg
Caplets: 200 mg◇
Oral suspension: 100 mg/5 ml

ACTION

Mechanism: Produces anti-inflammatory, analgesic, and antipyretic effects, possibly through inhibition of prostaglandin synthesis.
Absorption: Rapidly and completely absorbed from the GI tract.
Distribution: Highly protein-bound.
Metabolism: Undergoes biotransformation in the liver.
Excretion: Mainly in urine, with some biliary excretion. Half-life: Plasma half-life ranges from 2 to 4 hours.
Onset, peak, duration: Effects are seen within 1 hour and last 4 to 8 hours.

INDICATIONS & DOSAGE

Mild-to-moderate pain, arthritis, primary dysmenorrhea, gout, postextraction dental pain–
Adults: 200 to 800 mg P.O. t.i.d. or q.i.d. not to exceed 3.2 g/day.

CONTRAINDICATIONS & PRECAUTIONS

Contraindicated in patients with hypersensitivity to the drug and in patients in whom aspirin or other NSAIDs induce symptoms of asthma, urticaria, or rhinitis.

Patients with known "triad" symptoms (aspirin hypersensitivity, rhinitis/nasal polyps, and asthma) are at high risk of bronchospasm.

Serious GI toxicity, especially ulceration or hemorrhage, can occur at any time in patients on chronic NSAID therapy. Ibuprofen should be administered cautiously to patients with a history of GI disease, hepatic or renal disease, cardiac decompensation, systemic lupus erythematosus, or bleeding abnormalities because the drug may worsen these conditions.

NSAIDs may mask the signs and symptoms of acute infection (fever, myalgia, erythema); carefully evaluate patients with high risk (for example, those with diabetes).

ADVERSE REACTIONS

Common reactions are in italics; life-threatening reactions are in bold italics.
Blood: prolonged bleeding time.
CNS: *headache, drowsiness, dizziness,* aseptic meningitis.
CV: *peripheral edema.*
EENT: visual disturbances, *tinnitus.*
GI: *epigastric distress, nausea, occult blood loss, peptic ulceration.*
GU: reversible renal failure.

†Available in Canada only. ‡Available in Australia only. ◇Available OTC.

Hepatic: elevated enzymes.
Skin: pruritus, rash, urticaria.
Other: ***bronchospasm,*** edema.

INTERACTIONS

Furosemide, thiazide diuretics: ibuprofen may decrease the effectiveness of diuretics.
Oral anticoagulants, lithium: ibuprofen may increase plasma levels or pharmacologic effects of these agents. Monitor for toxicity.

EFFECTS ON DIAGNOSTIC TESTS

Bleeding time: prolonged.
Blood glucose: decreased concentrations.
BUN: increased levels.
Prothrombin time: increased.
Serum alkaline phosphatase, serum lactic dehydrogenase, and serum transaminase: increased levels.
Serum creatinine and serum potassium: increased levels.
Serum uric acid, hemoglobin, and hematocrit levels: decreased levels.

NURSING CONSIDERATIONS

Besides those related universally to drug therapy (see "How to use this book"), consider the following specific recommendations:

Assessment

- Obtain a baseline assessment of the patient's pain before therapy.
- Be alert for adverse reactions and drug interactions throughout therapy.
- Evaluate the patient's and family's knowledge about ibuprofen therapy.

Nursing Diagnoses

- Pain related to the patient's underlying condition.
- High risk for trauma related to possible drowsiness or dizziness from adverse CNS reaction to ibuprofen.
- Knowledge deficit related to ibuprofen therapy.

Planning and Implementation

Preparation and Administration

- ***P.O. use:*** Give with meals or milk to reduce adverse GI reactions.

Monitoring

- Regularly monitor for relief of pain, keeping in mind that full therapeutic effects in arthritis may take 2 to 4 weeks of therapy.
- Test the patient's stool for occult blood.
- Regularly monitor renal and hepatic function in long-term therapy.
- Monitor for fluid retention, especially in elderly patients.

Supportive Care

- Notify the doctor if the patient's pain persists or worsens.
- If adverse CNS reactions occur, institute safety precautions: supervise ambulation and keep the bed rails up.
- Hold dose and notify the doctor if the patient develops renal or hepatic abnormalities, or experiences nausea, vomiting, or epigastric distress that is not relieved by taking drug with food or milk.

Patient Teaching

- Inform the patient that the full therapeutic effect for arthritis may be delayed for 2 to 4 weeks. Explain that the analgesic effect occurs at low dosage levels, but the anti-inflammatory effect requires dosages above 400 mg q.i.d.
- Advise the patient to notify the doctor if pain persists or becomes worse.
- Instruct the patient not to exceed 3.2 g daily, nor to self-medicate for extended periods without consulting the doctor.
- Advise the patient to avoid driving and other hazardous activities that require mental alertness until CNS effects of the drug are known.
- Tell the patient to take the drug with food or milk.
- Because serious GI toxicity can occur at any time in chronic NSAID therapy, teach the patient signs and symptoms of GI bleeding. Tell the patient to report these to the doctor immediately.

• Advise the patient to avoid aspirin and alcohol during therapy. Concomitant use with aspirin, alcohol, or steroids may increase the risk of adverse GI reactions.

Evaluation

In the patient receiving ibuprofen, appropriate evaluation statements include:

• Patient states pain is relieved.
• Patient does not develop traumatic injuries as a result of adverse CNS reactions.
• Patient and family state an understanding of ibuprofen therapy.

idoxuridine (IDU)

(eye dox yoor´ i deen)

Herplex, Stoxil

• *Classification:* antiviral agent (halogenated pyrimidine)
• *Pregnancy Risk Category:* C

HOW SUPPLIED

Ophthalmic ointment: 0.5%
Ophthalmic solution: 0.1%

ACTION

Mechanism: A pyrimidine nucleoside that interferes with DNA synthesis. Drug is converted intracellularly to the triphosphate form, which is incorporated into viral DNA during replication instead of thymidine. This renders the DNA molecule more susceptible to breakage, resulting in an increased number of mutations, interference with protein synthesis, and inhibition of viral replication.

Absorption: After topical ophthalmic administration, absorption is poor.

Metabolism: Experimental evidence suggests that the drug is rapidly degraded to iodouracil and iodide in the liver.

INDICATIONS & DOSAGE

Herpes simplex keratitis–

Adults and children: instill 1 drop of solution into conjunctival sac q 1 hour during day and q 2 hours at night, or apply ointment to conjunctival sac q 4 hours or 5 times daily, with last dose at bedtime. A response should be seen in 7 days; if not, discontinue and begin alternate therapy. Therapy should not be continued longer than 21 days.

CONTRAINDICATIONS & PRECAUTIONS

Contraindicated in patients with hypersensitivity to idoxuridine or to any component of the preparation.

ADVERSE REACTIONS

Common reactions are in italics; life-threatening reactions are in bold italics.

Eye: *temporary visual haze; blurred vision (with ointment);* irritation, pain, burning, or inflammation of eye; mild edema of eyelid or cornea; photophobia; small punctate defects in corneal epithelium, corneal ulceration; slowed corneal wound healing (with ointment).

Other: hypersensitivity.

INTERACTIONS

Boric acid: precipitate formation; increased risk of ocular toxicity.

EFFECTS ON DIAGNOSTIC TESTS

None reported.

NURSING CONSIDERATIONS

Besides those related universally to drug therapy (see "How to use this book"), consider the following specific recommendations:

Assessment

• Obtain a baseline assessment of allergies and other eye medications currently being used before therapy.
• Be alert for adverse reactions and drug interactions throughout therapy.

• Evaluate the patient's and family's knowledge about idoxuridine therapy.

Nursing Diagnoses

• Altered protection related to ocular infection.

• Sensory/perceptual alteration (visual), related to idoxuridine-induced visual blurring.

• Knowledge deficit related to idoxuridine therapy.

Planning and Implementation

Preparation and Administration

• Refrigerate idoxuridine 0.1% solution. Store in a tightly sealed, light-resistant container.

• Wash hands before and after administration.

• Cleanse eye area of excess exudate before administration.

• Do not mix with other eye medications.

Monitoring

• Monitor effectiveness by culturing the eye to check for microorganisms.

• Observe color, amount, and consistency of exudate.

• Check the patient's vision.

• Observe for signs of hypersensitivity to drug.

Supportive Care

• Apply warm, moist compress to aid in removal of dried exudate.

• Use safety precautions if vision is impaired. Assist with activities.

• Do not use for long-term therapy or deep ulceration.

• Do not use old solution; causes ocular burning and has no antiviral activity.

Patient Teaching

• Teach the patient how to instill. Advise him to wash hands before and after administration. Warn him not to touch tip of dropper to eye or surrounding tissue.

• Instruct the patient to apply light finger pressure to lacrimal sac for 1 minute after drops are instilled. Caution him to avoid rubbing or scratching the eye area.

• Instruct the patient to watch for signs of hypersensitivity (itching lids, swelling, constant burning). If these occur, stop the drug and notify the doctor immediately.

• Warn patient to avoid sharing washcloths and towels with family members during infection.

• Advise the patient to wear sunglasses to minimize photophobia and avoid prolonged exposure to sunlight.

• Warn the patient not to share eye medications with family members. A family member who develops the same symptoms should contact the doctor.

Evaluation

In patients receiving idoxuridine, appropriate evaluation statements may include:

• Patient remains free from signs and symptoms of infection.

• Patient reports decrease or absence of visual blurring.

• Patient and family state an understanding of idoxuridine therapy.

---

ifosfamide

(eye foss´ fa mide)

Ifex

• *Classification:* antineoplastic (alkylating agent)

• *Pregnancy Risk Category:* D

HOW SUPPLIED

Injection: 1 g (supplied with 200-mg ampule of mesna), 2 g†, 3 g†

ACTION

Mechanism: An alkylating agent that cross-links strands of cellular DNA, and interferes with RNA transcription causing an imbalance of growth that leads to cell death. A synthetic analog of cyclophosphamide that is inactive, drug requires hepatic microsomal liver enzyme metabolism to the active form. Cell cycle–nonspecific.

Distribution: Crosses the blood-brain barrier but its metabolites do not; therefore, alkylating activity does not occur in the cerebrospinal fluid.
Metabolism: Dose-dependent; about 40% metabolized at doses of 5 g/m², while 80% to 90% is metabolized at lower doses (1.6 to 2.4 g/m²). Metabolism is required to generate the active form of the drug; alkylated metabolites interact with DNA. Metabolism is quite variable among patients.
Excretion: Ifosfamide and its metabolites are excreted primarily in the urine. Half-life: Elimination half-life is also dose-dependent; mean terminal half-life is about 15 hours at doses of 3.8 to 5 g/m², and drug disappears from the plasma in a biphasic manner. At lower doses (1.6 to 2.4 g/m²), drug elimination is monophasic, with a mean elimination half-life of about 7 hours.

INDICATIONS & DOSAGE

Testicular cancer–
Adults: 1.2 g/m²/day I.V. for 5 consecutive days. Treatment is repeated every 3 weeks or after the patient recovers from hematologic toxicity.

CONTRAINDICATIONS & PRECAUTIONS

No contraindications. Dosage adjustments are necessary in renal impairment.

ADVERSE REACTIONS

Common reactions are in italics; life-threatening reactions are in bold italics.
Blood: leukopenia, thrombocytopenia, ***myelosuppression.***
CNS: *lethargy, somnolence, confusion, depressive psychosis,* coma.
GI: *nausea, vomiting.*
GU: ***hemorrhagic cystitis*** *(dose-limiting adverse reaction occurring in up to 50% of patients), hematuria,* nephrotoxicity.
Hepatic: elevated liver enzymes.
Other: *alopecia.*

INTERACTIONS

Allopurinol: may produce excessive ifosfamide effect by prolonging half-life. Monitor for enhanced toxicity.
Barbiturates: induce hepatic enzymes, hastening the formation of toxic metabolites. Ifosfamide toxicity may be increased.
Corticosteroids: may inhibit hepatic enzymes, reducing ifosfamide's effect. Monitor for enhanced ifosfamide toxicity if concurrent steroid dosage is suddenly reduced or discontinued.
Myelosuppressants: enhanced hematologic toxicity. Dosage adjustment may be necessary.

EFFECTS ON DIAGNOSTIC TESTS

Serum AST (SGOT), ALT (SGPT), and alkaline phosphatase: increased concentrations.

NURSING CONSIDERATIONS

Besides those related universally to drug therapy (see "How to use this book"), consider the following specific recommendations:

Assessment
- Obtain a baseline assessment of CBC, platelets, liver enzymes, bilirubin, and urinalysis before initiating therapy.
- Be alert for adverse reactions and drug interactions throughout therapy.
- Evaluate the patient's and family's knowledge about ifosfamide therapy.

Nursing Diagnoses
- High risk for infection related to leukopenia and myelosuppression.
- Pain related to drug-induced hemorrhagic cystitis.
- Knowledge deficit related to ifosfamide therapy.

Planning and Implementation
Preparation and Administration
- Expect to administer antiemetics before giving this drug. Premedicating with antiemetics may help lessen nausea and vomiting.
- Avoid giving drug at bedtime, as in-

frequent voiding throughout night may lead to cystitis.

• ***I.V. use:*** Keep in mind that preparation of parenteral form is potentially risky. Follow institutional policy to prevent personal exposure and risk. Reconstitute the drug with sterile water or bacteriostatic water for injection to reach a final concentration of 50 mg/ml. It may be further diluted with 0.9% sodium chloride, dextrose 5% in water, or Ringer's lactated solution. Reconstituted solutions are stable for 1 week at 30° C. and 3 weeks at 5° C. However, use within 6 hours if reconstituted with sterile water without a preservative (such as benzyl alcohol or parabens.). Administer this drug slowly over 30 minutes and give with a protecting agent (mesna) to prevent hemorrhagic cystitis.

Monitoring

• Monitor effectiveness by noting results of follow-up diagnostic tests and overall physical status.

• Monitor CBC results, liver enzymes level, platelet count, and urinalysis during treatment.

• Monitor for CNS changes such as changes in mental status, cerebellar dysfunction, lethargy, and depression.

• Monitor intake and output; promote intake of up to 3 liters daily.

• Monitor patient's mouth for furry patches on the tongue and oral membranes.

• Monitor for the presence of light-colored stools, jaundice, or frothy dark urine.

• Monitor the patient for signs of infection (fever, sore throat, fatigue).

Supportive Care

• Provide adequate intake when the patient is given ifosfamide. It is essential that fluid intake of 2 liters/day, either P.O. or I.V. be maintained to help prevent hemorrhagic cystitis.

• Use cautiously with renal or hepatic impairment.

• Keep in mind that bladder irrigation with normal saline may decrease the possibility of cystitis. Notify the doctor if you suspect that cystitis has developed and expect to stop the drug.

• Do not give any I.M. injections if platelet count $< 100{,}000/mm^3$.

Patient Teaching

• Instruct patient to watch for signs of infection (fever, sore throat, fatigue) and bleeding (easy bleeding, nosebleeds, bleeding gums, and melena). Tell him to take his temperature daily.

• Stress the importance of adequate fluid intake when ifosfamide is administered. Explain that it may help prevent hemorrhagic cystitis.

• Warn the patient that hyperpigmentation may occur.

• Advise female patients to use contraception for 4 months after therapy. If the treatment is to last 6 months, advise that infertility may result.

• Ask the patient's family to help monitor for neurotoxic effects, which may elude the patient.

• Stress that normal wound healing may be delayed during treatment with ifosfamide.

• Explain to the patient that hair loss, nausea, and vomiting are frequent side effects.

• Tell the patient to avoid using OTC products that contain aspirin. Explain that use of these products can increase the possibility of bleeding problems.

Evaluation

In patients receiving ifosfamide, appropriate evaluation statements may include:

• Patient remains free of infection during and after ifosfamide therapy.

• Pain is alleviated by adequate hydration and prevention of cystitis.

• Patient and family state an understanding of ifosfamide therapy.

imipenem/cilastatin sodium
(i mi pen´ em)
Primaxin

• *Classification:* antibiotic (carbapenem, beta-lactam)
• *Pregnancy Risk Category:* C

HOW SUPPLIED
Injection: 250-ml, 500-ml vials

ACTION
Mechanism: Bactericidal and inhibits bacterial cell wall synthesis. Cilastatin inhibits the enzymatic breakdown of imipenem in the kidney, making it effective in the urinary tract.
Absorption: Imipenem/cilastatin must be given parenterally; incompletely absorbed after I.M. administration, with peak serum levels lower than after I.V. infusion. However, drug is present in the plasma longer after I.M. injection.
Distribution: Imipenem/cilastatin is distributed rapidly and widely. Approximately 20% of imipenem is protein-bound; 40% of cilastatin is protein-bound.
Metabolism: Imipenem is metabolized by kidneys to dehydropeptidase I, resulting in low urine concentration. Cilastatin inhibits this enzyme, thereby reducing imipenem's metabolism.
Excretion: About 70% of imipenem/cilastatin dose is excreted unchanged by the kidneys by tubular secretion and glomerular filtration. Imipenem is removed by hemodialysis. Half-life: About 1 hour.
Onset, peak, duration: After I.M. injection, peak plasma levels of imipenem occur within 2 hours, and peak levels of cilastatin occur within 1 hour.

INDICATIONS & DOSAGE
Treatment of serious infections of the lower respiratory and urinary tracts, intraabdominal and gynecologic infections, bacterial septicemia, bone and joint infections, skin and soft tissue infections, and endocarditis. Most known microorganisms susceptible: Staphylococcus, Streptococcus, Escherichia coli, Klebsiella, Proteus, Enterobacter, Pseudomonas aeruginosa, *and* Bacteroides, *including* B. fragilis–
Adults: 250 mg to 1 g by I.V. infusion q 6 to 8 hours. Maximum daily dosage is 50 mg/kg/day or 4 g/day, whichever is less.

CONTRAINDICATIONS & PRECAUTIONS
Contraindicated in patients with hypersensitivity to the drug.

Use cautiously in patients with a history of seizures, especially if they also have compromised renal function, because drug may induce seizures; and in patients who are allergic to penicillin or cephalosporins, because this drug is chemically similar to them. Chloramphenicol may impede the bactericidal effects of imipenem; give chloramphenicol a few hours after imipenem/cilastatin.

ADVERSE REACTIONS
Common reactions are in italics; life-threatening reactions are in bold italics.
CNS: *seizures,* dizziness.
CV: hypotension.
GI: nausea, vomiting, diarrhea, ***pseudomembranous colitis.***
Skin: rash, urticaria, pruritus.
Local: *thrombophlebitis, pain at injection site.*
Other: ***hypersensitivity.***

INTERACTIONS
None significant.

EFFECTS ON DIAGNOSTIC TESTS

AST (SGOT), ALT (SGPT), alkaline phosphatase, lactic dehydrogenase, and bilirubin: elevated serum levels.
CBC: reduced RBC, WBC, erythrocyte, and platelet counts.

NURSING CONSIDERATIONS

Besides those related universally to drug therapy (see "How to use this book"), consider the following specific recommendations:

Assessment

- Obtain a baseline assessment of infection before imipenem/cilastatin therapy.
- Be alert for adverse reactions and drug interactions throughout therapy.
- Evaluate the patient's and family's knowledge about imipenem/cilastatin therapy.

Nursing Diagnoses

- High risk for injury related to ineffectiveness of imipenem/cilastatin to eradicate the infection.
- High risk for fluid volume deficit related to adverse GI reactions caused by imipenem/cilastatin.
- Knowledge deficit related to imipenem/cilastatin.

Planning and Implementation

Preparation and Administration

- Obtain specimen for culture and sensitivity tests before first dose. Therapy may begin pending test results.
- Before giving first dose, ask patient about hypersensitivity reactions to either drug.
- Be aware that patients with impaired renal function may need lower dosage or longer intervals between doses.
- ***I.V. use:*** Don't administer by direct I.V. bolus injection. Each 250 or 500 mg dose should be infused over 20 to 30 minutes; each 1 g dose over 40 to 60 minutes. If nausea develops, the infusion may be slowed further. When reconstituting powder, shake until the solution is clear. Solutions may range from colorless to yellow and; color variations within this range don't affect the drug's potency. After reconstitution, solution is stable for 10 hours at room temperature and for 48 hours when refrigerated.

Monitoring

- Monitor effectiveness by regularly assessing for improvement in the infection.
- Monitor hydration status if adverse GI reactions occur.
- Monitor patient for bacterial or fungal superinfections and resistant infections during and after therapy.

Supportive Care

- Institute safety and seizure precautions. If patient develops seizures despite anticonvulsant therapy, notify doctor. The drug should then be discontinued.

Patient Teaching

- Instruct the patient and family about imipenem/cilastatin, including the dose, frequency, action, and adverse reactions.

Evaluation

In patients receiving imipenem/cilastatin, appropriate evaluation statements may include:

- Patient is free from infection.
- Patient's maintains adequate hydration throughout imipenem/cilastatin therapy.
- Patient and family state an understanding of imipenem/cilastatin therapy.

---

imipramine hydrochloride

(im ip´ ra meen)

Apo-Imipramine†, Impirin‡, Impril†, Janimine**, Novo-Pramine†, Tripramine, Tofranil**

imipramine pamoate

Tofranil-PM**

- *Classification:* tricyclic antidepressant (dibenzazepine)

*Liquid form contains alcohol.

**May contain tartrazine.

• *Pregnancy Risk Category:* D

HOW SUPPLIED

Tablets: 10 mg, 25 mg, 50 mg
Injection: 12.5 mg/ml

ACTION

Mechanism: Increases the amount of norepinephrine or serotonin, or both, in the CNS by blocking their reuptake by the presynaptic neurons.
Absorption: Rapidly absorbed from the GI tract and muscle tissue after oral and I.M. administration.
Distribution: Widely distributed into the body, including the CNS and breast milk. Drug is 90% protein-bound. Therapeutic plasma levels (parent drug and metabolite) are thought to range from 150 to 300 ng/ml.
Metabolism: By the liver to the active metabolite desipramine. A significant first-pass effect may explain variability of serum concentrations in different patients taking the same dosage.
Excretion: Most of drug is excreted in urine. Half-life: 6 to 12 hours.
Onset, peak, duration: Peak plasma levels are seen in 30 minutes to 2 hours; steady state is achieved with 2 to 5 days of daily administration. Optimal antidepressant effect may take several weeks.

INDICATIONS & DOSAGE

Treatment of depression–
Adults: 75 to 100 mg P.O. or I.M. daily in divided doses, with 25- to 50-mg increments up to 200 mg. Maximum dosage is 300 mg daily. Alternatively, the entire dosage may be given at bedtime. (I.M. route rarely used.)
Childhood enuresis–
Children 6 years and older:
25 mg P.O. 1 hour before bedtime. If no response within 1 week, increase to 50 mg if the child is under 12 years; increase to 75 mg for children 12 years and over. In either case, do not exceed 2.5 mg/kg/day.

CONTRAINDICATIONS & PRECAUTIONS

Contraindicated in patients with hypersensitivity to tricyclic antidepressants, trazodone, and related compounds; in the acute recovery phase of myocardial infarction (MI) because of arrhythmogenic potential; in patients in coma or severe respiratory depression because of additive CNS depression; and during or within 14 days of therapy with MAO inhibitors.

Use cautiously in patients with other cardiac disease (arrhythmias, CHF, angina pectoris, valvular disease, increased QRS intervals, or heart block); respiratory disorders; seizure disorders; scheduled electroconvulsive therapy; bipolar disease; glaucoma; hyperthyroidism, or in those taking thyroid replacement; Type I and Type II diabetes; prostatic hypertrophy, paralytic ileus, or urinary retention; hepatic or renal dysfunction; Parkinson's disease; and in those undergoing surgery with general anesthesia.

Some formulations contain tartrazine and may provoke asthma in patients with aspirin allergy.

ADVERSE REACTIONS

Common reactions are in italics; life-threatening reactions are in bold italics.
CNS: *drowsiness, dizziness,* excitation, tremors, weakness, confusion, headache, nervousness.
CV: *orthostatic hypotension, tachycardia, ECG changes,* hypertension.
EENT: *blurred vision,* tinnitus, mydriasis.
GI: *dry mouth, constipation,* nausea, vomiting, anorexia, paralytic ileus.
GU: *urine retention.*
Skin: rash, urticaria.
Other: *sweating,* allergy.
After abrupt withdrawal of long-term

therapy: nausea, headache, malaise. (Does not indicate addiction.)

INTERACTIONS

Barbiturates: decrease TCA blood levels. Monitor for decreased antidepressant effect.
Cimetidine: may increase imipramine serum levels. Monitor for increased adverse reactions.
Epinephrine, norepinephrine: increase hypertensive effect. Use with caution.
MAO inhibitors: may cause severe excitation, hyperpyrexia, or seizures, usually with high dose. Use together cautiously.
Methylphenidate: increases TCA blood levels. Monitor for enhanced antidepressant effect.

EFFECTS ON DIAGNOSTIC TESTS

CBC: decreased WBC counts.
ECG: elongated Q-T and PR intervals; flattened T waves.
Liver function tests: elevated results.
Serum glucose: decreased or increased levels.

NURSING CONSIDERATIONS

Besides those related universally to drug therapy (see "How to use this book"), consider the following specific recommendations:

Assessment

- Obtain a baseline assessment of depression before therapy.
- Be alert for adverse reactions and drug interactions throughout therapy.
- Evaluate the patient's and family's knowledge about imipramine therapy.

Nursing Diagnoses

- Ineffectve individual coping related to the patient's underlying condition.
- High risk for injury related to imipramine-induced CNS and cardiovascular adverse reactions.
- Knowledge deficit related to imipramine therapy.

Planning and Implementation

Preparation and Administration

- Expect reduced dosage in elderly patients, debilitated patients, adolescents and patients with aggravated psychotic symptoms.
- For treatment of "early night" bedwetting, drug may be more effective in divided dosage, with the first dose administered earlier in the day (such as late afternoon). If necessary, discuss the dosage schedule with the doctor.

Monitoring

- Monitor effectiveness by having the patient discuss his feelings (ask broad, open-ended questions) and by evaluating his behavior; or the drug is given to treat enuresis, by noting decreased bedwetting.
- Monitor blood pressure (supine and standing), ECG for changes, and heart rate for tachycardia.
- Monitor bowel patterns for constipation.
- Monitor for suicidal tendencies.

Supportive Care

- Institute safety precautions if adverse CNS reactions occur.
- Do not withdraw drug abruptly.
- If psychotic signs increase, notify doctor and expect dosage to be reduced.
- If not contraindicated, increase the patient's fluid and fiber intake to prevent constipation; if needed, obtain an order for a stool softener or laxative.
- Assist the patient in changing positions slowly to minimize orthostatic hypotension.
- I.M. route is rarely used.

Patient Teaching

- Tell the patient to relieve dry mouth with sugarless hard candy or gum, but explain that saliva substitutes may be necessary.
- Advise patient to minimize constipation by increasing fluid intake. Suggest stool softener or high-fiber diet, if needed.

• Warn the patient to avoid driving and other hazardous activities that require alertness and good psychomotor coordination until CNS effects of the drug are known. Inform the patient that drug has strong sedative effects. Warn against combining with alcohol or other CNS depressants.
• Tell the patient that drowsiness and dizziness usually subside after first few weeks.
• Tell the patient that treatment must continue for 2 weeks or more before noticeable effect, and for 4 weeks or more for effect. Encourage the patient to continue taking medication until it achieves full therapeutic effect.
• Advise the patient not to take any other drugs (prescription or OTC) without first consulting the doctor.
• Warn the patient about possible morning orthostatic hypotension. Instruct the patient to rise slowly and to sit for several minutes before standing up.

Evaluation
In patients receiving imipramine, appropriate evaluation statements may include:
• Patient behavior and communication indicate improvement of depression.
• Patient has not experienced injury from adverse CNS or cardiovascular reactions.
• Patient and family state an understanding of imipramine therapy.

immune globulin intramuscular (IGIM, IG, gamma globulin)
Gamastan, Gammar

immune globulin intravenous (IGIV)
Gamimine N, Gammagard, Sandoglobulin, Venoglobulin-I

• *Classification:* immune serum
• *Pregnancy Risk Category:* C

HOW SUPPLIED
intramuscular
Injection: 2-ml, 10-ml vials
intravenous
Injection: 5% in 10-ml, 50-ml, 100-ml vials (Gamimune N)
Powder for injection: 50 mg protein/ml in 0.5-g, 2.5-g, 5-g, 10-g vials (Gammagard); 1-g, 3-g, 6-g vials (Sandoglobulin); 2.5-g, 5-g vials (Venoglobulin-I)

ACTION
Mechanism: Provides passive immunity by increasing antibody titer.
Distribution: Gamma globulin evenly distributed between intravascular and extravascular spaces.
Metabolism: Unknown.
Excretion: Half-life: Serum half-life of gamma globulin is reportedly 21 to 24 days in immunocompetent patients.
Onset, peak, duration: After slow I.M. absorption, serum concentrations of gamma globulin peak within 2 days.

INDICATIONS & DOSAGE
Agammaglobulinemia or hypogammaglobulinemia –
Adults: 30 to 50 ml I.M. monthly. Alternatively, administer 100 mg/kg I.V. (Gamimune N) once a month. Infuse at 0.01 to 0.02 ml/kg/min for 30 minutes. For Sandoglobulin, administer 200 mg/kg I.V. once a month. Infuse at 0.5 to 1 ml/min. After 15 to 30 minutes, increase infusion rate to 1.5 to 2.5 ml/min.
Children: 20 to 40 ml I.M. monthly.
Hepatitis A exposure –
Adults and children: 0.02 to 0.04 ml/kg I.M. as soon as possible after exposure. Up to 0.1 ml/kg may be given after prolonged or intense exposure.

Post-transfusion hepatitis B–
Adults and children: 10 ml I.M. within 1 week after transfusion and 10 ml I.M. 1 month later.
Measles exposure–
Adults and children: 0.02 ml/kg I.M. within 6 days after exposure.
Modification of measles–
Adults and children: 0.04 ml/kg I.M. within 6 days after exposure.
Measles vaccine complications–
Adults and children: 0.02 to 0.04 ml/kg I.M.
Poliomyelitis exposure–
Adults and children: 0.3 to 0.4 ml/kg I.M. within 7 days after exposure.
Chicken pox exposure–
Adults and children: 0.2 to 1.3 ml/kg I.M. as soon as exposed.
Rubella exposure in first trimester of pregnancy–
Women: 0.2 to 0.4 ml/kg I.M. as soon as exposed.
Prophylaxis in primary immunodeficiencies–
Adults and children: 100 mg/kg by I.V. infusion monthly (Gamimune only). Infusion rate is 0.01 to 0.02 ml/kg/minute for 30 minutes. Rate can then be increased to 0.04 ml/minute for remainder of infusion.
Idiopathic thrombocytopenic purpura–
Adults: 0.4 g/kg Gamimune N or Sandoglobulin I.V. for 5 consecutive days; or 1,000 mg/kg Gammagard. Additional doses may be given based on response. Give up to three doses (every other day) if necessary. Or, give Venoglobulin-1,500 mg/kg/day for 2 to 7 days.

CONTRAINDICATIONS & PRECAUTIONS

Contraindicated in patients known to have had an anaphylactic or severe systemic response to immune globulin and in patients with hypersensitivity to thimerosal, maltose, or any component of the formulation.

ADVERSE REACTIONS

Common reactions are in italics; life-threatening reactions are in bold italics.
Skin: urticaria.
Systemic: angioedema, headache, malaise, fever, nephrotic syndrome, ***anaphylaxis.***
Local: pain, erythema, muscle stiffness.

INTERACTIONS

Live virus vaccines: don't administer within 3 months after administration of immune globulin.

EFFECTS ON DIAGNOSTIC TESTS

None reported.

NURSING CONSIDERATIONS

Besides those related universally to drug therapy (see "How to use this book"), consider the following specific recommendations:

Assessment
- Obtain a baseline assessment of the patient's allergies and reaction to immunization before therapy.
- Be alert for adverse reactions and drug interactions throughout therapy.
- Evaluate the patient's and family's knowledge about immune globulin therapy.

Nursing Diagnoses
- Altered protection related to lack or decreased immunity.
- Ineffective breathing pattern related to immunization-induced anaphylaxis.
- Knowledge deficit related to immune globulin immunization.

Planning and Implementation
Preparation and Administration
- ***I.V. use:*** Infuse slowly, once a month.
- ***I.M. use:*** Inject into different sites, preferably anterolateral aspect of thigh or deltoid muscle for adults and anterolateral aspect of thigh for neonates and children under 3 years.
- Do not inject more than 3 ml per injection site.

Monitoring
• Monitor effectiveness by checking the patient's antibody titers after immunization.
• Observe the patient for signs of anaphylaxis immediately after injection.
• Check vital signs.
• Observe injection site for local reaction (pain, erythema, muscle stiffness).
Supportive Care
• Keep epinephrine 1:1000 available in case of anaphylaxis. Have oxygen and resuscitation equipment nearby.
• Do not give for hepatitis A exposure if 6 weeks or more have elapsed since exposure or after onset of clinical illness.
Patient Teaching
• Instruct the patient to report respiratory difficulty immediately.
• Tell the patient that headache, fever, malaise, and local soreness may occur after immunization with immune globulin.
Evaluation
In patients receiving immune globulin, appropriate evaluation statements may include:
• Patient exhibits increased passive immunity.
• Patient demonstrates no signs of anaphylaxis.
• Patient and family state an understanding of immune globulin immunization.

indapamide
(in dap´ a mide)
Lozide†, Lozol, Natrilix‡

• *Classification:* antihypertensive, diuretic (thiazide)
• *Pregnancy Risk Category:* B

HOW SUPPLIED
Tablets: 2.5 mg

ACTION
Mechanism: A thiazidelike diuretic that inhibits sodium reabsorption in the cortical diluting site of the nephron. Also has a direct vasodilating effect that may be a result of calcium channel-blocking action.
Absorption: Completely absorbed from the GI tract.
Distribution: Widely distributed into body tissues as a result of its lipophilicity; drug is 71% to 79% plasma protein-bound.
Metabolism: Significant hepatic metabolism.
Excretion: About 60% of a dose of indapamide is excreted in urine within 48 hours; approximately 16% to 23% is excreted in feces.
Onset, peak, duration: Peak serum levels occur at 2 to 2½ hours.

INDICATIONS & DOSAGE
Edema, hypertension–
Adults: 2.5 mg P.O. as a single daily dose taken in the morning. Dosage may be increased to 5 mg daily.

CONTRAINDICATIONS & PRECAUTIONS
Contraindicated in patients with anuria or in those with sensitivity to the drug or to sulfonamide derivatives.
Use cautiously in patients with: severe renal disease because it may decrease glomerular filtration rate and precipitate azotemia; impaired hepatic function or liver disease because electrolyte changes may precipitate coma; and in those taking digoxin because hypokalemia may predispose them to digitalis toxicity.

ADVERSE REACTIONS
Common reactions are in italics; life-threatening reactions are in bold italics.
CNS: headache, irritability, nervousness.
CV: *volume depletion and dehydration,* orthostatic hypotension.
GI: anorexia, nausea, pancreatitis.

Metabolic: *hypokalemia; asymptomatic hyperuricemia;* fluid and electrolyte imbalances, including dilutional hyponatremia and hypochloremia; metabolic alkalosis; gout.
Skin: dermatitis, photosensitivity, rash.
Other: muscle cramps and spasms.

INTERACTIONS

Diazoxide: increased antihypertensive, hyperglycemic, and hyperuricemic effects. Use together cautiously.
NSAIDs: decreased diuretic effectiveness. Avoid concomitant use.

EFFECTS ON DIAGNOSTIC TESTS

Parathyroid function tests: test interference. Drug should be discontinued before such tests.
Serum electrolytes: altered levels.
Serum urate, glucose, cholesterol, and triglyceride: increased levels.

NURSING CONSIDERATIONS

Besides those related universally to drug therapy (see "How to use this book"), consider the following specific recommendations:

Assessment

- Obtain a baseline assessment of blood pressure, serum electrolytes, urine output, weight, and peripheral edema before initiating indapamide therapy.
- Be alert for adverse reactions and drug interactions throughout therapy.
- Evaluate the patient's and family's knowledge about indapamide therapy.

Nursing Diagnoses

- Fluid volume excess related to the patient's underlying condition as evidenced by edema.
- Altered urinary elimination related to indapamide therapy.
- Knowledge deficit related to indapamide therapy.

Planning and Implementation

Preparation and Administration

- ***P.O. use:*** If possible, give drug early in the day to prevent nocturia.

Monitoring

- Monitor effectiveness by regularly checking blood pressure, urine output, and weight.
- Monitor serum electrolytes, BUN, creatinine, glucose, and uric acid levels.
- Monitor the patient receiving concomitant digitalis therapy for increased risk of digitalis toxicity.
- Monitor for signs of hypokalemia (for example, muscle weakness and cramps).
- Monitor the diabetic patient's insulin requirements because hydrochlorothiazide has hyperglycemic effects.
- Monitor skin turgor and mucous membranes for signs of fluid volume deficit.
- Monitor elderly patients closely because they are especially susceptible to excessive diuresis.

Supportive Care

- Hold drug and notify the doctor if hypersensitivity reactions occur.
- Keep accurate records of intake and output, blood pressure, and weight.
- Provide frequent skin and mouth care to relieve dryness from diuretic therapy.
- Answer the patient's call bells promptly; make sure patient's bathroom or bedpan is easily accessible.
- Use safety precautions to minimize risk of falling due to hypotension.
- In the patient undergoing tests of parathyroid function, hold thiazide and thiazide-like drugs before these tests are performed.
- Be aware that optimal antihypertensive effect may not occur for several days after beginning of therapy with indapamide.
- Elevate the patient's legs to aid reduction of peripheral edema.
- Administer potassium supplements as indicated.

Patient Teaching

- Teach the patient and family to identify and report signs of hypersensitivity reaction and hypokalemia.

• Teach the patient and family to monitor the patient's fluid volume by recording daily weight and intake and output.
• Inform the patient that optimal therapeutic response may not occur until several days after beginning indapamide therapy.
• Teach the patient to avoid high-sodium foods and to choose high-potassium foods.
• Advise the patient to change positions slowly, especially when rising to standing position, to avoid dizziness and fainting due to orthostatic hypotension.
• Advise the patient to minimize risks of photosensitivity reaction by using a sunscreen when outdoors.
• Advise the diabetic patient that insulin dosage may require adjustment.
• Advise the patient who is taking digitalis that the drug's potassium-depleting effect may increase the risk of digitalis toxicity.
• Advise the patient to take indapamide early in the day to avoid interruptions of sleep due to nocturia.

Evaluation

In patients receiving indapamide, appropriate evaluation statements may include:
• Patient is free of edema.
• Patient demonstrates adjustment of life-style to deal with altered patterns of urinary elimination.
• Patient and family state an understanding of indapamide therapy.

indomethacin

(in doe meth´ a sin)

Apo-Indomethacin†, Arthrexin‡, Indameth, Indocid†‡, Indocid SR†, Indocin, Indocin SR, Indomed, Novomethacin†, Rheumacin‡, Zendole

indomethacin sodium trihydrate

Apo-Indomethacin†, Indocid†, Indocin I.V., Indometh, Novomethacin

• *Classification:* nonnarcotic analgesic, antipyretic, (nonsteroidal anti-inflammatory agent)
• *Pregnancy Risk Category:* B (D in 3rd trimester)

HOW SUPPLIED

Capsules: 10 mg, 25 mg, 50 mg, 75 mg
Capsules (sustained-release): 75 mg
Oral suspension: 25 mg/5 ml
Injection: 1-mg vials
Suppositories: 50 mg

ACTION

Mechanism: Produces anti-inflammatory, analgesic, and antipyretic effects, possibly through inhibition of prostaglandin synthesis.
Absorption: Rapidly and completely absorbed from the GI tract.
Distribution: Indomethacin is highly protein-bound.
Metabolism: Indomethacin is metabolized in the liver.
Excretion: Indomethacin is excreted mainly in urine, with some biliary excretion. Half-life: In healthy adults, terminal elimination half-life ranges from 2.6 to 11.2 hours. Half-life is 20 to 28 hours in neonates 1 week of age and less; 12 to 19 hours after the first week.
Onset, peak, duration: Peak serum levels are seen within 30 minutes to 2 hours of an immediate-release capsule and within 12 hours of a timed-release capsule.

INDICATIONS & DOSAGE

Moderate-to-severe arthritis, ankylosing spondylitis–
Adults: 25 mg P.O. or rectally b.i.d. or t.i.d. with food or antacids; may increase dosage by 25 mg daily q 7 days up to 200 mg daily. Alterna-

tively, sustained-release capsules (75 mg) may be given: 75 mg to start, in the morning or h.s., followed, if necessary, by 75 mg b.i.d.
Acute gouty arthritis–
Adults: 50 mg P.O. t.i.d. Reduce dose as soon as possible, then stop. Sustained-release capsules shouldn't be used for this condition.
To close a hemodynamically significant patent ductus arteriosus in premature infants (I.V. form only)–
Neonates under 48 hours: 0.2 mg/kg I.V. followed by 2 doses of 0.1 mg/kg at 12- to 24-hour intervals.
Neonates 2 to 7 days: 0.2 mg/kg I.V. followed by 2 doses of 0.2 mg/kg at 12- to 24-hour intervals.
Over 7 days: 0.2 mg/kg I.V. followed by 2 doses of 0.25 mg/kg at 12- to 24-hour intervals.

CONTRAINDICATIONS & PRECAUTIONS

Contraindicated in patients with hypersensitivity to the drug; in patients in whom aspirin or other NSAIDs induce symptoms of asthma, urticaria, or rhinitis; in patients with active GI disorders because it may cause GI upset; in infants with untreated infection; and in patients with active bleeding; in coagulation defects or thrombocytopenia, in necrotizing enterocolitis or impaired renal function. Rectal form of indomethacin is contraindicated in patients with a history of recent rectal bleeding, proctitis, or ulcerative colitis.

Use cautiously in patients with epilepsy, parkinsonism, hepatic or renal disease, cardiovascular disease, intrinsic coagulation defects, infection, or a history of mental illness because it may exacerbate the symptoms of these disorders.

Patients with "triad" symptoms (aspirin hypersensitivity, rhinitis/nasal polyps, and asthma) are at high risk of bronchospasm. NSAIDs may mask the signs and symptoms of acute infection (fever, myalgia, erythema); carefully evaluate patients with high risk (such as those with diabetes).

ADVERSE REACTIONS

Common reactions are in italics; life-threatening reactions are in bold italics.
Oral form:
Blood: ***hemolytic anemia, aplastic anemia, agranulocytosis,*** leukopenia, *thrombocytopenic purpura,* iron deficiency anemia.
CNS: *headache, dizziness,* depression, drowsiness, confusion, peripheral neuropathy, seizures, psychic disturbances, syncope, *vertigo.*
CV: hypertension, *edema.*
EENT: *blurred vision, corneal and retinal damage,* hearing loss, tinnitus.
GI: *nausea, vomiting,* anorexia, *diarrhea, peptic ulceration,* ***severe GI bleeding.***
GU: hematuria, hyperkalemia, acute renal failure.
Hepatic: elevated enzymes.
Skin: pruritus, urticaria, ***Stevens-Johnson syndrome.***
Other: ***hypersensitivity (shocklike symptoms, rash, respiratory distress, angioedema).***
I.V. form:
Blood: decreased platelet aggregation.
GI: *bleeding,* vomiting.
GU: *renal dysfunction.*
Metabolic: *hyponatremia, hyperkalemia,* hypoglycemia.

INTERACTIONS

Antihypertensive agents: reduced antihypertensive effect.
Aspirin: decreased blood levels of indomethacin.
Diflunisal, probenecid: decreases indomethacin excretion; watch for increased incidence of indomethacin adverse reactions.
Lithium: increased plasma lithium levels. Monitor for toxicity.
Thiazide diuretics, furosemide: im-

paired response to both drugs. Avoid using together if possible.
Triamterene: possible nephrotoxicity. Don't use together.

EFFECTS ON DIAGNOSTIC TESTS

Dexamethasone suppression test: interference.
Urine 5-HIAA: interference.

NURSING CONSIDERATIONS

Besides those related universally to drug therapy (see "How to use this book"), consider the following specific recommendations:

Assessment

- Obtain a baseline assessment of pain before starting therapy.
- Be alert for adverse reactions and drug interactions throughout therapy.
- Evaluate the patient's and family's knowledge about indomethacin therapy.

Nursing Diagnoses

- Pain related to the patient's underlying condition.
- High risk for trauma related to possible adverse CNS reactions.
- Knowledge deficit related to indomethacin therapy.

Planning and Implementation

Preparation and Administration

- ***I.V. use:*** Don't administer the second or third scheduled dose if anuria or marked oliguria is evident.
- ***I.V. use:*** Administer the drug by direct injection over 5 to 10 seconds through the tubing of a compatible I.V. solution. Avoid extravasation because the drug irritates tissues. Remember that this drug is not recommended for intermittent or continuous infusion.

Monitoring

- Monitor effectiveness by regularly evaluating the patient's pain relief.

Oral form:

- Monitor for visual and hearing changes and CNS adverse reactions, such as dizziness and vertigo. CNS adverse reactions are more common and serious in elderly patients.
- Monitor for bleeding if the patient is receiving anticoagulants.
- Monitor for weight gain (especially in elderly patients) and for increased blood pressure in patients with hypertension because this drug causes sodium retention.

I.V. form:

- Monitor carefully for bleeding and for reduced urine output. Discontinue drug and notify the doctor if either occurs.

Supportive Care

Oral form:

- Notify the doctor if the patient's pain is not relieved or if it worsens.
- If adverse CNS reactions occur, institute safety precautions, such as supervising ambulation and keeping the bed rails up.
- Keep in mind that because of high incidence of adverse reactions to chronic use, indomethacin should not be used routinely as an analgesic or antipyretic.

I.V. form:

- Keep in mind that if ductus arteriosus reopens, a second course of one to three doses may be given. If ineffective, surgery may be necessary.

Patient Teaching

Oral form:

- Because serious GI toxicity can occur at any time in chronic NSAID therapy, teach the patient signs and symptoms of GI bleeding. Tell the patient to report these to the doctor immediately.
- Advise the patient to avoid aspirin and alcohol. Concomitant use with aspirin, alcohol, or steroids may increase the risk of adverse GI reactions.
- Advise the patient to notify the doctor if pain persists or becomes worse.
- Explain the importance of regular eye examinations, hearing tests, CBC, and renal fuction tests to help moni-

tor for toxicity during prolonged therapy.

Evaluation

In patients receiving indomethacin, appropriate evaluation statements may include:

• Patient states pain is relieved.

• Patient does not develop traumatic injuries as a result of adverse CNS reactions.

• Patient and family state an understanding of indomethacin therapy.

---

influenza virus vaccine, 1992-1993 trivalent types A & B (purified surface antigen)

(in floo en´ za)

Flu-Imune

influenza virus vaccine, 1992-1993 trivalent types A & B (subvirion or split virion)

Fluogen Split, Fluzone Split, Influenza Virus Vaccine (Split)

influenza virus vaccine, 1992-1993 trivalent types A & B (whole virion)

Fluzone (Whole)

• *Classification:* influenza prophylaxis (viral vaccine)

• *Pregnancy Risk Category:* C

HOW SUPPLIED

Injection: 15 mcg A/Texas/36/91-like (H1N1), 15 mcg A/Beijing/353/89-like (H3N2), and 15 mcg B/Panama/45/90-like hemagglutinin antigens per 0.5 ml

ACTION

Mechanism: Promotes immunity to influenza by inducing production of antibodies to influenza A and B.

Pharmacokinetics: Unknown.

Onset, peak, duration: A protective effect is achieved in most patients 10 to 14 days after administration. The duration of immunity varies widely but usually lasts about 1 year; infecting virus strains vary from flu season to flu season, making annual immunization necessary.

INDICATIONS & DOSAGE

Influenza prophylaxis–

Adults and children over 12 years: 0.5 ml whole or split virus I.M. Only one dose is required.

Children 3 to 12 years: 0.5 ml split virus I.M. Repeat dose in 4 weeks unless child has been previously vaccinated.

Children 6 to 35 months: 0.25 ml split virus I.M. Repeat dose in 4 weeks unless child has been previously vaccinated.

CONTRAINDICATIONS & PRECAUTIONS

Contraindicated in patients with a sensitivity to egg or chick embryo protein, in patients with an acute respiratory infection or any other active infection, and in patients with a history of Guillain-Barré syndrome or hypersensitivity to thimerosal, a component of the vaccine.

ADVERSE REACTIONS

Common reactions are in italics; life-threatening reactions are in bold italics.

Systemic: fever, malaise, myalgia, ***Guillain-Barré syndrome*** (rare), ***anaphylaxis.***

Local: erythema, induration, soreness at the injection site.

Fever and malaise reactions occur most often in children and in others not exposed to influenza viruses. Severe reactions in adults are rare.

INTERACTIONS

Theophylline, warfarin: clearance may be impaired.

EFFECTS ON DIAGNOSTIC TESTS

None report.

NURSING CONSIDERATIONS

Besides those related universally to drug therapy (see "How to use this book"), consider the following specific recommendations:

Assessment

• Obtain a baseline assessment of allergies (especially to eggs and sulfites), immunization history, and reaction to immunization before therapy.

• Be alert for adverse reactions and drug interactions throughout therapy.

• Evaluate the patient's and family's knowledge about influenza virus vaccine therapy.

Nursing Diagnoses

• Altered protection related to lack of immunity to influenza virus.

• Hyperthermia related to vaccine-induced fever.

• Knowledge deficit related to influenza virus vaccine.

Planning and Implementation

Preparation and Administration

• Ideally vaccinations should be performed in November, since outbreaks of influenza generally don't occur until December. Try to avoid administering the vaccine too early in the season because antibody titer may begin to decline prior to the flu season.

• ***I.M. use:*** Give injections for adults and older children in deltoid muscle; in anterolateral aspect of thigh for infants and children under 3 years old.

• Note that the combination of antigens used to create influenza vaccine changes annually even though some of the antigens may be the same as the previous year. Leftover supplies of 1991-1992 vaccine should not be used to immunize patients for the 1992-1993 flu season.

Monitoring

• Monitor effectiveness by checking the patient's antibody titers to influenza virus.

• Check patient's temperature; fever may occur after immunization.

• Observe the injection site for localized reaction.

• Assess patient's neurological status. Paralysis associated with Guillain-Barré syndrome is rare and has only been associated with the 1976 vaccine.

Supportive Care

• Contraindicated in egg allergy; use with caution in patients with a history of sulfite allergy. Defer in acute respiratory or other active infection.

• Keep epinephrine 1:1000 available; anaphylaxis is rare but may occur immediately after injection.

• Obtain order for antipyretics as needed.

• Children under 12 years of age may require two injections of split dosage; the second dose should be given in December, if possible.

• Vaccines can be given to both children and adults throughout the flu season, even as late as April.

• Children should not receive pertussis vaccine within 3 days of influenza virus vaccine. However they may receive *Haemophilus* b vaccine, oral polio vaccine, measles-mumps-rubella, or pneumococcal vaccine at the same time. Injections should be made at different sites.

• Split virus and purified surface antigen vaccines cause somewhat fewer adverse reactions than whole virus in children.

Patient Teaching

• Tell the patient that fever, malaise, and myalgia may begin 6 to 12 hours after vaccination and persist 1 to 2 days.

• Inform the patient that annual vaccination using the current vaccine is necessary because immunity to influenza decreases in the year after injection.

• Advise the patient that the vaccine is strongly recommended for anyone over 6 months, and patients with chronic disease, metabolic disorders, or medical conditions that put them

at risk of complications from influenza. Also strongly recommended for health care workers and household members who may contact persons at high risk of medical complications of influenza.
• Make the patient aware of the risks associated with the vaccine as compared to the risk of influenza and its complications.

Evaluation

In patients receiving influenza virus vaccine, appropriate evaluation statements may include:
• Patient exhibits immunity to influenza virus.
• Patient's temperature remains within the normal range.
• Patient and family state an understanding of influenza virus vaccine.

insulins
(in´ su lin)

insulin injection (regular insulin, crystalline zinc insulin)
Actrapid HM‡, Actrapid HM Penfill‡, Actrapid MC‡, Actrapid MC Penfill‡, Beef Regular Iletin II◊, Humulin R◊, Hypurin Neutral‡, Insulin 2‡, Novolin R◊, Novolin R Penfill◊, Pork Regular Iletin II◊, Regular (Concentrated) Iletin II, Regular Iletin I◊, Regular Purified Pork Insulin◊, Velosulin◊, Velosulin Human‡, Velosulin Insuject◊

insulin zinc suspension, prompt (semilente)
Semilente Iletin I◊, Semilente Insulin◊, Semilente MC Pork‡, Semilente Purified Pork◊

isophane insulin suspension (neutral protamine Hagedorn insulin, NPH)
Beef NPH Iletin II◊, Humulin N◊, Humulin NPH‡, Hypurin Isophane‡, Insulatard‡, Insulatard Human‡, Insulatard NPH◊, Isotard MC‡, Novolin N◊, NPH Iletin I◊, NPH Insulin◊, NPH Purified Pork◊, Pork NPH Iletin II◊, Protaphane HM‡, Protaphane HM Penfill‡, Protaphane MC‡

isophane insulin suspension with insulin injection
Actraphane HM‡, Actraphane HM Penfill‡, Actraphane MC‡, Mixtard◊, Mixtard Human‡, Novolin 70/30

insulin zinc suspension (lente)
Humulin L◊, Lente Iletin I◊, Lente Iletine II◊, Lente Insulin◊, Lente MC‡, Lente Purified Pork Insulin◊, Monotard HM‡, Monotard MC‡, Novolin L◊

protamine zinc suspension (PZI)
Protamine, Zinc & Iletin I◊; Protamine, Zinc & Iletin II (Beef)◊; Protamine, Zinc & Iletin II (Pork)◊; Protamine Zinc Insulin MC‡

insulin zinc suspension, extended (ultralente)
Ultralente Iletin I◊, Ultralente Insulin◊, Ultralente Purified Beef◊, Ultratard HM‡, Ultratard MC‡

• *Classification:* antidiabetic agent (pancreatic hormone)
• *Pregnancy Risk Category:* B

HOW SUPPLIED

insulin injection
Injection (from beef and pork): 40 units/ml◊, 100 units/ml◊ (Regular Iletin I◊)
Injection (human): 100 units/ml (Actrapid HM‡, Humulin R◊, Novolin R◊, Velosulin◊, Velosulin Human‡); 100 units/ml in 1.5-ml cartridge system◊ (Actrapid HM Penfill‡, Novolin R Penfill◊)
Injection (from pork): 100 units/ml◊
Injection (purified beef): 100 units/ml (Beef Regular Iletin II◊, Hypurin Neutral‡, Insulin 2‡)

Injection (purified pork): 100 units/ml (Actrapid MC‡, Pork Regular Iletin II◇, Regular Purified Pork Insulin◇, Velosulin◇); 100 units/ml in 1.5-ml cartridge system‡ (Actrapid MC Penfill‡); 100 units/ml in 2-ml cartridge system‡ (Velosulin Insuject‡); 500 units/ml (Regular [Concentrated] Iletin II)

insulin zinc suspension, prompt
Injection (from beef): 100 units/ml◇ (Semilente Insulin◇)
Injection (from beef and pork): 40 units/ml◇, 100 units/ml◇ (Semilente Iletin◇)
Injection (purified pork): 100 units/ml◇ (Semilente MC‡, Semilente Purified Pork◇)

isophane insulin suspension
Injection (from beef): 100 units/ml◇ (NPH Insulin◇)
Injection (from beef and pork): 40 units/ml◇, 100 units/ml◇ (NPH Iletin I◇)
Injection (human, recombinant): 100 units/ml (Humulin N◇, Humulin NPH‡, Insulatard Human†, Insulatard NPH◇, Novolin N◇, Protaphane HM‡); 100 units/ml in 1.5-ml cartridge system‡ (Protaphane HM Penfill‡)
Injection (purified beef): 100 units/ml (Beef NPH Iletin II◇, Hypurin Isophane†, Isotard MC†)
Injection (purified pork): 100 units/ml (Insulatard‡, Insulatard NPH◇, NPH Purified Pork◇, Pork NPH Iletin II, Protaphane MC‡)

isophane insulin suspension with insulin injection
Injection (human): 100 units/ml (Actraphane HM‡, Mixtard Human‡, Novolin 70/30◇); 100 units/ml in 1.5-ml cartridge system‡ (Actraphane HM Penfill‡)
Injection (purified pork): 100 units/ml (Actraphane MC‡, Mixtard◇, Lente MC‡)

insulin zinc suspension
Injection (beef): 100 units/ml (Lente Insulin◇, Lente MC‡)
Injection (from beef and pork): 40 units/ml◇, 100 units/ml◇ (Lente Iletin I◇)
Injection (purified beef): 100 units/ml (Lente Iletin II◇, Lente MC‡)
Injection (purified pork): 100 units/ml (Monotard MC‡, Lente Purified Pork Insulin◇)
Injection (human): 100 units/ml◇ (Humulin L◇, Monotard HM◇, Novolin L◇)

protamine zinc suspension
Injection (from beef and pork): 40 units/ml◇, 100 units/ml◇ (Protamine, Zinc & Iletin I◇)
Injection (purified beef): 100 units/ml◇ (Protamine, Zinc & Iletin II [Beef]◇)
Injection (purified pork): 100 units/ml (Protamine, Zinc & Iletin II [Pork]◇, Protamine Zinc Insulin MC‡)

insulin zinc suspension, extended
Injection (from beef): 100 units/ml◇ (Ultralente Purified Beef◇)
Injection (from beef and pork): 40 units/ml◇, 100 units/ml◇ (Ultralente Iletin I◇)
Injection (human): 100 units/ml‡ (Ultratard HM‡)
Injection (purified pork): 100 units/ml‡ (Ultralente MC‡)

ACTION

Mechanism: Increases glucose transport across muscle and fat cell membranes to reduce blood glucose level. Promotes conversion of glucose to its storage form, glycogen; triggers amino acid uptake and conversion to protein in muscle cells and inhibits protein degradation; stimulates triglyceride formation and inhibits release of free fatty acids from adipose tissue; and stimulates lipoprotein lipase activity, which converts circulating lipoproteins to fatty acids.
Absorption: Insulin must be given parenterally because it is destroyed in the GI tract. It is completely absorbed after I.M. or S.C. administra-

tion; rate of absorption varies depending on the injection route, site, volume, concentration, and type of insulin. Absorption may also be delayed or decreased if the patient has insulin-binding antibodies, which develop in most patients after 2 or 3 months of treatment.
Distribution: Widely distributed throughout the extracellular space.
Metabolism: Some insulin is bound and inactivated by peripheral tissues, but most appears to be degraded in the liver and kidneys.
Excretion: Insulin is filtered by the renal glomeruli and undergoes some tubular reabsorption. Half-life: Plasma half-life is about 9 minutes after I.V. administration but can be considerably longer if the patient has insulin-binding antibodies.
Onset, peak, duration: Commercially available preparations are formulated to differ in onset, peak, and duration after S.C. administration. They are classified as rapid-acting (30 minutes to 1 hour onset), intermediate-acting (1 to 2 hour onset), and long-acting (4 to 8 hour onset). The accompanying table summarizes major pharmacokinetic differences.

INDICATIONS & DOSAGE

Diabetic ketoacidosis (use regular insulin only)–
Adults: 25 to 150 units I.V. immediately, then additional doses may be given q 1 hour based on blood sugar level until patient is out of acidosis; then give S.C. q 6 hours thereafter. Alternative dosage schedule: 50 to 100 units I.V. and 50 to 100 units S.C. stat; additional doses may be given q 2 to 6 hours based on blood sugar levels; or 0.33 units/kg I.V. bolus, followed by 7 to 10 units/hour I.V. by continuous infusion. Continue infusion until blood sugar drops to 250 mg/dl, then start S.C. insulin q 6 hours.
Children: 0.5 to 1 unit/kg in two divided doses, 1 given I.V. and the other S.C., followed by 0.5 to 1 unit/kg I.V. q 1 to 2 hours; or 0.1 unit/kg I.V. bolus, then 0.1 unit/kg hourly continuous I.V. infusion until blood sugar drops to 250 mg/dl, then start S.C. insulin. Preparation of infusion: add 100 units regular insulin and 1 g albumin to 100 ml 0.9% saline solution. Insulin concentration will be 1 unit/ml. (The albumin will adsorb to plastic, preventing loss of the insulin to plastic.)
Type I (insulin-dependent) diabetes mellitus, ketosis-prone diabetics, diabetes mellitus inadequately controlled by diet and oral hypoglycemics–
Adults and children: therapeutic regimen prescribed by doctor and adjusted according to patient's blood and urine glucose concentrations.

CONTRAINDICATIONS & PRECAUTIONS

Use only regular insulin in patients with circulatory collapse, diabetic ketoacidosis, or hyperkalemia. Do not administer regular insulin concentrated by I.V. Do not use intermediate- or long-acting insulins for coma or other emergency requiring rapid drug action.

ADVERSE REACTIONS

Common reactions are in italics; life-threatening reactions are in bold italics.
Metabolic: *hypoglycemia, hyperglycemia (rebound, or Somogyi, effect).*
Skin: urticaria.
Local: *lipoatrophy, lipohypertrophy,* itching, swelling, redness, stinging, warmth at site of injection.
Other: ***anaphylaxis.***

INTERACTIONS

Alcohol, beta blockers, clofibrate, fenfluramine, MAO inhibitors, salicylates, tetracycline: prolonged hypoglycemic effect. Monitor blood glucose level carefully.
Corticosteroids, thiazide diuretics: di-

COMPARING INSULIN PREPARATIONS

The chart below lists the various forms of insulin and their times of onset, peak, and duration.

PREPARATION	PURIFIED*	ONSET	PEAK	DURATION
Rapid-acting Insulins				
Insulin injection (regular, crystalline zinc)				
Regular Iletin I	No	½ to 1 hr	2 to 4 hr	6 to 8 hr
Regular Insulin	No	½ hr	2½ to 5 hr	8 hr
Pork Regular Iletin II	Yes	½ to 1 hr	2 to 4 hr	6 to 8 hr
Beef Regular Iletin II	Yes	½ to 1 hr	2 to 4 hr	6 to 8 hr
Regular (concentrated) Iletin II	Yes	½ hr	varies	24 hr
Velosulin	Yes	½ hr	1 to 3 hr	8 hr
Purified Pork Insulin	Yes	½ hr	2½ to 5 hr	8 hr
Humulin R	N.A.	½ to 1 hr	2 to 4 hr	6 to 8 hr
Humulin B.R.	N.A.	½ hr	2 to 4 hr	6 to 8 hr
Novolin R	N.A.	½ hr	2½ to 5 hr	6 to 8 hr
Prompt insulin zinc suspension (semilente)				
Semilente Iletin I	No	1 to 2 hr	3 to 8 hr	10 to 16 hr
Semilente Insulin	No	1½ hr	5 to 10 hr	16 hr
Semilente Purified Pork Prompt Insulin	Yes	1½ hr	5 to 10 hr	16 hr
Intermediate-acting Insulins				
Isophane insulin suspension (NPH)				
NPH Iletin I	No	2 hr	6 to 12 hr	18 to 26 hr
NPH Insulin	No	1½ hr	4 to 12 hr	24 hr
Beef NPH Iletin II	Yes	2 hr	6 to 12 hr	18 to 26 hr
Pork NPH Iletin II	Yes	2 hr	6 to 12 hr	18 to 26 hr
NPH Purified Pork Isophane Insulin	Yes	1½ hr	4 to 12 hr	24 hr
Insulatard NPH	Yes	1½ hr	4 to 12 hr	24 hr
Humulin N	N.A.	1 to 2 hr	6 to 12 hr	18 to 24 hr
Novolin N	N.A.	1½ hr	4 to 12 hr	24 hr
Insulin zinc suspension (lente)				
Lente Iletin I	No	2 to 4 hr	6 to 12 hr	18 to 26 hr
Lente Insulin	No	2½ hr	7 to 15 hr	24 hr
Beef Lente Iletin II	Yes	2 to 4 hr	6 to 12 hr	18 to 36 hr
Pork Lente Iletin II	Yes	2 to 4 hr	6 to 12 hr	18 to 36 hr
Lente Purified Pork Insulin	Yes	2½ hr	7 to 15 hr	22 hr
Humulin L	N.A.	1 to 3 hr	6 to 12 hr	18 to 21 hr
Novolin L	N.A.	2½ hr	7 to 15 hr	22 hr
Isophane (NPH) 70%, regular insulin 30%				
Humulin 70/30	N.A.	½ hr	4 to 8 hr	24 hr
Mixtard	Yes	½ hr	4 to 8 hr	24 hr
Mixtard Human	N.A.	½ hr	4 to 8 hr	24 hr
Novolin 70/30	N.A.	½ hr	2 to 12 hr	24 hr

(continued)

COMPARING INSULIN PREPARATIONS *(continued)*

PREPARATION	PURIFIED*	ONSET	PEAK	DURATION
Long-acting Insulins				
Protamine zinc insulin suspension				
Protamine Zinc & Iletin I	No	4 to 8 hr	14 to 24 hr	28 to 36 hr
Beef Protamine Zinc & Iletin II	Yes	4 to 8 hr	14 to 24 hr	28 to 36 hr
Pork Protamine Zinc & Iletin II	Yes	4 to 8 hr	14 to 24 hr	28 to 36 hr
Extended insulin zinc suspension (ultralente)				
Ultralente Iletin I	No	4 to 8 hr	14 to 24 hr	28 to 36 hr
Ultralente Insulin	No	4 hr	10 to 30 hr	36 hr
Ultralente Purified Beef Insulin	Yes	4 hr	10 to 30 hr	36 hr

N.A. indicates not applicable
*Purified insulins contain <10 ppm proinsulin.

minished insulin response. Monitor for hyperglycemia.

EFFECTS ON DIAGNOSTIC TESTS

Serum magnesium, potassium, or inorganic phosphate: decreased concentrations.

NURSING CONSIDERATIONS

Besides those related universally to drug therapy (see "How to use this book"), consider the following specific recommendations:

Assessment

- Obtain a baseline assessment of the patient's blood glucose level before initiating insulin therapy.
- Be alert for adverse reactions and drug interactions throughout therapy.
- Evaluate the patient's and family's knowledge about insulin therapy as well as other aspects of diabetes treatment that may affect insulin therapy.

Nursing Diagnoses

- Altered nutrition: More than body requirements related to inability to produce insulin to maintain blood gluocose at normal levels.
- High risk for injury related to insulin-induced hypoglycemia.
- Knowledge deficit related to insulin therapy.

Planning and Implementation

Preparation and Administration

- Accuracy of measurement is very important, especially with regular insulin concentrated. Use aids, such as a magnifying sleeve or dose magnifiers to improve accuracy.
- Be aware that the dosage is always expressed in USP units.
- Do not interchange beef, pork, or human insulins; a dosage adjustment may be required.
- Regular insulin may be mixed with NPH or lente insulins in any proportion. However, in vitro binding will occur over time until an equilibrium is reached. Administer these mixtures immediately after preparation or after stability occurs (15 minutes for NPH regular, 24 hours for lente regular) to minimize variability in patient response. Note that switching from separate injections to a prepared mixture also may alter the patient's response.
- Store insulin in cool area. Refrigeration is desirable but not essential, except with regular insulin concentrated.

*Liquid form contains alcohol.

**May contain tartrazine.

• Do not use insulin that has changed color or becomes clumped or granular in appearance.
• Check expiration date on vial before using contents.
• Some patients may develop insulin resistance and require large insulin doses to control symptoms of diabetes. U-500 insulin is available as Regular (Concentrated) Iletin I for such patients. Never store U-500 insulin in same area with other insulin preparations because of danger of severe overdose if given accidentally to other patients. U-500 insulin must be administered with a U-100 syringe because no syringes are made for this drug.
• Human insulin may be advantageous in patients who are allergic to pork or beef forms.
• Patients with juvenile-onset diabetes mellitus, as well as ketosis-prone, severely ill, and newly diagnosed diabetics with very high blood glucose levels may require hospitalization and I.M. or I.V. treatment with regular fast-acting insulin.
• ***I.V. use:*** Only regular insulin should be administered I.V. Inject directly into vein, through an intermittent infusion device, or into a port close to I.V. access site at ordered rate. Intermittent infusion is not recommended. If given by continuous infusion infuse drug diluted in 0.9% sodium chloride at a rate sufficient to reverse ketoacidosis.
• ***S.C. use:*** Insulin is usually administered by S.C. route. When injecting insulin S.C., insert needle at a 90° angle unless 1 inch of subcutaneous tissue cannot be bunched together; then insert at a 45° angle. You do not need to aspirate before injection. Press but do not rub site after injection. Rotate injection sites. Record sites to avoid overuse of one area. However, some diabetics may achieve better control if injection site is rotated within the same anatomic region.

Monitoring
• Monitor effectiveness by regularly checking the patient's blood glucose levels. Monitor blood glucose levels more frequently if the patient is under stress, unstable, pregnant, or is recently diagnosed.
• Monitor the patient for signs and symptoms of both hyperglycemia and hypoglycemia; note time and circumstances associated with each.
• Monitor the patient's hemoglobin A1C regularly, as ordered.
• Monitor the patient's urine ketone levels when blood glucose levels are elevated.
• Monitor injection sites for local reactions, such as lipoatrophy or lipohypertrophy.

Supportive Care
• Notify the doctor if sudden changes in blood glucose levels occur, if they are dangerously high or low, or if ketosis is present.
• Be prepared to provide supportive measures if diabetic ketoacidosis or hyperglycemic hyperosmolar nonketotic coma occurs.
• Treat a hypoglycemic reaction with an oral form of rapid-acting glucose if the patient is awake or with glucagon or I.V. glucose if the patient cannot be aroused. Follow up treatment with a complex carbohydrate snack when patient is awake, and determine cause of reaction.
• Be sure that other treatment measures, such as diet and exercise programs are being used appropriately. Expect to adjust insulin dosage when other aspects of treatment regimen are altered.
• Discuss with the doctor how to deal with issues of noncompliance.
• Treat lipoatrophy or lipohypertrophy according to prescribed protocol.

Patient Teaching
• Teach the patient how to draw up insulin and self-administer S.C. dose.

• Teach the patient the preferred injection sites, the importance of site rotation, and how to rotate sites.
• Teach the patient how to store insulin and injection equipment.
• Advise the patient not to change the order of mixing insulins nor the model or brand of syringe or needle used.
• Be sure the patient knows that insulin therapy relieves symptoms but does not cure the disease.
• Tell the patient about the nature of the disease and the importance of following the therapeutic regimen (specific diet, weight reduction, and exercise programs; maintaining personal hygiene; avoiding infection; and timing injection and eating properly).
• Emphasize the importance of regular mealtimes and that meals must not be omitted.
• Teach the patient that blood glucose testing is an essential guide to correct dosage and to therapeutic success. Instruct patient how to self-test blood glucose.
• Emphasize the importance of recognizing hypoglycemic symptoms because insulin-induced hypoglycemia is hazardous and may cause brain damage if prolonged.
• Advise the patient to always wear a medical alert bracelet or pendant, to carry ample insulin supply and syringes on trips, to have carbohydrates (sugar or candy) on hand for emergency, and to note any time-zone changes for dosage schedule when traveling.
• Tell the patient that use of marijuana may increase insulin requirements.
• Cigarette smoking decreases the absorption of insulin administered subcutaneously. Advise the patient not to smoke within 30 minutes after insulin injection.

Evaluation
In patients receiving insulin injection, appropriate evaluation statements may include:
• Patient's blood glucose level is normal.
• Patient recognizes hypoglycemia early and treats hypoglycemic episodes effectively before injury occurs.
• Patient and family state an understanding of insulin therapy and demonstrate correct insulin administration.

interferon alfa-2a, recombinant (rIFN-A)
(in ter ferr´ on)
Roferon-A

• *Classification:* antineoplastic (biological response modifier)
• *Pregnancy Risk Category:* C

HOW SUPPLIED
Injection: 3 million IU/vial; 18 million IU/multiple-dose vial

ACTION
Mechanism: A protein synthesized using recombinant DNA techniques that has complex antiviral, antineoplastic, and immunomodulating effects. Mimics the action of the naturally occurring protein produced and secreted by peripheral blood leukocytes, epithelial cells, and fibroblasts in response to certain inducers, such as a viral infection. Its mechanism of action appears to involve direct action against tumor cells or viral cells to inhibit replication and modulation of host immune response by enhancing the phagocytic activity of macrophages, and by augmenting specific cytotoxicity of lymphocytes against target cells. Interferon alfa-2a and interferon alfa-2b are similar; each has a molecular weight of 19,000 daltons and is made of 165 amino acids.

They differ at position 23, where interferon alfa-2a has a lysine group, while interferon alfa-2b has an arginine group.
Absorption: Because the drug is subject to degradation by enzymes within the GI tract, it must be administered parenterally. More than 80% of the dose is absorbed after I.M. or S.C. injection.
Distribution: Rapidly cleared from plasma after I.V. administration. Limited data suggest that highest levels are found in the kidney, liver, spleen, and lung. Small amounts enter the CSF. Unknown if drug crosses placenta or enters breast milk.
Metabolism: By the kidney. The drug undergoes rapid proteolytic degradation within the brush border of the renal tubule or by lysosomes of the tubular epithelium.
Excretion: By the kidney, with minor biliary elimination. Half-life: 3.7 to 8.5 hours (mean 5.1 hours)
Onset, peak, duration: Peak serum levels occur within 15 minutes to 1 hour of I.V. injection and are higher than those following I.M. or S.C. administration; however, serum levels are maintained longer after I.M. or S.C. administration. Serum interferon levels are detectable for 4 to 8 hours after I.V. injection or 16 to 30 hours after I.M. or S.C. administration.

INDICATIONS & DOSAGE

Treatment of hairy-cell leukemia –
Adults: for induction, give 3 million units S.C. or I.M. daily for 16 to 24 weeks. For maintenance, 3 million units S.C. or I.M. three times a week.
Treatment of AIDS-related Kaposi's sarcoma –
Adults: for induction, give 36 million units S.C. or I.M. daily for 10 to 12 weeks. For maintenance, 36 million units S.C. or I.M. three times a week.

CONTRAINDICATIONS & PRECAUTIONS

Contraindicated in patients with hypersensitivity to interferon or to any components of the product. Use cautiously in patients with severe hepatic or renal function impairment, seizure disorders, compromised CNS function, cardiac disease, or myelosuppression because the drugs may worsen these conditions.

ADVERSE REACTIONS

Common reactions are in italics; life-threatening reactions are in bold italics.
Blood: leukemia, mild thrombocytopenia.
CNS: *dizziness,* confusion, paresthesias, numbness, lethargy, depression, nervousness, difficulty in thinking or concentrating, insomnia, sedation, apathy, anxiety, irritability, fatigue, vertigo, gait disturbances, poor coordination.
CV: hypotension, chest pain, dysrhythmias, palpitations, syncope, ***CHF,*** hypertension, edema.
EENT: visual disturbances, dryness or inflammation of the oropharynx, rhinorrhea, sinusitis, conjunctivitis, earache, eye irritation, rhinitis.
GI: *anorexia, nausea, diarrhea,* vomiting, abdominal fullness, abdominal pain, flatulence and constipation, hypermotility, gastric distress, dysgeusia.
GU: transient impotence.
Hepatic: hepatitis.
Respiratory: ***bronchospasm,*** coughing, dyspnea, tachypnea.
Skin: *rash,* dryness, *pruritus,* partial alopecia, urticaria, flushing.
Local: inflammation at injection site (rare).
Other: *flulike syndrome (fever, fatigue, myalgias, headache, chills, arthralgia),* diaphoresis, hot flashes, excessive salivation, cyanosis.

INTERACTIONS

Aminophylline: may reduce the clearance of aminophylline.

CNS depressants: enhanced CNS effects.

EFFECTS ON DIAGNOSTIC TESTS

ALT (SGPT), AST (SGOT), LDH, and alkaline phosphatase: increased levels (dose-related and reversible on withdrawal of interferon).
Blood pressure: mild and trasient hypotension is likely.
Hemoglobin, hematocrit, leukocyte counts, platelets, and neutrophils: decreased (dose-related; recovery within days or weeks after withdrawal of interferon).
Prothrombin time and partial thromboplastin time: increased (dose-related).
Serum calcium, serum phosphorus, and fasting blood glucose: increased levels.

NURSING CONSIDERATIONS

Besides those related universally to drug therapy (see "How to use this book"), consider the following specific recommendations:

Assessment
- Obtain a baseline assessment of the patient's CBC with differential, platelet count, blood chemistry, electrolytes studies, liver function studies, and ECG before therapy.
- Be alert for adverse reactions and drug interactions throughout therapy.
- Evaluate the patient's and family's knowledge about interferon alfa-2a therapy.

Nursing Diagnoses
- Altered protection related to proliferation of tumor or viral cells.
- Altered cardiovascular tissue perfusion related to interferon-induced CHF.
- Knowledge deficit related to interferon alfa-2a therapy.

Planning and Implementation
Preparation and Administration
- Consult most recent source of clinical information about the drug. Dosage, indications, and adverse reaction profile may change with additional clinical experience.
- Store drug in the refrigerator.
- Read label carefully. Different brands of interferon may not be equivalent and require different dosage.
- ***S.C. use:*** Give S.C. in patients whose platelet count is below 50,000 mm^3.
- Administer at bedtime to diminish daytime drowsiness.

Monitoring
- Monitor effectiveness by evaluating the proliferation of tumor or viral cells and patient's immune response.
- Monitor CBC count with differential, coagulation time, and platelet count.
- Monitor blood chemistry, electrolytes, liver function studies, and ECG (if the patient has a preexisting advanced stage of cancer or cardiac disorder).
- Monitor temperature, pulse, blood pressure, and respiration regularly.
- Monitor for signs and symptoms of infection.
- Observe for signs and symptoms of CHF. Monitor daily weight and fluid balance. Auscultate lungs and check extremities for peripheral edema.
- Observe for CNS adverse reactions, such as decreased mental status and dizziness. Periodic neuropsychiatric monitoring is recommended during drug therapy.
- Monitor for bleeding: test urine, emesis fluid, stool, and secretions for occult blood; inspect skin for bruising and petechiae.

Supportive Care
- Premedicate with acetaminophen to relieve flulike symptoms induced by drug.
- Use reverse isolation procedure. Because interferon may decrease antibody response and potentiate replication of viruses, the patient is at special risk for infection during therapy.
- Severe adverse reactions may re-

quire reduction of dosage to one-half or discontinuation of the drug until reactions subside.
• Special precautions are necessary for patients who develop thrombocytopenia: exercise extreme care in performing invasive procedures, limit frequency of I.M. injection, and avoid I.V. infiltration.
• Make sure the patient is well hydrated especially during the initial stages of therapy.
• Provide frequent mouth care. Use a soft toothbrush and a mild mouth wash.
• Be aware that interferons may decrease hemoglobin, hematocrit, leukocytes, platelet, and neutrophils; increase prothrombin and partial thromboplastin time; and increase serum levels of AST (SGOT), ALT (SGPT), LDH, alkaline phosphatase calcium, phosphorous, and fasting glucose. These effects are dose-related and reversible; recovery occurs within several days or weeks after withdrawal of interferon.
• Use seizure precautions. Have airway or padded tongue blade nearby.
• Be aware that use with blood dyscrasia-causing medications, bone marrow suppressant therapy, or radiation therapy may increase bone marrow suppressant effects. Dosage reduction may be required.
• Neurotoxicity and cardiotoxicity occur most commonly in elderly patients, especially those with underlying CNS or cardiac impairment.
• Be aware that concurrent use with a live virus vaccine may potentiate replication of vaccine virus, increase adverse reactions, and decrease patient's antibody response.

Patient Teaching
• Advise patient that flulike symptoms usually occur at the beginning of therapy. These effects tend to diminish with continued therapy.
• Advise the patient that drug may cause temporary hair loss. Reassure him that normal hair growth should return when the drug is withdrawn.
• Advise the patient that laboratory tests will be performed before and periodically during therapy.
• Teach patient to practice meticulous oral hygiene during treatment; bone marrow suppressant effects of interferon may lead to microbial infection, delayed healing, and gingival bleeding. Interferon may also decrease salivary flow.
• Teach patient to self-administer and to use disposable syringes correctly. Provide patient with written information on drug stability.
• Emphasize need to follow doctor's instructions about taking temperature, and how and when to take acetaminophen.
• Warn patient not to have any immunization without doctor's approval and to avoid contact with persons who have taken oral polio vaccine.
• Advise the patient to check with the doctor for further instructions after missing a dose.

Evaluation
In patients receiving interferon alfa-2a, appropriate evaluation statements may include:
• Patient exhibits signs of decreased tumor or viral cell activity and modulation of immune response.
• Patient remains free from signs and symptoms of CHF.
• Patient and family state an understanding of interferon alfa-2a therapy.

interferon alfa-2b recombinant (IFN-alpha 2)

(in ter ferr´ on)
Intron A

• *Classification:* antineoplastic (biological response modifier)
• *Pregnancy Risk Category:* C

HOW SUPPLIED

Injection: 3 million IU/vial with diluent, 5 million IU/vial with diluent, 10 million IU/vial with diluent, 25 million IU/vial with diluent, 50 million IU/vial with diluent

ACTION

Mechanism: A protein synthesized using recombinant DNA techniques that has complex antiviral, antineoplastic, and immunomodulating effects. Mimics the action of the naturally occuring protein produced and secreted by peripheral blood leukocytes in response to certain inducers, such as a viral infection. Its mechanism of action appears to involve a direct effect against tumor cells or viral cells to inhibit replication, and modulation of host immune response by enhancing the phagocytic activity of macrophages, and by augmenting specific cytotoxicity of lymphocytes against target cells. Interferon alfa-2a and interferon alfa-2b are similar; each has a molecular weight of 19,000 daltons and is made of 165 amino acids. They differ at position 23, where interferon alfa-2a has a lysine group, while interferon alfa-2b has an arginine group.
Absorption: Because the drug is subject to degradation by enzymes within the GI tract, it must be administered parenterally. More than 80% of the dose is absorbed after I.M. or S.C. injection.
Distribution: Rapidly cleared from plasma after I.V. administration. Limited data suggest that highest levels are found in the kidney, liver, spleen and lung. Small amounts enter the CSF. Unknown if drug crosses placenta or enters breast milk.
Metabolism: By the kidney. The drug undergoes rapid proteolytic degradation within the brush border of the renal tubule or by lysosomes of the tubular epithelium.
Excretion: By the kidney, with minor biliary elimination. Half-life: About 2 hours.
Onset, peak, duration: Peak serum levels occur within 15 minutes to1 hour of I.V. injection and are higher than those following I.M. or S.C. administration; however, serum levels are maintained longer after I.M. or S.C. administration. Serum interferon levels are detectable for 4 to 8 hours after I.V. injection or 16 to 30 hours after I.M. or S.C. administration.

INDICATIONS & DOSAGE

Treatment of hairy-cell leukemia –
Adults: 2 million units/m² I.M. or S.C. three times a week.
Treatment of condylomata acuminata (genital or venereal warts) –
Adults: 1 million units/lesion intralesionally three times a week for 3 weeks.
Treatment of AIDS-related Kaposi's sarcoma –
Adults: 30 million units/m² S.C. or I.M. three times a week.
Treatment of chronic hepatitis B –
Adults: 5 million units S.C. daily for up to 4 months.

CONTRAINDICATIONS & PRECAUTIONS

Contraindicated in patients with hypersensitivity to interferon or to any components of the product.

Use cautiously in patients with severe hepatic or renal function impairment, seizure disorders, compromised CNS function, cardiac disease, or myelosuppression because the drugs may worsen these conditions.

ADVERSE REACTIONS

Common reactions are in italics; life-threatening reactions are in bold italics.
Blood: leukemia, mild thrombocytopenia.
CNS: dizziness, confusion, paresthesias, lethargy, depression, difficulty in thinking or concentrating, insomnia, sedation, anxiety, *fatigue,* hypoes-

thesia, amnesia, agitation, weakness, ***seizures.***
CV: hypotension, chest pain.
EENT: visual disturbances, hearing disorders, stye, pharyngitis, nasal congestion, sinusitis, rhinitis.
GI: *anorexia, nausea,* diarrhea, vomiting, abdominal pain, dyspepsia, constipation, loose stools, eructation, dry mouth, dysgeusia.
GU: transient impotence, gynecomastia.
Respiratory: dyspnea, coughing.
Skin: rash, dryness, pruritus, partial alopecia, urticaria, moniliasis, flushing, dermatitis.
Other: *flu-like symptoms (fever, fatigue, headache, chills, muscle aches), arthralgia,* asthenia, rigors, leg cramps, arthrosis, bone disorders, back pain, increased sweating, stomatitis, gingivitis, decreased libido, hypertonia, migraine, thirst.

INTERACTIONS

CNS depressants: CNS effects enhanced.

EFFECTS ON DIAGNOSTIC TESTS

ALT (SGPT), AST (SGOT), LDH, and alkaline phosphatase: increased levels (dose-related and reversible on withdrawal of interferon).
Blood pressure: mild and trasient hypotension is likely.
Hemoglobin, hematocrit, leukocyte counts, platelets, and neutrophils: decreased (dose-related; recovery within days or weeks after withdrawal of interferon).
Prothrombin time and partial thromboplastin time: increased (dose-related).
Serum calcium, serum phosphorus, and fasting blood glucose: increased levels.

NURSING CONSIDERATIONS

Besides those related universally to drug therapy (see "How to use this book"), consider the following specific recommendations:

Assessment
- Obtain a baseline assessment of the patient's CBC with differential, platelet count, coagulation time, electrolyte studies, blood chemistry, liver-function studies, and ECG before therapy.
- Be alert for adverse reactions and drug interactions throughout therapy.
- Evaluate the patient's and family's knowledge about interferon alfa-2b therapy.

Nursing Diagnoses
- Altered protection related to proliferation of tumor or viral cells.
- Altered nutrition: Less than body requirements related to interferon-induced anorexia and nausea.
- Knowledge deficit related to interferon alfa-2b therapy.

Planning and Implementation

Preparation and Administration
- Consult most recent source of clinical information about the drug. Dosage, indications, and adverse reaction profile may change with additional clinical experience.
- Store drug in the refrigerator.
- Read label carefully. Different brands of interferon may not be equivalent and require different dosage.
- ***S.C. use:*** Give S.C. in patients whose platelet count is below 50,000 mm^3.
- Administer at bedtime to diminish daytime drowsiness.
- When administering interferon for condylomata acuminata, use only 10-million-IU vial since dilution of other strengths required for intralesional use results in hypertonic solution.
- Do not reconstitute 10-million-IU vial with more than 1 ml of diluent. Use tuberculin or similar syringe and 25G to 30G needle.
- Avoid injecting too superficially be-

neath the condylomata acuminata lesion.

• As many as five lesions may be treated at one time. To ease discomfort, administer in the evening with acetaminophen.

Monitoring

• Monitor effectiveness by evaluating the proliferation of tumor or viral cells and patient's immune response.

• Monitor CBC count with differential, coagulation time, and platelet count.

• Monitor blood chemistry, electrolytes, liver function studies, and if the patient has a preexisting advanced stage of cancer or cardiac disorder ECGs.

• Monitor temperature, pulse, blood pressure, and respiration regularly.

• Monitor for signs and symptoms of infection.

• Monitor daily weight and fluid balance.

• Observe for CNS adverse reactions, such as decreased mental status and dizziness. Periodic neuropsychiatric monitoring is recommended during drug therapy.

• Monitor for bleeding: test urine, emesis fluid, stool, and secretions for occult blood; inspect skin for bruising and petechiae.

Supportive Care

• Premedicate with acetaminophen to alleviate flulike symptoms induced by drug.

• Use reverse isolation procedure. Because interferon may decrease antibody response and potentiate replication of viruses, the patient is at special risk for infection during therapy.

• Severe adverse reactions may require reduction of dosage to one-half or discontinuation of the drug until reactions subside.

• Special precautions are necessary for patients who develop thrombocytopenia: exercise extreme care in performing invasive procedures, limit frequency of I.M. injection, and avoid I.V. infiltration.

• Make sure the patient is well hydrated especially during the initial stages of therapy.

• Provide frequent mouth care. Use a soft toothbrush and a mild mouth wash.

• Offer frequent, small, bland meals. Obtain order for medication to relieve nausea.

• Be aware that interferons may decrease hemoglobin, hematocrit, leukocytes, platelet, and neutrophils; increase prothrombin and partial thromboplastin time; and increase serum levels of AST (SGOT), ALT (SGPT), LDH, alkaline phosphatase, calcium, phosphorous, and fasting glucose. These effects are dose-related and reversible; recovery occurs within several days or weeks after withdrawal of interferon.

• Use seizure precautions. Have airway or padded tongue blade nearby.

• Use with caution in patient with history of cardiovascular disease, pulmonary disease, diabetes mellitus, coagulation disorders, and severe myelosuppression.

• Use with blood dyscrasia-causing medications, bone marrow suppressant therapy, or radiation therapy may increase bone marrow suppressant effects. Dosage reduction may be required.

• Neurotoxicity and cardiotoxicity occur most commonly in elderly patients, especially those with underlying CNS or cardiac impairment.

• Be aware that concurrent use with a live-virus vaccine may potentiate replication of vaccine virus, increase adverse reactions and decrease patient's antibody response.

• For patients receiving interferon for condylomata acuminata, maximum response usually occurs 4 to 8 weeks after initiation of therapy. If results are not satisfactory after 12 to 16

weeks, a second course of therapy may be instituted.
Patient Teaching
• Advise patient that flulike symptoms usually occur at the start of therapy. These effects tend to diminish with continued therapy.
• Advise the patient that drug may cause temporary loss of hair. Reassure him that normal hair growth should return when the drug is withdrawn.
• Advise the patient that laboratory tests will be performed before and periodically during therapy.
• Teach the patient to practice meticulous oral hygiene during treatment; bone marrow suppressant effects of interferon may lead to microbial infection, delayed healing, and gingival bleeding. Interferon may also decrease salivary flow.
• Teach patient to self-administer and to use disposable syringes correctly. Provide written information on drug stability.
• Emphasize need to follow doctor's instructions about taking temperature, and how and when to take acetaminophen.
• Advise the patient to check with the doctor after missing a dose.
• Warn patient not to have any immunization without doctor's approval and to avoid contact with persons who have taken oral polio vaccine.
Evaluation
In patients receiving interferon, appropriate evaluation statements may include:
• Patient exhibits signs of decreased tumor or viral cell activity and modulation of immune response.
• Patient reports decrease or absence in drug-induced anorexia and nausea.
• Patient and family state an understanding of interferon alfa-2b therapy.

interferon alfa-n3
(in ter feer′ on)
Alferon N

• *Classification:* antineoplastic (biological response modifier)
• *Pregnancy Risk Category:* C

HOW SUPPLIED
Injection: 5 million units/ml in 1-ml vials

ACTION
Mechanism: Interferon alfa-n3 is a naturally occurring antiviral agent derived from human leukocytes. It attaches to membrane receptors and causes cellular changes, including increased protein synthesis.
Absorption: After intralesional injection, plasma concentrations are below detectable levels, but systemic effects indicate that some systemic absorption does occur.

INDICATIONS & DOSAGE
Treatment of condylomata acuminata –
Adults: 0.05 ml/wart by intralesional injection. Treatment usually continues twice weekly for 8 weeks. Dosage should not exceed 0.5 ml (2.5 million units)/session.

CONTRAINDICATIONS & PRECAUTIONS
Contraindicated in patients with hypersensitivity to human interferon alfa or any component of the injection and in patients who have anaphylactic sensitivity to mouse immunoglobulin G, egg protein, or neomycin. Use cautiously in patients with debilitating medical conditions, such as cardiac disease, severe pulmonary disease, diabetes mellitus with ketoacidosis, coagulation disorders, seizure disorders, or severe myelosuppression because drug may worsen these con-

ditions due to the association of interferon with flulike syndrome.

ADVERSE REACTIONS

Common reactions are in italics; life-threatening reactions are in bold italics.

CNS: dizziness, light-headedness.

GI: dyspepsia, heartburn, vomiting, nausea.

Other: *mild to moderate flu-like syndrome (myalgia, fever, headache), arthralgia, back pain, malaise.*

INTERACTIONS

None reported.

EFFECTS ON DIAGNOSTIC TESTS

CBC: decreased WBC count.

Hemoglobin, WBC count, platelet counts, gamma-glutamyltransferase, AST (SGOT), alkaline phosphatase, and total bilirubin: abnormal values in cancer patients.

NURSING CONSIDERATIONS

Besides those related universally to drug therapy (see "How to use this book"), consider the following specific recommendations:

Assessment

- Obtain a baseline assessment of extent of skin lesions, allergies, and overall health status before therapy.
- Be alert for adverse reactions and drug interactions throughout therapy.
- Evaluate the patient's and family's knowledge about interferon alfa-n3 therapy.

Nursing Diagnoses

- Impaired skin integrity related to lesions induced by condylomata acuminata.
- Pain related to interferon-induced headache, backache, and arthralgia.
- Knowledge deficit related to interferon alfa-n3 therapy.

Planning and Implementation

Preparation and Administration

- Read labels carefully; dosage may change with different brands of interferon. Do not change brands during course of therapy.
- ***Intralesional use:*** Inject into each lesion at the base of the wart using 30G needle.

Monitoring

- Monitor effectiveness by observing the extent of lesions and warts present.
- Observe for signs of anaphylactic reactions.
- Monitor for signs of CNS adverse reactions (dizziness, lightheadedness).
- Observe for hypersensitivity reaction.

Supportive Care

- Keep epinephrine available. Have oxygen and resuscitation equipment nearby.
- Treat flulike symptoms with acetaminophen.
- Obtain an order for medication to relieve drug-induced headache, backache, or arthralgia.
- Obtain order for antiemetics. Offer frequent, small, bland meals.
- Do not give to patients hypersensitive to interferon alfa and in patients with a history of anaphylactic reactions to murine immunoglobulin, egg protein, or neomycin.

Patient Teaching

- Explain to the patient that the warts will continue to disappear after the 8 weeks of therapy are completed and the drug has been discontinued.
- Teach patients to recognize symptoms of hypersensitivity (hives, urticaria, wheezing, chest tightness, shortness of breath). Instruct them to notify the doctor immediately.
- Advise the patient that flulike symptoms usually occur.
- Teach the patient good hand-washing technique. Caution him to avoid scratching, rubbing, or picking lesions or warts.

Evaluation
In patients receiving interferon alfa-n3, appropriate evaluation statements may include:
- Patient exhibits decrease or absence of lesion and warts.
- Patient remains pain free.
- Patient and family state an understanding of interferon alfa-n3 therapy.

interferon gamma-1b
(in ter feer´ on)
Actimmune

- *Classification:* antineoplastic (biological response modifier)
- *Pregnancy Risk Category:* C

HOW SUPPLIED
injection: 100 mcg (3 million units)/vial

ACTION
Mechanism: Acts as an interleukin-type lymphokine. It has potent phagocyte-activating properties and enhances the oxidative metabolism of tissue macrophages.
Absorption: About 90% is absorbed after S.C. injection.
Excretion: Half-life: Elimination half-life is 5.9 hours.
Onset, peak, duration: Peak plasma concentrations are reached after 7 hours; no accumulation is noted after 12 consecutive daily doses.

INDICATIONS & DOSAGE
Chronic granulomatous disease –
Adults with a body surface area > 0.5 m²: 50 mcg/m² (1.5 million units/m²) I.M. three times weekly, preferably h.s. The preferred injection site is the deltoid or anterior thigh.
Adults with a body surface area ≤ 0.5 m²: 1.5 mcg/kg/dose three times weekly.

CONTRAINDICATIONS & PRECAUTIONS
Contraindicated in patients with hypersensitivity to interferon gamma, *Escherichia coli*–derived products, or any component of the formulation.
Use cautiously in patients with preexisting cardiac disease, including ischemia, CHF, or arrhythmia; with seizure disorders or compromised CNS function; and with myelosuppression.

ADVERSE REACTIONS
Common reactions are in italics; life-threatening reactions are in bold italics.
Blood: ***myelosuppression*** (at high doses).
CNS: *headache, chills (flulike syndrome),* fatigue, decreased mental status, gait disturbance.
GI: nausea, vomiting, diarrhea.
Local: erythema or tenderness at the injection site.
Metabolic: elevated hepatic enzymes (at high doses).
Skin: rash.
Other: fever, myalgia, arthralgia.

INTERACTIONS
Myelosuppressive agents: possible additive myelosuppression. Use together with caution.

EFFECTS ON DIAGNOSTIC TESTS
Blood glucose, liver function tests: elevated levels during high dose therapy.
Serum sodium: decreased levels during high dose therapy.

NURSING CONSIDERATIONS
Besides those related universally to drug therapy (see "How to use this book"), consider the following specific recommendations:
Assessment
- Obtain a baseline assessment of patient's overall physical status, CBC, and liver enzymes before initiating therapy.

• Be alert for adverse reactions and drug interactions throughout therapy.
• Evaluate the patient's and familiy's knowledge about interferon gamma-1b therapy.

Nursing Diagnoses
• Hyperthermia associated with interferon gamma-1b–induced fever.
• Pain associated with interferon gamma-1b–induced flulike symptoms.
• Knowledge deficit related to interferon gamma-1b therapy.

Planning and Implementation
Preparation and Administration
• Refrigerate drug immediately. Vials must be stored in refrigerator (36°F to 46° F [2° C to 8° C]); do not freeze. Discard vials that have been left at room temperature for more than 12 hours.
• Do not shake vial and avoid excessive agitation.
• Each vial is for single use only. Because the drug does not contain a preservative, discard the unused contents safely.
Monitoring
• Monitor effectiveness by noting results of follow-up diagnostic tests and patient's overall physical status.
• Monitor for pain, fever, chills, and other flulike symptoms; these are commonly seen with high-dose therapy.
• Monitor hepatic enzymes for elevations (at high doses).
• Monitor CBC for myelosuppression at high doses. Also monitor patient for evidence of infection or bleeding.
Supportive Care
• Administer the drug at bedtime to reduce discomfort from flulike symptoms.
• Administer acetaminophen, as ordered, to relieve pain and reduce fever.
Patient Teaching
• Ensure the patient who will self-administer the drug has a copy of the patient information leaflet, which will aid in the safe and effective use of the medication. Be sure the patient understands the correct methods of drug administration and waste disposal.
• Warn patients to watch for and report signs of infection (sore throat, fever, fatigue) or bleeding.
• Tell patients that acetaminophen may reduce discomfort and fever associated with flulike symptoms, and that taking the medication at bedtime may also reduce discomfort.

Evaluation
In patients receiving interferon gamma-1b, appropriate evaluation statements may include:
• Temperature is within normal limits or returned to normal limits.
• Pain is relieved.
• Patient and family state an understanding of interferon gamma-1b therapy.

ipecac syrup*
(ip´ e kak)

• *Classification:* emetic (alkaloid)
• *Pregnancy Risk Category:* C

HOW SUPPLIED
Syrup: 70 mg powdered ipecac/ml* ◇

ACTION
Mechanism: Induces vomiting by producing gastric irritation. Also acts in the CNS on the chemoreceptor trigger zone.
Absorption: Usually not absorbed; absorption may occur when drug fails to produce emesis.
Excretion: Slowly in urine over 60 days.
Onset, peak, duration: Onset of action usually occurs in 20 minutes. Duration of effect is 30 minutes to 2 hours.

INDICATIONS & DOSAGE

To induce vomiting in poisoning–
Adults and children over 12 years: 30 ml P.O., followed by 200 to 300 ml of water.
Children 1 year or older: 15 ml P.O., followed by about 200 ml of water or milk.
Children under 1 year: 5 to 10 ml P.O., followed by 100 to 200 ml of water or milk. May repeat dose once after 20 minutes, if necessary.

CONTRAINDICATIONS & PRECAUTIONS

Contraindicated in patients with poisoning caused by alkalies or corrosive agents because of hazard of further esophageal or mediastinal injury; poisoning from petroleum distillates; in patients who are semiconscious, unconscious, comatose, or in shock; with seizures, severe inebriation, depressed gag reflexes, or strychnine poisoning because of hazards of aspiration: pneumonitis, bronchospasm, or pulmonary edema; and in patients with heart disease because ipecac is potentially cardiotoxic.

ADVERSE REACTIONS

Common reactions are in italics; life-threatening reactions are in bold italics.
CNS: depression.
CV: ***cardiac arrhythmias,*** *bradycardia, hypotension, atrial fibrillation, or* ***fatal myocarditis after ingestion of excessive dose.***
GI: diarrhea.

INTERACTIONS

Activated charcoal: neutralized emetic effect. Don't give together but may give activated charcoal after vomiting has occurred.

EFFECTS ON DIAGNOSTIC TESTS

None reported.

NURSING CONSIDERATIONS

Besides those related universally to drug therapy (see "How to use this book"), consider the following specific recommendations:

Assessment

- Obtain a baseline assessment of circumstances surrounding situation, substance reportedly ingested, gag reflex, and cardiac status before using ipecac.
- Be alert for adverse reactions and drug interactions throughout therapy.
- Evaluate the patient's and family's knowledge about the use of ipecac therapy.

Nursing Diagnoses

- High risk for injury related to ingestion of poisonous substance.
- Decreased cardiac output related to ipecac syrup–induced cardiac arrhythmias.
- Knowledge deficit related to the use of ipecac syrup.

Planning and Implementation

Preparation and Administration

- Read label and order carefully. *Note:* ipecac syrup is not the same as single word "ipecac" (fluidextract). Fluidextract is 14 times more concentrated and if inadvertently used instead of ipecac syrup may cause death. Ipecac fluidextract is no longer commercially available in the United States.
- ***P.O. use:*** Follow dose with 200 to 300 ml of water.
- If two doses do not induce vomiting, gastric lavage is necessary.

Monitoring

- Monitor effectiveness by observing the patient for vomiting, which usually begins within 30 minutes in more than 90% of patients; average time of onset is usually less than 20 minutes.
- Monitor blood pressure and ECG.
- Monitor fluid and electrolyte balance.

Supportive Care

• Do not give after ingestion of caustic substances, such as lye; additional injury to the esophagus and mediastinum can occur.
• Be aware that stomach is usually emptied completely; vomitus may contain some intestinal material as well.
• In antiemetic toxicity, ipecac syrup is usually effective if less than 1 hour has passed since ingestion of antiemetic.
• No systematic toxicity occurs with doses of 30 ml or less.
• Be aware that ipecac syrup is now commonly abused by bulimics who practice "binge-purge."
• Position patient on side to prevent aspiration of vomitus. Have airway and suction equipment nearby.
• Provide mouth care when emesis is completed.

Patient Teaching

• Advise parents of children 1 year and over to keep 1 oz (30 ml) of ipecac syrup available in the home for immediate use in case of emergency.
• Encourage proper storage of medications and hazardous substances to avoid accidental poisonings.
• Advise patient and family to keep poison control phone number on or near telephone.
• Provide "Mr. Yuk" labels to parents of small children.

Evaluation

In patients receiving ipecac syrup, appropriate evaluation statements may include:
• Patient remains free from injury related to ingestion of poisonous substance.
• Patient's cardiac output remains adequate.
• Patient and family state an understanding of the use of ipecac syrup.

ipratropium bromide

(i pra troe´ pee um)
Atrovent

• *Classification:* bronchodilator (anticholinergic)
• *Pregnancy Risk Category:* B

HOW SUPPLIED

Inhaler: each metered dose supplies 18 mcg
Solution (for nebulizer): 0.025% (250 mcg/ml)‡

ACTION

Mechanism: Inhibits vagally mediated reflexes by antagonizing acetylcholine. An anticholinergic.
Absorption: Not readily absorbed into the systemic circulation either from the surface of the lung or from the GI tract as confirmed by blood levels and renal excretion studies. Much of an inhaled dose is swallowed as shown by fecal excretion studies.
Distribution: Acts locally in the respiratory tract.
Metabolism: Hepatic.
Excretion: Most is excreted unchanged in feces. Absorbed drug is excreted in urine and bile. Half-life: About 2 hours.
Onset, peak, duration: Drug action peaks in 1 to 2 hours, and persists for 3 to 4 hours in most patients and up to 6 hours in some patients.

INDICATIONS & DOSAGE

Maintenance treatment of bronchospasm associated with chronic obstructive pulmonary disease–
Adults: 2 inhalations (26 mcg) q.i.d. Additional inhalations may be needed. However, total inhalations should not exceed 12 in 24 hours.

CONTRAINDICATIONS & PRECAUTIONS

Contraindicated in patients allergic to atropine or its derivatives.

Use cautiously in patients with narrow-angle glaucoma, prostatic hypertrophy, or bladder neck obstruction, because anticholinergics can worsen the symptoms associated with these disorders.

Warning: Ipratropium is not indicated for the initial treatment of acute episodes of bronchospasm when rapid response is required.

ADVERSE REACTIONS

Common reactions are in italics; life-threatening reactions are in bold italics.
CNS: nervousness, dizziness, headache.
CV: palpitations.
EENT: cough, blurred vision.
GI: nausea, GI distress, dry mouth.
Skin: rash.

INTERACTIONS

None significant.

EFFECTS ON DIAGNOSTIC TESTS

None reported.

NURSING CONSIDERATIONS

Besides those related universally to drug therapy (see "How to use this book"), consider the following specific recommendations:

Assessment

- Obtain a baseline assessment of the patient's bronchospasms before therapy.
- Be alert for adverse reactions and drug interactions throughout therapy.
- Evaluate the patient's and family's knowledge about ipratropium therapy.

Nursing Diagnoses

- Ineffective airway clearance related to patient's underlying condition.
- Sensory/perceptual alterations (visual) related to adverse reactions to ipratropium.
- Knowledge deficit related to ipratropium therapy.

Planning and Implementation

Preparation and Administration

- ***Inhalation:*** The inhalations are usually given q.i.d. Additional inhalations may be needed, but total inhalations should not exceed 12 in 24 hours. If the bronchodilator is administered via inhalant and more than one inhalation is ordered, 2 minutes should elapse between inhalations. If more than one type of inhalant is ordered, always administer the bronchodilator first and wait 5 minutes before administering the other.
- Be sure to give the medication on time to ensure maximal effect.

Monitoring

- Monitor effectiveness by regularly assessing the patient's lung fields for bronchospasm.
- Monitor for blurred vision and dizziness. Remember that dizziness occurs more often in elderly patients at the start of treatment.

Supportive Care

- Notify the doctor if bronchospasms are not relieved with ipratropium.
- Institute safety precautions if blurred vision or dizziness occurs.
- Remember that ipratropium is not effective for treatment of acute episodes of bronchospasm when rapid response is required.

Patient Teaching

- Tell the patient to always take the medication exactly as prescribed and to take it around the clock.
- Instruct the patient to perform oral inhalation correctly as follows: Clear nasal passages and throat. Breathe out, expelling as much air from the lungs as possible. Place the mouthpiece well into the mouth as the dose from the inhaler is released, and inhale deeply. Hold breath for several seconds, remove the mouthpiece, and exhale slowly.
- If more than 1 inhalation is ordered, tell the patient to wait at least

2 minutes before repeating the procedure for a second dose.
• Explain why it is necessary to use the bronchodilator first if other inhalants such as a steroid inhaler are prescribed. This allows the bronchodilator to open air passages for maximum effectiveness. Tell the patient to allow 5 minutes between the inhalant treatments.
• Warn the patient to avoid accidentally spraying the inhalant into the eyes, which may cause temporary blurring of vision.
• Tell the patient to reduce the intake of foods containing caffeine, such as coffee, colas, and chocolates, when taking a bronchodilator.
• Warn the patient to contact the doctor immediately if he experiences a fluttering of the heart, rapid beating of the heart, shortness of breath, or chest pain.
• Warn elderly patients that dizziness may occur at the start of therapy. Therefore, they should take precautions to avoid injury from falls.
• Tell the patient not to self-medicate with any OTC drugs without medical approval while taking this drug.
• Warn the patient against increasing the dosage or frequency of administration. Advise the patient to notify the doctor if prescribed dosage does not relieve symptoms.
• Show the patient how to check the pulse. Instruct the patient to check his pulse before and after using a bronchodilator and to call the doctor if his pulse increases more than 20 to 30 beats per minute.
• Teach patient how to perform self-injection of ipratropium in case of an acute hypersensitivity reaction at home.
• Warn the patient that this drug is not effective in the treatment of acute episodes of bronchospasm when rapid response is required.

Evaluation
In patients receiving ipratropium, appropriate evaluation statements may include:
• Patient's bronchospasms are relieved by ipratropium.
• Patient's vision is unaffected by ipratropium therapy.
• Patient and family state an understanding of ipratropium therapy.

iron dextran
Hydextran, Imferon, K-FeRON

• *Classification:* hematinic (parenteral iron supplement)
• *Pregnancy Risk Category:* C

HOW SUPPLIED
Injection: 50 mg elemental iron/ml

ACTION
Mechanism: Provides elemental iron, an essential component in the formation of hemoglobin; 1 ml iron dextran provides 50 mg elemental iron.
Absorption: I.M. doses are absorbed in two stages: 60% after 3 days and up to 90% by 3 weeks. Remainder is absorbed over several months or longer.
Distribution: During first 3 days, local inflammation facilitates passage of drug into the lymphatic system; drug is then ingested by macrophages, which enter lymph and blood.
Metabolism: After I.M. or I.V. administration, iron dextran is cleared from plasma by reticuloendothelial cells of the liver, spleen, and bone marrow.
Excretion: Traces are excreted in breast milk, urine, bile, and feces. Drug cannot be removed by hemodialysis. Half-life: In doses of 500 mg or less, half-life is 6 hours.

INDICATIONS & DOSAGE

Iron deficiency anemia –
Adults: I.M. or I.V. injections of iron are advisable only for patients for whom oral administration is impossible or ineffective. Test dose (0.5 ml) required before administration.
I.M. (by Z-track): inject 0.5 ml test dose. If no reactions next daily dose should ordinarily not exceed 0.5 ml (25 mg) for infants under 5 kg; 1 ml (50 mg) for children under 9 kg; 2 ml (100 mg) for patients under 50 kg; 5 ml (250 mg) for patients over 50 kg.
I.V. push: inject 0.5 ml test dose. If no reaction, within 2 to 3 days the dosage may be raised to 2 ml daily I.V., 1 ml/minute undiluted and infused slowly until total dose is achieved. No single dose should exceed 100 mg.
I.V. infusion: dosages are expressed in terms of elemental iron. Dilute in 250 to 1,000 ml of normal saline solution; dextrose increases local vein irritation. Infuse test dose of 25 mg slowly over 5 minutes. If no reaction occurs in 5 minutes, infusion may be started. Infuse total dose slowly over approximately 6 to 12 hours.

CONTRAINDICATIONS & PRECAUTIONS

Contraindicated in patients with hypersensitivity to any of the components; in patients with any anemia other than iron-deficiency anemia; and for simultaneous use with oral iron. Use cautiously in patients with rheumatoid arthritis because I.V. injections may exacerbate joint pain and swelling; and in patients with a significant history of allergies or asthma. Administer with extreme caution to patients with serious hepatic impairment because of potential for additional liver damage.

ADVERSE REACTIONS

Common reactions are in italics; life-threatening reactions are in bold italics.
CNS: headache, transitory paresthesias, arthralgia, myalgia, dizziness, malaise, syncope.
CV: *hypotensive reaction, peripheral vascular flushing with overly rapid I.V. administration, tachycardia.*
GI: nausea, vomiting, metallic taste, transient loss of taste perception.
Local: *soreness and inflammation at injection site (I.M.); brown skin discoloration at injection site (I.M.); local phlebitis at injection site (I.V.).*
Skin: rash, urticaria.
Other: ***anaphylaxis.***

INTERACTIONS

None significant.

EFFECTS ON DIAGNOSTIC TESTS

Note: Large doses (over 100 mg iron) may color the serum brown.
Serum bilirubin: false elevations.
Serum calcium: falsely reduced levels.
Serum iron concentration and total iron binding capacity: misleading results for up to 3 weeks.
Bone scans using technetium 99m diphosphonate: dense areas of activity for 1 to 6 days after I.M. injection.

NURSING CONSIDERATIONS

Besides those related universally to drug therapy (see "How to use this book"), consider the following specific recommendations:
Assessment
- Obtain a baseline assessment of hemoglobin concentration, hematocrit, and reticulocyte counts before therapy.
- Be alert for adverse reactions and drug interactions throughout therapy.
- Evaluate the patient's and family's knowledge about iron dextran therapy.

Nursing Diagnoses

- Activity intolerance related to iron deficency.
- Altered tissue perfusion (renal, cerebral, cardiopulmonary, GI, peripheral) related to iron dextran therapy.
- Knowledge deficit related to iron dextran therapy.

Planning and Implementation

Preparation and Administration

- Keep in mind that I.M. or I.V. iron injections are advisable only for patients for whom oral administration is impossible or ineffective.
- ***I.M. use:*** Administer undiluted. Administer 0.5 ml test dose (Z-track) and observe for reactions. If no reaction, the next daily dose should be appropriate to age and weight. Give injection deep I.M. using Z-track method to avoid leakage into subcutaneous tissue and skin staining. Use the upper outer quadrant of the buttock—never the arm or other exposed area—and a 2- to 3-inch 19G or 20G needle. Skin staining may be minimized by using a separate needle to withdraw the drug from its container.
- ***I.V. use:*** Use this route only when oral route is unsatisfactory or impossible or when rapid replenishment of iron stores is necessary. Because of risk of anaphylaxis, inject a test dose of 0.5 ml (25 mg) over 5 minutes. Observe patient for 1 hour and, if no adverse reactions occur, proceed with full dose. After initial test dose: for direct injection, give undiluted dose of 2 ml or less over at least 2 minutes; for intermittent infusion, infuse solution over 1 to 6 hours or more using an appropriate diluting solution. On completion, infuse 0.9% sodium chloride solution to flush vein. This drug should not be administered by continuous I.V. infusion.

Monitoring

- Monitor effectiveness by evaluating hemoglobin concentration, hematocrit, and reticulocyte count and the patient's health status.
- Monitor the patient for symptoms of adverse reactions and anaphylaxis. Reactions vary, ranging from pain, myalgia, and inflammation to hypotension, shock, and death. Check the patient's vital signs.
- Monitor the patient for symptoms of drug toxicity. Evaluate serum ferritin, hemoglobin, hematocrit, and reticulocyte counts. Late signs of toxicity include bluish lips, fingernails, and palms; drowsiness; pale, clammy skin; tachycardia; and unusual tiredness or weakness.
- Observe the patient for delayed reactions (1 to 2 days), which are more common with parenteral administration. Reactions may include arthralgia, backache, chills, dizziness, headache, malaise, moderate-to-high fever, myalgia, nausea, and vomiting.

Supportive Care

- Be aware that iron toxicity may occur and check that the diagnosis of iron deficiency anemia is definitive before giving the drug.
- Keep epinephrine and resuscitation equipment readily available to treat anaphlylaxis.
- Keep in mind that the patient should rest for 15 to 30 minutes after I.V. administration.

Patient Teaching

- Warn the patient to avoid OTC vitamins that include iron.
- Teach the patient symptoms of reaction or toxicity and to report them.

Evaluation

In patients receiving iron dextran, appropriate evaluation statements may include:

- Activity level is within normal limits; hemoglobin, hematocrit and reticulocyte counts are within normal parameters.
- Patient has not experienced an adverse reaction to therapy.
- Patient and family state an understanding of iron dextran therapy.

iron supplements, oral

ferrous fumarate
Eldofe◇, Feostat◇, Ferranol◇, Fersamal†, Fumasorb◇, Fumerin◇, Hemocyte◇, Ircon◇, Maniron◇, Novofumar†, Palafer†, Span-FF◇

ferrous gluconate
Fergon*◇, Ferralet◇, Fertinic†, Novoferrogluc†

ferrous sulfate
Feosol*◇, Fer-In-Sol*◇, Feritard‡, Fero-Grad†, Fero-Gradumet◇, Ferolix*◇, Ferospace◇, Ferralyn◇, Fespan‡, Irospan◇, Mol-Iron*◇, Novoferrosulfa†, Slow-Fe, Telefon◇

• *Classification:* hematinic (iron supplement)
• *Pregnancy Risk Category:* A

HOW SUPPLIED
fumarate
Each 100 mg provides 33 mg of elemental iron.
Tablets◇*:* 63 mg, 195 mg, 200 mg, 324 mg, 325 mg
Tablets (chewable): 100 mg◇
Capsules (controlled-release): 325 mg◇
Oral suspension: 100 mg/5 ml◇
Drops: 45 mg/0.6 ml◇
gluconate
Each 100 mg provides 11.6 mg of elemental iron.
Tablets: 300 mg◇, 320 mg◇, 325 mg◇
Capsules: 86 mg◇, 325 mg◇, 435 mg◇
Elixir: 300 mg/5 ml◇
sulfate
Each 100 mg provides 20 mg of elemental iron; dried and powdered (exsiccated), provides about 32 mg of elemental iron.
Tablets: 195 mg◇, 300 mg◇, 325 mg◇; 200 mg (exsiccated)◇
Tablets (extended-release): 160 mg (exsiccated)◇
Capsules◇*:* 150 mg, 225 mg, 250 mg, 390 mg, 190 mg (exsiccated)
Capsules (extended-release): 525 mg◇, 150 mg◇, 167 mg (exsiccated)◇
Elixir: 220 mg/5 ml*◇
Liquid: 75 mg/0.6 ml◇
Syrup: 90 mg/5 ml◇

ACTION
Mechanism: Provides elemental iron, an essential component in the formation of hemoglobin.
Absorption: Absorbed from the entire length of the GI tract, but primary absorption sites are the duodenum and proximal jejunum. Up to 10% of iron is absorbed by healthy individuals; patients with iron-deficiency anemia may absorb up to 60%. Enteric coating and some extended-release formulas decrease absorption because they are designed to release iron past the points of highest absorption; food may decrease absorption by 33% to 50%.
Distribution: Transported through GI mucosal cells directly into the blood, where it is immediately bound to a carrier protein, transferrin, and transported to the bone marrow for incorporation into hemoglobin. Iron is highly protein-bound.
Metabolism: Liberated by the destruction of hemoglobin but conserved and reused by the body.
Excretion: Healthy individuals lose only small amounts of iron each day. Men and postmenopausal women lose about 1 mg/day, and premenopausal women about 1.5 mg/day. The loss usually occurs in nails, hair, feces, and urine; trace amounts are lost in bile and sweat.

INDICATIONS & DOSAGE
Iron deficiency–
Adults: 200 mg (fumarate) P.O. t.i.d. or q.i.d.; or 300 to 325 mg (gluconate) P.O. q.i.d., increased to 650 mg q.i.d. as needed and tolerated; or 325 mg (sulfate) P.O. t.i.d. or q.i.d.

Alternatively, give (sulfate) as 1 delayed-release capsule (160 or 525 mg) P.O. b.i.d.
Children 2 years or over: 3 mg/kg (fumarate or gluconate) P.O. t.i.d., increased to 6 mg/kg P.O. t.i.d. as needed and tolerated; or 5 mg/kg (sulfate) P.O. t.i.d., increased to 10 mg/kg P.O. t.i.d. as needed and tolerated.
Prophylaxis for iron-deficiency anemia –
Pregnant women: 150 to 300 mg (sulfate) P.O. daily in divided doses.
Premature or undernourished infants: 1 to 2 mg/kg (sulfate) P.O. daily (as elemental iron) in divided doses.

CONTRAINDICATIONS & PRECAUTIONS

Contraindicated in patients with hemochromatosis, hemosiderosis, hemolytic anemia, or hypersensitivity to any components of the product.

Use with extreme caution in patients with peptic ulcer, regional enteritis, ulcerative colitis, or hepatitis because iron has irritant effects on the GI mucosa and with caution in patients requiring prolonged therapy.

ADVERSE REACTIONS

Common reactions are in italics; life-threatening reactions are in bold italics.
GI: *nausea,* vomiting, *constipation, black stools.*
Other: elixir may stain teeth.

INTERACTIONS

Antacids, cholestyramine resin, pancreatic extracts, vitamin E: decreased iron absorption. Separate doses if possible.
Chloramphenicol: watch for delayed response to iron therapy.
Vitamin C: concurrent administration may increase iron absorption. Beneficial drug interaction.

EFFECTS ON DIAGNOSTIC TESTS

Fecal occult blood: test interference (Guaiac test and orthotoluidine test may yield false-positive results; benzidine test usually not affected.)
Skeletal imaging: test interference. Iron overload may decrease uptake of technetium 99m.

NURSING CONSIDERATIONS

Besides those related universally to drug therapy (see "How to use this book"), consider the following specific recommendations:

Assessment
- Obtain a baseline assessment of hemoglobin and reticulocyte counts before therapy.
- Be alert for adverse reactions and drug interactions throughout therapy.
- Evaluate the patient's and family's knowledge about oral iron supplement therapy.

Nursing Diagnoses
- Activity intolerance related to patient's underlying condition.
- Constipation related to adverse reactions to oral iron supplements.
- Knowledge deficit related to therapy with oral iron supplements.

Planning and Implementation
Preparation and Administration
- ***P.O. use:*** Administer between meals; if GI upset occurs, give with food. Dilute liquids with orange juice or water, and give tablets with orange juice; this promotes iron absorption. Do not use milk or antacids to dilute the liquid preparations. Use a straw to administer iron elixir to help prevent staining the teeth.

Monitoring
- Monitor effectiveness by regularly evaluating the patient's hemoglobin level and reticulocyte count.
- Monitor the patient for constipation; record the color and amount of stools.
- Monitor the patient for GI upset.

Supportive Care
• Notify the doctor of changes in the hemoglobin level and reticulocyte count.
• Encourage the patient to use measures to prevent constipation; increase fiber and fluids and regular exercise if they are not contraindicated. If constipation occurs and persists, notify the doctor; combination products with a stool softener are available but should be avoided if possible.
• Notify the doctor of persistent GI upset not relieved by taking drug with food. Combination product with antacid is available, but its use should be avoided because it decreases iron absorption.
Patient Teaching
• Tell the patient to take iron supplements between meals and to take them with food if GI upset occurs. Mix the liquid with orange juice or water, but not in milk or antacids. The tablets may also be taken with orange juice since this promotes iron absorption. A straw should be used to take the iron elixir to help prevent dental stains.
• Teach the patient measures to prevent constipation. Inform him that the drug may turn his stools black but that this effect is harmless; however, tell him that melena may be masked.
• Teach parents to keep iron supplements out of children's reach and to administer to children carefully. Iron is toxic.
Evaluation
In patients receiving oral iron supplements, appropriate evaluation statements may include:
• Patient's activity level is within normal range, and his hemoglobin level and reticulocyte count are within normal parameters.
• Patient does not report GI upset.
• Patient and family state an understanding of therapy with oral supplements.

isocarboxazid
(eye soe kar box´ a zid)
Marplan

• *Classification:* antidepressant (monoamine oxidase inhibitor)
• *Pregnancy Risk Category:* C

HOW SUPPLIED
Tablets: 10 mg

ACTION
Mechanism: Promotes accumulation of neurotransmitters by inhibiting their breakdown.
Absorption: Rapidly and completely absorbed from the GI tract.
Distribution: Not yet determined; dosage adjustments are determined by therapeutic response and adverse reaction profile.
Metabolism: Hepatic.
Excretion: Primarily in urine within 24 hours; some in feces via the biliary tract. Half-life: 2½ hours (relatively short), but enzyme inhibition is prolonged and unrelated to half-life.
Onset, peak, duration: Peak therapeutic effect may not be seen for several weeks.

INDICATIONS & DOSAGE
Treatment of depression–
Adults: 30 mg P.O. daily in divided doses. Reduce to 10 to 20 mg daily when condition improves. Not recommended for children under 16 years.

CONTRAINDICATIONS & PRECAUTIONS
Contraindicated in patients with uncontrolled hypertension and seizure disorders because the drug may precipitate hypertensive reactions and lower the seizure threshold.

Use cautiously in patients with angina pectoris or other cardiovascular diseases, Type I and Type II diabetes, Parkinson's disease and other motor disorders, hyperthyroidism, pheochromocytoma, renal or hepatic insufficiency, and bipolar disease (reduce dosage during manic phase).

ADVERSE REACTIONS

Common reactions are in italics; life-threatening reactions are in bold italics.
CNS: *dizziness,* vertigo, weakness, headache, overactivity, hyperreflexia, tremors, muscle twitching, mania, *insomnia,* confusion, memory impairment, fatigue.
CV: *orthostatic hypotension,* arrhythmias, paradoxical hypertension.
EENT: blurred vision.
GI: dry mouth, *anorexia,* nausea, diarrhea, constipation.
Skin: rash.
Other: peripheral edema, sweating, weight changes, altered libido.

INTERACTIONS

Alcohol, barbiturates, and other sedatives; narcotics; dextromethorphan; TCAs: unpredictable interaction. Use with caution and in reduced dosage.
Amphetamines, antihistamines, ephedrine, levodopa, meperidine, metaraminol, methotrimeprazine, methylphenidate, phenylephrine, phenylpropanolamine: pressor effects of these drugs are enhanced by isocarboxazid. Use together very cautiously.
Insulin, oral hypoglycemic agents: isocarboxazid may alter requirements for antidiabetic medications.

EFFECTS ON DIAGNOSTIC TESTS

Liver function tests: elevated results.
Urine catecholamine: elevated levels.

NURSING CONSIDERATIONS

Besides those related universally to drug therapy (see "How to use this book"), consider the following specific recommendations:

Assessment

- Obtain a baseline assessment of severity of depression and baseline blood pressure readings, CBC, and liver function tests before therapy.
- Be alert for adverse reactions and drug interactions throughout therapy.
- Evaluate the patient's and family's knowledge about isocarboxazid therapy.

Nursing Diagnoses

- Ineffective individual coping related to the patient's underlying condition.
- High risk for injury related to isocarboxazid-induced adverse reactions.
- Knowledge deficit related to isocarboxazid therapy.

Planning and Implementation

Preparation and Administration

- Expect dosage to be reduced to maintenance levels as soon as possible.

Monitoring

- Monitor effectiveness by having the patient discuss his feelings (ask broad, open-ended questions) and by evaluating his behavior.
- Monitor blood pressure (supine and standing), ECG for changes, and heart rate for tachycardia.
- Monitor results of CBC and liver function tests throughout therapy.
- Monitor for signs of overdosage (palpitations, frequent headaches, or severe orthostatic hypotension).
- Monitor for edema and urine retention.
- Monitor for suicidal tendencies.

Supportive Care

- Expect this drug to be used only when electroconvulsive therapy or TCA is ineffective or contraindicated.
- Hold dose and notify the doctor if the patient develops signs of overdosage.
- Weigh the patient biweekly to help detect edema.
- Assist the patient in changing positions slowly to minimize orthostatic hypotension and supervise the patient when walking to prevent injury.
- Have phentolamine (Regitine) available to counteract severe hypertension.

• Do not withdraw the drug abruptly.
• Continue safety precautions for 10 days after the drug is discontinued because it has long-lasting effects.
Patient Teaching
• Teach the patient how to check for edema and urine retention.
• Warn the patient to avoid foods high in tyramine or tryptophan (aged cheese, Chianti wine, beer, avocados, chicken livers, chocolate, bananas, soy sauce, meat tenderizers, salami, bologna); large amounts of caffeine; and self-medication with OTC cold, hay fever, or diet preparations.
• Tell the patient that drug commonly causes orthostatic hypotension. Advise him to get out of bed slowly, waiting for 1 minute before attempting to stand.
• Tell the patient therapy must continue for 2 weeks or more before noticeable effect, and for 4 weeks or more before full effect. Encourage the patient to continue to take medication until it achieves full therapeutic effect.
• Warn against combining drug with alcohol or other CNS depressants.
Evaluation
In patients receiving isocarboxazid, appropriate evaluation statements may include:
• Patient behavior and communication indicate improvement of depression.
• Patient does not experience injury from adverse CNS or CV reactions.
• Patient and family state an understanding of isocarboxazid therapy.

---

isoetharine hydrochloride
(eye soe eth´ a reen)
Arm-a-Med Isoetharine, Beta-2, Bisorine, Bronkosol, Dey-Dose Isoetharine, Dey-Dose Isoetharine S/F, Dey-Lute Isoetharine, Dispos-a-Med Isoetharine

isoetharine mesylate
Bronkometer

• *Classification:* bronchodilator (adrenergic)
• *Pregnancy Risk Category:* C

HOW SUPPLIED
Aerosol inhaler: 340 mcg/metered spray
Nebulizer inhaler: 0.062%, 0.08%, 0.1%, 0.125%, 0.14%, 0.167%, 0.17%, 0.2%, 0.25%, 0.5%, 1% solution

ACTION
Mechanism: Relaxes bronchial smooth muscle by acting on $beta_2$-adrenergic receptors.
Absorption: Rapidly absorbed from the respiratory tract after oral inhalation.
Metabolism: Metabolized in lungs, liver, GI tract, and other tissues by the enzyme catechol-O-methyltransferase.
Excretion: In urine as unchanged drug (10%) and metabolites (90%).
Onset, peak, duration: Bronchodilation occurs immediately, peaks in 5 to 15 minutes, and persists 1 to 4 hours.

INDICATIONS & DOSAGE
Bronchial asthma and reversible bronchospasm that may occur with bronchitis and emphysema –
Adults: *(hydrochloride) administered by oxygen aerosolization* – 0.5 to 1 ml of a 0.5%, or 0.5 ml (range 0.25 to 0.5 ml) of a 1% solution diluted 1.3; or undiluted, 4 ml (range 2 to 4 ml) of a 0.125% solution, 2.5 ml of a 0.2% solution, or 2 ml of a 0.25% solution. *Administered by IPPB solution* – 0.5 to 1 ml of a 0.5% solution, or 0.5 ml (range 0.25 to 1 ml) of a 1% solution diluted 1:3; or undiluted, 4 ml (range 2 to 4 ml) of a 0.125% solution, 2.5 of 0.2% solution, or 2 ml of a 0.25% solution. *Adminis-*

tered by hand nebulizer–4 inhalations (range 3 to 7 inhalations) of undiluted 0.5% or 1% solution.

(mesylate) administered by metered aerosol–1 to 2 inhalations. Occasionally, more may be required.

CONTRAINDICATIONS & PRECAUTIONS

Contraindicated in patients with hypersensitivity to the drug or any ingredients in the formulation. Use cautiously in patients with hyperthyroidism, hypertension, acute coronary disease, angina, cardiac asthma, limited cardiac reserve, and cerebral arteriosclerosis because the drug may worsen these conditions and to patients with sulfite sensitivity because some formulations contain sulfite preservatives.

ADVERSE REACTIONS

Common reactions are in italics; life-threatening reactions are in bold italics.

CNS: *tremor, headache,* dizziness, excitement.

CV: *palpitations,* increased heart rate.

GI: nausea, vomiting.

INTERACTIONS

Propranolol and other beta blockers: blocked bronchodilating effect of isoetharine. Monitor patient carefully if used together.

EFFECTS ON DIAGNOSTIC TESTS

None reported.

NURSING CONSIDERATIONS

Besides those related universally to drug therapy (see "How to use this book"), consider the following specific recommendations:

Assessment

- Obtain a baseline assessment of the patient's pulmonary status by taking vital signs, noting ECG results, and auscultating lung fields.
- Be alert for adverse reactions or drug interactions throughout therapy.
- Evaluate the patient and family's knowledge about isoetharine therapy.

Nursing Diagnoses

- Ineffective airway clearance related to patient's underlying respiratory condition.
- Pain related to isoetharine-induced headache.
- Knowledge deficit related to isoetharine therapy.

Planning and Implementation

Preparation and Administration

- ***Inhalation:*** If the bronchodilator is administered via inhalant and more than one inhalation is ordered, 2 minutes should elapse between inhalations. If more than one type of inhalant is ordered, always administer bronchodilator first and wait 5 minutes before administering the other.

Monitoring

- Monitor effectiveness by regularly auscultating the lungs, noting respiratory rate and results of laboratory studies such as arterial blood gases.
- Monitor for severe paradoxic bronchoconstriction after excessive use.

Supportive Care

- Discontinue use immediately if bronchoconstriction occurs.
- Remember that excessive use can lead to decreased effectiveness.
- Notify the doctor if headache occurs.

Patient Teaching

- Instruct the patient to perform oral inhalation correctly as follows: Clear nasal passages and throat. Breathe out, expelling as much air from the lungs as possible. Place the mouthpiece well into the mouth as the dose from the inhaler is released, and inhale deeply. Hold breath for several seconds, remove the mouthpiece, and exhale slowly.
- If more than one inhalation is ordered, tell the patient to wait at least 2 minutes before repeating the procedure for a second dose.
- Explain why it is necessary to use the bronchodilator first if other in-

halants such as a steroid inhaler are prescribed. This allows the bronchodilator to open air passages for maximum effectiveness. Tell the patient to allow 5 minutes between the inhalant treatments.
• Tell the patient not to be concerned if pink sputum mimicking hemoptysis occurs after inhalation. This is due to oxidation of drug when diluted with water.
• Tell the patient that excessive use can lead to decreased effectiveness.
• Warn the patient to avoid accidentally spraying the inhalant into the eyes, which may cause temporary blurring of vision.
• Tell the patient to reduce the intake of foods containing caffeine, such as coffee, colas, and chocolates, when taking a bronchodilator.

Evaluation

In the patient receiving isoetharine, appropriate evaluation statements include:
• Patient reports relief from respiratory symptoms.
• Patient does not report headache.
• Patient and family state understanding of isoetharine therapy.

isoniazid (INH)

(eye soe nye´ a zid)

DOW-Isoniazid, Isotamine†, Laniazid, Nydrazid**, PMS-Isoniazid†

• *Classification:* antitubercular (isonicotinic acid hydrazine)
• *Pregnancy Risk Category:* C

HOW SUPPLIED

Tablets: 50 mg, 100 mg, 300 mg
Oral solution: 50 mg/5 ml
Injection: 100 mg/ml

ACTION

Mechanism: Inhibits cell wall biosynthesis by interfering with lipid and DNA synthesis (bactericidal).

Absorption: Completely and rapidly absorbed from the GI tract after oral administration, but food reduces extent of absorption and peak levels. Also absorbed readily after I.M. injection.

Distribution: Widely distributed into body tissues, CSF, and other body fluids, including ascitic, synovial, and pleural; lungs and other organs; and sputum and saliva. Drug crosses the placenta and reaches concentrations in breast milk that are comparable to plasma.

Metabolism: Inactivated primarily in the liver by acetylation. Rate of metabolism varies individually because of genetic makeup; fast acetylators metabolize drug five times faster than slow acetylators. About 50% of blacks and whites are slow acetylators; over 80% of Chinese, Japanese, and Inuits are fast acetylators.

Excretion: About 75% of a dose is excreted in urine as unchanged drug and metabolites in 24 hours; some is excreted in saliva, sputum, feces, and breast milk. Isoniazid is removed by peritoneal dialysis or hemodialysis. Half-life: 1 to 8 hours in adults, depending on metabolic rate.

Onset, peak, duration: Peak serum concentrations occur 1 to 2 hours after ingestion; peak plasma levels in fast acetylators are 50% of those of slow acetylators.

INDICATIONS & DOSAGE

Primary treatment against actively growing tubercle bacilli –

Adults: 5 mg/kg P.O. or I.M. daily single dose, up to 300 mg/day, continued for 6 months to 2 years.

Infants and children: 10 to 20 mg/kg P.O. or I.M. daily single dose, up to 300 to 500 mg/day, continued for 18 months to 2 years. Concomitant administration of at least one other effective antitubercular drug is recommended.

Preventive therapy against tubercle bacilli of those closely exposed or those with positive skin test whose chest X-rays and bacteriologic studies are consistent with nonprogressive tuberculous disease–
Adults: 300 mg P.O. daily single dose, continued for 1 year.
Infants and children: 10 mg/kg P.O. daily single dose, up to 300 mg/day, continued for 1 year.

CONTRAINDICATIONS & PRECAUTIONS

Contraindicated in patients with hypersensitivity to isoniazid and a history of isoniazid-induced hepatic disease or other severe reactions, including arthralgia, fever, chills, or acute hepatic disease. Use cautiously in patients who ingest alcohol daily and in patients with chronic hepatic or renal disease or a history of seizures.

ADVERSE REACTIONS

Common reactions are in italics; life-threatening reactions are in bold italics.
Blood: ***agranulocytosis, hemolytic anemia, aplastic anemia,*** eosinophilia, leukopenia, neutropenia, thrombocytopenia, methemoglobinemia, pyridoxine-responsive hypochromic anemia.
CNS: *peripheral neuropathy* (especially in the malnourished, alcoholics, diabetics, and slow acetylators), usually preceded by paresthesias of hands and feet, psychosis.
GI: nausea, vomiting, epigastric distress, constipation, dryness of the mouth.
Hepatic: ***hepatitis, occasionally severe and sometimes fatal, especially in elderly patients.***
Metabolic: hyperglycemia, metabolic acidosis.
Local: irritation at injection site.
Other: rheumatic syndrome and systemic lupus erythematosus–like syndrome; hypersensitivity (fever, rash, lymphadenopathy, vasculitis).

INTERACTIONS

Aluminum-containing antacids and laxatives: may decrease the rate and amount of isoniazid absorbed. Give isoniazid at least 1 hour before antacid or laxative.
Carbamazepine: increased risk of isoniazid hepatotoxicity. Use together very cautiously.
Corticosteroids: may decrease therapeutic effectiveness. Monitor need for larger isoniazid dose.
Disulfiram: neurologic symptoms, including changes in behavior and coordination, may develop with concomitant isoniazid use. Avoid concomitant use.

EFFECTS ON DIAGNOSTIC TESTS

Liver function studies: elevated results in about 15%; most abnormalities are mild and transient but may persist throughout treatment.
Urine glucose tests with copper sulfate (Benedict's reagent or Clinitest): false-positive results.

NURSING CONSIDERATIONS

Besides those related universally to drug therapy (see "How to use this book"), consider the following specific recommendations:

Assessment
- Obtain a baseline assessment of patient's infection before INH therapy.
- Be alert for adverse reactions and drug interactions throughout therapy.
- Evaluate the patient's and family's knowledge about INH therapy.

Nursing Diagnoses
- High risk for injury related to ineffectiveness of isoniazid to eradicate the infection.
- Sensory/perceptual alterations (tactile) related to isoniazid induced peripheral neuropathy.
- Knowledge deficit related to isoniazid.

*Liquid form contains alcohol.

**May contain tartrazine.

Planning and Implementation
Preparation and Administration
• Obtain specimen for culture and sensitivity testing before administering the first dose.
• ***P.O. use:*** Administer the drug with food if GI irritation occurs.
Monitoring
• Monitor effectiveness by regularly assessing patient for improvement of infection and by evaluating culture and sensitivity tests.
• Monitor patient for parasthesia of hands and feet, which usually precede peripheral neuropathy, especially in patients who are malnourished, alcoholic, or diabetic or who are slow acetylators.
• Monitor hepatic function.
Supportive Care
• Expect to give pyridoxine to prevent peripheral neuropathy, especially in malnourished patients.
Patient Teaching
• Tell patient to take the drug with food if GI irritation occurs.
• Instruct patient to take this drug exactly as prescribed; warn against discontinuing drug without doctor's approval.
• Encourage patient to fully comply with treatment, which may take months or years.
• Tell patient to notify doctor immediately of loss of appetite, fatigue, malaise, jaundice, or dark urine, which may signal liver toxicity.
• Advise patient to avoid alcohol, which may be associated with greater risk of isoniazid-related hepatitis.
• Advise patient to notify the doctor promptly if paresthesia of the hands or feet develop.
Evaluation
In patients receiving isoniazid, appropriate evaluation statements may include:
• Patient is free of infection.
• Patient maintains normal peripheral nervous system function throughout therapy.
• Patient and family state an understanding of isoniazid therapy.

---

isoproterenol
(eye soe proe ter´ e nole)
Aerolone, Dey-Dose Isoproterenol, Dispos-a-Med Isoproterenol, Isuprel, Vapo-Iso

isoproterenol hydrochloride
Isuprel, Isuprel Mistometer, Norisodrine Aerotrol

isoproterenol sulfate
Medihaler-Iso

• *Classification:* bronchodilator, cardiac stimulant (adrenergic)
• *Pregnancy Risk Category:* C

HOW SUPPLIED
isoproterenol
Nebulizer inhaler: 0.25%, 0.5%, and 1%
isoproterenol hydrochloride
Tablets (sublingual): 10 mg, 15 mg
Aerosol inhaler: 120 mcg or 131 mcg/metered spray
Injection: 200 mcg/ml
isoproterenol sulfate
Aerosol inhaler: 80 mcg/metered spray

ACTION
Mechanism: Relaxes bronchial smooth muscle by acting on $beta_2$-adrenergic receptors. As a cardiac stimulant, acts on $beta_1$-adrenergic receptors in the heart.
Absorption: Rapidly absorbed after injection or oral inhalation. After sublingual administration, absorption is variable and often unreliable.
Metabolism: Metabolized in liver, lungs, and other tissues by the enzyme catechol-O-methyltransferase and by conjugate formation in the liver.
Excretion: Primarily in urine as un-

changed drug (40% to 50%) and metabolites.
Onset, peak, duration: Onset of action is prompt after oral inhalation and persists up to 1 hour. Effects persist for a few minutes after I.V. injection, up to 2 hours after S.C. or sublingual administration, and up to 4 hours after rectal administration of sublingual tablet.

INDICATIONS & DOSAGE

Bronchial asthma and reversible bronchospasm–
Adults: 10 to 20 mg (hydrochloride) S.L. q 6 to 8 hours.
Children: 5 to 10 mg (hydrochloride) S.L. q 6 to 8 hours. Not recommended for children under 6 years.
Bronchospasm–
Adults and children: (sulfate) acute dyspneic episodes: 1 inhalation initially. May repeat if needed after 2 to 5 minutes.

Maintenance dosage is 1 to 2 inhalations q.i.d. to 6 times daily. May repeat once more 10 minutes after second dose. Not more than 3 doses should be administered for each attack.
Heart block and ventricular arrhythmias–
Adults: (hydrochloride) initially, 0.02 to 0.06 mg I.V. Subsequent doses 0.01 to 0.2 mg I.V. or 5 mcg/minute I.V.; or 0.2 mg I.M. initially, then 0.02 to 1 mg, p.r.n.
Children: (hydrochloride) may give half of initial adult dose.
Shock–
Adults and children: (hydrochloride) 0.5 to 5 mcg/ minute by continuous I.V. infusion. Usual concentration is 1 mg (5 ml) in 500 ml dextrose 5% in water. Adjust rate according to heart rate, central venous pressure, blood pressure, and urine flow.

CONTRAINDICATIONS & PRECAUTIONS

Contraindicated in patients with preexisting cardiac arrhythmias, especially tachycardia (including tachycardia caused by digitalis toxicity), because of the drug's cardiac stimulant effects; and in those with hypersensitivity to this drug or other sympathomimetics.

Administer cautiously to elderly patients, diabetic patients, those with renal or cardiovascular disease (hypertension, coronary insufficiency, angina, degenerative heart disease), or hyperthyroidism, because drug may worsen these conditions; and to sulfite-sensitive patients, because some formulations contain sulfite preservatives.

ADVERSE REACTIONS

Common reactions are in italics; life-threatening reactions are in bold italics.
CNS: *headache*, mild tremor, weakness, dizziness, nervousness, insomnia.
CV: *palpitations, tachycardia, anginal pain;* blood pressure may rise and then fall.
GI: nausea, vomiting.
Metabolic: hyperglycemia.
Other: sweating, flushing of face, ***bronchial edema*** and inflammation.

INTERACTIONS

Epinephrine: increased risk of arrhythmias.
Propranolol and other beta blockers: blocked bronchodilating effect of isoproterenol. Monitor patient carefully if used together.

EFFECTS ON DIAGNOSTIC TESTS

Spirometry (in the diagnosis of asthma): reduced sensitivity.

NURSING CONSIDERATIONS

Besides those related universally to drug therapy (see "How to use this

book"), consider the following specific recommendations:

Assessment

• Obtain a baseline assessment of the patient's cardiopulmonary status by taking vital signs, noting ECG results, and auscultating the heart and lungs.
• Be alert for adverse reactions or drug interactions during therapy.
• Evaluate the patient and family's knowledge about isoproterenol therapy.

Nursing Diagnoses

• Ineffective airway clearance related to patient's underlying respiratory condition.
• Pain related to isoproterenol-induced adverse reactions.
• Knowledge deficit related to isoproterenol therapy.

Planning and Implementation

Preparation and Administration

• Replace volume deficit before administering vasopressors. Isoproterenol is not a substitute for blood or fluid replacement.
• ***P.O. use:*** Oral and sublingual tablets are poorly and erratically absorbed.
• ***Inhalation:*** Be sure that when isoproterenol inhalant is ordered with oxygen that the oxygen concentration will not suppress the respiratory drive. If more than one inhalation is ordered, 2 minutes should elapse between inhalations. If more than one type of inhalant is ordered, always administer bronchodilator first and wait 5 minutes before administering the other. Discard inhalation solution if it is discolored or contains precipitate.
• ***I.V. use:*** Use a continuous infusion pump to regulate infusion flow rate. Be aware that it is advisable to decrease the infusion rate or temporarily stop the infusion if the heart rate exceeds 110 beats per minute. Doses sufficient to increase heart rate to more than 130 beats per minute may induce ventricular arrhythmias.
• Avoid giving at bedtime, if possible. This drug can interrupt sleep patterns.

Monitoring

• Monitor effectiveness by regularly auscultating lungs and heart, noting vital signs, and evaluating laboratory studies such as arterial blood gas (ABG) measurements. Drug may cause a slight rise in systolic blood pressure and a slight to marked drop in diastolic blood pressure.
• Closely monitor blood pressure, central venous pressure, ECG, ABG measurements, and urine output when administering this drug for treatment of shock. Expect to adjust infusion rate carefully according to these measurements.

Supportive Care

• Notify doctor if adverse reactions occur. Dosage adjustment or discontinuation of drug may be required.
• Stop drug immediately if precordial distress or anginal pain occurs.
• Keep in mind that this drug may aggravate ventilation and perfusion abnormalities; even while ease of breathing is improved, arterial oxygen tension may fall paradoxically.

Patient Teaching

• Teach patient how to take sublingual tablets properly. Tell him to hold tablet under tongue until it dissolves and is absorbed and not to swallow saliva until that time. Prolonged use of sublingual tablets can cause tooth decay. Instruct patient to rinse mouth with water between doses. This will also help prevent dryness of oropharynx.
• Tell patient to discontinue the drug if it increases chest tightness or dyspnea.
• Warn against overuse of drug. Tell the patient that tolerance can develop.
• Warn patient using oral inhalant that this drug may turn sputum and saliva pink.
• Instruct the patient to perform oral inhalation correctly as follows: Clear

nasal passages and throat. Breathe out, expelling as much air from the lungs as possible. Place the mouthpiece well into the mouth as the dose from the inhaler is released, and inhale deeply. Hold breath for several seconds, remove the mouthpiece, and exhale slowly. Keep in mind that instructions for a metered-dose inhaler are the same, except that deep inhalation is not necessary.
• If more than one inhalation is ordered, tell the patient to wait at least 2 minutes before repeating the procedure for a second dose.
• Explain why it is necessary to use the bronchodilator first if other inhalants such as a steroid inhaler are prescribed. Tell the patient that this allows the bronchodilator to open air passages for maximum effectiveness. Tell the patient to allow 5 minutes between the inhalant treatments.
• Warn the patient to avoid accidentally spraying the inhalant into the eyes, which may cause temporary blurring of vision.
• Tell the patient to reduce the intake of foods containing caffeine, such as coffee, colas, and chocolates, when taking a bronchodilator.
• Warn the patient to contact the doctor immediately if he experiences a "fluttering" of the heart, rapid beating of the heart, shortness of breath, or chest pain.
• Tell the patient not to self-medicate with any OTC drugs without medical approval while taking this drug.
• Warn the patient against increasing the dosage or frequency of administration. Advise the patient to notify the doctor if prescribed dosage does not relieve symptoms.
• Show the patient how to check the pulse. Instruct the patient to check his pulse before and after using a bronchodilator and to call the doctor if the pulse increases more than 20 to 30 beats per minute.

Evaluation
In patients receiving isoproterenol, appropriate evaluation statements may include:
• Patient's does not experience respiratory symptoms.
• Patient does not experience isoproterenol-induced headache or anginal pain.
• Patient and family state an understanding of isoproterenol therapy.

isosorbide dinitrate
(eye soe sor´ bide)
Apo-ISDN†, Cedocard-SR†, Coronex†, Dilatrate-SR, Iso-Bid, Isonate, Isorbid, Isordil, Isotrate, Nitro-Spray‡, Novosorbide†, Sorbitrate, Sorbitrate SA

• *Classification:* antiglaucoma agent (osmotic diuretic)
• *Pregnancy Risk Category:* C

HOW SUPPLIED
Tablets: 5 mg, 10 mg, 20 mg, 30 mg, 40 mg
Tablets (chewable): 5 mg, 10 mg
Tablets (sublingual): 2.5 mg, 5 mg, 10 mg
Tablets (sustained-release): 40 mg
Capsules: 40 mg
Capsules (sustained-release): 40 mg
Topical spray: 10% w/w‡, 12.5 mg/metered spray‡

ACTION
Mechanism: Reduces cardiac oxygen demand by decreasing left ventricular end-diastolic pressure (preload) and, to a lesser extent, systemic vascular resistance (afterload). Also increases blood flow through the collateral coronary vessels.
Absorption: Well absorbed from the GI tract but undergoes first-pass metabolism, resulting in bioavailability of about 50% (depending on dosage form used). Sublingual administra-

tion bypasses the portal circulation; and allows lower dosage and faster onset of action.
Distribution: Widely distributed throughout the body. Limited information is available on drug's plasma protein binding.
Metabolism: In the liver to active metabolites.
Excretion: About 80% to 100% of absorbed dose is excreted in the urine within 24 hours. Metabolites are excreted. Half-life: Elimination half-life of the parent compound is about 45 minutes. Active metabolites are cleared slowly, with half-lives of 2 to 5 hours.
Onset, peak, duration: With sublingual and chewable forms, onset of action is 3 minutes; with other oral forms, 30 minutes; with extended-release form, 1 hour. Duration of effect of oral preparation is longer than of sublingual preparations. With sublingual and chewable forms, duration of effect is 30 minutes to 2 hours; with other oral forms, 5 to 6 hours.

INDICATIONS & DOSAGE

Treatment of acute anginal attacks (sublingual and chewable tablets only); prophylaxis in situations likely to cause anginal attacks; treatment of chronic ischemic heart disease (by preload reduction)–
Adults: *Sublingual form*–2.5 to 10 mg under the tongue for prompt relief of anginal pain, repeated q 5 to 10 minutes (maximum of three doses per 30-minute period). For prophylaxis, 2.5 to 10 mg under the tongue q 2 to 3 hours.
Chewable form–5 to 10 mg, p.r.n., for acute attack or q 2 to 3 hours for prophylaxis but only after initial test dose of 5 mg to determine risk of severe hypotension.
Oral form–5 to 30 mg P.O. q.i.d. for prophylaxis only (use smallest effective dose); sustained-release forms 40 mg P.O. q 6 to 12 hours.
Topical form (where available)–initially, 2 sprays to the chest in the morning from a distance of about 20 cm. Rub solution in. Dosage is gradually increased as needed to 2 to 5 sprays, daily or b.i.d. (in the morning and h.s.).
Adjunct with other vasodilators, such as hydralazine and prazosin, in treatment of severe chronic CHF–
Adults: *Oral or chewable form*–20 to 40 mg q 4 hours.

CONTRAINDICATIONS & PRECAUTIONS

Contraindicated in patients with a history of hypersensitivity or idiosyncratic reaction to nitrates; and in patients with severe anemia, because nitrate ions readily oxidize hemoglobin to methemoglobin.

Use cautiously in patients with increased intracranial pressure or recent head trauma because the drug dilates meningeal vessels; open- or closed-angle glaucoma, although intraocular pressure is increased only briefly and aqueous humor drainage from the eye is impeded; diuretic-induced fluid depletion or low systolic blood pressure (below 90 mm Hg) because of the drug's hypotensive effect; and during the initial days after acute MI because the drug may cause excessive hypotension and tachycardia.

Use of extended-release preparations in patients with malabsorption syndromes or GI hypermotility is not recommended. Lack of response to three or more S.L. tablets may indicate acute M.I.; this situation mandates immediate medical attention.

ADVERSE REACTIONS

Common reactions are in italics; life-threatening reactions are in bold italics.
CNS: *headache, sometimes with throbbing; dizziness;* weakness.
CV: *orthostatic hypotension, tachy-*

cardia, palpitations, ankle edema, fainting.
GI: nausea, vomiting.
Skin: cutaneous vasodilation, *flushing.*
Local: sublingual burning.
Other: hypersensitivity reactions.

INTERACTIONS

Antihypertensives: possibly increased hypotensive effects. Monitor closely during initial therapy.

EFFECTS ON DIAGNOSTIC TESTS

Serum cholesterol (Zlatkis-Zak color reaction): falsely decreased value.

NURSING CONSIDERATIONS

Besides those related universally to drug therapy (see "How to use this book"), consider the following specific recommendations:

Assessment

- Obtain a baseline assessment of the patient's anginal state before therapy.
- Be alert for adverse reactions and drug interactions throughout therapy.
- Evaluate the patient's and family's knowledge about isosorbide therapy.

Nursing Diagnoses

- Pain related to ineffectiveness of isosorbide therapy.
- High risk for injury related to isosorbide-induced dizziness or orthostatic hypotension.
- Knowledge deficit related to isosorbide therapy.

Planning and Implementation

Preparation and Administration

- ***Sublingual use:*** Administer at first sign of attack. Have patient wet the tablet with saliva, place it under his tongue until completely absorbed, and sit down and rest. Dose may be repeated every 10 to 15 minutes for a maximum of three doses.
- ***P.O. use:*** Administer oral tablet on empty stomach, either 30 minutes before or 1 to 2 hours after meals, and have patient swallow oral tablets whole. Have patient chew chewable tablets thoroughly before swallowing.
- Provide additional dose at bedtime if nocturnal angina occurs or before anticipated stress as ordered.
- Do not discontinue drug abruptly as coronary vasospasm may occur.
- Store drug in cool place, in a tightly closed container, away from light.

Monitoring

- Monitor effectiveness by regularly evaluating the severity and frequency of the patient's anginal pain.
- Monitor patient's heart rate and rhythm regularly.
- Monitor blood pressure and intensity and duration of response to drug.

Supportive Care

- Consult the doctor if the patient does not experience pain relief.
- Obtain an order for a mild analgesic if headache occurs. Be aware that dosage may need to be reduced temporarily but tolerance usually develops.
- To minimize orthostatic hypotension, have patient change to upright position slowly, go up and down stairs carefully, and lie down at the first sign of dizziness.
- Maintain safety precautions if dizziness occurs; assist the patient with daily activities to minimize energy expenditure.
- Obtain an order for an antiemetic agent as needed.

Patient Teaching

- Teach patient how to take drug form prescribed. Stress importance of taking the drug exactly as prescribed and to keep it easily accessible at all times.
- Tell patient to take additional dose before anticipated stress or at bedtime if angina is nocturnal.
- Teach patient to take sublingual tablet at first sign of attack and to sit down and rest. Dose may be repeated every 10 to 15 minutes for a maximum of three doses. If no relief, pa-

tient should call doctor or go to hospital emergency room. If patient complains of tingling sensation with drug placed sublingually, tell him he may try holding tablet in buccal pouch.
• Warn patient that discontinuing drug abruptly may cause coronary vasospasm.
• Tell the patient to schedule activities to allow adequate rest.
• Reassure patient that if headache occurs it is usually temporary and to take a mild analgesic until tolerance occurs. However, if headache is severe, tell patient to notify doctor as dosage may need to be reduced temporarily until tolerance occurs.
• Advise patient to avoid alcoholic beverages; may produce increased hypotension.
• Tell patient how to minimize effects of orthostatic hypotension.
• Instruct patient to store drug in cool place, in a tightly closed container, away from light. To ensure freshness, tell patient to replace supply every 3 months.

Evaluation

In patients receiving isosorbide, appropriate evaluation statements may include:
• Patient states anginal pain relief occurs with isosorbide therapy.
• Patient does not experience injury as a result of dizziness or orthostatic hypotension caused by isosorbide therapy.
• Patient and family state an understanding of isosorbide therapy.

isotretinoin

(eye soe tret´ i noyn)
Accutane, Roaccutane‡

• *Classification:* antiacne agent, keratinization stabilizer (retinoic acid derivative)
• *Pregnancy Risk Category:* X

HOW SUPPLIED

Capsules: 10 mg, 20 mg, 40 mg

ACTION

Mechanism: Normalizes keratinization, reversibly decreases the size of sebaceous glands, and alters the composition of sebum to a less viscous form that's less likely to cause follicular plugging.
Absorption: Rapidly absorbed after oral administration.
Distribution: Widely distributed. In animals, found in most organs and known to cross the placenta. In humans, degree of placental transfer and degree of secretion in breast milk are unknown. Isotretinoin is 99.9% protein-bound, primarily to albumin.
Metabolism: In the liver and possibly the gut wall. The major metabolite is 4-oxo-isotretinoin, with tretinoin and 4-oxo-tretinoin also found in the blood and urine.
Excretion: Not fully understood, but renal and biliary pathways are known to be used.
Onset, peak, duration: Peak concentrations occur in 3 hours; peak concentrations of the metabolite 4-oxo-isotretinoin occur in 6 to 12 hours.

INDICATIONS & DOSAGE

Severe cystic acne unresponsive to conventional therapy–
Adults and adolescents: 0.5 to 2 mg/kg P.O. daily given in two divided doses and continued for 15 to 20 weeks.

CONTRAINDICATIONS & PRECAUTIONS

Contraindicated in patients with sensitivity to isotretinoin, vitamin A, or other retinoids, and in those with sensitivity to parabens, which are used as preservatives in this drug. Do not use in pregnant women because of possible teratogenic effects, including hydrocephalus and microcephaly. Start therapy only after confirmation that patient is not pregnant and appropriate contraceptive measures have been instituted. Frequent check of blood chemistry during therapy is also recommended.

ADVERSE REACTIONS

Common reactions are in italics; life-threatening reactions are in bold italics.
Blood: anemia, elevated platelet count.
CNS: headache, fatigue, ***pseudotumor cerebri*** (benign intracranial hypertension).
EENT: *conjunctivitis,* corneal deposits, dry eyes.
Endocrine: hyperglycemia.
GI: nonspecific GI symptoms, gum bleeding and inflammation.
Hepatic: elevated AST (SGOT), ALT (SPGT), and alkaline phosphatase.
Skin: *cheilosis, rash, dry skin,* peeling of palms and toes, skin infection, photosensitivity.
Other: *hypertriglyceridemia, musculoskeletal pain (skeletal hyperostosis),* thinning of hair.

INTERACTIONS

Abrasives, medicated soaps and cleansers, acne preparations containing peeling agents, topical alcohol preparations (including cosmetics, after-shave, cologne): cumulative irritation of skin or excessive drying of skin. Use together cautiously.
Alcohol: increased risk of hypertriglyceridemia
Tetracyclines: increased risk of pseudotumor cerebri.
Vitamin A and vitamin supplements containing vitamin A: increase in isotretinoin's toxic effects. Don't use together without doctor's permission.

EFFECTS ON DIAGNOSTIC TESTS

Erythrocyte sedimentation rate: elevations.
Liver function tests, blood counts, and blood glucose, uric acid, cholesterol, and triglyceride levels: altered results due to physiologic effects of the drug.

NURSING CONSIDERATIONS

Besides those related universally to drug therapy (see "How to use this book"), consider the following specific recommendations:

Assessment

- Obtain a baseline assessment of the patient's skin condition before therapy.
- Be alert for adverse reactions and drug interactions throughout therapy.
- Evaluate the patient's and family's knowledge about isotretinoin therapy.

Nursing Diagnoses

- Impaired skin integrity related to underlying condition.
- Impaired tissue integrity related to adverse effects of the drug.
- Knowledge deficit related to isotretinoin therapy.

Planning and Implementation

Preparation and Administration

- Affirm that female patient has a negative pregnancy test within 2 weeks before initiating therapy. If patient is not pregnant, begin drug therapy on the second or third day of the next menstrual cycle.
- Perform lipid and liver function tests before initiating therapy.
- Check the patient for hypersensitivity to parabens.
- Begin second course of therapy, if needed, at least 8 weeks after completion of the first course.
- Administer the drug with meals or shortly thereafter to enhance absorption.

Monitoring

- Monitor effectiveness by evaluating the severity of the underlying disorder and the condition of the skin.
- Assess the patient for photosensitivity.
- Screen the patient with headache,

nausea, and vomiting for papilledema.
• Evaluate blood glucose levels regularly.
• Monitor CPK levels in patients who undergo vigorous physical activity.
• Check for corneal abrasions in a patient wearing contact lenses who complains of eye pain.
• Monitor for dose-related adverse reactions.
• Continue to monitor lipid studies and liver function tests at regular intervals until response to drug is established, usually about 4 weeks.

Supportive Care

• Notify the doctor if signs of pseudotumor cerebri develop. These signs usually indicate immediate discontinuance of therapy and prompt neurologic intervention.
• Keep in mind that a second course of therapy should not be started until at least 8 weeks after completion of the first course because improvement may continue after withdrawal of the drug.

Patient Teaching

• Tell the patient to take the drug with or shortly after meals to enhance absorption.
• Explain the need for follow-up laboratory studies.
• Instruct the patient to notify the doctor immediately is headache, nausea, and vomiting develop.
• Instruct the patient to immediately report any visual disturbances and bone or skeletal pain.
• Warn patients that contact lenses may feel uncomfortable during isotretinoin therapy.
• Explain that many adverse reactions are dose-related and are generally reversible if dosage is reduced or therapy is discontinued.
• Tell patient to refrain from donating blood for at least 30 days after therapy has been discontinued.

Evaluation

In patients receiving isotretinoin, appropriate evaluation statements may include:
• Patient reports a decrease in the severity of the underlying disorder and improved skin condition.
• Patient is free of conjunctivitis, corneal deposits, and dry eyes.
• Patient and family state an understanding of isotretinoin therapy.

---

isoxsuprine hydrochloride

(eye sox´ syoo preen)
Duvadilan‡, Vasodilan, Vasoprine

• *Classification:* peripheral vasodilator (beta-adrenergic agonist)
• *Pregnancy Risk Category:* C

HOW SUPPLIED

Tablets: 10 mg, 20 mg

ACTION

Mechanism: Stimulates beta receptors and may also be a direct-acting peripheral vasodilator.
Absorption: Almost completely absorbed from the GI tract.
Distribution: Widely distributed; drug crosses the placenta.
Metabolism: Partially metabolized in the liver.
Excretion: Primarily in urine; fecal excretion is insignificant. Half-life: About 1¼ hours.
Onset, peak, duration: After oral administration, action begins in 1 hour; effects persist for about 3 hours.

INDICATIONS & DOSAGE

Adjunct for relief of symptoms associated with cerebrovascular insufficiency, peripheral vascular diseases (such as arteriosclerosis obliterans, thromboangiitis obliterans, Raynaud's disease) –
Adults: 10 to 20 mg P.O. t.i.d. or q.i.d.

CONTRAINDICATIONS & PRECAUTIONS

Contraindicated in patients immediately postpartum and in the presence of arterial bleeding because of its uterine vasodilating relaxant effects. Also contraindicated for I.V. use because it increases the risk of adverse reactions; parenteral administration is not recommended for patients with hypotension or tachycardia because the drug may exacerbate these symptoms. Because efficacy in the treatment of peripheral vascular disease has not been established, do not use drug as a substitute for appropriate medical or surgical therapy for peripheral or cerebrovascular disease.

ADVERSE REACTIONS

Common reactions are in italics; life-threatening reactions are in bold italics.
CV: tachycardia, hypotension.
GI: vomiting, abdominal distress, intestinal distention.
Skin: severe rash.

INTERACTIONS

None significant.

EFFECTS ON DIAGNOSTIC TESTS

Blood glucose and free fatty acids: altered serum concentrations.

NURSING CONSIDERATIONS

Besides those related universally to drug therapy (see "How to use this book"), consider the following specific recommendations:

Assessment
- Obtain a baseline assessment of the patient's underlying condition before therapy.
- Be alert for adverse reactions and drug interactions throughout therapy.
- Evaluate the patient's and family's knowledge about isoxsuprine therapy.

Nursing Diagnoses
- Altered tissue perfusion (cerebral, peripheral areas) related to the patient's underlying condition.
- Impaired skin integrity related to adverse reactions.
- Knowledge deficit related to isoxsuprine therapy.

Planning and Implementation

Preparation and Administration
- Drug has been used to inhibit contractions in premature labor, although safe use in pregnancy and breast-feeding has not been established. It has also been used to minimize cramping in patients with severe primary dysmenorrhea.
- Discontinue if a rash develops.

Monitoring
- Observe the patient's skin for the development of a rash.
- Monitor the patient's blood pressure and heart rate and rhythm.

Supportive Care
- Withhold dose and notify the doctor immediately of any changes in patient's health status occur.
- Obtain an order for a mild analgesic if patient experiences a rash.

Patient Teaching
- Teach the patient to notify the doctor if he develops a rash.
- Instruct the patient to avoid sudden position changes to minimize the risk of orthostasis.
- Advise the patient to have blood pressure checked regularly and to promptly report signs and symptoms of hypotension.

Evaluation

In patients receiving isoxspurine, appropriate evaluation statements may include:
- Patient maintains tissue perfusion and cellular oxygenation.
- Patient does not develop a rash.
- Patient and family state an understanding of isoxsuprine therapy.

isradipine

(is ra´ di peen)
DynaCirc

• *Classification:* antihypertensive (calcium channel blocker)
• *Pregnancy Risk Category:* C

HOW SUPPLIED

Capsules: 2.5 mg, 5 mg

ACTION

Mechanism: A calcium channel blocking agent that inhibits calcium ion influx across cardiac and smooth muscle cells, thus decreasing arteriolar resistance and reducing blood pressure.
Absorption: 90% to 95% of oral dose is absorbed and is subject to extensive first-pass metabolism resulting in a bioavailability of about 15% to 24%. Administering with food delays absorption but does not affect total amount absorbed.
Distribution: 95% is bound to plasma protein.
Metabolism: Completely metabolized by the liver.
Excretion: About 60% to 65% of an administered dose is excreted in the urine and 25% to 30% in the feces. Half-life: Biphasic elimination with an early half-life of 1½ to 2 hours, and a terminal half-life of about 8 hours.
Onset, peak, duration: Detectable in plasma within 20 minutes, and peak concentrations occur about 1½ hours after drug administration.

INDICATIONS & DOSAGE

Essential hypertension–
Adults: initially, 2.5 mg P.O. b.i.d given alone or with a thiazide diuretic. Adjust dosage based on tolerance and response to a maximum of 20 mg daily.

CONTRAINDICATIONS & PRECAUTIONS

Contraindicated in patients allergic to the drug. Use cautiously in patients with CHF especially when given with a beta-adrenergic blocking agent.

ADVERSE REACTIONS

Common reactions are in italics; life-threatening reactions are in bold italics.
CNS: dizziness.
CV: edema, flushing, palpitations, tachycardia.
GI: nausea, diarrhea.
GU: pollakiuria.
Skin: rash.
Other: dyspnea.

INTERACTIONS

Fentanyl anesthesia: severe hypotension has been reported with concomitant use of a beta blocker and a calcium channel blocker. Be sure to inform anesthesiologist that the patient is taking a calcium channel blocker.

EFFECTS ON DIAGNOSTIC TESTS

None reported.

NURSING CONSIDERATIONS

Besides those related universally to drug therapy (see "How to use this book"), consider the following specific recommendations:
Assessment
• Obtain a baseline assessment of the patient's blood pressure before beginning therapy.
• Be alert for adverse reactions and drug interactions throughout therapy.
• Evaluate the patient's and family's knowledge about isradipine therapy.
Nursing Diagnoses
• Altered tissue perfusion (renal, cerebral, cardiopulmonary, and peripheral) related to the patient's underlying condition.
• High risk for injury related to isradipine-induced hypotension and adverse CNS reactions.

• Knowledge deficit related to isradipine therapy.

Planning and Implementation

Preparation and Administration

• Remember that dosage is increased by gradual titration. If response is inadequate after the first 2 to 4 weeks, the doctor increases the dosage to 5 mg b.i.d. The dosage may continue to be increased at intervals of 5 mg/day every 2 to 4 weeks to a maximum of 10 mg daily (5 mg b.i.d.). Most patients show no additional response at dosages over 10 mg daily (5 mg b.i.d.).

• Keep in mind that the bioavailability of isradipine is increased in elderly patients and those with impaired hepatic function but the starting doage should still be 2.5 mg b.i.d..

Monitoring

• Monitor effectiveness by regularly checking blood pressure, pulse, and ECG. Initial therapy produces an antihypertensive effect in 2 to 3 hours; however, maximal response usually develops after 2 to 4 weeks of continuous therapy.

• Monitor urine output. Isradipine has diuretic activity.

• Monitor patient's blood pressure in both the supine and standing positions during dosage adjustment to check for orthostatic hypotension. Remember that symptomatic hypotension may occur with this drug, but most adverse reactions are mild and transient.

• Monitor for adverse CNS reactions, such as dizziness and weakness. Syncope and severe dizziness have not been reported with use of this drug.

Supportive Care

• If the patient experiences dizziness, weakness, or hypotension, institute safety precautions, including continuous use of side rails.

Patient Teaching

• Tell the patient that he may notice an increased need to void because of this drug's diuretic effect.

• Explain that most adverse reactions are mild and transient and usually cause symptoms related to vasodilation, such as dizziness, edema, flushing, palpitations, and tachycardia.

• Teach patient and family member how to take blood pressure measurements. Stress the importance of monitoring blood pressure at least once weekly during antihypertensive treatment.

• Tell the patient to report significant changes in blood pressure to the doctor.

Evaluation

In patients receiving isradipine, appropriate evaluation statements may include:

• Patient's blood pressure is controlled within normal limits.

• Patient does not experience injury, hypotension, and adverse CNS reactions.

• Patient and family state an understanding of isradipine therapy.

kanamycin sulfate

(kan a mye´ sin)

Kanasig‡, Kantrex, Klebcil

• *Classification:* antibiotic (aminoglycoside)

• *Pregnancy Risk Category:* D

HOW SUPPLIED

Capsules: 500 mg

Injection: 37.5 mg/ml (pediatric), 250 mg/ml, 333 mg/ml

ACTION

Mechanism: Inhibits protein synthesis by binding directly to the 30S ribosomal subunit. Generally bactericidal.

Absorption: Poorly absorbed after oral administration (only about 1% of a dose in normal patients). Oral absorption is enhanced in patients with impaired GI motility or mucosal ulcerations. Drug is usually given par-

enterally, but may be administered orally for bowel sterilization.
Distribution: Widely distributed after parenteral administration; intraocular penetration is poor; CSF penetration is low, even in patients with inflamed meninges. Intraventricular administration produces high concentrations throughout the CNS. Protein binding is minimal. Kanamycin crosses the placenta.
Metabolism: Not metabolized.
Excretion: Orally administered drug is primarily excreted in the feces. Kanamycin that reaches the bloodstream is excreted primarily in urine by glomerular filtration. Small amounts may be excreted in bile and breast milk. Half-life: 2 to 4 hours in adults; in severe renal damage, up to 80 hours.
Onset, peak, duration: Peak serum concentrations occur 60 minutes after I.M. administration and immediately after completion of I.V. infusion.

INDICATIONS & DOSAGE

Serious infections caused by sensitive Escherichia coli, Proteus, Enterobacter aerogenes, Klebsiella pneumoniae, Serratia marcescens, Acinetobacter–
Adults and children with normal renal function: 15 mg/kg daily divided q 8 to 12 hours deep I.M. into upper outer quadrant of buttocks or I.V. infusion (diluted 500 mg/200 ml of normal saline solution or dextrose 5% in water infused at 60 to 80 drops/minute). Maximum daily dosage is 1.5 g.
Neonates: 15 mg/kg daily I.M. or I.V. divided q 12 hours.
Adjunctive treatment in hepatic coma–
Adults: 8 to 12 g daily P.O. in divided doses.
Preoperative bowel sterilization–
Adults: 1 g P.O. q 1 hour for 4 doses, then q 4 hours for 4 doses; or 1 g P.O. q 1 hour for 4 doses, then q 6 hours for 36 to 72 hours.
Intraperitoneal irrigation–
500 mg in 20 ml sterile distilled water instilled via catheter into wound after patient is fully recovered from anesthesia and neuromuscular blocking agent effects.
Wound irrigation–
Up to 2.5 mg/ml in normal saline solution irrigant.

CONTRAINDICATIONS & PRECAUTIONS

Contraindicated in patients with hypersensitivity to kanamycin or any aminoglycoside and, when given orally, in patients with intestinal obstruction. Use cautiously in patients with intestinal mucosal ulcerations because of increased potential for pseudomembranous colitis; in patients with decreased renal function, tinnitus, vertigo, and high-frequency hearing loss who are susceptible to ototoxicity; in those with dehydration, myasthenia gravis, parkinsonism, and hypocalcemia because the drug can exacerbate these symptoms or illnesses; and in neonates, infants, and elderly patients.

ADVERSE REACTIONS

Common reactions are in italics; life-threatening reactions are in bold italics.
CNS: headache, lethargy, ***neuromuscular blockade.***
EENT: *ototoxicity (tinnitus, vertigo, hearing loss).*
GU: *nephrotoxicity (cells or casts in the urine, oliguria, proteinuria, decreased creatinine clearance, increased BUN and serum creatinine levels).*
Other: ***hypersensitivity reactions.***

INTERACTIONS

Cephalothin: increases nephrotoxicity. Use together cautiously.
Dimenhydrinate: may mask symptoms of ototoxicity. Use with caution.

General anesthetics, neuromuscular blocking agents: may potentiate neuromuscular blockade.
I.V. loop diuretics (e.g., furosemide): increase ototoxicity. Use cautiously.
Other aminoglycosides, amphotericin B, cisplatin, methoxyflurane: increases nephrotoxicity. Don't use together.
Parenteral penicillins (e.g., carbenicillin, ticarcillin): kanamycin inactivation in vitro. Don't combine in I.V.

EFFECTS ON DIAGNOSTIC TESTS

Renal function tests: elevated BUN, nonprotein nitrogen, or serum creatinine levels and increased excretion of casts.

NURSING CONSIDERATIONS

Besides those related universally to drug therapy (see "How to use this book"), consider the following specific recommendations:

Assessment

• Obtain a baseline assessment of infection before therapy.
• Be alert for adverse reactions and drug interactions throughout therapy.
• Evaluate the patient's and family's knowledge about kanamycin therapy.

Nursing Diagnoses

• High risk for injury related to ineffectiveness of kanamycin to eradicate the infection.
• Altered urinary elimination related to kanamycin-induced nephrotoxicity.
• Knowledge deficit related to kanamycin therapy.

Planning and Implementation

Preparation and Administration

• Obtain specimen for culture and sensitivity tests before first dose. Therapy may begin pending test results.
• Weigh patient and obtain baseline renal function studies before therapy.
• ***I.M. use:*** Administer deep I.M. into upper outer quadrant of buttocks.
• ***I.V. use:*** Dilute 500 mg of the drug per 200 ml of normal saline solution or dextrose 5% in water and infuse at 60 to 80 drops/minute.

Monitoring

• Monitor effectiveness by regularly assessing for improvement of infection.
• Monitor serum kanamycin level. Peak blood levels > 30 mcg/ml and trough levels > 10 mcg/ml may be associated with increased incidence of toxicity.
• Monitor renal function (intake and output, specific gravity, urinalysis, BUN, creatinine, and creatinine clearance).

Supportive Care

• Be aware that if no response occurs in 3 to 5 days, drug may be stopped and new specimens obtained for culture and sensitivity.
• Notify doctor if patient develops signs of decreased renal function, tinnitus, vertigo, or hearing loss.
• Encourage patient to consume 2,000 ml of fluid daily during drug therapy (if not contraindicated) to minimize chemical irritation of the renal tubules.

Patient Teaching

• Tell patient to drink 2,000 ml of fluid each day, not including coffee, tea, or other caffeinated beverages.
• Instruct the patient to notify the doctor immediately if changes in hearing or urinary elmination patterns occur.
• Tell the patient to call the doctor if infection worsens or does not improve.
• Stress the importance of recommended blood tests to monitor kanamycin level and renal function, to determine the effectiveness of therapy, and to detect adverse drug reactions.
• Teach patient to watch for and promptly report the signs and symptoms of superinfection (continued fever and other signs of new infection, especially of upper respiratory tract).

Evaluation

In patients receiving kanamycin, ap-

propriate evaluation statements may include:
• Patient is free of infection.
• Patient's renal function studies remain normal throughout therapy.
• Patient and family state an understanding of kanamycin therapy.

kaolin and pectin mixtures

(kay´ o lin/pek´ tin)
Donnagel-MB*†, Kao-Con†, Kaopectate◇, Kaopectate Concentrate◇, Kao-tin◇, Kapectolin◇, K-P◇, K-Pek◇

• *Classification:* antidiarrheal (adsorbent)
• *Pregnancy Risk Category:* C

HOW SUPPLIED

Oral suspension: 5.2 mg kaolin and 260 mg pectin per 30 ml◇ (K-P◇); 5.85 g kaolin and 130 mg pectin per 30 ml◇ (Kaopectate◇, Kao-tin◇, Kapectolin◇, K-Pek◇); 5.91 g kaolin and 132 mg pectin per 30 ml◇ (Kaopectate◇), 6 g kaolin and 130 mg pectin per 30 ml◇ (Kaopectate†◇); 6 g kaolin and 143 mg pectin per 30 ml◇, with 3.8% alcohol (Donnagel-MB*†); 8.7 g kaolin and 195 mg pectin per 30 ml◇ (Kaopectate Concentrate◇); 8.8 g kaolin and 195 mg pectin per 30 ml◇ (Kaopectate Concentrate†◇, Kao-Con†)

ACTION

Mechanism: Adsorbents and protectants that decrease the stool's fluid content, although *total* water loss seems to remain the same.
Absorption: None.
Distribution: None.
Metabolism: None.
Excretion: In feces.

INDICATIONS & DOSAGE

Mild, nonspecific diarrhea –
Adults: 60 to 120 ml P.O. after each bowel movement.
Children over 12 years: 60 ml P.O. after each bowel movement.
Children 6 to 12 years: 30 to 60 ml P.O. after each bowel movement.
Children 3 to 6 years: 15 to 30 ml P.O. after each bowel movement.

CONTRAINDICATIONS & PRECAUTIONS

Contraindicated in patients with bowel obstruction because it may exacerbate this condition. Do not administer continuously for more than 48 hours.

ADVERSE REACTIONS

Common reactions are in italics; life-threatening reactions are in bold italics.
GI: drug absorbs nutrients, drugs, and enzymes; fecal impaction or ulceration in infants and elderly or debilitated patients after chronic use; constipation.

INTERACTIONS

None significant.

EFFECTS ON DIAGNOSTIC TESTS

None reported.

NURSING CONSIDERATIONS

Besides those related universally to drug therapy (see "How to use this book"), consider the following specific recommendations:
Assessment
• Obtain a baseline assessment of history of bowel disorders, GI status, and frequency of loose stools before therapy.
• Be alert for adverse reactions and drug interactions throughout therapy.
• Evaluate the patient's and family's knowledge about kaolin and pectin mixtures therapy.

Nursing Diagnoses
• Diarrhea related to interruption in normal pattern of elimination characterized by frequent loose stools.
• Colonic constipation related to chronic use of kaolin and pectin mixtures.
• Knowledge deficit related to therapy with kaolin and pectin mixture.

Planning and Implementation
Preparation and Administration
• Read label carefully. Check dosage and strength.
• ***P.O. use:*** Administer dose after each loose bowel movement.
• Do not use in place of specific therapy for underlying cause of diarrhea.
Monitoring
• Monitor effectiveness by monitoring the frequency and characteristics of stools.
• Auscultate bowel sounds at least once a shift. Assess for pain and cramping.
• Monitor fluid and electrolyte balance.
• Weigh patient daily until diarrhea is controlled to detect fluid loss or retention.
• Check skin in perianal area to detect and prevent breakdown.
Supportive Care
• Make sure that the patient is well hydrated. Correct fluid and electrolyte disturbances.
• Provide good skin care, especially in the perianal area. Use soothing lotion and powder.
• Consult with dietitian to modify diet to help control diarrhea.
• Do not give to patients with suspected obstructive bowel lesions.
• Be aware that drug is a GI absorbent and may reduce absorption of other P.O. drugs, requiring dosage adjustments.
Patient Teaching
• Instruct the patient not to use kaolin and pectin mixtures for more than 2 days.
• Encourage proper storage to keep the drug out of children's hands.

Evaluation
In patients receiving kaolin and pectin mixtures, appropriate evaluation statements may include:
• Patient reports decrease or absence of loose stools.
• Patient remains free from signs and symptoms of colonic constipation.
• Patient and family state an understanding of therapy with kaolin and pectin mixtures.

ketamine hydrochloride
(keet´ a meen)
Ketalar

• *Classification:* intravenous anesthetic (dissociative anesthetic)
• *Pregnancy Risk Category:* C

HOW SUPPLIED
Injection: 10 mg/ml, 50 mg/ml, 100 mg/ml

ACTION
Mechanism: Interrupts association pathways in the brain, causing dissociative anesthesia, a feeling of dissociation from the environment.
Absorption: Rapidly absorbed after I.M. injection.
Distribution: Rapidly distributes to body fat, liver, lung, and brain. Not significantly bound to plasma proteins.
Metabolism: By the liver to an active metabolite with one-third to one-sixth the potency of the parent drug.
Excretion: Over 90% of the drug is excreted in the urine.
Onset, peak, duration: Drug induces surgical anesthesia in 30 seconds after I.V. administration, which lasts 5 to 10 minutes. After I.M. injection, anesthesia begins in 3 to 4 minutes and lasts 12 to 25 minutes.

INDICATIONS & DOSAGE

Induce anesthesia for procedures, especially short-term diagnostic or surgical, not requiring skeletal muscle relaxation; before giving other general anesthetics or to supplement low-potency agents, such as nitrous oxide—

Adults and children: 1 to 4.5 mg/kg I.V., administered over 60 seconds; or 6.5 to 13 mg/kg I.M. To maintain anesthesia, repeat in increments of half to full initial dose.

CONTRAINDICATIONS & PRECAUTIONS

Contraindicated in patients with schizophrenia or other acute psychosis because drug may exacerbate the condition; in patients with cardiovascular disease in which a sudden rise in blood pressure would be harmful; and in those allergic to ketamine.

ADVERSE REACTIONS

Common reactions are in italics; life-threatening reactions are in bold italics.

CNS: *tonic and clonic movements resembling seizures,* ***respiratory depression, apnea when administered too rapidly.***

CV: *increased blood pressure and pulse rate,* hypotension, bradycardia.

EENT: diplopia, nystagmus, slight increase in intraocular pressure, ***laryngospasms, salivation.***

GI: mild anorexia, nausea, vomiting.

Skin: transient erythema, measles-like rash.

Other: *dream-like states, hallucinations, confusion, excitement,* irrational behavior, psychic abnormalities.

INTERACTIONS

Thyroid hormones: may elevate blood pressure and cause tachycardia. Give cautiously.

Barbiturates: chemically incompatible. Do not administer together.

EFFECTS ON DIAGNOSTIC TESTS

None significant.

NURSING CONSIDERATIONS

Besides those related universally to drug therapy (see "How to use this book"), consider the following specific recommendations:

Assessment

- Obtain a baseline assessment of the patient's vital signs, mental status, and overall physical status before anesthesia.
- Be alert for adverse reactions and drug interactions throughout anesthesia.
- Evaluate the patient's and family's knowledge about ketamine therapy.

Nursing Diagnoses

- High risk for injury related to ketamine-induced dissociative reaction.
- Ineffective breathing pattern related to ketamine-induced respiratory depression.
- Knowledge deficit related to ketamine.

Planning and Implementation

Preparation and Administration

- ***I.V. use:*** Keep in mind that only staff specially trained in giving I.V. anesthetics and managing potential adverse reactions should administer this drug.
- Because of rapid induction, patient should be physically supported during administration.
- Do not inject barbiturates and ketamine from same syringe because they are chemically incompatible.

Monitoring

- Monitor effectiveness by evaluating anesthesia effect after administration of ketamine.
- Monitor patient's vital signs before, during, and after anesthesia.
- Monitor respiratory status frequently. Be aware that respiratory depression may occur; apnea also may occur when drug is administered too rapidly.
- Monitor ECG during administra-

tion, especially in patients with hypertension or cardiac depression.

Supportive Care

- Notify the doctor immediately if CNS, respiratory, or cardiovascular status changes.
- Maintain airway.
- Have resuscitative equipment available and ready for use.
- Start supportive respiration if respiratory depression occurs. Use mechanical support if possible rather than administering analeptics.
- Implement safety measures to protect the unconscious patient. Before giving drug, make sure patient hasn't eaten because of the risk of aspirating vomitus.
- Keep verbal, tactile, and visual stimulation at a minimum during recovery phase to reduce incidence of emergent reactions.
- Keep in mind that hallucinations and excitement can occur on emergence from anesthesia; they can be abated by administering diazepam.
- Be aware that ketamine is a potent hallucinogen that can readily produce dissociative anesthesia (patient feels detached from environment). Dissociative effect and hallucinatory adverse reactions have made this a popular drug of abuse among young people.
- After use of ketamine, do not release an outpatient until effects wear off and then only if patient is accompanied by a responsible adult.

Patient Teaching

- Explain that this drug is used to induce anesthesia, especially for short-term procedures or surgery.
- Tell the patient what to expect during induction of anesthesia and during recovery from anesthesia. As needed, clarify any other information provided by the anesthesiologist, including risks.
- Warn patient not to drive or perform other tasks that require alertness for 24 hours after use of ketamine because of the risk of psychomotor impairment.

Evaluation

In patients receiving ketamine, appropriate evaluation statements may include:

- Patient experiences effective anesthesia; patient safety is maintained.
- Patient's airway is patent and adequate ventilatory status is maintained.
- Patient and family state an understanding of ketamine anesthesia.

ketoconazole (systemic)

(kee toe koe´ na zole)

Nizoral

- *Classification:* antifungal (imidazole derivative)
- *Pregnancy Risk Category:* C

HOW SUPPLIED

Tablets: 200 mg

Oral suspension: 100 mg/5 ml

ACTION

Mechanism: Inhibits purine transport and DNA, RNA, and protein synthesis; increases cell wall permeability, making the fungus more susceptible to osmotic pressure.

Absorption: Rapid but erratic; decreased by raised gastric pH. Converted to the hydrochloride salt by hydrochloric acid in the stomach before absorption. Administering the drug with food may slow gastric emptying, resulting in increased absorption and more consistent plasma levels.

Distribution: Distributed into bile, saliva, cerumen, synovial fluid, and sebum; CSF penetration is erratic and considered minimal. Drug is 84% to 99% bound to plasma proteins.

Metabolism: Converted into several inactive metabolites in the liver.

*Liquid form contains alcohol.

**May contain tartrazine.

Excretion: Over 50% of a dose is excreted in feces within 4 days; drug and metabolites are secreted in bile. About 13% is excreted unchanged in urine. Drug is probably excreted in breast milk. Half-life: Biphasic; initially 2 hours, with a terminal half-life of 8 hours.
Onset, peak, duration: Peak plasma concentrations occur at 1 to 4 hours.

INDICATIONS & DOSAGE

Treatment of systemic candidiasis, chronic mucocandidiasis, oral thrush, candiduria, coccidioidomycosis, histoplasmosis, chromomycosis, and paracoccidioidomycosis; severe cutaneous dermatophyte infections resistant to therapy with topical or oral griseofulvin—
Adults and children over 40 kg: initially, 200 mg P.O. daily single dose. Dosage may be increased to 400 mg once daily in patients who don't respond to lower dosage.
Children less than 20 kg: 50 mg (¼ tablet) daily single dose.
Children 20 to 40 kg: 100 mg (½ tablet) daily single dose.

CONTRAINDICATIONS & PRECAUTIONS

Contraindicated in patients with hypersensitivity to the drug. Use cautiously in patients with hepatic disease and in those taking other hepatotoxic drugs. Because of the potential for serious hepatic toxicity, use drug only for severe systemic fungal infections, not for fungal infections of the skin and nails.

ADVERSE REACTIONS

Common reactions are in italics; life-threatening reactions are in bold italics.
CNS: headache, nervousness, dizziness.
GI: *nausea, vomiting,* abdominal pain, diarrhea, constipation.
Hepatic: elevated liver enzymes, ***fatal hepatotoxicity.***
Skin: itching.
Other: gynecomastia with breast tenderness in men.

INTERACTIONS

Antacids, anticholinergics, H_2 blockers: decreased absorption of ketoconazole. Wait at least 2 hours after ketoconazole dose before administering these drugs.
Rifampin, isoniazid: increases ketoconazole metabolism. Monitor for decreased antifungal effect.

EFFECTS ON DIAGNOSTIC TESTS

AST (SGOT), ALT (SGPT), and alkaline phosphatase levels: transient elevations.
Serum cholesterol and triglycerides: transiently increased levels.

NURSING CONSIDERATIONS

Besides those related universally to drug therapy, (see "How to use this book"), consider the following specific recommendations:

Assessment
- Obtain a baseline assessment of infection, including appropriate specimens for identifying fungi, before therapy.
- Be alert for adverse reactions and drug interactions throughout therapy.
- Evaluate the patient's and family's knowledge about ketoconazole therapy.

Nursing Diagnoses
- High risk for injury related to ineffectiveness of ketoconazole to eradicate the fungus infection.
- High risk for fluid volume deficit related to ketoconazole-induced adverse GI reactions.
- Knowledge deficit related to ketoconazole therapy.

Planning and Implementation
Preparation and Administration
- ***P.O. use:*** To minimize nausea, divide the daily dosage b.i.d. and administer with meals.
- When administering the drug to a

patient with achlorhydria, dissolve each tablet in 4 ml aqueous solution of 0.2 N hydrochloric acid and have patient sip the mixture through a straw to avoid contact with teeth. Have patient drink a full glass (8 oz) of water afterward.

Monitoring

• Monitor effectiveness by regularly assessing for improvement of infection and by evaluating laboratory studies for eradication of fungi.

• Monitor patient's hydration status if adverse GI reactions occur.

• Monitor for signs of hepatotoxicity: elevated liver enzymes, persistent nausea, unusual fatigue, jaundice, dark urine, or pale stools.

Supportive Care

• Institute safety precautions if dizziness occurs.

• Obtain an order for an antiemetic, antidiarrheal, or laxative agent as needed.

Patient Teaching

• Stress importance of continuing treatment until clinical and laboratory tests indicate eradication of fungal infection. Tell patient that infection will recur if drug is discontinued too soon. Minimum treatment is 7 to 14 days for candidiasis, 6 months for other systemic fungal infections, and at least 4 weeks for resistant dermatophyte infections.

• Reassure patient that nausea is common in early therapy, but will subside. To minimize nausea, patient may, with doctor's permission, divide the daily dosage into two doses and take the drug with meals.

• Teach patient with achlorhydria how to take the drug. Drug requires acidity for dissolution and absorption.

• Warn patient to avoid hazardous activities if dizziness occurs.

• Warn male patients that gynecomastia with breast tenderness may occur.

Evaluation

In patients receiving ketoconazole, appropriate evaluation statements may include:

• Patient's infection is controlled.

• Patient remains adequately hydrated throughout therapy.

• Patient and family state an understanding of ketoconazole therapy.

ketoconazole (topical)

(kee toe koe´ na zole)

Nizoral

• *Classification:* topical antifungal (imidazole derivative)

• *Pregnancy Risk Category:* C

HOW SUPPLIED

Cream: 2%

ACTION

Mechanism: Inhibits fungal growth by altering the permeability of the cell membrane.

Absorption: Not absorbed when applied topically; minimal systemic absorption when applied intravaginally.

INDICATIONS & DOSAGE

Treatment of tinea corporis, tinea cruris, and tinea versicolor caused by susceptible organisms; seborrheic dermatitis–

Adults: apply once daily to cover the affected and immediate surrounding area. Apply twice daily, if necessary, in the more resistant cases.

CONTRAINDICATIONS & PRECAUTIONS

Contraindicated in patients with hypersensitivity to the drug.

ADVERSE REACTIONS

Common reactions are in italics; life-threatening reactions are in bold italics.

Skin: severe irritation, pruritus, stinging.

Systemic: localized allergic reaction.

INTERACTIONS

None reported.

EFFECTS ON DIAGNOSTIC TESTS

AST (SGOT), ALT (SGPT), and alkaline phosphatase: transiently elevated levels.
Serum cholesterol and triglyceride levels: transient alterations.

NURSING CONSIDERATIONS

Besides those related universally to drug therapy (see "How to use this book"), consider the following specific recommendations:

Assessment

- Obtain a baseline assessment of the patient's skin for redness and swelling before therapy.
- Be alert for adverse reactions and drug interactions throughout therapy.
- Evaluate the patient's and family's knowledge about ketoconazole therapy.

Nursing Diagnoses

- Impaired skin integrity related to patient's underlying condition.
- High risk for impaired skin integrity related to ketoconazole-induced irritation and pruritus.
- Knowledge deficit related to topical ketoconazole therapy.

Planning and Implementation

Preparation and Administration

- ***Topical use:*** Apply once daily to cover the affected and immediate surrounding area.

Monitoring

- Monitor effectiveness by observing the condition of affected skin.
- Observe for sensitivity or chemical irritation and discontinue use if it occurs.
- Check with doctor if condition worsens. Drug may have to be discontinued and the diagnosis reevaluated.
- Monitor for adverse reactions by frequently assessing the patient's skin for pruritus and irritation.

Supportive Care

- Notify the doctor if sensitivity or chemical irritation occurs.
- Most patients show improvement soon after treatment begins. However, treatment of tinea cruris or tinea corporis should continue for at least 2 weeks to reduce the possibility of recurrence.

Patient Teaching

- Teach patient to apply medication.
- Tell the patient that most patients show improvement soon after treatment begins but that treatment should continue for at least 2 weeks to prevent recurrence.

Evaluation

In patients receiving ketoconazole, appropriate evaluation statements may include:

- Patient states impaired skin integrity has resolved.
- Patient does not experience irritation and pruritus of affected area.
- Patient and family state an understanding of topical ketoconazole therapy.

---

ketoprofen

(kee toe proe´ fen)
Orudis, Orudis E†, Orudis SR†‡

- *Classification:* nonnarcotic analgesic, antipyretic (nonsteroidal anti-inflammatory drug)
- *Pregnancy Risk Category:* B (D in 3rd trimester)

HOW SUPPLIED

Tablets (sustained-release): 200 mg†
Capsules: 25 mg, 50 mg, 75 mg
Suppositories: 100 mg†

ACTION

Mechanism: Produces anti-inflammatory, analgesic, and antipyretic effects,

possibly through inhibition of prostaglandin synthesis.
Absorption: Rapidly and completely absorbed from the GI tract.
Distribution: Highly protein-bound. The extent of body tissue fluid distribution is not known, but therapeutic levels appear to range from 0.4 to 6 mcg/ml.
Metabolism: Extensively metabolized in the liver.
Excretion: In urine as the parent drug and metabolites. Half-life: Terminal elimination half-life ranges from 1.1 to 4 hours.
Onset, peak, duration: Analgesic effects are seen within 1 to 2 hours and last 3 to 4 hours.

INDICATIONS & DOSAGE

Rheumatoid arthritis and osteoarthritis–
Adults: 150 to 300 mg P.O. in three or four divided doses. Usual dosage is 75 mg t.i.d. Maximum dosage is 300 mg/day.
Alternatively, may use suppository where available–
Adults: 100 mg P.R. b.i.d.; or 1 suppository h.s. (in conjunction with oral ketoprofen during the day).
Mild to moderate pain; dysmenorrhea–
Adults: 25 to 50 mg P.O. q 6 to 8 hours p.r.n.

CONTRAINDICATIONS & PRECAUTIONS

Contraindicated in patients with hypersensitivity to the drug or in patients in whom aspirin or other NSAIDs induce symptoms of asthma, urticaria, or rhinitis.

Serious GI toxicity, such as ulceration or hemorrhage, can occur at any time in patients on chronic NSAID therapy. Use cautiously in patients with a history of peptic ulcer disease, renal dysfunction, or hepatic dysfunction because the drug may worsen these conditions; and in patients predisposed to fluid retention, such as those with CHF and hypertension, because ketoprofen may increase the risk of fluid retention and edema.

Patients with known "triad" symptoms (aspirin hypersensitivity, rhinitis/nasal polyps, and asthma) are at high risk for bronchospasm. Patients may experience an exacerbation of rectal or anal conditions when rectal suppository is used; use cautiously. NSAIDs may mask the signs and symptoms of acute infection (fever, myalgia, erythema); carefully evaluate patients with high risk for infection (such as those with diabetes).

ADVERSE REACTIONS

Common reactions are in italics; life-threatening reactions are in bold italics.
Blood: prolonged bleeding time.
CNS: *headache,* dizziness, *CNS inhibition or excitation.*
EENT: tinnitus, visual disturbances.
GI: *nausea, abdominal pain, diarrhea, constipation, flatulence, peptic ulceration,* anorexia, vomiting, stomatitis.
GU: nephrotoxicity, *elevated BUN.*
Hepatic: elevated enzymes.
Skin: rash.

INTERACTIONS

Oral anticoagulants: increased risk of bleeding.
Probenecid, aspirin: decreased plasma levels of ketoprofen.

EFFECTS ON DIAGNOSTIC TESTS

Blood glucose determinations (glucose enzymatic and peroxidase methods): altered results.
Serum iron: falsely increased or decreased levels.
Serum bilirubin: These in vitro interactions were reported with drug concentrations above those seen clinically (60 mg/ml).

NURSING CONSIDERATIONS

Besides those related universally to drug therapy (see "How to use this book"), consider the following specific recommendations:

Assessment

- Obtain a baseline assessment of the patient's pain before therapy.
- Be alert for adverse reactions and drug interactions throughout therapy.
- Evaluate the patient's and family's knowledge about ketoprofen therapy.

Nursing Diagnoses

- Pain related to patient's underlying condition.
- High risk for trauma related to possible adverse CNS reactions.
- Knowledge deficit related to ketoprofen therapy.

Planning and Implementation

Preparation and Administration

- ***PO use:*** Give dose 30 minutes before or 2 hours after meals. If adverse GI reactions occur, give with milk or meals.

Monitoring

- Regularly monitor for relief of pain, keeping in mind that full therapeutic effects for arthritis may require 2 to 4 weeks of therapy.
- Monitor the patient for adverse CNS reactions.
- Monitor the patient's renal and hepatic function every 6 months during prolonged therapy.
- Assess for GI toxicity.

Supportive Care

- Notify the doctor if the patient's pain is not relieved or if it worsens.
- If adverse CNS reactions occur, notify the doctor and institute safety precautions, which may include supervising ambulation and keeping the bed rails up.

Patient Teaching

- Tell the patient that the full therapeutic effect for arthritis may be delayed for 2 to 4 weeks.
- Advise the patient to notify the doctor if pain persists or worsens.
- Tell the patient to promptly report CNS or other adverse reactions, such as visual or auditory disturbances.
- Advise the patient to avoid driving and other hazardous activities that require mental alertness until CNS effects of the drug are known.
- Tell the patient to take the drug with food or milk if adverse GI reactions occur.
- Because serious GI toxicity can occur at any time in chronic NSAID therapy, teach the patient signs and symptoms of GI bleeding. Tell the patient to report these to the doctor immediately.
- Concomitant use with aspirin, alcohol, or steroids may increase the risk of adverse GI reactions. Advise the patient to avoid aspirin and alcohol.

Evaluation

In patients receiving ketoprofen, appropriate evaluation statements may include:

- Patient states pain is relieved.
- Patient does not develop traumatic injuries as a result of adverse CNS reactions.
- Patient and family state an understanding of ketoprofen therapy.

ketorolac tromethamine

(kee´ toe role ak)

Toradol

- *Classification:* analgesic (nonsteroidal anti-inflammatory)
- *Pregnancy Risk Category:* B

HOW SUPPLIED

Injection: 15 mg, 30 mg, 60 mg

ACTION

Mechanism: Produces anti-inflammatory and analgesic effects by inhibiting the synthesis of prostaglandins.

Absorption: Completely absorbed after I.M. administration.

Distribution: More than 99% protein-bound.

Metabolism: Primarily hepatic; a para hydroxy metabolite and conjugates have been identified; less than 50% of a dose is metabolized. Liver impairment does not substantially alter drug clearance.
Excretion: Primarily in urine (greater than 90%); the remainder, in feces. Half-life: Terminal plasma half-life is 3.8 to 6.3 hours (average 4½ hours) in young adults; substantially prolonged in patients with renal failure.
Onset, peak, duration: Mean peak plasma levels occur about 30 minutes after a 50-mg dose and range from 2.2 to 3 mcg/ml.

INDICATIONS & DOSAGE

Short-term management of pain–
Adults: initially, give 30 or 60 mg I.M as a loading dose, followed by half of the loading dose (15 or 30 mg) q 6 hours on a regular schedule or p.r.n. Subsequent dosage should be based on patient response. If pain returns before 6 hours, dosage may be increased by as much as 50% (up to 60 mg); if pain relief continues for 8 to 12 hours, increase interval between doses to q 8 to 12 hours, or reduce dose. The recommended maximum dosage is 150 mg on the first day and 120 mg daily thereafter.

CONTRAINDICATIONS & PRECAUTIONS

Contraindicated in patients with hypersensitivity to the drug and in those with the complete or partial triad syndrome (nasal polyps, angioedema, and bronchospasm after use of aspirin or other NSAIDs). Because NSAIDs can cause fluid retention and edema, use cautiously in patients with cardiac disease or hypertension. NSAIDs can also cause serious GI toxicity, especially ulceration or hemorrhage, in patients on chronic therapy. Use cautiously in patients with a history of GI disease, especially peptic ulcer disease, even for short-term management of pain.

ADVERSE REACTIONS

Common reactions are in italics; life-threatening reactions are in bold italics.
CNS: *drowsiness,* dizziness, headache, sweating.
CV: edema.
GI: *nausea, dyspepsia, GI pain,* diarrhea.
Local: pain at the injection site.

INTERACTIONS

Lithium: NSAIDs increase lithium levels.
Methotrexate: NSAIDs decrease methotrexate clearance and increase its toxicity.
Salicylates, warfarin: ketorolac may increase the levels of free (unbound) salicylates or warfarin in the blood. Clinical significance is unknown.

EFFECTS ON DIAGNOSTIC TESTS

AST (SGOT) or ALT (SGPT) levels: significant elevations.
Bleeding times: prolonged.
Liver function tests: borderline elevations.

NURSING CONSIDERATIONS

Besides those related universally to drug therapy (see "How to use this book"), consider the following specific recommendations:

Assessment

- Obtain a baseline assessment of the patient's pain before therapy.
- Be alert for adverse reactions and drug interactions throughout therapy.
- Evaluate the patient's and family's knowledge about ketorolac tromethamine therapy.

Nursing Diagnoses

- Pain related to the patient's underlying condition.
- High risk for trauma related to drowsiness or dizziness caused by CNS reaction to ketorolac.

• Knowledge deficit related to ketorolac therapy.

Planning and Implementation

Preparation and Administration

• Use lower initial doses in patients who are over age 65 or who weigh less than 110 lb (50 kg).

Monitoring

• Regularly monitor the patient for relief of pain.

• Monitor for adverse CNS reactions.

• Carefully observe patients with coagulopathies and those who are taking anticoagulants. Ketorolac inhibits platelet aggregation and can prolong bleeding time. This effect will disappear within 48 hours of discontinuing the drug. Drug will not alter platelet count, PTT or PT.

• Monitor for fluid retention, especially in patients with cardiac disease or hypertension.

Supportive Care

• Notify the doctor if the patient's pain persists or worsens.

• If adverse CNS reactions occur, notify the doctor and institute safety precautions, such as supervising ambulation and keeping the bed rails up.

• Carefully observe patients with coagulopathies and those receiving anticoagulants because drug inhibits platelet aggregation and can prolong bleeding time. This effect disappears within 48 hours of discontinuing the drug. It will not alter platelet count, partial thromboplastin time (PTT), or prothrombin time (PT).

Patient Teaching

• Advise the patient to report persistent or worsening pain.

• Explain that this drug is intended solely for short-term management of pain and that this should decrease the rate and severity of adverse reactions. However, tell the patient to report adverse CNS reactions and explain relevant precautions. Also teach the patient the signs and symptoms of GI bleeding, and tell the patient to report these immediately.

Evaluation

In patients receiving ketorolac, apppropriate evaluation statements may include:

• Patient states pain is relieved.

• Patient does not develop traumatic injuries as a result of adverse CNS reactions.

• Patient and family state an understanding of ketorolac therapy.

L

labetalol hydrochloride

(la bet´ a lole)
Normodyne, Presolol‡, Trandate

• *Classification:* antihypertensive (alpha- and beta-adrenergic blocking agent)
• *Pregnancy Risk Category:* C

HOW SUPPLIED

Tablets: 100 mg, 200 mg, 300 mg
Injection: 5 mg/ml

ACTION

Mechanism: Blocks response to alpha and beta stimulation and depresses renin secretion.
Absorption: Oral absorption of labetalol is high (90% to 100%); however, drug undergoes extensive first-pass metabolism in the liver and only about 25% of an oral dose reaches systemic circulation unchanged.
Distribution: Widely distributed throughout the body; drug is approximately 50% protein-bound.
Metabolism: Extensively metabolized in the liver. Oral form may also be metabolized in GI mucosa.
Excretion: About 5% of a dose is excreted unchanged in urine; remainder is excreted as metabolites in urine and feces. Half-life: About 5½ hours after I.V. administration; 6 to 8 hours after oral administration.
Onset, peak, duration: Antihypertensive effect is apparent in 20 minutes to 2 hours, peaks in 1 to 4 hours, and persists for 8 to 24 hours. After direct I.V. administration, antihypertensive effect occurs in 2 to 5 minutes, peaks in 5 to 15 minutes, and lasts 2 to 4 hours.

INDICATIONS & DOSAGE

Treatment of hypertension–
Adults: 100 mg P.O. b.i.d. with or without a diuretic. Dose may be increased to 200 mg b.i.d. after 2 days. Further dose increases may be made q 1 to 3 days until optimum response is reached. Usual maintenance dosage is 200 to 400 mg b.i.d.
For severe hypertension and hypertensive emergencies–
Adults: Dilute 200 mg to 200 ml with dextrose 5% in water. Infuse at 2 mg/minute until satisfactory response is obtained. Then stop the infusion. May repeat q 6 to 8 hours.

Alternatively, administer by repeated I.V. injection: Initially, give 20 mg I.V. slowly over 2 minutes. May repeat injections of 40 to 80 mg q 10 minutes until maximum dose of 300 mg is reached.

CONTRAINDICATIONS & PRECAUTIONS

Contraindicated in patients with hypersensitivity to the drug; and in patients with overt cardiac failure, severe bradycardia, second- or third-degree atrioventricular block, bronchial asthma, or cardiogenic shock because the drug may worsen these conditions.

Use cautiously in patients with cardiomyopathy because beta blockade may precipitate CHF; pheochromocytoma because paradoxical hypertensive responses have been reported; diabetes mellitus or hyperthyroidism because labetalol may mask tachycardia (but not sweating or dizziness) caused by hypoglycemia or hyperthyroidism; and impaired hepatic function caused by increased metabolism (lower dosage may be necessary).

ADVERSE REACTIONS

Common reactions are in italics; life-threatening reactions are in bold italics.
CNS: vivid dreams, fatigue, headache.
CV: *orthostatic hypotension and dizziness,* peripheral vascular disease, bradycardia.
EENT: nasal stuffiness.
Endocrine: hypoglycemia without tachycardia.
GI: nausea, vomiting, diarrhea.
GU: sexual dysfunction, urine retention.
Skin: rash.
Other: increased airway resistance, transient scalp tingling.

INTERACTIONS

Cimetidine: may enhance labetalol's effect. Give together cautiously.
Halothane: additive hypotensive effect.
Insulin, hypoglycemic drugs (oral): can alter dosage requirements in previously stabilized diabetics. Observe patient carefully.

EFFECTS ON DIAGNOSTIC TESTS

Urine free and total catecholamine level: false-positive increase with fluorometric method.

NURSING CONSIDERATIONS

Besides those related universally to drug therapy (see "How to use this book"), consider the following specific recommendations:

Assessment

- Obtain a baseline assessment of the patient's blood pressure before therapy.
- Be alert for adverse reactions and drug interactions throughout therapy.
- Evaluate the patient's and family's knowledge about labetalol therapy.

Nursing Diagnoses

- Altered tissue perfusion (renal, cerebral, cardiopulmonary, and peripheral) related to the patient's underlying condition.
- High risk for injury related to labetalol-induced adverse reactions.
- Knowledge deficit related to labetalol therapy.

Planning and Implementation

Preparation and Administration

- Discuss schedule changes with the doctor if patient experiences dizziness. Taking a dose at bedtime or taking smaller doses t.i.d. can help minimize this adverse reaction.
- ***I.V. use:*** Administer labetalol injection with a controlled infusion pump.

Monitoring

- Monitor effectiveness by frequently checking the patient's blood pressure, pulse, and ECG. Remember that, unlike other beta blockers, labetalol does not decrease heart rate or cardiac output.
- Monitor blood pressure closely after initial I.V. dose for a hypertensive emergency: every 5 minutes for first 30 minutes, every 30 minutes for the next 2 hours, then hourly for 6 hours. Keep the patient supine for 3 hours after the infusion. When administered I.V. for hypertensive emergencies, labetalol produces a rapid, predictable fall in blood pressure within 5 to 10 minutes.
- Monitor the patient for dizziness, especially in the early stages of treatment.

Supportive Care

- Keep in mind that this drug masks common signs of shock and hypoglycemia.
- Institute safety measures, such as continuous use of side rails, if dizziness or orthostatic hypotension occurs.

Patient Teaching

- Explain the importance of taking this drug as prescribed, even when feeling well.
- Tell the patient not to discontinue this drug suddenly even if unpleasant adverse reactions occur. Tell the patient to call the doctor and discuss the problem with him. Explain that

abrupt discontinuation of the drug can exacerbate angina and myocardial infarction.
• Instruct the patient to check with the doctor or pharmacist before taking any OTC medications.
• Tell the patient that dizziness, the most troublesome reaction to this drug, tends to occur in the early stages of treatment. Advise patient to minimize dizziness by rising slowly and avoiding sudden position changes.
• Tell the patient that transient scalp tingling sometimes occurs at the beginning of therapy but usually subsides quickly.
• Teach the patient and family caregiver to take frequent blood pressure measurements and to report significant changes to the doctor.

Evaluation

In patients receiving labetalol, appropriate evaluation statements may include:
• Patient's blood pressure is controlled within normal limits.
• Patient does not experience injury from adverse reactions to labetalol.
• Patient and family state an understanding of labetalol therapy.

lactulose

(lak´ tyoo lose)

Cephulac, Cholac, Chronulac, Constilac, Duphalac, Enulose, Lactulax†

• *Classification:* laxative (disaccharide)
• *Pregnancy Risk Category:* B

HOW SUPPLIED

Syrup: 10 g/15 ml

ACTION

Mechanism: A disaccharide sugar that produces an osmotic effect in the colon. Resultant distention promotes peristalsis. Also decreases blood ammonia, probably as a result of bacterial degradation, which decreases the pH of colon contents.
Absorption: Less than 3% of a dose is absorbed.
Distribution: Locally distributed, primarily in the colon.
Metabolism: Metabolized by colonic bacteria (absorbed portion is not metabolized).
Excretion: Most in feces; absorbed portion is excreted in urine.
Onset, peak, duration: Peak effect may not be seen for 24 to 48 hours.

INDICATIONS & DOSAGE

Treatment of constipation–
Adults: 15 to 30 ml P.O. daily.
To prevent and treat portal-systemic encephalopathy, including hepatic precoma and coma in patients with severe hepatic disease–
Adults: initially, 20 to 30 g P.O. (30 to 45 ml) t.i.d. or q.i.d., until two or three soft stools are produced daily. Usual dosage is 60 to 100 g daily in divided doses. Can also be given by retention enema in at least 100 ml of fluid.

CONTRAINDICATIONS & PRECAUTIONS

Lactulose is contraindicated in patients who must restrict galactose intake and in patients with appendicitis, acute surgical abdomen, fecal impaction, or intestinal obstruction, because drug may aggravate symptoms of these disorders.

Lactulose should be used with caution in diabetic patients because of sugar content (lactose and galactose). Because of a theoretical potential for accumulation of hydrogen gas in the GI tract, patients receiving lactulose who undergo electrocautery procedures during proctoscopy and colonoscopy should receive a thorough bowel cleansing before the procedure to minimize the risk of explosion.

ADVERSE REACTIONS

Common reactions are in italics; life-threatening reactions are in bold italics.
GI: abdominal cramps, belching, diarrhea, gaseous distention, flatulence.
Metabolic: hypernatremia.

INTERACTIONS

None significant.

EFFECTS ON DIAGNOSTIC TESTS

None reported.

NURSING CONSIDERATIONS

Besides those related universally to drug therapy (see "How to use this book"), consider the following specific recommendations:

Assessment

- Obtain a baseline assessment of history of bowel disorder, GI status, fluid intake, nutritional status, exercise habits, and normal pattern of elimination before therapy.
- Be alert for adverse reactions and drug interactions throughout therapy.
- Evaluate the patient's and family's knowledge about lactulose therapy.

Nursing Diagnoses

- Constipation related to interruption of normal pattern of elimination characterized by infrequent or absent stools.
- Pain related to abdominal cramping.
- Knowledge deficit related to lactulose therapy.

Planning and Implementation

Preparation and Administration

- Store at room temperature, preferably below 86° F (30° C). Do not freeze.
- ***P.O. use:*** Minimize drug's sweet taste by diluting with water or fruit juice or giving with food.

Monitoring

- Monitor effectiveness by monitoring the frequency and characteristics of stools.
- Monitor serum sodium for possible hypernatremia, especially when giving higher doses to treat hepatic encephalopathy.
- Auscultate bowel sounds at least once a shift. Assess for pain and cramping.
- Monitor nutritional status and fluid intake.

Supportive Care

- Do not give in low-galactose diet. Use with caution in patients with diabetes mellitus.
- Reduce dosage if diarrhea occurs. Replace fluid loss.
- Provide privacy for elimination.
- Unless contraindicated encourage fluid intake up to 2,500 ml a day.
- Consult with a dietitian to modify diet to increase fiber and bulk.

Patient Teaching

- Discourage excessive use of laxatives by patient to prevent dependence.
- Teach the patient about the relationship between fluid intake, dietary fiber, exercise, and constipation.
- Teach patient that dietary sources of fiber include bran and other cereals, fresh fruit, and vegetables.
- Warn patient that abdominal cramping may occur.

Evaluation

In patients receiving lactulose, appropriate evaluation statements may include:

- Patient reports return of normal pattern of elimination.
- Patient remains free from abdominal cramping.
- Patient and family state an understanding of lactulose therapy.

---

leucovorin calcium (citrovorum factor or folinic acid)

(loo koe vor´ in)
Wellcovorin

- *Classification:* vitamin, antidote (folic acid derivative)

• *Pregnancy Risk Category:* C

HOW SUPPLIED

Tablets: 5 mg, 25 mg
Injection: 1-ml ampule (3 mg/ml with 0.9% benzyl alcohol or 5 mg/ml, with methyl and propyl parabens); 50-mg vial (10 mg/ml after reconstitution, contains no preservatives); 5-ml ampule (5 mg/ml, with methyl and propyl parabens)

ACTION

Mechanism: A derivative of tetrahydrofolic acid, the reduced form of folic acid that is involved in the synthesis of purines, pyrimidines, and nucleic acids. It is readily converted to other folic acid derivatives.
Absorption: Rapidly absorbed after oral administration. The increase in plasma and serum folate activity after oral administration is mainly from 5-methyltetrahydrofolate (the major transport and storage form of folate in the body).
Distribution: Tetrahydrofolic acid and its derivatives are distributed throughout the body; the liver contains approximately half of the total body folate stores.
Metabolism: In the liver.
Excretion: By the kidneys as 10-formyl tetrahydrofolate and 5,10-methenyl tetrahydrofolate. Duration of action is 3 to 6 hours. Half life is 6.2 hours after parenteral administration; 5.7 hours after oral administration.
Onset, peak, duration: After oral administration, peak serum folate concentrations occur in about 2 hours; after I.V. administration, within 10 minutes; after I.M. administration, within 1 hour.

INDICATIONS & DOSAGE

Overdose of folic acid antagonist–
Adults and children: P.O., I.M., or I.V. dose equivalent to the weight of the antagonist given.
Leucovorin rescue after high methotrexate dose in treatment of malignancy–
Adults and children: dose at doctor's discretion within 6 to 36 hours of last dose of methotrexate.
Toxic effects of methotrexate used to treat severe psoriasis–
Adults and children: 4 to 8 mg I.M. 2 hours after methotrexate dose.
Hematologic toxicity caused by pyrimethamine therapy–
Adults and children: 5 mg P.O. or I.M. daily.
Hematologic toxicity caused by trimethoprim therapy–
Adults and children: 400 mcg to 5 mg P.O. or I.M. daily.
Megaloblastic anemia caused by congenital enzyme deficiency–
Adults and children: 3 to 6 mg I.M. daily, then 1 mg P.O. daily for life.
Folate-deficient megaloblastic anemia –
Adults and children: up to 1 mg of leucovorin I.M daily. Duration of treatment depends on hematologic response.

CONTRAINDICATIONS & PRECAUTIONS

Contraindicated in patients with allergic reactions after oral and parenteral administration of folic acid. In patients with undiagnosed pernicious anemia, leucovorin may mask the anemia by relieving its hematologic effects while allowing neurologic complications to progress.

ADVERSE REACTIONS

Common reactions are in italics; life-threatening reactions are in bold italics.
Skin: allergic reactions (rash, pruritus, erythema).
Other: ***allergic bronchospasms.***

INTERACTIONS

None significant.

EFFECTS ON DIAGNOSTIC TESTS

Red cell indices: false normal levels. Leucovorin may mask the diagnosis of pernicious anemia.

NURSING CONSIDERATIONS

Besides those related universally to drug therapy (see "How to use this book"), consider the following specific recommendations:

Assessment

• Obtain a baseline assessment of patient's underlying condition before therapy.

• Be alert for adverse reactions and drug interactions throughout therapy.

• Evaluate the patient's and family's knowledge about leucovorin therapy.

Nursing Diagnoses

• Altered protection related to the patient's underlying condition.

• Ineffective breathing pattern related to adverse respiratory reactions.

• Knowledge deficit related to leucovorin therapy.

Planning and Implementation

Preparation and Administration

• Protect from light and heat, especially reconstituted parenteral preparations.

• ***I.V. use:*** Inject directly into vein or I.V. tubing containing a free-flowing compatible solution over 5 minutes. For intermittent infusion, infuse the solution over 15 minutes; for continuous infusion, infuse over 24 hours at a rate of about 40 ml/hour.

Monitoring

• Monitor effectiveness by assessing for the reduction of myelosupression.

• Monitor for adverse reactions and interactions by assessing respiratory status. Drug may cause allergic bronchospasm.

• Monitor the patient's skin for allergic reactions (rash, pruritus, erythema).

• Monitor for allergic reactions because severe allergic reactions to folic acid have been reported.

Supportive Care

• For overdose of folic acid antagonists, administer within 1 hour if possible; usually ineffective after 4-hour delay.

• Follow leucovorin rescue schedule and protocol closely to maximize therapeutic response. Generally, leucovorin should not be administered simultaneously with systemic methotrexate.

• Do not confuse leucovorin (folinic acid) with folic acid.

Patient Teaching

• Tell the patient that this drug should not be confused with folic acid.

Evaluation

In patients receiving leucovorin, appropriate evaluation statements may include:

• Patient's myelosupression improves.

• Patient does not develop drug-induced allergic bronchospasm.

• Patient and family state an understanding of leucovorin therapy.

leuprolide acetate

(loo proe´ lide)

Lucrin‡, Lupron, Lupron Depot

• *Classification:* antineoplastic (gonadotropic hormone)

• *Pregnancy Risk Category:* B

HOW SUPPLIED

Injection: 1 mg/0.2 ml (5 mg/ml) in 2.8-ml multiple-dose vials

Depot injection: 7.5 mg/ml

ACTION

Mechanism: Initially stimulates but then inhibits the release of follicle-stimulating and luteinizing hormones, resulting in testosterone suppression.

Absorption: Leuprolide is a polypeptide molecule that is destroyed in the GI tract. After S.C. or I.M. adminis-

tration, the drug is rapidly, and essentially completely, absorbed.
Distribution: High concentrations distribute into kidney, liver, pineal, and pituitary tissue. Approximately 7% to 15% of a dose is bound to plasma proteins.
Metabolism: May be metabolized in the anterior pituitary and hypothalamus, similar to endogenous gonadotropin-releasing hormone.
Excretion: Half-life: The plasma elimination half-life has been reported to be 3 hours.

INDICATIONS & DOSAGE

Management of advanced prostate cancer–
Adults: 1 mg S.C. daily. Alternatively, give 7.5 mg I.M. (depot injection) monthly.

CONTRAINDICATIONS & PRECAUTIONS

No contraindications. Use cautiously in patients with sensitivity to benzyl alcohol, a preservative used in some formulations.

ADVERSE REACTIONS

Common reactions are in italics; life-threatening reactions are in bold italics.
Endocrine: *hot flashes.*
GI: nausea, vomiting.
Local: skin reactions at injection site.
Other: ***pulmonary embolus,*** peripheral edema, decreased libido, transient bone pain during first week of treatment.

INTERACTIONS

None significant.

EFFECTS ON DIAGNOSTIC TESTS

None reported.

NURSING CONSIDERATIONS

Besides those related universally to drug therapy (see "How to use this book"), consider the following specific recommendations:

Assessment
- Obtain a baseline assessment of patient's underlying condition before therapy.
- Be alert for adverse reactions and drug interactions throughout therapy.
- Evaluate the patient's and family's knowledge about leuprolide therapy.

Nursing Diagnoses
- High risk for impaired skin integrity related to drug-induced skin reactions.
- Sexual dysfunction related to drug-induced decreased libido.
- Knowledge deficit related to leuprolide therapy.

Planning and Implementation
Preparation and Administration
- Never administer by I.V. injection.
- May be stored at room temperature under 86° F (30° C), but protected from light and heat sources.
- The injection should be administered using only the syringe provided by the manufacturer. If another syringe must be substituted, a low-dose insulin syringe (U-100, 0.5 ml) may be appropriate.
- A depot injection should be given monthly under the supervision of a doctor. Use the supplied diluent to reconstitute drug. Draw 1 mg into syringe with a 22G needle; discard any extra diluent. Inject into vial and shake well. Suspension will appear milky.
- The depot injection will remain stable for 24 hours after reconstitution; however, it should be used immediately, as there is no preservative in the drug.
- Never use a needle smaller that 22G for depot injection.
- Patients may be maintained on this drug for long-term treatment.

Monitoring
- Monitor effectiveness by assessing renal and hepatic functioning.
- Monitor for signs of pulmonary embolus or peripheral edema.

• Monitor hydration status if patient develops nausea and vomiting.
• Monitor the patient's skin integrity at the injection site–drug may cause skin reactions.
• Monitor effectiveness by noting results of follow-up diagnostic tests and overall physical status.
• Monitor for bone pain, which is common during the first week of therapy.

Supportive Care

• Know that leuprolide is a nonsurgical alternative to orchiectomy for prostate cancer.
• Know that studies show that this drug is therapeutically equivalent to diethylstilbestrol in "medical castration" palliation treatment but has significantly milder and fewer adverse reactions.
• Provide the patient with fluids if he develops nausea and vomiting.
• Obtain an order for a mild analgesic if the patient develops transient bone pain.
• Encourage the patient to discuss his fears and concerns about sexual dysfunction.
• Encourage the patient to seek professional evaluation and therapy for sexual dysfunction.

Patient Teaching

• Teach patient correct administration technique for self-administration. Advise patient to use only the syringe supplied with the drug. If another syringe must be substituted, a low-dose insulin syringe (U-100, 0.5 ml) may be an appropriate choice.
• Reassure patient that adverse effects of leuprolide are often less severe than with other endocrine therapies.
• Reassure patient that bone pain is transient and should last no longer than the first week.

Evaluation

In patients receiving leuprolide, appropriate evaluation statements may include:

• Patient's skin integrity is not impaired.
• Patient and significant other adjust to drug-induced sexual dysfunction.
• Patient and family state an understanding of leuprolide therapy.

levamisole hydrochloride

(lee vam´ i sole)
Ergamisol

• *Classification:* antineoplastic (immunomodulator)
• *Pregnancy Risk Category:* C

HOW SUPPLIED

Tablets: 50 mg (base)

ACTION

Mechanism: An immunomodulator; action is unknown. The effects of the drug on the immune system are complex. It appears to restore depressed immune function and may potentiate the actions of monocytes and macrophages and enhance T-cell responses.
Absorption: Rapidly absorbed from the GI tract.
Metabolism: Extensively metabolized by the liver.
Excretion: 70% of metabolites are excreted in urine over 3 days; 5%, in feces; less than 5% of unchanged drug is excreted in urine; less than 2%, in feces. Half-life: 3 to 4 hours.
Onset, peak, duration: Peak plasma levels are obtained within 1½ to 2 hours.

INDICATIONS & DOSAGE

Adjuvant treatment of Dukes' stage C colon cancer (with fluorouracil) after surgical resection–
Adults: 50 mg P.O. q 8 hours for 3 days. Therapy should begin no sooner than 7 days and no later than 30 days after surgery, providing that the patient is out of the hospital, ambulating, maintaining normal oral nutri-

tion, has well-healed wounds, and has recovered from any postoperative complications. Fluorouracil (450 mg/m^2/day I.V.) is given daily for 5 days starting 21 to 34 days after surgery.

Maintenance dosage is 50 mg P.O. q 8 hours for 3 days q 2 weeks for 1 year. Given in conjunction with fluorouracil maintenance therapy (450 mg/m^2/day by rapid I.V. push, once a week beginning 28 days after the initial 5-day course) for 1 year.

CONTRAINDICATIONS & PRECAUTIONS

Contraindicated in patients with hypersensitivity to levamisole or its components. Use cautiously in patients with impaired renal or hepatic function.

ADVERSE REACTIONS

Common reactions are in italics; life-threatening reactions are in bold italics.
Blood: ***agranulocytosis,*** *leukopenia,* ***thrombocytopenia, granulocytopenia.***
CNS: *dizziness, headache, paresthesia, somnolence, depression, nervousness, insomnia, anxiety, fatigue, fever.*
CV: chest pain, edema.
EENT: blurred vision, conjunctivitis.
GI: *nausea, diarrhea, stomatitis, vomiting, anorexia, abdominal pain, constipation, flatulence, dyspepsia.*
Metabolic: hyperbilirubinemia.
Skin: *dermatitis, alopecia,* ***exfoliative dermatitis,*** *pruritus, urticaria.*
Other: rigors, *infection, dysgeusia, altered sense of smell, arthralgia, myalgia.*

INTERACTIONS

Alcohol: may precipitate a disulfiram-like (Antabuse) reaction. Avoid concomitant use.
Phenytoin: plasma levels may be elevated when administered with levamisole and fluorouracil. Monitor phenytoin plasma levels.

EFFECTS ON DIAGNOSTIC TESTS

Serum AST (SGOT), lactate dehydrogenase: increased levels.
Serum high-density lipoproteins, serum estrogen: decreased levels.
Serum triglycerides, total cholesterol, low-density-lipoprotein cholesterol: increased levels.

NURSING CONSIDERATIONS

Besides those related universally to drug therapy (see "How to use this book"), consider the following specific recommendations:

Assessment
- Obtain a baseline assessment of condition of colon after resection before therapy.
- Be alert for adverse reactions and drug interactions throughout therapy.
- Evaluate the patient's and family's knowledge about levamisole therapy.

Nursing Diagnoses
- Altered protection related to the patient's underlying condition.
- High risk for injury related to hematologic effects of levamisole.
- Knowledge deficit related to levamisole therapy.

Planning and Implementation
Preparation and Administration
- Obtain a baseline CBC with differential, platelet count, electrolytes, and liver function studies immediately before starting levamisole therapy.
- If levamisole therapy begins 7 to 20 days after surgery, fluorouracil should be started with the second course of levamisole therapy. It should begin no sooner than 21 days and no later than 35 days after surgery. If levamisole is deferred until 21 to 30 days after surgery, fluorouracil therapy should begin with the first course of levamisole.
- Do not exceed recommended doses. Higher doses are associated with a greater incidence of agranulocytosis.
- Dosage modifications are based on hematologic parameters. If WBC

count is 2500/mm³ to 3500/mm³, don't administer fluorouracil until WBC count is above 3500/mm³. When fluorouracil is restarted, reduce dosage by 20%. If WBC count stays below 2500/mm³ for over 10 days after fluorouracil is withdrawn, discontinue levamisole.

• Discontinue therapy with both levamisole and fluorouracil if platelet count is below 100,000/mm³.

Monitoring

• Monitor effectiveness by assessing tumor size and rate of growth.

• Monitor hematologic status closely because of the association with agranulocytosis, which is sometimes fatal. Neutropenia is usually reversible when levamisole therapy is discontinued.

• Monitor CBC with differential and platelet at weekly intervals before treatment with fluorouracil.

• Repeat liver function studies and electrolytes every 3 months for a year.

• Observe for signs of bleeding and infection.

• Observe patient for signs of levamisole-induced CNS disturbances, such as dizziness, insomnia, headache, depression, somnolence, and anxiety.

Supportive Care

• Discontinue drug if stomatitis or diarrhea develops during the initial course of fluorouracil therapy; the drug may be restarted 28 days after the start of the initial course.

• Defer fluorouracil therapy if stomatitis and diarrhea develop during the weekly doses. Fluorouracil may be restarted at a 20% reduction in dosage when the symptoms subside.

• Obtain orders for antidiarrheal or antiemetics, as needed.

• Provide good skin care to alleviate levamisole-induced skin reactions.

Patient Teaching

• Advise the patient to immediately report any flulike symptoms, such as fever and chills.

• Instruct patients undergoing fluorouracil therapy to immediately report stomatitis or diarrhea.

• Instruct patients to report bruising, bleeding, and petechiae immediately to their doctor.

Evaluation

In patients receiving levamisole, appropriate evaluation statements may include:

• Patient demonstrates no new tumor growth.

• Patient's hematologic parameters remain stable.

• Patient and family state an understanding of levamisole therapy.

levobunolol hydrochloride

(lee voe byoo´ noe lole)

Betagan

• *Classification:* antiglaucoma agent (beta-adrenergic blocking agent)

• *Pregnancy Risk Category:* C

HOW SUPPLIED

Ophthalmic solution: 0.5%

ACTION

Mechanism: Reduces formation and possibly increases outflow of aqueous humor.

Absorption: Some systemic absorption follows topical application to the eye.

Distribution: In animals, distributed widely throughout ocular tissues.

Metabolism: Extensively metabolized, probably in the liver.

Excretion: In urine and feces.

Onset, peak, duration: Onset of activity usually occurs within 1 hour, with peak effect in 2 to 6 hours. Duration of effect is 24 hours.

INDICATIONS & DOSAGE

Chronic open-angle glaucoma and ocular hypertension–
Adults: instill 1 drop in eyes once daily or b.i.d..

CONTRAINDICATIONS & PRECAUTIONS

Contraindicated in patients with hypersensitivity to any component of the preparation and in patients with bronchial asthma, severe COPD, sinus bradycardia, second- or third-degree AV block, cardiac failure, or cardiogenic shock because it may worsen these symptoms or disorders. Use cautiously in patients with angle-closure glaucoma (use with a miotic), in patients with muscle weakness (myasthenic-like symptoms), and in those with a history of heart failure, restricted pulmonary function, or diabetes mellitus.

ADVERSE REACTIONS

Common reactions are in italics; life-threatening reactions are in bold italics.
CNS: headache, dizziness, depression.
CV: slight reduction in resting heart rate.
Eye: *transient stinging and burning.* Long-term use may decrease corneal sensitivity.
GI: nausea.
Skin: urticaria.
Other: evidence of beta blockade and systemic absorption *(hypotension, bradycardia, syncope, exacerbation of asthma,* and *congestive heart failure).*

INTERACTIONS

Propranolol, metoprolol, and other oral beta-adrenergic blocking agents: increased ocular and systemic effect. Use together cautiously.
Reserpine and other catecholomine-depleting drugs: enhanced hypotensive and bradycardiac effects.

EFFECTS ON DIAGNOSTIC TESTS

None reported with ophthalmic use of beta blockers.

NURSING CONSIDERATIONS

Besides those related universally to drug therapy, (see "How to use this book"), consider the following specific recommendations:

Assessment
• Obtain a baseline assessment of the patient's visual status, ocular pressure, and vital signs before therapy.
• Be alert for adverse reactions and drug interactions throughout therapy.
• Evaluate the patient's and family's knowledge about levobunolol therapy.

Nursing Diagnoses
• Sensory/perceptual alterations (visual) related to the patient's underlying condition.
• Pain related to levobunolol-induced transient eye stinging and burning.
• Knowledge deficit related to levobunolol therapy.

Planning and Implementation
Preparation and Administration
• Instill in lacrimal sac; remove excess solution from around eyes with a clean tissue or gauze and apply light finger pressure to lacrimal sac for 1 minute.
Monitoring
• Monitor effectiveness by assessing the patient's visual status and intraocular pressure. The onset of action is usually within 1 hour, peaking between 2 to 6 hours.
• Monitor blood pressure and apical rate for drug-induced hypotension or bradycardia; obtain ECG as indicated.
• Monitor respiratory status closely in patients with underlying chronic bronchitis or emphysema.
Supportive Care
• Notify the doctor immediately of any changes in the patient's health status.
• Obtain an order for a mild analge-

*Liquid form contains alcohol.

**May contain tartrazine.

sic if the patient experiences a headache.

• Notify the doctor if eye stinging or burning persists after instillation.

Patient Teaching

• Teach the patient how to instill and advise him to wash his hands before and after administering the drug.

• Advise patient to continue with regular medical supervision, especially if he has underlying diabetes or thyroid disease.

• Warn patient that instillation of the solution may cause transient stinging or burning.

Evaluation

In patients receiving levobunolol, appropriate evaluation statements may include:

• Patient experiences therapeutic reduction in intraocular pressure.

• Patient can cope with transient eye stinging or burning.

• Patient and family state an understanding of levobunolol therapy.

levodopa

(lee voe doe´ pa)

Dopar, Larodopa, Levopa, Parda, Rio-Dopa

• *Classification:* antiparkinsonian agent (precursor of dopamine)
• *Pregnancy Risk Category:* C

HOW SUPPLIED

Tablets: 100 mg, 250 mg, 500 mg
Capsules: 100 mg, 250 mg, 500 mg

ACTION

Mechanism: Levodopa is decarboxylated to dopamine, countering the depletion of striatal dopamine in extrapyramidal centers, which is thought to produce parkinsonism.

Absorption: Rapidly absorbed from small intestine by an active amino acid transport system, with 30% to 50% reaching general circulation.

Distribution: Widely distributed to most body tissues, but less than 1% reaches the CNS because of extensive metabolism in the periphery.

Metabolism: 95% is converted to dopamine by L-aromatic amino acid decarboxylase in the lumen of the stomach and intestines and on the first pass through the liver.

Excretion: Primarily in urine; 80% of dose is excreted within 24 hours as dopamine metabolites. Half-life: About 1 hour.

Onset, peak, duration: Most patients experience a short-duration improvement (lasting about 5 hours after a dose) and a long-duration improvement (beginning only after repeated doses, and lasting more than 10 hours). The long-duration response usually lasts for 3 to 5 days after discontinuation.

INDICATIONS & DOSAGE

Treatment of idiopathic parkinsonism, postencephalitic parkinsonism, and symptomatic parkinsonism after carbon monoxide or manganese intoxication; or in association with cerebral arteriosclerosis–

Adults and children over 12 years: initially, 0.5 to 1 g P.O. daily, given b.i.d., t.i.d., or q.i.d. with food; increase by no more than 0.75 g daily q 3 to 7 days, until usual maximum of 8 g is reached. Carefully adjust dosage to individual requirements, tolerance, and response. Higher dosage requires close supervision.

CONTRAINDICATIONS & PRECAUTIONS

Contraindicated in patients with hypersensitivity and in patients receiving monoamine oxidase (MAO) inhibitors. Because levodopa may activate a malignant melanoma, do not use in patients with suspicious undiagnosed skin lesions or history of melanoma.

Use cautiously in patients with cardiovascular, renal, hepatic, or endocrine disease; in patients with history of myocardial infarction with residual arrhythmias, peptic ulcer, convulsions, psychiatric disorders, chronic wide-angle glaucoma, diabetes, pulmonary diseases, or bronchial asthma; and in patients receiving antihypertensives.

ADVERSE REACTIONS

Common reactions are in italics; life-threatening reactions are in bold italics.
Blood: ***hemolytic anemia,*** leukopenia.
CNS: *aggressive behavior, choreiform, dystonic, and dyskinetic movements, involuntary grimacing, head movements, myoclonic body jerks, ataxia, tremors, muscle twitching, bradykinetic episode, psychiatric disturbances, memory loss, mood changes, nervousness, anxiety, disturbing dreams, euphoria, malaise, fatigue, severe depression,* ***suicidal tendencies,*** *dementia, delirium, hallucinations (may necessitate reduction or withdrawal of drug).*
CV: *orthostatic hypotension,* cardiac irregularities, flushing, hypertension, phlebitis.
EENT: blepharospasm, blurred vision, diplopia, mydriasis or miosis, widening of palpebral fissures, activation of latent Horner's syndrome, oculogyric crises, nasal discharge.
GI: *nausea, vomiting, anorexia,* weight loss may occur at start of therapy, constipation, flatulence, diarrhea, epigastric pain, hiccups, sialorrhea, dry mouth, bitter taste.
GU: urinary frequency, urine retention, incontinence, darkened urine, excessive and inappropriate sexual behavior, priapism.
Hepatic: hepatotoxicity.
Other: dark perspiration, hyperventilation.

INTERACTIONS

Antacids: increased absorption of levodopa.
Antihypertensives: additive hypertensive effect.
High-protein foods: decreased absorption of levodopa.
Metoclopramide: accelerated gastric emptying of levodopa.
Papaverine, phenothiazines and other antipsychotics, phenytoin: watch for decreased levodopa effect.
Pyridoxine: reduced efficacy of levodopa. Examine vitamin preparations and nutritional supplements for content of vitamin B_6 (pyridoxine).
Sympathomimetics: increased risk of cardiac arrhythmias.

EFFECTS ON DIAGNOSTIC TESTS

Coombs' test: occasionally becomes positive (during chronic therapy).
Uric acid (colorimetric test): false elevations.
Urine glucose with copper sulfate method: false-positive results.
Urine glucose with glucose enzymatic method: false-negative results.
Urine ketones: test interference.

NURSING CONSIDERATIONS

Besides those related universally to drug therapy (see "How to use this book"), consider the following specific recommendations:

Assessment

- Obtain a baseline assessment of the patient's parkinsonian signs and symptoms before therapy.
- Be alert for adverse reactions and drug interactions throughout therapy.
- Evaluate the patient's and family's knowledge about levodopa therapy.

Nursing Diagnoses

- Impaired physical mobility related to underlying parkinsonian syndrome.
- Altered thought processes related to adverse CNS reactions to levodopa.
- Fluid volume deficit related to high risk of adverse GI reactions.
- Knowledge deficit related to levodopa therapy.

Planning and Implementation

Preparation and Administration

• Adjust dosage according to patient's response and tolerance.

• Crush tablets and mix with applesauce or baby food fruits for patients who have difficulty swallowing tablets.

• Withdraw MAO inhibitors at least 2 weeks before levodopa therapy.

• Administer with food to prevent GI discomfort.

• If therapy is interrupted for a long time, resumed dosage should be adjusted gradually to previous level.

• Patient who must undergo surgery should continue levodopa as long as oral intake is permitted, generally 6 to 24 hours before surgery. After surgery, administer drug as soon as patient is able to take oral medication.

• Protect levodopa from heat, light, and moisture. If preparation darkens, it has lost potency and should be discarded.

Monitoring

• Monitor effectiveness by regularly checking body movements for signs of improvement; therapeutic response usually follows each dose and disappears within 5 hours but varies considerably.

• Carefully monitor the patient who is also receiving an antihypertensive and a hypoglycemic agent.

• Monitor for signs of overdose; muscle twitching and blepharospasm (twitching of eyelids) may be early signs of drug overdosage; report them to the doctor immediately.

• Monitor for CNS and other adverse drug reactions.

• Regularly test the patient on long-term therapy for diabetes and acromegaly; periodically repeat blood tests and liver and kidney function studies.

• Monitor dietary intake of protein because high-protein foods can decrease absorption of levodopa.

• Monitor for dystonic, choreiform, and dyskinetic movements.

• Monitor vital signs closely, especially during dosage adjustment.

Supportive Care

• Withhold dose and notify the doctor if significant changes in vital signs or mental status occur. Reduced dosage or discontinuation of levodopa may be necessary.

• Institute safety precautions.

• Keep in mind that a doctor-supervised period of drug discontinuation (a drug holiday) may reestablish the effectiveness of a lower dosage regimen.

• Evaluate test results carefully: Coombs' test occasionally becomes positive during extended use. Expect uric acid elevations with colorimetric method but not with uricase method. Alkaline phosphatase, AST (SGOT), ALT (SGPT), lactate dehydrogenase, bilirubin, BUN, and protein-bound iodine levels show transient elevations in patients receiving levodopa; WBC counts, hemoglobin, and hematocrit show occasional reduction.

• Assist the patient with daily activities as needed.

• Be aware that levodopa-carbidopa combination usually reduces amount of levodopa needed by 75%, thereby reducing incidence of adverse reactions.

Patient Teaching

• Warn the patient of possible dizziness and orthostatic hypotension, especially at start of therapy. The patient should change position slowly and dangle legs briefly before getting out of bed. Inform the patient that elastic stockings may control this adverse reaction.

• Advise the patient and family that multivitamin preparations, fortified cereals, and certain OTC medications may contain pyridoxine (vitamin B_6), which can reverse the effects of levodopa.

• Warn the patient and family not to

increase dosage without the doctor's orders (they may be tempted to do this as disease symptoms of parkinsonism progress). Daily dosage should not exceed 8 g.

• Instruct the patient's family to notify the doctor if they notice changes in the patient's behavior or mental status.
• Advise the patient to avoid hazardous activities that require mental alertness until adverse CNS reactions are known.
• Instruct the patient to take levodopa with food.

Evaluation

In patients receiving levodopa, appropriate evaluation statements may include:

• Patient exhibits improved mobility with reduction of muscular rigidity and tremor.
• Patient remains mentally alert throughout levodopa therapy.
• Patient and family state an understanding of levodopa therapy.

levodopa-carbidopa

(lee voe doe´ pa/kar bi doe´ pa)
Sinemet

• *Classification:* antiparkinsonian agent (decarboxylase inhibitor and dopamine precursor)
• *Pregnancy Risk Category:* C

HOW SUPPLIED

Tablets: carbidopa 10 mg with levodopa 100 mg (Sinemet 10-100), carbidopa 25 mg with levodopa 100 mg (Sinemet 25-100), carbidopa 25 mg with levodopa 250 mg (Sinemet 25-250)

ACTION

Mechanism: Because dopamine does not enter the CNS, the precursor levodopa is administered. Levodopa is decarboxylated to dopamine, countering the depletion of striatal dopamine in extrapyramidal centers. Carbidopa inhibits the peripheral decarboxylation of levodopa without affecting levodopa's metabolism within the CNS. Therefore, more levodopa is available to be decarboxylated to dopamine in the brain.

Absorption: When levodopa is administered orally it is rapidly converted to dopamine in extracerebral tissues so that only a small portion of a given dose is transported unchanged to the CNS. About 40% to 70% of a dose of carbidopa is absorbed. Carbidopa enhances levodopa's absorption by preventing its breakdown in the GI tract. Levodopa absorption is decreased by meals, particularly high-protein meals.

Distribution: Carbidopa inhibits decarboxylation of peripheral levodopa. It does not cross the blood-brain barrier and does not affect the metabolism of levodopa within the CNS. Levodopa enters the CNS.

Metabolism: Converted to dopamine in the basal ganglia.

Excretion: Simultaneous administration of carbidopa and levodopa produces greater urinary excretion of levodopa in proportion to the excretion of dopamine than administration of the two drugs at separate times. Half-life: Carbidopa, about 2 hours; levodopa, about 1 hour; levodopa in the presence of carbidopa, about 2 hours. Carbidopa reduces the amount of levodopa required by about 75% and, when administered with levodopa, increases both plasma levels and the plasma half-life of levodopa, and decreases plasma and urinary dopamine and homovanillic acid.

Onset, peak, duration: Most patients experience a short-duration improvement (lasting about 5 hours after a dose) and a long-duration improvement (beginning only after repeated doses, and lasting more than 10 hours). The long-duration response usually lasts for 3 to 5 days after discontinuation.

INDICATIONS & DOSAGE

Treatment of idiopathic Parkinson's disease, postencephalitic parkinsonism, and symptomatic parkinsonism resulting from carbon monoxide or manganese intoxication–
Adults: 3 to 6 tablets of 25 mg carbidopa/250 mg levodopa daily given in divided doses. Do not exceed 8 tablets of 25 mg carbidopa/250 mg levodopa daily. Optimum daily dosage must be determined by careful titration for each patient.

CONTRAINDICATIONS AND PRECAUTIONS

Contraindicated in patients hypersensitive to either drug and in patients with bronchial asthma, emphysema, or other severe pulmonary disorders; severe cardiovascular disease; narrow-angle glaucoma; history of or suspected melanoma; or history of myocardial infarction, because the drug may exacerbate symptoms of these disorders.

ADVERSE REACTIONS

Common reactions are in italics; life-threatening reactions are in bold italics.
Blood: ***hemolytic anemia.***
CNS: *choreiform, dystonic, dyskinetic movements; involuntary grimacing, head movements, myoclonic body jerks, ataxia,* tremors, muscle twitching; bradykinetic episodes; psychiatric disturbances, memory loss, nervousness, anxiety, disturbing dreams, euphoria, malaise, fatigue; severe depression, ***suicidal tendencies,*** dementia, delirium, hallucinations (may necessitate reduction or withdrawal of drug).
CV: *orthostatic hypotension,* cardiac irregularities, flushing, hypertension, phlebitis.
EENT: blepharospasm, blurred vision, diplopia, mydriasis or miosis, widening of palpebral fissures, activation of latent Horner's syndrome, oculogyric crises, nasal discharge.
GI: *nausea, vomiting, anorexia,* weight loss may occur at start of therapy; constipation; flatulence; diarrhea; *epigastric pain;* hiccups; sialorrhea; *dry mouth;* bitter taste.
GU: urinary frequency, urine retention, urinary incontinence, darkened urine, excessive and inappropriate sexual behavior, priapism.
Hepatic: hepatotoxicity.
Other: dark perspiration, hyperventilation.

INTERACTIONS

Antihypertensives: additive hypotensive effects.
Papaverine, phenothiazines and other antipsychotics, phenytoin: may antagonize antiparkinsonian actions. Use together cautiously.
Sympathomimetics: increased risk of cardiac arrhythmias.

EFFECTS ON DIAGNOSTIC TESTS

BUN, ALT (SGPT), alkaline phosphatase, AST (SGOT), serum bilirubin, lactate dehydrogenase, and serum protein-bound iodine: elevated levels resulting from drug's systemic effects.
Coombs' test: occasional positive results after long-term use.
Serum gonadotropin: elevated levels.
Serum uric acid determinations: false elevations.
Urine glucose (copper sulfate method): false-positive results.
Urine glucose (glucose enzymatic method): false-negative results.
Urine ketone test (dipstick method): test interference.
Urine protein (Lowery method): false-positive results.

NURSING CONSIDERATIONS

Besides those related universally to drug therapy, (see "How to use this

book"), consider the following specific recommendations:

Assessment

• Obtain a baseline assessment of the patient's parkinsonian signs and symptoms before therapy.

• Be alert for adverse reactions and drug interactions throughout therapy.

• Evaluate the patient's and family's knowledge about levodopa-carbidopa therapy.

Nursing Diagnoses

• Impaired physical mobility related to underlying parkinsonian syndrome.

• Altered thought processes related to adverse CNS reactions to levodopa-carbidopa.

• Knowledge deficit related to levodopa-carbidopa therapy.

Planning and Implementation

Preparation and Administration

• Adjust dosage according to patient's response and tolerance.

• Withdraw MAO inhibitors at least 2 weeks before therapy.

• Administer with food to prevent GI discomfort.

• If therapy is interrupted temporarily, give the usual dosage as soon as the patient resumes oral medication.

• If patient is being treated with levodopa, discontinue at least 8 hours before starting levodopa-carbidopa.

• Keep in mind that the different ratios of levodopa-carbidopa facilitate dosage adjustments. At least 70 mg of the carbidopa component should be given daily to effectively block peripheral dopa decarboxylase.

• Be aware that carbidopa as a single agent is available from Merck Sharp & Dohme on doctor's request.

Monitoring

• Monitor effectiveness by regularly checking body movements for signs of improvement; therapeutic response usually follows each dose and disappears within 5 hours but varies considerably.

• Carefully monitor the patient who is also receiving an antihypertensive and a hypoglycemic agent.

• Monitor for signs of overdose; muscle twitching and blepharospasm (twitching of eyelids) may be early signs of drug overdosage; report them to the doctor immediately.

• Monitor for CNS and other adverse reactions, which occur more rapidly than with levodopa alone.

• During chronic therapy, regularly test the patient for diabetes and acromegaly; periodically repeat blood tests and liver and kidney function studies.

• Monitor for dystonic, choreiform, and dyskinetic movements.

• Monitor vital signs closely, especially during dosage adjustment.

Supportive Care

• Withhold dose and notify the doctor if significant changes in vital signs or mental status occur. Reduced dosage or discontinuation of levodopa-carbidopa may be necessary.

• Institute safety precautions.

• Assist the patient with daily activities as needed.

• Keep in mind that pyridoxine (vitamin B_6) does not reverse the beneficial effects of levodopa-carbidopa. Multivitamins can be taken without fear of losing control of symptoms.

• Be aware that levodopa-carbidopa combination usually reduces amount of levodopa needed by 75%, thereby reducing incidence of adverse reactions.

Patient Teaching

• Warn the patient of possible dizziness and orthostatic hypotension, especially at start of therapy. Advise patient to change position slowly and dangle legs briefly before getting out of bed. Inform the patient that elastic stockings may control this adverse reaction.

• Warn the patient and family not to increase dosage without the doctor's order.

• Instruct the patient's family to no-

tify the doctor if they notice changes in the patient's behavior or mental status.
• Advise the patient to avoid hazardous activities that require mental alertness until adverse CNS reactions are known.
• Instruct the patient to take levodopa with food.

Evaluation

In patients receiving levodopa-carbidopa, appropriate evaluation statements may include:
• Patient exhibits improved mobility with reduction of muscular rigidity and tremor.
• Patient remains mentally alert throughout levodopa-carbidopa therapy.
• Patient and family state an understanding of levodopa-carbidopa therapy.

levonorgestrel

(lee´ voe nor jess trel)
Norplant System

• *Classification:* contraceptive (progestin)
• *Pregnancy Risk Category:* X

HOW SUPPLIED

Implants: 36 mg per capsule; each kit contains six capsules

ACTION

Mechanism: Slowly releases the synthetic progestin levonorgestrel into the bloodstream. Contraceptive effect is not fully understood, but progestins alter the mucus covering the cervix, prevent implantation of the egg, and in some patients prevent ovulation.
Absorption: Slowly and steadily absorbed from the silastic capsule implant.
Distribution: Bound by the circulating protein sex hormone-binding globulin (SHBG).
Metabolism: Metabolized by the liver.
Excretion: Metabolites are excreted in the urine. Half life: 11 to 45 hours.
Onset, peak, duration: Maximum or near-maximum concentrations are reached within 24 hours of implantation. Levonorgestrel is 100% bioavailable. Plasma concentrations average 0.3 ng/ml over 5 years but are highly variable as a function of individual metabolism and body weight.

INDICATIONS & DOSAGE

Prevention of pregnancy—
Women: six capsules implanted subdermally in the midportion of the upper arm, about 8 cm above the elbow crease, during the first 7 days of the onset of menses. Capsules should be placed fanlike, 15 degrees apart (total of 75 degrees). Contraceptive efficacy lasts for 5 years.

CONTRAINDICATIONS & PRECAUTIONS

Contraindicated in women with active thrombophlebitis, thromboembolic disorders, undiagnosed abnormal genital bleeding, known or suspected pregnancy, acute liver disease, benign or malignant liver tumors, and known or suspected breast carcinoma.

Use with caution in women with cardiac or renal disease, seizure disorders, migraines, or other conditions that might be aggravated by fluid and electrolyte retention. Also use with caution in women who become significantly depressed or have a history of depression or emotional disorders, because these conditions may worsen as a result of levonorgestrel; monitor such patients closely.

ADVERSE REACTIONS

Common reactions are in italics; life-threatening reactions are in bold italics.

CNS: headache, nervousness, dizziness, change of appetite.
GI: nausea, *abdominal discomfort.*
GU: *amenorrhea, many bleeding days or prolonged bleeding, spotting, irregular onset of bleeding, frequent onset of bleeding, scanty bleeding, cervicitis, vaginitis, leukorrhea.*
Skin: dermatitis, acne, hirsutism, hypertrichosis, scalp hair loss.
Local: infection at implant site, transient pain or itching at implant site.
Other: adnexal enlargement, mastalgia, weight gain, *musculoskeletal pain, breast discharge.*

INTERACTIONS

Carbamazepine, phenytoin: may reduce the contraceptive efficacy of levonorgestrel implants.

EFFECTS ON DIAGNOSTIC TESTS

SHBG and thyroxine: decreased concentrations.
Triiodothyronine uptake: increased.

NURSING CONSIDERATIONS

Besides those related universally to drug therapy (see "How to use this book"), consider the following specific recommendations:

Assessment

- Determine patient's pregnancy status before therapy.
- Be alert for adverse reactions and drug interactions throughout therapy.
- Evaluate the patient's and family's knowledge about levonorgestrel therapy.

Nursing Diagnoses

- Pain related to levonorgestrel-induced abdominal and musculoskeletal discomfort.
- Impaired tissue integrity related to high risk for levonorgestrel-induced cervicitis and vaginitis.
- Knowledge deficit related to levonorgestrel therapy.

Planning and Implementation

Preparation and Administration

- Follow institutional guidelines for care required before and after levonorgestrel implants are performed.

Monitoring

- Monitor effectiveness by noting the patient's pregnancy status.
- Monitor patient for thromboemboli formation by noting any changes in cerebral or cardiopulmonary function or peripheral circulation.
- Monitor patient for variations in menstrual bleeding patterns.
- Monitor patient for jaundice because if it occurs, capsules will have to be removed.
- Closely monitor patients with conditions that may be aggravated by fluid retention because steroid hormones may cause fluid retention.
- Ask the patient regularly if she has experienced any abdominal or musculoskeletal discomfort or pain after drug therapy begins.

Supportive Care

- Withhold drug and notify the doctor if a thromboembolic event is suspected; be prepared to provide supportive care as indicated.
- Institute safety measures if adverse CNS reactions occur.
- Notify doctor of irregular bleeding as it may mask symptoms of cervical or endometrial cancer.
- Have a pregnancy test done as ordered if patient develops amenorrhea that lasts 6 weeks or longer.
- Prepare patient for removal of implants if pregnancy occurs, if patient develops active thrombophlebitis or thromboembolic disease, becomes immobilized for a significant length of time, or develops jaundice.
- Notify the doctor if vaginitis or cervicitis develops.
- If fluid retention occurs, limit sodium intake if not contraindicated.
- Report sudden unexplained vision problems. For example, if users of contact lenses develop vision changes

or changes in lens tolerance, they should be immediately evaluated by an ophthalmologist.
• Be aware that laboratory tests for SHBG and thyroxine concentrations may show decreased values; for triiodothyronine uptake, increased values.
Patient Teaching
• Inform patient that most patients develop variations in menstrual bleeding patterns, including irregular bleeding, prolonged bleeding, spotting, and amenorrhea. Reassure patient that these irregularities usually diminish over time. Tell patient to notify the doctor if they do not.
• Warn patients that missed menstrual periods are not an accurate indicator of early pregnancy because the drug may induce amenorrhea. Advise patients that amenorrhea that lasts 6 weeks or longer (after a pattern of regular menstrual periods) could indicate pregnancy and the doctor should be notified.
• Inform patient about the conditions that would require removal of the implants.
• Encourage patient to have regular (at least annual) physical examinations.
• Instruct patient to report to the doctor immediately if one of the implant capsules falls out (before skin heals over the implant). Contraceptive efficacy may be impaired.
• Stress the importance of reporting immediately any sudden unexplained vision problems, including those associated with contact lens use.

Evaluation
In patients receiving levonorgestrel, appropriate evaluation statements may include:
• Patient does not experience abdominal or musculoskeletal discomfort.
• Patient's vaginitis and cervicitis responds to treatment.
• Patient and family state an understanding of levonorgestrel therapy.

levorphanol tartrate
(lee vor′ fa nole)
Levo-Dromoran

• Controlled Substance Schedule II
• *Classification:* analgesic, adjunct to anesthesia (opioid)
• *Pregnancy Risk Category:* B (D for prolonged use or use of high doses at term)

HOW SUPPLIED
Tablets: 2 mg
Injection: 2 mg/ml

ACTION
Mechanism: Binds with opiate receptors at many sites in the CNS (brain, brain stem, and spinal cord), altering both perception of and emotional response to pain through an unknown mechanism.
Absorption: Well absorbed after oral or S.C. administration.
Distribution: Distributed widely throughout the body. Drug crosses the placenta and enters breast milk.
Metabolism: Primarily in the liver, where it undergoes conjugation with glucuronic acid.
Excretion: Principally in the urine as the glucuronide conjugate. Half-life: 12 to 16 hours.
Onset, peak, duration: Onset of action is 20 to 90 minutes after parenteral administration. Duration of action is 4 to 8 hours.

INDICATIONS & DOSAGE
Moderate to severe pain—
Adults: 2 to 3 mg P.O. or S.C.

CONTRAINDICATIONS & PRECAUTIONS
Contraindicated in patients with hypersensitivity to the drug or other phenanthrene opioids (codeine, hydrocodone, morphine, oxymorphone, or oxycodone).

Use with extreme caution in patients with supraventricular arrhythmias; avoid or use drug with extreme caution in patients with head injury or increased intracranial pressure because drug obscures neurologic parameters; and during pregnancy and labor because drug readily crosses placenta (premature infants are especially sensitive to respiratory and CNS depressant effects).

Also use cautiously in patients with renal or hepatic dysfunction because drug accumulation or prolonged duration of action may occur; in patients with pulmonary disease (asthma, chronic obstructive pulmonary disease) because drug depresses respiration and suppresses cough reflex; in patients undergoing biliary tract surgery because drug may cause biliary spasm; in patients with seizure disorders because drug may precipitate seizures; in elderly or debilitated patients, who are more sensitive to this drug's effects; and in patients prone to physical or psychological addiction because of the high risk of addiction to this drug.

ADVERSE REACTIONS

Common reactions are in italics; life-threatening reactions are in bold italics.

CNS: *sedation, somnolence, clouded sensorium,* dizziness, *euphoria,* seizures with large doses.

CV: *hypotension,* bradycardia.

GI: *nausea, vomiting, constipation,* ileus.

GU: urine retention.

Other: ***respiratory depression,*** physical dependence.

INTERACTIONS

Alcohol, CNS depressants: additive effects. Use together cautiously.

EFFECTS ON DIAGNOSTIC TESTS

Plasma amylase: increased levels.

NURSING CONSIDERATIONS

Besides those related universally to drug therapy (see "How to use this book"), consider the following specific recommendations:

Assessment

Obtain a baseline assessment of the patient's pain before therapy.

- Be alert for adverse reactions and drug interactions throughout therapy.
- Evaluate the patient's and family's knowledge about levorphanol therapy.

Nursing Diagnoses

- Pain related to patient's underlying condition.
- Ineffective breathing pattern related to levorphanol-induced respiratory depression.
- Knowledge deficit related to levorphanol therapy.

Planning and Implementation

Preparation and Administration

- Reduce levorphanol dose, as ordered, if used with other narcotic analgesics, general anesthetics, tranquilizers, alcohol, sedatives, hypnotics, tricyclic antidepressants, or MAO inhibitors because such use increases CNS depression. Use together with extreme caution, and monitor patient response.
- For better analgesic effect, administer before patient has intense pain.
- Protect drug from light.

Monitoring

- Monitor effectiveness by evaluating degree of pain relief.
- Monitor for evidence of respiratory depression, such as decreased rate or depth of respirations.
- Monitor circulatory status and bowel function.

Supportive Care

- Notify the doctor if pain is not relieved.
- Notify the doctor if the patient's rate of respirations is below 12/minute.
- Keep narcotic antagonist (naloxone) available.
- When used postoperatively, encour-

age turning, coughing, and deep breathing to avoid atelectasis.

Patient Teaching

• Tell the patient or family caregiver to notify the doctor if respiration rate decreases or if other adverse reactions develop.
• Warn patient that drug has bitter taste.
• Warn ambulatory patient to avoid hazardous activities that require alertness.
• Tell patient to request medication before pain becomes intense.

Evaluation

In patients receiving levorphanol, appropriate evaluation statements may include:

• Patient reports relief of pain after administration of levorphanol.
• Patient's respiratory rate and pattern are within normal limits after administration of levorphanol.
• Patient and family state an understanding of levorphanol therapy.

levothyroxine sodium (T_4 or L-thyroxine sodium)

(lee voe thye rox´ een)

Eltroxin†, Levoid, Levothroid, Levoxine, Oroxine‡, Synthroid**, Synthrox

• *Classification:* thyroid hormone replacement agent (thyroid hormone)
• *Pregnancy Risk Category:* A

HOW SUPPLIED

Tablets: 25 mcg, 50 mcg, 75 mcg, 100 mcg, 112 mcg, 125 mcg, 150 mcg, 175 mcg, 200 mcg, 300 mcg
Injection: 200 mcg/vial, 500 mcg/vial

ACTION

Mechanism: Stimulates the metabolism of all body tissues by accelerating the rate of cellular metabolism.
Absorption: About 50% to 80% is absorbed from the GI tract. After I.M. administration, absorption is variable and poor.
Distribution: Not fully described; however, the drug is distributed into most body tissues and fluids, with highest levels in the liver and kidneys. Levothyroxine is 99% protein-bound.
Metabolism: Metabolized in peripheral tissues, primarily in the liver, kidneys, and intestines. About 85% of metabolized levothyroxine is deiodinated.
Excretion: Fecal excretion eliminates 20% to 40% of levothyroxine. Half-life: 6 to 7 days.
Onset, peak, duration: Full effects occur 1 to 3 weeks after oral therapy begins. After an I.V. dose in patients with myxedema coma, increased responsiveness may occur within 6 to 8 hours, but maximum therapeutic effect may not occur for up to 24 hours.

INDICATIONS & DOSAGE

Cretinism–
Children under 1 year: initially, 0.025 to 0.05 mg P.O. daily, increased by 0.05 mg P.O. q 2 to 3 weeks to total daily dosage of 0.1 to 0.4 mg P.O.
Myxedema coma–
Adults: 0.2 to 0.5 mg I.V. If no response in 24 hours, additional 0.1 to 0.3 mg I.V. After condition stabilized, oral maintenance.
Thyroid hormone replacement–
Adults: initially, 0.025 to 0.1 mg P.O. daily, increased by 0.05 to 0.1 mg P.O. q 1 to 4 weeks until desired response. Maintenance dosage is 0.1 to 0.4 mg daily. May be administered I.V. or I.M. when P.O. ingestion is precluded for long periods.
Adults over 65 years: 0.025 mg P.O. daily. May be increased by 0.025 mg at 3- to 4-week intervals depending on response.
Children: initially, maximum 0.05 mg P.O. daily, gradually increased by

0.025 to 0.05 mg P.O. q 1 to 4 weeks until desired response.

CONTRAINDICATIONS & PRECAUTIONS

Contraindicated in patients with thyrotoxicosis, acute myocardial infarction, and uncorrected adrenal insufficiency because drug increases tissue metabolic demands; and for treating obesity because it is ineffective and can cause life-threatening adverse reactions.

Use cautiously in patients with angina or other cardiovascular disease because of the risk of increased metabolic demands; diabetes mellitus because of reduced glucose tolerance; malabsorption states because of decreased absorption; and long-standing hypothyroidism or myxedema because these patients may be more sensitive to the drug's effects.

ADVERSE REACTIONS

Common reactions are in italics; life-threatening reactions are in bold italics.

Adverse reactions of thyroid hormones are extensions of their pharmacologic properties and reflect patient sensitivity to them.

Signs of overdosage:

CNS: *nervousness, insomnia, tremor.*

CV: *tachycardia, palpitations, arrhythmias, angina pectoris,* hypertension.

GI: change in appetite, nausea, diarrhea.

Other: headache, leg cramps, weight loss, sweating, heat intolerance, fever, menstrual irregularities.

INTERACTIONS

Cholestyramine and colestipol: levothyroxine absorption impaired. Separate doses by 4 to 5 hours.

I.V. phenytoin: free thyroid released. Monitor for tachycardia.

EFFECTS ON DIAGNOSTIC TESTS

Radioactive iodine (^{131}I) thyroid uptake, protein-bound iodine levels, and liothyronine uptake: altered results.

NURSING CONSIDERATIONS

Besides those related universally to drug therapy, (see "How to use this book"), consider the following specific recommendations:

Assessment

- Obtain a baseline assessment of the patient's thyroid status before therapy.
- Be alert for adverse reactions and drug interactions throughout therapy.
- Evaluate the patient's and family's knowledge about levothyroxine therapy.

Nursing Diagnoses

- High risk for activity intolerance related to the patient's underlying condition.
- Decreased cardiac output related to high risk for adverse CV reactions.
- Knowledge deficit related to levothyroxine therapy.

Planning and Implementation

Preparation and Administration

- Be aware that when changing from levothyroxine to liothyronine, the doctor will stop levothyroxine and begin liothyronine. Liothyronine will be increased in small increments after residual effects of levothyroxine have disappeared. When changing from liothyronine to levothyroxine, the doctor will start levothyroxine several days before withdrawing liothyronine to avoid relapse.
- ***I.V. use:*** Prepare I.V. dose immediately before injection. Do not mix with other I.V. solutions. Inject into vein over 1 to 2 minutes.
- ***P.O. use:*** Administer as a single dose before breakfast.
- Protect drug from moisture and light.

Monitoring

- Monitor effectiveness by regularly checking thyroid function studies and

assessing the patient for signs and symptoms of thyroid dysfunction.
- Monitor the patient for signs of overdosage.
- Monitor the patient's temperature, pulse rate, and blood pressure regularly for alterations such as fever, tachycardia, or hypertension.
- Monitor the patient with a history of lactose intolerance, who may be sensitive to Levothroid, which contains lactose.
- Monitor for hypersensitivity. Synthroid 100- and 300-mcg tablets contain tartrazine, a dye that causes allergic reactions in susceptible individuals.

Supportive Care
- Withhold drug and notify the doctor if the patient develops signs of overdosage. Be prepared to treat overdosage with antithyroid drugs.
- Assist the patient with activities as needed until a euthyroid state is achieved.
- Obtain an order for an antiemetic or antidiarrheal agent, as needed.
- Administer a mild analgesic as prescribed if drug-induced headache occurs.
- Keep the patient dry if profuse sweating occurs.

Patient Teaching
- Instruct the patient to take the medication at the same time each day; encourage morning dosing to avoid insomnia.
- Tell the patient to notify doctor if he experiences headache, diarrhea, nervousness, excessive sweating, heat intolerance, chest pain, increased pulse rate, or palpitations.
- Advise the patient not to store the drug in warm, humid areas, such as the bathroom, to prevent deterioration of the drug.
- Tell the patient who has achieved a stable response not to change product brands, because they are not all bioequivalent.
- Warn female patients that levothyroxine may cause menstrual irregularities.
- Stress the importance of taking the drug exactly as prescribed and of receiving follow-up care.

Evaluation

In patients receiving levothyroxine, appropriate evaluation statements may include:
- Patient is able to perform self-care and other activities without becoming overtired.
- Patient does not exhibit signs and symptoms of cardiac problems.
- Patient and family state an understanding of levothyroxine therapy.

lidocaine hydrochloride (lignocaine hydrochloride)

(lye´ doe kane)

Lido Pen Auto-Injector, Xylocaine, Xylocard†‡

- *Classification:* ventricular antiarrhythmic, local anesthetic (amide derivative)
- *Pregnancy Risk Category:* B

HOW SUPPLIED

Injection (for direct I.V. use): 1% (10 mg/ml) in 5-ml (50-mg), 10-ml (100-mg) syringes; 2% (20 mg/ml) in 5-ml (100-mg) vials, syringes, and ampules
Injection (for I.M. use): 10% (100 mg/ml) in 3-ml automatic injection device or 5-ml ampules
Injection (for I.V. admixtures): 4% (40 mg/ml) in 25-ml (1-g) vials and syringes and 50-ml (2-g) vials and syringes; 10% (100 mg/ml) in 10-ml (1-g) vials; 20% (200 mg/ml) in 5-ml (1-g) vials and syringes and 10-ml (2-g) vials and syringes
Infusion (premixed): 0.2% (2 mg/ml) in 500-ml vials; 0.4% (4 mg/ml) in 250-ml, 500-ml, 1,000-ml vials; 0.8% (8 mg/ml) in 250-ml, 500-ml vials

ACTION

Mechanism: A local anesthetic, lidocaine is a class Ib antiarrhythmic that depresses phase O. It shortens the action potential. All class I drugs have membrane stabilizing effects.
Absorption: Not effective orally because most of the drug is metabolized by the liver before reaching the systemic circulation (first-pass effect); usually administered I.V.; when given I.M., highest peak plasma levels are seen after injection into the deltoid muscle.
Distribution: Widely distributed throughout the body; high affinity for adipose tissue. After I.V. bolus administration, an early, rapid decline in plasma levels occurs; this is associated mainly with distribution into highly perfused tissues, such as the kidneys, lungs, liver, and heart, followed by a slower elimination phase in which metabolism and redistribution into skeletal muscle and adipose tissue occur. The first (early) distribution phase occurs rapidly, calling for initiation of a constant infusion after an initial bolus dose. Distribution volume declines in patients with liver or hepatic disease, resulting in toxic concentrations with usual doses. About 60% to 80% of circulating drug is bound to plasma proteins. Usual therapeutic drug level is 1.5 to 5 mcg/ml. Although toxicity may occur within this range, levels higher than 5 mcg/ml are considered toxic and warrant dosage reduction.
Metabolism: Hepatic conversion to two active metabolites. Metabolism is affected by hepatic blood flow, which may decrease after myocardial infarction and with CHF or liver disease.
Excretion: Metabolites are excreted by the kidneys; less than 3% of a dose is excreted unchanged. in the urine. Half-life: Elimination is biphasic, with an initial phase of 7 to 30 minutes followed by a terminal half-life of 1½ to 2 hours; may be prolonged in patients with CHF or liver disease. Continuous infusions longer than 24 hours also may cause an apparent half-life increase.
Onset, peak, duration: Immediate onset (30 to 90 seconds) after I.V. bolus administration and a brief duration (10 to 20 minutes). After I.M. injection, onset is slower (5 to 15 minutes) and duration is longer (up to 2 hours).

INDICATIONS & DOSAGE

Ventricular arrhythmias from myocardial infarction, cardiac manipulation, or cardiac glycosides; ventricular tachycardia –
Adults: 50 to 100 mg (1 to 1.5 mg/kg) I.V. bolus at 25 to 50 mg/minute. Give half this amount to elderly patients or patients under 50 kg, and to those with CHF or hepatic disease. Repeat bolus q 3 to 5 minutes until arrhythmias subside or adverse reactions develop. Don't exceed 300-mg total bolus during a 1-hour period. Simultaneously, begin constant infusion of 1 to 4 mg/minute. If single bolus has been given, repeat smaller bolus 15 to 20 minutes after start of infusion to maintain therapeutic serum level. After 24 hours of continuous infusion, decrease rate by half.
I.M. administration: 200 to 300 mg in deltoid muscle only.
Children: 1mg/kg by I.V. bolus, followed by infusion of 30 mcg/kg/minute.

CONTRAINDICATIONS & PRECAUTIONS

Contraindicated in patients with Stokes-Adams syndrome or severe degrees of sinoatrial, atrioventricular, or intraventricular heart block who do not have an artificial pacemaker, because the drug may worsen these conditions; and in patients with hypersensitivity to this drug or other amide-type anesthetic agents; in patients with inflammation or infection in puncture region, septicemia, severe hypertension, spinal deformities, and neurologic disorders. Use cautiously in debilitated, elderly, acutely ill, or obstetric patients; and in those with severe shock, heart block, general drug allergies, and paracervical block; in patients with Wolff-Parkinson-White syndrome, bradycardia, or incomplete heart block because the drug may exacerbate these conditions and precipitate other serious arrhythmias; and in patients with atrial fibrillation because the drug may increase the ventricular rate.

ADVERSE REACTIONS

Common reactions are in italics; life-threatening reactions are in bold italics.
CNS: *confusion, tremors,* lethargy, somnolence, *stupor, restlessness,* slurred speech, euphoria, depression, *light-headedness,* paresthesias, muscle twitching, *seizures.*
CV: *hypotension,* bradycardia, further arrhythmias.
EENT: *tinnitus, blurred or double vision.*
Other: ***anaphylaxis,*** soreness at injection site, sensations of cold, diaphoresis.

INTERACTIONS

Cimetidine, beta blockers: decreased metabolism of lidocaine. Monitor for toxicity.
Phenytoin: additive cardiac depressant effects. Monitor carefully.

EFFECTS ON DIAGNOSTIC TESTS

CPK: increased levels after I.M. use. Isoenzyme tests should be performed for differential diagnosis of acute myocardial infarction.

NURSING CONSIDERATIONS

Besides those related universally to drug therapy (see "How to use this book"), consider the following specific recommendations:

Assessment

- Obtain a baseline assessment of the patient's heart rate and rhythm before therapy.
- Be alert for adverse reactions and drug interactions throughout therapy.
- Evaluate the patient's and family's knowledge about lidocaine therapy.

Nursing Diagnoses

- Decreased cardiac output related to ineffectiveness of lidocaine therapy.
- Altered thought processes related to lidocaine-induced confusion.
- Knowledge deficit related to lidocaine therapy.

Planning and Implementation

Preparation and Administration

- Be aware that patients over age 65 should initially receive half the recommended dosage.
- Do not use lidocaine with epinephrine (for local anesthesia) to treat arrhythmias.
- ***I.M. use:*** Administer drug in deltoid muscle only.
- ***I.V. use:*** Administer an I.V. bolus slowly (no faster than 25 to 50 mg/minute). Expect to give drug I.V. push q 3 to 5 minutes until arrhythmia has disappeared or adverse reactions develop. Be aware that a bolus dose not followed by infusion will have a transient effect. Administer continuous infusion at a rate that does not exceed 4 mg/minute as ordered because a faster rate increases risk of toxicity. Use an infusion pump to administer the dose precisely. Attend patients receiving an infusion at all times and keep on a cardiac monitor.

Monitoring

- Monitor effectiveness by frequently assessing ECG recording.
- Monitor patient for toxicity. In many severely ill patients, seizures may be the first sign of toxicity. However, severe reactions usually are preceded by somnolence, confusion, and paresthesias.

• Monitor serum electrolyte, BUN, and creatinine levels.
• Monitor serum lidocaine levels, if indicated. Normal therapeutic blood levles are 2 to 5 mcg/ml.
Supportive Care
• If ECG disturbances occur, withhold the drug, obtain a rhythm strip, and notify the doctor immediately.
• Keep emergency equipment nearby.
• Maintain seizure precautions.
• If signs of toxicity occur, stop administration at once and notify the doctor. Continued infusion could lead to seizures and coma. Give oxygen via nasal cannula, if not contraindicated.
• Institute safety precautions if adverse CNS reactions occur.
Patient Teaching
• Inform the patient that continuous ECG monitoring is required during lidocaine therapy.

Evaluation
In patients receiving lidocaine, appropriate evaluation statements may include:
• Patient's ECG reveals arrhythmia has been corrected.
• Patient remains alert and oriented to person, place, and time throughout lidocaine therapy.
• Patient and family state an understanding of lidocaine therapy.

lidocaine hydrochloride (lignocaine hydrochloride)
(lye´ doe kane)
Caine-2, Dalcaine, Dilocaine, Duo-Trach Kit, Lidoject-2, Nervocaine 2%, Octocaine, Xylocaine

• *Classification:* local anesthetic (amide derivative)
• *Pregnancy Risk Category:* B

HOW SUPPLIED
Injection: 2%, 4%, 10%, 20%
Injection (with dextrose 7.5%): 1.5%, 5%
Injection (with epinephrine 1:50,000): 2% (for dental use)
Injection (with epinephrine 1:100,000): 1%, 2%
Injection (with epinephrine 1:200,000): 1%, 1.5%, 2%

ACTION
Mechanism: Blocks depolarization by interfering with sodium-potassium exchange across the nerve cell membrane, preventing generation and conduction of the nerve impulse. When combined with epinephrine, action is prolonged because epinephrine restricts blood flow to the area, preventing metabolism or absorption of the drug.
Absorption: Rapidly absorbed from parenteral administration sites.
Distribution: Rapidly distributes to the tissues; protein binding is both variable and concentration-dependent. Drug crosses the placenta.
Metabolism: In the liver.
Excretion: In the urine, mostly as metabolites.
Onset, peak, duration: When used as a 2% solution without epinephrine, a lumbar epidural block will last about 100 minutes. When used as a caudal block, duration is 75 to 150 minutes.

INDICATIONS & DOSAGE
Doses cited are for drug without *epinephrine except where indicated.*
For anesthesia other than spinal–
maximum single adult dose is 4.5 mg/kg or 300 mg.
With epinephrine for anesthesia other than spinal–
maximum single adult dose is 7 mg/kg or 500 mg. Don't repeat dose more often than q 2 hours.

Caudal (obstetrics) or epidural (thoracic):

Sol.	Vol. (ml)	Dose (mg)
1%	20 to 30	200 to 300

Caudal (surgery):

Sol.	Vol. (ml)	Dose (mg)
1.5%	15 to 20	225 to 300

Epidural (lumbar anesthesia):

Sol.	Vol. (ml)	Dose (mg)
1.5%	15 to 20	225 to 300
2%	10 to 15	200 to 300

Maximum dose 200 to 300 mg/hour.

Spinal surgical anesthesia:

Sol.	Vol. (ml)	Dose (mg)
5% with 7.5% dextrose	1.5 to 2	75 to 100

Dosage and interval are increased with epinephrine.

For anesthesia other than spinal–maximum single adult dose is 4.5 mg/kg or 300 mg.

With epinephrine for anesthesia other than spinal–maximum single adult dose is 7 mg/kg or 500 mg. Don't repeat dose more often than q 2 hours.

CONTRAINDICATIONS & PRECAUTIONS

Contraindicated in patients with hypersensitivity to the drug or other amide-type anesthetics; in patients with inflammation or infection in puncture region, septicemia, severe hypertension, spinal deformities, and neurologic disorders. Use cautiously in debilitated, elderly, acutely ill, or obstetric patients; in those with severe shock or heart block; and in atopic individuals.

ADVERSE REACTIONS

Common reactions are in italics; life-threatening reactions are in bold italics.

Skin: dermatologic reactions.

Other: edema, ***status asthmaticus, anaphylaxis,*** anaphylactoid reactions.

The following systemic effects may result from high blood levels of the drug:

CNS: anxiety, nervousness, seizures followed by drowsiness, unconsciousness, tremors, twitches, shivering, ***respiratory arrest.***

CV: myocardial depression, ***arrhythmias, cardiac arrest.***

EENT: blurred vision, tinnitus.

GI: nausea, vomiting.

INTERACTIONS

Enflurane, halothane, isoflurane, and related drugs: cardiac arrhythmias when used with lidocaine *with* epinephrine. Use with extreme caution.

MAO inhibitors, cyclic antidepressants: severe, sustained hypertension when used with lidocaine *with* epinephrine. Use with extreme caution.

EFFECTS ON DIAGNOSTIC TESTS

None reported.

NURSING CONSIDERATIONS

Besides those related universally to drug therapy (see "How to use this book"), consider the following specific recommendations:

Assessment

- Obtain a baseline assessment of the patient's sensory status status before therapy.
- Be alert for adverse reactions and drug interactions throughout therapy.
- Evaluate the patient's and family's knowledge about lidocaine therapy.

Nursing Diagnoses

- Pain related to inadequate block.
- Decreased cardiac output related to adverse reaction to lidocaine.
- Knowledge deficit related to lidocaine therapy.

Planning and Implementation

Preparation and Administration

- Use solutions with epinephrine cautiously in cardiovascular disorders and in body areas with limited blood supply (ears, nose, fingers, toes).
- ***Epidural use:*** Be aware that for epidural use, test doses are administered to verify needle or catheter placement. Initially, 2 to 3 ml is given to

check for subarachnoid injection (which would cause extensive motor paralysis of the lower limbs and extensive sensory deficit). After about 5 minutes and in the absence of symptoms, a second, larger test dose of about 5 ml is given to check for intravascular injection (which would cause tinnitus, numbness around the lips, metallic taste, dysphoria, lethargy, or hypotension).
• Don't use solution with preservative for spinal, caudal, or epidural block.
• Discard partially used vials without preservatives.
• Check solution for particles.

Monitoring
• Monitor effectiveness by evaluating pain relief. Continue to monitor sensory level every 15 minutes after completion of surgery or treatment until sympathetic innervation returns.
• Monitor for signs of anaphylaxis after administration of drug.
• Monitor for signs of myocardial depression, respiratory depression, seizures, and other adverse reactions that may result from high blood levels of the drug.

Supportive Care
• Keep resuscitative equipment and drugs available.
• Consult with the doctor if pain relief is ineffective.
• Notify the doctor immediately if the patient's CNS, cardiac, or respiratory status deteriorates.

Patient Teaching
• Explain that the drug will cause a local loss of sensation providing pain relief in the selected body area, but, unlike general anesthetics, will not cause unconsciousness.
• Describe the route of administration, such as epidural, caudal, or spinal.

Evaluation
In patients receiving lidocaine, appropriate evaluation statements include:
• Patient experiences adequate anesthesia.
• Patient's cardiac status remains within normal limits.
• Patient and family state an understanding of lidocaine therapy.

lincomycin hydrochloride
(lin koe mye´ sin)
Lincocin

• *Classification:* antibiotic (lincosamide)
• *Pregnancy Risk Category:* B

HOW SUPPLIED
Capsules: 500 mg
Pediatric capsules: 250 mg
Syrup: 250 mg/5 ml
Injection: 300 mg/ml in 2-ml and 10-ml vials and 2-ml U-Ject

ACTION
Mechanism: Inhibits bacterial protein synthesis by binding to the 50S subunit of the ribosome.
Absorption: With oral administration, only about 20% to 30% of dose is absorbed; food delays and decreases absorption.
Distribution: Distributed in pleural fluid, synovial fluid, peritoneal fluid, bone, bile, and aqueous humor. CSF penetration is poor. Plasma protein-binding is concentration-dependent and ranges from about 57% to 72%.
Metabolism: Partially metabolized in the liver.
Excretion: Primarily by the kidneys and liver; some is also excreted in breast milk. Half-life: 4 to 6 hours in patients with normal renal function; may be prolonged in patients with impaired renal or hepatic function.
Onset, peak, duration: Peak levels occur within 2 hours after oral administration and within 30 minutes after I.M. injection; after I.V. administration, slightly less than for I.M.

INDICATIONS & DOSAGE

Respiratory tract, skin and soft tissue, and urinary tract infections; osteomyelitis, septicemia caused by sensitive group A beta-hemolytic streptococci, pneumococci, and staphylococci –

Adults: 500 mg P.O. q 6 to 8 hours (not to exceed 8 g daily); or 600 mg I.M. daily or q 12 hours; or 600 mg to 1 g I.V. q 8 to 12 hours (not to exceed 8 g daily).

Children over 1 month: 30 to 60 mg/kg P.O. daily, divided q 6 to 8 hours; or 10 mg/kg I.M. daily or divided q 12 hours; or 10 to 20 mg/kg I.V. daily, divided q 6 to 8 hours. For I.V. infusion, dilute to 100 ml; infuse over 1 hour to avoid hypotension.

CONTRAINDICATIONS & PRECAUTIONS

Contraindicated in patients with hypersensitivity to lincomycin or clindamycin. Use cautiously in atopic patients because of potential for allergic reactions; in patients with preexisting hepatic disease because the drug may cause cholestatic jaundice; and in those with a history of colitis because the drug may cause pseudomembranous colitis.

ADVERSE REACTIONS

Common reactions are in italics; life-threatening reactions are in bold italics.

Blood: *neutropenia, leukopenia,* thrombocytopenic purpura.

CNS: dizziness, headache.

CV: hypotension with rapid I.V. infusion.

EENT: glossitis, tinnitus.

GI: nausea, vomiting, ***pseudomembranous colitis,*** *persistent diarrhea,* abdominal cramps, stomatitis, pruritus ani.

GU: vaginitis.

Hepatic: cholestatic jaundice.

Skin: rashes, urticaria.

Local: pain at injection site.

Other: ***hypersensitivity,*** angioedema.

INTERACTIONS

Antidiarrheal medication (kaolin, pectin, attapulgite): reduce oral absorption of lincomycin by as much as 90%. Antidiarrheals should be avoided or given at least 2 hours before lincomycin.

Neuromuscular blocking agents: lincomycin may potentiate neuromuscular blockade.

EFFECTS ON DIAGNOSTIC TESTS

CBC: decreased counts.

Liver function tests: abnormal results.

NURSING CONSIDERATIONS

Besides those related universally to drug therapy (see "How to use this book"), consider the following specific recommendations:

Assessment

- Obtain a baseline assessment of infection before therapy.
- Be alert for adverse reactions and drug interactions throughout therapy.
- Evaluate the patient's and family's knowledge about lincomycin therapy.

Nursing Diagnoses

- High risk for injury related to ineffectiveness of lincomycin to eradicate the infection.
- High risk for fluid volume deficit related to lincomycin-induced adverse GI reactions.
- Knowledge deficit related to lincomycin therapy.

Planning and Implementation

Preparation and Administration

- Obtain specimen for culture and sensitivity tests before first dose. Therapy may begin pending test results.
- ***P.O. use:*** Administer drug with a full glass of water 1 hour before or 2 hours after meals to enhance absorption.
- ***I.M. use:*** Give deep I.M. Rotate sites. Be aware that injection may be painful.
- ***I.V. use:*** Administer as an infusion.

Do not administer rapidly because it may result in hypotension and syncope. Dilute drug with 100 to 400 ml of dextrose 5% or 10% in water, 0.9% sodium chloride, or Ringer's lactate. Solution remains stable for 24 hours at room temperature.

Monitoring

• Monitor effectiveness by regularly assessing for improvement in the infection.
• Monitor patient's blood pressure when administering drug parenterally.
• Monitor hydration status if adverse GI reactions occur.
• Monitor hepatic function as well as CBC and platelets.
• Monitor for signs of bacterial and fungal superinfection, especially when therapy exceeds 10 days.
• When giving drug I.V. monitor site daily for phlebitis and irritation.

Supportive Care

• Obtain an order for an antiemetic or antidiarrheal agent as needed. Don't give diphenoxylate compound (Lomotil) to treat drug-induced diarrhea. May prolong and worsen diarrhea.
• Discontinue drug immediately if neutropenia, leukopenia, or other blood disorders develop.
• Rotate I.V. infusion sites regularly.

Patient Teaching

• Advise patient taking oral form to take with a full glass of water 1 hour before or 2 hours after meals.
• Tell the patient to take medication for as long as prescribed, exactly as directed, and even after feeling better and to take entire amount prescribed.
• Warn patient that I.M. injection may be painful.
• Instruct patient to report diarrhea and to avoid self-treatment.
• Advise patient to tell the nurse promptly about any discomfort at the infusion site.

Evaluation

In patients receiving lincomycin, appropriate evaluation statements may include:

• Patient is free from infection.
• Patient maintains adequate hydration throughout lincomycin therapy.
• Patient and family state an understanding of lincomycin therapy.

lindane

(lin´ dane)

gBh†, Kwell, Kwellada†, Scabene

• *Classification:* scabicide, pediculicide (chlorinated hydrocarbon)
• *Pregnancy Risk Category:* C

HOW SUPPLIED

Cream: 1%
Lotion: 1%
Shampoo: 1%

ACTION

Mechanism: Appears to inhibit neuronal membrane function in arthropods, causing seizures and death. A cyclic chlorinated hydrocarbon originally developed as an agricultural pesticide.
Absorption: Slowly and incompletely absorbed through intact skin. 10% of topical dose may be absorbed in 24 hours.
Distribution: Stored in body fat.
Metabolism: In the liver.
Excretion: In urine and feces.

INDICATIONS & DOSAGE

Parasitic infestation (scabies, pediculosis)–

Adults and children: scrub entire body with soap and water.
Cream or lotion–apply thin layer over entire skin surface (with special attention to folds, creases, interdigital spaces, and genital area) for scabies, or to hairy areas for pediculosis. Af-

ter 12 hours, wash off drug. If second application is needed, wait 1 week before repeating, but never more than twice in a week.
Shampoo—apply 30 ml undiluted to affected area and work into lather for 4 to 5 minutes. Rinse thoroughly and rub with dry towel.

CONTRAINDICATIONS & PRECAUTIONS

Contraindicated in patients with sensitivity to the drug. Use cautiously in pregnant women, because drug can be absorbed systemically. Avoid contact with face, eyes and mucous membranes, and urethral meatus. Because drug can be absorbed through the skin, the potential for CNS toxicity exists; therefore, use cautiously in children.

ADVERSE REACTIONS

Common reactions are in italics; life-threatening reactions are in bold italics.
CNS: dizziness, seizures.
Skin: *irritation* with repeated use.

INTERACTIONS

None significant.

EFFECTS ON DIAGNOSTIC TESTS

None reported.

NURSING CONSIDERATIONS

Besides those related universally to drug therapy (see "How to use this book"), consider the following specific recommendations:

Assessment

- Obtain a baseline assessment of skin and genital area before therapy.
- Be alert for adverse reactions throughout therapy.
- Evaluate the patient's and family's knowledge about lindane therapy.

Nursing Diagnoses

- Body image disturbance related to patient's underlying condition.
- Altered (cerebral) tissue perfusion related to lindane-induced adverse CNS reactions.
- Knowledge deficit related to lindane therapy.

Planning and Implementation

Preparation and Administration

- ***Topical use:*** Apply thin layer over entire skin surface (with special attention to folds, creases, interdigital spaces, and genital area) for scabies, or to hairy areas for pediculosis. After 12 hours, wash off drug. If second application is needed, wait 1 week before repeating, but don't repeat more than twice in a week.
- Shampoo—apply undiluted to affected area and work into lather for 4 or 5 minutes. Rinse thoroughly.

Monitoring

- Monitor effectiveness by examining skin and genital area for mites and irritation.
- Monitor skin for irritation or hypersensitivity; if it develops, tell patient to discontinue drug and to wash it off skin.
- Monitor for adverse reactions by observing the patient for dizziness or seizures.

Supportive Care

- Do not apply to open areas or acutely inflamed skin, or to face, eyes, mucous membranes, or urethral meatus. If accidental contact with eyes does occur, flush with water and notify doctor. Avoid inhaling vapors.
- Obtain an order for topical corticosteroids or oral antihistamines if itching becomes severe.
- After application, use a fine comb dipped in white vinegar to remove nits from hair.
- Hospitalized patients should be placed in isolation with special linen-handling precautions until treatment is completed.
- While assisting the patient with self-care, encourage him to express fears and concerns about body image disturbance.
- Be cautious; this drug is extremely

toxic to CNS if accidentally swallowed.

Patient Teaching

- Teach patient to apply medication.
- Inform patient that repeated use can lead to skin irritation and systemic toxicity. Repeat only if live lice or nits are found after 1 week.
- Warn patient that itching may continue for several weeks after effective treatment, especially in scabies.
- Instruct patient to change and sterilize (boil, launder, dry clean, or apply very hot iron) all clothing and bed linen after drug is washed off, and to wash combs and brushes thoroughly after cleaning them with lindane shampoo.
- Warn patient not to use lindane shampoo routinely to clean combs or brushes.
- Instruct patient to reapply if drug is washed off during treatment.

Evaluation

In patients receiving lindane, appropriate evaluation statements may include:

- Patient states that body image disturbance has been resolved.
- Patient does not develop drug-induced adverse CNS reactions.
- Patient and family state an understanding of lindane therapy.

liothyronine sodium (T_3)

(lye oh thye´ roe neen)

Cyronine, Cytomel, Tertroxin‡

- *Classification:* thyroid hormone replacement agent (thyroid hormone)
- *Pregnancy Risk Category:* A

HOW SUPPLIED

Tablets: 5 mcg, 25 mcg, 50 mcg

ACTION

Mechanism: Stimulates the metabolism of all body tissues by accelerating the rate of cellular metabolism.
Absorption: Approximately 95% absorbed from the GI tract.
Distribution: Highly protein-bound.
Metabolism: Not fully understood.
Excretion: Half-life: 1 to 2 days.
Onset, peak, duration: Peak effect occurs within 24 to 72 hours.

INDICATIONS & DOSAGE

Cretinism–
Children 3 years and older: 50 to 100 mcg P.O. daily.
Children under 3 years: 5 mcg P.O. daily, increased by 5 mcg q 3 to 4 days until desired response occurs.
Myxedema–
Adults: initially, 5 mcg P.O. daily, increased by 5 to 10 mcg q 1 or 2 weeks. Maintenance dosage is 50 to 100 mcg daily.
Nontoxic goiter–
Adults: initially, 5 mcg P.O. daily; may be increased by 12.5 to 25 mcg daily q 1 to 2 weeks. Usual maintenance dosage is 75 mcg daily.
Adults over 65 years: initially, 5 mcg P.O. daily, increased by 5-mcg increments at weekly intervals until desired response.
Children: initially, 5 mcg P.O. daily, increased by 5-mcg increments at weekly intervals until desired response.
Thyroid hormone replacement–
Adults: initially, 25 mcg P.O. daily, increased by 12.5 to 25 mcg q 1 to 2 weeks until satisfactory response. Usual maintenance dosage is 25 to 75 mcg daily.
T_3 suppression test to differentiate hyperthyroidism from euthyroidism–
Adults: 75 to 100 mcg P.O. daily for 7 days.

CONTRAINDICATIONS & PRECAUTIONS

Contraindicated in patients with thyrotoxicosis, acute myocardial infarction, and uncorrected adrenal insufficiency because the drug increases tissue metabolic demands; and for treatment of obesity because it is ineffective and can cause life-threatening adverse reactions.

Use cautiously in patients with angina or other cardiovascular disease because of the risk of increased metabolic demands; diabetes mellitus because of reduced glucose tolerance; malabsorption states caused by decreased absorption; and long-standing hypothyroidism or myxedema because these patients may be more sensitive to the drug's effects.

ADVERSE REACTIONS

Common reactions are in italics; life-threatening reactions are in bold italics.

Adverse reactions of thyroid hormones are extensions of their pharmacologic properties and reflect patient sensitivity to them.

CNS: hyperirritability, *nervousness, insomnia,* twitching, *tremors,* headache.
CV: increased cardiac output, *tachycardia,* cardiac arrhythmias, *angina pectoris,* increased blood pressure, ***cardiac decompensation and collapse.***
GI: diarrhea, abdominal cramps, vomiting.
Other: weight loss, heat intolerance, hyperhidrosis, menstrual irregularities; in infants and children—accelerated rate of bone maturation.

INTERACTIONS

Cholestyramine and colestipol: liothyronine absorption impaired. Separate doses by 4 to 5 hours.
I.V. phenytoin: free thyroid released. Monitor for tachycardia.

EFFECTS ON DIAGNOSTIC TESTS

Radioactive iodine (^{131}I) uptake, protein-bound iodine levels, and liothyronine uptake: altered results.

NURSING CONSIDERATIONS

Besides those related universally to drug therapy (see "How to use this book"), consider the following specific recommendations:

Assessment
- Obtain a baseline assessment of the patient's thyroid status before therapy.
- Be alert for adverse reactions and drug interactions throughout therapy.
- Evaluate the patient's and family's knowledge about liothyronine therapy.

Nursing Diagnoses
- High risk for activity intolerance related to ineffective dosage of liothyronine.
- Altered (myocardial) tissue perfusion related to liothyronine-induced angina pectoris.
- Knowledge deficit related to liothyronine therapy.

Planning and Implementation

Preparation and Administration
- Be aware that when changing from levothyroxine to liothyronine, the doctor will stop levothyroxine and begin liothyronine. Liothyronine will be increased in small increments after residual effects of levothyroxine have disappeared. When changing from liothyronine to levothyroxine, the doctor will start levothyroxine several days before withdrawing liothyronine to avoid relapse.
- ***P.O. use:*** Administer daily dose in morning to prevent insomnia.
- Be aware that patients who need radioactive iodine uptake studies must discontinue drug 7 to 10 days before testing.

Monitoring
- Monitor effectiveness by regularly checking thyroid function studies and assessing the patient for signs and symptoms of thyroid dysfunction.

• Monitor the patient for signs of overdosage.
• Monitor the patient's temperature, pulse rate, and blood pressure regularly for alterations such as fever, tachycardia, or hypertension.
• Monitor patients with coronary artery disease who must receive thyroid hormones carefully for possible coronary insufficiency if catecholamines must be given.
• Monitor patients with myxedema closely because these patients are unusually sensitive to thyroid hormone.

Supportive Care

• Withhold drug and notify the doctor if the patient develops signs of overdosage. Be prepared to treat overdosage with antithyroid drugs.
• Assist the patient with activities as needed until a euthyroid state is achieved.
• Obtain an order for an antiemetic or antidiarrheal agent, as needed.
• Administer a mild analgesic as prescribed if drug-induced headache occurs.
• Keep the patient dry if profuse sweating occurs.
• Be aware that thyroid hormones alter results of thyroid function tests.

Patient Teaching

• Instruct the patient to take the medication at the same time each day; encourage morning dosing to avoid insomnia.
• Tell the patient to notify doctor if he experiences headache, diarrhea, nervousness, excessive sweating, heat intolerance, chest pain, increased pulse rate, or palpitations; and to notify doctor immediately of any signs of aggravated cardiovascular disease.
• Tell the patient who has achieved a stable response not to change product brands because they are not all bioequivalent.
• Stress the importance of taking the drug exactly as prescribed and of receiving follow-up care.

Evaluation

In patients receiving liothyronine, appropriate evaluation statements may include:
• Patient is able to perform activities without overtiring.
• Patient does not exhibit signs and symptoms of angina.
• Patient and family state an understanding of liothyronine therapy.

lisinopril

(lyse in´ oh pril)
Prinivil, Zestril

• *Classification:* antihypertensive (angiotensin-converting enzyme inhibitor)
• *Pregnancy Risk Category:* C (D in second and third trimesters)

HOW SUPPLIED

Tablets: 5 mg, 10 mg, 20 mg

ACTION

Mechanism: Inhibits angiotensin-converting enzyme (ACE), preventing pulmonary conversion of angiotensin I to angiotensin II, a potent vasoconstrictor. This decreases peripheral arterial resistance and aldosterone secretion, thereby reducing sodium and water retention and blood pressure.
Absorption: Variable after oral administration; an average of about 25% of an oral dose has been absorbed by test subjects.
Distribution: Widely distributed in tissues. Plasma protein binding appears insignificant. Minimal amounts enter the brain. Preclinical studies indicate that it crosses the placenta.
Metabolism: Not metabolized.
Excretion: Unchanged in the urine. Half-life: About 12 hours.
Onset, peak, duration: Peak serum levels occur in about 7 hours. Onset of antihypertensive activity occurs in

about 1 hour, peaks in 6 hours, and persists for 24 hours.

INDICATIONS & DOSAGE

Mild to severe hypertension–
Adults: initially, 10 mg P.O. daily. Most patients are well controlled on 20 to 40 mg daily as a single dose.

CONTRAINDICATIONS & PRECAUTIONS

Contraindicated in patients hypersensitive to the drug. Use cautiously in patients with impaired renal function because accumulation of the drug may occur, and patients with severe CHF (because renal function may depend on the renin-angiotensin system, lisinopril may worsen oliguria or progressive azotemia).

ADVERSE REACTIONS

Common reactions are in italics; life-threatening reactions are in bold italics.
Blood: neutropenia.
CNS: *dizziness, headache, fatigue,* depression, somnolescence, paresthesia.
CV: hypotension, *orthostasis,* chest pain.
EENT: *nasal congestion.*
GI: *diarrhea,* nausea, dyspepsia, dysgeusia.
GU: impotence.
Metabolic: hyperkalemia.
Skin: rash.
Other: *upper respiratory symptoms, cough, muscle cramps, angiodema,* decreased libido.

INTERACTIONS

Diuretics: excessive hypotension.
Indomethacin: attenuated hypotensive effect.
Potassium-sparing diuretics, potassium supplements, potassium-containing salt substitutes: possible hyperkalemia.

EFFECTS ON DIAGNOSTIC TESTS

Hemoglobin and hematocrit: minor reductions and changes in liver enzymes.
Serum potassium, serum creatinine, BUN, and bilirubin: elevated levels.

NURSING CONSIDERATIONS

Besides those related universally to drug therapy (see "How to use this book"), consider the following specific recommendations:

Assessment

- Obtain a baseline assessment of the patient's blood pressure before beginning therapy.
- Be alert for adverse reactions and drug interactions throughout therapy.
- Evaluate the patient's and family's knowledge about lisinopril therapy.

Nursing Diagnoses

- Altered tissue perfusion (renal, cerebral, cardiopulmonary, and peripheral) related to the patient's underlying condition.
- High risk for injury related to lisinopril-induced adverse reactions.
- Knowledge deficit related to lisinopril therapy.

Planning and Implementation

Preparation and Administration

- Keep in mind that a lower dosage should be ordered for the patient with impaired renal function.
- If the patient is taking a diuretic, the diuretic should be discontinued 2 to 3 days before beginning lisinopril therapy or lisinopril dosage should be reduced to 5 mg once daily.

Monitoring

- Monitor effectiveness by frequently checking the patient's blood pressure, pulse, and ECG.
- Monitor the patient for light-headedness, facial swelling, and difficulty breathing. Ask about any loss of taste.
- Review WBC and differential counts before treatment, every 2 weeks for 3 months, and periodically thereafter.

Supportive Care
• Notify the doctor if patient experiences light-headedness or loss of taste. Light-headedness may require dosage adjustment; loss of taste may necessitate discontinuation of the drug.
• Keep in mind that the doctor may add a diuretic if drug does not adequately control blood pressure.
• Monitor the patient for dizziness and hypotension.
• Institute safety measures, such as continuous use of side rails, if the patient experiences dizziness or hypotension.
Patient Teaching
• Explain the importance of taking this drug as prescribed, even when feeling well.
• Tell the patient not to discontinue this drug suddenly, even if unpleasant adverse reactions occur. Tell the patient to discuss the problem with the doctor.
• Instruct the patient to check with the doctor or pharmacist before taking any OTC medications.
• Tell the patient that the beneficial effects of lisinopril may not appear until after several weeks of therapy.
• Tell the patient to report light-headedness, especially in the first few days of treatment, so dosage can be adjusted. Also tell patient to report facial swelling because the drug can cause angioedema and loss of taste, which may necessitate discontinuation of the drug.
• Advise the patient to avoid sudden position changes to minimize orthostatic hypertension.
• Teach the patient and family caregiver how to take blood pressure measurements. Tell the patient to report any significant changes.
Evaluation
In patients receiving lisinopril, appropriate evaluation statements may include:
• Patient's blood pressure is controlled within normal limits for this patient.
• Patient does not experience injury from possible adverse reactions, such as dizziness and hypotension.
• Patient and family state an understanding of lisinopril therapy.

lithium carbonate
(lith´ ee um)
Camcolit‡, Carbolith†, Duralith†, Eskalith, Eskalith CR, Lithane**, Lithicarb‡, Lithizine†, Lithobid, Lithonate, Lithotabs, Priadel‡

lithium citrate
Cibalith-S*

• *Classification:* antimanic, antipsychotic (alkali metal)
• *Pregnancy Risk Category:* D

HOW SUPPLIED
Tablets: 250 mg‡, 300 mg (300 mg = 8.12 mEq lithium)
Tablets (sustained-release): 300 mg, 400 mg‡, 450 mg
Capsules: 300 mg
Syrup (sugarless): 300 mg/5 ml (0.3% alcohol)

ACTION
Mechanism: Alters chemical transmitters in the CNS, possibly by interfering with ionic pump mechanisms by substituting for sodium in brain cells.
Absorption: Rate and extent of absorption vary with dosage form. Absorption is complete within 6 hours of oral administration. Food does not interfere with absorption.
Distribution: Widely distributed into the body, including breast milk; concentrations in thyroid gland, bone, and brain tissue exceed serum levels. Steady-state serum level is achieved in 12 hours, at which time, trough levels should be drawn; therapeutic

effect begins in 5 to 10 days and is maximal within 3 weeks. Therapeutic and toxic serum levels and therapeutic effects show good correlation. Therapeutic range is 0.6 to 1.2 mEq/liter; adverse reactions increase as level reaches 1.5 to 2 mEq/liter–such concentrations may be necessary in acute mania. Toxicity usually occurs at levels above 2 mEq/liter.
Metabolism: Not metabolized.
Excretion: 95% excreted unchanged in urine; about 50% to 80% of a given dose is excreted within 24 hours. Level of renal function determines elimination rate. Half-life: Terminal half-life is about 24 hours; half-life increases in renal failure and in patients on chronic therapy (longer than 1 year).
Onset, peak, duration: Peak serum levels are seen in 30 minutes to 3 hours after administration of tablets and capsules; after liquid form is administered, serum levels peak at 15 minutes to 1 hour. Extended-release preparations cause peak serum levels in 4 to 12 hours.

INDICATIONS & DOSAGE

Prevention or control of mania –
Adults: 300 to 600 mg P.O. up to q.i.d., increasing on the basis of blood levels to achieve optimal dosage. Recommended therapeutic lithium blood levels: 1 to 1.5 mEq/liter for acute mania; 0.6 to 1.2 mEq/liter for maintenance therapy; and 2 mEq/liter as maximum.

Note: 5 ml lithium citrate (liquid) contains 8 mEq lithium equal to 300 mg lithium carbonate.

CONTRAINDICATIONS & PRECAUTIONS

Contraindicated in patients with hypersensitivity to lithium.

Use cautiously in patients with cardiovascular disease because drug causes ECG changes (including T-wave depression in 20% to 30% of patients), heart block, and premature ventricular contractions; renal dysfunction because delayed elimination may induce lithium toxicity and diabetes insipidus (characterized by extreme thirst and excessive urination in 30% to 50% of patients); hypovolemia, sodium depletion, or dehydration, which increase drug's effects; hypothyroidism because of risk of disease exacerbation or goiter formation; psoriasis because lithium may exacerbate condition; and seizure disorders because drug may induce seizures. Many oral lithium products contain tartrazine, which may exacerbate asthma or respiratory disorders in aspirin-allergic patients.

Lithium has caused pseudotumor cerebri with papilledema and increased intracranial pressure in some patients. If this occurs, the drug should be discontinued, if possible; however, some clinicians may elect to treat the patient with acetazolamide.

ADVERSE REACTIONS

Common reactions are in italics; life-threatening reactions are in bold italics.
Blood: *leukocytosis of 14,000 to 18,000 (reversible).*
CNS: tremors, drowsiness, headache, confusion, restlessness, dizziness, psychomotor retardation, stupor, lethargy, coma, blackouts, ***epileptiform seizures,*** EEG changes, worsened organic brain syndrome, impaired speech, ataxia, muscle weakness, incoordination, hyperexcitability.
CV: *reversible ECG changes,* arrhythmias, hypotension, peripheral circulatory collapse, allergic vasculitis, ankle and wrist edema.
EENT: tinnitus, impaired vision.
GI: nausea, vomiting, anorexia, diarrhea, dry mouth, *thirst,* metallic taste.
GU: *polyuria,* glycosuria, incontinence, renal toxicity with long-term use.
Metabolic: transient hyperglycemia, goiter, hypothyroidism (lowered T_3,

T_4, and protein-bound iodine, but elevated ^{131}I uptake), hyponatremia.
Skin: pruritus, rash, diminished or lost sensation, drying and thinning of hair.

INTERACTIONS

Aminophylline, sodium bicarbonate, sodium chloride: ingestion of these salts increases lithium excretion. Avoid salt loads and monitor lithium levels.
Carbamazepine, probenecid, indomethacin, methyldopa, piroxicam: increased effect of lithium. Monitor for lithium toxicity.
Diuretics: increased reabsorption of lithium by kidneys, with possible toxic effect. Use with extreme caution, and monitor lithium and electrolyte levels (especially sodium).
Haloperidol, thioridazine: encephalopathic syndrome (lethargy, tremors, extrapyramidal symptoms). Watch for syndrome, and stop drug if it occurs.
Thyroid hormones: lithium may induce hypothyroidism.

EFFECTS ON DIAGNOSTIC TESTS

CBC: elevated neutrophil count.
Thyroid function tests: false-positive test results.

NURSING CONSIDERATIONS

Besides those related universally to drug therapy (see "How to use this book"), consider the following specific recommendations:

Assessment
- Obtain a baseline assessment of the patient's mental status before therapy.
- Be alert for adverse reactions and drug interactions throughout therapy.
- Evaluate the patient's and family's knowledge about lithium therapy.

Nursing Diagnoses
- Altered thought processes related to patient's underlying psychiatric disorder.
- High risk for trauma related to adverse CNS reactions to lithium therapy.
- Knowledge deficit related to lithium therapy.

Planning and Implementation
Preparation and Administration
- Administer with plenty of water and after meals to minimize GI upset.
- Before leaving the bedside, make sure the patient has swallowed medication.
- Ensure that patient can have regular checks of lithium blood levels because this is crucial to the safe use of the drug. If regular follow-up is doubtful, confer with doctor before administering the drug.

Monitoring
- Regularly monitor effectiveness by interacting with the patient and observing the patient's behavior.
- Monitor WBC count for leukocytosis. Also monitor renal and thyroid studies, and electrolyte levels. Palpate thyroid to check for enlargement.
- Monitor ECG for changes or arrhythmias and blood pressure for hypotension.
- Check fluid intake and output, especially when surgery is scheduled.
- Check urine for specific gravity, and report level below 1.005, which may indicate diabetes insipidus syndrome.
- Monitor blood glucose closely for hyperglycemia because lithium may alter glucose tolerance.
- Monitor mental status and level of consciousness throughout lithium therapy.
- Weigh patient daily; check for signs of edema or sudden weight gain.
- Monitor lithium blood levels 8 to 12 hours after first dose, usually before morning dose, two or three times weekly first month, then weekly to monthly during maintenance. When blood levels of lithium are below 1.5 mEq/liter, adverse reactions usually remain mild.

Supportive Care

- Expect delay of 1 to 3 weeks before drug's beneficial effects are noticed. However, notify the doctor if the patient's behavior does not improve in 3 weeks or if it worsens.
- Withhold one dose if lithium toxicity is suspected (diarrhea, vomiting, drowsiness, muscular weakness, ataxia) and notify the doctor promptly.
- Adjust fluid and sodium intake to compensate if excessive loss occurs through protracted sweating or diarrhea. Under normal conditions, patients should have fluid intake of 2,500 to 3,000 ml daily and a balanced diet with adequate sodium intake.
- Have outpatient follow-up of thyroid and renal functions every 6 to 12 months.
- If adverse CNS reactions occur, institute safety precautions, such as supervising ambulation.
- Identify a responsible family member or friend to oversee the patient's compliance with drug therapy.
- Institute seizure precautions as needed.
- Be aware that this drug may be used investigationally to increase white cells in patients undergoing cancer chemotherapy; it may also be used to treat cluster headaches, aggression, organic brain syndrome, and tardive dyskinesia. Has been used to treat SIADH.

Patient Teaching

- Warn the patient and family to watch for signs of toxicity (diarrhea, vomiting, drowsiness, muscular weakness, ataxia) and to expect transient nausea, polyuria, thirst, and discomfort during first few days of therapy. Tell the patient to withhold one dose and call the doctor if toxic symptoms appear but not to discontinue drug abruptly.
- Tell the patient to expect delay of 1 to 3 weeks before drug's beneficial effects are noticed.
- Explain the importance of having lithium blood levels checked regularly. Stress that lithium has a narrow therapeutic margin of safety. Warn patient that a blood level that is even slightly too high can be dangerous.
- Instruct the patient to carry an identification card (available from pharmacy) with toxicity and emergency information.
- Warn the ambulatory patient to avoid hazardous activities that require alertness and good psychomotor coordination until CNS effects of the drug are known.
- Tell the patient not to switch brands of lithium or to take other drugs (prescription or OTC) without doctor's guidance.
- Stress the importance of compliance with lithium therapy.
- Explain the importance of having laboratory and other diagnostic studies done when ordered.
- Tell the patient to take the drug with plenty of water and after meals to minimize GI upset.
- Tell the patient to increase fluid and salt intake if excessive sweating or diarrhea occurs.
- Tell the patient to notify the doctor if CNS or other adverse reactions develop.

Evaluation

In patients receiving lithium, appropriate evaluation statements may include:

- Patient exhibits improved behavior and thought processes.
- Patient's safety is maintained.
- Patient and family state an understanding of lithium therapy.

lomustine (CCNU)

(loe mus´ teen)
CeeNU

• *Classification:* antineoplastic (alkylating agent, nitrosourea)
• *Pregnancy Risk Category:* D

HOW SUPPLIED

Capsules: 10 mg, 40 mg, 100 mg, dose pack (2 100-mg, 2 40-mg, 2 10-mg capsules)

ACTION

Mechanism: An alkylating agent that cross-links strands of cellular DNA and interferes with RNA transcription, causing an imbalance of growth that leads to cell death. Cell cycle–nonspecific.
Absorption: Rapidly and well absorbed across the GI tract after oral administration; also absorbed topically.
Distribution: Widely distributed into body tissues. Metabolites are found in the CSF within 30 minutes of administration; they may reach 50% or more of concurrent blood levels.
Metabolism: All of the drug is metabolized by the liver within 1 hour of administration. Some of the metabolites have cytotoxic activity.
Excretion: Metabolites are excreted primarily in urine, with smaller amounts excreted in feces and through the lungs. Half-life: Biphasic, plasma elimination: the initial half-life is about 6 hours; terminal elimination half-life is 1 to 2 days. The extended half-life of the terminal phase is attributed to enterohepatic circulation and protein-binding.

INDICATIONS & DOSAGE

Brain tumors, Hodgkin's disease–
Adults and children: 130 mg/m² P.O. as a single dose q 6 weeks. Reduce dosage according to degree of bone marrow suppression. Repeat doses should not be given until WBC is more than 4,000/mm³ and platelet count is more than 100,000/mm³.

CONTRAINDICATIONS & PRECAUTIONS

Contraindicated in patients with a history of hypersensitivity to the drug. Use cautiously in patients with renal and hepatic dysfunction because drug accumulation may occur; and in patients with hematologic compromise and those who have recently received cytotoxic or radiation therapy because the drug's adverse hematologic effects may be exacerbated. Use cautiously in patients with infection because the drug is myelosuppressive and may exacerbate infections.

ADVERSE REACTIONS

Common reactions are in italics; life-threatening reactions are in bold italics.
Blood: *leukopenia, delayed up to 6 weeks, lasting 1 to 2 weeks;* ***thrombocytopenia,*** *delayed up to 4 weeks, lasting 1 to 2 weeks.*
GI: *nausea and vomiting beginning within 4 to 5 hours, lasting 24 hours;* stomatitis.
GU: ***nephrotoxicity,*** progressive azotemia.

INTERACTIONS

None significant.

EFFECTS ON DIAGNOSTIC TESTS

Liver function tests: transient elevations.

NURSING CONSIDERATIONS

Besides those related universally to drug therapy (see "How to use this book"), consider the following specific recommendations:
Assessment
• Obtain a baseline assessment of the patient's underlying condition and CBC, platelet, and uric acid levels before therapy.

*Liquid form contains alcohol.

**May contain tartrazine.

• Be alert for adverse reactions throughout therapy.
• Evaluate the patient's and family's knowledge about lomustine therapy.

Nursing Diagnoses

• High risk for infection related to adverse reactions to lomustine.
• Altered nutrition: Less than body requirements related to prolonged episodes of nausea and vomiting.
• Knowledge deficit related to lomustine therapy.

Planning and Implementation

Preparation and Administration

• Premedicate patient with an antiemetic, as ordered, before giving lomustine.
• Keep in mind that dosage modification may be required in patients with decreased platelets, leukocytes, or erythrocytes and in patients receiving other myelosuppressive drugs.
• Remember that lomustine may be given alone or in combination with other drugs and that it is usually not administered more often than every 6 weeks because bone marrow toxicity is cumulative and delayed.
• ***P.O. use:*** Give 2 to 4 hours after meals as it will be more completely absorbed when taken on an empty stomach. Store drug below 40° C.

Monitoring

• Monitor effectiveness by noting results of follow-up diagnostic tests and overall physical status.
• Monitor CBC, platelet, and uric acid levels weekly during therapy.
• Monitor liver function periodically.
• Monitor for signs of bleeding (bruising, hematuria, petechiae, melena) and signs of infection (sore throat, fever, malaise).

Supportive Care

• Do not give any I.M. injections when the platelet count is below 100,000/mm³.
• Keep in mind that this drug may be useful in cancer involving the CNS, because CSF level equals 30% to 50% of plasma level 1 hour after administration. Since lomustine crosses the blood-brain barrier, it may be used to treat primary brain tumors.
• Anticoagulants and aspirin products should be used with caution.
• Expect therapeutic effects of the drug to be accompanied by toxicity.

Patient Teaching

• Instruct patient to take daily temperatures and watch for signs of infection or bleeding.
• Explain to the patient that intervals of 6 weeks are necessary between treatments for optimal effect with minimal toxicity.
• Encourage the patient to eat frequent, small meals to lessen the nausea and vomiting associated with therapy.

Evaluation

In patients receiving lomustine, appropriate evaluation statements may include:
• Patient remains infection-free while undergoing lomustine therapy.
• Patient maintains adequate nutrition and healing capabilities with little nausea and vomiting during drug treatments.
• Patient and family state an understanding of lomustine therapy.

loperamide

(loe per´ a mide)

Imodium, Imodium A-D◇

• *Classification:* antidiarrheal (piperidine derivative)
• *Pregnancy Risk Category:* B

HOW SUPPLIED

Tablets: 2 mg
Capsules: 2 mg
Oral liquid: 1 mg/5 ml◇

ACTION

Mechanism: Inhibits peristaltic activity, prolonging transit time of intestinal contents.

Absorption: About 40% of a dose is absorbed from the GI tract.
Distribution: Not known if drug crosses placenta; does not enter CNS.
Metabolism: Hepatic; 75% metabolized to glucuronide conjugate.
Excretion: primarily in feces; less than 2% is excreted in urine. Half-life: 10.8 hours.
Onset, peak, duration: Peak plasma levels are similar after administration of either capsule or oral liquid formulation; peak levels occur 2½ hours after liquid and 5 hours after capsule form.

INDICATIONS & DOSAGE

Acute, nonspecific diarrhea –
Adults: initially, 4 mg P.O., then 2 mg after each unformed stool. Maximum 16 mg daily.
Children 8 to 12 years: 10 ml t.i.d. P.O. on first day. (Subsequent doses of 5 ml per 10 kg of body weight may be administered after each unformed stool.)
Children 5 to 8 years: 10 ml P.O. b.i.d. on first day.
Children 2 to 5 years: 5 ml P.O. t.i.d. on first day.
Chronic diarrhea –
Adults: initially, 4 mg P.O., then 2 mg after each unformed stool until diarrhea subsides. Adjust dosage to individual response.

CONTRAINDICATIONS & PRECAUTIONS

Contraindicated in patients with diarrhea from pseudomembranous colitis or ulcerative colitis because drug may precipitate toxic megacolon; in patients with diarrhea resulting from poisoning or infection by microbes that can penetrate the intestinal mucosa because expulsion of intestinal contents may be a protective mechanism; and in patients with known hypersensitivity to the drug. Use cautiously in patients with a history of narcotic dependence, and in patients with severe prostatic hypertrophy or hepatic disease because the drug may worsen the symptoms of this disorder.

ADVERSE REACTIONS

Common reactions are in italics; life-threatening reactions are in bold italics.
CNS: drowsiness, fatigue, dizziness.
GI: dry mouth; abdominal pain, distention, or discomfort; *constipation;* nausea; vomiting.
Skin: rash.

INTERACTIONS

None significant.

EFFECTS ON DIAGNOSTIC TESTS

None reported.

NURSING CONSIDERATIONS

Besides those related universally to drug therapy (see "How to use this book"), consider the following specific recommendations:

Assessment
• Obtain a baseline assessment of history of bowel disorders, GI status, and frequency of loose stools before therapy.
• Be alert for adverse reactions throughout therapy.
• Evaluate the patient's and family's knowledge about loperamide therapy.

Nursing Diagnoses
• Diarrhea related to interruption of normal pattern of elimination characterized by frequent loose stools.
• Colonic constipation related to excessive use of loperamide.
• Knowledge deficit related to loperamide therapy.

Planning and Implementation
Preparation and Administration
• Read drug label carefully.
• ***P.O. use:*** Available in liquid, capsule, and tablet forms.
Monitoring
• Monitor effectiveness by monitoring the frequency and characteristics of stool.

• Auscultate bowel sounds at least once a shift. Assess for pain and cramping.
• Monitor closely for fluid and electrolyte balance.
• Weigh patient daily until diarrhea is controlled to detect fluid loss or retention.
• Check skin in perianal area to detect and prevent breakdown.
• Monitor for adverse CNS reactions (drowsiness, dizziness).

Supportive Care
• Encourage oral fluid intake to maintain hydration and prevent fluid loss.
• Consult with dietitian to modify diet to help control diarrhea.
• Provide good skin care, especially in the perianal area. Use soothing lotion and powder.
• Stop the drug immediately if abdominal distention or other symptoms develop in acute colitis.
• Discontinue drug if no improvement occurs after giving 16 mg daily for at least 10 days.
• Be aware that loperamide produces antidiarrheal action similar to diphenoxylate but without as many adverse CNS reactions.

Patient Teaching
• Warn patient not to exceed the recommended dosage. In acute diarrhea instruct the patient to stop drug and notify doctor if no improvement occurs within 48 hours.
• Encourage proper storage to keep drug out of the reach of children.

Evaluation
In patients receiving loperamide, appropriate evaluation statements may include:
• Patient reports decrease or absence of loose stools.
• Patient remains free from signs and symptoms of colonic constipation.
• Patient and family state an understanding of loperamide therapy.

lorazepam
(lor a´ ze pam)
Alzapam, Apo-Lorazepam†, Ativan, Loraz, Novolorazem†

• Controlled Substance Schedule IV
• *Classification:* anxiolytic (benzodiazepine)
• *Pregnancy Risk Category:* D

HOW SUPPLIED
Tablets: 0.5 mg, 1 mg, 2 mg
Tablets (sublingual): 1 mg†, 2 mg†
Injection: 2 mg/ml, 4 mg/ml

ACTION
Mechanism: Depresses the CNS at the limbic and subcortical levels of the brain.
Absorption: When administered orally, well absorbed through the GI tract; also well absorbed from I.M. injection sites.
Distribution: Widely distributed throughout the body. About 85% protein-bound.
Metabolism: In the liver to inactive metabolites.
Excretion: Metabolites are excreted in urine as glucuronide conjugates. Half-life: 10 to 20 hours.
Onset, peak, duration: Peak serum levels occur in 2 hours after an oral dose.

INDICATIONS & DOSAGE
Anxiety, tension, agitation, irritability, especially in anxiety neuroses or organic (especially GI or CV) disorders–
Adults: 2 to 6 mg P.O. daily in divided doses. Maximum dosage is 10 mg daily.
Insomnia–
Adults: 2 to 4 mg P.O. h.s.
Premedication before operative procedure–
Adults: 0.05 mg/kg I.M. or I.V., not to exceed 4 mg.

CONTRAINDICATIONS & PRECAUTIONS

Contraindicated in patients with hypersensitivity to the drug or any ingredients in its formulation; in patients with acute narrow-angle glaucoma or untreated open-angle glaucoma because of the drug's possible anticholinergic effect; in those in coma because the drug's hypnotic or hypotensive effect may be prolonged or intensified; and in patients with acute alcohol intoxication who have depressed vital signs, because the drug will worsen CNS depression.

Use cautiously in patients with psychoses because the drug is rarely beneficial in such patients and may induce paradoxical reactions; in patients with myasthenia gravis or Parkinson's disease because drug may exacerbate the disorder; in those with impaired hepatic function, which prolongs elimination of the drug; in elderly or debilitated patients, who are usually more sensitive to the drug's CNS effects; in those prone to addiction or drug abuse; and in those with impaired respiratory function, such as COPD.

ADVERSE REACTIONS

Common reactions are in italics; life-threatening reactions are in bold italics.

CNS: *drowsiness, lethargy, hangover,* fainting.

CV: transient hypotension.

GI: dry mouth, abdominal discomfort.

INTERACTIONS

Alcohol, other CNS depressants: increased CNS depression. Avoid concomitant use.

EFFECTS ON DIAGNOSTIC TESTS

Liver function tests: elevated results.

NURSING CONSIDERATIONS

Besides those related universally to drug therapy (see "How to use this book"), consider the following specific recommendations:

Assessment

- Obtain a baseline assessment of the patient's anxiety before therpay.
- Be alert for adverse reactions and drug interactions throughout therapy.
- Evaluate the patient's and family's knowledge about lorazepam therapy.

Nursing Diagnoses

- Anxiety related to the patient's underlying condition.
- High risk for injury related to drug-induced CNS reactions.
- Knowledge deficit related to lorazepam therapy.

Planning and Implementation

Preparation and Administration

- Reduce the dosage in elderly or debilitated patients who may be more susceptible to CNS reactions from the drug.
- Preoperative I.V. dose should not exceed 2 mg in patients over age 50.
- ***I.M. use:*** When administering I.M., inject deep into the muscle mass. Do not dilute.
- ***I.V. use:*** Dilute with an equal volume of sterile water for injection, sodium chloride injection, or dextrose 5% injection.
- Drug may be used as a premedication before surgery as it provides substantial amnestic effects.
- Drug has a short half-life; therefore, it has fewer cumulative effects than other benzodiazepines.
- Store parenteral form in refrigerator to prolong shelf-life.

Monitoring

- Monitor for adverse reactions or drug interactions to lorazepam by frequently checking the patient's vital signs for hypotension.
- Regularly monitor effectiveness by asking the patient about feelings of anxiety and by observing the patient's behavior.
- Monitor the degree of dry mouth.
- Monitor for drug interactions by observing for excessive sedation due

to potentiation with other CNS drugs.

Supportive Care

• Provide frequent sips of water or ice chips for dry mouth.

• If patient experiences drowsiness, light-headedness, lethargy, or fainting, institute safety measures, such as supervising patient activities. Reorient patient as needed and ensure a safe environment.

• Be aware that drug should not be prescribed for everyday stress.

• Do not withdraw drug abruptly. Abuse or addiction is possible and withdrawal symptoms may occur.

Patient Teaching

• Suggest sugarless hard candy, ice chips, or gum to relieve dry mouth.

• Warn the patient not to combine drug with alcohol or other CNS depressants and to avoid driving and other hazardous activities that require alertness and psychomotor coordination until adverse CNS effects of the drug are known.

• Warn the patient against giving medication to others.

• Warn the patient to take this drug only as directed and not discontinue it without the doctor's approval. Inform the patient of the drug's potential for dependence if taken longer than directed.

Evaluation

In patients receiving lorazepam, appropriate evaluation statements may include:

• Patient states he is less anxious.

• Patient does not experience injury as a result of adverse CNS reactions.

• Patient and family state an understanding of lorazepam therapy.

lovastatin

(loe´ va sta tin)

Mevacor

• *Classification:* cholesterol-lowering agent (lactone)

• *Pregnancy Risk Category:* X

HOW SUPPLIED

Tablets: 20 mg

ACTION

Mechanism: Inhibits 3-hydroxy-3-methylglutaryl-coenzyme A (HMG-CoA) reductase. This enzyme is an early (and rate-limiting) step in the synthetic pathway of cholesterol.

Absorption: Animal studies indicate that about 30% of an oral dose is absorbed. Administration with food improves plasma concentrations of total inhibitors by about 30%.

Distribution: Less than 5% of an oral dose reaches the systemic circulation because of extensive first-pass hepatic extraction; the liver is the drug's principal site of action. Both the parent compound and its principal metabolite are highly bound (more than 95%) to plasma proteins. Animal studies indicate that lovastatin can cross the placenta and the blood-brain barrier.

Metabolism: Converted to the active beta hydroxy acid form (mevinolinic acid) in the liver. Other metabolites include the 6′ hydroxy derivative and two unidentified compounds.

Excretion: About 80% is excreted primarily in feces; about 10% in urine. Half-life: Elimination half-life of unchanged drug is not known. Plasma half-life of mevinolinic acid is 1.1 to 1.7 hours.

Onset, peak, duration: Onset of action is about 3 days, with maximal therapeutic effects seen in 4 to 6 weeks.

INDICATIONS & DOSAGE

Reduction of low-density lipoprotein and total cholesterol levels in patients with primary hypercholesterolemia (types IIa and IIb) –
Adults: initially, 20 mg P.O. once daily with the evening meal. For patients with severely elevated cholesterol levels (for example, over 300 mg/dl), the initial dose should be 40 mg. The recommended range is 20 to 80 mg in single or divided doses.

CONTRAINDICATIONS & PRECAUTIONS

Contraindicated in patients hypersensitive to the drug; patients with active liver disease or unexplained persistent elevations of liver transaminase levels because the drug may be hepatotoxic; and in pregnant or breast-feeding women because the drug is teratogenic in animals.

Because marked persistent elevations in serum transaminase levels have been noted, liver function tests should be performed every 4 to 6 weeks during the first 15 months of therapy and periodically thereafter.

Use cautiously in patients with a history of liver disease and those who consume substantial quantities of alcohol; in patients at risk of developing renal failure secondary to rhabdomyolysis; in trauma patients; in patients undergoing major surgery; and in patients with severe acute infection, hypotension, severe metabolic, endocrine, or electrolyte disorders, or uncontrolled seizures.

ADVERSE REACTIONS

Common reactions are in italics; life-threatening reactions are in bold italics.
CNS: headache, dizziness.
EENT: blurred vision, dysgeusia.
GI: constipation, diarrhea, dyspepsia, flatus, abdominal pain or cramps, heartburn, nausea.
Metabolic: elevated serum transaminase levels, abnormal liver test results.
Skin: rash, pruritus.
Other: peripheral neuropathy, muscle cramps, myalgia, myositis, ***rhabdomyolysis.***

INTERACTIONS

Cholestyramine, clofibrate: enhanced lipid-reducing effects.
Immunosuppressive agents, gemfibrozil: possible increased risk of polymyositis and rhabdomyolysis. Maximum recommended lovastatin dosage is 20 mg daily; monitor patient closely.

EFFECTS ON DIAGNOSTIC TESTS

Serum creatinine phosphokinase: elevated levels.
Serum transaminase: elevated levels.

NURSING CONSIDERATIONS

Besides those related universally to drug therapy (see "How to use this book"), consider the following specific recommendations:

Assessment

- Obtain a baseline assessment of the patient's serum lipoprotein and total cholesterol levels before drug therapy.
- Be alert for adverse reactions and drug interactions throughout therapy.
- Evaluate the patient's and family's knowledge about lovastatin therapy.

Nursing Diagnoses

- High risk for injury related to ineffectiveness of lovastatin to lower LDL and total cholesterol levels.
- Sensory/perceptual alteration (visual) related to adverse drug reaction.
- Knowledge deficit related to lovastatin therapy.

Planning and Implementation

Preparation and Administration

- Store tablets at room temperature in a light-resistant container.
- Administer with evening meal. Absorption is enhanced and biosynthesis is greater in the evening.

Monitoring
• Monitor effectiveness by regularly checking the patient's serum lipoprotein and total cholesterol levels.
• Regularly monitor serum transaminase levels and other liver function studies.
• Monitor the patient for adverse drug reactions.
• Monitor the patient for drug interactions if he is taking cholestyramine, clofibrate, immunosuppressive agents, or gemfibrozil.
Supportive Care
• Institute safety precautions if CNS reactions occur.
• Obtain an order for a mild analgesic if drug-induced headache occurs.
• Assist the patient in and out of bed if dizziness or blurred vision occurs.
Patient Teaching
• Teach the patient appropriate dietary management (restricting total fat and cholesterol intake), weight control, and exercise. Explain their importance in controlling elevated serum lipids.
• Advise the patient to restrict alcohol intake, which can affect cholesterol profile.
• Instruct the patient to store drug at room temperature in a light-resistant container.
• Advise the patient to have regular eye examinations; lovastatin can cause blurred vision.
• Instruct the patient to take lovastatin with evening meal.

Evaluation

In patients receiving lovastatin, appropriate evaluation statements may include:
• Patient's serum lipoprotein and total cholesterol levels are within normal limits.
• Patient does not develop blurred vision or dizziness.
• Patient and family state an understanding of lovastatin therapy.

loxapine hydrochloride
(lox´ a peen)
Loxapac†, Loxitane C, Loxitane I.M.

loxapine succinate
Loxapac†, Loxitane

• *Classification:* antipsychotic (dibenzoxazepine)
• *Pregnancy Risk Category:* C

HOW SUPPLIED
Capsules: 5 mg, 10 mg, 25 mg, 50 mg
Oral concentrate: 25 mg/ml
Injection: 50 mg/ml

ACTION
Mechanism: A dibenzoxazepine that blocks postsynaptic dopamine receptors in the brain.
Absorption: Rapidly and completely absorbed from the GI tract; also completely absorbed after I.M. injection.
Distribution: Widely distributed into the body, including breast milk. Drug is 91% to 99% protein-bound.
Metabolism: Extensively metabolized by the liver, forming a few active metabolites.
Excretion: Most is excreted as metabolites in urine; some is excreted in feces via the biliary tract. About 50% of drug is excreted in urine and feces within 24 hours. Half-life: Biphasic; first phase about 5 hours; second phase is 19 hours.
Onset, peak, duration: Sedation occurs in 30 minutes. Peak effect occurs at 1½ to 3 hours; steady-state serum level is achieved within 3 to 4 days. Duration of action is 12 hours.

INDICATIONS & DOSAGE
Psychotic disorders–
Adults: 10 mg P.O. or I.M. b.i.d. to q.i.d., rapidly increasing to 60 to 100 mg P.O. daily for most patients; dosage varies from patient to patient.

CONTRAINDICATIONS & PRECAUTIONS

Contraindicated in patients with hypersensitivity to loxapine and in patients with disorders accompanied by coma, CNS depression, brain damage, circulatory collapse, or cerebrovascular disease because of the potential hypotensive effects.

Use cautiously in patients with cardiac disease (arrhythmias, CHF, angina pectoris, valvular disease, or heart block), encephalitis, Reye's syndrome, head injury, respiratory disease, epilepsy and other seizure disorders, glaucoma, prostatic hypertrophy, urine retention, hepatic or renal dysfunction, Parkinson's disease, pheochromocytoma, or hypocalcemia.

ADVERSE REACTIONS

Common reactions are in italics; life-threatening reactions are in bold italics.

Blood: transient leukopenia.
CNS: *extrapyramidal reactions (moderate incidence), sedation (moderate incidence), tardive dyskinesia,* pseudoparkinsonism, EEG changes, dizziness.
CV: *orthostatic hypotension,* tachycardia, ECG changes.
EENT: *blurred vision.*
GI: *dry mouth, constipation.*
GU: *urine retention,* dark urine, menstrual irregularities, gynecomastia.
Skin: *mild photosensitivity,* dermal allergic reactions.
Other: weight gain; increased appetite; rarely, ***neuroleptic malignant syndrome*** (fever, tachycardia, tachypnea, profuse diaphoresis).

INTERACTIONS

Alcohol, other CNS depressants: increased CNS depression. Avoid concomitant use.

EFFECTS ON DIAGNOSTIC TESTS

ECG: quinidine-like effects.
Liver enzymes and protein-bound iodine: elevated results.
Urine porphyrins, urobilinogen, amylase, and 5-hydroxyindoleacetic acid: false-positive results because of darkening of urine by metabolites.
Urine pregnancy test using human chorionic gonadotropin: false-positive results.

NURSING CONSIDERATIONS

Besides those related universally to drug therapy (see "How to use this book"), consider the following specific recommendations:

Assessment
- Obtain baseline assessment of patient's mental status, including psychotic symptoms, before therapy.
- Be alert for adverse reactions and drug interactions throughout therapy.
- Evaluate the patient's and family's knowledge about loxapine therapy.

Nursing Diagnoses
- Impaired thought processes related to the patient's underlying condition.
- Urinary retention related to adverse reactions.
- Knowledge deficit related to loxapine therapy.

Planning and Implementation

Preparation and Administration
- Dose of 10 mg is therapeutic equivalent of 100 mg of chlorpromazine.
- ***P.O. use:*** Dilute liquid concentrate with orange or grapefruit juice just before giving.

Monitoring
- Monitor effectiveness of therapy by regularly observing the patient's behavior and noting chnges in psychotic symptoms.
- Monitor for extrapyramidal and anticholinergic effects (blurred vision, dry mouth, constipation, urine retention) and tardive dyskinesia during prolonged therapy.
- Watch for orthostatic hypotension,

especially after parenteral administration.
• Monitor therapy by weekly bilirubin tests during the first month; periodic blood tests (CBC and liver function); and ophthalmic tests (long-term use).
• Monitor for neuroleptic malignant syndrome. This rare, potentially fatal reaction is not necessarily related to type of neuroleptic or duration of drug. It usually occurs in men (60% of affected patients).
• Monitor the patient's blood pressure frequently.

Supportive Care

• Obtain baseline blood pressure reading before beginning therapy.
• Keep the patient supine for 1 hour after I.M. administration. Then assist patient to get up slowly to avoid orthostatic hypotension.
• Do not discontinue drug abruptly unless required by severe adverse reactions.
• Increase the patient's fluid and fiber intake–if not contraindicated–to prevent constipation. If necessary, request doctor's order for a laxative.
• Give the patient sugarless gum, sour hard candy, ice chips, or a mouthwash rinse to relieve dryness.
• Be prepared to give I.V. diphenhydramine, as ordered, to treat acute dystonic reactions.
• Hold dose if patient develops jaundice, symptoms of blood dyscrasias (fever, sore throat, infection, cellulitis, weakness), persistent (longer than a few hours) extrapyramidal reactions or any such reactions during pregnancy.

Patient Teaching

• Tell the patient to avoid exposure to direct sunlight and to use a sunscreen when going outdoors to prevent photosensitivity reactions. (*Note:* Sunlamps and tanning beds may cause burning of the skin or skin discoloration.)
• Tell the patient not to stop taking the drug suddenly.
• Encourage the patient to report difficult urination, sore throat, dizziness, or fainting.
• Advise the patient to increase fluid and fiber intake, if appropriate.
• Tell the patient to avoid driving and other hazardous activities that require alertness until the effect of the drug is established. Excessive sedative effects tend to subside after several weeks.
• Explain which fluids are appropriate for diluting the concentrate, and show the dropper technique for measuring dose.
• Tell the patient that sugarless hard candy, chewing gum, or ice chips can alleviate dry mouth.
• Recommend periodic eye examinations.

Evaluation

In patients receiving loxapine, appropriate evaluation statements may include:
• Patient demonstrates a decrease in psychotic behavior.
• Patient voids without difficulty.
• Patient and family state an understanding of loxapine therapy.

lypressin

(lye press´ in)
Diapid

• *Classification:* antidiuretic hormone (posterior pituitary hormone)
• *Pregnancy Risk Category:* B

HOW SUPPLIED

Nasal spray: 0.185 mg/ml

ACTION

Mechanism: Promotes reabsorption of water through renal tubular epithelium and produces a concentrated urine (antidiuretic hormone effect).
Absorption: Because drug is destroyed by trypsin in the GI tract, it

is given intranasally; rapidly absorbed from the nasal mucosa.
Distribution: Into the extracellular fluid.
Metabolism: By the kidneys and liver.
Excretion: A small amount of active drug and its inactive metabolites are excreted in urine. Half-life: About 15 minutes.
Onset, peak, duration: Duration of action is 3 to 8 hours.

INDICATIONS & DOSAGE

Nonnephrogenic diabetes insipidus—
Adults and children: 1 or 2 sprays (approximately 2 USP posterior pituitary pressor units/spray) in either or both nostrils q.i.d. and an additional dose at bedtime, if needed, to prevent nocturia. If usual dosage is inadequate, increase frequency rather than number of sprays.

CONTRAINDICATIONS & PRECAUTIONS

Contraindicated in patients with hypersensitivity to the drug. Use large doses cautiously in patients with coronary artery disease because lypressin may cause coronary artery constriction. Although drug's pressor effects are minimal, also use cautiosuly in patients in whom blood pressure elevation is hazardous.

ADVERSE REACTIONS

Common reactions are in italics; life-threatening reactions are in bold italics.
CNS: headache, dizziness.
EENT: nasal congestion or ulceration, irritation, pruritus of nasal passages, rhinorrhea, conjunctivitis.
GI: heartburn due to drip of excess spray into pharynx, abdominal cramps, frequent bowel movements.
GU: possible transient fluid retention from overdose.
Skin: hypersensitivity reaction.

INTERACTIONS

None significant.

EFFECTS ON DIAGNOSTIC TESTS

None reported.

NURSING CONSIDERATIONS

Besides those related universally to drug therapy (see "How to use this book"), consider the following specific recommendations:

Assessment

- Obtain a baseline assessment of the patient's nonnephrogenic diabetes insipidus condition before initiating lypressin therapy.
- Be alert for adverse reactions throughout therapy.
- Evaluate the patient's and family's knowledge about lypressin therapy.

Nursing Diagnoses

- Fluid volume deficit related to increased urine output.
- Impaired tissue integrity related to drug-induced nasal congestion or ulceration.
- Knowledge deficit related to lypressin therapy.

Planning and Implementation

Preparation and Administration

- Be aware that nasal congestion, allergic rhinitis, or upper respiratory infections may diminish drug absorption and require larger dose or adjunctive therapy.
- Test patient sensitive to antidiuretic hormone for sensitivity to lypressin.
- ***Nasal use:*** To administer a uniform, well-diffused spray, hold bottle upright with patient in vertical position holding head upright.

Monitoring

- Monitor effectiveness by regularly checking the patient's intake and output, serum and urine osmolality, and urine specific gravity.
- Monitor for early signs of water intoxication: drowsiness, listlessness, headache, confusion, anuria, and weight gain to prevent seizures, coma, and death.
- Monitor the patient's weight daily and observe for edema.

• Monitor patient's nasal passages for ulceration or irritation.

Supportive Care

• Adjust the patient's fluid intake to reduce risk of water intoxication and of sodium depletion, especially in young or elderly patients.

• Overdose may cause oxytoxic or vasopressor activity. Withhold drug as prescribed until effects subside.

• Administer a mild analgesic for drug-induced headache, if not contraindicated.

Patient Teaching

• Teach patient how to administer drug. Instruct the patient to clear nasal passages before administering drug.

• Warn patient to avoid inhalation of spray as chest tightness, coughing, and transient dyspnea may occur.

• Emphasize that the patient should not increase or decrease dosage unless instructed by doctor.

• Review fluid intake measurement and methods for measuring fluid output with patient.

• Tell the patient to contact doctor if signs of water intoxication (drowsiness, listlessness, headache, or shortness of breath) develop.

• Nasal congestion, allergic rhinitis, or upper respiratory infections may impair drug absorption. Advise the patient to report such conditions to the doctor because they may require dosage adjustment.

• Instruct patient to wear medical alert identification.

Evaluation

In patients receiving lypressin, appropriate evaluation statements may include:

• Patient achieves normal fluid and electrolyte balance.

• Patient does not experience impaired nasal tissue.

• Patient and family state an understanding of lypressin therapy.

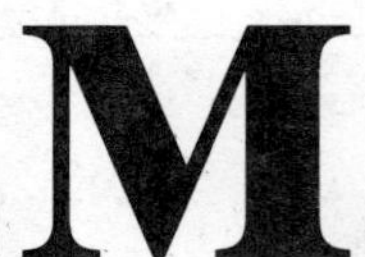

M

mafenide acetate

(ma´ fe nide)
Sulfamylon

- *Classification:* topical antibacterial
- *Pregnancy Risk Category:* C

HOW SUPPLIED

Cream: 8.5%

ACTION

Mechanism: Interferes with bacterial cellular metabolism.
Absorption: Drug diffuses through the burn eschar and is absorbed quickly.
Distribution: Rapidly distributed after topical application.
Metabolism: Rapidly and extensively metabolized in the plasma to a metabolite with weak carbonic anhydrase inhibitor activity. This metabolite can increase bicarbonate and ammonia excretion through the kidneys; if compensatory hyperventilation is inadequate, drug can cause acidosis.
Excretion: In the urine.

INDICATIONS & DOSAGE

Adjunctive treatment of second- and third-degree burns–
Adults and children: apply 1/16″ thickness of cream daily or b.i.d. to cleansed, debrided wounds. Reapply p.r.n. to keep burned area covered.

CONTRAINDICATIONS & PRECAUTIONS

Contraindicated in patients with hypersensitivity to mafenide acetate or to other sulfonamide derivatives (including furosemide, thiazide diuretics, carbonic anhydrase inhibitors, sulfites, parabens) and in women of childbearing age, unless benefit outweighs risk of hazard to fetus. Use with caution in patients with renal failure.

Drug is intended for topical use only; avoid contact with eyes and mucous membranes; use of mafenide may be followed by fungal colonization in and below eschar.

ADVERSE REACTIONS

Common reactions are in italics; life-threatening reactions are in bold italics.
Blood: eosinophilia.
Skin: pain, *burning sensation,* rash, itching, swelling, hives, blisters, erythema, facial edema.
Other: *metabolic acidosis.*

INTERACTIONS

None significant.

EFFECTS ON DIAGNOSTIC TESTS

None reported.

NURSING CONSIDERATIONS

Besides those related universally to drug therapy (see "How to use this book"), consider the following specific recommendations:

Assessment

- Obtain a baseline assessment of burn wounds before therapy.
- Be alert for adverse reactions and drug interactions throughout therapy.
- Evaluate the patient's and family's knowledge about mafenide acetate therapy.

Nursing Diagnoses

- Altered tissue perfusion (peripheral) related to patient's underlying condition.
- Impaired gas exchange related to

mafenide acetate-induced metabolic acidosis.
• Knowledge deficit related to mafenide acetate therapy.

Planning and Implementation

Preparation and Administration
• ***Topical use:*** Cleanse area before applying. Mafenide washes off with water. Keep burn areas medicated at all times.

Monitoring
• Monitor effectiveness by observing burn wounds frequently.
• Monitor for adverse reactions and interactions by closely assessing for acid-base balance, especially in the presence of pulmonary or renal dysfunction. If acidosis occurs, discontinue use for 24 to 48 hours.

Supportive Care
• Remember to use with caution in acute renal failure and in patients with hypersensitivity to sulfonamides.
• Using reverse isolation technique with sterile gloves and instruments to apply cream minimizes risk of further wound contamination.
• Notify doctor if patient reports pain and burning at application site. Severe and prolonged pain may indicate allergy. If other allergic reactions occur, treatment may have to be temporarily discontinued.
• Be aware it is sometimes difficult to distinguish between adverse reactions and effects of severe burn.

Patient Teaching
• Teach patient how to apply medication.

Evaluation

In patients receiving mafenide acetate, appropriate evaluation statements may include:
• Burn wounds have healed.
• Metabolic acidosis did not occur.
• Patient and family state an understanding of mafenide therapy.

magaldrate (aluminum-magnesium complex)

(mag´ al drate)

Antiflux†, Lowsium◇, Riopan◇

• *Classification:* antiulcer agent, antacid (magnesium/aluminum salt)
• *Pregnancy Risk Category:* C

HOW SUPPLIED

Tablets: 480 mg◇
Tablets (chewable): 480 mg◇
Oral suspension: 540 mg/5 ml◇, 1,080 mg/5 ml◇

ACTION

Mechanism: An antacid that reacts with gastric hydrochloric acid to form aluminum chloride, magnesium chloride, carbon dioxide, and water. Reduces total acid load in the GI tract and elevates gastric pH to reduce pepsin activity.
Absorption: Small amounts of aluminum or magnesium may be absorbed systemically, posing a risk to patients with renal failure.
Metabolism: None.
Excretion: Most is excreted in feces; absorbed aluminum and magnesium are excreted in the urine. Some aluminum and magnesium may be excreted in breast milk.

INDICATIONS & DOSAGE

Antacid–

Adults: suspension: 540 to 1,080 mg (5 to 10 ml) P.O. between meals and h.s. with water. Tablet: 480 to 960 mg (1 to 2 tablets) P.O. with water between meals and h.s. Chewable tablet: 480 to 960 mg (1 to 2 tablets) P.O. chewed before swallowing, between meals and h.s.

CONTRAINDICATIONS & PRECAUTIONS

Contraindicated in patients with a colostomy or an ileostomy, renal failure or any degree of renal impairment, hypophosphatemia, appendicitis, undiagnosed rectal or GI bleeding, ulcerative colitis, diverticulitis, chronic diarrhea, or intestinal or gastric outlet obstruction, because this drug may exacerbate the symptoms of these conditions.

Use cautiously in patients with decreased GI motility, such as elderly patients and those taking anticholinergics or antidiarrheals.

ADVERSE REACTIONS

Common reactions are in italics; life-threatening reactions are in bold italics.

GI: mild constipation or diarrhea.

INTERACTIONS

Allopurinol, antibiotics (including quinolones and tetracyclines), corticosteroids, diflunisal, digoxin, iron, isoniazid, penicillamine, phenothiazines, ranitidine: decreased pharmacologic effect because absorption may be impaired. Separate administration times.

EFFECTS ON DIAGNOSTIC TESTS

Gastric acid secretion test: antagonism of pentagastrin's effect.

Serum gastrin and urine pH: increased levels.

Serum potassium: decreased levels.

NURSING CONSIDERATIONS

Besides those related universally to drug therapy (see "How to use this book"), consider the following specific recommendations:

Assessment

• Obtain a baseline assessment of the patient's pain or discomfort before beginning therapy.

• Be alert for adverse reactions and drug interactions throughout therapy.

• Evaluate the patient's and family's knowledge about magaldrate therapy.

Nursing Diagnoses

• Pain related to gastric hyperacidity.

• Constipation related to adverse reactions to magaldrate.

• Knowledge deficit related to magaldrate therapy.

Planning and Implementation

Preparation and Administration

• ***P.O. use:*** Administer drug 1 hour after meals and at bedtime. Do not give other oral medications within 1 to 2 hours of antacid administration. May cause enteric-coated drugs to be released prematurely in stomach.

• ***Suspension:*** Shake suspension well; give with small amount of water or milk to ensure passage to stomach. When administering through nasogastric tube, make sure tube is placed correctly and is patent. After instilling antacid, flush tube with water.

• ***Chewable tablets:*** This form of the medication should be chewed completely before swallowing and followed by a glass of water or milk.

Monitoring

• Monitor effectiveness by regularly assessing pain relief.

• Monitor the patient's bowel pattern. Watch for development of constipation, especially in the elderly patient.

• Periodically monitor serum magnesium levels in patients with mild renal impairment. Symptomatic hypermagnesemia usually occurs only in severe renal failure.

Supportive Care

• If the patient develops constipation, notify the doctor and obtain an order for a laxative or stool softener and monitor its effectiveness. Also, if not contraindicated, encourage the patient to eat a high-fiber diet and to drink 8 to 13 8-oz glasses (2 to 3 liters) of water per day to help prevent constipation. Keep in mind that magaldrate usually causes only mild constipation.

• Encourage the patient to discuss any emotional factors or dietary hab-

its that may be contributing to the patient's GI problems.
• Keep in mind that therapy with this drug may interfere with imaging techniques using sodium pertechnetate Tc 99m and thus impair evaluation of Meckel's diverticulum. It may also interfere with reticuloendothelial imaging of liver, spleen, and bone marrow using technetium Tc 99m sulfur colloid. Drug may antagonize pentagastrin's effect during gastric acid secretion tests. This drug may also elevate serum gastrin levels and reduce serum phosphate levels.
• Don't expect this drug to be used in patients with renal failure (although it contains aluminum) to help control hypophosphatemia, because it contains magnesium, which may accumulate in renal failure.

Patient Teaching

• Warn the patient to take magaldrate only as directed; to shake suspension well, and to follow with sips of water or juice.
• Tell the patient receiving the chewable tablet form of the drug to chew the tablets completely before swallowing and, after swallowing, to drink a glass of milk or water.
• Tell the patient that this drug has a very low sodium content and that Riopan, Riopan Plus liquid, and Riopan Swallow Tablets contain no sugar. Point out that the chewable tablets contain sugar.
• Advise the patient not to switch to another antacid without consulting the doctor.
• Teach the patient how to prevent constipation during therapy, if necessary.
• Warn the patient not to take magaldrate indiscriminately.

Evaluation

In patients receiving magaldrate, appropriate evaluation statements may include:
• Patient's pain subsides or is relieved.
• Patient experiences no constipation; maintains normal bowel function during therapy.
• Patient and family state an understanding of magaldrate therapy.

magnesium chloride

(mag nee´ zhum)
Slow-Mag◇

magnesium sulfate

• *Classification:* anticonvulsant, electrolyte supplement, antiarrhythmic (mineral/electrolyte)
• *Pregnancy Risk Category:* B

HOW SUPPLIED

chloride
Tablets (delayed-release): 64 mg
sulfate
Injectable solutions: 10%, 12.5%, 25%, 50% in 2-ml, 5-ml, 10-ml, 20-ml, and 30-ml ampules, vials, and prefilled syringes

ACTION

Mechanism: Divalent cation that is necessary for the function of several enzymes; also involved in calcium and potassium metabolism in a poorly understood fashion. As an I.V. additive, used to replace and maintain serum magnesium (Mg^{++}) levels. In pharmacologic doses, depresses neuronal function and may be used as an anticonvulsant. Also reduces muscle contractions by interfering with the release of acetylcholine at the neuromuscular junction.
Distribution: Widely distributed throughout the body. Only about 1% is found in the extracellular fluid; about 50% is found in bone and this fraction is not exchangable with extracellular Mg^{++}. The rest is intracellular. Serum Mg^{++} levels are not closely related to body stores or in-

tracellular Mg^{++} levels; however, low Mg^{++} serum levels indicate low Mg^{++} stores.
Metabolism: None.
Excretion: Mainly unchanged in urine; some, in breast milk.
Onset, peak, duration: I.V. magnesium sulfate acts immediately; effects last about 30 minutes. After I.M. injection, it acts within 60 minutes and lasts for 3 to 4 hours. Effective anticonvulsant serum levels are 2.5 to 7.5 mEq/liter.

INDICATIONS & DOSAGE

Hypomagnesemia –
Adults: 1 g, or 8.12 mEq, of 50% solution (2 ml) I.M. q 6 hours for 4 doses, depending on serum magnesium level.
Severe hypomagnesemia (serum magnesium 0.8 mEq/liter or less, with symptoms) –
Adults: 6 g, or 50 mEq, of 50% solution I.V. in 1 liter of solution over 4 hours.

Subsequent doses depend on serum magnesium levels.
Magnesium supplementation –
Adults: 64 mg (1 tablet) P.O. t.i.d.
Magnesium supplementation in total parenteral nutrition (TPN) –
Adults: 8 to 24 mEq I.V. daily added to TPN solution.
Children over 6 years: 2 to 10 mEq I.V. daily added to TPN solution.

Each 2 ml of 50% solution contains 1 g, or 8.12 mEq, magnesium sulfate.
Acute treatment of preeclampsia and eclampsia –
Adults: loading dose: 2 to 4 g (4 to 8 ml of 50% solution) given by slow I.V. bolus (over 5 minutes).
Maintenance dosage: 1 to 2 g hourly as a constant infusion. Prepare by adding 8 ml of 50% solution to 250 ml dextrose 5% in water.
Hypomagnesemic seizures –
Adults: 1 to 2 g (as 10% solution) I.V. over 15 minutes, then 1 g I.M. q 4 to 6 hours, based on patient response and magnesium blood level.
Seizures secondary to hypomagnesemia in acute nephritis –
Adults: 0.2 ml/kg of 50% solution I.M. q 4 to 6 hours, p.r.n. or 100 mg/kg of 10% solution I.V. very slowly. Titrate dosage according to magnesium blood level and seizure response.
Paroxysmal atrial tachycardia –
Adults: 3 to 4 g I.V. (as a 10% solution) over 30 seconds, with close monitoring of ECG.

CONTRAINDICATIONS & PRECAUTIONS

Contraindicated in patients with known heart block, myocardial damage, respiratory depression, renal failure, and in eclampsia for 2 hours preceding induced delivery to prevent toxicity and respiratory and CNS depression in neonates. Patient's urine output should be maintained at 100 ml/4 hours; use magnesium sulfate cautiously in patients with decreased renal function.

ADVERSE REACTIONS

Common reactions are in italics; life-threatening reactions are in bold italics.
CNS: toxicity, *weak or absent deep tendon reflexes,* flaccid paralysis, hypothermia, drowsiness, hypocalcemia (perioral paresthesias, twitching carpopedal spasm, tetany, and seizures).
CV: slow, weak pulse; cardiac arrhythmias (hypocalcemia); *hypotension.*
Skin: flushing, sweating.
Other: ***respiratory paralysis,*** hypocalcemia.

INTERACTIONS

Neuromuscular blocking agents: may cause increased neuromuscular blockage. Use cautiously.

EFFECTS ON DIAGNOSTIC TESTS

None reported.

*Liquid form contains alcohol. **May contain tartrazine.

NURSING CONSIDERATIONS

Besides those related universally to drug therapy (see "How to use this book"), consider the following specific recommendations:

Assessment

• Obtain a baseline assessment of patient's serum magnesium level and renal function before therapy.
• Be alert for adverse reactions and drug interactions throughout therapy.
• Evaluate the patient's and family's knowledge about magnesium therapy.

Nursing Diagnoses

• High risk for injury related to the patient's seizures.
• Impaired mobility related to magnesium-induced adverse CNS reactions.
• Knowledge deficit related to magnesium therapy.

Planning and Implementation

Preparation and Administration

• ***I.V. use:*** When administering as a direct injection, inject directly into vein not exceeding 150 mg/minute to avoid respiratory or cardiac arrest.. When giving as an intermittent infusion, administer diluted drug over 1 to 3 hours. When administering as a continuous infusion, give by infusion pump, not exceeding 150 mg/minute (1.2 mEq/minute).
• Test knee jerk and patellar reflexes before each additional dose. If absent, do not give more magnesium until reflexes return.

Monitoring

• Monitor effectiveness by evaluating magnesium levels frequently and, if the drug was given as an anticonvulsant, by noting the number and severity of seizures.
• Monitor vital signs every 15 minutes when giving I.V. for severe hypomagnesemia. Watch for respiratory depression and signs of heart block. Respirations should be more than 16/minute before dose is given.
• Monitor intake and output. Output should be 100 ml or more during the 4-hour period before dose.
• If toxemic mother received drug within 24 hours of delivery, watch neonate for signs of magnesium toxicity, including neuromuscular and respiratory depression.

Supportive Care

• Keep I.V. calcium available to reverse magnesium intoxication.
• Institute safety precautions if adverse CNS reactions occur.

Patient Teaching

• Stress the importance of follow-up care and regular blood tests to monitor magnesium levels.
• Warn patient to avoid hazardous activities that require mental alertness until adverse CNS effects are known.

Evaluation

In patients receiving magnesium, appropriate evaluation statements may include:

• Patient does not experience injury and patient's magnesium level is normal.
• Patient does not exhibit adverse reactions during magnesium therapy.
• Patient and family state an understanding of magnesium therapy.

---

magnesium citrate (citrate of magnesia)

(mag nee´ zhum)

Citroma◇, Citro-Nesia◇

magnesium hydroxide (milk of magnesia)

M.O.M.◇

magnesium sulfate (epsom salts)◇

• *Classification:* antacid, antiulcer agent, laxative (magnesium salt)
• *Pregnancy Risk Category:* B

HOW SUPPLIED

citrate

Oral solution: approximately 168 mEq magnesium/240 ml◇

hydroxide
Oral suspension: 7% to 8.5% (approximately 80 mEq magnesium/30 ml)◇
sulfate
Granules: approximately 40 mEq magnesium/5 g◇

ACTION
Mechanism: A saline laxative that produces an osmotic effect in the small intestine by drawing water into the intestinal lumen.
Absorption: About 15% to 30% of magnesium may be absorbed systemically (posing a potential risk to patients with renal failure).
Excretion: Unabsorbed drug is excreted in feces; absorbed drug is excreted rapidly in urine.
Onset, peak, duration: Produces an effect in 3 to 6 hours.

INDICATIONS & DOSAGE
Constipation, to evacuate bowel before surgery–
Adults and children over 6 years: 15 g magnesium sulfate P.O. in glass of water; or 10 to 20 ml concentrated milk of magnesia P.O.; or 15 to 60 ml milk of magnesia P.O.; or 5 to 10 oz magnesium citrate h.s.
Children 2 to 6 years: 5 to 15 ml milk of magnesia P.O.
Antacid–
Adults: 5 to 15 ml milk of magnesia P.O. t.i.d. or q.i.d.

CONTRAINDICATIONS & PRECAUTIONS
Contraindicated in patients with renal failure because of decreased excretion of absorbed magnesium, which may lead to hypermagnesemia, and in patients with an ileostomy, a colostomy, abdominal pain, nausea, vomiting, fecal impaction, or intestinal obstruction or perforation, because the drug may worsen the symptoms associated with these conditions.

ADVERSE REACTIONS
Common reactions are in italics; life-threatening reactions are in bold italics.
GI: *abdominal cramping, nausea.*
Metabolic: fluid and electrolyte disturbances if used daily.
Other: laxative dependence in long-term or excessive use.

INTERACTIONS
None significant.

EFFECTS ON DIAGNOSTIC TESTS
None reported.

NURSING CONSIDERATIONS
Besides those related universally to drug therapy (see "How to use this book"), consider the following specific recommendations:
Assessment
- Obtain a baseline assessment of history of bowel disorder, GI status, fluid intake, nutritional status, exercise habits, and normal pattern of elimination.
- Be alert for adverse reactions and drug interactions throughout therapy.
- Evaluate the patient's and family's knowledge about magnesium citrate, magnesium hydroxide, or magnesium sulfate therapy.

Nursing Diagnoses
- Constipation related to interruption of normal pattern of elimination characterized by infrequent or absent stools.
- Pain related to drug-induced abdominal cramping.
- Knowledge deficit related to magnesium citrate, magnesium hydroxide, or magnesium sulfate therapy.

Planning and Implementation
Preparation and Administration
- ***P.O. use:*** Shake suspension well; give with large amount of water when used as a laxative.
- ***Nasogastric tube administration:*** Check tube position and patency. After instilling, flush tube with water to

*Liquid form contains alcohol. **May contain tartrazine.

ensure passage to stomach and to maintain tube patency.
• Reschedule other oral drugs 1 to 2 hours before or after administration.
• Schedule administration of drug to avoid interference with scheduled activities or sleep. Be aware that as a saline laxative, drug produces watery stool in 3 to 6 hours.

Monitoring
• Monitor effectiveness by checking frequency and characteristics of stools.
• Monitor serum electrolytes during prolonged use.
• Auscultate bowel sounds at least once a shift. Assess for pain and cramping.
• Monitor nutritional status and fluid intake.

Supportive Care
• Do not give in patients with abdominal pain, nausea, vomiting, or other symptoms of appendicitis or acute surgical abdomen; and in those with myocardial damage, heart block, imminent delivery, fecal impaction, rectal fissures, intestinal obstruction or perforation, or renal disease.
• Use with caution in rectal bleeding.
• Be aware that these drugs are for short-term therapy and should not be used for longer than 1 week.
• Provide privacy for elimination.
• Unless contraindicated, encourage fluid intake up to 2,500 ml a day.
• Consult with a dietitian to modify diet to increase fiber and bulk.

Patient Teaching
• Discourage excessive use of laxatives to avoid dependence.
• Teach the patient about the relationship between fluid intake, dietary fiber, exercise, and constipation.
• Teach the patient that dietary sources of fiber include bran and other cereals, fresh fruit, and vegetables.
• Advise the patient that chilling before use may make magnesium citrate more palatable.
• Warn the patient that abdominal cramping may occur, but will subside when the bowel is emptied.

Evaluation
In patients receiving magnesium citrate, magnesium hydroxide, or magnesium sulfate, appropriate evaluation statements may include:
• Patient reports return of normal pattern of elimination.
• Patient remains free from abdominal cramping.
• Patient and family state an understanding of magnesium citrate, magnesium hydroxide, or magnesium sulfate therapy.

magnesium oxide
(mag nee´ zhum)
Mag-Ox 400◇, Maox◇, Par-Mag◇, Uro-Mag◇

• *Classification:* antacid (magnesium salt)
• *Pregnancy Risk Category:* C

HOW SUPPLIED
Tablets: 400 mg◇, 420 mg◇
Capsules: 140 mg◇
Oral suspension: 7.75%◇

ACTION
Mechanism: In water, magnesium oxide readily forms magnesium hydroxide, which reacts with gastric hydrochloric acid to form magnesium chloride and water. Reduces total acid load in the GI tract and elevates gastric pH to reduce pepsin activity.
Absorption: Small amounts are absorbed from the GI tract.
Metabolism: None.
Excretion: Most is excreted in the feces. Absorbed magnesium is excreted in urine, and may also be excreted in breast milk.

INDICATIONS & DOSAGE

Antacid–
Adults: 140 mg P.O. with water or milk after meals and h.s.
Laxative–
Adults: 4 g P.O. with water or milk, usually h.s.
Oral replacement therapy in mild hypomagnesemia–
Adults: 400 mg to 840 mg P.O. daily. Monitor serum magnesium response.

CONTRAINDICATIONS & PRECAUTIONS

Contraindicated in patients with renal failure because of decreased excretion of absorbed magnesium, which may lead to hypermagnesemia, and in patients with an ileostomy, a colostomy, abdominal pain, nausea, vomiting, fecal impaction, or intestinal obstruction or perforation, because the drug may worsen the symptoms associated with these disorders.

ADVERSE REACTIONS

Common reactions are in italics; life-threatening reactions are in bold italics.
GI: *diarrhea,* nausea, abdominal pain.
Metabolic: hypermagnesemia.

INTERACTIONS

Allopurinol, antibiotics (including quinolones and tetracyclines), corticosteroids, diflunisal, digoxin, iron, isoniazid, penicillamine, phenothiazines, ranitidine: decreased pharmacologic effect because absorption may be impaired. Separate administration times.

EFFECTS ON DIAGNOSTIC TESTS

Serum gastrin: elevated levels.
Serum phosphate: reduced levels.
Systemic and urine pH: increased.

NURSING CONSIDERATIONS

Besides those related universally to drug therapy (see "How to use this book"), consider the following specific recommendations:

Assessment
- Obtain a baseline assessment of the patient's pain or discomfort before beginning therapy.
- Be alert for adverse reactions and drug interactions throughout therapy.
- Evaluate the patient's and family's knowledge about magnesium oxide therapy.

Nursing Diagnoses
- Pain related to gastric hyperacidity.
- Diarrhea related to adverse reactions to magnesium oxide.
- Knowledge deficit related to magnesium oxide therapy.

Planning and Implementation
Preparation and Administration
- When used as a laxative do not give other oral drugs 1 to 2 hours before or after giving this drug. May cause entric-coated drugs to be released prematurely in the stomach.

Monitoring
- Monitor effectiveness by regularly assessing reduction or relief of the patient's pain.
- If the drug is given for its laxative effect, note increased number of stools.
- Monitor the patient's bowel pattern. Watch for development of diarrhea. If diarrhea occurs on antacid doses, an alternative preparation shoud be considered.
- Watch for symptoms of hypermagnesemia (hypotension, nausea, vomiting, depressed reflexes, respiratory depression, and coma) and monitor serum magnesium in patients with renal impairment and in those taking the drug for a prolonged time.

Supportive Care
- Notify the doctor if diarrhea occurs on an antacid dosage. He may want to order an alternative preparation.
- Encourage the patient to modify any emotional factors or dietary habits that may be contributing to GI problems.

Patient Teaching
• Teach the patient how to take the medication.
• Advise the patient not to switch to another antacid without consulting the doctor.
• Warn the patient not to take magnesium oxide indiscriminately.
• Explain the importance of taking the medications as prescribed, and not taking other medications at the same time.

Evaluation
In patients receiving magnesiun oxide, appropriate evaluation statements may include:
• Patient's pain subsides or is relieved.
• Patient experiences no diarrhea; maintains normal bowel function during therapy.
• Patient and family state an understanding of magnesium oxide therapy.

magnesium salicylate
(mag nee´ zhum)
Extra-Strength Doan's◇, Magan◇, Mobidin◇, Original Doan's◇

• *Classification:* non-narcotic analgesic, antipyretic, anti-inflammatory agent (salicylate)
• *Pregnancy Risk Category:* C

HOW SUPPLIED
Tablets: 545 mg, 600 mg
Caplets: 325 mg◇, 500 mg◇

ACTION
Mechanism: Inhibits prostaglandin synthesis. Produces antipyretic effect by acting on the hypothalamus. Produces analgesia by blocking generation of pain impulses or decreasing inflammation.
Absorption: Rapidly and completely absorbed from the GI tract.
Distribution: Highly protein-bound.
Metabolism: Hydrolyzed in the liver.
Excretion: Metabolites are excreted in urine.
Onset, peak, duration: Peak levels occur within 2 hours of a dose.

INDICATIONS & DOSAGE
Arthritis–
Adults: 545 mg to 1.2 g P.O. t.i.d. or q.i.d. not to exceed 4.8 g daily.
Mild pain or fever–
Adults: 300 to 600 mg P.O. q 4 hours, not to exceed 3.5 g/24 hours.

CONTRAINDICATIONS & PRECAUTIONS
Contraindicated in patients with hypersensitivity to salicylate or other nonsteroidal anti-inflammatory drugs (NSAIDs) and in patients with GI ulcer, GI bleeding, or renal insufficiency, because of the risk of magnesium toxicity.

Use cautiously in patients with a history of GI disease, increased risk of GI bleeding, or decreased renal function.

Patients with known "triad" symptoms (aspirin hypersensitivity, rhinitis/nasal polyps, and asthma) are at high risk of bronchospasm. Salicylates may mask the signs and symptoms of acute infection (fever, myalgia, erythema); carefully evaluate patients with high risk (such as those with diabetes).

ADVERSE REACTIONS
Common reactions are in italics; life-threatening reactions are in bold italics.
EENT: *tinnitus and hearing loss.*
GI: *nausea, vomiting, GI distress.*
Hepatic: abnormal liver function studies, hepatitis.
Skin: *rash,* bruising.
Other: ***hypersensitivity manifested by anaphylaxis*** or asthma.

INTERACTIONS
Ammonium chloride (and other urine acidifiers): increased blood levels of

salicylates. Monitor for salicylate toxicity.
Antacids in high doses (and other urine alkalinizers): decreased levels of salicylates. Monitor for decreased salicylate effect.
Corticosteroids: enhance salicylate elimination. Monitor for decreased salicylate effect.
Oral anticoagulants, heparin: increased risk of bleeding. Avoid using together if possible.

EFFECTS ON DIAGNOSTIC TESTS

Serum AST (SGOT), ALT (SGPT), alkaline, phosphatase, and bilirubin: increased levels.
Serum uric acid: false increases.
Urine aceto-acetic acid test (Gerhardt test): test interference.
Urine glucose (copper sulfate method): false-positive results.
Urine glucose (glucose enzymatic method): false-negative results.
Urine VMA tests: false increases or decreases.

NURSING CONSIDERATIONS

Besides those related universally to drug therapy (see "How to use this book"), consider the following specific recommendations:

Assessment
- Obtain a baseline assessment of pain before therapy.
- Be alert for adverse reactions and drug interactions throughout therapy.
- Evaluate the patient's and family's knowledge about magnesium salicylate therapy.

Nursing Diagnoses
- Pain related to the patient's underlying condition.
- Sensory/perceptual alterations related to adverse drug reaction.
- Knowledge deficit related to magnesium salicylate therapy.

Planning and Implementation

Preparation and Administration
- Do not give to children or teenagers with chicken pox or influenza-like illness because of epidemiologic association with Reye's syndrome.
- Give with food, milk, antacid or large glass of water to reduce adverse GI reactions.
- If GI problems occur, patient should take the drug with meals and take an antacid 2 hours after meals.

Monitoring
- Monitor effectiveness by regularly evaluating the degree of pain relief.
- Monitor the patient for toxicity. Keep in mind that febrile dehydrated children can rapidly develop toxicity.
- Monitor the patient's blood salicylate level. Therapeutic blood salicylate level in arthritis is 10 to 30 mg/dl. With chronic therapy, mild toxicity may occur at plasma levels of 20 mg/dl. Tinnitus may occur at plasma levels of 30 mg/dl and above, but is not a reliable indicator of toxicity, especially in very young patients and those over age 60.
- Obtain hemoglobin and prothrombin times in patients receiving long-term therapy with large doses.

Supportive Care
- Notify the doctor if the patient develops signs of adverse reactions such as salicylism (tinnitus, hearing loss), GI problems, or skin rash.
- Keep in mind that drug may cause increased serum levels of AST (SGOT), ALT (SGPT), alkaline phosphatase, and bilirubin, and abnormal results of liver function tests.
- Know that, unlike aspirin, this drug does not inhibit platelet aggregation.

Patient Teaching
- Tell the patient to take the drug with food, milk, an antacid, or a large glass of water to help reduce adverse GI reactions. If GI reactions occur, tell the patient to take the drug with meals and to take an antacid 2 hours after meals.
- Explain the importance of monitoring serum levels of AST, ALT, alkaline phosphatase, and bilirubin, as well as blood salicylate levels, hemo-

*Liquid form contains alcohol.

**May contain tartrazine.

globin levels, and prothrombin times. Also explain that liver function studies may become abnormal during treatment with this drug.
- Tell the patient to notify the doctor of tinnitus or hearing loss, which may be an adverse reaction to the drug.

Evaluation

In patients receiving magnesium salicylate, appropriate evaluation statements may include:
- Patient states pain is relieved.
- Patient denies tinnitus, and hearing loss has not occurred.
- Patient and family state an understanding of magnesium salicylate therapy.

magnesium sulfate
(mag nee´ zhum)

- *Classification:* anticonvulsant (mineral/electrolyte)
- *Pregnancy Risk Category:* B

HOW SUPPLIED
Injection: 10% (0.8 mEq/ml), 12.5% (1 mEq/ml), 25% (2 mEq/ml), 50% (4 mEq/ml)

ACTION
Mechanism: May decrease acetylcholine released by nerve impulse, but its anticonvulsant mechanism is unknown.
Absorption: Slowly absorbed from I.M. injection sites.
Distribution: Widely distributed throughout the body.
Metabolism: None.
Excretion: Unchanged in urine; some is excreted in breast milk.
Onset, peak, duration: I.V. magnesium sulfate acts immediately; effects last about 30 minutes. After I.M. injection, it acts within 60 minutes and lasts for 3 to 4 hours. Effective anticonvulsant serum levels are 2.5 to 7.5 mEq/liter.

INDICATIONS & DOSAGE
Hypomagnesemic seizures–
Adults: 1 to 2 g (as 10% solution) I.V. over 15 minutes, then 1 g I.M. q 4 to 6 hours, based on patient response and blood magnesium levels.
Seizures secondary to hypomagnesemia in acute nephritis–
Children: 0.2 ml/kg of 50% solution I.M. q 4 to 6 hours, p.r.n. or 100 mg/kg of 10% solution I.V. very slowly. Titrate dosage according to blood magnesium levels and seizure response.
Prevention or control of seizures in preeclampsia or eclampsia –
Women: initially, 4 g I.V. in 250 ml dextrose 5% in water and 4 g deep I.M. each buttock; then 4 g deep I.M. into alternate buttock q 4 hours, p.r.n. Alternatively, 4 g I.V. loading dose followed by 1 to 4 g hourly as an I.V. infusion.

CONTRAINDICATIONS & PRECAUTIONS
Contraindicated in patients with heart block, myocardial damage, respiratory depression, or renal failure; and for 2 hours before induced delivery in patients with eclampsia, to prevent toxicity and respiratory and CNS depression in the newborn.

Patient's urine output should be maintained at 100 ml/4 hours; use with caution in patients with decreased renal function.

ADVERSE REACTIONS
Common reactions are in italics; life-threatening reactions are in bold italics.
CNS: *sweating,* drowsiness, *depressed reflexes,* flaccid paralysis, hypothermia.
CV: *hypotension, flushing,* ***circulatory collapse,*** depressed cardiac function, *heart block.*
Other: ***respiratory paralysis,*** hypocalcemia.

INTERACTIONS

Neuromuscular blocking agents: may cause increased neuromuscular blockade. Use cautiously.

EFFECTS ON DIAGNOSTIC TESTS

None reported.

NURSING CONSIDERATIONS

Besides those related universally to drug therapy (see "How to use this book"), consider the following specific recommendations:

Assessment

- Obtain a baseline assessment of seizure activity before beginning therapy.
- Be alert for adverse reactions and drug interactions throughout therapy.
- Evaluate the patient's and family's knowledge about magnesium sulfate therapy.

Nursing Diagnoses

- High risk for injury related to the underlying seizure disorder or seizure possibility.
- Ineffective breathing pattern related to magnesium sulfate-induced respiratory depression.
- Knowledge deficit related to magnesium sulfate therapy.

Planning and Implementation

Preparation and Administration

- ***I.V. use:*** Keep in mind that the maximum infusion rate is 150 mg/minute. Rapid administration will induce uncomfortable feeling of heat.
- ***I.M. use:*** Be aware that I.M. administration precedes I.V. administration in pediatric hypertension and encephalopathy.

Monitoring

- Monitor effectiveness by evaluating seizure activity.
- Monitor vital signs every 15 minutes when giving drug I.V.
- Watch for respiratory depression and signs of heart block. Respirations should be approximately 16 breaths per minute before each dose is given.
- Monitor intake and output. Urine output should be 100 ml or more in 4-hour period before each dose.
- Monitor blood magnesium levels after repeated doses. Keep in mind that signs of hypermagnesemia begin to appear at blood levels of 4 mEq/liter. At higher levels, life-threatening reactions, such as cardiac arrest, respiratory paralysis, severe hypotension, and severe bradycardia are possible.
- Check knee-jerk and patellar reflexes. Disappearance of these reflexes signals pending magnesium toxicity.
- Especially when given to toxemic mothers within 24 hours before delivery, observe neonates for signs of magnesium toxicity, including neuromuscular or respiratory depression.

Supportive Care

- Notify the doctor immediately if respiratory rate decreases, if patellar reflexes disappear, or if other adverse reactions occur.
- Maintain seizure precautions.
- If CNS reactions occur, institute safety precautions.
- Keep I.V. calcium gluconate available to reverse magnesium intoxication; however, use cautiously in patients receiving digitalis glycosides due to danger of arrhythmias. In severe overdose, peritoneal dialysis or hemodialysis may be necessary.
- Be aware that magnesium sulfate can decrease the frequency and force of uterine contractions. This drug has been used as a tocolytic agent to inhibit premature labor.

Patient Teaching

- Explain that magnesium sulfate does have adverse effects but that vital signs, reflexes, and blood levels will be checked frequently to ensure patient safety.

Evaluation

In patients receiving magnesium sulfate, appropriate evaluation statments may include:

- Patient remains free of seizure activity.

• Patient's respiratory rate and pattern remain within normal range.
• Patient and family state an understanding of magnesium sulfate therapy.

mannitol

(man´ i tole)
Osmitrol†

• *Classification:* diuretic, reduction of intracranial or intraocular pressure, treatment of drug intoxication (osmotic diuretic)
• *Pregnancy Risk Category:* C

HOW SUPPLIED

Injection: 5%, 10%, 15%, 20%, 25%

ACTION

Mechanism: Increases the osmotic pressure of glomerular filtrate, inhibiting tubular reabsorption of water and electrolytes. Also elevates blood plasma osmolality, resulting in enhanced flow of water from tissues (such as the brain and the eye) into extracellular fluid.
Absorption: Absorbed from the GI tract. Administered I.V.
Distribution: In the extracellular compartment. Does not cross the blood-brain barrier.
Metabolism: Minimally metabolized to glycogen in the liver.
Excretion: Filtered by the glomeruli. Half-life: About 100 minutes in adults with normal renal function.
Onset, peak, duration: I.V. mannitol lowers intracranial pressure in 15 minutes and intraocular pressure in 30 to 60 minutes; it produces diuresis in 1 to 3 hours.

INDICATIONS & DOSAGE

Test dose for marked oliguria or suspected inadequate renal function –
Adults and children over 12 years: 200 mg/kg or 12.5 g as a 15% or 20% solution I.V. over 3 to 5 minutes. Response adequate if 30 to 50 ml urine/hour is excreted over 2 to 3 hours.
Treatment of oliguria –
Adults and children over 12 years: 50 to 100 g I.V. as a 15% to 20% solution over 90 minutes to several hours.
Prevention of oliguria or acute renal failure –
Adults and children over 12 years: 50 to 100 g I.V. of a concentrated (5% to 25%) solution. Exact concentration is determined by fluid requirements.
Edema –
Adults and children over 12 years: 100 g I.V. as a 10% to 20% solution over 2- to 6-hour period.
To reduce intraocular pressure or intracranial pressure –
Adults and children over 12 years: 1.5 to 2 g/kg as a 15% to 25% solution I.V. over 30 to 60 minutes.
To promote diuresis in drug intoxication –
Adults and children over 12 years: 5% to 10% solution continuously up to 200 g I.V., while maintaining 100 to 500 ml urine output/hour and a positive fluid balance.

CONTRAINDICATIONS & PRECAUTIONS

Contraindicated in patients with established anuria who do not respond to a test dose and in those with severe pulmonary congestion, pulmonary edema, severe CHF, or severe dehydration, because of the risk of circulatory overload. Do not administer mannitol until adequate renal function and urine flow are determined by a test dose. Evaluate patient's CV status before and during drug administration; sudden expansion of extracellular fluid may precipitate congestive heart failure.

ADVERSE REACTIONS

Common reactions are in italics; life-threatening reactions are in bold italics.
CNS: rebound increase in intracranial pressure 8 to 12 hours after diuresis, headache, confusion.
CV: *transient expansion of plasma volume during infusion causing **circulatory overload and pulmonary edema,*** tachycardia, angina-like chest pain.
EENT: blurred vision, rhinitis.
GI: thirst, nausea, vomiting.
GU: urine retention.
Metabolic: *fluid and electrolyte imbalance, water intoxication, cellular dehydration.*

INTERACTIONS

None significant.

EFFECTS ON DIAGNOSTIC TESTS

Electrolyte levels: altered results.
Inorganic phosphorus or blood ethylene glycol concentrations: test interference.

NURSING CONSIDERATIONS

Besides those related universally to drug therapy (see "How to use this book"), consider the following specific recommendations:

Assessment

- Obtain a baseline assessment of hourly urine output; vital signs, including central venous pressure; breath sounds; serum electrolyte levels; and peripheral edema before therapy.
- Be alert for adverse reactions and drug interactions throughout therapy.
- Evaluate the patient's and family's knowledge about mannitol therapy.

Nursing Diagnoses

- Fluid volume excess related to the patient's underlying condition as evidenced by edema.
- Altered urinary elimination related to diuretic therapy.
- Knowledge deficit related to mannitol therapy.

Planning and Implementation

Preparation and Administration

- Be aware that drug may be used to test for marked oliguria or suspected inadequate renal function (see "Indications & Dosage").
- For maximum intraocular pressure reduction before surgery, give 1 to 1½ hours preoperatively.
- Solution often crystallizes, especially at low temperatures. To redissolve, warm bottle in hot water and shake vigorously. Cool to body temperature before giving. Concentrations more than 15% have greater tendency to crystallize. Do not use solution with undissolved crystals.
- Do not administer with whole blood; agglutination will occur.
- Be aware that rapid administration of large doses may lead to drug accumulation and circulatory overload.
- ***I.V. use:*** Always give mannitol infusions via an in-line filter and with an infusion pump. Direct injection is not recommended. Administer drug as an intermittent or continuous infusion at prescribed rate. Check I.V. line patency infusion site before and during administration.

Monitoring

- Monitor effectiveness by checking hourly urine output, vital signs, breath sounds, and CVP readings.
- Regularly monitor serum and urine levels of sodium and potassium.
- Weigh the patient daily, if possible.
- Monitor renal function studies.
- Monitor for signs of rebound increased intracranial pressure (headache and confusion) as indicated.
- Monitor I.V. line patency and infusion site to prevent infiltration of mannitol and possible local edema and tissue necrosis.
- Monitor skin turgor and mucous membranes for signs of fluid volume deficit.
- Monitor the patient's extremities for peripheral edema.

Supportive Care
• Hold dose and notify the doctor immediately if adverse reactions occur.
• Keep accurate record of intake and output, vital signs, and CVP measurement.
• Provide frequent skin and mouth care to relieve dryness due to mannitol therapy.
• If extravasation of mannitol occurs, elevate the extremity, apply warm moist compress, and notify the doctor.
• Use safety precautions to avoid risk of injury due to falls.
• Be aware that the comatose or incontinent patient requires insertion of a urethral catheter because therapy is based on strict evaluation of intake and output. In the patient with a urethral catheter, use an hourly urometer collection bag to facilitate accurate evaluation of output.
• Reorient the confused patient to person, time, and place.
• If peripheral edema is present, elevate the patient's extremities.
Patient Teaching
• Teach the patient to avoid foods high in sodium.
• Tell the patient he may feel thirsty or experience mouth dryness and emphasize importance of drinking only the amount of fluids provided, as ordered by the doctor.
• With initial doses, warn the patient to change positions slowly, especially when rising from a lying or sitting position, to prevent dizziness from orthostatic hypotension.
• Instruct the patient to tell the doctor immediately if he experiences pain in the chest, back, or legs or shortness of breath.

Evaluation
In patients receiving mannitol, appropriate evaluation statements may include:
• Patient is free of edema.
• Patient demonstrates coping behaviors and comfort in dealing with altered patterns of urinary elimination.
• Patient and family state an understanding of mannitol therapy.

maprotiline hydrochloride
(ma proe´ ti leen)
Ludiomil

• *Classification:* tricyclic antidepressant
• *Pregnancy Risk Category:* B

HOW SUPPLIED
Tablets: 25 mg, 50 mg, 75 mg

ACTION
Mechanism: Increases the amount of norepinephrine or serotonin, or both, in the CNS by blocking their reuptake by presynaptic neurons. This allows these neurotransmitters to accumulate.
Absorption: Slowly but completely absorbed from the GI tract after oral administration.
Distribution: Widely distributed into the body, including the CNS and breast milk. Drug is 88% protein-bound. Proposed therapeutic serum levels range between 200 and 300 ng/ml.
Metabolism: Slowly metabolized by the liver to the active metabolite desmethylmaprotiline; a significant first-pass effect may account for variability of serum concentrations in different patients taking the same dosage.
Excretion: Most is excreted in urine as metabolites within 3 weeks. About 30% is excreted in feces via the biliary tract. Half-life: About 50 hours.
Onset, peak, duration: Peak serum concentration levels occur 8 to 24 hours after oral dose; steady-state plasma levels and peak therapeutic effect usually occur within 2 weeks.

INDICATIONS & DOSAGE

Treatment of depression–
Adults: initial dose of 75 mg P.O. daily for patients with mild to moderate depression. The dosage may be increased as required to a dose of 150 mg daily. Maximum dosage is 225 mg in patients who are not hospitalized. Severely depressed, hospitalized patients may receive up to 300 mg daily.

CONTRAINDICATIONS & PRECAUTIONS

Contraindicated in patients with hypersensitivity to tricyclic antidepressants, trazodone, and related compounds; in the acute recovery phase of myocardial infarction because of arrhythmogenic potential; in coma or severe respiratory depression because of additive CNS depression; and during or within 14 days of therapy with MAO inhibitors because the combination can precipitate hyperpyrexia, hypertension, and seizures.

Use cautiously in patients with other cardiac disease (arrhythmias, CHF, angina pectoris, valvular disease, or heart block); respiratory disorders; alcoholism, other seizure disorders; scheduled electroconvulsive therapy; bipolar disease; glaucoma; hyperthyroidism or in those taking thyroid replacement; Type I and Type II diabetes; prostatic hypertrophy, paralytic ileus, or urine retention; hepatic or renal dysfunction; or Parkinson's disease; and in those undergoing surgery with general anesthesia.

ADVERSE REACTIONS

Common reactions are in italics; life-threatening reactions are in bold italics.
CNS: *drowsiness, dizziness,* excitation, ***seizures,*** tremors, weakness, confusion, headache, nervousness.
CV: orthostatic hypotension, tachycardia, *ECG changes,* hypertension.
EENT: *blurred vision,* tinnitus, mydriasis.
GI: *dry mouth, constipation,* nausea, vomiting, anorexia, paralytic ileus.
GU: *urine retention.*
Skin: rash, urticaria.
Other: *sweating,* allergy.
After abrupt withdrawal of long-term therapy: nausea, headache, malaise. (Does not indicate addiction.)

INTERACTIONS

Barbiturates: decrease maprotiline blood levels. Monitor for decreased antidepressant effect.
Cimetidine: may increase maprotiline serum levels. Monitor for increased adverse reactions.
Epinephrine, norepinephrine: increase hypertensive effect. Use with caution.
MAO inhibitors: may cause severe excitation, hyperpyrexia, or seizures, usually with high dose. Use together cautiously.
Methylphenidate: increases maprotiline blood levels. Monitor for enhanced antidepressant effect.

EFFECTS ON DIAGNOSTIC TESTS

CBC: decreased WBC counts.
ECG: elongated Q-T and PR intervals, flattened T waves.
Liver function tests: elevated results.
Serum glucose: decreased or increased levels.

NURSING CONSIDERATIONS

Besides those related universally to drug therapy (see "How to use this book"), consider the following specific recommendations:

Assessment
- Obtain a baseline assessment of depression before therapy.
- Be alert for adverse reactions and drug interactions throughout therapy.
- Evaluate the patient's and family's knowledge about maprotiline therapy.

Nursing Diagnoses
- Altered individual coping related to the patient's underlying condition.

• Constipation related to maprotiline-induced adverse GI reactions.
• Knowledge deficit related to maprotiline therapy.

Planning and Implementation

Preparation and Administration
• Whenever possible, patient should take full dose at bedtime.
• Expect reduced dosage in elderly or debilitated patients and adolescents.

Monitoring
• Monitor effectiveness by having the patient discuss his feelings (ask broad, open-ended questions) and by evaluating his behavior.
• Monitor blood pressure (supine and standing), ECG for changes, and heart rate for tachycardia.
• Monitor bowel patterns for constipation and check for urine retention.
• Note mood changes and monitor for suicidal tendencies.

Supportive Care
• Institute safety precautions if adverse CNS reactions occur.
• Do not withdraw drug abruptly.
• If psychotic signs increase, notify doctor and expect dosage to be reduced.
• If not contraindicated, increase the patient's fluid and fiber intake to prevent constipation; if needed, obtain an order for a stool softener or a laxative.

Patient Teaching
• Tell the patient to relieve dry mouth with sugarless hard candy or gum. However, maprotiline has a low potential for inducing anticholinergic effects.
• Teach the patient to minimize constipation by increasing fluid intake. Suggest stool softener or high-fiber diet, if needed.
• Warn the patient to avoid driving and other hazardous activities that require alertness and good psychomotor coordination until CNS effects of the drug are known. Tell the patient that drowsiness and dizziness usually subside after first few weeks.

Evaluation

In patients receiving maprotiline, appropriate evaluation statements may include:
• Patient behavior and communication indicate improvement of depression.
• Constipation has not occurred.
• Patient and family state an understanding of maprotiline therapy.

measles, mumps, and rubella virus vaccine, live

M-M-RII

• *Classification:* viral vaccine
• *Pregnancy Risk Category:* X

HOW SUPPLIED

Injection: single-dose vial containing not less than 1,000 $TCID_{50}$ (tissue culture infective doses) of attenuated measles virus derived from Enders' attenuated Edmonston strain (grown in chick embryo culture), 5,000 $TCID_{50}$ of the Jeryl Lynn (B level) mumps strain (grown in chick embryo culture), and the Wistar RA 27/3 strain of rubella virus (propagated in human diploid cell culture)

ACTION

Mechanism: Promotes immunity to measles, mumps, and rubella virus by inducing production of antibodies.
Pharmacokinetics: Unknown.
Onset, peak, duration: Antibodies are usually evident 2 to 3 weeks after injection. The duration of vaccine-induced immunity is unknown.

INDICATIONS & DOSAGE

Routine vaccination—
Children: administer 1 vial S.C. A two-dose schedule is recommended, with the first dose given at 15 months (12 months in high-risk areas) and the second dose given at

the entry of school (kindergarten or first grade).

Measles outbreak control–

Children: if cases are occurring in children under 1 year, vaccinate children as young as 6 months. All students and their siblings should be revaccinated if they are without documentation of measles immunity.

Adults: school personnel born in or after 1957 should be revaccinated if they are without proof of measles immunity. If the outbreak is in a medical facility, all workers born in or after 1957 should be revaccinated if they are without proof of immunity. Revaccination should be considered for persons born before 1957 as well.

CONTRAINDICATIONS & PRECAUTIONS

Contraindicated in patients with infections, blood dyscrasia, cancers of or affecting the bone marrow or lymphatic systems, primary immunodeficiency states; in pregnant patients; and in those receiving corticotropin, corticosteroids, irradiation, or other immunosuppressant therapy.

Use cautiously in patients with hypersensitivity (other than dermatitis) to neomycin, a component of the vaccine; in children with a history of febrile seizures or cerebral injury; or in any febrile situation.

ADVERSE REACTIONS

Common reactions are in italics; life-threatening reactions are in bold italics.

Systemic: fever, rash, regional lymphadenopathy, urticaria, ***anaphylaxis.***

Local: erythema.

INTERACTIONS

Immune serum globulin, whole blood, plasma: antibodies in serum may interfere with immune response. Don't use vaccine within 3 months of transfusion.

EFFECTS ON DIAGNOSTIC TESTS

Tuberculin skin testing: temporary decreased response.

NURSING CONSIDERATIONS

Besides those related universally to drug therapy (see "How to use this book"), consider the following specific recommendations:

Assessment

- Obtain a baseline assessment of allergies (especially to ducks, rabbits, and antibiotics), immunization history, and immunization reaction before administering vaccine.
- Be alert for adverse reactions and drug interactions throughout therapy.
- Evaluate the patient's and family's knowledge about measles, mumps, and rubella virus vaccine therapy.

Nursing Diagnoses

- Altered protection related to lack of immunity to measles, mumps, and rubella virus.
- Hyperthermia related to vaccine-induced fever.
- Knowledge deficit related to live measles, mumps, and rubella virus vaccine.

Planning and Implementation

Preparation and Administration

- Store vaccine in the refrigerator protect from light. Solution may be used if it is red, yellow, or pink, but it must be clear.
- Use only diluent supplied. Discard 8 hours after reconstituting.
- ***S.C. use:*** Inject in outer aspect of upper arm.
- Do not give I.V.
- If a tuberculin skin test is necessary, administer it either before or simultaneously with this vaccine.

Monitoring

- Monitor effectiveness by checking the patient's antibody titers to measles, mumps, and rubella virus.
- Observe the patient for signs of anaphylaxis immediately after injecting vaccine.
- Check the patient's temperature; fe-

ver commonly occurs after immunization.

Supportive Care

• Keep epinephrine 1:1,000 available to treat possible anaphylaxis.

• Treat fever with antipyretics.

• Apply ice or cold compresses to localized erythema.

• Defer immunization in acute illness.

• Presence of maternal antibodies may prevent immune response in children under 12 months.

• Clinical trials have shown that vitamin A supplementation reduces morbidity and mortality in children with measles. Studies have used 100,000 to 400,000 IU daily.

• The Centers for Disease Control recommends that, during a measles outbreak in a health care facility, susceptible personnel exposed to the measles virus (whether or not they received the measles vaccine or immunoglobulin) avoid patient contact for days 5 through 21 after such exposure. If they become ill, they should avoid patient contact for at least 7 days after developing rash.

Patient Teaching

• Inform the patient or parents that fever and local erythema may occur after immunization.

• Inform the patient or parents that, because of a recent rise in the incidence of measles, the Immunization Practices Advisory Committee (ACIP) recommends that colleges and other post–high school educational institutions, as well as medical institutions employing health care providers, obtain documentation confirming two doses of vaccine after age 1 (or other proof of immunity, such as infection, documented by a doctor). Combined measles, mumps, and rubella vaccine is preferred.

Evaluation

In patients receiving live measles, mumps, and rubella virus vaccine, appropriate evaluation statements may include:

• Patient exhibits immunity to measles, mumps, and rubella viruses.

• Patient's temperature remains within the normal range.

• Patient and family state an understanding of live measles, mumps, and rubella virus vaccine therapy.

mebendazole

(me ben´ da zole)

Vermox

• *Classification:* anthelmintic (benzimidazole)

• *Pregnancy Risk Category:* C

HOW SUPPLIED

Tablets (chewable): 100 mg

Oral suspension: 100 mg/5 ml‡

ACTION

Mechanism: Selectively and irreversibly inhibits uptake of glucose and other nutrients in susceptible helminths.

Absorption: Most of the drug remains at its site of action within the intestinal lumen. Absorption varies widely but an estimated 5% to 10% of dose is absorbed. Administering the drug with food does not appear to impair its effectiveness.

Distribution: Highly bound to plasma proteins; it crosses the placenta.

Metabolism: Mebendazole is metabolized to inactive 2-amino 5(6)-benzimidazolyl phenyketone.

Excretion: Most of a dose is excreted in the feces; 2% to 10% is excreted in urine in 48 hours as the unchanged drug or its inactive metabolite. Unknown if it's excreted in breast milk. Half-life: 3 to 9 hours.

Onset, peak, duration: Peak plasma concentrations occur at 2 to 4 hours.

INDICATIONS & DOSAGE

Pinworm–

Adults and children over 2 years: 100 mg P.O. as a single dose. If infection persists 3 weeks later, repeat treatment.

Roundworm, whipworm, hookworm–

Adults and children over 2 years: 100 mg P.O. b.i.d. for 3 days. If infection persists 3 weeks later, repeat treatment.

CONTRAINDICATIONS & PRECAUTIONS

Contraindicated in patients with hypersensitivity to the drug.

ADVERSE REACTIONS

Common reactions are in italics; life-threatening reactions are in bold italics.

GI: occasional, transient abdominal pain and diarrhea in massive infection and expulsion of worms.

INTERACTIONS

None significant.

EFFECTS ON DIAGNOSTIC TESTS

None reported.

NURSING CONSIDERATIONS

Besides those related universally to drug therapy (see "How to use this book"), consider the following specific recommendations:

Assessment

- Obtain a baseline assessment of infection, including appropriate specimens for analysis before therapy.
- Be alert for adverse reactions and drug interactions throughout therapy.
- Evaluate the patient's and family's knowledge about mebendazole therapy.

Nursing Diagnoses

- Altered health maintenance related to ineffectiveness of mebendazole.
- Diarrhea related to an adverse GI reaction to mebendazole therapy.
- Knowledge deficit related to mebendazole.

Planning and Implementation

Preparation and Administration

- ***P.O. use:*** Mebendazole tablets may be chewed, swallowed whole, or crushed and mixed with food.

Monitoring

- Monitor effectiveness by regularly assessing for improvement of infection and by obtaining specimens for laboratory analysis as prescribed.
- Monitor number and characteristics of stools daily.

Supportive Care

- Obtain an order for an antidiarrheal agent as needed.
- Ensure that patient's family and suspected contacts are treated to prevent reinfection.

Patient Teaching

- Teach the patient and family about the need for meticulous personal hygiene, especially good hand-washing technique. To avoid reinfection, teach the patient to wash perianal area, to change undergarments and bed clothes daily, and to wash hands and clean fingernails before meals and after bowel movements.
- Tell the patient to avoid preparing food during infection.
- Inform the patient and family that no dietary restriction, laxatives, or enemas are necessary.
- Tell the patient the tablets may be chewed, swallowed whole, or crushed and mixed with food.

Evaluation

In patients receiving mebendazole, appropriate evaluation statements may include:

- Patient is free of infection and maintains normal health status.
- Patient does not experience diarrhea during therapy.
- Patient and family state an understanding of mebendazole therapy.

mechlorethamine hydrochloride (nitrogen mustard)

(me klor eth´ a meen)
Mustargen

- *Classification:* antineoplastic (alkylating agent)
- *Pregnancy Risk Category:* D

HOW SUPPLIED

Injection: 10-mg vials

ACTION

Mechanism: An alkylating agent that cross-links strands of cellular DNA and interferes with RNA transcription, causing an imbalance of growth that leads to cell death. Cell cycle–nonspecific.
Absorption: Well absorbed after oral administration; however, because the drug is very irritating to tissue, it must be administered I.V. After intracavitary administration, drug is only partially absorbed, probably because of deactivation by body fluids in the cavity.
Distribution: Does not cross the blood-brain barrier.
Metabolism: Rapidly converted to its active form. Parent drug is undetectable in the bloodstream within a few minutes of administration.
Excretion: Metabolites are excreted in urine. Less than 0.01% of an I.V. dose is excreted unchanged in urine.

INDICATIONS & DOSAGE

Breast, lung, and ovarian cancer; Hodgkin's disease; non-Hodgkin's lymphomas; diffuse lymphocytic lymphoma–
Adults: 0.4 mg/kg or 10 mg/m^2 I.V. as a single dose or in divided doses q 3 to 6 weeks. Give through running I.V. infusion. Dosage reduced in prior radiation or chemotherapy to 0.2 to 0.4 mg/kg. Dosage based on ideal or actual body weight, whichever is less.
Neoplastic effusions–
Adults: 0.4 mg/kg intracavitarily.

CONTRAINDICATIONS & PRECAUTIONS

Contraindicated in patients with foci of chronic or suppurative inflammation because of the potential for extensive and rapid development of amyloidosis. It may be necessary to adjust dosage or discontinue therapy in patients with infections, hematologic compromise, or bone marrow infiltration with malignant cells because of the drug's adverse hematologic effects.

ADVERSE REACTIONS

Common reactions are in italics; life-threatening reactions are in bold italics.
Blood: *nadir of myelosuppression occurring by days 4 to 10, lasting 10 to 21 days;* mild anemia begins in 2 to 3 weeks, possibly lasting 7 weeks.
CNS: headache.
EENT: tinnitus; *metallic taste* (immediately after dose); deafness with high doses.
GI: *nausea, vomiting, and anorexia* begin within minutes, last 8 to 24 hours.
Metabolic: hyperuricemia.
Skin: rash.
Local: ***thrombophlebitis,*** *sloughing, severe irritation if drug extravasates or touches skin.*
Other: *alopecia,* may precipitate herpes zoster, ***anaphylaxis.***

INTERACTIONS

Procarbazine, cyclophosphamide: possible increased risk of hepatotoxicity.

EFFECTS ON DIAGNOSTIC TESTS

Blood and urine uric acid: increased levels.
Serum pseudocholinesterase: decreased activity.

NURSING CONSIDERATIONS

Besides those related universally to drug therapy (see "How to use this book"), consider the following specific recommendations:

Assessment

• Obtain a baseline assessment of the patient's underlying condition and CBC, platelet, uric acid, BUN, creatinine, liver enzyme and total bilirubin levels before therapy.

• Be alert for adverse reactions and drug interactions throughout therapy.

• Evaluate the patient's and family's knowledge about mechlorethamine therapy.

Nursing Diagnoses

• High risk for infection related to mechlorethamine-induced adverse reactions.

• Altered nutrition: Less than body requirements, related to drug-induced severe nausea and vomiting.

• Knowledge deficit related to mechlorethamine therapy.

Planning and Implementation

Preparation and Administration

• Exercise caution when preparing and administering this drug to avoid mutagenic, teratogenic, and carcinogenic risks. Use a biological containment cabinet, wear gloves and a mask, and avoid contaminating work surfaces. If skin contact occurs, wash with copious amounts of water. Any equipment used in the preparation and administration of this drug should be disposed of properly according to institutional policy.

• This solution is very unstable; therefore, prepare it immediately before use and use within 15 minutes. Unused solution should be neutralized with an equal volume of 5% sodium chloride and 5% sodium thiosulfate.

• Expect antiemetics to be given preceding or during infusion of this drug to decrease severe nausea and vomiting, which usually begins 1 to 3 hours after administration.

• ***I.V. use:*** Administer with hydrocortisone to decrease risk of phlebitis and painful administration. Take all possible precautions to avoid infiltration. In direct injection, use one sterile needle to aspirate reconstituted drug from the vial and another for direct injection. Inject the reconstituted solution directly into a vein or, prefereably, into a free-flowing I.V. solution over a few minutes or according to protocol. After administration, flush the vein with I.V. solution for a few minutes.

• ***Intracavitary use:*** When given intracavitarily for sclerosing effect, turn patient from side to side every 15 minutes to 1 hour to distribute drug.

Monitoring

• Monitor effectiveness by noting results of follow-up diagnostic tests and overall physical status.

• Monitor CBC, platelet, serum uric acid, BUN, creatinine, liver enzyme, and bilirubin levels throughout therapy.

• Monitor for signs of bleeding (hematuria, ecchymosis, petechiae, epistaxis, melena).

• Closely monitor for signs of potentially fatal infections or hemorrhagic complications noted by temperature elevation, sore throat, malaise, or unusual bruising or bleeding.

• Monitor vital signs frequently during I.V. infusion of this drug.

• Monitor intake and output during drug therapy.

• Monitor for extravasation during administration. If it occurs, immediately treat as described above.

Supportive Care

• If drug infiltrates, discontinue the drug, inject the area with sterile isotonic sodium thiosulfate (1/6 M), and apply ice compresses for 6 to 12 hours. Use 4.14 g of sodium thiosulfate per 100 ml of sterile water for injection, or dilute 4 ml of sodium thiosulfate (10%) with 6 ml of sterile water for injection. Mechlorethamine

is a potent vesicant; if infiltration occurs, immediate treatment is required.
- Use anticoagulants and aspirin products with extreme caution.
- Give antibiotics, as ordered, to patients with leukopenia who develop infections.
- Give antiemetics, as required, to reduce severity of nausea and vomiting, which occurs in almost all patients.
- Avoid contact with skin. If contact occurs, wash the area liberally with soap and water.
- To prevent hyperuricemia with resulting uric acid nephropathy, allopurinol may be administered with adequate hydration.
- Expect some evidence of toxicity with a therapeutic response. Mechlorethamine is highly toxic and has a low therapeutic index.
- Do not give any I.M. injections when the platelet count is below 100,000/mm³.

Patient Teaching
- Explain all the adverse reactions that may occur with this drug and teach patient actions to take to help prevent or alleviate each reaction.
- Warn patient to watch for signs of infection (sore throat, fever, fatigue), and bleeding (easy bruising, nosebleeds, bleeding gums). Tell patient to take his temperature daily, and to avoid exposure to people with infections.
- Teach patient to avoid the use of all OTC products containing aspirin.

Evaluation
In patients receiving mechlorethamine, appropriate evaluation statements may include:
- Patient remains free from infection during and after chemotherapy.
- Patient's nutritional status improves and remains stable without compromise from the effects of nausea and vomiting.
- Patient and family state an understanding of mechlorethamine therapy.

meclizine hydrochloride (meclozine hydrochloride)
(mek′ li zeen)
Ancolan‡, Antivert, Antivert/25◇, Antivert/50, Bonamine†, Bonine◇, Dizmiss◇, Meni-D, Ru-Vert M

- *Classification:* antiemetic and antivertigo agent (piperazine-derivative antihistamine)
- *Pregnancy Risk Category:* B

HOW SUPPLIED
Tablets: 12.5 mg, 25 mg◇, 50 mg
Tablets (chewable): 25 mg◇
Capsules: 15 mg, 25 mg, 30 mg

ACTION
Mechanism: Drug has anticholinergic and antihistaminergic properties. May block neural pathways originating in the labyrinth of the ear projecting to the vomiting center or chemoreceptor trigger zone in the medulla to inhibit nausea and vomiting, but the exact mechanism of action is unknown.
Absorption: Rapidly absorbed from the GI tract.
Distribution: Well distributed throughout the body and crosses the placenta.
Metabolism: In the liver.
Excretion: Unchanged in feces; metabolites are found in urine. Half-life: About 6 hours.
Onset, peak, duration: Action persists for 8 to 24 hours.

INDICATIONS & DOSAGE
Dizziness–
Adults: 25 to 100 mg P.O. daily in divided doses. Dosage varies with patient response.
Motion sickness–
Adults: 25 to 50 mg P.O. 1 hour before travel, repeated daily for duration of journey.

CONTRAINDICATIONS & PRECAUTIONS

Contraindicated in patients with hypersensitivity to this drug or other antiemetic antihistamines with a similar chemical structure, such as cyclizine, buclizine, or dimenhydrinate.

Use with caution in patients with narrow-angle glaucoma, asthma, prostatic hypertrophy, or GU or GI obstruction because of anticholinergic effects. Drug may mask signs of intestinal obstruction or brain tumor.

ADVERSE REACTIONS

Common reactions are in italics; life-threatening reactions are in bold italics.
CNS: *drowsiness,* fatigue.
EENT: dry mouth, blurred vision.
Other: may mask symptoms of ototoxicity, brain tumor, or intestinal obstruction.

INTERACTIONS

CNS depressants: increased drowsiness.

EFFECTS ON DIAGNOSTIC TESTS

Diagnostic skin tests: test interference.

NURSING CONSIDERATIONS

Besides those related universally to drug therapy (see "How to use this book"), consider the following specific recommendations:

Assessment
- Obtain a baseline assessment of mental status and fluid balance before therapy.
- Be alert for adverse reactions and drug interactions throughout therapy.
- Evaluate the patient's and family's knowledge about meclizine therapy.

Nursing Diagnoses
- High risk for fluid volume deficit related to nausea and vomiting induced by motion sickness.
- Altered thought processes related to meclizine-induced drowsiness.
- Knowledge deficit related to meclizine therapy.

Planning and Implementation

Preparation and Administration
- Check order carefully and read drug label. Drug available in different forms and strengths.

Monitoring
- Monitor effectiveness by monitoring the patient for nausea and vomiting.
- Monitor fluid balance.
- Observe for signs of adverse CNS reactions.

Supportive Care
- Use cautiously in glaucoma, GU or GI obstruction, and in elderly males with possible prostatic hypertrophy.
- Be aware that this antihistamine has a slower onset and longer duration of action than other antihistamine antiemetics.
- If patient is alert, encourage intake of adequate fluids to prevent fluid deficit.
- Use safety precautions if CNS adverse reactions develop.

Patient Teaching
- Warn the patient to avoid driving and other hazardous activities that require alertness until CNS adverse reactions are known.
- Advise the patient to take drug 1 hour before travel and repeated daily during journey.

Evaluation

In patients receiving meclizine, appropriate evaluation statements may include:
- Patient exhibits no signs of fluid deficit.
- Patient demonstrates no signs of altered thought processes.
- Patient and family state an understanding of meclizine therapy.

meclofenamate sodium

(me kloe fen am´ ate)
Meclomen

- *Classification:* nonnarcotic analgesic, antipyretic, anti-inflammatory (nonsteroidal anti-inflammatory)
- *Pregnancy Risk Category:* B (D in 3rd trimester)

HOW SUPPLIED

Tablets: 50 mg, 100 mg
Capsules: 50 mg, 100 mg

ACTION

Mechanism: Produces anti-inflammatory, analgesic, and antipyretic effects, possibly through inhibition of prostaglandin synthesis.
Absorption: Rapidly and completely absorbed from the GI tract.
Distribution: Highly bound (more than 99%) to plasma proteins.
Metabolism: Oxidized in the liver to active and inactive metabolites.
Excretion: Excreted in urine, with some biliary excretion. Half-life: Plasma half-life after repeated doses is about 3 hours.
Onset, peak, duration: Peak plasma levels are seen in 30 minutes to 2 hours.

INDICATIONS & DOSAGE

Rheumatoid arthritis and osteoarthritis–
Adults: 200 to 400 mg/day P.O. in three or four equally divided doses.
Mild to moderate pain–
Adults: 50 to 100 mg P.O. q 4 to 6 hours. Maximum dose is 400 mg/day.

CONTRAINDICATIONS & PRECAUTIONS

Contraindicated in patients with hypersensitivity to the drug, and in patients in whom aspirin or other nonsteroidal anti-inflammatory drugs (NSAIDs) induce symptoms of asthma, urticaria, or rhinitis. Serious GI toxicity, including ulceration or hemorrhage, can occur at any time with NSAID use, especially in patients on chronic therapy.

Use cautiously in patients with a history of GI bleeding, hepatic or renal disease, blood dyscrasias, or diabetes mellitus, because the drug may worsen these disorders; and in asthmatic patients with nasal polyps, because patients with known "triad" symptoms (aspirin hypersensitivity, rhinitis/nasal polyps, and asthma) are at high risk of bronchospasm resulting from cross-sensitivity to meclofenamate.

ADVERSE REACTIONS

Common reactions are in italics; life-threatening reactions are in bold italics.
Blood: leukopenia, thrombocytopenia, ***agranulocytosis, aplastic anemia.***
CNS: fatigue, malaise, insomnia, *dizziness,* nervousness, *headache.*
CV: edema.
EENT: blurred vision, eye irritation.
GI: *abdominal pain, flatulence, peptic ulceration,* nausea, vomiting, *diarrhea,* hemorrhage.
GU: dysuria, hematuria, nephrotoxicity.
Hepatic: hepatotoxicity.
Skin: rash, urticaria.

INTERACTIONS

Aspirin: decreased plasma levels of meclofenamate.
Oral anticoagulants: enhanced anticoagulant effect. Monitor for toxicity.

EFFECTS ON DIAGNOSTIC TESTS

Urine bilirubin (Di-Azo method): false-positive results.

NURSING CONSIDERATIONS

Besides those related universally to drug therapy (see "How to use this book"), consider the following specific recommendations:

Assessment
• Obtain a baseline assessment of the patient's pain before therapy.
• Be alert for adverse reactions and drug interactions throughout therapy.
• Evaluate the patient's and family's knowledge about meclofenamate therapy.
Nursing Diagnoses
• Pain related to patient's underlying condition.
• High risk for trauma related to adverse CNS reactions.
• Knowledge deficit related to meclofenamate therapy.
Planning and Implementation
Preparation and Administration
• Administer with food to minimize adverse GI reactions.
Monitoring
• Regularly monitor the patient for relief of pain.
• Monitor for CNS and other adverse reactions, including GI toxicity.
• Regularly monitor the patient's CBC and renal and hepatic function in long-term therapy.
Supportive Care
• Notify the doctor if the patient's pain persists or worsens.
• If adverse CNS reactions occur, notify the doctor and institute safety precautions: supervise ambulation and keep the bed rails up.
• Discontinue drug if patient develops rash, visual disturbances, or diarrhea.
Patient Teaching
• Advise the patient to notify the doctor if pain persists or becomes worse.
• Instruct the patient not to self-medicate for extended periods without consulting the doctor.
• Advise the patient to avoid driving and other hazardous activities that require mental alertness until CNS effects of the drug are known.
• Tell the patient to take the drug with food or milk.
• Because serious GI toxicity can occur at any time in chronic NSAID therapy, teach the patient signs and symptoms of GI bleeding. Tell the patient to report these to the doctor immediately.
• Concomitant use with aspirin, alcohol, or steroids may increase the risk of adverse GI reactions. Advise the patient to avoid aspirin and alcohol.
Evaluation
In patients receiving meclofenamate, appropriate evaluation statements may include:
• Patient states pain is relieved.
• Patient does not develop traumatic injuries as a result of adverse CNS reactions.
• Patient and family state an understanding of meclofenamate therapy.

medroxyprogesterone acetate
(me drox´ ee proe jess´ te rone)
Amen, Curretab, Cycrin, Depo-Provera, Provera

• *Classification:* progestin, antineoplastic (progestin)
• *Pregnancy Risk Category:* X

HOW SUPPLIED
Tablets: 2.5 mg, 5 mg, 10 mg
Injection (suspension): 100 mg/ml, 400 mg/ml

ACTION
Mechanism: Suppresses ovulation, possibly by inhibiting pituitary gonadotropin secretion. Also forms a thick cervical mucus.
Absorption: Slow absorption after I.M. administration.
Metabolism: Primarily hepatic.
Excretion: Primarily renal.

INDICATIONS & DOSAGE
Abnormal uterine bleeding due to hormonal imbalance–
Women: 5 to 10 mg P.O. daily for 5 to 10 days beginning on the 16th day of menstrual cycle. If patient has re-

*Liquid form contains alcohol.

**May contain tartrazine.

ceived estrogen – 10 mg P.O. daily for 10 days beginning on 16th day of cycle.
Secondary amenorrhea –
Women: 5 to 10 mg P.O. daily for 5 to 10 days.
Endometrial or renal carcinoma –
Adults: 400 to 1,000 mg/week I.M.

CONTRAINDICATIONS & PRECAUTIONS

Contraindicated in patients with hypersensitivity to progestins, a history of thromboembolic disorders, severe hepatic disease, breast or genital cancer, or undiagnosed abnormal vaginal bleeding because it may worsen these disorders; and in pregnant or breast-feeding women.

Use cautiously in patients with existing conditions that might be aggravated by fluid and electrolyte retention, such as cardiac or renal disease, epilepsy, or migraine, because drug may worsen these conditions. Caution is also advised in administering this agent to diabetic patients (because decreased glucose tolerance may occur) or to patients with a history of mental depression (because drug may induce depression).

ADVERSE REACTIONS

Common reactions are in italics; life-threatening reactions are in bold italics.
CNS: dizziness, migraine headache, lethargy, depression.
CV: hypertension, thrombophlebitis, ***pulmonary embolism,*** *edema.*
GI: nausea, vomiting, abdominal cramps.
GU: breakthrough bleeding, dysmenorrhea, amenorrhea, cervical erosion, or abnormal secretions, uterine fibromas, vaginal candidiasis.
Hepatic: cholestatic jaundice.
Metabolic: hyperglycemia.
Skin: melasma, rash.
Local: pain, induration, sterile abscesses.
Other: breast tenderness, enlargement, or secretion; decreased libido.

INTERACTIONS

Rifampin: decreased progestogen effects. Monitor for diminished therapeutic response.

EFFECTS ON DIAGNOSTIC TESTS

Glucose tolerance tests: depressed response.
Pregnanediol excretion: decreased.
Serum alkaline phosphatase and amino acid: decreased levels in a small percentage of patients.

NURSING CONSIDERATIONS

Besides those related universally to drug therapy (see "How to use this book"), consider the following specific recommendations:

Assessment

- Obtain a baseline assessment of the patient's underlying condition, including her menstrual history, before initiating therapy with medroxyprogesterone.
- Be alert for adverse reactions and drug interactions throughout therapy.
- Evaluate the patient's and family's knowledge about medroxyprogesterone therapy.

Nursing Diagnoses

- Sexual dysfunction related to the patient's underlying condition.
- Fluid volume excess related to medroxyprogesterone-induced edema.
- Knowledge deficit related to therapy with medroxyprogesterone.

Planning and Implementation

Preparation and Administration

- FDA regulations require that, before receiving first dose, patients read package insert explaining possible progestin adverse reactions. Provide verbal explanation as well.
- ***I.M. use:*** Be aware that I.M. injection may be painful. Rotate injection sites to prevent muscle atrophy.
- Be aware that drug should not be used for pregnancy; drug may cause

birth defects and masculinization of female fetus.

Monitoring

• Monitor effectiveness by regularly assessing underlying condition for signs of improvement.
• Monitor for edema; weigh patient daily.
• Monitor injection sites for evidence of sterile abscess.

Supportive Care

• Withhold drug and notify the doctor if visual disturbances, migraine headache, or pulmonary emboli is suspected; be prepared to provide supportive care as indicated.
• Institute safety measures if adverse CNS reactions occur.
• Obtain an order for an antiemetic agent, as needed.
• Notify doctor if hyperglycemia occurs, especially in a diabetic patient, because therapy may need to be adjusted.
• Limit patient's sodium intake if not contraindicated.

Patient Teaching

• Instruct patients to report any unusual symptoms immediately and to stop taking the drug and call the doctor if visual disturbances or migraine occurs.
• Check patient's understanding of the package insert information.
• Tell diabetic patients to report symptoms of hyperglycemia or glycosuria.
• Tell patients who become pregnant during therapy with medroxyprogesterone to stop taking the drug immediately, because it may adversely affect the fetus.
• Warn patient that edema and weight gain are likely. Advise them to restrict sodium intake.

Evaluation

In patients receiving medroxyprogesterone, appropriate evaluation statements may include:

• Sexual dysfunction is relieved; patient exhibits improved health as a result of medroxyprogesterone therapy.
• Patient does not exhibit fluid excess.
• Patient and family state an understanding of medroxyprogesterone therapy.

mefenamic acid

(me fe nam´ ik)

Ponstan†, Ponstel

• *Classification:* nonnarcotic analgesic, antipyretic anti-inflammatory (nonsteroidal anti-inflammatory)
• *Pregnancy Risk Category:* C

HOW SUPPLIED

Capsules: 250 mg

ACTION

Mechanism: Produces anti-inflammatory, analgesic, and antipyretic effects, possibly through inhibition of prostaglandin synthesis.
Absorption: Rapidly and completely absorbed from the GI tract.
Distribution: Drug is highly protein-bound.
Metabolism: Hepatic.
Excretion: Mainly in urine, with some biliary excretion. Half-life: Around 2 hours.
Onset, peak, duration: Peak levels are seen in about 2 hours.

INDICATIONS & DOSAGE

Mild to moderate pain, dysmenorrhea –

Adults and children over 14 years: Initially 500 mg P.O., then 250 mg q 6 hours, p.r.n. Maximum therapy 1 week.

CONTRAINDICATIONS & PRECAUTIONS

Contraindicated in patients with hypersensitivity to this drug or in patients in whom aspirin or other nonsteroidal anti-inflammatory drugs

(NSAIDs) induce symptoms of asthma, urticaria, or rhinitis. Patients with known "triad" symptoms (aspirin hypersensitivity, rhinitis/nasal polyps, and asthma) are at high risk of bronchospasm.

Serious GI toxicity, especially ulceration or hemorrhage, can occur at any time with NSAID use, especially in patients on chronic therapy. Use cautiously in patients with a history of GI disease, cardiac disease, hepatic or renal disease, blood dyscrasias, or diabetes mellitus, because it may worsen these conditions. Because NSAIDs may mask the signs and symptoms of acute infection (fever, myalgia, erythema), carefully evaluate patients with high risk (such as those with diabetes).

ADVERSE REACTIONS

Common reactions are in italics; life-threatening reactions are in bold italics.

Blood: leukopenia, thrombocytopenia, ***agranulocytosis, aplastic anemia.***

CNS: *drowsiness, dizziness,* nervousness, headache.

CV: edema.

EENT: blurred vision, eye irritation.

GI: nausea, vomiting, *diarrhea, peptic ulceration,* hemorrhage.

GU: dysuria, hematuria, nephrotoxicity.

Hepatic: hepatotoxicity.

Skin: rash, urticaria.

INTERACTIONS

Oral anticoagulants, sulfonylureas, and other drugs that are highly protein bound: increased risk of toxicity.

EFFECTS ON DIAGNOSTIC TESTS

Hematocrit: decreased.

Prothrombin time: increased.

Serum BUN, transaminase, and potassium: increased levels.

Urine bilirubin (Di-Azo method): false-positive results.

NURSING CONSIDERATIONS

Besides those related universally to drug therapy (see "How to use this book"), consider the following specific recommendations:

Assessment

- Obtain a baseline assessment of the patient's pain before therapy.
- Be alert for adverse reactions and drug interactions throughout therapy.
- Evaluate the patient's and family's knowledge about mefenamic acid therapy.

Nursing Diagnoses

- Pain related to patient's underlying condition.
- High risk for trauma related to drowsiness or dizziness caused by CNS reaction to mefenamic acid.
- Knowledge deficit related to mefenamic acid therapy.

Planning and Implementation

Preparation and Administration

- Administer with food to minimize adverse GI reactions.
- Drug should not be administered for longer than 1 week at a time, because prolonged use increases risk of toxicity.

Monitoring

- Regularly monitor the patient for relief of pain.
- Monitor the patient for CNS and other adverse reactions, especially GI toxicity.
- Monitor CBC every 4 to 6 months, as indicated. Severe hemolytic anemia may occur with prolonged use.

Supportive Care

- Notify the doctor if the patient's pain persists or worsens.
- If adverse CNS reactions occur, notify the doctor and institute safety precautions, such as supervising ambulation and keeping the bed rails up.
- Discontinue drug if patient develops rash, visual disturbances, or diarrhea.

Patient Teaching
• Advise the patient to notify the doctor if pain persists or becomes worse.
• Advise the patient to avoid hazardous activities that require mental alertness until CNS effects of the drug are known.
• Because serious GI toxicity can occur at any time in chronic NSAID therapy, teach the patient signs and symptoms of GI bleeding. Tell the patient to report these to the doctor immediately.
• Advise the patient to avoid aspirin and alcohol because concomitant use with aspirin, alcohol, or steroids may increase the risk of adverse GI reactions.
• Tell the patient to take drug with food to minimize GI adverse reactions.

Evaluation
In patients receiving mefenamic acid, appropriate evaluation statements may include:
• Patient states pain is relieved.
• Patient does not develop traumatic injuries as a result of adverse CNS reactions.
• Patient and family state an understanding of mefenamic acid therapy.

mefloquine hydrochloride
(me´ floe kwin)
Lariam

• *Classification:* antimalarial (quinine derivative)
• *Pregnancy Risk Category:* C

HOW SUPPLIED
Tablets: 250 mg

ACTION
Mechanism: Exact mechanism unknown. Mefloquine is a structural analog of quinine. Antimalarial activity may be related to its ability to form complexes with hemin.
Absorption: Well absorbed from the GI tract after oral administration.
Distribution: Concentrates in the red blood cells and is approximately 98% protein-bound.
Metabolism: By the liver.
Excretion: Primarily excreted via the liver. Small amounts are excreted in the urine and breast milk. Half-life: Approximately 21 days in normal adults.

INDICATIONS & DOSAGE
Treatment of acute malaria infections caused by mefloquine-sensitive strains of Plasmodium falciparum *or Plasmodium vivax–*
Adults: 1,250 mg P.O. as a single dose. Patients with *P. vivax* infections should receive subsequent therapy with primaquine or other 8-aminoquinolones to avoid relapse after treatment of the initial infection.
Malaria prophylaxis–
Adults: 250 mg P.O. once weekly. Initiate prophylaxis 1 week before entering endemic area, and continue prophylaxis for 4 weeks after return from such areas. When returning to an area without malaria after a prolonged stay in an endemic area, prophylaxis ends after three doses.

CONTRAINDICATIONS & PRECAUTIONS
Contraindicated in patients with hypersensitivity to mefloquine or related compounds.

ADVERSE REACTIONS
Common reactions are in italics; life-threatening reactions are in bold italics.
CNS: dizziness, syncope, headache, transient emotional disturbances (rare).
CV: extrasystoles.
EENT: tinnitus.
GI: loss of appetite, vomiting, *nausea,* loose stools, diarrhea, GI discomfort.

Skin: rash.
Other: fatigue, fever, chills.

INTERACTIONS

Quinine, chloroquine: increased risk of seizures.
Quinine, quinidine, beta-adrenergic blocking agents: ECG abnormalities and cardiac arrest may occur.
Valproic acid: decreased valproic acid blood levels and loss of seizure control at start of mefloquine therapy. Monitor anticonvulsant blood levels.

EFFECTS ON DIAGNOSTIC TESTS

None reported.

NURSING CONSIDERATIONS

Besides those related universally to drug therapy (see "How to use this book"), consider the following specific recommendations:

Assessment

- Obtain a baseline assessment of infection before therapy.
- Be alert for adverse reactions and drug interactions throughout therapy.
- Evaluate the patient's and family's knowledge about mefloquine therapy.

Nursing Diagnoses

- High risk for injury related to ineffective dosage regimen.
- High risk for fluid volume deficit related to mefloquine-induced adverse GI reactions.
- Knowledge deficit related to mefloquine.

Planning and Implementation

Preparation and Administration

- ***P.O. use:*** Administer with food and a full glass (at least 8 oz [240 ml]) of water.
- Because of the great health risks from concomitant administration of quinine and mefloquine, remember that mefloquine therapy should not begin sooner than 12 hours after the last dose of quinine or quinidine.

Monitoring

- Monitor effectiveness by regularly assessing patient for improvement of infectious process.
- Monitor patient for visual disturbances during prolonged therapy. Periodic ophthalmic examinations are recommended.
- Monitor liver function tests.
- Monitor patient's hydration status if adverse GI reactions occur.

Supportive Care

- Withhold drug and notify doctor if toxic signs and symptoms occur.
- Obtain an order for an antiemetic or antidiarrheal agent as needed.
- Institute safety precautions if visual or other CNS reactions occur.
- In suspected overdose, induce vomiting and notify doctor immediately because there is potential for cardiotoxicity.

Patient Teaching

- Tell patient to take the drug on the same day of the week when using it for prophylaxis.
- Instruct the patient to take the drug with food and with a full glass (at least 8 oz [240 ml]) of water.
- Advise caution during hazardous activites that require alertness and good coordination.
- Instruct patient to discontinue the drug if unexplained anxiety, depression, confusion, or restlessness occurs. These symptoms may indicate impending toxicity.
- Alert patients with infections caused by *Plasmodium vivax* that they are at high risk for relapse because the drug does not eliminate the hepatic phase (Exoerythrocytic parasites), and stress importance of follow-up care.

Evaluation

In patients receiving mefloquine, appropriate evaluation statements may include:

- Patient is free of infection.
- Patient maintains adequate hydration throughout therapy.

• Patient and family state an understanding of therapy.

megestrol acetate

(me jess´ trole)
Megace, Megostat‡

• *Classification:* antineoplastic (progestin)
• *Pregnancy Risk Category:* X

HOW SUPPLIED

Tablets: 20 mg, 40 mg

ACTION

Mechanism: A synthetic progestin that may inhibit pituitary function and suppress luteinizing hormone. Changes the tumor's hormonal environment and alters the neoplastic process.
Absorption: Well absorbed across the GI tract after oral administration.
Distribution: Stored in fatty tissue; highly bound to plasma proteins.
Metabolism: Completely metabolized in the liver.
Excretion: Metabolites are primarily eliminated through the kidneys. Half-life: Average 34.2 hours.
Onset, peak, duration: Peak drug levels range from 10 to 56 ng/ml (mean 27.6 ng/ml) and occur 1 to 3 hours (mean 2.2 hours) after a dose.

INDICATIONS & DOSAGE

Breast cancer–
Women: 40 mg P.O. q.i.d.
Endometrial cancer–
Women: 40 to 320 mg P.O. daily in divided doses.

CONTRAINDICATIONS & PRECAUTIONS

Contraindicated in patients with hypersensitivity to progestins, a history of thromboembolic disorder because the drug may be associated with thromboembolic disease, severe hepatic disease because drug accumulation may occur, undiagnosed abnormal vaginal bleeding because drug may stimulate growth of some tumors, and in pregnant or breast-feeding women because of the potential for adverse effects on the fetus or neonate.

Use cautiously in patients with conditions that might be aggravated by fluid and electrolyte retention such as cardiac or renal disease, seizure disorder, or migraine. Also, use caution in administering this agent to diabetic patients because decreased glucose tolerance may occur or to patients with a history of mental depression because drug may exacerbate these effects.

ADVERSE REACTIONS

Common reactions are in italics; life-threatening reactions are in bold italics.
GU: dysfunctional uterine bleeding when drug is discontinued.
Other: carpal tunnel syndrome, thrombophlebitis, alopecia, hirsutism, breast tenderness.

INTERACTIONS

None significant.

EFFECTS ON DIAGNOSTIC TESTS

Glucose tolerance: decreased in a small percentage of patients.
Pregnanediol excretion: decreased.
Serum alkaline phosphatase and amino acid: increased concentrations.

NURSING CONSIDERATIONS

Besides those related universally to drug therapy (see "How to use this book"), consider the following specific recommendations:

Assessment

• Obtain a baseline assessment of patient's underlying condition before therapy.
• Be alert for adverse reactions and drug interactions throughout therapy.

• Evaluate the patient's and family's knowledge about megesterol therapy.
Nursing Diagnoses
• Impaired physical mobility related to drug-induced adverse reaction.
• Body image disturbance related to drug-induced masculinizing adverse effects.
• Knowledge deficit related to megestrol therapy.
Planning and Implementation
Preparation and Administration
• ***P.O. use:*** Endometrial cancer may require up to 320 mg daily in divided doses.
• Continue drug therapy for at least 2 months to determine efficacy.
Monitoring
• Monitor effectiveness by evaluating prothrombin and bleeding times and by noting the results of follow-up diagnostic tests and overall physical status.
• Monitor for signs of thrombophlebitis.
• Monitor patient's menstrual cycle; drug may cause dysfunctional uterine bleeding when drug is discontinued.
• Monitor for masculinizing effects such as hirsutism, which may be manifested during drug therapy.
Supportive Care
• Arrange for the patient to obtain a wig or hairpiece if hair loss is a problem.
• Encourage the patient to wear a supportive bra to help alleviate breast tenderness.
• Encourage the patient to enhance her self-image by the use of cosmetics and clothes.
• Assist the patient with activities that may be difficult if she develops carpal tunnel syndrome.
Patient Teaching
• Reassure patient that response to therapy is not immediate.
• Teach patient signs and symptoms of thrombophlebitis, and to report any to the doctor immediately.
• Tell patient to keep track of her menstrual cycle and amount of bleeding when drug is discontinued.
Evaluation
In patients receiving megestrol, appropriate evaluation statements may include:
• Patient does not develop impaired physical mobility.
• Patient can cope with alterations in body image.
• Patient and family state an understanding of megesterol therapy.

melphalan (L-phenylalanine mustard)
(mel´ fa lan)
Alkeran

• *Classification:* antineoplastic (alkylating agent)
• *Pregnancy Risk Category:* D

HOW SUPPLIED
Tablets (scored): 2 mg

ACTION
Mechanism: An alkylating agent that cross-links strands of cellular DNA and interferes with RNA transcription, causing an imbalance of growth that leads to cell death. Cell cycle–nonspecific.
Absorption: Incomplete and variable from the GI tract. In one study, absorption ranged from 25% to 89% after an oral dose of 0.6 mg/kg.
Distribution: Rapidly and widely distributed into total body water. Drug initially is 50% to 60% bound to plasma proteins and increases to 80% to 90% over 4 to 12 hours.
Metabolism: Extensively deactivated by spontaneous hydrolysis.
Excretion: Parent drug and metabolites are excreted primarily in urine, with 10% of an oral dose excreted as unchanged drug. Half-life: Biphasic; initial half-life is 8 minutes; terminal elimination half-life is 2 hours.

INDICATIONS & DOSAGE

Multiple myeloma –
Adults: initially, 6 mg P.O. daily for 2 to 3 weeks, then stop drug for up to 4 weeks or until WBC and platelets stop dropping and begin to rise again; resume with maintenance dosage of 2 mg daily. Stop drug if WBC is below 3,000/mm³ or platelets are below 100,000/mm³. Alternate therapy: 0.15 mg/kg P.O. daily for 7 days, or 0.25 mg/kg for 4 days; repeat q 4 to 6 weeks.
Nonresectable advanced ovarian cancer–
Adults: 0.2 mg/kg P.O. daily for 5 days. Repeat q 4 to 5 weeks, depending on bone marrow recovery.

CONTRAINDICATIONS AND PRECAUTIONS

Contraindicated in hypersensitivity to the drug or resistance to previous therapy with it. Cross-sensitivity with other alkylating agents may occur. Not recommended in severe leukopenia, thrombocytopenia, or anemia; or in chronic lymphophatic leukemia. Use with caution in hemotologic dysfunction, recent exposure to cytotoxic drugs or radiation, and renal dysfunction.

ADVERSE REACTIONS

Common reactions are in italics; life-threatening reactions are in bold italics.
Blood: ***thrombocytopenia,*** *leukopenia,* ***agranulocytosis.***
Skin: rash, alopecia.
Other: ***pneumonitis and pulmonary fibrosis, anaphylaxis.***

INTERACTIONS

None significant.

EFFECTS ON DIAGNOSTIC TESTS

Blood and urine studies: increased uric acid levels.

NURSING CONSIDERATIONS

Besides those related universally to drug therapy (see "How to use this book"), consider the following specific recommendations:

Assessment
- Obtain a baseline assessment of the patient's underlying condition and CBC and serum uric acid levels before therapy.
- Be alert for adverse reactions throughout therapy.
- Evaluate the patient's and family's knowledge about melphalan therapy.

Nursing Diagnoses
- High risk for injury related to hemorrhage secondary to thrombocytopenia and myelosuppression.
- High risk for infection related to the immunosupressant effects of drug therapy.
- Knowledge deficit related to melphalan therapy.

Planning and Implementation
Preparation and Administration
- ***P.O. use:*** Administer on an empty stomach because absorption is decreased by food.

Monitoring
- Monitor effectiveness by noting results of follow-up diagnostic tests and overall physical status.
- Monitor chest X-ray and assess lung sounds for signs of pulmonary changes or infection.

Supportive Care
- Expect this drug to be discontinued if severe leukopenia, thrombocytopenia or anemia occurs. Also expect that therapy may be resumed when these problems resolve.
- Use anticoagulants and aspirin products cautiously and watch for bleeding if they are used.
- Do not give any I.M. injections when platelet count is below 100,000/mm³. May need dosage adjustment in renal-impaired patients.

Patient Teaching
- Warn patient to watch for signs of infection (sore throat, cough, fever, fatigue) and bleeding (easy bruising, nosebleeds, bleeding gums). Tell the

patient to take his temperature daily.
• Tell the patient to avoid the use of all OTC products containing aspirin.
• Review all possible adverse reactions with the patient, explaining how to treat or prevent them and when to notify the doctor. This is especially important with this drug because adverse reactions commonly occur.

Evaluation

In patients receiving melphalan, appropriate evaluation statements may include:
• High risk for injury from hemorrhage did not occur during therapy.
• Respiratory and other infections did not occur during therapy.
• Patient and family state an understanding of melphalan therapy.

menotropins

(men oh troe´ pins)
Pergonal

• *Classification:* ovulation stimulant, spermatogenesis stimulant (gonadotropin)
• *Pregnancy Risk Category:* C

HOW SUPPLIED

Injection: 75 IU of luteinizing hormone (LH) and 75 IU of follicle-stimulating hormone (FSH) activity/ampule; 150 IU of LH and 150 IU of FSH activity/ampule

ACTION

Mechanism: A mixture of human FSH and LH that has been isolated from the urine of postmenopausal women. When given to a woman who does not have primary ovarian failure, FSH aids follicular development and LH aids follicular maturation.
Absorption: Because the drug is a polypeptide, it is destroyed in the GI tract after oral administration. Administered I.M.
Excretion: About 8% excreted unchanged in the urine. Half-life: Biphasic for both components; initial phase is 4 hours; terminal phase is 70 hours for FSH; initial phase is 20 minutes and terminal phase is 4 hours for LH.
Onset, peak, duration: Administration for 9 to 12 consecutive days usually produces follicular maturation; a single large dose of human chorionic gonadotropin (HCG), which has LH activity, is administered at the appropriate time to induce ovulation.

INDICATIONS & DOSAGE

Anovulation–
Women: 75 IU each FSH and LH I.M. daily for 9 to 12 days, followed by 10,000 units chorionic gonadotropin I.M. 1 day after last dose of menotropins. Repeat for one to three menstrual cycles until ovulation occurs.
Infertility with ovulation–
Women: 75 IU each of FSH and LH I.M. daily for 9 to 12 days followed by 10,000 units chorionic gonadotropin I.M. 1 day after last dose of menotropins. Repeat for two menstrual cycles and then increase to 150 IU each FSH and LH I.M. daily for 9 to 12 days, followed by 10,000 units chorionic gonadotropin I.M. 1 day after last dose of menotropins. Repeat for two menstrual cycles.
Infertility–
Men: 1 ampule I.M. three times weekly (given concomitantly with HCG 2,000 units twice weekly) for at least 4 months.

Menotropins are available in ampules containing 75 IU each FSH and LH.

CONTRAINDICATIONS & PRECAUTIONS

Contraindicated in women with primary ovarian failure and infertility not resulting from anovulation because therapy will not correct infertility; in women with overt adrenal or thyroid disease, pituitary tumors, undiagnosed abnormal vaginal bleeding, or ovarian cysts; and in pregnant or breast-feeding women. Also contraindicated in men with normal pituitary function, primary testicular failure, or infertility from any cause other than hypogonadotropic hypogonadism because therapy will not correct infertility.

Use cautiously in initiating therapy with menotropins. In women, primary ovarian failure or early pregnancy must be ruled out, and anovulation confirmed, before treatment may begin. In men, primary testicular failure must be ruled out, and abnormally low gonadotropin levels must be present.

ADVERSE REACTIONS

Common reactions are in italics; life-threatening reactions are in bold italics.
Blood: hemoconcentration with fluid loss into abdomen.
GI: nausea, vomiting, diarrhea.
GU: in women–*ovarian enlargement with pain and abdominal distention,* multiple births, ovarian hyperstimulation syndrome (sudden ovarian enlargement, ascites with or without pain, or pleural effusion); in men–*gynecomastia.*
Other: fever.

INTERACTIONS

None significant.

EFFECTS ON DIAGNOSTIC TESTS

None reported.

NURSING CONSIDERATIONS

Besides those related universally to drug therapy (see "How to use this book"), consider the following specific recommendations:

Assessment
- Obtain a baseline assessment of the patient's infertility problems before therapy.
- Be alert for adverse reactions and drug interactions throughout therapy.
- Evaluate the patient's and family's knowledge about menotropins therapy.

Nursing Diagnoses
- Sexual dysfunction related to the patient's underlying condition.
- Pain related to ovarian enlargement induced by menotropins.
- Knowledge deficit related to therapy with menotropins.

Planning and Implementation

Preparation and Administration
- ***I.M. use:*** Reconstitute with 1 to 2 ml sterile saline injection. Use immediately. Rotate injection sites to prevent muscle atrophy.

Monitoring
- Monitor effectiveness by determining if monthly conception has occurred.
- Closely monitor the patient response; this is critical to ensure adequate ovarian stimulation without hyperstimulation (sudden ovarian enlargement, ascites, or pleural effusion).
- Monitor for abdominal pain and discomfort, which may indicate ovarian enlargement.

Supportive Care
- Menotropins should be discontinued if ovarian hyperstimulation syndrome or abdominal pain occurs or if ovaries become abnormally enlarged.
- Obtain an order for an antiemetic or antidiarrheal as needed.

Patient Teaching
- Teach the patient signs and tests that indicate time of ovulation, such as increase in basal body temperature and change in the appearance and volume of cervical mucus.
- Warn the patient to report immediately symptoms of ovarian hyperstimulation syndrome: abdominal distention and pain, dyspnea, and vaginal bleeding.
- Tell the patient that multiple births are possible.

• In patient being treated for infertility, encourage daily intercourse from day before HCG is given until ovulation occurs.
• Advise the patient that she should be examined at least every other day for signs of excessive ovarian stimulation during therapy and for 2 weeks after treatment is discontinued.

Evaluation

In patients receiving menotropins, appropriate evaluation statements may include:
• In females, follicular maturation occurs; in males, spermatogenesis increases.
• Patient does not experience ovarian enlargement and pain.
• Patient and family state an understanding of menotropins therapy.

meperidine hydrochloride (pethidine hydrochloride)

(me per´ i deen)
Demerol

• Controlled Substance Schedule II
• *Classification:* analgesic, adjunct to anesthesia (opioid)
• *Pregnancy Risk Category:* B (D for prolonged use or use of high doses at term)

HOW SUPPLIED

Tablets: 50 mg, 100 mg
Syrup: 50 mg/ml
Injection: 10 mg/ml, 25 mg/ml, 50 mg/ml, 75 mg/ml, 100 mg/ml

ACTION

Mechanism: Binds with opiate receptors at many sites in the CNS (brain, brain stem, and spinal cord), altering both perception of and emotional response to pain through an unknown mechanism.
Absorption: Well absorbed from the GI tract; however, drug undergoes a substantial first-pass effect.
Distribution: Widely distributed throughout the body. Crosses placenta.
Metabolism: Primarily in the liver.
Excretion: About 30% of a dose is excreted in the urine as the N-demethylated derivative; about 5% is excreted unchanged. Excretion is enhanced by acidifying the urine. Half-life: About 3 to 4 hours.
Onset, peak, duration: Onset of analgesia occurs within 10 to 45 minutes. Duration of action is 2 to 4 hours.

INDICATIONS & DOSAGE

Moderate to severe pain–
Adults: 50 to 150 mg P.O., I.M., or S.C. q 3 to 4 hours, p.r.n. or around the clock; or 15 to 35 mg/hour by continuous I.V. infusion.
Children: 1 to 1.8 mg/kg P.O., I.M., or S.C. q 4 to 6 hours. Maximum dosage is 100 mg q 4 hours, p.r.n. or around the clock.
Preoperatively–
Adults: 50 to 100 mg I.M. or S.C. 30 to 90 minutes before surgery.
Children: 1 to 2.2 mg/kg I.M. or S.C. 30 to 90 minutes before surgery.

CONTRAINDICATIONS & PRECAUTIONS

Contraindicated in patients with hypersensitivity to the drug or any phenylpiperidine opioid (meperidine or its analogues). Administer with extreme caution to patients with supraventricular arrhythmias; avoid, or administer drug with extreme caution to patients with head injury or increased intracranial pressure, because drug obscures neurologic parameters; and during pregnancy and labor, because drug readily crosses placenta (premature infants are especially sensitive to respiratory and CNS depressant effects of narcotic agonists).

Use cautiously in patients with renal or hepatic dysfunction, because drug accumulation or prolonged duration of action may occur; asthma or chronic obstructive pulmonary disease, because drug depresses respiration and suppresses cough reflex; glaucoma, because drug has atropine-like effects; seizure disorders, because drug may precipitate seizures; in patients undergoing biliary tract surgery, because drug may cause biliary spasm; in elderly or debilitated patients, who are more sensitive to drug's effects; and in patients prone to physical or psychic addiction, because of the high risk of addiction to this drug.

ADVERSE REACTIONS

Common reactions are in italics; life-threatening reactions are in bold italics.

CNS: *sedation, somnolence, clouded sensorium, euphoria,* paradoxical excitement, tremors, dizziness, seizures with large doses.

CV: *hypotension,* bradycardia, tachycardia.

GI: *nausea, vomiting, constipation,* ileus.

GU: *urine retention.*

Local: pain at injection site, local tissue irritation and induration after S.C. injection; phlebitis after I.V. injection.

Other: ***respiratory depression,*** physical dependence, muscle twitching.

INTERACTIONS

Alcohol, CNS depressants: additive effects. Use together cautiously.

MAO inhibitors, barbiturates, isoniazid: increased CNS excitation or depression can be severe or fatal. Don't use together.

Phenytoin: decreased blood levels of meperidine. Monitor for decreased analgesia.

EFFECTS ON DIAGNOSTIC TESTS

Plasma amylase or lipase: increased levels.

NURSING CONSIDERATIONS

Besides those related universally to drug therapy (see "How to use this book"), consider the following specific recommendations:

Assessment

- Obtain a baseline assessment of the patient's pain before therapy.
- Be alert for adverse reactions and drug interactions throughout therapy.
- Evaluate the patient's and family's knowledge about meperidine therapy.

Nursing Diagnoses

- Pain related to patient's underlying condition.
- Ineffective breathing pattern related to meperidine-induced respiratory depression.
- Knowledge deficit related to meperidine therapy.

Planning and Implementation

Preparation and Administration

- Reduce meperidine dose, as ordered, for use with other narcotic analgesics, general anesthetics, phenothiazines, alcohol, sedatives, hypnotics, or tricyclic antidepressants, and use together with extreme caution because such combinations may cause respiratory depression, hypotension, profound sedation, and coma.
- For better analgesic effect, give before patient has intense pain. Initially, administration on a fixed schedule may provide better pain control with a smaller daily dose by reducing patient anxiety. Once good pain control has been achieved, adjust scheduling per individual requirements.
- Chemically incompatible with barbiturates. Don't mix together.
- Recognize that the oral form is less effective than parenteral use. Therefore, when changing from parenteral to P.O. route, dose should be increased. Give I.M., if possible. S.C. injection is not recommended because it is very painful.
- Be aware that alternating administration of a centrally active (opiate

narcotic) with a peripherally active nonnarcotic analgesic (aspirin, acetaminophen, or NSAID) may improve pain control while requiring lower narcotic doses.
• *P.O. use:* Be aware that meperidine syrup has local anesthetic effect. Give with a full glass of water.
• *I.V. use:* Carefully check access site before administration. Keep in mind that inadvertent injection arround a nerve trunk may cause transient sensorimotor paralysis. Administer I.V. meperidine slowly, preferably as a diluted solution. Give meperidine with the patient lying down to minimize hypotension.

Monitoring
• Monitor effectiveness by evaluating pain relief.
• Monitor respirations of neonates exposed to drug during labor. Have resuscitative equipment and naloxone available.
• Monitor for signs of respiratory depression, such as decreased rate or depth of respirations.
• Monitor cardiovascular status carefully.
• Monitor bladder function in postoperative patients.
• Monitor bowel function.
• Watch for withdrawal symptoms if drug is discontinued abruptly after long-term use.
• Keep in mind that meperidine and an active metabolite, normeperidine, accumulate. Monitor for increased toxic effect, especially in patients with impaired renal function.

Supportive Care
• Notify the doctor if pain is not relieved.
• Keep resuscitation equipment and naloxone available when giving the drug I.V. If respirations drop below 8 breaths/minute, arouse patient to stimulate breathing and notify the doctor.
• *Treatment of overdose:* Maintain airway patency and provide respiratory support. To reverse respiratory depression, give 0.4 mg of naloxone by I.V. push; repeat as necessary. Maintain blood pressure with I.V. fluids and vasopressors, as ordered.
• Remember that meperidine may be used in some patients allergic to morphine.
• Keep in mind that long-term use can lead to dependence.
• Know that because meperidine toxicity often appears after several days of treatment, it is not recommended for treatment of chronic pain.

Patient Teaching
• When used postoperatively, encourage turning, coughing, deep breathing, and use of incentive spirometer to avoid atelectasis.
• Tell the patient or family to notify the doctor if patient's respiratory rate decreases.
• Warn ambulatory patient to avoid hazardous activities that require alertness.
• If not contraindicated, instruct the patient to increase fluid and fiber intake, to prevent or treat constipation. A laxative or stool softener may also be needed.

Evaluation

In patients receiving meperidine, appropriate evaluation statements may include:
• Patient reports relief of pain.
• Respiratory rate and pattern are within normal limits after administration of meperidine.
• Patient and family state an understanding of meperidine therapy.

meprobamate

(me proe ba´ mate)

Apo-Meprobamate†, Equanil**, Meditran, Meprospan, Miltown, Neuramate, Novo-Mepro†, Sedabamate, Tranmep

• Controlled Substance Schedule IV

• *Classification:* anxiolytic (carbamate)
• *Pregnancy Risk Category:* D

HOW SUPPLIED
Tablets: 200 mg, 400 mg, 600 mg
Capsules: 200 mg, 400 mg
Capsules (sustained-release): 200 mg, 400 mg

ACTION
Mechanism: Depresses the CNS at the limbic and subcortical levels of the brain.
Absorption: Well absorbed after oral administration.
Distribution: Distributed throughout the body; 20% is protein-bound. The drug occurs in breast milk at two to four times the serum concentration; and crosses the placenta.
Metabolism: Rapidly metabolized in the liver to inactive glucuronide conjugates.
Excretion: Metabolites and 10% to 20% of a single dose as unchanged drug are excreted in urine. Half-life: 6 to 16 hours.
Onset, peak, duration: Peak serum levels occur in 1 to 3 hours. Sedation usually occurs within 1 hour.

INDICATIONS & DOSAGE
Anxiety and tension–
Adults: 1.2 to 1.6 g P.O. in three or four equally divided doses. Maximum dosage is 2.4 g daily.
Children 6 to 12 years: 100 to 200 mg P.O. b.i.d. or t.i.d. Not recommended for children under 6 years.

CONTRAINDICATIONS & PRECAUTIONS
Contraindicated in patients with hypersensitivity to the drug or other carbamates and in patients with intermittent porphyria. Some formulations contain tartrazine, which is contraindicated in patients allergic to aspirin because significant cross-reactivity has been demonstrated.

Use cautiously in patients with impaired renal or hepatic function, and in patients with depression, suicidal tendencies, or a history of drug abuse or addiction. Because it may precipitate seizures or lower seizure threshold, use cautiously, if at all, in patients with a history of seizures or an active seizure disorder.

ADVERSE REACTIONS
Common reactions are in italics; life-threatening reactions are in bold italics.
Blood: *thrombocytopenia.*
CNS: *drowsiness,* ataxia, dizziness, slurred speech, headache, vertigo.
CV: palpitation, tachycardia, hypotension.
GI: anorexia, nausea, vomiting, diarrhea, stomatitis.
Skin: pruritus, urticaria, erythematous maculopapular rash.

INTERACTIONS
Alcohol, other CNS depressants: increased CNS depression. Avoid concomitant use.

EFFECTS ON DIAGNOSTIC TESTS
Urine 17-ketosteroids, 17-ketogenic steroids (Zimmerman reaction), and 17-hydroxycorticosteroids (Glenn-Nelson technique): falsely elevated levels.

NURSING CONSIDERATIONS
Besides those related universally to drug therapy (see "How to use this book"), consider the following specific recommendations:
Assessment
• Obtain a baseline assessment of the patient's anxiety level before drug therapy.
• Be alert for adverse reactions and drug interactions throughout therapy.
• Evaluate the patient's and family's knowledge about meprobamate therapy.
Nursing Diagnoses
• Anxiety related to the patient's underlying condition.
• Altered tissue perfusion (venous)

*Liquid form contains alcohol.
**May contain tartrazine.

related to adverse reactions to meprobamate.
• Knowledge deficit related to meprobamate therapy.

Planning and Implementation

Preparation and Administration

• Dosage should be reduced in elderly or debilitated patients, who may be more susceptible to drug's CNS effects.
• Give drug with meals to prevent GI distress.
• Know that this drug should not be used for everyday stress.

Monitoring

• Monitor for adverse reactions or drug interactions by frequently checking the patient's vital signs for hypotension and tachycardia.
• Regularly monitor effectiveness by asking the patient about feelings of anxiety and by observing the patient's behavior.
• Monitor for nausea, vomiting, and diarrhea.
• Monitor hydration status if nausea, vomiting, and diarrhea occurs.
• Monitor for drug interactions by observing for excessive sedation due to potentiation with other CNS drugs.
• Observe the patient's skin for possible drug-induced urticaria or maculopapular rash.
• Periodic evaluation of CBC and liver function tests is indicated in patients receiving high doses.
• Monitor blood levels. Therapeutic blood levels are 0.5 to 2 mg/ 100 ml. Levels above 20 mg/100 ml may cause coma and death.

Supportive Care

• If drowsiness, dizziness, slurred speech, or headache occurs, institute safety measures, such as supervising patient activities. Reorient patient as needed and ensure a safe environment.
• Obtain an order for a mild analgesic if drug-induced headache develops.
• Do not withdraw drug abruptly. Abuse or addiction is possible, and withdrawal symptoms may occur.
• Provide additional fluids if the patient develops nausea, vomiting, and diarrhea.
• Withdraw drug gradually (over 2 weeks) to avoid withdrawal symptoms, which include severe generalized tonic-clonic seizures.

Patient Teaching

• Warn the patient to avoid concurrent use of drug with alcohol or other CNS depressants and also to avoid driving and other hazardous activities that require alertness and psychomotor coordination until adverse CNS effects of the drug are known.
• Warn the patient against giving medication to others.
• Warn the patient to take this drug only as directed and not to discontinue taking it without the doctor's approval. Inform the patient of the drug's potential for dependence if taken longer than directed.
• Tell the patient to take the drug with meals to reduce GI distress.

Evaluation

In patients receiving meprobamate, appropriate evaluation statements may include:
• Patient states he is less anxious.
• Patient's blood values remain within established limits.
• Patient and family state an understanding of meprobamate therapy.

mercaptopurine (6-MP, 6-mercaptopurine)

(mer kap toe pyoor´ een)
Purinethol

• *Classification:* antineoplastic (antimetabolite)
• *Pregnancy Risk Category:* D

HOW SUPPLIED

Tablets (scored): 50 mg

ACTION

Mechanism: An antimetabolite, drug is converted intracellularly to a ribonucleotide, which functions as a purine antagonist. Inhibits RNA and DNA synthesis. Also acts as an immunosuppressant, primarily blocking the humoral response.
Absorption: Incomplete and variable after an oral dose; approximately 50% of a dose is absorbed.
Distribution: Widely distributed into total body water. Drug crosses the blood-brain barrier, but the CSF concentration is too low for treatment of meningeal leukemias.
Metabolism: Extensively metabolized in the liver; xanthine oxidase may oxidize the drug to 6-thiouric acid. Drug appears to undergo extensive first-pass metabolism, contributing to its low bioavailability.
Excretion: Mercaptopurine and its metabolites are excreted in urine; about 11% of a dose appears in the urine within 6 hours.
Onset, peak, duration: Peak serum levels occur 2 hours after a dose.

INDICATIONS & DOSAGE

Acute lymphoblastic leukemia (in children), acute myeloblastic leukemia, chronic myelocytic leukemia –
Adults: 80 to 100 mg/m² P.O. daily as a single dose up to 5 mg/kg daily.
Children: 70 mg/m² P.O. daily.
Usual maintenance for adults and children: 1.5 to 2.5 mg/kg daily.

CONTRAINDICATIONS & PRECAUTIONS

Contraindicated in patients whose disease has shown resistance to therapy with this drug.

ADVERSE REACTIONS

Common reactions are in italics; life-threatening reactions are in bold italics.
Blood: *decreased RBC; leukopenia,* ***thrombocytopenia,*** *and anemia; all may persist several days after drug is stopped.*
GI: *nausea, vomiting, and anorexia in 25% of patients;* painful oral ulcers.
Hepatic: *jaundice,* ***hepatic necrosis.***
Metabolic: hyperuricemia.
Skin: rash, hyperpigmentation.

INTERACTIONS

Allopurinol: slowed inactivation of mercaptopurine. Decrease mercaptopurine to ¼ or ⅓ normal dose.
Hepatotoxic drugs: may enhance liver toxicity of mercaptopurine.
Warfarin: enhanced anticoagulant effect.

EFFECTS ON DIAGNOSTIC TESTS

Serum glucose and uric acid: falsely elevated values (sequential multiple analyzer).

NURSING CONSIDERATIONS

Besides those related universally to drug therapy (see "How to use this book"), consider the following specific recommendations:

Assessment
- Obtain a baseline assessment of patient's overall physical status, CBC, serum uric acid, renal panel, and hepatic profile before therapy.
- Be alert for adverse reactions and drug interactions throughout therapy.
- Evaluate the patient's and family's knowledge about mercaptopurine therapy.

Nursing Diagnoses
- Altered protection related to mercaptopurine-induced myelosuppression and immunosuppression.
- Altered oral mucous membrane related to mercaptopurine-induced stomatitis.
- Knowledge deficit related to mercaptopurine therapy.

Planning and Implementation

Preparation and Administration
- Dosage modification may be required after chemotherapy or radiation therapy, in depressed neutrophil

or platelet count, and in impaired hepatic or renal function.
• Be aware that this drug is sometimes ordered as 6-mercaptopurine. The numeral 6 is part of the drug name and does not signify number of dosage units.
Monitoring
• Monitor effectiveness by noting results of follow-up diagnostic tests and patient's overall physical status.
• Monitor weekly blood counts; watch for precipitous fall.
• Monitor hepatic function; watch for clay-colored stools, jaundice, and frothy, dark urine.
• Monitor for signs of infection (cough, fever, sore throat) and bleeding (easy bruising, nosebleeds, bleeding gums).
• Monitor intake and output.
• Monitor serum uric acid. If allopurinol is necessary, use cautiously.
• Monitor for adverse GI reactions, including nausea, vomiting, anorexia, and painful oral lesions. Keep in mind that GI adverse reactions are less common in children than adults.
Supportive Care
• Increase oral fluids to 3 liters daily.
• Be aware that drug should be discontinued if hepatic tenderness occurs.
• Provide meticulous mouth care to help prevent stomatitis.
• To help prevent infection, maintain the patient's optimal health and protect him from undue exposure to environmental contagions. If signs of infection occur, notify doctor promptly; administer antibiotics, as ordered.
• Provide a safe environment to minimize risk of bleeding.
• Avoid all I.M. injections when platelet count is below 100,000/mm^3.
Patient Teaching
• Warn the patient that improvement may take 2 to 4 weeks or longer.
• Warn patient to watch for signs of infection (sore throat, fever, fatigue, and bleeding (easy bruising, nosebleeds, bleeding gums). Tell patient to take temperature daily and to report signs of infection or bleeding promptly.
• Encourage the patient to drink at least 3 liters of fluids daily and to void as often as possible.
• Instruct patient about need for protective measures, including conservation of energy, balanced diet, adequate rest, personal cleanliness, clean environment, and avoidance of exposure to persons with infections.
• Instruct patient about safety precautions to reduce risks of bleeding from falls, cuts, or other injuries.
• Instruct patient about the need for frequent oral hygiene. Tell the patient to use a soft-bristled toothbrush and nonalcoholic mouthwash. If oral lesions are present, tell the patient to avoid drinking alcohol, smoking, and eating extremely hot or spicy foods. If lesions are painful, tell the patient to consult with the doctor about using a topical oral anesthetic.

Evaluation

In patients receiving mercaptopurine, appropriate evaluation statements may include:
• Patient does not demonstrate signs and symptoms of infection or bleeding.
• Oral lesions are absent, or, if present, complications are avoided or minimized.
• Patient and family state an understanding of mercaptopurine therapy.

mesalamine
(me sal´ a meen)
Rowasa

• *Classification:* anti-inflammatory (salicylate)
• *Pregnancy Risk Category:* B

HOW SUPPLIED

Rectal suspension: 4 g/60 ml.

ACTION

Mechanism: Exact mechanism unknown; mesalamine is one of the metabolites of sulfasalazine. Probably acts topically by inhibiting prostaglandin synthesis in the colon.
Absorption: Administered rectally as a suspension enema but is poorly absorbed from the colon. The extent of absorption depends on the retention time and varies considerably.
Distribution: At steady state, approximately 10% to 30% of the daily 4-g dose can be recovered in cumulative 24-hour urine collections. Distribution to other organs and other bioavailabilities of absorbed mesalamine are unknown.
Metabolism: Undergoes acetylation, but whether this takes place at colonic or systemic sites is unknown. Most absorbed mesalamine is excreted in urine as the N-acetyl-5-ASA metabolite. Patients demonstrated plasma levels of 2 mcg/ml 10 to 12 hours after administration. About two-thirds of this was the N-acetyl metabolite.
Excretion: Most is excreted in the feces. The elimination half-life of mesalamine is 0.5 to 1.5 hour; half-life of the acetylated metabolite is 5 to 10 hours. Steady-state plasma levels showed no accumulation of either free or metabolized drug during repeated daily administrations.

INDICATIONS & DOSAGE

Treatment of active mild to moderate distal ulcerative colitis, proctitis, or proctosigmoiditis–
Adults: 1 rectal unit as a retention enema once daily (preferably h.s.). Drug should be retained overnight (for about 8 hours). Usual course of therapy is 3 to 6 weeks.

CONTRAINDICATIONS & PRECAUTIONS

Contraindicated in patients with hypersensitivity to the drug or any component of the formulation including sulfites. Mesalamine has been associated with an acute intolerance syndrome, marked by cramping, acute abdominal pain and bloody diarrhea; sometimes fever, headache, and a rash. This reaction requires prompt withdrawal of the drug. The patient's history of sulfasalazine intolerance, if any, should be re-evaluated. Rechallenge to validate the hypersensitivity should be attempted only if clearly necessary, under close medical supervision, and with due consideration of reduced dosage.

Because preclinical studies showed the kidneys to be the major target organ for mesalamine toxicity, consider the possibility of increased absorption and renal tubular damage. Monitor urinalysis, BUN, and creatinine levels, especially in patients receiving concurrent drugs that liberate mesalamine, and in those with preexisting renal disease. When mesalamine is given rectally, absorption is poor and limited to the distal colon; overt renal toxicity has not been observed with such use.

Most patients hypersensitive to sulfasalazine are able to tolerate mesalamine enemas without any allergic reaction. Nevertheless, exercise caution when mesalamine is initially used in patients allergic to sulfasalazine. Instruct these patients to discontinue therapy at the first sign of rash or fever.

While using mesalamine some patients have developed pancolitis. However, extension of upper disease boundary or flare-ups occurred less often in mesalamine patients than in those recieving placebos.

In patients with sulfite sensitivity, mesalamine may cause allergic reactions (hives, itching, wheezing, and anaphylaxis). Sulfite sensitivity is more common in asthmatics and in atopic nonasthmatic persons.

Epinephrine is the preferred treatment for serious allergic emergencies even though epinephrine injection contains sodium or potassium metabisulfite. The alternatives to epinephrine may not be satisfactory in a life-threatening situation. The presence of a sulfite in epinephrine injection should not deter the use of the drug for treatment of serious allergy or other emergency.

ADVERSE REACTIONS

Common reactions are in italics; life-threatening reactions are in bold italics.
CNS: headache, dizziness, fatigue, malaise.
GI: abdominal pain, cramps, discomfort, flatulence, diarrhea, rectal pain, bloating, nausea, *pancolitis.*
Skin: itching, rash, urticaria, hair loss.
Other: wheezing, ***anaphylaxis*** (rare), fever.

INTERACTIONS

None significant.

EFFECTS ON DIAGNOSTIC TESTS

None reported.

NURSING CONSIDERATIONS

Besides those related universally to drug therapy (see "How to use this book"), consider the following specific recommendations:

Assessment

- Obtain a baseline assessment of the patient's GI system and pain related to the underlying condition before therapy.
- Be alert for adverse reactions and drug interactions throughout therapy.
- Evaluate the patient's and family's knowledge about mesalamine therapy.

Nursing Diagnoses

- Pain related to the underlying condition.
- Diarrhea related to adverse effects of the medication.
- Knowledge deficit related to mesalamine.

Planning and Implementation

Preparation and Administration

- Check for hypersensitivity to sulfasalazine.
- ***Rectal use:*** Shake suspension well before administration. Prepare enema equipment and administer as a retention enema, preferably at bedtime. Have patient retain drug at least 8 hours.

Monitoring

- Monitor effectiveness by evaluating the patient's pain.
- Evaluate the character of the patient's stools.
- Monitor the patient's hydration status.
- Monitor the renal status of the patient on long-term therapy. Note results of periodic renal function studies.

Supportive Care

- Administer analgesics as ordered.
- Monitor the patient's nutritional status.
- Call the doctor immediately if signs of anaphylaxis develop.

Patient Teaching

- Explain the importance of retaining the medication for at least 8 hours.
- Tell patient to follow the administration directions supplied with the medication.
- Instruct the patient to discontinue the medication if fever or a rash develops.

Evaluation

In patients receiving mesalamine, appropriate evaluation statements may include:

- Patient reports relief of GI pain.
- Patient has normal bowel movements.
- Patient and family state an understanding of mesalamine therapy.

mesna
(mess´ na)
Mesnex

• *Classification:* uroprotectant (thiol derivative)
• *Pregnancy Risk Category:* B

HOW SUPPLIED
Injection: 100 mg/ml

ACTION
Mechanism: Prevents ifosfamide-induced hemorrhagic cystitis by reacting with urotoxic ifosfamide metabolites.
Distribution: Rapidly distributed to extracellular space.
Metabolism: Rapidly metabolized to mesna disulfide, its only metabolite.
Excretion: In the kidneys, 33% of the dose is eliminated in the urine in 24 hours. Half-life: Of mesna and mesna disulfide are 0.36 and 1.17 hours respectively.

INDICATIONS & DOSAGE
Prophylaxis of hemorrhagic cystitis in patients receiving ifosfamide–
Adults: dosage varies with amount of ifosfamide administered. Usual dosage is 240 mg/m² administered as an I.V. bolus with administration of ifosfamide. Repeat dosage at 4 hours and 8 hours after administration of ifosfamide.

CONTRAINDICATIONS & PRECAUTIONS
Contraindicated in patients with hypersensitivity to mesna or other thiol compounds.

Note that the drug does not reduce the other toxicities associated with ifosfamide therapy, nor is it effective in all patients.

ADVERSE REACTIONS
Common reactions are in italics; life-threatening reactions are in bold italics.
Note: Because it is used concomitantly with ifosfamide and other chemotherapeutic agents, it is difficult to determine adverse reactions attributable solely to mesna.
EENT: dysgeusia.
GI: soft stools, nausea, vomiting, diarrhea.

INTERACTIONS
None reported.

EFFECTS ON DIAGNOSTIC TESTS
Urine ketones: false-positive result. Red-violet color returns to violet with the addition of acetic acid.

NURSING CONSIDERATIONS
Besides those related universally to drug therapy (see "How to use this book"), consider the following specific recommendations:
Assessment
• Obtain a baseline assessment of renal status before therapy.
• Be alert for adverse reactions and drug interactions throughout therapy.
• Evaluate the patient's and family's knowledge about mesna therapy.
Nursing Diagnoses
• Decreased renal perfusion due to ifosfamine-induced hemorrhage.
• Diarrhea related to adverse effects of the drug.
• Knowledge deficit related to mesna.
Planning and Implementation
Preparation and Administration
• ***I.V. use:*** Dilute with dextrose 5% in water, dextrose 5% and normal saline injection, normal saline injection, or lactated Ringer's solution. Administer as a bolus with administration of ifosfamide. Refrigerate after preparation and use within 6 hours.

Discard any unused drug. Remember that drug is administered only intravenously.

• Do not give mesna I.V. if the patient is receiving cisplatin. The two drugs are incompatible.
Monitoring
• Monitor effectiveness by checking urine output for hematuria.
• Assess the patient's intake and output.
• Evaluate vital signs for indications of severe hemorrhage.
• Monitor the patient's level of activity and fatigue.
Supportive Care
• Notify the doctor immediately if urine is grossly bloody.
• Provide periods of rest following activity.
• Keep in mind that up to 6% of patient's may not respond to the drug's protective effects.
• Keep in mind that this drug may interfere with diagnostic tests for urine ketones.
Patient Teaching
• Explain the action of the medication as it relates to ifosfamide.
• Tell the patient to report any changes in color and consistency of urinary output.
• Instruct the patient in the mechanics of measuring output.
Evaluation
In patients receiving mesna, appropriate evaluation statements may include:
• Patient's urinary output will be free of hematuria.
• Patient stools are normal in consistency and frequency.
• Patient and family state an understanding of mesna therapy.

mesoridazine besylate
(mez oh rid´ a zeen)
Serentil* **

• *Classification:* antipsychotic (phenothiazine)
• *Pregnancy Risk Category:* C

HOW SUPPLIED
Tablets: 10 mg, 25 mg, 50 mg, 100 mg
Oral concentrate: 25 mg/ml (0.6% alcohol)
Injection: 25 mg/ml

ACTION
Mechanism: Blocks postsynaptic dopamine receptors in the brain. Apiperidine phenothiazine and the major sulfoxide metabolite of thioridazine.
Absorption: Rate and extent vary with administration route. Oral tablet absorption is erratic and variable, with onset ranging from 30 minutes to 1 hour. Oral liquids are much more predictable; I.M. dosage form is absorbed rapidly.
Distribution: Widely distributed into the body, including breast milk. Drug is 91% to 99% protein-bound.
Metabolism: Extensively metabolized by the liver; no active metabolites are formed.
Excretion: Most as metabolites in urine; some is excreted in feces via the biliary tract. Half-life: 24 to 48 hours.
Onset, peak, duration: Peak effects occur at 2 to 4 hours; steady-state serum level is achieved within 4 to 7 days. Duration of action is 4 to 6 hours. Onset with oral tablet ranges from 30 minutes to 1 hour.

INDICATIONS & DOSAGE
Alcoholism–
Adults and children over 12 years: 25 mg P.O. b.i.d. up to maximum of 200 mg daily.
Behavioral problems associated with chronic brain syndrome–
Adults and children over 12 years: 25 mg P.O. t.i.d. up to maximum of 300 mg daily.

Psychoneurotic manifestations (anxiety) –
Adults and children over 12 years: 10 mg P.O. t.i.d. up to maximum of 150 mg daily.
Schizophrenia –
Adults and children over 12 years: initially, 50 mg P.O. t.i.d. or 25 mg I.M. repeated in 30 to 60 minutes, p.r.n.

CONTRAINDICATIONS & PRECAUTIONS

Contraindicated in patients with hypersensitivity to phenothiazines and related compounds, including allergic reactions involving hepatic function, because it is potentially hepatotoxic; blood dyscrasias and bone marrow depression, because it may induce agranulocytosis; disorders accompanied by coma, brain damage, or CNS depression because of additive CNS depression; in patients with circulatory collapse or cerebrovascular disease because of its hypotensive effects; and for use with adrenergic-blocking agents or spinal or epidural anesthetics because of its alpha-blocking activity.

Use cautiously in patients with cardiac disease (arrhythmias, congestive heart failure, angina pectoris, valvular disease, or heart block), encephalitis, Reye's syndrome, head injury, respiratory disease, epilepsy and other seizure disorders, glaucoma, prostatic hypertrophy, urine retention, hepatic or renal dysfunction, Parkinson's disease, pheochromocytoma, or hypocalcemia.

Oral dosage forms may contain tartrazine; dye may cause allergic reaction in aspirin-allergic patients.

ADVERSE REACTIONS

Common reactions are in italics; life-threatening reactions are in bold italics.
Blood: transient leukopenia, ***agranulocytosis.***
CNS: extrapyramidal reactions (low incidence), *tardive dyskinesia, sedation (high incidence),* EEG changes, dizziness.
CV: *orthostatic hypotension,* tachycardia, ECG changes.
EENT: *ocular changes, blurred vision,* pigmentary retinopathy.
GI: *dry mouth, constipation.*
GU: *urine retention,* dark urine, menstrual irregularities, gynecomastia, inhibited ejaculation.
Hepatic: cholestatic jaundice, abnormal liver function tests.
Metabolic: hyperprolactinemia.
Skin: *mild photosensitivity,* dermal allergic reactions.
Local: pain at I.M. injection site, sterile abscess.
Other: weight gain; increased appetite; rarely, ***neuroleptic malignant syndrome*** (fever, tachycardia, tachypnea, profuse diaphoresis).
After abrupt withdrawal of long-term therapy: gastritis, nausea, vomiting, dizziness, tremors, feeling of warmth or cold, sweating, tachycardia, headache, insomnia.

INTERACTIONS

Alcohol, other CNS depressants: increased CNS depression. Avoid concomitant use.
Antacids: inhibit absorption of oral phenothiazines. Separate antacid and phenothiazine doses by at least 2 hours.
Barbiturates: may decrease mesoridazine effect. Observe patient.

EFFECTS ON DIAGNOSTIC TESTS

ECG: quinidine-like effects.
Liver function tests: elevated results.
Protein-bound iodine: elevated levels.
Urine porphyrins, urobilinogen, amylase, and 5-hydroxyindoleacetic acid: false-positive results because of darkening of urine by metabolites.
Urine pregnancy tests using human chorionic gonadotropin: false-positive results.

NURSING CONSIDERATIONS

Besides those related universally to drug therapy (see "How to use this book"), consider the following specific recommendations:

Assessment

• Obtain a baseline assessment of the patient's underlying condition before therapy.
• Be alert for adverse reactions and drug interactions throughout therapy.
• Evaluate the patient's and family's knowledge about mesoridazine therapy.

Nursing Diagnoses

• Altered health maintenance related to the patient's underlying condition.
• Sensory/perceptual alterations (visual) related to adverse drug reaction.
• Knowledge deficit related to mesoridazine therapy.

Planning and Implementation

Preparation and Administration

• Protect medication from light. Slight yellowing of injection or concentrate is common and does not affect potency. Discard markedly discolored solutions.
• Dose of 50 mg is therapeutic equivalent of 100 mg of chlorpromazine.
• ***P.O. use:*** Dilute liquid concentrate with 60 ml tomato or fruit juice, carbonated beverages, coffee, tea, milk, water, or semisolid food just before giving.
• ***I.M. use:*** Give injection deeply only in upper outer quadrant of buttocks. Massage slowly afterward to prevent sterile abscess.
• Avoid skin contact with the injectable or liquid form because it may cause a rash.

Monitoring

• Monitor effectiveness by regularly observing the patient's behavior and noting changes in symptoms.
• Monitor for adverse reactions, especially extrapyramidal and anticholinergic effects (blurred vision, dry mouth, constipation, urine retention), and tardive dyskinesia, during prolonged therapy.
• Frequently check the patient's blood pressure for orthostatic hypotension, especially after parenteral administration.
• Monitor therapy by weekly bilirubin tests during the first month; periodic blood tests (CBC and liver function); and ophthalmic tests (long-term use).
• Monitor for neuroleptic malignant syndrome. This rare, potentially fatal reaction is not necessarily related to duration of treatment or type of neuroleptic drug, but usually occurs in men. (60% of affected patients).

Supportive Care

• Obtain baseline measurements of the patient's blood pressure before therapy starts.
• Keep the patient supine for 1 hour after I.M. administration. Then assist patient to get up slowly to avoid orthostatic hypotension.
• Do not discontinue drug abruptly unless required by severe adverse reactions.
• Increase the patient's fluid and fiber intake—if not contraindicated—to prevent constipation. If necessary, request doctor's order for a laxative.
• Give the patient sugarless gum, sour hard candy, ice chips, or mouthwash rinse to relieve dryness.
• Be prepared to give I.V. diphenhydramine, as ordered, to treat acute dystonic reactions.
• Hold the dose if patient develops jaundice, symptoms of blood dyscrasias (fever, sore throat, infection, cellulitis, weakness), persistent (longer than a few hours) extrapyramidal reactions, or any such reactions during pregnancy.

Patient Teaching

• Warn the patient that injections may sting.
• Tell the patient to avoid exposure to direct sunlight and to use a sunscreen when going outdoors to prevent photosensitivity reactions. (*Note:*

Sun lamps and tanning beds may cause burning of the skin or skin discoloration.)
• Tell the patient not to stop taking the drug suddenly.
• Encourage the patient to report difficult urination, sore throat, dizziness, or fainting.
• Advise the patient to increase fluid and fiber in the diet, if appropriate.
• Tell the patient to avoid driving and other hazardous activities that require alertness until the effect of the drug is established. Excessive sedation subsides after several weeks.
• Warn the patient to avoid spilling liquid on skin because rash and irritation may occur.
• Tell the patient that sugarless hard candy, chewing gum, or ice chips can alleviate dry mouth.

Evaluation

In patients receiving mesoridazine, appropriate evaluation statements may include:
• Patient is able to perform activities of daily living without assistance.
• Patient voids without difficulty.
• Patient and family state an understanding of mesoridazine therapy.

methadone hydrochloride

(meth′ a done)

Dolophine, Methadose, Physeptone‡

• Controlled Substance Schedule II
• *Classification:* analgesic, opiate detoxification adjunct (opioid)
• *Pregnancy Risk Category:* B (D for prolonged use or use of high doses at term)

HOW SUPPLIED

Tablets: 5 mg, 10 mg
Dispersible tablets (for methadone maintenance therapy): 40 mg
Oral solution: 5 mg/5 ml, 10 mg/5 ml, 10 mg/ml (concentrate)
Injection: 10 mg/ml

ACTION

Mechanism: Binds with opiate receptors at many sites in the CNS (brain, brain stem, and spinal cord), altering both perception of and emotional response to pain through an unknown mechanism.
Absorption: Well absorbed after S.C. or I.M. injection, and from the GI tract. Oral administration delays onset and prolongs duration of action.
Distribution: Highly bound to tissue protein, which may explain its cumulative effects and slow elimination.
Metabolism: Primarily in the liver by N-demethylation.
Excretion: Urinary excretion, the major route, is dose-dependent. Metabolites are also excreted in the feces via the bile. Half-life: 15 to 30 hours.
Onset, peak, duration: Onset of action occurs within 30 minutes to 1 hour; peak effect is seen at 30 minutes to 1 hour. Duration of action is 4 to 6 hours.

INDICATIONS & DOSAGE

Severe pain–
Adults: 2.5 to 10 mg P.O., I.M., or S.C. q 6 to 8 hours, p.r.n. or around the clock.
Narcotic abstinence syndrome–
Adults: 15 to 40 mg P.O. daily (highly individualized). Maintenance dosage is 20 to 120 mg P.O. daily. Adjust dose as needed. Daily dosages greater than 120 mg require special state and federal approval.

CONTRAINDICATIONS & PRECAUTIONS

Contraindicated in patients with hypersensitivity to the drug.

Administer with extreme caution to patients with supraventricular arrhythmias; avoid, or administer with extreme caution to patients with head injury or increased intracranial pressure, because drug obscures neurologic parameters; and during pregnancy and labor, because drug readily crosses placenta (premature infants are especially sensitive to respiratory and CNS depressant effects).

Use cautiously in patients with renal or hepatic dysfunction, because drug accumulation or prolonged duration of action may occur; asthma or chronic obstructive pulmonary disease, because drug depresses respiration and suppresses cough reflex; or seizure disorders, because drug may precipitate seizures; to those undergoing biliary surgery, because drug may cause biliary spasm; to elderly or debilitated patients, who are more sensitive to both therapeutic and adverse drug effects; and to patients prone to physical or psychological addiction, because of the high risk of addiction to this drug.

ADVERSE REACTIONS

Common reactions are in italics; life-threatening reactions are in bold italics.

CNS: *sedation, somnolence, clouded sensorium, euphoria,* dizziness, seizures with large doses.

CV: *hypotension,* bradycardia.

GI: *nausea, vomiting, constipation,* ileus.

GU: *urine retention.*

Local: pain at injection site, tissue irritation, induration following S.C. injection.

Other: ***respiratory depression,*** decreased libido, sweating, physical dependence.

INTERACTIONS

Alcohol, CNS depressants: additive effects. Use together cautiously.

Ammonium chloride and other urine acidifiers, phenytoin: may reduce methadone effect. Monitor for decreased pain control.

Rifampin: withdrawal symptoms; reduced blood levels of methadone. Use together cautiously.

EFFECTS ON DIAGNOSTIC TESTS

Plasma amylase: increased levels.

NURSING CONSIDERATIONS

Besides those related universally to drug therapy (see "How to use this book"), consider the following specific recommendations:

Assessment

- Obtain a baseline assessment of pain before therapy.
- Be alert for adverse reactions and drug interactions throughout therapy.
- Evaluate the patient's and family's knowledge about methadone therapy.

Nursing Diagnoses

- Pain related to the patient's underlying condition.
- Ineffective breathing pattern related to methadone-induced respiratory depression.
- Knowledge deficit related to methadone therapy.

Planning and Implementation

Preparation and Administration

- ***P.O. use:*** Be aware that the oral liquid form is legally required in maintenance programs. Completely dissolve tablets in 120 ml of orange juice or powdered citrus drink.
- ***I.M. or S.C. use:*** Rotate injection sites.
- Be aware that the oral dose is half as potent as injected dose.
- Keep in mind that once-daily dosage is adequate for maintenance. No advantage to divided doses.
- Remember that regimented scheduling (around the clock) is beneficial in severe, chronic pain. However, tolerance may develop with long-term use, requiring a higher dose to achieve the same degree of analgesia. This is not a sign of addiction.

Monitoring

- Monitor effectiveness by evaluating pain relief after administration of methadone.
- Monitor respiratory status throughout methadone therapy, noting any evidence of respiratory depression, such as decreased rate or depth of respiration.

• Monitor circulatory status and bowel and bladder function.
Supportive Care
• Notify the doctor and discuss increase of dosage or frequency if pain persists.
• Hold dose and notify the doctor if patient's respirations are below 12 breaths/minute.
• Keep in mind that when used as an adjunct in the treatment of narcotic addiction ("maintenance"), withdrawal will usually be delayed and mild.
• Be aware that combined use with general anesthetics, tranquilizers, sedatives, hypnotics, alcohol, tricyclic antidepressants, or MAO inhibitors may cause respiratory depression, hypotension, profound sedation, or coma. Administer such drugs with extreme caution and monitor patient response.
• Keep in mind that safety of maintenance use in adolescent addicts is not established.
• Be aware that the patient treated for narcotic abstinence syndrome usually requires an additional analgesic if pain control is necessary.
• Marked sedation can follow repeated doses; drug has cumulative effect.
Patient Teaching
• Tell the patient or family to notify the nurse or doctor if respiratory rate decreases.
• Warn ambulatory patient to avoid activities that require alertness.
• Suggest high-fiber diet and liberal fluid intake to prevent constipation during maintenance regimen. Patient may also need laxatives or stool softeners.
Evaluation
In patients receiving methadone, appropriate evaluation statements may include:
• Patient reports relief of pain after administration of methadone.
• Patient's respiratory status remains within normal limits.
• Patient and family state an understanding of methadone therapy.

methantheline bromide
(meth an´ tha leen)
Banthine

• *Classification:* antimuscarinic, GI antispasmodic (anticholinergic)
• *Pregnancy Risk Category:* C

HOW SUPPLIED
Tablets: 50 mg

ACTION
Mechanism: A quarternary anticholinergic that competitively blocks acetylcholine's effects at parasympathetic (muscarinic) sites, decreasing GI motility and inhibiting gastric acid secretion.
Absorption: Only 10% to 25% of a dose is absorbed.
Distribution: Quarternary compounds do not cross the blood-brain barrier; little else is known about its distribution.
Excretion: In urine as metabolites and unchanged drug and in feces in large percentages as unabsorbed drug.

INDICATIONS & DOSAGE
Adjunctive therapy in peptic ulcer, pylorospasm, spastic colon, biliary dyskinesia, pancreatitis, and certain forms of gastritis–
Adults: 50 to 100 mg P.O. q 6 hours.
Children over 1 year: 12.5 to 50 mg P.O. q.i.d.
Children under 1 year: 12.5 to 25 mg P.O. q.i.d.
Neonates: 12.5 mg P.O. b.i.d.

CONTRAINDICATIONS & PRECAUTIONS

Contraindicated in patients with narrow-angle glaucoma, because drug-induced cycloplegia and mydriasis may increase intraocular pressure; obstructive uropathy, obstructive GI tract disease, severe ulcerative colitis, myasthenia gravis, paralytic ileus, intestinal atony, or toxic megacolon, because the drug may exacerbate these conditions; and hypersensitivity to anticholinergics or bromides.

Administer cautiously to patients with autonomic neuropathy, hyperthyroidism, coronary artery disease, cardiac arrhythmias, CHF, or ulcerative colitis, because the drug may exacerbate the symptoms of these disorders; hepatic or renal disease, because toxic accumulation may occur; hiatal hernia associated with reflux esophagitis, because the drug may decrease lower esophageal sphincter tone; to patients over age 40, because the drug increases the glaucoma risks; and in hot or humid environments, because the drug may predispose the patient to heatstroke.

ADVERSE REACTIONS

Common reactions are in italics; life-threatening reactions are in bold italics.

CNS: headache, insomnia, drowsiness, dizziness, *confusion or excitement in elderly patients,* nervousness, weakness.

CV: *palpitations,* tachycardia.

EENT: *blurred vision,* mydriasis, increased ocular tension, cycloplegia, photophobia.

GI: *dry mouth,* dysphagia, *constipation,* heartburn, loss of taste, nausea, vomiting, *paralytic ileus.*

GU: *urinary hesitancy, urine retention,* impotence.

Skin: urticaria, decreased sweating or possible anhidrosis, other dermal manifestations.

Other: fever, allergic reactions.

Overdosage may cause curare-like symptoms.

INTERACTIONS

None significant.

EFFECTS ON DIAGNOSTIC TESTS

None reported.

NURSING CONSIDERATIONS

Besides those related universally to drug therapy (see "How to use this book"), consider the following specific recommendations:

Assessment

- Obtain a baseline assessment of the patient's pain related to his underlying condition before drug therapy.
- Be alert for adverse reactions and drug interactions throughout therapy.
- Evaluate the patient's and family's knowledge about methantheline therapy.

Nursing Diagnoses

- Pain related to the patient's underlying condition.
- Urinary retention related to adverse drug reaction.
- Knowledge deficit related to methantheline therapy.

Planning and Implementation

Preparation and Administration

- ***P.O. use:*** Give this drug 30 minutes to 1 hour before meals and at bedtime.
- Bedtime dose can be larger and should be given at least 2 hours after the last meal of the day.

Monitoring

- Monitor effectiveness by regularly assessing the patient's pain related to his underlying condition.
- Monitor for adverse reactions or drug interactions by checking intake and output.
- Monitor vital signs frequently for tachycardia.
- Monitor the patient's degree of dry mouth, especially if he is also taking antihistamines, which may cause additional dryness of mouth.

• Know that the therapeutic effects of the drug appear in 30 to 45 minutes and persist for 4 to 6 hours after oral administration.
• Monitor the patient's bowel habits because drug may cause constipation.
Supportive Care
• Help the patient to get in and out of bed if he has dizziness or blurred vision.
• Institute safety precautions if he experiences dizziness or confusion.
• Provide gum or sugarless hard candy to relieve dry mouth.
• If constipation occurs, obtain an order for a laxative.
• Provide the patient with fluids to help prevent constipation.
• Have the patient void before taking this medication.
Patient Teaching
• Instruct the patient to avoid driving and other hazardous activities that require alertness if he is drowsy, dizzy, or has blurred vision.
• Encourage the patient to drink plenty of fluids to avoid constipation.
• Tell him to report any rash or skin eruptions.
• Tell the patient to take this drug 30 minutes to 1 hour before meals and to take the bedtime dose at least 2 hours after the last meal of the day.
Evaluation
In patients receiving methantheline, appropriate evaluation statements may include:
• Patient states that pain related to his underlying condition is reduced.
• Patient does not develop urine retention.
• Patient and family state an understanding of methantheline therapy.

methazolamide
(meth a zoe´ la mide)
Neptazane

• *Classification:* adjunctive treatment for open-angle glaucoma, perioperative adjunct for acute angle-closure glaucoma (carbonic anhydrase inhibitor)
• *Pregnancy Risk Category:* C

HOW SUPPLIED
Tablets: 25 mg, 50 mg

ACTION
Mechanism: A carbonic anhydrase inhibitor that decreases secretion of aqueous humor in the eye, thereby lowering intraocular pressure.
Distribution: Into plasma, erythrocytes, extracellular fluid, bile, aqueous humor, and CSF.
Metabolism: Partially metabolized by the liver.
Excretion: About 20% to 30% of a dose is excreted in urine.

INDICATIONS & DOSAGE
Glaucoma (open-angle, or preoperatively in obstructive or narrow-angle) –
Adults: 50 to 100 mg b.i.d. or t.i.d.

CONTRAINDICATIONS & PRECAUTIONS
Contraindicated in patients with hepatic insufficiency, low potassium or sodium levels, hyperchloremic acidosis, or severe renal impairment because of the potential for enhanced electrolyte imbalances.

Use cautiously in patients with respiratory acidosis or other severe respiratory problems because the drug may produce acidosis; in patients with diabetes because it may cause hyperglycemia and glycosuria; in patients taking digitalis glycosides because they are more susceptible to digitalis toxicity from methazolamide-induced hypokalemia; and in those taking other diuretics.

ADVERSE REACTIONS
Common reactions are in italics; life-threatening reactions are in bold italics.

Blood: ***aplastic anemia, hemolytic anemia,*** leukopenia.
CNS: drowsiness, paresthesias.
EENT: transient myopia.
GI: nausea, vomiting, anorexia.
GU: crystalluria, renal calculi.
Metabolic: *hyperchloremic acidosis,* hypokalemia, asymptomatic hyperuricemia.
Skin: rash.

INTERACTIONS

NSAIDs: decreased diuretic effectiveness. Avoid concomitant use.

EFFECTS ON DIAGNOSTIC TESTS

Thyroid function tests: decreased iodine uptake.
Urine protein tests (with Albustix or Albutest): false-positive.

NURSING CONSIDERATIONS

Besides those related universally to drug therapy (see "How to use this book"), consider the following specific recommendations:

Assessment

- Obtain a baseline assessment of patient's intraocular pressure before methazolamide therapy.
- Be alert for adverse reactions and drug interactions throughout therapy.
- Evaluate the patient's and family's knowledge about methazolamide therapy.

Nursing Diagnoses

- High risk for injury related to intraocular pressure above normal.
- Altered protection related to methazolamide-induced blood disorders.
- Knowledge deficit related to methazolamide therapy.

Planning and Implementation

Preparation and Administration

- Anticipate that drug will be given every day.

Monitoring

- Monitor effectiveness by evaluating patient for eye pain and having intraocular pressure checked regularly. Be aware that diuretic effect decreases in acidosis.
- Monitor intake and output, vital signs, and weight regularly.
- Monitor electrolytes, especially serum potassium, in initial treatment.
- Monitor CBC routinely for alterations.

Supportive Care

- Notify doctor if adverse reactions occur to determine if drug should be discontinued and another drug substituted.
- Interpret urine protein test results carefully because drug may cause false-positive results.
- Institute safety precautions if adverse CNS reactions occur.
- Obtain an order for an antiemetic if vomiting occurs with drug use.

Patient Teaching

- Instruct patient to notify the doctor if eye pain occurs.
- Tell patient not to perform activities that require mental alertness until CNS effect of drug is known.
- Stress importance of having regular follow-up care and laboratory studies performed as ordered.

Evaluation

In patients receiving methazolamide, appropriate evaluation statements may include:

- Patient's intraocular pressure is normal.
- Patient's CBC is normal.
- Patient and family state an understanding of methazolamide therapy.

methdilazine hydrochloride

(meth dill´ a zeen)
Dilosyn†, Tacaryl*

- *Classification:* antihistamine (H_1-receptor antagonist), antipruritic (phenothiazine)
- *Pregnancy Risk Category:* C

HOW SUPPLIED

Tablets: 8 mg
Tablets (chewable): 3.6 mg methdilazine (equal to 4 mg methdilazine hydrochloride)
Syrup: 4 mg/5 ml*

ACTION

Mechanism: Competes with histamine for H_1-receptor sites on effector cells. Prevents but does not reverse histamine-mediated responses.
Pharmacokinetics: Unknown.

INDICATIONS & DOSAGE

Allergic rhinitis; pruritus–
Adults: 8 mg P.O. b.i.d. to q.i.d. or (chewable tablets) 7.2 mg P.O. b.i.d. to q.i.d.
Children over 3 years: 4 mg P.O. b.i.d. to q.i.d. or (chewable tablets) 3.6 mg P.O. b.i.d. to q.i.d.

CONTRAINDICATIONS & PRECAUTIONS

Contraindicated in patients with hypersensitivity to this medication or other antihistamines or phenothiazines with a similar chemical structure, such as promethazine or trimeprazine; during acute asthmatic attack, because it thickens bronchial secretions; in acutely ill or dehydrated children, because they are at increased risk of developing dystonias; and in patients who have taken monoamine oxidase (MAO) inhibitors within the preceding 2 weeks.

Use cautiously in patients with narrow-angle glaucoma; pyloroduodenal obstruction or urinary bladder obstruction from prostatic hypertrophy or narrowing of the bladder neck, because of its significant anticholinergic effects; or cardiovascular disease or hypertension, because of risks of palpitations and tachycardia; in patients with acute or chronic respiratory dysfunction (especially children) because methdilazine may suppress the cough reflex; and in children with a history of sleep apnea, a family history of sudden infant death syndrome, or Reye's syndrome.

ADVERSE REACTIONS

Common reactions are in italics; life-threatening reactions are in bold italics.
CNS: (especially in elderly patients) *drowsiness,* dizziness, headache.
GI: nausea, *dry mouth and throat.*
GU: urine retention.
Hepatic: cholestatic jaundice.
Skin: rash.

INTERACTIONS

CNS depressants: increased sedation. Use together cautiously.
MAO inhibitors: increased anticholinergic effects. Don't use together.
Phenothiazines: increased effects. Don't use together.

EFFECTS ON DIAGNOSTIC TESTS

Diagnostic skin tests: interference.

NURSING CONSIDERATIONS

Besides those related universally to drug therapy (see "How to use this book"), consider the following specific recommendations.

Assessment

- Obtain a baseline assessment of the patient's respiratory status and signs and symptoms before beginning therapy.
- Be alert for adverse reactions and drug interactions throughout therapy.
- Evaluate the patient's and family's knowledge about methdilazine therapy.

Nursing Diagnoses

- Ineffective airway clearance related to the patient's underlying condition.
- High risk for injury related to methdilazine-induced drowsiness.
- Knowledge deficit related to methdilazine therapy.

Planning and Implementation

Preparation and Administration

- ***P.O. use:*** Give with food or milk to reduce G.I. distress.

*Liquid form contains alcohol.

**May contain tartrazine.

• Instruct children to chew tablets completely and swallow promptly as methdilazine may cause a local anesthetic effect in the mouth, which increases the risk of choking.

Monitoring

• Monitor effectiveness by regularly assessing the patient's condition for relief of symptoms.

• Monitor patient for adverse CNS reactions such as drowsiness.

• Monitor elderly patients carefully because they are especially vulnerable to reactions such as drowsiness, dizziness, and headaches.

• Monitor lung sounds and characteristics of the secretions if bronchial secretions are present.

• Monitor the patient's intake and output for possible urine retention.

Supportive Care

• Ensure adequate fluid intake to decrease the viscosity of the secretions in patients with bronchial secretions.

• Take safety precautions with all patients, particularly during ambulation.

• Keep in mind that if tolerance develops, another antihistamine may be substituted.

Patient Teaching

• Explain that drug interactions are likely with simultaneous use of CNS depressants. The patient should seek medical approval before taking any OTC medication.

• Warn the patient against drinking alcoholic beverages during therapy.

• Warn the patient to avoid driving and other hazardous activities that require alertness until the CNS effects of the drug are established.

• Tell the patient that coffee or tea may reduce drowsiness and that dry mouth may be relieved with sugarless gum, hard candy, or ice chips.

• Encourage the patient to notify the doctor of any dysuria or urine retention.

• Tell the patient to notify the doctor if allergy symptoms persist.

• Tell the patient to discontinue the medication for 4 days before allergy skin tests to preserve the accuracy of the tests.

Evaluation

In patients receiving methdilazine, appropriate evaluation statements may include:

• Patient's symptoms are relieved.

• Injury did not occur; patient did not experience adverse CNS reactions.

• Patient and family state an understanding of methdilazine therapy.

methenamine hippurate

(meth en´ a meen)

Hiprex**, Hip-Rex†, Urex

methenamine mandelate

Mandameth, Mandelamine, Sterine†

• *Classification:* urinary tract antiseptic (formaldehyde pro-drug)

• *Pregnancy Risk Category:* C

HOW SUPPLIED

hippurate

Tablets: 1 g

mandelate

Tablets: 500 mg, 1 g

Tablets (enteric-coated): 250 mg, 500 mg, 1 g

Tablets (film-coated): 500 mg, 1 g

Oral suspension: 250 mg/5 ml

Granules: 500 mg, 1 g

ACTION

Mechanism: In acid urine, methenamines are hydrolyzed to ammonia and to formaldehyde, which is responsible for antibacterial action against gram-positive and gram-negative organisms. Mandelic and hippuric acids, with which methenamines are combined, are also antibacterial by unknown mechanisms.

Absorption: About 10% to 30% of an oral dose is hydrolyzed by gastric acid to ammonia and formaldehyde; enteric-coated tablets undergo less

degradation, but extent and rate of absorption is slowed.
Distribution: Crosses the placenta and enters breast milk.
Metabolism: About 10% to 25% of methenamine is metabolized in the liver.
Excretion: Primarily excreted by the kidneys via glomerular filtration and tubular secretion. In the urine, methenamine is converted to formaldehyde. Half-life: Plasma half-life of parent drug is 3 to 6 hours.
Onset, peak, duration: Peak formaldehyde concentrations occur in approximately 2 hours.

INDICATIONS & DOSAGE

Long-term prophylaxis or suppression of chronic urinary tract infections–
Adults and children over 12 years: 1 g (hippurate) P.O. q 12 hours.
Children 6 to 12 years: 500 mg to 1 g (hippurate) P.O. q 12 hours.
Urinary tract infections, infected residual urine in patients with neurogenic bladder–
Adults: 1 g (mandelate) P.O. q.i.d. after meals.
Children 6 to 12 years: 500 mg (mandelate) P.O. q.i.d. after meals.
Children under 6 years: 50 mg/kg (mandelate) P.O. divided in four doses after meals.

CONTRAINDICATIONS & PRECAUTIONS

Contraindicated in patients with severe renal or hepatic dysfunction because the drug may worsen these conditions; in patients who are severely dehydrated because crystalluria may occur in patients with reduced urine flow rates; and in patients with hypersensitivity to the drug.

ADVERSE REACTIONS

Common reactions are in italics; life-threatening reactions are in bold italics.
GI: nausea, vomiting, diarrhea.
GU: with high doses, urinary tract irritation, dysuria, frequency, albuminuria, hematuria.
Hepatic: elevated liver enzymes.
Skin: rashes.

INTERACTIONS

Acetazolamide: antagonizes methenamine effect. Use together cautiously.
Urine alkalinizing agents: inhibit methenamine action. Don't use together.

EFFECTS ON DIAGNOSTIC TESTS

Catecholamine and 17-hydroxycorticosteroids: false elevations.
5-hydroxyindoleacetic acid and estriol: falsely decreased.
Liver function tests: abnormal results.

NURSING CONSIDERATIONS

Besides those related universally to drug therapy (see "How to use this book"), consider the following specific recommendations:

Assessment
- Obtain a baseline assessment of infection before therapy.
- Be alert for adverse reactions and drug interactions throughout therapy.
- Evaluate the patient's and family's knowledge about methenamine therapy.

Nursing Diagnoses
- High risk for injury related to ineffectiveness of methenamine to eradicate the infection.
- High risk for fluid volume deficit related to methenamine induced adverse GI reactions.
- Knowledge deficit related to methenamine.

Planning and Implementation
Preparation and Administration
- Obtain a clean-catch urine specimen for culture and sensitivity tests before first dose. Therapy may begin pending test results.
- ***P.O. use:*** Administer after meals to minimize GI upset. Administer oral

suspension cautiously to elderly or debilitated patients because it contains vegetable oil and could cause lipid pneumonia if aspirated.

Monitoring

• Monitor effectiveness by regularly assessing for improvement in infection.
• Monitor intake/output.
• Monitor urine pH using Nitrazine paper.
• Monitor liver function studies periodically during long-term therapy.
• Monitor hydration status if adverse GI reactions occur.

Supportive Care

• If rash appears, withhold dose and notify doctor.
• Encourage fluid intake of at least 1,500 to 2,000 ml daily.
• Limit intake of alkaline foods, such as vegetables, milk, and peanuts. If urine pH is above 5.5 encourage patient to drink acidifying juices (cranberry, plum, and prune juices). If necessary, large doses of ascorbic acid (12 g/day) may be used to acidify urine.
• Obtain an order for an antiemetic or antidiarrheal agent as needed.

Patient Teaching

• Tell patient to take drug after meals to minimize GI upset.
• Instruct patient to discontinue drug and notify doctor if rash appears.
• Teach patient how to test urine pH with Nitrazine paper.
• Advise patient to limit intake of alkaline foods while increasing intake of acidic foods and increasing fluid intake to at least 1,500 to 2,000 ml of fluids daily.
• Warn patient not to take antacids including Alka-Seltzer and sodium bicarbonate.

Evaluation

In patients receiving methenamine, appropriate evaluation statements may include:

• Patient is free from infection.
• Patient maintains adequate hydration throughout methenamine therapy.
• Patient and family state an understanding of methenamine therapy.

methicillin sodium

(meth i sill′ in)

Metin‡, Staphcillin

• *Classification:* antibiotic (penicillinase-resistant penicillin)
• *Pregnancy Risk Category:* B

HOW SUPPLIED

Injection: 1 g, 4 g, 6 g
I.V. infusion piggyback: 1 g, 4 g
Pharmacy bulk package: 10 g

ACTION

Mechanism: Bactericidal by inhibiting cell wall synthesis during active multiplication. Bacteria resist penicillins by producing penicillinases—enzymes that inactivate penicillins. Methicillin resists these enzymes.
Absorption: Inactivated in gastric acid secretions and must be administered parenterally. Well absorbed after I.M. administration, but peak serum levels are higher after an I.V. infusion.
Distribution: Widely distributed; CSF penetration is poor but enhanced by meningeal inflammation. Methicillin crosses the placenta; it is 30% to 50% protein-bound.
Metabolism: Partially metabolized.
Excretion: Methicillin and metabolites are excreted in urine by renal tubular secretion and glomerular filtration; also excreted in breast milk and in bile. Half-life: About ½ hour in adults; 2½ hours in severe renal impairment; 4 to 6 hours in anuric patients.
Onset, peak, duration: Peak plasma concentrations occur 30 to 60 minutes after I.M. injection.

INDICATIONS & DOSAGE

Systemic infections caused by penicillinase-producing staphylococci–
Adults: 4 to 12 g I.M. or I.V. daily, divided into doses given q 4 to 6 hours.
Children: 100 to 200 mg/kg I.M. or I.V. daily, divided into doses given q 4 to 6 hours.

CONTRAINDICATIONS & PRECAUTIONS

Contraindicated in patients with hypersensitivity to any other penicillin or to cephalosporins.

ADVERSE REACTIONS

Common reactions are in italics; life-threatening reactions are in bold italics.
Blood: ***agranulocytosis,*** *eosinophilia,* hemolytic anemia, transient neutropenia.
CNS: neuropathy, ***seizures with high doses.***
GI: glossitis, stomatitis.
GU: interstitial nephritis.
Local: *vein irritation, thrombophlebitis.*
Other: *hypersensitivity (chills, fever, edema, rash, urticaria,* ***anaphylaxis***), overgrowth of nonsusceptible organisms.

INTERACTIONS

Probenecid: increases blood levels of methicillin and other penicillins. Probenecid may be used for this purpose.

EFFECTS ON DIAGNOSTIC TESTS

Aminoglycoside serum levels: falsely decreased concentrations.
CBC: transient reductions in RBC, WBC, and platelet counts.
Coombs' test: positive.
Methicillin Serum uric acid: falsely increased concentration levels (copper-chelate method). 17-hydroxycorticosteroids (Porter-Silber test): interference.
Urinalysis: Abnormal result indicating drug-induced interstitial nephritis.

NURSING CONSIDERATIONS

Besides those related universally to drug therapy (see "How to use this book"), consider the following specific recommendations:

Assessment

- Obtain a baseline assessment of infection before therapy.
- Be alert for adverse reactions and drug interactions throughout therapy.
- Evaluate the patient's and family's knowledge about methicillin therapy.

Nursing Diagnoses

- High risk for injury related to ineffectiveness of methicillin to eradicate the infection.
- Impaired tissue integrity related to methicillin-induced thrombophlebitis at the injection site.
- Knowledge deficit related to methicillin therapy.

Planning and Implementation

Preparation and Administration

- Obtain specimen for culture and sensitivity tests before first dose. Therapy may begin pending test results.
- Before first dose, ask the patient about previous allergic reactions to this drug or other penicillins. However, a negative history of penicillin allergy does not guarantee future safety.
- Give methicillin at least 1 hour before bacteriostatic antibiotics.
- If ordered q.i.d., be sure to give every 6 hours, around the clock.
- ***I.V. use:*** Do not add or mix other drugs with I.V. infusions–they may be chemically and physically incompatible. If other drugs must be given I.V., temporarily stop infusion of primary drug. When giving I.V., mix with 0.9% sodium chloride solution. Initial dilution must be made with sterile water for injection. Give I.V. intermittently to prevent vein irritation.

Monitoring
• Monitor effectiveness by regularly assessing for improvement of infectious process.
• Monitor renal function closely with frequent urinalysis to detect interstitial nephritis.
• Monitor hepatic and hematopoietic function closely during prolonged therapy.
• Monitor for bacterial and fungal superinfections during prolonged or high-dose therapy, especially in elderly, debilitated, or immunosuppressed patients.
Supportive Care
• Discontinue the drug immediately if the patient develops signs of anaphylactic shock (rapidly developing dyspnea and hypotension). Notify the doctor and prepare to administer immediate treatment, such as epinephrine, corticosteroids, antihistamines, and other resuscitative measures as indicated.
• Change I.V. site every 48 hours. If signs of thrombophlebitis occur change site immediately and apply warm compresses.
• If the patient develops a rash, notify the doctor and expect to discontinue the drug.
• Institute seizure precautions; high blood level of the drug may induce seizures.
Patient Teaching
• Advise the patient who becomes allergic to methicillin to wear medical alert identification stating this information.
Evaluation
In patients receiving methicillin, appropriate evaluation statements may include:
• Patient is free of infection.
• Patient does not experience impaired tissue integrity as a result of therapy.
• Patient and family state an understanding of methicillin therapy.

methimazole
(meth im´ a zole)
Tapazole

• *Classification:* antihypertensive agent (thyroid hormone antagonist)
• *Pregnancy Risk Category:* D

HOW SUPPLIED
Tablets: 5 mg, 10 mg

ACTION
Mechanism: Inhibits oxidation of iodine in the thyroid gland, blocking iodine's ability to combine with tyrosine to form thyroxine. May also prevent the coupling of monoiodotyrosine and diiodotyrosine to form thyroxine and triiodothyronine.
Absorption: Rapidly absorbed from the GI tract (70% to 80% bioavailable).
Distribution: Readily crosses the placenta and is distributed into breast milk. Concentrated in the thyroid; not protein-bound.
Metabolism: Hepatic.
Excretion: About 80% of the drug and its metabolites are excreted by the kidney; 7% is excreted unchanged. Half-life: 5 to 13 hours.
Onset, peak, duration: Peak plasma levels are reached within 1 hour.

INDICATIONS & DOSAGE
Hyperthyroidism—
Adults: 5 mg P.O. t.i.d. if mild; 10 to 15 mg P.O. t.i.d. if moderately severe; and 20 mg P.O. t.i.d. if severe. Continue until patient is euthyroid, then start maintenance dosage of 5 mg daily to t.i.d. Maximum dosage 150 mg daily.
Children: 0.4 mg/kg P.O. daily divided q 8 hours. Continue until patient is euthyroid, then start maintenance dosage of 0.2 mg/kg daily divided q 8 hours.

Preparation for thyroidectomy–
Adults and children: same doses as for hyperthyroidism until patient is euthyroid; then iodine may be added for 10 days before surgery.
Thyrotoxic crisis–
Adults and children: same doses as for hyperthyroidism, with concomitant iodine therapy and propranolol.

CONTRAINDICATIONS & PRECAUTIONS

Contraindicated in patients with hypersensitivity to the drug and in breast-feeding women. Use cautiously in patients over age 40, and at dosages greater than 40 mg/day because of increased risk of agranulocytosis; in patients receiving other agents known to cause agranulocytosis; and in those with infection or hepatic dysfunction.

ADVERSE REACTIONS

Common reactions are in italics; life-threatening reactions are in bold italics.
Blood: ***agranulocytosis,*** leukopenia, granulopenia, thrombocytopenia (appear to be dose-related).
CNS: headache, drowsiness, vertigo.
GI: diarrhea, nausea, vomiting (may be dose-related).
Hepatic: jaundice.
Skin: rash, urticaria, skin discoloration.
Other: arthralgia, myalgia, salivary gland enlargement, loss of taste, drug fever, lymphadenopathy.

INTERACTIONS

None significant.

EFFECTS ON DIAGNOSTIC TESTS

^{123}I or ^{131}I uptake by the thyroid: altered results.
Prothrombin time: prolonged.
Selenomethionine (^{75}Se) uptake by the pancreas: altered results.
Serum ALT (SGPT), serum AST (SGOT), bilirubin, alkaline phosphatase, and lactate dehydrogenase: elevated levels (signs of hepatotoxicity).

NURSING CONSIDERATIONS

Besides those related universally to drug therapy (see "How to use this book"), consider the following specific recommendations:

Assessment
• Obtain a baseline assessment of the patient's thyroid function before therapy.
• Be alert for adverse reactions and drug interactions throughout therapy.
• Evaluate the patient's and family's knowledge about methimazole therapy.

Nursing Diagnoses
• Activity intolerance related to increased metabolic rate.
• High risk for infection related to methimazole-induced blood reaction.
• Knowledge deficit related to methimazole therapy.

Planning and Implementation
Preparation and Administration
• Store in light-resistant container.
• ***P.O. use:*** Give with meals to reduce adverse GI reactions.
Monitoring
• Monitor effectiveness by regularly reviewing results of thyroid function studies and assessing patient's signs and symptoms for hyperthyroidism. Be aware that euthyroidism may take several months to develop.
• Monitor for signs of hypothyroidism (mental depression; cold intolerance; hard, nonpitting edema). Dosage adjustment may be required.
• Monitor CBC periodically to detect impending leukopenia, thrombocytopenia, and agranulocytosis. Dosage that exceeds 30 mg/day increases the risk of agranulocytosis.
• Monitor hydration status if GI reactions occur.
Supportive Care
• Withhold methimazole therapy if patient develops severe rash or enlarged cervical lymph nodes.

• Notify the doctor if the patient shows signs and symptoms of hypothyroidism; if so, dosage reduction will be required.
• Institute safety precautions if adverse CNS reactions occur.
• Obtain an order for an antiemetic or antidiarrheal, as needed.

Patient Teaching

• Tell the patient to take drug at regular intervals around-the-clock and to take it at the same time each day in relation to meals.
• If GI upset occurs, tell the patient to take drug with meals.
• Tell the patient to ask the doctor whether he should use iodized salt or eat shellfish during treatment, because their iodine content can interfere with the drug's effectiveness.
• Warn the patient not to use OTC cough medicines; many contain iodine.
• Tell the patient to notify doctor promptly if fever, sore throat, malaise, unusual bleeding, yellowing of eyes, nausea, or vomiting occurs.
• Advise the patient not to store drug in bathroom; heat and humidity cause it to deteriorate.
• Have the patient check with the doctor before undergoing surgery (including dental surgery).
• Teach the patient how to recognize the signs of hyperthyroidism and hypothyroidism and what to do if they occur.

Evaluation

In patients receiving methimazole, appropriate evaluation statements may include:

• Patient is euthyroid with methimazole therapy and able to maintain normal activity level.
• Patient maintains WBC count within normal levels.
• Patient and family state an understanding of methimazole therapy.

methocarbamol

(meth oh kar´ ba mole)

Delaxin, Marbaxin-750, Robaxin, Robomol-500, Robomol-750

• *Classification:* skeletal muscle relaxant (carbonate derivative of guiaifenesin)
• *Pregnancy Risk Category:* C

HOW SUPPLIED

Tablets: 500 mg, 750 mg
Injection: 100 mg/ml

ACTION

Mechanism: Reduces transmission of impulses from the spinal cord to skeletal muscle.
Absorption: Rapidly and completely absorbed from the GI tract.
Distribution: Widely distributed throughout the body.
Metabolism: Extensively metabolized in liver via dealkylation and hydroxylation.
Excretion: Rapidly and almost completely excreted in urine, mainly as its glucuronide and sulfate metabolites (40% to 50%), with 10% to 15% as unchanged drug, and the rest as unidentified metabolites. Half-life: 1 to 2 hours.
Onset, peak, duration: Onset of action after single oral dose is within 30 minutes; immediate after I.V. injection.

INDICATIONS & DOSAGE

As an adjunct in acute, painful musculoskeletal conditions–
Adults: 1.5 g P.O. for 2 to 3 days, then 1 g P.O. q.i.d., or not more than 500 mg (5 ml) I.M. into each gluteal region. May repeat q 8 hours. Or 1 to 3 g daily (10 to 30 ml) I.V. directly into vein at 3 ml/minute, or 10 ml may be added to no more than 250 ml of dextrose 5% in water or

normal saline solution. Maximum dosage is 3 g daily.
Supportive therapy in tetanus management–
Adults: 1 to 2 g into tubing of running I.V. or 1 to 3 g in infusion bottle q 6 hours.
Children: 15 mg/kg I.V. q 6 hours.

CONTRAINDICATIONS & PRECAUTIONS

Contraindicated in patients with hypersensitivity to the drug.

Administer injectable methocarbamol with caution, if at all, to patients with seizure disorders, because of the potential for seizures; and to those with impaired renal function because athe propylene glycol vehicle may irritate the kidneys.

ADVERSE REACTIONS

Common reactions are in italics; life-threatening reactions are in bold italics.
Blood: ***hemolysis,*** increased hemoglobin (I.V. only).
CNS: drowsiness, dizziness, lightheadedness, headache, syncope, mild muscular incoordination (I.M. or I.V. only), seizures (I.V. only).
CV: hypotension, bradycardia (I.M. or I.V. only).
GI: nausea, anorexia, GI upset, metallic taste.
GU: hematuria (I.V. only), discoloration of urine.
Skin: urticaria, pruritus, rash.
Local: thrombophlebitis, extravasation (I.V. only).
Other: fever, flushing, ***anaphylactic reactions (I.M. or I.V. only).***

INTERACTIONS

Alcohol and CNS depressants: increased CNS depression.

EFFECTS ON DIAGNOSTIC TESTS

5-HIAA using Udenfriend and urine vanillylmandelic acid (Gitlow screening test): falsely elevated results.

NURSING CONSIDERATIONS

Besides those related universally to drug therapy (see "How to use this book"), consider the following specific recommendations:

Assessment

- Obtain a baseline assessment of the patient's pain and muscle spasm related to underlying condition before drug therapy.
- Be alert for adverse reactions and drug interactions during methocarbamol therapy.
- Evaluate the patient's and family's knowledge about methocarbamol therapy.

Nursing Diagnoses

- Pain related to the patient's underlying condition.
- High risk for injury related to drug-induced drowsiness.
- Knowledge deficit related to methocarbamol therapy.

Planning and Implementation

Preparation and Administration

- ***P.O. use:*** Give with milk or meals to prevent GI distress.
- Prepare liquid by crushing tablets into water or sodium chloride solution. Give through nasogastric tube.
- ***I.V. use:*** I.V. irritates the vein. Give I.V. slowly. Maximum rate 300 mg (3 ml)/minute.
- ***I.M. use:*** Give I.M. deeply, only in upper outer quadrant of buttocks, with maximum of 5 ml in each buttock, and inject slowly. Do not give subcutaneously.
- Avoid combining with alcohol or other CNS depressants.

Monitoring

- With I.V. use, monitor for vein irritation and phlebitis.
- Monitor for fainting if drug is administered rapidly by I.V. route.
- Monitor effectiveness by evaluating degree of pain and muscle spasms.
- Monitor for seizures, which may be aggravated by I.V. administration.
- Watch for sensitivity reactions such as fever and skin eruptions.

• Monitor for mild muscular incoordination with I.M. or I.V. use.
• Monitor patient's vital signs for orthostatic hypotension and bradycardia, especially with parenteral administration.
• Obtain CBC periodically during prolonged therapy; drug may cause increased hemoglobin and hemolysis with I.V. use.
• Monitor the patient's urine for hematuria after I.V. administration.

Supportive Care

• Institute safety precautions if patient develops blurred vision, confusion, or dizziness.
• To reduce GI distress give the drug with milk or meals.
• Keep patient supine for 15 minutes after parenteral administration, and supervise ambulation, making sure the patient rises slowly.
• Have epinephrine, antihistamines, and corticosteroids available.
• Know that drug interferes with urine tests for 5-hydroxyindoleacetic acid (5-HIAA) and vanillylmandelic acid (VMA).
• When drug is used in tetanus management, it will be used with tetanus antitoxin, penicillin, tracheotomy, and aggressive supportive care. Long course of I.V. methocarbamol is required.

Patient Teaching

• Warn the patient to avoid driving and other hazardous activities that require alertness until CNS effects of drug are known.
• Advise the patient to follow the doctor's orders regarding rest and physical therapy.
• Advise the patient to take the drug with food or milk to prevent GI distress.
• Tell the patient to remain supine for 15 minutes after parenteral administration of the drug and then to rise from this position slowly to prevent orthostatic hypotension.
• Tell the patient that this drug may turn his urine green, black, or brown.
• Tell the patient to avoid alcohol or other CNS depressants.
• Tell the patient that he may take the drug with milk or food if he develops GI distress.
• Tell the patient that he may experience a metallic taste with the use of this drug.

Evaluation

In patients receiving methocarbamol, appropriate evaluation statements may include:
• Patient reports pain and muscle spasms have ceased.
• Patient does not experience injury as a result of drug-induced drowsiness.
• Patient and family state an understanding of methocarbamol therapy.

methohexital sodium (methohexitone sodium)

(meth oh hex´ i tal)

Brévital Sodium, Brietal Sodium†‡

• Controlled Substance Schedule IV
• *Classification:* I.V. anesthetic (barbiturate)
• *Pregnancy Risk Category:* D

HOW SUPPLIED

Powder for injection: 500 mg, 2.5 g, 5 g

ACTION

Mechanism: Inhibits the firing of neurons within the ascending reticular activating system.
Distribution: Throughout the body; highest initial concentrations occur in vascular areas of the brain, primarily gray matter. 80% protein-bound. Termination of anesthetic effect is dependent upon drug redistribution to peripheral tissues.
Metabolism: Extensively metabolized in the liver.

Excretion: In the urine, mostly as metabolites.
Onset, peak, duration: Peak concentrations in the brain occur between 30 seconds and 2 minutes after administration.

INDICATIONS & DOSAGE

General anesthetic for short-term procedures (oral surgery, gynecologic and genitourinary examinations); reduction of fractures; before electroconvulsive therapy; for prolonged anesthesia when used with gaseous anesthetics–
Adults and children: 5 to 12 ml 1% solution (50 to 120 mg) I.V. at 1 ml/5 seconds. Dose required for induction may vary from 50 to 120 mg or more; average about 70 mg. Induction dose provides anesthesia for 5 to 7 minutes.
Maintenance–
Intermittent injection: 2 to 4 ml 1% solution (20 to 40 mg) q 4 to 7 minutes.
Continuous I.V. drip: administer 0.2% solution (1 drop/second).

CONTRAINDICATIONS & PRECAUTIONS

Contraindicated in patients with acute intermittent or variegate porphyria; in patients with hypersensitivity to the drug; and whenever general anesthesia is contraindicated.

Use cautiously in patients with respiratory obstruction; circulatory, cardiac, renal, or hepatic dysfunction; severe anemia; marked obesity or status asthmaticus (use *extreme* caution), because the drug worsens these conditions; and in patients with a full stomach because it blocks airway reflexes and may predispose to aspiration.

ADVERSE REACTIONS

Common reactions are in italics; life-threatening reactions are in bold italics.
CNS: *muscular twitching,* headache, emergence delirium.
CV: *transient hypotension, tachycardia,* circulatory depression, ***peripheral vascular collapse.***
GI: excessive salivation, *nausea, vomiting.*
Respiratory: ***laryngospasm, bronchospasm, respiratory depression, apnea.***
Skin: tissue necrosis with extravasation.
Local: thrombophlebitis, pain at injection site, injury to nerves adjacent to injection site.
Other: hiccups, coughing, acute allergic reactions. Extended use may cause cumulative effect.

INTERACTIONS

None significant.

EFFECTS ON DIAGNOSTIC TESTS

EEG: dose-dependent alteration of patterns.

NURSING CONSIDERATIONS

Besides those related universally to drug therapy (see "How to use this book"), consider the following specific recommendations:

Assessment
• Obtain a baseline assessment of the patient's vital signs, and overall physical status before therapy.
• Be alert for adverse reactions and drug interactions throughout therapy.
• Evaluate the patient's and family's knowledge about methohexital therapy.

Nursing Diagnoses
• High risk for injury related to methohexital-induced unconsciousness.
• Ineffective breathing pattern related to possible methohexital-induced respiratory depression.
• Knowledge deficit related to methohexital therapy.

Planning and Implementation
Preparation and Administration
• Keep in mind that only staff specially trained in giving I.V. anesthetics and managing potential adverse reactions should administer this drug.
• Avoid extravascular or intra-arterial injections.
• Incompatible with silicone; avoid contact with rubber stoppers or parts of syringes that have been treated with silicone.
• Keep in mind that this drug is incompatible with Ringer's solution. Diluents recommended are 5% dextrose solution or 0.9% sodium chloride solution instead of distilled water.
• Do not mix with acid solutions, such as atropine sulfate.
• Adjust the flow rate individually for each patient.
• Solutions may be stored and used as long as they remain clear and colorless. Solutions cannot be heated for sterilization.
Monitoring
• Monitor effectiveness by evaluating level of unconsciousness after administration of methohexital.
• Monitor patient's vital signs before, during, and after anesthesia.
• Monitor respiratory status frequently. Be aware that respiratory depression or apnea may occur.
Supportive Care
• Notify the doctor immediately if CNS, respiratory, or cardiovascular status changes.
• Maintain pulmonary ventilation.
• Have resuscitative equipment and drugs ready.
• To reduce postoperative nausea and prevent aspiration, have the patient fast before administration.
• Implement safety measures to protect the unconscious patient.
Patient Teaching
• Explain that this drug provides general anesthesia. The patient will not experience pain during surgery or other procedures.
• Tell the patient what to expect during induction of and recovery from anesthesia. As needed, clarify any other information provided by the anesthesiologist, including risks.
• Warn ambulatory patient to avoid driving or other hazardous tasks that require alertness for 24 hours after anesthesia because of the risk of psychomotor impairment.

Evaluation
In patients receiving methohexital, appropriate evaluation statements may include:
• Effective anesthesia achieved; patient safety maintained.
• Patent airway and adequate ventilatory status maintained.
• Patient and family state an understanding of methohexital therapy.

methotrexate
(meth oh trex´ ate)

methotrexate sodium
Folex, Mexate, Rheumatrex

• *Classification:* antineoplastic (antimetabolite)
• *Pregnancy Risk Category:* D

HOW SUPPLIED
Tablets (scored): 2.5 mg
Injection: 20-mg, 25-mg, 50-mg, 100-mg, 250-mg vials, lyophilized powder, preservative-free; 25-mg/ml vials, preservative-free solution; 2.5-mg/ml, 25-mg/ml vials, lyophilized powder, preserved

ACTION
Mechanism: An antimetabolite that prevents reduction of folic acid to tetrahydrofolate by binding to dihydrofolate reductase.
Absorption: From GI tract, appears to be dose-related. Absorption of

lower doses is essentially complete; of larger doses, incomplete and variable. I.M. doses are absorbed completely.
Distribution: Widely distributed throughout the body, with the highest concentrations in the kidneys, gallbladder, spleen, liver, and skin. Drug crosses the blood-brain barrier but does not achieve therapeutic levels in the CSF. Approximately 50% of the drug is bound to plasma protein. Crosses the placenta and enters breast milk.
Metabolism: A small proportion is metabolized in the liver.
Excretion: Primarily into urine as unchanged drug; small amounts in the feces, probably as a result of biliary excretion. Elimination is biphasic, with 90% or more of the drug excreted within the first 24 hours, followed by 1% to 2% daily. However, with large doses (10 mg/kg P.O.), the excretion pattern changes: only 15% of the drug is excreted in the first 24 hours, about 50% in 5 days, and nearly 40% is found in the feces. Half-life: Initial phase elimination half-life is 45 minutes; terminal elimination half-life is 4 hours.
Onset, peak, duration: Peak serum levels are achieved 30 minutes to 2 hours after an I.M. dose and 1 to 4 hours after an oral dose.

INDICATIONS & DOSAGE

Trophoblastic tumors (choriocarcinoma, hydatidiform mole) –
Adults: 15 to 30 mg P.O. or I.M. daily for 5 days. Repeat after 1 or more weeks, according to response or toxicity.
Acute lymphoblastic and lymphatic leukemia –
Adults and children: 3.3 mg/m² P.O., I.M., or I.V. daily for 4 to 6 weeks or until remission occurs; then 20 to 30 mg/m² P.O. or I.M. twice weekly.
Meningeal leukemia –
Adults and children: 10 to 15 mg/m² intrathecally q 2 to 5 days until cerebrospinal fluid is normal. Use only 20-, 50-, or 100-mg vials of powder with no preservatives; dilute using 0.9% sodium chloride injection *without* preservatives or Elliot's B solution. Use only new vials of drug and diluent. Use immediately.
Burkitt's lymphoma (Stage I or Stage II) –
Adults: 10 to 25 mg P.O. daily for 4 to 8 days with 1-week rest intervals.
Lymphosarcoma (Stage III) –
Adults: 0.625 to 2.5 mg/kg daily P.O., I.M., or I.V.
Mycosis fungoides –
Adults: 2.5 to 10 mg P.O. daily or 50 mg I.M. weekly; or 25 mg I.M. twice weekly.
Psoriasis –
Adults: 10 to 25 mg P.O., I.M., or I.V. as single weekly dose.
Rheumatoid arthritis –
Adults: Initially 7.5 mg P.O. weekly, either in a single dose or divided as 2.5 mg P.O. q 12 hours for three doses once a week. Dosage may be gradually increased to a maximum of 20 mg weekly.

CONTRAINDICATIONS & PRECAUTIONS

Contraindicated in patients with impaired renal, hepatic, or hematologic status because of the drug's adverse hematologic effects and in pregnant patients because the drug may be fetotoxic. Immunizations may not be effective when given during methotrexate therapy. Because of the risk of disseminated infections, live virus vaccines are generally not recommended during therapy.

ADVERSE REACTIONS

Common reactions are in italics; life-threatening reactions are in bold italics.
Blood: WBC and platelet nadir occurring on day 7; anemia, *leukopenia, thrombocytopenia* (all dose-related).
CNS: ***arachnoiditis*** *within hours of intrathecal use;* ***subacute neurotoxic-***

*Liquid form contains alcohol. **May contain tartrazine.

ity which may begin a few weeks later; necrotizing demyelinating leukoencephalopathy a few years later.
GI: *stomatitis; diarrhea leading to* ***hemorrhagic enteritis and intestinal perforation;*** *nausea; vomiting.*
GU: nephropathy, ***tubular necrosis.***
Hepatic: acute toxicity (elevated transaminases), *chronic toxicity* (cirrhosis, ***hepatic fibrosis).***
Metabolic: hyperuricemia.
Skin: exposure to sun may aggravate psoriatic lesions, rash, photosensitivity.
Other: alopecia; ***pulmonary interstitial infiltrates;*** long-term use in children may cause osteoporosis.

INTERACTIONS

Folic acid derivatives: antagonized methotrexate effect.
Probenecid, phenylbutazone, NSAIDs, salicylates, sulfonamides: increased methotrexate toxicity; don't use together if possible.
Vaccines: immunizations may be ineffective; risk of disseminated infection with live virus vaccines.

EFFECTS ON DIAGNOSTIC TESTS

Folate concentration: altered results interfering with the detection of folic acid deficiency.
Uric acid: increased concentrations in blood and urine.

NURSING CONSIDERATIONS

Besides those related universally to drug therapy (see "How to use this book"), consider the following specific recommendations:

Assessment

- Obtain a baseline assessment of patient's overall physical status, CBC, serum uric acid concentration, and hepatic profile before therapy.
- Be alert for adverse reactions and drug interactions throughout therapy.
- Evaluate the patient's and family's knowledge about methotrexate therapy.

Nursing Diagnoses

- Altered protection related to methotrexate-induced myelosuppression and immunosuppression.
- Altered oral mucous membrane related to methotrexate-induced stomatitis.
- Knowledge deficit related to methotrexate therapy.

Planning and Implementation

Preparation and Administration

- Follow institutional policy for administration to avoid mutagenic, teratogenic, and carcinogenic risks.
- ***I.V. use:*** Keep in mind that methotrexate may be administered undiluted by I.V. push injection.
- ***Intrathecal use:*** Use preservative-free formulations only. Dilute with unpreserved 0.9% sodium chloride solution and further dilute with either lactated Ringer's or Elliott's B solution, to a final concentration of 1 mg/ml.
- Use reconstituted solutions of preservative-free drug within 24 hours after mixing.
- Expect to administer lower doses in renal, hepatic, or hematopoietic impairment.
- Expect to reduce dosage by 25% if serum bilirubin level falls between 3 and 5 mg/dl or AST (SGOT) level is greater than 180 units/liter. Omit therapy if bilirubin level rises above 5 mg/dl.
- Do not repeat drug unless WBC count rises above 1,500/mm^3; neutrophil count rises above 200/mm^3; platelet count rises above 75,000/mm^3; ALT (SGPT) concentration is above 450 units/liter; serum creatinine level is normal; creatinine clearance is at least 60 mg/minute; and the patient shows evidence of healing (if he has mucositis). Also do not repeat therapy if the patient experiences pleural effusion.
- Administer only under the supervision of a doctor who is experienced

with the use of chemotherapeutic agents.

Monitoring

• Monitor effectiveness by noting results of follow-up diagnostic tests and the patient's overall physical status.

• Expect toxic reactions with therapeutic doses. Monitor for type and severity of reactions. Rash, redness, or ulcerations in mouth or adverse pulmonary reactions (cough, dyspnea, cyanosis) may signal serious complications.

• Monitor for signs of bleeding (hematuria, ecchymosis, petechiae, epistaxis, melena).

• Monitor for signs of infection (temperature elevation, sore throat, malaise). Take temperature daily.

• Monitor intake and output daily during drug therapy.

• Monitor serum creatinine and BUN levels daily during high-dose therapy.

• Monitor CBC, serum uric acid, ALT (SGPT), and AST (SGOT) concentrations.

• Monitor serum methotrexate levels. Continue monitoring until serum level falls below 5×10^{-8} moles/liter.

Supportive Care

• Antiemetics may be given before or during infusion of this drug to decrease severe nausea and vomiting. Be aware that nausea and vomiting occur in almost all patients.

• Leucovorin calcium is used in high-dose methotrexate therapy to minimize adverse hematologic and GI reactions.

• Keep in mind that methotrexate is commonly used with other antineoplastics.

• Encourage fluid intake to 3 liters daily. Report the first signs of oliguria. Keep in mind that administration of large volumes of fluid, alkalinization of urine by giving sodium bicarbonate tablets, or administration of allopurinol may prevent uric acid nephropathy.

• Avoid all I.M. injections in patients with thrombocytopenia.

• To help prevent infection, maintain the patient's optimal health and protect him from undue exposure to environmental contagions. If signs of infection occur, notify the doctor promptly; administer antibiotics, as ordered.

• Provide a safe environment to minimize risk of bleeding.

• Provide meticulous mouth care to prevent stomatitis.

Patient Teaching

• Warn patient to watch for signs of infection (sore throat, fever, fatigue) and bleeding (easy bruising, nosebleeds, bleeding gums). Take temperature daily. Have patient report such signs, as well as any cough, dyspnea, or cyanosis.

• Advise male patients to practice contraception during therapy and for at least 3 months after chemotherapy.

• Advise female patients to avoid becoming pregnant during therapy and for at least one ovulatory cycle after methotrexate therapy ends.

• Advise women not to breast-feed while on methotrexate therapy because of the potential for serious adverse effects in the infant.

• Advise patient to avoid alcoholic beverages during therapy with methotrexate.

• Explain the importance of continuing leucovorin rescue even if the patient experiences severe nausea and vomiting. Parenteral therapy may be necessary.

• Teach patient to use good, frequent oral care to prevent superinfection of the oral cavity. Tell the patient to use a soft-bristled toothbrush and nonalcoholic mouthwash. If oral lesions are present, tell the patient to avoid drinking alcohol, smoking, and eating extremely hot or spicy foods. If lesions are painful, tell the patient to consult with the doctor about using a topical oral anesthetic.

• Encourage the patient to drink at least 3 liters of fluids daily and to void as often as possible.
• Advise patient that hair should grow back after treatment has ended.
• Advise patient to avoid prolonged exposure to direct sunlight and to use a highly protective sunscreening agent when exposed to sunlight.
• Instruct patient about need for protective measures, including conservation of energy, balanced diet, adequate rest, personal cleanliness, clean environment, and avoidance of exposure to persons with infections.
• Teach patient to avoid the use of all OTC products containing aspirin. Instruct patient about safety precautions to reduce risks of bleeding from falls, cuts, or other injuries.

Evaluation

In patients receiving methotrexate, appropriate evaluation statements may include:
• Patient does not demonstrate signs and symptoms of infection or bleeding.
• Oral lesions are absent, or if present, complications are avoided or minimized.
• Patient and family state an understanding of methotrexate therapy.

methoxsalen

(meth ox´ a len)
Oxsoralen, Oxsoralen-Ultra

• *Classification:* pigmenting, antipsoriatic (psoralen derivative)
• *Pregnancy Risk Category:* C

HOW SUPPLIED

Capsules: 10 mg
Lotion: 1%

ACTION

Mechanism: May enhance melanogenesis, either directly or secondary, to an inflammatory process.

Absorption: After oral administration, well but variably absorbed, with peak serum concentrations in 1½ to 3 hours. Food increases both absorption and peak concentration. The extent of topical absorption has not been determined. Skin sensitivity to UV light occurs in about 1 to 2 hours, reaches a maximum effect in 1 to 4 hours, and persists for 3 to 8 hours. Topical administration yields a UV sensitivity in 1 to 2 hours, which may persist for several days.

Distribution: Throughout the body, with epidermal cells preferentially taking up the drug. It is 75% to 91% bound to serum proteins, most commonly albumin. Distribution across the placenta or in breast milk is unknown.

Metabolism: Activated by long-wavelength UV light and is metabolized in the liver.

Excretion: Almost entirely as metabolites in the urine, with 80% to 90% eliminated within the first 8 hours.

INDICATIONS & DOSAGE

To induce repigmentation in vitiligo; psoriasis–

Adults and children over 12 years: 0.6 mg/kg P.O. 1.5 to 2 hours before measured periods of high-intensity long-wave ultraviolet exposure, 2 to 3 times weekly at least 48 hours apart.

Topical solution:

Apply to small, well-defined vitiliginous lesions and allow to dry (1 to 2 minutes) and reapply: 2 to 2.5 hours before measured periods of long-wave ultraviolet exposure. After exposure, wash lesions with soap and water. Protect area with opaque sunscreen. Although manufacturer recommends treatment weekly, some clinicians may treat q 3 to 5 days.

CONTRAINDICATIONS & PRECAUTIONS

Contraindicated in patients hypersensitive to psoralens and in those with diseases associated with photosensitivity because of the drug's photosensitization. Do not use in patients with melanoma, history of melanoma, or invasive squamous cell carcinoma, because the drug may be a photocarcinogen. Oral methoxsalen is contraindicated in patients with aphakia, because increased retinal damage may occur.

Oxsoralen capsules contain tartrazine; therefore, use cautiously in patients with tartrazine or aspirin sensitivity.

ADVERSE REACTIONS

Common reactions are in italics; life-threatening reactions are in bold italics.
CNS: nervousness, insomnia, depression, vertigo, headache.
GI: *discomfort, nausea, diarrhea.*
Skin: edema, erythema, painful blistering, burning, peeling, pruritus.

INTERACTIONS

Photosensitizing agents: do not use together. May increase toxicity.

EFFECTS ON DIAGNOSTIC TESTS

Liver function tests: abnormal results.

NURSING CONSIDERATIONS

Besides those related universally to drug therapy (see "How to use this book"), consider the following specific recommendations:

Assessment

• Obtain a baseline assessment of vitiliginous lesions of the skin before therapy.
• Be alert for adverse reactions and drug interactions throughout therapy.
• Evaluate the patient's and family's knowledge about methoxsalen therapy.

Nursing Diagnoses

• Impaired skin integrity related to underlying condition.
• Pain related to headache from adverse reactions to drug.
• Knowledge deficit related to methoxsalen.

Planning and Implementation

Preparation and Administration

• Check patient and family history for sunlight allergies.
• ***P.O. use:*** Administer 1.5 to 2 hours before measured periods of high-intensity long-wave UV exposure. Administer with meals or milk.
• ***Topical use:*** Apply to small area and allow to dry (1 to 2 minutes), 2 to 2.5 hours before exposure to long-wave UV light. After exposure, wash lesions with soap and water.
• Regulate therapy carefully. Overdosage and overexposure to light can cause serious burning or blistering.

Monitoring

• Monitor effectiveness by evaluating repigmentation of the vitiliginous skin lesions.
• Evaluate oral mucosa for possible damage from light treatments.
• Assess liver function tests on a monthly basis in patients with vitiligo (especially at the beginning of therapy).

Supportive Care

• Regulate therapy carefully.
• Notify the doctor immediately of any excessive skin pain or blistering.
• Apply sunscreen to affected areas following light treatment.
• Protect the patient's eyes and lips during light exposure treatments.

Patient Teaching

• Remind the patient to protect affected areas by using sunscreen or covering with clothing. Tell the patient to avoid excessive sunlight during therapy.
• Tell the patient taking the drug orally to avoid eating limes, figs, parsley, parsnips, mustard, carrots, and celery during therapy with this drug.
• Tell the patient to report any pain or burning that follows the light treatment or inadvertent sun exposure.

*Liquid form contains alcohol.

**May contain tartrazine.

Evaluation
In patients receiving methoxsalen, appropriate evaluation statements may include:
• Patients relates improved skin integrity and pigmentation.
• Patient denies headaches related to drug effects.
• Patient and family state an understanding of methoxsalen therapy.

methylcellulose
(meth ill sell′ yoo lose)
Citrucel◊, Cologel◊

• *Classification:* bulk-forming laxative (absorbent)
• *Pregnancy Risk Category:* C

HOW SUPPLIED
Oral liquid: 450 mg/5 ml◊
Powder: 2 g/heaping tablespoon◊

ACTION
Mechanism: A bulk-forming laxative. Absorbs water and expands to increase bulk and moisture content of the stool. The increased bulk encourages peristalsis and bowel movement.
Absorption: Not absorbed.
Distribution: Locally distributed, in the intestine.
Metabolism: None.
Excretion: In feces.
Onset, peak, duration: Action begins in 12 to 24 hours, but full effect may not occur for 2 to 3 days.

INDICATIONS & DOSAGE
Chronic constipation–
Adults: 5 to 20 ml liquid P.O. t.i.d. with a glass of water; or 15 ml syrup P.O. morning and evening.
Children: 5 to 10 ml P.O. daily or b.i.d.

CONTRAINDICATIONS & PRECAUTIONS
Contraindicated in patients with abdominal pain, acute surgical abdomen, or intestinal obstruction or perforation, because the drug may exacerbate the symptoms of these conditions.

ADVERSE REACTIONS
Common reactions are in italics; life-threatening reactions are in bold italics.
GI: *nausea,* vomiting, diarrhea (all after excessive use); esophageal, gastric, small intestinal, or colonic strictures when drug is chewed or taken in dry form; *abdominal cramps,* especially in severe constipation.
Other: laxative dependence in long-term or excessive use.

INTERACTIONS
None significant.

EFFECTS ON DIAGNOSTIC TESTS
None reported.

NURSING CONSIDERATIONS
Besides those related universally to drug therapy (see "How to use this book"), consider the following specific recommendations:
Assessment
• Obtain a baseline assessment of history of bowel disorder, gastrointestinal status, fluid intake, nutritional status, exercise habits, and normal pattern of elimination.
• Be alert for adverse reactions and drug interactions throughout therapy.
• Evaluate the patient's and family's knowledge about methylcellulose therapy.
Nursing Diagnoses
• Constipation related to interruption of normal pattern of elimination characterized by infrequent or absent stools.
• Pain related to methylcellulose-induced abdominal cramping.

• Knowledge deficit related to methylcellulose therapy.

Planning and Implementation

Preparation and Administration

• Check drug label and order, two forms of methylcellulose available.

• ***P.O. use:*** Give with 8 oz (240 ml) fruit juice or carbonated beverage to mask grittiness.

Monitoring

• Monitor effectiveness by checking the frequency and characteristics of stools.

• Auscultate bowel sounds at least once a shift. Assess for pain and cramping.

• Monitor nutritional status and fluid intake.

Supportive Care

• Do not give in abdominal pain, nausea, vomiting, or other symptoms of appendicitis or acute surgical abdomen; and in intestinal obstruction or ulceration, disabling adhesion, or difficulty swallowing.

• Be aware that laxative effect usually takes 12 to 24 hours, but may be delayed 3 days.

• Especially useful in patients with postpartum constipation, irritable bowel syndrome, diverticular disease, or colostomy; in debilitated patients; in those who chronically abuse laxatives; and to empty colon before barium enema.

• Methylcellulose is not absorbed systematically and is nontoxic.

• Provide privacy for elimination.

• Unless contraindicated, encourage fluid intake up to 2,500 ml a day.

• Consult with a dietitian to modify diet to increase fiber and bulk.

Patient Teaching

• Tell the patient to take drug with at least 8 oz (240 ml) of pleasant-tasting liquid to mask grittiness.

• Discourage excessive use of laxatives.

• Teach the patient about the relationship between fluid intake, dietary fiber, exercise, and constipation.

• Teach patient that dietary sources of fiber include bran and other cereals, fresh fruit, and vegetables.

• Warn patient that abdominal cramping may occur.

Evaluation

In patients receiving methylcellulose, appropriate evaluation statements may include:

• Patient reports return of normal pattern of elimination.

• Patient remains free from abdominal cramping.

• Patient and family state an understanding of methylcellulose therapy.

methyldopa

(meth ill doe´ pa)

Aldomet, Aldomet M‡, Apo-Methyldopa†, Dopamet†, Hydopa‡, Novomedopa†

methyldopate hydrochloride

(meth ill doe´ pate)

Aldomet, Aldomet Ester Injection‡

• *Classification:* antihypertensive (centrally acting antiadrenergic agent)

• *Pregnancy Risk Category:* B

HOW SUPPLIED

methyldopa

Tablets: 125 mg, 250 mg, 500 mg

Oral suspension: 250 mg/5 ml

methyldopate hydrochloride

Injection: 250 mg/5 ml in 5-ml vials

ACTION

Mechanism: After conversion to alpha-methyl norepinephrine in the CNS, drug probably stimulates alpha$_2$-adrenergic receptors in the vasomotor centers, decreasing sympathetic outflow.

Absorption: Partially absorbed from the GI tract. Absorption varies, but usually about 50% of an oral dose is absorbed.

Distribution: Widely distributed

throughout the body and is bound weakly to plasma proteins.
Metabolism: Extensively metabolized in the liver and intestine.
Excretion: Methyldopa and its metabolites are excreted in urine; unabsorbed drug is excreted unchanged in feces. Half-life: Elimination half-life is approximately 2 hours. Antihypertensive activity usually persists up to 24 hours after oral administration and 10 to 16 hours after I.V. administration.
Onset, peak, duration: After oral administration, maximal decline in blood pressure occurs in 3 to 6 hours; however, full effect is not evident for 2 to 3 days. No correlation exists between plasma concentration and antihypertensive effect. After I.V. administration, blood pressure usually begins to fall in 4 to 6 hours.

INDICATIONS & DOSAGE

For sustained mild to severe hypertension; should not be used for acute treatment of hypertensive emergencies–
Adults: initially, 250 mg P.O. b.i.d. to t.i.d. in first 48 hours. Then increase as needed q 2 days. May give entire daily dosage in the evening or h.s. Dosages may need adjustment if other antihypertensive drugs are added to or deleted from therapy. Maintenance dosage is 500 mg to 2 g daily in two to four divided doses. Maximum recommended daily dosage is 3 g.
I.V.–250 to 500 mg q 6 hours, diluted in dextrose 5% in water and administered over 30 to 60 minutes. Maximum dosage is 1 g q 6 hours. Switch to oral antihypertensives as soon as possible.
Children: initially, 10 mg/kg P.O. daily in two to three divided doses; or 20 to 40 mg/kg I.V. daily in four divided doses. Increase dose daily until desired response occurs. Maximum daily dose is 65 mg/kg, 2 g/m^2, or 3 g/day, whichever is least.

CONTRAINDICATIONS & PRECAUTIONS

Contraindicated in patients with hypersensitivity to the drug and in patients with active hepatic disease, such as hepatitis or cirrhosis; in patients who developed hepatic dysfunction during previous methyldopa therapy, because such patients may have impaired drug metabolism and may be predisposed to methyldopa-induced hepatic dysfunction.

Use cautiously in patients taking diuretics and other antihypertensive drugs; in patients with renal failure, because accumulation of active metabolites may lead to prolonged hypotension; in patients with hepatic dysfunction, who may be predisposed to methyldopa-induced hepatic dysfunction; and in patients taking levodopa, because an additive antihypertensive effect may occur.

ADVERSE REACTIONS

Common reactions are in italics; life-threatening reactions are in bold italics.
Blood: ***hemolytic anemia,*** reversible granulocytopenia, thrombocytopenia.
CNS: *sedation,* headache, asthenia, weakness, dizziness, *decreased mental acuity,* involuntary choreoathetotic movements, psychic disturbances, depression, nightmares.
CV: bradycardia, *orthostatic hypotension,* aggravated angina, myocarditis, *edema, and weight gain.*
EENT: *dry mouth, nasal stuffiness.*
GI: diarrhea, pancreatitis.
Hepatic: ***hepatic necrosis.***
Other: gynecomastia, lactation, skin rash, *drug-induced fever,* impotence.

INTERACTIONS

Levodopa: additive hypotensive effects; possible increased CNS adverse reactions.
Norepinephrine, phenothiazines, tri-

cyclic antidepressants, amphetamines: possible hypertensive effects. Monitor carefully.

EFFECTS ON DIAGNOSTIC TESTS

Direct antiglobulin (Coombs' test): positive results.
Urine catecholamines: falsely high levels (interference with diagnosis of pheochromocytoma).
Urine uric acid, serum creatinine, and AST (SGOT): altered levels.

NURSING CONSIDERATIONS

Besides those related universally to drug therapy (see "How to use this book"), consider the following specific recommendations:

Assessment
- Obtain a baseline assessment of the patient's blood pressure before beginning therapy.
- Be alert for adverse reactions and drug interactions throughout therapy.
- Evaluate the patient's and family's knowledge about methyldopa therapy.

Nursing Diagnoses
- Altered tissue perfusion (renal, cerebral, cardiopulmonary, peripheral) related to the patient's underlying condition.
- High risk for injury related to methyldopa-induced adverse reactions.
- Knowledge deficit related to methyldopa therapy.

Planning and Implementation
Preparation and Administration
- ***P.O. use:*** If drowsiness is a problem, discuss the time of administration with the doctor. Once-daily dosage given at bedtime will minimize daytime drowsiness.
- ***I.V. use:*** Drug is available in concentrations of 50 mg/ml. For infusion add the required dose to 100 ml of dextrose 5% in water for a concentration of 100 mg/10 ml. Drug remains stable for 24 hours in most I.V. solutions; however, exposure to air may accelerate decomposition.

Monitoring
- Monitor effectiveness by frequently checking blood pressure, pulse rate, and ECG. Expect the doctor to order a change from I.V. form to the oral form as soon as blood pressure is normal.
- Check the patient's blood pressure in the supine and standing position to monitor for orthostatic hypotension.
- Monitor blood studies (CBC) before and during therapy.
- Monitor hepatic function periodically, especially during the first 6 to 12 weeks of therapy.
- Weigh the patient daily. Sodium and water retention may occur.
- Monitor for unexplained fever and for other adverse reactions, including involuntary choreoathetoid movements.
- Note the results of direct Coombs' test on the patient who has received this drug for several months. In this case a positive direct Coombs' test indicates hemolytic anemia.
- Monitor the patient who's had dialysis closely for hypertension. Patient may need an extra dose of methyldopa.
- Monitor elderly patients closely, because they are more likely to experience sedation and hypertension.
- Monitor pregnant patients who are receiving this drug very closely. Hypertension in pregnant patients has been successfully treated with this drug without ill effects to the fetus when the patient is closely monitored. Some clinicians recommend that therapy not begin between 16 and 20 weeks' gestation, if possible.

Supportive Care
- Notify the doctor of any weight increase. Sodium and water retention may be relieved with diuretics.
- Notify the doctor of involuntary choreoathetoid movements, which may cause discontinuation of the drug.

• If the patient requires blood transfusion, make sure he gets direct and indirect Coombs' tests to avoid cross-matching problems.
• If the patient experiences CNS reactions or orthostatic hypotension, institute safety measures such as continuous use of side rails and assistance when moving from a supine to a standing position.

Patient Teaching
• Explain the importance of taking this drug as prescribed, even when feeling well.
• Tell the patient not to discontinue this drug suddenly even if unpleasant adverse reactions occur, but to discuss the problem with the doctor.
• Instruct the patient to check with the doctor or pharmacist before taking OTC medications.
• Warn the patient that this drug may impair ability to perform tasks that require mental alertness, particularly at the start of therapy. Tell patient to avoid driving and other hazardous tasks until the CNS effects of the drug are known.
• Inform the patient that orthostatic hypotension may occur but that it can be minimized by rising slowly and avoiding sudden position changes.
• Advise the patient to relieve dry mouth with sugarless chewing gum, sour hard candy, or ice chips.
• Warn the patient that urine may turn dark in toilet bowls treated with bleach.
• Teach the patient or a family member how to take blood pressure measurements. Tell them to notify the doctor of a significant change in blood pressure.

Evaluation
In patients receiving methyldopa, appropriate evaluation statements may include:
• Blood pressure controlled within normal limits for this patient.
• Injury from adverse reactions to methyldopa did not occur.
• Patient and family state an understanding of methyldopa therapy.

methylene blue
(meth´ i leen)
Urolene Blue

• *Classification:* urinary tract antiseptic, cyanide poisoning antidote, treatment of methemoglobinemia (thiazine dye)
• *Pregnancy Risk Category:* C (D if injected intra-amniotically)

HOW SUPPLIED
Tablets: 55 mg, 65 mg
Injection: 10 mg/ml

ACTION
Mechanism: Methylene blue is a mildly antiseptic dye. High concentrations convert the ferrous iron of reduced hemoglobin to ferric iron to form methemoglobin. This mechanism is the basis for its use as an antidote in cyanide poisoning. Low concentrations of methylene blue can hasten conversion of methemoglobin to hemoglobin.
Absorption: When administered orally, methylene blue is well absorbed from the GI tract.
Metabolism: Reduced to leukomethylene blue (which is colorless) by the tissues.
Excretion: Mainly excreted in urine and bile; approximately 70% of oral dose is excreted in urine as leukomethylene blue. On exposure to air, the urine will turn blue or green because the metabolites will form methylene azure, an oxidation product.

INDICATIONS & DOSAGE
Cystitis, urethritis–
Adults: 55 to 130 mg P.O. b.i.d. or t.i.d. after meals with glass of water.

Methemoglobinemia and cyanide poisoning–
Adults and children: 1 to 2 mg/kg of 1% sterile solution slow I.V.

CONTRAINDICATIONS & PRECAUTIONS

Contraindicated in patients with renal insufficiency because drug accumulation may occur; in patients with glucose-6-phosphate dehydrogenase (G6PD) deficiency because the drug may cause hemolysis; and in patients with hypersensitivity to the drug.

ADVERSE REACTIONS

Common reactions are in italics; life-threatening reactions are in bold italics.
Blood: anemia (long-term use).
GI: nausea, vomiting, diarrhea, blue-green stool.
GU: dysuria, bladder irritation, blue-green urine.
Other: fever (large doses).

INTERACTIONS

None significant.

EFFECTS ON DIAGNOSTIC TESTS

CBC: decreased erythrocytes (high-dose therapy).

NURSING CONSIDERATIONS

Besides those related universally to drug therapy (see "How to use this book"), consider the following specific recommendations:

Assessment
- Obtain a baseline assessment of infection before therapy.
- Be alert for adverse reactions and drug interactions throughout therapy.
- Evaluate the patient's and family's knowledge about methylene blue therapy.

Nursing Diagnoses
- High risk for injury related to ineffectiveness of methylene blue to eradicate the infection.
- High risk for fluid volume deficit related to methylene blue-induced adverse GI reactions.
- Knowledge deficit related to methylene blue.

Planning and Implementation
Preparation and Administration
- Obtain specimen for culture and sensitivity tests before first dose. Therapy may begin pending test results.
- ***P.O. use:*** Administer drug after meals with a full glass of water.
- ***I.V. use:*** Use caution when handling injectable form, because the liquid can stain the skin. Administer over several minutes directly into vein or through an I.V. line containing a free-flowing compatible solution. Too rapid injection causes additional production of methemoglobin. Don't exceed recommended dosage. Avoid extravasation.

Monitoring
- Monitor effectiveness by regularly assessing for improvement in the infection.
- Monitor intake/output carefully.
- Monitor hemoglobin; possibility of anemia from accelerated destruction of erythrocytes
- Monitor hydration status if adverse GI reactions occur.

Supportive Care
- Encourage patient to drink at least 2,000 ml of fluid daily.
- Be aware that drug turns urine and stool blue-green.
- Obtain an order for an antiemetic or antidiarrheal agent as needed.

Patient Teaching
- Tell patient to take oral drug after meals with a full glass of water.
- Teach patient how to measure intake/output. Stress the importance of drinking at least 2,000 ml of fluid daily.
- Warn patient that drug will turn urine and stool blue-green.

Evaluation
In patients receiving methylene blue, appropriate evaluation statements may include:
- Patient is free from infection.
- Patient maintains adequate hydration throughout methylene blue therapy.
- Patient and family state an understanding of methylene blue therapy.

methylergonovine maleate
(meth ill er goe noe´ veen)
Methergine

- *Classification:* oxytocic (ergot alkaloid)

HOW SUPPLIED
Tablets: 0.2 mg
Injection: 0.2 mg/ml

ACTION
Mechanism: An ergot alkaloid that increases the strength, duration, and frequency of uterine contractions by direct stimulation.
Absorption: Rapid, with 60% of an oral dose appearing in the bloodstream.
Distribution: The distribution of this drug is not fully known.
Metabolism: Extensive first-pass metabolism precedes hepatic metabolism.
Excretion: Primarily in the feces, with a small amount in urine. Half-life: Biphasic, with an initial half life of 2 to 3 minutes and a terminal half-life of 20 to 30 minutes.
Onset, peak, duration: Peak plasma concentrations occur in approximately 3 hours. Onset of action is immediate for I.V., 2 to 5 minutes for I.M., and 5 to 15 minutes for oral doses.

INDICATIONS & DOSAGE
Prevent and treat postpartum hemorrhage caused by uterine atony or subinvolution–
Adults: 0.2 mg I.M. q 2 to 5 hours for maximum of 5 doses; or I.V. (excessive uterine bleeding or other emergencies) over 1 minute while blood pressure and uterine contractions are monitored. I.V. dose may be diluted to 5 ml with normal saline solution. Following initial I.M. or I.V. dose, may give 0.2 to 0.4 mg P.O. q 6 to 12 hours for 2 to 7 days. Decrease dosage if severe cramping occurs.

CONTRAINDICATIONS & PRECAUTIONS
Contraindicated in patients sensitive to ergot preparations and in threatened spontaneous abortion, induction of labor, and before delivery of placenta. Use cautiously in patients with hypertension, sepsis, obliterative vascular disease, and hepatic, renal, and cardiac disease, because of the potential for adverse cardiovascular effects.

ADVERSE REACTIONS
Common reactions are in italics; life-threatening reactions are in bold italics.
CNS: dizziness, headache.
CV: ***hypertension,*** transient chest pain, dyspnea, palpitation.
EENT: tinnitus.
GI: *nausea, vomiting.*
Other: sweating, hypersensitivity.

INTERACTIONS
Regional anesthetics, vasoconstrictors, dopamine, I.V. oxytocin: excessive vasoconstriction.

EFFECTS ON DIAGNOSTIC TESTS
Serum prolactin: decreased concentrations.

NURSING CONSIDERATIONS
Besides those related universally to drug therapy (see "How to use this

book"), consider the following specific recommendations:

Assessment

- Obtain a baseline assessment of the patient's hemodynamic status and condition of uterine musculature before therapy.
- Be alert for adverse reactions and drug interactions throughout therapy.
- Evaluate the patient's and family's knowledge about methylergonovine therapy.

Nursing Diagnoses

- Fluid volume deficit related to postpartum hemorrhage.
- Pain related to methylergonovine-induced uterine cramping.
- Knowledge deficit related to methylergonovine therapy.

Planning and Implementation

Preparation and Administration

- ***I.V. use:*** Do not routinely administer I.V. because of the risk of hypertension and CVA. If it must be given by this route, administer slowly over 1 minute with careful blood pressure monitoring. Store I.V. solutions below 46.4° F (8° C). Daily stock may be kept at room temperature for 60 to 90 days.
- Store in tightly closed, light-resistant containers. Discard if discolored.

Monitoring

- Monitor effectiveness by evaluating blood pressure, pulse rate, contractions, uterine tone, and character and amount of bleeding after administration of the drug.
- Be especially vigilant in monitoring for hypertension after I.V. administration.
- Be aware that contractions begin 5 to 15 minutes after P.O. administration; 2 to 5 minutes after I.M injection; immediately after I.V. injection. May continue 3 hours or more after P.O. or I.M. injection; 45 minutes after I.V. injection.

Supportive Care

- Report sudden changes in vital signs, frequent periods of uterine relaxation, or character and amount of vaginal bleeding.
- Maintain or restore adequate blood volume.
- Keep in mind that if hypertension occurs, it may respond to chlorpromazine or hydralazine.
- Administer analgesics as ordered. Assist patient with relaxation techniques, as needed. Reduce dosage, as ordered if severe uterine cramping occurs.

Patient Teaching

- Explain that this drug stimulates uterine musculature, controlling postpartum bleeding and atonia.
- Tell the patient to report pain, dizziness or other adverse reactions to the drug.

Evaluation

In patients receiving methylergonovine maleate, appropriate evaluation statements include:

- Vital signs stable; reduction in amount or absence of uterine bleeding; effective uterine contractions.
- Patient's pain is effectively relieved.
- Patient and family state an understanding of methyergonovine maleate therapy.

methylphenidate hydrochloride

(meth ill fen´ i date)

Ritalin, Ritalin SR

- Controlled Substance Schedule II
- *Classification:* CNS stimulant, analeptic (piperidine)
- *Pregnancy Risk Category:* C

HOW SUPPLIED

Tablets: 5 mg, 10 mg, 20 mg
Tablets (sustained-release): 20 mg

ACTION

Mechanism: Promotes nerve impulse transmission by releasing stored norepinephrine from nerve terminals in

the brain. Main site of activity appears to be the cerebral cortex and the reticular activating system. In children with hyperkinesia, amphetamines have a paradoxical calming effect.
Absorption: Rapidly absorbed and completely after oral administration.
Metabolism: Hepatic.
Excretion: In urine.
Onset, peak, duration: Peak plasma concentrations occur at 1 to 2 hours. Duration of action is usually 4 to 6 hours (with considerable individual variation); sustained-release tablets may act for up to 8 hours.

INDICATIONS & DOSAGE

Attention deficit disorder with hyperactivity (ADDH)–
Children 6 years and older: initial dose 5 to 10 mg P.O. daily before breakfast and lunch, with 5- to 10-mg increments weekly as needed, up to 60 mg daily.
Narcolepsy–
Adults: 10 mg P.O. b.i.d. or t.i.d. half hour before meals. Dosage varies with patient needs. Dosage range is 5 to 50 mg daily.

CONTRAINDICATIONS & PRECAUTIONS

Contraindicated in patients with hypersensitivity to sympathomimetic amines; symptomatic cardiovascular disease, hyperthyroidism, angina pectoris, moderate to severe hypertension, or advanced arteriosclerosis because it may cause dangerous arrhythmias and blood pressure changes; severe exogenous or endogenous depression, glaucoma, parkinsonism, or agitated states; a history of marked anxiety, tension, or agitation, because it can exacerbate such conditions; or a history of substance abuse.

Use cautiously in patients with a history of diabetes mellitus, cardiovascular disease, motor tics, seizures, or Gilles de la Tourette's syndrome (drug may precipitate disorder); and in elderly, debilitated, or hyperexcitable patients.

ADVERSE REACTIONS

Common reactions are in italics; life-threatening reactions are in bold italics.
Blood: thrombocytopenia.
CNS: *nervousness, insomnia,* dizziness, headache, akathisia, dyskinesia, *Tourette's disorder.*
CV: *palpitations,* angina, *tachycardia,* changes in blood pressure and pulse rate.
EENT: difficulty with accommodation and blurring of vision.
GI: nausea, dry throat, abdominal pain, anorexia, weight loss.
Skin: rash, urticaria, ***exfoliative dermatitis,*** erythema multiforme, thrombocytopenic purpura.
Other: growth suppression.

INTERACTIONS

Anticonvulsants, tricyclic antidepressants, oral anticoagulants: methylphenidate may increase plasma levels of these drugs and enhance their pharmacologic effects.
Centrally acting antihypertensives: decreased antihypertensive effect.
MAO inhibitors: severe hypertension; possible hypertensive crisis. Don't use together.

EFFECTS ON DIAGNOSTIC TESTS

None reported.

NURSING CONSIDERATIONS

Besides those related universally to drug therapy (see "How to use this book"), consider the following specific recommendations:
Assessment
- Obtain a baseline assessment of the patient's CNS status and behavior.
- Be alert for adverse reactions and drug interactions throughout therapy.
- Evaluate the patient's and family's

knowledge about methylphenidate therapy.

Nursing Diagnoses

• High risk for injury related to patient's underlying disorder.
• Sleep pattern disturbance related to methylphenidate-induced insomnia.
• Knowledge deficit related to methylphenidate therapy.

Planning and Implementation

Preparation and Administration

• Administer drug at least 6 hours before bedtime to avoid interference with sleep. Administer after meals to reduce appetite-suppressant effects.
• Avoid prolonged administration because of high abuse potential. After long-term use, reduce dosage gradually to prevent acute rebound depression.
• Be aware that the drug is now available in a sustained-release form (duration, 6 to 8 hours).

Monitoring

• Monitor effectiveness by regularly observing the patient's behavior and CNS status.
• Monitor pulse for tachycardia and closely monitor for blood pressure changes; question the patient regularly about palpitations.
• Monitor sleeping pattern for insomnia, and observe for other signs of excessive stimulation.
• May precipitate Gilles de la Tourette's syndrome. Monitor children, especially at the start of therapy.
• Observe for drug interactions, which may affect treatment of other disease states. For example, monitor blood glucose because drug may alter daily insulin needs in diabetic patients. May decrease seizure threshold in patients with seizure disorders.
• Periodically monitor CBC, differential, and platelet counts with long-term use.
• Monitor height and weight in children on prolonged therapy because drug has been associated with growth suppression. Recent evidence suggests it may delay "growth spurt," but children will attain normal height after drug is discontinued.

Supportive Care

• Provide frequent rest periods and assistance with activities as needed; fatigue may result as drug effects wear off.
• Institute safety precautions, by making environment safe and providing supervision of patient's activities.
• Keep in mind that this is the drug of choice for attention deficit disorder with hyperactivity (ADDH). Treatment usually is discontinued after puberty.
• Be aware that tolerance or psychic dependence may develop, especially in patients with history of drug addiction.

Patient Teaching

• Warn the patient to avoid activities that require alertness or good psychomotor coordination until effects of the drug are known.
• Tell the patient to avoid beverages containing caffeine, which increase the stimulant effects of amphetamines and related amines.
• Have the patient report insomnia and other signs of excessive stimulation.
• Tell the diabetic patient to monitor blood glucose levels closely.
• Teach the patient how to take the drug to minimize insomnia and enhance effectiveness.
• Tell the patient the drug should not be used to prevent fatigue.

Evaluation

In patients receiving methylphenidate, appropriate evaluation statements may include:

• Patient demonstrates clinical improvement; safety is maintained.
• Patient is able to sleep without difficulty.
• Patient and family state an understanding of methylphenidate therapy.

methylprednisolone (systemic)
(meth ill pred niss´ oh lone)
Medrol**, Meprolone

methylprednisolone acetate
depMedalone, Depoject, Depo-Medrol, Depopred, Depo-Predate, D-Med, Duralone, Durameth, Medralone, Medrol Enpak, Medrone, Methylone, M-Prednisol, Rep-Pred

methylprednisolone sodium succinate
A-Metha-pred, Medrol†, Solu-Medrol

• *Classification:* anti-inflammatory, immunosuppressant (glucocorticoid)
• *Pregnancy Risk Category:* C

HOW SUPPLIED
methylprednisolone
Tablets: 2 mg, 4 mg, 8 mg, 16 mg, 24 mg, 32 mg
methylprednisolone acetate
Injection (suspension): 20 mg/ml, 40 mg/ml, 80 mg/ml
methylprednisolone sodium succinate
Injection: 40 mg, 125 mg, 500 mg, 1,000 mg, 2,000 mg/vial

ACTION
Mechanism: Decreases inflammation, mainly by stabilizing leukocyte lysosomal membranes. Also suppresses the immune response, stimulates bone marrow, and influences protein, fat, and carbohydrate metabolism.
Absorption: Readily absorbed after oral or I.M. administration.
Distribution: Rapidly distributed to muscle, liver, skin, intestines, and kidneys. Adrenocorticoids are distributed into breast milk and through the placenta.
Metabolism: In the liver to inactive glucuronide and sulfate metabolites.
Excretion: The inactive metabolites and small amounts of unmetabolized drug are excreted by the kidneys. Insignificant amounts are excreted in feces. Half-life: 18 to 36 hours.
Onset, peak, duration: After oral and I.V. administration, peak effects occur in about 1 to 2 hours. The acetate suspension for injection has a variable absorption over 24 to 48 hours, depending on site of injection (intra-articular space, muscle, or blood supply to that muscle).

INDICATIONS & DOSAGE
Severe inflammation or immunosuppression–
Adults: 2 to 60 mg P.O. in four divided doses; or 40 to 80 mg (acetate) daily, I.M. or 10 to 250 mg (succinate) I.M. or I.V. q 4 hours; or 4 to 30 mg (acetate) into joints and soft tissue, p.r.n.
Children: 117 mcg to 1.66 mg/kg (succinate) I.V. in three or four divided doses.
Shock–
Adults: 100 to 250 mg (succinate) I.V. at 2- to 6-hour intervals.
To decrease residual damage following spinal cord trauma–
Adults: 30 mg/kg I.V. as a bolus injection within 8 hours of the injury, followed by a continous infusion of 5.4 mg/hour for the next 23 hours.

CONTRAINDICATIONS & PRECAUTIONS
Contraindicated in patients with hypersensitivity to ingredients of adrenocorticoid preparations, and in those with systemic fungal infections (except in adrenal insufficiency). Patients who are receiving methylprednisolone should not be given live virus vaccines because methylprednisolone suppresses the immune response.

Use with extreme caution in patients with GI ulceration, renal disease, hypertension, osteoporosis, diabetes mellitus, thromboembolic disorders, seizures, myasthenia gravis, CHF, tuberculosis, hypoalbuminemia, hypothyroidism, cirrhosis of the liver, emotional instability, psychotic tendencies, hyperlipidemias, glaucoma, or cataracts, because the drug may exacerbate these conditions.

Because adrenocorticoids increase the susceptibility to and mask symptoms of infection, methylprednisolone should not be used (except in life-threatening situations) in patients with viral or bacterial infections not controlled by anti-infective agents.

ADVERSE REACTIONS

Common reactions are in italics; life-threatening reactions are in bold italics. Most adverse reactions of corticosteroids are dose- or duration-dependent.

CNS: *euphoria, insomnia,* psychotic behavior, pseudotumor cerebri.
CV: ***CHF,*** hypertension, edema.
EENT: cataracts, glaucoma.
GI: *peptic ulcer,* GI irritation, increased appetite.
Metabolic: *possible hypokalemia, hyperglycemia and carbohydrate intolerance,* growth suppression in children.
Skin: delayed wound healing, acne, various skin eruptions.
Other: muscle weakness, pancreatitis, hirsutism, susceptibility to infections.
Acute adrenal insufficiency may occur with increased stress (infection, surgery, or trauma) or abrupt withdrawal after long-term therapy.
Withdrawal symptoms: rebound inflammation, fatigue, weakness, arthralgia, fever, dizziness, lethargy, depression, fainting, orthostatic hypotension, dyspnea, anorexia, hypoglycemia. ***Sudden withdrawal may be fatal.***

INTERACTIONS

Barbiturates, phenytoin, rifampin: decreased corticosteroid effect. Corticosteroid dose may need to be increased.
Indomethacin, aspirin: increased risk of GI distress and bleeding. Give together cautiously.

EFFECTS ON DIAGNOSTIC TESTS

Diagnostic skin tests: suppresses reactions.
Nitroblue tetrazolium test for systemic bacterial infections: false-negative results.
Serum glucose and cholesterol: increased levels.
Serum potassium, calcium, thyroxine, and triiodothyronine: decreased levels.
Thyroid function tests: decreased ^{131}I uptake and protein-bound iodine concentrations.
Urine glucose and calcium: increased levels.

NURSING CONSIDERATIONS

Besides those related universally to drug therapy (see "How to use this book"), consider the following specific recommendations:

Assessment
- Obtain a baseline assessment of the patient's underlying condition before initiating drug therapy.
- Be alert for adverse reactions and drug interactions throughout therapy.
- Evaluate the patient's and family's knowledge about methylprednisolone therapy.

Nursing Diagnoses
- Impaired tissue integrity related to the patient's underlying condition.
- High risk for injury related to adverse reactions to methylprednisolone.
- Knowledge deficit related to methylprednisolone therapy.

Planning and Implementation

Preparation and Administration

• May be used for alternate-day therapy.

• Gradually reduce drug dosage after long-term therapy. Never abruptly discontinue therapy as sudden withdrawal can be fatal.

• Always titrate to lowest effective dose, as prescribed.

• Give daily dosage in the morning for better results and less toxicity.

• Expect to increase dosage as prescribed during times of physiologic stress (surgery, trauma, or infection).

• Do not confuse Solu-Medrol with Solu-Cortef.

• Don't use acetate salt when immediate onset of action is needed.

• ***P.O. use:*** Give with food when possible to avoid GI upset. Critically ill patients may require concomitant antacid therapy.

• ***I.M. use:*** Give injection deep into gluteal muscle. Rotate injection sites to prevent muscle atrophy. Avoid S.C. injection, because atrophy and sterile abscesses may occur. Dermal atrophy may occur with large doses of acetate salt. Use multiple small injections rather than a single large dose.

• ***I.V. use:*** When administering as direct injection, inject diluted drug into a vein or free-flowing compatible I.V. solution over at least 1 minute. In shock, give massive doses over at least 10 minutes to prevent cardiac arrhythmias and circulatory collapse. When administering as an intermittent or continuous infusion, dilute solution according to manufacturer's instructions and give over the prescribed duration. If used for continuous infusion, change solution every 24 hours. Do not use acetate form for I.V. use.

• Discard reconstituted solutions after 48 hours.

Monitoring

• Monitor for adverse reactions because drug can cause serious or even life-threatening multisystem dysfunction.

• Monitor the patient's weight, blood pressure, blood glucose level, and serum electrolyte levels regularly.

• Monitor the patient for infection. Drug may mask or exacerbate infections.

• Monitor the patient's stress level. Stress (fever, trauma, surgery, or emotional problems) may increase adrenal insufficiency. Increased dose may be needed.

• Monitor the patient for depression or psychotic episodes, especially with high-dose therapy.

• Monitor patient's sleep patterns because drug may initially cause euphoria that may interfere with sleep, but patient generally adjusts to the medication after 1 to 3 weeks.

• Monitor patients receiving immunizations for decreased antibody response.

• Monitor for early signs of adrenal insufficiency or cushingoid symptoms.

Supportive Care

• Notify the doctor immediately if serious adverse drug reactions occur and be prepared to administer supportive care.

• Unless contraindicated, give the patient a low-sodium diet high in potassium and protein. Potassium supplement may be needed.

• Be aware that diabetic patients may have increased insulin requirements.

Patient Teaching

• Be sure that the patient understands the need to take the drug as prescribed. Give the patient instructions on what to do if a dose is inadvertently missed.

• Warn the patient not to discontinue the drug abruptly or without the doctor's approval.

• Advise the patient to take oral form with meals to minimize adverse GI reactions.

• Inform the patient of the possible therapeutic and adverse effects of the

drug, so that he may report complications to the doctor as soon as possible.
• Tell the patient to carry a medical alert card indicating the need for supplemental adrenocorticoids during stress.
• Teach the patient to recognize signs of early adrenal insufficiency (fatigue, muscular weakness, joint pain, fever, anorexia, nausea, dyspnea, dizziness, and fainting) and to notify the doctor promptly if they occur.
• Warn patients on long-term therapy about cushingoid symptoms, which may develop regardless of route of administration.

Evaluation

In patients receiving methylprednisolone, appropriate evaluation statements may include:
• Patient's condition shows improvement.
• Patient does not experience serious adverse reactions associated with methylprednisolone.
• Patient and family state an understanding of methylprednisolone therapy.

methylprednisolone acetate (topical)

(meth ill pred niss′ oh lone)
Medrol Acetate

• *Classification:* anti-inflammatory, immunosuppressant (glucocorticoid)
• *Pregnancy Risk Category:* C

HOW SUPPLIED

Ointment: 0.25%, 1%

ACTION

Mechanism: Produces local anti-inflammatory, vasoconstrictor, and antipruritic actions. Diffuses across cell membranes to form complexes with specific cytoplasmic receptors, influencing cellular metabolism. Corticosteroids stabilize leukocyte lysosomal membranes, inhibit local actions and accumulation of macrophages, decrease local edema, and reduce the formation of scar tissue.

Absorption: Depends on the potency of the preparation, the amount applied, and the nature of the skin at the application site. Absorption is lowest in areas with a thick stratum corneum (on the palms, soles, elbows, and knees) and higher in thinner areas (face, eyelids, and genitals). Absorption increases in areas of skin damage, inflammation, or occlusion. Some systemic absorption occurs, especially through the oral mucosa.

Distribution: After topical application, distributed throughout the local skin. Any drug absorbed into circulation is distributed rapidly into muscle, liver, skin, intestines, and kidneys.

Metabolism: After topical administration, metabolized primarily in the skin. The small amount absorbed into systemic circulation is metabolized primarily in the liver to inactive compounds.

Excretion: Inactive metabolites are excreted by the kidneys, primarily as glucuronides and sulfates, but also as unconjugated products. Small amounts of the metabolites are also excreted in feces.

INDICATIONS & DOSAGE

Inflammation of corticosteroid-responsive dermatoses–

Adults and children: clean area; apply ointment daily to q.i.d.

CONTRAINDICATIONS & PRECAUTIONS

Contraindicated in patients who are hypersensitive to any component of the preparation and in patients with viral, fungal, or tubercular skin lesions. Use with extreme caution in patients with impaired circulation because it may increase the risk of skin ulceration.

ADVERSE REACTIONS

Common reactions are in italics; life-threatening reactions are in bold italics.
Skin: burning, itching, irritation, dryness, folliculitis, hypertrichosis, hypopigmentation, acneiform eruptions, allergic contact dermatitis. With occlusive dressings: *maceration of skin, secondary infection, atrophy, striae, miliaria.*

INTERACTIONS

None significant.

EFFECTS ON DIAGNOSTIC TESTS

None significant.

NURSING CONSIDERATIONS

Besides those related universally to drug therapy (see "How to use this book"), consider the following specific recommendations:

Assessment

- Obtain a baseline assessment of skin integrity before topical methylprednisolone therapy.
- Be alert for adverse reactions and drug interactions throughout therapy.
- Evaluate the patient's and family's knowledge about topical methylprednisolone therapy.

Nursing Diagnoses

- Impaired skin integrity related to the patient's underlying condition.
- High risk for infection related to adverse drug reaction.
- Knowledge deficit related to topical methylprednisolone therapy.

Planning and Implementation

Preparation and Administration

- Avoid application near eyes, mucous membranes, or in ear canal.
- Before applying, gently wash the skin. To prevent skin damage, rub medication in gently, leaving a thin coat.
- When treating hairy sites, part hair and apply directly to lesion.
- Wear gloves when administering drug.
- To apply an occlusive dressing (only if ordered by doctor), apply cream heavily, then cover with a thin, pliable, nonflammable plastic film; seal to adjacent normal skin with hypoallergenic tape.
- To prevent recurrence, treatment should continue for a few days after clearing of lesions.

Monitoring

- Monitor effectiveness by regularly assessing skin for extent and severity of inflammation.
- Know that systemic absorption is especially likely with occlusive dressings, prolonged treatment, or extensive body-surface treatment.
- Monitor for signs of secondary infection.
- Frequently assess the patient's skin for burning, itching, and dryness.
- Monitor patients who must use occlusive dressings for maceration of the skin and secondary infection.

Supportive Care

- When using on diaper area of young children, avoid the use of plastic pants or tight-fitting diapers.
- Be prepared to stop the drug and notify the doctor if patient develops systemic absorption, skin irritation or ulceration, hypersensitivity, or infection. (If antifungals or antibiotics are being used with corticosteroids and infection does not respond immediately, corticosteroids should be discontinued until infection is controlled.)
- To minimize adverse reactions, use occlusive dressing intermittently. Don't use occlusive dressings in the presence of infection or on weeping or exudative lesions. Don't leave them in place longer than 16 hours each day.
- For patients with eczematous dermatitis who may develop irritation with adhesive material, hold dressing in place with gauze, elastic bandage, or stockings.
- Notify the doctor and remove occlusive dressing if fever develops.

• Have the patient's fingernails cut short to minimize skin trauma from scratching.
• Apply cool, moist compresses to involved areas to relieve itching and burning.
Patient Teaching
• Instruct the patient to cleanse involved area before applying methylprednisolone in a thin layer to cover the entire surface.
• Teach the patient how to apply an occlusive dressing.
• Instruct the patient to complete the entire treatment regimen as prescribed, even if the lesions appear to have healed.
• Tell the patient and family not to share the prescription with others.
Evaluation
In patients receiving topical methylprednisolone, appropriate evaluation statements may include:
• The patient regains skin integrity.
• Patient does not develop secondary infection.
• Patient and family state an understanding of topical methylprednisolone therapy.

methyltestosterone
(meth ill tess toss´ te rone)
Android, Metandren**, Metandren Linguets, Oreton Methyl, Testomet‡, Testred, Virilon

• Controlled Substance Schedule III
• *Classification:* androgen replacement (androgen)
• *Pregnancy Risk Category:* X

HOW SUPPLIED
Tablets: 5 mg‡, 10 mg, 25 mg, 50 mg‡
Tablets (buccal): 5 mg, 10 mg
Capsules: 10 mg

ACTION
Mechanism: An androgen that stimulates cytosol steroid receptors in tissues to effect protein synthesis. Stimulates target tissues to develop normally in androgen-deficient males.
Pharmacokinetics: Unknown.

INDICATIONS & DOSAGE
Breast engorgement of nonnursing mothers–
Adults: 80 mg P.O. daily, or 40 mg buccal daily for 3 to 5 days.
Breast cancer in women 1 to 5 years postmenopausal–
Adults: 200 mg P.O. daily; or 100 mg buccal daily.
Eunuchoidism and eunuchism, male climacteric symptoms–
Adults: 10 to 40 mg P.O. daily; or 5 to 20 mg buccal daily.
Postpubertal cryptorchidism–
Adults: 30 mg P.O. daily; or 15 mg buccal daily.

CONTRAINDICATIONS & PRECAUTIONS
Contraindicated in patients with sensitivity to the drug; severe renal or cardiac disease, which may be aggravated by fluid and electrolyte retention caused by this drug; hepatic disease, because impaired elimination may cause toxic accumulation of drug; prostate or breast cancer or benign prostatic hypertrophy with obstruction because this drug can stimulate the growth of cancerous breast or prostate tissue in males; undiagnosed abnormal genital bleeding, as this drug can stimulate the growth of malignant neoplasms; in pregnant and breast-feeding women because animal studies have shown that administration of androgens during pregnancy causes masculinization of the female fetus. Metandren 10-mg Linguets and 25-mg tablets contain tartrazine, which may cause allergic reactions in sensitive patients. Use with caution.

*Liquid form contains alcohol.

**May contain tartrazine.

ADVERSE REACTIONS

Common reactions are in italics; life-threatening reactions are in bold italics.
Androgenic: in women–*acne, edema, oily skin, weight gain, hirsutism, hoarseness,* clitoral enlargement, changes in libido. In men–prepubertal: premature epiphyseal closure, acne, priapism, growth of body and facial hair, phallic enlargement; postpubertal: testicular atrophy, oligospermia, decreased ejaculatory volume, impotence, gynecomastia, epididymitis.
CV: edema.
GI: gastroenteritis, constipation, nausea, vomiting, diarrhea, change in appetite.
GU: bladder irritability.
Hepatic: reversible jaundice.
Hypoestrogenic: in women–flushing; sweating; vaginitis with itching, drying, burning, or bleeding; menstrual irregularities.
Local: irritation of oral mucosa with buccal administration.
Other: hypercalcemia.

INTERACTIONS

None significant.

EFFECTS ON DIAGNOSTIC TESTS

Fasting plasma glucose, glucose tolerance test (GTT), and metyrapone test: abnormal results.
17-ketosteroids: decreased levels.
Liver function tests and serum creatinine: elevated results.
Prothrombin time (especially in patients on anticoagulant therapy): prolonged.
Serum sodium, potassium, calcium, phosphate, and cholesterol: increased levels.
Sulfobromophthalein (BSP) retention: increased.
Thyroid function tests (protein-bound iodine, ^{131}I uptake, thyroid-binding capacity): decreased.

NURSING CONSIDERATIONS

Besides those related universally to drug therapy (see "How to use this book"), consider the following specific recommendations:

Assessment

- Obtain a baseline assessment of the patient's underlying condition before initiating therapy.
- Be alert for adverse reactions and drug interactions throughout therapy.
- Evaluate the patient's and family's knowledge about methyltestosterone therapy.

Nursing Diagnoses

- Sexual dysfunction related to hormonal dysfunction.
- Body image disturbance related to adverse androgenic reactions associated with methyltestosterone.
- Knowledge deficit related to methyltestosterone therapy.

Planning and Implementation

Preparation and Administration

- Be aware that treatment of breast cancer with this drug is usually restricted to patients who are 1 to 5 years' postmenopausal.
- Know that therapeutic response of drug used in breast cancer is usually apparent within 3 months. Expect therapy to be stopped if signs of disease progression appear.
- ***P.O. use:*** Administer with food or meals if GI upset occurs.
- Be aware that buccal tablets are twice as potent as oral tablets. Be sure patient does not swallow buccal tablets. When administering buccal tablets, place tablet in upper or lower buccal pouch between cheek and gum. Tablet requires 30 minutes to 1 hour to dissolve. Change absorption site with each dose to minimize risk of buccal irritation.

Monitoring

- Monitor effectiveness by regularly assessing the patient's condition for signs of improvement.
- Monitor the patient for hypercalcemia and obtain calcium levels regu-

larly. Hypercalcemia is particularly likely in patients with metastatic breast cancer and may indicate bone metastases.
• Monitor female patients for signs of virilization.
• Monitor the patient for symptoms of jaundice, which may be reversed by dosage adjustment. Periodic liver function tests should be performed.
• Monitor the patient on concomitant anticoagulant therapy for ecchymotic areas, petechiae, or abnormal bleeding. Monitor prothrombin time.
• Monitor the patient's weight routinely for fluid retention.
• Monitor for signs of hypoglycemia in patients with diabetes. Check blood glucose levels frequently.
• Monitor serum cholesterol and cardiac function studies periodically as ordered.

Supportive Care
• Report signs of hypercalcemia and virilization in females to the doctor.
• Give the patient a diet high in calories and protein unless contraindicated. Give small, frequent feedings. Also implement salt restriction if edema occurs; expect to administer a diuretic concurrently, if needed.
• Carefully evaluate results of laboratory studies. Many laboratory results may be altered during therapy and for 2 to 3 weeks after therapy ends.
• Obtain an order for an antiemetic, antidiarrheal, or laxative, as indicated.
• Prepare patient for altered body image if androgenic adverse reactions occur.
• Be prepared to treat hypoglycemia in the diabetic patient and report to doctor; it may require an adjustment in antidiabetic regimen.

Patient Teaching
• Tell the patient to take drug with food or meals if GI upset occurs.
• Instruct patient how to take buccal tablets if appropriate. Tell him to avoid eating, drinking, chewing, or smoking while buccal tablet is in place and not to swallow it as it takes up to 30 to 60 minutes for drug to dissolve.
• Explain to female patients that virilization may occur. Tell these patients to report such effects immediately as they may be irreversible.
• Tell patient to eat a diet high in calories and protein and low in sodium if not contraindicated and to eat small, frequent meals.
• Warn the diabetic patient about the potential for hypoglycemia, and instruct him how to manage symptoms and to notify doctor if it occurs.
• Correct any misconception about methyltestosterone, because it is erroneously thought the drug enhances athletic ability.

Evaluation
In patients receiving methyltestosterone, appropriate evaluation statements may include:
• Patient's underlying condition exhibits improvement.
• Patient states acceptance of body image changes caused by methyltestosterone therapy.
• Patient and family state an understanding of methyltestosterone therapy.

methysergide maleate
(meth i ser´ jide)
Deseril‡, Sansert**

• *Classification:* vasoconstrictor (ergot alkaloid)
• *Pregnancy Risk Category:* C

HOW SUPPLIED
Tablets: 1 mg‡, 2 mg

ACTION
Mechanism: A semisynthetic ergot alkaloid that blocks serotonin (5-HT) in the periphery, but may act as a 5-HT agonist in the CNS. Probably

*Liquid form contains alcohol.

**May contain tartrazine.

acts by preventing increased blood vessel permeability by preventing 5-HT release from platelets and blocking histamine release from mast cells.
Absorption: Rapidly absorbed from the GI tract.
Distribution: Widely distributed; enters CNS and probably enters breast milk.
Metabolism: In the liver to methylergonovine and glucuronide metabolites.
Excretion: 56% of a dose is excreted in urine as unchanged drug and its metabolites. Half-life: 10 hours.
Onset, peak, duration: Not effective during an acute attack; used only for prophylaxis.

INDICATIONS & DOSAGE

Prevention of frequent, severe, uncontrollable, or disabling migraine or vascular headache–
Adults: 4 to 8 mg P.O. daily with meals.
To control diarrhea caused by carcinoid disease–
Adults: initially, 2 mg P.O. t.i.d., increased p.r.n. to 4 to 16 mg t.i.d.

CONTRAINDICATIONS & PRECAUTIONS

Contraindicated in patients with peripheral vascular disease, severe arteriosclerosis, severe hypertension, coronary artery disease, phlebitis or cellulitis of lower limbs, pulmonary disease, collagen disease, and valvular heart disease, because of the potential for adverse cardiovascular effects; impaired renal or hepatic function or fibrotic processes, because of the potential for accumulation after chronic administration; or peptic ulcer or serious infections; in patients who have shown previous sensitivity to ergot drugs; those in debilitated states; and during pregnancy.

Long-term, uninterrupted therapy is associated with fibrosis in pulmonary, cardiac, and retroperitoneal tissues. Methysergide must not be administered continuously for longer than 6 months, and a drug-free interval of 3 to 4 weeks must follow each 6-month course of therapy. Administer cautiously to patients sensitive to tartrazine dye because tablets contain tartrazine. Tartrazine sensitivity often occurs in patients sensitive to aspirin.

ADVERSE REACTIONS

Common reactions are in italics; life-threatening reactions are in bold italics.
Blood: neutropenia, eosinophilia.
CNS: insomnia, drowsiness, *euphoria, vertigo,* ataxia, *light-headedness,* hyperesthesia, weakness, *hallucinations or feelings of dissociation.*
CV: *fibrotic thickening of cardiac valves and aorta, inferior vena cava, and common iliac branches* ***(retroperitoneal fibrosis);*** vasoconstriction, causing chest pain, abdominal pain, vascular insufficiency of lower limbs; cold, numb, painful extremities with or without paresthesias and diminished or absent pulses; postural hypotension; tachycardia; peripheral edema; murmurs; bruits.
EENT: nasal stuffiness.
GI: nausea, vomiting, diarrhea, constipation, epigastric pain.
Skin: hair loss, dermatitis, sweating, flushing, rash.
Other: ***retroperitoneal fibrosis,*** causing general malaise, fatigue, weight gain, backache, low-grade fever, urinary obstruction; ***pulmonary fibrosis,*** causing dyspnea, tightness and pain in chest, pleural friction rubs and effusion, arthralgia, myalgia.

INTERACTIONS

None significant.

EFFECTS ON DIAGNOSTIC TESTS

None reported.

NURSING CONSIDERATIONS

Besides those related universally to drug therapy (see "How to use this book"), consider the following specific recommendations:

Assessment

- Obtain a baseline assessment of the patient's pain before drug therapy.
- Be alert for adverse reactions and drug interactions throughout therapy.
- Evaluate the patient's and family's knowledge about methysergide therapy.

Nursing Diagnoses

- Pain related to the patient's underlying condition.
- High risk for injury related to adverse drug reaction.
- Knowledge deficit related to methysergide therapy.

Planning and Implementation

Preparation and Administration

- Gradually introduce medication and administer with meals to prevent GI effects.
- Give drug for 3 weeks before evaluating effectiveness.

Monitoring

- Frequently check the patient's vital signs, especially respirations and breath sounds.
- Obtain studies of cardiac and renal function studies, blood count, and sedimentation rate before and during therapy.
- Monitor the patient's bowel pattern; drug may cause diarrhea or constipation.
- Monitor the patient's vital signs frequently.
- Monitor for altered sensation by asking patient if he experiences any cold, numb, or painful hands and feet; leg cramps when walking; or chest, flank, or pelvic pain.
- Monitor effectiveness by frequently monitoring the patient's level of pain.
- Monitor sensation level, especially in the patient's hands and feet.
- Monitor the patient's weight daily.
- Monitor hydration status if patient develops nausea, vomiting, and diarrhea.

Supportive Care

- Provide fluids if the patient develops nausea, vomiting, and diarrhea.
- Obtain an order for a mild laxative if he develops constipation.
- Know that this drug is not for the treatment of migraine or vascular headaches in progress or for treatment of tension (muscle contraction) headaches.
- Institute safety precautions if the patient develops vertigo, dizziness, or hallucinations.
- Know that this drug is indicated only for patients who are unresponsive to other drugs and who can be kept under close medical supervision.
- If the patient develops GI effects, give the drug with meals.
- Be prepared to gradually discontinue the drug over 2 to 3 weeks. Do not discontinue it abruptly.

Patient Teaching

- Tell the patient to take this drug with meals to prevent GI distress.
- Tell the patient not to stop taking the drug abruptly; may cause rebound headaches. Drug must be discontinued gradually over 2 to 3 weeks.
- Tell the patient to notify the doctor promptly if he experiences cold, numb, or painful hands and feet; leg cramps when walking; or pelvic, chest, or flank pain.

Evaluation

In patients receiving methysergide, appropriate evaluation statements may include:

- Patient states his pain has diminished.
- Patient does not experience any injury related to adverse drug reactions.
- Patient and family state an understanding of methysergide therapy.

metoclopramide hydrochloride

(met oh kloe´ pra mide)
Maxeran†, Maxolon‡, Maxolon High Dose‡, Reglan

- *Classification:* antiemetic, GI stimulant (para-aminobenzoic acid derivative)
- *Pregnancy Risk Category:* B

HOW SUPPLIED

Tablets: 5 mg, 10 mg
Syrup: 5 mg/5 ml
Injection: 5 mg/ml

ACTION

Mechanism: Stimulates motility of the upper GI tract by increasing lower esophageal sphincter tone. Also blocks dopamine receptors at the chemoreceptor trigger zone.
Absorption: Absorbed rapidly and thoroughly from the GI tract after oral administration.
Distribution: Well distributed to most body tissues and fluids, including the brain. It crosses the placenta and is distributed in breast milk.
Metabolism: Extensively metabolized; a small amount is metabolized in the liver.
Excretion: Mostly in urine and feces. Hemodialysis and renal dialysis remove minimal amounts. Half-life: 5 to 6 hours.
Onset, peak, duration: After oral administration, action begins in 30 to 60 minutes. After I.M. administration, about 74% to 96% of the drug is bioavailable; action begins in 10 to 15 minutes. After I.V. administration, onset of action occurs in 1 to 3 minutes. Duration of effect is 1 to 2 hours.

INDICATIONS & DOSAGE

Preventing or reducing nausea and vomiting induced by cisplatin and other chemotherapy–
Adults: 2 mg/kg I.V. q 2 hours for 5 doses, beginning 30 minutes prior to cisplatin administration.
To facilitate small-bowel intubation and to aid in radiologic examinations–
Adults: 10 mg (2 ml) I.V. as a single dose over 1 to 2 minutes.
Children 6 to 14 years: 2.5 to 5 mg I.V. (0.5 to 1 ml).
Children under 6 years: 0.1 mg/kg I.V.
Delayed gastric emptying secondary to diabetic gastroparesis–
Adults: 10 mg P.O. 30 minutes before meals and h.s. for 2 to 8 weeks, depending on response.
Treatment of gastroesophageal reflux–
Adults: 10 to 15 mg P.O. q.i.d., p.r.n. Take 30 minutes before meals.

CONTRAINDICATIONS & PRECAUTIONS

Contraindicated in patients with hypersensitivity to the drug or to sulfonamides; pheochromocytoma, because it may induce hypertensive crisis; and seizure disorders, renal failure, liver failure, Parkinson's disease, GI hemorrhage, or intestinal obstruction or perforation, because the drug may exacerbate symptoms of these disorders.

Use cautiously in children because they may have a higher incidence of adverse CNS effects and in patients with a history of breast cancer because the drug stimulates prolactin secretion.

Do not use the drug for longer than 12 weeks.

ADVERSE REACTIONS

Common reactions are in italics; life-threatening reactions are in bold italics.
CNS: *restlessness, anxiety, drowsiness,* fatigue, *lassitude,* insomnia, headache, dizziness, *extrapyramidal symptoms, tardive dyskinesia, dystonic reactions,* sedation.

CV: transient hypertension.
GI: nausea, bowel disturbances.
Skin: rash.
Other: fever, prolactin secretion, loss of libido.

INTERACTIONS

Anticholinergics, narcotic analgesics: antagonize effects of metoclopramide. Use together cautiously.

EFFECTS ON DIAGNOSTIC TESTS

Serum aldosterone and prolactin: increased levels.

NURSING CONSIDERATIONS

Besides those related universally to drug therapy (see "How to use this book"), consider the following specific recommendations:

Assessment

- Obtain a baseline assessment of blood pressure, mental status, GI status, and history of seizure disorder or pheochromocytoma before therapy.
- Be alert for adverse reactions or drug interactions during therapy.
- Evaluate the patient's and family's knowledge about metoclopramide.

Nursing Diagnoses

- High risk for fluid volume deficit related to nausea and vomiting induced by chemotherapy.
- Altered thought processes related to adverse CNS reactions to metoclopramide.
- Knowledge deficit related to metoclopramide therapy.

Planning and Implementation

Preparation and Administration

- ***P.O. use:*** Administer 30 minutes before meals and at hour of sleep.
- ***I.V. use:*** Infuse slowly over 15 minutes. Protection from light is unnecessary if the infusion mixture is administered within 24 hours.
- Be aware that safety and effectiveness have not been established for therapy that continues longer than 12 weeks.

Monitoring

- Monitor effectiveness by observing the patient for nausea and vomiting.
- Monitor fluid balance.
- Monitor blood pressure frequently in patients receiving I.V. doses.
- Observe for changes in mental status, mood, and behavior. Observe for extrapyramidal symptoms and tardive dyskinesia.

Supportive Care

- Contraindicated whenever stimulation of GI motility might be dangerous (hemorrhage, obstruction, or perforation) and in pheochromocytoma or epilepsy.
- Diphenhydramine 25 mg I.V. may be prescribed to counteract the extrapyramidal effects associated with high doses of metoclopramide.
- Be aware that elderly patients are more likely to experience extrapyramidal symptoms and tardive dyskinesia.
- Oral form is being used experimentally to treat nausea and vomiting.
- Use safety precautions for patients who develop adverse CNS reactions.
- If patient is alert, encourage adequate intake of fluids to prevent fluid volume deficit.

Patient Teaching

- Warn patient to avoid activities requiring alertness for 2 hours after taking each dose.
- Advise patient that changes in mood and behavior may accompany therapy with metoclopramide.

Evaluation

In patients receiving metoclopramide, appropriate evaluation statements may include:

- Patient exhibits no signs of fluid volume deficit.
- Patient demonstrates no signs of altered thought processes.
- Patient and family state an understanding of metoclopramide therapy.

metolazone

(me tole´ a zone)
Diulo, Mykrox, Zaroxolyn**

- *Classification:* diuretic, antihypertensive (quinazoline [thiazide-like])
- *Pregnancy Risk Category:* D

HOW SUPPLIED

Tablets: 0.5 mg, 2.5 mg, 5 mg, 10 mg

ACTION

Mechanism: Although not a thiazide diuretic, metolazone acts in a similar fashion. It increases urine excretion of sodium and water by inhibiting sodium reabsorption in the cortical diluting site of the ascending loop of Henle.
Absorption: About 65% of a given dose is absorbed after oral administration to healthy subjects; in cardiac patients, absorption falls to 40%. Rate and extent of absorption vary among preparations.
Distribution: Metolazone is 50% to 70% erythrocyte-bound and about 33% protein-bound.
Metabolism: Insignificant.
Excretion: About 70% to 95% is excreted unchanged in urine. Half-life: About 5½ hours in healthy subjects; may be prolonged in patients with decreased creatinine clearance.

INDICATIONS & DOSAGE

Edema (heart failure)–
Adults: 5 to 10 mg P.O. daily.
Edema (renal disease)–
Adults: 5 to 20 mg P.O. daily.
Hypertension–
Adults: 2.5 to 5 mg (Diulo and Zaroxolyn) P.O. daily. Maintenance dosage determined by patient's blood pressure.
Adults: 0.5 mg (Mykrox) once daily in the a.m. Increase to 1 mg P.O. daily as needed. If response is inadequate, add another antihypertensive agent.

CONTRAINDICATIONS & PRECAUTIONS

Contraindicated in patients with anuria and in those with sensitivity to the drug. Use cautiously in patients with severe renal disease because it may decrease glomerular filtration rate and precipitate azotemia; in patients with impaired hepatic function or liver disease because electrolyte changes may precipitate coma; and in those taking digoxin because hypokalemia may predispose them to digitalis toxicity.

ADVERSE REACTIONS

Common reactions are in italics; life-threatening reactions are in bold italics.
Blood: ***aplastic anemia, agranulocytosis,*** leukopenia, thrombocytopenia.
CV: *volume depletion and dehydration,* orthostatic hypotension.
GI: anorexia, nausea, pancreatitis.
Hepatic: hepatic encephalopathy.
Metabolic: *hypokalemia, asymptomatic hyperuricemia, hyperglycemia and impairment of glucose tolerance,* fluid and electrolyte imbalances including dilutional hyponatremia and hypochloremia, metabolic alkalosis, hypercalcemia, gout.
Skin: dermatitis, photosensitivity, rash.
Other: ***hypersensitivity, such as pneumonitis and vasculitis.***

INTERACTIONS

Cholestyramine, colestipol: intestinal absorption of thiazides decreased. Keep doses as separate as possible.
Diazoxide: increased antihypertensive, hyperglycemic, and hyperuricemic effects. Use together cautiously.
NSAIDs: decreased diuretic effect. Avoid concomitant use.

EFFECTS ON DIAGNOSTIC TESTS

Parathyroid function tests: test interference. Drug should be discontinued before such tests.
Serum electrolytes: altered levels.
Serum urate, glucose, cholesterol, and triglycerides: increased levels.

NURSING CONSIDERATIONS

Besides those related universally to drug therapy (see "How to use this book"), consider the following specific recommendations:

Assessment

- Obtain a baseline assessment of blood pressure, serum electrolytes, urine output, weight, and peripheral edema before therapy.
- Be alert for adverse reactions and drug interactions throughout therapy.
- Evaluate the patient's and family's knowledge about metolazone therapy.

Nursing Diagnoses

- Fluid volume excess related to sodium and water retention.
- Altered urinary elimination related to metolazone therapy.
- Knowledge deficit related to metolazone therapy.

Planning and Implementation

Preparation and Administration

- ***P.O. use:*** If possible, give drug early in the day to prevent nocturia.

Monitoring

- Monitor effectiveness by regularly checking blood pressure, urine output, and weight.
- Monitor serum electrolyte, BUN, creatinine, glucose, and uric acid levels.
- Monitor CBC, differential, and platelet count.
- Monitor the patient receiving concomitant digitalis therapy for increased risk of digitalis toxicity.
- Monitor for signs of hypokalemia (for example, muscle weakness and cramps).
- Monitor the diabetic patient's insulin requirements because metolazone has hyperglycemic effects.
- Monitor skin turgor and mucous membranes for signs of fluid volume deficit.
- Monitor elderly patients closely because they are especially susceptible to excessive diuresis.

Supportive Care

- Hold drug and notify the doctor if hypersensitivity reactions occur.
- Keep accurate records of intake and output, blood pressure, and weight.
- Provide frequent skin and mouth care to relieve dryness from diuretic therapy.
- Answer the patient's call bell promptly; make sure bathroom or bedpan is easily accessible.
- Use safety precautions to minimize risk of falling due to hypotension.
- In the patient undergoing tests of parathyroid function, hold thiazide and thiazide-like drugs before these tests are performed.
- Be aware that optimal antihypertensive effect may not occur for several days after beginning of therapy with metolazone.
- Elevate the patient's legs to aid reduction of peripheral edema.
- Administer potassium supplements as indicated.

Patient Teaching

- Teach the patient and family to identify and report signs of hypersensitivity reaction and hypokalemia.
- Teach the patient and family to monitor the patient's fluid volume by recording daily weight and intake and output.
- Inform the patient that optimal therapeutic response may not occur until several days after beginning metolazone therapy.
- Teach the patient to avoid high-sodium foods and to choose high-potassium foods.
- Advise the patient to change positions slowly, especially when rising to standing position, to avoid dizziness and fainting due to orthostatic hypotension.

• Advise the patient to minimize risks of photosensitivity reaction by using a sunscreen when outdoors.
• Advise the diabetic patient that insulin dosage may require adjustment.
• Advise the patient who is taking digitalis that the drug's potassium-depleting effect may increase the risk of digitalis toxicity.
• Advise the patient to take drug early in the day to avoid interruption of sleep by nocturia.

Evaluation

In patients receiving metolazone, appropriate evaluation statements may include:
• Patient is free of edema.
• Patient demonstrates adjustment of life-style to deal with altered patterns of urinary elimination.
• Patient and family state an understanding of metolazone therapy.

metoprolol tartrate

(me toe´ proe lole)

Apo-Metoprolol†, Betaloc†‡, Betaloc Durules†, Lopresor†, Lopresor SR†, Lopressor, Novometoprol†

• *Classification:* antihypertensive, adjunctive treatment of acute MI (beta-adrenergic blocking agent)
• *Pregnancy Risk Category:* B

HOW SUPPLIED

Tablets: 50 mg, 100 mg
Tablets (sustained-release): 100 mg†, 200 mg†
Injection: 1 mg/ml in 5-ml ampules or refilled syringes

ACTION

Mechanism: Blocks cardiac $beta_1$ receptors and depresses renin secretion.
Absorption: Rapidly and almost completely absorbed from GI tract; food enhances absorption.
Distribution: Widely distributed throughout the body; drug is about 12% protein-bound.
Metabolism: Hepatic.
Excretion: About 95% of a given dose is excreted in urine. Half-life: 3 to 7 hours.
Onset, peak, duration: After oral administration, peak plasma concentrations occur in 90 minutes, and beta blockade persists for about 24 hours. At start of therapy, maximum effect appears after 1 week of daily use. After I.V. administration, maximum beta blockade occurs in 20 minutes and lasts for 5 to 8 hours.

INDICATIONS & DOSAGE

For hypertension; may be used alone or in combination with other antihypertensives—
Adults: 50 mg b.i.d. or 100 mg once daily P.O. initially. Up to 200 to 400 mg daily in two to three divided doses. No dosage recommendations for children.
Early intervention in acute myocardial infarction—
Adults: Three injections of 5-mg I.V. boluses q 2 minutes. Then, 15 minutes after last dose, administer 50 mg P.O. q 6 hours for 48 hours. Maintenance dosage is 100 mg P.O. b.i.d.

CONTRAINDICATIONS & PRECAUTIONS

Contraindicated in patients with hypersensitivity to the drug; and in patients with overt cardiac failure, second- or third-degree atrioventricular block, and cardiogenic shock, because the drug may worsen these conditions.

Use cautiously in patients with coronary insufficiency because beta-adrenergic blockade may precipitate congestive heart failure (CHF); impaired hepatic function (dosage reduction may be necessary); diabetes mellitus or hyperthyroidism, because metoprolol may mask the tachycardia associated with hypoglycemia and hyperthyroidism (drug will not mask dizziness and sweating from hypoglycemia); bronchospastic disease (dosages higher than 100 mg/day may inhibit bronchodilating effects of endogenous catecholamines [at lower doses, metoprolol selectively inhibits $beta_1$-receptors]); and sinus node dysfunction because depression of sinoatrial node automaticity may occur.

ADVERSE REACTIONS

Common reactions are in italics; life-threatening reactions are in bold italics.
CNS: fatigue, lethargy, dizziness.
CV: *bradycardia, hypotension, CHF,* peripheral vascular disease.
GI: nausea, vomiting, diarrhea.
Skin: rash.
Respiratory: dyspnea, ***bronchospasm.***
Other: fever, arthralgias.

INTERACTIONS

Barbiturates, rifampin: increased metabolism of metoprolol. Monitor for decreased effect.
Chlorpromazine, cimetidine, verapamil: decreased hepatic clearance. Monitor for greater beta-blocking effect.
Digitalis glycosides: excessive bradycardia and increased depressant effect on myocardium. Use together cautiously.
Indomethacin: decrease in antihypertensive effect. Monitor blood pressure and adjust dosage.
Insulin, oral hypoglycemic drugs: can alter dosage requirements in previously stabilized diabetics. Observe patient carefully.

EFFECTS ON DIAGNOSTIC TESTS

Serum transaminase, alkaline phosphatase, lactic dehydrogenase, and uric acid: elevated levels.

NURSING CONSIDERATIONS

Besides those related universally to drug therapy (see "How to use this book"), consider the following specific recommendations:

Assessment
• Obtain a baseline assessment of the patient's blood pressure and pulse before beginning therapy.
• Be alert for adverse reactions and drug interactions throughout therapy.
• Evaluate the patient's and family's knowledge about metoprolol therapy.

Nursing Diagnoses
• Altered tissue perfusion (renal, cerebral, cardiopulmonary and peripheral) related to the patient's underlying condition.
• High risk for injury related to adverse reactions to metoprolol.
• Knowledge deficit related to metoprolol therapy.

Planning and Implementation

Preparation and Administration
• Always check the patient's apical pulse rate before giving this drug. If it's slower than 60 beats/minute, hold drug and call doctor immediately.
• Keep in mind that although most patients with asthma and bronchitis can take this drug without fear of worsening their condition, doses over 100 mg daily should be used cautiously.
• ***P.O. use:*** Give consistently with meals. Food may increase absorption of the drug.
• ***I.V. use:*** Store the drug at room temperature and protect from light. Discard solution if discolored or if particulates form.

Monitoring
• Monitor effectiveness by frequently checking the patient's blood pressure, apical pulse rate, and ECG.
• Monitor the patient for hypotension, and CNS and other adverse reactions.

Supportive Care
• Keep in mind that this drug masks the common signs of shock and hypoglycemia; however, it doesn't potentiate insulin-induced hypoglycemia or

delay recovery of blood glucose to normal levels.
• Notify the doctor if the patient develops hypotension or bradycardia. Doctor may adjust the drug dosage.
• Institute safety precautions, such as continuous use of side rails, if the patient experiences hypotension or adverse CNS reactions.

Patient Teaching
• Tell the patient to always take the oral drug with meals because food increases drug absorption.
• Explain the importance of taking this drug as prescribed, even when feeling well.
• Tell the patient not to discontinue this drug suddenly even if unpleasant adverse reactions occur, but to discuss the problem with the doctor. Explain that abrupt discontinuation of the drug can exacerbate angina and myocardial infarction.
• Instruct the patient to check with the doctor or pharmacist before taking OTC medications.
• Teach the patient and family caregiver how to take blood pressure measurements. Tell them to notify the doctor of any significant change in blood pressure.
• Tell the patient that periodic eye examinations are recommended during therapy with this drug.

Evaluation
In patients receiving metoprolol, appropriate evaluation statements may include:
• Blood pressure controlled within normal limits for this patient.
• Injury related to adverse reactions to metoprolol did not occur.
• Patient and family state an understanding of metoprolol therapy.

metronidazole (topical)
(me troe ni´ da zole)
MetroGel

• *Classification:* antibacterial, antiprotozoal (nitroimidazole)
• *Pregnancy Risk Category:* B

HOW SUPPLIED
Topical gel: 0.75%

ACTION
Mechanism: Exact mechanism of action is unknown. Probably exerts an anti-inflammatory effect through its antibacterial and antiprotozoal actions, which result from disruption of DNA and nucleic acid synthesis.
Absorption: Not appreciably absorbed through intact skin.
Distribution: Unknown after topical application; drug is less than 20% bound to plasma proteins.
Metabolism: Probably in the liver.
Excretion: In urine.
Onset, peak, duration: Under normal conditions, serum levels are negligible after topical administration.

INDICATIONS & DOSAGE
Topical treatment of acne rosacea –
Adults: apply a thin film b.i.d. to affected area during the morning and evening. Significant results should appear within 3 weeks and continue for the first 9 weeks of therapy.

CONTRAINDICATIONS & PRECAUTIONS
Contraindicated in patients allergic to the drug or other ingredients of the formulation (such as parabens). Use cautiously in patients with history or evidence of blood dyscrasias, because chemically related compounds are associated with blood dyscrasias.

ADVERSE REACTIONS

Common reactions are in italics; life-threatening reactions are in bold italics.
EENT: lacrimation (if drug applied in area around the eyes).

INTERACTIONS

Oral anticoagulants: may potentiate anticoagulant effect. Monitor patient for potential adverse reactions.

EFFECTS ON DIAGNOSTIC TESTS

None reported.

NURSING CONSIDERATIONS

Besides those related universally to drug therapy (see "How to use this book"), consider the following specific recommendations:

Assessment
- Obtain a baseline assessment of papules before therapy.
- Be alert for adverse reactions and drug interactions throughout therapy.
- Evaluate the patient's and family's knowledge about topical metronidazole therapy.

Nursing Diagnoses
- Impaired skin integrity related to patient's underlying condition.
- Sensory/perceptual alterations (visual) related to metronidazole-induced lacrimation.
- Knowledge deficit related to metronidazole therapy.

Planning and Implementation

Preparation and Administration
- ***Topical use:*** Cleanse affected area before application. Apply drug in a thin film.

Monitoring
- Monitor effectiveness by regularly examining patient's papules.
- Observe for local reaction; if it occurs, apply less frequently or discontinue.
- Frequently observe the patient for increased lacrimation.

Supportive Care
- Notify doctor if local irritation occurs.

Patient Teaching
- Teach patient how to apply medication.
- Advise patient to cleanse area thoroughly before use. Patient may use cosmetics after applying the drug.
- Instruct patient to avoid use of the drug around the eyes.

Evaluation

In patients receiving topical metronidazole, appropriate evaluation statements may include:
- Patient states that papules have healed.
- The patient did not develop increased lacrimation.
- Patient and family state an understanding of topical metronidazole therapy.

---

metronidazole (systemic)

(me troe ni´ da zole)

Apo-Metronidazole†, Flagyl, Metizol, Metrogyl‡, Metrozine‡, Metryl, Neo-Metric†, Novonidazol†, PMS Metronidazole†, Protostat

metronidazole hydrochloride

Flagyl I.V., Flagyl I.V. RTU, Metro I.V., Novonidazol†

- *Classification:* amebicide and trichomonacide
- *Pregnancy Risk Category:* B

HOW SUPPLIED

Tablets: 200 mg‡, 250 mg, 400 mg‡, 500 mg
Oral suspension (benzoyl metronidazole): 200 mg/5 ml‡
Injection: 500 mg/100 ml ready to use
Powder for injection: 500-mg single-dose vials

ACTION

Mechanism: A direct-acting trichomonacide and amebicide that works at both intestinal and extraintestinal

sites. The drug disrupts both DNA and nucleic acid synthesis.
Absorption: Well absorbed after oral administration. About 80% of a dose is absorbed.
Distribution: Widely distributed into most body tissues and fluids, including cerebrospinal fluid, bone, bile, saliva, pleural and peritoneal fluids, vaginal secretions, seminal fluids, middle ear fluid, and hepatic and cerebral abscesses. Less than 20% of metronidazole is bound to plasma proteins. It readily crosses the placenta.
Metabolism: In the liver to the 2-hydroxymethyl metabolite, which has some antibacterial and antiprotozoal activity; other metabolites are inactive.
Excretion: Both active drug and metabolites are excreted; about 60% to 80% is excreted in the urine, and 15% in the feces; also excreted in breast milk. Half-life: 6 to 8 hours in adults with normal renal function; may be prolonged in patients with impaired hepatic function.
Onset, peak, duration: Peak serum concentrations of metronidazole occur in about 1 to 3 hours after oral administration; food slows absorption and delays peak levels, but does not affect total amount absorbed.

INDICATIONS & DOSAGE

Amebic hepatic abscess–
Adults: 500 to 750 mg P.O. t.i.d. for 5 to 10 days.
Children: 35 to 50 mg/kg daily (in three doses) for 10 days.
Intestinal amebiasis–
Adults: 750 mg P.O. t.i.d. for 5 to 10 days.
Children: 35 to 50 mg/kg daily (in three doses) for 10 days. Follow this therapy with oral iodoquinol.
Trichomoniasis–
Adults (both male and female): 250 mg P.O. t.i.d. for 7 days or 2 g P.O. in single dose; 4 to 6 weeks should elapse between courses of therapy.
Refractory trichomoniasis–
Women: 250 mg P.O. b.i.d. for 10 days.
Treatment of bacterial infections caused by anaerobic microorganisms–
Adults: Loading dose is 15 mg/kg I.V. infused over 1 hour (approximately 1 g for a 70-kg adult). Maintenance dose is 7.5 mg/kg I.V. or P.O. q 6 hours (approximately 500 mg for a 70-kg adult). The first maintenance dose should be administered 6 hours following the loading dose. Maximum dosage not to exceed 4 g daily.
Giardiasis–
Adults: 250 mg P.O. t.i.d. for 5 days.
Children: 5 mg/kg P.O. t.i.d. for 5 days.
Prevention of postoperative infection in contaminated or potentially contaminated colorectal surgery–
Adults: 15 mg/kg infused over 30 to 60 minutes and completed approximately 1 hour before surgery. Then, 7.5 mg/kg infused over 30 to 60 minutes at 6 and 12 hours after the initial dose.

CONTRAINDICATIONS & PRECAUTIONS

Contraindicated in patients with hypersensitivity to nitroimidazole derivatives, and in pregnancy during the first trimester because its safety for such use has not been studied.

Use cautiously in patients with a history of blood dyscrasia, because the drug can cause leukopenia; in patients receiving corticosteroids; and in those with edema from the sodium content of the injection. Use with extreme caution (and at lower than recommended doses) in patients with severe hepatic impairment because metronidazole and its metabolites accumulate in the plasma. Metronidazole should not be used indiscriminately because animal studies suggest carcinogenicity.

ADVERSE REACTIONS

Common reactions are in italics; life-threatening reactions are in bold italics.

Blood: transient leukopenia, neutropenia.

CNS: vertigo, *headache,* ataxia, incoordination, confusion, irritability, depression, restlessness, weakness, fatigue, drowsiness, insomnia, sensory neuropathy, paresthesias of extremities, psychic stimulation, neuromyopathy.

CV: ECG change (flattened T wave), edema (with I.V. RTU preparation).

GI: abdominal cramping, stomatitis, *nausea, vomiting, anorexia,* diarrhea, constipation, proctitis, dry mouth.

GU: darkened urine, polyuria, dysuria, pyuria, incontinence, cystitis, decreased libido, dyspareunia, dryness of vagina and vulva, sense of pelvic pressure.

Skin: pruritus, flushing.

Local: thrombophlebitis after I.V. infusion.

Other: overgrowth of nonsusceptible organisms, especially *Candida* (glossitis, furry tongue), metallic taste, fever, gynecomastia.

INTERACTIONS

Alcohol: disulfiram-like reaction (nausea, vomiting, headache, cramps, flushing). Don't use together.

Disulfiram: acute psychoses and confusional states. Don't use together.

EFFECTS ON DIAGNOSTIC TESTS

Aminotransferases and triglycerides: falsely decreased values.

ECG: flattened T waves.

NURSING CONSIDERATIONS

Besides those related universally to drug therapy (see "How to use this book"), consider the following specific recommendations:

Assessment

- Obtain a baseline assessment of infection, including appropriate specimen for culture and sensitivity, before therapy.
- Be alert for adverse reactions and drug interactions throughout therapy.
- Evaluate the patient's and family's knowledge about metronidazole therapy.

Nursing Diagnoses

- High risk for injury related to dosage regimen inadequate to alleviate infection.
- Alteration in nutrition: Less than body requirements, related to anorexia, nausea, and vomiting.
- Knowledge deficit related to metronidazole.

Planning and Implementation

Preparation and Administration

- Be aware that metronidazole should be used only after *Trichomonas vaginalis* or *Entamoeba histolytica* has been identified.
- ***P.O. use:*** Give oral form with meals to minimize GI distress.
- ***I.V. use:*** Follow package instructions carefully when mixing the I.V. solution. Don't refrigerate Flagyl I.V. RTU.

  Administer the I.V. form by slow infusion either as a continuous or intermittent infusion. Additives should not be introduced into solution. If used with a primary I.V. fluid system, discontinue the primary fluid during the infusion; do not give by I.V. push. Do not use equipment containing aluminum (for example, needles, cannulas) that would contact the drug solution. Solution should be clear, pale yellow-green. Do not use cloudy or precipitated solutions.

Monitoring

- Monitor effectiveness by regularly assessing for improvement of infectious process.
- Monitor nutritional status, including body weight if GI adverse reactions occur.

Supportive Care

- When treating amebiasis, record number and character of stools; send

fecal specimens to laboratory promptly because amebiasis is detectable only in warm specimens.
• If the patient develops nausea or vomiting, obtain an order for an antiemetic.
Patient Teaching
• Tell the patient to avoid alcohol or alcohol-containing medications (for example, cough syrups) during therapy and for at least 48 hours after therapy ends.
• Tell the patient that drug may cause metallic taste and discolored (red-brown) urine.
• Tell patient to take tablets with meals to minimize GI distress and that tablets may be crushed to facilitate swallowing.
• Emphasize the need for medical follow-up after discharge.
• For the patient with amebiasis, explain that follow-up examinations of stool specimens are necessary for 3 months after treatment is discontinued, to ensure elimination of amebae. To prevent reinfection, instruct the patient and family in proper hygiene, including: disposal of feces; meticulous hand washing after defecation and before handling, preparing, or eating food; the risks of eating raw food; and control of contamination by flies. Encourage other household members and suspected contacts to be tested and, if necessary, treated.
• Teach correct personal hygiene, including perineal care for the patient with trichomoniasis. Explain that asymptomatic sexual partner should be treated simultaneously to prevent reinfection. The patient should avoid intercourse during therapy or have partner use condom.

Evaluation
In patients receiving metronidazole, appropriate evaluation statements may include:
• Patient is free of infection.
• Patient maintains normal nutritional status.
• Patient and family state an understanding of metronidazole therapy.

mexiletine hydrochloride
(mex´ i le teen)
Mexitil

• *Classification:* ventricular antiarrhythmic (lidocaine analogue)
• *Pregnancy Risk Category:* C

HOW SUPPLIED
Capsules: 50 mg‡, 100 mg†, 150 mg, 200 mg, 250 mg
Injection: 250 mg/10 ml‡

ACTION
Mechanism: A class Ib antiarrhythmic that depresses phase O, it shortens the action potential. All class I drugs have membrane-stabilizing effects.
Absorption: When administered orally, about 90% of drug is absorbed from the GI tract. Absorption rate decreases with conditions that speed gastric emptying.
Distribution: Widely distributed throughout the body. Distribution volume declines in patients with hepatic disease, resulting in toxic serum drug levels with usual doses. About 50% to 60% of circulating drug is bound to plasma proteins. Usual therapeutic drug level is 0.5 to 2 mcg/ml. Although toxicity may occur within this range, levels above 2 mcg/ml are considered toxic and are associated with a higher incidence of adverse CNS effects, warranting dosage reduction.
Metabolism: In the liver to relatively inactive metabolites. Metabolism is affected by hepatic blood flow, which may be reduced in patients who are recovering from myocardial infarction and in those with CHF or liver disease.
Excretion: Less than 10% of a dose

is excreted unchanged. Urinary excretion increases with urine acidification and slows with urine alkalinization. Half-life: In healthy patients, 10 to 12 hours; may be prolonged in patients with CHF or hepatic disease. **Onset, peak, duration:** Peak serum levels occur 2 to 3 hours after oral administration.

INDICATIONS & DOSAGE

Treatment of refractory ventricular arrhythmias, including ventricular tachycardia and premature ventricular contractions–

Adults: 200 to 400 mg P.O. followed by 200 mg q 8 hours. May increase dose to 400 mg q 8 hours if satisfactory control is not obtained. Some patients may respond well to an every-12-hour schedule. May give up to 450 mg q 12 hours.

Where available, mexiletine may be given I.V.–

Adults: following a loading dose of 200 to 250 mg I.V. at a rate of 25 mg/minute, prepare an infusion solution of 250 mg mexiletine/500 ml dextrose 5% in water. Administer the first 120 ml (60 mg) over 1 hour. If clinical response is inadequate, give another bolus of 200 mg over 10 to 20 minutes. Maintenance dose is 0.5 mg/minute (1 ml/minute of prepared solution).

CONTRAINDICATIONS & PRECAUTIONS

Contraindicated in patients with cardiogenic shock, because the drug has a mild negative inotropic effect and may increase systemic vascular resistance slightly, thereby exacerbating this condition; in patients with preexisting second- or third-degree heart block without an artificial pacemaker, because the drug may further depress cardiac conduction; and in patients with hypersensitivity to the drug.

Use cautiously in patients with severe degrees of SA, AV, or intraventricular heart block who do not have an artificial pacemaker, because the drug may worsen these conditions; hepatic or myocardial failure, because the drug may accumulate and cause toxicity; seizure disorders, because the drug may induce seizures; and bradycardia or hypotension, because the drug may worsen these conditions.

ADVERSE REACTIONS

Common reactions are in italics; life-threatening reactions are in bold italics.

CNS: *tremor, dizziness,* blurred vision, ataxia, diplopia, confusion, nystagmus, nervousness, headache.

CV: hypotension, bradycardia, widened QRS complex, arrhythmias.

GI: nausea, vomiting.

Skin: rash.

INTERACTIONS

Cimetidine: increased mexiletine blood levels. Monitor carefully.

Phenytoin, rifampin, phenobarbital: decreased mexiletine blood levels. Monitor carefully.

EFFECTS ON DIAGNOSTIC TESTS

Liver function tests: transiently altered results.

NURSING CONSIDERATIONS

Besides those related universally to drug therapy (see "How to use this book"), consider the following specific recommendations:

Assessment

- Obtain a baseline assessment of the patient's heart rate and rhythm before mexiletine therapy.
- Be alert for adverse reactions and drug interactions throughout therapy.
- Evaluate the patient's and family's knowledge about mexiletine therapy.

Nursing Diagnoses

- Decreased cardiac output related to ineffectiveness of mexiletine.
- High risk for injury related to mexiletine-induced CNS reactions.

• Knowledge deficit related to mexiletine.

Planning and Implementation

Preparation and Administration

• ***P.O. use:*** Administer drug with meals to lessen GI distress. Patients who respond well to mexiletine can often be maintained on a q 12 hour schedule. Notify doctor if you feel the patient is a good candidate for q 12 hour therapy.

• ***I.V. use:*** Administer a loading dose of 200 to 250 mg I.V. at a rate of 25 mg/minute as ordered. Follow this with an infusion. Prepare the infusion solution with 250 mg mexiletine in 500 ml dextrose 5% in water. Administer the first 120 ml (60 mg) over 1 hour. If clinical response is inadequate, expect to give another bolus of 200 mg over 10 to 20 minutes. Administer maintenance dose at 0.5 mg/minute (1 ml/minute of prepared solution). Mexiletine injection is compatible with 0.9% sodium chloride, 5% dextrose in water, 5% sodium bicarbonate, 1/6M sodium lactate, and 10% fructose (laevulose).

• When changing from lidocaine to mexiletine, stop the infusion when the first mexiletine dose is given. Keep the infusion line open, however, until the arrhythmia appears to be controlled.

Monitoring

• Monitor effectiveness by regularly assessing ECG recordings and the patient's heart rate and rhythm.

• Monitor patient for early signs of mexiletine toxicity, such as a fine tremor of the hands. This progresses to dizziness and later to ataxia and nystagmus as the drug's blood level increases.

• Monitor therapeutic blood levels of mexiletine. Therapeutic levels range from 0.75 to 2 mcg/ml.

• Monitor hydration status if adverse GI disturbances occur.

Supportive Care

• If ECG disturbances occur, withhold the drug, obtain a rhythm strip, and notify the doctor immediately.

• Notify the doctor immediately if mexiletine toxicity is suspected and be prepared to draw a blood sample for a mexiletine level.

• Obtain an order for an antiemetic agent as needed.

• Institute safety precautions if adverse CNS reactions occur.

Patient Teaching

• Tell patient to take the drug with meals to minimize adverse GI reactions.

• Stress importance of taking the drug exactly as prescribed.

• Emphasize the importance of close follow-up care that includes frequent ECGs and blood tests.

• Instruct patient to notify the doctor if a fine tremor of the hands occur.

• Warn patient to avoid hazardous activities that require mental alertness until CNS effects of drug are known.

• Tell patient how to handle troublesome GI reactions.

Evaluation

In patients receiving mexiletine, appropriate evaluation statements may include:

• Patient's ECG reveals arrhythmia has been corrected.

• Patient does not experience injury as a result of adverse CNS reactions to mexiletine therapy.

• Patient and family state an understanding of mexiletine therapy.

mezlocillin sodium

(mez loe sill´ in)

Mezlin

• *Classification:* antibiotic (extended-spectrum penicillin)

• *Pregnancy Risk Category:* B

HOW SUPPLIED

Injection: 1 g, 2 g, 3 g, 4 g

ACTION

Mechanism: Bactericidal against microorganisms by inhibiting cell wall synthesis during active multiplication. Bacteria resist mezlocillin by producing penicillinases–enzymes that hydrolyze mezlocillin.
Absorption: Not absorbed after oral administration and must be administered parenterally. After I.M. administration, about 63% of a dose is rapidly absorbed. Peak levels of the drug are higher after I.V. administration.
Distribution: After parenteral administration, the apparent volume of distribution is approximately equal to the extracellular fluid volume. Mezlocillin is distributed widely. It penetrates minimally into CSF with uninflamed meninges; it crosses the placenta, and is 16% to 42% protein-bound.
Metabolism: About 15% of a dose is metabolized to inactive metabolites.
Excretion: Primarily excreted in urine (39% to 72%) by glomerular filtration and renal tubular secretion; up to 30% of a dose is excreted in bile; some is excreted in breast milk. Half-life: Elimination half-life in adults is dose dependent–the half-life is longer with increasing doses and averages ¾ to 1½ hours; in extensive renal impairment half-life is extended to 2 to 14 hours.

INDICATIONS & DOSAGE

Systemic infections caused by susceptible strains of gram-positive and especially gram-negative organisms (including Proteus, Pseudomonas aeruginosa)–
Adults: 200 to 300 mg/kg daily I.V. or I.M. given in 4 to 6 divided doses. Usual dose is 3 g q 4 hours or 4 g q 6 hours. For very serious infections, up to 24 g daily may be administered.
Children to age 12: 50 mg/kg q 4 hours by I.V. infusion or direct I.V. injection.

CONTRAINDICATIONS & PRECAUTIONS

Contraindicated in patients with hypersensitivity to any penicillin or cephalosporins. Use cautiously in patients with renal impairment because drug is excreted by the kidneys; decreased dosage is required in moderate to severe renal failure.

ADVERSE REACTIONS

Common reactions are in italics; life-threatening reactions are in bold italics.
Blood: ***bleeding with high doses,*** neutropenia, eosinophilia, leukopenia, ***thrombocytopenia.***
CNS: neuromuscular irritability.
GI: nausea, diarrhea.
Metabolic: *hypokalemia.*
Local: pain at injection site, vein irritation, phlebitis.
Other: *hypersensitivity (edema, fever, chills, rash, pruritus, urticaria, **anaphylaxis**),* overgrowth of nonsusceptible organisms.

INTERACTIONS

Aminoglycoside antibiotics (e.g., gentamicin, tobramycin): chemically incompatible. Don't mix together in I.V. solution. Give 1 hour apart, especially in patients with renal insufficiency.
Probenecid: increases blood levels of mezlocillin. Probenecid may be used for this purpose.

EFFECTS ON DIAGNOSTIC TESTS

Aminoglycoside serum levels: falsely decreased concentrations.
CBC: transient reductions in RBC, WBC, and platelet counts.
Coombs' test: positive results.
Liver function tests: transient elevations.
Prothrombin time: prolonged.
Serum electrolytes: hypokalemia and hypernatremia.

Urine or serum protein tests: altered results, chemical interference with methods that use sulfosalicylic acid, trichloroacetic acid, acetic acid, or nitric acid, but not with tests using bromo-phenol blue (Albustix, Albutest, MultiStix).

NURSING CONSIDERATIONS

Besides those related universally to drug therapy (see "How to use this book"), consider the following specific recommendations:

Assessment

- Obtain a baseline assessment of infection before therapy.
- Be alert for adverse reactions and drug interactions throughout therapy.
- Evaluate the patient's and family's knowledge about mezlocillin therapy.

Nursing Diagnoses

- High risk for injury related to ineffectiveness of mezlocillin to eradicate the infection.
- Impaired tissue integrity related to mezlocillin induced thrombophlebitis at the injection site.
- Knowledge deficit related to mezlocillin therapy.

Planning and Implementation

Preparation and Administration

- Obtain specimen for culture and sensitivity tests before first dose. Therapy may begin pending test results.
- Before first dose, ask the patient about previous allergic reactions to this drug or other penicillins. However, a negative history of penicillin allergy does not guarantee future safety.
- Give mezlocillin at least 1 hour before bacteriostatic antibiotics.
- Expect to administer with another antibiotic, such as gentamicin.
- Be aware that dosage should be reduced in patients with impaired renal function.
- ***I.V. use:*** When giving I.V., mix with dextrose 5% in water or other suitable I.V. fluids, and infuse intermittently to prevent vein irritation.

Monitoring

- Monitor effectiveness by regularly assessing for improvement of infectious process.
- Monitor CBC, platelets, and serum potassium regularly as ordered.
- Monitor for bacterial and fungal superinfections during prolonged or high-dose therapy, especially in elderly, debilitated, or immunosuppressed patients.

Supportive Care

- Discontinue the drug immediately if the patient develops signs of anaphylactic shock (rapidly developing dyspnea and hypotension). Notify the doctor and prepare to administer immediate treatment, such as epinephrine, corticosteroids, antihistamines, and other resuscitative measures.
- Change I.V. site every 48 hours. If signs of thrombophlebitis occur, change site immediately and apply warm compresses.
- If the patient develops a rash, notify the doctor and expect to discontinue the drug.
- Institute seizure precautions; high blood levels may induce seizures.
- Limit patient's salt intake because drug contains 1.85 mEq Na/g.

Patient Teaching

- Advise the patient who becomes allergic to mezlocillin to wear medical alert identification stating this information.
- Tell patient to limit salt intake during mezlocillin therapy.

Evaluation

In patients receiving mezlocillin, appropriate evaluation statements may include:

- Patient is free of infection.
- Patient does not experience impaired tissue integrity as a result of therapy.
- Patient and family state an understanding of mezlocillin therapy.

miconazole (systemic)
(mi kon´ a zole)
Monistat I.V.

- *Classification:* antifungal (imidazole derivative)
- *Pregnancy Risk Category:* B

HOW SUPPLIED
Injection: 10 mg/ml

ACTION
Mechanism: Inhibits purine transport and DNA, RNA, and protein synthesis; increases cell wall permeability, making the fungus more susceptible to osmotic pressure.
Absorption: About 50% of a dose is absorbed after oral administration. (An oral form of the drug is not available in the U.S.)
Distribution: Penetrates well into inflamed joints, vitreous humor, and the peritoneal cavity. Distribution into sputum and saliva is poor, and CSF penetration is unpredictable. Miconazole is over 90% bound to plasma proteins.
Metabolism: Predominantly to inactive metabolites in the liver.
Excretion: 14% to 22% of an I.V. dose is excreted in urine. It is unknown whether it is excreted in breast milk. Half-life: Triphasic; 0.4 hours, 2.1 hours; and terminal half-life is about 24 hours.
Onset, peak, duration: Doses above 9 mg/kg produce peak blood levels above 1 mcg/ml in most cases.

INDICATIONS & DOSAGE
Treatment of systemic fungal infections (coccidioidomycosis, candidiasis, cryptococcosis, paracoccidioidomycosis), chronic mucocutaneous candidiasis–
Adults: 200 to 3,600 mg/day. Dosages may vary with diagnosis and with infective agent. May divide daily dosage over 3 infusions, 200 to 1,200 mg per infusion. Dilute in at least 200 ml of 0.9% sodium chloride. Repeated courses may be needed because of relapse or reinfection.
Children 1 year and older: 20 to 40 mg/kg/day. Do not exceed 15 mg/kg per infusion.
Fungal meningitis–
Adults: 20 mg intrathecally as an adjunct to intravenous administration, q 3 to 7 days.

CONTRAINDICATIONS & PRECAUTIONS
Contraindicated in patients with hypersensitivity to the drug. Use cautiously in patients with hepatic disease.

ADVERSE REACTIONS
Common reactions are in italics; life-threatening reactions are in bold italics.
Blood: transient decreases in hematocrit, thrombocytopenia.
CNS: dizziness, drowsiness.
GI: *nausea, vomiting,* diarrhea.
Metabolic: *transient decrease in serum sodium.*
Skin: *pruritic rash.*
Local: *phlebitis at injection site.*

INTERACTIONS
None significant.

EFFECTS ON DIAGNOSTIC TESTS
CBC: transient decrease in hematocrit; increased or decreased platelet counts; erythrocyte aggregation.
Electrolytes: hyponatremia.
Lipids: hyperlipidemia and hypertriglyceridemia; abnormalities in lipoprotein and immunoelectrophoretic patterns from the polyoxyl 35 castor oil vehicle.

NURSING CONSIDERATIONS
Besides those related universally to drug therapy (see "How to use this book"), consider the following specific recommendations:

Assessment
- Obtain a baseline assessment of infection, including appropriate specimens to identify fungi, before therapy.
- Be alert for adverse reactions and drug interactions throughout therapy.
- Evaluate the patient's and family's knowledge about miconazole therapy.

Nursing Diagnoses
- High risk for infection related to ineffectiveness of miconazole to eradicate the fungal infection.
- Impaired tissue integrity related to miconazole-induced pruritic rash.
- Knowledge deficit related to miconazole.

Planning and Implementation
Preparation and Administration
- First I.V. dose should be administered under continuous medical supervision with emergency resuscitative equipment immediately available. Acute cardiorespiratory arrest has occurred with the first dose. Be prepared for anaphylaxis.
- Avoid administering the drug at mealtime in order to lessen GI adverse reactions.
- ***I.V. use:*** Dilute infusion with at least 200 ml of 0.9% sodium chloride and infuse over 30 to 60 minutes because rapid injection of undiluted miconazole may produce arrhythmias.
- Expect to supplement treatment with intrathecal administration for fungal meningitis and bladder irrigation for urinary bladder infections.

Monitoring
- Monitor effectiveness by regularly assessing for improvement of infection and by evaluating the appropriate tests for eradication of fungi.
- Monitor patient's skin for a pruritic rash.
- Regularly monitor patient's levels of hemoglobin, hematocrit, electrolytes, and lipids. Transient elevations in serum cholesterol and triglycerides may be due to castor oil vehicle.

Supportive Care
- Have emergency resuscitative equipment readily available.
- Be aware that premedication with an antiemetic may minimize nausea and vomiting. Consult with the patient's doctor if nausea and vomiting occur.
- Institute safety precautions if adverse CNS reactions occur.
- If phlebitis occurs, change injection site and apply warm compresses to site.

Patient Teaching
- Inform patient that pruritic rash may persist for weeks after drug is discontinued, but pruritus may be controlled with oral or I.V. diphenhydramine.
- Tell patient that adequate therapeutic response may take weeks or months.
- Inform patient that supplemental treatment with intrathecal administration will be necessary for fungal meningitis or bladder irrigation for urinary bladder infections.
- Advise patient who develops adverse reactions to seek help when ambulating.
- Instruct patient to request an antiemetic before drug is given if nausea or vomiting occurred with previous dose.
- Emphasize the need for frequent laboratory studies to monitor for effectiveness and adverse reactions.

Evaluation
In patients receiving miconazole, appropriate evaluation statements may include:
- Patient's infection is alleviated.
- Patient's skin remains intact despite presence of pruritic rash.
- Patient and family state an understanding of miconazole therapy.

miconazole nitrate (topical)

(mi kon´ a zole)

Micatin◇, Monistat-Derm Cream and Lotion, Monistat 7 Vaginal Cream◇, Monistat 7 Vaginal Suppository◇, Monistat 3 Vaginal Suppository

- *Classification:* antifungal (imidazole derivative)
- *Pregnancy Risk Category:* C

HOW SUPPLIED

Cream: 2%◇
Lotion: 2%◇
Powder: 2%◇
Spray: 2%◇
Vaginal cream: 2%◇
Vaginal suppositories: 100 mg◇, 200 mg

ACTION

Mechanism: Controls or destroys fungus by disrupting fungal cell membrane permeability.
Absorption: A small amount of drug is systemically absorbed after vaginal administration.
Distribution: Penetrates well into inflamed joints, vitreous humor, and the peritoneal cavity. Distribution into sputum and saliva is poor, and CSF penetration is unpredictable. Over 90% bound to plasma proteins.
Metabolism: In the liver, predominantly to inactive metabolites.
Excretion: Up to 1% of a vaginal dose is excreted in urine. Half-life: About 24 hours.

INDICATIONS & DOSAGE

Tinea pedis, tinea cruris, tinea corporis, tinea versicolor, cutaneous candidiasis (moniliasis), infections from common dermatophytes–
Adults and children: apply or spray sparingly b.i.d. for 2 to 4 weeks.
Vulvovaginal candidiasis–
Adults: insert 1 applicatorful or suppository (Monistat 7) intravaginally for 7 days at bedtime; repeat course if necessary. Alternatively, insert suppository (Monistat 3) intravaginally for 3 days at bedtime.

CONTRAINDICATIONS & PRECAUTIONS

Contraindicated in patients with hypersensitivity to the drug. Concurrent use of latex contraceptive diaphragms is not recommended because the base contained in the suppository formulation may interact with latex. Use cautiously in patients with hepatic disease.

ADVERSE REACTIONS

Common reactions are in italics; life-threatening reactions are in bold italics.
Skin: isolated reports of irritation, burning, maceration.
Other: (with vaginal cream) vulvovaginal burning, itching, or irritation.

INTERACTIONS

None significant.

EFFECTS ON DIAGNOSTIC TESTS

None reported.

NURSING CONSIDERATIONS

Besides those related universally to drug therapy (see "How to use this book"), consider the following specific recommendations:

Assessment
- Obtain a baseline assessment of vaginal infection before therapy.
- Be alert for adverse reactions and drug interactions throughout therapy.
- Evaluate the patient's and family's knowledge about miconazole nitrate therapy.

Nursing Diagnoses
- Impaired skin integrity related to patient's underlying condition.
- High risk for impaired skin integrity related to maceration induced by miconazole nitrate therapy.
- Knowledge deficit related to miconazole nitrate therapy.

Planning and Implementation
Preparation and Administration
• ***Intravaginal use:*** Apply or spray sparingly. Insert 1 applicatorful or suppository, as ordered.
Monitoring
• Monitor effectiveness by regularly evaluating vaginal infection, drainage, and discomfort.
• Monitor for adverse reactions and interactions by assessing the patient's skin for sensitivity or chemical irritation and maceration.
Supportive Care
• Be prepared to discontinue drug and notify doctor if adverse reactions occur.
• Do not use occlusive dressings.
• Be aware that concurrent use of intravaginal forms and certain latex products, such as vaginal contraceptive diaphragms, is not recommended because of possible interaction.
Patient Teaching
• Teach patient how to apply medication.
• Tell patient to continue using for full treatment period prescribed, even if condition has improved.
• Inform patient, when using intravaginal forms, cautiously insert high into the vagina with applicator provided.
• Tell patient that drug may stain clothing.
Evaluation
In patients receiving miconazole nitrate, appropriate evaluation statements may include:
• Vaginal infection has resolved.
• Maceration did not occur.
• Patient and family state an understanding of miconazole nitrate therapy.

midazolam hydrochloride
(mid´ ay zoe lam)
Versed

• Controlled Substance Schedule IV
• *Classification:* preoperative sedative, agent for conscious sedation, adjunct for induction of general anesthesia, amnesic agent (benzodiazepine)
• *Pregnancy Risk Category:* D

HOW SUPPLIED
Injection: 1 mg/ml, 5 mg/ml

ACTION
Mechanism: Depresses the CNS at the limbic and subcortical levels of the brain.
Absorption: After I.M. administration, 80% to 100% absorbed.
Distribution: Large volume of distribution; approximately 97% protein-bound. The drug crosses the placenta and enters fetal circulation.
Metabolism: Hepatic.
Excretion: Metabolites are excreted in urine. Half-life: 2 to 6 hours.
Onset, peak, duration: Peak serum concentrations occur in 45 minutes and are about one half of those after I.V. administration. Sedation begins within 15 minutes after an I.M. dose and within 2 to 5 minutes after I.V. injection. After I.V. administration, induction of anesthesia occurs in 1½ to 2½ minutes. Duration of sedation is usually 1 to 4 hours.

INDICATIONS & DOSAGE
Preoperative sedation (to induce sleepiness or drowsiness and relieve apprehension) –
Adults: 0.07 mg to 0.08 mg/kg I.M. approximately 1 hour before surgery. May be administered with atropine or scopolamine and reduced doses of narcotics.

Conscious sedation before short diagnostic or endoscopic procedures– **Adults:** initially, 0.035 mg/kg slowly I.V.(not to exceed 2.5 mg). Dose is then titrated in small amounts to a total dosage of 0.1 mg/kg.
Induction of general anesthesia– **Adults:** 0.3 to 0.35 mg/kg I.V. over 20 to 30 seconds. Additional increments of 25% of the initial dose may be needed to complete induction. Up to 0.6 mg/kg total dosage may be given.

CONTRAINDICATIONS & PRECAUTIONS

Contraindicated in patients with hypersensitivity to benzodiazepines. Do not administer to patients with severe hypotension or shock, or to patients with alcohol intoxication and depressed vital signs.

Use cautiously in patients with severe hepatic dysfunction, renal failure, or CHF, because these patients eliminate the drug more slowly and increased toxic effects may occur, and in patients with glaucoma, because midazolam may elevate intraocular pressure. Use cautiously in debilitated patients and elderly patients, especially those with chronic obstructive pulmonary disease (COPD), who are at greatly increased risk for hypotension or respiratory depression.

ADVERSE REACTIONS

Common reactions are in italics; life-threatening reactions are in bold italics.
CNS: headache, oversedation, involuntary movements, combativeness.
CV: variations in blood pressure and pulse rate.
GI: nausea, vomiting, hiccups.
Local: pain and tenderness at injection site.
Other: ***decreased respiratory rate, apnea.***

INTERACTIONS

CNS depressants: may increase the risk of apnea. Prepare to adjust drug dosage.

EFFECTS ON DIAGNOSTIC TESTS

None reported.

NURSING CONSIDERATIONS

Besides those related universally to drug therapy (see "How to use this book"), consider the following specific recommendations:

Assessment

- Obtain a baseline assessment of CNS and respiratory status before therapy.
- Be alert for adverse reactions and drug interactions throughout therapy.
- Evaluate the patient's and family's knowledge about midazolam therapy.

Nursing Diagnoses

- Anxiety related to upcoming surgery or diagnostic procedure.
- Ineffective breathing pattern related to midazolam-induced respiratory depression.
- Knowledge deficit related to midazolam therapy.

Planning and Implementation

Preparation and Administration

- ***I.M. use:*** Inject deeply into a large muscle mass.
- ***I.V. use:*** Take care to avoid extravasation. Do not administer rapidly. Excessive dosage or rapid infusion has been associated with respiratory arrest, particularly in elderly or debilitated patients.
- May be mixed in the same syringe with morphine sulfate, meperidine, atropine sulfate, or scopolamine.

Monitoring

- Monitor effectiveness by evaluating the patient's state of sedation.
- Monitor for evidence of respiratory depression, such as decreased rate or depth of respirations.
- Monitor blood pressure during supine procedures, especially in pa-

tients who have also been premedicated with opiates (narcotics).

Supportive Care

• After administration, institute safety precautions, such as keeping bed rails up.
• Notify the doctor if the patient's respirations are below 12 breaths/minute.
• Before administering I.V. midazolam, have oxygen and resuscitative equipment available in case of severe respiratory depression.
• Be aware that midazolam has a beneficial amnesic effect, which diminishes patient's recall of perioperative events. This drug offers advantages over diazepam, hydroxyzine, and barbiturates.

Patient Teaching

• Explain that midazolam will provide sedation and relieve anxiety before surgery or a short diagnostic or endoscopic procedure.
• Instruct the patient to remain in bed after taking drug.

Evaluation

In patients receiving midazolam, appropriate evaluation statements may include:
• Patient's anxiety relieved; sedation obtained.
• Patient's respiratory status remained within normal limits.
• Patient and family state an understanding of midazolam therapy.

---

mineral oil (liquid petrolatum)

Agoral Plain◇, Fleet Mineral Oil◇, Kondremul Plain◇, Liqui-Doss◇, Milkinol◇, Neo-Cultol◇, Zymenol◇

• *Classification:* laxative (lubricant oil)
• *Pregnancy Risk Category:* C

HOW SUPPLIED

Emulsion: 50%◇
Jelly: 55%◇
Oral liquid: in pints, quarts, gallons◇

ACTION

Mechanism: A lubricant laxative that increases water retention in the stool by creating a barrier between colon wall and feces that prevents colonic reabsorption of fecal water.
Absorption: Minimally absorbed; significant absorption with emulsified drug form.
Distribution: Locally distributed, primarily in the colon.
Metabolism: None.
Excretion: In feces.
Onset, peak, duration: Action begins in 6 to 8 hours.

INDICATIONS & DOSAGE

Constipation; preparation for bowel studies or surgery–
Adults: 15 to 30 ml P.O. h.s.; or 120 ml enema.
Children: 5 to 15 ml P.O. h.s.; or 30 to 60 ml enema.

CONTRAINDICATIONS & PRECAUTIONS

Contraindicated in patients with fluid and electrolyte disturbances, appendicitis, acute surgical abdomen, fecal impaction, or intestinal obstruction or perforation, because the drug may exacerbate these symptoms or these conditions.

The enema form is contraindicated in children under age 2 because of potential for adverse effects.

Oral forms should be avoided in elderly bedridden patients and in children under age 6 because of the risk of oil droplet aspiration. Repeated use is not recommended in pregnant patients because the drug may cause hypoprothrombinemia and hemorrhagic disease of the neonate.

ADVERSE REACTIONS

Common reactions are in italics; life-threatening reactions are in bold italics.
GI: *nausea;* vomiting; diarrhea in ex-

cessive use; *abdominal cramps,* especially in severe constipation; decreased absorption of nutrients and fat-soluble vitamins, resulting in deficiency; and slowed healing after hemorrhoidectomy.
Other: laxative dependence in long-term or excessive use, pruritus.

INTERACTIONS

Docusate salts: may increase mineral oil absorption and cause lipid pneumonia. Don't administer together.
Fat-soluble vitamins (A, D, E, and K): absorption may be decreased after prolonged administration.

EFFECTS ON DIAGNOSTIC TESTS

None reported.

NURSING CONSIDERATIONS

Besides those related universally to drug therapy (see "How to use this book"), consider the following specific recommendations:

Assessment
- Obtain a baseline assessment of history of bowel disorder, GI status, fluid intake, nutritional status, exercise habits, and normal pattern of elimination.
- Be alert for adverse reactions and drug interactions throughout therapy.
- Evaluate the patient's and family's knowledge about mineral oil therapy.

Nursing Diagnoses
- Constipation related to interruption of normal pattern of elimination characterized by infrequent or absent stools.
- Pain related to mineral oil–induced abdominal cramping.
- Knowledge deficit related to mineral oil therapy.

Planning and Implementation

Preparation and Administration
- Check drug order because mineral oil is available in three forms.
- ***P.O. use:*** Give with fruit juice or carbonated drinks to disguise taste.
- Do not administer with meals or immediately after, because mineral oil delays passage of food from the stomach. Mineral oil is more active on an empty stomach.
- Give at bedtime only.

Monitoring
- Monitor effectiveness by checking the frequency and characteristics of stools.
- Auscultate bowel sounds at least once a shift. Assess for pain and cramping.
- Monitor nutritional status and fluid intake.

Supportive Care
- Do not give enema to children under age 2.
- Use when patient needs to ease strain of evacuation.
- Provide privacy for elimination.
- Unless contraindicated, encourage fluid intake up to 2,500 ml a day.
- Consult with a dietitian to modify diet to increase fiber and bulk.

Patient Teaching
- Discourage excessive use of laxatives by patient. Warn patient not to take mineral oil for more than 1 week.
- Teach the patient about the relationship between fluid intake, dietary fiber, exercise, and constipation.
- Teach patient that dietary sources of fiber include bran and other cereals, fresh fruit, and vegetables.
- Warn patient of possible rectal leakage from excessive dosage so he can avoid soiling clothing.
- Warn the patient that abdominal cramping may occur.

Evaluation

In patients receiving mineral oil, appropriate evaluation statements may include:
- Patient reports return of normal pattern of elimination.
- Patient remains free from abdominal cramping.
- Patient and family state an understanding of mineral oil therapy.

minocycline hydrochloride

(mi noe sye´ kleen)

Minocin*, Minomycin‡, Minomycin IV‡

- *Classification:* antibiotic (tetracycline)
- *Pregnancy Risk Category:* D

HOW SUPPLIED

Tablets: 50 mg, 100 mg
Capsules: 50 mg, 100 mg
Oral suspension: 50 mg/5 ml
Injection: 100 mg‡

ACTION

Mechanism: Exerts bacteriostatic effect by binding to the 30S ribosomal subunit of microorganisms, thus inhibiting protein synthesis.
Absorption: 90% to 100% absorbed after oral administration.
Distribution: Widely distributed into body tissues and fluids, including synovial, pleural, prostatic, and seminal fluids, bronchial secretions, saliva, and aqueous humor; CSF penetration is poor. Minocycline crosses the placenta; it is 55% to 88% protein-bound.
Metabolism: Partially metabolized.
Excretion: Primarily excreted unchanged in urine by glomerular filtration; is excreted in breast milk. Half-life: 11 to 26 hours in adults with normal renal function.
Onset, peak, duration: Peak serum levels occur at 2 to 3 hours after an oral dose.

INDICATIONS & DOSAGE

Infections caused by sensitive gram-negative and gram-positive organisms, trachoma, amebiasis–
Adults: 200 mg I.V., then 100 mg I.V. q 12 hours. Do not exceed 400 mg/day. Or, give 200 mg P.O. initially, then 100 mg P.O. q 12 hours. Some clinicians use 100 or 200 mg P.O. initially, followed by 50 mg q.i.d.
Children over 8 years: initially, 4 mg/kg P.O. or I.V., followed by 2 mg/kg q 12 hours.
Give I.V. in 500- to 1,000-ml solution without calcium, and administer over 6 hours.
Gonorrhea in patients sensitive to penicillin–
Adults: initially, 200 mg P.O., then 100 mg q 12 hours for 4 days.
Syphilis in patients sensitive to penicillin–
Adults: initially, 200 mg P.O., then 100 mg q 12 hours for 10 to 15 days.
Meningococcal carrier state–
100 mg P.O. q 12 hours for 5 days.
Uncomplicated urethral, endocervical, or rectal infection caused by Chlamydia trachomatis *or* Ureaplasma urealyticam–
Adults: 100 mg P.O. b.i.d. for at least 7 days.
Uncomplicated gonoccocal urethritis in men–
Adults: 100 mg P.O. b.i.d. for 5 days.

CONTRAINDICATIONS & PRECAUTIONS

Contraindicated in patients with hypersensitivity to any tetracycline; during the second half of pregnancy; and in children under age 8 because of the risk of permanent discoloration of teeth, enamel defects, and retardation of bone growth. Use cautiously in patients likely to be exposed to direct sunlight or ultraviolet light because of the risk of photosensitivity reactions.

ADVERSE REACTIONS

Common reactions are in italics; life-threatening reactions are in bold italics.
Blood: neutropenia, eosinophilia.
CNS: *light-headedness, dizziness from vestibular toxicity.*
CV: pericarditis.
EENT: dysphagia, glossitis.
GI: *anorexia,* epigastric distress, *nausea,* vomiting, *diarrhea,* enterocolitis,

inflammatory lesions in anogenital region.
Metabolic: increased BUN.
Skin: *maculopapular and erythematous rashes, photosensitivity, increased pigmentation, urticaria.*
Local: *thrombophlebitis.*
Other: ***hypersensitivity.***

INTERACTIONS

Antacids (including sodium bicarbonate) and laxatives containing aluminum, magnesium, or calcium: decrease antibiotic absorption. Give antibiotic 1 hour before or 2 hours after any of the above.
Ferrous sulfate and other iron products, zinc: decrease antibiotic absorption. Tetracyclines should be given 3 hours after or 2 hours before iron administration.
Methoxyflurane: may cause severe nephrotoxicity with tetracyclines. Monitor carefully.
Oral contraceptives: decreased contraceptive effectiveness and increased risk of breakthrough bleeding.

EFFECTS ON DIAGNOSTIC TESTS

Urine glucose tests with glucose enzymatic reagent (Clinistix or Tes-Tape): false-negative results.

NURSING CONSIDERATIONS

Besides those related universally to drug therapy (see "How to use this book"), consider the following specific recommendations:

Assessment
- Obtain a baseline assessment of infection before therapy.
- Be alert for adverse reactions and drug interactions throughout therapy.
- Evaluate the patient's and family's knowledge about minocycline therapy.

Nursing Diagnoses
- High risk for infection related to ineffectiveness of minocycline to eradicate the infection.
- High risk for fluid volume deficit related to adverse GI reactions to minocycline therapy.
- Knowledge deficit related to minocycline.

Planning and Implementation
Preparation and Administration
- Obtain specimen for culture and sensitivity tests before first dose. Therapy may begin pending test results.
- Check expiration date. Outdated or deteriorated tetracyclines have been associated with reversible nephrotoxicity (Fanconi's syndrome).
- Do not expose drug to light or heat. Keep container tightly closed.
- ***P.O. use:*** May administer drug with food.
- ***I.V. use:*** Reconstitute 100 mg powder with 5 ml sterile water for injection with further dilution of 500 to 1,000 ml for I.V. infusion. Stable for 24 hours at room temperature.

Monitoring
- Monitor effectiveness by regularly assessing for improvement of infection.
- Monitor patient for tooth discoloration if a young adult.
- Monitor for signs and symptoms of superinfections.
- Monitor hydration status if adverse GI reactions occur.
- Monitor I.V. site for phlebitis.

Supportive Care
- If the patient develops a superinfection, or new infection, notify the doctor. Prepare to discontinue the drug and substitute another antibiotic. If the patient develops oral thrush, provide good mouth care.
- If patient develops brown pigmentation on teeth notify the doctor.
- If the patient develops diarrhea, nausea, or vomiting, request an antiemetic or antidiarrheal agent, if needed. Expect to substitute a parenteral form of minocycline or another antibiotic as prescribed.
- For patient receiving I.V. therapy, rotate site to minimize irritation.

• Be aware that minocycline may alter urine glucose test results. Monitor diabetic patient's blood glucose level instead.

Patient Teaching

• Tell the patient to take oral minocycline with food if desired.
• Emphasize importance of completing prescribed regimen exactly as ordered and keeping follow-up appointments.
• Instruct patient to inform doctor if brown pigmentation occurs on teeth.
• Tell the patient to check expiration dates and discard any outdated minocycline as it may become toxic.
• Teach the patient to report signs of superinfection (furry overgrowth on tongue, vaginal itch or discharge, foul-smelling stool). Stress good oral hygiene.
• Advise female patient taking an oral contraceptive to use an alternative means of contraception during minocycline therapy and for 1 week after it is discontinued.

Evaluation

In patients receiving minocycline, appropriate evaluation statements may include:
• Patient is free of infection.
• Patient maintains adequate hydration throughout minocycline therapy.
• Patient and family state an understanding of minocycline therapy.

minoxidil

(mi nox´ i dill)
Loniten, Minodyl

• *Classification:* antihypertensive (peripheral vasodilator)
• *Pregnancy Risk Category:* C

HOW SUPPLIED

Tablets: 2.5 mg, 10 mg, 25 mg‡

ACTION

Mechanism: Produces direct arteriolar vasodilation.
Absorption: Rapidly absorbed from the GI tract.
Distribution: Widely distributed into body tissues; it is not bound to plasma proteins.
Metabolism: Approximately 90% of a dose is metabolized.
Excretion: Drug and metabolites are excreted primarily in urine. Half-life: Averages 4.2 hours.
Onset, peak, duration: Antihypertensive effect occurs in 30 minutes, peaking at 2 to 8 hours. Antihypertensive action persists for 2 to 5 days.

INDICATIONS & DOSAGE

Treatment of severe hypertension—
Adults: 5 mg P.O. initially as a single dose. Effective dosage range is usually 10 to 40 mg daily. Maximum dosage is 100 mg daily.
Children under 12 years: 0.2 mg/kg as a single daily dose. Effective dosage range usually is 0.25 to 1 mg/kg daily. Maximum dosage is 50 mg.

CONTRAINDICATIONS & PRECAUTIONS

Contraindicated in patients with hypersensitivity to the drug, and in patients with pheochromocytoma because it may stimulate catecholamine secretion from the tumor.

Use cautiously in patients with recent myocardial infarction because vasodilation may increase myocardial oxygen demand via reflex tachycardia; and in patients with pulmonary hypertension, CHF, or significant renal impairment, because pulmonary artery pressure may increase.

ADVERSE REACTIONS

Common reactions are in italics; life-threatening reactions are in bold italics.
CV: *edema, tachycardia,* ***pericardial effusion and tamponade, CHF,*** ECG changes.

Skin: rash, ***Stevens-Johnson syndrome.***
Other: *hypertrichosis* (elongation, thickening, and enhanced pigmentation of fine body hair), breast tenderness.

INTERACTIONS

Guanethidine: severe orthostatic hypotension. Advise patient to stand up slowly.

EFFECTS ON DIAGNOSTIC TESTS

Antinuclear antibody (ANA) titer: increased titers.
ECG: altered direction and magnitude of T waves.
Hemoglobin and hematocrit: transiently decreased levels.
Serum alkaline phosphatase, serum creatinine, and BUN: elevated levels.

NURSING CONSIDERATIONS

Besides those related universally to drug therapy (see "How to use this book"), consider the following specific recommendations:

Assessment
• Obtain a baseline assessment of the patient's blood pressure before beginning therapy.
• Be alert for adverse reactions and drug interactions throughout therapy.
• Evaluate the patient's and family's knowledge about minoxidil therapy.

Nursing Diagnoses
• Altered tissue perfusion (renal, cerebral, cardiopulmonary, peripheral) related to the patient's underlying condition.
• Fluid volume excess related to minoxidil-induced adverse reactions.
• Knowledge deficit related to minoxidil therapy.

Planning and Implementation
Preparation and Administration
• Keep in mind that dosage adjustments should usually be made at no less than 3-day intervals to allow the full effect of the new dose.
• Expect patients with malignant hypertension to be hospitalized during initial therapy.
Monitoring
• Monitor effectiveness by frequently taking the patient's blood pressure, pulse, and ECG. Monitor blood pressure and pulse very carefully at beginning of therapy. Remember that elderly patients are especially sensitive to drug's hypotensive effects.
• Monitor intake and output and check for weight gain and edema throughout therapy. Most patients retain water and sodium.
Supportive Care
• Expect the doctor to order minoxidil only when other antihypertensives have failed.
• Be sure to administer a dose of this drug after hemodialysis because it removes minoxidil from the body.
• Expect the doctor to order a beta-blocking drug to control tachycardia and a diuretic to combat fluid retention at start of minoxidil therapy.
Patient Teaching
• Teach the patient how to take his own pulse. Tell patient to report increases greater than 20 beats/minute to the doctor.
• Tell the patient to weigh himself at least weekly and to report substantial weight gain (more than 5 lb per week).
• Explain the importance of following prescribed treatment regimen.
• Tell the patient that unwanted hair growth occurs in many patients taking this drug within 3 to 6 weeks of beginning treatment. Tell the patient that he can remove unwanted hair with a depilatory or by shaving. Assure the patient that this effect will disappear within 1 to 6 months after minoxidil is discontinued.
• Explain the importance of taking drug as prescribed, even when not feeling well.
• Tell the patient not to discontinue this drug suddenly even if unpleasant

adverse reactions occur, but to discuss the problem with the doctor.
• Instruct the patient to check with the doctor or pharmacist before taking OTC medications.
• Advise the patient to thoroughly read the manufacturer's package insert that describes this drug and its adverse reactions.
• Teach the patient and a family caregiver to take blood pressure measurements. Tell them to report a significant change in measurements.

Evaluation

In patients receiving minoxidil, appropriate evaluation statements may include:
• Blood pressure controlled within normal limits for this patient.
• Fluid retention controlled with prescribed diuretic.
• Patient and family state an understanding of minoxidil therapy.

---

misoprostol

(mye soe prost´ ole)
Cytotec

• *Classification:* antiulcer agent, gastric mucosal protectant (prostaglandin E_1 analogue)
• *Pregnancy Risk Category:* X

HOW SUPPLIED

Tablets: 200 mcg

ACTION

Mechanism: A synthetic prostaglandin E_1 analogue, that replaces gastric prostaglandins depleted by NSAID therapy. It also decreases basal and stimulated gastric acid secretion, and may increase gastric mucus and bicarbonate production.
Absorption: Rapid after oral administration.
Distribution: Highly bound (about 90%) to plasma proteins.
Metabolism: Rapidly de-esterified to misoprostol acid, the biologically active metabolite. The de-esterified metabolite undergoes further oxidation in several body tissues.
Excretion: About 15% of an oral dose appears in the feces; the balance is excreted in the urine. Half-life: Terminal half-life is 20 to 40 minutes.
Onset, peak, duration: Peak levels are reached in about 12 minutes.

INDICATIONS & DOSAGE

Prevention of NSAID-induced gastric ulcers in elderly or debilitated patients at high risk of complications from gastric ulcer, and patients with a history of NSAID-induced ulcers–
Adults: 200 mcg P.O. q.i.d. with food. If this dosage isn't tolerated, it may be decreased to 100 mcg P.O. q.i.d.

CONTRAINDICATIONS & PRECAUTIONS

Contraindicated during pregnancy because of abortifacient property. Drug should not be used in women of childbearing age unless they require NSAID therapy, are at high risk of developing gastric ulcers, and are aware of risks of using the drug during pregnancy.

Also contraindicated in patients allergic to prostaglandin derivatives.

ADVERSE REACTIONS

Common reactions are in italics; life-threatening reactions are in bold italics.
CNS: headache.
GI: diarrhea, abdominal pain, nausea, flatulence, dyspepsia, vomiting, constipation.
GU: hypermenorrhea, dysmenorrhea, spotting, cramps, menstrual disorders.

INTERACTIONS

Antacids: reduced plasma levels when administered concomitantly. Not considered significant.

EFFECTS ON DIAGNOSTIC TESTS

Basal pepsin secretion: modestly decreased.

NURSING CONSIDERATIONS

Besides those related universally to drug therapy (see "How to use this book"), consider the following specific recommendations:

Assessment

• Obtain a baseline assessment of the patient's pain or disconfort before beginning therapy.

• Be alert for adverse reactions and drug interactions throughout therapy.

• Evaluate the patient's and family's knowledge about misoprostol therapy.

Nursing Diagnoses

• Pain related to the patient's underlying condition.

• Diarrhea related to adverse GI reactions to misoprostol.

• Knowledge deficit related to misoprostol therapy.

Planning and Implementation

Preparation and Administration

• Expect misoprostol therapy to be started at the same time as NSAID therapy.

• ***P.O. use:*** Give the drug with or after meals and at bedtime for maximum effectiveness.

Monitoring

• Monitor effectiveness by regularly assessing for relief of GI pain.

• Monitor the patient's stool for type, amount, and color.

Supportive Care

• Administer antacids before or after misoprostol, as ordered, for the relief of pain. Keep in mind that magnesium-containing antacids are not recommended because they may aggravate misoprostol-induced diarrhea.

• Expect to take special precautions to prevent use of the drug during pregnancy in women with childbearing potential. These include making the patient fully aware of the dangers of misoprostol to a fetus, giving the patient verbal and written warnings regarding these dangers, ensuring that the patient is capable of complying with effective contraceptive means, having the patient undergo a pregnancy test with negative results within 2 weeks of initiating therapy and, finally, starting the drug therapy only on the second or third day of the next normal menstrual period.

Patient Teaching

• Tell the patient to continue taking the medication for the prescribed period.

• Tell the patient to notify the doctor if diarrhea deveops and continues for more than 1 week.

• Instruct the patient not to share the medication with anyone else. Explain that if this drug is taken by a pregnant patient it may cause miscarriage, often with potentially life-threatening bleeding.

• Urge the patient to avoid smoking cigarettes, which may increase gastric acid secretion and worsen disease.

• Instruct the patient to avoid sources of GI irritation, such as alcohol, certain foods, and drugs containing aspirin.

• Tell the patient that he should take the drug for only 4 weeks unless the doctor tells him to continue the therapy. The doctor may wish to continue treatment for a second 4 weeks if ulcers have not completely healed.

Evaluation

In patients receiving misoprostol, appropriate evaluation statements may include:

• Patient has decrease in or relief of GI pain.

• Patient maintains normal bowel habits and does not experience diarrhea.

• Patient and family state an understanding of misoprostol therapy.

mitomycin (mitomycin-C)
(mye to mye´ sin)
Mutamycin

• *Classification:* antineoplastic (antibiotic)
• *Pregnancy Risk Category:* D

HOW SUPPLIED
Injection: 5-mg, 20-mg vials

ACTION
Mechanism: An antineoplastic antibiotic that acts like an alkylating agent, cross-linking strands of DNA. This causes an imbalance of cell growth, leading to cell death. Also shows some antiviral and antimicrobial activity (especially against gram-positive bacteria), but the drug's toxicity precludes its use as an anti-infective.
Absorption: Because of its toxicity to tissues, must be administered I.V.
Distribution: Widely distributed into body tissues; animal studies show that the highest concentrations are found in the kidneys, muscle, eyes, lungs, intestines, and stomach. The drug does not cross the blood-brain barrier.
Metabolism: By microsomal enzymes of the liver. Similar enzymes are found in the kidneys, spleen, brain, and heart. There is an inverse relationship between the ability of tumor tissues to deactivate the drug and antitumor efficacy.
Excretion: Drug and its metabolites are excreted in urine, with less than 10% excreted as parent compound. A small portion is eliminated in bile and feces.

INDICATIONS & DOSAGE
Dosage and indications may vary. Check patient's protocol with doctor.

Breast, colon, head, neck, lung, pancreatic, and stomach cancer; malignant melanoma –
Adults: 2 mg/m^2 I.V. daily for 5 days. Stop drug for 2 days, then repeat dosage for 5 more days; or 20 mg/m^2 as a single dose. Repeat cycle 6 to 8 weeks. Stop drug if WBC less than 4,000/mm^3 or platelets less than 75,000/mm^3.

CONTRAINDICATIONS & PRECAUTIONS
Contraindicated in patients with a history of hypersensitivity to the drug; in patients with a WBC count below 3,000/mm^3, platelet count below 75,000/mm^3, or serum creatinine level above 1.7 mg/dl; and in those with coagulation disorders, prolonged prothrombin time, or serious infections because of the potential for adverse effects.

ADVERSE REACTIONS
Common reactions are in italics; life-threatening reactions are in bold italics.
Blood: ***thrombocytopenia,*** *leukopenia (may be delayed up to 8 weeks and may be cumulative with successive doses).*
CNS: paresthesias.
GI: *nausea, vomiting,* anorexia, stomatitis.
Local: desquamation, induration, pruritus, *pain at injection site.* Extravasation causes cellulitis, ulceration, sloughing.
Other: *reversible alopecia; purple coloration of nail beds;* fever; ***microangiopathic hemolytic anemia; syndrome characterized by thrombocytopenia, renal failure, and hypertension; interstitial pneumonitis.***

INTERACTIONS
None significant.

EFFECTS ON DIAGNOSTIC TESTS
Serum creatinine and BUN: increased levels.

NURSING CONSIDERATIONS

Besides those related universally to drug therapy (see "How to use this book"), consider the following specific recommendations:

Assessment

• Obtain a baseline assessment of the patient's overall physical status, CBC, and pulmonary and renal function tests before therapy.

• Be alert for adverse reactions and drug interactions throughout therapy.

• Evaluate the patient's and family's knowledge about mitomycin therapy.

Nursing Diagnoses

• Impaired tissue integrity related to extravasation of mitomycin.

• Altered protection related to myelosuppression.

• Knowledge deficit related to mitomycin therapy.

Planning and Implementation

Preparation and Administration

• ***I.V. use:*** Follow institutional policy when preparing and administering this drug to avoid mutagenic, teratogenic, and carcinogenic risks.

• Avoid extravasation because of the potential for severe ulceration and necrosis.

• Keep in mind that dosage modification is required when WBC count is below 4,000/mm³ and platelet count is less than 75,000/mm³; and in coagulation or bleeding disorders, serious infections, and impaired renal function.

• Be aware that reconstituted solution is stable for 1 week at room temperature and 2 weeks if refrigerated.

• Keep in mind that mitomycin has been administered topically by bladder instillation and has been given intra-arterially through the hepatic artery.

Monitoring

• Monitor effectiveness by noting results of follow-up diagnostic tests and patient's overall physical status.

• Monitor hematologic studies weekly during therapy and for at least 7 weeks after cessation of mitomycin therapy.

• Monitor for signs of bleeding (hematuria, ecchymosis, petechiae, epistaxis, melena).

• Monitor for signs of infection (temperature elevation, sore throat, malaise).

• Monitor pulmonary and renal function.

• Monitor I.V. site for signs of extravasation.

Supportive Care

• If the patient complains of discomfort at the I.V. site, extravasation may have occurred. Immediately stop infusion, restart at another site, and notify the doctor. Extravasation of this drug can cause severe tissue necrosis.

• Administer antiemetics, as ordered, before or during infusion of this drug to decrease severe nausea and vomiting.

• Avoid all I.M. injections in patients with thrombocytopenia.

• To help prevent infection, maintain the patient's optimal health and protect him from undue exposure to environmental contagion. If signs of infection occur, notify doctor promptly; and administer antibiotics, as ordered.

• Provide a safe environment to minimize risk of bleeding.

Patient Teaching

• Warn the patient to watch for signs of infection (sore throat, fever, fatigue) and bleeding (easy bruising, nosebleeds, bleeding gums). Tell patient to take temperature daily and to report signs of infection or bleeding.

• Instruct patient about need for protective measures, including conservation of energy, balanced diet, adequate rest, personal cleanliness, clean environment, and avoidance of exposure to persons with infections.

• Instruct patient about safety precautions to reduce risks of bleeding from falls, cuts, or other injuries.

• Instruct patient about the need for frequent oral hygiene.
• Teach patient to avoid the use of all OTC products containing aspirin.
• Inform the patient that hair loss is possible, but is usually reversible.

Evaluation

In patients receiving mitomycin, appropriate evaluation statements may include:
• Patient does not exhibit evidence of local tissue damage.
• Patient does not demonstrate signs and symptoms of infection or bleeding.
• Patient and family state an understanding of mitomycin therapy.

mitotane

(mye´ toe tane)
Lysodren

• *Classification:* antineoplastic, antiadrenal agent (chlorophenothane [DDT] analogue)
• *Pregnancy Risk Category:* C

HOW SUPPLIED

Tablets (scored): 500 mg

ACTION

Mechanism: Selectively destroys adrenocortical tissue and hinders extraadrenal metabolism of cortisol. Structurally related to chlorophenothane (DDT).
Absorption: After oral administration, 35% to 40% of a dose is absorbed from the GI tract.
Distribution: Widely distributed into body tissue; fatty tissue is the primary storage site. Slow release of mitotane from fatty tissue into the plasma occurs after the drug is discontinued. A metabolite has been detected in the CSF.
Metabolism: In the liver and other tissues.
Excretion: Drug and metabolites are excreted in urine and bile. Half-life: Plasma elimination half-life is reported to be 18 to 159 days.
Onset, peak, duration: Peak serum levels are seen after about 8 weeks of continuous therapy.

INDICATIONS & DOSAGE

Inoperable adrenocortical cancer–
Adults: initially, 1 to 6 g P.O. daily divided t.i.d. or q.i.d.; increased to 9 to 10 g P.O. daily, divided t.i.d. or q.i.d. Dosage is adjusted until maximum tolerated dosage is achieved (varies from 2 to 16 g daily but is usually 8 to 10 g daily).
Children: initially, 0.5 to 1 g P.O. daily in divided doses. Increase dosage based upon patient tolerance and response.

CONTRAINDICATIONS & PRECAUTIONS

Contraindicated in patients with a history of hypersensitivity to the drug. Use cautiously in patients with impaired liver function; the drug may accumulate in the body because of impaired metabolism.

ADVERSE REACTIONS

Common reactions are in italics; life-threatening reactions are in bold italics.
CNS: *depression, somnolence, vertigo;* brain damage and dysfunction in long-term, high-dose therapy.
GI: *severe nausea, vomiting,* diarrhea, anorexia.
Metabolic: adrenal insufficiency.
Skin: dermatitis.

INTERACTIONS

None significant.

EFFECTS ON DIAGNOSTIC TESTS

Urine 17-hydroxycorticosteroid, plasma cortisol, protein-bound iodine, and serum uric acid: decreased levels.

NURSING CONSIDERATIONS

Besides those related universally to drug therapy (see "How to use this book"), consider the following specific recommendations:

Assessment

• Obtain a baseline assessment of patient's underlying disease before therapy.
• Be alert for adverse reactions and drug interactions throughout therapy.
• Evaluate the patient's and familiy's knowledge about mitotane therapy.

Nursing Diagnoses

• High risk for fluid volume deficit related to drug-induced adverse reactions
• High risk for impaired skin integrity related to drug-induced adverse reactions.
• Knowledge deficit related to mitotane therapy.

Planning and Implementation

Preparation and Administration

• Give antiemetics before administering mitotane to reduce severe nausea.
• Dosage may be reduced if adverse GI reactions are severe.
• Obese patients may need higher dosage and may have longer-lasting adverse reactions since drug distribution is mostly in body fat.

Monitoring

• Monitor effectiveness by noting the results of follow-up diagnostic tests and overall physical status and by evaluating adrenal cortex function.
• Monitor for weakness, increased fatigue, lethargy, and GI effects.
• Monitor behavioral and neurologic performance daily.
• Monitor the patient's hydration status if he develops severe nausea, vomiting, diarrhea, and anorexia.
• Assess the patient's skin since drug may cause dermatitis.
• Monitor obese patients for potential longer-lasting adverse reactions since drug distribution is mostly in body fat.
• Assess the patient's mental status because the drug may cause depression.

Supportive Care

• Provide the patient with fluids if he develops severe nausea, vomiting, diarrhea, and anorexia.
• Institute safety precautions and assist the patient with ambulation if he develops vertigo.
• Administer an antiemetic, as ordered, before administration of drug to reduce nausea.

Patient Teaching

• Warn ambulatory patients of adverse CNS reactions; advise patients to avoid hazardous tasks requiring mental alertness or physical coordination.

Evaluation

In patients receiving mitotane, appropriate evaluation statements may include:

• Patient does not develop fluid volume deficit.
• Patient does not develop drug-induced dermatitis.
• Patient and family state an understanding of mitotane therapy.

mitoxantrone hydrochloride

(mye toe zan´ trone)

Novantrone

• *Classification:* antineoplastic (antibiotic)
• *Pregnancy Risk Category:* D

HOW SUPPLIED

Injection: 2 mg/ml in 10-ml, 12.5-ml, 15-ml vials

ACTION

Mechanism: An antineoplastic antibiotic that exerts a non-cell-cycle–specific cytotoxicity by reacting with DNA.
Distribution: Mitoxantrone is 78% plasma protein-bound.
Metabolism: By the liver.

Excretion: Via renal and hepatobiliary systems; 6% to 11% of dose is excreted in urine within 5 days: 65% is unchanged drug; 35% is two inactive metabolites. Within 5 days, 25% of dose is excreted in feces. Half-life is about 6 days.

INDICATIONS & DOSAGE

Combination initial therapy for acute nonlymphocytic leukemia (ANL)– **Adults:** 12 mg/m² I.V. daily on days 1 through 3, in combination with cytosine arabinoside 100 mg/m² daily on days 1 through 7. If a repeat course is necessary, mitoxantrone should be given on days 1 and 2 with cytosine arabinoside administered on days 1 through 5.

CONTRAINDICATIONS & PRECAUTIONS

Contraindicated in patients with hypersensitivity to the drug and in patients with preexisting myelosuppression resulting from prior drug therapy unless possible benefit warrants risk of further myelosuppression. Use cautiously in patients with hepatic or renal impairment, preexisting cardiac disease, or previous exposure to cardiotoxic drugs.

ADVERSE REACTIONS

Common reactions are in italics; life-threatening reactions are in bold italics.
Blood: ***myelosuppression.***
CNS: seizures, headache.
CV: CHF, arrhythmias, tachycardia.
GI: *bleeding, abdominal pain, diarrhea, nausea, mucositis, stomatitis, vomiting.*
Respiratory: dyspnea, cough.
Other: alopecia, jaundice, fever, hyperuricemia.

INTERACTIONS

Heparin: incompatible when mixed together.

EFFECTS ON DIAGNOSTIC TESTS

CBC: abnormal values, reflecting hematologic toxicity.
Liver function tests: abnormal values, reflecting hepatotoxicity.
Serum uric acid: increased levels.

NURSING CONSIDERATIONS

Besides those related universally to drug therapy (see "How to use this book"), consider the following specific recommendations:

Assessment

- Obtain a baseline assessment of the patient's underlying condition before therapy.
- Be alert for adverse reactions and drug interactions throughout therapy.
- Evaluate the patient's and family's knowledge about mitoxantrone therapy.

Nursing Diagnoses

- High risk for fluid volume deficit related to adverse drug reactions.
- Altered protection related to drug-induced myelosuppression.
- Knowledge deficit related to mitoxantrone therapy.

Planning and Implementation

Preparation and Administration

- ***I.V. use:*** Exercise caution when preparing and administering this drug to avoid mutagenic, teratogenic, and carcinogenic risks. Use a biological containment cabinet, wear gloves and mask, and avoid contaminating work surfaces. Do not inhale dust or vapors and avoid contact with skin or mucous membranes. Use luer-lock syringes and needles to prevent leakage of solution. Dispose of unused drug and all supplies in biohazardous waste containers, according to hospital policy.
- Available as an aqueous solution of 2 mg/ml in volumes of 10, 12.5, and 15 ml. The dose should be diluted in at least 50 ml of 0.9% sodium chloride injection or 5% dextrose in water (D_5W) injection. Drug should be administered by direct injection

into a free-flowing I.V. of 0.9% sodium chloride or D_5W injection over at least 3 minutes. Mixing with other drugs is not recommended.
• Undiluted solution is stable at room temperature. Once diluted, the solution is stable for 48 hours at room temperature.
• Take care to prevent infiltration. If it occurs, discontinue infusion and apply ice for 2 minutes at infusion site. Mixing with other drugs is not recommended.
• Administer only under the supervision of a doctor who is experienced with the use of chemotherapeutic agents.

Monitoring
• Obtain baseline CBC, liver enzymes, uric acid levels, and ECG before therapy.
• Monitor effectiveness by checking tumor size and rate of growth through appropriate studies.
• Monitor effectiveness by noting the results of follow-up diagnostic tests and overall physical status.
• Monitor for signs of bleeding (hematuria, ecchymosis, petechiae, epistaxis, melena).
• Monitor for signs of infection (temperature elevation, sore throat, malaise).
• Monitor serum uric acid level.
• Monitor CBC, hepatic function, and bone marrow depression.
• Monitor vital signs (especially blood pressure) frequently during I.V. infusion of this drug.
• Monitor left ventricular ejection fraction during administration.
• Monitor hydration status if patient develops nausea, vomiting, and diarrhea.

Supportive Care
• Provide the patient with fluids if he develops severe nausea, vomiting, and diarrhea.
• Use anticoagulants and aspirin products with extreme caution.
• Avoid contact with skin. If contact occurs, wash the area liberally with soap and water.
• To prevent hyperuricemia with resulting uric acid nephropathy, allopurinol may be administered with adequate hydration.
• Be prepared to administer epinephrine, corticosteroids, or antihistamines for anaphylactoid reactions, which usually respond to immediate treatment.
• Know that therapeutic effects are often accompanied by toxicity.
• Be prepared to treat infections with antibiotics. If severe nonhematologic toxicity occurs during the first treatment, the second treatment should be delayed until the patient recovers.

Patient Teaching
• Inform patient that urine may appear bluish green within 24 hours after administration and some bluish discoloration of the sclera may occur. These effects are not harmful.
• Warn patient to watch for signs of infection (sore throat, fever, fatigue), and for signs of bleeding (easy bruising, nosebleeds, bleeding gums). Advise him to take his temperature daily.
• Teach patient to avoid the use of all OTC products containing aspirin.

Evaluation

In patients receiving mitoxantrone, appropriate evaluation statements may include:
• Patient does not develop fluid volume deficit.
• Patient's immune system response improves with therapy.
• Patient and family state an understanding of mitoxantrone therapy.

molindone hydrochloride

(moe lin´ done)
Moban

• *Classification:* antipsychotic (dihydroindolone)

• *Pregnancy Risk Category:* C

HOW SUPPLIED

Tablets: 5 mg, 10 mg, 25 mg, 50 mg, 100 mg
Oral solution: 20 mg/ml

ACTION

Mechanism: Blocks postsynaptic dopamine receptors in the brain. A dihydroindolone.
Absorption: Rapidly absorbed after oral administration.
Distribution: Widely distributed; enters CSF and probably enters breast milk.
Metabolism: Rapidly and extensively metabolized by the liver.
Excretion: Most is excreted as metabolites in urine; some is excreted in feces via the biliary tract. Overall, 90% of a given dose is excreted within 24 hours. Half-life: 1.5 hours.
Onset, peak, duration: Peak blood levels are seen within 1 hour. Peak effects occur within 1½ hours. Drug effects persist for 24 to 36 hours.

INDICATIONS & DOSAGE

Psychotic disorders–
Adults: 50 to 75 mg P.O. daily, increasing to maximum of 225 mg daily. Doses up to 400 mg may be required.

CONTRAINDICATIONS & PRECAUTIONS

Contraindicated in patients with hypersensitivity to molindone and in patients with disorders accompanied by coma, CNS depression, brain damage, circulatory collapse, or cerebrovascular disease because of additive CNS depression and adverse effects on blood pressure. Use cautiously in patients with cardiac disease (arrhythmias, CHF, angina pectoris, valvular disease, or heart block); Reye's syndrome; encephalitits, head injury, or related conditions because drug may mask signs and symptoms; respiratory disease because molindone may cause respiratory depression; glaucoma, because the autonomic effects of the drug may elevate intraocular pressure; prostatic hypertrophy; urine retention; hepatic or renal dysfunction because decreased metabolism and excretion may cause the drug to accumulate in the plasma of these patients; Parkinson's disease; and pheochromocytoma, because drug may cause excessive buildup of transmitters, resulting in adverse cardiovascular effects.

Molindone lowers seizure threshold and may cause seizures in patients with seizure disorders.

Patients with hypocalcemia are more likely to develop extrapyramidal reactions. Administration of molindone may influence the CNS thermoregulatory center and predispose the patient to hyperthermia or hypothermia.

Sulfite preservatives in oral solution could induce acute asthmatic attack in asthma patients.

ADVERSE REACTIONS

Common reactions are in italics; life-threatening reactions are in bold italics.
Blood: transient leukopenia.
CNS: *extrapyramidal reactions (moderate incidence), tardive dyskinesia, sedation (moderate incidence),* pseudoparkinsonism, EEG changes, dizziness.
CV: *orthostatic hypotension,* tachycardia, ECG changes.
EENT: *blurred vision.*
GI: *dry mouth, constipation.*
GU: *urine retention,* dark urine, menstrual irregularities, gynecomastia, inhibited ejaculation.
Hepatic: cholestatic jaundice, abnormal liver function tests.
Metabolic: hyperprolactinemia.
Skin: *mild photosensitivity,* dermal allergic reactions.
Other: rarely, ***neuroleptic malignant***

syndrome (fever, tachycardia, tachypnea, profuse diaphoresis).

INTERACTIONS

Alcohol, other CNS depressants: increased CNS depression. Avoid concomitant use.

EFFECTS ON DIAGNOSTIC TESTS

AST (SGOT) and ALT (SGPT), free fatty acids, and BUN: elevated results.
CBC: altered WBC counts.
Metrizamide myelography: additive potential for causing seizures.
Serum glucose: increased or decreased levels.
Urine pregnancy tests using human chorionic gonadotropin: false-positive results.

NURSING CONSIDERATIONS

Besides those related universally to drug therapy (see "How to use this book"), consider the following specific recommendations:

Assessment

• Obtain a baseline assessment of the patient's mental status, including psychotic symptoms, before drug therapy.
• Be alert for adverse reactions and drug interactions throughout therapy.
• Evaluate the patient's and family's knowledge about molindone therapy.

Nursing Diagnoses

• Impaired thought processes related to the patient's underlying condition.
• Constipation related to adverse reactions to molindone.
• Knowledge deficit related to molindone therapy.

Planning and Implementation

Preparation and Administration

• Drug may be administered in a single daily dose.
• Dose of 20 mg is therapeutic equivalent of 100 mg of chlorpromazine.
• Drug is the only dihydroindolone derivative.

Monitoring

• Monitor effectiveness by regularly observing the patient's behavior and noting changes in psychotic symptoms.
• Monitor the patient for adverse reactions, especially extrapyramidal and anticholinergic effects (blurred vision, dry mouth, constipation, urine retention), and tardive dyskinesia, during prolonged therapy.
• Frequently check the patient's blood pressure for orthostatic hypotension.
• Monitor therapy by weekly bilirubin tests during the first month; periodic blood tests (CBC and liver function); and ophthalmic tests (long-term use).
• Monitor for neuroleptic malignant syndrome. This rare, potentially fatal reaction is not necessarily related to length of drug therapy or type of neuroleptic, but usually occurs in men (60% of affected patients).

Supportive Care

• Do not discontinue drug abruptly unless required by severe adverse reactions.
• Increase the patient's fluid and fiber intake–if not contraindicated–to prevent constipation. If necessary, request doctor's order for a laxative.
• Give the patient sugarless gum, sour hard candy, ice chips, or a mouthwash rinse to relieve dryness.
• Be prepared to give I.V. diphenhydramine, as ordered, to treat acute dystonic reactions.

Patient Teaching

• Tell the patient not to stop taking the drug suddenly.
• Encourage the patient to report difficulty urinating, sore throat, dizziness, or fainting.
• Advise the patient to increase fluid and fiber in the diet, if appropriate.
• Tell the patient to avoid driving and other hazardous activities that require alertness until the effect of the drug is established. Excessive sedation tends to subside after several weeks.

• Tell the patient that sugarless hard candy, chewing gum, or ice chips can alleviate dry mouth.

Evaluation

In patients receiving molindone, appropriate evaluation statements may include:

• Patient demonstrates a decrease in psychotic behavior.
• Patient does not develop constipation.
• Patient and family state an understanding of molindone therapy.

mometasone furoate

(moe met´ a sone)
Elocon

• *Classification:* anti-inflammatory, antipruritic (glucocorticoid)
• *Pregnancy Risk Category:* C

HOW SUPPLIED

Cream: 0.1%
Ointment: 0.1%
Lotion: 0.1%

ACTION

Mechanism: Produces local anti-inflammatory, vasoconstrictor, and antipruritic actions. Diffuses across cell membranes to form complexes with specific cytoplasmic receptors, influencing cellular metabolism. Corticosteroids stabilize leukocyte lysosomal membranes, inhibit local actions and accumulation of macrophages, decrease local edema, and reduce the formation of scar tissue.

Absorption: Depends on the potency of the preparation, the amount applied, and the nature of the skin at the application site. Absorption is lowest in areas with a thick stratum corneum (on the palms, soles, elbows, and knees) and higher in thinner areas (face, eyelids, and genitals). Absorption increases in areas of skin damage, inflammation, or occlusion. Some systemic absorption occurs, especially through the oral mucosa.

Distribution: Bound to plasma protein in varying degrees.

Metabolism: Primarily in the liver.

Excretion: By the kidneys. Some drug and metabolites are also excreted into the bile.

INDICATIONS & DOSAGE

Inflammatory and pruritic manifestations of corticosteroid-responsive dermatoses–

Adults: apply cream or ointment to affected areas once daily. Do not use occlusive dressings.

CONTRAINDICATIONS & PRECAUTIONS

Contraindicated in patients hypersensitive to the drug, other corticosteroids, or any product in the formulation. Also contraindicated in patients with viral, fungal, or tubercular skin lesions. Use with extreme caution in patients with impaired circulation because it may increase the risk of skin ulceration.

Because of the risk of absorption of the drug into the systemic circulation, evaluate the patient periodically for evidence of hypothalamic-pituitary-adrenal (HPA) axis suppression.

ADVERSE REACTIONS

Common reactions are in italics; life-threatening reactions are in bold italics.

Skin: burning, pruritus, atrophy, irritation, acneiform eruptions, hypopigmentation, allergic contact dermatitis.

Other: HPA axis suppression, Cushing's syndrome.

INTERACTIONS

None reported.

EFFECTS ON DIAGNOSTIC TESTS

None reported.

NURSING CONSIDERATIONS

Besides those related universally to drug therapy (see "How to use this book"), consider the following specific recommendations:

Assessment

- Obtain a baseline assessment of patient's skin integrity before mometasone therapy.
- Be alert for adverse reactions and drug interactions throughout therapy.
- Evaluate the patient's and family's knowledge about mometasone therapy.

Nursing Diagnoses

- Impaired skin integrity related to the patient's underlying condition.
- Impaired tissue integrity related to drug-induced adverse reaction.
- Knowledge deficit related to mometasone therapy.

Planning and Implementation

Preparation and Administration

- Read order and drug labels carefully.
- Wear gloves when administering drug.
- Before applying, gently wash the patient's skin. Apply a thin layer of medication and rub in gently.
- When treating hairy sites, part hair and apply directly to lesion.
- To prevent recurrence, treatment should continue for a few days after clearing of lesions.

Monitoring

- Monitor effectiveness by regularly assessing skin for extent and severity of inflammation.
- Monitor for hypersensitivity reaction to mometasone.
- Frequently assess the patient's skin for burning, atrophy, and hyperpigmentation.

Supportive Care

- Withhold the drug and notify the doctor if hypersensitivity reaction or infection occurs.
- Have the patient's fingernails cut short to minimize skin trauma from scratching.
- Apply cool, moist compresses to involved areas to relieve itching and burning.

Patient Teaching

- Instruct the patient to cleanse involved area before applying mometasone in a thin layer to cover the entire surface.
- Teach the patient and family how to recognize signs of a hypersensitivity reaction or infection. Advise them to discontinue the drug and notify the doctor immediately if such reactions occur.
- Instruct the patient to complete the entire treatment regimen as prescribed, even if the lesions appear to have healed.
- Tell the patient and family not to share the prescription with others.

Evaluation

In patients receiving mometasone, appropriate evaluation statements may include:

- Patient's skin maintains integrity.
- Patient remains free of tissue integrity impairment related to adverse drug reactions.
- Patient and family state an understanding of mometasone therapy.

PHARMACOLOGIC CLASS

monoamine oxidase inhibitors

isocarboxazid
pargyline hydrochloride
phenelzine sulfate
selegiline hydrochloride
tranylcypromine sulfate

OVERVIEW

Antidepressant effects of monoamine oxidase (MAO) inhibitors were first noted in 1952. All four have antihypertensive activity and antidepressant effects; only pargyline is used (rarely) to treat severe hypertension.

MAO inhibitors can cause serious adverse reactions and interact adversely with many foods and drugs. They are useful drugs for treating affective illness, especially "atypical" major depression disorders (particularly depression with hypersomnia, hyperphagia, or severe anxiety) or depression unresponsive to tricyclic antidepressants. They are also useful for panic disorder.

Some forms of depression are thought to result from low CNS levels of neurotransmitters, including norepinephrine and serotonin. MAO inhibitors, as their name implies, depress the effects of MAO, an enzyme that is present principally in the CNS and inactivates the neurotransmitters. Many adverse effects from MAO inhibitors are attributed to gradual buildup and increased activity of neurotransmitters after enzyme inhibition.

CLINICAL INDICATIONS AND ACTIONS

Depression

MAO inhibitors are used to treat severe, atypical depression refractory to tricyclic antidepressants. Data suggest that depressed patients with coexisting obsessive-compulsive behavior, histrionic personality, or phobia respond more favorably to MAO inhibitors than to tricyclic antidepressants.

Hypertension

Pargyline is used to treat moderate to severe hypertension. Although rarely used, it may be effective in some patients refractory to other agents.

Parkinson's disease

Selegiline is used as an adjunct to carbidopa-levodopa in the treatment of Parkinson's disease.

OVERVIEW OF ADVERSE REACTIONS

MAO inhibitors' most serious adverse reactions involve blood pressure. Hypotensive reactions appear to follow gradual accumulation of false neurotransmitters (phenylethylamines) in adrenergic nerve terminals; normal breakdown of these agents is also inhibited by MAO. Severe hypertension also may result from interaction with drugs with sympathomimetic activity, such as pseudoephedrine, phenylephrine, and phenylpropanolamine, other false neurotransmitters, and other drugs with vasoconstrictive effects.

Ingestion of food or beverages containing tyramine may provoke hypertensive crisis—a rapid and severe increase in blood pressure. Prodromal symptoms of hypertensive crisis include severe occipital headache, tachycardia, sweating, and visual disturbances.

All MAO inhibitors cause CNS adverse reactions, including restlessness, hyperexcitability, insomnia, and headache. Over time, tolerance develops to most adverse reactions.

REPRESENTATIVE COMBINATIONS

Pargyline hydrochloride with methylclothiazide: Eutron.

---

moricizine hydrochloride

(mor´ siz een)

Ethmozine

- *Classification:* antiarrhythmic (sodium channel blocker)
- *Pregnancy Risk Category:* B

HOW SUPPLIED

Tablets: 200 mg, 250 mg, 300 mg

ACTION

Mechanism: A class I antiarrhythmic that reduces the fast inward current carried by sodium ions. All class I antiarrhythmics have membrane-stabilizing (local anesthetic) effects.

Absorption: Administration within 30 minutes of food ingestion delays absorption and lowers peak plasma levels but does not affect extent of absorption.

Distribution: 95% plasma protein-bound.
Metabolism: Undergoes significant first-pass metabolism and at least 26 metabolites have been identified with no single one representing more than 1% of the administered dose. Moricizine has been shown to induce its own metabolism.
Excretion: 56% is excreted in feces; 39%, in urine; some is also recycled through enterohepatic circulation. Half-life: Plasma half life of the parent compound is about 2 hours.
Onset, peak, duration: Peak plasma concentrations are usually reached within 0.5 to 2 hours.

INDICATIONS & DOSAGE

Treatment of life-threatening ventricular arrhythmias–
Adults: individualized dosage is based on clinical response and patient tolerance. Therapy should begin in the hospital. Most patients respond to 600 to 900 mg P.O. daily, given in divided doses q 8 hours. Increase daily dosage q 3 days by 150 mg until the desired clinical effect is seen.
Patients with hepatic or renal function impairment–
Adults: start therapy at 600 mg P.O. daily or less. Monitor closely and adjust dosage carefully.

CONTRAINDICATIONS & PRECAUTIONS

Contraindicated in patients with known hypersensitivity to the drug and in those with preexisting second- or third-degree AV block, with right bundle branch block when associated with left hemiblock (unless a pacemaker is present), and in cardiogenic shock. Use with extreme caution in patients with sick sinus syndrome as it may cause sinus bradycardia, sinus pause, or sinus arrest. Use with caution in patients with hepatic or renal impairment, CHF, and preexisting conduction abnormalities and when concomitant medications that affect cardiac conduction are initiated; monitor such patients carefully.

ADVERSE REACTIONS

Common reactions are in italics; life-threatening reactions are in bold italics.
CNS: *dizziness, headache, fatigue,* anxiety, hypoesthesia, asthenia, nervousness, paresthesia, sleep disorders.
CV: *proarrhythmic events, ECG abnormalities (including conduction defects, sinus pause, junctional rhythm, or AV block), CHF, palpitations,* ***sustained ventricular tachycardia,*** *chest pain, sinus bradycardia, sinus arrest.*
EENT: blurred vision.
GI: *nausea, vomiting, abdominal pain, dyspepsia, diarrhea, dry mouth.*
GU: urine retention.
Skin: rash.
Other: dyspnea, drug fever, sweating, musculoskeletal pain.

INTERACTIONS

Cimetidine: increased plasma levels of and decreased clearance of moricizine. Begin moricizine therapy at low dosage (not more than 600 mg daily) and monitor plasma levels and therapeutic effect closely.
Propranolol, digoxin: additive prolongation of the PR interval. Monitor closely.
Theophylline: increased theophylline clearance and reduced plasma levels. Monitor plasma levels and therapeutic response; adjust theophylline dosage as needed.

EFFECTS ON DIAGNOSTIC TESTS

None reported.

NURSING CONSIDERATIONS

Besides those related universally to drug therapy (see "How to use this book"), consider the following specific recommendations:

Assessment

• Obtain a baseline assessment of the patient's heart rate and rhythm before moricizine therapy.

• Be alert for adverse reactions and drug interactions throughout therapy.

• Evaluate the patient's and family's knowledge about moricizine therapy.

Nursing Diagnoses

• Decreased cardiac output related to ineffectivenss of moricizine to correct arrhythmia.

• Altered protection related to moricizine-induced proarrhythmias.

• Knowledge deficit related to moricizine.

Planning and Implementation

Preparation and Administration

• Be aware that the drug should be initially administered in the hospital with continuous ECG monitoring.

• Be aware that drug should only be used for patients with life-threatening ventricular arrhythmias and individual dosage is based on clinical response and patient tolerance.

• Correct electrolyte imbalances as ordered before administering drug, because hypokalemia, hyperkalemia, and hypomagnesemia may alter the drug's effects.

• Expect to administer reduced dosage to patients with hepatic or renal dysfunction.

• When substituting for another antiarrhythmic, withdraw previous antiarrhythmic therapy for one to two half-lives of the drug, as prescribed, before starting moricizine at recommended dosage. Patients who develop life-threatening arrhythmias after withdrawal of drug therapy should be hospitalized during withdrawal and adjustment to moricizine. Start moricizine therapy 6 to 12 hours after the last dose of disopyramide, 8 to 12 hours after the last dose of mexiletine, 3 to 6 hours after the last dose of procainamide, 8 to 12 hours after the last dose of propafenone, 6 to 12 hours after the last dose of quinidine, and 8 to 12 hours after the last dose of tocainide.

• ***P.O. use:*** Expect to start therapy with 600 mg daily or less and to give in divided doses q 8 hours.

Monitoring

• Monitor effectiveness by continuous ECG recordings in a coronary care setting initially, followed by regular ECG assessments.

• Monitor patient for proarrhythmic events and other ECG abnormalities throughout therapy.

• Monitor for elctrolyte disturbances before and regularly throughout therapy.

Supportive Care

• Notify the doctor immediately and obtain further administration guidelines if the patient develops a drug fever, proarrhythmias, or other ECG abnormalities.

• Keep emergency equipment nearby and be prepared to use other methods to treat arrhythmia if moricizine is ineffective or causes other life-threatening arrhythmias.

• Institute safety precautions if CNS reactions occur.

• Correct electrolyte imbalances as they arise throughout drug therapy.

• Administer a mild analgesic if a headache or musculoskeletal pain occurs.

• Assist the patient with daily activities if fatigue develops.

• Obtain an order for an antiemetic or antidiarrheal agent if needed. Ensure that patient maintains an adequate intake if GI upset occurs.

• Use measures to minimize CHF, such as fluid and sodium restriction, unless adverse GI effects are present.

Patient Teaching

• Inform breast-feeding mothers that because the drug is excreted in breast milk a decision will need to be made to discontinue breast-feeding or discontinue the drug.

• Warn the patient to avoid hazardous activities that require mental

alertness until CNS effects are known.
• Stress the importance of close follow-up care.

Evaluation

In patients receiving moricizine, appropriate evaluation statements may include:
• Patient's ventricular arrhythmia is abolished.
• Patient's ECG does not exhibit proarrhythmic activity.
• Patient and family state an understanding of moricizine therapy.

morphine hydrochloride

(mor´ feen)

Morphitec†, M.O.S.†, M.O.S.-S.R.†

morphine sulfate

Astramorph, Astramorph P.F., Duramorph PF, Epimorph†, Morphine H.P.†, MS Contin, MSIR, RMS Uniserts, Roxanol, Roxanol SR, Statex†
• Controlled Substance Schedule II

• *Classification:* narcotic analgesic (opioid)
• *Pregnancy Risk Category:* B (D for prolonged use or use of high doses at term)

HOW SUPPLIED

hydrochloride

Tablets: 10 mg†, 20 mg†, 40 mg†, 60 mg†
Oral solution†*:* 1 mg/ml, 5 mg/ml, 10 mg/ml, 20 mg/ml, 50 mg/ml
Syrup: 1 mg/ml†, 5 mg/ml†
Suppositories: 20 mg†, 30 mg†

sulfate

Tablets: 15 mg, 30 mg
Tablets (controlled-release): 30 mg, 60 mg
Soluble tablets: 10 mg, 15 mg, 30 mg
Oral solution: 10 mg/5 ml, 20 mg/5 ml, 20 mg/ml (concentrate)
Syrup: 1 mg/ml, 5 mg/ml
Injection (with preservative): 1 mg/ml, 2 mg/ml, 3 mg/ml, 4 mg/ml, 5 mg/ml, 8 mg/ml, 10 mg/ml, 15 mg/ml
Injection (without preservative): 500 mcg/ml, 1 mg/ml
Suppositories: 5 mg, 10 mg, 20 mg, 30 mg

ACTION

Mechanism: Binds with opiate receptors at many sites in the CNS (brain, brain stem, and spinal cord), altering both perception of and emotional response to pain through an unknown mechanism.
Absorption: Well absorbed from S.C. and I.M. injection sites; variably from the GI tract.
Distribution: Widely distributed throughout the body. Drug crosses the placenta.
Metabolism: Primarily in the liver.
Excretion: In the urine and bile. Half-life: Reportedly varies between 2 and 4 hours.
Onset, peak, duration: Onset of analgesia occurs within 15 minutes to 1 hour. Peak analgesia occurs 30 minutes to 1 hour after dosing. Duration of action is 3 to 7 hours.

INDICATIONS & DOSAGE

Severe pain–
Adults: 4 to 15 mg S.C. or I.M.; or 30 to 60 mg P.O. or rectally q 4 hours, p.r.n. or around the clock. May be injected slow I.V. (over 4 to 5 minutes) diluted in 4 to 5 ml water for injection. May also administer controlled-release tablets q 8 to 12 hours. As an epidural injection, 5 mg via an epidural catheter q 24 hours.
Children: 0.1 to 0.2 mg/kg dose S.C. or I.M. q 4 hours. Maximum dosage is 15 mg.

In some situations, morphine may be administered by continuous I.V. infusion or by intraspinal and intrathecal injection.

CONTRAINDICATIONS & PRECAUTIONS

Contraindicated in patients with hypersensitivity to the drug or other phenanthrene opioids (codeine, hydrocodone, hydromorphone, oxycodone, oxymorphone).

Use with extreme caution in patients with supraventricular arrhythmias and in those with head injury or increased intracranial pressure, because it obscures neurologic parameters; and during pregnancy and labor, because drug readily crosses placenta (premature infants are especially sensitive to respiratory and CNS depressant effects).

Administer cautiously to patients with renal or hepatic dysfunction, because drug accumulation or prolonged duration of action may occur; asthma or chronic obstructive pulmonary disease, because drug depresses respiration and suppresses cough reflex; or seizure disorders, because drug may precipitate seizures; to patients undergoing biliary tract surgery, because drug may cause biliary spasm; to elderly or debilitated patients, who are more sensitive to both therapeutic and adverse drug effects; and to patients prone to physical or psychological addiction, because of the high risk of addiction to this drug.

ADVERSE REACTIONS

Common reactions are in italics; life-threatening reactions are in bold italics.

CNS: *sedation, somnolence, clouded sensorium, euphoria,* ***seizures*** with large doses, dizziness, *nightmares* (with long-acting oral forms).

CV: *hypotension,* bradycardia.

GI: *nausea, vomiting, constipation,* ileus.

GU: *urine retention.*

Other: ***respiratory depression,*** *physical dependence, pruritus and skin flushing (with epidural administration).*

INTERACTIONS

Alcohol, CNS depressants: additional effects. Use together cautiously.

EFFECTS ON DIAGNOSTIC TESTS

Plasma amylase: increased levels.

NURSING CONSIDERATIONS

Besides those related universally to drug therapy (see "How to use this book"), consider the following specific recommendations:

Assessment

- Obtain a baseline assessment of the patient's pain before therapy.
- Be alert for adverse reactions and drug interactions throughout therapy.
- Evaluate the patient's and family's knowledge about morphine therapy.

Nursing Diagnoses

- Pain related to patient's underlying condition.
- Ineffective breathing pattern related to morphine-induced respiratory depression.
- Knowledge deficit related to morphine therapy.

Planning and Implementation

Preparation and Administration

- ***P.O. use:*** Oral solutions (sulfate) of various concentrations are available, as well as a concentrated oral solution (20 mg/ml). Be sure to note the strength you are administering. Do not crush or break controlled-release tablets.
- If S.L. administration is ordered, measure out oral solution with tuberculin syringe; administer dose a few drops at a time to allow maximal S.L. absorption and to minimize swallowing.
- ***Rectal use:*** Be aware that rectal suppository is available in 5-, 10-, 20- and 30-mg dosages. Refrigeration is not necessary. Note that, in some patients, rectal and oral absorption may not be equivalent.
- ***Epidural and intrathecal use:*** Preservative-free preparations are now available for epidural and intrathecal

administration. Epidural is becoming more common.

• ***I.V. use:*** Administer drug slowly with patient lying down to minimize hypotension. Rapid administration can result in life-threatening adverse reactions. Generic preparations may contain sulfites.

• Around-the-clock administration is beneficial in severe, chronic pain.

• Be aware that respiratory depression, hypotension, profound sedation, or coma may occur if used with general anesthetics, tranquilizers, sedatives, hypnotics, alcohol, tricyclic antidepressants, or MAO inhibitors. Morphine should be used with such drugs at reduced dosage and with extreme caution.

Monitoring

• Monitor effectiveness after each dose by evaluating degree of pain relief.

• Monitor respiratory status throughout morphine therapy, noting any evidence of respiratory depression, such as decreased rate or depth of respiration. Continue monitoring for respiratory depression every 15 minutes for 1 hour after I.V. infusion; after epidural administration, monitor closely for up to 24 hours.

• Regularly monitor blood pressure for hypotension and heart rate for bradycardia.

• Monitor bowel and bladder function daily for constipation or ileus, or urine retention.

Supportive Care

• Notify the doctor and discuss increase of dosage or frequency if pain is not relieved.

• Hold dose and notify the doctor if patient's respirations are below 12 breaths/minute or if significant hypotension occurs.

• Keep narcotic antagonist (naloxone) and resuscitative equipment available.

• Because adverse CNS reactions are possible, institute safety precautions, such as supervising ambulation and keeping bed rails up.

• If not contraindicated, obtain an order for a stool softener or other laxative and increase the patient's fluid and fiber intake to prevent or treat constipation, which can become severe during maintenance use of morphine.

• Be aware that morphine may worsen or mask gallbladder pain.

• Morphine is the drug of choice in relieving pain of myocardial infarction; during such use, be alert for a transient decrease in blood pressure.

• Recognize that habituation and physical dependence may result from long-term use.

Patient Teaching

• Warn the ambulatory patient who is taking oral maintenance doses to avoid driving and other hazardous activities that require alertness.

• Teach the patient to remain in bed for 1 hour after I.M. injection and to obtain assistance before getting out of bed. Tell the patient to get up slowly following I.V. administration to minimize dizziness and fainting.

• When used postoperatively, encourage turning, coughing, and deep breathing and use of the incentive spirometer to avoid atelectasis.

• Suggest high-fiber diet and liberal fluid intake to prevent constipation in the patient on a maintenance regimen.

• Encourage the patient to ask for medication or to activate a patient-controlled analgesia (PCA) device before pain becomes severe.

• Tell the patient or family to notify the nurse or doctor if respiratory rate decreases.

Evaluation

In the patient receiving morphine, appropriate evaluation statements include:

• Patient reports relief of pain after administration of morphine.

• Respiratory status remains within normal limits.
• Patient and family state an understanding of morphine therapy.

moxalactam disodium (latamoxef disodium)

(mox´ a lak tam)
Moxalactam‡, Moxam

• *Classification:* antibiotic (third-generation cephalosporin)
• *Pregnancy Risk Category:* C

HOW SUPPLIED

Parenteral: 1 g, 2 g

ACTION

Mechanism: Inhibits cell wall synthesis during bacterial replication, promoting osmotic instability. Usually bactericidal.
Absorption: Not absorbed from the GI tract and must be given parenterally. Because it is well absorbed from I.M. injection sites, serum levels 1 hour after injection are similar to those 1 hour after I.V. injection.
Distribution: Widely distributed into most body tissues, and fluids, including the gallbladder, liver, kidneys, bone, sputum, bile, and pleural and synovial fluids; unlike most other cephalosporins, it has good CSF penetration. Moxalactam crosses the placenta; it is 45% to 60% protein-bound.
Metabolism: Not metabolized.
Excretion: Primarily excreted in urine by renal tubular secretion and glomerular filtration; small amounts are excreted in breast milk. Half-life: 2 to 3½ hours in normal adults; 5 to 10 hours in severe renal disease.
Onset, peak, duration: Peak serum levels occur ½ to 1 hour after an I.M. dose.

INDICATIONS & DOSAGE

Treatment of serious infections of lower respiratory and urinary tract, CNS infections, intraabdominal infections, gynecologic infections, bacteremia, septicemia, and skin infections.
Susceptible microorganisms include Streptococcus pneumoniae *and* pyogenes; Staphylococcus aureus *(penicillinase- and nonpenicillinase-producing)* and epidermidis; Escherichia coli; Klebsiella; Hemophilus influenzae; Enterobacter; Proteus; *some* Pseudomonas; *and* Peptostreptococcus—
Adults: Usual daily dose is 2 to 6 g I.M. or I.V. administered in divided doses q 8 hours for 5 to 10 days, or up to 14 days. Up to 12 g daily may be needed in life-threatening infections or in infections due to less susceptible organisms.
Children: 50 mg/kg I.M. or I.V. q 6 to 8 hours.
Neonates: 50 mg/kg I.M. or I.V. q 8 to 12 hours.

Total daily dosage is same for I.M. or I.V. administration and depends on susceptibility of organism and severity of infection. In patients with impaired renal function, doses or frequency of administration must be modified according to degree of impairment, severity of infection, and susceptibility of organism. Should be injected deep I.M. into the gluteus or lateral aspect of thigh.

CONTRAINDICATIONS & PRECAUTIONS

Contraindicated in patients with hypersensitivity to any cephalosporin. Use with caution in patients with penicillin allergy, who are usually more susceptible to such reactions; and in patients with coagulopathy and elderly, debilitated, or malnourished patients, who are usually at greater risk of bleeding complications.

ADVERSE REACTIONS

Common reactions are in italics; life-threatening reactions are in bold italics.

Blood: transient neutropenia, eosinophilia, ***hemolytic anemia,*** *hypoprothrombinemia, bleeding.*

CNS: headache, malaise, paresthesias, dizziness.

GI: ***pseudomembranous colitis,*** nausea, anorexia, vomiting, *diarrhea,* glossitis, dyspepsia, abdominal cramps, tenesmus, pruritus ani, oral candidiasis (thrush).

GU: genital moniliasis.

Skin: *maculopapular and erythematous rashes, urticaria.*

Local: *pain at injection site, induration, sterile abscesses, tissue sloughing; phlebitis and thrombophlebitis with I.V. injection.*

Other: ***hypersensitivity,*** dyspnea, elevated temperature.

INTERACTIONS

Ethyl alcohol: may cause a disulfiram-like reaction. Warn patients not to drink alcohol for several days after discontinuing moxalactam.

Oral anticoagulants, aspirin: increased risk of bleeding.

EFFECTS ON DIAGNOSTIC TESTS

Coombs' test: positive results.

Liver function tests: elevated results.

Prothrombin time: prolonged.

NURSING CONSIDERATIONS

Besides those related universally to drug therapy (see "How to use this book"), consider the following specific recommendations:

Assessment

- Obtain a baseline assessment of infection before therapy.
- Be alert for adverse reactions and drug interactions throughout therapy.
- Evaluate the patient's and family's knowledge about moxalactam therapy.

Nursing Diagnoses

- High risk for injury related to ineffectiveness of moxalactam to eradicate the infection.
- High risk for fluid volume deficit related to adverse GI reactions to moxalactam.
- Knowledge deficit related to moxalactam therapy.

Planning and Implementation

Preparation and Administration

- Obtain specimen for culture and sensitivity tests before first dose. Therapy may begin pending test results.
- Before giving first dose, ask patient about reactions to previous cephalosporin or penicillin therapy.
- ***I.M. use:*** Reconstitute according to manufacturer's instructions. Inject deep I.M. into the gluteus or lateral aspect of thigh.
- ***I.V. use:*** For direct intermittent I.V. administration, add 10 ml of sterile water for injection, dextrose 5% injection, or 0.9% NaCl injection/g of moxalactam.

Monitoring

- Monitor effectiveness by regularly assessing for improvement of infection.
- Monitor for adverse reactions or drug interactions to moxalactam.
- During prolonged or high-dose therapy, monitor for superinfection, especially in high-risk patients.
- Monitor hydration status if adverse GI reactions occur.
- Monitor prothrombin time because this drug's chemical structure includes the methylthiotetrazole side chain that has been associated with bleeding disorders.

Supportive Care

- Obtain an order for an antiemetic or antidiarrheal agent as needed.
- If bleeding occurs be prepared to administer vitamin K as prescribed. Doctor may order 10 mg vitamin K per week to be given prophylactically.

Patient Teaching
• Instruct the patient and family about moxalactam, including the dose, frequency, action, and adverse reactions.

Evaluation
In patients receiving moxalactam, appropriate evaluation statements may include:
• Patient is free of infection.
• Patient maintains adequate hydration throughout moxalactam therapy.
• Patient and family state an understanding of moxalactam therapy.

mumps virus vaccine, live
Mumpsvax

• *Classification:* viral vaccine
• *Pregnancy Risk Category:* X

HOW SUPPLIED
Injection: single-dose vial containing not less than 5,000 $TCID_{50}$ (tissue culture infective doses) of attenuated mumps virus derived from Jeryl Lynn mumps strain (grown in chick embryo culture), and vial of diluent.

ACTION
Mechanism: Promotes active immunity to mumps.
Pharmacokinetics: Unknown.
Onset, peak, duration: Antibodies are usually evident 2 to 3 weeks after injection. The duration of vaccine-induced immunity is unknown.

INDICATIONS & DOSAGE
Immunization–
Adults and children over 1 year: 1 vial (5,000 units) S.C.

CONTRAINDICATIONS & PRECAUTIONS
Contraindicated in patients with hypersensitivity (other than dermatitis) to neomycin, a component of the vaccine; infections, blood dyscrasia, or cancers of or affecting the bone marrow or lymphatic systems; primary immunodeficiency; in pregnant patients; and in those receiving corticotropin, corticosteroids, irradiation, or other immunosuppressant therapy. Use cautiously in patients with hypersensitivity to neomycin, chickens, eggs, ducks, or feathers.

ADVERSE REACTIONS
Common reactions are in italics; life-threatening reactions are in bold italics.
Systemic: *slight fever,* rash, malaise, mild allergic reactions, febrile seizures (rare).

INTERACTIONS
Immune serum globulin, whole blood, plasma: antibodies in serum may interfere with immune response. Don't use vaccine within 3 months of transfusion.

EFFECTS ON DIAGNOSTIC TESTS
Tuberculin skin test: temporarily decreased response.

NURSING CONSIDERATIONS
Besides those related universally to drug therapy (see "How to use this book"), consider the following specific recommendations:

Assessment
• Obtain a baseline assessment of the patient's allergies (especially to antibiotics), immunization history, and immunization reaction before therapy.
• Be alert for adverse reactions and drug interactions throughout therapy.
• Evaluate the patient's and family's knowledge about mumps virus vaccine therapy.

Nursing Diagnoses
• Altered protection related to lack of immunity to mumps virus.
• Hyperthermia related to vaccine-induced fever.
• Knowledge deficit related to live mumps virus vaccine.

Planning and Implementation

Preparation and Administration

• Store in the refrigerator and protect from light. Solution may be used if red, pink, or yellow, but it must be clear.

• Use only diluent supplied. Discard 8 hours after reconstituting.

• ***S.C. use*** Give by S.C. route only. Do not give by I.V. route.

• If a tuberculin skin test is necessary, administer it either before or simultaneously with vaccine.

Monitoring

• Monitor effectiveness by evaluating the patient's antibody titers to mumps virus.

• Observe the patient for signs of anaphylaxis immediately after administration of the vaccine.

• Check the patient's temperature.

Supportive Care

• Keep epinephrine 1:1,000 available in case of anaphylactic reaction.

• Treat fever with antipyretics.

• Defer in acute or febrile illness and for 3 months after transfusions or treatment with immune serum globulin.

• Live mumps virus vaccine should not be given less than 1 month before or after immunization with other live virus vaccines, with the exception of Attenuvax, Meruvax, or monovalent or trivalent live oral polio virus vaccine, which may be administered simultaneously.

• The virus vaccine will not protect after exposure to natural mumps.

• The vaccine is not recommended for infants under age 12 months because of retained maternal mumps antibodies, which may interfere with the immune response.

Patient Teaching

• Warn the patient to avoid conception for 3 months after immunization. Provide contraceptive information if necessary.

• Advise the patient or parents that a slight fever may occur after immunization.

Evaluation

In patients receiving live mumps virus vaccine, appropriate evaluation statements may include:

• Patient exhibits active immunity to the mumps virus.

• Patient's temperature remains within the normal range.

• Patient and family state an understanding of live mumps virus vaccine therapy.

mupirocin

(myoo peer´ oh sin)

Bactroban

• *Classification:* topical antibacterial (antibiotic)

• *Pregnancy Risk Category:* C

HOW SUPPLIED

Ointment: 2%

ACTION

Mechanism: Inhibits bacterial protein and RNA synthesis.

Absorption: None seen in normal patients after 24-hour application under occlusive dressings.

Distribution: Highly protein-bound (about 95%). A substantial decrease in activity can be expected in the presence of serum (as in exudative wounds.)

Metabolism: Locally metabolized in the skin to monic acid.

Excretion: Eliminated locally by desquamation of the skin.

INDICATIONS & DOSAGE

Treatment of common bacterial skin infections caused by susceptible bacteria –

Adults and children: apply to affected areas b.i.d. to t.i.d.

CONTRAINDICATIONS & PRECAUTIONS

Contraindicated in any patient who is sensitive to the drug or ingredients in the formulation. This drug should not be used in the eyes.

ADVERSE REACTIONS

Common reactions are in italics; life-threatening reactions are in bold italics.

Local: burning, itching, stinging, rash.

INTERACTIONS

None reported.

EFFECTS ON DIAGNOSTIC TESTS

None reported.

NURSING CONSIDERATIONS

Besides those related universally to drug therapy (see "How to use this book"), consider the following specific recommendations:

Assessment

• Obtain a baseline assessment of skin infection before therapy.
• Be alert for adverse reactions and drug interactions throughout therapy.
• Evaluate the patient's and family's knowledge about mupirocin therapy.

Nursing Diagnoses

• Impaired skin integrity related to patient's underlying condition.
• High risk for impaired skin integrity related to mupirocin-induced rash.
• Knowledge deficit related to mupirocin therapy.

Planning and Implementation

Preparation and Administration

• ***Topical use:*** Cleanse affected area, then apply.

Monitoring

• Monitor effectiveness by regularly examining the skin of the affected area.
• Monitor the patient's condition. If no improvement is seen or condition worsens, notify doctor immediately.
• Monitor for adverse reactions and interactions by frequently assessing the patient's skin for rash, itching, and burning.

Supportive Care

• Be aware that mupirocin has proven especially useful in the treatment of impetigo in early clinical trials.
• Local reactions appear to result from the polyethylene glycol vehicle.
• Keep in mind that prolonged use may cause overgrowth of nonsusceptible bacteria and fungi.
• Avoid use on burns.
• Do not use on eyes.

Patient Teaching

• Teach patient how to apply medication.
• Advise the patient not to use the drug around his eyes.

Evaluation

In patients receiving mupirocin, appropriate evaluation statements may include:

• Patient states that the impaired skin integrity is resolved.
• Patient did not develop a drug-induced rash.
• Patient and family state an understanding of mupirocin therapy.

---

muromonab-CD3

(myoo roe moe´ nab-CD3)
Orthoclone OKT3

• *Classification:* immunosuppressant (monoclonal antibody)
• *Pregnancy Risk Category:* C

HOW SUPPLIED

Injection: 5 mg/5 ml in 5-ml ampules

ACTION

Mechanism: A murine (mouse) monoclonal antibody that reacts with an antigen recognition site (CD3) within the T-lymphocyte membrane. Depletes the blood of CD3-positive T cells, which leads to restoration of allograft function and reversal of rejection.

Pharmacokinetics: Unknown.

INDICATIONS & DOSAGE

Treatment of acute allograft rejection in renal transplant patients–

Adults: 5 mg I.V. bolus once daily for 10 to 14 days.

Children: 2.5 mg I.V. bolus once daily for 10 to 14 days.

CONTRAINDICATIONS & PRECAUTIONS

Contraindicated in patients allergic to muromonab-CD3 and in patients with fluid overload. Use with extreme caution in patients allergic to products of murine origin.

This drug contains polysorbate 80 and should not be used for the *in vitro* treatment of bone marrow. Because this drug is a heterologous protein, it induces antibodies, which could limit its efficacy and may cause serious reactions upon readministration. A second course should be administered with caution.

Monitor patient closely for 48 hours after the first dose. Administration of methylprednisolone sodium succinate 1 mg/kg I.V. before muromonab-CD3 and I.V. hydrocortisone sodium succinate 100 mg 30 minutes after is strongly recommended to minimize the first-dose reaction. Acetaminophen and antihistamines given concomitantly may reduce early reactions.

The most serious first-dose reaction, potentially fatal severe pulmonary edema, has occurred infrequently (in fewer than 5% of the first 107 patients and in none of the subsequent 311 patients treated with first-dose restrictions). In every patient who developed pulmonary edema, fluid overload was present before treatment. Therefore, carefully evaluate patients for fluid overload by chest X-ray or weight gain of greater than 3%. The patient's weight should be less than 3% above minimum weight the week before treatment begins.

ADVERSE REACTIONS

Common reactions are in italics; life-threatening reactions are in bold italics.

CV: *chest pain.*

GI: *nausea, vomiting,* diarrhea.

Other: ***severe pulmonary edema,*** *fever, chills, tremor, dyspnea, infection.*

INTERACTIONS

None reported.

EFFECTS ON DIAGNOSTIC TESTS

None reported.

NURSING CONSIDERATIONS

Besides those related universally to drug therapy (see "How to use this book"), consider the following specific recommendations:

Assessment

- Obtain a baseline assessment of the patient's immune status before therapy.
- Be alert for adverse reactions and drug interactions throughout therapy.
- Evaluate the patient's and family's knowledge about muromonab-CD3 therapy.

Nursing Diagnoses

- Altered protection related to organ rejection.
- Altered tissue perfusion (cardiopulmonary) related to muromonab-CD3 therapy.
- Knowledge deficit related to muromonab-CD3 therapy.

Planning and Implementation

Preparation and Administration

- Begin treatment with muromonab-CD3 only in a facility in which the patient can be monitored closely and that is equipped and staffed for cardiopulmonary resuscitation.
- Assess for signs of fluid overload before starting treatment with the drug. Do not start treatment in pa-

tients with fluid overload as evidenced by chest X-ray or a weight gain greater than 3% within the week before treatment.
• Obtain a baseline chest X-ray 24 hours before starting treatment with muromonab-CD3.
• ***I.V. use:*** Administer muromonab-CD3 in an I.V. bolus once daily.

Monitoring

• Monitor effectiveness by observing the patient for signs of organ rejection.
• Assess the patient for signs of fluid overload, auscultate lungs, and check for peripheral edema.
• Monitor the patient's daily weight and fluid intake and output.
• Monitor vital signs and be alert for dyspnea, tachycardia, and hypotension, which may indicate the development of pulmonary edema.
• Monitor for signs of infection (fever, chills, sore throat, malaise).
• Observe the patient for tremor, which may indicate adverse CNS reactions.

Supportive Care

• Keep resuscitation equipment nearby in case of severe pulmonary edema.
• Administer an antipyretic before the drug to decrease the incidence of expected fever and chills.
• Corticosteroids may also be administered before the first dose of muromonab-CD3 to help decrease the incidence of adverse reactions.
• Offer emotional support and reassurance.
• Obtain an order for medication to relieve muromonab-CD3–induced chest pain.
• Obtain an order for antiemetics and antidiarrheals as needed.

Patient Teaching

• Inform the patient about the expected adverse reactions.
• Reassure the patient that most adverse reactions develop within 30 minutes to 6 hours after the first dose and then gradually subside.
• Advise the patient to immediately report chest pain, dyspnea, or respiratory difficulty.

Evaluation

In patients receiving muromonab-CD3, appropriate evaluation statements may include:
• Patient exhibits no signs of organ rejection.
• Patient demonstrates no signs of altered cardiopulmonary tissue perfusion.
• Patient and family state an understanding of muromonab-CD3 therapy.

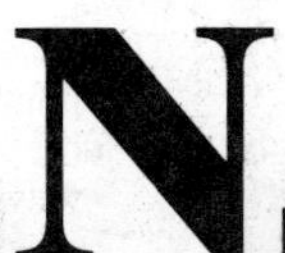

nadolol

(nay doe´ lole)
Corgard

• *Classification:* beta-adrenergic blocking agent
• *Pregnancy Risk Category:* C

HOW SUPPLIED

Tablets: 20 mg, 40 mg, 80 mg, 120 mg, 160 mg

ACTION

Mechanism: A beta-adrenergic blocker that reduces cardiac oxygen demand by blocking catecholamine-induced increases in heart rate, blood pressure, and force of myocardial contraction. Depresses renin secretion.
Absorption: From 30% to 40% of a dose is absorbed from the GI tract. Absorption is not affected by food.
Distribution: Widely distributed throughout the body; drug is about 30% protein-bound.
Metabolism: None.
Excretion: Most of a given dose is excreted unchanged in urine, the remainder in feces. Half-life: Plasma half-life is about 20 hours.
Onset, peak, duration: Peak plasma concentrations occur in 2 to 4 hours. Antihypertensive and antianginal effects persist for about 24 hours.

INDICATIONS & DOSAGE

Management of angina pectoris–
Adults: 40 mg P.O. once daily, initially. Dosage may be increased in 40- to 80-mg increments until optimum response occurs. Usual maintenance dosage range is 40 to 240 mg once daily.
Treatment of hypertension–
Adults: 40 mg P.O. once daily, initially. Dosage may be increased in 40- to 80-mg increments until optimum response occurs. Usual maintenance dosage range is 40 to 320 mg once daily. Doses of 640 mg may be necessary in rare cases.

CONTRAINDICATIONS & PRECAUTIONS

Contraindicated in patients with hypersensitivity to the drug and in patients with sinus bradycardia, overt cardiac failure, second- or third-degree atrioventricular block, or bronchial asthma, because the drug may worsen these conditions.

Use cautiously in patients with impaired hepatic or renal function (decrease dose if creatinine clearance falls below 50 ml/minute); coronary insufficiency, because beta-adrenergic blockade may precipitate CHF; diabetes mellitus and hyperthyroidism, because drug may mask tachycardia (it does not mask sweating and dizziness caused by hypoglycemia); and bronchospastic diseases. High doses may inhibit bronchodilating effects of endogenous catecholamines.

ADVERSE REACTIONS

Common reactions are in italics; life-threatening reactions are in bold italics.
CNS: fatigue, lethargy.
CV: *bradycardia, hypotension,* ***CHF,*** peripheral vascular disease.
GI: nausea, vomiting, diarrhea.
Metabolic: hypoglycemia without tachycardia.
Skin: rash.

Other: ***increased airway resistance,*** fever.

INTERACTIONS

Antihypertensive agents: enhanced antihypertensive effect.
Digitalis glycosides: excessive bradycardia and increased depressant effect on myocardium. Use together cautiously.
Epinephrine: severe vasoconstriction and reflex bradycardia. Monitor blood pressure and observe patient carefully.
Indomethacin: decreased antihypertensive effect. Monitor blood pressure and adjust dosage.
Insulin, oral hypoglycemic drugs: can alter dosage requirements in previously stabilized diabetics. Observe patient carefully.

EFFECTS ON DIAGNOSTIC TESTS

None reported.

NURSING CONSIDERATIONS

Besides those related universally to drug therapy (see "How to use this book"), consider the following specific recommendations:

Assessment

- Obtain a baseline assessment of the patient's anginal state before nadolol therapy.
- Be alert for adverse drug reactions or drug interactions throughout nadolol therapy.
- Evaluate the patient's and family's knowledge about nadolol therapy.

Nursing Diagnoses

- Pain related to ineffectiveness of nadolol therapy.
- Fluid volume excess related to nadolol-induced CHF.
- Knowledge deficit related to nadolol.

Planning and Implementation

Preparation and Administration

- Check the patient's apical pulse for bradycardia before each dose.
- Don't discontinue drug abruptly; can exacerbate angina and MI. Expect to gradually reduce dosage over 1 to 2 weeks.

Monitoring

- Monitor effectiveness by regularly evaluating the severity and frequency of the patient's anginal pain.
- Monitor for signs of CHF (shortness of breath, abnormal heart and breath sounds, weight gain, or changes in patient's skin color).
- Be aware that this drug masks common signs of shock, hyperthyroidism, and hypoglycemia. Monitor vital signs, thyroid function studies, and blood glucose levels regularly.

Supportive Care

- If pulse is slower than 60 beats/minute, withhold drug and call the doctor.
- Consult the doctor if the patient does not experience pain relief.
- Maintain safety precautions if bradycardia and hypotension occur; assist the patient with daily activities to minimize energy expenditure.
- Alert the doctor if dyspnea or abnormal breath sounds occur.
- Restrict the patient's fluid and sodium intake to minimize CHF.

Patient Teaching

- Stress importance of taking the drug exactly as prescribed even when the patient is feeling well.
- Teach patient how to check pulse rate, and to do so before each dose. If pulse rate is below 60 beats/minute, tell the patient to notify the doctor.
- Tell outpatients not to discontinue this drug suddenly; abrupt discontinuation can exacerbate angina and MI.
- Tell the patient to schedule activities to allow adequate rest if fatigue becomes troublesome.
- Encourage the patient to restrict fluid and sodium intake to minimize CHF.

Evaluation

In patients receiving nadolol, appropriate evaluation statements may include:

- Patient states anginal pain is relieved with nadolol therapy.
- Patient does not experience fluid retention with nadolol use.
- Patient and family state an understanding of nadolol therapy.

nafarelin acetate

(naf´ a re lin)

Synarel

- *Classification:* gonadotropin-releasing hormone analog (synthetic decapeptide)
- *Pregnancy Risk Category:* X

HOW SUPPLIED

Nasal solution: 200 mcg/spray in metered-dose spray bottle (2 mg/ml)

ACTION

Mechanism: A gonadotropin-releasing hormone (GnRH) analog that acts on the pituitary to decrease the release of follicle-stimulating hormone (FSH) and luteinizing hormone (LH). The result is decreased ovarian stimulation, lowered circulating estrogens, and improvement of the symptoms associated with endometriosis.
Absorption: After intranasal administration, rapidly absorbed through the nasal mucosa into systemic circulation.
Distribution: 80% is bound to plasma proteins.
Metabolism: Degraded by peptidase.
Excretion: Unknown. Half-life: Average serum half-life is about 3 hours.
Onset, peak, duration: Maximum serum concentrations are achieved in 10 to 40 minutes.

INDICATIONS & DOSAGE

Management of endometriosis–
Women 18 years and older: 1 spray in one nostril b.i.d. Maximum duration of therapy is 6 months.

CONTRAINDICATIONS & PRECAUTIONS

Contraindicated in patients with hypersensitivity to GnRH and GnRH-agonist analogs; with undiagnosed abnormal vaginal bleeding; and in patients who are or may become pregnant or who are breast-feeding.

Because of the risk of pregnancy, patients should use nonhormonal methods of contraception. Pregnancy must be excluded before starting treatment. If patient becomes pregnant during therapy, discontinue drug and inform patient of potential risk to fetus.

ADVERSE REACTIONS

Common reactions are in italics; life-threatening reactions are in bold italics.
CNS: *headaches, emotional lability, insomnia,* depression.
CV: edema.
EENT: *nasal irritation.*
GU: *vaginal dryness.*
Skin: *acne,* seborrhea, hirsutism.
Other: *hot flashes, decreased libido, myalgia,* reduced breast size, weight gain or loss, increased libido, decreased bone density.

INTERACTIONS

None reported.

EFFECTS ON DIAGNOSTIC TESTS

Pituitary gonadotropin and gonadal functions tests: misleading results during treatment and for 4 to 8 weeks after treatment.

NURSING CONSIDERATIONS

Besides those related universally to drug therapy (see "How to use this

book"), consider the following specific recommendations:

Assessment

- Obtain a baseline assessment of the patient's endometriosis condition before therapy.
- Be alert for adverse reactions and drug interactions throughout therapy.
- Evaluate the patient's and family's knowledge about nafarelin acetate therapy.

Nursing Diagnoses

- Sexual dysfunction related to the patient's underlying condition.
- Impaired tissue integrity related to nafarelin-induced adverse reactions.
- Knowledge deficit related to nafarelin therapy.

Planning and Implementation

Preparation and Administration

- If a topical nasal decongestant is used concurrently, administer it at least 30 minutes after nafarelin treatment to reduce the possibility of interference with nafarelin absorption.

Monitoring

- Monitor effectiveness by regularly assessing patient for improvement.
- Monitor nasal tissue for evidence of dryness and irritation.

Supportive Care

- Notify doctor if patient develops nasal dryness or irritation.
- Institute safety precautions to prevent patient from falling because bone density may decrease with drug use, predisposing patient to fractures.

Patient Teaching

- Advise the patient that she should contact her doctor if she develops a cold or rhinitis during therapy. If she requires a topical nasal decongestant, tell her the manufacturer suggests that it be used at least 30 minutes after nafarelin treatment.
- Advise the patient to use a nonhormonal form of contraception (such as barrier contraception). Although the drug will usually inhibit ovulation and stop menstruation, tell the patient it is not a reliable contraceptive, particularly if the patient misses a few doses.
- Tell the patient to stop taking the drug immediately and contact her doctor if she suspects that she is pregnant.
- Teach the patient that menstruation will stop with regular use of the drug. She should contact her doctor if menstruation persists or breakthrough bleeding occurs.

Evaluation

In patients receiving nafarelin, appropriate evaluation statements may include:

- Sexual function impaired by dyspareunia is restored.
- Impaired tissue integrity did not occur.
- Patient and family state an understanding of nafarelin therapy.

nafcillin sodium

(naf sill´ in)

Nafcil, Nallpen, Unipen

- *Classification:* antibiotic (penicillinase-resistant penicillin)
- *Pregnancy Risk Category:* B

HOW SUPPLIED

Tablets: 500 mg
Capsules: 250 mg
Oral solution: 250 mg/5 ml (after reconstitution)
Injection: 500 mg, 1 g, 2 g
I.V. infusion piggyback: 1 g, 1.5 g, 2 g, 4 g
Pharmacy bulk package: 10 g

ACTION

Mechanism: Bactericidal against microorganisms by inhibiting cell wall synthesis during active multiplication. Nafcillin resists the effects of penicillinases—enzymes that inactivate penicillin.

Absorption: More resistant to gastric acid than some other penicillinase-

resistant penicillins, but it is absorbed erratically and poorly from the GI tract. Rapidly absorbed after I.M. administration; however, I.V. administration produces higher blood levels.
Distribution: Widely distributed; CSF penetration is poor but enhanced by meningeal inflammation. Nafcillin crosses the placenta and is 70% to 90% protein-bound.
Metabolism: Primarily in the liver; drug undergoes enterohepatic circulation. No dosage adjustment is necessary for renal failure.
Excretion: Nafcillin and metabolites are excreted primarily in breast milk. Half-life: 30 minutes to 1½ hours in adults.
Onset, peak, duration: Peak serum levels occur at 30 minutes to 2 hours after an oral dose and 30 minutes to 1 hour after an I.M. dose.

INDICATIONS & DOSAGE

Systemic infections caused by penicillinase-producing staphylococci –
Adults: 2 to 4 g P.O. daily, divided into doses given q 6 hours; 2 to 12 g I.M. or I.V. daily, divided into doses given q 4 to 6 hours.
Children: 50 to 100 mg/kg P.O. daily, divided into doses given q 4 to 6 hours; or 100 to 200 mg/kg I.M. or I.V. daily, divided into doses given q 4 to 6 hours.

CONTRAINDICATIONS & PRECAUTIONS

Contraindicated in patients with hypersensitivity to any penicillin or cephalosporins.

ADVERSE REACTIONS

Common reactions are in italics; life-threatening reactions are in bold italics.
Blood: transient leukopenia, neutropenia, granulocytopenia, ***thrombocytopenia*** with high doses.
GI: *nausea,* vomiting, diarrhea.
Local: *vein irritation, thrombophlebitis.*
Other: *hypersensitivity (chills, fever, rash, pruritus, urticaria,* ***anaphylaxis****).*

INTERACTIONS

None significant.

EFFECT ON DIAGNOSTIC TESTS

CBC: transient reductions in RBCs, WBCs, and platelet counts.
Urinalysis: abnormal results may indicate drug-induced interstitial nephritis.
Urine and serum proteins: false-positive or elevated in tests using sulfosalicylic acid or trichloroacetic acid.

NURSING CONSIDERATIONS

Besides those related universally to drug therapy (see "How to use this book"), consider the following specific recommendations:

Assessment
- Obtain a baseline assessment of infection before nafcillin therapy.
- Be alert for adverse reactions and drug interactions throughout therapy.
- Evaluate the patient's and family's knowledge about nafcillin therapy.

Nursing Diagnoses
- High risk for injury related to ineffectiveness of nafcillin to eradicate the infection.
- High risk for fluid volume deficit related to nafcillin-induced adverse GI reactions.
- Knowledge deficit related to nafcillin therapy.

Planning and Implementation

Preparation and Administration
- Obtain specimen for culture and sensitivity tests before first dose. Therapy may begin pending test results.
- Before first dose, ask the patient about previous allergic reactions to this drug or other penicillins. However, a negative history of penicillin allergy does not guarantee future safety.

• Give nafcillin at least 1 hour before bacteriostatic antibiotics.
• ***P.O. use:*** Oral drug may cause GI disturbances. Food may interfere with absorption, so give 1 to 2 hours before meals or 2 to 3 hours after.
• ***I.V. use:*** Infuse I.V. drug intermittently to prevent vein irritation. Mix with dextrose 5% in water or a saline solution.
Monitoring
• Monitor effectiveness by regularly assessing for improvement of infection process.
• Monitor compliance with oral nafcillin therapy.
• Allergic reactions are the major adverse reactions to penicillin, especially with large doses, parenteral administration, or prolonged therapy. Keep in mind that the previously nonallergic patient may become sensitized to penicillin during therapy.
• Monitor hydration status if adverse GI reactions occur.
• Monitor for bacterial and fungal superinfections during high dose or prolonged therapy, especially in elderly, debilitated, or immunosuppressed patients.
Supportive Care
• Discontinue the drug immediately if the patient develops signs of anaphylactic shock (rapidly developing dyspnea and hypotension). Notify the doctor and prepare to administer immediate treatment, such as epinephrine, corticosteroids, antihistamines, and other resuscitative measures as indicated.
• Change I.V. site every 48 hours.
• Obtain an order for an antiemetic or antidiarrheal agent as needed.
• If the patient develops a rash, notify the doctor and expect to discontinue the drug.
Patient Teaching
• Advise the patient who becomes allergic to nafcillin to wear medical alert identification stating this information.
• Tell the patient to take medication exactly as prescribed and to complete the entire prescription even after he feels better.
• Tell the patient to call the doctor if rash, fever, or chills develop. A rash is the most common allergic reaction.
• Tell the patient to take oral nafcillin 1 hour before or 2 hours after meals to ensure an optimal serum concentration.
Evaluation
In patients receiving nafcillin, appropriate evaluation statements may include:
• Patient is free of infection.
• Patient maintains adequate hydration throughout therapy.
• Patient and family state an understanding of therapy.

naftifine
(naf′ te feen)
Naftin

• *Classification:* pediculicide; antifungal (synthetic allylamine derivative)
• *Pregnancy Risk Category:* B

HOW SUPPLIED
Cream: 1%

ACTION
Mechanism: Inhibits sterol biosynthesis in susceptible fungi by blocking the actions of the enzyme squalene 2,3 epoxidase. A broad-spectrum fungicidal agent.
Absorption: After single topical application of ^{3}H-labeled naftifine gel 1% to the skin of healthy subjects, up to 4.2% of the applied dose was absorbed.
Excretion: Naftifine and/or its metabolites are excreted in urine and feces. Half-life: Approximately 2 to 3 days.

INDICATIONS & DOSAGE

Treatment of tinea corporis and tinea cruris–
Adults: Apply to affected area b.i.d.

CONTRAINDICATIONS & PRECAUTIONS

Contraindicated in patients hypersensitive to the drug. This drug is for external use only and should not be applied to the eye or ingested.

ADVERSE REACTIONS

Common reactions are in italics; life-threatening reactions are in bold italics.
Local: burning, dryness, itching, stinging, local irritation.

INTERACTIONS

None significant.

EFFECTS ON DIAGNOSTIC TESTS

None reported.

NURSING CONSIDERATIONS

Besides those related universally to drug therapy (see "How to use this book"), consider the following specific recommendations:

Assessment

- Obtain a baseline assessment of skin in affected area before therapy.
- Be alert for adverse reactions and drug interactions throughout therapy.
- Evaluate the patient's and family's knowledge about naftifine therapy.

Nursing Diagnoses

- Impaired skin integrity related to patient's underlying condition.
- High risk for impaired skin integrity related to naftifine-induced dryness and local irritation.
- Knowledge deficit related to naftifine therapy.

Planning and Implementation

Preparation and Administration

- Clean affected area and apply medication.

Monitoring

- Monitor effectiveness by examining the skin in the affected area regularly.
- Monitor for adverse reactions and interactions by frequently assessing the patient's skin for irritation or sensitivity.

Supportive Care

- Remember therapy should be reevaluated if no improvement after 4 weeks.
- Be aware that cultures should be done to confirm diagnosis before therapy.
- Be prepared to discontinue drug and notify doctor if adverse reactions occur.

Patient Teaching

- Teach patient how to apply medication.
- Instruct patient to keep cream away from mucous membranes (eyes, nose, and mouth).
- Tell patient to wash hands after application.

Evaluation

In patients receiving naftifine, appropriate evaluation statements may include:

- Infection has resolved.
- Dryness and local irritation did not occur.
- Patient and family state an understanding of naftifine therapy.

nalbuphine hydrochloride

(nal´ byoo feen)
Nubain

- *Classification:* analgesic, adjunct to anesthesia (opioid partial agonist; narcotic agonist-antagonist)
- *Pregnancy Risk Category:* B (D for prolonged use or use of high doses at term)

HOW SUPPLIED

Injection: 10 mg/ml, 20 mg/ml

ACTION

Mechanism: An opiate agonist-antagonist that binds with opiate receptors at many sites in the CNS (brain, brain stem, and spinal cord), altering both perception of and emotional response to pain through an unknown mechanism.
Absorption: Well absorbed from I.M. and S.C. injection sites. Not given orally because of "first-pass" metabolism in the GI tract and liver.
Distribution: Not appreciably bound to plasma proteins.
Metabolism: In the liver; duration of action is 3 to 6 hours.
Excretion: In urine and to some degree in bile. Half-life: About 5 hours.
Onset, peak, duration: Onset of action is within 15 minutes, with peak effect seen at 30 minutes to 1 hour.

INDICATIONS & DOSAGE

Moderate to severe pain–
Adults: 10 to 20 mg S.C., I.M., or I.V. q 3 to 6 hours, p.r.n. or around the clock. Maximum daily dosage is 160 mg.

CONTRAINDICATIONS & PRECAUTIONS

Contraindicated in patients with hypersensitivity to the drug or other phenanthrene opioids (codeine, hydrocodone, hydromorphone, morphine, oxycodone, oxymorphone).

Administer with extreme caution to patients with supraventricular arrhythmias; avoid, or administer with extreme caution to patients with head injury or increased intracranial pressure, because drug obscures neurologic parameters; and during pregnancy and labor, because drug readily crosses placenta (premature infants are especially sensitive to respiratory and CNS depressant effects of opioids).

Nalbuphine contains sulfites as preservatives and should not be used in patients who are allergic to sulfites.

Administer cautiously to patients with MI who are nauseated or vomiting because it may induce nausea and vomiting; renal or hepatic dysfunction, because drug accumulation or prolonged duration of action may occur; asthma or chronic obstructive pulmonary disease, because drug depresses respiration and suppresses cough reflex; or seizure disorders, because drug may precipitate seizures; to patients undergoing biliary tract surgery, because drug may cause biliary spasm; to elderly or debilitated patients, who are more sensitive to both therapeutic and adverse drug effects; and to patients prone to physical or psychic addiction, because of the high risk of addiction. However, this drug has a lower potential for abuse than narcotic agonists.

ADVERSE REACTIONS

Common reactions are in italics; life-threatening reactions are in bold italics.
CNS: *headache, sedation,* dizziness, nervousness, depression, restlessness, crying, euphoria, hostility, unusual dreams, confusion, hallucinations, delusions.
GI: cramps, dyspepsia, bitter taste, *nausea, vomiting,* constipation.
GU: urinary urgency.
Skin: itching; burning; urticaria; *sweaty, clammy feeling.*
Other: ***respiratory depression.***

INTERACTIONS

Alcohol, CNS depressants: additive effects. Use together cautiously.
Narcotic analgesics: avoid concomitant use. Possible decreased analgesic effect.

EFFECTS ON DIAGNOSTIC TESTS

None reported.

NURSING CONSIDERATIONS

Besides those related universally to drug therapy (see "How to use this

book"), consider the following specific recommendations:

Assessment

• Obtain a baseline assessment of the patient's pain before therapy.
• Be alert for adverse reactions and drug interactions throughout therapy.
• Evaluate the patient's and family's knowledge about nalbuphine therapy.

Nursing Diagnoses

• Pain related to patient's underlying condition.
• Ineffective breathing pattern related to nalbuphine-induced respiratory depression.
• Knowledge deficit related to nalbuphine therapy.

Planning and Implementation

Preparation and Administration

• When administering to patients who have received chronic opiate therapy, give 25% of the usual dose initially. Observe for signs of withdrawal.
• ***I.V. use:*** Administer drug with patient lying down to minimize hypotension. Reduce dosage for the elderly.
• Drug may contain sulfites.

Monitoring

• Monitor effectiveness by evaluating pain relief after each dose.
• Monitor respiratory status throughout nalbuphine therapy, noting any evidence of respiratory depression, such as decreased rate or depth of respiration. Continue monitoring for respiratory depression every 15 minutes for 1 hour following I.V. infusion. Keep in mind that respiratory depression at 10 mg is equal to the respiratory depression produced by 10 mg of morphine.
• Monitor respirations of neonates exposed to the drug during labor.
• Monitor circulatory status.
• Monitor bowel function for constipation, which is often severe during maintenance therapy.

Supportive Care

• Notify the doctor and discuss increase of dosage or frequency if pain is not relieved.
• Hold dose and notify the doctor if the patient's respirations are below 12 breaths/minute. Keep in mind that respiratory depression can be reversed with naloxone. Keep resuscitative equipment available, particularly when administering I.V.
• Recognize that psychological and physical dependence may occur. Also be aware that nalbuphine acts as a narcotic antagonist; may precipitate abstinence syndrome.
• If not contraindicated, obtain an order for a stool softener or other laxative and increase the patient's fluid and fiber intake to prevent or treat constipation.

Patient Teaching

• Warn the ambulatory patient to avoid driving and other hazardous activities that require alertness until CNS effects of the drug are known.
• Tell the patient to get up slowly following I.V. administration to lessen dizziness and fainting.
• Suggest high-fiber diet and liberal fluid intake to prevent constipation in the patient on a maintenance regimen.
• Tell the patient or family to notify the nurse or doctor if respiratory rate decreases.

Evaluation

In patients receiving nalbuphine, appropriate evaluation statements may include:

• Patient reports relief of pain after administration of nalbuphine.
• Patient does not develop significant respiratory depression.
• Patient and family state an understanding of nalbuphine therapy.

nalidixic acid

(nal i dix´ ik)
NegGram

• *Classification:* antibiotic, urinary tract antiseptic (quinolone)
• *Pregnancy Risk Category:* B

HOW SUPPLIED

Tablets: 250 mg, 500 mg, 1 g
Oral suspension: 250 mg/5 ml

ACTION

Mechanism: Inhibits microbial DNA synthesis by inhibiting DNA-gyrase.
Absorption: Well absorbed from the GI tract.
Distribution: Concentrates in renal tissue and seminal fluid; does not penetrate prostate tissues; only minimal amounts appear in CSF and the placenta. The drug is highly protein-bound (82% to 97%).
Metabolism: Metabolized to hydroxynalidixic acid and inactive conjugates in the liver.
Excretion: Metabolites and 2% to 3% of unchanged drug are excreted via the kidneys. Nalidixic acid (and probably metabolites) are found in breast milk. Half-life: Plasma half-life is 1 to 2½ hours in patients with normal renal function. In anuric patients, up to 21 hours.
Onset, peak, duration: Peak serum levels occur about 1 to 2 hours after an oral dose.

INDICATIONS & DOSAGE

Acute and chronic urinary tract infections caused by susceptible gram-negative organisms (Proteus, Klebsiella, Enterobacter, *and* Escherichia coli) –
Adults: 1 g P.O. q.i.d. for 7 to 14 days; 2 g daily for long-term use.
Children over 3 months: 55 mg/kg P.O. daily divided q.i.d. for 7 to 14 days; 33 mg/kg daily for long-term use.

CONTRAINDICATIONS & PRECAUTIONS

Contraindicated in patients with: a history of seizure disorders because the drug may induce seizures; glucose-6-phosphate dehydrogenase deficiency because drug may induce hemolytic anemia; and in those with hypersensitivity to the drug.

Use cautiously in patients with renal or hepatic dysfunction because of potential for drug accumulation, and in patients with severe cerebral arteriosclerosis because of potential for CNS toxicity. Cross-resistance with cinoxacin has been reported.

ADVERSE REACTIONS

Common reactions are in italics; life-threatening reactions are in bold italics.
Blood: eosinophilia.
CNS: drowsiness, weakness, headache, dizziness, vertigo, seizures in epileptics, confusion, hallucinations.
EENT: sensitivity to light, change in color perception, diplopia, blurred vision.
GI: *abdominal pain, nausea, vomiting,* diarrhea.
Skin: pruritus, photosensitivity, urticaria, rash.
Other: angioedema, fever, chills, ***increased intracranial pressure in children and infants (bulging fontanelles).***

INTERACTIONS

Oral anticoagulants: Increased anticoagulant effect.

EFFECTS ON DIAGNOSTIC TESTS

CBC: transiently decreased RBC, WBC, and platelet counts.
Urine glucose tests with copper sulfate (Benedict's test, Fehling's test, and Clinitest): false-positive reactions.
Urine 17-ketosteroid and urine

17-ketogenic steroid: falsely elevated levels.

NURSING CONSIDERATIONS

Besides those related universally to drug therapy (see "How to use this book"), consider the following specific recommendations:

Assessment

• Obtain a baseline assessment of infection before nalidixic acid therapy.
• Be alert for adverse reactions and drug interactions throughout therapy.
• Evaluate the patient's and family's knowledge about nalidixic therapy.

Nursing Diagnoses

• High risk for injury related to ineffectiveness of nalidixic acid to eradicate the infection.
• High risk for fluid volume deficit related to adverse GI reactions caused by nalidixic acid.
• Knowledge deficit related to nalidixic acid.

Planning and Implementation

Preparation and Administration

• Obtain specimen for culture and sensitivity tests before first dose. Therapy may begin pending test results.

Monitoring

• Monitor effectiveness by regularly assessing for improvement in infection and evaluating results of specimens for culture and sensitivity, as ordered.
• Monitor hydration status if adverse GI reactions occur.
• Monitor CBC, renal and liver function studies during long-term therapy.

Supportive Care

• Obtain an order for an antiemetic or antidiarrheal agent as needed.
• Impose safety precautions if the patient experiences adverse CNS reactions.
• Report visual disturbances; these usually disappear with reduced dose.
• Use Clinistix or Tes-Tape to monitor urine glucose because drug may cause false-positive reactions to Clinitest.

Patient Teaching

• May cause dizziness or drowsiness. Warn the patient to avoid driving and other hazardous tasks that require alertness until CNS effects of the drug are known.
• Instruct patient to notify the doctor if visual disturbances occur because dosage adjustment may be needed.
• Remind patient to continue taking this drug, even when feeling better, and to take entire amount prescribed.
• Instruct diabetic patients to monitor urine glucose with Clinistix or Tes-Tape.
• Tell patient to avoid prolonged exposure to direct sunlight because drug may cause photosensitivity. Inform patient that photosensitivity may last as long as 3 months after drug is discontinued.

Evaluation

In patients receiving nalidixic acid, appropriate evaluation statements may include:

• Patient is free of infection.
• Patient maintains adequate hydration throughout nalidixic acid therapy.
• Patient and family state an understanding of nalidixic acid therapy.

naloxone hydrochloride

(nal ox´ one)

Narcan

• *Classification:* narcotic antagonist (opioid antagonist)
• *Pregnancy Risk Category:* B

HOW SUPPLIED

Injection: 0.4 mg/ml, 1 mg/ml

ACTION

Mechanism: Competitively binds to opiate receptors, preventing the ac-

tion of opiate agonists. Has no agonist activity of its own.
Absorption: Rapidly inactivated after oral administration; therefore, it is given parenterally.
Distribution: Rapidly distributed into body tissues and fluids; readily enters the CNS.
Metabolism: Rapidly metabolized in the liver, primarily by conjugation.
Excretion: In urine. Plasma half-life is reportedly from 30 to 90 minutes in adults, and 3 hours in neonates.
Onset, peak, duration: Onset of action is 1 to 2 minutes after I.V. administration, and 2 to 5 minutes after I.M. or S.C. administration. Duration of action is approximately 45 minutes, depending on route and dose. The duration of action is longer after I.M. use and higher doses than after I.V. use and lower doses.

INDICATIONS & DOSAGE

Known or suspected narcotic-induced respiratory depression, including that caused by pentazocine and propoxyphene–
Adults: 0.4 to 2 mg I.V., S.C., or I.M. May repeat q 2 to 3 minutes, p.r.n. If no response is observed after 10 mg has been administered, the diagnosis of narcotic-induced toxicity should be questioned.
Postoperative narcotic depression–
Adults: 0.1 to 0.2 mg I.V. q 2 to 3 minutes, p.r.n. Adult concentration is 0.4 mg/ml.
Children: 0.01 mg/kg dose I.M., I.V., or S.C. May repeat q 2 to 3 minutes.

Note: If initial dose of 0.01 mg/kg does not result in clinical improvement, up to 10 times this dose (0.1 mg/kg) may be needed to be effective.
Neonates (asphyxia neonatorum): 0.01 mg/kg I.V. into umbilical vein. May repeat q 2 to 3 minutes for 3 doses.

CONTRAINDICATIONS & PRECAUTIONS

Contraindicated in patients with hypersensitivity to the drug. Use with extreme caution in patients with supraventricular arrhythmias; patients with a head injury or increased intracranial pressure, because drug obscures neurologic parameters; and during pregnancy and labor, because drug readily crosses the placenta (premature infants appear especially sensitive to its respiratory and CNS depressant effects when the drug is used during delivery).

Use cautiously in patients with seizure disorders, because naloxone can precipitate seizures; in elderly or debilitated patients, who are more sensitive to the drug's therapeutic and adverse effects; and in narcotic addicts, including newborns of women with narcotic dependence, in whom it may produce an acute abstinence syndrome.

Because the duration of action of naloxone is shorter than that of most opiates, continued surveillance of the patient is mandatory, and repeated naloxone doses are often necessary. Other supportive therapy, with attention to maintenance of adequate respiratory and cardiovascular function, is imperative.

ADVERSE REACTIONS

Common reactions are in italics; life-threatening reactions are in bold italics.
With higher-than-recommended doses:
CV: tachycardia, hypertension.
GI: nausea, vomiting.
Other: tremors, withdrawal symptoms (in narcotic-dependent patients).

INTERACTIONS

None significant.

EFFECTS ON DIAGNOSTIC TESTS

None reported.

NURSING CONSIDERATIONS

Besides those related universally to drug therapy (see "How to use this book"), consider the following specific recommendations:

Assessment

- Obtain a baseline assessment of narcotic reportedly taken, respiratory status, and blood pressure before therapy.
- Be alert for adverse reactions and drug interactions throughout therapy.
- Evaluate the patient's and family's knowledge about naloxone therapy.

Nursing Diagnoses

- Ineffective breathing pattern related to known or suspected narcotic induced respiratory depression.
- Decreased cardiac output related to naloxone-induced tachycardia.
- Knowledge deficit related to naloxone therapy.

Planning and Implementation

Preparation and Administration

- Available in 1 ml prefilled disposable syringes, 1 ml ampules, and 10 ml vials.
- ***I.V. use:*** May be given by continuous I.V. infusion, which may be necessary to control the adverse effects of epidurally administered morphine.
- Dilute adult concentration (0.4 mg) by mixing 0.5 ml with 9.5 ml sterile water or saline solution for injection to make neonatal concentration (0.02 mg/ml).
- Be aware that dosage may have to be repeated every 20 minutes.

Monitoring

- Monitor effectiveness by checking for decreasing signs and symptoms of repiratory depression. Respiratory rate increases within 1 to 2 minutes. Effects last 1 to 4 hours.
- Monitor respiratory rate and depth closely for 24 hours. Duration of narcotic may exceed that of naloxone. Patient may relapse into respiratory depression.
- Be alert for "overshoot effect" when respiratory rate exceeds rate before respiratory depression.
- Monitor ECG for cardiac arrhythmias.
- Monitor blood pressure frequently until stable.

Supportive Care

- Use with caution in cardiac irritability and narcotic addiction.
- Be aware that naloxone is only effective in reversing respiratory depression caused by opiates. It is not effective against other drug-induced respiratory depression (barbiturates, sedatives). However, recent reports indicate that naloxone may reverse coma induced by alcohol intoxication.
- Note that naloxone does *not* reverse respiratory depression second to diazepam.
- Have oxygen, ventilation, and resuscitation equipment available.
- Naloxone has also been used investigationally to treat senile dementia in Alzheimer's disease, to relieve certain kinds of chronic constipation, and to improve circulation in refractory shock.

Patient Teaching

- Instruct patient to report return of respiratory difficulties immediately.
- Encourage proper storage of medications to prevent accidental poisoning.

Evaluation

In patients receiving naloxone, appropriate evaluation statements may include:

- Patient exhibits no signs of ineffective breathing pattern.
- Patient's cardiac output remains adequate.
- Patient and family state an understanding of naloxone hydrochloride therapy.

naltrexone hydrochloride

(nal trex´ one)
Trexan

• *Classification:* narcotic detoxification adjunct (opioid antagonist)
• *Pregnancy Risk Category:* C

HOW SUPPLIED

Tablets: 50 mg

ACTION

Mechanism: Competitively binds to opiate receptors, preventing the action of opiate agonists. Has no agonist activity of its own. Reversibly blocks the subjective effects of intravenously administered opioids by occupying opiate receptors in the brain.
Absorption: Well absorbed after oral administration, reaching peak plasma levels after 1 hour, although it does undergo extensive first-pass hepatic metabolism (only 5% to 20% of an oral dose reaches the systemic circulation unchanged).
Distribution: Extent and duration of the antagonist activity of naltrexone appear directly related to plasma and tissue concentrations of the drug. It is widely but variably distributed throughout the body.
Metabolism: Undergoes extensive first-pass hepatic metabolism. Its major metabolite is believed to be a pure antagonist also and may contribute to its efficacy. Drug and hepatic metabolites may undergo enterohepatic recirculation.
Excretion: Primarily by the kidneys. Half-life: Elimination half-life is about 10 hours; half-life of major active metabolite is about 14 hours.
Onset, peak, duration: Peak effect occurs within 1 hour.

INDICATIONS & DOSAGE

As an adjunct for maintenance of an opioid-free state in detoxified individuals–
Adults: initially, 25 mg P.O. If no withdrawal signs occur within 1 hour, give an additional 25 mg. Once patient has been started on 50 mg q 24 hours, flexible maintenance schedule may be used. From 50 to 150 mg may be given daily, depending on the schedule prescribed.

CONTRAINDICATIONS & PRECAUTIONS

Contraindicated in patients with hypersensitivity to the drug. Use with extreme caution in patients with allergy to another drug in the same chemical class; in patients receiving narcotic analgesics or those who are narcotic dependent or are undergoing narcotic withdrawal; in any individual who fails a naloxone challenge or who has a positive urinary screen for opioids; and in patients with acute hepatitis or liver failure (naltrexone can cause dose-related hepatocellular injury.)

Naltrexone is a potent antagonist with a prolonged pharmacologic effect (48 to 72 hours), but the blockade produced is surmountable; any attempt by a patient to overcome the antagonism by taking narcotics is very dangerous and could lead to fatal overdose.

ADVERSE REACTIONS

Common reactions are in italics; life-threatening reactions are in bold italics.
CNS: *insomnia, anxiety, nervousness, headache,* depression.
GI: *nausea, vomiting,* anorexia, *abdominal pain.*
Hepatic: hepatotoxicity.
Other: *muscle and joint pain.*

INTERACTIONS

None significant.

EFFECTS ON DIAGNOSTIC TESTS

Liver function tests: abnormal results reflecting hepatotoxicity.

NURSING CONSIDERATIONS

Besides those related universally to drug therapy (see "How to use this book"), consider the following specific recommendations:

Assessment

• Obtain a baseline assessment of drug history, hepatic function, and CNS status before therapy.
• Be alert for adverse reactions and drug interactions throughout therapy.
• Evaluate the patient's and family's knowledge about naltrexone therapy.

Nursing Diagnoses

• High risk for aspiration related to opioid dependence.
• Pain related to drug-induced muscle and joint pain.
• Knowledge deficit related to naltrexone hydrochloride therapy.

Planning and Implementation

Preparation and Administration

• Administer Narcan challenge (a provocative test of opioid dependence) before initiating treatment with naltrexone. If signs of opioid withdrawal persist after Narcan challenge, do not administer naltrexone.
• Consider a flexible maintenance dosage regimen: 100 mg on Monday and Wednesday; 150 mg on Friday. This schedule would be preferred for those expected to show poor compliance.

Monitoring

• Monitor effectiveness by observing the patient for absence of signs of opioid withdrawal.
• In patients who must receive opioid analgesics, monitor for respiratory depression from the opioid which may be longer and deeper.
• Monitor liver function studies.
• Observe for signs of CNS adverse reactions (insomnia, anxiety, depression, nervousness).

Supportive Care

• Do not give to patients receiving opioid analgesics, opioid-dependent patients, patients with acute opioid withdrawal, and in those with a positive urine screen for opioids or acute hepatic or liver failure.
• Use with caution in patients with mild liver disease or history of recent liver disease.
• Be aware that patients must be completely free of opioids before taking naltrexone, or they may experience severe withdrawal symptoms. Those who have been addicted to short-acting opioids (heroin, meperidine) must wait at least 7 days after the last dose before starting naltrexone. Those who have been addicted to longer-acting opioids (methadone) should wait at least 10 days.
• In an emergency that requires opioid analgesics, a patient receiving naltrexone can be given an opioid analgesic. However, the dose must be higher than usual to surmount naltrexone.
• Naltrexone should be used only as a part of a comprehensive rehabilitation program.
• Obtain an order for nonopioid analgesic to relieve drug-induced muscle and joint pain.

Patient Teaching

• Advise the patient to carry a medical identification card, and to tell medical personnel that he is taking naltrexone whenever he needs treatment.
• Recommend nonopioid drugs the patient can continue to take for pain, diarrhea, or cough.
• Stress the importance of not taking opioids while receiving naltrexone therapy.
• Encourage compliance with the dosing schedule.

Evaluation

In patients receiving naltrexone, appropriate evaluation statements may include:

• Patient remains free from danger of aspiration.
• Patient remains free from drug induced muscle and joint pain.
• Patient and family state an understanding of naltrexone hydrochloride therapy.

nandrolone decanoate

(nan´ droe lone)
Anabolin LA, Androlone-D, Deca-Durabolin, Decolone, Hybolin Decanoate, Kabolin, Nandrobolic L.A., Neo-Durabolic

nandrolone phenpropionate

Anabolin IM, Androlone, Durabolin, Hybolin Improved, Nandrobolic

• Controlled Substance Schedule III
• *Classification:* erythropoietic steroid (decanoate), anabolic steroid (decanoate), antineoplastic (phenproprionate) (anabolic steroid)
• *Pregnancy Risk Category:* X

HOW SUPPLIED

decanoate
Injection (in oil): 50 mg/ml, 100 mg/ml, 200 mg/ml
phenpropionate
Injection (in oil): 25 mg/ml, 50 mg/ml

ACTION

Mechanism: An anabolic steroid that stimulates cytosol steroid receptors in tissues to effect protein synthesis. Also stimulates erythropoiesis.
Pharmacokinetics: Unknown.

INDICATIONS & DOSAGE

Severe debility or disease states, refractory anemias (decanoate)–
Adults: 100 to 200 mg I.M. weekly. Therapy should be intermittent.
Tissue-building (decanoate)–
Adults: 50 to 100 mg I.M. q 3 to 4 weeks.
Children 2 to 13 years: 25 to 50 mg I.M. q 3 to 4 weeks.
Control of metastatic breast cancer (phenpropionate)–
Adults: 25 to 50 mg I.M. weekly.
Children 2 to 13 years: 12.5 to 25 mg I.M. every 2 to 4 weeks.

CONTRAINDICATIONS & PRECAUTIONS

Contraindicated in patients with severe renal or cardiac disease because fluid and electrolyte retention caused by this agent may aggravate these disorders; hepatic disease, because impaired elimination of the drug may cause toxic accumulation; prostatic or breast cancer or benign prostatic hypertrophy with obstruction and undiagnosed abnormal genital bleeding because this drug can stimulate the growth of cancerous breast or prostate tissue in males; and in pregnant or breast-feeding women, because animal studies have shown that administration of anabolic steroids during pregnancy causes masculinization of the female fetus. Administer cautiously in patients with a history of coronary artery disease, because the drug has hypercholesterolemic effects.

ADVERSE REACTIONS

Common reactions are in italics; life-threatening reactions are in bold italics.
Androgenic: in women–*acne, edema, oily skin, weight gain, hirsutism, hoarseness,* clitoral enlargement, decreased or increased libido. In men–prepubertal: premature epiphyseal closure, acne, priapism, growth of body and facial hair, phallic enlargement; postpubertal: testicular atrophy, oligospermia, decreased ejaculatory volume, impotence, gynecomastia, epididymitis.
CV: edema.
GI: gastroenteritis, nausea, vomiting, diarrhea, change in appetite.
GU: bladder irritability.

Hepatic: reversible jaundice, hepatotoxicity.
Hypoestrogenic: in women–flushing; sweating; vaginitis with itching, drying, burning, or bleeding; menstrual irregularities with large doses.
Local: pain at injection site, induration.
Other: hypercalcemia, hypercalciuria.

INTERACTIONS

None significant.

EFFECTS ON DIAGNOSTIC TESTS

Fasting plasma glucose, glucose tolerance test (GTT), and metyrapone test: abnormal results.
17-ketosteroids: decreased results.
Liver function tests, serum creatinine levels: elevated results.
Prothrombin time (especially in patients on anticoagulant therapy): prolonged.
Serum sodium, potassium, calcium, phosphate, and cholesterol: increased levels.
Sulfobromophthalein (BSP) retention: increased.
Thyroid function test results (protein-bound iodine, radioactive iodine uptake, thyroid-binding capacity): decreased.

NURSING CONSIDERATIONS

Besides those related universally to drug therapy (see "How to use this book"), consider the following specific recommendations:

Assessment

- Obtain a baseline assessment of patient's underlying condition before initiating nandrolone therapy.
- Be alert for adverse reactions and drug interactions throughout therapy.
- Evaluate the patient's and family's knowledge about nandrolone therapy.

Nursing Diagnoses

- High risk for injury related to the patient's underlying condition.
- Body image disturbance related to adverse androgenic reactions associated with nandrolone.
- Knowledge deficit related to nandrolone therapy.

Planning and Implementation

Preparation and Administration

- Check that in children, therapy is preceded by X-ray of wrist bones to establish level of bone maturation. During treatment, bone maturation may proceed more rapidly than linear growth; dosage should be intermittent and X-rays taken periodically.
- ***I.M. use:*** Inject drug deep I.M., preferably into upper outer quadrant of gluteal muscle in adults. Rotate injection sites to prevent muscle atrophy.

Monitoring

- Monitor effectiveness by regularly assessing the patient's condition for signs of improvement.
- Monitor the patient for hypercalcemia and obtain quantitative urine and serum calcium levels regularly. Hypercalcemia is most likely in patients with mammary carcinoma.
- Monitor female patients for signs of virilization or menstrual irregularities.
- Monitor the patient for symptoms of jaundice, which may be reversed by dosage adjustment. Periodic liver function tests should be performed.
- Monitor the patient receiving concomitant anticoagulant therapy for ecchymotic areas, petechiae, or abnormal bleeding. Monitor prothrombin time.
- Monitor boys under age 7 for precocious sexual development.
- Monitor the patient's weight routinely for fluid retention.
- Monitor for hypoglycemia in the diabetic patient and check blood glucose levels regularly.

Supportive Care

- Report signs of menstrual irregularities and virilization in females to the doctor because they may require discontinuation of therapy. Be aware

that virilization effects may be irreversible despite prompt discontinuation of therapy.
• Give the patient a diet high in calories and protein unless contraindicated. Give small, frequent feedings. Also implement salt restriction if edema occurs; expect to administer a diuretic concurrently, if needed.
• Carefully evaluate results of laboratory studies. Many laboratory results may be altered during therapy and for 2 to 3 weeks after therapy ends.
• Obtain an order for an antiemetic, antidiarrheal, or laxative, as indicated.
• Prepare patient for altered body image if androgenic adverse reactions occur.
• Be prepared to treat hypoglycemia and notify doctor if it occurs in the diabetic patient; it requires adjustment of antidiabetic treatment.

Patient Teaching
• Tell female patients to report menstrual irregularities; therapy should be discontinued pending etiologic determination.
• Explain to female patients that virilization may occur. Tell them to report such effects immediately.
• Stress importance of not abusing drug to enhance athletic performance.
• Instruct patient to eat a diet high in calories and protein and low in sodium, unless contraindicated, and to eat small frequent meals.
• Instruct diabetic patient how to manage hypoglycemia and to report it to doctor.
• Correct any misconception about drug. It is erroneously thought to enhance athletic ability.

Evaluation
In patients receiving nandrolone, appropriate evaluation statements may include:
• Patient's underlying condition being treated with nandrolone improves.
• Patient states acceptance of body image changes caused by nandrolone therapy.
• Patient and family state an understanding of nandrolone therapy.

naphazoline hydrochloride (nasal)
(nuh fay´ zoe leen)
Privine◇

• *Classification:* nasal agent
• *Pregnancy Risk Category:* C

HOW SUPPLIED
Nasal drops: 0.05% solution
Nasal spray: 0.05% solution

ACTION
Mechanism: An alpha-adrenergic agonist that produces local vasoconstriction of dilated arterioles to reduce blood flow and nasal congestion.
Pharmacokinetics: Unknown.
Onset, peak, duration: Onset occurs within 10 minutes and persists for 2 to 6 hours.

INDICATIONS & DOSAGE
Nasal congestion–
Adults: apply 2 drops or sprays of 0.05% solution to nasal mucosa q 3 to 4 hours.
Children 6 to 12 years: 1 to 2 drops or sprays of 0.05% solution. Repeat q 3 to 6 hours, p.r.n. Use no longer than 3 to 5 days.

CONTRAINDICATIONS & PRECAUTIONS
Contraindicated in narrow-angle glaucoma. Use cautiously in hyperthyroidism, heart disease, hypertension, or diabetes mellitus, because systemic absorption can occur.

ADVERSE REACTIONS
Common reactions are in italics; life-threatening reactions are in bold italics.
EENT: rebound nasal congestion with

†Available in Canada only. ‡Available in Australia only. ◇Available OTC

excessive or long-term use, sneezing, stinging, dryness of mucosa.
Other: systemic effects in children after excessive or long-term use; marked sedation.

INTERACTIONS

Tricyclic antidepressants, MAO inhibitors: hypertensive crisis if naphazoline is systemically absorbed. Use together cautiously.

EFFECTS ON DIAGNOSTIC TESTS

None reported.

NURSING CONSIDERATIONS

Besides those related universally to drug therapy (see "How to use this book"), consider the following specific recommendations.

Assessment

- Obtain a baseline assessment of the patient's breathing pattern and degree of nasal congestion.
- Be alert for adverse reactions and drug interactions throughout therapy.
- Evaluate the patient's and family's knowledge about naphazoline therapy.

Nursing Diagnoses

- Ineffective breathing pattern related to the patient's underlying condition.
- High risk for poisoning (systemic effects).
- Knowledge deficit related to naphazoline hydrochloride therapy.

Planning and Implementation

Preparation and Administration

- Have patient hold head upright. Hold spray container upright and insert nozzle into nostril (point away from septum) and spray nasal mucosa. If drops are used, apply to nasal mucosa.
- Do not shake container.

Monitoring

- Monitor effectiveness by assessing the patient's breathing pattern and degree of nasal congestion; or by assessing the patient's visual status and conjunctival appearance.
- Monitor for systemic absorption, especially in children or patients with underlying cardiac disease, thyroid disease, or diabetes mellitus.
- Monitor for drug-induced sedation.

Supportive Care

- Notify the doctor immediately of any changes in the patient's health status.

Patient Teaching

- Teach patient how to administer the solution and tell him the medicine should be used by one person only.
- Warn patient not to exceed recommended dosage.
- Advise patient to notify the doctor if symptoms persist for more than 5 days; drug is for short-term use only and therapy should not continue beyond 5 days.

Evaluation

In patients receiving naphazoline hydrochloride, appropriate evaluation statements may include:

- Patient obtains relief from nasal congestion.
- Patient remains free of systemic effects.
- Patient and family state an understanding of naphazoline hydrochloride therapy.

naphazoline hydrochloride (ophthalmic)

(nuh fay´ zoe leen)

AK-Con, Albalon Liquifilm, Allerest◇, Clear Eyes◇, Degest 2◇, Estivin II, Naphcon◇, Naphcon Forte, Optazine‡, Vasoclear◇, Vasocon Regular

- *Classification:* decongestant, vasoconstrictor (sympathomimetic agent)
- *Pregnancy Risk Category:* C

HOW SUPPLIED

Ophthalmic solution: 0.012%◇, 0.02%, 0.03%, 0.05%, 0.1%

Liquid form contains alcohol. **May contain tartrazine.

ACTION

Mechanism: Produces vasoconstriction by stimulating alpha-receptors on the blood vessels and arterioles of the conjunctiva.
Pharmacokinetics: Unknown.
Onset, peak, duration: Onset of action is within 10 minutes, with effects lasting 2 to 6 hours.

INDICATIONS & DOSAGE

Ocular congestion, irritation, itching–
Adults: instill 1 to 2 drops of 0.1% solution in eye q 3 to 4 hours or 1 drop of 0.012% to 0.05% solution up to q.i.d.

CONTRAINDICATIONS & PRECAUTIONS

Contraindicated in patients with hypersensitivity to any component of the preparation and in patients with narrow-angle glaucoma. Use with caution in patients with hyperthyroidism, cardiac disease, hypertension, or diabetes mellitus and in elderly patients.

ADVERSE REACTIONS

Common reactions are in italics; life-threatening reactions are in bold italics.
Eye: transient stinging, pupillary dilation, irritation, photophobia.
Other: dizziness, headache, increased sweating, nausea, nervousness, weakness.

INTERACTIONS

Tricyclic antidepressants, MAO inhibitors: hypertensive crisis if naphazoline is systemically absorbed. Use together cautiously.

EFFECTS ON DIAGNOSTIC TESTS

None reported.

NURSING CONSIDERATIONS

Besides those related universally to drug therapy, (see "How to use this book"), consider the following specific recommendations:

Assessment
- Obtain a baseline assessment of the patient's vision and ocular appearance.
- Be alert for adverse reactions and drug interactions throughout therapy.
- Evaluate the patient's and family's knowledge about naphazoline hydrochloride therapy.

Nursing Diagnoses
- Sensory/perceptual alterations (visual) related to the patient's underlying condition.
- High risk for poisoning related to possible systemic effects of the drug.
- Knowledge deficit related to naphazoline hydrochloride therapy.

Planning and Implementation
Preparation and Administration
- Solution should be stored in a tightly closed container.
- Instill in lacrimal sac; remove excess solution from around eyes with a clean tissue or gauze and apply light finger pressure to lacrimal sac for 1 minute.

Monitoring
- Monitor effectiveness by assessing the patient's visual status and conjunctival appearance.
- Monitor the patient for systemic effects.
- Monitor the patient for blurred vision, pain, or lid edema.

Supportive Care
- Notify the doctor immediately if changes in the patient's health or visual status occur.

Patient Teaching
- Teach the patient how to instill the solution and advise him to wash his hands before and after administering the drug.
- Warn the patient that the drug may cause brief, transient stinging when instilled.
- Warn the patient with young children that the drug can cause serious

sedation – even coma – if accidentally ingested by children.
• Warn patient not to exceed the recommended dosage or use a nonprescription preparation for more than 72 hours: rebound congestion may result from prolonged use.
• Advise the patient that photophobia may develop in individuals sensitive to the drug, and tell him to report this effect to his doctor if it occurs.

Evaluation

In patients receiving naphazoline hydrochloride, appropriate evaluation statements may include:
• Patient experiences relief of ocular irritation.
• Patient remains free of systemic effects.
• Patient and family state an understanding of naphazoline hydrochloride therapy.

naproxen

(na prox´ en)

Apo-Naproxen†, Naprosyn, Naxen†‡, Novonaprox†

naproxen sodium

Anaprox, Anaprox DS, Naprogesic‡

• *Classification:* nonnarcotic analgesic, antipyretic, anti-inflammatory (nonsteroidal anti-inflammatory)
• *Pregnancy Risk Category:* B (D in 3rd trimester)

HOW SUPPLIED

naproxen
Tablets: 250 mg, 375 mg, 500 mg
Oral suspension: 125 mg/5 ml
Suppositories: 500 mg‡
naproxen sodium
Tablets (film-coated): 275 mg, 550 mg
Note: 275 mg naproxen sodium = 250 mg naproxen

ACTION

Mechanism: Produces anti-inflammatory, analgesic, and antipyretic effects, possibly through inhibition of prostaglandin synthesis.
Absorption: Rapidly and completely absorbed from the GI tract.
Distribution: Highly protein bound.
Metabolism: Hepatic.
Excretion: In urine. Half-life: Elimination half-life is about 13 hours.
Onset, peak, duration: Plasma levels peak at 2 to 4 hours.

INDICATIONS & DOSAGE

Arthritis, primary dysmenorrhea (free base) –
Adults: 250 to 500 mg P.O. b.i.d.
Alternatively, may use suppository where available –
Adults: 500 mg P.R. h.s. with oral naproxen during the day.
Maximum dosage is 1,250 mg daily.
Mild to moderate pain and treatment of primary dysmenorrhea (naproxen sodium) –
Adults: 2 tablets (275 mg each tablet) P.O. to start, followed by 275 mg q 6 to 8 hours as needed. Maximum daily dosage should not exceed 1,375 mg.

CONTRAINDICATIONS & PRECAUTIONS

Contraindicated in patients with hypersensitivity and in patients in whom aspirin or other nonsteroidal anti-inflammatory drugs (NSAIDs) induce symptoms of asthma, urticaria, or rhinitis. Patients with known "triad" symptoms (aspirin hypersensitivity, rhinitis/nasal polyps, and asthma) are at high risk of cross-sensitivity to naproxen with precipitation of bronchospasm. Avoid use during pregnancy (especially the third trimester) because these drugs may prolong labor.

Serious GI toxicity, especially ulceration or hemorrhage, can occur at any time in patients on chronic NSAID therapy. Use cautiously in patients with a history of angioedema or of GI disease, peptic ulcer, or renal or cardiovascular disease, because the drug may worsen these conditions.

Because the drug may mask signs and symptoms of acute infection (fever, myalgias, erythema), carefully evaluate patients with high risk of infection (such as diabetic patients).

ADVERSE REACTIONS

Common reactions are in italics; life-threatening reactions are in bold italics.
Blood: prolonged bleeding time, ***agranulocytosis,*** neutropenia.
CNS: *headache,* drowsiness, *dizziness,* tinnitus.
CV: peripheral edema, dyspnea.
EENT: visual disturbances.
GI: *epigastric distress, occult blood loss, nausea, peptic ulceration.*
GU: nephrotoxicity.
Hepatic: elevated enzymes.
Skin: *pruritus, rash,* urticaria.

INTERACTIONS

Oral anticoagulants, sulfonylureas, and drugs that are highly protein bound: increased risk of toxicity.

EFFECTS ON DIAGNOSTIC TESTS

Bleeding time: increased (may persist for 4 days after withdrawal of drug).
BUN, serum creatinine, potassium, and transaminase: increased levels.
Urinary 5-HIAA and 17-hydroxycorticosteroid: test interference.

NURSING CONSIDERATIONS

Besides those related universally to drug therapy (see "How to use this book"), consider the following recommendations:

Assessment
- Obtain a baseline assessment of the patient's pain before therapy.
- Be alert for adverse reactions and drug interactions throughout therapy.
- Evaluate the patient's and family's knowledge about naproxen or naproxen sodium therapy.

Nursing Diagnoses
- Pain related to the patient's underlying condition.
- High risk for trauma related to drowsiness or dizziness caused by CNS reaction to naproxen or naproxen sodium.
- Knowledge deficit related to naproxen or naproxen sodium therapy.

Planning and Implementation
Preparation and Administration
- ***P.O. use:*** Give with food or milk to minimize GI upset.

Monitoring
- Regularly monitor for relief of pain, keeping in mind that full therapeutic effects may be delayed 2 to 4 weeks.
- Monitor CBC and renal and hepatic function every 4 to 6 months or as indicated in long-term therapy.

Supportive Care
- If adverse CNS reactions occur, notify the doctor and institute safety precautions, such as supervising ambulation and keeping the bed rails up.
- Expect naproxen sodium to be absorbed more rapidly than naproxen.

Patient Teaching
- Tell the patient that the full therapeutic effect may be delayed for 2 to 4 weeks.
- Advise the patient to notify the doctor if pain persists or becomes worse.
- Advise the patient to avoid hazardous activities that require mental alertness until CNS effects of the drug are known.
- Tell the patient to take the drug with food or milk.
- Because serious GI toxicity can occur at any time in chronic NSAID therapy, teach the patient signs and symptoms of GI bleeding. Tell the patient to report these to the doctor immediately.
- Advise the patient to avoid aspirin

and alcohol because concomitant use with aspirin, alcohol, or steroids may increase the risk of adverse GI reactions.
• Recommend periodic eye examinations during therapy.
• Warn patient against taking naproxen and naproxen sodium at the same time because both circulate in the blood as the naproxen anion.
Evaluation
In patients receiving naproxen or naproxen sodium, appropriate evaluation statements may include:
• Patient states pain is relieved.
• Patient does not develop traumatic injuries as a result of adverse CNS reactions.
• Patient and family state an understanding of naproxen or naproxen sodium therapy.

natamycin
(na ta mye´ sin)
Natacyn

• *Classification:* antifungal (macrolide)
• *Pregnancy Risk Category:* C

HOW SUPPLIED
Ophthalmic suspension: 5%
Limited availability requires that orders be placed with manufacturer directly.

ACTION
Mechanism: A polyene macrolide antibiotic related to nystatin and amphotericin B. Binds to sterols in the cell membrane of fungi, increasing permeability.
Absorption: Systemic absorption is unlikely after topical ophthalmic administration. Drug is not absorbed from the GI tract.
Distribution: Topical ophthalmic administration produces effective concentrations within the corneal stroma but not in intraocular fluid. Drug appears to concentrate within areas of epithelial ulceration.

INDICATIONS & DOSAGE
Treatment of fungal keratitis–
Adults: initial dosage is 1 drop instilled in conjunctival sac q 1 to 2 hours. After 3 to 4 days, reduce dosage to 1 drop 6 to 8 times daily.
Treatment of blepharitis or fungal conjunctivitis–
Adults: instill 1 drop q 4 to 6 hours.

CONTRAINDICATIONS & PRECAUTIONS
Contraindicated in patients with hypersensitivity to any component of the formulation. If keratitis fails to improve after a 7- to 10-day course, the infection may be caused by nonsusceptible organism. Monitor tolerance to natamycin twice weekly. Determine initial and sustained therapy by laboratory diagnosis and response to the drug.

ADVERSE REACTIONS
Common reactions are in italics; life-threatening reactions are in bold italics.
Eye: ocular edema, hyperemia.

INTERACTIONS
None significant.

EFFECTS ON DIAGNOSTIC TESTS
None reported.

NURSING CONSIDERATIONS
Besides those related universally to drug therapy (see "How to use this book"), consider the following specific recommendations:
Assessment
• Obtain a baseline assessment of the patient's allergies before therapy.
• Be alert for adverse reactions and drug interactions throughout therapy.
• Evaluate the patient's and family's knowledge about natamycin therapy.

Nursing Diagnoses
• Altered protection related to ocular fungal infection.
• Impaired tissue integrity related to natamycin-induced ocular edema.
• Knowledge deficit related to natamycin therapy.
Planning and Implementation
Preparation and Administration
• Wash hands before and after administration.
• Shake well before using. May be kept in refrigerator or at room temperature.
• Clean eye area of excess exudate before administration.
• Reduce dosage gradually at 4- to 7-day intervals to ensure that organism has been eliminated.
Monitoring
• Monitor effectiveness by culturing the eye to check for microorganisms.
• Observe color, amount, and consistency of exudate.
• Monitor extent of ocular edema and for signs of hypersensitivity.
• Check patient's vision.
Supportive Care
• Apply warm, moist compresses to aid in removal of dried exudate.
• Use safety precautions if vision is impaired. Assist with activities.
• Only antifungal available as an ophthalmic preparation.
• Treatment of choice for fungal keratitis. May also be used to treat fungal blepharitis and conjunctivitis.
• Continue therapy for 14 to 21 days or until active disease subsides.
• Clinical and laboratory reevaluation is recommended if infection does not improve with 7 to 10 days of therapy.
Patient Teaching
• Teach patient how to instill the drops. Advise him to wash hands before and after administration. Do not touch tip of dropper to eye or surrounding tissue.
• Instruct the patient to apply light finger pressure to lacrimal sac for 1 minute after administering drops. Caution him to avoid rubbing or scratching the eye area.
• Warn patient to avoid sharing washcloths and towels with family members during infection.
• Warn the patient not to share eye medication with family members. A family member who develops the same symptoms should contact the doctor.
Evaluation
In patients receiving natamycin, appropriate evaluation statements may include:
• Patient remains free from signs and symptoms of infection.
• Patient reports decrease or absence of ocular edema.
• Patient and family state an understanding of natamycin therapy.

neomycin sulfate (oral)
(nee oh mye´ sin)
Mycifradin, Neosulf‡

• *Classification:* antibiotic (aminoglycoside)
• *Pregnancy Risk Category:* C

HOW SUPPLIED
Tablets: 500 mg
Oral solution: 125 mg/ml

ACTION
Mechanism: Inhibits protein synthesis in susceptible bacteria by binding directly to the 30S ribosomal subunit. Generally bactericidal.
Absorption: Poorly absorbed (about 3%) after oral administration; may be given for bowel sterilization. Oral absorption is enhanced in patients with impaired GI motility or intestinal ulcerations. Plasma levels are similar after oral or rectal administration. Because of the risk of toxicity, the drug is not administered parenterally.
Distribution: Oral administration re-

stricts distribution to the intestine. Small amounts of absorbed drug are widely distributed; plasma protein binding is minimal.
Metabolism: Not metabolized.
Excretion: Primarily excreted in urine by glomerular filtration. After oral administration, excreted primarily unchanged in feces. Half-life: 2 to 3 hours in adults; 24 hours in severe renal damage.
Onset, peak, duration: After oral administration peak serum levels occur at 1 to 4 hours.

INDICATIONS & DOSAGE

Infectious diarrhea caused by enteropathogenic Escherichia coli –
Adults: 50 mg/kg daily P.O. in four divided doses for 2 to 3 days.
Children: 50 to 100 mg/kg daily P.O. divided q 4 to 6 hours for 2 to 3 days.
Suppression of intestinal bacteria preoperatively –
Adults: 1 g P.O. q 1 hour for four doses, then 1 g q 4 hours for the balance of the 24 hours. A saline cathartic should precede therapy.
Children: 40 to 100 mg/kg daily P.O. divided q 4 to 6 hours. First dose should follow saline cathartic.
Adjunctive treatment in hepatic coma –
Adults: 1 to 3 g P.O. q.i.d. for 5 to 6 days; or 200 ml of 1% or 100 ml of 2% solution as enema retained for 20 to 60 minutes q 6 hours.

CONTRAINDICATIONS & PRECAUTIONS

Contraindicated in patients with hypersensitivity to neomycin or any aminoglycoside and, when given orally, in patients with intestinal obstruction. Otic form is contraindicated in perforated eardrum.

Use cautiously in patients with intestinal mucosal ulcerations; large skin wounds; decreased renal function; tinnitus, vertigo, and high-frequency hearing loss, who are susceptible to ototoxicity; dehydration, myasthenia gravis, parkinsonism, and hypocalcemia; and in neonates and other infants and elderly patients.

ADVERSE REACTIONS

Common reactions are in italics; life-threatening reactions are in bold italics.
CNS: headache, lethargy.
EENT: *ototoxicity (tinnitus, vertigo, hearing loss).*
GI: nausea, vomiting.
GU: *nephrotoxicity (cells or casts in the urine, oliguria, proteinuria, decreased creatinine clearance, increased BUN and serum creatinine levels).*
Skin: rash, urticaria.
Other: ***hypersensitivity.***

INTERACTIONS

Cephalothin: increases nephrotoxicity. Use together cautiously.
Dimenhydrinate: may mask symptoms of ototoxicity. Use with caution.
I.V. loop diuretics (e.g. furosemide): increase ototoxicity. Use cautiously.
Oral anticoagulants: oral neomycin inhibits vitamin K–producing bacteria and may potentiate anticoagulant effect.
Other aminoglycosides, amphotericin B, cisplatin, methoxyflurane: increases nephrotoxicity. Use together cautiously.

EFFECTS ON DIAGNOSTIC TESTS

BUN, nonprotein nitrogen, or serum creatinine: elevated levels and increased excretion of casts, if systemic absorption occurs.

NURSING CONSIDERATIONS

Besides those related universally to drug therapy (see "How to use this book"), consider the following specific recommendations:
Assessment
• Obtain a baseline assessment of infection before therapy.

• Be alert for adverse reactions and drug interactions throughout therapy.
• Evaluate the patient's and family's knowledge about neomycin therapy.

Nursing Diagnoses

• High risk for injury related to ineffectiveness of neomycin to eradicate the infection.
• Altered urinary elimination related to neomycin-induced nephrotoxicity.
• Knowledge deficit related to neomycin.

Planning and Implementation

Preparation and Administration

• Obtain specimen for culture and sensitivity tests before first dose. Therapy may begin pending test results.
• Weigh patient and determine baseline renal function before therapy.
• For preoperative disinfection, provide a low-residue diet and a cathartic immediately before oral administration of neomycin.

Monitoring

• Monitor effectiveness by regularly assessing patient for improvement of infection.
• Monitor renal function (intake and output, specific gravity, urinalysis, BUN, and creatinine levels, and creatinine clearance).
• Monitor patients with renal disease, hypocalcemia, or neuromuscular diseases such as myasthenia gravis for respiratory depression.
• Closely monitor neurologic status when neomycin is used to decrease ammonia-producing flora in the GI tract.

Supportive Care

• Notify doctor promptly if signs of decreased renal function occur or complaints of tinnitus, vertigo, or hearing loss. Deafness may occur several weeks after drug is discontinued.
• Encourage patient to consume 2,000 ml of fluid daily (if not contraindicated) during therapy to minimize chemical irritation of the renal tubules.
• During use to decrease ammonia-producing flora in the GI tract, decrease the patient's dietary intake of protein.

Patient Teaching

• Emphasize the need to drink 2,000 ml of fluid each day, not including coffee, tea, or other caffeinated beverages.
• Instruct the patient to notify the doctor immediately of changes in urine elimination patterns or changes in hearing.
• Tell the patient to alert the doctor if infection worsens or does not improve.
• Stress the importance of recommended blood tests to monitor renal function and to detect adverse reactions.
• Teach patient to recognize and promptly report the signs and symptoms of superinfection (continued fever and other signs of new infection, especially of upper respiratory tract).
• Teach patient receiving neomycin to decrease ammonia-producing flora in the GI tract to decrease dietary intake of protein.
• Inform the patient receiving neomycin for preoperative disinfection that he will receive a low-residue diet and a cathartic immediately before oral administration of the drug.

Evaluation

In patients receiving neomycin, appropriate evaluation statements may include:

• Patient is free of infection.
• Patient's renal function studies remain normal throughout therapy.
• Patient and family state an understanding of therapy.

neomycin sulfate (topical)

(nee oh mye´ sin)
Mycifradin†, Myciguent◇

• *Classification:* antibiotic (aminoglycoside)
• *Pregnancy Risk Category:* C

HOW SUPPLIED

Cream: 0.5%◇
Ointment: 0.5%◇

ACTION

Mechanism: Binds to the 30S subunit of bacterial ribosomes and disrupts protein synthesis.
Absorption: Not absorbed through intact skin, but may be absorbed from wounds, burns, or skin ulcers.

INDICATIONS & DOSAGE

Topical bacterial infections, minor burns, wounds, skin grafts, following surgical procedure, primary pyodermas, pruritus, trophic ulcerations, otitis externa –
Adults and children: rub in small quantity gently b.i.d., t.i.d., or as directed.

CONTRAINDICATIONS & PRECAUTIONS

Chronic application to inflamed skin increases hazard of sensitization to neomycin.

ADVERSE REACTIONS

Common reactions are in italics; life-threatening reactions are in bold italics.
Skin: *rashes, contact dermatitis,* urticaria.
Other: *possible* ***nephrotoxicity,*** *ototoxicity, and* ***neuromuscular blockade;*** *possible systemic absorption when used on extensive areas of the body.*

INTERACTIONS

None significant.

EFFECTS ON DIAGNOSTIC TESTS

None reported.

NURSING CONSIDERATIONS

Besides those related universally to drug therapy (see "How to use this book"), consider the following specific recommendations:
Assessment
• Obtain a baseline assessment of wound before therapy.
• Be alert for adverse reactions and drug interactions throughout therapy.
• Evaluate the patient's and family's knowledge about neomycin therapy.
Nursing Diagnoses
• Impaired skin integrity related to wounds.
• Sensory/perceptual alterations, auditory, related to neomycin-induced ototoxicity.
• Knowledge deficit related to neomycin therapy.
Planning and Implementation
Preparation and Administration
• ***Topical use:*** Cleanse area and rub in small quantity gently.
Monitoring
• Monitor effectiveness by regularly examining wounds for erythema and inflammation.
• Watch for signs of hypersensitivity and contact dermatitis.
• Monitor for adverse reactions or interactions by frequently evaluating the patient for signs of ototoxicity during prolonged use.
• Monitor patient's condition; if no improvement or if condition worsens, stop using and report to doctor.
Supportive Care
• Remember, don't use on more than 20% of the body surface and on patent with impaired renal function unless risk/benefit ratio has been assessed.
• Keep in mind that prolonged use may result in overgrowth of nonsusceptible organisms.
• Be aware, in combination products that contain corticosteroids, use of

occlusive dressings increases corticosteroid absorption and the risk of systemic effects.
• Application on denuded or abraded areas enhances systemic absorption.

Patient Teaching
• Teach patient to apply medication.
• Instruct patient to inform doctor of any adverse reactions.

Evaluation

In patients receiving neomycin, appropriate evaluation statements may include:
• Patient shows improvement of infection.
• Patient did not develop drug-induced ototoxicity.
• Patient and family state an understanding of neomycin therapy.

---

neostigmine bromide
(nee oh stig´ meen)
Prostigmin Bromide

neostigmine methylsulfate
Prostigmin

• *Classification:* muscle stimulant (cholinesterase inhibitor)
• *Pregnancy Risk Category:* C

HOW SUPPLIED
Tablets: 15 mg
Injection: 0.25 mg/ml, 0.5 mg/ml, 1 mg/ml

ACTION
Mechanism: Inhibits the destruction of acetylcholine released from the parasympathetic and somatic efferent nerves. Acetylcholine accumulates, promoting increased stimulation of the receptor.
Absorption: Poorly absorbed (1% to 2%) from the GI tract after oral administration. It is well absorbed from I.M. and S.C. sites.
Distribution: About 15% to 25% bound to plasma proteins. In usual doses, drug probably does not cross placenta or enter breast milk. As a quaternary ammonium compound, drug is not expected to enter the CNS.
Metabolism: Hydrolyzed by cholinesterases to 3-hydroxyphenyltrimethylammonium (3-OH PTM) which has some pharmacologic activity; also metabolized by microsomal liver enzymes.
Excretion: About 50% of dose is excreted in urine as unchanged drug; 80% of an I.M. dose appears in urine in the first 24 hours after administration. Half-life: About 50 minutes.
Onset, peak, duration: Action usually begins 2 to 4 hours after oral administration and 10 to 30 minutes after injection. Duration of effect varies, depending on patient's physical and emotional status and on disease severity.

INDICATIONS & DOSAGE
Antidote for nondepolarizing neuromuscular blocking agents–
Adults: 0.5 to 2 mg I.V. slowly. Repeat p.r.n. to a total of 5 mg. Give 0.6 to 1.2 mg atropine sulfate I.V. before antidote dose.
Postoperative abdominal distention and bladder atony–
Adults: 0.5 to 1 mg I.M. or S.C. q 4 to 6 hours.
Postoperative ileus–
Adults: 0.25 to 1 mg I.M. or S.C. q 4 to 6 hours.
Diagnosis of myasthenia gravis–
Adults: 0.022 mg/kg I.M. 30 minutes after 0.011 mg of atropine sulfate.
Treatment of myasthenia gravis–
Adults: 15 to 30 mg P.O. t.i.d. (range is 15 to 375 mg daily); or 0.5 to 2 mg I.M. or I.V. q 1 to 3 hours. Dosage must be individualized, depending on response and tolerance of adverse reactions. Therapy may be required day and night.

Children: 7.5 to 15 mg P.O. t.i.d. to q.i.d.

Note: 1:1,000 solution of injectable solution contains 1 mg/ml; 1:2,000 solution contains 0.5 mg/ml.

CONTRAINDICATIONS & PRECAUTIONS

Contraindicated in patients with mechanical obstruction of the urinary or intestinal tract, because of its stimulatory effect on smooth muscle; bradycardia or hypotension, because the drug may exacerbate these conditions; and hypersensitivity to cholinergics or bromides.

Administer with extreme caution to patients with bronchial asthma, because the drug may precipitate bronchospasm. Administer cautiously to patients with seizure disorders, because it may stimulate the CNS; peritonitis, vagotonia, hyperthyroidism, or cardiac arrhythmias, because it may exacerbate these conditions; peptic ulcer disease, because it may increase gastric acid secretion; and recent coronary occlusion, because drug stimulates the cardiovascular system.

ADVERSE REACTIONS

Common reactions are in italics; life-threatening reactions are in bold italics.

CNS: dizziness, muscle weakness, mental confusion, jitters, sweating, ***respiratory depression.***

CV: bradycardia, hypotension.

EENT: miosis.

GI: *nausea, vomiting, diarrhea, abdominal cramps,* excessive salivation.

GU: urinary frequency.

Skin: rash (bromide).

Other: bronchospasm, *muscle cramps,* muscle fasciculations, ***bronchoconstriction.***

INTERACTIONS

Atropine, anticholinergic agents, procainamide, aminoglycosides, quinidine: may reverse cholinergic effect on muscle. Observe for lack of drug effect.

EFFECTS ON DIAGNOSTIC TESTS

None reported.

NURSING CONSIDERATIONS

Besides those related universally to drug therapy (see "How to use this book"), consider the following specific recommendations:

Assessment

- Obtain a baseline assessment of the patient's underlying condition before initiating drug therapy.
- Be alert for adverse reactions and drug interactions throughout neostigmine therapy.
- Evaluate the patient's and family's knowledge about neostigmine therapy.

Nursing Diagnoses

- Impaired physical mobility related to the patient's underlying condition.
- Diarrhea related to adverse reaction to neostigmine.
- Knowledge deficit related to neostigmine therapy.

Planning and Implementation

Preparation and Administration

- Make sure that all other cholinergics have been discontinued before administering this drug.
- In myasthenia gravis, schedule the dose before periods of fatigue. For example, if patient has dysphagia, schedule dose 30 minutes before each meal.
- Give the drug with milk or food to reduce adverse GI reactions.
- Hospitalized patient with chronic myasthenia gravis may request bedside supply of tablets for self-administration. This will enable patient to take each dose precisely as ordered. Seek approval for self-medication program according to hospital policy, but continue to oversee medication.
- Be prepared to administer I.M. neostigmine instead of edrophonium to diagnose myasthenia gravis; may

be preferable to edrophonium when limb weakness is the only symptom.

Monitoring

• Monitor effectiveness by regularly assessing signs and symptoms of the underlying disorder for evidence of relief or diminished severity; patients may develop resistance to this drug.

• Monitor for adverse reactions and drug interactions by checking vital signs frequently; check respirations carefully.

• Monitor and document the patient's response after each dose because it is difficult to determine optimal dosage.

• Monitor closely for improvement in strength, vision, and ptosis 45 to 60 minutes after each dose.

• Monitor for diarrhea and other adverse GI reactions; if present, monitor hydration status.

• Monitor for abdominal or muscle cramping.

Supportive Care

• Have atropine injection readily available and be prepared to give as ordered to reverse toxicity.

• Provide respiratory support as needed if adverse reactions occur.

• Insert a rectal tube to help passage of gas, if used to prevent abdominal distention.

• Report severe muscle weakness to doctor, who will determine if it reflects drug-induced toxicity or exacerbation of myasthenia gravis. Test dose of edrophonium I.V. will worsen drug-induced weakness but will temporarily relieve weakness caused by disease.

• Obtain an order for an antidiarrheal or antiemetic as needed.

• Consult with the doctor to manage abdominal or muscle cramping.

Patient Teaching

• Tell the patient how to handle troublesome GI reactions and abdominal or muscle cramping.

• Tell the patient to take the drug with food or milk to reduce adverse GI reactions.

Evaluation

In patients receiving neostigmine, appropriate evaluation statements may include:

• Patient is able to perform activities of daily living without assistance.

• Patient's bowel patterns are unaffected by neostigmine therapy.

• Patient and family state an understanding of neostigmine chloride therapy.

netilmicin sulfate

(ne til mye´ sin)

Netromycin

• *Classification:* antibiotic (aminoglycoside)

• *Pregnancy Risk Category:* C

HOW SUPPLIED

Injection: 10 mg/ml, 25 mg/ml, 100 mg/ml

ACTION

Mechanism: Inhibits protein synthesis by binding directly to the 30S ribosomal subunit of susceptible bacteria. Generally bactericidal.

Absorption: Poorly absorbed after oral administration and is given parenterally. Rapidly and completely absorbed after I.M. administration; peak levels are similar to those after a 1-hour I.V. infusion of the same dose.

Distribution: Widely distributed after parenteral administration; intraocular penetration is poor; CSF penetration is low, even in patients with inflamed meninges. Protein binding is minimal. Netilmicin crosses the placenta.

Metabolism: Not metabolized.

Excretion: Primarily excreted in urine by glomerular filtration; small amounts may be excreted in bile and breast milk. Half-life: 2 to 2½ hours in adults; over 30 hours in severe renal damage.

Onset, peak, duration: Peak serum concentrations occur 30 to 60 minutes after I.M. administration.

INDICATIONS & DOSAGE

Serious infections caused by sensitive Pseudomonas aeruginosa, Escherichia coli, Proteus, Klebsiella, Serratia, Enterobacter, Citrobacter, Staphylococcus–

Adults and children over 12 years: 3 to 6.5 mg/kg/day by I.M. injection or I.V. infusion. May be given q 12 hours to treat serious urinary tract infections and q 8 to 12 hours to treat serious systemic infections.

Infants and children 6 weeks to 12 years: 5.5 to 8 mg/kg/day by I.M. injection or I.V. infusion given either as 1.8 to 2.7 mg/kg q 8 hours or as 2.7 to 4 mg/kg q 12 hours.

Neonates under 6 weeks: 4 to 6.5 mg/kg/day by I.M. injection or I.V. infusion given as 2 to 3.25 mg/kg q 12 hours.

Patients with impaired renal function: Initial dose is the same as for patients with normal renal function. Subsequent doses and frequency are determined by renal function and serum concentration of netilmicin.

CONTRAINDICATIONS & PRECAUTIONS

Contraindicated in patients with hypersensitivity to netilmicin, any aminoglycoside, or bisulfites. Use cautiously in patients with decreased renal function; tinnitus, vertigo, and high-frequency hearing loss who are susceptible to ototoxicity; dehydration, myasthenia gravis, parkinsonism, and hypocalcemia; and in neonates and other infants, and elderly patients.

ADVERSE REACTIONS

Common reactions are in italics; life-threatening reactions are in bold italics.

CNS: headache, lethargy, ***neuromuscular blockade.***

EENT: *ototoxicity (tinnitus, vertigo, hearing loss).*

GU: ***nephrotoxicity*** *(cells or casts in the urine; oliguria; proteinuria; decreased creatinine clearance; increased BUN, nonprotein nitrogen, and serum creatinine levels).*

Other: ***hypersensitivity.***

INTERACTIONS

Cephalothin: increases nephrotoxicity. Use together cautiously.

Dimenhydrinate: may mask symptoms of ototoxicity. Use with caution.

General anesthetics, neuromuscular blocking agents: may potentiate neuromuscular blockade.

I.V. loop diuretics (e.g., furosemide): increase ototoxicity. Use cautiously.

Other aminoglycosides, amphotericin B, cisplatin, methoxyflurane: increases nephrotoxicity. Use together cautiously.

Parenteral penicillins (e.g., carbenicillin, ticarcillin): netilmicin inactivation. Don't mix together in I.V.

EFFECTS ON DIAGNOSTIC TESTS

BUN, nonprotein nitrogen, or serum creatinine: elevated levels and increased urinary excretion of casts.

NURSING CONSIDERATIONS

Besides those related universally to drug therapy (see "How to use this book"), consider the following specific recommendations:

Assessment

• Obtain a baseline assessment of infection before therapy.

• Be alert for adverse reactions and drug interactions throughout therapy.

• Evaluate the patient's and family's knowledge about netilmicin therapy.

Nursing Diagnoses

• Injury related to potential ineffectiveness of netilmicin to eradicate the infection.

• Altered urinary elimination related to netilmicin-induced nephrotoxicity.

• Knowledge deficit related to netilmicin.

Planning and Implementation

Preparation and Administration

• Obtain specimen for culture and sensitivity tests before first dose. Therapy may begin pending test results.

• Weigh patient and determine baseline renal function before therapy.

• ***I.V. use:*** After completing I.V. infusion, flush the line with normal saline solution or dextrose 5% in water.

Monitoring

• Monitor effectiveness by regularly assessing for improvement of infection.

• Monitor serum netilmicin level. Draw blood for peak netilmicin level 1 hour after I.M. injection and 30 minutes to 1 hour after I.V. infusion ends; for trough levels, draw blood just before next dose. Don't use a heparinized tube because heparin is incompatible with aminoglycosides. Peak blood levels over 16 μg/ml and trough levels over 4 μg/ml may be associated with increased toxicity.

• Monitor renal function (intake and output, specific gravity, urinalysis, BUN, and creatinine levels, and creatinine clearance).

Supportive Care

• Be aware that usual duration of therapy is 7 to 10 days. If no response occurs in 3 to 5 days, therapy may be discontinued and new specimens obtained for culture and sensitivity.

• Notify doctor if patient shows signs of decreased renal function or complains of tinnitus, vertigo, or hearing loss.

• Encourage patient to consume 2,000 ml of fluid daily (if not contraindicated) during therapy to minimize chemical irritation of the renal tubules.

Patient Teaching

• Emphasize the need to drink 2,000 ml of fluid each day, not including coffee, tea, or other caffeinated beverages.

• Instruct the patient to notify the doctor immediately of changes in urine elimination patterns or hearing.

• Tell the patient to alert the doctor if infection worsens or does not improve.

• Stress the importance of recommended blood tests to monitor netilmicin level and renal function, to determine the effectiveness of therapy, or detect increased risk of adverse drug reactions.

• Teach patient to recognize and repeat the signs and symptoms of superinfection (continued fever and other signs of new infection, especially of upper respiratory tract).

Evaluation

In patients receiving netilmicin, appropriate evaluation statements may include:

• Patient is free of infection.

• Patient's renal function studies remain normal throughout therapy.

• Patient and family state an understanding of therapy.

nicardipine

(nye kar´ de peen)

Cardene

• *Classification:* antianginal, antihypertensive (calcium channel blocker)

• *Pregnancy Risk Category:* C

HOW SUPPLIED

Capsules: 20 mg, 30 mg

ACTION

Mechanism: Inhibits calcium ion influx across cardiac and smooth muscle cells, thus decreasing myocardial contractility and oxygen demand, and dilates coronary arteries and arterioles.

Absorption: Completely absorbed after oral administration. Absorption may be decreased if drug is taken with food.
Distribution: Extensively (>95%) bound to plasma proteins.
Metabolism: A substantial first-pass effect reduces absolute bioavailability to about 35%. The drug is extensively metabolized in the liver, and the process is saturable. Increasing dosage yields nonlinear increases in plasma levels.
Excretion: In the urine. Half-life: Elimination half-life is about 8.6 hours after steady-state levels are reached.
Onset, peak, duration: Plasma levels are detectable within 20 minutes and peak in about 1 hour.

INDICATIONS & DOSAGE

Chronic stable angina (used alone or in combination with beta blockers)–
Adults: initially, 20 mg P.O. t.i.d. Titrate dosage according to patient response. Usual dosage range is 20 to 40 mg P.O. t.i.d.
Hypertension–
Adults: initially, 20 to 40 mg P.O. t.i.d. Increase dosage according to patient response.

CONTRAINDICATIONS & PRECAUTIONS

Contraindicated in patients hypersensitive to the drug, and in patients with advanced aortic stenosis because the decrease in afterload produced by the drug may worsen myocardial oxygen balance in these patients. Some patients experience worsened severity, frequency, or duration of angina at start of therapy.

Use cautiously in patients with CHF because the drug has a negative inotropic effect. Careful monitoring of blood pressure is recommended during initiation of therapy.

ADVERSE REACTIONS

Common reactions are in italics; life-threatening reactions are in bold italics.
CNS: ***dizziness*** or light-headedness, *headache*, paresthesias, drowsiness, *asthenia.*
CV: *pedal edema,* palpitations, *angina,* tachycardia.
GI: nausea, abdominal discomfort, dry mouth.
Skin: rash, *flushing.*

INTERACTIONS

Antihypertensive agents: enhanced antihypertensive effect.
Beta-adrenergic blocking agents: may increase cardiac depressant effects. Monitor patient closely.
Cimetidine: may decrease metabolism of calcium channel blocking agents. Monitor for increased pharmacologic effect.
Cyclosporine: may increase plasma levels of cyclosporine. Monitor for toxicity.
Theophylline: pharmacologic effects of theophylline may be enhanced. Monitor for toxicity.

EFFECTS ON DIAGNOSTIC TESTS

None reported.

NURSING CONSIDERATIONS

Besides those related universally to drug therapy (see "How to use this book"), consider the following specific recommendations:

Assessment
- Obtain a baseline assessment of the patient's anginal status before nicardipine therapy.
- Be alert for adverse reactions and drug interactions throughout nicardipine therapy.
- Evaluate the patient's and family's knowledge about nicardipine therapy.

Nursing Diagnoses
- Pain related to ineffectiveness of nicardipine therapy.
- High risk for injury related to ni-

cardipine-induced CNS reactions or orthostatic hypotension.
• Knowledge deficit related to nicardipine.

Planning and Implementation

Preparation and Administration

• Expect patients with renal impairment to be titrated slowly to optimal response and patients with hepatic impairment to receive lower initial doses and to be carefully titrated to optimal response.
• Be aware that there should be a 3-day interval between dosage adjustments to achieve steady plasma levels.

Monitoring

• Monitor effectiveness by regularly evaluating the severity and frequency of the patient's anginal pain.
• Monitor patient for chest pain, especially at beginning of therapy or during dosage adjustment, because some patients may experience increased frequency, severity, or duration of chest pain at this time.
• Monitor blood pressure frequently during initial therapy. Maximum blood pressure response occurs about 1 hour after dosing. Monitor for potential orthostatic hypotension 1 to 2 hours after first dose.
• Monitor patient's heart rate and rhythm regularly.

Supportive Care

• Consult the doctor if the patient does not experience pain relief.
• Maintain safety precautions if adverse CNS reactions occur; assist the patient with daily activities to minimize energy expenditure.
• To minimize orthostatic hypotension have patient change to upright position slowly, go up and down stairs carefully, and lie down at the first sign of dizziness.
• Obtain an order for a mild analgesic if a headache occurs.
• Restrict the patient's fluid and sodium intake to minimize edema.
• Obtain an order for an antiemetic agent as needed.

Patient Teaching

• Stress importance of taking the drug exactly as prescribed even when feeling well.
• Advise patient to report chest pain immediately because some patients may experience increased frequency, severity, or duration of chest pain at beginning of therapy or during dosage adjustments.
• Instruct patient how to minimize orthostatic hypotension.
• Tell the patient to schedule activities to allow adequate rest.
• Encourage the patient to restrict fluid and sodium intake to minimize edema.

Evaluation

In patients receiving nicardipine, appropriate evaluation statements may include:
• Patient states anginal pain relief occurs with nicardipine therapy.
• Patient does not experience injury as a result of adverse CNS reactions or orthostatic hypotension caused by nicardipine therapy.
• Patient and family state an understanding of nicardipine therapy.

nicotine polacrilex (nicotine resin complex)

(nik´ oe teen)

Nicorette

• *Classification:* smoking cessation aid (nicotinic agonist)
• *Pregnancy Risk Category:* X

HOW SUPPLIED

Chewing gum: 2 mg/square

ACTION

Mechanism: Stimulates receptors in the CNS and causes the release of catecholamines from the adrenal medulla.

Absorption: The nicotine is bound to ion-exchange resin and is released

only during chewing; drug is not released if gum is swallowed. The blood level depends upon the vigor with which the gum is chewed.
Distribution: Distribution into tissues has not been fully characterized. Crosses the placenta and is distributed into the breast milk.
Metabolism: Primarily by the liver and somewhat by the kidney and lung. The main metabolites are cotinine and nicotine-1′-N-oxide.
Excretion: Both nicotine and its metabolites are excreted in urine, with approximately 10% to 20% excreted unchanged. Excretion of nicotine is increased in acid urine and by high urine output. Half life: About 1 hour.

INDICATIONS & DOSAGE

Temporary aid to the cigarette smoker seeking to give up smoking while participating in a behavior modification program under medical supervision–
Adults: chew one piece of gum slowly and intermittently for 30 minutes whenever the urge to smoke occurs. Most patients require approximately 10 pieces of gum daily during the first month. Don't exceed 30 pieces of gum daily.

CONTRAINDICATIONS & PRECAUTIONS

Contraindicated in nonsmokers; in patients recovering from a myocardial infarction, in those with life-threatening arrhythmias, and in those with severe or worsening angina pectoris (Buerger's disease, Prinzmetal variant angina), because it may exacerbate the symptoms of these disorders; in patients with active temporomandibular joint disease, because the drug is released by vigorous chewing; and in pregnant women because nicotine resin complex may cause fetal harm.

Use with caution in patients having pharyngeal inflammation and in those with a history of peptic ulcer or esophagitis; and in patients with dental problems that may be exacerbated by vigorous chewing.

To minimize the risk of dependence to Nicorette gum, encourage patient to stop using it after 3 months; longer use is not associated with further success in smoking cessation.

ADVERSE REACTIONS

Common reactions are in italics; life-threatening reactions are in bold italics.
CNS: dizziness, light-headedness.
CV: atrial fibrillation.
EENT: throat soreness, jaw muscle ache (from chewing).
GI: nausea, vomiting, indigestion.
Other: hiccups.

INTERACTIONS

None significant.

EFFECTS ON DIAGNOSTIC TESTS

None significant.

NURSING CONSIDERATIONS

Besides those related universally to drug therapy (see "How to use this book"), consider the following specific recommendations:

Assessment
- Obtain a baseline assessment of smoking history and cardiovascular status before therapy.
- Be alert for adverse reactions and drug interactions throughout therapy.
- Evaluate the patient's and family's knowledge about nicotine polacrilex therapy.

Nursing Diagnoses
- Altered health maintenance related to negative health habits.
- Decreased cardiac output related to drug induced atrial fibrillation.
- Knowledge deficit related to nicotine polacrilex.

Planning and Implementation
Preparation and Administration
• Determine patient's smoking history and habits.
• Have the patient chew the gum slowly and intermittently (chew several times then place between cheek and gums) for about 30 minutes to promote slow and even buccal absorption of nicotine.
Monitoring
• Monitor effectiveness by evaluating the patient's tolerance of smoking abstinence.
• Assess cardiovascular status of the patient on a weekly basis.
• Observe the patient for signs of nicotine overdose.
• Review duration of therapy. Drug should not be used longer than 6 months.
Supportive Care
• Encourage the patient to attend concurrent behavior modification classes.
• Review lifestyle changes that may result from cessation of smoking, (weight gain, increased energy, improved sleep pattern).
Patient Teaching
• Provide the instruction sheet which accompanies the drug. Instruct the patient to chew the gum slowly, then place between cheek and gum for 30 minutes to promote slow and even buccal absorption.
• Tell the patient the gum is sugarfree and won't stick to dental work.
• Review the importance of gradual withdrawal of the gum which can be done by cutting the gum in halves or quarters, and by mixing it with other sugarfree gum.
• Remind the patient that abstinence from smoking may require dosage adjustments in other medications (such as theophylline).
Evaluation
In patients receiving nicotine polacrilex, appropriate evaluation statements may include:
• Patient is no longer smoking.
• Patient denies palpitations related to adverse drug effects.
• Patient and family state an understanding of nicotine polacrilex therapy.

nifedipine
(nye fed´ i peen)
Adalat, Adalat P.A.†, Apo-Nifed, Novo-Nifedin, Procardia, Procardia XL

• *Classification:* antianginal (calcium channel blocker)
• *Pregnancy Risk Category:* C

HOW SUPPLIED
Tablets (sustained-release): 30 mg, 60 mg, 90 mg
Capsules: 10 mg, 20 mg

ACTION
Mechanism: A calcium channel blocker that inhibits calcium ion influx across cardiac and smooth muscle cells, decreasing myocardial contractility and oxygen demand, and dilates coronary arteries and arterioles.
Absorption: Approximately 90% of a dose is absorbed rapidly from the GI tract after oral administration; however, only about 65% to 70% of drug reaches the systemic circulation because of a significant first-pass effect in the liver.
Distribution: About 92% to 98% of circulating nifedipine is bound to plasma proteins.
Metabolism: Hepatic.
Excretion: In the urine and feces as inactive metabolites. Half-life: Elimination half-life is 2 to 5 hours.
Onset, peak, duration: Peak serum levels occur in about 30 minutes to 2 hours. Hypotensive effects may occur 5 minutes after sublingual administration. Duration of effect ranges from 4 to 12 hours.

INDICATIONS & DOSAGE

Management of vasospastic (also called Prinzmetal's or variant) angina and classic chronic stable angina pectoris; Raynaud's disease–
Adults: starting dose is 10 mg P.O. t.i.d. Usual effective dose range is 10 to 20 mg t.i.d. Some patients may require up to 30 mg q.i.d. Maximum daily dosage is 180 mg.
Hypertension–
Adults: 30 or 60 mg P.O. (sustained release form only) once daily. Titrate over a 7- to 14-day period.

CONTRAINDICATIONS & PRECAUTIONS

Contraindicated in patients with hypersensitivity to the drug. Use with caution in patients with CHF or aortic stenosis (especially if they are receiving concomitant beta blockers), because the drug may precipitate or worsen heart failure and cause excessive hypotension (from its peripheral vasodilatory effects), possibly exacerbating angina symptoms when therapy begins or dosage is increased.

ADVERSE REACTIONS

Common reactions are in italics; life-threatening reactions are in bold italics.
CNS: *dizziness, light-headedness, flushing, headache,* weakness, syncope.
CV: peripheral edema, hypotension, palpitations.
EENT: nasal congestion.
GI: *nausea, heartburn,* diarrhea.
Metabolic: hypokalemia.
Other: muscle cramps, dyspnea.

INTERACTIONS

Cimetidine, ranitidine: decreased nifedipine metabolism.
Propranolol (and other beta blockers): may cause hypotension and heart failure. Use together cautiously.

EFFECTS ON DIAGNOSTIC TESTS

Serum alkaline phosphate, LDH, AST (SGOT), and ALT (SGPT): mild to moderately increased concentration.

NURSING CONSIDERATIONS

Besides those related universally to drug therapy (see "How to use this book"), consider the following specific recommendations:

Assessment
- Obtain a baseline assessment of the patient's anginal status before therapy.
- Be alert for adverse reactions and drug interactions throughout nifedipine therapy.
- Evaluate the patient's and family's knowledge about nifedipine therapy.

Nursing Diagnoses
- Pain related to ineffectiveness of nifedipine therapy.
- High risk for injury related to nifedipine-induced CNS reactions.
- Knowledge deficit related to nifedipine.

Planning and Implementation

Preparation and Administration
- Do not break, crush, or have patient chew the capsules. Instead have patient swallow the capsule whole. The sustained-release tablets should never be chewed, crushed, or broken.
- Protect capsules from direct light and moisture and store at room temperature.
- No sublingual form of nifedipine is available. However, during an emergency the liquid in the oral capsule can be withdrawn by puncturing the capsule with a needle. The contents can then be instilled into the buccal pouch.
- Although a rebound effect hasn't been observed after withdrawal of the drug, expect dosage to be reduced slowly under a doctor's supervision.

Monitoring
• Monitor effectiveness by regularly evaluating the severity and frequency of the patient's anginal pain.
• Monitor blood pressure regularly, especially in patients who are also taking beta blockers or antihypertensives.
• Monitor serum potassium level regularly for hypokalemia.
Supportive Care
• Consult the doctor if the patient does not experience pain relief.
• Maintain safety precautions if adverse CNS reactions occur; assist the patient with daily activities to minimize energy expenditure.
• Obtain an order for a mild analgesic if a headache occurs.
• Restrict the patient's fluid and sodium intake to minimize edema.
• Obtain an order for an antiemetic agent as needed.
Patient Teaching
• Stress importance of taking the drug exactly as prescribed even when feeling well.
• If the patient is continuing nitrate therapy while drug dosage is being titrated, urge continued compliance. Sublingual nitroglycerin, especially, may be taken as needed when anginal symptoms are acute.
• Instruct the patient to swallow the capsule whole without breaking, crushing, or chewing it. Tell the patient that the sustained-release tablets should never be chewed, crushed, or broken.
• Advise patient to report chest pain immediately as some patients may experience anginal exacerbation at beginning of therapy or during dosage adjustments. Reassure the patient that this symptom is temporary.
• Advise the patient to notify a doctor if nifedipine does not relieve anginal pain.
• Advise the patient how to handle adverse GI reactions.
• Warn the patient to avoid hazardous activities that require mental alertness until CNS effects are known.
• Tell the patient to schedule activities to allow adequate rest.
• Encourage the patient to restrict fluid and sodium intake to minimize edema.

Evaluation
In patients receiving nifedipine, appropriate evaluation statements may include:
• Patient states anginal pain relief occurs with nifedipine therapy.
• Patient does not experience injury as a result of adverse CNS reactions to nifedipine therapy.
• Patient and family state an understanding of nifedipine therapy.

nimodipine
(nye moe´ di peen)
Nimotop

• *Classification:* cerebral vasodilator (calcium channel blocker)
• *Pregnancy Risk Category:* C

HOW SUPPLIED
Capsules: 30 mg

ACTION
Mechanism: A calcium channel blocking agent that inhibits calcium ion influx across cardiac and smooth muscle cells, thus decreasing myocardial contractility and oxygen demand, and dilates coronary arteries and arterioles. Initially thought to relieve vasospasm in patients after subarachnoid hemorrhage; its mechanism of action in the treatment of stroke is not fully known.
Absorption: Well absorbed after oral administration. However, because of extensive first-pass metabolism, bioavailability is only about 3% to 30%.
Distribution: Greater than 95% protein bound.

Metabolism: Extensively metabolized in the liver. The drug and metabolites undergo enterohepatic recycling.
Excretion: Less than 1% as the parent drug. Half-life: Elimination half-life is 1 to 9 hours.
Onset, peak, duration: Peak plasma levels are seen within 1 hour of an oral dose.

INDICATIONS & DOSAGE

Improvement of neurologic deficits in patients after subarachnoid hemorrhage from ruptured congenital aneurysms–
Adults: 60 mg P.O. q 4 hours for 21 days. Therapy should begin within 96 hours after subarachnoid hemorrhage.

CONTRAINDICATIONS & PRECAUTIONS

No known contraindications to nimodipine therapy. Drug was relatively well tolerated in clinical trials. Nimodipine should be reserved for patients who are in good neurologic condition postictus (for example, Hunt and Hess grades I to III).

ADVERSE REACTIONS

Common reactions are in italics; life-threatening reactions are in bold italics.
CNS: headaches.
CV: decreased blood pressure, flushing, edema.

INTERACTIONS

Antihypertensives: possible enhanced hypotensive effect.
Calcium channel blockers: possible enhanced cardiovascular effects.

EFFECTS ON DIAGNOSTIC TESTS

None reported.

NURSING CONSIDERATIONS

Besides those related universally to drug therapy (see "How to use this book"), consider the following recommendations:

Assessment
- Obtain a baseline assessment of the patient's underlying neurologic condition before drug therapy.
- Be alert for adverse reactions and drug interactions throughout nimodipine therapy.
- Evaluate the patient's and family's knowledge about nimodipine therapy.

Nursing Diagnoses
- Altered health maintenance related to the patient's underlying condition.
- Pain related to adverse drug reaction.
- Knowledge deficit related to nimodipine therapy.

Planning and Implementation

Preparation and Administration
- Patients with hepatic failure should receive lower doses. Begin therapy at 30 mg P.O. every 4 hours, with close monitoring of blood pressure and heart rate.

Monitoring
- Monitor blood pressure and heart rate in all patients, especially at the start of therapy.
- Monitor for drug interactions in patient receiving antihypertensives and calcium channel blockers.
- Monitor the patient for drug-induced headache.

Supportive Care
- Obtain an order for a mild analgesic if the patient develops a drug-induced headache.
- At the beginning of therapy, have the patient avoid any sudden position changes and to rise from the supine position slowly to avoid dizziness and hypotension.

Patient Teaching
- Teach the patient to avoid sudden position changes, which may cause dizziness and orthostatic hypotension.
- Tell patient to take a mild analgesic if headache develops.

Evaluation
In patients receiving nimodipine, appropriate evaluation statements may include:
• Patient is able to perform activities of daily living without assistance.
• Patient does not develop a headache.
• Patient and family state an understanding of nimodipine therapy.

PHARMACOLOGIC CLASS

nitrates
amyl nitrate
erythrityl tetranitrate
isosorbide dinitrate
nitroglycerin
pentaerythritol tetranitrate

OVERVIEW
Nitrates have been recognized as effective vasodilators for over 100 years. The best known drug of this group, nitroglycerin, remains the therapeutic mainstay for classic and variant angina. With the availability of a commercial I.V. nitroglycerin form, the drug's use in reducing afterload and preload in various cardiac disorders has generated renewed enthusiasm. Various other dosage forms of nitroglycerin and of the other nitrates also are available, thereby improving and extending their clinical usefulness.

Nitrates' major pharmacologic property is vascular smooth muscle relaxation, resulting in generalized vasodilation. Venous effects predominate; however, nitroglycerin produces dose-dependent dilation of both arterial and venous beds. Decreased peripheral venous resistance results in venous pooling of blood and decreased venous return to the heart (preload); decreased arteriolar resistance reduces systemic vascular resistance and arterial pressure (afterload). These vascular effects lead to reduction of myocardial oxygen consumption. In the coronary circulation, nitrates redistribute circulating blood flow along collateral channels and preferentially increase subendocardial blood flow, improving perfusion to the ischemic myocardium.

Nitrates relax all smooth muscle—not just vascular smooth muscle—regardless of autonomic innervation, including bronchial, biliary, gastrointestinal, ureteral, and uterine smooth muscle.

CLINICAL INDICATIONS AND ACTIONS
Angina pectoris
By relaxing vascular smooth muscle in both the venous and arterial beds, nitrates cause a net decrease in myocardial oxygen consumption; by dilating coronary vessels, they lead to redistribution of blood flow to ischemic tissue. Although systemic and coronary vascular effects may vary slightly, depending on which nitrate is used, both smooth muscle relaxation and vasodilation probably account for nitrates' value in treating angina. Because individual nitrates have similar pharmacologic and therapeutic properties, the best nitrate to use in a specific situation depends mainly on the onset of action and duration of effect required.

Sublingual nitroglycerin is considered the drug of choice to treat acute angina pectoris because of its rapid onset of action, relatively low cost, and well-established effectiveness. Lingual or buccal nitroglycerin and other rapidly acting nitrates (amyl nitrate and sublingual or chewable isosorbide dinitrate) also may prove useful for this indication. Amyl nitrate is rarely used because it is expensive, inconvenient, and carries a high risk of adverse effects. Sublingual, lingual, or buccal nitroglycerin or sublingual or chewable isosorbide dinitrate or erythritol tetranitrate typically prove effective in circumstances likely to provoke an angina attack.

Long-acting nitrates and/or beta-adrenergic blockers usually are considered the drugs of choice in the prophylactic management of angina pectoris. Nitrates with a relatively long duration of effect include oral preparations of erythrityl tetranitrate, isosorbide dinitrate, pentaerythritol tetranitrate, and oral or topical nitroglycerin.

The effectiveness of oral nitrates is debatable, although isosorbide dinitrate and nitroglycerin generally are now considered effective. However, the effectiveness of erythrityl tetranitrate, pentaerythritol tetranitrate, and topical nitroglycerin preparations has not been fully determined. Some experts believe oral nitrates are ineffective or less effective than rapidly acting I.V. nitrates in reducing frequency of angina and increasing exercise tolerance. Also, prolonged use of oral nitrates may cause cross-tolerance to sublingual nitrates.

I.V. nitroglycerin may be used to treat unstable angina pectoris, Prinzmetal's angina, and angina pectoris in patients who have not responded to recommended doses of nitrates and/or a beta-adrenergic blocker.

Sedatives may be useful in the adjunctive management of angina pectoris associated with psychogenic factors. However, if combination therapy is required, each drug should be adjusted individually; fixed combinations of oral nitrates and sedatives should be avoided.

Acute myocardial infarction

The hemodynamic effects of I.V., sublingual, or topical nitroglycerin may prove beneficial in treating left ventricular failure and pulmonary congestion associated with acute myocardial infarction. However, the drugs' effects on morbidity and mortality in patients with these conditions is controversial.

I.V., sublingual, and topical nitroglycerin and isosorbide dinitrate are effective adjunctive agents in managing acute and chronic heart failure. Sublingual administration can quickly reverse the signs and symptoms of pulmonary congestion in acute pulmonary edema; however, the I.V. form may control hemodynamic status more accurately.

OVERVIEW OF ADVERSE REACTIONS

Headache, the most common adverse effect, is most common early in therapy. Possibly severe, it usually diminishes rapidly. Postural hypotension may occur and may result in dizziness and/or weakness. Patients who are especially sensitive to hypotensive effects may experience nausea, vomiting, weakness, restlessness, pallor, cold sweats, tachycardia, syncope, or cardiovascular collapse. Alcohol may intensify these effects. Transient flushing may occur; GI upset may be controlled by a temporary dosage reduction. If blurred vision, dry mouth, or rash develops, therapy should be discontinued (rash occurs more commonly with pentaerythritol). Both tolerance and dependence to these agents can occur with repeated, prolonged use.

Tolerance to both the vascular and antianginal effects of the drugs can develop, and cross-tolerance between the nitrates and nitrites has been demonstrated. Tolerance is associated with a high or sustained plasma drug concentration and occurs most frequently with oral, I.V., and topical therapy. It rarely occurs with intermittent sublingual use. However, patients taking oral isosorbide dinitrate or topical nitroglycerin have not exhibited cross-tolerance to sublingual nitroglycerin.

Development of tolerance can be prevented by using the lowest effective dose and maintaining an intermittent dosing schedule. A nitrate-free interval of 10 to 12 hours daily (for example, by removing the transdermal nitroglycerin patch in the early evening and not reapplying until the next morning) may also help prevent tolerance.

REPRESENTATIVE COMBINATIONS
None.

---

nitrofurantoin macrocrystals
(nye troe fyoor an´ toyn)
Macrodantin

nitrofurantoin microcrystals
Apo-Nitrofurantoin†, Furadantin, Furalan, Furan, Furanite, Macrodantin, Nephronex†, Nitrofan, Novofuran†

• *Classification:* urinary tract antiseptic (nitrofuran)
• *Pregnancy Risk Category:* B

HOW SUPPLIED
macrocrystals
Capsules: 25 mg, 50 mg, 100 mg
Oral suspension: 25 mg/5 ml
microcrystals
Tablets: 50 mg, 100 mg
Capsules: 50 mg, 100 mg
Oral suspension: 25 mg/5 ml

ACTION
Mechanism: Bacteriostatic in low concentration and possibly bactericidal in high concentration by interference with bacterial enzyme systems.
Absorption: When administered orally, nitrofurantoin is well absorbed (mainly by the small intestine) from the GI tract. Presence of food aids drug's dissolution and speeds absorption, especially with the macrocrystal form. Microcrystal form is absorbed more rapidly, but may be more irritating to the GI tract.
Distribution: Crosses into bile and placenta; 20% to 60% binds to plasma proteins.
Metabolism: Partially metabolized in the liver.
Excretion: About 30% to 50% of dose is eliminated by glomerular filtration and tubular excretion to urine as unchanged drug within 24 hours. Some drug may be excreted in breast milk. Half-life: Approximately 20 minutes.
Onset, peak, duration: Peak urine concentrations occur in about 30 minutes when drug is given as microcrystals; later when given as macrocrystals.

INDICATIONS & DOSAGE
Pyelonephritis, pyelitis, and cystitis due to susceptible Escherichia coli, Staphylococcus aureus, *enterococci; certain strains of* Klebsiella, Proteus, *and* Enterobacter–
Adults and children over 12 years: 50 to 100 mg P.O. q.i.d. with milk or meals.
Children 1 month to 12 years: 5 to 7 mg/kg P.O. daily, divided q.i.d.
Long-term suppression therapy–
Adults: 50 to 100 mg P.O. daily at bedtime.
Children: 1 to 2 mg/kg P.O. daily at bedtime.

CONTRAINDICATIONS & PRECAUTIONS
Contraindicated in patients with severe renal dysfunction (creatinine clearance less than 40 ml/minute) because urine concentrations of the drug will be ineffective and toxicity may occur; in infants under age 1 month, in pregnant patients, and in patients with glucose-6-phosphate dehydrogenase (G6PD) deficiency because of the potential for hemolytic anemias; and in patients with hypersensitivity to the drug. Use cautiously in patients with diabetes mellitus, asthma, anemia, vitamin B deficiency, or electrolyte imbalance, because it

increases the risk of peripheral neuropathy.

ADVERSE REACTIONS

Common reactions are in italics; life-threatening reactions are in bold italics.

Blood: ***hemolysis in patients with G6PD deficiency*** (reversed after stopping drug), ***agranulocytosis,*** thrombocytopenia.

CNS: peripheral neuropathy, headache, dizziness, drowsiness, *ascending polyneuropathy with high doses or renal impairment.*

GI: *anorexia, nausea, vomiting,* abdominal pain, *diarrhea.*

Hepatic: hepatitis.

Skin: maculopapular, erythematous, or eczematous eruption; pruritus; urticaria; *exfoliative dermatitis;* ***Stevens-Johnson syndrome.***

Other: asthmatic attacks in patients with history of asthma; ***anaphylaxis;*** hypersensitivity; transient alopecia; drug fever; overgrowth of nonsusceptible organisms in the urinary tract; *pulmonary sensitivity reactions (cough, chest pains, fever, chills, dyspnea).*

INTERACTIONS

Magnesium-containing antacids: decreased nitrofurantoin absorption. Separate administration times by 1 hour.

Nalidixic acid, norfloxacin: possible decreased effectiveness. Avoid using together.

Probenecid, sulfinpyrazone: increased blood levels and decreased urine levels. May result in increased toxicity and lack of therapeutic effect. Don't use together.

EFFECTS ON DIAGNOSTIC TESTS

CBC: decreased RBC (anemia).

Liver function tests: abnormal results.

Urine glucose tests with copper sulfate (Benedict's test, Fehling's test, or Clinitest): false-positive results.

NURSING CONSIDERATIONS

Besides those related universally to drug therapy (see "How to use this book"), consider the following specific recommendations:

Assessment

- Obtain a baseline assessment of infection before therapy.
- Be alert for adverse reactions and drug interactions throughout therapy.
- Evaluate the patient's and family's knowledge about nitrofurantoin therapy.

Nursing Diagnoses

- High risk for injury related to ineffectiveness of nitrofurantoin to eradicate the infection.
- High risk for fluid volume deficit related to nitrofurantoin induced adverse GI reactions.
- Knowledge deficit related to nitrofurantoin.

Planning and Implementation

Preparation and Administration

- Obtain specimen for culture and sensitivity tests before first dose. Therapy may begin pending test results.
- Administer with food or milk to minimize GI distress.
- Store in amber container. Keep away from metals other than stainless steel or aluminum to avoid precipitate formation.
- Expect to continue treatment for 3 days after sterile urine specimens have been obtained.

Monitoring

- Monitor effectiveness by regularly assessing for improvement in the infection.
- Be aware that some patients may experience fewer GI adverse effects with nitrofurantoin macrocrystals.
- Monitor intake/output carefully.
- Monitor patient for hypersensitivity with long-term use.
- Monitor urine culture and sensitivity tests, pulmonary status, and CBC regularly, as ordered.

• Monitor hydration status if adverse GI reactions occur.
Supportive Care
• Obtain an order for an antiemetic or antidiarrheal agent as needed.
• Do not use copper sulfate reduction method (Clinitest) to determine urine glucose because drug may cause false-positive results.
• Be aware that drug may turn urine brown or darker.
Patient Teaching
• Tell patient to take the drug with food or milk to minimize GI distress.
• Stress importance of frequent urine and blood tests to monitor effectiveness of therapy and detect adverse reactions.
• Teach patient how to measure intake/output. Warn patient that the drug will turn urine brown or darker.
• Instruct patient to store drug in original container and to keep it away from metals except stainless steel or aluminum to avoid precipitate formation.
• Tell diabetic patients not to use Clinitest to determine urine glucose because drug may cause false-positive result.
Evaluation
In patients receiving nitrofurantoin, appropriate evaluation statements may include:
• Patient is free from infection.
• Patient maintains adequate hydration throughout nitrofurantoin therapy.
• Patient and family state an understanding of nitrofurantoin therapy.

nitrofurazone
(nye troe fu´ rah zone)
Furacin

• *Classification:* topical antibacterial (nitrofuran derivative)
• *Pregnancy Risk Category:* C

HOW SUPPLIED
Cream: 0.2%
Ointment: 0.2% (soluble dressing)
Topical solution: 0.2%

ACTION
Mechanism: Inhibits bacterial enzymes responsible for carbohydrate metabolism.
Pharmacokinetics: Unknown.

INDICATIONS & DOSAGE
Adjunctive treatment of second- and third-degree burns (especially when resistance to other antibiotics and sulfonamides occurs); prevention of skin allograft rejection–
Adults and children: apply directly to lesion daily or every few days, depending on severity of burn.

CONTRAINDICATIONS & PRECAUTIONS
Contraindicated in patients with hypersensitivity to the drug. Use may result in bacterial or fungal overgrowth of nonsusceptible organisms, which may lead to secondary infections. Use with caution in patients with renal impairment.

ADVERSE REACTIONS
Common reactions are in italics; life-threatening reactions are in bold italics.
GU: possible renal toxicity.
Skin: *erythema, pruritus,* burning, edema, severe reactions (vesiculation, denudation, ulceration), *allergic contact dermatitis.*

INTERACTIONS
None significant.

EFFECTS ON DIAGNOSTIC TESTS
None reported.

NURSING CONSIDERATIONS
Besides those related universally to drug therapy (see "How to use this book"), consider the following specific recommendations:

Assessment
- Obtain a baseline assessment of burn wounds before therapy.
- Be alert for adverse reactions and drug interactions throughout therapy.
- Evaluate the patient's and family's knowledge about nitrofurazone therapy.

Nursing Diagnoses
- High risk for infection related to burn wounds.
- Impaired skin integrity related to nitrofurazone-induced allergic contact dermatitis.
- Knowledge deficit related to nitrofurazone therapy.

Planning and Implementation
Preparation and Administration
- Clean wound as indicated by doctor before reapplying dressings. When using wet dressing, protect skin around wound with zinc oxide.
- Store solution in tight light-resistant containers (brown bottles). Avoid exposure of solution at all times to direct light, prolonged heat, and alkaline materials.

Monitoring
- Monitor effectiveness by regularly examining burn wounds.
- Monitor serum creatinine regularly.
- Monitor for adverse reactions and interactions by frequently examining the patient's skin for irritation, sensitization, or infection.

Supportive Care
- Be prepared to discontinue the drug and notify doctor if adverse reactions occur.
- Use cautiously in patients with known or susceptible renal impairment.
- Remember, drug may discolor in light but is still usable because it retains its potency.
- Discard cloudy solutions if warming to 131° to 140° F. (55° to 60° C.) does not restore clarity.
- Use reverse isolation and/or sterile application technique to prevent further wound contamination.

Patient Teaching
- Teach patient to apply medication.
- Instruct patient to notify doctor of any adverse reactions.

Evaluation
In patients receiving nitrofurazone therapy, appropriate evaluation statements may include:
- Burn wounds have healed.
- Allergic dermatitis did not occur.
- Patient and family state an understanding of nitrofurazone therapy.

nitroglycerin (glyceryl trinitrate)
(nye troe gli´ ser in)
Deponit, Klavikordal, Niong, Nitradisc‡, Nitro-Bid, Nitro-Bid I.V., Nitrocap, Nitrocap T.D., Nitrocine, Nitrodisc, Nitro-Dur, Nitro-Dur II, Nitrogard, Nitrogard SR, Nitrol, Nitrolate Ointment‡, Nitrolin, Nitrolingual, Nitrol TSAR, Nitronet, Nitrong, Nitrong S.R., Nitrospan, Nitrostat, Nitrostat I.V., NTS, Transderm-Nitro, Tridil

- *Classification:* antianginal, vasodilator (nitrate)
- *Pregnancy Risk Category:* C

HOW SUPPLIED
Tablets (buccal): 1 mg, 2 mg, 3 mg
Tablets (sublingual): 0.15 mg (1/400 gr), 0.3 mg (1/200 gr), 0.4 mg (1/150 gr), 0.6 mg (1/100 gr)
Tablets (sustained-release): 2.6 mg, 6.5 mg, 9 mg
Capsules (sustained-release): 6.5 mg, 9 mg
I.V.: 0.5 mg/ml, 0.8 mg/ml, 5 mg/ml
Aerosol (translingual): 0.4 mg/metered spray
Topical: 2% ointment
Transdermal: 2.5 mg, 5 mg, 7.5 mg, 10 mg, 15 mg/24 hour systems

ACTION

Mechanism: Reduces cardiac oxygen demand by decreasing left ventricular end-diastolic pressure (preload) and, to a lesser extent, systemic vascular resistance (afterload). Also increases blood flow through the collateral coronary vessels.

Absorption: Well absorbed from the GI tract. However, because it undergoes first-pass metabolism in the liver, the drug is incompletely absorbed into the systemic circulation. After sublingual administration, absorption from the oral mucosa is relatively complete; also well absorbed after topical administration as an ointment or transdermal system.

Distribution: Widely distributed throughout the body. About 60% of circulating drug is bound to plasma proteins.

Metabolism: In the liver and serum to 1,3 glyceryl dinitrate, 1,2 glyceryl dinitrate, and glyceryl mononitrate. Dinitrate metabolites have a slight vasodilatory effect.

Excretion: Metabolites are excreted in the urine. Half-life: About 1 to 4 minutes.

Onset, peak, duration: Onset of action for oral preparations is slow (except for sublingual tablets). Onset of action for various preparations is as follows: I.V., 1 to 2 minutes; sublingual, 1 to 3 minutes; translingual spray, 2 minutes; transmucosal tablet, 3 minutes; ointment, 20 to 60 minutes; oral (sustained-release), 40 minutes; transdermal, 40 to 60 minutes. Duration of effect is as follows: I.V., 30 minutes; sublingual, up to 30 minutes; translingual spray, 30 to 60 minutes; transmucosal tablet, 5 hours; ointment, 3 to 6 hours; oral (sustained-release), 4 to 8 hours; transdermal, 18 to 24 hours.

INDICATIONS & DOSAGE

Prophylaxis against chronic anginal attacks–

Adults: 2.5 mg sustained-release (capsule) q 8 to 12 hours; or 2% ointment: Start with ½″ ointment, increasing by ½″ increments until headache occurs, then decreasing to previous dose. Range of dosage with ointment is 2″ to 5″. Usual dose is 1″ to 2″. Alternatively, transdermal disc or pad (Nitrodisc, Nitro-Dur, or Transderm-Nitro) may be applied to hairless site once daily.

Relief of acute angina pectoris, prophylaxis to prevent or minimize anginal attacks when taken immediately before stressful events–

Adults: 1 sublingual tablet (gr 1/400, 1/200, 1/150, 1/100) dissolved under the tongue or in the buccal pouch immediately upon indication of anginal attack. May repeat q 5 minutes for 15 minutes. Or, using Nitrolingual spray, spray one or two doses into mouth, preferably onto or under the tongue. May repeat q 3 to 5 minutes to a maximum of 3 doses within a 15-minute period. Or, transmucosally, 1 to 3 mg q 3 to 5 hours during waking hours.

To control hypertension associated with surgery; to treat CHF associated with myocardial infarction (MI); to relieve angina pectoris in acute situations; to produce controlled hypotension during surgery (by I.V. infusion)–

Adults: initial infusion rate is 5 mcg/minute. May be increased by 5 mcg/minute q 3 to 5 minutes until a response is noted. If a 20 mcg/minute rate doesn't produce a response, dosage may be increased by as much as 20 mcg/minute q 3 to 5 minutes.

CONTRAINDICATIONS & PRECAUTIONS

Contraindicated in patients with head trauma or cerebral hemorrhage, because of potential for increased intracranial pressure (ICP); severe anemia, because nitrate ions can readily oxidize hemoglobin to methemoglobin; and in patients with a history of hypersensitivity or idiosyncratic reaction to nitrates; contraindicated in patients with hypotension or uncorrected hypovolemia, because the drug may cause severe hypotension and shock; and constrictive pericarditis and pericardial tamponade, because the drug may cause hypotension, reduce preload, and decrease cardiac output.

Use with caution in patients with ICP, because the drug dilates meningeal vessels; open- or closed-angle glaucoma, although intraocular pressure is increased only briefly and drainage of aqueous humor from the eye is unimpeded; diuretic-induced fluid depletion or low systolic blood pressure (less than 90 mm Hg), because of the drug's hypotensive effect; and during the initial days after acute MI because the drug may cause excessive hypotension and tachycardia. (However, nitroglycerin has been used with some success to decrease myocardial ischemia and possibly reduce the extent of infarction.)

Tolerance to both the vascular and antianginal effects of the drugs can develop, and cross-tolerance between the nitrates and nitrites has been demonstrated. Tolerance is associated with a high or sustained plasma drug concentration and occurs most frequently with oral, I.V., and topical therapy. It rarely occurs with intermittent sublingual use. However, patients taking oral isosorbide dinitrate or topical nitroglycerin have not exhibited cross-tolerance to sublingual nitroglycerin.

Tolerance can be prevented by using the lowest effective dose and maintaining an intermittent dosing schedule. A nitrate-free interval of 10 to 12 hours daily (for example, by removing the transdermal nitroglycerin patch in the early evening and not reapplying until the next morning) may also help prevent tolerance.

ADVERSE REACTIONS

Common reactions are in italics; life-threatening reactions are in bold italics.
CNS: *headache, sometimes with throbbing; dizziness;* weakness.
CV: *orthostatic hypotension, tachycardia, flushing, palpitations,* fainting.
GI: nausea, vomiting.
Skin: cutaneous vasodilation.
Local: sublingual burning.
Other: hypersensitivity.

INTERACTIONS

Antihypertensives: possibly enhanced hypotensive effect. Monitor closely.

EFFECTS ON DIAGNOSTIC TESTS

Serum cholesterol (Zlatkis-Zak color reaction): falsely decreased values.

NURSING CONSIDERATIONS

Besides those related universally to drug therapy (see "How to use this book"), consider the following specific recommendations:

Assessment

- Obtain a baseline assessment of patient's angina or blood pressure (if used to control hypertension or produce controlled hypotension) before nitroglycerin therapy.
- Be alert for adverse reactions or drug interactions throughout therapy.
- Evaluate patient's and family's knowledge about nitroglycerin therapy.

Nursing Diagnoses

- Pain related to ineffectiveness of nitroglycerin.
- Potential for injury related to nitroglycerin-induced dizziness or orthostatic hypotension.
- Knowledge deficit related to nitroglycerin.

Planning and Implementation

Preparation and Administration

• ***Topical use:*** Spread ointment in a uniform, thin layer on any hairless body area. Do not rub in. Cover with plastic film to aid absorption and protect clothing.

• If using Tape-Surrounded Appli-Ruler (TSAR) system, keep the TSAR on skin to protect patient's clothing and to ensure that ointment remains in place. Remove all excess ointment from previous site before applying the next dose. Avoid getting ointment on fingers.

• Transdermal dosage forms can be applied to any hairless part of the skin except distal parts of the arms or legs, because absorption will not be maximal at these sites.

• When terminating transdermal treatment for angina, gradually reduce the dosage and frequency of application over 4 to 6 weeks as ordered.

• ***Sublingual use:*** Place the tablet under the patient's tongue. Dose may be repeated every 10 to 15 minutes for a maximum of three doses. The patient who complains of tingling sensation with drug administration may try holding tablet in buccal pouch. Sublingual nitroglycerin tablets are still potent if they cause a burning sensation under the tongue. However, not all currently available preparations produce this sensation.

• ***Buccal use:*** Have patient place the tablet between his lip and gum above the incisors or between his cheek and gum. Make sure the patient doesn't swallow or chew the tablet, as this will make it ineffective.

• ***Lingual spray use:*** Nitroglycerin lingual spray should not be swallowed immediately after administering. Have the patient wait about 10 seconds or so before swallowing.

• ***P.O. use:*** Administer oral tablets on an empty stomach, either 30 minutes before or 1 to 2 hours after meals.

• ***I.V. use:*** Infuse diluted drug at the rate required for therapeutic effect. Always administer with an infusion pump and titrate the dose to desired patient response. Always mix in glass bottles and avoid use of I.V. filters because the drug binds to plastic. Regular polyvinyl chloride (PVC) tubing can bind up to 80% of the drug, requiring infusions of higher dosages. A special nonabsorbing (non-PVC) tubing is available from the manufacturer; patients receive more drug when these infusion sets are used. Always use the same type of infusion set when changing I.V. lines.

• Tolerance may develop rather quickly, especially with the long-acting forms of nitrates. To prevent tolerance, the patient should have a daily nitrate-free interval of 6 to 12 hours. Nitroglycerin patches should be applied in the morning and removed at bedtime. Sustained-release capsules should be taken morning, noon, and night as opposed to every 8 hours. Nitrate-free intervals help maintain responsiveness to the drug's clinical effects.

Monitoring

• Monitor effectiveness to prevent or relieve anginal pain by assessing patient's degree and frequency of pain.

• Monitor for headache, which may be throbbing but usually subsides in a few days as tolerance develops.

• Monitor blood pressure, heart rate, and intensity and duration of response to drug; ask the patient about palpitations.

• Closely monitor vital signs during infusion of nitroglycerin. Be particularly aware of blood pressure, especially if the drug is being used in a patient with an MI. Excessive hypotension may worsen the MI.

Supportive Care

• Alert the doctor immediately if nitroglycerin is ineffective; keep patient at rest during anginal attacks.

• Be sure to remove transdermal

patch before defibrillation. Because the patch has an aluminum backing, the electric current may cause it to explode.
• Treat headache with a mild analgesic as ordered.
• Assist the patient to a sitting or standing position gradually to minimize effects of orthostatic hypotension.
• Maintain safety precautions during nitroglycerin therapy. Keep bed rails up and assist patient with activities such as walking if dizziness occurs (with long-acting forms of nitrates).

Patient Teaching
• Tell the patient to take medication regularly, even long-term, as prescribed, and to keep it easily accessible at all times.
• Tell the patient that an additional dose may be taken before anticipated stress or at bedtime if angina is nocturnal.
• Teach the patient how to administer the prescribed form of nitroglycerin.
• Instruct patient taking sublingual tablets that dose may be repeated every 10 to 15 minutes for a maximum of three doses. If this provides no relief the patient should call a doctor or go to a hospital emergency room.
• Instruct patient to use caution when wearing a transdermal patch near a microwave oven. Leaking radiation may heat the patch's metallic backing and cause burns.
• Tell the patient to store nitroglycerin sublingual tablets in their original container or another container specifically approved for this use; also tell the patient to store drug in cool, dark place in a tightly closed container. To ensure freshness, the patient should replace the supply of sublingual tablets every 3 months. Tell the patient to remove cotton from container, because it absorbs drug.
• Advise the patient not to carry bottle containing sublingual or submucosal tablets close to the body because body heat may accelerate decomposition of the tablets; patient should carry it in a jacket pocket or purse, and never store it in a closed car or glove compartment.
• Inform the patient that headache usually subsides in a few days as tolerance develops; tell the patient to take a mild analgesic for headache relief until tolerance ccours.
• Nitroglycerin may cause orthostatic hypotension. Teach the patient how to minimize it by changing to an upright position slowly, going up and down the stairs carefully, and lying down at the first sign of dizziness.

Evaluation
In patients receiving nitroglycerin, appropriate evaluation statements may include:
• Patient reports nitroglycerin relieves anginal pain.
• Patient does not experience injury as a result of dizziness or orthostatic hypotension.
• Patient and family state an understanding of nitroglycerin therapy.

nitroprusside sodium
(nye troe pruss´ ide)
Nipride, Nitropress

• *Classification:* antihypertensive (vasodilator)
• *Pregnancy Risk Category:* C

HOW SUPPLIED
Injection: 50 mg/vial in 2-ml, 5-ml vials

ACTION
Mechanism: Relaxes both arteriolar and venous smooth muscle.
Absorption: Drug is administered I.V.
Distribution: Drug distributes to extracellular space.
Metabolism: Rapidly metabolized in

erythrocytes and tissues and is converted to thiocyanate.
Excretion: Thiocyanate is excreted primarily in urine. Half-life: Circulating half-life of nitroprusside is about 2 minutes; elimination half-life of thiocyanate is about 3 days in patients with normal renal function.
Onset, peak, duration: I.V. infusion reduces blood pressure almost immediately. Blood pressure returns to pretreatment level 1 to 10 minutes after infusion ends.

INDICATIONS & DOSAGE

To lower blood pressure quickly in hypertensive emergencies; to control hypotension during anesthesia; to reduce preload and afterload in cardiac pump failure or cardiogenic shock; may be used with or without dopamine–
Adults: 50-mg vial diluted with 2 to 3 ml of dextrose 5% in water I.V. and then added to 250, 500, or 1,000 ml dextrose 5% in water. Infuse at 0.5 to 10 mcg/kg/minute. Average dose is 3 mcg/kg/minute. Maximum infusion rate is 10 mcg/kg/minute.

Patients taking other antihypertensive drugs along with nitroprusside are very sensitive to this drug. Adjust dosage accordingly.

CONTRAINDICATIONS & PRECAUTIONS

Contraindicated in patients with hypersensitivity to the drug and in patients with compensatory hypertension secondary to arteriovenous shunt or coarctation of the aorta, because a decrease in blood pressure may be harmful to these patients.

Use cautiously in patients with renal insufficiency because thiocyanate, one of the metabolic products of nitroprusside, is excreted by the kidneys, and may accumulate; hepatic insufficiency because drug metabolism may be impaired; hypothyroidism because thiocyanate inhibits iodine uptake and binding; and low vitamin B_{12} concentrations because the drug may interfere with vitamin B_{12} distribution and metabolism.

ADVERSE REACTIONS

Common reactions are in italics; life-threatening reactions are in bold italics.
The following adverse reactions usually indicate overdosage:
CNS: *headache, dizziness,* ataxia, loss of consciousness, coma, weak pulse, absent reflexes, widely dilated pupils, *restlessness, muscle twitching, diaphoresis.*
CV: distant heart sounds, palpitations, dyspnea, shallow breathing.
GI: *vomiting, nausea, abdominal pain.*
Metabolic: acidosis.
Skin: pink color.

INTERACTIONS

None significant.

EFFECTS ON DIAGNOSTIC TESTS

Serum creatinine: increased concentration.

NURSING CONSIDERATIONS

Besides those related universally to drug therapy (see "How to use this book"), consider the following specific recommendations:

Assessment

- Obtain a baseline assessment of the patient's blood pressure before beginning therapy.
- Be alert for adverse reactions or drug interactions during therapy.
- Evaluate the patient's and family's knowledge about nitroprusside sodium therapy.

Nursing Diagnoses

- Altered tissue perfusion (renal, cerebral, cardiopulmonary, peripheral) related to the patient's underlying condition.
- Pain related to nitroprusside-induced adverse reactions such as headache and abdominal discomfort.

• Knowledge deficit related to nitroprusside therapy.

Planning and Implementation

Preparation and Administration

• Keep the patient supine when initiating and titrating nitroprusside therapy.

• Obtain baseline vital signs before giving this drug, and find out what parameters the doctor wants to achieve.

• ***I.V. use:*** When preparing this drug don't use bacteriostatic water for injection or sterile 0.9% sodium chloride solution for reconstitution. Because of light sensitivity, wrap I.V. solution in foil; it is not necessary to wrap the tubing. Fresh solutions should have a faint brownish tint. Discard the solution after 24 hours. It's best to run the drug piggyback through a peripheral line with no other medication using a continuous infusion pump. Don't adjust the rate of the main I.V. line while the drug is running.

Monitoring

• Monitor effectiveness by checking the patient's blood pressure every 5 minutes at the start of the infusion and every 15 minutes thereafter.

• Keep in mind that even small bolus doses of nitroprusside can cause severe hypotension.

• Check serum thiocyanate levels every 72 hours because excessive doses or rapid infusion (> 15 mcg/kg/minute) of this drug can cause cyanide toxicity. Thiocyanate levels over 100 mcg/ml are associated with toxicity. Watch for signs of thiocyanate toxicity: profound hypotension, metabolic acidosis, dyspnea, headache, loss of consciousness, ataxia, and vomiting.

Supportive Care

• If severe hypotension occurs, stop the infusion of nitroprusside; effects of the drug quickly reverse. Notify the doctor and prepare for insertion of an arterial line. Then regulate the drug flow to the specified level.

• Keep in mind that this drug is sometimes used with a direct-acting cardiac stimulant such as dopamine in patients with refractory heart failure.

• If signs of thiocyanate toxicity occur, discontinue the drug immediately and notify the doctor.

Patient Teaching

• Explain that this drug will rapidly reduce the patient's blood pressure.

• Advise the patient to tell you immediately if he experiences headache, dizziness, or abdominal pain.

Evaluation

In patients receiving nitroprusside, appropriate evaluation statements may include:

• Blood pressure controlled within normal limits for this patient.

• Pain from headache and abdominal discomfort did not occur.

• Patient and family state an understanding of nitroprusside sodium therapy.

nizatidine

(ni za´ ti deen)

Axid

• *Classification:* antiulcer (histamine H_2-receptor antagonist)

• *Pregnancy Risk Category:* C

HOW SUPPLIED

Capsules: 150 mg, 300 mg

ACTION

Mechanism: Competitively inhibits the action of histamine at H_2-receptor sites of the parietal cells, decreasing gastric acid secretion.

Absorption: Well absorbed (> 90%) after oral administration. Absorption may be slightly enhanced by food and slightly impaired by antacids.

Distribution: Approximately 35% is bound to plasma protein.
Metabolism: Probably undergoes hepatic metabolism. About 40% of excreted drug is metabolized; the remainder is excreted unchanged.
Excretion: More than 90% of an oral dose of nizatidine is excreted in the urine within 12 hours. Renal clearance is about 500 ml/minute, which indicates excretion by active tubular secretion. Less than 6% of an administered dose is eliminated in the feces. Half-life: 1 to 2 hours. Moderate to severe renal impairment significantly prolongs the half-life and decreases the clearance of nizatidine. In anephric persons, the half-life is 3.5 to 11 hours; the plasma clearance is 7 to 14 liters per hour.
Onset, peak, duration: Peak plasma concentrations occur from 0.5 to 3 hours after a dose.

INDICATIONS & DOSAGE

Active duodenal ulcer treatment–
Adults: 300 mg P.O. once daily at bedtime. Alternatively, patient may receive 150 mg b.i.d.
Maintenance therapy of duodenal ulcer–
Adults: 150 mg once daily h.s.

CONTRAINDICATIONS & PRECAUTIONS

Contraindicated in patients with hypersensitivity to the drug. Use with caution in patients with hypersensitivity to other H_2-receptor antagonists.

ADVERSE REACTIONS

Common reactions are in italics; life-threatening reactions are in bold italics.
Blood: ***thrombocytopenia.***
CNS: *somnolence.*
CV: arrhythmias.
Skin: *sweating,* rash, urticaria, ***exfoliative dermatitis.***
Other: hepatic damage, hyperuricemia, gynecomastia.

INTERACTIONS

Aspirin: nizatidine may elevate serum salicylate levels in patients taking high doses of aspirin.

EFFECTS ON DIAGNOSTIC TESTS

Alkaline phosphatase, serum ALT, serum AST: increased levels.
Urobilinogen: false-positive results.

NURSING CONSIDERATIONS

Besides those related universally to drug therapy (see "How to use this book"), consider the following specific recommendations:

Assessment
- Obtain a baseline assessment of the patient's GI pain before initiating nizatidine therapy.
- Be alert for adverse reactions or drug interactions during therapy.
- Evaluate the patient's and family's knowledge about nizatidine therapy.

Nursing Diagnoses
- Pain related to the patient's underlying condition.
- High risk for impaired skin integrity related to nizatidine-induced dermatitis.
- Knowledge deficit related to nizatidine therapy.

Planning and Implementation
Preparation and Administration
- Expect reduced dosage in patient with impaired renal function. Patients with a creatinine clearance of 20 to 50 ml/minute should receive 150 mg daily for treatment of active duodenal ulcer, or 150 mg every other day for maintenance therapy. Patients with a creatinine clearance below 20 ml/minute should receive 150 mg every other day for treatment or 150 mg every third day for maintenance.

Monitoring
- Monitor effectiveness by regularly assessing for relief of GI pain.
- Evaluate hematologic studies for signs of abnormalities, such as granulocytopenia.
- Check the patient's skin for rashes

and frequently ask about skin problems.

Supportive Care

• Notify the doctor if a skin problem or other adverse reactions develop.

Patient Teaching

• Urge the patient to avoid smoking cigarettes, which may increase gastric acid secretion and worsen disease.

• Instruct the patient to avoid sources of GI irritation, such as alcohol, certain foods, and drugs containing aspirin.

• Warn the patient to take drug as directed and to continue taking it even after pain subsides, to allow for adequate healing.

Evaluation

In patients receiving nizatidine, appropriate evaluation statements may include:

• Patient has decrease in or relief of GI pain.

• Patient's skin remains normal with no evidence of rash.

• Patient and family state an understanding of nizatidine therapy.

PHARMACOLOGIC CLASS

nonsteroidal anti-inflammatory drugs (NSAIDs)

diflunisal
diclofenac sodium
etodolac
fenoprofen calcium
flurbiprofen
ibuprofen
indomethacin
indomethacin sodium trihydrate
ketoprofen
ketorolac tromethamine
meclofenamate
mefenamic acid
nabumetone
naproxen
naproxen sodium
oxyphenbutazone
phenylbutazone
piroxicam
sulindac
tolmetin sodium

OVERVIEW

Nonsteroidal anti-inflammatory drugs (NSAIDs) are a growing class of drugs that are prescribed widely for their analgesic and anti-inflammatory effects; some members of this class have an antipyretic effect.

The analgesic effect of NSAIDs may result from interference with the prostaglandins involved in pain. Prostaglandins appear to sensitize pain receptors. NSAIDs inhibit synthesis of prostaglandins peripherally and possibly centrally. Their anti-inflammatory action may also contribute indirectly to their analgesic effect.

Like the salicylates, the anti-inflammatory effects of NSAIDs may result in part from inhibition of prostaglandin synthesis.

CLINICAL INDICATIONS AND ACTIONS

Pain, inflammation, and fever

NSAIDs are used principally for symptomatic relief of mild to moderate pain and inflammation. These agents usually provide temporary relief of mild to moderate pain, especially that associated with inflammation. NSAIDs are used to treat low-intensity pain of headache, arthralgia, myalgia, neuralgia, and mild to moderate pain from dental or surgical procedures or dysmenorrhea.

Oral NSAIDs are also used for long-term treatment of rheumatoid arthritis, juvenile arthritis, and osteoarthritis. In osteoarthritis, NSAIDs are used primarily for analgesia. NSAIDs offer only symptomatic treatment for rheumatoid conditions, and do not reverse or arrest the disease process. NSAIDs reduce pain, stiffness, swelling, and tenderness.

OVERVIEW OF ADVERSE REACTIONS

Adverse reactions to oral NSAIDs chiefly involve the GI tract, particularly erosion of the gastric mucosa. Most common symptoms are dyspepsia, heartburn, epigastric distress, nausea, and abdominal pain. GI symptoms usually occur in the first few days of therapy, and often subside with continuous treatment. They can be minimized by administering NSAIDs with meals or food, antacids, or large quantities of water or milk.

CNS side effects (headache, dizziness, drowsiness) may also occur. Flank pain with other signs and symptoms of nephrotoxicity has occasionally been reported. Fluid retention may aggravate preexisting hypertension or CHF. NSAIDs should not be used in patients with renal insufficiency.

REPRESENTATIVE COMBINATIONS

None.

norepinephrine injection (levarterenol bitartrate)

(nor ep i nef′ rin)

Levophed

- *Classification:* vasopressor (adrenergic, direct acting)
- *Pregnancy Risk Category:* D

HOW SUPPLIED

Injection: 1 mg/ml

ACTION

Mechanism: Stimulates alpha- and beta-adrenergic receptors within the sympathetic nervous system.

Absorption: Orally administered drug is destroyed in the GI tract. Poor absorption occurs with S.C. administration. The drug is usually given I.V.

Distribution: Localizes in sympathetic nerve tissues. Crosses the placenta, but does not enter the CNS.

Metabolism: In the liver and other tissues by the enzymes monoamine oxidase (MAO) or catechol-o-methyl transferase (COMT) to inactive compounds.

Excretion: In urine primarily as sulfate and glucuronide conjugates. Small amounts are excreted unchanged.

Onset, peak, duration: Pressor effect occurs rapidly after start of infusion, and ends 1 to 2 minutes after infusion is stopped.

INDICATIONS & DOSAGE

To restore blood pressure in acute hypotensive states—

Adults: initially, 8 to 12 mcg/minute I.V. infusion, then adjust to maintain normal blood pressure. Average maintenance dosage is 2 to 4 mcg/minute.

CONTRAINDICATIONS & PRECAUTIONS

Contraindicated in patients with peripheral or mesenteric vascular thrombosis, because it may increase ischemia and extend area of infarction; profound hypoxia or hypercapnea, hypovolemia; and in those undergoing general anesthesia with cyclopropane and other inhalation hydrocarbon anesthetics because of risk of inducing cardiac arrhythmias; also contraindicated for use with local anesthetics in fingers, toes, ears, nose, or genitalia.

Administer cautiously to hypertensive or hyperthyroid patients because they are at increased risk of adverse reactions. Also administer cautiously to patients with hypersensitivity to sulfites; commercially available formulation contains sodium metabisulfite.

ADVERSE REACTIONS

Common reactions are in italics; life-threatening reactions are in bold italics.

CNS: *headache,* anxiety, weakness, dizziness, tremor, restlessness, insomnia.
CV: bradycardia, severe hypertension, marked increase in peripheral resistance, decreased cardiac output, arrhythmias, ***ventricular tachycardia, fibrillation,*** bigeminal rhythm, ***atrioventricular dissociation,*** precordial pain.
GU: *decreased urine output.*
Metabolic: *metabolic acidosis,* hyperglycemia, increased glycogenolysis.
Local: irritation with extravasation.
Other: fever, ***respiratory difficulty.***

INTERACTIONS

Alpha-adrenergic blocking agents: may antagonize drug effects.
MAO inhibitors: increased risk of hypertensive crisis.
Tricyclic antidepressants: when given with sympathomimetics, may cause severe hypertension (hypertensive crisis). Don't give together.

EFFECTS ON DIAGNOSTIC TESTS

None reported.

NURSING CONSIDERATIONS

Besides those related universally to drug therapy (see "How to use this book"), consider the following specific recommendations:

Assessment
- Obtain a baseline assessment of the patient's hypotension before drug therapy.
- Be alert for adverse reactions and drug interactions during therapy.
- Evaluate the patient's and family's knowledge about norepinephrine therapy.

Nursing Diagnoses
- Altered tissue perfusion (cardiopulmonary, renal, GI, peripheral, cerebral) related to the patient's underlying condition.
- Altered urinary elimination related to adverse reaction to norepinephrine.
- Knowledge deficit related to norepinephrine therapy.

Planning and Implementation
Preparation and Administration
- Norepinephrine solutions deteriorate after 24 hours.
- Use large vein, as in the anticubital fossa, to minimize the risk of extravasation.
- ***I.V. use:*** Direct and intermittent infusion is not recommended. Use a continuous infusion pump to regulate infusion flow rate.
- Use a piggyback setup so that I.V. can be continued if norepinephrine is stopped.
- Administer in dextrose 5% in water and 0.9% sodium chloride solution; 0.9% sodium chloride solution alone is not recommended.

Monitoring
- Monitor the patient's blood pressure during the infusion. Check blood pressure every 2 minutes until stabilized; then every 5 minutes. Also check pulse rates, urine output, and color and temperature of extremities.
- Monitor the patient's ECG for possible drug-induced arrhythmias
- Monitor fluid volume. Know that this drug cannot replace blood or fluid volume deficit. Volume deficit should be replaced before vasopressors are administered.
- Check the infusion site for extravasation and superficial sloughing.
- Monitor the patient's vital signs even after the drug is stopped. Watch for severe drop in blood pressure.

Supportive Care
- Be prepared to stop the infusion and call the doctor immediately if extravasation occurs.
- Expect the doctor to order treatment of the extravasation by infiltrating the area with 5 to 10 mg phentolamine and 10 to 15 ml 0.9% sodium chloride solution.
- Titrate the infusion rate according to the assessment findings, using the doctor's guidelines. Know that the

blood pressure in previously hypertensive patients should not be raised more than 40 mm Hg below preexisting systolic pressure.
• Never leave the patient unattended during the infusion.
• Change the injection site frequently if prolonged therapy is necessary.
• Report decreased urine output to the doctor immediately.
• Keep emergercy drugs on hand to reverse effects of norepinephrine: atropine for reflex bradycardia; phentolamine for increased vasopressor effects; and propranolol for arrhythmias.
• Be prepared to slow the infusion gradually when discontinuing the drug.
• Institute safety precautions if the patient develops dizziness or weakness.

Patient Teaching
• Tell the patient to immediately report any discomfort at the infusion site.
• Tell the patient to report any difficulties in breathing.
• Have the patient report a drug-induced headache.

Evaluation
In patients receiving norepinephrine, appropriate evaluation statements may include:
• The patient maintains tissue perfusion and cellular oxygenation.
• The patient does not develop decreased urine ouput.
• Patient and family state an understanding of norepinephrine therapy.

norethindrone
(nor eth in´ drone)
Micronor, Norlutin, Nor-Q.D.

norethindrone acetate
Aygestin, Aygestin Cycle Pack, Norlutate

• *Classification:* contraceptive (progestin)
• *Pregnancy Risk Category:* X

HOW SUPPLIED
norethindrone:
Tablets: 0.35 mg, 5 mg
norethindrone acetate:
Tablets: 5 mg

ACTION
Mechanism: Suppresses ovulation, possibly by inhibiting pituitary gonadotropin secretion. Also forms a thick cervical mucus. Norethindrone and norethindrone acetate differ only in potency; the acetate is about twice as potent.
Absorption: Well absorbed after oral administration, although there is considerable variation in peak plasma levels.
Distribution: Widely distributed. It is about 80% protein-bound and distributes into bile and breast milk.
Metabolism: Primarily hepatic; it undergoes extensive first-pass metabolism.
Excretion: Primarily in feces. Half-life: Elimination half-life is 5 to 14 hours.
Onset, peak, duration: Peak levels occur in 0.5 to 4 hours after an oral dose. Peak levels are more delayed as the dose increases.

INDICATIONS & DOSAGE
Norethindrone
Amenorrhea, abnormal uterine bleeding–
Adults: 5 to 20 mg P.O. daily on days 5 to 25 of menstrual cycle.
Endometriosis–
Adults: 10 mg P.O. daily for 14 days, then increase by 5 mg P.O. daily q 2 weeks up to 30 mg daily.
Contraception–
Adults: initiate therapy with 0.35 mg P.O. on the first day of menstruation. Then, 0.35 mg P.O. daily.

norethindrone acetate
Amenorrhea, abnormal uterine bleeding–
Women: 2.5 to 10 mg P.O. daily on days 5 to 25 of menstrual cycle.
Endometriosis–
Women: 5 mg P.O. daily for 14 days, then increase by 2.5 mg daily q 2 weeks up to 15 mg daily.

CONTRAINDICATIONS & PRECAUTIONS

Contraindicated in patients with hypersensitivity to progestins, a history of thromboembolic disorders, severe hepatic disease, breast cancer, or undiagnosed abnormal vaginal bleeding; and in pregnant and breast-feeding women.

Use cautiously in patients with existing conditions that might be aggravated by fluid and electrolyte retention, such as cardiac or renal disease, epilepsy, or migraine; in diabetic patients because decreased glucose tolerance may occur; and in patients with a history of mental depression because norethindrone may worsen this condition.

ADVERSE REACTIONS

Common reactions are in italics; life-threatening reactions are in bold italics.
CNS: dizziness, migraine headache, lethargy, depression.
CV: hypertension, thrombophlebitis, ***pulmonary embolism,*** edema.
GI: nausea, vomiting, abdominal cramps.
GU: breakthrough bleeding, dysmenorrhea, amenorrhea, cervical erosion, or abnormal secretions, uterine fibromas, vaginal candidiasis.
Hepatic: cholestatic jaundice.
Metabolic: hyperglycemia.
Skin: melasma, rash.
Other: breast tenderness, enlargement, or secretion; decreased libido.

INTERACTIONS

Rifampin: decreased progestogen effects. Monitor for diminished therapeutic response.

EFFECTS ON DIAGNOSTIC TESTS

Glucose tolerance: decreased in a small percentage of patients.
Pregnanediol excretion: decreased.
Serum alkaline phosphatase and amino acid: increased levels.

NURSING CONSIDERATIONS

Besides those related universally to drug therapy, (see "How to use this book"), consider the following specific recommendations:

Assessment
- Obtain a baseline assessment of the patient's underlying condition before initiating therapy with norethindrone or norethindrone acetate.
- Be alert for common adverse reactions and drug interactions.
- Evaluate the patient's and family's knowledge about norethindrone therapy.

Nursing Diagnoses
- High risk for fluid volume deficit related to abnormal uterine bleeding.
- Fluid volume excess related to norethindrone-induced edema.
- Knowledge deficit related to therapy with norethindrone.

Planning and Implementation
Preparation and Administration
- FDA regulations require that, before receiving first dose, patients read package insert explaining possible progestin adverse reactions. Provide verbal explanation as well.
- Be aware that drug should not be used to sustain a pregnancy; drug may cause birth defects and masculinization of female fetus.
- Be aware that norethindrone acetate is twice as potent as norethindrone.

Monitoring
- Monitor for edema; weigh patient daily.

Supportive Care
• Withhold drug and notify the doctor if visual disturbances, migraine headache, or pulmonary emboli is suspected; be prepared to provide supportive care as indicated.
• Institute safety measures if adverse CNS reactions occur.
• Obtain an order for an antiemetic agent, as needed.
• Notify doctor if hyperglycemia occurs, especially in a diabetic patient, because therapy may need to be adjusted.
• Limit patient's sodium intake, if not contraindicated, to combat edema.
• Check patient's understanding of the package insert information.

Patient Teaching
• Instruct patients to report any unusual symptoms immediately and to stop taking the drug and call the doctor immediately if visual disturbances or migraine occurs.
• Tell diabetic patients to report symptoms of hyperglycemia or glycosuria.
• Tell patients who become pregnant during therapy with norethindrone to stop taking the drug immediately, because it may adversely affect the fetus.
• Warn patient that edema and weight gain are likely. Advise patient to restrict sodium intake.
• Teach patient how to perform monthly breast self-examination.

Evaluation
In patients receiving norethindrone, appropriate evaluation statements may include:
• Abnormal uterine bleeding is relieved.
• Edema is controlled with treatment.
• Patient states an understanding of norethindrone therapy.

norfloxacin
(nor flox´ a sin)
Noroxin

• *Classification:* antibiotic (fluoroquinolone)
• *Pregnancy Risk Category:* C

HOW SUPPLIED
Tablets: 400 mg

ACTION
Mechanism: Inhibits bacterial DNA synthesis, mainly by inhibiting DNA gyrase. Bactericidal.
Absorption: About 30% to 90% of norfloxacin dose is absorbed from GI tract (as dose increases, percentage of absorbed drug decreases). Food may reduce absorption.
Distribution: Into renal tissue, liver, gallbladder, prostatic fluid, testicles, seminal fluid, bile, and sputum. Biliary levels may be 10 times higher than serum levels. The drug is 10% to 15% bound to plasma proteins.
Metabolism: Six metabolites have been identified; all are less active than the parent drug.
Excretion: Most systemically absorbed drug is excreted by the kidneys; about 30% appears in bile. Half-life: 2½ to 4 hours in patients with normal renal function; up to 8 hours in severe renal impairment. It is not known if the drug is excreted in breast milk.
Onset, peak, duration: Peak levels occur 1 to 2 hours after an oral dose.

INDICATIONS & DOSAGE
Treatment of complicated or uncomplicated urinary tract infections caused by susceptible strains of Escherichia coli, Klebsiella, Enterobacter, Proteus, Pseudomonas aeruginosa, Citrobacter, Staphylococcus aureus *(and* epidermidis*), and group D streptococci–*

Adults: For uncomplicated infections, 400 mg P.O. b.i.d. for 7 to 10 days. For complicated infections, 400 mg b.i.d. for 10 to 21 days.

CONTRAINDICATIONS & PRECAUTIONS

Contraindicated in pregnant women because it has demonstrated embryotoxic effects in animals; in children because it has exhibited neurotoxic effects in young animals; and in patients with hypersensitivity to other quinolones (nalidixic acid or cinoxacin). Use cautiously in patients with a history of seizures because drug's CNS effects are unknown.

ADVERSE REACTIONS

Common reactions are in italics; life-threatening reactions are in bold italics.
Blood: eosinophilia.
CNS: fatigue, somnolence, headache, dizziness.
GI: nausea, constipation, flatulence, heartburn, dry mouth.
Hepatic: transient elevations of AST (SGOT) and ALT (SGPT).
Skin: rash.
Other: ***hypersensitivity*** (rash, anaphylactoid reactions).

INTERACTIONS

Antacids containing magnesium or aluminum: decreased absorption of norfloxacin. Separate administration times by at least 2 hours.
Nitrofurantoin: decreases norfloxacin's effectiveness. Don't use together.
Probenecid: may increase serum levels of norfloxacin by decreasing its excretion.

EFFECTS ON DIAGNOSTIC TESTS

Blood urea nitrogen (BUN), serum creatinine, and ALT (SGPT), AST (SGOT), and alkaline phosphatase: increased levels.
CBC: eosinophilia, neutropenia.
Hematocrit: decreased.

NURSING CONSIDERATIONS

Besides those related universally to drug therapy (see "How to use this book"), consider the following specific recommendations:

Assessment
- Obtain a baseline assessment of infection before therapy.
- Be alert for adverse reactions and drug interactions throughout therapy.
- Evaluate the patient's and family's knowledge about norfloxacin therapy.

Nursing Diagnoses
- High risk for injury related to ineffectiveness of norfloxacin to eradicate the infection.
- Constipation related to adverse effect of norfloxacin on GI tract.
- Knowledge deficit related to norfloxacin.

Planning and Implementation

Preparation and Administration
- Obtain clean-catch urine specimen for culture and sensitivity tests before first dose. Therapy may begin pending test results.
- Administer drug 1 hour before or 2 hours after meals because food may hinder absorption.

Monitoring
- Monitor effectiveness by regularly assessing for improvement in infection and by evaluating results of urine specimens ordered.
- Monitor patient for constipation throughout norfloxacin therapy.

Supportive Care
- Obtain an order for a laxative as needed.
- Ensure that patient drinks several glasses of water throughout the day to maintain hydration and adequate urine output.
- Impose safety precautions if the patient experiences adverse CNS reactions.

Patient Teaching
- Drug may cause dizziness or drowsiness. Warn the patient to avoid driving and other hazardous tasks that

require alertness, until CNS effects of the drug are known.
• Tell patient to take drug 1 hour before or 2 hours after meals because food may hinder absorption.
• Warn patient not to exceed dose prescribed.
• Remind patient to continue taking this drug, even when feeling better, and to take entire amount prescribed.

Evaluation

In patients receiving norfloxacin, appropriate evaluation statements may include:
• Patient is free of infection.
• Patient maintains normal bowel patterns throughout therapy.
• Patient and family state an understanding of therapy.

norgestrel

(nor jess´ trel)
Ovrette**

• *Classification:* contraceptive (progestin)
• *Pregnancy Risk Category:* X

HOW SUPPLIED

Tablets: 0.075 mg

ACTION

Mechanism: Suppresses ovulation, possibly by inhibiting pituitary gonadotropin secretion. Also forms a thick cervical mucus.
Absorption: Well-absorbed after oral administration.
Distribution: About 80% bound to plasma proteins. Distributes into bile.
Metabolism: Probably hepatic.
Excretion: In urine and feces.

INDICATIONS & DOSAGE

Contraception–
Women: 0.075 mg P.O. daily.

CONTRAINDICATIONS & PRECAUTIONS

Contraindicated in thromboembolic disorders, breast cancer, undiagnosed abnormal vaginal bleeding, severe hepatic disease, missed abortion, or in pregnant women. Used cautiously in diabetes mellitus, seizure disorders, migraine, cardiac or renal disease, asthma, and mental illness.

ADVERSE REACTIONS

Common reactions are in italics; life-threatening reactions are in bold italics.
CNS: cerebral thrombosis or hemorrhage, migraine headache, lethargy, depression.
CV: hypertension, thrombophlebitis, ***pulmonary embolism,*** edema.
GI: nausea, vomiting, abdominal cramps, gallbladder disease.
GU: *breakthrough bleeding, change in menstrual flow,* dysmenorrhea, spotting, amenorrhea, cervical erosion, vaginal candidiasis.
Hepatic: cholestatic jaundice.
Skin: melasma, rash.
Other: breast tenderness, enlargement, or secretion.

INTERACTIONS

Rifampin: decreased progestogen effects. Monitor for diminished therapeutic response.

EFFECTS ON DIAGNOSTIC TESTS

BSP test: increased retention.
Metgrapone test: decreased response.
Nitro blue tetrazolium (NBT): false positive results.
SGOT (AST) and alkaline phosphatase: increased levels.

NURSING CONSIDERATIONS

Besides those related universally to drug therapy (see "How to use this book"), consider the following specific recommendations:

Assessment

• Obtain a baseline assessment of the patient's pregnancy status before initiating oral contraceptive therapy.

• Be alert for adverse reactions and drug interactions throughout therapy.

• Evaluate the patient's and family's knowledge about oral contraceptive therapy.

Nursing Diagnoses

• High risk for fluid volume deficit related to drug-induced excessive uterine bleeding.

• Altered tissue perfusion (pulmonary) related to drug-induced thromboembolism.

• Knowledge deficit related to oral conceptive therapy.

Planning and Implementation

Preparation and Administration

• FDA regulations require that, before receiving first dose, patients read package insert explaining possible progestin adverse reactions. Provide verbal explanations as well.

• Check to be sure a negative pregnancy test has been obtained before drug is initiated.

Monitoring

• Monitor effectiveness by regularly assessing that pregnancy has not occurred; have pregnancy test performed if menstruation does not occur when expected.

• Monitor the patient's mental status for CNS changes such as depression.

• Regularly monitor blood pressure and weight.

• Regularly monitor the patient for breakthrough bleeding or abnormal vaginal secretions.

Supportive Care

• Alert the doctor immediately if visual disturbances, migraine headache, tingling in limbs, or a thromboembolic event is suspected and be prepared to provide supportive care as indicated.

Patient Teaching

• Instruct patient how to take the drug. Tell patient to take pill every day, even if menstruating. Pill should be taken at the same time every day.

• Tell patient that risk of pregnancy increases with each tablet missed. Teach patient that if one tablet is missed, she should take it as soon as she remembers; she should then take the next tablet at the regular time. A patient who misses two tablets should take one as soon as she remembers and then take the next regular dose at the usual time; she should use a nonhormonal method of contraception in addition to norgestrel until 14 tablets have been taken. If she misses three or more tablets she should discontinue the drug and use a nonhormonal method of contraception until after her menses. If her menstrual period does not occur within 45 days, pregnancy testing is necessary.

• Many doctors recommend that women not become pregnant within 2 months after stopping oral contraceptive therapy. Advise the patient to check with her doctor about how soon pregnancy may be safely attempted after oral contraceptive therapy is stopped.

• Inform the patient that oral contraceptives decrease viscosity of the cervical mucus and increase susceptibility to vaginal infections. Good hygienic practices are essential.

• Teach patient how to perform a monthly breast self-examination.

• Advise the patient of the increased risk of serious adverse cardiovascular reactions associated with heavy cigarette smoking (15 or more cigarettes per day). These risks are quite marked in women over age 35.

• Instruct patient to immediately report excessive bleeding or bleeding between menstrual cycles.

Evaluation

In patients receiving norgestrel, appropriate evaluation statements may include:

• Excessive uterine bleeding did not occur.

• Patient does not experience a thromboembolic event during oral contraceptive therapy.
• Patient states an understanding of oral contraceptive therapy.

nortriptyline hydrochloride

(nor trip´ ti leen)
Aventyl*, Pamelor*

• *Classification:* tricyclic antidepressant
• *Pregnancy Risk Category:* D

HOW SUPPLIED

Capsules: 10 mg, 25 mg, 75 mg
Oral solution: 10 mg/5ml (4% alcohol)

ACTION

Mechanism: Increases the amount of norepinephrine or serotonin, or both, in the CNS by blocking their reuptake by the presynaptic neurons.
Absorption: Rapidly absorbed from the GI tract after oral administration.
Distribution: Widely distributed into the body, including the CNS and breast milk. Drug is 95% protein-bound. Therapeutic serum level ranges from 50 to 150 ng/ml.
Metabolism: By the liver; a significant first-pass effect may account for variability of serum concentrations in different patients taking the same dosage.
Excretion: Most excreted in urine; some in feces, via the biliary tract. Half-life: 16 to 90 hours.
Onset, peak, duration: Peak plasma levels occur within 8 hours after a given dose; steady-state serum levels are achieved within 2 to 4 weeks. Peak antidepressant effect may not be seen for several weeks.

INDICATIONS & DOSAGE

Treatment of depression–
Adults: 25 mg P.O. t.i.d. or q.i.d., gradually increasing to maximum of 150 mg daily. Alternatively, entire dose may be given h.s.

CONTRAINDICATIONS & PRECAUTIONS

Contraindicated in patients with hypersensitivity to tricyclic antidepressants, trazodone, and related compounds; in the acute recovery phase of myocardial infarction (MI) because it can cause arrhythmias and depress cardiac function; in patients in coma or severe respiratory depression because of additive CNS depression; and during or within 14 days of therapy with MAO inhibitors because this combination may cause excessive sympathetic stimulation with hypertensive crisis, high fevers, and seizures.

Use cautiously in patients with other cardiac disease (arrhythmias, CHF, angina pectoris, valvular disease, or heart block); respiratory disorders; alcoholism, or seizure disorders because this drug may lower the seizure threshold; bipolar disease; glaucoma because drug may increase intraocular pressure, even in normal doses; hyperthyroidism or in those taking thyroid replacement; Type I and Type II diabetes; in patients with prostatic hypertrophy, paralytic ileus, or urine retention because drug may worsen these conditions; in patients with hepatic or renal dysfunction because impaired metabolism and excretion may result in drug accumulation; Parkinson's disease; in those undergoing surgery with general anesthesia; and in patients receiving electroconvulsive therapy because of added risk of hypomania and delirium.

ADVERSE REACTIONS

Common reactions are in italics; life-threatening reactions are in bold italics.
CNS: *drowsiness, dizziness,* excitation, seizures, tremors, weakness, confusion, headache, nervousness.

CV: *tachycardia, ECG changes,* hypertension.
EENT: *blurred vision,* tinnitus, mydriasis.
GI: *dry mouth, constipation,* nausea, vomiting, anorexia, paralytic ileus.
GU: *urine retention.*
Skin: rash, urticaria.
Other: *sweating,* allergy.
After abrupt withdrawal of long-term therapy: nausea, headache, malaise. (Does not indicate addiction.)

INTERACTIONS

Barbiturates: decrease TCA blood levels. Monitor for decreased antidepressant effect.
Cimetidine: may increase nortriptyline serum levels. Monitor for increased adverse reactions.
Epinephrine, norepinephrine: increase hypertensive effect. Use with caution.
MAO inhibitors: may cause severe excitation, hyperpyrexia, or seizures, usually with high dose. Use together cautiously.
Methylphenidate: increases TCA blood levels. Monitor for enhanced antidepressant effect.

EFFECTS ON DIAGNOSTIC TESTS

CBC: decreased WBC count.
ECG: elongated Q-T and PR intervals, flattened T waves.
Liver function tests: elevated results.
Serum glucose: decreased or increased levels.

NURSING CONSIDERATIONS

Besides those related universally to drug therapy (see "How to use this book"), consider the following specific recommendations:

Assessment
- Obtain a baseline assessment of depression before therapy.
- Be alert for adverse reactions or drug interactions during therapy.
- Evaluate the patient's and family's knowledge about nortriptyline hydrochloride therapy.

Nursing Diagnoses
- Ineffective individual coping related to the patient's underlying condition.
- Constipation related to nortriptyline-induced adverse GI reactions.
- Knowledge deficit related to nortriptyline therapy.

Planning and Implementation

Preparation and Administration
- Whenever possible, patient should take full dose at bedtime.
- Expect reduced dosage in elderly or debilitated patients and adolescents.

Monitoring
- Monitor effectiveness by having the patient discuss his feelings (ask broad, open-ended questions) and by evaluating his behavior.
- Monitor blood pressure for alterations, heart rate for tachycardia, and ECG for changes. This drug has a low potential for orthostatic hypotension.
- Monitor bowel patterns for constipation and check for urine retention.
- Monitor for suicidal tendencies.

Supportive Care
- Institute safety precautions if adverse CNS reactions occur.
- Do not withdraw drug abruptly.
- If psychotic signs increase, notify doctor and expect dosage to be reduced. Allow only a minimum supply of tablets to lessen suicide risk.
- If not contraindicated, increase the patient's fluid and fiber intake to prevent constipation; if needed, obtain an order for a stool softener or laxative.

Patient Teaching
- Tell the patient to relieve dry mouth with sugarless hard candy or gum but explain that saliva substitutes may be necessary.
- Teach the patient to increase fluids to lessen constipation. Suggest stool softener or high-fiber diet, if needed.
- Warn the patient to avoid driving and other hazardous activities that

require alertness and good psychomotor coordination until CNS effects of the drug are known. Tell the patient that drowsiness and dizziness usually subside after first few weeks. Warn against combining with alcohol or other CNS depressants.
• Tell the patient that therapy must continue for 2 weeks or more before noticeable effect, and for 4 weeks or more before full effect. Encourage the patient to continue taking the medication until it achieves full therapeutic effect.
• Advise the patient not to take any other drugs (prescription or OTC) without first consulting the doctor.

Evaluation

In patients receiving nortriptyline, appropriate evaluation statements may include:
• Patient behavior and communication indicate improvement of depression.
• Constipation from adverse GI reactions to nortriptyline has not occurred.
• Patient and family state an understanding of nortriptyline therapy.

nystatin (topical)

(nye stat´ in)

Mycostatin, Nadostine†, Nilstat

• *Classification:* antifungal (macrolide)
• *Pregnancy Risk Category:* B

HOW SUPPLIED

Cream: 100,000 units/g
Ointment: 100,000 units/g
Powder: 100,000 units/g
Vaginal tablets: 100,000 units

ACTION

Mechanism: Binds to sterols in the cell walls of susceptible fungi and alters cellular permeability.
Absorption: Not absorbed from the GI tract or through the intact skin or mucous membranes.

INDICATIONS & DOSAGE

Infant eczema, pruritus ani and vulvae, localized forms of candidiasis–
Adults and children: apply to affected area b.i.d. for 2 weeks.
Vulvovaginal candidiasis–
Adults: one vaginal tablet daily or b.i.d. for 14 days.

CONTRAINDICATIONS & PRECAUTIONS

Contraindicated in patients with hypersensitivity to the drug.

ADVERSE REACTIONS

Common reactions are in italics; life-threatening reactions are in bold italics.
Skin: occasional contact dermatitis from preservatives present in some formulations.

INTERACTIONS

None significant.

EFFECTS ON DIAGNOSTIC TESTS

None reported.

NURSING CONSIDERATIONS

Besides those related universally to drug therapy (see "How to use this book"), consider the following specific recommendations:

Assessment
• Obtain a baseline assessment of eczema before therapy.
• Be alert for adverse reactions throughout therapy.
• Evaluate the patient's and family's knowledge about topical nystatin therapy.

Nursing Diagnoses
• Impaired skin integrity related to patient's underlying condition.
• High risk for impaired skin integrity related to nystatin-induced contact dermatitis.
• Knowledge deficit related to topical nystatin therapy.

Planning and Implementation

Preparation and Administration

• Clean and apply to affected area. Cream is recommended for intertriginous areas; powder, for very moist areas; ointment, for dry areas.

• ***Vaginal use:*** Insert vaginal tablets high into the vagina. Vaginal tablets may be used by pregnant women up to 6 weeks before term to treat maternal infection that may cause thrush in neonates. Continue therapy during menstruation.

• Store vaginal tablets in the refrigerator.

Monitoring

• Monitor effectiveness by regularly examining the patient's skin for eczema.

• Monitor for adverse reactions by observing the skin and questioning the patient about increased irritation and burning.

Supportive Care

• Keep in mind drug is generally tolerated by all age-groups, including debilitated infants.

• Remember: do not use occlusive dressings.

• Wash vaginal applicator thoroughly after each use.

• Notify doctor if adverse reactions occur.

Patient Teaching

• Teach patient to apply medication.

• Tell patient to continue using for full treatment period prescribed, even if condition has improved. Immunosuppressed patients may use the drug constantly.

• Inform patient that preparation does not stain skin or mucous membranes.

• Tell the patient not to use occlusive dressings.

• Inform pregnant women that the vaginal tablets can be used up to 6 weeks before term.

• Stress importance of continuing therapy during menstruation if vaginal application is prescribed. Instruct patient to wash applicator thoroughly after each use.

• Explain factors that predispose to vaginal infection: use of antibiotics, oral contraceptives, and corticosteroids; diabetes; reinfection by sexual partner; and tight-fitting synthetic pantyhose, and underpants.

Evaluation

In patients receiving topical nystatin, appropriate evaluation statements may include:

• Patient states an improvement in condition.

• Patient does not develop drug-induced contact dermatitis.

• Patient and family state an understanding of topical nystatin therapy.

nystatin (oral)

(nye stat´ in)

Mycostatin*, Nadostine†, Nilstat, Nystex*

• *Classification:* antifungal (macrolide)
• *Pregnancy Risk Category:* B

HOW SUPPLIED

Oral tablets: 500,000 units
Oral suspension: 100,000 units/ml

ACTION

Mechanism: Probably acts by binding to sterols in the fungal cell membrane, altering cell permeability and allowing leakage of intracellular components.

Absorption: Not absorbed from the GI tract or through the intact skin or mucous membranes. Used for a local effect in the oral cavity or vagina.

Excretion: Orally administered nystatin is excreted almost entirely unchanged in feces.

Onset, peak, duration: Inhibitory levels of drug persist for about 2 hours after dissolution of an oral tablet.

*Liquid form contains alcohol. **May contain tartrazine.

INDICATIONS & DOSAGE

Gastrointestinal infections–
Adults: 500,000 to 1 million units as oral tablets, t.i.d.
Treatment of oral, vaginal, and intestinal infections caused by Candida albicans (Monilia) *and other* Candida *species–*
Adults: 400,000 to 600,000 units oral suspension q.i.d. for oral candidiasis.
Children and infants over 3 months: 250,000 to 500,000 units oral suspension q.i.d.
Newborn and premature infants: 100,000 units oral suspension q.i.d.

CONTRAINDICATIONS & PRECAUTIONS

Contraindicated in patients with hypersensitivity to the drug.

ADVERSE REACTIONS

Common reactions are in italics; life-threatening reactions are in bold italics.
GI: transient nausea, vomiting, diarrhea (usually with large oral dosage).

INTERACTIONS

None significant.

EFFECTS ON DIAGNOSTIC TESTS

None reported.

NURSING CONSIDERATIONS

Besides those related universally to drug therapy (see "How to use this book"), consider the following specific recommendations:

Assessment
- Obtain a baseline assessment of patient's fungal infection, including appropriate specimens to identify presence of fungi, before therapy.
- Be alert for adverse reactions throughout therapy.
- Evaluate the patient's and family's knowledge about nystatin therapy.

Nursing Diagnoses
- Injury related to high risk of ineffectiveness of nystatin to eradicate the fungus infection.
- Fluid volume deficit related to potential nystatin-induced adverse GI reactions.
- Knowledge deficit related to nystatin.

Planning and Implementation
Preparation and Administration
- ***P.O. use:*** Be sure mouth is clean and free of food debris before administering drug. Have patient hold suspension in mouth for several minutes before swallowing. When treating infants, swab medication on oral mucosa.

Monitoring
- Monitor effectiveness by regularly assessing for improvement of infectious process.
- Be aware that large oral dosages of nystatin may cause adverse GI reactions.
- Monitor hydration status if adverse GI reactions occur.

Supportive Care
- Provide good oral hygiene for patient who is unable to perform self care.
- Obtain an order for an antiemetic or antidiarrheal agent as needed.

Patient Teaching
- Although nystatin is virtually nontoxic and nonsensitizing when used orally, vaginally, or topically, advise patient to report redness, swelling, or irritation.
- Instruct patient to clean mouth of food debris before taking nystatin and to hold suspension (if prescribed) in mouth for several minutes before swallowing.
- Instruct mothers of infants being treated with oral nystatin to swab medication on oral mucosa.
- Teach patient good oral hygiene techniques. Explain that excessive use of mouthwash and poorly fitting dentures, may alter flora and promote

infection, especially in older patients.

• Advise patient to continue medication for 1 to 2 weeks after symptoms subside to ensure against reinfection. Tell patient to consult doctor for exact length of therapy.

• Instruct patient in careful hygiene of other affected areas, including cleansing perineal area from front to back after defecation.

Evaluation

In patients receiving nystatin, appropriate evaluation statements may include:

• Patient's infection is alleviated.

• Patient maintains adequate hydration throughout therapy.

• Patient and family state an understanding of therapy.

O

octreotide acetate
(ock tree´ oh tyde)
Sandostatin

• *Classification:* somatotropic hormone (synthetic octapeptide)
• *Pregnancy Risk Category:* B

HOW SUPPLIED
Injection: 0.05 mg, 0.1 mg, 0.5 mg

ACTION
Mechanism: Mimics the action of naturally occurring somatostatin, which inhibits the secretion of several hormones, including gastrin, secretin, motilin, insulin, glucagon, and vasoactive intestinal peptide.
Absorption: Rapidly and completely absorbed after S.C. injection.
Distribution: About 65% bound to serum lipoprotein and albumin.
Metabolism: Eliminated from the plasma at a slower rate than the naturally occuring hormone.
Excretion: About 35% of the drug appears unchanged in the urine. Half-life: About 1.5 hours.
Onset, peak, duration: Peak plasma levels occur in less than 30 minutes, with a duration of effect of up to 12 hours.

INDICATIONS & DOSAGE
Symptomatic treatment of flushing and diarrhea associated with carcinoid tumors–
Adults: initially, 0.1 to 0.6 mg daily S.C. in two to four divided doses for the first 2 weeks of therapy (usual daily dosage is 0.3 mg). Subsequent dosage is based upon individual response.
Symptomatic treatment of watery diarrhea associated with vasoactive intestinal peptide secreting tumors (VIPomas)–
Adults: initially, 0.2 to 0.3 mg daily S.C. in two to four divided doses for the first 2 weeks of therapy. Subsequent dosage is based upon individual response, but usually will not exceed 0.45 mg daily.

CONTRAINDICATIONS & PRECAUTIONS
Contraindicated in patients allergic to the drug or any of its components.

Octreotide therapy may be associated with the development of cholelithiasis by altering gallbladder motility or fat absorption. Monitor patient regularly for gallbladder disease.

ADVERSE REACTIONS
Common reactions are in italics; life-threatening reactions are in bold italics.
CNS: dizziness, light-headedness, fatigue.
GI: *nausea, diarrhea, abdominal pain or discomfort,* loose stools, vomiting, fat malabsorption.
Metabolic: hyperglycemia, hypoglycemia, hypothyroidism.
Skin: flushing, edema, wheal, erythema or pain at injection site.

INTERACTIONS
Cyclosporine: may decrease plasma levels of cyclosporine.

EFFECTS ON DIAGNOSTIC TESTS
Gastrin, vasoactive intestinal peptide (VIP), insulin, glucagon, secretin, motilin, and pancreatic polypeptide: decreased secretions.
Growth hormone: decreased secretions.

NURSING CONSIDERATIONS

Besides those related universally to drug therapy (see "How to use this book"), consider the following specific recommendations:

Assessment

• Obtain a baseline assessment of history of bowel disorders, GI status, allergies, thyroid function, and frequency of loose stools before therapy.
• Be alert for adverse reactions or drug interactions during therapy.
• Evaluate the patient's and family's knowledge about octreotide therapy.

Nursing Diagnoses

• Diarrhea related to interruption of normal pattern of elimination characterized by frequent loose stools.
• Pain related to octreotide-induced abdominal pain or discomfort.
• Knowledge deficit related to octreotide therapy.

Planning and Implementation

Preparation and Administration

• ***S.C. use:*** Administer in divided doses for first 2 weeks of therapy. Subsequent daily dosage depends on patient's response.
• Read drug label carefully and check dosage and strength.

Monitoring

• Monitor effectiveness by monitoring the frequency and characteristics of stools.
• Monitor thyroid function; urine 5-hydroxyindoleacetic acid (5-HIAA), plasma serotonin, and plasma substance P levels (for carcinoid tumors); and plasma VIP for VIPomas during therapy.
• Monitor closely for symptoms of glucose imbalance during therapy; mild, transient hypoglycemia or hyperglycemia may occur.
• Monitor fluid and electrolyte balance.
• Weigh daily until diarrhea is controlled to detect fluid loss or retention.
• Auscultate bowel sounds at least once a shift. Assess for pain and cramping.
• Check skin in perianal area to detect and prevent breakdown.
• Monitor for signs of gallbladder disease, because octreotide may be associated with the development of cholelithiasis by either altering gallbladder motility or fat absorption.

Supportive Care

• Do not give to patients with hypersensitivity to the drug or any of its components.
• Be aware that drug's half-life may be altered in patients with end-stage renal failure who are receiving dialysis.
• Insulin-dependent diabetics and patients receiving oral hypoglycemics (sulfonylureas) or oral diazoxide may require dosage adjustment during therapy.
• Be aware that octreotide therapy may require adjustment of other drugs used to control symptoms of the disease (such as beta blockers).
• Obtain order for pain medication to relieve abdominal discomfort.
• Provide good skin care, especially in the perianal area; apply soothing lotions and powder.

Patient Teaching

• Instruct patient to report any signs of abdominal discomfort immediately.
• Advise patient that periodic laboratory testing will be necessary during octreotide therapy.

Evaluation

In patients receiving octreotide, appropriate evaluation statements may include:

• Patient reports decrease or absence of loose stools.
• Patient is pain-free.
• Patient and family state an understanding of octreotide therapy.

ofloxacin

(oh floks´ a sin)
Floxin

• *Classification:* antibiotic (fluoroquinolone)
• *Pregnancy Risk Category:* C

HOW SUPPLIED

Tablets: 200 mg, 300 mg, 400 mg

ACTION

Mechanism: Bactericidal effects may result from ability to inhibit bacterial DNA gyrase and to prevent DNA replication in susceptible bacteria.
Absorption: Well absorbed (about 98% bioavailable). The amount of drug absorbed increases proportionately with the dose.
Distribution: Widely distributed to body tissues and fluids including blister fluid, cervix, lung tissue, ovary, prostatic fluid, prostatic tissue, skin, and sputum.
Metabolism: Not significant. Less than 5% of an administered dose is recovered as metabolites.
Excretion: Mainly by renal excretion; between 70% to 80% of drug is excreted unchanged in urine within 36 hours of dosing; 4% to 8% is excreted in feces. Half-life: About 5 hours in most patients; 8 hours, in elderly patients.
Onset, peak, duration: Maximum serum concentrations are achieved 1 to 2 hours after an oral dose.

INDICATIONS & DOSAGE

Lower respiratory tract infections caused by susceptible organisms–
Adults: 400 mg P.O. q 12 hours for 10 days.
Cervicitis or urethritis caused by Chlamydia trachomatis *or* Neisseria gonorrhoeae–
Adults: 300 mg P.O. q 12 hours for 7 days.
Acute, uncomplicated gonorrhea–
Adults: 400 mg P.O. as a single dose.
Mild-to-moderate skin and skin structure infections caused by susceptible strains of Haemophilus influenzae *or* Streptococcus pneumoniae–
Adults: 400 mg P.O. q 12 hours for 10 days.
Cystitis caused by Escherichia coli *or* Klebsiella pneumoniae–
Adults: 200 mg. P.O. q 12 hours for 3 days.
Urinary tract infections caused by susceptible strains of Citrobacter diversus, Enterobacter aeorgenes, E. coli, Proteus mirabilis, *or* Pseudomonas aeruginosa–
Adults: 200 mg P.O. q 12 hours for 7 days. Complicated infections may require therapy for 10 days.
Prostatitis caused by E. coli–
Adults: 200 mg P.O. q 12 hours for 6 weeks.
Dosage adjustment for patients with renal failure–
If creatinine clearance is 10 to 50 ml/minute, decrease dosage interval to once q 24 hours. If creatinine clearance is <10 ml/minute, give half the recommended dose q 24 hours.

CONTRAINDICATIONS & PRECAUTIONS

Contraindicated in patients with a history of or sensitivity to quinolone antibiotics (including cinoxacin, ciprofloxacin, nalidixic acid, and norfloxacin). Use with caution in patients with known or suspected CNS disorders, such as cerebral arteriosclerosis, seizure disorders, or other factors that predispose to seizures because seizures have been linked with the use of other quinolone derivatives.

ADVERSE REACTIONS

Common reactions are in italics; life-threatening reactions are in bold italics.

CNS: headache, dizziness, fatigue, lethargy, malaise, drowsiness, sleep disorders, nervousness, light-headedness, insomnia, seizures.
CV: chest pain.
GI: anorexia, nausea, abdominal pain or discomfort, diarrhea, vomiting, dry mouth, flatulence, dysgeusia.
GU: vaginitis, vaginal discharge, genital pruritus.
Skin: rash, pruritus, photosensitivity.
Other: ***hypersensitivity (anaphylactoid)*** reaction, visual disturbances, fever.

INTERACTIONS

Antacids containing aluminum or magnesium hydroxide, iron salts, sucralfate, products containing zinc: may interfere with the GI absorption of ofloxacin. Separate administration times by at least 2 hours.
Anticoagulants: increased effect. Monitor for bleeding and altered prothrombin time.
Antineoplastic agents: may lower serum levels of quinolones.
Theophylline: some quinolones may decrease clearance of theophylline. Monitor theophylline levels.

EFFECTS ON DIAGNOSTIC TESTS

None reported.

NURSING CONSIDERATIONS

Besides those related universally to drug therapy (see "How to use this book"), consider the following specific recommendations:

Assessment

- Obtain a baseline assessment of infection before therapy.
- Be alert for adverse reactions and drug interactions throughout therapy.
- Evaluate the patient's and family's knowledge about ofloxacin therapy.

Nursing Diagnoses

- High risk for injury related to ineffectiveness of ofloxacin to eradicate the infection.
- High risk for fluid volume deficit related to adverse GI reactions caused by ofloxacin.
- Knowledge deficit related to ofloxacin.

Planning and Implementation

Preparation and Administration

- Obtain specimen for culture and sensitivity tests before first dose. Therapy may begin pending test results.
- Expect dosage adjustment for patients with renal failure.
- Be aware that patients treated for gonorrhea should have a serologic test for syphilis because drug is not effective against syphilis and treatment of gonorrhea may mask or delay symptoms of syphilis.
- ***P.O. use:*** Administer drug on an empty stomach with plenty of water and do not administer with antacids and products containing iron or zinc for at least 2 hours before or after each dose.

Monitoring

- Monitor effectiveness by regularly assessing for improvement in infection and by evaluating results of specimen cultures and sensitivity tests as ordered.
- Monitor hydration status if adverse GI reactions occur.
- Monitor regular blood studies and hepatic and renal function tests during prolonged therapy.

Supportive Care

- Obtain an order for an antiemetic or antidiarrheal agent as needed.
- Impose safety precautions if the patient experiences CNS adverse reactions.
- Report CNS adverse reactions to the doctor immediately.
- Take seizure precautions, such as padding bed rails, if needed. Notify the doctor if seizures occur.
- Withhold the drug and notify the doctor if a rash or other signs of hypersensitivity develop.

Patient Teaching
• Drug may cause dizziness or drowsiness. Warn the patient to avoid hazardous tasks that require alertness, such as driving, until CNS effects of the drug are known.
• Instruct patient to notify the doctor if adverse CNS reactions occur.
• Tell patient to take drug with plenty of fluids, but not with meals, and to avoid antacids and products containing iron or zinc for at least 2 hours before or after each dose.
• Remind patient to continue taking this drug, even when feeling better, and to take entire amount prescribed.
• Tell patient to withhold drug and notify doctor if a rash or other signs of hypersensitivity develop.
• Advise patient to use sunscreens and protective clothing to avoid photosensitivity reactions.
Evaluation
In patients receiving ofloxacin, appropriate evaluation statements may include:
• Patient is free of infection.
• Patient maintains adequate hydration throughout ofloxacin therapy.
• Patient and family state an understanding of ofloxacin therapy.

olsalazine sodium
(ole sal´ a zeen)
Dipentum

• *Classification:* anti-inflammatory (salicylate)
• *Pregnancy Risk Category:* C

HOW SUPPLIED
Capsules: 250 mg

ACTION
Mechanism: Presumably diminishes inflammation by blocking cyclooxygenase and inhibiting prostaglandin production in the colon.
Absorption: After oral administration, approximately 2.4% of a single dose is absorbed; maximum concentrations appear in about 2 hours.
Distribution: Liberated mesalamine is absorbed slowly from the colon, resulting in very high local concentrations.
Metabolism: 0.1% is metabolized in the liver; remainder will reach the colon, where it is rapidly converted to mesalamine by colonic bacteria.
Excretion: Less than 1% is recovered in urine.

INDICATIONS & DOSAGE
Maintenance of remission of ulcerative colitis in patients intolerant of sulfasalazine–
Adults: 500 mg P.O. b.i.d. with meals.

CONTRAINDICATIONS & PRECAUTIONS
Contraindicated in patients with hypersensitivity to salicylates.

ADVERSE REACTIONS
Common reactions are in italics; life-threatening reactions are in bold italics.
CNS: headache, depression, vertigo, dizziness.
GI: *diarrhea,* nausea, abdominal pain, heartburn.
Skin: rash, itching.
Other: arthralgia.

INTERACTIONS
None reported.

EFFECTS ON DIAGNOSTIC TESTS
None reported.

NURSING CONSIDERATIONS
Besides those related universally to drug therapy (see "How to use this book"), consider the following specific recommendations:
Assessment
• Obtain a baseline assessment of GI system before therapy.
• Be alert for adverse reactions or drug interactions during therapy.

• Evaluate the patient's and family's knowledge about olsalazine sodium.

Nursing Diagnoses

• Pain related to underlying disorder.
• Diarrhea related to olsalazine-induced adverse effects.
• Knowledge deficit related to olsalazine.

Planning and Implementation

Preparation and Administration

• ***P.O. use:*** Administer the drug in evenly divided doses. Give the medication with food.

Monitoring

• Monitor effectiveness by evaluating GI pain.
• Note any diarrhea related to painful episodes.
• Monitor the BUN and creatinine levels in the patient with renal disease. Although problems have not been reported for this drug, the possibility of renal tubular damage from absorbed mesalamine or its metabolites must be considered.
• Assess the hydration level of the patient experiencing severe diarrhea.

Supportive Care

• Notify the doctor of acute episodes of pain and of the occurrence of diarrhea.
• Provide adequate amounts of I.V. fluid intake if the patient has diarrhea and notify the doctor.
• Administer analgesics as ordered.

Patient Teaching

• Teach the patient to take the drug in evenly divided doses with food.
• Tell the patient to report diarrhea or increased levels of pain.

Evaluation

In patients receiving olsalazine sodium, appropriate evaluation statements may include:

• Patient is free of GI pain.
• Patient has not experienced diarrhea.
• Patient and family state an understanding of olsalazine sodium therapy.

omeprazole

(oh me´ pray zol)
Prilosec

• *Classification:* gastric acid suppressant (benzimidazole)
• *Pregnancy Risk Category:* C

HOW SUPPLIED

Capsules (delayed-release): 20 mg

ACTION

Mechanism: Inhibits the activity of the acid (proton) pump, H^+/K^+ ATPase, located at the secretory surface of the gastric parietal cell. This blocks the formation of gastric acid.
Absorption: Acid-labile; bioavailability is about 40% because of a substantial first-pass effect and instability in gastric acid. The formulation contains enteric-coated granules that permit absorption after the drug leaves the stomach. Absorption is rapid. Bioavailability increases slightly with repeated dosing, possibly because of the drug's action to decrease gastric acidity.
Distribution: Protein binding is about 95%.
Metabolism: Primarily hepatic.
Excretion: Primarily renal. Half-life: Plasma half-life is 0.5 to 1 hour, but drug effects may persist for days.
Onset, peak, duration: Peak levels occur in less than 3.5 hours.

INDICATIONS & DOSAGE

Severe erosive esophagitis; symptomatic, poorly responsive gastroesophageal reflux disease (GERD) –
Adults: 20 mg P.O. daily for 4 to 8 weeks. Patients with GERD should have failed initial therapy with a histamine H_2 antagonist.
Pathologic hypersecretory conditions (such as Zollinger-Ellison syndrome) –
Adults: initially, 60 mg P.O. daily,

with dosage titrated according to patient response. Daily dosage exceeding 80 mg should be administered in divided doses. Dosages up to 120 mg t.i.d. have been administered. Therapy should continue as long as clinically indicated.

CONTRAINDICATIONS & PRECAUTIONS

Contraindicated in patients hypersensitive to the drug or any component of the enteric formulation. Prolonged (2-year) studies in rats revealed a dose-related increase in gastric carcinoid tumors; studies in humans have not detected a risk from short-term exposure to the drug. Further study is needed to assess the impact of sustained hypergastrinemia and hypochlorhydria. The manufacturer recommends that duration of omeprazole therapy not exceed the recommended period.

ADVERSE REACTIONS

Common reactions are in italics; life-threatening reactions are in bold italics.
CNS: headache, dizziness.
GI: diarrhea, abdominal pain, nausea, vomiting, constipation, flatulence.
Respiratory: cough.
Skin: rash.
Other: back pain.

INTERACTIONS

Diazepam, warfarin, phenytoin: decreased hepatic clearance possibly leading to increased serum levels. Monitor closely.
Ketoconazole, iron derivatives, ampicillin esters: may exhibit poor bioavailability in patients taking omeprazole because optimal absorption of these drugs requires a low gastric pH.

EFFECTS ON DIAGNOSTIC TESTS

Serum gastrin: increased levels in most patients during the first 2 weeks of therapy.

NURSING CONSIDERATIONS

Besides those related universally to drug therapy (see "How to use this book"), consider the following specific recommendations:

Assessment
- Obtain a baseline assessment of the patient's disease, especially his GI symptoms, before initiating omeprazole therapy.
- Be alert for common adverse reactions and drug interactions.
- Evaluate the patient's and family's knowledge about omeprazole therapy.

Nursing Diagnoses
- Pain related to the patient's underlying condition.
- Diarrhea related to omeprazole-induced GI adverse reactions.
- Knowledge deficit related to omeprazole therapy.

Planning and Implementation

Preparation and Administration
- ***P.O. use:*** Administer the drug before meals and do not open or crush capsules to administer them. They should be swalllowed whole. Keep in mind that omeprazole increases its own bioavailability with repeated administration. The drug is labile in gastric acid, and less drug is lost to hydrolysis as the drug increases gastric pH.
- Dosage adjustments are not required for renal or hepatic impairment.

Monitoring
- Monitor effectiveness by regularly assessing for decreased GI reflux (heartburn).
- Monitor the patient's stool for amount, type, and color.
- Monitor diagnostic test results. Serum gastrin levels rise in most patients during the first 2 weeks of therapy.

Supportive Care
• If the patient's stool becomes black and tarry, perform a test for occult blood and notify the doctor of results.
Patient Teaching
• Explain the importance of taking the drug exactly as prescribed.
• Tell patient to take drug before meals and not to crush the capsule.
Evaluation
In patients receiving omeprazole, appropriate evaluation statements may include:
• Patient obtains relief of or decrease in GI reflux (heartburn).
• Patient maintains normal elimination patterns.
• Patient and family state an understanding of omeprazole therapy.

ondansetron hydrochloride
(on dan´ se tron)
Zofran

• *Classification:* antiemetic serotonin ([5-HT_3] receptor antagonist)
• *Pregnancy Risk Category:* B

HOW SUPPLIED
Injection: 2 mg/ml

ACTION
Mechanism: A selective antagonist of a specific type of serotonin receptor (5-HT_3), which is located in the CNS at the area postrema (chemoreceptor trigger zone) and in the peripheral nervous system on nerve terminals of the vagus nerve. The drug's blocking action may occur at both sites. Chemotherapy-induced nausea and vomiting may be related to release of serotonin (5-HT) from enterochromaffin cells located in the small intestine, where it stimulates vagal efferent nerve endings to initiate the vomiting reflex.
Absorption: Oral bioavailability is 50% to 60%; however, an oral dosage form is not yet available in the U.S.
Distribution: Plasma protein binding of ondansetron as measured *in vitro* was 70% to 76%, with binding constant over the pharmacologic concentration range (10 to 500 ng/ml). Circulating drug also distributed into RBCs.
Metabolism: Extensively metabolized, with approximately 5% of a radiolabeled dose recovered as the parent compound from the urine.
Excretion: Urinary 5-HIAA excretion increases after cisplatin administration in parallel with the onset of emesis. Half-life: In patients ages 19 to 40, mean elimination half-life is 3.5 hours; in patients ages 61 to 74, half-life is 4.7 hours, and in those over age 75, half-life is 5.5 hours.
Onset, peak, duration: Variable; drug is most effective if therapy begins before emetogenic chemotherapy.

INDICATIONS & DOSAGE
Prevention of nausea and vomiting associated with emetogenic chemotherapy (including high-dose cisplatin) –
Adults and children over 4 years: administered in three doses of 0.15 mg/kg I.V. Give first dose 30 minutes before administration of chemotherapy; administer subsequent doses 4 and 8 hours after the first dose. Infuse drug over 15 minutes.

CONTRAINDICATIONS & PRECAUTIONS
Contraindicated in patients with hypersensitivity to the drug. Use with caution in patients with hepatic impairment.

ADVERSE REACTIONS
Common reactions are in italics; life-threatening reactions are in bold italics.
CNS: *headache.*
GI: diarrhea, *constipation.*

Metabolic: transient elevations in AST and ALT levels.
Skin: rash.
Other: ***bronchospasm (rare).***

INTERACTIONS

Drugs that alter hepatic drug metabolizing enzymes, such as phenobarbital or cimetidine: may alter pharmacokinetics of ondansetron. No dosage adjustment appears necessary.

EFFECTS ON DIAGNOSTIC TESTS

SGOT (AST), SGPT (ALT): increased levels.

NURSING CONSIDERATIONS

Besides those related universally to drug therapy (see "How to use this book"), consider the following specific recommendations:

Assessment
• Obtain a baseline assessment of allergies, liver function studies (AST and ALT levels), and GI status before therapy.
• Be alert for adverse reactions or drug interactions during therapy.
• Evaluate the patient's and family's knowledge about ondansetron therapy.

Nursing Diagnoses
• High risk for fluid volume deficit related to chemotherapy-induced nausea and vomiting.
• Constipation related to infrequent or absent bowel movements induced by ondansetron.
• Knowledge deficit related to ondansetron therapy.

Planning and Implementation
Preparation and Administration
• ***I.V. use:*** Dilute the drug in 50 ml of dextrose 5% in water injection or 0.9% sodium chloride injection before administration. The drug is also stable for up to 48 hours after dilution in 5% dextrose in 0.9% sodium chloride injection, 5% dextrose in 0.45% sodium chloride injection, and 3% sodium chloride injection.
• Inspect solutions for particulate matter or discolorations before giving.
• Give first dose 30 minutes before beginning chemotherapy.
Monitoring
• Monitor effectiveness by observing the patient for nausea and vomiting.
• Observe for hypersensitivity reaction.
• Monitor AST and ALT levels.
• Monitor fluid balance and nutritional status.
• Monitor for signs of constipation.
Supportive Care
• Be aware that decreased ondansetron clearance and prolonged half-life have been reported in patients over age 75. However, there are no recommendations for reducing dosage in these patients because these pharmokinetic changes have not been associated with reduced safety or efficacy.
• Encourage the patient to maintain an adequate fluid intake to prevent fluid volume deficit.
• Obtain an order for a stool softener or laxative to relieve constipation.
• Consult with dietitian to modify diet to include increased fiber to help alleviate constipation.
Patient Teaching
• Instruct the patient to report signs of hypersensitivity immediately.
• Advise patient to report constipation immediately in order to provide treatment as soon as possible.

Evaluation
In patients receiving ondansetron, appropriate evaluation statements may include:
• Patient exhibits no signs of fluid deficit.
• Patient is free from constipation.
• Patient and family state an understanding of ondansetron therapy.

PHARMACOLOGIC CLASS

opioid (narcotic) antagonists

naloxone
naltrexone

OVERVIEW

The narcotic antagonists naloxone and naltrexone do not produce analgesia; they produce few effects in the absence of an opioid agonist.

The pharmacologic actions depend on whether an opioid agonist has been administered previously, the actions of that opioid, and the extent of physical dependence to it. At higher dosages, naloxone and naltrexone may have some agonistic effects, but these are clinically insignificant.

CLINICAL INDICATIONS AND ACTIONS

Opioid-induced respiratory depression

Narcotic antagonists are used to reverse or block the effects of narcotic agonists (and, acutely, narcotic agonist-antagonists). Naloxone is used in acute, emergency situations, primarily to treat opioid-induced respiratory depression, though naloxone-treated patients may not show complete reversal of the opiate sedative effects.

Adjunct in treating opiate addiction

Naltrexone is used as part of long-term treatment for opioid addiction. By preventing the euphoria that normally results from the use of opioids, use of naltrexone helps discourage their illicit use.

OVERVIEW OF ADVERSE REACTIONS

Nausea and vomiting may occur with high doses. Abrupt reversal of narcotic agonist effects may result in nausea, vomiting, sweating, tachycardia, increased blood pressure, and tremulousness. In postoperative patients, excessive dosage may reverse analgesia and cause excitement, with arrhythmias and fluctuations in blood pressure. When given to a narcotic addict, opioid antagonists may produce an acute abstinence syndrome. Drug should be discontinued if signs of a severe acute abstinence syndrome appear.

REPRESENTATIVE COMBINATIONS

None.

PHARMACOLOGIC CLASS

opioids

alfentanil hydrochloride
codeine phosphate
codeine sulfate
difenoxin
diphenoxylate
fentanyl citrate
hydromorphone hydrochloride
levorphanol tartrate
meperidine hydrochloride
methadone hydrochloride
morphine sulfate
oxycodone hydrochloride
oxymorphone hydrochloride
propoxyphene hydrochloride
propoxyphene napsylate
sufentanil citrate

OVERVIEW

Opioids, previously called narcotic agonists, are usually understood to include natural and semisynthetic alkaloid derivatives from opium and their synthetic surrogates, whose actions mimic those of morphine. Except for propoxyphene, which is Schedule IV, these drugs are classified as Schedule II by the federal Drug Enforcement Agency, because they have a high potential for addiction and abuse. Until relatively recently, opioids were used indiscriminately for analgesia and sedation and to control diarrhea and cough.

Opioids act as agonists at specific opiate receptor binding sites in the CNS and other tissues; these are the same receptors occupied by endoge-

COMPARING OPIOIDS

DRUG	ROUTE	ONSET	PEAK	DURATION
codeine	I.M., P.O., S.C.	15 to 30 min	30 to 60 min	4 to 6 hours
hydrocodone	P.O.	30 min	60 min	4 to 6 hours
hydromorphone	I.M., I.V., S.C.	15 min	30 min	4 to 5 hours
	P.O., rectal	30 min	60 min	4 to 5 hours
levorphanol	I.V.	15 min	20 min	4 to 8 hours
	P.O.	≤60 min	90 min	4 to 8 hours
	S.C.	≤60 min	60 to 90 min	4 to 8 hours
meperidine	I.M.	10 to 15 min	30 to 50 min	2 to 4 hours
	P.O.	15 to 30 min	60 min	2 to 4 hours
	S.C.	10 to 15 min	40 to 60 min	2 to 4 hours
methadone	I.M., P.O., S.C.	30 to 60 min	30 to 60 min	4 to 6 hours †
morphine	I.M.	≤20 min	30 to 60 min	3 to 7 hours
	P.O., rectal	≤20 min	≤60 min	3 to 7 hours
	S.C.	≤20 min	50 to 90 min	3 to 7 hours
oxycodone	P.O.	15 to 30 min	30 to 60 min	4 to 6 hours
oxymorphone	I.M., S.C.	10 to 15 min	30 to 60 min	3 to 6 hours
	I.V.	5 to 10 min	30 to 60 min	3 to 6 hours
	rectal	15 to 30 min	30 to 60 min	3 to 6 hours
propoxyphene	P.O.	20 to 60 min	2 to 2½ hours	4 to 6 hours

†Due to cumulative effects, duration of action increases with repeated doses.

nous opioid peptides (enkephalins and endorphins) to alter CNS response to painful stimuli. Opiate agonists do not alter the cause of pain, but only the patient's perception of the pain; they relieve pain without affecting other sensory functions. Opiate receptors are present in highest concentrations in the limbic system, thalamus, striatum, hypothalamus, midbrain, and spinal cord.

Opioids produce respiratory depression by a direct effect on the respiratory centers in the brain stem, resulting in decreased sensitivity and responsiveness to increases in carbon dioxide tension. These drugs' antitussive effects are mediated by a direct suppression of the cough reflex center. They cause nausea, probably by stimulation of the chemoreceptor trigger zone in the medulla oblongata; through orthostatic hypotension, which causes dizziness; and possibly by increasing vestibular sensitivity.

Some of the opioids are well absorbed after oral or rectal administration; others must be administered parenterally. Intravenous dosing is the most rapidly effective and reliable; absorption after I.M. or S.C. dosing may be erratic. Opioids vary in onset and duration of action; they are removed rapidly from the bloodstream and distributed, in decreasing order of concentration, into skeletal muscle, kidneys, liver, intestinal tract, lungs, spleen, and brain; they readily cross the placenta.

Opioids are metabolized mainly in

the liver (first-pass effect) and also in the CNS, kidneys, lungs, and placenta. They are excreted primarily in the urine; small amounts are excreted in the feces.

CLINICAL INDICATIONS AND ACTIONS

The opioids produce varying degrees of analgesia and have antitussive, antidiarrheal, and sedative effects. Clinical response is dose-related and varies with each patient.

Analgesia

Opioids may be used in the symptomatic management of moderate to severe pain associated with acute and some chronic disorders, including renal or biliary colic, myocardial infarction, acute trauma, postoperative pain, or terminal cancer. They also may be used to provide analgesia during diagnostic and orthopedic procedures and during labor. Drug selection, route of administration, and dosage depend on a variety of factors. For example, in mild pain, oral therapy with codeine or oxycodone usually suffices. In acute pain of known short duration, such as that associated with diagnostic procedures or orthopedic manipulation, a short-acting drug such as meperidine, or fentanyl is effective. These drugs are often given to alleviate postoperative pain, but because they influence CNS function require special care to monitor the course of recovery and to detect early signs of complications. Opioids are commonly used to manage severe, chronic pain associated with terminal cancer; this requires careful evaluation and titration of drug used and dosage and route of administration.

Pulmonary edema

Morphine, meperidine, oxymorphone, hydromorphone, and other similar drugs have been used to relieve anxiety in patients with dyspnea associated with acute pulmonary edema and acute left ventricular failure. These drugs should not be used to treat pulmonary edema resulting from a chemical respiratory stimulant. Opioids decrease peripheral resistance, causing pooling of blood in the extremities and decreased venous return, cardiac work load, and pulmonary venous pressure; blood is thus shifted from the central to the peripheral circulation.

Preoperative sedation

Routine use of opioids for preoperative sedation in patients without pain is not recommended, because it may cause complications during and after surgery. To allay preoperative anxiety, a barbiturate or benzodiazepine is equally effective, with a lower incidence of postoperative vomiting.

Anesthesia

Certain opioids, including alfentanil, fentanyl, and sufentanil, may be used for induction of anesthesia, as an adjunct in the maintenance of general and regional anesthesia, or as a primary anesthetic agent in surgery.

Cough suppression

Some opioids, most commonly codeine and its derivative, hydrocodone, are used as antitussives to relieve dry, nonproductive cough.

Diarrhea

Diphenoxylate and other opioids are used as antidiarrheal agents. All opioids cause constipation to some degree; however, only a few are indicated for this use. Usually, opiate antidiarrheals are empirically combined with antacids, absorbing agents, and belladonna alkaloids in commercial preparations.

OVERVIEW OF ADVERSE REACTIONS

Respiratory depression and, to a lesser extent, circulatory depression (including orthostatic hypotension) are the major hazards of treatment with opioids. Rapid I.V. administration increases the incidence and severity of these serious adverse effects. Respiratory arrest, shock, and cardiac arrest have occurred. It is likely that equianalgesic doses of individual opiates produce a comparable degree of respiratory depression, but its duration may vary. Other adverse CNS effects include dizziness, visual disturbances, mental clouding or depression, sedation, coma, euphoria, dysphoria, weakness, faintness, agitation, restlessness, nervousness, seizures, and, rarely, delirium and insomnia. Adverse effects seem to be more prevalent in ambulatory patients and those not experiencing severe pain. Adverse GI effects include nausea, vomiting, and constipation, as well as increased biliary tract pressure that may result in biliary spasm or colic. Tolerance, psychological dependence, and physical dependence (addiction) may follow prolonged, high-dose therapy (more than 100 mg of morphine daily for more than 1 month).

Use opiate agonists with extreme caution during pregnancy and labor, because they readily cross the placenta. Premature infants appear especially sensitive to their respiratory and CNS depressant effects when used during delivery.

Opiate agonists have a high potential for addiction and should always be administered with caution in patients prone to physical or psychic dependence. The agonist-antagonists have a lower potential for addiction and abuse, but the liability still exists.

REPRESENTATIVE COMBINATIONS

Codeine with acetaminophen: Tylenol with codeine, Empracet with codeine, Emtec*, Phenaphen with codeine, Rovnox with codeine*, Ty-tab with codeine, Acetaco, Aceta with codeine

Codeine phosphate with guaifenesin: Baytussin A.C., Cheracol, Guiatuss A.C., Guiatussin with codeine Liquid, Robitussin AC; with iodinated glycerol: Iophen-C Liquid, Tussi-Organidin Liquid; with phenylephrine hydrochloride, chlorpheniramine maleate, and ammonium chloride: Ru-Tuss; with tripolodine hydrochloride and pseudoephedrine hydrochloride: Actifed-C; with ephedrine and theophylline: Co-Xan; with pheniramine maleate and alcohol: Partuss AC. Empirin with codeine.

Codeine and aspirin with caffeine: Fiorinal with codeine; with phenacetin and caffeine: APC with codeine; with magnesium hydroxide and aluminum hydroxide: Ascriptin with codeine; with butalbital and caffeine: Buff-a-comp No. 3.

Dihydrocodeine with acetaminophen and caffeine: Compal, Synalgos-DC-A.

Fentanyl with droperidol: Innovar.

Hydrocodone bitartrate with acetaminophen: Bancap-HC, Dolacet, Hydrocet, Lorcet HD, Propain-HC, Zydone, Lortab; with aspirin, acetaminophen, and caffeine: Diagesic, Hyco-pap; with guaifenesin: Entuss tablets, Hycotuss liquid (with alcohol); with guaifenesin and pseudoephedrine hydrochloride: Detussin expectorant, Entuss-D, Tussero expectorant (with alcohol); with guaifenesin and phenindamine tartrate: P-V Tussin tablets; with guaifenesin and phenylephrine: Donatussin DC; with potassium guaiacosulfonate: Codiclear DH, Entuss Liquid; with pseudoephedrine hydrochloride: Detussin Liquid, Tussero; with homatropine methylbromide: Hycodan; with phenylephrine hydrochloride and pyrilamine maleate: Codimal DH syrup; with phenylpropanolamine hydrochloride: Hycomine; with phenylephrine hydrochloride, pyrilamine maleate, chlorpheniramine maleate salicylamide, citric acid, and caffeine: Citra forte capsules; with phenindamine tartrate, ammonium chloride, and alcohol: P-V Tussin syrup; with pheniramine maleate, pyrilamine maleate, potassium citrate, and ascorbic acid: Citra forte; with phenylephrine hydrochloride, phenylpropanolamine hydrochloride, pheniramine maleate, pyrilamine maleate, and alcohol: Ru-Tuss with hydrocodone; with guaifenesin and alcohol: S-T forte; with phenyl toloxamine: Tussionex.

Meperidine with acetaminophen: Demerol-APAP; with promethazine: Mepergan, Mepergan fortis.

Methadone with aspirin, phenacetin, and caffeine: Nodalin.

Oxycodone hydrochloride with acetaminophen: Tylox, Roxicet, Oxycocet*, Percocet, with oxycodone terephthalate and aspirin: Percodan, Percodan-Demi.

Propoxyphene with acetaminophen: Dolene AP-65, Dolene-AP, Lorcet, Wygesic, Darvocet-N, Propacet SK; with aspirin and caffeine: Darvon Compound, Darvon Compound-65, Dolene Compound 65, Propoxyphene Compound 65, Ropoxy Compound 65; with aspirin, phenacetin, and caffeine: Doraphen Compound 65, Procomp-65.

opium tincture*

(oh´ pee um)

• Controlled Substance Schedule II

opium tincture, camphorated*

Paregoric

• Controlled Substance Schedule III

• *Classification:* antidiarrheal (opiate)
• *Pregnancy Risk Category:* B (D for prolonged use or high doses at term)

HOW SUPPLIED

opium tincture
Oral solution: equivalent to morphine 10 mg/ml*
opium tincture, camphorated
Oral solution: Each 5 ml contains morphine, 2 mg; anise oil, 0.2 ml; benzoic acid, 20 mg; camphor, 20 mg; glycerin, 0.2 ml; and ethanol to make 5 ml

ACTION

Mechanism: A mixture of several alkaloids, including morphine, codeine, and papaverine. Increases smooth muscle tone in the GI tract, inhibits motility and propulsion, and diminishes secretions of digestive juices.
Absorption: Variably absorbed from the gut.
Distribution: Although the alkaloids are distributed widely in the body, the low doses used to treat diarrhea act primarily within the GI tract. Camphor crosses the placenta.
Metabolism: In the liver.
Excretion: In urine; alkaloids (especially morphine) enter the CNS and are found in breast milk. Half-life: Plasma half-life is about 2.5 to 3 hours in young adults; in older patients, the half-life may be prolonged.
Onset, peak, duration: Drug effect persists 4 to 5 hours.

INDICATIONS & DOSAGE

Acute, nonspecific diarrhea –
Adults: 0.6 ml opium tincture (range 0.3 to 1 ml) P.O. q.i.d. Maximum dosage 6 ml daily; or 5 to 10 ml camphorated opium tincture daily b.i.d., t.i.d., or q.i.d. until diarrhea subsides.
Children: 0.25 to 0.5 ml/kg camphorated opium tincture P.O. daily, b.i.d., t.i.d., or q.i.d. until diarrhea subsides.

CONTRAINDICATIONS & PRECAUTIONS

Contraindicated in patients with hypersensitivity to morphine alkaloids; acute respiratory depression, because opium tincture may worsen this condition; diarrhea resulting from pseudomembranous colitis or ulcerative colitis because of the potential for toxic megacolon; and diarrhea resulting from poisoning or from certain bacterial or parasitic infections, because expulsion of intestinal contents may be beneficial (until toxic agent has been eliminated from the GI tract).

Use cautiously in patients with asthma or severe prostatic hypertrophy, because the drugs may exacerbate symptoms associated with these disorders; hepatic disease because of the potential for drug accumulation; and narcotic or alcohol dependence because the drugs contain alcohol and opiates.

ADVERSE REACTIONS

Common reactions are in italics; life-threatening reactions are in bold italics.
GI: nausea, vomiting.
Other: physical dependence after long-term use.

INTERACTIONS

None significant.

EFFECTS ON DIAGNOSTIC TESTS

Hepatobiliary imaging (with technetium-99m disofenin): test interference.
Serum amylase and lipase: increased levels.

NURSING CONSIDERATIONS

Besides those related universally to drug therapy (see "How to use this book"), consider the following specific recommendations:

Assessment

- Obtain a baseline assessment of history of bowel disorder, GI status, and frequency of loose stools before therapy.
- Be alert for adverse reactions or drug interactions during therapy.
- Evaluate the patient's and family's knowledge about opium tincture therapy.

Nursing Diagnoses

- Diarrhea related to interruption of normal pattern of elimination characterized by frequent loose stools.
- Altered nutrition: Less than body requirements, related to drug-induced nausea and vomiting.
- Knowledge deficit related to opium tincture therapy.

Planning and Implementation

Preparation and Administration

- Read drug label carefully. Opium content of opium tincture is 25 times greater than camphorated opium tincture.
- Use a teaspoon to measure camphorated opium, which is more dilute than opium tincture.
- ***P.O. use:*** Mix with enough water to ensure passage to stomach. Milky fluid forms when camphorated opium tincture is mixed with water.
- Store in tightly capped, light, resistant container.

Monitoring

- Monitor effectiveness by checking the frequency and characteristics of stools.
- Monitor fluid and electrolyte balance.
- Weigh daily until diarrhea is controlled to detect fluid loss or retention.
- Auscultate bowel sounds at least once a shift. Assess for pain and cramping.
- Check skin in perianal area to detect and prevent breakdown.
- Observe for signs of respiratory depression, which indicates overdosage.

Supportive Care

- Keep naloxone on hand to reverse respiratory depression. Have an airway nearby.
- Obtain order for antiemetics to relieve nausea and vomiting.
- Be aware that opium tincture is an effective and prompt-acting antidiarrheal; it is unique because dosage can be adjusted precisely to patient's needs.
- Provide good skin care, especially in the perianal area; apply soothing lotions and powder.
- Encourage patient to drink sufficient quantities to prevent fluid loss.

• Consult with dietitian to modify diet to control diarrhea, nausea, and vomiting.

Patient Teaching

• Advise patient not to use longer than 2 days. Risk of physical dependence increases with long-term use.
• Encourage proper storage to keep drug out of children's hands.

Evaluation

In patients receiving opium tincture, appropriate evaluation statements may include:

• Patient reports decrease or absence of loose stools.
• Patient reports decrease or absence of nausea and vomiting.
• Patient and family state an understanding of opium tincture therapy.

orphenadrine citrate

(or fen´ a dreen)

Banflex, Flexoject, Flexon, K-Flex, Marflex, Myolin, Neocyten, Noradex, Norflex, O-Flex, Orflagen, Orphenate

• *Classification:* skeletal muscle relaxant (diphenhydramine analog)
• *Pregnancy Risk Category:* C

HOW SUPPLIED

Tablets: 100 mg
Tablets (sustained-release): 100 mg
Injection: 30 mg/ml

ACTION

Mechanism: Reduces transmission of impulses from the spinal cord to skeletal muscle.
Absorption: Rapidly absorbed from the GI tract.
Distribution: Drug may cross placenta; highest concentrations are found in highly perfused organs (such as the lungs).
Metabolism: Almost completely metabolized to at least eight metabolites.
Excretion: In urine, mainly as its metabolites. Small amounts are excreted unchanged. Half-life: About 14 hours.
Onset, peak, duration: Onset of action occurs within 1 hour, peaks within 2 hours, and persists for 4 to 6 hours.

INDICATIONS & DOSAGE

Adjunctive treatment in painful, acute musculoskeletal conditions–
Adults: 100 mg P.O. b.i.d., or 60 mg I.V. or I.M. q 12 hours, p.r.n. For maintenance, switch to oral therapy beginning 12 hours after last parenteral dose.

CONTRAINDICATIONS & PRECAUTIONS

Contraindicated in patients with hypersensitivity to the drug, and in patients in whom anticholinergic and antimuscarinic effects are undesirable: those with achalasia, bladder neck obstruction, glaucoma, myasthenia gravis, peptic ulcer, prostate hypertrophy, or pyloric or duodenal obstruction. Use cautiously in patients with cardiac, hepatic, or renal function impairment.

ADVERSE REACTIONS

Common reactions are in italics; life-threatening reactions are in bold italics.
Blood: ***aplastic anemia.***
CNS: disorientation, restlessness, irritability, weakness, *drowsiness,* headache, dizziness.
CV: palpitations, tachycardia.
EENT: dilated pupils, blurred vision, difficulty swallowing.
GI: constipation, *dry mouth,* nausea, vomiting, paralytic ileus, epigastric distress.
GU: urinary hesitancy or urine retention.

INTERACTIONS

Alcohol, other CNS depressants: increased CNS depression.

EFFECTS ON DIAGNOSTIC TESTS

None reported.

NURSING CONSIDERATIONS

Besides those related universally to drug therapy (see "How to use this book"), consider the following specific recommendations:

Assessment

- Obtain a baseline assessment of the patient's pain before drug therapy.
- Be alert for adverse reactions and drug interactions during orphenadrine citrate therapy.
- Evalute the patient's and family's knowledge about orphenadrine therapy.

Nursing Diagnoses

- Pain related to the patient's underlying condition.
- Altered oral mucous membrane related to adverse drug reactions.
- Knowledge deficit related to orphenadrine therapy.

Planning and Implementation

Preparation and Administration

- Check all dosages carefully because even a slight overdose can lead to toxicity.
- ***I.V. use:*** Inject the drug over approximately 5 minutes while patient is supine.
- Continuous and intermittent infusion is not recommended.

Monitoring

- Monitor the degree of dry mouth.
- Monitor effectiveness by frequently evaluating the patient's level of pain.
- Monitor for adverse reactions or drug interactions by frequently monitoring the patient's vital signs for tachycardia.
- Evaluate the patient's vision by asking if he has experienced blurred vision.
- Monitor for early signs of drug toxicity (excessive dry mouth, dilated pupils, blurred vision, skin flushing and fever).
- Monitor CBC and urinalysis in patients receiving the drug over extended periods.
- Monitor the patient's pulse while giving the drug I.V.; may cause paradoxical bradycardia, which usually disappears in 2 minutes.

Supportive Care

- Provide sugarless hard candy, ice chips (unless contraindicated), or sugarless gum to relieve dry mouth.
- After I.V. administration, wait 5 to 10 minutes before assisting the patient to rise slowly from the supine position.
- Encourage patient to void before taking this drug. Orphenadrine is an anticholinergic.
- Institute safety precautions if the patient develops blurred vision or dizziness. Assist the patient with ambulation.
- Obtain an order for a stool softener if constipation becomes bothersome.

Patient Teaching

- Tell the patient that sugarless gum, ice chips, or sugarless hard candy will help to relieve dry mouth.
- Tell the patient to immediately report excessive dry mouth, blurred vision, skin flushing, and fever. These may indicate drug toxicity.
- Tell the patient to report urinary hesitancy and urine retention.
- Tell patient to avoid hazardous tasks that require alertness (such as driving or operating heavy machinery) until the CNS effects of the drug are known.
- Tell the patient to avoid alcohol or other CNS depressants.

Evaluation

In patients receiving orphenadrine, appropriate evaluation statements may include:

- Patient states his pain is relieved.
- Patient does not develop dry mouth.
- Patient and family state an understanding of orphenadrine therapy.

oxacillin sodium

(ox a sill′ in)
Bactocill, Prostaphlin

- *Classification:* antibiotic (penicillinase-resistant penicillin)
- *Pregnancy Risk Category:* B

HOW SUPPLIED

Capsules: 250 mg, 500 mg
Oral solution: 250 mg/5 ml (after reconstitution)
Injection: 250 mg, 500 mg, 1 g, 2 g, 4 g, 10 g
I.V. infusion: 1 g, 2 g, 4 g
Pharmacy bulk package: 4 g, 10 g

ACTION

Mechanism: Bactericidal against microorganisms by inhibiting cell wall synthesis during active multiplication. Oxacillin resists penicillinases, enzymes that inactivate penicillins.
Absorption: Rapidly but incompletely absorbed from the GI tract; it is stable in an acid environment. Food decreases rate and extent of absorption. Rapidly absorbed after I.M. injection, but the peak plasma levels are lower than those seen following I.V. injection.
Distribution: Widely distributed; CSF penetration is poor but enhanced by meningeal inflammation. Oxacillin crosses the placenta; it is 89% to 94% protein-bound.
Metabolism: Partially metabolized.
Excretion: Primarily excreted in urine by renal tubular secretion and glomerular filtration; also excreted in breast milk and in small amounts in bile. Half-life: 30 minutes to 1 hour in adults; 2 hours in severe renal impairment. Dosage adjustments are not required in patients with renal impairment.
Onset, peak, duration: Peak serum concentrations occur within ½ to 2 hours after an oral dose, 30 minutes after an I.M. dose, and immediately after an I.V. injection.

INDICATIONS & DOSAGE

Systemic infections caused by penicillinase-producing staphylococci –
Adults: 2 to 4 g P.O. daily, divided into doses given q 6 hours; 2 to 12 g I.M. or I.V. daily, divided into doses given q 4 to 6 hours.
Children: 50 to 100 mg/kg P.O. daily, divided into doses given q 6 hours; 100 to 200 mg/kg I.M. or I.V. daily, divided into doses given q 4 to 6 hours.

CONTRAINDICATIONS & PRECAUTIONS

Contraindicated in patients with hypersensitivity to any penicillin or cephalosporin.

ADVERSE REACTIONS

Common reactions are in italics; life-threatening reactions are in bold italics.
Blood: granulocytopenia, thrombocytopenia, eosinophilia, ***hemolytic anemia,*** transient neutropenia.
CNS: neuropathy, neuromuscular irritability, ***seizures.***
GI: oral lesions.
GU: interstitial nephritis, transient hematuria, proteinuria.
Hepatic: hepatitis, elevated enzymes.
Local: *thrombophlebitis.*
Other: *hypersensitivity (fever, chills, rash, urticaria, **anaphylaxis**),* overgrowth of nonsusceptible organisms.

INTERACTIONS

Probenecid: increases blood levels of oxacillin and other penicillins. Probenecid may be used for this purpose.

EFFECTS ON DIAGNOSTIC TESTS

Aminoglycoside serum levels: falsely decreased concentrations.
CBC: transient reductions in RBCs, WBCs, and platelet counts.
Liver function tests: elevations may

indicate drug-induced hepatitis or cholestasis.
Urinalysis: abnormal results may indicate drug-induced interstitial nephritis.
Urine and serum proteins: falsely positive turbidimetric urine and serum proteins are often in tests using sulfosalicylic acid or trichloroacetic acid.

NURSING CONSIDERATIONS

Besides those related universally to drug therapy (see "How to use this book"), consider the following specific recommendations:

Assessment

• Obtain a baseline assessment of infection before therapy.
• Be alert for adverse reactions and drug interactions throughout therapy.
• Evaluate the patient's and family's knowledge about oxacillin therapy.

Nursing Diagnoses

• High risk for injury related to ineffectiveness of oxacillin to eradicate the infection.
• Impaired tissue integrity related to oxacillin-induced thrombophlebitis when administered I.V.
• Knowledge deficit related to oxacillin therapy.

Planning and Implementation

Preparation and Administration

• Obtain specimen for culture and sensitivity tests before first dose. Therapy may begin pending test results.
• Before first dose, ask the patient about previous allergic reactions to this drug and other penicillins. However, a negative history of penicillin allergy does not guarantee future safety.
• Give oxacillin at least 1 hour before bacteriostatic antibiotics.
• ***P.O. use:*** When given orally, drug may cause GI disturbances. Food may interfere with absorption, so give 1 to 2 hours before meals or 2 to 3 hours after.
• Don't give I.M. or I.V. unless infection is severe or patient can't take oral dose.
• ***I.V. use:*** Infuse I.V. drug intermittently to prevent vein irritation. Mix with dextrose 5% in water or a saline solution.

Monitoring

• Monitor effectiveness by regularly assessing for improvement of infection.
• Mainly, allergic reactions especially with large doses, parenteral administration, or prolonged therapy. Keep in mind that the previously non-allergic patient may become sensitized to penicillin during therapy.
• Monitor patient for bacterial and fungal superinfections during high-dose prolonged therapy, especially in elderly, debilitated, or immunosuppressed patients.
• Monitor liver function studies periodicly; watch for elevated AST (SGOT) and ALT (SGPT).

Supportive Care

• Discontinue the drug immediately if the patient develops signs of anaphylactic shock (rapidly developing dyspnea and hypotension). Notify the doctor and prepare to administer immediate treatment, such as epinephrine, corticosteroids, antihistamines, and other resuscitative measures as indicated.
• Change I.V. site every 48 hours. If patient develops thrombphlebitis change site immediately and apply warm compresses to the affected area.

Patient Teaching

• Advise the patient who becomes allergic to oxacillin to wear medical alert identification stating this information.
• Tell the patient to take medication exactly as prescribed and to complete the entire prescription even after feeling better.
• Tell the patient to call the doctor if

rash, fever, or chills develop. A rash is the most common allergic reaction.

• Tell the patient to take oral oxacillin 1 hour before or 2 hours after meals to ensure an optimal serum concentration.

Evaluation

In patients receiving oxacillin appropriate evaluation statements may include:

• Patient is free of infection.
• Patient does not develop thrombophlebitis with I.V. administration of oxacillin.
• Patient and family state an understanding of therapy.

oxazepam

(ox a´ ze pam)

Apo-Oxazepam†, Novoxapam†, Ox-Pam†, Serax**, Zapex†

• Controlled Substance Schedule IV
• *Classification:* anxiolytic, sedative-hypnotic (benzodiazepine)
• *Pregnancy Risk Category:* C

HOW SUPPLIED

Tablets: 10 mg, 15 mg, 30 mg
Capsules: 10 mg, 15 mg, 30 mg

ACTION

Mechanism: Depresses the CNS at the limbic and subcortical levels of the brain.
Absorption: Well absorbed from the GI tract after oral administration.
Distribution: Widely distributed throughout the body. Drug is 85% to 95% protein-bound.
Metabolism: In the liver to inactive metabolites.
Excretion: Metabolites are excreted in urine as glucuronide conjugates. Half-life: Ranges from 5 to 13 hours.
Onset, peak, duration: Peak levels occur in 1 to 4 hours. Onset of action occurs at 60 to 120 minutes.

INDICATIONS & DOSAGE

Alcohol withdrawal–
Adults: 15 to 30 mg P.O. t.i.d. or q.i.d.
Severe anxiety–
Adults: 15 to 30 mg P.O. t.i.d. or q.i.d.
Tension, mild to moderate anxiety–
Adults: 10 to 15 mg P.O. t.i.d. or q.i.d.

CONTRAINDICATIONS & PRECAUTIONS

Contraindicated in patients with hypersensitivity to the drug; acute narrow-angle glaucoma or untreated open-angle glaucoma, because of the drug's possible anticholinergic effects; in coma, because the drug's hypnotic effect may be prolonged or intensified; and acute alcohol intoxication who have depressed vital signs, because the drug will worsen CNS depression. Oxazepam tablets contain tartrazine, which may induce allergic reaction in hypersensitive individuals. Patients allergic to aspirin exhibit a high incidence of cross-sensitivity.

Use cautiously in patients with psychoses, because the drug is rarely beneficial in such patients and may induce paradoxic reactions; myasthenia gravis or Parkinson's disease, because it may exacerbate the disorder; or impaired renal or hepatic function, which prolongs elimination of the drug; in elderly or debilitated patients, who are usually more sensitive to the drug's CNS effects; and in individuals prone to addiction or drug abuse.

ADVERSE REACTIONS

Common reactions are in italics; life-threatening reactions are in bold italics.
Blood: *leukopenia* (rare).
CNS: *drowsiness, lethargy, hangover,* fainting.
CV: transient hypotension.
GI: nausea, vomiting, abdominal discomfort.
Metabolic: hepatic dysfunction.

*Liquid form contains alcohol. **May contain tartrazine.

INTERACTIONS

Alcohol, other CNS depressants: increased CNS depression. Avoid concomitant use.

EFFECTS ON DIAGNOSTIC TESTS

EEG: changes in patterns, (low-voltage, fast activity) during and after therapy.

Liver function tests: increased results.

NURSING CONSIDERATIONS

Besides those related universally to drug therapy (see "How to use this book"), consider the following specific recommendations:

Assessment

- Obtain a baseline assessment of the patient's anxiety before drug therapy.
- Be alert for adverse reactions and drug interactions during oxazepam therapy.
- Evaluate the patient's and family's knowledge about oxazepam therapy.

Nursing Diagnoses

- Anxiety related to the patient's underlying condition.
- High risk for injury related to drug-induced CNS reactions.
- Knowledge deficit related to oxazepam therapy.

Planning and Implementation

Preparation and Administration

- Reduce the dosage in elderly or debilitated patients who may be more susceptible to CNS reactions to the drug.
- Drug has a short half-life and therefore fewer cumulative effects than other benzodiazepines.

Monitoring

- Frequently monitor the patient's vital signs for hypotension.
- Regularly monitor effectiveness by asking the patient about feelings of anxiety and by observing the patient's behavior.
- Monitor for excessive sedation due to potentiation with other CNS drugs.
- Monitor CBC and hepatic function periodically in patients on long-term therapy.

Supportive Care

- Provide additional fluids if the patient develops nausea, vomiting, and diarrhea.
- If drowsiness, light-headedness, lethargy or fainting occurs, institute safety measures, such as supervising patient activities. Reorient patient as needed and ensure a safe environment.
- Be aware that drug should not be prescribed for everyday stress.
- Do not withdraw drug abruptly. Abuse or addiction is possible and withdrawal symptoms may occur.

Patient Teaching

- Warn the patient not to combine drug with alcohol or other CNS depressants and to avoid driving and other hazardous activities that require alertness and psychomotor coordination until adverse CNS effects of the drug are known.
- Warn the patient against giving medication to others.
- Warn the patient to take this drug only as directed and not discontinue it without the doctor's approval. Inform the patient of the drug's potential for dependence if taken longer than directed.

Evaluation

In patients receiving oxazepam, appropriate evaluation statements may include:

- Patient states he is less anxious.
- Patient does not experience injury as a result of adverse CNS reactions.
- Patient and family state an understanding of oxazepam therapy.

oxiconazole nitrate

(ox i kon´ a zole)
Oxistat

• *Classification:* antifungal (ergosterol synthesis inhibitor)
• *Pregnancy Risk Category:* B

HOW SUPPLIED

Cream: 1%

ACTION

Mechanism: Inhibits ergosterol synthesis in susceptible fungal organisms, thereby weakening cell wall integrity.
Absorption: Systemic absorption is low. Less than 0.3% is recovered in the urine up to 5 days after application.
Distribution: Most of the drug concentrates in the epidermis, with smaller amounts in the upper and deeper corneum.
Excretion: In urine. Unknown if the drug is excreted in feces.

INDICATIONS & DOSAGE

Topical treatment of dermal infections caused by tinea rubrum and tinea mentagrophytes (tinea pedis, tinea cruris, and tinea corporis)–
Adults: apply to affected area once daily (in the evening) for 2 weeks (1 month for tinea pedis).

CONTRAINDICATIONS & PRECAUTIONS

Contraindicated in patients hypersensitive to oxiconazole nitrate. This drug is not for ophthalmic use. Use cautiously in breast-feeding women because animal studies report that oxiconazole is excreted in breast milk.

ADVERSE REACTIONS

Common reactions are in italics; life-threatening reactions are in bold italics.
Skin: itching, burning, irritation, maceration, erythema, fissuring.

INTERACTIONS

None reported.

EFFECTS ON DIAGNOSTIC TESTS

None reported.

NURSING CONSIDERATIONS

Besides those related universally to drug therapy (see "How to use this book"), consider the following specific recommendations:

Assessment
• Obtain a baseline assessment of the dermal infection before therapy.
• Be alert for adverse reactions or drug interactions during therapy.
• Evaluate the patient's and family's knowledge about oxiconazole therapy.

Nursing Diagnoses
• Impaired skin integrity related to dermal infections.
• High risk for impaired skin integrity related to oxiconazole-induced maceration.
• Knowledge deficit related to oxiconazole therapy.

Planning and Implementation
Preparation and Administration
• ***Topical use:*** Apply to affected area.
Monitoring
• Monitor effectiveness by regularly examining the dermal infection.
• Monitor for adverse reactions or interactions by frequently observing the patient's skin for itching, burning, or maceration.
Supportive Care
• Be prepared to discontinue the drug and notify the doctor if adverse reactions occur.
Patient Teaching
• Teach patient to apply medication.
• Be sure patient understands that drug is for external use only. Instruct him to avoid using it near the eyes.

Evaluation
In patients receiving oxiconazole, appropriate evaluation statements may include:
• Dermal infection has healed.
• Maceration did not occur.
• Patient and family state an understanding of oxiconazole therapy.

oxtriphylline (choline theophyllinate)
(ox trye´ fi lin)
Choledyl*

• *Classification:* bronchodilator (xanthine derivative)
• *Pregnancy Risk Category:* C

HOW SUPPLIED
Tablets: 100 mg, 200 mg
Tablets (sustained-release): 400 mg, 600 mg
Elixir: 100 mg/5 ml
Syrup: 50 mg/5 ml

ACTION
Mechanism: The choline salt of theophylline that releases theophylline in the stomach. Pharmacologic activity is caused by theophylline, which inhibits phosphodiesterase, the enzyme that degrades cyclic 3′, 5′ adenosine monophosphate (cyclic AMP). Increased cellular cAMP levels alters intracellular calcium movement, resulting in relaxation of smooth muscle of the bronchial airways and pulmonary blood vessels.
Absorption: Dissolution of the drug into free theophylline in the stomach is the rate-limiting step in oral absorption. Food alters the rate, but not the extent, of absorption.
Distribution: Theophylline is distributed in all tissues and extracellular fluids except fatty tissue.
Metabolism: Metabolized to inactive compounds.
Excretion: Small amounts (8% to 12%) are excreted in the urine; only about 10% is excreted in the feces unchanged. Half-life: Variable; averages 7 to 9 hours in healthy adults, 1.5 to 9.5 hours in children, and 15 to 58 hours in neonates. The half-life in smoking adults is shorter (4 to 5 hours); longer in adults with CHF, cor pulmonale, COPD, or liver disease.
Onset, peak, duration: Dependent on serum concentration of drug; serum theophylline concentrations of 10 to 20 mcg/ml are usually required for optimum response.

INDICATIONS & DOSAGE
To relieve acute bronchial asthma and reversible bronchospasm associated with chronic bronchitis and emphysema –
Adults and children over 12 years: 200 mg P.O. q 6 hours; or 400 to 600 mg sustained-release form P.O. q 12 hours, then adjust dosage based upon serum theophylline levels.
Children 2 to 12 years: 4 mg/kg P.O. q 6 hours. Adjust as needed to maintain therapeutic levels of theophylline (10 to 20 mcg/ml).

CONTRAINDICATIONS & PRECAUTIONS
Contraindicated in patients with hypersensitivity to xanthines. Use cautiously in patients with compromised cardiac or circulatory function, diabetes, glaucoma, hypertension, hyperthyroidism, peptic ulcer, or gastroesophageal reflux, because drug may worsen these symptoms or conditions.

ADVERSE REACTIONS
Common reactions are in italics; life-threatening reactions are in bold italics.
CNS: *restlessness, dizziness,* headache, *insomnia,* light-headedness, *seizures,* muscle twitching.
CV: *palpitations, sinus tachycardia,*

extrasystoles, flushing, marked hypotension, increase in respiratory rate.
GI: *nausea, vomiting, anorexia,* bitter aftertaste, dyspepsia, heavy feeling in stomach.
Skin: urticaria.

INTERACTIONS

Barbiturates, phenytoin, rifampin: enhanced metabolism and decreased theophylline blood levels. Monitor for decreased effect.
Beta-adrenergic blockers: antagonism. Propranolol and nadolol, especially, may cause bronchospasms in sensitive patients. Use together cautiously.
Erythromycin, troleandomycin, cimetidine, influenza virus vaccine, oral contraceptives: decreased hepatic clearance of theophylline; increased plasma level. Monitor for signs of toxicity.

EFFECTS ON DIAGNOSTIC TESTS

Serum uric acid (measured by colorimetric methods): falsely elevated.
Theophylline: falsely elevated levels in patients using furosemide, phenylbutazone, probenecid, some cephalosporins, sulfa medications, theobromine, caffeine, tea, chocolate, cola beverages, and acetaminophen, depending on assay method.

NURSING CONSIDERATIONS

Besides those related universally to drug therapy (see "How to use this book"), consider the following specific recommendations.

Assessment
- Obtain a baseline assessment of cardiopulmonary status before oxtriphylline therapy by taking vital signs, noting ECG results and auscultating heart and lung fields.
- Be alert for adverse reactions or drug interactions during therapy.
- Evaluate the patient's and family's knowledge about oxtriphylline therapy.

Nursing Diagnoses
- Ineffective airway clearance related to patients underlying condition.
- High risk for injury related to adverse CNS reactions to oxtriphylline.
- Knowledge deficit related to oxtriphylline therapy.

Planning and Implementation
Preparation and Administration
- ***P.O. use:*** Administer drug after meals and at bedtime.
- Store at 15° to 30° C (59° to 86 °F). Protect elixir from light and tablets from moisture.

Monitoring
- Monitor effectiveness by monitoring respiratory rate, auscultating lung fields, and following laboratory studies such as arterial blood gases.
- Monitor vital signs, noting heart rate and rhythm.
- Measure intake and output.
- Observe the patient for signs of restlessness, dizziness, and complaints of insomnia.

Supportive Care
- If adverse CNS reactions develop in the hospitalized patient, notify the doctor, who may alter the dose or change medications.
- Institute safety precautions if adverse CNS effects occur.
- Institute seizure precautions until adverse CNS reactions are known.
- Obtain an order for antiemetic or antidiarrheal if GI reactions occur.
- Remember that oxytriphylline is equivalent to 64% anhydrous theophylline.

Patient Teaching
- Tell the patient to report GI distress, palpitations, irritability, restlessness, nervousness, or insomnia as this may indicate excessive CNS stimulation.
- Tell the patient to check with his doctor or pharmacist before taking any other medications, because OTC remedies may contain ephedrine and excessive CNS stimulation may result.

Evaluation
In patients receiving oxtriphylline, appropriate evaluation statements may include:
• Patient experiences improved respiratory status.
• Patient does not develop adverse CNS reactions as a result of oxtriphylline therapy.
• Patient and family state an understanding of oxtriphylline therapy.

oxybutynin chloride
(ox i byoo´ ti nin)
Ditropan

• *Classification:* antispasmodic (synthetic tertiary amine)
• *Pregnancy Risk Category:* C

HOW SUPPLIED
Tablets: 5 mg
Syrup: 5 mg/5 ml

ACTION
Mechanism: Has both a direct spasmolytic effect and an atropine-like effect on urinary tract smooth muscles. It has about 20% of the anticholinergic activity of atropine, but 4 to 10 times the antispasmotic activity. It increases urinary bladder capacity and provides some local anesthesia and mild analgesia.
Absorption: Rapidly absorbed.
Metabolism: By the liver.
Excretion: Principally in urine.
Onset, peak, duration: Peak levels in 3 to 6 hours. Action begins in 30 to 60 minutes and persists for 6 to 10 hours.

INDICATIONS & DOSAGE
Antispasmodic for neurogenic bladder–
Adults: 5 mg P.O. b.i.d. to t.i.d., to maximum of 5 mg q.i.d.
Children over 5 years: 5 mg P.O. b.i.d., to maximum of 5 mg t.i.d.

CONTRAINDICATIONS & PRECAUTIONS
Contraindicated in patients with partial or complete GI tract obstruction, glaucoma, myasthenia gravis, adynamic ileus, megacolon, or severe or ulcerative colitis, because it may worsen these symptoms or disorders; in debilitated and elderly patients with intestinal atony; in hemorrhaging patients with unstable cardiovascular status; and in patients with obstructive uropathy.

Use with caution in elderly patients, in patients with autonomic neuropathy or hepatic or renal disease, and in patients with reflux esophagitis because drug may aggravate these conditions.

ADVERSE REACTIONS
Common reactions are in italics; life-threatening reactions are in bold italics.
CNS: *drowsiness,* dizziness, insomnia, *dry mouth,* flushing.
CV: *palpitations, tachycardia.*
EENT: *transient blurred vision,* mydriasis, cycloplegia.
GI: nausea, vomiting, *constipation,* bloated feeling.
GU: impotence, *urinary hesitance or urine retention.*
Skin: urticaria, ***severe allergic reactions in patients sensitive to anticholinergics.***
Other: decreased sweating, fever, suppression of lactation.

INTERACTIONS
None significant.

EFFECTS ON DIAGNOSTIC TESTS
None reported.

NURSING CONSIDERATIONS
Besides those related universally to drug therapy (see "How to use this book"), consider the following specific recommendations:

Assessment
• Obtain a baseline urologic assessment focusing on frequency and intensity of bladder spasms before therapy.
• Be alert for adverse reactions or drug interactions during therapy.
• Evaluate the patient's and family's knowledge about oxybutynin chloride.

Nursing Diagnoses
• Pain (bladder spasms) related to patient's underlying condition.
• High risk for injury related to oxybutynin chloride induced blurred vision and drowsiness.
• Knowledge deficit related to oxybutynin chloride therapy.

Planning and Implementation

Preparation and Administration
• Store in tightly closed containers at 59° to 86° F. (15° to 30° C.).
• Be sure that partial intestinal obstruction has been ruled out in patients with diarrhea, especially those with colostomy or ileostomy, before giving oxybutynin chloride.
• Administer antibiotics concomitantly, as ordered, in patients who also have urinary tract infections.
• Neurogenic bladder should be confirmed by cystometry administering before oxybutynin chloride.

Monitoring
• Monitor effectiveness by determining patient's level of discomfort and through periodically monitoring cystometry results to determine the presence of neurogenic bladder.
• Monitor for signs of CNS adverse effects.
• Monitor intake and output, particularly if GI adverse effects develop.
• Monitor for increased temperature and heat stroke during hot weather. Oxybutynin chloride suppresses sweating and may precipitate fever or heat stroke.

Supportive Care
• Institute safety measures such as assisting the patient out of bed and using side rails at all times if CNS adverse reactions develop.
• Stop therapy periodically, as ordered, to determine whether patient can get along without it. This may minimize tendency toward tolerance.
• Evaluate patient's response to therapy by periodically noting cystometry results.
• Notify the doctor if a skin rash develops; this may require discontinuation of the drug.

Patient Teaching
• Warn patient that drug may impair alertness or vision. Patient should avoid driving and other hazardous activities until the adverse CNS effects of the drug are known.
• Tell patient to notify doctor if CNS side effects develop.
• Inform the patient that oxybutynin chloride has a rapid onset of action. It peaks at 3 to 4 hours, and lasts 6 to 10 hours.

Evaluation
In patients receiving oxybutynin chloride, appropriate evaluation statements may include:
• Patient expresses pain relief from bladder spasms.
• Patient does not sustain injuries resulting from oxybutynin chloride therapy.
• Patient and family state an understanding of oxybutynin chloride therapy.

oxycodone hydrochloride
(ox i koe´ done)
Endone‡, Roxicodone, Supeudol†
• Controlled Substance Schedule II

oxycodone pectinate
Proladone‡

• *Classification:* analgesic (opioid)

• *Pregnancy Risk Category:* B (D for prolonged use or use of high doses at term)

HOW SUPPLIED

hydrochloride
Tablets: 5 mg
Oral solution: 5 mg/5 ml
Suppositories: 10 mg, 20 mg
pectinate
Suppositories: 30 mg‡

ACTION

Mechanism: Binds with opiate receptors at many sites in the CNS (brain, brain stem, and spinal cord), altering both perception of and emotional response to pain through an unknown mechanism.
Absorption: Rapidly absorbed from the GI tract.
Distribution: Drug crosses placenta.
Metabolism: Hepatic.
Excretion: Oxycodone and metabolites are excreted principally by the kidneys.
Onset, peak, duration: After oral administration, the onset of analgesic effect occurs within 15 to 30 minutes and peak effect is reached within 1 hour. Duration of analgesia is 4 to 6 hours.

INDICATIONS & DOSAGE

Moderate to severe pain–
Adults: available in combination with other drugs, such as aspirin (Percodan, Percodan-Demi) or acetaminophen (Percocet, Tylox). One to 2 tablets P.O. q 6 hours, p.r.n. or around the clock. Or 5 mg (5 ml) of oxycodone oral solution P.O. q 6 hours.
Adults: (Supeudol) 1 to 3 suppositories rectally daily, p.r.n. or around the clock.
Children: (Percodan-Demi) ¼ to ½ tablet P.O. q 6 hours, p.r.n. or around the clock.

CONTRAINDICATIONS & PRECAUTIONS

Contraindicated in patients with hypersensitivity to the drug or other phenanthrene opioids (codeine, hydrocodone, hydromorphone, or oxymorphone).

Administer with extreme caution to patients with supraventricular arrhythmias; avoid, or administer with extreme caution to patients with head injury or increased intracranial pressure, because drug obscures neurologic parameters; and during pregnancy and labor, because drug readily crosses placenta (premature infants are especially sensitive to respiratory and CNS depressant effects of opioids).

Administer cautiously to patients with renal or hepatic dysfunction, because drug accumulation or prolonged duration of action may occur; asthma or chronic obstructive pulmonary disease, because drug depresses respiration and suppresses cough reflex; seizure disorders, because drug may precipitate seizures; or to patients undergoing biliary tract surgery, because drug may cause biliary spasm; elderly or debilitated patients, who are more sensitive to both therapeutic and adverse drug effects; and to patients prone to physical or psychic addiction, because of the high risk of addiction to this drug.

ADVERSE REACTIONS

Common reactions are in italics; life-threatening reactions are in bold italics.
CNS: *sedation, somnolence, clouded sensorium, euphoria,* dizziness, seizures with large doses.
CV: *hypotension,* bradycardia.
GI: *nausea, vomiting, constipation,* ileus.
GU: *urine retention.*
Other: ***respiratory depression,*** physical dependence.

INTERACTIONS

Alcohol, CNS depressants: additive effects. Use together cautiously.
Anticoagulants: products containing aspirin may increase anticoagulant effect. Monitor clotting times. Use together cautiously.

EFFECTS ON DIAGNOSTIC TESTS

Liver function tests: elevated levels.
Plasma amylase and lipase: increased levels.

NURSING CONSIDERATIONS

Besides those related universally to drug therapy (see "How to use this book"), consider the following specific recommendations:

Assessment

- Obtain a baseline assessment of the patient's pain before therapy.
- Be alert for common adverse reactions and drug interactions during therapy.
- Evaluate the patient's and family's knowledge about oxycodone.

Nursing Diagnoses

- Pain related to patient's underlying condition.
- Ineffective breathing pattern related to oxycodone-induced respiratory depression.
- Knowledge deficit related to oxycodone therapy.

Planning and Implementation

Preparation and Administration

- ***P.O. use:*** Give after meals or with milk. Keep in mind that single-agent oxycodone solution or tablets are especially good for patients who shouldn't take aspirin or acetaminophen.
- For full analgesic effect, give before patient has intense pain.
- Be aware that use with general anesthetics, tranquilizers, sedatives, hypnotics, alcohol, tricyclic antidepressants, or MAO inhibitors increase CNS depression. Reduce oxycodone dose and use together with extreme caution. Monitor patient's response.
- Don't give to children, except for the combination product, Percodan-Demi.

Monitoring

- Monitor effectiveness by assessing pain relief after each dose.
- Monitor patient's rate and pattern of breathing for evidence of respiratory depression.
- Monitor circulatory status and bowel and bladder function.

Supportive Care

- Notify the doctor if pain is not relieved.
- Hold drug and notify the doctor if the patient's respirations are below 12 breaths/minute.
- If not contraindicated, increase the patient's fluid and fiber intake to prevent or treat constipation. Obtain an order for a laxative or stool softener, as needed.

Patient Teaching

- Warn the ambulatory patient to avoid driving and other hazardous activities that require mental alertness.
- Tell the patient or family to notify the nurse or doctor if respiratory rate decreases.
- Suggest high-fiber diet and liberal fluid intake to prevent constipation.

Evaluation

In the patient receiving oxycodone, appropriate evaluation statements include:

- Patient reports pain relief.
- Patient's respiratory rate and pattern remain within normal limits.
- Patient and family state an understanding of oxycodone therapy.

---

oxymetazoline hydrochloride

(ox i met az´ oh leen)

Afrin◇, Afrin Children's Strength Nose Drops◇, Allerest 12-Hour Nasal◇, Chlorphed-LA◇, Coricidin Nasal

Mist◇, Dristan Long Lasting◇, Drixine Nasal‡, Duramist Plus◇, Duration◇, 4-Way Long-Acting Nasal, Genasal Spray◇, Neo-Synephrine 12 Hour◇, Nostrilla◇, NTZ Long Acting Nasal◇, Sinarest 12-Hour◇, Sinex Long-Acting◇, Twice-A-Day Nasal◇

• *Classification:* decongestant, vasoconstrictor (sympathomimetic agent)
• *Pregnancy Risk Category:* C

HOW SUPPLIED

Nasal solution: 0.025%◇, 0.05%◇

ACTION

Mechanism: An alpha-adrenergic agonist that produces local vasoconstriction of dilated arterioles to reduce blood flow and nasal congestion.
Pharmacokinetics: Unknown.
Onset, peak, duration: Onset is 5 to 10 minutes, and persists for about 6 hours. Effects gradually diminish over the next 6 hours, making twice a day dosing possible.

INDICATIONS & DOSAGE

Nasal congestion–
Adults and children over 6 years: apply 2 to 4 drops or sprays of 0.05% solution to nasal mucosa b.i.d.
Children 2 to 6 years: apply 2 to 3 drops 0.025% solution to nasal mucosa b.i.d. Use no longer than 3 to 5 days. Dosage for younger children has not been established.

CONTRAINDICATIONS & PRECAUTIONS

Contraindicated in patients with narrow-angle glaucoma or hypersensitivity to any components of the preparation. Use cautiously in patients with hyperthyroidism, cardiac disease, hypertension, diabetes mellitus, and advanced arteriosclerosis.

ADVERSE REACTIONS

Common reactions are in italics; life-threatening reactions are in bold italics.
CNS: headache, drowsiness, dizziness, insomnia, possible sedation.
CV: palpitations, ***hypotension with cardiovascular collapse,*** hypertension.
EENT: rebound nasal congestion or irritation with excessive or long-term use, dryness of nose and throat, increased nasal discharge, stinging, sneezing.
Other: systemic effects in children with excessive or long-term use.

INTERACTIONS

None significant.

EFFECTS ON DIAGNOSTIC TESTS

None reported.

NURSING CONSIDERATIONS

Besides those related universally to drug therapy, (see "How to use this book"), consider the following recommendations.

Assessment

• Obtain a baseline assessment of the patient's breathing pattern and degree of nasal congestion.
• Be alert for adverse reactions or drug interactions during therapy.
• Evaluate the patient's and family's knowledge about oxymetazoline hydrochloride therapy.

Nursing Diagnoses

• Ineffective breathing pattern related to the patient's underlying condition.
• Decreased cardiac output related to systemic absorption of oxymetazoline hydrochloride.
• Knowledge deficit related to oxymetazoline hydrochloride therapy.

Planning and Implementation

Preparation and Administration
• ***Inhalation:*** Have patient hold head upright and sniff spray briskly.
Monitoring
• Monitor effectiveness by assessing the patient's breathing pattern and degree of nasal congestion.

• Monitor blood pressure and apical rate for drug-induced cardiac effects; obtain ECG as indicated.
• Closely monitor use in patients with underlying cardiac or thyroid disease or diabetes mellitus.

Supportive Care

• Notify the doctor immediately if changes in the patient's health status occur.

Patient Teaching

• Teach the patient how to administer the drug, and tell him it should be used by one person only.
• Warn the patient not to exceed the recommended dose, and to use the drug only when needed.
• Warn the patient that excessive use may cause cardiac effects, dizziness or sedation.

Evaluation

In patients receiving oxymetazoline hydrochloride, appropriate evaluation statements may include:

• Patient obtains relief from nasal congestion.
• Patient remains free of systemic cardiac effects.
• Patient and family state an understanding of oxymetazoline hydrochloride therapy.

oxymorphone hydrochloride

(ox i mor´ fone)

Numorphan

• Controlled Substance Schedule II
• *Classification:* analgesic (opioid)
• *Pregnancy Risk Category:* B (D for prolonged use or use of high doses at term)

HOW SUPPLIED

Injection: 1 mg/ml, 1.5 mg/ml
Suppositories: 5 mg

ACTION

Mechanism: Binds with opiate receptors at many sites in the CNS (brain, brain stem, and spinal cord), altering both perception of and emotional response to pain through an unknown mechanism.
Absorption: Well absorbed after rectal, S.C., or I.M. administration.
Distribution: Widely distributed.
Metabolism: Primarily in the liver.
Excretion: Primarily in the urine as oxymorphone hydrochloride.
Onset, peak, duration: Onset of action usually occurs within 15 to 30 minutes. Peak analgesic effect is seen at 30 minutes to 1 hour. Duration of action is 3 to 6 hours.

INDICATIONS & DOSAGE

Moderate to severe pain–
Adults: 1 to 1.5 mg I.M. or S.C. q 4 to 6 hours, p.r.n. or around the clock; or 0.5 mg I.V. q 4 to 6 hours, p.r.n. or around the clock; or 2.5 to 5 mg rectally q 4 to 6 hours, p.r.n. or around the clock.

CONTRAINDICATIONS & PRECAUTIONS

Contraindicated in patients with hypersensitivity to the drug or any phenanthrene opioid (codeine, hydrocodone, hydromorphone, morphine, oxycodone). Administer with extreme caution to patients with supraventricular arrhythmias; avoid, or administer with extreme caution to patients with head injury or increased intracranial pressure, because drug obscures neurologic parameters; and during pregnancy and labor, because drug readily crosses placenta (premature infants are especially sensitive to respiratory and CNS depressant effects).

Administer cautiously to patients with renal or hepatic dysfunction, because drug accumulation or prolonged duration of action may occur; asthma or chronic obstructive pulmonary disease because drug depresses respiration and suppresses cough reflex; or seizure disorders, because drug may precipitate seizures; to patients undergoing biliary tract surgery, because drug may cause biliary spasm; elderly or debilitated patients, who are more sensitive to both therapeutic and adverse effects; and to patients prone to physical or psychic addiction, because of the high risk of addiction to this drug.

ADVERSE REACTIONS

Common reactions are in italics; life-threatening reactions are in bold italics.
CNS: *sedation, somnolence, clouded sensorium, euphoria,* dizziness, seizures with large doses.
CV: *hypotension,* bradycardia.
GI: *nausea, vomiting, constipation,* ileus.
GU: *urine retention.*
Other: ***respiratory depression,*** physical dependence.

INTERACTIONS

Alcohol, CNS depressants: additive effects. Use together cautiously.

EFFECTS ON DIAGNOSTIC TESTS

Plasma amylase: increased levels.

NURSING CONSIDERATIONS

Besides those related universally to drug therapy (see "How to use this book"), consider the following specific recommendations:

Assessment

- Obtain a baseline assessment of the patient's pain before therapy.
- Be alert for common adverse reactions and drug interactions during therapy.
- Evaluate the patient's and family's knowledge about oxymorphone.

Nursing Diagnoses

- Pain related to patient's underlying condition.
- Ineffective breathing pattern related to oxymorphone-induced respiratory depression.
- Knowledge deficit related to oxymorphone therapy.

Planning and Implementation

Preparation and Administration

- ***I.V. use:*** Keep patient supine during administration to minimize hypotension.
- For better analgesic effect, give before patient has intense pain.
- Be aware that CNS depression is increased if used with general anesthetics, tranquilizers, sedatives, hypnotics, alcohol, tricyclic antidepressants, or MAO inhibitors. Reduce oxymorphone use. Use together with extreme caution. Monitor patient's response.

Monitoring

- Monitor effectiveness by assessing the patient's degree of pain relief after each dose.
- Monitor patient's rate and pattern of breathing for evidence of respiratory depression. Remember to monitor respirations for at least 1 hour after I.V. dose.
- Monitor patient's cardiovascular status and bowel and bladder function.

Supportive Care

- Notify the doctor if pain is not relieved.
- Hold drug and notify the doctor if the patient's respirations are below 12 breaths/minute.
- Be aware that the drug is well absorbed rectally. Alternative to narcotics with more limited dosage forms.
- Keep narcotic antagonist (naloxone) and resuscitative equipment available.
- Keep in mind that dependence can develop with long-term use.
- Be aware that this drug is not intended for mild to moderate pain. May worsen gallbladder pain.
- Unless contraindicated, increase the patient's fluid and fiber intake to prevent or treat constipation. Obtain order for laxative or stool softener, if needed.

Patient Teaching

- Warn the ambulatory patient to avoid driving and other hazardous

activities that require mental alertness.
• Tell the patient to rise slowly following I.V. administration to reduce faintness and dizziness.
• Tell the patient or family to notify the nurse or doctor if respiratory rate decreases.
• During postoperative use, encourage turning, coughing, and deep breathing and use of the incentive spirometer to avoid atelectasis.
• Instruct the patient to request medication before pain becomes intense.
• Suggest high-fiber diet and liberal fluid intake to prevent constipation in the patient.

Evaluation

In the patient receiving oxymorphone, appropriate evaluation statements include:
• Patient reports pain relief.
• Patient's respiratory status within normal limits.
• Patient and family state an understanding of oxymorphone therapy.

oxytetracycline hydrochloride
(ox i tet ra sye´ kleen)
E.P. Mycin, Terramycin

• *Classification:* antibiotic (tetracycline)
• *Pregnancy Risk Category:* D

HOW SUPPLIED
Tablets: 250 mg
Capsules: 250 mg
Injection for I.M. use: 50 mg/ml, 125 mg/ml (with lidocaine 2%)

ACTION
Mechanism: Exerts bacteriostatic effect by binding to the 30S ribosomal subunit of microorganisms, thus inhibiting protein synthesis.
Absorption: After oral administration in fasting adults, oxytetracycline is 60% absorbed from GI tract. Absorption after I.M. injection is erratic and incomplete, and usually produces peak levels lower than those after oral administration.
Distribution: Widely distributed into body tissues and fluids, including synovial, pleural, prostatic, and seminal fluids, bronchial secretions, saliva, and aqueous humor; CSF penetration is poor. Oxytetracycline crosses the placenta; it is 10% to 14% protein-bound.
Metabolism: Not metabolized.
Excretion: Primarily excreted unchanged in urine by glomerular filtration; some may be excreted in breast milk. Half-life: 6 to 10 hours in adults with normal renal function.
Onset, peak, duration: Peak serum levels occur at 2 to 4 hours after oral administration.

INDICATIONS & DOSAGE
Infections caused by sensitive gram-negative and gram-positive organisms, trachoma, rickettsiae–
Adults: 250 mg P.O. q 6 hours; 100 mg I.M. q 8 to 12 hours; 250 mg I.M. as a single dose.
Children over 8 years: 25 to 50 mg/kg P.O. daily, divided q 6 hours; 15 to 25 mg/kg I.M. daily, divided q 8 to 12 hours
Brucellosis–
Adults: 500 mg P.O. q.i.d. for 3 weeks with streptomycin 1 g I.M. q 12 hours first week, once daily second week.
Syphilis in patients sensitive to penicillin–
Adults: 30 to 40 g total dosage P.O., divided equally over 10 to 15 days.
Gonorrhea in patients sensitive to penicillin–
Adults: initially, 1.5 g P.O. followed by 0.5 g q.i.d. for a total of 9 g.

CONTRAINDICATIONS & PRECAUTIONS
Contraindicated in patients with hypersensitivity to any tetracycline; during the second half of pregnancy; and

in children under age 8 because of the risk of permanent discoloration of teeth, enamel defects, and retardation of bone growth.

Use with caution in patients with decreased renal function because drug may elevate BUN levels and exacerbate dysfunction; and in patients apt to be exposed to sunlight or ultraviolet light because of the risk of photosensitivity reactions.

ADVERSE REACTIONS

Common reactions are in italics; life-threatening reactions are in bold italics.
Blood: neutropenia, eosinophilia.
CNS: ***intracranial hypertension.***
CV: pericarditis.
EENT: dysphagia, glossitis.
GI: *anorexia, nausea,* vomiting, *diarrhea,* enterocolitis, anogenital inflammation.
Metabolic: *increased BUN.*
Skin: *maculopapular and erythematous rashes, urticaria, photosensitivity, increased pigmentation.*
Local: *irritation after I.M. injection, thrombophlebitis.*
Other: ***hypersensitivity.***

INTERACTIONS

Antacids (including sodium bicarbonate) and laxatives containing aluminum, magnesium, or calcium; food, milk, or other dairy products: decrease antibiotic absorption. Give antibiotic 1 hour before or 2 hours after.
Ferrous sulfate and other iron products, zinc: decrease antibiotic absorption. Give tetracyclines 3 hours after or 2 hours before iron administration.
Methoxyflurane: may cause severe nephrotoxicity with tetracyclines.
Oral contraceptives: decreased contraceptive effectiveness and increased risk of breakthrough bleeding.

EFFECTS ON DIAGNOSTIC TESTS

BUN: elevated levels with decreased renal function.
Urine catecholamines: false elevations in fluorometric tests.
Urine glucose tests with glucose enzymatic (Clinistix or Tes-Tape): false-negative results.
Urine glucose tests with Clinitest: false-negative results with parenteral use.

NURSING CONSIDERATIONS

Besides those related universally to drug therapy (see "How to use this book"), consider the following specific recommendations:

Assessment

- Obtain a baseline assessment of infection before therapy.
- Be alert for adverse reactions and drug interactions throughout therapy.
- Evaluate the patient's and family's knowledge about oxytetracycline therapy.

Nursing Diagnoses

- High risk for infection related to ineffectiveness of oxytetracycline to eradicate the infection.
- High risk for fluid volume deficit related to adverse GI reactions caused by oxytetracycline therapy.
- Knowledge deficit related to oxytetracycline.

Planning and Implementation

Preparation and Administration

- Obtain specimen for culture and sensitivity tests before first dose. Therapy may begin pending test results.
- Check expiration date. Outdated or deteriorated tetracyclines have been associated with reversible nephrotoxicity (Fanconi's syndrome).
- Be aware that use of oxytetracycline during the last half of pregnancy and in children under 8 years may cause permanent discoloration of teeth, enamel defects, and retardation of bone growth. Question an order

for oxytetracycline before administering the first dose to a child.
• Do not expose drug to light or heat.
• ***P.O. use:*** Giving with milk or other dairy products, food, antacids, or iron products reduces effectiveness. Administer with a full glass of water on an empty stomach, at least 1 hour before meals or 2 hours afterward. Give at least 1 hour before bedtime to prevent esophagitis.
• ***I.M. use:*** Administer drug deep I.M. Be aware that injection may be painful. Rotate sites. I.M. preparations contain a local anesthetic; ask patient about hypersensitivity to local anesthetics before administering first dose.
• ***I.V. use:*** Reconstitute 250 mg and 500 mg powder for injection with 10 ml sterile water. Dilute to at least 100 ml in dextrose 5% in water, normal saline solution or Ringer's solution. Do not mix with any other drug. Store reconstituted solutions in refrigerator. Stable for 48 hours.
Monitoring
• Monitor effectiveness by regularly assessing for improvement of infection.
• Monitor for signs and symptoms of superinfections.
• Monitor hydration status if adverse GI reactions occur.
• Monitor I.V. site for phlebitis.
Supportive Care
• If the patient develops a superinfection, or new infection, notify the doctor. Prepare to discontinue the drug and substitute another antibiotic. If the patient develops oral thrush, provide good mouth care.
• If the patient develops diarrhea, nausea, or vomiting, request an antiemetic or antidiarrheal agent, if needed. Expect to substitute a parenteral form of oxytetracycline or another antibiotic as prescribed.
• Rotate I.V. site to minimize irritation.
• Monitor diabetic patient's blood glucose levels because drug can alter test results for urine glucose.
Patient Teaching
• Advise the patient to avoid direct exposure to sunlight and ultraviolet light and to use a sunscreen with a sun protection factor of 15 or higher to help prevent photosensitivity reactions. Remind the patient that photosensitivity persists for some time after discontinuation of drug.
• Tell the patient to take oral oxytetracycline with a full glass of water (To facilitate passage to the stomach), 1 hour before or 2 hours after meals for maximum absorption, and not less than 1 hour before bedtime (to prevent irritation from esophageal reflux).
• Tell the patient not to take the drug with food, milk or other dairy products, antacids, or iron compounds as it may interfere with absorption.
• Emphasize importance of completing prescribed regimen exactly as ordered and keeping follow-up appointments.
• Tell the patient to check expiration dates and discard any outdated oxytetracycline as it may become toxic.
• Teach the patient to report signs of superinfection (furry overgrowth on tongue, vaginal itch or discharge, foul-smelling stool). Stress good oral hygiene.
• Inform diabetic patients that drug may alter urine glucose test results. Teach patient to monitor blood glucose levels instead.
• Advise female patient taking an oral contraceptive to use an alternative means of contraception during therapy and for 1 week after drug is discontinued.
Evaluation
In patients receiving oxytetracycline, appropriate evaluation statements may include:
• Patient is free of infection.
• Patient maintains adequate hydra-

tion throughout oxytetracycline therapy.
• Patient and family state an understanding of oxytetracycline therapy.

oxytocin, synthetic injection
(ox i toe´ sin)
Oxytocin, Pitocin, Syntocinon

• *Classification:* oxytocic, lactation stimulant (exogenous hormone)

HOW SUPPLIED
Injection: 10 units/ml

ACTION
Mechanism: A synthetic form of the naturally occurring posterior pituitary hormone. Causes potent and selective stimulation of uterine and mammary gland smooth muscle.
Distribution: Drug is distributed throughout the extracellular fluid; small amounts may enter the fetal circulation.
Metabolism: Oxytocin is metabolized rapidly in the kidneys and liver. In early pregnancy, a circulating enzyme, oxytocinase, can inactivate the drug.
Excretion: Only small amounts are excreted in the urine as oxytocin. Half-life: 3 to 5 minutes.
Onset, peak, and duration: Onset is immediate following I.V. injection and occurs within 3 to 5 minutes of an I.M. injection. Duration of action is 1 hour after I.V. infusion; 2 to 3 hours after I.M. injection.

INDICATIONS & DOSAGE
Induction or stimulation of labor–
Adults: initially, 1 ml (10 units) ampule in 1,000 ml of dextrose 5% injection or normal saline solution I.V. infused at 1 to 2 milliunits/minute. Increase rate at 15- to 30-minute intervals until normal contraction pattern is established. Maximum is 1 to 2 ml (20 milliunits)/minute. Decrease rate when labor is firmly established.
Reduction of postpartum bleeding after expulsion of placenta–
Adults: 10 to 40 units added to 1,000 ml of dextrose 5% in water or normal saline solution infused at rate necessary to control bleeding, usually 10 to 20 milliunits/minute. Also, 1 ml (10 units) can be given I.M. after delivery of the placenta.
Incomplete or inevitable abortion–
Adults: I.V. infusion with 10 units of oxytocin in 500 ml of normal saline solution or dextrose 5% in normal saline solution. Infuse at rate of 10 to 20 milliunits/minute.

CONTRAINDICATIONS & PRECAUTIONS
Contraindicated in patients with hypersensitivity to the drug. The nasal preparation is contraindicated during pregnancy. Oxytocin should not be used to induce labor when the benefit-to-risk ratio for the mother or child favors surgical intervention, when labor is progressing normally during the first and second stages of labor, when hypertonic patterns of labor occur, or when vaginal delivery is contraindicated.

ADVERSE REACTIONS
Common reactions are in italics; life-threatening reactions are in bold italics.
Maternal–
Blood: afibrinogenemia; may be related to increased postpartum bleeding.
CNS: ***subarachnoid hemorrhage resulting from hypertension; seizures or coma resulting from water intoxication.***
CV: hypotension; increased heart rate, systemic venous return, and cardiac output; arrhythmias.
GI: nausea, vomiting.
Other: hypersensitivity, tetanic contractions, abruptio placentae, *im-*

paired uterine blood flow, pelvic hematoma, *increased uterine motility,* ***anaphylaxis.***
Fetal–
Blood: hyperbilirubinemia.
CV: bradycardia, tachycardia, premature ventricular contractions.
Other: *anoxia,* ***asphyxia.***

INTERACTIONS

Cyclopropane anesthetics: less pronounced bradycardia; hypotension.
Thiopental anesthetics: delayed induction reported.
Vasoconstrictors: severe hypertension if oxytocin is given within 3 to 4 hours of vasoconstrictor in patient receiving caudal block anesthetic.

EFFECTS ON DIAGNOSTIC TESTS

None reported.

NURSING CONSIDERATIONS

Besides those related universally to drug therapy (see "How to use this book"), consider the following specific recommendations:

Assessment
- Obtain a baseline assessment of the patient's pregnancy status before therapy.
- Be alert for common adverse reactions or drug interactions during therapy.
- Evaluate the patient's and family's knowledge about oxytocin therapy.

Nursing Diagnoses
- Fluid volume deficit related to postpartum bleeding.
- Fluid volume excess related to oxytocin-induced antidiuretic effect.
- Knowledge deficit related to oxytocin therapy.

Planning and Implementation
Preparation and Administration
- ***I.V. use:*** Don't give by I.V. bolus injection. Must administer by infusion; give by piggyback infusion so the drug may be discontinued without interrupting the I.V. line. Use an infusion pump.
- Administer only in hospital where critical care facilities and doctor are immediately available.
- Never administer oxytocin simultaneously by more than one route.
- Be aware that I.M. route is not recommended. However, 10 units may be given I.M. after delivery of placenta to control postpartum uterine bleeding.

Monitoring
- Monitor effectiveness by continuously assessing frequency, duration, and force of uterine contractions, and, if appropriate, effect on postpartum uterine bleeding.
- Also frequently monitor resting uterine tone; fetal heart rate; maternal heart rate and blood pressure; and intrauterine pressure.
- Monitor fluid intake and output. Oxytocin may produce an antidiuretic effect; fluid overload can lead to seizures and coma.

Supportive Care
- If contractions occur less than 2 minutes apart and if contractions above 50 mm Hg are recorded, or if contractions last 90 seconds or longer, stop infusion, turn patient on her side, and notify doctor.
- Maintain adequate fluid volume if postpartum bleeding occurs.
- Notify doctor if signs of fluid overload occur; if vital signs or fetal heart rate change significantly, if postpartum bleeding persists, or if any other adverse effect occurs.
- To avoid antidiuretic effects, unless contraindicated, restrict fluid intake, as ordered; avoid prolonged infusion of low-sodium fluids and high oxytocin doses.
- Have magnesium sulfate (20% solution) available for relaxation of the myometrium.
- Keep in mind that oxytocin is used to induce labor only when pelvis is known to be adequate, when vaginal delivery is indicated, when fetal ma-

turity is assured, and when fetal position is favorable.

Patient Teaching

• Explain that this drug is used to induce or reinforce labor, or to reduce postpartum bleeding.

• Tell the patient to report any unusual feelings or adverse effects to the doctor or nurse immediately.

• Explain that uterine contractions, maternal and fetal heart rates, and maternal blood pressure will be monitored frequently.

Evaluation

In the patient receiving oxytocin, appropriate evaluation statements may include:

• Adequate fluid volume is maintained; amount of postpartum uterine bleeding is reduced.

• Urinary output is normal; no indications of fluid volume excess.

• Patient and family state an understanding of oxytocin therapy.

oxytocin, synthetic nasal solution

(ox i toe´ sin)

Syntocinon

• *Classification:* oxytocic (synthetic hormone)

HOW SUPPLIED

Nasal solution: 40 units/ml

ACTION

Mechanism: A synthetic form of the naturally occurring posterior pituitary hormone. Causes potent and selective stimulation of uterine and mammary gland smooth muscle. Stimulates impaired milk ejection.

Absorption: Through the nasal mucosa is rapid but may be erratic; it acts within a few minutes.

Distribution: Throughout the extracellular fluid.

Metabolism: In both kidneys and liver.

Excretion: Small amounts are excreted in the urine as unchanged drug.

INDICATIONS & DOSAGE

To promote initial milk ejection; may relieve postpartum breast engorgement–

Adults: 1 spray into one or both nostrils 2 or 3 minutes before breast-feeding or pumping breasts.

CONTRAINDICATIONS & PRECAUTIONS

Contraindicated in patients with hypersensitivity to the drug. The nasal preparation is contraindicated during pregnancy. Oxytocin should not be used to induce labor when the benefit-to-risk ratio for the mother or child favors surgical intervention, when labor is progressing normally during the first and second stages of labor, when hypertonic patterns of labor occur, or when vaginal delivery is contraindicated.

ADVERSE REACTIONS

None reported.

INTERACTIONS

None significant.

EFFECTS ON DIAGNOSTIC TESTS

None reported.

NURSING CONSIDERATIONS

Besides those related universally to drug therapy (see “How to use this book”), consider the following specific recommendations:

Assessment

• Obtain a baseline assessment of the patient’s breast-feeding status before therapy.

• Be alert for common adverse reactions or drug interactions during therapy.

• Evaluate the patient’s and family’s

knowledge about oxytocin nasal solution therapy.

Nursing Diagnoses

• Pain related to postpartum breast engorgement.

• Knowledge deficit related to oxytocin nasal solution therapy.

Planning and Implementation

Preparation and Administration

• First, have patient clear nasal passages. With patient's head in vertical position, hold squeeze bottle upright and eject solution into nostril.

Monitoring

• Monitor effectiveness by assessing milk ejection and relief of pain due to breast engorgement.

Supportive Care

• Use spray before breast feeding or pumping breasts. Assist patient with procedures initially.

Patient Teaching

• Inform the patient that no adverse reactions have been reported following use of oxytocin nasal solution.

• Teach patient correct administration of oxytocin nasal solution.

Evaluation

In patients receiving oxytocin nasal solution, appropriate evaluation statements may include:

• Patient states relief of pain; relief of breast engorgement.

• Patient and family state an understanding of oxytocin nasal solution therapy.

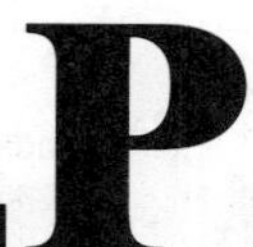

pancreatin

(pan´ kree a tin)

Dizymes Tablets◇, Hi-Vegi-Lip Tablets◇, Pancreatin Enseals◇, Pancreatin Tablets◇

• *Classification:* digestant (pancreatic enzyme)
• *Pregnancy Risk Category:* C

HOW SUPPLIED

Dizymes
Tablets (enteric-coated): 250 mg pancreatin, 6,750 units lipase, 41,250 units protease, 43,750 units amylase◇
Hi-Vegi-Lip
Tablets (enteric-coated): 2,400 mg pancreatin, 12,000 units lipase, 60,000 units protease, and 60,000 units amylase◇
Pancreatin Enseals
Tablets (enteric-coated): 1,000 mg pancreatin, 2,000 units lipase, 25,000 units protease, 25,000 units amylase◇
Pancreatin Tablets
Tablets (enteric-coated): 325 mg pancreatin, 650 units lipase, 8,125 units protease, 8,125 units amylase◇

ACTION

Mechanism: Replaces endogenous exocrine pancreatic enzymes and aids digestion of starches, fats, and proteins.
Absorption: Not absorbed; it acts locally in the GI tract.
Distribution: None.
Metabolism: None.
Excretion: In feces.

INDICATIONS & DOSAGE

Exocrine pancreatic secretion insufficiency, digestive aid in cystic fibrosis–
Adults and children: 1 to 3 tablets P.O. with meals.

CONTRAINDICATIONS & PRECAUTIONS

Contraindicated in patients with hypersensitivity to hog protein.

ADVERSE REACTIONS

Common reactions are in italics; life-threatening reactions are in bold italics.
GI: nausea, diarrhea with high doses.
Other: hyperuricosuria (with high doses).

INTERACTIONS

Antacids: may negate pancreatin's beneficial effect. Don't use together.

EFFECTS ON DIAGNOSTIC TESTS

Serum uric acid: increased concentrations.

NURSING CONSIDERATIONS

Besides those related universally to drug therapy (see "How to use this book"), consider the following specific recommendations:
Assessment
• Obtain a baseline assessment of the patient's digestive distress before initiating pancreatin therapy.
• Be alert for adverse reactions and drug interactions throughout therapy.
• Evaluate the patient's and family's knowledge about pancreatin therapy.
Nursing Diagnoses
• Altered health maintenance related to the patient's underlying condition.
• Noncompliance (medication admin-

istration) related to long-term therapy.
• Knowledge deficit related to pancreatin therapy.

Planning and Implementation

Preparation and Administration

• Use only after confirmed diagnosis of exocrine pancreatic insufficiency. Not effective in GI disorders unrelated to pancreatic enzyme deficiency.
• For maximal effect, administer dose just before or during a meal or snack.
• Tablets may not be crushed or chewed.
• For young children, mix powders (including content of capsule) with applesauce and give with meals. Older children may swallow capsules with food.
• Do not mix the drug with foods that contain proteins. Avoid inhalation of powder.
• Enteric coating on some products may reduce availability of enzyme in upper portion of jejunum.
• Dosage varies according to degree of maldigestion and malabsorption, amount of fat in diet, and enzyme activity of individual preparations.
• Store in airtight containers at room temperature.

Monitoring

• Monitor effectiveness by regularly assessing relief of digestive distress when the patient ingests proteins, carbohydrates, and fats.
• Monitor the patient's bowel habits. Adequate replacement decreases number of bowel movements and improves stool consistency.
• Monitor the patient's diet and eating habits. Diet should balance fat, protein, and carbohydrate intake properly to avoid indigestion.

Supportive Care

• Keep in mind that pancreatin, particularly in large doses, increases serum uric acid concentrations.

Patient Teaching

• Explain use of drug and advise storage away from heat and light.
• Be sure the patient or family understands special dietary instructions for the particular disease.
• Tell the patient that adequate replacement of the pancreatic enzyme will decrease the number of bowel movements and improve stool consistency.
• Tell the parents (if the patient is a child) or the patient that the pancreatic enzymes should be taken with all regular meals as well as snacks.
• Warn the patient that digestants interact with antacids, and should not be used together. Tell the patient not to self-medicate with an OTC antacid.
• Warn the patient that eating unbalanced amounts of fat, protein, and starch may cause indigestion.
• If the patient is a child, instruct the parents about the importance of watching the child's appetite and eating habits. The child's appetite will be dramatically decreased and a nutritional problem could develop.
• Tell the parents to clean the enzyme from the child's lips and skin to prevent skin breakdown.
• Tell the parents to notify the doctor if the child experiences diarrhea.
• Symptoms of inadequate pancreatic replacement and excessive intake of fat, such as abdominal cramps and distention; mushy, light-colored stools; foul-smelling gas; rectal seepage of oil; rectal prolapse; or continual weight loss despite a voracious appetite, should be reported to the doctor.
• Inform the patient that he will probably take this drug for the rest of his life.

Evaluation

In patients receiving pancreatin, appropriate evaluation statements may include:
• Patient maintains normal digestion and shows no signs of digestive distress when ingesting proteins, carbohydrates, and fats.

• Patient complies with prescribed drug regimen.
• Patient and family state an understanding of pancreatin therapy.

pancrelipase

(pan kre li´ pase)
Cotazym Capsules, Cotazym-S Capsules, Creon Capsules, Festal II Tablets◇, Ilozyme Tablets, Ku-Zyme HP Capsules, Pancrease Capsules, Pancrease MT4, Pancrease MT10, Pancrease MT16, Viokase Powder, Viokase Tablets

• *Classification:* digestant (pancreatic enzyme)
• *Pregnancy Risk Category:* C

HOW SUPPLIED

Cotazym
Capsules: 8,000 units lipase, 30,000 units protease, 30,000 units amylase, 25 mg calcium carbonate
Cotazym-S
Capsules (enteric-coated spheres): 5,000 units lipase, 20,000 units protease, 20,000 units amylase
Creon
Capsules (enteric-coated microspheres): 8,000 units lipase, 13,000 units protease, 30,000 units amylase
Festal II
Tablets (enteric-coated): 6,000 units lipase, 20,000 units protease, 30,000 units amylase◇
Ilozyme
Tablets: 11,000 units lipase, 30,000 units protease, 30,000 units amylase
Ku-Zyme HP
Capsules: 8,000 units lipase, 30,000 units protease, 30,000 units amylase
Pancrease
Capsules (enteric-coated microspheres): 4,000 units lipase, 25,000 units protease, 20,000 units amylase
Pancrease MT4
Capsules (enteric-coated microtablets): 4,000 units lipase, 12,000 units protease, 30,000 units amylase
Pancrease MT10
Capsules (enteric-coated microtablets): 10,000 units lipase, 30,000 units protease, 30,000 units amylase
Pancrease MT16
Capsules (enteric-coated microtablets): 16,000 units lipase, 48,000 units protease, 48,000 units amylase
Viokase
Tablets: 8,000 units lipase, 30,000 units protease, 30,000 units amylase
Powder: 16,800 units lipase, 70,000 units protease, 70,000 units amylase

ACTION

Mechanism: A combination of digestive enzymes that replaces endogenous exocrine pancreatic enzymes and aids digestion of starches, fats, and proteins.
Absorption: Not absorbed; acts locally in the GI tract.
Distribution: None.
Metabolism: None.
Excretion: In feces.

INDICATIONS & DOSAGE

Dose must be titrated to patient's response. Exocrine pancreatic secretion insufficiency, cystic fibrosis in adults and children, steatorrhea and other disorders of fat metabolism secondary to insufficient pancreatic enzymes–
Adults and children: dosage ranges from 1 to 3 capsules or tablets P.O. before or with meals and 1 capsule or tablet with snack; or 1 to 2 powder packets before meals or snacks.

CONTRAINDICATIONS & PRECAUTIONS

Contraindicated in patients with hypersensitivity to pork or pork derivatives. The powder is extremely irritating if inhaled.

ADVERSE REACTIONS

Common reactions are in italics; life-threatening reactions are in bold italics.
GI: *nausea,* diarrhea with high doses.

INTERACTIONS

Antacids: may negate pancrelipase's beneficial effect. Don't use together.

EFFECTS ON DIAGNOSTIC TESTS

Serum uric acid: increased concentrations.

NURSING CONSIDERATIONS

Besides those related universally to drug therapy (see "How to use this book"), consider the following specific recommendations:

Assessment

- Obtain a baseline assessment of the patient's digestive distress before initiating pancrelipase therapy.
- Be alert for adverse reactions and drug interactions throughout therapy.
- Evaluate the patient's and family's knowledge about pancrelipase therapy.

Nursing Diagnoses

- Altered nutrition: Less than body requirements related to the patient's underlying condition.
- Noncompliance (medication administration) related to long-term therapy.
- Knowledge deficit related to pancrelipase therapy.

Planning and Implementation

Preparation and Administration

- Use only after confirmed diagnosis of exocrine pancreatic insufficiency. Not effective in GI disorders unrelated to pancreatic enzyme deficiency.
- Give drug just before or with meals.
- Tablets may not be crushed or chewed to avoid irritation of the mouth, lips, and tongue and should be swallowed quickly with liquid.
- For young children, mix powders (including content of capsule) with applesauce and give with meals. Older children may swallow capsules with food.
- Do not mix the drug with foods that contain proteins. Avoid inhalation of powder.
- Enteric coating on some products may reduce availability of enzyme in upper portion of jejunum.
- Dosage varies according to degree of maldigestion and malabsorption, amount of fat in diet, and enzyme activity of individual preparations.

Monitoring

- Monitor effectiveness by regularly assessing relief of digestive distress when the patient ingests proteins, carbohydrates, and fats.
- Monitor the patient's bowel habits. Adequate replacement decreases number of bowel movements and improves stool consistency.
- Monitor the patient's diet and eating habits. Diet should balance fat, protein, and carbohydrate intake properly to avoid indigestion.

Supportive Care

- If the patient is unable to comply with therapy, discuss reasons why and suggest possible methods the patient may use to maintain compliance.

Patient Teaching

- Explain use of drug and how the form of the drug prescribed for the patient may be taken.
- Tell the patient that adequate replacement of the pancreatic enzyme will decrease the number of bowel movements and improve stool consistency.
- Tell the parents (if the patient is a child) or the patient that pancrelipase should be taken with all regular meals as well as snacks.
- Stress the importance of following the special diet that was prescribed with the medication.
- Warn the patient that digestants interact with antacids and should not be used together. Tell the patient not to self-medicate with an OTC antacid.

• Warn the patient that eating unbalanced amounts of fat, protein, and starch may cause indigestion.
• If the patient is a child, instruct the parents about the importance of watching the child's appetite and eating habits.
• Tell the parents to clean the enzyme from the child's lips and skin to prevent skin breakdown.
• Tell the parents to notify the doctor if the child experiences diarrhea.
• Tell patients or parents that symptoms of inadequate pancreatic replacement and excessive intake of fat, such as abdominal cramps and distention; mushy, light-colored stools; foul-smelling gas; rectal seepage of oil; rectal prolapse; or continual weight loss despite a voracious appetite, should be reported to the doctor.

Evaluation

In patients receiving pancrelipase, appropriate evaluation statements may include:
• Patient maintains normal digestion and shows no signs of digestive distress when ingesting proteins, carbohydrates, and fats.
• Patient complies with prescribed drug regimen.
• Patient and family state an understanding of pancrelipase therapy.

pancuronium bromide

(pan kyoo roe´ nee um)
Pavulon

• *Classification:* skeletal muscle relaxant (nondepolarizing neuromuscular blocking agent)
• *Pregnancy Risk Category:* C

HOW SUPPLIED

Injection: 1 mg/ml, 2 mg/ml

ACTION

Mechanism: Prevents acetylcholine from binding to the receptors on the muscle end plate, thus blocking depolarization. Nondepolarizing agent.
Distribution: Protein binding characteristics are complex, and may be concentration-dependent. Small amounts cross the placenta. Redistribution is responsible for termination of pharmacologic activity.
Metabolism: Small amounts may be metabolized by the liver.
Excretion: Mainly excreted unchanged in urine; small amounts may appear in the feces as a result of biliary excretion. Half-life: Terminal elimination half-life is about 2 hours.
Onset, peak, duration: Dose-related. After usual doses, onset of action occurs within 30 to 45 seconds, with peak effects seen in 3 to 4½ minutes. Effects begin to subside in 35 to 45 minutes. Repeated doses may shorten onset and increase the duration of action.

INDICATIONS & DOSAGE

Adjunct to anesthesia to induce skeletal muscle relaxation; facilitate intubation; lessen muscle contractions in pharmacologically or electrically induced seizures; assist with mechanical ventilation–
Dosage depends on anesthetic used, individual needs, and response. Dosages are representative and must be adjusted.
Adults: initially, 0.04 to 0.1 mg/kg I.V.; then 0.01 mg/kg q 30 to 60 minutes.
Children over 10 years: initially, 0.04 to 0.1 mg/kg I.V., then ⅕ initial dose q 30 to 60 minutes.

CONTRAINDICATIONS & PRECAUTIONS

Contraindicated in patients with hypersensitivity to the drug or to bromides, and in patients with preexisting tachycardia or in whom minor elevation in heart rate is undesirable. Administer with extreme caution to patients with poor renal perfusion or severe renal disease; with caution to patients with bronchogenic carcinoma, dehydration or electrolyte imbalances, hepatic or pulmonary function impairment, hyperthermia, hypothermia, or myasthenia gravis; and at reduced dosage in pregnant women receiving magnesium sulfate.

ADVERSE REACTIONS

Common reactions are in italics; life-threatening reactions are in bold italics.
CV: tachycardia, increased blood pressure.
Skin: transient rashes.
Local: burning sensation.
Other: excessive sweating and salivation, ***prolonged dose-related apnea,*** wheezing, residual muscle weakness, ***allergic or idiosyncratic hypersensitivity reactions.***

INTERACTIONS

Aminoglycoside antibiotics (including amikacin, gentamicin, kanamycin, neomycin, streptomycin); polymyxin antibiotics (polymyxin B sulfate, colistin); clindamycin; quinidine; general anesthetics (such as halothane, enflurane, isoflurane): potentiated neuromuscular blockade, leading to increased skeletal muscle relaxation and possible respiratory paralysis. Use cautiously during surgical and postoperative periods.
Lithium, narcotic analgesics: potentiated neuromuscular blockade, leading to increased skeletal muscle relaxation and possible respiratory paralysis. Use with extreme caution, and reduce dose of pancuronium.

EFFECTS ON DIAGNOSTIC TESTS

None significant.

NURSING CONSIDERATIONS

Besides those related universally to drug therapy (see "How to use this book"), consider the following specific recommendations:

Assessment
- Obtain a baseline assessment of skeletal muscle function and respiratory pattern before drug therapy.
- Be alert for adverse reactions and drug interactions throughout therapy.
- Evaluate the patient's and family's knowledge about pancuronium therapy.

Nursing Diagnoses
- Ineffective breathing pattern related to the patient's underlying condition.
- Impaired verbal communication related to drug-induced paralysis.
- Knowledge deficit related to pancuronium therapy.

Planning and Implementation
Preparation and Administration
- Pancuronium should be administered only by personnel experienced in airway management.
- Have emergency respiratory support equipment (endotracheal equipment, ventilator, oxygen, atropine, edrophonium, epinephrine, and neostigmine) on hand before administration.
- Dose of 1 mg is the approximate therapeutic equivalent of 5 mg d-tubocurarine.
- Store in refrigerator. Do not store in plastic containers or syringes, but plastic syringes may be used for administration.
- Do not mix with barbiturate solutions (precipitate will form); use only fresh solutions.
- Usually administered together with a cholinergic blocker (such as atropine or glycopyrrolate).
- If succinylcholine is used, allow effects to subside before giving pancuronium.
- ***I.V. use:*** Continuous infusion is not recommended.

Monitoring
- Monitor effectiveness by regularly checking relaxation state of the patient's skeletal muscles; close observation of the patient is mandatory.
- Closely monitor baseline electrolyte determinations (electrolyte imbalance

can potentiate neuromuscular effects) and vital signs (watch respiration and heart rate).
• Measure intake and output (renal dysfunction may prolong duration of action, since 25% of the drug is excreted unchanged).
• Monitor respirations and respiratory status closely until patient recovers fully from neuromuscular blockade, as evidenced by tests of muscle strength (hand grip, head lift, and ability to cough).
• Frequently check the patient's vital signs for tachycardia and increased blood pressure.
Supportive Care
• Maintain adequate ventilation through respiratory support equipment throughout drug therapy and provide pulmonary care as indicated.
• Once spontaneous recovery starts, pancuronium-induced neuromuscular blockade may be reversed with an anticholinesterase agent (such as neostigmine or edrophonium).
• Provide emotional support for the intubated patient who is awake.
• Administer pain medication on regular basis (as condition dictates) because the patient will be unable to communicate that pain is present.
• Anticipate the patient's needs and try to meet them. Explain everything thoroughly before performing any procedure. Use nonverbal communication, especially eye contact.
• Protect the patient from injury when moving him in bed.
• Provide meticulous eye care because patient's blink reflex will be absent.
Patient Teaching
• Reassure the patient that necessary pain management will be provided regularly.
• Inform the patient that drug-induced paralysis will inhibit his ability to communicate but that he will receive continuous monitoring and care.
• Reassure the patient that as soon as the need for neuromuscular blockade is no longer necessary, the drug-induced paralysis will be reversed.
• Tell the patient that he may feel a burning sensation at the injection site.
Evaluation
In patients receiving pancuronium, appropriate evaluation statements may include:
• Patient maintains adequate ventilation.
• Patient's basic needs are anticipated and met.
• Patient and family state an understanding of pancuronium therapy.

papaverine hydrochloride
(pa pav´ er een)
Cerespan, Genabid, Pavabid, Pavabid HP Capsulets, Pavabid Plateau Caps, Pavarine Spancaps, Pavasule, Pavatine, Pavatym, Paverolan Lanacaps

• *Classification:* peripheral vasodilator (benzylisoquinoline derivative, opiate alkaloid)
• *Pregnancy Risk Category:* C

HOW SUPPLIED
Tablets: 30 mg, 60 mg, 100 mg, 150 mg, 200 mg, 300 mg
Tablets (timed-release): 200 mg
Capsules (timed-release): 150 mg
Injection: 30 mg/ml

ACTION
Mechanism: Directly relaxes smooth muscle by inhibiting phosphodiesterase, resulting in increased levels of cyclic adenosine monophosphate (cyclic AMP), which alters calcium movement.
Absorption: Well absorbed after I.M. injection; 54% bioavailable after oral administration. Sustained-release forms are sometimes absorbed poorly and erratically.
Distribution: Tends to localize in adi-

pose tissue and in the liver; the remainder is distributed throughout the body. About 90% of the drug is protein-bound.
Metabolism: Hepatic.
Excretion: In urine as metabolites. Half-life: Varies from 30 minutes to 24 hours, but levels can be maintained by giving drug at 6-hour intervals.
Onset, peak, duration: Peak plasma levels occur 1 to 2 hours after an oral dose of regular tablets.

INDICATIONS & DOSAGE

Relief of cerebral and peripheral ischemia associated with arterial spasm and myocardial ischemia; treatment of smooth muscle spasm (coronary occlusion, angina pectoris, sequelae of peripheral and pulmonary embolism, certain cerebral angiospastic states) and visceral spasms (biliary, ureteral, or GI colic) –
Adults: 60 to 300 mg P.O. 1 to 5 times daily, or 150- to 300-mg sustained-release preparations q 8 to 12 hours; 30 to 120 mg I.M. or I.V. q 3 hours, as indicated.

CONTRAINDICATIONS & PRECAUTIONS

Contraindicated in patients with complete atrioventricular (AV) heart block because large doses may depress AV and intraventricular conduction, causing serious arrhythmias. Use cautiously in patients with glaucoma.

Papaverine is not recommended as a substitute for nitroglycerin during anginal attacks.

ADVERSE REACTIONS

Common reactions are in italics; life-threatening reactions are in bold italics.
CNS: *headache.*
CV: *increased heart rate, increased blood pressure* (with parenteral use), depressed AV and intraventricular conduction, hypotension, arrhythmias.
GI: constipation, *nausea.*
Other: *sweating, flushing,* malaise, hepatic damage, increased depth of respiration.

INTERACTIONS

Levodopa: papaverine may interfere with the therapeutic effects of levodopa in patients with Parkinson's disease.

EFFECTS ON DIAGNOSTIC TESTS

CBC: altered eosinophils.
Serum ALT (SGPT) and alkaline phosphatase: altered concentrations.
Serum bilirubin: elevated levels (a sign of hepatic hypersensitivity).

NURSING CONSIDERATIONS

Besides those related universally to drug therapy (see "How to use this book"), consider the following specific recommendations:

Assessment
- Obtain a baseline assessment of the patient's underlying condition before drug therapy.
- Be alert for adverse reactions and drug interactions throughout therapy.
- Evaluate the patient's and family's knowledge about papaverine therapy.

Nursing Diagnoses
- Altered tissue perfusion (cerebral, peripheral) related to patient's underlying condition.
- Pain related to adverse drug reaction.
- Knowledge deficit related to papaverine therapy.

Planning and Implementation

Preparation and Administration
- Drug is rarely used parenterally, except when immediate effect is desired.
- ***I.V. use:*** Give I.V. slowly (over 1 to 2 minutes) to avoid serious adverse reactions.
- Do not add lactated Ringer's injec-

tion to the injectable form because drug will precipitate.

Monitoring

• Frequently monitor the patient's blood pressure and heart rate and rhythm, especially in patients with cardiac disease.

• Monitor the patient for drug-induced headache.

• Monitor for adverse hepatic reactions in patients during long-term therapy.

• Know that objective evidence of drug efficacy is lacking.

Supportive Care

• Withhold dose and notify the doctor immediately if changes in patient's health status occur.

• Obtain an order for a mild analgesic if patient experiences a headache.

Patient Teaching

• Tell patient to take the medication regularly; long-term therapy is required.

• Advise the patient to have blood pressure checked regularly and to notify the doctor promptly about signs and symptoms of hypertension (throbbing headache, visual changes).

• Tell the patient to take a mild analgesic for drug-induced headache.

• Encourage increased fluid and fiber intake (if not contraindicated) to prevent constipation.

• Advise patient to avoid hazardous tasks that require mental alertness (such as driving or operating heavy machinery) until CNS effects of the drug are known.

• Instruct patient to avoid sudden position changes to minimize the risks of orthostatic hypotension.

Evaluation

In patients receiving papaverine, appropriate evaluation statements may include:

• Patient maintains tissue perfusion and cellular oxygenation.

• Patient does not experience a headache.

• Patient and family state an understanding of papaverine therapy.

pemoline

(pem´ oh leen)

Cylert, Cylert Chewable

• Controlled Substance Schedule IV

• *Classification:* analeptic (oxazolidinedione derivative, CNS stimulant)

• *Pregnancy Risk Category:* B

HOW SUPPLIED

Tablets: 18.75 mg, 37.5 mg, 75 mg

Tablets (chewable and containing povidine): 37.5 mg

ACTION

Mechanism: Promotes nerve impulse transmission by releasing stored norepinephrine from nerve terminals in the brain. Main site of activity appears to be the cerebral cortex and the reticular activating system.

Absorption: Well absorbed after oral administration.

Distribution: Drug is 50% protein-bound.

Metabolism: Metabolized by the liver to active and inactive metabolites.

Excretion: Drug and metabolites are excreted in urine; 75% of an oral dose is excreted within 24 hours. Half-life: 9 to 14 hours.

Onset, peak, duration: Peak therapeutic effects occur at 4 hours and persist about 8 hours.

INDICATIONS & DOSAGE

Attention deficit disorder with hyperactivity (ADDH)–

Children 6 years and older: initially, 37.5 mg P.O. given in the morning. Daily dose can be raised by 18.75 mg weekly. Effective dosage range is 56.25 to 75 mg daily; maximum dosage is 112.5 mg daily.

CONTRAINDICATIONS & PRECAUTIONS

Contraindicated in patients with hypersensitivity to pemoline; in those with impaired hepatic function because it may have an adverse effect on liver function; and in children under age 6. Use with caution in patients with decreased renal function and in patients with a history of Gilles de la Tourette's syndrome because it may precipitate this disorder.

ADVERSE REACTIONS

Common reactions are in italics; life-threatening reactions are in bold italics.
CNS: *insomnia,* malaise, irritability, fatigue, mild depression, dizziness, headache, drowsiness, hallucinations, nervousness (large doses), seizures, *Tourette's disorder,* psychosis.
CV: *tachycardia (large doses).*
GI: anorexia, abdominal pain, nausea, diarrhea.
Hepatic: elevated liver enzymes.
Skin: rash.

INTERACTIONS

Insulin, oral hypoglycemics: pemoline may alter requirements of antidiabetic agents.

EFFECTS ON DIAGNOSTIC TESTS

Liver function tests: elevated levels.

NURSING CONSIDERATIONS

Besides those related universally to drug therapy (see "How to use this book"), consider the following specific recommendations:

Assessment
- Obtain a baseline assessment of the patient's attention span and behavior.
- Be alert for adverse reactions and drug interactions throughout therapy.
- Evaluate the patient's and family's knowledge about pemoline therapy.

Nursing Diagnoses
- High risk for injury related to patient's underlying attention deficit disorder with hyperactivity (ADDH).
- Sleep pattern disturbance related to pemoline-induced insomnia.
- Knowledge deficit related to pemoline therapy.

Planning and Implementation

Preparation and Administration
- Administer drug at least 6 hours before bedtime to avoid interference with sleep.

Monitoring
- Monitor effectiveness by observing the patient's behavior and attention span. Keep in mind that therapeutic effects may not be evident for up to 3 or 4 weeks.
- Monitor pulse for evidence of tachycardia, especially with large doses.
- Monitor sleeping pattern for insomnia, and observe for other adverse CNS reactions. Drug is structurally dissimilar to amphetamines or methylphenidate, but may produce similar adverse reactions, including lowered seizure threshold.
- May precipitate Gilles de la Tourette's syndrome. Monitor children, especially at the start of therapy.
- Closely monitor patients on long-term therapy for possible blood abnormalities or hepatic dysfunction and for growth suppression.

Supportive Care
- Institute safety precautions, making environment safe and providing supervision of patient's activities.
- Be aware that drug is now considered to have a more significant potential for drug abuse and dependence than previously thought.

Patient Teaching
- Warn the patient to avoid hazardous activities that require alertness or good psychomotor coordination until effects of the drug are known.
- Have the patient report insomnia and other adverse effects.
- Teach the patient how to take the drug to minimize insomnia and enhance effectiveness.

Evaluation
In patients receiving pemoline, appropriate evaluation statements may include:
• Patient demonstrates clinical improvement; safety is maintained.
• Patient is able to sleep without difficulty.
• Patient and family state an understanding of pemoline therapy.

penbutolol sulfate
(pen byoo´ toe lole)
Levatol

• *Classification:* antihypertensive (beta-adrenergic blocking agent)
• *Pregnancy Risk Category:* C

HOW SUPPLIED
Tablets: 20 mg

ACTION
Mechanism: Blocks both $beta_1$- and $beta_2$-adrenergic receptors; decreases heart rate and cardiac output.
Absorption: Almost completely absorbed after oral administration.
Distribution: 80% to 98% bound to plasma proteins.
Metabolism: Hepatic. Several metabolites have been identified; some retain partial pharmacologic activity.
Excretion: Most metabolites are excreted in the urine. Half-life: Average elimination half-life of the parent drug is 5 hours; some metabolites persist for 20 hours or more.
Onset, peak, duration: Peak plasma levels occur 2 to 3 hours after administration.

INDICATIONS & DOSAGE
Treatment of mild to moderate hypertension—
Adults: 20 mg P.O. once daily. Usually given with other antihypertensive agents, such as thiazide diuretics.

CONTRAINDICATIONS & PRECAUTIONS
Contraindicated in patients allergic to this drug or other beta blockers; in those with sinus bradycardia, cardiogenic shock, CHF, or overt cardiac failure; and in patients with greater than first-degree heart block. Avoid in patients with pheochromocytoma unless alpha-adrenergic blocking agents are also used; and in patients with chronic airway disease, such as chronic bronchitis or emphysema. Administer cautiously to patients with a history of CHF controlled by digitalis glycosides and diuretics.

ADVERSE REACTIONS
Common reactions are in italics; life-threatening reactions are in bold italics.
CNS: syncope, *dizziness,* vertigo, headache, fatigue, mental depression, paresthesias, hypoesthesia or hyperesthesia, lethargy, anxiety, nervousness, diminished concentration, sleep disturbances, nightmares, bizarre or frequent dreams, sedation, changes in behavior, reversible mental depression, catatonia, hallucinations, alteration of time perception, memory loss, emotional lability, light-headedness.
CV: ***bradycardia,*** chest pain, *CHF,* asymptomatic hypotension, peripheral ischemia, worsening of angina or arterial insufficiency, peripheral vascular insufficiency, claudication, edema, ***pulmonary edema,*** vasodilation, symptomatic postural hypotension, tachycardia, palpitations, conduction disturbances, first-degree and third-degree heart block, intensification of AV block.
EENT: dry mouth.
GI: gastric pain, flatulence, nausea, constipation, heartburn, vomiting, taste alteration.
GU: impotence, nocturia, urine retention.
Metabolic: hyperglycemia, hypoglycemia.

Respiratory: pharyngitis, laryngospasm, ***respiratory distress,*** shortness of breath.
Skin: pallor, flushing, rash.
Other: allergic reactions, eye discomfort, decreased libido.

INTERACTIONS

Clonidine: may cause paradoxical hypertension when combined with beta-adrenergic blocking agents. Also, beta blockers may enhance rebound hypertension when clonidine is withdrawn.
Insulin, oral hypoglycemic agents: beta-adrenergic blocking agents may alter the hypoglycemic response to these drugs. Monitor patient closely.
NSAIDs: possibly decreased antihypertensive effects.
Prazosin, terazosin: beta blockers may enhance the "first dose" orthostatic hypotension seen with these drugs.
Sympathomimetics, including isoproterenol, dopamine, dobutamine, or norepinephrine: decreased hypotensive response.
Theophylline: possibly decreased bronchodilator effect.

EFFECTS ON DIAGNOSTIC TESTS

None reported.

NURSING CONSIDERATIONS

Besides those related universally to drug therapy (see "How to use this book"), consider the following specific recommendations:

Assessment

- Obtain a baseline assessment of the patient's blood pressure before beginning therapy.
- Be alert for adverse reactions and drug interactions throughout therapy.
- Evaluate the patient's and family's knowledge about penbutolol therapy.

Nursing Diagnoses

- Altered tissue perfusion (renal, cerebral, cardiopulmonary, peripheral) related to the patient's underlying condition.
- Potential for injury related to CNS adverse reactions to penbutolol.
- Knowledge deficit related to penbutolol therapy.

Planning and Implementation

Preparation and Administration

- Always check the patient's apical pulse before giving this drug. If you detect extremes in pulse rates, hold drug and call doctor immediately.
- Administer with caution to patients with a history of bronchospastic disease.

Monitoring

- Monitor effectiveness by frequently checking the patient's blood pressure, ECG, and heart rate and rhythm.
- Monitor for signs and symptoms of CHF. Listen to breath sounds and check for edema.
- Monitor the patient for CNS reactions such as dizziness and weakness and for other adverse reactions.

Supportive Care

- Notify the doctor if signs of CHF become apparent.
- If the patient experiences dizziness or weakness, institute safety precautions such as continuous use of side rails.

Patient Teaching

- Teach the patient the signs and symptoms of CHF (edema and pulmonary congestion) and advise him to report them to the doctor.
- Explain the importance of taking this drug as prescribed, even when feeling well.
- Tell the patient not to discontinue this drug suddenly even if unpleasant adverse reactions occur, but to discuss the problem with the doctor. Explain that sudden withdrawal may precipitate angina and myocardial infarction.
- Instruct the patient to check with the doctor or pharmacist before taking OTC medications.
- Teach the patient and family caregiver how to take blood pressure measurements. Tell them to notify

the doctor of significant changes in blood pressure.

Evaluation

In patients receiving penbutolol, appropriate evaluation statements may include:

• Blood pressure is controlled within normal limits for this patient.

• Patient does not experience adverse CNS reactions to penbutolol.

• Patient and family state an understanding of penbutolol therapy.

penicillamine

(pen i sill′ a meen)

Cuprimine, Depen, D-Penamine‡

• *Classification:* heavy metal antagonist, antirheumatic agent (chelating agent)

• *Pregnancy Risk Category:* D

HOW SUPPLIED

Tablets: 125 mg‡, 250 mg

Capsules: 125 mg, 250 mg

ACTION

Mechanism: Probably acts in rheumatoid arthritis by inhibition of collagen formation. Also chelates heavy metals and cysteine.

Absorption: Absorbed after oral administration; food and mineral supplements, especially those containing iron, decrease absorption by complexing in the gut.

Distribution: Limited data suggest that the drug may cross the placenta.

Metabolism: Uncomplexed drug is metabolized in the liver to inactive disulfides.

Excretion: Small amounts are excreted unchanged after 24 hours; 50% of the drug is excreted in urine; 20% in feces, and 30% is unaccounted for.

Onset, peak, duration: Peak serum levels occur at 1 hour.

INDICATIONS & DOSAGE

Wilson's disease–

Adults: 250 mg P.O. q.i.d. 30 to 60 minutes before meals. Adjust dosage to achieve urinary copper excretion of 0.5 to 1 mg daily.

Children: 20 mg/kg P.O. daily divided q.i.d. before meals. Adjust dosage to achieve urinary copper excretion of 0.5 to 1 mg daily.

Cystinuria–

Adults: 250 mg to 1 g P.O. q.i.d. before meals. Adjust dosage to achieve urinary cystine excretion of less than 100 mg daily when renal calculi present, or 100 to 200 mg daily when no calculi present. Maximum dosage is 5 g daily.

Children: 30 mg/kg P.O. daily divided q.i.d. before meals. Adjust dosage to achieve urinary cystine excretion of less than 100 mg daily when renal calculi present, or 100 to 200 mg daily when no calculi present.

Rheumatoid arthritis–

Adults: 125 to 250 mg P.O. daily initially, with increases of 250 mg q 2 to 3 months if necessary. Maximum dosage is 1.5 g daily.

CONTRAINDICATIONS & PRECAUTIONS

Contraindicated in patients hypersensitive to the drug. Also contraindicated in patients with a history of penicillamine-related aplastic anemia, bone marrow depression, or agranulocytosis; in patients with renal insufficiency; and during pregnancy or breast-feeding.

Penicillamine has been associated with a number of severe, potentially life-threatening syndromes, including aplastic anemia, thrombocytopenia, agranulocytosis, myasthenia gravis, and Goodpasture's syndrome. Frequent monitoring of CBC, platelet counts, and hemoglobin levels, as well as close monitoring of the patient's clinical symptoms, are necessary, especially during the first 6 months of therapy.

ADVERSE REACTIONS

Common reactions are in italics; life-threatening reactions are in bold italics.
Blood: *leukopenia, eosinophilia,* ***thrombocytopenia,*** monocytosis, granulocytopenia, ***agranulocytosis, aplastic anemia,*** elevated sedimentation rate, lupus-like syndrome.
EENT: tinnitus.
GU: *nephrotic syndrome, Goodpasture's syndrome, glomerulonephritis, proteinuria.*
Hepatic: hepatotoxicity.
Metabolic: *decreased pyridoxine (may cause optic neuritis),* decreased zinc and mercury.
Skin: friability, especially at pressure spots; wrinkling; erythema; urticaria; ecchymoses.
Other: ***pancreatitis;*** reversible taste impairment, especially of salts and sweets; hair loss. *About ⅓ of patients develop allergic reactions (rash, pruritus, fever), arthralgia, lymphadenopathy, or pneumonitis.* With long-term use, myasthenia gravis syndrome.

INTERACTIONS

Antacids, oral iron: decreased effectiveness of penicillamine. If used together, give at least 2 hours apart.

EFFECTS ON DIAGNOSTIC TESTS

None reported.

NURSING CONSIDERATIONS

Besides those related universally to drug therapy (see "How to use this book"), consider the following specific recommendations:

Assessment
- Obtain a baseline assessment of allergies, CBC, platelets, and renal and hepatic function before therapy.
- Be alert for adverse reactions and drug interactions throughout therapy.
- Evaluate the patient's and family's knowledge about penicillamine therapy.

Nursing Diagnoses
- Impaired physical mobility related to Wilson's disease.
- Altered urinary elimination related to penicillamine-induced glomerulonephritis.
- Knowledge deficit related to penicillamine therapy.

Planning and Implementation

Preparation and Administration
- Give dose 1 hour before or 3 hours after meals to facilitate absorption.

Monitoring
- Monitor effectiveness by monitoring patient's urinary copper or cysteine excretion.
- Observe for signs of toxicity (rash, fever).
- Monitor CBC, platelet count, and renal and hepatic function regularly throughout therapy (every 2 weeks for the first 6 months and then monthly).
- Monitor urinalysis regularly for protein loss and hematuria.
- Monitor urine output. Weigh patient daily to detect fluid volume deficit or retention.
- Observe patient for signs of bruising and check bleeding times to detect granulocytopenia.
- Check patient's ROM and joint mobility.

Supportive Care
- Do not give to pregnant women with cystinuria.
- Use with caution in penicillin allergy; cross-sensitivity may occur. However, most penicillin-allergic patients can receive penicillamine.
- Give supplemental pyridoxine daily.
- Use extreme care when handling patient to avoid skin damage if patient has a skin reaction. Use antihistamines to manage skin reaction.
- Encourage the patient to drink large amounts of fluid, especially at night.
- Withhold drug and notify the doc-

tor if WBC count falls below 3,500/mm^3 and/or platelet count falls below 100,000/mm^3 (indications to stop drug). A progressive decline in platelet or WBC count in three successive blood tests may necessitate temporary discontinuation of therapy, even if these counts are within normal limits.
• Provide good skin care with mild soap and soothing lotion. Turn and position patient frequently; use padding and supportive measures to promote comfort.
• If patient's physical mobility is limited, assist with activities.
Patient Teaching
• Instruct patient to report rash, fever, chills, sore throat, and bleeding immediately.
• Inform the patient that the drug's therapeutic effect may be delayed up to 3 months in the treatment of rheumatoid arthritis.
• Advise the patient that taste impairment may occur and usually subsides itself in about 6 weeks.
• Provide appropriate health teaching for patients with Wilson's disease and cystinuria.
Evaluation
In patients receiving penicillamine, appropriate evaluation statements may include:
• Patient reports decrease in mobility impairment.
• Patient reports no disruption in normal urinary elimination pattern.
• Patient and family state an understanding of penicillamine therapy.

penicillin G benzathine (benzylpenicillin benzathine)

(pen i sill′ in)
Bicillin L-A, Megacillin

• *Classification:* antibiotic (natural penicillin)
• *Pregnancy Risk Category:* B

HOW SUPPLIED

Tablets: 200,000 units
Injection: 300,000 units/ml, 600,000 units/ml

ACTION

Mechanism: Bactericidal against microorganisms by inhibiting cell wall synthesis during active multiplication.
Absorption: After oral administration, is hydrolyzed by gastric acid. After I.M. injection, the benzathine salt of the drug forms a tissue depot from which penicillin G is slowly absorbed.
Distribution: Widely distributed into synovial, pleural, pericardial, and ascitic fluids, into bile, and into liver, skin, lungs, kidneys, muscle, intestines, tonsils, maxillary sinuses, saliva, and erythrocytes. CSF penetration is poor but is enhanced in patients with inflamed meninges. Drug crosses the placenta; it is 45% to 68% protein-bound.
Metabolism: Between 16% and 30% of an I.M. dose is metabolized to inactive compounds.
Excretion: Primarily excreted in urine by tubular secretion; 20% to 60% of dose is recovered in 6 hours; some is excreted in breast milk. Half-life: 30 minutes to 1 hour in adults; prolonged in severe renal impairment.
Onset, peak, duration: Peak serum concentrations occur 13 to 24 hours after injection, with serum concentrations detectable for 1 to 4 weeks.

INDICATIONS & DOSAGE

Congenital syphilis–
Children under age 2: 50,000 units/kg I.M. as a single dose.
Group A streptococcal upper respiratory infections–
Adults: 1.2 million units I.M. in a single injection.

Children over 27 kg: 900,000 units I.M. in a single injection.
Children under 27 kg: 300,000 to 600,000 units I.M. in a single injection.
Prophylaxis of poststreptococcal rheumatic fever–
Adults and children: 1.2 million units I.M. once a month or 600,000 units twice a month.
Syphilis of less than 1 year's duration–
Adults: 2.4 million units I.M. in a single dose.
Syphilis of more than 1 year's duration–
Adults: 2.4 million units I.M. weekly for 3 successive weeks.

CONTRAINDICATIONS & PRECAUTIONS

Contraindicated in patients with hypersensitivity to any penicillin or cephalosporin. Use cautiously in patients with renal impairment because drug is excreted by kidneys; decreased dosage is required in patient with moderate to severe renal failure.

ADVERSE REACTIONS

Common reactions are in italics; life-threatening reactions are in bold italics.
Blood: eosinophilia, ***hemolytic anemia,*** thrombocytopenia, leukopenia.
CNS: neuropathy, seizures with high doses.
Local: pain and sterile abscess at injection site.
Other: *hypersensitivity (maculopapular and **exfoliative dermatitis,*** chills, fever, edema, ***anaphylaxis***).

INTERACTIONS

Probenecid: increases blood levels of penicillin. Probenecid may be used for this purpose.

EFFECTS ON DIAGNOSTIC TESTS

Aminoglycoside serum levels: falsely decreased concentrations.
Coombs' test: positive results.
CSF protein: false-positive (Folin-Ciocalteau method).
17-ketogenic steroids: falsely elevated Norymberski and Zimmermann test results.
Urine and serum protein tests: chemical interference with methods using sulfosalicylic acid, trichloracetic acid, acetic acid, and nitric acid; not with tests using bromophenol blue (Albustix, Albutest, Multistix).
Urine glucose with copper sulfate (Benedict's reagent): interference; use Clinistix or Tes-Tape.
Urine specific gravity: falsely elevated results in patients with low urine output and dehydration.

NURSING CONSIDERATIONS

Besides those related universally to drug therapy (see "How to use this book"), consider the following specific recommendations:

Assessment

- Obtain a baseline assessment of infection before therapy.
- Be alert for adverse reactions and drug interactions throughout therapy.
- Evaluate the patient's and family's knowledge about penicillin G benzathine therapy.

Nursing Diagnoses

- High risk for injury related to ineffectiveness of penicillin G benzathine to eradicate the infection.
- Altered protection related to allergic reactions to pencillin G benzathine.
- Knowledge deficit related to penicillin G benzathine therapy.

Planning and Implementation

Preparation and Administration

- Obtain specimen for culture and sensitivity tests before first dose. Therapy may begin pending test results.
- Before first dose, ask the patient about previous allergic reactions to this drug or other penicillins. However, a negative history of penicillin

allergy does not guarantee future safety.
• Give penicillin G benzathine at least 1 hour before bacteriostatic antibiotics.
• ***I.M. use:*** Shake medication well before injection; administer deep into upper outer quadrant of buttocks in adults; into midlateral thigh in infants and small children. Rotate injection sites to minimize tissue injury. Apply ice to injection site for pain.
• *Never administer drug I.V.* Inadvertent I.V. administration has caused cardiac arrest and death.

Monitoring
• Monitor effectiveness by regularly assessing for improvement of infection.
• Allergic reactions are the major adverse reactions to penicillin, especially with large doses, parenteral administration, or prolonged therapy. Keep in mind that the previously nonallergic patient may become sensitized to penicillin during therapy.
• Monitor for bacterial and fungal superinfectins during high-dose or prolonged therapy, especially in elderly, debilitated, or immunosuppressed patients.

Supportive Care
• Discontinue the drug immediately if the patient develops signs of anaphylactic shock (rapidly developing dyspnea and hypotension). Notify the doctor and prepare to administer immediate treatment, such as epinephrine, corticosteroids, antihistamines, and other resuscitative measures as indicated.

Patient Teaching
• Advise the patient who becomes allergic to penicillins to wear medical alert identification stating this information.
• Warn the patient receiving penicillin G benzathine I.M that the injection may be painful but that ice applied to the site may ease discomfort.
• Tell patient to call the doctor if rash, fever, or chills develop. Fever and eosinophilia are the most common allergic reactions.
• Instruct patient to take oral penicillin G benzathine exactly as prescribed, even if feeling better.

Evaluation
In patients receiving penicillin G benzathine, appropriate evaluation statements may include:
• Patient is free of infection.
• Patient does not exhibit allergy to pencillin G benzathine therapy.
• Patient and family state an understanding of therapy.

penicillin G potassium (benzylpenicillin potassium)

(pen i sill´ in)
Megacillin†, NovoPen-G†, P-50†, Pentids**, Pfizerpen

• *Classification:* antibiotic (natural penicillin)
• *Pregnancy Risk Category:* B

HOW SUPPLIED

Tablets: 200,000 units, 250,000 units, 400,000 units, 500,000 units, 800,000 units
Oral suspension: 200,000 units/5 ml, 250,000 units/5 ml, 400,000 units/5 ml (after reconstitution)
Injection: 200,000 units, 500,000 units, 1 million units, 5 million units, 10 million units, 20 million units

ACTION

Mechanism: Bactericidal against microorganisms by inhibiting cell wall synthesis during active multiplication.
Absorption: Only 15% to 30% of an oral dose of penicillin G potassium is absorbed; the remainder is hydrolyzed by gastric secretions. Penicillin G potassium is absorbed rapidly after I.M. injection, but highest peak plasma levels follow after I.V. injection.

Distribution: Widely distributed into synovial, pleural, pericardial, and ascitic fluids and bile, and into liver, skin lungs, kidneys, muscle, intestines, tonsils, maxillary sinuses, saliva, and erythrocytes. CSF penetration is poor but is enhanced in patients with inflamed meninges. Penicillin G crosses the placenta; it is 45% to 68% protein-bound.
Metabolism: Between 16% and 30% of a dose of penicillin G is metabolized to inactive compounds.
Excretion: Primarily excreted in urine by tubular secretion; 20% to 60% of dose is recovered in 6 hours; some is excreted in breast milk. Half-life: About 30 minutes to 1 hour in adults; prolonged in severe renal impairment.
Onset, peak, duration: Peak serum concentrations after oral penicillin G potassium occur at 30 minutes; after I.M. injections peak at 15 to 30 minutes; after I.V. administration immediately after the completion of an infusion.

INDICATIONS & DOSAGE

Moderate to severe systemic infections–
Adults: 1.6 to 3.2 million units P.O. daily in divided doses given q 6 hours (1 mg = 1,600 units); 1.2 to 24 million units I.M. or I.V. daily in divided doses given q 4 hours.
Children: 25,000 to 100,000 units/kg P.O. daily in divided doses given q 6 hours; or 25,000 to 300,000 units/kg I.M. or I.V. daily in divided doses given q 4 hours.

CONTRAINDICATIONS & PRECAUTIONS

Contraindicated in patients with hypersensitivity to any other penicillin or to cephalosporins. Use cautiously in patients with renal impairment because it is excreted in urine; decreased dosage is required in patients with moderate to severe renal failure.

ADVERSE REACTIONS

Common reactions are in italics; life-threatening reactions are in bold italics.
Blood: ***hemolytic anemia,*** leukopenia, thrombocytopenia.
CNS: neuropathy, seizures with high doses.
Metabolic: possible severe potassium poisoning with high doses (hyperreflexia, seizures, ***coma***).
Local: *thrombophlebitis, pain at injection site.*
Other: *hypersensitivity (rash, urticaria, maculopapular eruptions, exfoliative dermatitis, chills, fever, edema,* ***anaphylaxis****),* overgrowth of nonsusceptible organisms.

INTERACTIONS

Probenecid: increases blood levels of penicillin. Probenecid may be used for this purpose.

EFFECTS ON DIAGNOSTIC TESTS

Aminoglycoside serum levels: falsely decreased concentrations.
Coombs' test: positive results.
CSF protein: false-positive (Folin-Ciocalteau method).
17-ketogenic steroids: falsely elevated Norymberski and Zimmermann test results.
Urine glucose with copper sulfate (Benedict's reagent): interference; use Clinistix or Tes-Tape.
Urine and serum protein tests: chemical interference with methods using sulfosalicyclic acid, tricholoracetic acid, acetic acid, and nitric acid; not with tests using bromophenol blue (Albustix, Albutest, Multistix).
Urine specific gravity: falsely elevated results in patients with low urine output and dehydration.

NURSING CONSIDERATIONS

Besides those related universally to drug therapy (see "How to use this book"), consider the following specific recommendations:

Assessment

• Obtain a baseline assessment of infection before therapy.

• Be alert for adverse reactions and drug interactions throughout therapy.

• Evaluate the patient's and family's knowledge about penicillin G potassium therapy.

Nursing Diagnoses

• High risk for injury related to ineffectiveness of penicillin G potassium to eradicate the infection.

• Altered protection related to allergic reaction to pencillin G potassium.

• Knowledge deficit related to penicillin G potassium therapy.

Planning and Implementation

Preparation and Administration

• Obtain specimen for culture and sensitivity tests before first dose. Therapy may begin pending test results.

• Before giving penicillin, ask the patient about previous allergic reactions to this drug. However, a negative history of penicillin allergy is no guarantee against a future allergic reaction.

• Give penicillin G potassium at least 1 hour before bacteriostatic antibiotics.

• ***P.O. use:*** Food may interfere with absorption, so give 1 to 2 hours before meals or 2 to 3 hours after.

• ***I.M. use:*** Administer deep into large muscle; extremely painful when given I.M. Rotate injection sites to minimize tissue injury. Apply ice to injection site for pain.

• ***I.V. use:*** When giving I.V., mix with dextrose 5% in water or sodium chloride solution. Give intermittently to prevent vein irritation.

Monitoring

• Monitor effectiveness by regularly assessing for improvement of infection.

• Allergic reactions are the major adverse reactions to penicillin, especially with large doses, parenteral administration, or prolonged therapy. Keep in mind that the patient may become sensitized to penicillin through exposure.

• Monitor patient for bacterial and fungal superinfections with large doses or prolonged therapy, especially in elderly, debilitated, or immunosuppressed patients.

• Monitor renal function closely as patients with poor renal function are predisposed to high blood levels.

Supportive Care

• Discontinue the drug at once if the patient develops anaphylactic shock (exhibited by rapidly developing dyspnea and hypotension). Notify the doctor and prepare to administer immediate treatment, such as epinephrine, corticosteroids, antihistamines, and other resuscitative measures as indicated.

• If the patient develops an adverse reaction, notify the doctor for appropriate treatment and provide supportive care as appropriate.

• Institute seizure precautions as a patient with high blood level of the drug may have seizures.

Patient Teaching

• Advise the patient who becomes allergic to penicillins to wear medical alert identification stating this information.

• Warn the patient receiving penicillin G potassium I.M. that the injection may be painful but that ice applied to the site may help alleviate discomfort.

• Tell patient to call the doctor if rash, fever, or chills develop. A rash is the most common allergic reaction.

• Instruct patient to take oral penicillin G potassium exactly as prescribed, even if feeling better, and to take entire amount prescribed.

• Tell patient receiving oral penicillin G potassium to take the drug 1 to 2 hours before meals or 2 to 3 hours after as food may interfere with absorption.

- Warn patient never to use leftover penicillin for a new illness or to share penicillin with family and friends.
- Instruct patient to notify the nurse or doctor if adverse reactions develop, or concerns or questions arise about penicillin G potassium therapy.

Evaluation

In patients receiving penicillin G potassium, appropriate evaluation statements may include:

- Patient is free of infection.
- Patient does not exhibit an allergic response to pencillin G potassium therapy.
- Patient and family state an understanding of penicillin G potassium therapy.

penicillin G procaine (benzylpenicillin procaine)

(pen i sill′ in)

Ayercillin†, Crysticillin A.S., Duracillin A.S., Pfizerpen-AS, Wycillin

- *Classification:* antibiotic (natural penicillin)
- *Pregnancy Risk Category:* B

HOW SUPPLIED

Injection: 300,000 units/ml, 500,000 units/ml, 600,000 units/ml

ACTION

Mechanism: Bactericidal against microorganisms by inhibiting cell wall synthesis during active multiplication.
Absorption: The procaine salt of penicillin G is insoluble; it forms a tissue depot after I.M. injection that slowly releases penicillin G to the systemic circulation.
Distribution: Widely distributed into synovial, pleural, pericardial, and ascitic fluids and bile, and into liver, skin, lungs, kidneys, muscle, intestines, tonsils, maxillary sinuses, saliva, and erythrocytes. CSF penetration is poor but is enhanced in patients with inflamed meninges. Penicillin G crosses the placenta; it is 95% to 68% protein-bound.
Metabolism: Between 16% and 30% of a dose of penicillin G is metabolized to inactive compounds.
Excretion: Primarily excreted in urine by tubular secretion; 20% to 60% of dose is recovered in 6 hours; some is excreted in breast milk. Half-life: About 30 minutes to 1 hour in adults; prolonged in severe renal impairment.
Onset, peak, duration: Peak serum concentrations occur at 1 to 4 hours, with drug detectable in serum for 1 to 2 days.

INDICATIONS & DOSAGE

Moderate to severe systemic infections–
Adults: 600,000 to 1.2 million units I.M. daily given as a single dose.
Children: 300,000 units I.M. daily given as a single dose.
Uncomplicated gonorrhea–
Adults and children over 12 years: give 1 g probenecid; then 30 minutes later give 4.8 million units of penicillin G procaine I.M., divided into two injection sites.
Pneumococcal pneumonia–
Adults and children over 12 years: 300,000 to 600,000 units I.M. daily q 6 to 12 hours.

CONTRAINDICATIONS & PRECAUTIONS

Contraindicated in patients with hypersensitivity to any penicillin or cephalosporin. Use cautiously in patients with renal impairment because drug is excreted by kidneys; decreased dosage is required in patient with moderate to severe renal failure.

ADVERSE REACTIONS

Common reactions are in italics; life-threatening reactions are in bold italics.

Blood: thrombocytopenia, ***hemolytic anemia,*** leukopenia.
CNS: arthralgia, seizures.
Other: *hypersensitivity (rash, urticaria, chills, fever, edema, prostration,* ***anaphylaxis****),* overgrowth of nonsusceptible organisms.

INTERACTIONS

Probenecid: increases blood levels of penicillin. Probenecid may be used for this purpose.

EFFECTS ON DIAGNOSTIC TESTS

Aminoglycoside serum levels: falsely decrease concentrations.
Coombs' test: positive results.
CSF protein: false-positive (Folin-Ciocalteau method).
17-ketogenic steroids: falsely elevated Norymberski and Zimmermann test results.
Urine glucose with copper sulfate (Benedict's reagent): interference; use Clinistix or Tes-Tape.
Urine and serum protein tests: chemical interference with methods using sulfosalicylic acid, trichloracetic acid, acetic acid, and nitric acid; not with tests using bromophenol blue (Albustix, Albutest, Multistix).
Urine specific gravity: falsely elevated results in patients with low urine output and dehydration.

NURSING CONSIDERATIONS

Besides those related universally to drug therapy (see "How to use this book"), consider the following specific recommendations:

Assessment

- Obtain a baseline assessment of infection before penicillin G procaine therapy.
- Be alert for adverse reactions and drug interactions throughout therapy.
- Evaluate the patient's and family's knowledge about penicillin G procaine therapy.

Nursing Diagnoses

- High risk for injury related to ineffectiveness of penicillin G procaine to eradicate the infection.
- Altered protection related to penicillin G procaine induced allergic reaction.
- Knowledge deficit related to penicillin G procaine therapy.

Planning and Implementation

Preparation and Administration

- Obtain specimen for culture and sensitivity tests before first dose. Therapy may begin pending test results.
- Before first dose, ask the patient about previous allergic reactions to this drug or other penicillins. However, a negative history of penicillin allergy does not guarantee future safety.
- Give penicillin G procaine at least 1 hour before bacteriostatic antibiotics.
- ***I.M. use:*** Administer deep into upper outer quadrant of buttocks in adults; into midlateral thigh in small child. Don't massage injection site. Apply ice to injection site for pain.
- *Never administer drug I.V.* Inadvertent I.V. administration has caused fatal CNS toxicity from procaine.

Monitoring

- Monitor effectiveness by regularly assessing for improvement of infection.
- Allergic reactions are the major adverse reactions to penicillin, especially with large doses, parenteral administration, or prolonged therapy. Keep in mind that the previously non-allergic patient may become sensitized to penicillin during therapy.
- Monitor for bacterial and fungal superinfection during high-dose or prolonged therapy, especially in elderly, debilitated or immunosuppressed patients.
- Regularly monitor renal and hematopoietic function, as ordered.

Supportive Care

• Discontinue the drug immediately if the patient develops signs of anaphylactic shock (rapidly developing dyspnea and hypotension). Notify the doctor and prepare to administer immediate treatment, such as epinephrine, corticosteroids, antihistamines, and other resuscitative measures as indicated.

Patient Teaching

• Advise the patient who becomes allergic to penicillins to wear medical alert identification stating this information.

• Warn the patient that the injection may be painful but that ice applied to the site may help alleviate discomfort.

Evaluation

In patients receiving penicillin G procaine, appropriate evaluation statements may include:

• Patient is free of infection.

• Patient does not experience an allergic reaction to therapy.

• Patient and family state an understanding of therapy.

penicillin G sodium (benzylpenicillin sodium)

(pen i sill′ in)

Crystapen†

• *Classification:* antibiotic (natural penicillin)

• *Pregnancy Risk Category:* B

HOW SUPPLIED

Injection: 5 million units

ACTION

Mechanism: Bactericidal against microorganisms by inhibiting cell wall synthesis during active multiplication.

Absorption: Penicillin G sodium is absorbed rapidly after I.M. injection.

Distribution: Widely distributed into synovial, pleural, pericardial and ascitic fluids and bile, and into liver, skin, lungs, kidneys, muscle, intestines, tonsils, maxillary sinuses, saliva, and erythrocytes. CSF penetration is poor but is enhanced in patients with inflamed meninges. Penicillin G crosses the placenta; it is 45% to 68% protein-bound.

Metabolism: Between 16% and 30% of an I.M. dose of penicillin G is metabolized to inactive compounds.

Excretion: Primarily excreted in urine by tubular secretion; 20% to 60% of dose is recovered in 6 hours; some is excreted in breast milk. Half-life: About 30 minutes to 1 hour in adults; prolonged in severe renal impairment.

Onset, peak, duration: Peak serum concentrations after I.M. administration occur within 15 to 30 minutes.

INDICATIONS & DOSAGE

Moderate to severe systemic infections–

Adults: 1.2 to 24 million units daily I.M. or I.V., divided into doses given q 4 hours.

Children: 25,000 to 300,000 units/kg daily I.M. or I.V., divided into doses given q 4 hours.

Endocarditis prophylaxis for dental surgery–

Adults: 2 million units I.V. or I.M. 30 to 60 minutes before procedure, then 1 million units 6 hours later.

CONTRAINDICATIONS & PRECAUTIONS

Contraindicated in patients with hypersensitivity to any penicillin or cephalosporin. Use cautiously in patients with renal impairment because drug is excreted by kidneys; decreased dosage is required in patients with moderate-to-severe renal failure.

ADVERSE REACTIONS

Common reactions are in italics; life-threatening reactions are in bold italics.

Blood: ***hemolytic anemia,*** leukopenia, thrombocytopenia.
CNS: arthralgia, neuropathy, seizures.
CV: *congestive heart failure with high doses.*
Local: *vein irritation, pain at injection site, thrombophlebitis.*
Other: *hypersensitivity (chills, fever, edema, maculopapular rash, exfoliative dermatitis, urticaria,* ***anaphylaxis****),* overgrowth of nonsusceptible organisms.

INTERACTIONS

Probenecid: increases blood levels of penicillin. Probenecid may be used for this purpose.

EFFECTS ON DIAGNOSTIC TESTS

Aminoglycoside serum levels: falsely decrease concentrations.
Coombs' test: positive results.
CSF protein: false-positive (Folin-Ciocalteau method).
17-ketogenic steroids: falsely elevated Norymberski and Zimmermann test results.
Urine glucose with copper sulfate (Benedict's reagent): interference; use Clinistix or Tes-Tape.
Urine and serum protein tests: chemical interference with methods using sulfosalicylic acid, trichloracetic acid, acetic acid, and nitric acid; not with tests using bromophenol blue (Albustix, Albutest, Multistix).
Urine specific gravity: falsely elevated results in patients with low urine output and dehydration.

NURSING CONSIDERATIONS

Besides those related universally to drug therapy (see "How to use this book"), consider the following specific recommendations:

Assessment

- Obtain a baseline assessment of infection before penicillin G sodium therapy.
- Be alert for adverse reactions and drug interactions throughout therapy.
- Evaluate the patient's and family's knowledge about penicillin G sodium therapy.

Nursing Diagnoses

- High risk for injury related to ineffectiveness of penicillin G sodium to eradicate the infection.
- Impaired tissue integrity related to thrombophlebitis caused by I.V. administration of penicillin G sodium.
- Knowledge deficit related to penicillin G sodium therapy.

Planning and Implementation

Preparation and Administration

- Obtain specimen for culture and sensitivity tests before first dose. Therapy may begin pending test results.
- Before first dose, ask the patient about previous allergic reactions to this drug or other penicillins. However, a negative history of penicillin allergy does not guarantee future safety.
- Solutions should always be clear, colorless to pale yellow, and free of particles; do not give solutions containing precipitates or other foreign matter.
- Give penicillin G sodium at least 1 hour before bacteriostatic antibiotics.
- Expect to reduce dosage for a patient with impaired renal function. Because penicillins are dialyzable, patients undergoing hemodialysis may need dosage adjustments.
- ***I.M. use:*** Administer deep into large muscle mass (gluteal or midlateral thigh); rotate injection sites to minimize tissue injury; do not inject more than 2 g of drug per injection site. Apply ice to injection site for pain.
- ***I.V. use:*** Do not add or mix other drugs with I.V. infusions—particularly aminoglycosides, which will be inactivated if mixed with penicillins; they are chemically and physically incompatible. If other drugs must be given I.V., temporarily stop infusion of primary drug. Infuse I.V. drug continu-

ously or intermittently (over 30 minutes). Intermittent I.V. infusion may be diluted in 50 to 100 ml sterile water, 0.9% sodium chloride solution, dextrose 5% in water, dextrose 5% in water and 0.45% sodium chloride solution, or lactated Ringer's solution.

Monitoring

• Monitor effectiveness by regularly assessing for improvement of infectious process.

• Allergic reactions are the major adverse reactions to penicillin, especially with large doses, parenteral administration, or prolonged therapy. Keep in mind that the previously nonallergic patient may become sensitized to penicillin during therapy.

• Closely monitor I.V. site for thrombophlebitis.

• If a patient with decreased renal function is receiving more than 20 million units of penicillin G sodium daily, monitor closely for decreased level of consciousness or seizures.

Supportive Care

• Discontinue the drug immediately if the patient develops signs of anaphylactic shock (rapidly developing dyspnea and hypotension). Notify the doctor and prepare to administer immediate treatment, such as epinephrine, corticosteroids, antihistamines, and other resuscitative measures as indicated.

• Drug may induce seizures. Institute seizure precautions for the patient with a high blood level.

• Change I.V. site every 48 hours.

Patient Teaching

• Advise the patient who becomes allergic to penicillins to wear medical alert identification stating this information.

• Tell the patient to inform the nurse if pain or discomfort is felt at the I.V. site. Also warn the patient receiving penicillin G sodium I.M that the injection may be painful but that ice applied to the site may help alleviate discomfort.

Evaluation

In patients receiving penicillin G sodium, appropriate evaluation statements may include:

• Patient is free of infection.

• Patient maintains good tissue intergrity and exhibits no signs of thrombophlebitis.

• Patient and family state an understanding of therapy.

PHARMACOLOGIC CLASS

penicillins

Natural penicillin

penicillin G benzathine; potassium; procaine; sodium
penicillin V potassium

Aminopenicillin

amoxicillin trihydrate; clavulanate
ampicillin
ampicillin sodium; sulbactam
ampicillin sodium; trihydrate
bacampicillin hydrochloride

Penicillinase-resistant

cloxacillin sodium
dicloxacillin sodium
methicillin sodium
nafcillin sodium
oxacillin sodium

Extended-spectrum

azlocillin sodium
carbenicillin sodium; indanyl sodium
mezlocillin sodium
piperacillin sodium
ticarcillin clavulanate
ticarcillin disodium

OVERVIEW

Penicillins are very effective antibiotics with low toxicity. Their activity was first discovered by Sir Alexander Fleming in 1928, but they were not developed for use against systemic infections until 1940. Penicillin is naturally derived from *Penicillium chrysogenum.* New synthetic derivatives are created by chemical reactions that modify their structure, resulting in increased GI absorption, resistance to destruction by beta-lactamase (penicillinase), and a broader spectrum of susceptible organisms.

Penicillins are generally bactericidal. They inhibit synthesis of the bacterial cell wall, causing rapid cell lysis, and are most effective against fast-growing susceptible bacteria.

The sites of action for penicillins are enzymes known as penicillin-binding proteins (PBP). The affinity of certain penicillins for PBP in various microorganisms helps explain differing spectra of activity in this class of antibiotics.

Oral absorption of penicillin varies widely; the most acid labile is penicillin G. Side-chain modifications in penicillin V, ampicillin, amoxicillin, and other orally administered penicillins increase gastric acid stability and permit better absorption from the GI tract.

Penicillins are distributed widely throughout the body; CSF penetration is minimal but is enhanced in patients with inflamed meninges. Most penicillins are only partially metabolized. With the exception of nafcillin, penicillins are excreted primarily in urine; nafcillin undergoes enterohepatic circulation and is excreted chiefly through the biliary tract.

CLINICAL INDICATIONS AND ACTIONS

Infection caused by susceptible organisms

• *Natural penicillins:* Penicillin G is the prototype of this group; derivatives such as penicillin V are more acid stable and thus better absorbed by the oral route. All natural penicillins are vulnerable to inactivation by beta-lactamase producing bacteria. Natural penicillins act primarily against gram-positive organisms.

Clinical indications for natural penicillins include streptococcal pneumonia, enterococcal and nonenterococcal Group D endocarditis, diphtheria, anthrax, meningitis, tetanus, botulism, actinomycosis, syphilis, relapsing fever, Lyme disease, and others. Natural penicillins are used prophylactically against pneumococcal infections, rheumatic fever, bacterial endocarditis, and neonatal Group B streptococcal disease.

Susceptible aerobic gram-positive cocci include *Staphylococcus aureus* and *S. epidermidis;* nonenterococcal Group D streptococci, Groups A, B, D, G, H, K, L, and M streptococci, *S. viridans;* and enterococcus (usually in combination with an aminoglycoside). Susceptible aerobic gram-negative cocci include *Neisseria meningitidis* and non–penicillinase-producing *N. gonorrhoeae.*

Susceptible aerobic gram-positive bacilli include *Corynebacterium* (both diphtheria and opportunistic species), *Listeria,* and *Bacillus anthracis.* Susceptible anaerobes include *Peptococcus, Peptostreptococcus, Actinomyces, Clostridium, Fusobacterium, Veillonella,* and non–beta-lactamase–producing strains of *S. pneumoniae.*

Susceptible spirochetes include *Treponema pallidum, T. pertenue, Leptospira,* and *Borrelia recurrentis.*

• *Aminopenicillins* (amoxacillin, ampicillin, and bacampicillin) offer a broader spectrum of activity including many gram-negative organisms. Like natural penicillins, aminopenicillins are vulnerable to inactivation by penicillinase. They are primarily used to treat septicemia, gynecologic infections, and infections of the urinary, respiratory, and GI tracts, and skin, soft tissue, bones, and joints. Their activity spectrum includes *Escherichia coli, Proteus mirabilis,*

COMPARING PENICILLINS

DRUG	ROUTE	ADULT DOSAGE	FREQUENCY	PENICILLINASE RESISTANT
amoxicillin	P.O.	250 to 500 mg 3 g with 1 g probenecid for gonorrhea	q 8 hours single dose	No
amoxicillin/clavulanate potassium	P.O.	250 to 500 mg	q 8 hours	Yes
ampicillin	I.M., I.V.	2 to 14 g daily	divided doses given q 4 to 6 hours	No
	P.O.	250 to 500 mg 3.5 g with 1 g probenecid (for gonorrhea)	q 6 hours single dose	
ampicillin sodium/ sulbactum sodium	I.M., I.V.	1.5 to 3 g	q 6 to 8 hours	Yes
azlocillin	I.V.	200 to 350 mg/ kg daily	divided doses given q 4 to 6 hours	No
bacampicillin	P.O.	400 to 800 mg	q 12 hours	No
carbenicillin	I.M., I.V.	200 mg/kg daily (for urinary infections) 30 to 40 g daily (for systemic infections)	divided doses given q 4 to 6 hours divided doses given q 4 to 6 hours	No
	P.O.	382 to 764 mg	q 6 hours	No
cloxacillin	P.O.	250 mg to 1 g	q 6 hours	Yes
dicloxacillin	P.O.	125 to 500 mg	q 6 hours	Yes
methicillin	I.M., I.V.	1 to 2 g	q 4 to 6 hours	Yes
mezlocillin	I.M., I.V.	3 to 4 g	q 4 to 6 hours	No
nafcillin	I.M., I.V.	250 mg to 2 g	q 4 to 6 hours	Yes
	P.O.	500 mg to 1 g	q 6 hours	
oxacillin	I.M., I.V.	250 mg to 2 g	q 4 to 6 hours	Yes
	P.O.	500 mg to 1 g	q 6 hours	
penicillin G benzathine	I.M.	1.2 to 2.4 million units	single dose	No
penicillin G potassium	I.M., I.V.	200,000 to 4 million units	q 4 hours	No
	P.O.	400,000 to 800,000 units	q 6 hours	

(continued)

COMPARING PENICILLINS *(continued)*

DRUG	ROUTE	ADULT DOSAGE	FREQUENCY	PENICILLINASE RESISTANT
penicillin G procaine	I.M.	600,000 to 1.2 million units	q 1 to 3 days	No
		4.8 million units with 1 g probenecid (for syphilis)	single dose for primary, secondary, and early latent syphilis; weekly for 3 weeks for late latent syphilis	
penicillin G sodium	I.M., I.V.	200,000 to 4 million units	q 4 hours	No
penicillin V potassium	P.O.	250 to 500 mg	q 6 to 8 hours	No
piperacillin	I.M., I.V.	100 to 300 mg/kg daily	divided doses given q 4 to 6 hours	No
ticarcillin	I.M., I.V.	150 to 300 mg/kg daily	divided doses given q 3 to 6 hours	No
ticarcillin/clavulanate potassium	I.V.	3 g	q 4 to 6 hours	Yes

Shigella, Salmonella, S. pneumoniae, N. gonorrhoeae, Haemophilus influenzae, Staphylococcus aureus, Staphylococcus epidermidis, and *Listeria monocytogenes.*

• *Penicillinase-resistant penicillins* (cloxacillin, dicloxacillin, oxacillin, and nafcillin) are semisynthetic penicillins designed to remain stable against hydrolysis by most staphylococcal penicillinases and thus are the drugs of choice against susceptible penicillinase-producing staphylococci. They also retain activity against most organisms susceptible to natural penicillins. Clinical indications are much the same as for aminopenicillins.

• *Extended-spectrum penicillins* (azlocillin, carbenicillin, mezlocillin, piperacillin, and ticarcillin), as their name implies, offer a wider range of bactericidal action than the other three classes, are used in hard-to-treat gram-negative infections, and are usually given in combination with aminoglycosides. They are used most often against susceptible strains of *Enterobacter, Klebsiella, Citrobacter, Serratia, Bacteroides fragilis,* and *Pseudomonas aeruginosa;* their gram-negative spectrum also includes *Proteus vulgaris, Providencia rettgeri,* and *Morganella morganii.* These penicillins are also vulnerable to destruction by beta-lactamase or penicillinases.

OVERVIEW OF ADVERSE REACTIONS

• *Systemic reactions:* Hypersensitivity reactions occur with all penicillins; they range from mild rashes, fever and eosinophilia to fatal anaphylaxis. Hematologic reactions include hemolytic anemia, transient neutropenia, leukopenia, and thrombocytopenia.

Certain adverse reactions are more common with specific classes of penicillin: bleeding episodes are usually seen at high-dose levels of extended-spectrum penicillins; acute interstitial nephritis is reported most often with methicillin; GI adverse effects are most common with but not limited to ampicillin. High doses, especially of penicillin G, irritate the CNS in patients with renal disease, causing confusion, twitching, lethargy, dysphagia, seizures, and coma. Hepatotoxicity is most common with penicillinase-resistant penicillins; hyperkalemia and hypernatremia with extended-spectrum penicillins.

Jarisch-Herxheimer reaction can occur when penicillin G is used in secondary syphilis; it presents as chills, fever, headache, myalgia, tachycardia, malaise, sweating, hypotension, and sore throat and is attributed to release of endotoxin following spirochete death.

• *Local reactions:* Local irritation from parenteral therapy may be severe enough to require discontinuation of the drug or administration by subclavian catheter if drug therapy is to continue.

REPRESENTATIVE COMBINATIONS

Amoxicillin with clavulanate potassium: Augmentin.

Ampicillin trihydrate with probenecid: Polycillin PRB, Principen with Probenecid, Probampacin, Trojacillin-Plus.

Penicillin G benzathine with penicillin G procaine: Bicillin, Curacillin F.A., Duracillin Fortified, Bicillin C-R, Bicillin 900/300.

Penicillin G procaine with dihydrostreptomycin sulfate: Intramammary infusion USP XXI; with novobiocin sodium: USP XXI; with aluminum stearate: USP XXI.

penicillin V (phenoxymethyl penicillin)

penicillin V potassium (phenoxymethylpenicillin potassium)

(pen i sill´ in)

Abbocillin VK‡, Apo-Pen-VK†, Beepen-VK, Betapen-VK, Cilicane VK‡, Ledercillin VK, Nadopen-V†, NovoPen-VK†, PVK‡, Penapar VK, Pen Vee K, PVF K†, Robicillin VK, V-Cillin K, VC-K, Veetids**

• *Classification:* antibiotic (natural penicillin)
• *Pregnancy Risk Category:* B

HOW SUPPLIED

penicillin V
Tablets: 250 mg, 500 mg
Oral suspension: 125 mg/5 ml, 250 mg/5 ml (after reconstitution)
penicillin V potassium
Tablets: 125 mg, 250 mg, 500 mg
Tablets (film-coated): 250 mg, 500 mg
Capsules: 250 mg‡
Oral suspension: 125 mg/5 ml, 250 mg/5 ml (after reconstitution)

ACTION

Mechanism: Bactericidal against microorganisms by inhibiting cell wall synthesis during active multiplication.
Absorption: Penicillin V has greater acid stability and is absorbed more completely than penicillin G after oral administration. About 60% to 75% of an oral dose of penicillin V is absorbed.
Distribution: Widely distributed into synovial, pleural, pericardial, and ascitic fluids and bile, and into liver, skin, lungs, kidneys, muscle, intestines, tonsils, maxillary sinuses, saliva, and erythrocytes. CSF penetration is poor but is enhanced in patients with inflamed meninges. Peni-

*Liquid form contains alcohol.

**May contain tartrazine.

cillin V crosses the placenta; it is 75% to 89% protein-bound.
Metabolism: Between 35% and 70% of a penicillin V dose is metabolized to inactive compounds.
Excretion: Primarily excreted in urine by tubular secretion; 26% to 65% of dose is recovered in 6 hours; some is excreted in breast milk. Half-life: 30 minutes in adults; prolonged in severe renal impairment.
Onset, peak, duration: Peak serum concentrations occur at 60 minutes; food has no significant effect.

INDICATIONS & DOSAGE

Mild to moderate systemic infections–
Adults: 250 to 500 mg (400,000 to 800,000 units) P.O. q 6 hours.
Children: 15 to 50 mg/kg (25,000 to 90,000 units/kg) P.O. daily, divided into doses given q 6 to 8 hours.
Endocarditis prophylaxis for dental surgery–
Adults: 2 g P.O. 30 to 60 minutes before procedure, then 1 g 6 hours after.
Children under 30 kg: half of the adult dose.

CONTRAINDICATIONS & PRECAUTIONS

Contraindicated in patients with hypersensitivity to any penicillin or cephalosporins. Use cautiously in patients with renal impairment because drug is excreted by kidneys; decreased dosage is required in patients with moderate to severe renal failure.

ADVERSE REACTIONS

Common reactions are in italics; life-threatening reactions are in bold italics.
Blood: eosinophilia, ***hemolytic anemia,*** leukopenia, thrombocytopenia.
CNS: neuropathy.
GI: *epigastric distress,* vomiting, diarrhea, *nausea.*
Other: *hypersensitivity (rash, urticaria, chills, fever, edema, **anaphylaxis),*** overgrowth of nonsusceptible organisms.

INTERACTIONS

Neomycin: decreases absorption of penicillin. Give penicillin by injection.
Probenecid: increases blood levels of penicillin. Probenecid may be used for this purpose.

EFFECTS ON DIAGNOSTIC TESTS

Aminoglycoside serum levels: falsely decreased concentrations.
Urine and serum protein levels: interference with methods using sulfosalicylic acid, trichloracetic acid, acetic acid, and nitric acid; not with tests using bromophenol blue (Albustix, Albutest, MultiStix).

NURSING CONSIDERATIONS

Besides those related universally to drug therapy (see "How to use this book"), consider the following specific recommendations:

Assessment
- Obtain a baseline assessment of infection before therapy.
- Be alert for adverse reactions and drug interactions throughout therapy.
- Evaluate the patient's and family's knowledge about penicillin V therapy.

Nursing Diagnoses
- High risk for injury related to ineffectiveness of penicillin V to eradicate the infection.
- Altered protection related to penicillin V induced allergic reaction.
- Knowledge deficit related to penicillin V therapy.

Planning and Implementation
Preparation and Administration
- Obtain specimen for culture and sensitivity tests before first dose. Therapy may begin pending test results.
- Before first dose, ask the patient about previous allergic reactions to this drug or other penicillins. However, a negative history of penicillin

allergy does not guarantee future safety.
• Give penicillin V at least 1 hour before bacteriostatic antibiotics.
• ***P.O. use:*** Food may interfere with absorption, so give 1 to 2 hours before meals or 2 to 3 hours after. Administer with a full glass (8 oz) of water, not fruit juice or a carbonated beverage because acid inactivates the drug.
• Be aware that patients being treated for streptococcal infections should take the drug until the full 10-day course is completed.

Monitoring
• Monitor effectiveness by regularly assessing for improvement of infection.
• Keep in mind that the previously nonallergic patient may become sensitized to penicillin during therapy.
• Monitor for bacterial and fungal superinfections during high-dose or prolonged therapy, especially in elderly, debilitated, or immunosuppressed patients.
• Monitor renal and hematopoietic function studies during prolonged therapy.

Supportive Care
• Discontinue the drug immediately if the patient develops signs of anaphylactic shock (rapidly developing dyspnea and hypotension). Notify the doctor and prepare to administer immediate treatment, such as epinephrine, corticosteroids, antihistamines, and other resuscitative measures as indicated.

Patient Teaching
• Advise the patient who becomes allergic to penicillins to wear medical alert identification stating this information.
• Tell patient to call the doctor if rash,fever, or chills develop. A rash is the most common allergic reaction.
• Instruct patient to take penicillin V exactly as prescribed, even if feeling better, and to take entire amount prescribed.
• Tell patient receiving penicillin V to take the drug 1 to 2 hours before meals or 2 to 3 hours after as food may interfere with absorption. Also tell patient to take the drug with a full glass of water, not fruit juice or a carbonated beverage, because acid will inactivate the drug.
• Warn patient never to use leftover penicillin for a new illness or to share penicillin with family and friends.

Evaluation
In patients receiving penicillin V, appropriate evaluation statements may include:
• Patient is free of infection.
• Patient does not exhibit an allergic response to therapy.
• Patient and family state an understanding of penicillin V therapy.

pentaerythritol tetranitrate
(pen ta er ith´ ri tole)
Dilar, Duotrate, Naptrate, Pentritol, Pentylan, Peritrate, Peritrate Forte†, Peritrate SA, PETN

• *Classification:* antianginal, vasodilator (nitrate)
• *Pregnancy Risk Category:* C

HOW SUPPLIED
Tablets: 10 mg, 20 mg, 40 mg, 80 mg
Tablets (sustained-release): 80 mg
Capsules (sustained-release): 30 mg, 45 mg, 80 mg

ACTION
Mechanism: Reduces cardiac oxygen demand by decreasing left ventricular end-diastolic pressure (preload) and, to a lesser extent, systemic vascular resistance (afterload). Also increases blood flow through the collateral coronary vessels.
Absorption: Well absorbed from the

GI tract, with bioavailability of about 50%.
Distribution: Probably similar to that of nitroglycerin and other nitrates.
Metabolism: In the liver and serum to pentaerythritol mononitrate, pentaerythritol dinitrate, pentaerythritol trinitrate, and pentaerythritol.
Excretion: In the urine primarily as inactive metabolites. Half-life: Pentaerythritol trinitrate, the only active metabolite, has a plasma half-life of about 10 minutes.
Onset, peak, duration: Onset of action of hemodynamic effects is about 20 to 60 minutes. Duration of effect is 4 to 5 hours.

INDICATIONS & DOSAGE

Prophylaxis against angina pectoris– **Adults:** 10 to 20 mg P.O. q.i.d.; may be titrated upward to 40 mg P.O. q.i.d. half an hour before or 1 hour after meals and h.s.; 80 mg sustained-release preparations P.O. b.i.d.

CONTRAINDICATIONS & PRECAUTIONS

Contraindicated in patients with severe anemia, because nitrate ions can readily oxidize hemoglobin to methemoglobin; head trauma or cerebral hemorrhage, because it may increase intracranial pressure (ICP); severe anemia, because the hypotensive effects of the drug may further worsen tissue perfusion; and hypersensitivity or idiosyncratic reaction to nitrates.

Use cautiously in patients with hypotension, because the drug may worsen this condition; increased ICP, because drug dilates meningeal vessels; open-angle or narrow-angle glaucoma, although intraocular pressure is increased only briefly and drainage of aqueous humor from the eye is unimpeded; diuretic-induced fluid depletion or low systolic blood pressure (below 90 mm Hg), because of drug's hypotensive effect; and recent acute myocardial infarction (MI), because drug may cause excessive hypotension and tachycardia.

ADVERSE REACTIONS

Common reactions are in italics; life-threatening reactions are in bold italics.
CNS: *headache, sometimes with throbbing; dizziness;* weakness.
CV: *orthostatic hypotension, tachycardia, flushing, palpitations,* fainting.
GI: nausea, vomiting.
Skin: cutaneous vasodilation.
Other: hypersensitivity reactions.

INTERACTIONS

None significant.

EFFECTS ON DIAGNOSTIC TESTS

Serum cholesterol (Zlatkis-Zak color reaction): falsely decreased values.

NURSING CONSIDERATIONS

Besides those related universally to drug therapy (see "How to use this book"), consider the following specific recommendations:

Assessment

- Obtain a baseline assessment of the patient's angina status before pentaerythritol therapy.
- Be alert for adverse reactions and drug interactions throughout therapy.
- Evaluate the patient's and family's knowledge about pentaerythritol therapy.

Nursing Diagnoses

- Pain related to ineffectiveness of pentaerythritol therapy.
- High risk for injury related to adverse CNS reactions to pentaerythritol and pentaerythritol-induced orthostatic hypotension.
- Knowledge deficit related to pentaerythritol.

Planning and Implementation

Preparation and Administration

- Should never be used for relief of acute anginal attacks.
- Do not discontinue abruptly because coronary vasospasm may occur.
- Additional doses may be adminis-

tered before anticipated stress or at bedtime for nocturnal angina.
• *P.O. use:* Administer drug 30 minutes before or 1 hour after meals.
• Store drug in a cool place, in a tightly covered container away from light.

Monitoring
• Monitor effectiveness by regularly evaluating pain relief.
• Monitor blood pressure and intensity and duration of response to drug.

Supportive Care
• Institute safety precautions if adverse CNS reactions occur.
• To minimize orthostatic hypotension effects, have patient rise slowly to an upright position, go up and down stairs slowly, and lie down at the first sign of dizziness.
• Obtain an order for a mild analgesic if a headache occurs. Be aware that dosage may need to be reduced temporarily, so notify doctor. However, tolerance usually develops.

Patient Teaching
• Stress importance of taking the drug exactly as prescribed even when feeling well.
• Tell outpatients not to discontinue this drug suddenly; abrupt discontinuation can exacerbate angina and MI.
• Instruct patient to take drug 30 minutes before or 1 hour after a meal and at bedtime if ordered q.i.d.
• Tell patient how to minimize orthostatic hypotensive effects.
• Advise patient not to perform hazardous activities until CNS effects are known.
• Tell patient to take a mild analgesic if headache occurs and to notify the doctor because dosage may need to be reduced temporarily.
• Instruct patient to take additional dose before anticipated stress or at bedtime for nocturnal angina as prescribed.
• Stress the importance of not using drug for relief of acute anginal attacks.
• Advise patient to avoid alcoholic beverages; may exacerbate hypotension.

Evaluation
In patients receiving pentaerythritol, appropriate evaluation statements may include:
• Patient states anginal pain is relieved with pentaerythritol therapy.
• Patient does not experience injury from pentaerythritol-induced orthostatic hypotension or adverse CNS reactions to the drug.
• Patient and family state an understanding of pentaerythritol therapy.

pentamidine isethionate
(pen ta mi´ deen)
NebuPent, Pentam 300

• *Classification:* antiprotozoal (diamidine derivative)
• *Pregnancy Risk Category:* C

HOW SUPPLIED
Injection: 300 mg/vial
Aerosol: 300 mg/vial

ACTION
Mechanism: Interferes with biosynthesis of DNA, RNA, phospholipids, and proteins in susceptible organisms.
Absorption: Well absorbed after I.M. injection, but plasma levels are lower than after a 2-hour I.V. infusion. Absorption is limited after aerosol administration.
Distribution: Pentamidine appears to be extensively tissue-bound, with highest levels found in the liver, followed by kidneys, adrenals, spleen, lungs and pancreas. CNS penetration is poor.
Excretion: Most of drug is excreted unchanged in the urine. Drug's extensive tissue-binding may account

for its continued appearance in urine 6 to 8 weeks after therapy ends. Half-life: Biphasic elimination, with the initial phase 54 minutes after I.M. injection or 18 minutes after I.V. infusion; terminal phase is 9.4 hours after I.M. injection and 6.4 hours after I.V. administration.
Onset, peak, duration: Daily I.M. doses (4 mg/kg) produce surprisingly few plasma level fluctuations. Plasma levels usually increase slightly 1 hour after I.M. injection. In patients who received aerosolized pentamidine, the peak plasma levels of pentamidine were at or below the lower limit of detection of the assay (2.3 ng/ml). Higher plasma levels found in patients with elevated BUN levels.

INDICATIONS & DOSAGE

Treatment of pneumonia due to Pneumocystis carinii–
Adults and children: 4 mg/kg I.V. or I.M. once a day for 14 days.
Prevention of Pneumocystis carinii *pneumonia in high-risk individuals*–
Adults: 300 mg by inhalation (using a Respirgard II nebulizer) once every 4 weeks.

CONTRAINDICATIONS & PRECAUTIONS

Because of its potentially toxic effects, use only as a second-line agent for *Pneumocystis carinii* pneumonia. Administer cautiously to patients with hypertension, hypotension, hyperglycemia, hypoglycemia, hypocalcemia, leukopenia, thrombocytopenia, anemia, or hepatic or renal dysfunction because of risk of serious adverse effects.

Patients who have developed serious or life-threatening reactions to systemic pentamidine may not be good candidates for treatment with the aerosol form.

The Centers for Disease Control recommends against administering pentamidine prophylaxis to HIV-infected pregnant women because of the risk to the fetus; such treatment may be considered postpartum.

ADVERSE REACTIONS

Common reactions are in italics; life-threatening reactions are in bold italics.
Blood: *leukopenia,* thrombocytopenia, anemia.
CNS: confusion, hallucinations.
CV: ***hypotension,*** tachycardia.
Endocrine: *hypoglycemia,* hyperglycemia, hypocalcemia.
GI: nausea, anorexia, metallic taste.
GU: *elevated serum creatinine,* renal toxicity.
Hepatic: elevated liver enzymes.
Local: *sterile abscess, pain or induration at injection site.*
Skin: rash, facial flushing, pruritus.
Other: fever.

INTERACTIONS

Aminoglycosides, amphotericin B, cisplatin, vancomycin, zidovudine: increased risk of nephrotoxicity.

EFFECTS ON DIAGNOSTIC TESTS

BUN, serum creatinine, AST (SGOT), and ALT (SGPT): may increase levels.
Electrolytes: hyperkalemia and hypocalcemia.
Serum glucose: hypoglycemia initially (possibly from stimulation of endogenous insulin release); later, hyperglycemia from direct pancreatic cell damage.

NURSING CONSIDERATIONS

Besides those related universally to drug therapy (see "How to use this book"), consider the following specific recommendations:

Assessment

- Obtain a baseline assessment of respiratory status and appropriate culture and sensitivity tests before therapy.
- Be alert for adverse reactions and drug interactions throughout therapy.

• Evaluate the patient's and family's knowledge about pentamidine therapy.

Nursing Diagnoses

• Impaired gas exchange related to ineffectiveness of pentamidine to alleviate pneumonia due to *Pneumocystis carinii.*

• Decreased tissue perfusion (cerebral) related to pentamidine induced hypotension.

• Knowledge deficit related to pentamidine.

Planning and Implementation

Preparation and Administration

• Take patient's blood pressure several times during administration and have patient lie down when drug is administered because sudden severe hypotension may develop.

• ***Aerosol use:*** Use only the Respirgard II nebulizer manufactured by Marquest to administer the drug by aerosol. Mix the contents of one vial in 6 ml of sterile water for injection. Do not use saline because this will cause the drug to precipitate. Do not mix with other drugs. Do not use low pressure (< 20 psi) compressors. The flow rate should be 5 to 7 liters/minute from a 40 to 50 psi air or oxygen source. Administer until the chamber is empty, which may take up to 45 minutes.

• ***I.M. use:*** Administer by deep I.M. injection. Pain and induration occur universally with I.M. injection.

• ***I.V. use:*** Infuse the drug I.V. over 60 minutes to minimize risk of hypotension.

Monitoring

• Monitor effectiveness by performing a respiratory assessment every shift and obtaining culture and sensitivity studies as prescribed.

• Monitor blood pressure during administration and several times thereafter until blood pressure is stable.

• Monitor blood glucose, serum creatinine, and BUN daily. After parenteral administration, blood glucose may decrease initially; hypoglycemia may be severe in 5% to 10% of patients. This may be followed by hyperglycemia and insulin-dependent diabetes mellitus (which may be permanent).

Supportive Care

• Apply warm compresses to ease pain at injection site.

• Institute safety measures if adverse CNS reactions or endocrine imbalances occur.

• Be prepared to provide additional care as indicated by patient's reaction to the drug.

Patient Teaching

• Advise patient to lie down during administration of the drug because sudden severe hypotension may occur.

• Emphasize the importance of reporting lightheadness or signs and symptoms of hypoglycemia immediately to the nurse and of remaining recumbent until blood pressure or blood glucose returns to normal.

• Warn patient receiving the drug I.M. that pain or induration may occur at the injection site. Inform him that warm compresses applied to the site may help.

• Instruct the patient to use the aerosol device until the chamber is empty. (This may take up to 45 minutes.)

Evaluation

In patients receiving pentamidine, appropriate evaluation statements may include:

• Patient's respiratory status has returned to normal and no evidence of infection is present.

• Patient's blood pressure remains normal throughout therapy.

• Patient and family state an understanding of therapy.

pentazocine hydrochloride

(pen taz´ oh seen)

Fortral†‡, Talwin†

pentazocine hydrochloride and naloxone hydrochloride
Talwin Nx

pentazocine lactate
Fortral‡, Talwin

- Controlled Substance Schedule IV
- *Classification:* analgesic, adjunct to anesthesia (opioid partial agonist, narcotic agonist-antagonist)
- *Pregnancy Risk Category:* B (D for prolonged use or use of high doses at term)

HOW SUPPLIED

pentazocine hydrochloride
Tablets: 25 mg‡, 50 mg†‡
pentazocine hydrochloride and naloxone hydrochloride
Tablets: 50 mg pentazocine hydrochloride and 500 mcg naloxone hydrochloride
pentazocine lactate
Injection: 30 mg/ml

ACTION

Mechanism: An opiate agonist-antagonist that binds with opiate receptors at many sites in the CNS (brain, brain stem, and spinal cord), altering both perception of and emotional response to pain through an unknown mechanism.
Absorption: Well absorbed after oral or parenteral administration; however, orally administered drug undergoes first-pass metabolism in the liver and less than 20% of a dose reaches the systemic circulation unchanged. Bioavailability is increased in patients with hepatic dysfunction; patients with cirrhosis absorb 60% to 70% of the drug.
Distribution: Widely distributed in the body. Drug crosses placenta.
Metabolism: In the liver, mainly by oxidation and secondarily by glucuronidation. Metabolism may be prolonged in patients with impaired hepatic function.
Excretion: Variable urinary excretion. Very small amounts are excreted in the feces after oral or parenteral administration. Less than 5% excreted unchanged.
Onset, peak, duration: Onset of analgesia is 15 to 30 minutes, with peak effect at 15 to 60 minutes. Duration of effect is 3 hours.

INDICATIONS & DOSAGE

Moderate to severe pain–
Adults: 50 to 100 mg P.O. q 3 to 4 hours, p.r.n. or around the clock. Maximum oral dosage is 600 mg daily. Alternatively, may give 30 mg I.M., I.V., or S.C. q 3 to 4 hours, p.r.n. or around the clock. Maximum parenteral dosage is 360 mg daily. Single doses above 30 mg I.V. or 60 mg I.M. or S.C. not recommended.

CONTRAINDICATIONS & PRECAUTIONS

Contraindicated in patients with hypersensitivity to the drug or other opiate partial agonists.

Administer pentazocine with extreme caution after MI or to patients with supraventricular arrhythmias; avoid, or administer drug with extreme caution to patients with head injury or increased intracranial pressure, because drug obscures neurologic parameters; and during pregnancy and labor, because drug readily crosses placenta (premature infants are especially sensitive to respiratory and CNS depressant effects of narcotic agonist-antagonists).

Administer cautiously to patients with renal or hepatic dysfunction, because drug accumulation or prolonged duration of action may occur; asthma or chronic obstructive pulmonary disease, because drug depresses respiration and suppresses cough reflex; or seizure disorders, because drug may precipitate seizures; to patients undergoing biliary tract surgery, because drug may cause biliary spasm; to elderly or debilitated patients, who are more sensitive to both therapeutic and adverse drug effects; and to patients prone to physical or psychic addiction, because of the high abuse potential for this drug.

However, this drug has a lower potential for abuse than do narcotic agonists.

ADVERSE REACTIONS

Common reactions are in italics; life-threatening reactions are in bold italics.
CNS: *sedation,* visual disturbances, *hallucinations,* drowsiness, *dizziness, light-headedness,* confusion, euphoria, headache, *psychotomimetic effects.*
GI: *nausea, vomiting,* dry mouth, constipation.
GU: *urine retention.*
Local: induration, nodules, sloughing, and sclerosis of injection site.
Other: ***respiratory depression,*** physical and psychological dependence.

INTERACTIONS

Alcohol, CNS depressants: additive effects. Use together cautiously.
Narcotic analgesics: avoid concomitant use. Possible decreased analgesic effect.

EFFECTS ON DIAGNOSTIC TESTS

None reported.

NURSING CONSIDERATIONS

Besides those related universally to drug therapy (see "How to use this book"), consider the following specific recommendations:

Assessment
- Obtain a baseline assessment of the patient's pain before therapy.
- Be alert for adverse reactions and drug interactions throughout therapy.
- Evaluate the patient's and family's knowledge about pentazocine therapy.

Nursing Diagnoses
- Pain related to patient's underlying condition.
- Ineffective breathing pattern related to pentazocine-induced respiratory depression.
- Knowledge deficit related to pentazocine therapy.

Planning and Implementation
Preparation and Administration
- Do not mix in same syringe with soluble barbiturates.
- ***I.V. use:*** Keep patient supine during administration to minimize hypotension.

Monitoring
- Monitor effectiveness by assessing the patient's degree of pain relief after each dose.
- Monitor patient's rate and pattern of breathing for evidence of respiratory depression. Also monitor for other adverse effects.

Supportive Care
- Notify the doctor if pain is not relieved.
- Keep in mind that the oral pentazocine preparation available in the United States contains the narcotic antagonist naloxone. May precipitate abstinence syndrome in narcotic-dependent patients.
- Hold drug and notify the doctor if the patient's respiratory rate declines. Use naloxone, as ordered, to reverse respiratory depression.
- Be aware that tablets are not well absorbed.

Patient Teaching
- Warn the patient about the drug's potential for causing physical or psychological dependence.
- Warn the ambulatory patient to avoid driving and other hazardous activities that require mental alertness.
- Tell the patient to rise slowly after I.V. administration to reduce faintness and dizziness.
- Tell the patient or family caregiver

to notify the nurse or doctor if respiratory rate decreases.

Evaluation

In patients receiving pentazocine, appropriate evaluation statements may include:

- Patient reports pain relief.
- Patient's respiratory rate and pattern remain within normal limits.
- Patient and family state an understanding of pentazocine therapy.

pentobarbital

(pen toe bar′ bi tal)

Nembutal* **

pentobarbital sodium

Nembutal Sodium*, Novopentobarb†

- Controlled Substance Schedule II
- *Classification:* anitconvulsant, sedative-hypnotic (barbiturate)
- *Pregnancy Risk Category:* D

HOW SUPPLIED

pentobarbital

Elixir: 20 mg/5 ml

pentobarbital sodium

Capsules: 50 mg, 100 mg

Injection: 50 mg/ml

Suppositories: 30 mg, 60 mg, 120 mg, 200 mg

ACTION

Mechanism: Probably interferes with transmission of impulses from the thalamus to the cortex of the brain. A barbiturate.

Absorption: Rapidly absorbed after oral, I.M., or rectal administration.

Distribution: Widely distributed throughout the body. Approximately 35% to 45% is protein-bound.

Metabolism: In the liver by penultimate oxidation.

Excretion: 99% is eliminated as glucuronide conjugates and other metabolites in the urine. Half-life: Ranges from 35 to 50 hours.

Onset, peak, duration: Onset of action (oral or rectal administration) occurs in 10 to 15 minutes. Peak serum concentration occurs between 30 and 60 minutes after oral administration. After I.M. injection, the onset of action occurs within 10 to 25 minutes. After I.V. administration, the onset of action occurs immediately. Serum concentrations needed for sedation and hypnosis are 1 to 5 mcg/ml and 5 to 15 mcg/ml, respectively. After oral or rectal administration, duration of hypnosis is 1 to 4 hours. Duration of action is 3 to 4 hours.

INDICATIONS & DOSAGE

Sedation–

Adults: 20 to 40 mg P.O. b.i.d., t.i.d., or q.i.d.

Children: 6 mg/kg daily P.O. in divided doses.

Insomnia–

Adults: 100 to 200 mg P.O. h.s. or 150 to 200 mg deep I.M.; 100 mg initially, I.V., then additional doses up to 500 mg; 120 to 200 mg rectally.

Children: 3 to 5 mg/kg I.M. Maximum dosage is 100 mg. Rectal dosages are 2 months to 1 year, 30 mg; 1 to 4 years, 30 to 60 mg; 5 to 12 years, 60 mg; 12 to 14 years, 60 to 120 mg.

Preanesthetic medication–

Adults: 150 to 200 mg I.M. or P.O. in two divided doses.

CONTRAINDICATIONS & PRECAUTIONS

Contraindicated in patients with hypersensitivity to barbiturates and in patients with bronchopneumonia, status asthmaticus, or severe respiratory distress, because of the potential for respiratory depression. Do not use in patients who are depressed or have suicidal ideation because the drug can worsen depression; in patients with uncontrolled acute or chronic pain, because the drug can produce exacerbation of pain and paradoxical excitement; or in patients with porphyria, because this drug can trigger symptoms of this disease.

Use cautiously in patients who must perform hazardous tasks requiring mental alertness, because the drug causes drowsiness. Administer parenteral pentobarbital slowly and with extreme caution to patients with hypotension or severe pulmonary or cardiovascular disease because of potential adverse hemodynamic effects. Because tolerance and physical or psychological dependence may occur, prolonged use of high doses should be avoided. Pentobarbital capsules may contain tartrazine, which may cause an allergic reaction in certain individuals, especially those who are sensitive to aspirin. Prenatal exposure to barbiturates is associated with an increased incidence of fetal abnormalities and, possibly, brain tumors. Use of barbiturates in the third trimester may be associated with physical dependence in neonates.

ADVERSE REACTIONS

Common reactions are in italics; life-threatening reactions are in bold italics.
CNS: *drowsiness, lethargy, hangover,* paradoxical excitement in elderly patients.
GI: nausea, vomiting.
Skin: rash, urticaria.
Other: ***Stevens-Johnson syndrome,*** angioedema, exacerbation of porphyria.

INTERACTIONS

Alcohol or other CNS depressants, including narcotic analgesics: excessive CNS and respiratory depression. Use together cautiously.
Griseofulvin: decreased absorption of griseofulvin.
MAO inhibitors: inhibit metabolism of barbiturates; may cause prolonged CNS depression. Reduce barbiturate dosage.
Oral anticoagulants, estrogens and oral contraceptives, doxycycline, corticosteroids: may enhance the metabolism of these drugs. Monitor for decreased effect.
Rifampin: may decrease barbiturate levels. Monitor for decreased effect.

EFFECTS ON DIAGNOSTIC TESTS

EEG: persistent changes in low voltage, fast activity.
Phentolamine test: false-positive result.
Serum bilirubin: decreased in neonates, patients with seizure disorders, and those with congenital hyperbilirubinemia.

NURSING CONSIDERATIONS

Besides those related universally to drug therapy (see "How to use this book"), consider the following specific recommendations:

Assessment
- Obtain a baseline assessment of sleeping patterns and CNS status before therapy.
- Be alert for adverse reactions and drug interactions throughout therapy.
- Evaluate the patient's and family's knowledge about pentobarbital therapy.

Nursing Diagnoses
- Sleep pattern disturbance related to underlying patient problem.
- High risk for trauma related to adverse CNS reactions to pentobarbital.
- Knowledge deficit related to pentobarbital therapy.

Planning and Implementation
Preparation and Administration
- Use injectable solution within 30 minutes after opening container to minimize deterioration. Don't use cloudy solution.
- Keep in mind that parenteral solution is alkaline. Avoid extravasation; may cause tissue necrosis.
- Do not mix with other medications.
- ***P.O. use:*** Before leaving the bedside, make sure the patient has swallowed medication.

*Liquid form contains alcohol. **May contain tartrazine.

• ***Rectal use:*** To ensure accurate dosage, don't divide suppositories.
• ***I.V. use:*** Reserve I.V. use for emergency treatment and give under close supervision. Be prepared to give artificial respiration.
• ***I.M. use:*** Give I.M. injection deeply. Superficial injection may cause pain, sterile abscess, and sloughing.

Monitoring
• Regularly monitor the effectiveness of pentobarbital by evaluating the patient's ability to sleep after administration.
• Monitor the patient's CNS status for evidence of adverse reactions. Keep in mind that elderly patients are more sensitive to the drug's adverse CNS effects.
• Monitor for signs of barbiturate toxicity: coma, pupillary constriction, cyanosis, clammy skin, and hypotension. Overdose can be fatal.
• Carefully monitor respiratory and cardiovascular function after I.V. administration.
• After drug discontinuation, be alert for withdrawal symptoms.

Supportive Care
• After administration, institute safety precautions: remove cigarettes, keep bed rails up, and supervise or assist ambulation.
• Withhold the drug if barbiturate toxicity is suspected.
• Do not discontinue the drug abruptly after prolonged use. The drug may cause dependence and severe withdrawal symptoms. Always withdraw barbiturates gradually.
• Take precautions to prevent hoarding or self-overdosing, especially by a depressed or suicidal patient or one who has a history of drug abuse.
• Consult with the patient's doctor to obtain an analgesic order if the patient has pain. Barbiturates have no analgesic effect and may cause restlessness or delirium in presence of pain.
• During I.V. use, always keep resuscitation and mechanical ventilation equipment available.

Patient Teaching
• Explain that morning hangover is common after hypnotic dose. Encourage the patient to report severe hangover or oversedation so the doctor can be consulted for change of dose or drug.
• Explain that because hypnotic drugs suppress REM sleep, the patient may experience increased dreaming after the drug is discontinued.
• Instruct the patient to remain in bed after taking drug and to call for assistance to use the bathroom.
• Warn the patient that drug may cause physical dependence.
• Warn the patient to avoid hazardous activities that require mental alertness if adverse CNS reactions are present after awakening.
• Advise the patient to avoid alcoholic beverages during therapy with pentobarbital because they may cause excessive CNS depression.
• Tell the patient to notify the nurse or doctor if sleep pattern disturbances continue despite therapy.

Evaluation
In patients receiving pentobarbital, appropriate evaluation statements may include:
• Patient states drug was effective in inducing sleep.
• Patient's safety maintained.
• Patient and family state an understanding of pentobarbital therapy.

pentoxifylline
(pen tox´ i fi leen)
Trental

• *Classification:* hemorrheologic agent (xanthine derivative)
• *Pregnancy Risk Category:* C

HOW SUPPLIED
Tablets (extended-release): 400 mg

ACTION

Mechanism: Improves capillary blood flow by increasing erythrocyte flexibility and lowering blood viscosity.
Absorption: Almost completely absorbed from the GI tract but undergoes first-pass hepatic metabolism. Absorption is slowed by food.
Distribution: Bound to erythrocyte membrane.
Metabolism: Extensively metabolized by erythrocytes and the liver.
Excretion: Metabolites are excreted principally in urine; less than 4% of drug is excreted in feces. Half-life: Of unchanged drug, about 30 to 45 minutes; of metabolites, about 1 to 1½ hours.
Onset, peak, duration: Peak concentrations occur in 2 to 4 hours, but clinical effect requires 2 to 4 weeks of continuous therapy.

INDICATIONS & DOSAGE

Treatment of intermittent claudication caused by chronic occlusive vascular disease–
Adults: 400 mg P.O. t.i.d. with meals.

CONTRAINDICATIONS & PRECAUTIONS

Contraindicated in patients with hypersensitivity to this or other xanthine derivatives, such as caffeine, theophylline, or theobromine. Use cautiously in patients at high risk for hemorrhage, such as surgical patients or those with peptic ulcers.

ADVERSE REACTIONS

Common reactions are in italics; life-threatening reactions are in bold italics.
CNS: headache, dizziness.
GI: dyspepsia, nausea, vomiting.

INTERACTIONS

Anticoagulants: increased anticoagulant effect.
Antihypertensives: increased hypotensive effect. Dosage adjustments may be necessary.

EFFECTS ON DIAGNOSTIC TESTS

None reported.

NURSING CONSIDERATIONS

Besides those related universally to drug therapy (see "How to use this book"), consider the following specific recommendations:

Assessment
- Obtain a baseline assessment of cardiovascular status and activity levels before therapy.
- Be alert for adverse reactions and drug interactions throughout therapy.
- Evaluate the patient's and family's knowledge about pentoxifylline therapy.

Nursing Diagnoses
- Activity intolerance related to underlying disease.
- Pain related to drug-induced headache.
- Knowledge deficit related to pentoxifylline.

Planning and Implementation

Preparation and Administration
- ***P.O. use:*** Administer with meals to reduce gastric upset.
- Have the patient swallow the medication whole, without breaking, crushing, or chewing. Anticipate that therapy will last at least 8 weeks to be clinically effective.

Monitoring
- Monitor effectiveness by evaluating the patient's leg pain, especially with activity.

Supportive Care
- Provide short but frequent periods of activity.
- If patient smokes, encourage him to quit. Suggest a nicotine substitute and participation in a behavior modification program.
- Remember that elderly patients may be more sensitive to this drug's effects.

Patient Teaching
- Explain the needed duration of this therapy.
- Tell the patient *not* to discontinue

the drug unless specifically instructed by the doctor.
• Instruct the patient to take the drug with meals.
• Advise the patient to report any GI or CNS adverse reactions.
• Tell the patient to avoid smoking because nicotine causes vasoconstriction, which can worsen the condition.

Evaluation
In patients receiving pentoxifylline, appropriate evaluation statements may include:
• Patient reports increased level of pain-free activity.
• Patient denies presence of headache related to drug.
• Patient and family state an understanding of pentoxifylline therapy.

pergolide mesylate
(per´ go lide)
Permax

• *Classification:* antiparkinsonian agent (dopaminergic agonist)
• *Pregnancy Risk Category:* B

HOW SUPPLIED
Tablets: 0.05 mg, 0.25 mg, 1 mg

ACTION
Mechanism: Directly stimulates dopamine receptors in the nigrostriatal system.
Absorption: Well absorbed after oral administration.
Distribution: Approximately 90% bound to plasma proteins.
Metabolism: Metabolized to at least 10 different compounds, some of which retain some pharmacologic activity.
Excretion: Primarily in urine.

INDICATIONS & DOSAGE
Adjunctive treatment to levodopa-carbidopa in the management of the symptoms associated with Parkinson's disease –
Adults: initially, 0.05 mg P.O. daily for the first 2 days. Gradually increase dosage by 0.1 to 0.15 mg every third day over the next 12 days of therapy. Subsequent dosage can be increased by 0.25 mg every third day until optimum response is seen. The drug is usually administered in divided doses t.i.d. Gradual reductions in levodopa-carbidopa dosage may be made during dosage titration.

CONTRAINDICATIONS & PRECAUTIONS
Contraindicated in patients allergic to the drug or ergot alkaloids.

In premarketing trials, over 140 of approximately 2,300 patients died while taking pergolide. However, these deaths did not appear to be linked to use of the drug, since these patients were elderly and debilitated.

ADVERSE REACTIONS
Common reactions are in italics; life-threatening reactions are in bold italics.
CNS: headache, asthenia, *dyskinesia, dizziness, hallucinations,* dystonia, confusion, *somnolescence,* insomnia, anxiety, depression, tremor, abnormal dreams, personality disorder, psychosis, abnormal gait, akathisia, extrapyramidal syndrome, incoordination, paresthesias, akinesia, hypertonia, neuralgia, speech disorder.
CV: *orthostatic hypotension,* vasodilation, palpitations, hypotension, syncope, hypertension, arrhythmias, ***myocardial infarction.***
EENT: *rhinitis,* epistaxis, abnormal vision, diplopia, eye disorder.
GI: abdominal pain, *nausea, constipation,* diarrhea, dyspepsia, anorexia, vomiting, dry mouth, taste alteration.
GU: urinary frequency, urinary tract infection, hematuria.

Skin: rash, sweating.
Other: accident or injury; chest, neck, and back pain; flu-like syndrome; chills; infection; facial, peripheral, or generalized edema; weight gain; arthralgia; bursitis; myalgia; twitching.

Note: The above adverse reactions, although not always attributable to the drug, occurred in 1% of the study population.

INTERACTIONS

Phenothiazines, butyrophenones, thioxanthines, metoclopramide, and other dopamine antagonists: may antagonize the effects of pergolide.

EFFECTS ON DIAGNOSTIC TESTS

None reported.

NURSING CONSIDERATIONS

Besides those related universally to drug therapy (see "How to use this book"), consider the following specific recommendations:

Assessment
- Obtain a baseline assessment of the patient's parkinsonian signs and symptoms before therapy.
- Be alert for adverse reactions and drug interactions throughout therapy.
- Evaluate the patient's and family's knowledge about pergolide therapy.

Nursing Diagnoses
- Impaired physical mobility related to underlying parkinsonian syndrome.
- Altered thought processes related to CNS reactions to pergolide.
- Knowledge deficit related to pergolide therapy.

Planning and Implementation

Preparation and Administration
- Gradually increase dosage according to patient's response and tolerence.

Monitoring
- Monitor effectiveness by regularly checking the patient's body movements for signs of improvement.
- Monitor for signs of overdose, including unsteady gait, slurred speech, sustained nystagmus, somnolence, confusion, respiratory depression, pulmonary edema, areflexia, and coma. Report them to the doctor immediately.
- Monitor the patient for CNS and other adverse drug reactions. Hallucinations may occur in some patients. Tolerance to this adverse reaction was not seen in early clinical trials.
- Monitor for abnormal body movements, for example, dystonic and dyskinetic movements.
- Monitor vital signs closely, especially during dosage adjustment.

Supportive Care
- Notify the doctor if significant changes in vital signs or mental status occur. Keep in mind that in early clinical trials, 27% of patients who attempted pergolide therapy did not finish the trial because of adverse reactions (primarily confusion and hallucinations).
- Institute safety precautions.
- Assist the patient with daily activities, as needed.

Patient Teaching
- Warn the patient of possible dizziness and orthostatic hypotension, especially at start of therapy. The patient should change position slowly and dangle legs before getting out of bed. Inform the patient that elastic stockings may control this adverse reaction.
- Warn the patient and family not to increase dosage without the doctor's order.
- Instruct the family to notify the doctor if they notice changes in the patient's behavior or mental status. Tell the patient to notify the nurse or doctor if other adverse reactions develop.
- Advise the patient to avoid activities that could expose the patient to injury until adverse CNS and cardiovascular reactions are known.

Evaluation
In patients receiving pergolide, appropriate evaluation statements may include:
• Patient exhibits improved mobility with reduction of muscular rigidity and tremor.
• Patient remains mentally alert throughout pergolide therapy.
• Patient and family state an understanding of pergolide therapy.

permethrin
(per meth´ rin)
Nix

• *Classification:* pediculocide (synthetic pyrethroid)
• *Pregnancy Risk Category:* B

HOW SUPPLIED
Topical liquid: 1%

ACTION
Mechanism: Acts on the parasites' nerve cells to disrupt the sodium channel current, causing paralysis of the parasite.
Absorption: Less than 2% of a dose is absorbed.
Metabolism: Rapidly metabolized by ester hydrolysis to inactive metabolites.
Excretion: Metabolites are excreted in the urine. Residual drug is detectable on hair for up to 10 days.

INDICATIONS & DOSAGE
Treatment of infestation with Pediculus humanus capitis *(head lice) and its nits—*
Adults and children: use after hair has been washed with shampoo, rinsed with water, and towel-dried. Apply a sufficient amount (25 to 50 ml) of liquid to saturate the hair and scalp. Allow to remain on hair for 10 minutes before rinsing off with water.

CONTRAINDICATIONS & PRECAUTIONS
Contraindicated in persons with hypersensitivity to any synthetic pyrethroid or pyrethrin, to chrysanthemums, or to any component of the product, and in infants because their skin is more permeable than that of children or adults.

ADVERSE REACTIONS
Common reactions are in italics; life-threatening reactions are in bold italics.
Skin: itching, burning, stinging, tingling, numbness or scalp discomfort, mild erythema, rash on the scalp.

INTERACTIONS
None reported.

EFFECTS ON DIAGNOSTIC TESTS
None reported.

NURSING CONSIDERATIONS
Besides those related universally to drug therapy (see "How to use this book"), consider the following specific recommendations:
Assessment
• Obtain a baseline assessment of scalp and hair before therapy.
• Be alert for adverse reactions and drug interactions throughout therapy.
• Evaluate the patient's and family's knowledge about permethrin therapy.
Nursing Diagnoses
• Body image disturbance related to patient's underlying condition.
• Impaired skin integrity related to permethrin-induced rash on scalp.
• Knowledge deficit related to permethrin therapy.
Planning and Implementation
Preparation and Administration
• ***Topical use:*** Use after hair has been washed with shampoo, rinsed with water, and towel-dried. Apply a sufficient amount (25 to 50 ml) of liquid to saturate hair and scalp. Keep on hair 10 minutes before rinsing out with water.

Monitoring
• Monitor effectiveness by examining patient's scalp for lice.
• Frequently observe the patient's scalp for pruritus or irritation.
Supportive Care
• Keep in mind, a single treatment is usually all that is necessary. Combing of nits is not required for effectiveness, but drug package supplies a fine-toothed comb for cosmetic use as desired.
• Remember that drug is not indicated to treat scabies.
• Be aware permethrin is at least as effective as lindane (Kwell) in treating head lice.
• While assisting with self-care, encourage patient to express fears and concerns about body image disturbance.
Patient Teaching
• Teach patient how to apply medication.
• Inform patient that a second application may be necessary if lice are observed 7 days after the initial application.
Evaluation
In patients receiving permethrin, appropriate evaluation statements may include:
• Body image disturbance is resolved.
• Patient did not develop a drug-induced rash.
• Patient and family state an understanding of permethrin therapy.

perphenazine
(per fen´ a zeen)
Apo-Perphenazine†, Phenazine†, Trilafon

• *Classification:* antipsychotic, antiemetic (phenothiazine)
• *Pregnancy Risk Category:* C

HOW SUPPLIED
Tablets: 2 mg, 4 mg, 8 mg, 16 mg
Repetabs (sustained-release): 8 mg
Oral concentrate: 16 mg/5ml
Injection: 5 mg/ml

ACTION
Mechanism: Blocks postsynaptic dopamine receptors in the brain. As an antiemetic, inhibits the medullary chemoreceptor trigger zone.
Absorption: Rate and extent of absorption vary with administration route. Oral tablet absorption is erratic and variable; absorption of oral concentrate is more predictable. I.M. drug is absorbed rapidly.
Distribution: Widely distributed into the body, including breast milk. Drug is 91% to 99% protein-bound.
Metabolism: Extensively metabolized by the liver, but no active metabolites are formed.
Excretion: Most is excreted in urine via the kidneys; some is excreted in feces via the biliary tract.
Onset, peak, duration: After oral tablet administration, peak plasma levels are seen in 2 to 4 hours; steady-state serum levels are achieved within 4 to 7 days. Peak therapeutic effect may take several weeks.

INDICATIONS & DOSAGE
Hospitalized psychiatric patients–
Adults: initially, 8 to 16 mg P.O. b.i.d., t.i.d., or q.i.d., increasing to 64 mg daily.
Children over 12 years: 6 to 12 mg P.O. daily in divided doses.
Mental disturbances, acute alcoholism, nausea, vomiting, hiccups–
Adults and children over 12 years: 5 to 10 mg I.M., p.r.n. Maximum 15 mg daily in ambulatory patients, 30 mg daily in hospitalized patients.

CONTRAINDICATIONS & PRECAUTIONS
Contraindicated in patients with hypersensitivity to phenothiazines and

related compounds, including allergic reactions involving hepatic function, because perphenazine may be hepatotoxic; blood dyscrasias and bone marrow depression, because drug may have adverse effects on bone marrow and blood cell lines; coma, brain damage, or CNS depression, because of additive CNS and respiratory depression; circulatory collapse or cerebrovascular disease, because drug may adversely affect blood pressure through its alpha-blocking effects; and with adrenergic blocking agents or spinal or epidural anesthetics because of the potential for alpha blockade.

Use cautiously in patients with cardiac disease (arrhythmias, CHF, angina pectoris, valvular disease, or heart block); encephalitis; Reye's syndrome; head injury; respiratory disease; seizure disorders, because drug may lower seizure threshold; glaucoma, because drug may raise intraocular pressure; prostatic hypertrophy, Parkinson's disease, or urine retention, because drug may worsen these conditions; hepatic or renal dysfunction, because impaired metabolism and excretion may cause drug accumulation; pheochromocytoma; or hypocalcemia, because of increased risk of extrapyramidal reactions. Exposure to temperature extremes may predispose the patient to hyperthermia or hypothermia.

ADVERSE REACTIONS

Common reactions are in italics; life-threatening reactions are in bold italics.
Blood: transient leukopenia, ***agranulocytosis.***
CNS: *extrapyramidal reactions (high incidence), tardive dyskinesia,* sedation (low incidence), pseudoparkinsonism, EEG changes, dizziness.
CV: *orthostatic hypotension,* tachycardia, ECG changes.
EENT: ocular changes, *blurred vision.*
GI: *dry mouth, constipation.*
GU: *urine retention,* dark urine, menstrual irregularities, gynecomastia, inhibited ejaculation.
Hepatic: cholestatic jaundice, abnormal liver function tests.
Metabolic: hyperprolactinemia.
Skin: *mild photosensitivity,* dermal allergic reactions.
Local: pain at I.M. injection site, sterile abscess.
Other: weight gain; increased appetite; rarely, ***neuroleptic malignant syndrome*** (fever, tachycardia, tachypnea, profuse diaphoresis).
After abrupt withdrawal of long-term therapy: gastritis, nausea, vomiting, dizziness, tremors, feeling of warmth or cold, sweating, tachycardia, headache, insomnia.

INTERACTIONS

Alcohol, other CNS depressants: increased CNS depression. Avoid concomitant use.
Antacids: inhibit absorption of oral phenothiazines. Separate antacid and phenothiazine doses by at least 2 hours.
Barbiturates: may decrease phenothiazine effect. Observe patient.

EFFECTS ON DIAGNOSTIC TESTS

ECG: quinidine-like effects.
Liver enzymes: elevated results.
Protein-bound iodine: elevated results.
Urine porphyrins, urobilinogen, amylase, and 5-hydroxyindoleacetic acid: false-positive results because of darkening of urine by metabolites.
Urine pregnancy tests using human chorionic gonadotropin: false-positive results.

NURSING CONSIDERATIONS

Besides those related universally to drug therapy (see "How to use this book"), consider the following specific recommendations:

Assessment

- Obtain baseline assessment of patient's underlying condition before therapy.
- Be alert for adverse reactions and drug interactions throughout therapy.
- Evaluate the patient's and family's knowledge about perphenazine therapy.

Nursing Diagnoses

- Altered health maintenance related to patient's underlying condition.
- High risk for injury related to extrapyramidal adverse reactions to drug.
- Knowledge deficit related to perphenazine therapy.

Planning and Implementation

Preparation and Administration

- ***P.O. use:*** Dilute liquid concentrate with fruit juice, carbonated beverage, or semisolid food just before giving. Exceptions: Oral concentrate causes turbidity or precipitation in colas, black coffee, grape or apple juice, or tea. Do not mix with these liquids.
- ***I.V. use:*** Drug may be given by direct injection and intermittent infusion. Continuous infusion is not recommended.
- Protect medication from light. Slight yellowing of injection or concentrate is common and does not affect potency. Discard markedly discolored solutions.
- ***I.M. use:*** Give injection deeply only in upper outer quadrant of buttocks. Massage slowly afterward to prevent sterile abscess. The injection may sting.
- Avoid skin contact with the injectable or liquid form because it may cause a rash.
- Dose of 8 mg is therapeutic equivalent of 100 mg of chlorpromazine.

Monitoring

- Monitor effectiveness by regularly observing behavior and noting if symptoms have abated or diminished.
- Monitor for adverse reactions, especially extrapyramidal and anticholinergic effects (blurred vision, dry mouth, constipation, urine retention) and tardive dyskinesia during prolonged therapy. Tardive dyskinesia may not appear until months or years later and may disappear spontaneously or persist for life despite discontinuation of the drug.
- Frequently check blood pressure for orthostatic hypotension, especially after parenteral administration.
- Monitor therapy by weekly bilirubin tests during the first month, periodic blood tests (CBC and liver function), and ophthalmic tests (long-term use).
- Monitor for neuroleptic malignant syndrome. This rare, potentially fatal reaction is not necessarily related to type of neuroleptic or duration of drug therapy, but usually occurs in men (60% of affected patients).

Supportive Care

- Obtain baseline measures of blood pressure before starting therapy.
- Keep the patient supine for 1 hour after I.M. administration. Then assist patient to get up slowly to avoid orthostatic hypotension.
- Do not discontinue drug abruptly unless required by severe adverse reactions.
- Increase the patient's fluid and fiber intake—if not contraindicated—to prevent constipation. If necessary, request doctor's order for a laxative.
- Give the patient sugarless gum, sour hard candy, ice chips, or a mouthwash rinse to relieve dryness.
- Treat acute dystonic reactions with I.V. diphenhydramine, as ordered.
- Hold the patient's dose if he develops signs of jaundice, symptoms of blood dyscrasias (fever, sore throat, infection, cellulitis, weakness), persistent (longer than a few hours) extrapyramidal reactions, or any such reactions during pregnancy or in children.

Patient Teaching

- Warn the patient that the injection might sting.

• Tell the patient to avoid exposure to direct sunlight and to use a sunscreen when going outdoors to prevent photosensitivity reactions. (*Note:* Sun lamps and tanning beds may cause burning of the skin or skin discoloration.)
• Tell the patient not to stop taking the drug suddenly.
• Encourage the patient to report difficult urination, sore throat, dizziness, or fainting.
• Advise the patient to increase fluid and fiber in the diet, if appropriate.
• Tell the patient to avoid driving and other hazardous activities that require alertness until the effect of the drug is established. Excessive sedative effects (drowsiness and dizziness) tend to subside after several weeks.
• Explain which fluids are appropriate for diluting the concentrate and show the dropper technique for measuring dose. Warn the patient not to spill liquid preparation on skin because rash and irritation may occur.
• Tell the patient that sugarless hard candy, chewing gum, or ice chips can alleviate dry mouth.

Evaluation

In patients receiving perphenazine, appropriate evaluation statements may include:
• Patient is able to perform activities of daily living without assistance.
• Patient does not develop extrapyramidal symptoms.
• Patient and family state an understanding of perphenazine therapy.

phenazopyridine hydrochloride

(fen az oh peer´ i deen)

Azo-Standard◇, Baridium◇, Di-Azo◇, Eridium◇, Geridium◇, Phenazo†, Phenazodine◇, Pyrazodine◇, Pyridiate◇, Pyridin◇, Pyridium, Pyronium†, Urodine◇, Urogesic◇, Viridium◇

• *Classification:* urinary analgesic (azo dye)
• *Pregnancy Risk Category:* B

HOW SUPPLIED

Tablets: 100 mg◇, 200 mg

ACTION

Mechanism: Exerts local anesthetic action on urinary mucosa through unknown mechanism.
Absorption: Well absorbed after oral administration.
Metabolism: In the liver and other tissues.
Excretion: In the urine.
Onset, peak, duration: Maximum renal output occurs in 5 to 6 hours; most of the drug is eliminated within 24 hours.

INDICATIONS & DOSAGE

Pain with urinary tract irritation or infection–
Adults: 100 to 200 mg P.O. t.i.d.
Children: 100 mg P.O. t.i.d.

CONTRAINDICATIONS & PRECAUTIONS

Contraindicated in patients with hypersensitivity to phenazopyridine and in patients with renal and hepatic insufficiency because of the potential for drug accumulation.

ADVERSE REACTIONS

Common reactions are in italics; life-threatening reactions are in bold italics.
CNS: headache, vertigo.
GI: nausea.
Skin: rash.

INTERACTIONS

None significant.

EFFECTS ON DIAGNOSTIC TESTS

Phenolsulfonphthalein (PSP) excretion: test interference.
Sulfobromophthalein (BSP) excretion: test interference.

Urine urobilinogen (Ehrlich's test): test interference.
Urine glucose tests using copper sulfate method (Clinistix, Tes-Tape, Acetest, and Ketostix): altered results. Glucose enzymatic test (Clinitest) should be used to obtain accurate urine glucose test results.
Urine tests for protein, steroids, or bilirubin: test interference.

NURSING CONSIDERATIONS

Besides those related universally to drug therapy (see "How to use this book"), consider the following specific recommendations:

Assessment
- Obtain a baseline assessment of the patient's pain before therapy.
- Be alert for adverse reactions and drug interactions throughout therapy.
- Evaluate the patient's and family's knowledge about phenazopyridine therapy.

Nursing Diagnoses
- Pain related to the patient's underlying condition.
- High risk for injury related to phenazopyridine-induced vertigo.
- Knowledge deficit related to phenazopyridine therapy.

Planning and Implementation
Preparation and Administration
- Administer phenazopyridine with meals to minimize GI distress.

Monitoring
- Monitor effectiveness regularly by questioning the patient about pain in the urinary tract.

Supportive Care
- Notify the doctor if phenazopyridine does not relieve discomfort.
- Obtain urine samples for urinalysis and urine culture and sensitivity to detect infection as a source of the patient's dysuria.
- Keep in mind that this drug should be used only as an analgesic.
- Remember that this drug can be administered with antibiotics to treat urinary tract infection.
- Notify the doctor if the patient's skin or sclera becomes yellow-tinged. This may indicate accumulation of the drug caused by impaired renal excretion.
- Use copper sulfate test (Clinitest) for accurate urine glucose test results; drug may alter glucose enzymatic (Clinistix or Tes-Tape) results.
- Institute safety measures, such as supervising patient activities and keeping bed rails up, if the patient develops vertigo.

Patient Teaching
- Tell the patient the drug may be discontinued in 3 days if pain is relieved.
- Advise the diabetic patient to check urine glucose with copper sulfate test for accurate results.
- Warn the patient that the drug colors urine red or orange and that it may stain fabrics.
- Warn the patient to avoid hazardous activities that require mental alertness or physical ability if drug causes vertigo.

Evaluation
In patients receiving phenazopyridine, appropriate evaluation statements may include:
- Patient states pain has been relieved.
- Patient has not experienced injury.
- Patient and family state an understanding of phenazopyridine therapy.

---

phenelzine sulfate

(fen´ el zeen)
Nardil

- *Classification:* antidepressant (MAO inhibitor)
- *Pregnancy Risk Category:* C

HOW SUPPLIED

Tablets: 15 mg

ACTION

Mechanism: Promotes accumulation of neurotransmitters by inhibiting MAO.
Absorption: Rapidly and completely from the GI tract.
Distribution: Not yet determined; dose adjustments are determined by therapeutic response and adverse reaction profile.
Metabolism: Hepatic.
Excretion: Primarily in urine within 24 hours; some drug is excreted in feces via the biliary tract.
Onset, peak, duration: Enzyme inhibition is prolonged and unrelated to drug levels. Peak therapeutic effects may not be seen for several weeks.

INDICATIONS & DOSAGE

Treatment of depression–
Adults: 45 mg P.O. daily in divided doses, increasing rapidly to 60 mg daily. Then dosage can usually be reduced to 15 mg daily. Maximum is 90 mg daily.

CONTRAINDICATIONS & PRECAUTIONS

Contraindicated in patients with uncontrolled hypertension, because it may provoke hypertensive crisis, and in patients with seizure disorders, because it lowers the seizure threshold, even in patients controlled with anticonvulsant therapy.

Use cautiously in patients with angina pectoris and other cardiovascular disease; in patients with Type I and Type II diabetes; in patients with Parkinson's disease and other motor disorders or hyperthyroidism because it may worsen these conditions; in patients with pheochromocytoma because of risk of hypertensive crisis; in patients with renal or hepatic insufficiency because diminished metabolism and excretion can cause drug accumulation; and in patients with bipolar illness because drug may provoke sudden mood change from depression to mania (reduce dosage during manic phase).

ADVERSE REACTIONS

Common reactions are in italics; life-threatening reactions are in bold italics.
CNS: *dizziness,* vertigo, headache, overactivity, hyperreflexia, tremors, muscle twitching, mania, jitters, *insomnia,* confusion, memory impairment, drowsiness, weakness, fatigue.
CV: paradoxical hypertension, *orthostatic hypotension,* arrhythmias.
GI: dry mouth, *anorexia,* nausea, constipation.
Other: peripheral edema, sweating, weight changes.

INTERACTIONS

Alcohol, barbiturates, and other sedatives; narcotics; dextromethorphan; tricyclic antidepressants: unpredictable interaction. Use with caution and in reduced dosage.
Amphetamines, antihistamines, ephedrine, levodopa, meperidine, metaraminol, methotrimeprazine, methylphenidate, phenylephrine, phenylpropanolamine: enhance pressor effects. Use together cautiously.
Insulin, oral hypoglycemic agents: phenelzine may alter requirements for antidiabetic medications.

EFFECTS ON DIAGNOSTIC TESTS

CBC: elevated WBC count.
Liver function tests: elevated results.
Urine catecholamines: elevated levels.

NURSING CONSIDERATIONS

Besides those related universally to drug therapy (see "How to use this book"), consider the following specific recommendations:
Assessment
• Obtain a baseline assessment of severity of depression and baseline blood pressure readings and CBC and liver function tests before beginning therapy.

- Be alert for adverse reactions and drug interactions throughout therapy.
- Evaluate the patient's and family's knowledge about phenelzine sulfate therapy.

Nursing Diagnoses
- Ineffective individual coping related to the patient's underlying condition.
- High risk for injury related to adverse CNS and CV reactions to phenelzine.
- Knowledge deficit related to phenelzine therapy.

Planning and Implementation

Preparation and Administration
- Expect this medication to be ordered only when tricyclic antidepressants or electroconvulsive therapy is ineffective or contraindicated.
- Expect dosage reduction to maintenance levels as soon as possible.
- Store in a tight container away from heat and light.

Monitoring
- Monitor effectiveness by having the patient discuss his feelings (ask broad, open-ended questions) and by evaluating his behavior.
- Monitor blood pressure (supine and standing), ECG for changes, and heart rate for tachycardia.
- Monitor CBC results and results of liver function tests throughout therapy.
- Monitor the patient for signs of overdosage (palpitations, frequent headaches or severe hypotension).
- Monitor for suicidal tendencies.

Supportive Care
- Hold dose and notify the doctor if the patient develops signs of overdosage.
- Assist the patient in changing positions slowly to minimize orthostatic hypotension; to prevent injury supervise the patient when walking.
- Have phentolamine (Regitine) available to counteract severe hypertension.
- Continue precautions for 10 days after discontinuation of the drug because it has long-lasting effects.

Patient Teaching
- Warn the patient to avoid foods high in tyramine or tryptophan (aged cheese, Chianti wine, beer, avocados, chicken livers, chocolate, bananas, soy sauce, meat tenderizers, salami, bologna); large amounts of caffeine; and self-medication with OTC cold, hay fever, or diet preparations.
- Tell the patient that orthostatic hypotension is common. Advise him to get out of bed slowly, sitting up for 1 minute before attempting to stand to prevent dizziness.
- Tell the patient that therapy must continue for 2 weeks or more before noticeable effect, and for 4 weeks or more before full effect. Encourage the patient to continue taking medication until it achieves full therapeutic effect.
- Warn against combining drug with alcohol or other CNS depressants.

Evaluation

In patients receiving phenelzine, appropriate evaluation statements may include:
- Patient behavior and communication indicate improvement of depression.
- Patient has not experienced injury from adverse CNS or CV reactions.
- Patient and family state an understanding of phenelzine therapy.

---

phenobarbital (phenobarbitone)

(fee noe bar´ bi tal)

Barbita, Gardenal†, Luminal†, Solfoton

phenobarbital sodium (phenobarbitone sodium)

Luminal Sodium†

- Controlled Substance Schedule IV

• *Classification:* anticonvulsant, sedative-hypnotic (barbiturate)
• *Pregnancy Risk Category:* D

HOW SUPPLIED

Tablets: 8 mg, 15 mg, 16 mg, 30 mg, 32 mg, 60 mg, 65 mg, 100 mg
Capsules: 16 mg
Oral solution: 15 mg/5 ml, 20 mg/5 ml
Elixir: 20 mg/5 ml
Injection: 30 mg/ml, 60 mg/ml, 65 mg/ml, 130 mg/ml
Powder for injection: 120 mg/ampule

ACTION

Mechanism: Depresses neuronal transmission in the CNS and increases the threshold for seizure activity in the motor cortex. As a sedative, probably interferes with transmission of impulses from the thalamus to the cortex of the brain. A barbiturate.
Absorption: Well absorbed after oral and rectal administration, with 70% to 90% reaching the bloodstream. Absorption after I.M. administration is 100%. A serum concentration of 10 mcg/ml is needed to produce sedation; 40 mcg/ml usually produces sleep. Concentrations of 20 to 40 mcg/ml are considered necessary for anticonvulsant effect.
Distribution: Widely distributed throughout the body; approximately 25% to 30% protein-bound.
Metabolism: By the hepatic microsomal enzyme system.
Excretion: 25% to 50% of a dose is eliminated unchanged in urine. The remainder is excreted as metabolites of glucuronic acid. Half-life: 5 to 7 days.
Onset, peak, duration: After oral administration, peak serum levels are reached in 1 to 2 hours, and peak levels in the CNS are achieved at 1 to 3 hours. Onset of action occurs 1 hour or longer after oral dosing; onset after I.V. administration is about 5 minutes.

INDICATIONS & DOSAGE

All forms of epilepsy, febrile seizures in children–
Adults: 100 to 200 mg P.O. daily, divided t.i.d. or given as single dosage h.s.
Children: 4 to 6 mg/kg P.O. daily, usually divided q 12 hours. It can, however, be administered once daily, usually h.s.
Status epilepticus–
Adults: 10 mg/kg as I.V. infusion no faster than 50 mg/minute. May give up to 20 mg/kg total. Administer in acute care or emergency area only.
Children: 5 to 10 mg/kg I.V. May repeat q 10 to 15 minutes up to total of 20 mg/kg. I.V. injection rate should not exceed 50 mg/minute.
Sedation–
Adults: 30 to 120 mg P.O. daily in two or three divided doses.
Children: 6 mg/kg P.O. divided t.i.d.
Insomnia–
Adults: 100 to 320 mg P.O. or I.M.
Children: 3 to 6 mg/kg.
Preoperative sedation–
Adults: 100 to 200 mg I.M. 60 to 90 minutes before surgery.
Children: 16 to 100 mg I.M. 60 to 90 minutes before surgery.
Hyperbilirubinemia–
Neonates: 7 mg/kg daily P.O. from first to fifth day of life; or 5 mg/kg daily I.M. on first day, repeated P.O. on second to seventh days.
Chronic cholestasis–
Adults: 90 to 180 mg P.O. daily in two or three divided doses.
Children under 12 years: 3 to 12 mg/kg daily P.O. in two or three divided doses.

CONTRAINDICATIONS & PRECAUTIONS

Contraindicated in patients with hypersensitivity to barbiturates and in patients with bronchopneumonia, status asthmaticus, or other severe respiratory distress because of the potential for respiratory depression. Avoid use in patients who are depressed or have suicidal ideation, because the drug can worsen depression; in patients with uncontrolled acute or chronic pain, because exacerbation of pain or paradoxical excitement can occur; or in patients with porphyria, because this drug can trigger symptoms of this disease.

Use cautiously in patients who must perform hazardous tasks requiring mental alertness, because the drug causes drowsiness; and in patients with impaired renal function, because up to 50% of phenobarbital is excreted in urine. Administer parenteral phenobarbital slowly and with extreme caution to patients with hypotension or severe pulmonary or cardiovascular disease because of potential adverse hemodynamic effects. Because tolerance and physical or psychological dependence may occur, prolonged use of high doses should be avoided.

Prenatal exposure to barbiturates is associated with an increased incidence of fetal abnormalities and, possibly, brain tumors. Use of barbiturates in the third trimester may be associated with physical dependence in neonates. Risk-benefit must be considered.

ADVERSE REACTIONS

Common reactions are in italics; life-threatening reactions are in bold italics.
CNS: *drowsiness, lethargy, hangover,* paradoxical excitement in elderly patients.
GI: nausea, vomiting.
Skin: rash, ***Stevens-Johnson syndrome,*** urticaria.
Local: pain, swelling, thrombophlebitis, necrosis, nerve injury.
Other: angioedema.

INTERACTIONS

Alcohol and other CNS depressants, including narcotic analgesics: excessive CNS depression. Use cautiously.
Diazepam: increased effects of both drugs. Use together cautiously.
Griseofulvin: decreased absorption of griseofulvin.
MAO inhibitors: potentiated barbiturate effect. Monitor for increased CNS and respiratory depression.
Oral anticoagulants, estrogens and oral contraceptives, doxycycline, corticosteroids: may enhance the metabolism of these drugs. Monitor for decreased effect.
Primidone: monitor for excessive phenobarbital blood levels.
Rifampin: may decrease barbiturate levels. Monitor for decreased effect.
Valproic acid: increased phenobarbital levels. Monitor for toxicity.

EFFECTS ON DIAGNOSTIC TESTS

Cyanocobalamin ^{57}Co: impaired absorption.
EEG: changes in low-voltage, fast activity; changes persist for a time after therapy.
Phentolamine test: false-positive results.
Serum bilirubin: decreased concentrations in neonates, epileptics, and in patients with congenital nonhemolytic unconjugated hyperbilirubinemia.
Sulfobromophthalein excretion: increased retention.

NURSING CONSIDERATIONS

Besides those related universally to drug therapy (see "How to use this book"), consider the following specific recommendations:

Assessment

- Obtain a baseline assessment of the patient's seizure activity.
- Be alert for adverse reactions and drug interactions throughout therapy.
- Evaluate the patient's and family's

knowledge about phenobarbital therapy.

Nursing Diagnoses

• High risk for trauma related to patient's underlying seizure disorder.
• Noncompliance related to need for long-term use of phenobarbital anticonvulsant therapy.
• Knowledge deficit related to phenobarbital therapy.

Planning and Implementation

Preparation and Administration

• Do not use injectable solution if it contains a precipitate.
• Do not mix parenteral form with acidic solutions such as tetracyclines, metaraminol, or methyldopate hydrochloride; precipitation may result. Check with pharmacist before mixing.
• ***I.M use:*** Give I.M. injection deeply. Superficial injection may cause pain, sterile abscess, and tissue sloughing.
• ***I.V. use:*** I.V. injection should be reserved for emergency treatment and should be given slowly under close supervision. When administering I.V., do not give more than 60 mg/minute.

Monitoring

• Regularly monitor effectiveness by assessing seizure activity.
• Obtain baseline vital signs before administering phenobarbital I.V. Then closely monitor the patient's respiratory rate and depth for signs of respiratory depression when administering phenobarbital I.V. Also monitor blood pressure for signs of hypotension. Have resuscitative equipment readily available.
• Monitor for therapeutic blood levels (15 to 40 mcg/ml). If blood levels are not within normal range, check compliance.
• Monitor for signs of barbiturate toxicity: coma, asthmatic breathing, cyanosis, clammy skin, and hypotension. Overdose can be fatal.

Supportive Care

• Maintain seizure precautions; full therapeutic effect of phenobarbital is delayed 2 to 3 weeks, unless loading dose is used.
• Notify the doctor if seizure activity persists despite phenobarbital therapy.
• Withhold dose and notify the doctor if barbiturate toxicity is suspected, then expect to have the patient's barbiturate level determined; if confirmed, anticipate giving a different anticonvulsant.
• Consider and try to prevent possible noncompliance that may result from the patient's health belief system or life-style.
• If drowsiness or lethargy occurs, institute safety precautions, such as supervising activities.

Patient Teaching

• Warn the patient to avoid hazardous activities that require alertness and good psychomotor coordination until CNS effects of the drug are known.
• Warn the patient not to discontinue drug abruptly and to call the doctor immediately if adverse reactions develop or if seizure activity occurs.
• Make sure the patient is aware that phenobarbital is available in different milligram strengths. Tell the patient to check with pharmacist if a refill looks different from previous supply.
• Advise the patient to carry or wear medical alert identification indicating a seizure disorder and phenobarbital use.
• Warn the patient to avoid alcohol because it may cause excessive CNS depression when used concomitantly with phenobarbital.

Evaluation

In patients receiving phenobarbital, appropriate evaluation statements may include:

• Patient is free of seizure activity.
• Patient's phenobarbital blood level is within therapeutic range.
• Patient and family state an understanding of phenobarbital therapy.

phenolphthalein, white

(fee nole thay′ leen)
Alophen Pills◇, Medilax◇, Modane◇, Modane Mild◇, Phenolax Wafers**◇, Prulet◇

phenolphthalein, yellow

Evac-U-Gen◇, Evac-U-Lax◇, Ex-Lax◇, Feen-A-Mint Gum◇, Lax-Pills◇

- *Classification:* stimulant laxative (anthraquinone derivative)
- *Pregnancy Risk Category:* C

HOW SUPPLIED

phenolphthalein, white
Tablets: 60 mg◇
Tablets (chewable): 60 mg◇, 64.8 mg◇
phenolphthalein, yellow
Tablets (chewable): 80 mg◇, 90 mg◇, 97.2 mg◇
Chewing gum: 97.2 mg◇

ACTION

Mechanism: A stimulant laxative that increases peristalsis by direct effect on the smooth muscle of the intestine. Thought either to irritate the musculature or to stimulate the colonic intramural plexus. Also promotes fluid accumulation in the colon and small intestine.
Absorption: Approximately 15% of a dose is absorbed and enters the enterohepatic circulation.
Distribution: Primary site of action is the colon; drug enters breast milk.
Metabolism: Absorbed portion is metabolized in the liver.
Excretion: In feces, urine, and breast milk.
Onset, peak, duration: Action begins in 6 to 10 hours. Effect may last several days.

INDICATIONS & DOSAGE

Constipation–
Adults and children over 12 years: 30 to 270 mg P.O., preferably h.s.
Children 6 to 11 years: 30 to 60 mg P.O. h.s.
Children 2 to 5 years: 15 to 30 mg P.O. h.s.

CONTRAINDICATIONS & PRECAUTIONS

Contraindicated in patients with appendicitis, abdominal pain or cramps, nausea, vomiting, acute surgical abdomen, intestinal obstruction or perforation, or fecal impaction, because the drug may exacerbate these symptoms or conditions; and in patients with known hypersensitivity to the drug.

Use cautiously in patients with rectal bleeding because it may worsen this condition. Some formulations contain tartrazine, which may precipitate an allergic reaction, especially in persons allergic to aspirin.

ADVERSE REACTIONS

Common reactions are in italics; life-threatening reactions are in bold italics.
GI: diarrhea; *colic in large doses;* factitious nausea; vomiting; loss of normal bowel function in excessive use; *abdominal cramps,* especially in severe constipation; malabsorption of nutrients; "cathartic colon" (syndrome resembling ulcerative colitis radiologically and pathologically) in chronic misuse; reddish discoloration in alkaline feces or urine.
Skin: dermatitis, pruritus, rash, pigmentation.
Other: laxative dependence in long-term or excessive use, ***hypersensitivity.***

INTERACTIONS

None reported.

EFFECTS ON DIAGNOSTIC TESTS

Phenolsulfonphthalein (PSP) excretion tests: increased rate of excretion.
Urine urobilinogen and estrogen (Kolber procedure): false-positive results.

*Liquid form contains alcohol.

**May contain tartrazine.

NURSING CONSIDERATIONS

Besides those related universally to drug therapy (see "How to use this book"), consider the following specific recommendations:

Assessment

- Obtain a baseline assessment of history of bowel disorder, gastrointestinal status, fluid intake, nutritional status, exercise habits, and normal pattern of elimination.
- Be alert for adverse reactions and drug interactions throughout therapy.
- Evaluate the patient's and family's knowledge about phenolphthalein therapy.

Nursing Diagnoses

- Constipation related to interruption of normal pattern of elimination characterized by infrequent or absent stools.
- Pain related to phenolphthalein-induced abdominal cramping.
- Knowledge deficit related to phenolphthalein therapy.

Planning and Implementation

Preparation and Administration

- Check order carefully, because there are two forms of drug available. Phenolphthalein, yellow, is two to three times more potent than phenolphthalein, white.
- Schedule drug administration to avoid interference with scheduled activities. Produces semisolid stool within 6 to 8 hours.

Monitoring

- Monitor effectiveness by checking the frequency and characteristics of stools.
- Monitor for skin rash and other signs of hypersensitivity.
- Auscultate bowel sounds at least once a shift. Assess for pain and cramping.
- Monitor nutritional status and fluid intake.

Supportive Care

- Do not give to patients in abdominal pain, nausea, vomiting, or other symptoms of appendicitis or acute surgical abdomen; fecal impaction; or intestinal obstruction or perforation. Use cautiously in rectal bleeding.
- Provide privacy for elimination.
- Unless contraindicated, encourage fluid intake up to 2,500 ml a day.
- Consult with a dietitian to modify diet to increase fiber and bulk.

Patient Teaching

- Warn the patient with rash to avoid excessive sunlight and to discontinue drug, and to avoid using any other product containing phenolphthalein.
- Advise the patient that the drug may discolor alkaline urine red-pink and acidic urine yellow-brown.
- Warn the patient that abdominal cramping may occur, and that the laxative effect may last up to 3 to 4 days.
- Inform the patient that the tablet may be mistaken for candy. Encourage proper storage to keep drug out of the reach of children.
- Discourage excessive use of laxatives by patient to avoid dependence.
- Teach the patient about the relationship between fluid intake, dietary fiber, exercise, and constipation.
- Teach patient that dietary sources of fiber include bran and other cereals, fresh fruit, and vegetables.

Evaluation

In patients receiving phenolphthalein, appropriate evaluation statements may include:

- Patient reports return of normal pattern of elimination.
- Patient remains free from abdominal cramping.
- Patient and family state an understanding of phenolphthalein therapy.

PHARMACOLOGIC CLASS

phenothiazines

acetophenazine
chlorpromazine
chlorprothixene
ethopropazine
fluphenazine

mesoridazine
methdilazine
perphenazine
prochlorperazine
promazine
promethazine
propiomazine
thiethylperazine
thioridazine
thiothixene
trifluoperazine
triflupromazine
trimeprazine

OVERVIEW

The phenothiazines were originally synthesized by European scientists seeking aniline-like dyes in the late 1800s. Several decades later, in the 1930s, promethazine was identified and found to have sedative, antihistaminic, and narcotic-potentiating effects. Chlorpromazine was synthesized in the 1950s; this drug proved to have many effects, among them strong antipsychotic activity.

All antipsychotics have fundamentally similar mechanisms of action; they are believed to function as dopamine antagonists, blocking postsynaptic dopamine receptors in various parts of the CNS; their antiemetic effects result from blockage of the chemoreceptor trigger zone. They also produce varying degrees of anticholinergic and alpha-adrenergic receptor blocking actions. The drugs are structurally similar to tricyclic antidepressants (TCAs) and share many adverse reactions.

All antipsychotics have equal clinical efficacy when given in equivalent doses; choice of specific therapy is determined primarily by the individual patient's response and adverse reaction profile. A patient who does not respond to one drug may respond to another.

Onset of full therapeutic effects requires 6 weeks to 6 months of therapy; therefore, dosage adjustment is recommended at not less than weekly intervals.

CLINICAL INDICATIONS AND ACTIONS

Psychoses

The phenothiazines (except ethopropazine, methdilazine, promethazine, propiomazine, thiethylperazine, and trimeprazine) and thioxanthenes (chlorprothixene and thiothixene) are indicated to treat agitated psychotic states. They are especially effective in controlling hallucinations in schizophrenic patients, the manic phase of manic-depressive illness, and excessive motor and autonomic activity.

Nausea and vomiting

Chlorpromazine, perphenazine, prochlorperazine, thiethylperazine, and triflupromazine are effective in controlling severe nausea and vomiting induced by CNS disturbances. They do not prevent motion sickness or vertigo.

†Anxiety

Chlorpromazine, mesoridazine, promethazine, propiomazine, prochlorperazine, and trifluoperazine also may be used for short-term treatment of moderate anxiety in selected nonpsychotic patients, for example, to control anxiety before surgery.

Severe behavior problems

Chlorpromazine and thioridazine are indicated to control combativeness and hyperexcitability in children with severe behavior problems. They also are used in hyperactive children for short-term treatment of excessive motor activity with labile moods, impulsive behavior, aggressiveness, attention deficit, and poor tolerance of frustration. Mesoridazine is used to manage hypersensitivity and to promote cooperative behavior in patients with mental deficiency and chronic brain syndrome.

Tetanus

Chlorpromazine is an effective adjunct in treating tetanus.

*Liquid form contains alcohol.

**May contain tartrazine.

Porphyria
Because of its effects on the autonomic nervous system, chlorpromazine is effective in controlling abdominal pain in patients with acute intermittent porphyria.
Intractable hiccups
Chlorpromazine has been used to treat patients with intractable hiccups. The mechanism is unknown.
Neurogenic pain
Fluphenazine is a useful adjunct when managing selected chronic pain states (such as narcotic withdrawal).
Parkinson's disease
Ethopropazine, because of its potent anticholinergic effects, is useful in the adjunctive treatment of Parkinson's disease.
Allergies and pruritus
Because of their potent antihistaminic effects, many of these drugs (including methdilazine, promethazine, and trimeprazine) are used to relieve itching or symptomatic rhinitis.

OVERVIEW OF ADVERSE REACTIONS

Phenothiazines may produce extrapyramidal symptoms (dystonic movements, torticollis, oculogyric crises, parkinsonian symptoms) from akathisia during early treatment, to tardive dyskinesia after long-term use. In some cases, such symptoms can be alleviated by dosage reduction or treatment with diphenhydramine, trihexyphenidyl, or benztropine mesylate. Dystonia usually occurs on initial therapy or at increased dosage in children and younger adults; parkinsonian symptoms and tardive dyskinesia more often affect older patients, especially women.

A neuroleptic malignant syndrome resembling severe parkinsonism may occur (most often in young men taking fluphenazine); it consists of rapid onset of hyperthermia, muscular hyperreflexia, marked extrapyramidal and autonomic dysfunction, arrhythmias, sweating, and several other unpleasant reactions. Although rare, this condition carries a 10% mortality and requires immediate treatment, including cooling blankets, neuromuscular blocking agents, dantrolene, and supportive measures.

Other adverse reactions are similar to those seen with TCAs, including varying degrees of sedative and anticholinergic effects, orthostatic hypotension with reflex tachycardia, fainting and dizziness, and dysrhythmias; GI reactions including anorexia, nausea, vomiting, abdominal pain and local gastric irritation; seizures; endocrine effects; hematologic disorders; ocular changes and other visual disturbances; skin eruptions; and photosensitivity. Allergic manifestations are usually marked by elevation of liver enzymes progressing to obstructive jaundice.

Generally, the piperidine derivatives mesoridazine and thioridazine have the most pronounced cardiovascular effects, and piperazine derivatives have the least. As might be anticipated, parenteral administration is more often associated with cardiovascular effects because of more rapid absorption. Seizures are most common with aliphatic derivatives.

REPRESENTATIVE COMBINATIONS

None.

phenoxybenzamine hydrochloride

(fen ox ee ben´ za meen)
Dibenyline‡, Dibenzyline

• *Classification:* antihypertensive for pheochromocytoma, cutaneous vasodilator (alpha-adrenergic blocking agent)
• *Pregnancy Risk Category:* C

HOW SUPPLIED

Capsules: 10 mg

ACTION

Mechanism: An alpha-adrenergic blocker that non-competitively blocks the effect of catecholamines on alpha-adrenergic receptors.
Absorption: Variably absorbed from the GI tract after oral administration.
Distribution: Highly lipid-soluble; may accumulate in fat after large doses.
Metabolism: Dealkylation, probably in the liver.
Excretion: In urine and bile. Half-life: 24 hours.
Onset, peak, duration: Its effects begin gradually over several hours. Alpha-adrenergic blocking effects may persist for up to 7 days after therapy is discontinued.

INDICATIONS & DOSAGE

To control hypertension and sweating secondary to pheochromocytoma; may be used in combination with propranolol to control excessive tachycardia –
Adults: initially, 10 mg P.O. daily. Increase by 10 mg daily q 4 days. Maintenance dosage is 20 to 60 mg daily.
Children: initially, 0.2 mg/kg or 6 mg/m^2 P.O. daily in a single dose. Maintenance dosage is 12 to 36 mg/m^2 daily as a single dose or in divided doses.
To control Raynaud's disease, frostbite, acrocyanosis –
Adults: initially, 10 mg P.O., then increase by 10 mg q 4 days to a maximum of 60 mg daily.

CONTRAINDICATIONS & PRECAUTIONS

Contraindicated in patients with hypersensitivity to the drug.

Use cautiously in patients with cerebrovascular or coronary insufficiency, because decreased blood pressure may precipitate stroke or angina; CHF, coronary artery disease, or advanced renal disease, because hypotension may exacerbate these conditions; and shock, because additional fluid replacement will be needed.

ADVERSE REACTIONS

Common reactions are in italics; life-threatening reactions are in bold italics.
CNS: lethargy, drowsiness.
CV: *orthostatic hypotension, tachycardia,* shock.
EENT: *nasal stuffiness, dry mouth, miosis.*
GI: vomiting, abdominal distress.
Other: *impotence, inhibition of ejaculation.*

INTERACTIONS

Antihypertensives: excessive hypotension. Use together cautiously.

EFFECTS ON DIAGNOSTIC TESTS

None reported.

NURSING CONSIDERATIONS

Besides those related universally to drug therapy (see "How to use this book"), consider the following specific recommendations:

Assessment
- Obtain a baseline assessment of the patient's blood pressure before beginning therapy.
- Be alert for adverse reactions and drug interactions throughout therapy.
- Evaluate the patient's and family's knowledge about phenoxybenzamine therapy.

Nursing Diagnoses
- Altered tissue perfusion (renal, cerebral, cardiopulmonary, peripheral) related to the patient's underlying condition.
- High risk for injury related to phenoxybenzamine-induced orthostatic hypotension and CNS adverse reactions to the drug.
- Knowledge deficit related to phenoxybenzamine therapy.

Planning and Implementation

Preparation and Administration

• Keep in mind that small initial doses are increased gradually until the desired effect is obtained.

• To relieve GI distress, give the drug with milk or in divided doses.

Monitoring

• Monitor effectiveness by frequently checking the patient's blood pressure, heart rate, and ECG.

• Observe the patient for effectiveness of the therapy for at least 4 days after each dosage increase.

• Watch the patient taking this drug closely for side effects and call the doctor promptly if they occur. If severe hypotension occurs, the patient may require treatment with norepinephrine.

• Check the patient's blood pressure while he is in the supine and standing positions to identify orthostatic hypotension.

• Monitor respiratory status carefully. This drug may aggravate symptoms of pneumonia and asthma.

Supportive Care

• Keep in mind that patients with tachycardia may require concurrent propranolol therapy.

• If the patient experiences dizziness, weakness, or orthostatic hypotension, institute safety precautions such as continuous use of bed rails.

Patient Teaching

• Explain the importance of taking this drug as prescribed, even when feeling well.

• Tell the patient not to discontinue this drug suddenly even if unpleasant adverse reactions occur, but to discuss the problem with the doctor.

• Instruct the patient to check with the doctor or pharmacist before taking any OTC medications.

• Inform the patient that orthostatic hypotension can be minimized by rising slowly and avoiding sudden position changes.

• Tell the patient to relieve dry mouth with sugarless gum, sour hard candy, or ice chips.

• Tell the patient to relieve GI distress by taking the medication with milk or by asking the doctor to prescribe the medication in divided doses.

• Explain to the patient that this drug may have to be taken for several weeks to achieve optimal effect.

• Inform the patient that nasal congestion, inhibition of ejaculation, and impotence usually decrease with continued therapy.

Evaluation

In patients receiving phenoxybenzamine, appropriate evaluation statements may include:

• Blood pressure controlled within normal limits for this patient.

• Patient injury related to orthostatic hypotension and CNS adverse reactions to phenoxybenzamine did not occur.

• Patient and family state an understanding of phenoxybenzamine therapy.

phentermine hydrochloride

(fen´ ter meen)

Adipex-P, Dapex, Duromine‡, Fastin, Ionamin, Obe-Nix, Obephen, Obermine, Obestin, Oby-Trim, Parmine, Phentrol, Span R/D, Teramine, Unifast

• Controlled Substance Schedule IV
• *Classification:* short-term anorexigenic agent, indirect-acting sympathomimetic amine (amphetamine congener)
• *Pregnancy Risk Category:* C

HOW SUPPLIED

Tablets and capsules: 8 mg, 15 mg, 18.75 mg, 30 mg, 37.5 mg
Capsules (resin complex, sustained-release): 15 mg, 30 mg

ACTION

Mechanism: Main site of activity appears to be the cerebral cortex and the reticular activating system. Promotes nerve impulse transmission by releasing stored norepinephrine from nerve terminals in the brain.
Absorption: Readily absorbed after oral administration.
Distribution: Widely distributed throughout the body.
Excretion: In urine. Half-life: 19 to 24 hours.
Onset, peak, duration: Therapeutic effects persist for 4 to 6 hours.

INDICATIONS & DOSAGE

Short-term adjunct in exogenous obesity–
Adults: 8 mg P.O. t.i.d. half hour before meals; or 15 to 30 mg daily before breakfast (resin complex).

CONTRAINDICATIONS & PRECAUTIONS

Contraindicated in patients with hypersensitivity to phentermine; in patients with hyperthyroidism, all degrees of hypertension, angina pectoris or other severe cardiovascular disease, glaucoma, or advanced arteriosclerosis; and for use with monoamine oxidase (MAO) inhibitors or within 14 days of such use.

Use cautiously in patients with hypersensitivity to sympathomimetic amines; in hyperexcitability and agitated states; and in patients with a history of substance abuse. Habituation or psychic dependence may follow prolonged use.

ADVERSE REACTIONS

Common reactions are in italics; life-threatening reactions are in bold italics.
CNS: *nervousness,* dizziness, *insomnia.*
CV: *palpitations, tachycardia,* increased blood pressure.
GI: dry mouth, unpleasant taste, nausea, constipation, diarrhea.
Skin: urticaria.
Other: altered libido, impotence.

INTERACTIONS

Ammonium chloride, ascorbic acid: observe for decreased phentermine effects.
Antacids, sodium bicarbonate, acetazolamide: increased renal reabsorption. Monitor for enhanced effects.
MAO inhibitors: severe hypertension; possible hypertensive crisis. Don't use together.
Phenothiazines, haloperidol: observe for decreased effects.

EFFECTS ON DIAGNOSTIC TESTS

None reported.

NURSING CONSIDERATIONS

Besides those related universally to drug therapy (see "How to use this book"), consider the following specific recommendations:

Assessment
- Obtain a baseline assessment of the patient's weight and dietary intake.
- Be alert for adverse reactions and drug interactions throughout therapy.
- Evaluate the patient's and family's knowledge about phentermine therapy.

Nursing Diagnoses
- Altered nutrition: More than body requirements, related to obesity.
- Sleep pattern disturbance related to phentermine-induced insomnia.
- Knowledge deficit related to phentermine therapy.

Planning and Implementation
Preparation and Administration
- Administer drug at least 6 hours before bedtime to avoid interference with sleep.
- Administer drug 30 to 60 minutes before meals.
- Avoid prolonged administration because tolerance or dependence may occur.

Monitoring
• Monitor effectiveness by regularly assessing the patient's weight and monitoring dietary intake.
• Monitor vital signs for evidence of tachycardia or blood pressure changes; question the patient regularly about palpitations.
• Monitor sleeping pattern for insomnia, and observe for other signs of excessive CNS stimulation.
Supportive Care
• Provide frequent rest periods and assistance with activities as needed; fatigue may result as drug effects wear off.
• Institute safety precautions, as needed, by making environment safe and providing supervision of patient's activities.
• Make sure the patient is also following a weight-reduction program.
Patient Teaching
• Warn the patient to avoid hazardous activities that require alertness or good psychomotor coordination until CNS effects of the drug are known.
• Tell the patient to avoid beverages containing caffeine, which increase the stimulant effects of amphetamines and related amines.
• Have the patient report insomnia or other signs of excessive stimulation.
• Tell the patient to weigh himself weekly in the same clothes at the same time of day to evaluate effectiveness of drug therapy.
• Teach the patient how to take the drug to minimize insomnia and enhance effectiveness.
• Tell the patient to notify the nurse or doctor if palpitations or other adverse reactions develop.
Evaluation
In patients receiving phentermine, appropriate evaluation statements may include:
• Patient demonstrates safe, targeted weight loss.
• Patient is able to sleep without difficulty.
• Patient and family state an understanding of phentermine therapy.

phentolamine mesylate
(fen tole´ ah meen)
Regitine, Rogitine†

• *Classification:* antihypertensive agent for pheochromocytoma, cutaneous vasodilator (alpha-adrenergic blocking agent)
• *Pregnancy Risk Category:* C

HOW SUPPLIED
Injection: 5 mg/ml in 1-ml vials, 10 mg/ml‡

ACTION
Mechanism: An alpha-adrenergic blocker that competitively blocks the effects of catecholamines on alpha-adrenergic receptors.
Absorption: Not absorbed after oral administration. Antihypertensive effect is immediate after I.V. administration.
Excretion: About 10% of a given dose of phentolamine is excreted unchanged in urine; excretion of remainder is unknown. Half-life: Plasma half-life is 19 minutes after I.V. administration.
Onset, peak, duration: Onset is rapid after I.V. administration, and effects last for less than 30 minutes.

INDICATIONS & DOSAGE
To aid in diagnosis of pheochromocytoma; to control or prevent hypertension before or during pheochromocytomectomy–
Adults: I.V. diagnostic dose is 5 mg, with close monitoring of blood pressure.

Before surgical removal of tumor, give 2 to 5 mg I.M. or I.V. During surgery, patient may need small I.V.

doses (1 mg) or small I.M. doses (3 mg).
Children: I.V. diagnostic dose is 0.1 mg/kg or 3 mg/m² as single dose, with close monitoring of blood pressure.

Before surgical removal of tumor, give 1 mg I.V. or 3 mg I.M. During surgery, patient may need small I.V. doses (1 mg).
To treat extravasation–
Adults and children: infiltrate area with 5 to 10 mg phentolamine in 10 ml normal saline solution or give half the dosage through the infiltrated I.V. and the other half around the site. Must be done within 12 hours.

CONTRAINDICATIONS & PRECAUTIONS

Contraindicated in patients with hypersensitivity to the drug and in patients with coronary artery disease or recent myocardial infarction (MI), because the drug may exacerbate these conditions.

Drug should be given cautiously to patients with gastritis or peptic ulcer and to patients receiving other antihypertensives.

ADVERSE REACTIONS

Common reactions are in italics; life-threatening reactions are in bold italics.
CNS: *dizziness, weakness, flushing.*
CV: *hypotension,* shock, ***arrhythmias,*** palpitations, *tachycardia,* angina pectoris.
GI: *diarrhea,* abdominal pain, *nausea, vomiting,* hyperperistalsis.
Other: *nasal stuffiness,* hypoglycemia.

INTERACTIONS

Epinephrine: excessive hypotension. Don't use together.

EFFECTS ON DIAGNOSTIC TESTS

None reported.

NURSING CONSIDERATIONS

Besides those related universally to drug therapy (see "How to use this book"), consider the following specific recommendations:

Assessment

- Obtain a baseline assessment of the patient's blood pressure before beginning therapy.
- Be alert for adverse reactions and drug interactions throughout therapy.
- Evaluate the patient's and family's knowledge about phentolamine therapy.

Nursing Diagnoses

- Altered tissue perfusion (renal, cerebral, cardiopulmonary, peripheral) related to the patient's underlying condition.
- High risk for injury related to adverse reactions to phentolamine.
- Knowledge deficit related to phentolamine therapy.

Planning and Implementation

Preparation and Administration

- When using this drug as a diagnostic test for pheochromocytoma, also check blood pressure frequently during administration; every 30 seconds for 3 minutes, then every 60 seconds for 7 more minutes. Severe hypotension after test dose indicates pheochromocytoma.
- ***I.V. use:*** Drug is supplied as a powder. Reconstitute it for use and use it immediately after reconstitution. For infusion, dilute 5 to 10 mg of drug in 500 ml of 0.9% sodium chloride and use an infusion pump to control rate of infusion.
- ***Intercavernosal injection:*** Patients are taught to self-administer the drug using this route when the drug is used experimentally, alone or with papaverine, to treat impotence.

Monitoring

- Monitor effectiveness by frequently checking the patient's blood pressure, heart rate, and ECG.
- Monitor the patient for hypotension

and CNS reactions such as dizziness, as well as for other adverse reactions.

Supportive Care

• Remember that epinephrine should not be administered to treat phentolamine-induced hypotension because it may cause an additional fall in blood pressure ("epinephrine reversal"). Norepinephrine should be ordered instead.

• Don't give sedatives or narcotics 24 hours before diagnostic test. Rauwolfia alkaloids should be withdrawn at least 4 weeks before such testing.

• Institute safety measures such as continuous use of siderails if the adverse reactions that could result in patient injury occur.

Patient Teaching

• If the drug will be used as a diagnostic test, explain this to the patient.

• If the drug will be used experimentally to treat impotence as ordered, teach the patient how to administer the drug intercavernously.

Evaluation

In patients receiving phentolamine, appropriate evaluation statements may include:

• Blood pressure controlled within normal limits during pheochromocytomectomy.

• Patient injury due to orthostatic hypotension and CNS adverse reactions to phentolamine therapy did not occur.

• Patient and family state an understanding of phentolamine therapy.

phenylephrine hydrochloride (systemic)

(fen ill ef´ rin)

Neo-Synephrine

• *Classification:* vasoconstrictor (adrenergic)

• *Pregnancy Risk Category:* C

HOW SUPPLIED

Injection: 10 mg/ml

ACTION

Mechanism: Predominantly stimulates alpha-adrenergic receptors in the sympathetic nervous system.

Absorption: Slowly absorbed after I.M. or S.C. administration.

Metabolism: In the liver and intestine by the enzyme monoamine oxidase (MAO).

Excretion: Unknown. Drug action is partly terminated by uptake of the drug into tissues.

Onset, peak, duration: Pressor effects occur almost immediately after I.V. injection and persist 15 to 20 minutes; after I.M. injection, onset is within 10 to 15 minutes, persisting 30 minutes to 2 hours; after S.C. injection, onset is within 10 to 15 minutes, with effects persisting 50 to 60 minutes.

INDICATIONS & DOSAGE

Hypotensive emergencies during spinal anesthesia –

Adults: initially, 0.2 mg I.V., then subsequent doses of 0.1 to 0.2 mg.

Maintenance of blood pressure during spinal or inhalation anesthesia –

Adults: 2 to 3 mg S.C. or I.M. 3 or 4 minutes before anesthesia.

Children: 0.04 mg to 0.088 mg/kg S.C. or I.M.

Mild to moderate hypotension –

Adults: 2 to 5 mg S.C. or I.M.; 0.1 to 0.5 mg I.V. Not to be repeated more often than 10 to 15 minutes.

Paroxysmal supraventricular tachycardia –

Adults: initially, 0.5 mg rapid I.V.; subsequent doses should not exceed the preceding dose by more than 0.1 to 0.2 mg and should not exceed 1 mg.

Prolongation of spinal anesthesia –

Adults: 2 to 5 mg added to anesthetic solution.

Severe hypotension and shock (including drug-induced) –
Adults: 10 mg in 500 ml dextrose 5% in water. Start 100 to 180 drops per minute I.V. infusion, then 40 to 60 drops per minute. Adjust to patient response.
Vasoconstrictor for regional anesthesia –
Adults: 1 mg phenylephrine added to 20 ml local anesthetic.

CONTRAINDICATIONS & PRECAUTIONS

Contraindicated in patients with severe coronary disease, cardiovascular disease including MI, or peripheral or mesenteric vascular thrombosis (may increase ischemia or extend area of infarction); in patients with severe hypertension or ventricular tachycardia; or for use with local anesthetics on fingers, toes, ears, nose, and genitalia.

Use with extreme caution in elderly or debilitated patients, and those with hyperthyroidism, bradycardia, partial heart block, myocardial disease, diabetes mellitus, narrow-angle glaucoma, severe arteriosclerosis, acute pancreatitis, or hepatitis (may increase ischemia in liver or pancreas).

Also administer cautiously to patients with hypersensitivity to sulfites because phenylephrine contains sulfite preservatives.

ADVERSE REACTIONS

Common reactions are in italics; life-threatening reactions are in bold italics.
CNS: anxiety, *headache, restlessness, light-headedness, weakness,* ***cerebral hemorrhage, seizures.***
CV: palpitations, ventricular extrasystoles, ***hypertension,*** anginal pain, ***decreased cardiac output, ventricular tachycardia, severe bradycardia.***
EENT: blurred vision.
GI: vomiting.
GU: ***decreased renal perfusion,*** decreased urine output.
Skin: goose bumps, feeling of coolness.
Local: tissue sloughing with extravasation; paresthesia in extremity after injection.
Other: ***tachyphylaxis*** may occur with continued use; ***respiratory distress,*** metabolic acidosis.

INTERACTIONS

MAO inhibitors: may cause severe hypertension (hypertensive crisis). Don't use together.
Oxytocics, tricyclic antidepressants: increased pressor response. Observe patient.

EFFECTS ON DIAGNOSTIC TESTS

Tonometry: false-normal or low readings.

NURSING CONSIDERATIONS

Besides those related universally to drug therapy (see "How to use this book"), consider the following specific recommendations:

Assessment

- Obtain a baseline assessment of the patient's underlying condition before drug therapy.
- Be alert for adverse reactions and drug interactions throughout therapy.
- Evaluate the patient's and family's knowledge about phenylephrine therapy.

Nursing Diagnoses

- Altered tissue (cardiopulmonary, cerebral, renal, gastrointestinal, peripheral) perfusion related to the patient's underlying condition.
- Pain related to adverse drug reaction.
- Knowledge deficit related to phenylephrine hydrochloride therapy.

Planning and Implementation

Preparation and Administration

- ***I.V. use:*** Intermittent infusion is not recommended.
- Infuse diluted drug by continuous infusion at a rate required to main-

tain adequate blood pressure and tissue perfusion.

Monitoring

- Monitor for adverse reactions or drug interactions to phenylephrine hydrochloride by monitoring the patient's blood pressure frequently.
- Monitor the patient for drug-induced headache.
- Monitor for extravasation and sloughing at the infusion site.
- Monitor intake and output. Drug may cause decreased urine output.

Supportive Care

- Know that the drug is longer acting than ephedrine and epinephrine.
- Know that the drug causes little or no CNS stimulation.
- Maintain patient's blood pressure slightly below the patient's normal level. In previously normotensive patients, maintain systolic blood pressure at 80 to 100 mm Hg; in previously hypertensive patients, maintain systolic blood pressure at 30 to 40 mm Hg below their usual level.
- Be prepared to give phentolamine, as ordered, to reverse severe increase in blood pressure.
- Avoid abrupt withdrawal of I.V. infusion; instead, gradually reduce the infusion rate.
- Institute safety precautions if the patient develops light-headedness or weakness.

Patient Teaching

- Tell the patient to immediately report discomfort at the infusion site.

Evaluation

In patients receiving phenylephrine, appropriate evaluation statements may include:

- Patient maintains tissue perfusion and cellular oxygenation.
- Patient does not experience drug-induced headache.
- Patient and family state an understanding of phenylephrine hydrochloride therapy.

phenylephrine hydrochloride (ophthalmic)

(fen il ef´ rin)

AK-Dilate, AK-Nefrin Ophthalmic◇, I-Phrine 2.5%, Isopto Frin◇, Mydfrin, Neo-Synephrine, Prefrin Liquifilm

- *Classification:* mydriatic agent (adrenergic)
- *Pregnancy Risk Category:* C

HOW SUPPLIED

Ophthalmic solution: 0.12%◇, 2.5%, 10%

ACTION

Mechanism: Activates alpha-receptors on the arterioles of the conjunctiva and on the dilator muscle of the pupil. A mydriatic agent; drug produces only slight effects on the ciliary muscle so substantial cycloplegia will not occur.

Absorption: Some drug may be absorbed from the ocular mucosa.

Metabolism: In the liver, by monoamnine oxidase (MAO).

Onset, peak, duration: Peak effects for mydriasis are 15 to 60 minutes for the 2.5% solution; 10 to 90 minutes for the 10% solution. Mydriasis recovery time is 3 hours for the 2.5% solution; 3 to 7 hours for the 10% solution. Nasal or conjunctival decongestant effects persist 30 minutes to 4 hours.

INDICATIONS & DOSAGE

Mydriasis (without cycloplegia)–
Adults and children: instill 1 drop of 2.5% or 10% solution in eye before examination.

Mydriasis and vasoconstriction–
Adults and adolescents: instill 1 drop of 2.5% or 10% solution in eye; repeat in 1 hour if needed.
Children: instill 1 drop of 2.5% solution in eye; repeat in 1 hour if needed.

To relieve eye redness–
Adults: instill 1 to 2 drops of 0.12% solution in eye daily up to q.i.d.
Chronic mydriasis–
Adults and adolescents: instill 1 drop of 2.5% or 10% solution in eye b.i.d. or t.i.d.
Children: instill 1 drop of 2.5% solution in eye b.i.d. or t.i.d.
Posterior synechia (adhesion of iris)–
Adults and children: instill 1 drop of 10% solution in eye.

Do not use 10% concentration in infants; use cautiously in elderly patients.

CONTRAINDICATIONS & PRECAUTIONS

Contraindicated in patients with severe coronary disease, cardiovascular disease including MI, or peripheral or mesenteric vascular thrombosis (may increase ischemia or extend area of infarction); severe hypertension or ventricular tachycardia; or for use with local anesthetics on fingers, toes, ears, nose, and genitalia.

Use with extreme caution in elderly or debilitated patients, and those with hyperthyroidism, bradycardia, partial heart block, myocardial disease, diabetes mellitus, narrow-angle glaucoma, severe arteriosclerosis, acute pancreatitis, or hepatitis (may increase ischemia in liver or pancreas). Also use cautiously in patients with hypersensitivity to sulfites because phenylephrine contains sulfite preservatives.

ADVERSE REACTIONS

Common reactions are in italics; life-threatening reactions are in bold italics.
CNS: headache, brow ache.
CV: *hypertension* (with 10% solution), tachycardia, palpitations, premature ventricular contractions.
Eye: transient burning or stinging on instillation, blurred vision, reactive hyperemia, allergic conjunctivitis, iris floaters, narrow-angle glaucoma, rebound miosis, dermatitis.
Other: pallor, trembling, sweating.

INTERACTIONS

Guanethidine: increased mydriatic and pressor effects of phenylephrine. Use together cautiously.
Levodopa (systemic): reduced mydriatic effect of phenylephrine. Use together cautiously.
MAO inhibitors and beta blockers: may cause arrhythmias due to increased pressor effect. Use together cautiously.
Tricyclic antidepressants: potentiated cardiac effects of epinephrine. Use together cautiously.

EFFECTS ON DIAGNOSTIC TESTS

Tonometry: false-normal readings.

NURSING CONSIDERATIONS

Besides those related universally to drug therapy (see "How to use this book"), consider the following specific recommendations:

Assessment
- Obtain a baseline assessment of the patient's vision and pupil size.
- Be alert for adverse reactions and drug interactions throughout therapy.
- Evaluate the patient's and family's knowledge about ophthalmic phenylephrine therapy.

Nursing Diagnoses
- Sensory/perceptual alterations (visual) related to the patient's underlying condition.
- High risk for poisoning related to the drug's systemic adrenergic effects.
- Knowledge deficit related to ophthalmic phenylephrine therapy.

Planning and Implementation
Preparation and Administration
- Protect solution from heat and light; do not use if it is brown or contains a precipitate.
- Instill in lacrimal sac; remove excess solution from around eyes with a clean tissue or gauze and apply light

finger pressure to lacrimal sac for 1 minute.

Monitoring

• Monitor effectiveness by assessing the patient's visual status and pupil size.

• Monitor for systemic adrenergic effects, which are more likely with 10% solution but may also occur with 2.5%.

• Monitor blood pressure and apical rate for drug-induced hypertension, tachycardia and arrhythmias: obtain ECG as indicated.

Supportive Care

• Notify the doctor immediately of any changes in the patient's health status.

• Obtain an order for a mild analgesic if the patient experiences headache or brow ache.

Patient Teaching

• Teach the patient how to instill the solution and advise him to wash his hands before and after administering the drug.

• Warn patient not to exceed recommended dosage.

• Warn patient to avoid hazardous activities such as driving until blurring of vision subsides.

• Advise the patient to wear dark glasses to ease any discomfort from photophobia.

• Advise the patient to continue with regular medical supervision during therapy.

Evaluation

In patients receiving ophthalmic phenylephrine, appropriate evaluation statements may include:

• Patient experiences therapeutic mydriasis.

• Patient remains free of systemic adrenergic effects.

• Patient and family state an understanding of ophthalmic phenylephrine hydrochloride therapy.

phenylephrine hydrochloride (nasal)

(fen ill ef′ rin)

Alconefrin 12◇, Alconefrin 25◇, Alconefrin 50◇, Doktors◇, Duration◇, Neo-Synephrine◇, Nostril◇, Rhinall◇, Rhinall-10◇, Sinex◇, St. Joseph Measured Dose Nasal Decongestant◇

• *Classification:* vasoconstrictor, decongestant (adrenergic)
• *Pregnancy Risk Category:* C

HOW SUPPLIED

Nasal jelly: 0.5%
Nasal solution: 0.125%, 0.16%, 0.2%, 0.25%, 0.5%, 1%

ACTION

Mechanism: An alpha-adrenergic agonist that produces local vasoconstriction of dilated arterioles to reduce blood flow and nasal congestion.
Absorption: Variable; small amounts can be absorbed.
Metabolism: In the plasma and liver by monoamine oxidase.
Excretion: In the urine.
Onset, peak, duration: Onset within 10 minutes; duration, about 4 hours.

INDICATIONS & DOSAGE

Nasal congestion–
Adults: 1 to 2 drops or sprays of 0.125% to 1% solution; apply jelly or spray to nasal mucosa.
Children 6 to 12 years: apply 1 to 2 drops or sprays of 0.25% solution.
Children under 6 years: apply 2 to 3 drops or sprays of 0.125% solution.

Drops, spray, or jelly can be given q 4 hours, p.r.n.

CONTRAINDICATIONS & PRECAUTIONS

Contraindicated in patients with severe coronary disease, cardiovascular disease including MI, or peripheral or mesenteric vascular thrombosis (may increase ischemia or extend area of infarction); in patients with severe hypertension or ventricular tachycardia; or for use with local anesthetics on fingers, toes, ears, nose, and genitalia.

Use with extreme caution in elderly or debilitated patients, and those with hyperthyroidism, bradycardia, partial heart block, myocardial disease, diabetes mellitus, narrow-angle glaucoma, severe arteriosclerosis, acute pancreatitis, or hepatitis (may increase ischemia in liver or pancreas). Also use cautiously in patients with hypersensitivity to sulfites because phenylephrine contains sulfite preservatives.

ADVERSE REACTIONS

Common reactions are in italics; life-threatening reactions are in bold italics.
CNS: headache, tremors, dizziness, nervousness.
CV: *palpitations, tachycardia,* premature ventricular contractions, hypertension, pallor.
EENT: transient burning, stinging; dryness of nasal mucosa; rebound nasal congestion may occur with continued use.
GI: nausea.

INTERACTIONS

None significant.

EFFECTS ON DIAGNOSTIC TESTS

Tonometry: false-normal readings.

NURSING CONSIDERATIONS

Besides those related universally to drug therapy (see "How to use this book"), consider the following specific recommendations:

Assessment

- Obtain a baseline assessment of the patient's breathing pattern and degree of nasal congestion.
- Be alert for adverse reactions and drug interactions throughout therapy.
- Evaluate the patient's and family's knowledge about nasal phenylephrine therapy.

Nursing Diagnoses

- Ineffective airway clearance related to the patient's underlying condition.
- Decreased cardiac output related to systemic absorption of nasal phenylephrine hydrochloride.
- Knowledge deficit related to nasal phenylephrine hydrochloride therapy.

Planning and Implementation

Preparation and Administration

- ***Inhalation:*** Apply solution or jelly to nasal mucosa; have patient hold head erect to minimize swallowing of medication.

Monitoring

- Monitor effectiveness by assessing the patient's breathing pattern and degree of nasal congestion.
- Monitor blood pressure and apical rate for drug-induced cardiac effects; obtain ECG as indicated.
- Closely monitor use in patients with underlying cardiac or thyroid disease or diabetes mellitus.

Supportive Care

- Notify the doctor immediately of any changes in the patient's health status.

Patient Teaching

- Teach the patient how to administer the drug and tell him it should be used by one person only.
- Warn the patient not to exceed the recommended dose and to use the drug only as needed.
- Warn the patient he may experience transient burning or stinging upon administration.

Evaluation

In patients receiving nasal phenylephrine, appropriate evaluation statements may include:

- Patient obtains relief from nasal congestion.
- Patient remains free of drug-related cardiac effects.
- Patient and family state an understanding of nasal phenylephrine hydrochloride therapy.

phenytoin
(fen´ i toyn)
Dilantin, Dilantin Infatabs, Dilantin-30 Pediatric, Dilantin-125

phenytoin sodium
Dilantin

phenytoin sodium (extended)
Dilantin Kapseals

phenytoin sodium (prompt)
Diphenylan

- *Classification:* anticonvulsant (hydantoin derivative)
- *Pregnancy Risk Category:* D

HOW SUPPLIED
phenytoin
Tablets (chewable): 50 mg
Oral suspension: 30 mg/5 ml, 125 mg/5 ml
phenytoin sodium
Capsules: 30 mg (27.6-mg base), 100 mg (92-mg base)
Injection: 50 mg/ml (46-mg base)
phenytoin sodium (extended)
Capsules: 30 mg (27.6-mg base), 100 mg (92-mg base)
phenytoin sodium (prompt)
Capsules: 30 mg (27.6-mg base), 100 mg (92 mg-base)

ACTION
Mechanism: Stabilizes neuronal membranes and limits seizure activity by either increasing efflux or decreasing influx of sodium ions across cell membranes in the motor cortex during generation of nerve impulses. Produces antiarrhythmic effect by normalizing sodium influx to Purkinje's fibers when used to treat digitalis-induced arrhythmias. A hydantoin derivative.
Absorption: Slowly absorbed from the small intestine; absorption is formulation-dependent and bioavailability may differ among products.
Distribution: Widely distributed throughout the body; therapeutic plasma levels are 10 to 20 mcg/ml, although in some patients, they occur at 5 to 10 mcg/ml. Lateral nystagmus may occur at levels above 20 mcg/ml; ataxia usually occurs at levels above 30 mcg/ml; significantly decreased mental capacity occurs at 40 mcg/ml. Phenytoin is about 90% protein-bound, less so in uremic patients.
Metabolism: Metabolized by the liver to inactive metabolites.
Excretion: In urine and exhibits dose-dependent (zero-order) elimination kinetics; above a certain dosage level, small increases in dosage disproportionately increase serum levels. Half-life: 6 to 24 hours when plasma levels are 10 mcg/ml or less; 20 to 60 hours at therapeutic levels.
Onset, peak, duration: Therapeutic levels are 10 to 20 mcg/ml. Extended-release capsules give peak serum concentrations at 4 to 12 hours; prompt-release products peak at 1½ to 3 hours. I.M. doses are absorbed erratically; about 50% to 75% of I.M. dose is absorbed in 24 hours.

INDICATIONS & DOSAGE
Generalized tonic-clonic seizures, status epilepticus, nonepileptic seizures (post–head trauma, Reye's syndrome) –
Adults: loading dose is 900 mg to 1.5 g I.V. at 50 mg/minute or P.O. divided t.i.d., then start maintenance dosage of 300 mg P.O. daily (extended only) or divided t.i.d. (extended or prompt).
Children: loading dose is 15 mg/kg I.V. at 50 mg/minute or P.O. divided q 8 to 12 hours, then start maintenance dosage of 5 to 7 mg/kg P.O. or I.V. daily, divided q 12 hours.

If patient has not received phenytoin previously or has no detectable blood level, use loading dose–
Adults: 900 mg to 1.5 g I.V. divided into t.i.d. at 50 mg/minute. Do not exceed 500 mg each dose.
Children: 15 mg/kg I.V. at 50 mg/minute.
If patient has been receiving phenytoin but has missed one or more doses and has subtherapeutic levels–
Adults: 100 to 300 mg I.V. at 50 mg/minute.
Children: 5 to 7 mg/kg I.V. at 50 mg/minute. May repeat lower dose in 30 minutes if needed.
Neuritic pain (migraine, trigeminal neuralgia, Bell's palsy)–
Adults: 200 to 400 mg P.O. daily.
Ventricular arrhythmias unresponsive to lidocaine or procainamide; supraventricular and ventricular arrhythmias induced by digitalis glycosides–
Adults: loading dose is 1 g P.O. divided over first 24 hours, followed by 500 mg daily for 2 days, then maintenance dose of 300 mg P.O. daily; 250 mg I.V. over 5 minutes until arrhythmias subside, adverse reactions develop, or 1 g has been given. Infusion rate should never exceed 50 mg/minute (slow I.V. push).
Alternative method: 100 mg I.V. q 15 minutes until adverse reactions develop, arrhythmias are controlled, or 1 g has been given. May also administer entire loading dose of 1 g I.V. slowly at 25 mg/minute. Can be diluted in normal saline solution. I.M. dose not recommended because of pain and erratic absorption.
Children: 3 to 8 mg/kg P.O. or slow I.V. daily or 250 mg/m^2 daily given as single dose or in two divided doses.

CONTRAINDICATIONS & PRECAUTIONS

Contraindicated in patients with hypersensitivity to hydantoins or phenacemide; I.V. phenytoin is contraindicated in patients with sinus bradycardia, sinoatrial or atrioventricular block, or Stokes-Adams syndrome.

Use with caution in patients with acute intermittent porphyria, hepatic or renal dysfunction (especially in uremic patients, who have higher serum drug levels from decreased protein-binding), myocardial insufficiency, or respiratory depression; in elderly or debilitated patients; and in patients taking other hydantoin derivatives.

ADVERSE REACTIONS

Common reactions are in italics; life-threatening reactions are in bold italics.
Blood: thrombocytopenia, leukopenia, ***agranulocytosis,*** pancytopenia, macrocytosis, megaloblastic anemia.
CNS: *ataxia, slurred speech, confusion,* dizziness, insomnia, nervousness, twitching, headache.
CV: hypotension, ***ventricular fibrillation.***
EENT: *nystagmus, diplopia,* blurred vision.
GI: *nausea, vomiting, gingival hyperplasia (especially children).*
Hepatic: toxic hepatitis.
Skin: scarlatiniform or morbilliform rash; bullous, ***exfoliative,*** or ***purpuric dermatitis; Stevens-Johnson syndrome;*** lupus erythematosus; *hirsutism;* ***toxic epidermal necrolysis;*** photosensitivity.
Local: pain, necrosis, and inflammation at injection site; purple glove syndrome.
Other: periarteritis nodosa, lymphadenopathy, hyperglycemia, osteomalacia, hypertrichosis.

INTERACTIONS

Alcohol, dexamethasone, folic acid: monitor for decreased phenytoin activity.
Oral anticoagulants, antihistamines, amiodarone, chloramphenicol, cimetidine, cycloserine, diazepam, diazoxide, disulfiram, influenza vaccine, isoniazid, phenylbutazone, salicylates,

sulfamethizole, valproate: monitor for increased phenytoin activity and toxicity.
Oral tube feedings with Osmolite or Isocal: may interfere with absorption of oral phenytoin. Schedule feedings as far as possible from drug administration.

EFFECTS ON DIAGNOSTIC TESTS

Blood glucose: increased levels (by inhibition of insulin release).
Dexamethasone suppression test: interference.
Serum protein-bound iodine: decreased levels.

NURSING CONSIDERATIONS

Besides those related universally to drug therapy (see "How to use this book"), consider the following specific recommendations:

Assessment

• Obtain a baseline assessment of seizure activity before therapy.
• Be alert for adverse reactions and drug interactions throughout therapy.
• Evaluate the patient's and family's knowledge about phenytoin therapy.

Nursing Diagnoses

• High risk for injury related to patient's underlying seizure activity.
• Altered oral mucous membrane related to phenytoin-induced gingival hyperplasia.
• Knowledge deficit related to phenytoin therapy.

Planning and Implementation

Preparation and Administration

• Be aware that this drug was formerly known as diphenylhydantoin (DPH).
• Elderly patients may require lower dosages because they tend to metabolize phenytoin slowly.
• Use only clear solution for parenteral injection. Slight yellow color is acceptable. Don't refrigerate.
• ***P.O. use:*** Phenytoin sodium (extended) capsules are the only form that can be given once daily. Patients should be stabilized on the prompt formulation before switching to the extended form.
• Oral suspension is available as 30 mg/5 ml or 125 mg/5 ml. Read label carefully; shake oral suspension well before each dose.
• Use solid forms (tablets or capsules) if possible; give divided doses with or after meals to minimize GI reactions.
• ***I.V. use:*** Avoid administering I.V. push phenytoin injections into veins in the back of the hand. Inject into larger veins to avoid discoloration known as purple glove syndrome.
• Don't mix drug with dextrose 5% in water because it will precipitate. Clear I.V. tubing first with 0.9% sodium chloride solution. Never use cloudy solution. May mix with 0.9% sodium chloride solution, if necessary, and give as an infusion.
• Administer infusion over 30 to 60 minutes when possible. Infusion must begin within 1 hour after preparation and should run through an in-line filter. Discard 4 hours after preparation. Preferably, administer slowly (50 mg/minute) as an I.V. bolus.
• ***I.M. use:*** Do not give I.M. unless dosage adjustments are made. Drug may precipitate at injection site, cause pain, and be erratically absorbed.

Monitoring

• Monitor effectiveness by evaluating seizure activity.
• Monitor phenytoin blood levels regularly. Therapeutic blood level of phenytoin is 10 to 20 mcg/ml.
• Monitor the patient (especially child) for gingival hyperplasia and other adverse drug reactions.
• Monitor CBC and serum calcium levels every 6 months, and periodically monitor blood glucose levels and hepatic function.
• Be aware that phenytoin dosage requirements usually increase during pregnancy. Monitor serum levels closely and assess for seizures.
• Phenytoin levels may be decreased

in mononucleosis. Monitor for increased seizure activity.
• Monitor ECG, blood pressure, and respiratory status with I.V. therapy.
Supportive Care
• Don't withdraw drug suddenly. Call the doctor immediately if adverse reactions develop.
• Drug should be discontinued if rash appears. If rash is scarlet or measles-like, drug may be resumed after rash clears; if rash is exfoliative, purpuric, or bullous, drug should not be resumed. If rash reappears, drug should be discontinued.
• Folic acid and vitamin B_{12} may be prescribed if megaloblastic anemia is evident.
• Maintain seizure precautions.
• If adverse CNS reactions or visual disturbances occur, institute safety measures, such as assisting patient with ambulation and keeping bed rails up.
Patient Teaching
• Warn the patient to avoid hazardous activities that require alertness and good psychomotor coordination until CNS effects of the drug are known.
• Tell the patient to carry identification stating use of phenytoin.
• Stress importance of good oral hygiene and regular dental examinations. Gingivectomy may be necessary periodically if dental hygiene is poor.
• Advise the patient not to change brands or dosage forms once stabilized on therapy.
• Inform the patient that heavy use of alcoholic beverages may diminish benefits of drug.
• Tell the patient to take oral phenytoin with or after meals to minimize adverse GI reactions.
• Advise the patient to withhold the drug and notify the doctor at once if skin rash appears.
• Inform the patient that phenytoin may color the urine pink, red, or reddish brown but that this effect is harmless.

Evaluation
In patients receiving phenytoin, appropriate evaluation statements may include:
• Patient is free of seizure activity.
• Patient's oral mucous membrane is unaffected by phenytoin.
• Patient and family state an understanding of phenytoin therapy.

physostigmine
(fye zoe stig´ meen)
Eserine, Isopto-Eserine

• *Classification:* antiglaucoma agent (cholinergic agonist)
• *Pregnancy Risk Category:* C

HOW SUPPLIED
Ophthalmic ointment: 0.25%
Ophthalmic solution: 0.25%, 0.5%

ACTION
Mechanism: Inhibits the enzymatic destruction of acetylcholine by inactivating cholinesterase, leaving the acetylcholine free to act on effector cells of iridic sphincter and ciliary muscles, causing pupillary constriction and accommodation spasm. Contraction of the ciliary muscle widens the trabecular meshwork, facilitating the outflow of aqueous humor and decreases intraocular pressure. A miotic agent.
Pharmacokinetics: Unknown.
Onset, peak, duration: Onset of activity is within 10 to 30 minutes, and persists for 24 to 48 hours.

INDICATIONS & DOSAGE
Treatment of open-angle glaucoma – **Adults and children:** 1 drop of 0.25% to 0.5% solution b.i.d. to t.i.d. or thin strip of ointment once daily to t.i.d.

CONTRAINDICATIONS & PRECAUTIONS

Contraindicated in patients with narrow-angle glaucoma because it may cause pupillary blockage, resulting in increased intraocular pressure; hypersensitivity to cholinesterase inhibitors. Administer cautiously to patients with vagotonia, because they may experience enhanced drug effects; diabetes, because it may change insulin requirements; mechanical obstruction of the intestine or urinary tract, because of the drug's stimulatory effect on smooth muscle; bradycardia and hypotension, because the drug may exacerbate these conditions; and to patients receiving depolarizing neuromuscular blocking agents, because physostigmine may enhance and prolong the effects of such drugs.

Use cautiously in patients with seizure disorders, because of the drug's possible CNS stimulatory effects; recent coronary occlusion or cardiac arrhythmias, because of the drug's stimulatory effects on the cardiovascular system; peptic ulcer disease, because the drug may stimulate gastric acid secretion; and bronchial asthma, because the drug may precipitate asthma attacks.

ADVERSE REACTIONS

Common reactions are in italics; life-threatening reactions are in bold italics.
CNS: headache, weakness.
CV: slow or irregular heartbeats.
Eye: blurred vision, eye pain, burning, redness, stinging, eye irritation, twitching of eyelids, watering of eyes.
GI: nausea, vomiting, diarrhea.
GU: loss of bladder control.
Other: increased sweating, muscle weakness, shortness of breath.

INTERACTIONS

Echothiophate, isoflurophate: duration of action may be shortened.
Ophthalmic belladonna alkaloids: may antagonize miotic actions.

EFFECTS ON DIAGNOSTIC TESTS

None reported.

NURSING CONSIDERATIONS

Besides those related universally to drug therapy (see "How to use this book"), consider the following specific recommendations:

Assessment

- Obtain a baseline assessment of the patient's vision, especially ocular pressure.
- Be alert for adverse reactions and drug interactions throughout therapy.
- Evaluate the patient's and family's knowledge about physostigmine therapy.

Nursing Diagnoses

- Sensory/perceptual alterations (visual) related to the patient's underlying condition.
- High risk for poisoning related to the drug's systemic adverse effects.
- Knowledge deficit related to physostigmine therapy.

Planning and Implementation

Preparation and Administration

- ***Topical use:*** Apply thin strip of ointment to conjunctival sac; avoid touching applicator tip to any surface. Wipe tip with clean tissue or gauze before recapping. Instill drops in lacrimal sac; remove excess solution around eyes with clean tissue or gauze. Ointment form may be applied at h.s. to prolong contact with the drug.

Monitoring

- Monitor effectiveness by assessing the patient's vision and intraocular pressure.
- Monitor the patient's apical rate for drug-induced bradycardia or arrhythmia; obtain ECG as indicated.
- Monitor for systemic effects (nausea, vomiting, diarrhea, urinary incontinence).
- Monitor for tolerance to the drug

in long-term therapy, which may be restored by briefly substituting another miotic.

Supportive Care

• Notify doctor immediately of any changes in the patient's health status.
• Obtain an order for a mild analgesic if the patient experiences a headache.

Patient Teaching

• Teach the patient how to apply the ointment or drops, and advise him to wash his hands before and after administering the drug.
• Warn the patient not to exceed the recommended dosage.
• Advise the patient to continue with regular medical supervision during therapy.

Evaluation

In patients receiving physostigmine, appropriate evaluation statements may include:

• Patient experiences a reduction in intraocular pressure.
• Patient remains free of systemic side effects.
• Patient and family state an understanding of physostigmine therapy.

physostigmine salicylate (eserine)

(fye zoe stig´ meen)

Antilirium

• *Classification:* antimuscarinic antidote (cholinesterase inhibitor)
• *Pregnancy Risk Category:* C

HOW SUPPLIED

Injection: 1 mg/ml

ACTION

Mechanism: Inhibits the destruction of acetylcholine released from the parasympathetic and somatic efferent nerves. Acetylcholine accumulates, promoting increased stimulation of the receptor.

Absorption: Well absorbed after oral or I.M. administration.

Distribution: Widely distributed; crosses the blood-brain barrier.

Metabolism: Hydrolyzed relatively quickly by cholinesterase.

Excretion: Only a small amount is excreted in urine. Exact mode of excretion is unknown. Half-life: 15 to 40 minutes.

Onset, peak, duration: Onset after parenteral administration is 3 to 5 minutes. Duration of effect is 30 minutes to 5 hours.

INDICATIONS & DOSAGE

To reverse the CNS toxicity associated with tricyclic antidepressant and anticholinergic poisoning–

Adults: 0.5 to 2 mg I.M. or I.V. (1 mg/minute I.V.) repeated as necessary if life-threatening signs recur (coma, seizures, arrhythmias).

CONTRAINDICATIONS & PRECAUTIONS

Contraindicated in patients with narrow-angle glaucoma because it may cause pupillary blockage, resulting in increased intraocular pressure, and in patients with hypersensitivity to cholinesterase inhibitors. Administer cautiously to patients with vagotonia, because they may experience enhanced drug effects; diabetes, because it may change insulin requirements; mechanical obstruction of the intestine or urinary tract, because of the drug's stimulatory effect on smooth muscle; bradycardia and hypotension, because the drug may exacerbate these conditions; and to those receiving depolarizing neuromuscular blocking agents, because physostigmine may enhance and prolong the effects of such drugs.

Also use cautiously in patients with seizure disorders, because of the drug's possible CNS stimulatory effects; recent coronary occlusion or cardiac arrhythmias, because of the drug's stimulatory effects on the cardiovascular system; peptic ulcer disease, because the drug may stimulate gastric acid secretion; and bronchial asthma, because the drug may precipitate asthma attacks.

ADVERSE REACTIONS

Common reactions are in italics; life-threatening reactions are in bold italics.

CNS: ***seizures,*** hallucinations, muscular twitching, muscle weakness, ataxia, *restlessness, excitability, sweating.*

CV: irregular pulse, palpitations.

EENT: miosis.

GI: nausea, vomiting, epigastric pain, *diarrhea, excessive salivation.*

Other: ***bronchospasm, bronchial constriction,*** dyspnea.

INTERACTIONS

Atropine, anticholinergic agents, procainamide, quinidine: may reverse cholinergic effects. Observe for lack of drug effect.

EFFECTS ON DIAGNOSTIC TESTS

None reported.

NURSING CONSIDERATIONS

Besides those related universally to drug therapy (see "How to use this book"), consider the following specific recommendations:

Assessment

- Obtain a baseline assessment of the patient's anxiety before drug therapy.
- Be alert for adverse reactions and drug interactions throughout therapy.
- Evaluate the patient's and family's knowledge about physostigmine salicylate therapy.

Nursing Diagnoses

- Anxiety related to patient's underlying condition.
- Diarrhea related to adverse reaction to drug.
- Knowledge deficit related to physostigmine salicylate therapy.

Planning and Implementation

Preparation and Administration

- Use only clear solutions. Darkening may indicate loss of potency.
- This drug is uniquely useful in treating CNS effects of anticholinergic or tricyclic antidepressant toxicity.
- Effectiveness often immediate and dramatic but may be transient and may require repeat dose.
- May be used investigationally to improve cognitive function in patients with Alzheimer's disease. Investigators have used 0.5 mg P.O. q 2 hours, increasing to 2 to 2.5 mg P.O. q 2 hours, six or seven times a day. Maximum dose is 16 mg/day.
- ***I.V. use:*** Give at a controlled rate; use slow, direct injection at no more than 1 mg/minute.

Monitoring

- Monitor effectiveness by evaluating the reduction of symptoms of CNS toxicity.
- Monitor for adverse reactions and drug interactions by frequently checking vital signs, especially respirations.

Supportive Care

- Use side rails if patient becomes restless or hallucinates.
- Position patient to make breathing easier and provide respiratory support as needed if adverse reactions occur.
- Always have atropine injection readily available and be prepared to give 0.5 mg subcutaneously or slow I.V. push, as ordered.

Patient Teaching

- Instruct the patient about underlying disease condition requiring treatment with physostigmine salicylate.

Evaluation

In patients receiving physostigmine salicylate, appropriate evaluation statements may include:

- Patient's anxiety is relieved.
- Patient's bowel pattern is unaffected by physostigmine salicylate therapy.
- Patient and family state an under-

standing of physostigmine salicylate therapy.

pilocarpine hydrochloride

(pye lo kar´ peen)

Adsorbocarpine, Isopto Carpine, Miocarpine†, Ocusert Pilo, Pilocar, Pilocel, Pilomiotin, Pilopine HS, Pilopt‡

pilocarpine nitrate

P.V. Carpine Liquifilm

- *Classification:* miotic (cholinergic agonist)
- *Pregnancy Risk Category:* C

HOW SUPPLIED

hydrochloride

Ophthalmic solution: 0.25%, 0.5%, 1%, 2%, 3%, 4%, 5%, 6%, 8%, 10%
Ophthalmic gel: 4%
Releasing-system insert: 20 mcg/hr, 40 mcg/hr

nitrate

Ophthalmic solution: 1%, 2%, 4%

ACTION

Mechanism: Activates muscarinic acetylcholine receptors in the eye. Causes contraction of the sphincter muscles of the iris, resulting in miosis. Also produces ciliary spasm, deepening of the anterior chamber, and vasodilation of conjunctival vessels of the outflow tract.
Absorption: May be absorbed systemically from ocular mucosa.
Distribution: Animal studies show that the drug does not accumulate within ocular tissues.
Onset, peak, duration: Drops act within 10 to 30 minutes with peak effect at 2 to 4 hours. With the Ocusert Pilo System, 0.3 to 7 mg of pilocarpine are released during the initial 6-hour period; during the remainder of the 1-week insertion period, the release rate is within ±20% of the rated value. Effect is seen in 1½ to 2 hours and is maintained for the 1-week life of the insertion.

Duration of effect of pilocarpine drops is 4 to 6 hours.

INDICATIONS & DOSAGE

Primary open-angle glaucoma –
Adults and children: instill 1 to 2 drops in eye q.d. to q.i.d., as directed by doctor. Or, may apply 4% gel (Pilopine HS) once daily.

Alternatively, apply one Ocusert Pilo system (20 or 40 mcg/hour) q 7 days.

Emergency treatment of acute narrow-angle glaucoma –
Adults and children: 1 drop of 2% solution q 5 minutes for three to six doses, followed by 1 drop q 1 to 3 hours until pressure is controlled.

CONTRAINDICATIONS & PRECAUTIONS

Contraindicated in patients with acute iritis or hypersensitivity to the drug or any of the preparation's components. Use cautiously in patients with acute cardiac failure, bronchial asthma, urinary tract obstruction, GI spasm, peptic ulcer, hyperthyroidism, or Parkinson's disease.

ADVERSE REACTIONS

Common reactions are in italics; life-threatening reactions are in bold italics.
Eye: suborbital headache, *myopia,* ciliary spasm, *blurred vision,* conjunctival irritation, lacrimation, changes in visual field, *brow pain.*
GI: nausea, vomiting, abdominal cramps, diarrhea, salivation.
Other: hypersensitivity.

INTERACTIONS

Carbachol, echothiophate: additive effect. Don't use together.
Ophthalmic belladonna alkaloids (such as atropine, scopolamine), cyclopentolate: decreased antiglaucoma effects of pilocarpine; mydriatic ef-

fects of these agents blocked by pilocarpine.
Phenylephrine: decreased dilation by phenylephrine. Don't use together.

EFFECTS ON DIAGNOSTIC TESTS

None reported.

NURSING CONSIDERATIONS

Besides those related universally to drug therapy (see "How to use this book"), consider the following specific recommendations:

Assessment

- Obtain a baseline assessment of the patient's vision, especially ocular pressure.
- Be alert for adverse reactions and drug interactions throughout therapy.
- Evaluate the patient's and family's knowledge about pilocarpine therapy.

Nursing Diagnoses

- Sensory/perceptual alterations (visual) related to the patient's underlying condition.
- Pain related to the pilocarpine-induced brow discomfort.
- Knowledge deficit related to pilocarpine therapy.

Planning and Implementation

Preparation and Administration

- ***Topical use:*** Apply thin strip of gel to conjunctival sac; avoid touching applicator tip to any surface and wipe tip with clean tissue or gauze before recapping. Instill solution in lacrimal sac; remove excess solution around eyes with clean tissue or gauze and apply light finger pressure to lacrimal sac for 1 minute.
- May be used in combination with mannitol, urea, glycerol, or acetazolamide to treat acute narrow-angle glaucoma.
- May be used alternately with atropine to break adhesions.

Monitoring

- Monitor effectiveness by assessing the patient's visual status and intraocular pressure.
- Monitor for systemic cholinergic effects.

Supportive Care

- Notify the doctor immediately of any changes in the patient's health status.
- Obtain an order for a mild analgesic if the patient experiences headache or brow ache.

Patient Teaching

- Teach the patient how to instill the medication, and advise him to wash his hands before and after administering the drug.
- Warn the patient that his vision will be temporarily blurred. Patient should instill the drug at bedtime or avoid hazardous activities until the effect subsides.
- Reassure the patient that transient brow pain and myopia are common at the start of therapy and should subside within 2 weeks.
- Tell the patient what to do if the Ocusert system falls out during sleep; rinse the system in cool tap water, inspect the system for deformities, and, if it is intact, reinsert.

Evaluation

In patients receiving pilocarpine hydrochloride, appropriate evaluation statements may include:

- Patient experiences a reduction in intraocular pressure.
- Patient remains free of systemic effects.
- Patient and family state an understanding of pilocarpine hydrochloride therapy.

pindolol

(pin´ doe lole)
Barbloc‡, Visken

- *Classification:* antihypertensive (beta-adrenergic blocking agent)
- *Pregnancy Risk Category:* B

HOW SUPPLIED

Tablets: 5 mg, 10 mg, 15 mg‡

ACTION

Mechanism: Blocks response to beta stimulation.
Absorption: After oral administration, pindolol is absorbed rapidly from the GI tract. Food does not reduce bioavailability but may increase the rate of GI absorption.
Distribution: Widely distributed throughout the body and is 40% to 60% protein-bound.
Metabolism: About 60% to 65% of a given dose is metabolized by the liver.
Excretion: In adults with normal renal function, 35% to 50% of a given dose is excreted unchanged in urine. Half-life: About 3 to 4 hours.
Onset, peak, duration: Peak plasma concentrations occur in 1 to 2 hours. Effect on the heart rate usually occurs in 3 hours. Antihypertensive effect usually persists for 24 hours.

INDICATIONS & DOSAGE

Treatment of hypertension–
Adults: initially, 5 mg P.O. b.i.d. Dosage may be increased by 10 mg/day q 2 to 3 weeks up to a maximum of 60 mg/day.

CONTRAINDICATIONS & PRECAUTIONS

Contraindicated in patients with known hypersensitivity to the drug; and in patients with severe bradycardia, overt cardiac failure, second- or third-degree atrioventricular block, or bronchial asthma because the drug may worsen these conditions.

Use cautiously in patients with impaired hepatic or renal function or coronary insufficiency because beta-adrenergic blockade may precipitate CHF; in patients with hyperthyroidism or diabetes mellitus because the drug may mask tachycardia; in patients undergoing general anesthesia because severe hypotension or bradycardia may develop; and in patients with emphysema or other pulmonary disease.

ADVERSE REACTIONS

Common reactions are in italics; life-threatening reactions are in bold italics.
CNS: *insomnia, fatigue, dizziness, nervousness,* vivid dreams, hallucinations, lethargy.
CV: *edema,* bradycardia, CHF, peripheral vascular disease, hypotension.
EENT: visual disturbances.
GI: *nausea,* vomiting, diarrhea.
Metabolic: hypoglycemia without tachycardia.
Skin: rash.
Other: ***bronchospasm,*** *muscle pain, joint pain,* chest pain.

INTERACTIONS

Digitalis glycosides: excessive bradycardia and increased depressant effect on myocardium. Use together cautiously.
Epinephrine: severe vasoconstriction. Monitor blood pressure and observe patient carefully.
Indomethacin: decreased antihypertensive effect. Monitor blood pressure and adjust dosage.
Insulin, oral hypoglycemic drugs: can alter requirements for these drugs in previously stabilized diabetics. Monitor for hypoglycemia.

EFFECTS ON DIAGNOSTIC TESTS

Serum transaminase, alkaline phosphatase, lactic dehydrogenase, and uric acid: elevated levels.

NURSING CONSIDERATIONS

Besides those related universally to drug therapy (see "How to use this book"), consider the following specific recommendations:

Assessment
• Obtain a baseline assessment of the patient's blood pressure before beginning therapy.
• Be alert for adverse reactions and drug interactions throughout therapy.
• Evaluate the patient's and family's knowledge about pindolol therapy.
Nursing Diagnoses
• Altered tissue perfusion (renal, cerebral, cardiopulmonary, peripheral) related to the patient's underlying condition.
• Fatigue related to adverse CNS reactions to pindolol.
• Knowledge deficit related to pindolol therapy.
Planning and Implementation
Preparation and Administration
• Always check the patient's apical pulse rate before giving this drug. If you detect extremes in pulse rates, hold the medication and call the doctor immediately.
• ***P.O. use:*** Patient may take this drug without regard for meals. Many patients respond favorably to a dose of 5 mg t.i.d.
Monitoring
• Monitor effectiveness by frequently checking the patient's blood pressure, pulse, and ECG.
• Monitor for hypotension, and adverse CNS reactions such as fatigue and insomnia as well as other adverse reactions.
• Monitor blood glucose levels. This drug masks common signs of hypoglycemia and shock.
Supportive Care
• If the patient develops severe hypotension, notify the doctor, and be prepared to administer a vasopressor.
• Remember that the drug should be withdrawn gradually (over 1 to 2 weeks) after long-term administration.
• Keep in mind that pindolol is the first commercially available beta blocker with partial beta-agonist activity; in other words, pindolol stimulates and blocks beta-adrenergic receptors. Therefore, it decreases cardiac output less than other beta-adrenergic blockers. Drug may be helpful for patients who develop bradycardia with other beta blockers.
Patient Teaching
• Teach the patient how to take his pulse rate before taking the medication. Tell patient to notify the doctor before taking pindolol if his pulse rate varies significantly from its usual level.
• Explain the importance of taking this drug as prescribed, even when feeling well.
• Tell the patient not to discontinue this drug suddenly even if unpleasant adverse reactions occur, but to discuss the problem with the doctor.
• Explain that abrupt discontinuation of the drug can exacerbate angina and MI.
• Instruct the patient to check with the doctor or pharmacist before taking OTC medications.
• Teach the patient and family caregiver to take blood pressure measurements. Tell them to notify the doctor of any significant change in the blood pressure measurement.
Evaluation
In patients receiving pindolol, appropriate evaluation statements may include:
• Blood pressure is controlled within normal levels for this patient.
• Patient did not experience fatigue or insomnia.
• Patient and family state an understanding of pindolol therapy.

pipecuronium bromide
(pi pe kure oh´ nee um)
Arduan

• *Classification:* skeletal muscle relaxant (nondepolarizing neuromuscular blocking agent)

• *Pregnancy Risk Category:* C

HOW SUPPLIED

Powder for injection: 10 mg/vial

ACTION

Mechanism: Prevents acetylcholine from binding to the receptors on the muscle end plate, thus blocking depolarization. Nondepolarizing agent.
Distribution: Volume of distribution (V_D) is about 0.25 liters/kg and increases in patients with renal failure. Other conditions associated with increased V_D (including edema, old age, and cardiovascular disease) may delay onset.
Metabolism: Only about 20% to 40% of an administered dose is metabolized, probably in the liver. One metabolite (3-desacetyl pipecuronium) has about 50% of the neuromuscular blocking activity of the parent drug.
Excretion: Primarily renal. Half-life: Estimated at 1.7 hours; it may increase to 4 hours or more in patients with severe renal disease.
Onset, peak, duration: Maximum onset of action occurs within 5 minutes.

INDICATIONS & DOSAGE

To provide skeletal muscle relaxation during surgery as an adjunct to general anesthesia –
Adults and children: dosage is highly individualized. The following doses may serve as a guide for use in nonobese patients with normal renal function. Initially, 70 to 85 mcg/kg I.V. provides conditions considered ideal for endotracheal intubation and maintains paralysis for 1 to 2 hours. If succinylcholine is used for endotracheal intubation, initial doses of 50 mcg/kg I.V. provide good relaxation for 45 minutes or more. Maintenance doses of 10 to 15 mcg/kg provide relaxation for about 50 minutes.

CONTRAINDICATIONS & PRECAUTIONS

There are no known contraindications to the use of the drug. However, this drug should be used only under direct medical supervision by personnel familiar with the use of neuromuscular blocking agents and techniques involved in maintaining a patent airway. It should not be used unless facilities and equipment for artificial respiration, mechanical ventilation, oxygen therapy, and intubation and an antagonist are within reach.

Because of the lack of data supporting safety, this drug is not recommended for use in patients requiring prolonged mechanical ventilation in the intensive care unit; before or after use of other nondepolarizing neuromuscular blocking agents; or for use during cesarean section because safety to the neonate has not been established and because this drug's long duration of action exceeds the duration of the procedure.

Use cautiously in patients with renal failure because the drug is excreted by the kidneys. Patients with myasthenia gravis or myasthenic syndrome (Eaton-Lambert syndrome) are particularly sensitive to the effects of nondepolarizing agents. Shorter-acting agents are recommended for use in such patients.

Because the drug has minimal vagolytic action, bradycardia during anesthesia may be common, especially when administered with high doses of opioid narcotics for the induction and maintenance of anesthesia.

A nerve stimulator and train-of-four (T4) monitoring is recommended to document antagonism of neuromuscular blockade and recovery of muscle strength. Before pharmacologic reversal with neostigmine is attempted, some evidence of spontaneous recovery (T_4/T_1 ratio > 0, or $T_1 > 10\%$ of control) should be evident. Reversal with edrophonium is not recommended due to its short duration of action in comparison to neostigmine.

ADVERSE REACTIONS

Common reactions are in italics; life-threatening reactions are in bold italics.
CV: hypotension, bradycardia, hypertension, myocardial ischemia, ***CVA,*** thrombosis, atrial fibrillation, ***ventricular extrasystole.***
GU: anuria.
Metabolic: increased creatinine levels.
Respiratory: dyspnea, ***respiratory depression, respiratory insufficiency or apnea.***
Other: prolonged muscle weakness.

INTERACTIONS

Aminoglycosides (kanamycin, neomycin, streptomycin, dihydrostreptomycin, and gentamicin), bacitracin, colistin, polymyxin B, colistimethate, tetracyclines: increased muscle weakness. Use together cautiously.
Magnesium salts: may enhance neuromuscular blockade. Monitor for excessive weakness.
Quinidine, inhalational anesthetics: enhanced activity (or prolonged action) of nondepolarizing neuromuscular blocking agents.

EFFECTS ON DIAGNOSTIC TESTS

None reported.

NURSING CONSIDERATIONS

Besides those related universally to drug therapy (see "How to use this book"), consider the following specific recommendations:

Assessment

- Obtain a baseline assessment of the patient's breathing pattern and skeletal muscle function before drug therapy.
- Be alert for adverse reactions and drug interactions throughout therapy.
- Evaluate the patient's and family's knowledge about pipecuronium therapy.

Nursing Diagnoses

- Self-care deficit related to prolonged muscloskeletal effects.
- Ineffective breathing pattern related to adverse drug reaction.
- Knowledge deficit related to pipecuronium therapy.

Planning and Implementation

Preparation and Administration

- This drug should be used only under direct medical supervision by personnel familiar with the use of neuromuscular blocking agents and techniques involved in maintaining a patent airway.
- Dosage should be adjusted to ideal body weight in obese patients (patients 30% or more above their ideal weight) because prolonged neuromuscular blockade has been reported in these patients.
- After reconstitution with bacteriostatic water for injection, the drug is stable for 5 days at room temperature or in the refrigerator. Note that bacteriostatic water contains benzyl alcohol and is not intended for use in neonates.
- After reconstitution with any solution other than bacteriostatic water for injection, discard any unused portions of the drug.
- After reconstitution with sterile water for injection or other compatible I.V. solutions (such as dextrose 5% in water, 0.9% sodium chloride injection, lactated Ringer's injection, and dextrose 5% in lactated Ringer's injection), the drug is stable for 24 hours if refrigerated.
- Store the powder at room temperature or in the refrigerator (36° to 86° F [2° to 30° C]).
- Reconstitute with 10 ml solution before use to yield a solution of 1 mg/ml. Large volumes of diluent or addition of the drug to a hanging I.V. solution is not recommended.
- Know that because of its prolonged

duration of action, this drug is recommended only for procedures that take 90 minutes or longer.
• ***I.V. use:*** Intermittent and continuous infusions are not recommended.
• Know that pipecuronium may be administered after succinylcholine when the latter is used to facilitate intubation. However, there is no evidence to support the safe use of pipecuronium before succinylcholine to decrease the latter drug's adverse effects.

Monitoring
• A nerve stimulator and train-of-four monitoring are recommended to document antagonism of neuromuscular blockade and recovery of muscle strength. Before attempting pharmacologic reversal with neostigmine, some evidence of spontaneous recovery (T_4/T_1 ratio > 0 or $T_1 > 10\%$ of control) should be evident.
• Monitor obese patients for prolonged neuromuscular blockade.
• Monitor electrolyte and acid-base balances. These may influence the actions and response to nondepolarizing neuromuscular blocking agents. Acidosis may enhance the paralysis and alkalosis may counteract it.
• Monitor for adverse reactions and interactions by frequently checking the patient's blood pressure for hypertension or hypotension and heart rate for bradycardia.
• Monitor the ECG for atrial fibrillation or ventricular extrasystole.
• Monitor the patient's vital signs for bradycardia during anesthesia because the drug has minimal vagolytic action.
• Monitor the patient's respirations closely until patient is fully recovered from neuromuscular blockade as evidenced by tests of muscle strength (hand grip, head lift, and ability to cough).
• Monitor intake and output; drug may cause anuria.

Supportive Care
• Have equipment for mechanical ventilation, oxygen therapy, intubation, and an antagonist within reach while administering this drug.

Patient Teaching
• Teach the patient that this drug will be given as a part of anesthesia.
• Tell the patient that he may experience some residual muscle weakness.

Evaluation
In patients receiving pipecuronium, appropriate evaluation statements may include:
• Patient's breathing pattern remains normal.
• Patient and family state an understanding of pipecuronium therapy.

piperacillin sodium
(pi per´ a sill in)
Pipracil, Pipril‡

• *Classification:* antibiotic (extended-spectrum penicillin)
• *Pregnancy Risk Category:* B

HOW SUPPLIED
Injection: 2 g, 3 g, 4 g
Pharmacy bulk package: 40 g

ACTION
Mechanism: Bactericidal by inhibiting cell wall synthesis during active multiplication.
Absorption: Not absorbed after oral administration; about 70% to 80% of an I.M. dose is absorbed. Peak serum levels are higher after I.V. administration.
Distribution: Widely distributed after parenteral administration. It penetrates minimally into uninflamed meninges and slightly into bone and sputum. Piperacillin is 16% to 22% protein-bound; it crosses the placenta.
Metabolism: Probably not significantly metabolized.

Excretion: Primarily excreted (42% to 90%) in urine by renal tubular secretion and glomerular filtration; it is also excreted in bile and in breast milk. Half-life: Increases with increasing dose. In most patients, the half-life is about 30 minutes to 1½ hours; in extensive renal impairment, half-life is 2 to 6 hours; in hepatorenal dysfunction, 11 to 32 hours.
Onset, peak, duration: Peak plasma concentrations occur 30 to 50 minutes after an I.M. dose.

INDICATIONS & DOSAGE

Systemic infections caused by susceptible strains of gram-positive and especially gram-negative organisms (including Proteus, Pseudomonas aeruginosa*)–*
Adults and children over 12 years: 100 to 300 mg/kg daily divided q 4 to 6 hours I.V. or I.M. Doses for children under 12 years not established.
Prophylaxis of surgical infections–
Adults: 2 g I.V., given 30 to 60 minutes before surgery. Depending on type of surgery, dose may be repeated during surgery, and once or twice more after surgery.

CONTRAINDICATIONS & PRECAUTIONS

Contraindicated in patients with hypersensitivity to any penicillin or cephalosporins. Use cautiously in patients with renal impairment because drug is excreted by the kidneys; decreased dosage is required in moderate to severe renal failure. Use with caution in patients with bleeding tendencies, uremia, or hypokalemia.

ADVERSE REACTIONS

Common reactions are in italics; life-threatening reactions are in bold italics.
Blood: ***bleeding with high doses,*** neutropenia, eosinophilia, leukopenia, ***thrombocytopenia.***
CNS: neuromuscular irritability, seizures, headache, dizziness.
GI: nausea, diarrhea.
Local: pain at injection site, vein irritation, phlebitis.
Metabolic: *hypokalemia.*
Other: *hypersensitivity (edema, fever, chills, rash, pruritus, urticaria,* ***anaphylaxis****),* overgrowth of nonsusceptible organisms.

INTERACTIONS

Aminoglycoside antibiotics (e.g., gentamicin, tobramycin): chemically incompatible.
Probenecid: increases blood levels of piperacillin. Probenecid may be used for this purpose.

EFFECTS ON DIAGNOSTIC TESTS

Aminoglycoside serum levels: falsely decreased concentrations.
CBC: transient reductions in RBCs, WBCs, and platelet counts.
Coombs' test: positive results.
Electrolytes: hypokalemia, hypernatremia.
Liver function test: transient elevations.
Prothrombin times: prolonged.

NURSING CONSIDERATIONS

Besides those related universally to drug therapy (see "How to use this book"), consider the following specific recommendations:
Assessment
• Obtain a baseline assessment of infection before therapy.
• Be alert for adverse reactions and drug interactions throughout therapy.
• Evaluate the patient's and family's knowledge about piperacillin therapy.
Nursing Diagnoses
• High risk for injury related to ineffectiveness of piperacillin to eradicate the infection.
• Altered protection related to piperacillin-induced allergic reaction.
• Knowledge deficit related to piperacillin therapy.

Planning and Implementation
Preparation and Administration
• Obtain specimen for culture and sensitivity tests before first dose. Therapy may begin pending test results.
• Before giving penicillin, ask the patient about previous allergic reactions to this drug or other pencillins. However, a negative history of penicillin allergy does not guarantee future safety.
• Give piperacillin at least 1 hour before bacteriostatic antibiotics.
• Expect to reduce dosage for a patient with impaired renal function.
• Expect to give another antibiotic such as gentamicin concurrently.
• ***I.V. use:*** Administer intermittently to prevent vein irritation.
Monitoring
• Monitor effectiveness by regularly assessing for improvement of infection.
• Allergic reactions, especially with large doses, parenteral administration, or prolonged therapy. Keep in mind that the previously nonallergic patient may become sensitized to penicillin during therapy. Patients with cystic fibrosis tend to be most susceptible to fever or rash.
• Closely monitor I.V. site for thrombophlebitis.
• Monitor CBC, platelets, and serum potassium level frequently as ordered.
• Monitor for bacterial or fungal superinfections during high-dose or prolonged therapy, especially in elderly, debilitated, or immunosuppressed patients.
Supportive Care
• Discontinue the drug immediately if the patient develops signs of anaphylactic shock (rapidly developing dyspnea and hypotension). Notify the doctor and prepare to administer immediate treatment, such as epinephrine, corticosteroids, antihistamines, and other resuscitative measures as indicated.
• Drug may induce seizures. Institute seizure precautions for patient with high blood level.
• Change I.V. site every 48 hours.
• Limit patient's salt intake because piperacillin contains 1.98 mEq Na/g.
Patient Teaching
• Advise the patient who becomes allergic to penicillins to wear medical alert identification stating this information.
• Tell the patient to inform the nurse of pain or discomfort at the I.V. site.
• Instruct patient to limit salt intake while taking piperacillin.
Evaluation
In patients receiving piperacillin, appropriate evaluation statements may include:
• Patient is free of infection.
• Patient does not experience an allergic reaction to therapy.
• Patient and family state an understanding of therapy.

pirbuterol
(peer byoo´ ter ole)
Maxair

• *Classification:* bronchodilator (beta-adrenergic agonist)
• *Pregnancy Risk Category:* C

HOW SUPPLIED
Inhaler: 0.2 mg/metered dose

ACTION
Mechanism: Relaxes bronchial smooth muscle by acting on $beta_2$-adrenergic receptors.
Absorption: Poorly absorbed; acts locally in the respiratory tract. Negligible serum levels are achieved after inhalation of the usual dose.
Metabolism: Hepatic.
Excretion: About 50% of an inhaled dose is recovered in the urine as the parent drug and metabolites. Half-life: About 2 hours.

Onset, peak, duration: Onset of action is less than 5 minutes, and duration is about 5 hours.

INDICATIONS AND DOSAGE

Prevention and reversal of bronchospasm, asthma –
Adults: 1 or 2 inhalations (0.2 to 0.4 mg) repeated q 4 to 6 hours. Not to exceed 12 inhalations daily.

CONTRAINDICATIONS & PRECAUTIONS

Contraindicated in patients allergic to pirbuterol or other adrenergics, in patients with digitalis toxicity, and in patients with cardiac arrhythmias associated with tachycardia. Beta-adrenergic agonists may cause significant cardiovascular effects, as well as paradoxical bronchospasm in some patients.

Administer cautiously to patients with a history of exaggerated responses to sympathetic amines, and to patients with a history of seizure disorders.

ADVERSE REACTIONS

Common reactions are in italics; life-threatening reactions are in bold italics.
CNS: tremors, nervousness, dizziness, insomnia, headache.
CV: tachycardia, palpitations, increased blood pressure.
EENT: drying or irritation of throat.

INTERACTIONS

Propranolol and other beta-adrenergic blocking agents: decreased bronchodilating effects.

EFFECTS ON DIAGNOSTIC TESTS

None reported.

NURSING CONSIDERATIONS

Besides those related universally to drug therapy (see "How to use this book"), consider the following specific recommendations:

Assessment
- Obtain a baseline assessment of cardiopulmonary status before therapy by taking vital signs, obtaining an ECG (if ordered) and auscultating the heart and lung fields.
- Be alert for adverse reactions and drug interactions throughout therapy.
- Evaluate the patient's and family's knowledge about pirbuterol therapy.

Nursing Diagnoses
- Ineffective airway clearance related to patient's underlying condition.
- Sleep pattern disturbance related to pirbuterol-induced nervousness and insomnia.
- Knowledge deficit related to pirbuterol therapy.

Planning and Implementation
Preparation and Administration
- Shake the canister well before each use. Store the drug away from heat and direct sunlight.

Monitoring
- Monitor effectiveness by checking respiratory rate, auscultating lung fields, and following laboratory studies such as arterial blood gases.
- Observe patient for signs of restlessness and fatigue and complaints of insomnia.
- Be alert for adverse cardiovascular reactions during therapy.

Supportive Care
- Notify the doctor if previously effective dosage does not control symptoms, because this may signify worsening disease.
- Obtain an order for an antiemetic if adverse GI. reactions occur.
- Help the patient identify nonpharmacologic ways to manage insomnia; if ineffective, obtain an order for a hypnotic.

Patient Teaching
- Advise patient to seek medical attention if a previously effective dosage does not control symptoms, because this may signify a worsening of the disease.
- Tell patient to call the doctor

promptly if he experiences increased bronchospasm after using the drug.
• Teach patient to perform oral inhalation correctly. Give the following instructions for using a meter-dosed inhaler:
– Clear nasal passages and throat.
– Breathe out, expelling as much air from lungs as possible.
– Place mouthpiece well into mouth as inhaler is released, and inhale deeply.
– Hold breath for several seconds, remove mouthpiece, and exhale slowly.
• Tell the patient to wait at least 2 minutes between doses if more than one inhalation is ordered. Tell the patient who is also using a steroid inhaler to use the bronchodilator first, then wait about 5 minutes before using the steroid. This allows the bronchodilator to open passages for maximum effectiveness.

Evaluation

In patients receiving pirbuterol, appropriate evaluation statements may include:
• Patient experiences improved respiratory status.
• Patient is able to maintain an adequate sleep pattern.
• Patient and family state an understanding of pirbuterol therapy.

piroxicam

(peer ox´ i kam)
Apo-Piroxicam†, Feldene, Novopirocam†

• *Classification:* non-narcotic analgesic, antipyretic, anti-inflammatory (non-steroidal anti-inflammatory)
• *Pregnancy Risk Category:* C

HOW SUPPLIED

Capsules: 10 mg, 20 mg

ACTION

Mechanism: Produces anti-inflammatory, analgesic, and antipyretic effects, possibly through inhibition of prostaglandin synthesis.
Absorption: Rapidly absorbed from the GI tract. Food delays absorption.
Distribution: Highly protein-bound.
Metabolism: Hepatic.
Excretion: In urine. Half-life: Its long half-life (about 50 hours) allows for once-daily dosing.
Onset, peak, duration: Peak plasma levels are seen 3 to 5 hours after dosing.

INDICATIONS & DOSAGE

Osteoarthritis and rheumatoid arthritis–
Adults: 20 mg P.O. once daily. If desired, the dose may be divided.

CONTRAINDICATIONS & PRECAUTIONS

Contraindicated in patients with hypersensitivity to this drug, and in patients in whom aspirin or other nonsteroidal anti-inflammatory drugs (NSAIDs) induce symptoms of asthma, urticaria, or rhinitis. Patients with known "triad" symptoms (aspirin hypersensitivity, rhinitis/nasal polyps, and asthma) are at high risk of bronchospasm.

Serious GI toxicity, especially ulceration or hemorrhage, can occur at any time in patients on chronic NSAID therapy. Use cautiously in patients with a history of peptic ulcer disease, angioedema, or cardiac disease, because the drug may worsen these conditions; and in patients with decreased renal function because it may cause a further reduction in renal function.

NSAIDs may mask the signs and symptoms of acute infection (fever, myalgia, erythema); carefully evaluate patients with high risk of infection (such as those with diabetes).

ADVERSE REACTIONS

Common reactions are in italics; life-threatening reactions are in bold italics.

Blood: prolonged bleeding time, anemia.

CNS: headache, drowsiness, dizziness.

CV: peripheral edema.

GI: *epigastric distress, nausea, occult blood loss,* ***peptic ulceration, severe GI bleeding.***

GU: ***nephrotoxicity.***

Hepatic: elevated enzymes.

Skin: pruritus, rash, urticaria, *photosensitivity.*

INTERACTIONS

Aspirin: decreased plasma levels of piroxicam.

Lithium: increased plasma lithium levels.

Oral anticoagulants: enhanced risk of bleeding. Monitor patient closely.

Oral hypoglycemic agents: enhanced hypoglycemic effects. Monitor patient closely.

EFFECTS ON DIAGNOSTIC TESTS

Bleeding time: prolonged (may persist for 2 weeks after discontinuing drug).

BUN, serum creatinine and potassium levels: increased.

Hemoglobin, hematocrit: decreased.

Liver function tests: increased alkaline phosphatase, lactic dehydrogenase, or transaminase levels.

Prothrombin time: prolonged.

Serum glucose: decreased levels in diabetic patients.

Uric acid: decreased level.

NURSING CONSIDERATIONS

Besides those related universally to drug therapy (see "How to use this book"), consider the following specific recommendations:

Assessment

- Obtain a baseline assessment of the patient's pain before therapy.
- Be alert for adverse reactions and drug interactions throughout therapy.
- Evaluate the patient's and family's knowledge about piroxicam therapy.

Nursing Diagnoses

- Pain related to the patient's underlying condition.
- High risk for impaired skin integrity related to piroxicam-induced photosensitivity.
- Knowledge deficit related to piroxicam therapy.

Planning and Implementation

Preparation and Administration

- If adverse GI reactions occur, give with milk or meals.

Monitoring

- Regularly monitor the patient for relief of pain, keeping in mind that full therapeutic effects may be delayed for 2 to 4 weeks.
- Monitor for adverse skin reactions. This drug causes adverse skin reactions, especially photosensitivity, more often than other drugs in its class.
- Regularly monitor the patient's renal, hepatic, and auditory function during long-term therapy.
- Monitor the patient for GI toxicity.

Supportive Care

- Notify the doctor if the patient's pain is not relieved or if it worsens.
- Expect a longer duration of action than other similar drugs, because the drug's half-life is longer. Piroxicam is the first NSAID approved by the FDA for once-daily administration.
- Hold dose and notify the doctor if the patient develops nausea, vomiting, or epigastric distress that is not relieved by taking drug with food or milk or if auditory, renal, or hepatic abnormalities occur.

Patient Teaching

- Tell the patient that the full therapeutic effect of the drug may be delayed for 2 to 4 weeks.
- Advise the patient to notify the doctor if pain persists or becomes worse.
- Tell the patient to take the drug

with food or milk if GI distress occurs.
• Because serious GI toxicity can occur at any time in chronic NSAID therapy, teach the patient signs and symptoms of GI bleeding. Tell the patient to report these to the doctor immediately.
• Advise the patient to minimize exposure to direct sunlight and to use a sunscreen and to wear protective clothing when outdoors.

Evaluation

In patients receiving piroxicam, appropriate evaluation statements may include:
• Patient states pain is relieved.
• Patient's skin remains intact.
• Patient and family state an understanding of piroxicam therapy.

plasma protein fraction

(plaz´ ma proe´ teen frak´ shun)
Plasmanate, Plasma-Plex, Plasmatein, Protenate

• *Classification:* plasma volume expander (blood derivative)
• *Pregnancy Risk Category:* C

HOW SUPPLIED

Injection: 5% solution in 50-ml, 250-ml, 500-ml vials

ACTION

Mechanism: Supplies colloid to the blood and expands plasma volume. Albumin is the major constituent (83% to 90%).
Absorption: Not adequately absorbed from the GI tract.
Distribution: Accounts for approximately 50% of plasma proteins. Distributed into the intravascular space and extravascular sites, including skin, muscle, and lungs. In patients with reduced circulating blood volumes, hemodilution secondary to albumin administration persists for many hours; in patients with normal blood volume, excess fluid and protein are lost from the intravascular space within a few hours.
Metabolism: Although albumin is synthesized in the liver, the liver is not involved in clearance of albumin from the plasma in healthy individuals.
Excretion: Little is known about albumin excretion in healthy individuals. Administration of albumin decreases hepatic albumin synthesis and increases albumin clearance if plasma oncotic pressure is high. In certain pathologic states, the liver, kidneys, or intestines may provide elimination mechanisms.

INDICATIONS & DOSAGE

Shock–
Adults: varies with patient's condition and response, but usual dose is 250 to 500 ml I.V. (12.5 to 25 g protein), usually no faster than 10 ml/minute.
Children: 22 to 33 ml/kg I.V. infused at rate of 5 to 10 ml/minute.
Hypoproteinemia–
Adults: 1,000 to 1,500 ml I.V. daily. Maximum infusion rate 8 ml/minute.

CONTRAINDICATIONS & PRECAUTIONS

Contraindicated in patients with severe anemia or heart failure, in patients undergoing cardiac bypass surgery, and in those with increased blood volume. Use cautiously in patients with hepatic or renal failure, low cardiac reserve, or restricted sodium intake.

ADVERSE REACTIONS

Common reactions are in italics; life-threatening reactions are in bold italics.
CNS: headache.
CV: variable effects on blood pressure after rapid infusion or intraarterial administration; ***vascular overload after rapid infusion.***
GI: nausea, vomiting, hypersalivation.

Skin: erythema, urticaria.
Other: flushing, chills, fever, back pain, dyspnea.

INTERACTIONS

None significant.

EFFECTS ON DIAGNOSTIC TESTS

Plasma protein: slightly increased levels.

NURSING CONSIDERATIONS

Besides those related universally to drug therapy (see "How to use this book"), consider the following specific recommendations:

Assessment

- Obtain a baseline assessment of patient's vital signs, hemoglobin, and serum albumin levels before therapy.
- Be alert for adverse reactions and drug interactions throughout therapy.
- Evaluate the patient's and family's knowledge about plasma protein fraction therapy.

Nursing Diagnoses

- Fluid volume deficit related to the patient's underlying condition.
- Altered tissue perfusion related to the adverse side effects of plasma protein fraction.
- Knowledge deficit related to plasma protein fraction therapy.

Planning and Implementation

Preparation and Administration

- ***I.V. use:*** Administer by continuous infusion. Plasma protein fraction is ready for use. Solution varies from near colorless to straw to dark brown. Store at room temperature not over 86° F (30° C). Don't use if solution is cloudy, has been frozen, or contains sediment. Administer within 4 hours of opening container. Use bottle only once; it contains no preservatives. Discard unused portion. Infuse undiluted or in combination with other parenteral solutions, such as whole blood, plasma, 0.9% sodium chloride, glucose, or sodium lactate. Don't administer near site of infection or trauma. Infusion rate depends on response but should not exceed 10 ml/minute. Faster rates may result in sudden hypotension. As volume approaches normal, reduce rate to 5 to 8 ml/minute. In children, infuse at 5 to 10 ml/minute. Make sure administration set has adequate filter (provided by manufacturer).
- Direct injection or intermittent infusion is not recommended.

Monitoring

- Monitor effectiveness by carefully checking the patient's blood pressure, pulse, and respirations.
- Monitor hemoglobin; increased blood volume may cause significant fall. Transfusion of whole blood or packed RBCs may be necessary.
- Frequently check blood pressure of the patient in shock; widening pulse pressure correlates with increased stroke volume or cardiac output.
- Check for a sudden fall in blood pressure; if it occurs, stop the infusion and correct with vasopressors.
- Monitor serum albumin levels in patients with hypoproteinemia. Treating the underlying disorder and replacing amino acids and proteins restore albumin levels more effectively than plasma protein fraction or serum albumin infusions.
- Monitor injured or postoperative patients; elevated blood pressure may cause bleeding from severed blood vessels that may not have caused bleeding at lower blood pressure.

Supportive Care

- Remember that although plasma protein fraction is a pooled human plasma derivative, crossmatching is unnecessary.
- Keep in mind that if an allergic reaction occurs, discontinue and give antihistamines.

Patient Teaching

- Tell the patient to report headache, nausea, vomiting, hypersalivation, erythema, flushing, chills, fever, back pain, or dyspnea immediately.

Evaluation

In patients receiving plasma protein fraction, appropriate evaluation statements may include:

• Patient's fluid volume is within normal limits.
• Patient's hemoglobin and vital signs have remained within normal limits.
• Patient and family state an understanding of plasma protein fraction therapy.

plicamycin (mithramycin)

(plye kay mye´ sin)
Mithracin

• *Classification:* antineoplastic, hypocalcemic agent (antibiotic)
• *Pregnancy Risk Category:* X

HOW SUPPLIED

Injection: 2.5-mg vials

ACTION

Mechanism: An antineoplastic antibiotic that forms a complex with DNA, thus inhibiting RNA synthesis. Also inhibits osteocytic activity, blocking calcium and phosphorus resorption from bone. Pharmacologically similar to dactinomycin, drug is bacteriostatic against gram-positive bacteria; however, toxicity precludes its use as an antimicrobial. May lower serum calcium levels by blocking the effects of parathyroid hormone on osteoclasts.
Absorption: Not administered orally.
Distribution: Distributed mainly into the Kupffer's cells of the liver, into renal tubular cells, and along formed bone surfaces. Also crosses the blood-brain barrier and achieves appreciable concentrations in the CSF.
Excretion: Primarily through the kidneys.

INDICATIONS & DOSAGE

Dosage and indications may vary. Check patient's protocol with doctor.
Hypercalcemia associated with advanced malignancy–
Adults: 25 mcg/kg I.V. daily for 1 to 4 days.
Testicular cancer–
Adults: 25 to 30 mcg/kg I.V. daily for up to 10 days (based on ideal body weight or actual weight, whichever is less).

CONTRAINDICATIONS & PRECAUTIONS

Contraindicated in patients with impaired bone marrow function, thrombocytopenia, thrombocytopathy, coagulation disorders, or electrolyte imbalance because it may worsen the symptoms associated with these disorders. Use cautiously in patients with hepatic and renal dysfunction and in those who have previously received abdominal or mediastinal radiation because these patients may be more susceptible to the drug's toxic effects.

ADVERSE REACTIONS

Common reactions are in italics; life-threatening reactions are in bold italics.
Blood: ***thrombocytopenia; bleeding syndrome,*** *from epistaxis to* ***generalized hemorrhage;*** *facial flushing.*
GI: *nausea, vomiting,* anorexia, diarrhea, stomatitis, metallic taste.
GU: proteinuria; increased BUN, serum creatinine.
Metabolic: *decreased serum calcium,* potassium, and phosphorus; elevated liver enzymes.
Skin: periorbital pallor, usually the day before toxic symptoms occur.
Local: extravasation causes irritation, cellulitis.

INTERACTIONS

None significant.

EFFECTS ON DIAGNOSTIC TESTS

Serum alkaline phosphatase, AST (SGOT), ALT (SGPT), lactate dehydrogenase (LDH), and bilirubin: increased concentrations.
Serum creatinine and BUN: increased levels through nephrotoxicity.

NURSING CONSIDERATIONS

Besides those related universally to drug therapy (see "How to use this book"), consider the following specific recommendations:

Assessment

- Obtain a baseline assessment of the patient's overall physical status, CBC, platelet count, prothrombin time, serum calcium level, and hepatic and renal function tests before therapy.
- Be alert for adverse reactions and drug interactions throughout therapy.
- Evaluate the patient's and family's knowledge about plicamycin therapy.

Nursing Diagnoses

- Altered protection related to plicamycin-induced thrombocytopenia.
- Impaired tissue integrity related to extravasation of plicamycin.
- Knowledge deficit related to plicamycin therapy.

Planning and Implementation

Preparation and Administration

- Follow institutional policy when preparing and administering this drug to avoid mutagenic, teratogenic, and carcinogenic risks.
- Be aware that reconstituted solution is stable for 24 hours at room temperature or 48 hours if refrigerated. Store lyophilized powder in refrigerator.
- Avoid extravasation. Plicamycin is a vesicant.

Monitoring

- Monitor effectiveness by noting results of follow-up diagnostic tests and patient's overall physical status.
- Monitor serum calcium level for precipitous drop. Monitor patient for tetany, carpopedal spasm, Chvostek's sign, and muscle cramps.
- Monitor very carefully for signs of bleeding (hematuria, ecchymosis, petechiae, epistaxis, melena); generalized hemorrhaging is possible. Keep in mind that facial flushing is an early indicator of bleeding.
- Monitor platelet count and prothrombin time.
- Monitor for signs of infection (temperature elevation, sore throat, malaise).
- Monitor LDH, AST (SGOT), ALT (SGPT), alkaline phosphatase, BUN, creatinine, potassium, and phosphorus levels.
- Monitor liver and kidney function daily in patients with preexisting impairment.
- Monitor site for signs of extravasation.

Supportive Care

- Avoid contact with skin or mucous membranes.
- Be aware that therapeutic effect in hypercalcemia may not be seen for 24 to 48 hours; may last 3 to 15 days.
- Be aware that slow infusion reduces nausea that develops with I.V. push.
- Avoid all I.M. injections when the platelet count is below 100,000/mm^3.
- Administer antiemetics, as ordered, before or during infusion of this drug to decrease severe nausea and vomiting.
- If extravasation occurs, stop the infusion and restart it in another area. Apply cold to reduce pain and prevent swelling.
- Provide a safe environment to minimize risk of bleeding.
- If hemorrhage occurs, administer blood transfusion, vitamin K, and corticosteroids, as ordered. Use aminocaproic acid to counteract increased fibrinolytic activity, if indicated.

Patient Teaching

- Warn patient to watch for signs of infection (sore throat, fever, fatigue), and bleeding (easy bruising, nosebleeds, bleeding gums). Tell patient to

take temperature daily and to report signs of infection or bleeding.
• Instruct patient about need for protective measures, including conservation of energy, balanced diet, adequate rest, personal cleanliness, clean environment, and avoidance of exposure to persons with infections.
• Instruct patient about safety precautions to reduce risks of bleeding from falls, cuts, or other injuries.
• Instruct patient about the need for frequent oral hygiene.
• Teach patient to avoid the use of all OTC products containing aspirin.

Evaluation

In patients receiving plicamycin, appropriate evaluation statements may include:
• Patient does not exhibit evidence of local tissue damage.
• Patient does not demonstrate signs and symptoms of infection or bleeding.
• Patient and family state an understanding of plicamycin therapy.

pneumococcal vaccine, polyvalent

(new mo kock´ al)
Pneumovax 23, Pnu-Imune 23

• *Classification:* bacterial vaccine
• *Pregnancy Risk Category:* C

HOW SUPPLIED

Injection: 25 mcg each of 23 polysaccharide isolates/0.5 ml

ACTION

Mechanism: Promotes active immunity to infections caused by *Streptococcus pneumoniae.*
Pharmacokinetics: Unknown.
Onset, peak, duration: Protective antibodies are produced within 3 weeks after injection. The duration of vaccine-induced immunity is at least 5 years in adults.

INDICATIONS & DOSAGE

Pneumococcal immunization–
Adults and children over 2 years: 0.5 ml I.M. or S.C.

Not recommended for children under 2 years.

CONTRAINDICATIONS & PRECAUTIONS

Contraindicated in patients who previously received any polyvalent pneumococcal vaccine and those with a hypersensitivity to any component of the vaccine, such as thimerosal or phenol; in patients with Hodgkin's disease or those who have received extensive chemotherapy or radiation therapy (especially within the last 10 days); and in those with an acute respiratory infection or any active infection. Defer elective immunization during these situations.

ADVERSE REACTIONS

Common reactions are in italics; life-threatening reactions are in bold italics.
Systemic: *slight fever,* ***anaphylaxis.***
Local: soreness; severe, local reaction can occur when revaccination takes place within 3 years.

INTERACTIONS

None significant.

EFFECTS ON DIAGNOSTIC TESTS

None reported.

NURSING CONSIDERATIONS

Besides those related universally to drug therapy (see "How to use this book"), consider the following specific recommendations:

Assessment

• Obtain a baseline assessment of the patient's allergies, immunization history, and immunization reaction before therapy.
• Be alert for adverse reactions and drug interactions throughout therapy.
• Evaluate the patient's and family's

knowledge about pneumococcal vaccine therapy.

Nursing Diagnoses

- Altered protection related to lack of immunity to *Streptococcus pneumoniae.*
- Ineffective breathing pattern related to vaccine-induced anaphylaxis.
- Knowledge deficit related to pneumococcal vaccine.

Planning and Implementation

Preparation and Administration

- Keep refrigerated. Reconstitution or dilution not necessary.
- ***I.M. or S.C. use:*** Inject in deltoid or midlateral thigh.
- Do not give I.V.

Monitoring

- Monitor effectiveness by evaluating the patient's antibody titers to pneumococcal infection.
- Observe the patient for signs of anaphylaxis immediately after immunization.
- Check vital signs.
- Observe the injection site for local reaction.

Supportive Care

- Avoid revaccination within 3 years.
- Keep epinephrine 1:1000 available to treat possible anaphylaxis. Have oxygen and resuscitation equipment nearby.
- Treat fever with antipyretics.
- Vaccine protects against 23 pneumococcal types, which accounts for 90% of pneumococcal disease.

Patient Teaching

- Instruct the patient to report respiratory difficulty immediately.
- Warn the patient to avoid revaccination within 3 years.
- Advise the patient that slight fever and soreness at the injection site may occur after immunization.

Evaluation

In patients receiving pneumococcal vaccine, appropriate evaluation statements may include:

- Patient exhibits active immunity to pneumococcal bacteria.
- Patient demonstrates no signs of anaphylaxis.
- Patient and family state an understanding of pneumococcal vaccine.

poliovirus vaccine, live, oral, trivalent

(poe lee oh vye´ russ)

Orimune

- *Classification:* viral vaccine
- *Pregnancy Risk Category:* C

HOW SUPPLIED

Oral vaccine: mixture of three viruses (types 1, 2, and 3), grown in monkey kidney tissue culture, in 0.5-ml single-dose Dispettes

ACTION

Mechanism: Promotes immunity to poliomyelitis by inducing humoral antibodies and antibodies in the lymphatic tissue surrounding the intestinal tract.

Absorption: Live, attenuated virus multiplies in the lymphatic tissue surrounding the GI tract.

Onset, peak, duration: Antibody response to the presence of virus begins in about 7 days and peaks in about 3 weeks. Virus particles persist in the lymphatic tissue for 4 to 6 weeks. The duration of immunity is thought to be lifelong.

INDICATIONS & DOSAGE

Poliovirus immunization–

Children and nonimmunized adults: two 0.5-ml doses should be administered 8 weeks apart. Give third 0.5-ml dose 6 to 12 months after second dose. A reinforcing dose of 0.5 ml should be given before entry to school.

Infants: administer 0.5-ml dose at age 2 months, 4 months, and 18 months. Optional dose may be given at 6 months.

CONTRAINDICATIONS & PRECAUTIONS

Contraindicated in patients with persistent vomiting or diarrhea, immunodeficiency, or infection or those receiving immunosuppressants; severe debilitation, and severe allergy to sorbitol, streptomycin, or neomycin, components of the vaccine. Household contacts of an immunosuppressed child should not receive trivalent oral poliovirus vaccine.

ADVERSE REACTIONS

Common reactions are in italics; life-threatening reactions are in bold italics.
Systemic: ***paralytic poliomyelitis.***

INTERACTIONS

Immune serum globulin, whole blood, plasma: antibodies in serum may interfere with immune response. Don't use vaccine within 3 months of transfusion.

EFFECTS ON DIAGNOSTIC TESTS

Tuberculin skin test: skin test may be suppressed. Don't test for 6 weeks.

NURSING CONSIDERATIONS

Besides those related universally to drug therapy (see "How to use this book"), consider the following specific recommendations:

Assessment

• Obtain a baseline assessment of the patient's allergies, immunization history, and immunization reaction before therapy.
• Be alert for adverse reactions and drug interactions throughout therapy.
• Evaluate the patient's and family's knowledge about oral poliovirus vaccine therapy.

Nursing Diagnoses

• Altered protection related to lack of immunity to poliovirus.
• High risk for injury related to vaccine-induced paralytic poliomyelitis.
• Knowledge deficit related to trivalent oral poliovirus vaccine.

Planning and Implementation

Preparation and Administration

• Keep frozen until used. Once thawed, if unopened, may store refrigerated up to 30 days. Open vials may be refrigerated up to 7 days. Thaw before administration.
• Color change from pink to yellow does not reduce efficacy of the vaccine. Yellow color results from storage at lower temperatures.
• For P.O. use only. Not for parenteral use.

Monitoring

• Monitor effectiveness by evaluating the patient's antibody titers to poliovirus.
• Monitor neuromuscular status after immunization for signs of vaccine-induced poliomyelitis.
• Check vital signs.

Supportive Care

• Do not give to patients with immunosuppression, cancer, and immunoglobulin abnormalities and in patients undergoing radiation, antimetabolite, alkylating agent, or corticosteroid therapy.
• Defer in acute illness, vomiting, or diarrhea.
• Do not give to infants under 6 weeks.
• Vaccine is not effective in modifying or preventing existing or incubating poliomyelitis.

Patient Teaching

• Instruct the patient or parents to report any neuromuscular changes immediately.
• Inform the patient or parents that the vaccine must be given in two divided doses about 8 weeks apart with a booster a year later and before entry to school.
• Advise the parents of children receiving immunization to check their own immunization history in case a booster is needed.

Evaluation

In patients receiving trivalent oral poliovirus vaccine, appropriate evaluation statements may include:

- Patient exhibits immunity to poliovirus.
- Patient does not demonstrate signs of paralytic poliomyelitis.
- Patient and family state an understanding of poliovirus vaccine therapy.

polyethylene glycol-electrolyte solution

(pol i eth´ eye leen gly´ kol)

CoLyte, Glycoprep‡, GoLYTELY

- *Classification:* bowel preparation (isosmotic solution)
- *Pregnancy Risk Category:* C

HOW SUPPLIED

Powder for oral solution: polyethylene glycol (PEG) 3350 (120 g), sodium sulfate (3.36 g), sodium chloride (2.92 g), potassium chloride (1.49 g) per 2 liters (CoLyte); PEG 3350 (60 g), sodium chloride (1.46 g), potassium chloride (745 mg), sodium bicarbonate (1.68 g), sodium sulfate (5.68 g) per liter (Glycoprep‡); PEG 3350 (236 g), sodium sulfate (22.74 g), sodium bicarbonate (6.74g), sodium chloride (5.86 g), potassium chloride (2.97 g), per 4.8 liter (GoLYTELY)

ACTION

Mechanism: PEG 3350, a nonabsorbable solution, acts as an osmotic agent. Using sodium sulfate as the major sodium source, sodium absorption is greatly reduced.

Absorption: Results in virtually no net absorption or secretion of ions.

Excretion: In the feces.

Onset, peak, duration: Peak effect occurs within 4 hours.

INDICATIONS & DOSAGE

Bowel preparation before GI examination–

Adults: 240 ml P.O. q 10 minutes until 4 liters are consumed. Usually administered 4 hours before examination, allowing 3 hours for drinking and 1 hour for bowel evacuation.

CONTRAINDICATIONS & PRECAUTIONS

Contraindicated in patients with GI obstruction, gastric retention, bowel perforation, toxic colitis, and toxic megacolon or ileus. Use cautiously in patients with impaired gag reflex, unconscious or semiconscious patients or patients prone to vomiting.

ADVERSE REACTIONS

Common reactions are in italics; life-threatening reactions are in bold italics.

GI: *nausea, bloating, cramps, vomiting.*

INTERACTIONS

None significant.

EFFECTS ON DIAGNOSTIC TESTS

None reported.

NURSING CONSIDERATIONS

Besides those related universally to drug therapy (see "How to use this book"), consider the following specific recommendations:

Assessment

- Obtain a baseline assessment of history of bowel disorder and gastrointestinal status.
- Be alert for adverse reactions and drug interactions throughout therapy.
- Evaluate the patient's and family's knowledge about polyethylene glycol-electrolyte solution therapy.

Nursing Diagnoses

- High risk for injury related to underlying GI condition warranting bowel preparation.
- Pain related to polyethylene glycol-

electrolyte solution–induced abdominal cramping.
• Knowledge deficit related to polyethylene glycol-electrolyte solution therapy.

Planning and Implementation

Preparation and Administration
• Patient should fast for 3 to 4 hours before taking solution, and thereafter ingest only clear liquids until the examination is complete.
• Use tap water to reconstitute powder. Shake vigorously to ensure that all the powder is dissolved. Reconstituted solution may be refrigerated but should be used within 48 hours.
• Do not add flavoring or additional ingredients to the solution, and do not administer the solution chilled. Hypothermia has been reported after ingestion of large amounts of chilled solution.
• Administer solution in the early morning if the patient is scheduled for a mid-morning exam. Solution induces a diarrhea (onset, 30 to 60 minutes) that rapidly cleanses the bowel, usually within 4 hours.
• Administer to patients for barium enema the evening before the examination. Solution may interfere with the barium coating of the colonic mucosa.

Monitoring
• Monitor effectiveness by observing for the presence of diarrhea and the emptying of the bowel.
• Auscultate bowel sounds at least once a shift. Assess for pain, cramping, and abdominal distention.
• Monitor for nausea and vomiting.

Supportive Care
• Do not give to patients with GI obstruction or perforation, gastric retention, toxic colitis, or toxic megacolon or ileus.
• Use with caution in semiconscious patients or patients with impaired gag reflex. Take care to prevent aspiration.
• No major shifts in fluid and electrolyte balance have been reported.
• Provide privacy for elimination.

Patient Teaching
• Instruct the patient to fast 3 to 4 hours before taking the solution.
• Explain to the patient that 1 full glass (8 oz) of the solution must be taken every 10 minutes until 4 liters are consumed.
• Warn the patient that cramping, distension, and nausea may occur, but that they will subside as the bowel empties.

Evaluation

In patients receiving polyethylene glycol-electrolyte solution, appropriate evaluation statements may include:
• Patient reports emptying of the bowel.
• Patient is free from abdominal cramping.
• Patient and family state an understanding of polyethylene glycol-electrolyte solution therapy.

polymyxin B sulfate (systemic)

(pol i mix´ in)
Aerosporin

• *Classification:* antibiotic
• *Pregnancy Risk Category:* B

HOW SUPPLIED

Powder for injection: 500,000-unit vials

ACTION

Mechanism: Hinders bacterial cell wall synthesis, damaging the bacterial plasma membrane and making the cell more vulnerable to osmotic pressure.
Absorption: Not significantly absorbed from the GI tract in adults; infants may absorb up to 10% of a dose.
Distribution: With systemic adminis-

tration, drug is distributed widely except in CSF, aqueous humor, and placental and synovial fluids; minimally bound to plasma proteins.
Excretion: About 60% of dose is excreted renally. Half-life: 4 to 6 hours in patients with normal renal function; 2 to 3 days in patients with creatinine clearance below 10 ml/minute.
Onset, peak, duration: With I.M. administration, peak serum levels occur in 2 hours.

INDICATIONS & DOSAGE

Acute urinary tract infections or septicemia caused by sensitive Pseudomonas aeruginosa, *or when other antibiotics are ineffective or contraindicated; bacteremia caused by sensitive* Enterobacter aerogenes *and* Klebsiella pneumoniae, *or acute urinary tract infections caused by* Escherichia coli –
Adults and children: 15,000 to 25,000 units/kg daily I.V. infusion, divided q 12 hours; or 25,000 to 30,000 units/kg daily, divided q 4 to 8 hours. I.M. not advised due to severe pain at injection site.
Meningitis caused by sensitive P. aeruginosa *or* Hemophilus influenzae *when other antibiotics are ineffective or contraindicated–*
Adults and children over 2 years: 50,000 units intrathecally once daily for 3 to 4 days, then 50,000 units every other day for at least 2 weeks after cerebrospinal fluid tests are negative and cerebrospinal fluid sugar is normal.
Children under 2 years: 20,000 units intrathecally once daily for 3 to 4 days, then 25,000 units every other day for at least 2 weeks after cerebrospinal fluid tests are negative and cerebrospinal fluid sugar is normal.

CONTRAINDICATIONS & PRECAUTIONS

Contraindicated in patients with hypersensitivity to the drug. Use cautiously in patients with such neuromuscular diseases as myasthenia gravis because drug's neuromuscular blockade may exacerbate symptoms.

ADVERSE REACTIONS

Common reactions are in italics; life-threatening reactions are in bold italics.
CNS: irritability, drowsiness, facial flushing, weakness, ataxia, respiratory paralysis, headache and meningeal irritation with intrathecal administration, peripheral and perioral paresthesias, ***seizures, coma.***
EENT: blurred vision.
GU: ***nephrotoxicity*** (albuminuria, cylindruria, hematuria, proteinuria, decreased urine output, increased BUN).
Skin: urticaria.
Local: *pain at I.M. injection site.*
Other: hypersensitivity reactions with fever, ***anaphylaxis.***

INTERACTIONS

Aminoglycosides, amphotericin B, cisplatin, vancomycin, zidovudine: increased risk of nephrotoxicity.
Neuromuscular blocking agents: polymyxin B may potentiate neuromuscular blockade.

EFFECTS ON DIAGNOSTIC TESTS

BUN and serum creatinine levels: increased.
CSF protein and leukocyte levels: increased during intrathecal therapy.

NURSING CONSIDERATIONS

Besides those related universally to drug therapy (see "How to use this book"), consider the following specific recommendations:
Assessment
• Obtain a baseline assessment of infection before therapy.

• Be alert for adverse reactions and drug interactions throughout therapy.
• Evaluate the patient's and family's knowledge about polymyxin B sulfate therapy.

Nursing Diagnoses

• High risk for injury related to ineffectiveness of polymyxin B sulfate to eradicate the infection.
• Altered urinary elimination related to polymyxin B sulfate induced nephrotoxicity.
• Knowledge deficit related to polymyxin B sulfate.

Planning and Implementation

Preparation and Administration

• Obtain specimen for culture and sensitivity tests before first dose. Therapy may begin pending test results.
• Obtain specimens to evaluate renal function as ordered before administering the first dose
• ***I.M. use:*** Administer drug I.M. only when absolutely necessary because severe pain may occur at injection site. Give deep I.M. If patient isn't allergic to procaine, use 1% procaine (if hospital policy permits) as diluent to decrease pain. Rotate sites.
• ***I.V. use:*** Dilute each 500,000 units in 300 to 500 ml dextrose 5% in water; infuse over 60 to 90 minutes. Reconstituted solution should be refrigerated and used within 72 hours.

Monitoring

• Monitor effectiveness by regularly assessing for improvement in the infection.
• Monitor I.V. site daily for phlebitis and irritation.
• Monitor renal function including intake/output as ordered.

Supportive Care

• When administering I.V. change sites regularly to minimize risk of phlebitis and irritation.
• Encourage patient to drink enough fluid to maintain output at 1,500 ml/day (between 3,000 and 4,000 ml/day for adults).
• If patient is scheduled for surgery, notify anesthesiologist of preoperative treatment with this drug because it may prolong neuromuscular blockade.
• Notify doctor immediately if patient develops fever, CNS adverse effects, rash, or symptoms of nephrotoxicity.

Patient Teaching

• Warn the patient receiving the drug I.M. that it may cause pain at the injection site.
• Tell the patient to alert the nurse if pain or discomfort occurs at the site of I.V. injection, if prescribed.
• Tell the patient to drink at least 3,000 to 4,000 ml/day of fluid to maintain adequate output. Teach the patient how to measure his intake/output and to notify doctor if output is less than 1,500 ml/day despite adequate intake.

Evaluation

In patients receiving polymyxin B sulfate, appropriate evaluation statements may include:
• Patient is free from infection.
• Patient's maintains normal renal function throughout polymyxin B sulfate therapy.
• Patient and family state an understanding of polymyxin B sulfate therapy.

polymyxin B sulfate (ophthalmic)

(pol i mix′ in B)

• *Classification:* antibiotic (polymyxin)
• *Pregnancy Risk Category:* B

HOW SUPPLIED

Ophthalmic sterile powder for solution: 500,000-unit vials to be reconstituted to 20 to 50 ml

ACTION

Mechanism: Binds to phosphate groups of lipids within the cell wall of susceptible bacteria. Acts like a cationic detergent, causing leakage of essential cellular components. Bactericidal.

Absorption: No absorption after topical ophthalmic administration. Drug is not absorbed from conjunctival sac and does not penetrate into the aqueous humor. Also not absorbed from skin.

INDICATIONS & DOSAGE

Used alone or in combination with other agents for treating corneal ulcers resulting from Pseudomonas *infection or other gram-negative organism infections–*

Adults and children: instill 1 to 3 drops of 0.1% to 0.25% (10,000 to 25,000 units/ml) q 1 hour. Increase interval according to patient response; or up to 10,000 units subconjunctivally daily by doctor. Do not exceed 2,000,000 units daily.

CONTRAINDICATIONS & PRECAUTIONS

Contraindicated in patients with hypersensitivity to the drug.

ADVERSE REACTIONS

Common reactions are in italics; life-threatening reactions are in bold italics.

Eye: eye irritation, conjunctivitis.

Other: overgrowth of nonsusceptible organisms, hypersensitivity (local burning, itching).

INTERACTIONS

None significant.

EFFECTS ON DIAGNOSTIC TESTS

BUN and serum creatinine: increased levels.

CSF protein and leukocytes: increased levels.

NURSING CONSIDERATIONS

Besides those related universally to drug therapy (see "How to use this book"), consider the following specific recommendations:

Assessment

- Obtain a baseline assessment of the patient's allergies before therapy.
- Be alert for adverse reactions and drug interactions throughout therapy.
- Evaluate the patient's and family's knowledge about ophthalmic polymyxin B sulfate therapy.

Nursing Diagnoses

- Altered protection related to ocular infection.
- High risk for infection related to polymyxin B sulfate–induced overgrowth of nonsusceptible organisms.
- Knowledge deficit related to ophthalmic polymyxin B sulfate therapy.

Planning and Implementation

Preparation and Administration

- Reconstitute carefully to ensure the correct drug concentration in solution.
- Wash hands before and after administration.
- Clean the eye area of excess exudate before administration.
- In severe life-threatening *Pseudomonas* infections, polymyxin B sulfate is also administered as an ocular irrigant.

Monitoring

- Monitor effectiveness by culturing the eye to check for microorganisms.
- Observe the amount, color, and consistency of exudate.
- Check the patient's vision.

Supportive Care

- Apply warm, moist compresses to aid the removal of dried exudate.
- Use safety precautions if vision is impaired. Assist with activities.
- One of the most effective antibiotics against gram-negative organisms, especially *Pseudomonas.* Often used in combination with neomycin sulfate.

Patient Teaching

- Teach the patient how to instill the drops. Advise him to wash hands before and after administration. Warn him not to touch tip of dropper to

eye or surrounding tissue.
• Instruct the patient to apply light finger pressure to the lacrimal sac for 1 minute after the drops have been instilled. Warn him to avoid rubbing or scratching the eye area.
• Instruct the patient to watch for signs of hypersensitivity (itching lids, swelling, constant burning). If any of these signs occur, tell the patient to stop taking the drug and call the doctor immediately.
• Warn the patient to avoid sharing washcloths and towels with family members during infection.
• Instruct the patient not to share eye medications with family members. A family member who develops the same symptoms should contact the doctor.

Evaluation

In patients receiving ophthalmic polymyxin B sulfate, appropriate evaluation statements may include:
• Patient remains free from signs and symptoms of infection.
• Patient does not exhibit signs of polymyxin B sulfate–induced overgrowth of nonsusceptible organisms.
• Patient and family state an understanding of ophthalmic polymyxin B sulfate therapy.

potassium supplements
(poe tass´ e um)

• *Classification:* agent for electrolyte balance (potassium)

potassium acetate

potassium bicarbonate
K+Care ET, Klor-Con/EF

potassium chloride
K+10, K+Care, Kaochlor 10%*, Kaochlor S-F 10%*, Kaon-Cl, Kaon-Cl 20%*, Kato Powder, Kay Ciel*, K-Lease, K-Lor, Klor-10%*, Klor-Con, Klorvess, Klotrix, K-Lyte/Cl , K-Tab, Micro-K Extencaps, SK-Potassium Chloride, Slow-K, Ten-K

potassium gluconate
Kaon Liquid*, Kaon Tablets, Kayliker*, K-G Elixir*, Potassium Rougier†

• *Classification:* agent for electrolyte balance (potassium)
• *Pregnancy Risk Category:* A

HOW SUPPLIED

potassium acetate
Injection: 2 mEq/ml in 20-ml, 30-ml vials.
potassium bicarbonate
Effervescent tablets: 25 mEq
potassium chloride
Tablets: 1.22 mEq (99 mg), 8 mEq (600 mg), 10 mEq (750 mg), 20 mEq (1,500 mg), 25 mEq (1,875 mg)
Tablets (controlled-release): 6.7 mEq (500 mg), 8 mEq (600 mg), 10 mEq (750 mg), 20 mEq (1,500 mg)
Tablets (enteric-coated): 4 mEq (300 mg), 13.4 mEq (1,000 mg)
Capsules (controlled-release): 8 mEq (600 mg), 10 mEq (750 mg)
Oral liquid: 5% (10 mEq/15 ml), 7.5% (15 mEq/15 ml), 10% (20 mEq/15 ml), 15% (30 mEq/15 ml), 20% (40 mEq/15 ml)
Powder for oral use: 15 mEq/packet, 20 mEq/packet, 25 mEq/packet, 25 mEq/dose
Injection: 20 mEq, 40 mEq ampules; additive syringes containing 30 mEq or 40 mEq; 10 mEq, 20 mEq, 30 mEq, 40 mEq, 45 mEq, 60 mEq, 100 mEq, 200 mEq, 400 mEq, or 1,000 mEq vials.
potassium gluconate
Tablets: 500 mg (2mEq K^+), 1,170 mg (5 mEq K^+)†
Elixir: 4.68 g (20 mEq K^+)/15 ml*

ACTION

Mechanism: Primarily an intracellular cation, potassium influences the conduction and maintenance of the

*Liquid form contains alcohol. **May contain tartrazine.

electrical potential of excitable cells. Potassium salts are soluble forms of potassium used to maintain serum potassium levels.
Absorption: Well absorbed from the GI tract.
Distribution: The normal serum levels of potassium range from 3.8 to 5 mEq/liter. Plasma potassium concentrations up to 7.7 mEq/liter may be normal in neonates. Up to 60 mEq/liter of potassium may be found in gastric secretions and diarrhea fluid.
Metabolism: None significant.
Excretion: Largely by the kidneys. Small amounts may be excreted via the skin and intestinal tract, but intestinal potassium usually is reabsorbed. A healthy patient on a potassium-free diet will excrete 40 to 50 mEq of potassium daily.

INDICATIONS & DOSAGE

Potassium replacement–
I.V. potassium acetate, potassium chloride, or potassium gluconate should be used for life-threatening hypokalemia or when oral replacement not feasible. Give no more than 20 mEq hourly in concentration of 40 mEq/liter or less. Total 24-hour dosage should not exceed 150 mEq (3 mEq/kg in children). Potassium replacement should be done with ECG monitoring and frequent serum potassium determinations.
Prevention of hypokalemia–
Adults: dosage is individualized according to patient's needs. In most cases, dosage should not exceed 150 mEq/day.

Administer potassium acetate, potassium chloride, or potassium gluconate as an additive to I.V. infusions. Usual dose is 40 mEq/liter, and solutions are usually infused at a rate not to exceed 20 mEq/hour. Alternatively, administer oral potassium supplements
potassium bicarbonate
Adults: 25 to 50 mEq dissolved in ½ to a full glass of water (120 to 240 ml) once daily to q.i.d.
potassium chloride
Adults: 15 to 25 mEq dissolved in ½ to a full glass of water (120 to 240 ml) once daily to q.i.d.; or 1 to 25 mEq tablet, capsule, or controlled-release preparation P.O. daily.
potassium gluconate
Adults: 2 to 20 mEq P.O. daily.
potassium acetate
Adults: individualize dose. Usual dose should not exceed 3 mEq/kg/day. Administer as an additive to I.V. infusions.
potassium chloride
Adults: individualize dose. Usual dose should not exceed 3 mEq/kg/day.

CONTRAINDICATIONS & PRECAUTIONS

Contraindicated in patients with severe renal impairment, oliguria, anuria, or azotemia (unless patient is hypokalemic); hyperkalemia from any cause; untreated Addison's disease because of the potential for hyperkalemia; acute dehydration; or heat cramps because administration of potassium can worsen these conditions. Also contraindicated with potassium-sparing diuretics, unless patients are routinely monitored.

Use cautiously (particularly I.V.) in patients with cardiac disease, renal disease, or acidosis; conduct careful analysis of the acid-base balance, and monitor serum electrolytes, ECG, and clinical status of the patient. Acidosis can raise serum potassium levels to the normal range even when total body potassium is reduced.

ADVERSE REACTIONS

Common reactions are in italics; life-threatening reactions are in bold italics.
Signs of hyperkalemia:
CNS: paresthesias of the extremities, listlessness, mental confusion, weak-

ness or heaviness of legs, flaccid paralysis.
CV: ***peripheral vascular collapse with fall in blood pressure, cardiac arrhythmias, heart block, possible cardiac arrest,*** ECG changes (prolonged P-R intervals; wide QRS complex; ST segment depression; tall, tented T waves).
GI: nausea, vomiting, abdominal pain, diarrhea, bowel ulceration.
GU: oliguria.
Skin: cold skin, gray pallor.

INTERACTIONS

Anticholinergics, opiates, drugs that decrease GI motility: increased risk of GI ulceration from certain orally administered controlled or delayed release forms of potassium. Avoid concomitant use.

EFFECTS ON DIAGNOSTIC TESTS

None reported.

NURSING CONSIDERATIONS

Besides those related universally to drug therapy (see "How to use this book"), consider the following specific recommendations:

Assessment

- Obtain a baseline assessment of patient's potassium level before therapy.
- Be alert for adverse reactions and drug interactions throughout therapy.
- Evaluate the patient's and family's knowledge about potassium therapy.

Nursing Diagnoses

- Altered nutrition: Less than body requirements related to the patient's underlying condition.
- High risk for injury related to potassium-induced hyperkalemia.
- Knowledge deficit related to potassium therapy.

Planning and Implementation

Preparation and Administration

- Be aware that dosage is individualized according to the patient's needs.
- ***P.O. use:*** Dissolve effervescent tablets in 6 to 8 ounces of cold water. Dissolve completely to minimize GI irritation. Have patient take with meals and sip slowly over a 5- to 10-minute period.
- Potassium acetate is available in lime and orange flavors. Check for patient's flavor preference.
- ***I.V. use:*** Give as an infusion only through a large-bore needle; never give I.V. push or I.M. Give slowly as diluted solution; potentially fatal hyperkalemia may result from too-rapid infusion. Total 24-hour dosage should not exceed 150 mEq (3 mEq/kg in children).
- Never administer potassium postoperatively until urine flow is established.

Monitoring

- Monitor effectiveness by evaluating patient's serum potassium level regularly.
- Monitor ECG, renal function, intake/output, serum electrolytes, and creatinine and BUN levels during therapy.
- Monitor infusion site for redness.
- Monitor patient for signs of GI ulceration: obstruction, hemorrhage, pain, distention, severe vomiting, and bleeding.
- Monitor patient for signs and symptoms of hyperkalemia.

Supportive Care

- Withhold drug and notify doctor if hyperkalemia occurs. Be prepared to provide emergency supportive care until potassium level returns to normal.
- Change I.V. site at first sign of irritation.

Patient Teaching

- Teach patient the signs and symptoms of hyperkalemia and tell patient to notify doctor if present.
- Tell patient to notify the nurse if discomfort or pain is felt at the I.V. site.

Evaluation
In patients receiving potassium, appropriate evaluation statements may include:
- Patient's potassium level is normal.
- Patient does not experience hyperkalemia during potassium therapy.
- Patient and family state an understanding of potassium therapy.

potassium iodide
(poe tass´ e yum)
Pima

potassium iodide, saturated solution (SSKI)

strong iodine solution (Lugol's solution)

- *Classification:* antihyperthyroid agent, expectorant (electrolyte)
- *Pregnancy Risk Category:* D

HOW SUPPLIED
potassium iodide
Tablets (enteric-coated): 300 mg
Oral solution: 500 mg/15 ml
Syrup: 325 mg/5 ml
potassium iodide, saturated solution
Oral solution: 1 g/ml
strong iodine solution
Oral solution: iodine 50 mg/ml and potassium iodide 100 mg/ml

ACTION
Mechanism: Increases production of respiratory tract fluids to help liquefy and reduce the viscosity of thick secretions. Inhibits thyroid hormone formation by blocking synthesis of iodotyrosine and iodothyronine. It also limits iodide transport into the thyroid gland and blocks thyroid hormone release.
Absorption: Absorbed from the GI tract.
Distribution: Iodine concentrates within the thyroid gland.
Onset, peak, duration: Effects of the drug on thyroid function are usually evident within 24 hours, and effects peak after about 15 days of continued therapy.

INDICATIONS & DOSAGE
As expectorant, chronic bronchitis, chronic pulmonary emphysema, bronchial asthma –
Adults: 0.3 to 0.6 ml P.O. q 4 to 6 hours.
Children: 0.25 to 0.5 ml P.O. of saturated solution (1 g/ml) b.i.d. to q.i.d.
Preparation for thyroidectomy–
Adults and children: Strong Iodine Solution, USP, 0.1 to 0.3 ml P.O. t.i.d., or Potassium Iodide Solution, USP, 5 drops in water P.O. t.i.d. after meals for 2 to 3 weeks before surgery.
Thyrotoxic crisis–
Adults and children: Strong Iodine Solution, USP, 1 ml in water P.O. t.i.d. after meals.
Nuclear radiation protection–
Adults and children: 0.13 ml P.O. of SSKI immediately before or after initial exposure will block 90% of radioactive iodine. Same dose given 3 to 4 hours after exposure will provide 50% block. Should be administered for up to 10 days under medical supervision.
Infants under 1 year: ½ adult dose.

CONTRAINDICATIONS & PRECAUTIONS
Contraindicated in patients with hypersensitivity to iodides or iodine and during pregnancy because abnormal thyroid and goiter may occur. Use cautiously in patients with hyperkalemia, acute bronchitis, or tuberculosis; in children with cystic fibrosis because they are especially susceptible to the goitrogenic effects of iodides; and in iodide-sensitive hyperthyroid patients because of goitrogenic potential. Prolonged use of potassium iodide may cause hypothyroidism.

ADVERSE REACTIONS

Common reactions are in italics; life-threatening reactions are in bold italics.

GI: *nausea,* vomiting, *epigastric pain,* metallic taste.

Metabolic: goiter, hyperthyroid adenoma, hypothyroidism (with excessive use), collagen disease-like syndrome.

Skin: rash.

Other: drug fever.

Prolonged use: chronic iodine poisoning, soreness of mouth, coryza, sneezing, swelling of eyelids.

INTERACTIONS

Lithium carbonate: may cause hypothyroidism. Don't use together.

EFFECTS ON DIAGNOSTIC TESTS

Thyroid function tests: altered results.

NURSING CONSIDERATIONS

Besides those related universally to drug therapy (see "How to use this book"), consider the following specific recommendations:

Assessment

• Obtain a baseline assessment of the patient's cough and sputum production before initiating therapy.
• Be alert for adverse reactions and drug interactions throughout therapy.
• Evaluate the patient's and family's knowledge about potassium iodide therapy.

Nursing Diagnoses

• Ineffective airway clearance related to the patient's underlying condition.
• Pain (epigastric) related to potassium iodide–induced adverse GI effects.
• Knowledge deficit related to potassium iodide therapy.

Planning and Implementation

Preparation and Administration

• ***P.O. use:*** Dilute with milk, fruit juice, or broth to reduce GI distress and disguise taste. Potassium iodide has a strong salty, metallic taste.

Monitoring

• Monitor effectiveness by evaluating regularly the patient's cough and sputum production and his general respiratory status.
• Monitor hydration status; record intake and output.
• Observe the patient for epigastric pain, which may occur as an adverse reaction to this drug.

Supportive Care

• Provide the patient with the necessary tissues and waste receptacles for disposing of expectorated respiratory secretions.
• Provide for good oral hygiene for the patient receiving potassium iodide.
• Obtain an order for an antiemetic, as needed.
• Notify doctor if skin rash or other hypersensitivity reaction develops, because this may require stopping the drug.
• Notify the doctor if epigastric pain occurs. If severe, he may discontinue the drug.
• Expect the drug to be withdrawn gradually. Sudden withdrawal may precipitate thyroid storm.

Patient Teaching

• Tell the patient to avoid sources of respiratory irritants such as fumes, smoke, and dust.
• Encourage deep-breathing exercises.
• Tell the patient to increase fluid intake to at least 8 full (8-oz) glasses of fluid per 24 hours, if not contraindicated.

Evaluation

In patients receiving potassium iodide, appropriate evaluation statements may include:

• Patient's lungs are clear and respiratory secretions and cough are decreased.
• Patient tolerates therapy free of pain.
• Patient and family state an understanding of potassium iodide therapy.

pralidoxime chloride (pyridine-2-aldoxime methochloride; 2-PAM)

(pra li dox´ eem)
Protopam Chloride

- *Classification:* antidote (quaternary ammonium oxime)
- *Pregnancy Risk Category:* C

HOW SUPPLIED

Tablets: 500 mg
Injection: 1-g/20-ml vial without diluent or syringe; 1-g/20-ml vial with diluent, syringe, needle, alcohol swab (emergency kit); 600-mg/2-ml auto-injector, parenteral

ACTION

Mechanism: Reactives cholinesterase that has been inactivated by organophosphorus pesticides and related compounds. It permits degradation of accumulated acetylcholine and facilitates normal functioning of neuromuscular junctions.
Absorption: Variably and incompletely absorbed after oral administration.
Distribution: Throughout the extracellular water; not appreciably bound to plasma protein; does not readily pass into the CNS. Distribution into breast milk is unknown. Therapeutic concentrations are achieved in the eye after subconjunctival injection.
Metabolism: Exact mechanism is unknown, but hepatic metabolism is considered likely.
Excretion: Rapidly excreted in urine as unchanged drug and metabolite; 80% to 90% of I.V. or I.M. dose is excreted unchanged within 12 hours.
Onset, peak, duration: Peak plasma levels in 2 to 3 hours. After I.V. administration, peak plasma levels are reached in 5 to 15 minutes; after I.M., in 10 to 20 minutes.

INDICATIONS & DOSAGE

Antidote for organophosphate poisoning–
Adults: I.V. infusion of 1 to 2 g in 100 ml of saline solution over 15 to 30 minutes. If pulmonary edema is present, give drug by slow I.V. push over 5 minutes. Repeat in 1 hour if muscle weakness persists. Additional doses may be given cautiously. I.M. or S.C. injection can be used if I.V. is not feasible; or 1 to 3 g P.O. q 5 hours.
Children: 20 to 40 mg/kg I.V.
To treat cholinergic crisis in myasthenia gravis–
Adults: 1 to 2 g I.V., followed by increments of 250 mg I.V. q 5 minutes.

CONTRAINDICATIONS & PRECAUTIONS

Use cautiously in patients with myasthenia gravis who are receiving anticholinesterase agents because drug may precipitate a myasthenic crisis; and in patients with impaired renal function because accumulation of drug and metabolites may occur. Reduced dosage may be advisable in these patients. Use with extreme caution in renal insufficiency, asthma, or peptic ulcer.

ADVERSE REACTIONS

Common reactions are in italics; life-threatening reactions are in bold italics.
CNS: dizziness, headache, drowsiness, excitement, and manic behavior following recovery of consciousness.
CV: tachycardia.
EENT: blurred vision, diplopia, impaired accommodation, ***laryngospasm.***
GI: nausea.
Other: muscular weakness, muscle rigidity, hyperventilation.

INTERACTIONS

None significant.

EFFECTS ON DIAGNOSTIC TESTS

AST (SGOT), ALT (SGPT): return to normal in 2 weeks.
Creatine phosphokinase: transiently elevated levels.

NURSING CONSIDERATIONS

Besides those related universally to drug therapy (see "How to use this book"), consider the following specific recommendations:

Assessment
• Obtain a baseline assessment of medical history, chronology of poisoning, and serum cholinesterase levels before therapy.
• Be alert for adverse reactions and drug interactions throughout therapy.
• Evaluate the patient's and family's knowledge about pralidoxime therapy.

Nursing Diagnoses
• Ineffective breathing pattern related to organophosphate poisoning.
• Altered thought processes related to pralidoxime-induced manic behavior.
• Knowledge deficit related to pralidoxime therapy.

Planning and Implementation
Preparation and Administration
• Dilute with sterile water without preservative.
• ***I.V. use:*** Administer slowly, over at least 5 minutes, as a diluted solution.
• Give atropine I.V. 2 to 4 mg along with pralidoxime if cyanosis is not present. If cyanosis is present, atropine should be given I.M. Give atropine every 5 to 6 minutes until signs and symptoms of atropine toxicity appear (flushing, tachycardia, dry mouth, blurred vision, delirium, and hallucination); maintain atropinization for at least 48 hours.
Monitoring
• Monitor effectiveness by assessing the patient for improved respiratory status and serum cholinesterase levels.
• Monitor respiratory status, vital signs, intake and output, and mental status closely.
• Observe for development of atropine toxicity. Continue close monitoring for 48 to 72 hours after ingestion of poison. Difficult to distinguish between toxic effects of atropine and pralidoxime. Delayed absorption may occur from lower bowel.
Supportive Care
• Do not give in poisoning with Sevin, a carbamate insecticide, since it increases the drug's toxicity.
• Patients with myasthenia gravis treated for overdose of cholinergic drugs should be observed closely for signs of rapid weakening. These patients can pass quickly from cholinergic crisis to myasthenic crisis, and require more cholinergic drugs to treat the myasthenia. Keep edrophonium (Tensilon) available in such situations for establishing differential diagnosis.
• Use only in hospitalized patients. Give as soon as possible after ingestion of poison. Treatment is most effective if initiated within 24 hours of exposure.
• Have oxygen, suction, gastric lavage, and resuscitation equipment available. Initial measures include removal of secretions, maintenance of patent airway, and artificial ventilation if needed.
• After dermal exposure to organophosphate, remove patient's clothing and wash skin and hair with sodium bicarbonate soap, water and alcohol as soon as possible. A second washing may be necessary.
• Wear protective gloves and clothing while washing patient to avoid exposure.
• Use safety precautions for patients who develop manic behavior. Patient should be supervised at all times.
• Be aware that the drug relieves paralysis of respiratory muscles but is less effective in relieving depression of the respiratory center.
• Not effective against poisoning due

to phosphorous, inorganic phosphates, or organophosphates without anticholinesterase activity.

• Be aware that still unapproved subconjunctival injection of pralidoxime has been used to reverse ocular reactions resulting from splashing into the eye or systemic overdosage of organophosphates.

Patient Teaching

• Instruct the patient to report respiratory difficulty immediately.

• Caution patients treated for organophosphate poisoning to avoid contact with insecticides for several weeks.

• Encourage the proper storage of medications and hazardous substances to avoid accidental poisoning.

Evaluation

In patients receiving pralidoxime chloride, appropriate evaluation statements may include:

• Patient maintains patent and effective airway.

• Patient remains free from altered thought processes related to pralidoxime treatment.

• Patient and family state an understanding of pralidoxime chloride therapy.

---

prazepam

(pra´ ze pam)

Centrax

• Controlled Substance Schedule IV
• *Classification:* anxiolytic (benzodiazepine)
• *Pregnancy Risk Category:* C

HOW SUPPLIED

Tablets: 10 mg
Capsules: 5 mg, 10 mg, 20 mg

ACTION

Mechanism: Depresses the CNS at the limbic and subcortical levels of the brain.

Absorption: When administered orally, prazepam is well absorbed through the GI tract; undergoes nearly complete first-pass metabolism to desmethyldiazepam after absorption.

Distribution: Widely distributed throughout the body. Drug is 85% to 95% protein-bound.

Metabolism: In the liver to desmethyldiazepam and oxazepam.

Excretion: Metabolites are excreted in urine as glucuronide conjugates. Half-life: Of desmethyldiazepam is from 30 to 200 hours, and oxazepam is from 5 to 15 hours.

Onset, peak, duration: Peak levels occur in 2½ to 6 hours.

INDICATIONS & DOSAGE

Anxiety–

Adults: 20 to 60 mg P.O. daily in divided dose, or 20 mg h.s.

CONTRAINDICATIONS & PRECAUTIONS

Contraindicated in patients with hypersensitivity to the drug; in those with acute narrow-angle glaucoma or untreated open-angle glaucoma, because of the drug's possible anticholinergic effect; in patients in coma, because the drug's hypnotic or hypotensive effect may be prolonged or intensified; and in patients with acute alcohol intoxication who have depressed vital signs, because the drug will worsen CNS depression.

Use cautiously in patients with psychoses, because the drug is rarely beneficial in such patients and may induce paradoxical reactions; with myasthenia gravis or Parkinson's disease, because it may exacerbate the disorder; or impaired renal or hepatic function, which prolongs elimination of the drug; in elderly or debilitated patients, who are usually more sensitive to the drug's CNS effects; and in individuals prone to addiction or drug abuse.

ADVERSE REACTIONS

Common reactions are in italics; life-threatening reactions are in bold italics.
CNS: *drowsiness, lethargy, hangover,* dizziness, ataxia, fainting.
CV: transient hypotension.
GI: dry mouth, nausea, vomiting, abdominal discomfort.
Skin: rash.

INTERACTIONS

Alcohol, other CNS depressants: increased CNS depression. Avoid concomitant use.
Cimetidine: increased sedation. Monitor carefully.

EFFECTS ON DIAGNOSTIC TESTS

EEG: minor changes (usually low-voltage, fast activity) during and after therapy.
Liver function tests: elevated results.

NURSING CONSIDERATIONS

Besides those related universally to drug therapy (see "How to use this book"), consider the following specific recommendations:

Assessment

- Obtain a baseline assessment of the patient's anxiety before drug therapy.
- Be alert for adverse drug reactions and drug interactions throughout prazepam therapy.
- Evaluate the patient's and family's knowledge about prazepam therapy.

Nursing Diagnoses

- Anxiety related to the patient's underlying condition.
- High risk for injury related to adverse CNS reactions to prazepam.
- Knowledge deficit related to prazepam therapy.

Planning and Implementation

Preparation and Administration

- Dosage should be reduced in elderly or debilitated patients who may be more susceptible to adverse CNS reactions to the drug.

Monitoring

- Frequently check patient's vital signs for hypotension.
- Regularly monitor effectiveness by asking the patient about feelings of anxiety and by observing the patient's behavior.
- Monitor for adverse reactions by checking the degree of dry mouth.
- Observe for excessive sedation due to potentiation with other CNS drugs.

Supportive Care

- Provide frequent sips of water or ice chips for dry mouth.
- If drowsiness, light-headedness, lethargy, ataxia, or fainting occurs, institute safety measures, such as supervising patient activities. Reorient patient as needed and ensure a safe environment.
- Be aware that drug should not be prescribed for everyday stress.
- Do not withdraw drug abruptly. Abuse or addiction is possible and withdrawal symptoms may occur.
- Provide additional fluids if the patient develops nausea and vomiting.

Patient Teaching

- Suggest sugarless hard candy, ice chips, or sugarless chewing gum to relieve dry mouth.
- Warn the patient not to combine drug with alcohol or other CNS depressants and to avoid driving and other hazardous activities that require alertness and psychomotor coordination until adverse CNS effects of the drug are known.
- Warn the patient against giving medication to others.
- Warn the patient to take this drug only as directed and not to discontinue taking it without the doctor's approval. Inform the patient of the drug's potential for dependence if taken longer than directed.
- Advise the patient to notify the doctor if he develops a rash.

Evaluation
In patients receiving prazepam, appropriate evaluation statements may include:
• Patient states he is less anxious.
• Patient does not experience injury as a result of adverse CNS reactions.
• Patient and family state an understanding of prazepam therapy.

praziquantel
(pray zi kwon´ tel)
Biltricide

• *Classification:* anthelmintic (pyrazinoisoquinoline)
• *Pregnancy Risk Category:* B

HOW SUPPLIED
Tablets: 600 mg

ACTION
Mechanism: Kills schistosomes by a specific effect on the permeability of the cell membrane. This results in contraction and paralysis of the parasite's muscles, freeing them from their attachment sites.
Absorption: About 80% of praziquantel is absorbed.
Distribution: Not well documented; however, CSF levels are approximately 19% to 20% of plasma levels.
Metabolism: Significant first pass metabolism to hydroxylated metabolites in the liver.
Excretion: Drug is excreted in urine primarily as metabolites; also excreted in breast milk, reaching concentration levels about 25% of maternal serum levels. Half-life: Of parent drug, about 1 to 1½ hours; of metabolite, 4 to 5 hours.
Onset, peak, duration: Peak serum concentration occurs at 1 to 3 hours.

INDICATIONS & DOSAGE
Treatment of schistosomiasis caused by Schistosoma mekongi, S. japonicum, S. mansoni, *and* S. haematobium–
Adults and children 4 years and older: 20 mg/kg P.O. t.i.d. as a 1-day treatment. The interval between doses should be between 4 and 6 hours.

CONTRAINDICATIONS & PRECAUTIONS
Contraindicated in patients with hypersensitivity to the drug and in patients with ocular involvement of schistosomiasis, because destruction of parasites within eyes may cause irreversible ocular damage.

ADVERSE REACTIONS
Common reactions are in italics; life-threatening reactions are in bold italics.
CNS: *drowsiness, malaise,* headache, dizziness.
GI: abdominal discomfort, nausea.
Hepatic: minimal increase in liver enzymes.
Skin: urticaria.
Other: fever.

INTERACTIONS
None significant.

EFFECTS ON DIAGNOSTIC TESTS
CSF protein: increased concentrations.
Liver enzymes: increased concentrations.

NURSING CONSIDERATIONS
Besides those related universally to drug therapy (see "How to use this book"), consider the following specific recommendations:
Assessment
• Obtain a baseline assessment of infection including appropriate specimens to confirm schistosomiasis before therapy.

• Be alert for adverse reactions and drug interactions throughout therapy.
• Evaluate the patient's and family's knowledge about praziquantel therapy.

Nursing Diagnoses
• Altered health maintenance related to ineffectiveness of praziquantel.
• High risk for injury related to praziquantel induced CNS reactions.
• Knowledge deficit related to praziquantel.

Planning and Implementation

Preparation and Administration
• ***P.O. use:*** Administer during meals and have patient wash down the unchewed tablet with a liquid.

Monitoring
• Monitor effectiveness by assessing for improvement of infectious process and obtaining appropriate specimen for analysis.
• Adverse reactions may be more frequent or serious in patients with a heavy worm burden.

Supportive Care
• Institute safety measures if adverse CNS reactions occur during praziquantel therapy.
• In the event of overdose, give a fast-acting laxative.
• Obtain an order for an analgesic if patient develops a headache from praziquantel use.

Patient Teaching
• Advise patient to take the tablet during meals and to wash down the unchewed tablet with a liquid. Warn patient that tablets taste very bitter and that keeping them in the mouth may cause gagging or vomiting.
• Caution patient to avoid hazardous activities that require alertness on the day of treatment and the day after treatment.

Evaluation

In patients receiving praziquantel, appropriate evaluation statements may include:
• Patient is free of infection and maintains normal health status.
• Patient does not experience injury from adverse CNS reactions during therapy.
• Patient and family state an understanding of praziquantel therapy.

prazosin hydrochloride
(pra´ zoe sin)
Minipress

• *Classification:* antihypertensive (alpha-adrenergic blocking agent)
• *Pregnancy Risk Category:* C

HOW SUPPLIED
Capsules: 1 mg, 2 mg, 5 mg

ACTION
Mechanism: Relaxes both arteriolar and venous smooth muscle, probably by blocking postsynaptic alpha receptors.
Absorption: Variable absorption from the GI tract.
Distribution: Widely distributed throughout the body and is highly protein-bound (approximately 97%).
Metabolism: Extensively metabolized in the liver.
Excretion: Over 90% of a given dose is excreted in feces via bile; remainder is excreted in urine. Half-life: 2 to 4 hours.
Onset, peak, duration: Antihypertensive effect begins in about 2 hours, peaks in 2 to 4 hours, and lasts about 24 hours. At start of therapy, full antihypertensive effect may not occur for several weeks.

INDICATIONS & DOSAGE
For mild to moderate hypertension; used alone or in combination with a diuretic or other antihypertensive drugs; also used to decrease afterload in severe chronic congestive heart failure–
Adults: P.O. test dose is 1 mg given before bedtime to prevent "first-dose

syncope." Initial dose is 1 mg t.i.d. Increase dosage slowly. Maximum daily dosage is 20 mg. Maintenance dosage is 3 to 20 mg daily in three divided doses. A few patients have required dosages larger than this (up to 40 mg daily). If other antihypertensive drugs or diuretics are added to this drug, decrease prazosin dosage to 1 to 2 mg t.i.d. and retitrate.

CONTRAINDICATIONS & PRECAUTIONS

Contraindicated in patients with hypersensitivity to the drug. Use cautiously in elderly patients, in patients taking other antihypertensive drugs, and in patients with chronic renal failure.

ADVERSE REACTIONS

Common reactions are in italics; life-threatening reactions are in bold italics.
CNS: *dizziness,* headache, drowsiness, weakness, *"first-dose syncope,"* depression.
CV: orthostatic hypotension, *palpitations.*
EENT: blurred vision, dry mouth.
GI: vomiting, diarrhea, abdominal cramps, constipation, *nausea.*
GU: priapism, impotence.

INTERACTIONS

Propranolol and other beta blockers: syncope with loss of consciousness may occur more frequently. Advise patient to sit or lie down if he feels dizzy.

EFFECTS ON DIAGNOSTIC TESTS

Antinuclear antibody (ANA) titer: positive results.
CBC: transient fall in WBC count.
Liver function tests: abnormal results.
Pheochromocytoma screening tests: altered results.
Serum uric acid and BUN: increased levels.
Urinary metabolites of norepinephrine and vanillylmandelic acid: increased levels.

NURSING CONSIDERATIONS

Besides those related universally to drug therapy (see "How to use this book"), consider the following specific recommendations:

Assessment
- Obtain a baseline assessment of the patient's blood pressure before beginning therapy.
- Be alert for adverse reactions and drug interactions throughout therapy.
- Evaluate the patient's and family's knowledge about prazosin therapy.

Nursing Diagnoses
- Altered tissue perfusion (renal, cerebral, cardiopulmonary, peripheral) related to the patient's underlying condition.
- High risk for injury related to adverse CNS reactions to prazosin.
- Knowledge deficit related to prazosin therapy.

Planning and Implementation

Preparation and Administration
- Giving this drug once a day may improve compliance. If compliance is a problem, discuss frequency of medication with the doctor.
- Increase dosage slowly.

Monitoring
- Monitor effectiveness by frequently checking blood pressure and pulse rate.
- Monitor all patients for hypotension but be aware that elderly patients are more sensitive to the drug's hypotensive effects.
- If the initial dose is greater than 1 mg, patient may develop severe syncope with loss of consciousness (first-dose syncope). Monitor carefully.

Supportive Care
- If dizziness or first-dose syncope occur, have the patient lie down and institute safety measures such as continuously using the bed rails.

Patient Teaching
- Instruct the patient to sit or lie down if dizziness occurs.
- Explain the importance of taking this drug as prescribed, even when feeling well.
- Tell the patient not to discontinue this drug suddenly even if unpleasant adverse reactions occur, but to discuss the problem with the doctor.
- Instruct the patient to check with the doctor or the pharmacist before taking OTC medications.
- Inform the patient that orthostatic hypotension can be minimized by rising slowly and avoiding sudden position changes.
- Advise the patient to relieve dry mouth with sugarless chewing gum, sour hard candy, or ice chips.
- Teach the patient and family caregiver how to take blood pressure measurements. Tell the patient to notify the doctor of significant changes in blood pressure measurements.

Evaluation
In patients receiving prazosin, appropriate evaluation statements may include:
- Blood pressure is controlled within normal limits for this patient.
- Injury did not occur; patient did not experience adverse CNS reactions.
- Patient and family state an understanding of prazosin therapy.

---

prednisolone
(pred niss´ oh lone)
Cortalone, Delta-Cortef, Deltasolone‡, Novo-prednisolone†, Panafcortelone‡, Prelone, Solone‡

prednisolone acetate
Articulose, Key-Pred, Niscort, Predaject, Predalone, Predate, Predcor, Predicort

prednisolone sodium phosphate
Codesol, Hydeltrasol, Key-Pred-SP, Pediapred, Predate-S, Predicort RP, Predsol Retention Enema‡, Predsol Suppositories‡

prednisolone steaglate
Sintisone‡

prednisolone tebutate
Hydeltra-TBA, Metalone-TBA, Nor-Pred TBA, Predalone TBA, Predate TBA, Predcor TBA, Prednisol TBA

- *Classification:* anti-inflammatory, immunosuppressant (glucocorticoid, mineralocorticoid)
- *Pregnancy Risk Category:* B

HOW SUPPLIED
prednisolone
Tablets: 1 mg‡, 5 mg, 25 mg‡
Syrup: 15 mg/5 ml
prednisolone acetate
Injection (suspension): 25 mg/ml, 50 mg/ml, 100 mg/ml
prednisolone acetate and prednisolone sodium phosphate
Injection (suspension): 80 mg acetate and 20 mg sodium phosphate/ml
prednisolone sodium phosphate
Oral liquid: 6.7 mg (5-mg base)/5 ml
Injection: 20 mg/ml
Retention enema: 20 mg/100 ml‡
Suppositories: 5 mg‡
prednisolone steaglate
Tablets: 6.65 mg (equal to 3.5 mg prednisolone)‡
prednisolone tebutate
Injection (suspension): 20 mg/ml

ACTION
Mechanism: Decreases inflammation, mainly by stabilizing leukocyte lysosomal membranes. Also suppresses the immune response, stimulates bone marrow, and influences protein, fat, and carbohydrate metabolism.
Absorption: Readily absorbed after oral or I.M. administration. The ace-

tate and tebutate suspensions for injection have a variable absorption over 24 to 48 hours, depending on site of injection (intra-articular space, muscle, or blood supply to that muscle). Systemic absorption occurs slowly after intra-articular injection.
Distribution: Rapidly removed from the blood and distributed to muscle, liver, skin, intestines, and kidneys; extensively bound to plasma proteins (transcortin and albumin). Only the unbound portion is active. Distributed into breast milk and crosses the placenta.
Metabolism: In the liver to inactive glucuronide and sulfate metabolites.
Excretion: The inactive metabolites, and small amounts of unmetabolized drug, are excreted in urine. Insignificant amounts are excreted in feces. Half-life: 18 to 36 hours.
Onset, peak, duration: After oral and I.V. administration, peak effects occur in about 1 to 2 hours.

INDICATIONS & DOSAGE

Severe inflammation or immunosuppression–
Adults: 2.5 to 15 mg P.O. b.i.d., t.i.d., or q.i.d.; 2 to 30 mg I.M. (acetate, phosphate), or I.V. (phosphate) q 12 hours; or 2 to 30 mg (phosphate) into joints, lesions, and soft tissue; or 4 to 40 mg (tebutate) into joints and lesions; or 0.25 to 1 ml (acetate-phosphate suspension) into joints weekly, p.r.n.
Treatment of proctitis‡ –
Adults: 1 suppository b.i.d., preferably in the morning and h.s.
Treatment of ulcerative colitis‡ –
Adults: 1 retention enema h.s. nightly for 2 to 4 weeks. The contents of the enema should be retained overnight.

CONTRAINDICATIONS & PRECAUTIONS

Contraindicated in patients with hypersensitivity to ingredients of adrenocorticoid preparations or in those with systemic fungal infections (except in adrenal insufficiency). Patients who are receiving prednisolone should not receive live virus vaccines because prednisolone suppresses the immune response.

Use with extreme caution in patients with GI ulceration, renal disease, hypertension, osteoporosis, diabetes mellitus, thromboembolic disorders, seizures, myasthenia gravis, CHF, tuberculosis, hypoalbuminemia, hypothyroidism, cirrhosis of the liver, emotional instability, psychotic tendencies, hyperlipidemias, glaucoma, or cataracts, because the drug may exacerbate these conditions.

Because adrenocorticoids increase the susceptibility to and mask symptoms of infection, prednisolone should not be used (except in life-threatening situations) in patients with viral or bacterial infections not controlled by anti-infective agents.

ADVERSE REACTIONS

Common reactions are in italics; life-threatening reactions are in bold italics. Most adverse reactions to corticosteroids are dose- or duration-dependent.
CNS: *euphoria, insomnia,* psychotic behavior, pseudotumor cerebri.
CV: ***CHF,*** hypertension, edema.
EENT: cataracts, glaucoma.
GI: *peptic ulcer,* GI irritation, increased appetite.
Metabolic: *possible hypokalemia, hyperglycemia and carbohydrate intolerance,* growth suppression in children.
Skin: delayed wound healing, acne, various skin eruptions.
Other: muscle weakness, pancreatitis, hirsutism, susceptibility to infections. Acute adrenal insufficiency may occur with increased stress (infection, surgery, or trauma) or abrupt withdrawal after long-term therapy.
Withdrawal symptoms: rebound inflammation, fatigue, weakness, ar-

thralgia, fever, dizziness, lethargy, depression, fainting, orthostatic hypotension, dyspnea, anorexia, hypoglycemia. ***Sudden withdrawal may be fatal.***

INTERACTIONS

Barbiturates, phenytoin, rifampin: decreased corticosteroid effect. Corticosteroid dose may need to be increased.
Indomethacin, aspirin: increased risk of GI distress and bleeding. Give together cautiously.

EFFECTS ON DIAGNOSTIC TESTS

Diagnostic skin tests: suppressed reactions.
Glucose and cholesterol: increased levels.
Nitroblue tetrazolium test for systemic bacterial infections: false-negative results.
Serum potassium, calcium, thyroxine, and triiodothyronine: decreased levels.
Thyroid function tests (^{131}I uptake and protein-bound iodine concentrations): decreased.
Urine glucose and calcium: increased levels.

NURSING CONSIDERATIONS

Besides those related universally to drug therapy (see "How to use this book"), consider the following specific recommendations:

Assessment
- Obtain a baseline assessment of the patient's underlying condition before initiating drug therapy.
- Be alert for adverse reactions and drug interactions throughout therapy.
- Evaluate the patient's and family's knowledge about prednisolone therapy.

Nursing Diagnoses
- Impaired tissue integrity related to the patient's underlying condition.
- High risk for injury related to adverse reactions.
- Knowledge deficit related to prednisolone therapy.

Planning and Implementation
Preparation and Administration
- May be used for alternate-day therapy.
- Gradually reduce drug dosage after long-term therapy. Never abruptly discontinue therapy, as sudden withdrawal can be fatal.
- Always titrate to lowest effective dose, as prescribed.
- Expect to increase dosage as prescribed during times of physiologic stress (surgery, trauma, or infection).
- Don't confuse with prednisone.
- ***P.O. use:*** Give with food when possible to avoid GI upset.
- ***I.M. use:*** Give injection deep into gluteal muscle. Rotate injection sites to prevent muscle atrophy. Avoid S.C. injection, because atrophy and sterile abscesses may occur.
- ***I.V. use:*** When administering as direct injection, inject undiluted over at least 1 minute. When administering as an intermittent or continuous infusion, dilute solution according to manufacturer's instructions and give over the prescribed duration. Do not use acetate form for I.V. use.

Monitoring
- Monitor the patient for adverse drug reactions, because drug can cause serious or even life-threatening multisystem dysfunction.
- Monitor the patient's weight, blood pressure, blood glucose level, and serum electrolyte levels regularly.
- Monitor the patient for infection. Drug may mask or exacerbate infections.
- Monitor the patient's stress level. Stress (fever, trauma, surgery, or emotional problems) may increase adrenal insufficiency. Higher dose may be needed.
- Monitor the patient's mental status for depression or psychotic episodes, especially in high-dose therapy.
- Monitor patients receiving immuni-

zations for decreased antibody response.
• Monitor the patient for early signs of adrenal insufficiency or cushingoid symptoms.
Supportive Care
• Notify the doctor immediately if serious adverse drug reactions occur and be prepared to administer supportive care.
• Unless contraindicated, give the patient a low-sodium diet high in potassium and protein. Potassium supplement may be needed.
• Be aware that diabetic patients may have increased insulin requirements.
Patient Teaching
• Tell the patient to take the drug as prescribed. Give the patient instructions on what to do if a dose is inadvertently missed.
• Warn the patient not to discontinue the drug abruptly or without the doctor's approval.
• Advise the patient to take oral form with meals to minimize adverse GI reactions.
• Inform the patient of the possible therapeutic and adverse effects of the drug, so that he may report complications to the doctor as soon as possible.
• Tell the patient to carry a medical alert card indicating the need for supplemental adrenocorticoids during stress.
• Teach the patient to recognize signs of early adrenal insufficiency (fatigue, muscular weakness, joint pain, fever, anorexia, nausea, dyspnea, dizziness, and fainting) and to notify the doctor promptly if they occur.
• Warn patients on long-term therapy about cushingoid symptoms, which may develop regardless of route of administration.
• Tell patient to eat a low-sodium diet that is high in potassium and protein unless contraindicated.

Evaluation
In patients receiving prednisolone, appropriate evaluation statements may include:
• Patient's condition being treated with prednisolone therapy shows improvement.
• Patient does not experience serious adverse reactions to prednisolone.
• Patient and family state an understanding of prednisolone therapy.

prednisolone acetate (ophthalmic)
(pred niss´ oh lone)
Econopred Ophthalmic, Econopred Plus Ophthalmic, Pred-Forte, Pred Mild Ophthalmic

prednisolone sodium phosphate
AK-Pred, Hydeltrasol Ophthalmic, Inflamase Forte, Inflamase Ophthalmic, Ocu-Pred, Predsol Eye Drops‡

• *Classification:* ophthalmic anti-inflammatory agent (corticosteroid)
• *Pregnancy Risk Category:* C

HOW SUPPLIED
prednisolone acetate
Ophthalmic suspension: 0.12%, 0.125%, 0.25%, 1%
prednisolone sodium phosphate
Ophthalmic solution: 0.125%, 0.5%, 1%

ACTION
Mechanism: Decreases the inflammatory response. Exact mechanism unknown; drug inhibits edema formation, prevents fibrin deposition, and blocks infiltration of phagocytes and leukocytes at the site of inflammation.
Pharmacokinetics: Unknown.

INDICATIONS & DOSAGE

Inflammation of palpebral and bulbar conjunctiva, cornea, and anterior segment of globe–

Adults and children: instill 1 to 2 drops in eye of 0.12% to 1% suspension (acetate) or 0.125% to 1% solution (phosphate). In severe conditions, may be used hourly, tapering to discontinuation as inflammation subsides. In mild conditions, may be used up to four to six times daily.

CONTRAINDICATIONS & PRECAUTIONS

Contraindicated in patients with hypersensitivity to any component of the preparation; in patients with fungal infections of the eye; and in those with acute, untreated purulent bacterial, viral, or fungal ocular infections. Use cautiously in patients with corneal abrasions because they may be contaminated (especially with herpes).

ADVERSE REACTIONS

Common reactions are in italics; life-threatening reactions are in bold italics.

Eye: increased intraocular pressure; thinning of cornea, interference with corneal wound healing, increased susceptibility to viral or fungal corneal infection, corneal ulceration; with excessive or long-term use, glaucoma exacerbations, cataracts, visual acuity and visual field defects, optic nerve damage.

Other: systemic effects and adrenal suppression with excessive or long-term use.

INTERACTIONS

None significant.

EFFECTS ON DIAGNOSTIC TESTS

None reported.

NURSING CONSIDERATIONS

Besides those related universally to drug therapy (see "How to use this book"), consider the following specific recommendations:

Assessment

- Obtain a baseline assessment of the patient's allergies and culture and sensitivity of eye before therapy.
- Be alert for adverse reactions and drug interactions throughout therapy.
- Evaluate the patient's and family's knowledge about prednisolone therapy.

Nursing Diagnoses

- Altered protection related to ocular inflammatory process.
- High risk for injury related to prednisolone-induced increase in intraocular pressure.
- Knowledge deficit related to prednisolone therapy.

Planning and Implementation

Preparation and Administration

- Check dosage and label to ensure correct strength and preparation.
- Shake suspension before using and store in a tightly sealed container.
- Wash hands before and after administration.

Monitoring

- Monitor effectiveness by observing for decreased eye inflammation.
- Monitor the patient for signs of increased intraocular pressure.
- Measure intraocular pressure every 2 to 4 weeks for the first 2 months of ophthalmic corticosteroid therapy; if no increase in pressure has occurred, measure about every 1 to 2 months thereafter.
- Monitor the patient for changes in visual acuity and visual field defects.
- Observe the patient for signs of hypersensitivity.

Supportive Care

- Notify the doctor immediately of any changes in patient's health status.
- Be aware that a patient on long-term therapy may require a tapered dosage schedule if drug is stopped.

Patient Teaching

- Teach the patient how to instill drops. Advise him to wash hands be-

fore and after administration. Warn him not to touch the tip of the applicator to the eye or surrounding tissue.
• Instruct the patient to apply light finger pressure to the lacrimal sac for 1 minute after drops are instilled. Caution him to avoid scratching or rubbing the eye area.
• Advise the patient on long-term therapy to have frequent tonometric examinations.
• Warn the patient not to use leftover eye medication on a new eye inflammation.
• Instruct the patient not to share eye medications with family members. A family member who develops the same symptoms should contact the doctor.

Evaluation
In patients receiving prednisolone, appropriate evaluation statements may include:
• Patient exhibits decrease or absence in eye inflammation.
• Patient's intraocular pressure remains within normal range.
• Patient and family state an understanding of prednisolone therapy.

prednisone
(pred´ ni sone)
Apo-Prednisone†, Deltasone, Liquid Pred*, Meticorten, Novo-prednisone†, Orasone, Panafcort‡, Panasol, Prednicen-M, Prednisone Intensol*, Sone‡, Sterapred, Winpred†

• *Classification:* anti-inflammatory, immunosuppressant (glucocorticoid)
• *Pregnancy Risk Category:* B

HOW SUPPLIED
Tablets: 1 mg, 2.5 mg, 5 mg, 10 mg, 20 mg, 25 mg, 50 mg
Oral solution: 5 mg/5 ml*, 5 mg/ml (concentrate)*
Syrup: 5 mg/5 ml*

ACTION
Mechanism: Decreases inflammation, mainly by stabilizing leukocyte lysosomal membranes. Also suppresses the immune response, stimulates bone marrow, and influences protein, fat, and carbohydrate metabolism.
Absorption: Readily absorbed after oral administration.
Distribution: Rapidly distributed to muscle, liver, skin, intestines, and kidneys; extensively bound to plasma proteins (transcortin and albumin). Only the unbound portion is active. Distributed into breast milk and crosses the placenta.
Metabolism: In the liver to the active metabolite prednisolone, which is then metabolized to inactive glucuronide and sulfate metabolites.
Excretion: Inactive metabolites and small amounts of unmetabolized drug are excreted by the kidneys. Insignificant amounts are also excreted in feces. Half-life: 18 to 36 hours.
Onset, peak, duration: Peak effects occur in about 1 to 2 hours.

INDICATIONS & DOSAGE
Severe inflammation or immunosuppression–
Adults: 2.5 to 15 mg P.O. b.i.d., t.i.d., or q.i.d. Maintenance dosage given once daily or every other day. Dosage must be individualized.
Children: 0.14 to 2 mg/kg P.O. daily divided q.i.d.
Acute exacerbations of multiple sclerosis–
Adults: 200 mg P.O. daily for 1 week, then 80 mg every other day for 1 month.

CONTRAINDICATIONS & PRECAUTIONS
Contraindicated in patients with systemic fungal infections (except in adrenal insufficiency) and in those with hypersensitivity to ingredients of ad-

renocorticoid preparations. Patients receiving prednisone should not be given live virus vaccines because prednisone suppresses the immune response.

Use with extreme caution in patients with GI ulceration, renal disease, hypertension, osteoporosis, diabetes mellitus, thromboembolic disorders, seizures, myasthenia gravis, CHF, tuberculosis, hypoalbuminemia, hypothyroidism, cirrhosis of the liver, emotional instability, psychotic tendencies, hyperlipidemias, glaucoma, or cataracts, because the drug may exacerbate these conditions.

Because adrenocorticoids increase the susceptibility to and mask symptoms of infection, prednisone should not be used (except in life-threatening situations) in patients with viral or bacterial infections not controlled by anti-infective agents.

ADVERSE REACTIONS

Common reactions are in italics; life-threatening reactions are in bold italics.

Most adverse reactions to corticosteroids are dose- or duration-dependent.

CNS: *euphoria, insomnia,* psychotic behavior, pseudotumor cerebri.
CV: *CHF,* hypertension, edema.
EENT: cataracts, glaucoma.
GI: *peptic ulcer,* GI irritation, increased appetite.
Metabolic: *possible hypokalemia, hyperglycemia and carbohydrate intolerance,* growth suppression in children.
Skin: delayed wound healing, acne, various skin eruptions.
Other: muscle weakness, pancreatitis, hirsutism, susceptibility to infections. Acute adrenal insufficiency may occur with increased stress (infection, surgery, or trauma) or abrupt withdrawal after long-term therapy.
Withdrawal symptoms: rebound inflammation, fatigue, weakness, arthralgia, fever, dizziness, lethargy, depression, fainting, orthostatic hypotension, dyspnea, anorexia, hypoglycemia. ***Sudden withdrawal may be fatal.***

INTERACTIONS

Barbiturates, phenytoin, rifampin: decreased corticosteroid effect. Corticosteroid dose may need to be increased.
Indomethacin, aspirin: increased risk of GI distress and bleeding. Give together cautiously.

EFFECTS ON DIAGNOSTIC TESTS

Diagnostic skin tests: suppressed reactions.
Glucose and cholesterol: increased levels.
Nitroblue tetrazolium test for systemic bacterial infections: false-negative results.
Serum potassium, calcium, thyroxine, and triiodothyronine: decreased levels.
Thyroid function tests (^{131}I uptake and protein-bound iodine concentrations): decreased.
Urine glucose and calcium: increased levels.

NURSING CONSIDERATIONS

Besides those related universally to drug therapy (see "How to use this book"), consider the following specific recommendations:

Assessment
- Obtain a baseline assessment of the patient's underlying condition before initiating drug therapy.
- Be alert for adverse reactions and drug interactions throughout therapy.
- Evaluate the patient's and family's knowledge about prednisone therapy.

Nursing Diagnoses
- Impaired tissue integrity related to the patient's underlying condition.
- High risk for injury related to adverse reactions to prednisone.
- Knowledge deficit related to prednisone therapy.

Planning and Implementation

Preparation and Administration

- May be used for alternate-day therapy.
- Gradually reduce drug dosage after long-term therapy. Never abruptly discontinue therapy, as sudden withdrawal can be fatal.
- Always titrate to lowest effective dose, as prescribed.
- Give a daily dosage in the morning for better results and less toxicity.
- Expect to increase dosage as prescribed during times of physiologic stress (surgery, trauma, or infection).
- ***P.O. use:*** Give with food when possible to avoid GI upset.

Monitoring

- Monitor the patient for adverse reactions, as prednisone can cause serious or life-threatening multisystem dysfunction.
- Monitor the patient's weight, blood pressure, blood glucose level, and serum electrolyte levels regularly.
- Monitor the patient for infection. Drug may mask or exacerbate infections.
- Monitor the patient's stress level. Stress (fever, trauma, surgery, or emotional problems) may increase adrenal insufficiency. Higher dose may be needed.
- Monitor the patient's mental status for depression or psychotic episodes, especially in high-dose therapy.
- Monitor growth in infants and children on long-term therapy.
- Monitor patients receiving immunizations for decreased antibody response.
- Monitor the patient for early signs of adrenal insufficiency or cushingoid symptoms.

Supportive Care

- Notify the doctor immediately if serious adverse reactions occur, and be prepared to administer supportive care.
- Unless contraindicated, give the patient a low-sodium diet high in potassium and protein. Potassium supplement may be needed.
- Be aware that diabetic patients may have increased insulin requirements.

Patient Teaching

- Tell the patient to take the drug as prescribed. Give the patient instructions on what to do if a dose is inadvertently missed.
- Warn the patient not to discontinue the drug abruptly or without the doctor's approval.
- Advise the patient to take drug with meals to minimize adverse GI reactions.
- Inform the patient of the possible therapeutic and adverse effects of the drug, so that he may report complications to the doctor as soon as possible.
- Tell the patient to carry a medical alert card indicating the need for supplemental adrenocorticoids during stress.
- Teach the patient to recognize signs of early adrenal insufficiency (fatigue, muscular weakness, joint pain, fever, anorexia, nausea, dyspnea, dizziness, and fainting) and to notify the doctor promptly if they occur.
- Warn patients on long-term therapy about cushingoid symptoms, which may develop regardless of route of administration.
- Tell patient to eat a low-sodium diet that is high in potassium and protein, unless contraindicated.

Evaluation

In patients receiving prednisone, appropriate evaluation statements may include:

- Patient's condition shows signs of improvement.
- Patient does not experience serious adverse reactions to prednisone.
- Patient and family state an understanding of prednisone therapy.

primaquine phosphate

(prim´ a kween)

• *Classification:* antimalarial (8-aminoquinoline)
• *Pregnancy Risk Category:* C

HOW SUPPLIED

Tablets: 7.5 mg (base)‡, 15 mg (base)

ACTION

Mechanism: A gametocidal drug that destroys exoerythrocytic forms and prevents delayed primary attack. Its mechanism of action is unknown.
Absorption: Well absorbed from the GI tract.
Distribution: Widely distributed into the liver, lungs, heart, brain, skeletal muscle, and other tissues.
Metabolism: Carboxylated rapidly in the liver.
Excretion: Only a small amount of primaquine is excreted unchanged in urine. Half-life: 4 to 10 hours.
Onset, peak, duration: Peak concentration levels occur at 2 to 6 hours.

INDICATIONS & DOSAGE

Radical cure of relapsing vivax malaria, eliminating symptoms and infection completely; prevention of relapse–
Adults: 15 mg (base) P.O. daily for 14 days. (26.3 mg tablet = 15 mg of base).

CONTRAINDICATIONS & PRECAUTIONS

Contraindicated in patients receiving quinacrine because of possible additive toxicity, in patients predisposed to granulocytopenia, patients with lupus erythematosus or rheumatoid arthritis, and in patients receiving other drugs that might cause hemolysis or bone marrow depression.

Use cautiously in patients who have had an idiosyncratic reaction to primaquine and in patients with a history of favism, glucose-6-phosphate dehydrogenase (G6PD) deficiency, or NADH methemoglobin reductase deficiency, because hemolytic reactions may occur in these groups.

ADVERSE REACTIONS

Common reactions are in italics; life-threatening reactions are in bold italics.
Blood: leukopenia, ***hemolytic anemia in G6PD deficiency,*** methemoglobinemia in NADH methemoglobin reductase deficiency, leukocytosis, mild anemia, granulocytopenia, agranulocytosis.
CNS: headache.
EENT: disturbances of visual accommodation.
GI: nausea, vomiting, epigastric distress, abdominal cramps.
Skin: urticaria.

INTERACTIONS

Magnesium and aluminum salts: Decreased GI absorption. Separate administration times.

EFFECTS ON DIAGNOSTIC TESTS

CBC: decreased or increased WBCs, and RBCs; methemoglobinemia may occur.

NURSING CONSIDERATIONS

Besides those related universally to drug therapy (see "How to use this book"), consider the following specific recommendations:

Assessment

• Obtain a baseline assessment of the infection before therapy.
• Be alert for adverse reactions and drug interactions throughout therapy.
• Evaluate the patient's and family's knowledge about primaquine therapy.

Nursing Diagnoses

• High risk for injury related to ineffectiveness of primaquine to eradicate the infection.
• Altered protection related to prima-

quine induced hematologic abnormalities.
• Knowledge deficit related to primaquine.

Planning and Implementation

Preparation and Administration

• ***P.O. use:*** Administer drug with meals or with antacids.
• Expect to administer concurrently with a fast-acting antimalarial, such as chloroquine. Be aware that full dose should be used to reduce possibility of drug-resistant strains.

Monitoring

• Monitor effectiveness by regularly assessing patient for improvement in infectious process.
• Monitor blood studies and urine examinations frequently as ordered, especially in light-skinned patients taking more than 30 mg (base) daily, in dark-skinned patients taking more than 15 mg (base) daily, and in patients with severe anemia or suspected sensitivity. Sudden fall in hemoglobin concentration, erythrocyte or leukocyte count, or marked darkening of the urine suggests impending hemolytic reactions.
• Monitor closely for tolerance in patients with previous idiosyncrasy (manifested by hemolytic anemia, methemoglobinemia, or leukopenia); family or personal history of favism; erythrocytic G6PD deficiency or NADH methemoglobin reductase deficiency.

Supportive Care

• Withhold drug and notify doctor immediately if signs of an impending hemolytic reaction occur.
• Obtain an order for an analgesic if a primaquine induced headache occurs or for an antiemetic if GI reactions occur.
• Institute safety precautions if visual disturbances occur.

Patient Teaching

• Tell patient to take the drug with a meal or with an antacid.
• Teach patient to report marked darkening of urine immediately as this may signal an impending hemolytic reaction.
• Stress the importance of frequent blood tests and urine examinations throughout primaquine therapy.
• Tell patient to avoid hazardous activities if visual disturbances occur.

Evaluation

In patients receiving primaquine, appropriate evaluation statements may include:
• Patient is free of infection.
• Patient's blood tests and urine examinations remain normal throughout therapy.
• Patient and family state an understanding of therapy.

primidone

(pri´ mi done)

Apo-Primidone†, Myidone, Mysoline, Sertan†

• *Classification:* anticonvulsant (barbiturate)
• *Pregnancy Risk Category:* D

HOW SUPPLIED

Tablets: 50 mg, 250 mg
Oral suspension: 250 mg/5 ml

ACTION

Mechanism: Unknown, but some activity may be caused by phenobarbital, which is an active metabolite.
Absorption: Readily absorbed from the GI tract.
Distribution: Widely distributed throughout the body. Therapeutic levels are 5 to 12 mcg/ml for primidone and 10 to 30 mcg/ml for phenobarbital.
Metabolism: Slowly metabolized by the liver to phenylethylmalonamide (PEMA) and phenobarbital; PEMA is the major metabolite.
Excretion: In urine; substantial amounts are excreted in breast milk.

Half-life: Primidone, 5 to 15 hours; PEMA, 10 to 18 hours; phenobarbital, 53 to 140 hours.
Onset, peak, duration: Serum concentrations peak at about 3 hours. Phenobarbital appears in plasma after several days of continuous therapy.

INDICATIONS & DOSAGE

Generalized tonic-clonic seizures, complex-partial seizures–
Adults and children over 8 years: 250 mg P.O. daily. Increase by 250 mg weekly, up to maximum of 2 g daily, divided q.i.d.
Children under 8 years: 125 mg P.O. daily. Increase by 125 mg weekly, up to maximum of 1 g daily, divided q.i.d.

CONTRAINDICATIONS & PRECAUTIONS

Contraindicated in patients with hypersensitivity to barbiturates; in pregnancy because of hazard of respiratory depression and neonatal coagulation defects; in patients with severe respiratory disease or status asthmaticus because of respiratory depressant effects; in patients with por phyria because of potential for adverse hematologic effects; and in patients with markedly impaired hepatic function because of potential for enhanced hepatic impairment. Use caution in patients taking alcohol and other CNS depressants.

ADVERSE REACTIONS

Common reactions are in italics; life-threatening reactions are in bold italics.
Blood: leukopenia, eosinophilia.
CNS: *drowsiness, ataxia,* emotional disturbances, vertigo, hyperirritability, fatigue.
EENT: *diplopia,* nystagmus, edema of the eyelids.
GI: anorexia, *nausea, vomiting.*
GU: impotence, polyuria.
Skin: morbilliform rash, alopecia.
Other: edema, thirst.

INTERACTIONS

Carbamezepine: increased primidone levels. Observe for toxicity.
Phenytoin: stimulated conversion of primidone to phenobarbital. Observe for increased phenobarbital effect.

EFFECTS ON DIAGNOSTIC TESTS

Liver function tests: abnormal results.

NURSING CONSIDERATIONS

Besides those related universally to drug therapy (see "How to use this book"), consider the following specific recommendations:

Assessment
- Obtain a baseline assessment of seizure activity before therapy.
- Be alert for adverse reactions and drug interactions throughout therapy.
- Evaluate the patient's and family's knowledge about primidone therapy.

Nursing Diagnoses
- High risk for injury related to patient's underlying seizure disorder.
- Sensory/perceptual alterations (visual) related to primidone-induced diplopia.
- Knowledge deficit related to primidone therapy.

Planning and Implementation

Preparation and Administration
- Shake liquid suspension well.

Monitoring
- Monitor effectiveness by evaluating the patient's seizure activity. Full therapeutic response may take 2 weeks or more.
- Monitor CBC and routine blood chemistry every 6 months.
- Monitor for visual disturbances, such as diplopia.
- Monitor primidone blood levels regularly. The normal therapeutic blood level of primidone is 5 to 12 mcg/ml.

Supportive Care
- Don't withdraw drug suddenly. Call the doctor immediately if adverse reactions develop.
- If adverse CNS reactions or visual

disturbances occur, institute safety measures, such as assisting patient with ambulation and keeping bed rails up.

• Maintain seizure precautions.

Patient Teaching

• Warn the patient to avoid hazardous activities until CNS effects of the drug are known.

• Advise the patient not to discontinue drug suddenly.

Evaluation

In patients receiving primidone, appropriate evaluation statements may include:

• Patient is free of seizure activity.

• Patient states vision is unaffected by primidone.

• Patient and family state an understanding of primidone therapy.

probenecid

(proe ben´ e sid)

Benemid, Benn, Benuryl†, Probalan, Robenecid

• *Classification:* uricosuric agent (sulfonamide derivative)

• *Pregnancy Risk Category:* B

HOW SUPPLIED

Tablets: 500 mg

ACTION

Mechanism: Blocks renal tubular reabsorption of organic acids, such as uric acid, increasing their excretion. Also inhibits active renal tubular secretion of many weak organic acids (for example, penicillins and cephalosporins).

Absorption: Completely absorbed after oral administration.

Distribution: Drug is about 75% protein-bound. CSF levels are about 2% of serum levels.

Metabolism: In the liver to active metabolites, with some uricosuric effect.

Excretion: Drug and metabolites are excreted in urine; probenecid (but not metabolites) is actively reabsorbed.

Onset, peak, duration: Peak serum levels are reached at 2 to 4 hours.

INDICATIONS & DOSAGE

Adjunct to penicillin or cephalosporin therapy–

Adults and children over 50 kg: 500 mg P.O. q.i.d.

Children 2 to 14 years or under 50 kg: initially, 25 mg/kg P.O., then 40 mg/kg divided q.i.d.

Single-dose treatment of gonorrhea–

Adults: 3.5 g ampicillin P.O. with 1 g probenecid P.O. given together; or 1 g probenecid P.O. 30 minutes before dose of 4.8 million units of aqueous penicillin G procaine I.M., injected at two different sites.

Treatment of hyperuricemia of gout, gouty arthritis–

Adults: 250 mg P.O. b.i.d. for first week, then 500 mg b.i.d., to maximum of 2 g daily. Maintenance dosage is 500 mg daily for 6 months.

CONTRAINDICATIONS & PRECAUTIONS

Contraindicated in patients with hypersensitivity to the drug and in patients with acute gout, blood dyscrasias, or uric acid kidney stones because it may worsen these conditions. Use cautiously in patients with a history of peptic ulcer disease; renal impairment (drug is ineffective if glomerular filtration rate is lower than 30 ml/minute); and acute intermittent porphyria.

ADVERSE REACTIONS

Common reactions are in italics; life-threatening reactions are in bold italics.

Blood: ***hemolytic anemia.***

CNS: *headache,* dizziness.

CV: hypotension.

GI: anorexia, nausea, vomiting, *gastric distress.*

GU: urinary frequency, renal colic.
Skin: dermatitis, pruritus, alopecia.
Other: flushing, sore gums, fever.

INTERACTIONS

Indomethacin: decreased indomethacin excretion. Lower indomethacin dosages may be required.
Methotrexate: decreased methotrexate excretion. Lower methotrexate dosage may be required. Serum levels should be determined.
Oral hypoglycemic agents: enhanced hypoglycemic effect. Monitor blood glucose levels closely. Dosage adjustment may be required.
Salicylates: inhibited uricosuric effect of probenecid, causing urate retention. Do not use together.

EFFECTS ON DIAGNOSTIC TESTS

Urine glucose test using copper sulfate reagent (Benedict's reagent, Clinitest, and Fehling's test): false-positive results.
Urine 17-ketosteroids, sulfobromophthalein (BSP), aminohippuric acid, and iodine-related organic acids: decreased levels.

NURSING CONSIDERATIONS

Besides those related universally to drug therapy (see "How to use this book"), consider the following specific recommendations:

Assessment

- Obtain a baseline assessment of the patient's uric acid levels and his joint pain and stiffness.
- Be alert for adverse reactions and drug interactions throughout therapy.
- Evaluate the patient's and family's knowledge about probenecid therapy.

Nursing Diagnoses

- Pain (joint) related to patient's underlying condition.
- Altered tissue perfusion (cardiopulmonary, renal, GI, cerebral, peripheral) related to probenecid-induced hemolytic anemia.
- Knowledge deficit related to probenecid therapy.

Planning and Implementation

Preparation and Administration

- Start therapy after attack subsides as probenecid, when used for hyperuricemia associated with gout, has no analgesic or anti-inflammatory actions, and no effect on acute attacks.
- Expect to administer concomitant prophylactic doses of colchicine or an NSAID during the first 3 to 6 months of probenecid therapy because the drug may increase the frequency of acute attacks during the first 6 to 12 months of therapy.
- Give with food, milk, or prescribed antacids to lessen GI discomfort.
- Force fluids to maintain minimum daily output of 2 to 3 liters. Alkalinize urine with sodium bicarbonate or potassium citrate as ordered by the doctor. These measures will prevent hematuria, renal colic, urate stone development, and costovertebral pain.
- Expect adjustment of probenecid dosage to the lowest dosage that maintains normal uric acid levels.

Monitoring

- Monitor effectiveness by regularly assessing frequency and intensity of gouty arthritis attacks and monitoring uric acid level results.
- Monitor CBC results for evidence of hemolytic anemia, and assess patient for hemolytic anemia by noting symptoms of fatigue, tachycardia, pallor and dyspnea.
- Monitor for headache.
- Monitor blood pressure for hypotension and temperature for fever.
- Monitor BUN and serum creatinine level results closely. This drug is ineffective in patients with severe renal insufficiency.
- Monitor hydration status if adverse GI reactions occur.
- Monitor the patient's intake and output so that patient maintains minimum daily output of 2 to 3 liters.

Supportive Care
• Notify the doctor if the patient's uric acid level increases. Expect to alkalinize urine with sodium bicarbonate or potassium citrate as ordered by doctor. These measures will prevent hematuria, renal colic, urate calculi development, and costovertebral pain.
• Notify doctor of abnormal CBC results and if symptoms of hemolytic anemia develop.
• Maintain adequate hydration with high fluid intake to prevent formation of uric acid calculi.
• If the patient develops persistent GI distress, notify the doctor and expect to decrease dosage.
• If the patient develops a headache, obtain an order for a mild analgesic, such as acetaminophen. Avoid salicylate analgesics, which may prolong bleeding time.
• Remember that lower doses are indicated in elderly patients.
Patient Teaching
• Tell the patient and family that the drug must be taken regularly as ordered or gout attacks may result. Tell the patient not to discontinue drug without medical advice. Advise him to visit the doctor regularly so uric acid can be monitored and dosage can be adjusted if necessary. Lifelong therapy may be required in patients with hyperuricemia.
• Advise the patient to restrict foods high in purine: anchovies, liver, sardines, kidneys, sweetbreads, peas, and lentils.
• Tell the patient that probenecid may increase frequency, severity, and duration of acute gout attacks during the first 6 to 12 months of therapy. Prophylactic colchicine or another anti-inflammatory agent is given during the first 3 to 6 months.
• Tell the patient with gout to avoid alcohol because it increases the urate level.
• Advise diabetic patients to perform urine glucose tests with a glucose enzymatic reagent (Clinistix, Tes-Tape).
• Warn the patient not to use drug for pain or inflammation and not to increase dose during gout attack.
• Tell the patient to drink 8 to 10 glasses of fluid daily and to take drug with food to minimize GI upset.
• Advise female patients considering breast-feeding that it is unknown whether probenecid is excreted in breast milk. Therefore, an alternative feeding method is recommended during therapy with probenecid.
Evaluation
In patients receiving probenecid, appropriate evaluation statements may include:
• Patient expresses relief of gout-related pain.
• Patient maintains normal CBC counts.
• Patient and family state an understanding of probenecid therapy.

probucol
(proe´ byoo kole)
Lorelco, Lurselle ‡

• *Classification:* cholesterol-lowering agent (bis-phenol derivative)
• *Pregnancy Risk Category:* B

HOW SUPPLIED
Tablets: 250 mg, 500 mg

ACTION
Mechanism: Inhibits cholesterol transport from the intestine and may also decrease cholesterol synthesis. Appears to be more effective in patients with mild cholesterol elevations than in those with severe hypercholesterolemia.
Absorption: GI limited (2% to 8%) and variable. When taken with food, probucol produces high blood levels and is less variable.
Distribution: Lipid-soluble and accu-

mulates slowly in adipose tissue, persisting in fat and blood for at least 6 months after the last dose. Probucol blood level declines by 80% after 6 months; cholesterol-lowering effects disappear well before tissue level decrease.
Excretion: Eliminated via bile in feces. Half-life: Ranges from 12 hours to over 500 hours, as drug slowly leaches out of fat tissues.
Onset, peak, duration: Blood levels increase during first 3 to 4 months, then remain constant; clinical response usually occurs in 1 to 3 months.

INDICATIONS & DOSAGE

Primary hypercholesterolemia –
Adults: 500 mg P.O. b.i.d. with morning and evening meals. Do not exceed 1 g/day.
Not recommended for children.

CONTRAINDICATIONS & PRECAUTIONS

Contraindicated in patients with recent or progressive myocardial damage or cardiac arrhythmia because serious CV toxicity occurs in animals. Also contraindicated in patients hypersensitive to the drug and in pregnant patients. Patients wishing to conceive should discontinue the drug for at least 6 months before attempt to conceive and should use contraceptives throughout the waiting period because of persistent blood levels.

ADVERSE REACTIONS

Common reactions are in italics; life-threatening reactions are in bold italics.
CV: prolonged QT interval, arrhythmias.
GI: *diarrhea, flatulence, abdominal pain, nausea, vomiting.*
Other: *hyperhidrosis,* fetid sweat, angioneurotic edema.

INTERACTIONS

Clofibrate: additive pharmacologic effects.
Tricyclic antidepressants, Class Ia antiarrhythmics, phenothiazines, beta blockers, digitalis glycosides, calcium channel blocking agents: increased risk of arrhythmias.

EFFECTS ON DIAGNOSTIC TESTS

BUN: altered levels.
CBC: altered eosinophil count.
Hematocrit and hemoglobin: altered levels.
Serum bilirubin, glucose, creatine phosphokinase, AST (SGOT), ALT (SGPT), uric acid, alkaline phosphatase: altered levels.

NURSING CONSIDERATIONS

Besides those related universally to drug therapy (see "How to use this book"), consider the following specific recommendations:

Assessment
- Obtain a baseline assessment of the patient's cholesterol level before drug therapy.
- Be alert for adverse reactions and drug interactions throughout therapy.
- Evaluate the patient's and family's knowledge about probucol therapy.

Nursing Diagnoses
- High risk for injury related to elevated blood lipids and cholesterol levels.
- Diarrhea related to adverse drug reaction.
- Knowledge deficit related to probucol therapy.

Planning and Implementation
Preparation and Administration
- Drug's effect is enhanced when taken with food.

Monitoring
- Monitor the patient's vital signs.
- Monitor the patient's ECG periodically.
- Monitor the patient's intake and output if vomiting and diarrhea occur.

Supportive Care

• Provide fluids if the patient experiences vomiting and diarrhea.

• Discontinue the drug and notify the doctor if patient's ECG shows prolonged Q-T interval.

Patient Teaching

• Instruct the patient who wishes to become pregnant to discontinue the drug and use effective contraception for 6 months after drug withdrawal because drug persists in the body.

• Teach the patient dietary management (restricting total fat and cholesterol intake), weight control, and exercise. Explain their importance in controlling elevated serum lipids.

Evaluation

In patients receiving probucol, appropriate evaluation statements may include:

• Patient's blood lipid and cholesterol levels remain within normal limits.

• Patient does not develop diarrhea.

• Patient and family state an understanding of probucol therapy.

procainamide hydrochloride

(proe kane´ a mide)

Procan SR, Promine, Pronestyl**, Pronestyl-SR, Rhythmin

• *Classification:* ventricular supraventricular antiarrhythmic (procaine derivative)

• *Pregnancy Risk Category:* C

HOW SUPPLIED

Tablets: 250 mg, 375 mg, 500 mg
Tablets (sustained-release): 250 mg, 500 mg, 750 mg, 1,000 mg
Capsules: 250 mg, 375 mg, 500 mg
Injection: 100 mg/ml, 500 mg/ml

ACTION

Mechanism: A Class Ia antiarrhythmic that depresses phase O and prolongs the action potential. All class I drugs have membrane-stabilizing (local anesthetic) effects.

Absorption: Rate and extent of absorption from the intestines vary; usually, 75% to 95% of an orally administered dose is absorbed. Extended-release tablets are formulated to provide a sustained and relatively constant rate of release and absorption throughout the small intestine. After the drug's release, wax matrix is not absorbed and may appear in feces after 15 minutes to 1 hour. The drug is well absorbed after I.M. injection and peak plasma levels are seen in 15 to 60 minutes.

Distribution: Widely distributed in most body tissues, including cerebrospinal fluid, liver, spleen, kidneys, lungs, muscles, brain, and heart. Only about 15% binds to plasma proteins. Usual therapeutic range is 4 to 8 mcg/ml. Some experts suggest that a range of 10 to 30 mcg/ml for the sum of procainamide and N-acetylprocainamide (NAPA) serum concentrations are therapeutic.

Metabolism: Acetylated in the liver to form NAPA. Acetylation rate is determined genetically and affects NAPA formation. (NAPA also exerts antiarrhythmic activity.)

Excretion: Procainamide and NAPA metabolite are excreted in the urine. Half-life: Procainamide's half-life is about 2½ to 4¾ hours. NAPA's half-life is about 6 hours. In patients with CHF or renal dysfunction, half-life increases and dosage reduction is required to avoid toxicity.

Onset, peak, duration: Peak plasma levels occur in approximately 1 hour after oral administration. With I.M. injection, onset of action occurs in about 10 to 30 minutes, with peak levels in about 1 hour.

INDICATIONS & DOSAGE

Premature ventricular contractions, ventricular tachycardia, atrial arrhythmias unresponsive to quinidine, paroxysmal atrial tachycardia –
Adults: 100 mg q 5 minutes slow I.V. push, no faster than 25 to 50 mg/minute until arrhythmias disappear, adverse reactions develop, or 1 g has been given. (Usual effective dose is 500 to 600 mg.) When arrhythmias disappear, give continuous infusion of 2 to 6 mg/minute. If arrhythmias recur, repeat bolus as above and increase infusion rate; 0.5 to 1 g I.M. q 4 to 8 hours until oral therapy begins.
Loading dose for atrial fibrillation or paroxysmal atrial tachycardia –
Adults: 1 to 1.25 g P.O. If arrhythmias persist after 1 hour, give additional 750 mg. If no change occurs, give 500 mg to 1 g q 2 hours until arrhythmias disappear or adverse reactions occur.
Loading dose for ventricular tachycardia –
Adults: 1 g P.O. Maintenance dosage is 50 mg/kg daily q 3 hours; average is 250 to 500 mg q 3 hours.

Note: Sustained-release tablet may be used for maintenance dosing when treating ventricular tachycardia, atrial fibrillation, and paroxysmal atrial tachycardia. Dose is 500 mg to 1 g q 6 hours.

CONTRAINDICATIONS & PRECAUTIONS

Contraindicated in patients with complete AV block with AV junctional or idioventricular pacemaker without an operative artificial pacemaker, prolonged Q-T interval or QRS duration, because of potential for heart block; in patients with digitalis toxicity, because the drug may further depress conduction, which may result in ventricular asystole or fibrillation; torsades de pointes, because the drug may exacerbate this arrhythmia; myasthenia gravis, because the drug may exacerbate muscle weakness; and hypersensitivity to procainamide or related compounds (such as procaine).

Use with caution in patients with incomplete AV block or bundle branch block, because the drug may further depress conduction; CHF, because drug may worsen this condition; or renal or hepatic dysfunction, because the drug may accumulate, causing toxicity.

ADVERSE REACTIONS

Common reactions are in italics; life-threatening reactions are in bold italics.
Blood: thrombocytopenia, *neutropenia* (especially with sustained-release forms), ***agranulocytosis, hemolytic anemia,*** *increased antinuclear antibodies titer.*
CNS: hallucinations, confusion, seizures, depression.
CV: *severe hypotension,* ***bradycardia,*** AV block, ***ventricular fibrillation*** (after parenteral use).
GI: *nausea, vomiting, anorexia, diarrhea, bitter taste.*
Skin: *maculopapular rash.*
Other: *fever, lupus erythematosus syndrome (especially after prolonged administration),* myalgia.

INTERACTIONS

Amiodarone: increased procainamide levels and possible drug toxicity.
Anticholinergics: additive anticholinergic effects.
Anticholinesterase agents: anticholinesterase dosage may need to be increased.
Cimetidine: may increase procainamide blood levels. Monitor for toxicity.
Neuromuscular blocking agents: increased skeletal muscle relaxant effects. Monitor patient closely.

EFFECTS ON DIAGNOSTIC TESTS

ANA titers, direct antiglobulin (Coombs') tests: positive results.
Bentiromide test: invalidated results; discontinue at least 3 days before bentiromide test.
Bilirubin, LDH, alkaline phosphatase, ALT (SGPT), and AST (SGOT): increased levels.
CBC: decreased WBC and platelet counts.
ECG: possible changes.
Edrophonium test: altered results.

NURSING CONSIDERATIONS

Besides those related universally to drug therapy (see "How to use this book"), consider the following specific recommendations:

Assessment

- Obtain a baseline assessment of the patient's heart rate and rhythm before procainamide therapy.
- Be alert for adverse reactions and drug interactions throughout therapy.
- Evaluate the patient's and family's knowledge about procainamide therapy.

Nursing Diagnoses

- Decreased cardiac output related to ineffectiveness of drug or cardiovascular reactions to procainamide therapy.
- Altered protection related to procainamide-induced blood disorders.
- Knowledge deficit related to procainamide.

Planning and Implementation

Preparation and Administration

- Expect to decrease dosage in patients with hepatic and renal dysfunction, and give over 6 hours. Half-life of procainamide increases as much as threefold in these conditions.
- Be aware that patients with CHF have a lower volume of distribution and can be treated with lower dosage.
- ***I.V. use:*** Administer an I.V. bolus slowly (no faster than 25 to 50 mg/min.). Expect to give drug I.V. push q 5 minutes until arrhythmia has disappeared, adverse reactions develop, or 1 g has been given.
- Administer drug as a continuous infusion at 2 to 6 mg/minute as ordered. Use an infusion pump to administer the dose precisely.
- Keep patient supine for I.V. administration if hypotension occurs.
- Discard discolored procainamide solution for injection and obtain a new solution from pharmacy.

Monitoring

- Monitor effectiveness by frequently assessing ECG recording.
- Monitor the patient's serum electrolyte levels, especially potassium level. Hypokalemia predisposes patients to arrhythmias.
- Monitor blood pressure and ECG continuously during I.V. administration. Watch for prolonged Q-T and QRS intervals, heart block, or increased arrhythmias.
- Monitor CBC frequently during first 3 months of therapy, particularly in patients taking sustained-released dosage forms.
- Monitor serum creatinine levels because NAPA, an active metabolite, may accumulate when renal function is decreased, and may add to toxicity.
- Monitor hydration status if adverse GI disturbances occur.

Supportive Care

- If ECG disturbances occur, withhold the drug, obtain a rhythm strip, and notify the doctor immediately.
- After prolonged atrial fibrillation, restoration of normal rhythm may result in thromboembolism, due to dislodgement of thrombi from atrial wall. Be aware that anticoagulation is usually advised before restoration of normal sinus rhythm.
- Obtain an order for an antiemetic or antidiarrheal agent as needed.
- Maintain seizure precautions.
- Institute safety precautions if adverse CNS reactions occur.

Patient Teaching

• Stress importance of taking the drug exactly as prescribed. Patient may have to set an alarm clock for night doses.

• Reassure patients who are taking the extended-release form of procainamide that a wax matrix "ghost" from the tablet may be passed in the stool, and that the drug is completely absorbed before this occurs.

• Emphasize the importance of close follow-up care that includes frequent ECGs and blood tests.

• Warn patient to avoid hazardous activities that require mental alertness until CNS effects of drug are known.

• Tell patient how to handle troublesome GI reactions.

Evaluation

In patients receiving procainamide, appropriate evaluation statements may include:

• Patient's ECG reveals arrhythmia has been corrected.

• Patient's CBC remains normal throughout therapy.

• Patient and family state an understanding of procainamide therapy.

procaine hydrochloride

(pro kane´)

Novocain

• *Classification:* local anesthetic
• *Pregnancy Risk Category:* C

HOW SUPPLIED

Injection: 1%, 2%, 10%

ACTION

Mechanism: An ester-type local anesthetic that blocks depolarization by interfering with sodium-potassium exchange across the nerve cell membrane, preventing generation and conduction of the nerve impulse.

Absorption: Procaine is a vasodilator; therefore the addition of epinephrine or similar vasoconstrictor is necessary to retard absorption.

Distribution: Widely distributed; drug crosses the placenta.

Metabolism: In the plasma, by pseudocholinesterase, to para-amino benzoic acid (PABA) and diethylaminoethanol. These metabolites undergo further degradation in the liver.

Excretion: About 80% is excreted in the urine as PABA and metabolites.

Onset, peak, duration: Variable, but average onset is 2 to 5 minutes; duration of action, about 1 hour.

INDICATIONS & DOSAGE

Spinal anesthesia –

Maximum dose is 11 mg/kg (14 mg/kg when mixed with epinephrine).

Before using, dilute 10% solution with 0.9% sodium chloride injection, sterile distilled water, or cerebrospinal fluid.

For hyperbaric technique, use dextrose solution.

Perineum: use 0.5 ml 10% solution and 0.5 ml diluent injected at fourth lumbar interspace.

Perineum and lower extremities: use 1 ml 10% solution and 1 ml diluent injected at third or fourth lumbar interspace.

Up to costal margin: use 2 ml 10% solution and 1 ml diluent injected at second, third, or fourth lumbar interspace.

Epidural block:

Sol.	Vol. (ml)	Dose (mg)
1.5%	25	375

Peripheral nerve block:

Sol.	Vol. (ml)	Dose (mg)
1%	50	500
2%	25	500

Infiltration: use 250 to 600 mg 0.25% to 0.5% solution. Maximum initial dose 1 g. Dose and interval may be increased with epinephrine. Maximum dosage 11 mg/kg to 14 mg/kg or epinephrine.

CONTRAINDICATIONS & PRECAUTIONS

Contraindicated in patients with a traumatized urethra and in hypersensitivity to chloroprocaine, tetracaine, or other para-aminobenzoic acid derivatives. Use cautiously in hyperexcitable patients and in CNS diseases, infection at the puncture site, shock, profound anemia, cachexia, sepsis, GI hemorrhage, hypertension, bowel perforation or strangulation, peritonitis, cardiac decompensation, massive pleural effusions, and increased intra-abdominal pressure.

ADVERSE REACTIONS

Common reactions are in italics; life-threatening reactions are in bold italics.

Skin: dermatologic reactions.

Other: edema, ***status asthmaticus, anaphylaxis,*** anaphylactoid reactions.

The following systemic effects may result from high blood levels of the drug:

CNS: anxiety, nervousness, seizures followed by drowsiness, unconsciousness, tremors, twitches, shivering, *respiratory arrest.*

CV: myocardial depression, ***arrhythmias, cardiac arrest.***

EENT: blurred vision, tinnitus.

GI: nausea, vomiting.

INTERACTIONS

Echothiophate iodide: reduced hydrolysis of procaine. Use together cautiously.

EFFECTS ON DIAGNOSTIC TESTS

None reported.

NURSING CONSIDERATIONS

Besides those related universally to drug therapy (see "How to use this book"), consider the following specific recommendations:

Assessment

- Obtain a baseline assessment of the patient's sensory status before therapy.
- Be alert for adverse reactions and drug interactions throughout therapy.
- Evaluate the patient's and family's knowledge about procaine therapy.

Nursing Diagnoses

- Pain related to inadequate block.
- Decreased cardiac output related to adverse reaction to procaine.
- Knowledge deficit related to procaine therapy.

Planning and Implementation

Preparation and Administration

- ***Epidural use:*** Be aware that for epidural use, test doses are administered to verify needle or catheter placement. Initially, 2 to 3 ml is given to check for subarachnoid injection, which would cause extensive motor paralysis of the lower limbs and extensive sensory deficit. After about 5 minutes and in the absence of symptoms, a second, larger test dose of about 5 ml is given to check for intravascular injection, which would cause tinnitus, numbness around the lips, metallic taste, dysphoria, lethargy, or hypotension.
- Use solution without preservatives for epidural block.
- Discard partially used vials without preservatives.
- Check solution for particles.

Monitoring

- Monitor effectiveness by evaluating pain relief. Continue to monitor sensory level every 15 minutes after completion of surgery or treatment until sympathetic innervation returns.
- Monitor for signs of anaphylaxis after administration of drug.
- Monitor for signs of myocardial depression as well as unconsciousness, seizures, and other adverse reactions including cardiac and respiratory arrest, which may result from high blood levels of the drug.

Supportive Care
• Keep resuscitative equipment and drugs available.
• Consult with the doctor if pain relief is ineffective.
• Be aware that onset occurs in 2 to 5 minutes; duration is 60 minutes.
• Notify the doctor immediately if the patient's CNS, cardiac or respiratory status deteriorates.
• Keep patient supine until sympathetic return has been established in order to prevent hypotension.
Patient Teaching
• Explain that the drug will cause a local loss of sensation providing pain relief in the selected body area, but unlike general anesthesia will not cause unconsciousness.
• Describe the route of administration, such as spinal, epidural, infiltration or peripheral nerve block.

Evaluation

In patients receiving procaine, appropriate evaluation statements may include:
• Effective sensory block is achieved.
• Cardiac status is within normal limits.
• Patient and family state an understanding of procaine therapy.

procarbazine hydrochloride

(proe kar´ ba zeen)
Matulane, Natulan†‡

• *Classification:* antineoplastic (antibiotic)
• *Pregnancy Risk Category:* D

HOW SUPPLIED

Capsules: 50 mg

ACTION

Mechanism: Inhibits DNA, RNA, and protein synthesis, and may directly damage DNA. Effects are most prominent in rapidly proliferating cells. Also inhibits MAO.
Absorption: Rapidly and completely absorbed after oral administration.
Distribution: Widely distributed into body tissues, with the highest concentrations found in the liver, kidneys, intestinal wall, and skin. Readily crosses the blood-brain barrier and reaches equilibrium with plasma levels with repeated doses.
Metabolism: Extensively metabolized in the liver. Some of the metabolites have cytotoxic activity.
Excretion: Drug and metabolites are excreted primarily in urine. Half-life: About 1 hour.
Onset, peak, duration: Peak plasma levels occur within 1 hour of oral dosing and are similar to those achieved after I.V. administration.

INDICATIONS & DOSAGE

Dosage and indications may vary. Check patient's protocol with doctor.
Hodgkin's disease, lymphomas, brain and lung cancer–
Adults: 2 to 4 mg/kg P.O. daily in a single dose or divided doses for the first week. Then, 4 to 6 mg/kg daily until WBC falls below 4,000/mm^3 or platelets fall below 100,000/mm^3. After bone marrow recovers, resume maintenance dosage of 1 to 2 mg/kg/day.
Children: 50 mg/m^2 P.O. daily for first week, then 100 mg/m^2 until response or toxicity occurs. Maintenance dosage is 50 mg/m^2 P.O. daily after bone marrow recovery.

CONTRAINDICATIONS & PRECAUTIONS

Contraindicated in patients with a history of hypersensitivity to the drug and in those with poor bone marrow reserve because of potential for serious toxicity. Use cautiously in patients with hepatic or renal impairment because of potential for drug accumulation; in those with infections because of decreased immune response; and in those taking concurrent CNS depressants or MAO inhibitors because the drug has MAO-inhibiting activity.

ADVERSE REACTIONS

Common reactions are in italics; life-threatening reactions are in bold italics.
Blood: bleeding tendency, ***thrombocytopenia,*** *leukopenia,* anemia.
CNS: nervousness, depression, insomnia, nightmares, *hallucinations,* confusion.
EENT: retinal hemorrhage, nystagmus, photophobia.
GI: *nausea, vomiting, anorexia,* stomatitis, dry mouth, dysphagia, diarrhea, constipation.
Skin: dermatitis.
Other: reversible alopecia, pleural effusion.

INTERACTIONS

Alcohol: mild disulfiram-like reaction. Warn patient not to drink alcohol.
CNS depressants: additive depressant effects.
Meperidine: may cause severe hypotension and possible death. Don't give together.
Sympathomimetics, local anesthetics, antidepressants, foods high in tyramine content (chianti wine, cheese): possible tremors, palpitations, increased blood pressure.

EFFECTS ON DIAGNOSTIC TESTS

None reported.

NURSING CONSIDERATIONS

Besides those related universally to drug therapy (see "How to use this book"), consider the following specific recommendations:

Assessment

- Obtain a baseline assessment of patient's overall physical status, including CNS status, CBC, and renal and hepatic function before therapy.
- Be alert for adverse reactions and drug interactions throughout therapy.
- Evaluate the patient's and family's knowledge about procarbazine therapy.

Nursing Diagnoses

- Altered protection related to procarbazine-induced myelosupression.
- High risk for injury related to procarbazine-induced adverse CNS reactions.
- Knowledge deficit related to procarbazine therapy.

Planning and Implementation

Preparation and Administration

- Keep in mind that administering drug in divided doses may help to decrease nausea and vomiting.
- Do not administer procarbazine with other MAO inhibitors, tricyclic antidepressants, or foods with a high tyramine content since procarbazine inhibits MAO and can cause a disulfiram-like reaction.
- Do not administer with meperidine since severe hypertension and possible death may occur.

Monitoring

- Monitor effectiveness by noting results of follow-up diagnostic tests and patient's overall physical status.
- Monitor CBC and platelet count.
- Monitor for adverse CNS reactions, such as depression, hallucinations, and confusion.
- Monitor for signs of infection (cough, fever, sore throat) and bleeding (easy bruising, nosebleeds, bleeding gums).
- Monitor for adverse GI reactions.

Supportive Care

- To help prevent infection, maintain the patient's optimal health and protect him from undue exposure to environmental contagions. If signs of infection occur, notify the doctor promptly; administer antibiotics, as ordered.
- Provide a safe environment to minimize risk of bleeding and risk of injury if adverse CNS reactions occur. Assist patient with activities, if needed.
- Discontinue medication if disulfi-

ram-like reaction occurs (chest pains, rapid or irregular heartbeat, severe headache, stiff neck).
• Keep in mind that, since procarbazine crosses the blood-brain barrier, it may be used to treat primary brain tumors.
• Avoid all I.M. injections in patients with thrombocytopenia.
• Administer antiemetics to help control nausea and vomiting.

Patient Teaching
• Warn the patient to watch for signs of infection (sore throat, fever, fatigue) and bleeding (easy bruising, nosebleeds, bleeding gums). Tell patient to take temperature daily and to report signs of infection and bleeding.
• Teach patient to avoid the use of all OTC products containing aspirin.
• Inform the patient that hair loss is possible, but is usually reversible.
• Warn patient not to drink alcoholic beverages while taking this drug. Also instruct patient to avoid foods containing a high tyramine content, such as Chianti wine and cheese.
• Advise patient to inform any doctor that he is taking procarbazine since interactions with other medications can cause uncomfortable and harmful effects.
• Instruct patient to stop drug immediately and notify doctor if chest pain, rapid or irregular heart beat, severe headache, or stiff neck occurs.
• Warn patient to avoid hazardous tasks such as driving or operating heavy machinery until the adverse CNS effects are known.
• Inform patient that nausea and vomiting may be decreased if medication is taken at bedtime and in divided doses.

Evaluation

In patient's receiving procarbazine, appropriate evaluation statements may include:
• Patient does not demonstrate signs and symptoms of infection or bleeding.
• Patient's safety is maintained.
• Patient and family state an understanding of procarbazine therapy.

prochlorperazine
(proe klor per´ a zeen)
Compazine, Stemetil†‡

prochlorperazine edisylate
Compazine

1prochlorperazine maleate
Anti-Naus‡, Chlorpazine, Compazine, Stemetil†‡

• *Classification:* antipsychotic, antiemetic, anxiolytic (phenathiazine [piperazine derivative])
• *Pregnancy Risk Category:* C

HOW SUPPLIED
prochlorperazine
Injection: 5 mg/ml
Suppositories: 2.5 mg, 5 mg, 25 mg
prochlorperazine edisylate
Syrup: 1 mg/ml
prochlorperazine maleate
Tablets: 5 mg, 10 mg, 25 mg
Capsules (sustained-release): 10 mg, 15 mg, 30 mg

ACTION
Mechanism: A phenothiazine derivative that blocks dopamine receptors. Acts on the chemoreceptor trigger zone to inhibit nausea and vomiting, and in larger doses, partially depresses the vomiting center as well.
Absorption: Rate and extent of absorption vary with administration route; oral tablet absorption is erratic and variable, and I.M. injection is absorbed rapidly.
Distribution: Widely distributed into the body, including breast milk. Drug is 91% to 99% protein-bound.
Metabolism: Extensively metabolized

by the liver, but no active metabolites are formed; duration of action is about 4 to 6 hours.
Excretion: Most in urine via the kidneys; some in feces via the biliary tract.
Onset, peak, duration: Onset of action ranges from 30 minutes to 1 hour; oral concentrate absorption is more predictable. Peak effect occurs at 2 to 4 hours; steady-state serum levels are achieved within 4 to 7 days.

INDICATIONS & DOSAGE

Preoperative nausea control–
Adults: 5 to 10 mg I.M. 1 to 2 hours before induction of anesthetic, repeat once in 30 minutes, if necessary; or 5 to 10 mg I.V. 15 to 30 minutes before induction of anesthetic (repeat once if necessary); or 20 mg/liter dextrose 5% in water and 0.9% sodium chloride solution by I.V. infusion, added to infusion 15 to 30 minutes before induction. Maximum parenteral dosage is 40 mg daily.
Severe nausea, vomiting–
Adults: 5 to 10 mg P.O. t.i.d. or q.i.d.; or 15 mg sustained-release form P.O. on arising; or 10 mg sustained-release form P.O. q 12 hours; or 25 mg rectally b.i.d.; or 5 to 10 mg I.M. injected deeply into upper outer quadrant of gluteal region. Repeat q 3 to 4 hours, p.r.n. Maximum I.M. dosage is 40 mg daily.
Children 18 to 39 kg: 2.5 mg P.O. or rectally t.i.d.; or 5 mg P.O. or rectally b.i.d. Maximum dosage is 15 mg daily; or 0.132 mg/kg deep I.M. injection. (Control usually obtained with 1 dose.)
Children 14 to 17 kg: 2.5 mg P.O. or rectally b.i.d. or t.i.d. Maximum dosage is 10 mg daily; or 0.132 mg/kg deep I.M. injection. (Control usually obtained with 1 dose.)
Children 9 to 13 kg: 2.5 mg P.O. or rectally daily or b.i.d. Maximum dosage is 7.5 mg daily; or 0.132 mg/kg deep I.M. injection. (Control usually obtained with 1 dose.)
Symptomatic management of psychotic disorders–
Adults: 5 to 10 mg, P.O. t.i.d. or q.i.d.
Children 2 to 12 years: 2.5 mg P.O. or P.R. b.i.d. or t.i.d. Do not exceed 10 mg on day 1. Increase dosage gradually to recommended maximum (if necessary).
Children 6 to 10 years: maximum 25 mg P.O. daily.
Children 2 to 5 years: maximum 20 mg P.O. daily.
Symptomatic management of severe psychoses–
Adults: 10 to 20 mg I.M. May be repeated in 1 to 4 hours. Rarely, patients may receive 10 to 20 mg q 4 to 6 hours. Oral therapy should be instituted after symptoms are controlled.
Children: 0.13 mg/kg I.M.
Management of excessive anxiety–
Adults: 5 to 10 mg by deep I.M. injection every 3 to 4 hours, not to exceed 40 mg daily; or 5 to 10 mg P.O. t.i.d. or q.i.d.; alternatively, give 15 mg (as the extended-release capsule) once daily, or 10 mg (extended-release capsule) q 12 hours.

CONTRAINDICATIONS & PRECAUTIONS

Contraindicated in patients with hypersensitivity to phenothiazines and related compounds, including allergic reactions involving hepatic function; blood dyscrasias and bone marrow depression; and disorders accompanied by coma, brain damage, CNS depression, circulatory collapse, or cerebrovascular disease, because of adverse effects on blood pressure and possible additive CNS depression; also contraindicated for use with adrenergic-blocking agents or spinal or epidural anesthetics.

Use cautiously in patients with cardiac disease (arrhythmias, CHF, angina pectoris, valvular disease, or heart block) because of additive ar-rhythmic effects; encephalitis; Reye's syndrome, head injury, or respiratory disease, because of additive CNS and respiratory depression; seizure disorders, because of lowered seizure threshold; glaucoma, because of increased intraocular pressure; prostatic hypertrophy; urine retention; hepatic or renal dysfunction; Parkinson's disease; pheochromocytoma, because excessive buildup of neurotransmitters may have adverse cardiovascular effects; and hypocalcemia, which increases the risk of extrapyramidal symptoms.

ADVERSE REACTIONS

Common reactions are in italics; life-threatening reactions are in bold italics.
Blood: *transient leukopenia,* ***agranulocytosis.***
CNS: *extrapyramidal reactions,* sedation, pseudoparkinsonism, EEG changes, dizziness.
CV: *orthostatic hypotension,* tachycardia, ECG changes.
EENT: *ocular changes, blurred vision.*
GI: *dry mouth, constipation.*
GU: *urine retention,* dark urine, menstrual irregularities, gynecomastia, inhibited ejaculation.
Hepatic: *cholestatic jaundice.*
Metabolic: hyperprolactinemia.
Skin: *mild photosensitivity,* dermal allergic reactions, ***exfoliative dermatitis.***
Other: weight gain, increased appetite.

INTERACTIONS

Antacids: inhibited absorption of oral phenothiazines. Separate antacid and phenothiazine doses by at least 2 hours.
Anticholinergics, including antidepressants and antiparkinsonian agents: increased anticholinergic activity and aggravated parkinsonian symptoms. Use together cautiously.
Barbiturates: may decrease phenothiazine effect. Monitor patient for decreased antiemetic effect.

EFFECTS ON DIAGNOSTIC TESTS

ECG: quinidine-like effects.
Liver enzymes: elevated levels.
Protein-bound iodine: elevated value.
Urine porphyrins, urobilinogen, amylase, and 5-HIAA: false-positive results, because of darkening of urine by metabolites.
Urine pregnancy tests using human chorionic gonadotropin: false-positive results.

NURSING CONSIDERATIONS

Besides those related universally to drug therapy (see "How to use this book"), consider the following specific recommendations:

Assessment

- Obtain a baseline assessment of allergies, mental status, CBC, and liver function studies before therapy.
- Be alert for adverse reactions and drug interactions throughout therapy.
- Evaluate the patient's and family's knowledge about prochlorperazine therapy.

Nursing Diagnoses

- High risk for fluid volume deficit related to nausea and vomiting.
- Altered thought processes related to prochlorperazine-induced CNS depression.
- Knowledge deficit related to prochlorperazine therapy.

Planning and Implementation

Preparation and Administration

- Store in light-resistant container. Slight yellowing does not affect potency; discard very discolored solution.
- Avoid getting concentrate or injection solution on hands or clothing to prevent contact dermatitis.
- ***P.O. use:*** Dilute oral solution with tomato or fruit juice, carbonated beverage, milk, coffee, tea, water, soup, or pudding.

• ***I.V. use:*** Infuse slowly, never as a bolus injection.
• ***I.M. use:*** Give deep I.M. Never give S.C. or mix in syringe with another drug.
Monitoring
• Monitor effectiveness by monitoring patient for nausea and vomiting.
• Monitor CBC and liver function studies.
• Monitor blood pressure carefully in patients receiving I.V. doses.
• Monitor fluid balance.
• Observe for changes in mental status, mood, behavior, and visual acuity.
Supportive Care
• Use with cautioun in combination with other CNS depressants; in hepatic disease, arteriosclerosis or cardiovascular disease (may cause sudden drop in blood pressure), exposure to extreme heat or cold (including antipyretic therapy), respiratory disorders, hypocalcemia, seizure disorders or severe reactions to insulin or electroshock therapy, suspected brain tumor or intestinal obstruction, glaucoma, or prostatic hypertrophy; in acutely ill, dehydrated, or vomiting children; and in elderly or debilitated patients.
• Use only when vomiting can't be controlled by other measures, or when only a few doses are required. Notify the doctor if more than four doses are required in 24-hour period.
• Not effective in motion sickness.
• Be aware that elderly patients should usually receive dosages in the lower range.
Patient Teaching
• Warn patients to wear protective clothing when exposed to sunlight.
• Instruct patient to mix oral solution with pleasant-tasting liquid to mask taste.
• Advise patient that sugarless hard candy may reduce mouth dryness.

Evaluation
In patients receiving prochlorperazine, appropriate evaluation statements may include:
• Patient exhibits no signs of fluid volume deficit.
• Patient demonstrates no signs of altered thought processes.
• Patient and family state an understanding of prochlorperazine therapy.

progesterone
(proe jess´ ter one)
Gesterol 50, Progestaject, Progestilin†

• *Classification:* contraceptive (progestin)
• *Pregnancy Risk Category:* X

HOW SUPPLIED
Injection (in oil): 50 mg/ml

ACTION
Mechanism: Suppresses ovulation, possibly by inhibiting pituitary gonadotropin secretion. Also forms a thick cervical mucus.
Absorption: Must be administered parenterally, inactivated by the liver after oral administration. I.M. form is well absorbed.
Distribution: Widely distributed; drug crosses the placenta.
Metabolism: Reduced to pregnanediol in the liver, then conjugated with glucuronic acid.
Excretion: Glucuronide conjugate is excreted in urine. Half-life: Very short (several minutes).

INDICATIONS & DOSAGE
Amenorrhea –
Women: 5 to 10 mg I.M. daily for 6 to 8 days.
Dysfunctional uterine bleeding –
Women: 5 to 10 mg I.M. daily for 6 doses.

Management of premenstrual syndrome (PMS) –
Women: 200 to 400 mg as a suppository administered either rectally or vaginally.

CONTRAINDICATIONS & PRECAUTIONS

Contraindicated in patients with hypersensitivity to progestins or a history of thromboembolic disorder, severe hepatic disease, breast cancer, or undiagnosed abnormal vaginal bleeding; and in pregnant or breast-feeding women.

Use cautiously in patients with cardiac or renal disease, epilepsy, migraine, or other conditions that might be aggravated by fluid and electrolyte retention; in diabetic patients because glucose tolerance may occur; or in patients with a history of mental depression because the drug may worsen this condition.

ADVERSE REACTIONS

Common reactions are in italics; life-threatening reactions are in bold italics.
CNS: dizziness, migraine headache, lethargy, depression.
CV: hypertension, thrombophlebitis, ***pulmonary embolism,*** edema.
GI: nausea, vomiting, abdominal cramps.
GU: breakthrough bleeding, dysmenorrhea, amenorrhea, cervical erosion, or abnormal secretions, uterine fibromas, vaginal candidiasis.
Hepatic: cholestatic jaundice.
Local: pain at injection site.
Metabolic: hyperglycemia.
Skin: melasma, rash.
Other: breast tenderness, enlargement, or secretion; decreased libido.

INTERACTIONS

Rifampin: decreased progestogen effects. Monitor for diminished therapeutic response.

EFFECTS ON DIAGNOSTIC TESTS

Pregnanediol excretion: decreased.
Serum alkaline phosphatase and amino acid: increased levels.

NURSING CONSIDERATIONS

Besides those related universally to drug therapy (see "How to use this book"), consider the following specific recommendations:

Assessment
- Obtain a baseline assessment of the patient's uterine bleeding problem or PMS before initiating progesterone therapy.
- Be alert for adverse reactions and drug interactions throughout therapy.
- Evaluate the patient's and family's knowledge about progesterone therapy.

Nursing Diagnoses
- High risk for fluid volume deficit related to excessive abnormal uterine bleeding.
- Fluid volume excess related to progesterone-induced edema.
- Knowledge deficit related to progesterone therapy.

Planning and Implementation
Preparation and Administration
- FDA regulations require that before receiving their first dose, patients read the package insert describing possible adverse reactions to progesterone. Offer verbal explanations as well.
- Expect to administer preliminary estrogen treatment in patients with menstrual disorders.
- ***I.M. use:*** Give oil solutions (peanut oil or sesame oil) deep. Rotate injection sites.
- ***Intrauterine device (IUD):*** Prepare the patient for Progestasert insertion as directed by doctor.

Monitoring
- Monitor effectiveness by regularly assessing the degree and pattern of uterine bleeding or symptoms of PMS.

• Monitor injection sites frequently for evidence of irritation.
• Monitor the patient's blood pressure for elevation.
• Monitor frequently for breakthrough bleeding or abnormal vaginal secretions.
• Regularly monitor the patient's blood glucose level.
• Monitor the patient's weight for sudden increases suggestive of fluid retention.

Supportive Care

• Progesterone should be discontinued if hypersensitivity, thromboembolic or thrombotic disorders, visual disturbances, migraine headache, or severe depression occurs. Notify doctor immediately. Be prepared to provide supportive treatment as indicated.
• Expect to adjust diabetic patients' treatment regimen if hyperglycemia occurs.
• Limit patient's sodium intake if edema occur unless contraindicated.

Patient Teaching

• Advise the patient to discontinue therapy and call the doctor immediately if migraine or visual disturbances occur, or if sudden severe headache or vomiting develops.
• Teach the patient how perform breast self-examination.
• Tell patient receiving progesterone she should have a full physical examination, including a gynecologic exam and a Papanicolaou test, every 6 to 12 months.
• Tell the patient to check with her doctor promptly if period is missed or unusual bleeding occurs, and to discontinue drug immediately and check with her doctor if she suspects pregnancy.
• Advise the patient who misses a dose to take the missed dose as soon as possible or omit it, and not to double doses.
• Tell the patient that GI distress may subside after a few cycles.
• Inform the patient that progesterone may cause possible dental problems (tenderness, swelling, or bleeding of gums). Advise the patient to brush and floss teeth, massage gums, and have the dentist clean teeth regularly. The patient should check with the dentist if she has questions about care of teeth or gums or if tenderness, swelling or bleeding of gums occurs.

For the patient using Progestasert:

• Inform the patient that bleeding and cramping may occur for a few weeks after insertion.
• Advise the patient to contact the doctor if abnormal or excessive bleeding, severe cramping, abnormal vaginal discharge, fever, or flu-like syndrome occurs.
• Teach the patient how to check for proper placement of IUD.
• Tell the patient that the progesterone supply in the IUD is depleted in 1 year and the device must be changed at that time. Pregnancy risk increases if the patient relies on progesterone-depleted device for contraception.
• Inform the patient of the adverse reactions to IUD use: uterine perforation, increased risk of infection, pelvic inflammatory disease, ectopic pregnancy, abdominal cramping, increased menstrual flow, and expulsion of the device.

Evaluation

In patients receiving progesterone, appropriate evaluation statements may include:
• Abnormal uterine bleeding is controlled with progestrone therapy.
• Patient does not exhibit fluid retention.
• Patient and family states an understanding of progesterone therapy.

PHARMACOLOGIC CLASS

progestins

hydroxyprogesterone caproate
medroxyprogesterone acetate
megestrol acetate
norethindrone
norethindrone acetate
norgestrel
progesterone

OVERVIEW

Progesterone is the endogenous progestin, secreted by the ovary. Several synthetic progesterone derivatives with greater potency or duration of action have been synthesized. Some of these derivatives also possess weak androgenic or estrogenic activity.

Progesterone causes secretory changes in the endometrium, changes in the vaginal epithelium, increases in body temperature, relaxation of uterine smooth muscle, stimulation of growth of breast alveolar tissue, inhibition of gonadotropin release from the pituitary, and withdrawal bleeding (in the presence of estrogens). The synthetic progesterone derivatives have these properties as well.

CLINICAL INDICATIONS AND ACTIONS

Hormonal imbalance, female

Hydroxyprogesterone, medroxyprogesterone, norethindrone, and progesterone are indicated to treat amenorrhea and dysfunctional uterine bleeding resulting from hormonal imbalance. Hydroxyprogesterone also is indicated to produce desquamation and a secretory endometrium.

Endometriosis

Norethindrone and norethindrone acetate are indicated to treat endometriosis.

Carcinoma

Hydroxyprogesterone, medroxyprogesterone, and megestrol are indicated in the adjunctive and palliative treatment of certain types of metastatic tumors. They are not considered primary therapy. See individual agents for specific indications.

Contraception

Norethindrone and norgestrel are approved for use with estrogens or alone as oral contraceptives.

Medroxyprogesterone (parenteral) is not approved for use as a contraceptive in the United States but is used in other countries as a long-acting, effective contraceptive.

Progestins are no longer indicated to detect pregnancy (because of teratogenicity) or to treat threatened or habitual abortion, for which they are not effective.

OVERVIEW OF ADVERSE REACTIONS

The most common side effect of progestin administration is a change in menstrual bleeding pattern, ranging from spotting or breakthrough bleeding to complete amenorrhea. Breast tenderness and breast secretion may occur. Weight changes, increases in body temperature, edema, nausea, or acne also may occur. Somnolence, insomnia, hirsutism, hair loss, depression, cholestatic jaundice, and rare allergic reactions (ranging from rash to anaphylaxis) also have been reported. A few patients taking parenteral progestins have suffered localized reactions at the injection site.

REPRESENTATIVE COMBINATIONS

Hydroxyprogesterone caproate with estradiol valerate: Hy-Gestradol, Hylutin-Est.

Norethindrone acetate with ethinyl estradiol: Brevicon 21/28, Gestest, Loestrin, Modicon 21/28, Norinyl 1 + 35, Norlestrin, Norquest, Ortho 1/35*, Ortho 7/7/7*, Ortho 10/11*, Ortho-Novum 21/28, 7/7/7, 10/11, Ovcon-35, Ovcon-50, Tri-norinyl; with mestranol: Norinyl 1/50, Norinyl 1 + 80, Norinyl 1/80*, Norinyl 2, Ortho-Novum 0.5*, Ortho-Novum 1/

50, Ortho-Novum 1/80, Ortho-Novum 2, Program-20*, Program-40*, Program-80*; with mestranol and ferrous fumarate: Norinyl-1 Fe 28; with ethinyl estradiol and ferrous fumarate: Norlestrin Fe 1/50, 2.5/50.

Norgestrel with ethinyl estradiol: Lo/Ovral, Ovral-Prep, Lo/Ovral, Miss-Ovral*, Ovral.

Progesterone with estradiol benzoate: Pro-Estrone; with estradiol, testosterone and procaine hydrochloride: Hormo-Triad; with estrogenic substance: Profoygen Aqueous; with estrone: Proestrone.

promazine hydrochloride

(proe´ ma zeen)
Sparine**

• *Classification:* antipsychotic, antiemetic (phenothiazine)
• *Pregnancy Risk Category:* C

HOW SUPPLIED

Tablets: 25 mg, 50 mg, 100 mg
Syrup: 10 mg/5 ml
Injection: 25 mg/ml, 50 mg/ml

ACTION

Mechanism: Blocks postsynaptic dopamine receptors in the brain. Its antiemetic actions are probably related to dopamine receptor blockade in the chemoreceptor trigger zone in the medulla.
Absorption: Usually absorbed well from the GI tract. Liquid forms have the most predictable effect, whereas tablets have erratic and variable absorption. I.M. drug is absorbed rapidly.
Distribution: Widely distributed into the body, including breast milk. Drug is 91% to 99% protein-bound.
Metabolism: Extensively metabolized by the liver, but no active metabolites are formed.
Excretion: Most is excreted as metabolites in urine; some in feces via the biliary tract.
Onset, peak, duration: Onset of effect ranges from 30 minutes to 1 hour. Peak effect occurs at 2 to 4 hours; steady-state serum level is achieved within 4 to 7 days.

INDICATIONS & DOSAGE

Psychosis–
Adults: 10 to 200 mg P.O. or I.M. q 4 to 6 hours, up to 1 g daily. I.V. dose in concentrations no greater than 25 mg/ml for acutely agitated patients. Initial dose is 50 to 150 mg; repeat within 5 to 10 minutes if necessary.
Children over 12 years: 10 to 25 mg P.O. or I.M. q 4 to 6 hours.

CONTRAINDICATIONS & PRECAUTIONS

Contraindicated in patients with hypersensitivity to phenothiazines and related compounds, including allergic reactions involving hepatic function; blood dyscrasias and bone marrow depression, because of adverse hematologic effects; disorders accompanied by coma, CNS depression, or in patients with brain damage, because of additive CNS depression; in patients with circulatory collapse or cerebrovascular disease because of adverse effects on blood pressure; and in patients who are receiving adrenergic-blocking agents or spinal or epidural anesthetics, because of potential for excessive hypotensive response.

Use cautiously in patients with cardiac disease (arrhythmias, CHF, angina pectoris, valvular disease, or heart block), encephalitis, Reye's syndrome, head injury, respiratory disease, seizure disorders, glaucoma, prostatic hypertrophy, urine retention, hepatic or renal dysfunction, Parkinson's disease, pheochromocytoma, or hypocalcemia. Some oral preparations of promazine contain tartrazine; dyes may cause allergic reaction in aspirin-allergic patients.

ADVERSE REACTIONS

Common reactions are in italics; life-threatening reactions are in bold italics.
Blood: transient leukopenia, ***agranulocytosis.***
CNS: *extrapyramidal reactions (moderate incidence), tardive dyskinesia, sedation (high incidence),* pseudoparkinsonism, EEG changes, dizziness.
CV: *orthostatic hypotension,* tachycardia, ECG changes.
EENT: ocular changes, *blurred vision.*
GI: *dry mouth, constipation.*
GU: *urine retention,* dark urine, menstrual irregularities, gynecomastia, inhibited ejaculation.
Hepatic: cholestatic jaundice, abnormal liver function tests.
Metabolic: hyperprolactinemia.
Skin: *mild photosensitivity,* dermal allergic reactions.
Local: pain at I.M. injection site, sterile abscess.
Other: weight gain; increased appetite; ***rarely, neuroleptic malignant syndrome*** (fever, tachycardia, tachypnea, profuse diaphoresis).
After abrupt withdrawal of long-term therapy: gastritis, nausea, vomiting, dizziness, tremors, feeling of warmth or cold, sweating, tachycardia, headache, insomnia.

INTERACTIONS

Alcohol, other CNS depressants: increased CNS depression. Avoid concomitant use.
Antacids: inhibit absorption of oral phenothiazines. Separate antacid and phenothiazine doses by at least 2 hours.
Anticholinergics (including antidepressant and antiparkinsonian agents): increased anticholinergic activity, aggravated parkinsonian symptoms. Use with caution.
Barbiturates, lithium: may decrease phenothiazine effect. Observe patient.
Centrally acting antihypertensives: decreased antihypertensive effect.
Oral anticoagulants: decreased effectiveness.
Propranolol: increased serum levels of propranolol and promazine.

EFFECTS ON DIAGNOSTIC TESTS

ECG: quinidine-like effects.
Liver function tests: elevated results.
Protein-bound iodine: elevated results.
Urine porphyrins, urobilinogen, amylase, and 5-HIAA: false-positive results because of darkening of urine by metabolites.
Urine pregnancy tests using human chorionic gonadotropin: false-positive results.

NURSING CONSIDERATIONS

Besides those related universally to drug therapy (see "How to use this book"), consider the following specific recommendations:

Assessment

• Obtain baseline assessment of patient's mental status, including psychotic symptoms, before therapy.
• Be alert for adverse reactions and drug interactions throughout therapy.
• Evaluate the patient's and family's knowledge about promazine therapy.

Nursing Diagnoses

• Impaired thought processes related to patient's underlying condition.
• Urinary retention related to adverse drug reaction.
• Knowledge deficit related to promazine therapy.

Planning and Implementation

Preparation and Administration

• ***P.O. use:*** Dilute liquid concentrate with fruit juice, milk, semisolid food or chocolate-flavored drinks just before giving. For best taste, use at least 10 ml diluent per 25 mg drug.
• ***I.V. use:*** Drug is given by direct injection; not recommended for inter-

mittent or continuous infusion. Administer I.V. only to hospitalized patient and change to oral therapy as soon as possible.
• Administer drug promptly. Solutions prepared with 0.9% sodium chloride and left at room temperature in daylight lose 15% of potency within 24 hours.
• Protect medication from light. Slight yellowing of injection or concentrate is common and does not affect potency. Discard markedly discolored solutions.
• ***I.M. use:*** Give injection deeply only in upper outer quadrant of buttocks. Massage slowly afterward to prevent sterile abscess. The injection may sting.
• Avoid skin contact with the injectable or liquid form because it may cause a rash.

Monitoring
• Monitor effectiveness by regularly observing the patient's behavior and changes in psychotic symptoms.
• Monitor for adverse reactions, especially extrapyramidal and anticholinergic effects (blurred vision, dry mouth, constipation, urine retention), and tardive dyskinesia, during prolonged therapy. Tardive dyskinesia may not appear until months or years later and may disappear spontaneously or persist for life despite discontinuation of the drug.
• Monitor for adverse reactions by frequently checking the patient's blood pressure for orthostatic hypotension, especially after parenteral administration.
• Monitor therapy by weekly bilirubin tests during the first month; periodic blood tests (CBC and liver function); and ophthalmic tests (long-term use).
• Monitor for neuroleptic malignant syndrome. This rare, potentially fatal reaction is not necessarily related to type of neuroleptic or duration of drug therapy, but usually occurs in men (60% of affected patients).

Supportive Care
• Keep the patient supine for 1 hour after I.M. administration. Then assist patient to get up slowly to avoid orthostatic hypotension.
• Do not discontinue drug abruptly unless required by severe adverse reactions.
• Increase the patient's fluid and fiber intake – if not contraindicated – to prevent constipation. If necessary, request doctor's order for a laxative.
• Give the patient sugarless gum, sour hard candy, ice chips, or a mouthwash rinse to relieve dry mouth.
• Treat acute dystonic reactions with I.V. diphenhydramine, as ordered.
• Hold dose if patient develops jaundice, symptoms of blood dyscrasias (fever, sore throat, infection, cellulitis, weakness), persistent (longer than a few hours) extrapyramidal reactions, or any such reactions during pregnancy or in children.

Patient Teaching
• Warn the patient that the injection may sting.
• Tell the patient to avoid exposure to direct sunlight and to use a sunscreen when going outdoors to prevent photosensitivity reactions. (*Note:* Sun lamps and tanning beds may cause burning of the skin or skin discoloration.)
• Tell the patient not to stop taking the drug suddenly.
• Encourage the patient to report difficult urinating, sore throat, dizziness, or fainting.
• Advise the patient to increase fluid and fiber in the diet, if appropriate.
• Tell the patient to avoid driving and other hazardous activities that require alertness until the effect of the drug is established. Excessive sedative effects (drowsiness and dizziness) tend to subside after several weeks.
• Explain which fluids are appropriate for diluting the concentrate and show the dropper technique for measuring dose. Warn the patient to avoid spill-

ing liquid on skin because rash and irritation may occur.
• Tell the patient that sugarless hard candy, chewing gum or ice chips can alleviate dry mouth.

Evaluation

In patients receiving promazine, appropriate evaluation statements may include:
• Patient demonstrates a decrease in psychotic behavior.
• Patient voids without difficulty.
• Patient and family state an understanding of promazine therapy.

promethazine hydrochloride

(proe meth´ a zeen)

Anergan 25, Anergan 50, Histanil†, K-Phen, Mallergan, Pentazine, Phenameth, Phenazine 25, Phenazine 50, Phencen-50, Phenergan*, Phenergan-Fortis*, Phenergan-Plain*, Phenoject-50, PMS-Promethazine†, Pro-50, Prometh-25, Prometh-50, Promethegan, Prothazine‡*, Prothazine-25, Prothazine-50, Prothazine Plain, Remsed, V-Gan-25, V-Gan-50

• *Classification:* antiemetic, antivertigo agent, antihistamine (H_1-receptor antagonist); preoperative, postoperative, or obstetric sedative and adjunct to analgesics (phenothiazine derivative)
• *Pregnancy Risk Category:* C

HOW SUPPLIED

Tablets: 12.5 mg, 25 mg, 50 mg
Syrup: 5 mg/5 ml‡*, 6.25 mg/5 ml*, 10 mg/5 ml*, 25 mg/5 ml*
Injection: 25 mg/ml, 50 mg/ml
Suppositories: 12.5 mg, 25 mg, 50 mg

ACTION

Mechanism: Competes with histamine for H_1-receptor sites on effector cells. Prevents but does not reverse histamine-mediated responses.
Absorption: Well absorbed after oral or parenteral administration.
Distribution: Widely distributed throughout the body; drug crosses the placenta and enters the CNS. Drug is 70% to 90% protein-bound.
Metabolism: Hepatic.
Excretion: In urine and feces.
Onset, peak, duration: Onset begins 20 minutes after oral, rectal, or I.M. administration and within 3 to 5 minutes after I.V. administration. Effects usually last 4 to 8 hours but may persist for 12 hours.

INDICATIONS & DOSAGE

Motion sickness–
Adults: 25 mg P.O. b.i.d.
Children: 1 mg/kg P.O., I.M., or rectally b.i.d.
Nausea–
Adults: 12.5 to 25 mg P.O., I.M., or rectally q 4 to 6 hours, p.r.n.
Children: 1 mg/kg I.M. or rectally q 4 to 6 hours, p.r.n.
Rhinitis, allergy symptoms–
Adults: 12.5 mg P.O. q.i.d.; or 25 mg P.O. at bedtime.
Children: 6.25 to 12.5 mg P.O. t.i.d. or 25 mg P.O. or rectally at bedtime.
Sedation–
Adults: 25 to 50 mg P.O. or I.M. at bedtime or p.r.n.
Children: 12.5 to 25 mg P.O., I.M., or rectally at bedtime.
Routine preoperative or postoperative sedation or as an adjunct to analgesics–
Adults: 25 to 50 mg I.M., I.V., or P.O.
Children: 12.5 to 25 mg I.M., I.V., or P.O.

CONTRAINDICATIONS & PRECAUTIONS

Contraindicated in patients with hypersensitivity to promethazine or other antihistamines or phenothiazines; during asthmatic attacks, because it thickens bronchial secretions; in acutely ill or dehydrated children, because they are at increased risk of dystonias; in patients with bone marrow depression, because it may induce blood dyscrasias; in epilepsy, because it may worsen seizure disorder; in comatose patients; and in neonates.

Like other antihistamines, promethazine has significant anticholinergic effects. Use with caution in patients with narrow-angle glaucoma, peptic ulcer, or pyloroduodenal obstruction or urinary bladder obstruction from prostatic hypertrophy or narrowing of the bladder neck; cardiovascular disease or hypertension because of the risk of palpitations, tachycardia, and increased hypertension; acute or chronic respiratory dysfunction (especially in children), because drug may suppress the cough reflex; hepatic dysfunction; and in children with a history of sleep apnea or a family history of sudden infant death syndrome. The relationship between these conditions and the use of promethazine has not been studied; however, several deaths have occurred in children who received usual dosages of phenothiazines and antihistamines.

Antiemetic action may mask symptoms of undiagnosed diseases, drug overdose, and the ototoxic effects of aspirin – dizziness, vertigo, tinnitus – or other ototoxic drugs.

ADVERSE REACTIONS

Common reactions are in italics; life-threatening reactions are in bold italics.
Blood: leukopenia, ***agranulocytosis.***
CNS: (especially in elderly patients) *sedation,* confusion, restlessness, tremors, *drowsiness.*
CV: hypotension.
EENT: transient myopia, nasal congestion.
GI: anorexia, nausea, vomiting, constipation, *dry mouth.*
GU: urine retention.
Other: photosensitivity.

INTERACTIONS

CNS depressants: increased sedation. Use together cautiously.
MAO inhibitors: increased anticholinergic effects. Don't use together.
Phenothiazines: increased effects. Don't give together.

EFFECTS ON DIAGNOSTIC TESTS

ABO blood grouping: test interference.
Blood glucose: hyperglycemia.
Diagnostic skin tests: test interference.
Pregnancy tests: false-positive or false-negative.

NURSING CONSIDERATIONS

Besides those related universally to drug therapy (see "How to use this book"), consider the following specific recommendations:.

Assessment

- Obtain a baseline assessment of the patient's underlying condition before therapy.
- Be alert for adverse reactions and drug interactions throughout therapy.
- Evaluate the patient's and family's knowledge about promethazine therapy.

Nursing Diagnoses

- Altered nutrition: Less than body requirements, related to nausea and motion sickness.
- High risk for infection related to possible agranulocytosis induced by promethazine.
- Knowledge deficit related to promethazine therapy.

Planning and Implementation

Preparation and Administration

- ***P.O. use:*** Give with food or milk to reduce GI distress.
- ***I.V. use:*** Do not give in concentrations greater than 25 mg/ml, nor at a rate exceeding 25 mg/minute. Shield I.V. infusion from direct light.
- ***I.M. use:*** Inject deep into large muscle mass. Rotate injection sites.

• Do not administer this drug by the subcutaneous route.
• Keep in mind that parenteral forms of this drug may be mixed with meperidine (Demerol) in the same syringe.

Monitoring
• Monitor effectiveness by evaluating relief of nausea or motion sickness.
• Monitor the patient carefully for sedation. Pronounced sedative effect of the drug may limit use in many ambulatory patients. Elderly patients are especially sensitive to adverse CNS reactions to this drug.
• Monitor intake and output for possible urine retention.

Supportive Care
• Take safety precautions with all patients, particularly during ambulation.
• Remember that promethazine may be used as an adjunct to analgesics (usually to increase sedation), but has no analgesic effect alone.
• Keep in mind that promethazine may cause a false-positive immunologic urine pregnancy test (Gravindex) and also that it may interfere with blood grouping in ABO system.

Patient Teaching
• Warn patient to avoid alcoholic beverages during therapy and to avoid hazardous activities that require alertness until adverse CNS effects are known.
• Tell the patient to drink coffee or tea to reduce drowsiness.
• Tell patient that sugarless gum, sour hard candy, or ice chips may relieve dry mouth.
• Warn patient about possible photosensitivity and teach precautions to avoid it.
• When drug is used for motion sickness, tell the patient to take first dose 30 to 60 minutes before traveling. Instruct the patient to take dose upon arising and with the evening meal, on succeeding days of travel.
• Warn patient to discontinue promethazine 4 days before allergy skin testing to preserve the accuracy of the tests.

Evaluation
In patients receiving promethazine, appropriate evaluation statements may include:
• Patient's symptoms of motion sickness are relieved with promethazine.
• Patient does not experience injury, as well as severe drowsiness or other adverse reactions to promethazine.
• Patient and family state an understanding of promethazine therapy.

propafenone hydrochloride
(proe pa feen´ one)
Rythmol

• *Classification:* antiarrhythmic (sodium blocker; beta-adrenergic blocker)
• *Pregnancy Risk Category:* C

HOW SUPPLIED
Tablets: 150 mg, 300 mg

ACTION
Mechanism: A Class Ic antiarrhythmic agent that stabilizes cardiac cell membranes, probably by decreasing sodium influx (local anesthetic effect). It also has weak beta-adrenergic blocking properties.
Absorption: Well absorbed from the GI tract; absorption is not affected by food. Because of a significant first-pass effect, bioavailability is limited; however, it increases with dosage. Absolute bioavailability is 3.4% with the 150-mg tablet and 10.6% with the 300-mg tablet.
Distribution: Plasma levels following a dose are variable. Increases in plasma levels do not parallel increases in dosage. A threefold increase in dosage from 300 to 900 mg/day can result in a tenfold increase in plasma levels.
Metabolism: Hepatic, with a signifi-

cant first-pass effect. Two active metabolites have been identified: 5-hydroxypropafenone and N-depropylpropafenone. A few patients (10% of all patients and patients receiving quinidine) metabolize the drug more slowly. Little (if any) 5-hydroxypropafenone is present in the plasma.
Excretion: Metabolites are found in the urine. Half-life: Elimination half-life is 2 to 10 hours in normal metabolizers (about 90% of patients); it can be as long as 10 to 32 hours in slow metabolizers.
Onset, peak, duration: Peak plasma levels occur about 3.5 hours after oral administration.

INDICATIONS & DOSAGE

Suppression of life-threatening ventricular arrhythmias, such as episodic ventricular tachycardia –
Adults: initially, 150 mg P.O. q 8 hours. Dosage may be increased to 225 mg q 8 hours after 3 or 4 days; if necessary, increase dosage to 300 mg q 8 hours. Maximum daily dosage is 900 mg.

CONTRAINDICATIONS & PRECAUTIONS

Contraindicated in patients with uncontrolled CHF; cardiogenic shock; SA, AV, and intraventricular conduction disorders (such as sick sinus syndrome or AV block) in the absence of an artificial pacemaker; bradycardia; bronchospasm; significant hypotension; symptomatic electrolyte disturbances; and known hypersensitivity to the drug. Patients with bronchospastic disease should not receive this drug because of its beta-adrenergic blocking properties.

Use all Class Ic antiarrhythmics cautiously because of an association between other agents within the class and an increased cardiac morbidity and mortality as compared with placebo. The use of this drug should be limited to persons who have life-threatening arrhythmias. Because antiarrhythmic agents can cause new or worsened arrhythmias ranging from worsened premature ventricular contractions (PVCs) to ventricular tachycardia, frequently evaluate EEG. Propafenone may alter both the pacing and sensing thresholds of artificial pacemakers. Pacemakers should be monitored and reprogrammed as necessary.

Use cautiously in patients with a history of CHF because sympathetic stimulation may be important to continued function of the failing heart, and the beta-adrenergic blocking effects of propafenone may be detrimental to these patients; and in patients with hepatic or renal disease, because propafenone is extensively metabolized by the liver and excreted by the kidneys.

CBCs should be performed in patients with unexplained fever or decreased WBC count to rule out the possibility of agranulocytosis or granulocytopenia, especially during the first 3 months of therapy.

ADVERSE REACTIONS

Common reactions are in italics; life-threatening reactions are in bold italics.
CNS: anorexia, anxiety, ataxia, dizziness, drowsiness, fatigue, headache, insomnia, syncope, tremor, weakness.
CV: angina, atrial fibrillation, bradycardia, bundle branch block, *CHF,* chest pain, edema, first-degree AV block, hypotension, increased QRS duration, intraventricular conduction delay, palpitations, ***proarrhythmic events (ventricular tachycardia, premature ventricular contractions).***
EENT: blurred vision.
GI: abdominal pain or cramps, constipation, diarrhea, dyspepsia, flatulence, nausea, vomiting, dry mouth, unusual taste.
Respiratory: dyspnea.
Skin: rash.
Other: diaphoresis, joint pain.

INTERACTIONS

Antiarrhythmics: increased potential for CHF.
Cimetidine: decreased metabolism of propafenone.
Digitalis glycosides, oral anticoagulants: propafenone may increase serum levels of these agents, resulting in toxicity.
Local anesthetics: increased risk of CNS toxicity.
Propranolol, metoprolol: propafenone slows the metabolism of these agents. Dosage adjustments may be necessary.
Quinidine: slows the metabolism of propafenone. Avoid concomitant use.

EFFECTS ON DIAGNOSTIC TESTS

ECG: may slow conduction and increase PR interval and QRS duration.

NURSING CONSIDERATIONS

Besides those related universally to drug therapy (see "How to use this book"), consider the following specific recommendations:

Assessment

- Obtain a baseline assessment of the patient's heart rate and rhythm before therapy.
- Be alert for adverse reactions and drug interactions throughout therapy.
- Evaluate the patient's and family's knowledge about propafenone therapy.

Nursing Diagnoses

- Decreased cardiac output related to ineffectiveness of propafenone therapy.
- Altered protection related to propafenone-induced proarrhythmias.
- Knowledge deficit related to propafenone.

Planning and Implementation

Preparation and Administration

- ***P.O. use:*** Administer drug with food to minimize adverse GI reactions.
- Expect to make dosage adjustments stepwise at 3- to 4-day intervals because plasma levels do not increase linearly with dose.

Monitoring

- Monitor effectiveness by continuous cardiac monitoring during initiation of therapy and during dosage adjustments; then regularly evaluate ECG recordings as ordered and patient's heart rate and rhythm to assess for effectiveness of drug and for proarrhythmic events.
- If patient is receiving concomitant therapy with digoxin, frequently monitor ECG and serum digoxin levels because propafenone increases serum digoxin levels by 35% to 85%.

Supportive Care

- If ECG disturbances occur, withhold the drug, obtain a rhythm strip, and notify the doctor immediately. Be aware that if PR interval or QRS duration increase by more than 25%, dosage reduction may be necessary.
- Institute safety precautions if CNS disturbances occur.
- Obtain an order for an antiemetic if nausea and vomiting occur.
- Assist the patient with daily activities if joint pain occurs.

Patient Teaching

- Tell patient to take the drug with food to minimize adverse GI reactions.
- Stress importance of taking the drug exactly as prescribed.
- Emphasize the importance of close follow-up and regular diagnostic studies to monitor drug action and assess for adverse reactions.
- Warn the patient to avoid hazardous activities if adverse CNS disturbances occur.

Evaluation

In patients receiving propafenone, appropriate evaluation statements may include:

- Patient's ECG reveals arrhythmia has been corrected.
- Patient does not develop any proarrhythmic events during propafenone therapy.

• Patient and family state an understanding of propafenone therapy.

propantheline bromide

(proe pan´ the leen)

Norpanth, Pantheline‡, Pro-Banthine, Propanthel†

• *Classification:* antimuscarinic, GI antispasmodic (anticholinergic)
• *Pregnancy Risk Category:* C

HOW SUPPLIED

Tablets: 7.5 mg, 15 mg

ACTION

Mechanism: A quarternary anticholinergic that competitively blocks acetylcholine's effects at parasympathetic (muscarinic) sites, decreasing GI motility and inhibiting gastric acid secretion.
Absorption: Only 10% to 25% of a dose is absorbed.
Distribution: Does not cross the blood-brain barrier; little else is known about its distribution.
Excretion: In urine (mostly as metabolites) and in feces as unabsorbed drug.
Onset, peak, duration: Duration of action is about 6 hours.

INDICATIONS & DOSAGE

Adjunctive treatment of peptic ulcer, irritable bowel syndrome, and other GI disorders; to reduce duodenal motility during diagnostic radiologic procedures–
Adults: 15 mg P.O. t.i.d. before meals, and 30 mg h.s. up to 60 mg q.i.d. For elderly patients, 7.5 mg P.O. t.i.d. before meals.

CONTRAINDICATIONS & PRECAUTIONS

Contraindicated in patients with narrow-angle glaucoma, because drug-induced cycloplegia and mydriasis may increase intraocular pressure; obstructive uropathy, obstructive GI tract disease, severe ulcerative colitis, myasthenia gravis, paralytic ileus, intestinal atony, or toxic megacolon, because the drug may exacerbate these conditions; and hypersensitivity to anticholinergics or bromides.

Administer cautiously to patients with autonomic neuropathy, hyperthyroidism, coronary artery disease, cardiac arrhythmias, CHF, or ulcerative colitis, because the drug may exacerbate symptoms of these disorders; hepatic or renal disease, because toxic accumulation may occur; or hiatal hernia associated with reflux esophagitis, because the drug may decrease lower esophageal sphincter tone; to patients over age 40, because the drug increases the glaucoma risk; and in hot or humid environments, because the drug may predispose the patient to heatstroke.

ADVERSE REACTIONS

Common reactions are in italics; life-threatening reactions are in bold italics.
CNS: headache, insomnia, drowsiness, dizziness, *confusion or excitement in elderly patients,* nervousness, weakness.
CV: *palpitations,* tachycardia.
EENT: *blurred vision,* mydriasis, increased ocular tension, cycloplegia, photophobia.
GI: *dry mouth,* dysphagia, constipation, heartburn, loss of taste, nausea, vomiting, paralytic ileus.
GU: *urinary hesitancy, urine retention,* impotence.
Skin: urticaria, decreased sweating or possible anhidrosis, other dermal manifestations.
Other: fever, allergic reactions.

Overdosage may cause curare-like symptoms.

INTERACTIONS

None significant.

EFFECTS ON DIAGNOSTIC TESTS
None reported.

NURSING CONSIDERATIONS
Besides those related universally to drug therapy (see "How to use this book"), consider the following specific recommendations:

Assessment
- Obtain a baseline assessment of the patient's pain related to his underlying condition before drug therapy.
- Be alert for adverse reactions and drug interactions throughout therapy.
- Evaluate the patient's and family's knowledge about propantheline bromide therapy.

Nursing Diagnoses
- Pain related to the patient's underlying condition.
- High risk for injury related to drug-induced adverse reaction.
- Knowledge deficit related to propantheline therapy.

Planning and Implementation

Preparation and Administration
- ***P.O. use:*** Give this drug 30 minutes to 1 hour before meals and at bedtime.
- Bedtime dose can be larger and should be given at least 2 hours after the last meal of the day.

Monitoring
- Monitor effectiveness by regularly assessing pain related to his underlying condition.
- Monitor for adverse reactions or drug interactions by checking intake and output.
- Monitor vital signs frequently for tachycardia.
- Monitor the patient's degree of dry mouth.
- Monitor the patient's bowel habits, because drug may cause constipation.

Supportive Care
- Help the patient to get in and out of bed if he has dizziness or blurred vision.
- Institute safety precautions if he experiences dizziness or confusion.
- Provide gum or sugarless hard candy to relieve dry mouth.
- If constipation occurs, obtain an order for a laxative.
- Provide additional fluids to help prevent constipation.
- Encourage the patient to void before taking this medication.

Patient Teaching
- Instruct the patient to avoid driving and other hazardous activities that require alertness if he is drowsy, dizzy, or has blurred vision.
- Encourage the patient to drink plenty of fluids to avoid constipation.
- Tell him to report any rash or skin eruptions.
- Tell the patient to take this drug 30 minutes to 1 hour before meals and to take the bedtime dose at least 2 hours after the last meal of the day.

Evaluation
In patients receiving propantheline, appropriate evaluation statements may include:
- Patient states a reduction in pain related to his underlying condition.
- Patient does not experience injury related to adverse reactions.
- Patient and family state an understanding of propantheline therapy.

propofol
(proe´ po fole)
Diprivan

- *Classification:* anesthetic (phenol derivative)
- *Pregnancy Risk Category:* D

HOW SUPPLIED
Injection: 10 mg/ml in 20-ml ampules

ACTION
Mechanism: Produces a dose-dependent CNS depression similar to benzodiazepines and barbiturates. However, it can be used to maintain anes-

*Liquid form contains alcohol. **May contain tartrazine.

thesia through careful titration of infusion rate.
Distribution: Biphasic distribution phase: The rapid distribution phase has a half-life of 1.8 to 8.3 minutes; the slower phase, 34 to 64 minutes.
Metabolism: Within liver and tissues. Metabolites are not fully characterized.
Excretion: By the kidneys. However, termination of drug action is probably caused by redistribution out of the CNS as well as by metabolism. Half-life: With prolonged use, terminal elimination half-life is more than 11 hours.
Onset, peak, duration: Onset is rapid, usually less than 2 minutes. Termination of drug effect is also rapid; most patients are awake and responsive within 8 minutes after infusion ends.

INDICATIONS & DOSAGE

Induction of anesthesia –
Adults: doses must be individualized according to patient's condition and age. Most patients classified as American Society of Anesthesiologists (ASA) Physical Status category (PS) I or II under 55 years require 2 to 2.5 mg/kg I.V. The drug is usually administered in 40-mg boluses q 10 seconds until the desired response is obtained.

Elderly, debilitated, or hypovolemic patients, or patients in ASA PS III or IV should receive half of the usual induction dose (20 mg-boluses q 10 seconds).

Maintenance of anesthesia –
Adults: propofol may be given as a variable rate infusion, titrated to clinical effect. Most patients may be maintained with 0.1 to 0.2 mg/kg/minute (6 to 12 mg/kg/hr).

Elderly, debilitated, or hypovolemic patients, or patients in ASA PS III or IV should receive half of the usual maintenance dose (0.05 to 0.1 mg/kg/minute, or 3 to 6 mg/kg/hr).

CONTRAINDICATIONS & PRECAUTIONS

Contraindicated in patients with hypersensitivity to the drug or any components of the emulsion, including soybean oil, egg lecithin, and glycerol. Not recommended for use in obstetric anesthesia because the safety to the fetus has not been established or use in patients with increased intracranial pressure or impaired cerebral circulation because the reduction in systemic arterial pressure caused by the drug may substantially reduce cerebral perfusion pressure.

Use cautiously in patients with lipid metabolism disorders (such as pancreatitis, primary hyperlipoproteinemia, and diabetic hyperlipidemia), in elderly or debilitated patients, and in those with circulatory disorders. Although the hemodynamic effects of the drug can vary, its major effect in patients maintaining spontaneous ventilation is arterial hypotension (arterial pressure can decrease as much as 30%) with little or no change in heart rate and cardiac output. However, in patients undergoing assisted or controlled positive pressure ventilation, significant depression of cardiac output may occur.

ADVERSE REACTIONS

Common reactions are in italics; life-threatening reactions are in bold italics.
CNS: headache, dizziness, twitching, ***clonic/myoclonic movement.***
CV: hypotension, bradycardia, ***hypertension.***
GI: nausea, vomiting, abdominal cramping.
Respiratory: ***apnea,*** cough.
Skin: flushing.
Local: burning/stinging, pain, tingling or numbness, and coldness at injection site.
Other: fever, hiccups.

INTERACTIONS

Inhalational anesthetics (such as enflurane, isoflurane, and halothane) or supplemental anesthetics (such as nitrous oxide and opiates): may be expected to enhance the anesthetic and cardiovascular actions of propofol.
Opiate analgesics, sedatives: may cause a more pronounced decrease of systolic, diastolic, and mean arterial pressure and of cardiac output; may also decrease the induction dose requirements.

EFFECTS ON DIAGNOSTIC TESTS

None reported.

NURSING CONSIDERATIONS

Besides those related universally to drug therapy (see "How to use this book"), consider the following specific recommendations:

Assessment
• Obtain a baseline assessment of the patient's vital signs and overall physical status before anesthesia.
• Be alert for adverse reactions and drug interactions throughout anesthesia.
• Evaluate the patient's and family's knowledge about propofol.

Nursing Diagnoses
• High risk for injury related to propofol-induced CNS depression.
• Ineffective breathing pattern related to possible propofol-induced apnea.
• Knowledge deficit related to propofol.

Planning and Implementation
Preparation and Administration
• Keep in mind that propofol should be administered under direct medical supervision by persons familiar with airway management and the administration of I.V. anesthetics.
• Prepare under strict aseptic technique. The vehicle for propofol is fat emulsion, and it contains no preservative. Rapid microbial growth is possible if the solution is contaminated. It is intended for single use, and unused solution should be discarded at the end of the procedure. Postoperative fevers have been linked to the use of contaminated solutions.
• Do not mix propofol with other drugs or blood products. If it is to be diluted before infusion, use only dextrose 5% in water (D_5W), and do not dilute to a concentration less than 2 mg/ml. After dilution, it appears to be more stable in glass containers than in plastic.
• Be aware that, for administration into a running I.V. catheter, propofol emulsion is compatible with D_5W, lactated Ringer's injection, lactated Ringer's and 5% dextrose injection, 5% dextrose and 0.45% sodium chloride injection, and 5% dextrose and 0.9% sodium chloride injection.
• Store propofol emulsion above 40° F (4° C) and below 72° F (22° C). Refrigeration is not recommended.

Monitoring
• Monitor effectiveness by evaluating CNS depressant effect after administration.
• Monitor patient's vital signs before, during, and after anesthesia. Closely monitor for signs of significant hypotension or bradycardia. Also monitor for apnea, which may occur during induction.

Supportive Care
• Notify the doctor immediately if CNS, respiratory, or CV status changes.
• Keep in mind that apnea may persist for longer than 60 seconds. Ventilatory support may be required.
• Implement safety measures to protect the unconscious patient.
• Be aware that treatment for significant hypotension or bradycardia includes increased rate of fluid administration, pressor agents, elevation of lower extremities, or atropine.
• Know that drug's pharmacokinetics are not altered by chronic hepatic cirrhosis or chronic renal failure.

• Consider that propofol has no vagolytic activity. Premedication with anticholinergics, such as glycopyrrolate or atropine, may help manage potential increases in vagal tone caused by other drugs or surgical manipulations.
• Remember that propofol is excreted in breast milk and is not recommended for use by breast-feeding mothers.
Patient Teaching
• Explain that this drug is used to induce or maintain anesthesia during surgery.
• Tell the patient what to expect during induction of and recovery from anesthesia. As needed, clarify any other information provided by the anesthesiologist, including risks.
Evaluation
In patients receiving propofol, appropriate evaluation statements may include:
• Patient experiences adequate anesthesia and is not at risk for injury.
• Patient maintained patent airway and adequate ventilatory status.
• Patient and family state an understanding of propofol therapy.

---

propoxyphene hydrochloride (dextropropoxyphene hydrochloride)
(proe pox´ i feen)
Darvon, Dolene, Doraphen, Doxaphene, Novopropoxyn†, Pro-Pox, Propoxycon, 642†

propoxyphene napsylate (dextropropoxyphene napsylate)
Darvocet-N, Darvon-N, Doloxene‡, Doloxene Co‡

• Controlled Substance Schedule IV
• *Classification:* analgesic (opioid)
• *Pregnancy Risk Category:* C (D for prolonged use)

HOW SUPPLIED
hydrochloride
Capsules: 32 mg, 65 mg
napsylate
Tablets: 100 mg
Capsules: 50 mg, 100 mg
Oral suspension: 10 mg/ml

ACTION
Mechanism: Binds with opiate receptors at many sites in the CNS (brain, brain stem, and spinal cord), altering both perception of and emotional response to pain through an unknown mechanism.
Absorption: After oral administration, absorbed primarily in the upper small intestine. Equimolar doses of the hydrochloride and napsylate salts provide similar plasma concentrations.
Distribution: Enters the CSF. It is assumed that it crosses the placental; however, placental fluid and fetal blood concentrations have not been determined.
Metabolism: Degraded mainly in the liver; about one quarter of a dose is metabolized to norpropoxyphene, an active metabolite.
Excretion: In the urine. Half-life: 6 to 12 hours.
Onset, peak, duration: The onset of analgesia occurs in 20 to 60 minutes, and peak analgesic effects occur at 2 to 2½ hours. Duration of effect is 4 to 6 hours.

INDICATIONS & DOSAGE
Mild to moderate pain—
Adults: 65 mg (hydrochloride) P.O. q 4 hours p.r.n or 100 mg (napsylate) P.O. q 4 hours p.r.n.

CONTRAINDICATIONS & PRECAUTIONS
Contraindicated in patients with hypersensitivity to the drug or to methadone.

Administer with extreme caution to patients with supraventricular arrhythmias; avoid or administer with extreme caution to patients with head injury or increased intracranial pressure because drug obscures neurologic parameters and during pregnancy and labor because drug readily crosses placenta (premature infants are especially sensitive to respiratory and CNS depressant effects). Not recommended for use in suicidal or addiction-prone patients.

Administer cautiously to patients with renal or hepatic dysfunction, because drug accumulation or prolonged duration of action may occur; asthma or chronic obstructive pulmonary disease, because drug depresses respiration and suppresses cough reflex; or seizure disorders, because drug may precipitate seizures; to patients undergoing biliary tract surgery, because drug may cause biliary spasm; to elderly or debilitated patients, who are more sensitive to both therapeutic and adverse drug effects; and to patients prone to physical or psychic addiction, because of the high risk of addiction to this drug.

ADVERSE REACTIONS

Common reactions are in italics; life-threatening reactions are in bold italics.

CNS: *dizziness,* headache, sedation, euphoria, paradoxical excitement, insomnia.

GI: nausea, vomiting, constipation.

Other: psychological and physical dependence.

INTERACTIONS

Alcohol, CNS depressants: additive effects. Use together cautiously.

EFFECTS ON DIAGNOSTIC TESTS

Urinary steroids: falsely decreased excretion levels.

NURSING CONSIDERATIONS

Besides those related universally to drug therapy (see "How to use this book"), consider the following specific recommendations:

Assessment

• Obtain a baseline assessment of pain before therapy.

• Be alert for adverse reactions and drug interactions throughout therapy.

• Evaluate the patient's and family's knowledge about propoxyphene therapy.

Nursing Diagnoses

• Pain related to the patient's underlying condition.

• High risk for trauma related to possible sedation or dizziness from adverse CNS reaction to propoxyphene.

• Knowledge deficit related to propoxyphene therapy.

Planning and Implementation

Preparation and Administration

• Do not administer for maintenance purposes in narcotic addiction.

Monitoring

• Monitor effectiveness by assessing the patient's degree of pain relief after each dose.

Supportive Care

• Do not treat overdose with caffeine or amphetamines; may cause fatal seizures. Use narcotic antagonist instead.

• Keep in mind that this drug may falsely decrease results of urinary steroid excretion tests.

• Be aware that 65 mg propoxyphene hydrochloride equals 100 mg propoxyphene napsylate.

• Implement safety measures, such as assisting with ambulation, as needed to prevent trauma from possible CNS effects.

• Keep in mind that this drug can be considered a mild narcotic analgesic; pain relief is equivalent to that with aspirin. Often used with aspirin or acetaminophen to maximize analgesia.

Patient Teaching
- Advise patient to limit alcohol intake when taking this drug.
- Warn patient not to exceed recommended dosage.
- Warn ambulatory patient to avoid driving and other activities that require alertness until CNS effects of the drug are known.

Evaluation
In patients receiving propoxyphene, appropriate evaluation statements may include:
- Patient reports pain relief.
- Patient's safety is maintained.
- Patient and family state an understanding of propoxyphene therapy.

propranolol hydrochloride
(proe pran´ oh lole)
Apo-Propranolol†, Deralin‡, Detensol†, Inderal, Inderal LA, Ipran, Novopranol†, PMS-Propranolol†

- *Classification:* antihypertensive; antianginal, antiarrhythmic; adjunctive therapy of migraine or MI (beta-adrenergic blocking agent)
- *Pregnancy Risk Category:* C

HOW SUPPLIED
Tablets: 10 mg, 20 mg, 40 mg, 60 mg, 80 mg, 90 mg
Capsules (sustained-release): 60 mg, 80 mg, 120 mg, 160 mg
Oral solution: 4 mg/ml, 8 mg/ml, 80 mg/ml (concentrate)
Injection: 1 mg/ml

ACTION
Mechanism: A beta-adrenergic blocker that reduces cardiac oxygen demand by blocking catecholamine-induced increases in heart rate, blood pressure, and force of myocardial contraction. Depresses renin secretion. Also prevents vasodilation of the cerebral arteries.
Absorption: Almost completely absorbed from the GI tract; however, only a small portion of an oral dose reaches the systemic circulation because of a substantial first-pass effect. Absorption is enhanced when given with food.
Distribution: Widely distributed throughout the body; drug is more than 90% protein-bound.
Metabolism: Hepatic metabolism is almost total; oral dosage form undergoes extensive first-pass metabolism.
Excretion: Approximately 96% to 99% of a given dose is excreted in urine as metabolites; remainder is excreted in feces as unchanged drug and metabolites. Half-life: Biological half-life is about 4 hours.
Onset, peak, duration: Peak plasma concentrations occur 60 to 90 minutes after administration of regular-release tablets. After I.V. administration, peak concentrations occur in about 1 minute, with virtually immediate onset of action.

INDICATIONS & DOSAGE
Management of angina pectoris–
Adults: 10 to 20 mg P.O. t.i.d. or q.i.d. Or, 1 80-mg sustained-release capsule daily. Dosage may be increased at 7- to 10-day intervals. The average optimum dosage is 160 mg daily.
To reduce mortality following myocardial infarction–
Adults: 180 to 240 mg P.O. daily in divided doses. Usually administered t.i.d. to q.i.d.
Supraventricular, ventricular, and atrial arrhythmias; tachyarrhythmias caused by excessive catecholamine action during anesthesia, hyperthyroidism, and pheochromocytoma–
Adults: 1 to 3 mg by slow I.V. push, not to exceed 1 mg/minute. After 3 mg have been given, another dose may be given in 2 minutes; subsequent doses, no sooner than q 4 hours. Drug may be given by direct injection or diluted in 50 ml dextrose 5% in water or normal saline and in-

fused slowly. Usual maintenance dose is 10 to 80 mg P.O. t.i.d. to q.i.d.
Hypertension—
Adults: initial treatment of hypertension: 80 mg P.O. daily in two to four divided doses or the sustained-release form once daily. Increase at 3- to 7-day intervals to maximum daily dosage of 640 mg. Usual maintenance dosage for hypertension is 160 to 480 mg daily.
Prevention of frequent, severe, uncontrollable, or disabling migraine or vascular headache—
Adults: initially, 80 mg P.O. daily in divided doses or 1 sustained-release capsule daily. Usual maintenance dosage is 160 to 240 mg daily, divided t.i.d. or q.i.d.

CONTRAINDICATIONS & PRECAUTIONS

Contraindicated in patients with hypersensitivity to the drug; in patients with overt cardiac failure, sinus bradycardia, second- or third-degree AV block, bronchial asthma, cardiogenic shock, and Raynaud's syndrome, because drug may worsen these conditions.

Use cautiously in patients with coronary insufficiency, because beta-adrenergic blockade may precipitate CHF; pulmonary disease; diabetes mellitus, hypoglycemia, or hyperthyroidism because propranolol may mask tachycardia (it does not mask dizziness and sweating caused by hypoglycemia); and impaired hepatic function. Propranolol may also mask common signs of shock.

ADVERSE REACTIONS

Common reactions are in italics; life-threatening reactions are in bold italics.
CNS: *fatigue, lethargy,* vivid dreams, hallucinations.
CV: *bradycardia, hypotension, CHF,* peripheral vascular disease.
GI: nausea, vomiting, diarrhea.
Metabolic: hypoglycemia without tachycardia.
Skin: rash.
Other: ***increased airway resistance,*** fever, arthralgia.

INTERACTIONS

Aminophylline: antagonized beta-blocking effects of propranolol. Use together cautiously.
Cimetidine: inhibits propranolol's metabolism. Monitor for greater beta-blocking effect.
Digitalis glycosides, verapamil: excessive bradycardia and increased depressant effect on myocardium. Use together cautiously.
Epinephrine: severe vasoconstriction. Monitor blood pressure and observe patient carefully.
Insulin, oral hypoglycemic drugs: can alter requirements for these drugs in previously stabilized diabetics. Monitor for hypoglycemia.
Isoproterenol, glucagon: antagonized propranolol effect. May be used therapeutically and in emergencies.

EFFECTS ON DIAGNOSTIC TESTS

BUN: elevated levels.
Serum transaminase, alkaline phosphatase, and lactate dehydrogenase: elevated levels.

NURSING CONSIDERATIONS

Besides those related universally to drug therapy (see "How to use this book"), consider the following specific recommendations:

Assessment

- Obtain a baseline assessment of the patient's angina status before therapy.
- Be alert for adverse reactions and drug interactions throughout therapy.
- Evaluate the patient's and family's knowledge about propranolol therapy.

Nursing Diagnoses
• Pain related to ineffectiveness of propranolol therapy.
• Fluid volume excess related to propranolol-induced CHF.
• Knowledge deficit related to propranolol therapy.

Planning and Implementation

Preparation and Administration
• Double-check dose and route before administration. I.V. doses are much smaller than oral doses.
• ***P.O. use:*** Administer drug consistently with meals because food may increase the absorption of propranolol.
• ***I.V. use:*** Inject drug at a maximum rate of 1 mg/minute through an I.V. line containing a free-flowing compatible solution.

Monitoring
• Monitor effectiveness by regularly evaluating pain relief.
• Monitor patient's respiratory status, particularly for abnormal breath sounds and dyspnea suggestive of airway resistance.
• Monitor for fluid retention that could lead to CHF.
• Be aware that this drug masks common signs of shock and hypoglycemia. Monitor vital signs and blood glucose levels regularly.

Supportive Care
• If ECG disturbances or extremes in pulse rates occur, withhold the drug, obtain a rhythm strip, and notify the doctor immediately.
• After prolonged atrial fibrillation, restoration of normal rhythm may result in thromboembolism, due to dislodgement of thrombi from atrial wall. Be aware that anticoagulation is usually advised before restoration of normal sinus rhythm.
• Don't discontinue propranolol before surgery for pheochromocytoma. Before any surgical procedure, notify the anesthesiologist that the patient is receiving propranolol.
• Assist the patient with daily activities; schedule activities to promote adequate rest if fatigue occurs.
• Alert the doctor if dyspnea or abnormal breath sounds occur.
• Restrict the patient's fluid and sodium intake to minimize CHF.
• Have emergency drugs on hand to treat overdose.

Patient Teaching
• Stress importance of taking the drug exactly as prescribed even when feeling well. Teach patient how to check pulse rate, and to do so before each dose.
• Tell outpatients not to discontinue this drug suddenly; abrupt discontinuation can exacerbate angina and MI.
• Tell the patient to schedule activities to allow adequate rest if fatigue becomes troublesome.
• Encourage the patient to restrict fluid and sodium intake to minimize CHF.

Evaluation
In patients receiving propranolol, appropriate evaluation statements may include:
• Patient states anginal pain is relieved with propranolol therapy.
• Patient does not experience fluid retention with propranolol use.
• Patient and family state an understanding of propranolol therapy.

propylthiouracil (PTU)
(proe pill thye oh yoor´ a sill)
Propyl-Thyracil†

• *Classification:* antihyperthyroid agent (thyroid hormone antagonist)
• *Pregnancy Risk Category:* D

HOW SUPPLIED
Tablets: 50 mg, 100 mg†

ACTION
Mechanism: Inhibits oxidation of iodine in the thyroid gland, blocking

iodine's ability to combine with tyrosine to form thyroxine. May also prevent the coupling of monoiodotyrosine and diiodotyrosine to form thyroxine and triiodothyronine.
Absorption: About 80% of a dose is absorbed rapidly from the GI tract.
Distribution: Concentrates in the thyroid gland. Drug readily crosses the placenta and is distributed into breast milk. It is 75% to 80% protein-bound.
Metabolism: Rapidly metabolized in the liver.
Excretion: About 35% of a dose is excreted in urine. Half-life is 1 to 2 hours in patients with normal renal function and 8½ hours in anuric patients.
Onset, peak, duration: Peak levels occur at 1 to 1½ hours.

INDICATIONS & DOSAGE

Hyperthyroidism–
Adults: 100 mg P.O. t.i.d.; up to 300 mg q 8 hours have been used in severe cases. Continue until patient is euthyroid, then start maintenance dosage of 100 mg daily to t.i.d.
Children over 10 years: 100 mg P.O. t.i.d. Continue until patient is euthyroid, then start maintenance dosage of 25 mg t.i.d. to 100 mg b.i.d.
Children 6 to 10 years: 50 to 150 mg P.O. divided doses q 8 hours.
Preparation for thyroidectomy–
Adults and children: same doses as for hyperthyroidism, then iodine may be added 10 days before surgery.
Thyrotoxic crisis–
Adults and children: same doses as for hyperthyroidism, with concomitant iodine therapy and propranolol.

CONTRAINDICATIONS & PRECAUTIONS

Contraindicated in patients with hypersensitivity to the drug. Use cautiously in patients over 40 years because of an increased risk of agranulocytosis, in patients receiving other agents known to cause agranulocytosis, or in those with infection or hepatic dysfunction.

ADVERSE REACTIONS

Common reactions are in italics; life-threatening reactions are in bold italics.
Blood: ***agranulocytosis,*** leukopenia, thrombocytopenia (appear to be dose-related).
CNS: headache, drowsiness, vertigo.
EENT: visual disturbances.
GI: diarrhea, *nausea, vomiting* (may be dose-related).
Hepatic: jaundice, ***hepatotoxicity.***
Skin: rash, urticaria, skin discoloration, pruritus.
Other: arthralgia, myalgia, salivary gland enlargement, loss of taste, drug fever, lymphadenopathy, vasculitis.

INTERACTIONS

None significant.

EFFECTS ON DIAGNOSTIC TESTS

AST (SGOT), ALT (SGPT), and lactate dehydrogenase: altered levels.
Liothyronine uptake: altered results.
Prothrombin time: altered results.
Selenomethionine (^{75}Se) uptake: altered levels.

NURSING CONSIDERATIONS

Besides those related universally to drug therapy (see "How to use this book"), consider the following specific recommendations:
Assessment
- Obtain a baseline assessment of the patient's thyroid function before therapy.
- Be alert for adverse reactions throughout therapy.
- Evaluate the patient's and family's knowledge about propylthiouracil therapy.

Nursing Diagnoses
- Activity intolerance related to inceased metabolic rate.
- High risk for fluid volume deficit

related to propylthiouracil-induced GI reaction.
• Knowledge deficit related to propylthiouracil therapy.
Planning and Implementation
Preparation and Administration
• Store in light-resistant container.
• ***P.O. use:*** Give with meals to reduce adverse GI reactions.
Monitoring
• Monitor effectiveness by regularly reviewing results of thyroid function studies and assessing the patient's signs and symptoms for hyperthyroidism. Be aware that euthyroidism may take several months to develop.
• Monitor for signs of hypothyroidism (mental depression; cold intolerance; hard, nonpitting edema). Dosage adjustment may be required.
• Monitor CBC periodically to detect impending leukopenia, thrombocytopenia, and agranulocytosis.
• Monitor the patient's hydration status if GI reactions occur.
Supportive Care
• Withhold drug if fever, sore throat, mouth sores, or skin eruptions develop and notify the doctor.
• Notify the doctor if the patient shows signs and symptoms of hypothyroidism; if so, dosage reduction will be required.
• Institute safety precautions if adverse CNS reactions occur.
• Obtain an order for an antiemetic or antidiarrheal, as needed.
Patient Teaching
• Tell the patient to take drug at regular intervals around-the-clock and to take it at the same time each day in relation to meals.
• If GI upset occurs, tell the patient to take drug with meals.
• Tell the patient to ask the doctor whether he should use iodized salt or eat shellfish during treatment because their iodine content can interfere with the drug's effectiveness.
• Warn the patient not to use OTC cough medicines; many contain iodine.
• Tell the patient to notify the doctor promptly of fever, sore throat, mouth sores, or skin eruptions.
• Teach the patient how to recognize the signs of hyperthyroidism and hypothyroidism and what to do if they occur.
Evaluation
In patients receiving propylthiouracil, appropriate evaluation statements may include:
• Patient is euthyroid with propylthiouracil therapy and can tolerate normal activity level.
• Patient does not experience dehydration throughout therapy.
• Patient and family state an understanding of propylthiouracil therapy.

protamine sulfate
(proe´ ta meen)

• *Classification:* heparin antagonist, antidote (polypeptide)
• *Pregnancy Risk Category:* C

HOW SUPPLIED
Injection: 10 mg/ml

ACTION
Mechanism: Forms a physiologically inert complex with heparin sodium.
Metabolism: Fate of the heparin-protamine complex is unknown; however, it appears to be partially degraded, with release of some heparin.
Onset, peak, duration: Heparin-neutralizing effect of protamine occurs within 30 to 60 seconds.

INDICATIONS & DOSAGE
Heparin overdose–
Adults: dosage based on venous blood coagulation studies, usually 1 mg for each 90 to 115 units of heparin. Give diluted to 1% (10 mg/ml) slow I.V. injection over 1 to 3 min-

utes. Maximum dose is 50 mg/10 minutes.

CONTRAINDICATIONS & PRECAUTIONS

Use cautiously in patients allergic to fish; protamine is derived from sperm of salmon and other fish. Watch for spontaneous bleeding (heparin rebound), especially in patients undergoing dialysis and patients who have had cardiac surgery.

ADVERSE REACTIONS

Common reactions are in italics; life-threatening reactions are in bold italics.
CV: fall in blood pressure, bradycardia.
Other: transitory flushing, feeling of warmth, dyspnea, hypersensitivity.

INTERACTIONS

None significant.

EFFECTS ON DIAGNOSTIC TESTS

Partial thromboplastin time: shortens heparin-prolonged results.

NURSING CONSIDERATIONS

Besides those related universally to drug therapy (see "How to use this book"), consider the following specific recommendations:

Assessment
- Obtain a baseline assessment of vital signs, bleeding, and coagulation time before therapy.
- Be alert for adverse reactions throughout therapy.
- Evaluate the patient's and family's knowledge about protamine therapy.

Nursing Diagnoses
- High risk for injury related to heparin overdose.
- Decreased cardiac output related to hypotension and bradycardia induced by protamine.
- Knowledge deficit related to protamine therapy.

Planning and Implementation

Preparation and Administration
- ***I.V. use:*** Administer slowly by direct I.V. injection.
- Read label and calculate dosage carefully: 1 mg of protamine neutralizes 90 to 115 units of heparin depending on the salt (heparin calcium or heparin sodium) and the source of heparin (beef or pork).

Monitoring
- Monitor effectiveness by reviewing coagulation studies.
- Check vital signs frequently. Patient should be monitored continuously.
- Observe for spontaneous bleeding (heparin "rebound"), especially in patients undergoing dialysis and in those who have had cardiac surgery.
- Monitor fluid balance carefully; check intake and output and daily weight.
- Observe for hypersensitivity reaction.

Supportive Care
- Keep epinephrine 1:1000 available in case of hypersensitivity reaction. Have oxygen and resuscitation equipment nearby in case of shock.
- Before giving protamine, ensure adequate blood volume. Administer blood or I.V. fluids to correct hypovolemia.
- Be aware that protamine is a heparin antagonist, but it may act as an anticoagulant in high doses.

Patient Teaching
- Inform the patient that transitory flushing may accompany administration of protamine.

Evaluation

In patients receiving protamine, appropriate evaluation statements may include:
- Patient is free from injury related to heparin overdose.
- Patient does not exhibit signs of decreased cardiac output.
- Patient and family state an understanding of protamine therapy.

protriptyline hydrochloride
(proe trip´ ti leen)
Triptil†, Vivactil

• *Classification:* antidepressant (tricyclic)
• *Pregnancy Risk Category:* C

HOW SUPPLIED
Tablets: 5 mg, 10 mg

ACTION
Mechanism: Increases the amount of norepinephrine or serotonin, or both, in the CNS by blocking their reuptake by the presynaptic neurons. This allows these neurotransmitters to accumulate.
Absorption: Slowly absorbed from the GI tract after oral administration.
Distribution: Widely distributed into the body. Drug is 90% protein-bound.
Metabolism: By the liver; a significant first-pass effect may account for variability of serum concentrations in different patients taking the same dosage.
Excretion: Slowly excreted in urine; some in feces via the biliary tract. About 50% of a given dose is excreted as metabolites within 16 days.
Onset, peak, duration: Peak plasma levels occur in 24 to 30 hours. Proposed therapeutic drug levels range from 70 to 170 ng/ml. Steady-state plasma levels and peak therapeutic effect are achieved after several weeks of daily administration.

INDICATIONS & DOSAGE
Treatment of depression–
Adults: 15 to 40 mg P.O. daily in divided doses, increasing gradually to maximum of 60 mg daily.

CONTRAINDICATIONS & PRECAUTIONS
Contraindicated in patients with hypersensitivity to tricyclic antidepressants, trazodone, and related compounds; in the acute recovery phase of MI because of potential for cardiac arrhythmias; in coma or severe respiratory depression because of additive CNS depression; and during or within 14 days of therapy with MAO inhibitors because this combination may result in hypertensive response.

Use cautiously in patients with other cardiac disease (arrhythmias, CHF, angina pectoris, valvular disease, or heart block), because of additive antiarrhythmic effects; respiratory disorders, because of additive respiratory depression; alcoholism, seizure disorders, or during scheduled electroconvulsive therapy, because drug lowers seizure threshold; bipolar disease because drug may induce or worsen manic phase; glaucoma; hyperthyroidism or in patients taking thyroid replacement; Type I and Type II diabetes; prostatic hypertrophy, paralytic ileus, or urine retention, because drug may worsen these conditions; hepatic or renal dysfunction because diminished metabolism and excretion cause drug to accumulate; or Parkinson's disease, because drug may exacerbate tremors, expecially at high doses; and in patients undergoing surgery with general anesthesia, because of increased sensitivity to cardiac effects of general anesthetics or pressor agents.

ADVERSE REACTIONS
Common reactions are in italics; life-threatening reactions are in bold italics.
CNS: excitation, seizures, tremors, weakness, confusion, headache, nervousness.
CV: *orthostatic hypotension, tachycardia, ECG changes,* hypertension.
EENT: *blurred vision,* tinnitus, mydriasis.
GI: *dry mouth, constipation,* nausea, vomiting, anorexia, paralytic ileus.
GU: *urine retention.*
Skin: rash, urticaria.

Other: *sweating,* allergy.
After abrupt withdrawal of long-term therapy: nausea, headache, malaise. (Does not indicate addiction.)

INTERACTIONS

Barbiturates: decrease TCA blood levels. Monitor for decreased antidepressant effect.
Cimetidine: may increase protriptyline serum levels. Monitor for increased adverse reactions.
Epinephrine, norepinephrine: increase hypertensive effect. Use with caution.
MAO inhibitors: may cause severe excitation, hyperpyrexia, or seizures, and death, usually with high dose. Use together cautiously.
Methylphenidate: increases TCA blood levels. Monitor for enhanced antidepressant effect.

EFFECTS ON DIAGNOSTIC TESTS

CBC: decreased WBC counts.
ECG: elongation of Q-T and PR intervals, flattened T waves.
Liver enzymes: elevated levels.
Serum glucose: decreased and increased levels.

NURSING CONSIDERATIONS

Besides those related universally to drug therapy (see "How to use this book"), consider the following specific recommendations:

Assessment
- Obtain a baseline assessment of depression before therapy.
- Be alert for adverse reactions and drug interactions throughout therapy.
- Evaluate the patient's and family's knowledge about protriptyline therapy.

Nursing Diagnoses
- Ineffective individual coping related to the patient's underlying condition.
- Constipation related to adverse GI reactions to protriptyline.
- Knowledge deficit related to protriptyline therapy.

Planning and Implementation
Preparation and Administration
- Whenever possible, avoid late-day dosing to prevent insomnia.
- Expect reduced dosage in elderly or debilitated patients and adolescents.

Monitoring
- Monitor effectiveness by having the patient discuss his feelings (ask broad, open-ended questions) and by evaluating his behavior.
- Monitor blood pressure (supine and standing), ECG for changes, and heart rate for tachycardia.
- Monitor bowel patterns for constipation and check for urine retention.
- Note mood changes and monitor for suicidal tendencies.

Supportive Care
- Institute safety precautions if adverse CNS reactions occur.
- Do not withdraw drug abruptly.
- If psychotic signs, anxiety, agitation, or CV reactions increase, notify doctor and expect dosage to be reduced. Allow only a minimum supply of tablets to lessen suicide risk.
- If not contraindicated, increase the patient's fluid and fiber intake to prevent constipation; if needed, obtain an order for a stool softener or laxative.

Patient Teaching
- Tell the patient to relieve dry mouth with sugarless hard candy or gum, but explain that saliva substitutes may be necessary.
- Teach the patient to increase fluids to lessen constipation. Suggest stool softener or high-fiber diet, if needed.
- Warn the patient to avoid driving and other hazardous activities that require alertness and good psychomotor coordination until CNS effects of the drug are known. Tell the patient that this drug is less sedating than other similar drugs, and warn against combining with alcohol or other CNS depressants.
- Tell the patient that therapy must continue for 2 weeks or more before

noticeable effect, and for 4 weeks or more before full effect. Encourage the patient to continue to take medication until it achieves its full therapeutic effect.
• Advise the patient not to take any other drugs (prescription or OTC) without first consulting the doctor.

Evaluation

In patients receiving protriptyline, appropriate evaluation statements may include:
• Patient behavior and communication indicate improvement of depression.
• Constipation from adverse GI reaction does not occur.
• Patient and family state an understanding of protriptyline therapy.

pseudoephedrine hydrochloride

(soo doe e fed´ rin)

Cenafed◇, Children's Sudafed Liquid◇, Decofed◇, Dorcol Children's Decongestant◇, Eltor†◇, Genaphed◇, Halofed◇, NeoFed◇, Ornex Cold†◇, Pediacare Infant's Oral Decongestant Drops◇, Pseudofrin†◇, Pseudogest◇, Robidrine◇, Sinufed◇, Sudafed◇, Sudafed 12-Hour◇, Sudrin◇, Sufedrin◇

pseudoephedrine sulfate

Afrinol Repetabs

• *Classification:* decongestant (adrenergic)
• *Pregnancy Risk Category:* C

HOW SUPPLIED

Tablets: 30 mg◇, 60 mg◇
Tablets (extended-release): 120 mg◇
Oral solution: 15 mg/5 ml◇, 30 mg/5 ml◇, 7.5 mg/0.8 ml◇

ACTION

Mechanism: Stimulates both alpha- and beta-adrenergic receptors; may also stimulate norepinephrine release from adrenergic nerve terminals.
Absorption: Rapidly absorbed after oral administration.
Distribution: Widely distributed; probably enters CNS and crosses placenta.
Metabolism: Incompletely metabolized in liver by N-demethylation to inactive compounds
Excretion: 55% to 75% of a dose is excreted unchanged in urine; remainder is excreted as unchanged drug and metabolites.
Onset, peak, duration: Nasal decongestion occurs within 30 minutes and persists 4 to 6 hours after oral dose of 60-mg tablet or oral solution. Effects persist 8 hours after 60-mg dose and up to 12 hours after 120-mg dose of extended-release form.

INDICATIONS & DOSAGE

Nasal and eustachian tube decongestant–
Adults: 60 mg P.O. q 4 hours. Maximum dosage is 240 mg daily.
Children 6 to 12 years: 30 mg P.O. q 4 hours. Maximum dosage is 120 mg daily.
Children 2 to 6 years: 15 mg P.O. q 4 hours. Maximum dosage is 60 mg/day.
Extended-release tablets:
Adults and children over 12 years: 60 to 120 mg P.O. q 12 hours. This form is contraindicated for children under 12 years.
Relief of nasal congestion–
Adults: 120 mg q 12 hours.

CONTRAINDICATIONS & PRECAUTIONS

Contraindicated in patients with hypersensitivity to the drug and to other sympathomimetics, severe hypertension, or severe coronary artery disease and in those taking monoamine oxidase (MAO) inhibitors because of the potential for severe adverse cardiovascular effects.

Administer cautiously to patients

with hyperthyroidism, diabetes, ischemic heart disease, elevated intraocular pressure, or prostatic hypertrophy, because the drug may worsen these conditions.

ADVERSE REACTIONS

Common reactions are in italics; life-threatening reactions are in bold italics.
CNS: *anxiety,* transient stimulation, tremors, dizziness, headache, insomnia, *nervousness.*
CV: arrhythmias, *palpitations,* tachycardia.
EENT: dry mouth.
GI: anorexia, nausea, vomiting.
GU: difficulty in urinating.
Skin: pallor.

INTERACTIONS

Antihypertensives: hypotensive effect may be attenuated.
MAO inhibitors: may cause severe hypertension (hypertensive crisis). Don't use together.

EFFECTS ON DIAGNOSTIC TESTS

None reported.

NURSING CONSIDERATIONS

Besides those related universally to drug therapy (see "How to use this book"), consider the following specific recommendations:

Assessment
- Obtain a baseline assessment of the patient's underlying condition before drug therapy.
- Be alert for adverse reactions and drug interactions throughout therapy.
- Evaluate the patient's and family's knowledge about pseudoephedrine therapy.

Nursing Diagnoses
- Ineffective airway clearance related to the patient's underlying condition.
- Altered oral mucous membrane related to adverse drug reaction.
- Knowledge deficit related to pseudoephedrine therapy.

Planning and Implementation
Preparation and Administration
- Drug should not be given within 2 hours of bedtime.

Monitoring
- Monitor adverse reactions or drug interactions by checking the patient's vital signs for tachycardia.
- Monitor the patient's elimination pattern, because drug may cause difficult urination.
- Monitor hydration status if the patient develops nausea and vomiting.
- Monitor elderly patients who may be sensitive to the drug's effects.
- Monitor for adverse reactions by monitoring the patient's anxiety level after receiving the drug.

Supportive Care
- Provide the patient with sugarless gum, ice chips (unless contraindicated), or sour hard candy to relieve dry mouth.
- Institute safety precautions if the patient develops dizziness.
- Provide fluids if patient develops nausea and vomiting.
- Obtain an order for a mild analgesic if he develops a drug-induced headache.
- Be prepared to discontinue the drug and notify the doctor if the patient becomes unusually restless.

Patient Teaching
- Tell the patient not to take the drug within 2 hours of bedtime because the drug can cause insomnia.
- Tell the patient to relieve dry mouth with ice chips, sour hard candy, or sugarless gum.
- Tell the patient to take a mild analgesic if he experiences a drug-induced headache.
- Warn the patient against using OTC products containing other sympathomimetics.
- Tell the patient to stop the drug and notify the doctor if he becomes unusually restless.

Evaluation
In patients receiving pseudoephedrine, appropriate evaluation statements may include:
• Patient's airway remains patent.
• Patient does not develop a dry mouth.
• Patient and family state an understanding of pseudoephedrine therapy.

psyllium
(sill′ i yum)
Cillium◇, Konsyl◇, Metamucil◇, Metamucil Instant Mix◇, Metamucil Sugar Free◇, Naturacil◇, Perdiem Plain◇, Siblin◇, Syllact◇

• *Classification:* bulk laxative (absorbant)
• *Pregnancy Risk Category:* C

HOW SUPPLIED
Chewable pieces: 1.7 g/piece◇
Effervescent powder: 3.4 g/packet◇, 3.7 g/packet◇
Granules: 2.5 g/tsp, 4.03 g/tsp◇
Powder: 3.3 g/tsp◇, 3.4 g/tsp◇, 3.5 g/tsp◇, 4.94 g/tsp◇
Wafers: 3.4 g/wafer◇

ACTION
Mechanism: A bulk-forming laxative that absorbs water and expands to increase bulk and moisture content of the stool. The increased bulk encourages peristalsis and bowel movement.
Absorption: None.
Distribution: Locally distributed in the gut.
Metabolism: None.
Excretion: In feces.
Onset, peak, duration: Onset of action varies from 12 hours to 3 days.

INDICATIONS & DOSAGE
Constipation; bowel management—
Adults: 1 to 2 rounded teaspoonfuls P.O. in full glass of liquid daily, b.i.d. or t.i.d., followed by second glass of liquid; or 1 packet P.O. dissolved in water daily, b.i.d. or t.i.d.
Children over 6 years: 1 level teaspoonful P.O. in half a glass of liquid h.s.

CONTRAINDICATIONS & PRECAUTIONS
Contraindicated in patients with abdominal pain, fecal impaction, or intestinal obstruction or ulceration, because the drug may worsen these symptoms or conditions.

Use effervescent powder with caution in patients requiring sodium restriction because of the drug's high sodium content. Sugar-free drug preparations should be used with caution in patients who must restrict phenylalanine intake; these products may contain aspartame, which the GI tract metabolizes to phenylalanine.

ADVERSE REACTIONS
Common reactions are in italics; life-threatening reactions are in bold italics.
GI: nausea, vomiting, diarrhea, all after excessive use; esophageal, gastric, small intestinal, or colonic strictures when drug taken in dry form; abdominal cramps, especially in severe constipation.

INTERACTIONS
None significant.

EFFECTS ON DIAGNOSTIC TESTS
None reported.

NURSING CONSIDERATIONS
Besides those related universally to drug therapy (see "How to use this book"), consider the following specific recommendations:
Assessment
• Obtain a baseline assessment of history of bowel disorder, GI status, fluid intake, nutritional status, exercise habits, and normal pattern of elimination.

• Be alert for adverse reactions and drug interactions throughout therapy.
• Evaluate the patient's and family's knowledge about psyllium therapy.

Nursing Diagnoses

• Constipation related to interruption of normal pattern of elimination characterized by infrequent or absent stools.
• Pain related to psyllium-induced abdominal cramping.
• Knowledge deficit related to psyllium therapy.

Planning and Implementation

Preparation and Administration

• Mix with at least 240 ml (8 oz) of cold pleasant-tasting liquid such as orange juice to mask grittiness. Patient should drink it immediately or mixture will congeal. Follow with additional glass of liquid.
• Do not give before meals, because it may reduce appetite.

Monitoring

• Monitor effectiveness of therapy by checking the frequency and characteristics of stools.
• Auscultate bowel sounds at least once a shift. Assess for pain and cramping.
• Monitor nutritional status and fluid intake.

Supportive Care

• Do not give to patients with abdominal pain, nausea, vomiting, or other symptoms of appendicitis; and in intestinal obstruction or ulceration, disabling adhesion, or difficulty swallowing.
• In diabetic patients, use sugar-free brand of psyllium.
• Provide privacy for elimination.
• Be aware that laxative effect is usually seen in 12 to 24 hours, but may be delayed up to 3 days.
• Not absorbed systemically, nontoxic. Especially useful in postpartum constipation, debilitated patients, laxative abuse, irritable bowel syndrome, diverticular disease, and in combination with other laxatives to empty the colon before barium enema.
• Unless contraindicated, encourage fluid intake up to 2,500 ml a day.
• Consult with a dietitian to modify diet to increase fiber and bulk.

Patient Teaching

• Discourage excessive use of laxatives by patient.
• Teach the patient about the relationship between fluid intake, dietary fiber, exercise, and constipation.
• Teach patient that dietary sources of fiber include bran and other cereals, fresh fruit, and vegetables.
• Warn the patient that abdominal cramping may occur.
• Instruct the patient to mix granules with 8 oz fluid, drink it immediately, and follow with another full glass of fluid.

Evaluation

In patients receiving psyllium, appropriate evaluation statements may include:
• Patient reports return of normal pattern of elimination.
• Patient remains free from abdominal cramping.
• Patient and family state an understanding of psyllium therapy.

pyrazinamide

(peer a zin´ a mide)

PMS-Pyrazinamide†, Tebrazid†, Zinamide‡

• *Classification:* antitubercular (nicotinamide)
• *Pregnancy Risk Category:* C

HOW SUPPLIED

Tablets: 500 mg

ACTION

Mechanism: Unknown.
Absorption: Well absorbed after oral administration.
Distribution: Widely distributed into

body tissues and fluids, including lungs, liver, and CSF; drug is 50% protein-bound. Not known if drug crosses the placenta.
Metabolism: Hydrolyzed in the liver, with some hydrolysis in the stomach and possibly the bladder.
Excretion: Almost completely in urine by glomerular filtration. Only 4% to 14% is excreted as unchanged drug; the rest as metabolites. Not known if drug is excreted in breast milk. Half-life: 9 to 10 hours in adults; prolonged in renal and hepatic impairment. About 70% of a dose is excreted in urine within 24 hours.
Onset, peak, duration: Peak serum levels occur 2 hours after an oral dose.

INDICATIONS & DOSAGE

Adjunctive treatment of tuberculosis (when primary and secondary antitubercular drugs cannot be used or have failed) –
Adults: 20 to 35 mg/kg P.O. daily, divided in 3 to 4 doses. Maximum dosage is 3 g daily.

CONTRAINDICATIONS & PRECAUTIONS

Contraindicated in patients with hypersensitivity to pyrazinamide and in those with severe hepatic disease.

Use cautiously in patients with acute intermittent porphyria, decreased renal function, diabetes, or a history of peptic ulcer disease or gout.

ADVERSE REACTIONS

Common reactions are in italics; life-threatening reactions are in bold italics.
Blood: sideroblastic anemia, possible bleeding tendency due to thrombocytopenia.
CNS: ***neuromuscular blockade.***
GI: anorexia, nausea, vomiting.
GU: dysuria.
Hepatic: hepatitis.
Metabolic: interference with control in diabetes mellitus, hyperuricemia.
Skin: maculopapular rash, photosensitivity.
Other: malaise, fever, arthralgia.

INTERACTIONS

None significant.

EFFECTS ON DIAGNOSTIC TESTS

17-ketosteroid levels: transient decrease.
Liver function tests: elevated results.
Protein-bound iodine: increased levels.
Urate levels: increased.
Urine ketone determinations: chemical interference.

NURSING CONSIDERATIONS

Besides those related universally to drug therapy (see "How to use this book"), consider the following specific recommendations:

Assessment

- Obtain a baseline assessment of infection before therapy.
- Be alert for adverse reactions throughout therapy.
- Evaluate the patient's and family's knowledge about pyrazinamide therapy.

Nursing Diagnoses

- High risk for injury related to the ineffectiveness of pyrazinamide to eradicate the infection.
- Altered health maintenance related to pyrazinamide-induced gout.
- Knowledge deficit related to pyrazinamide therapy.

Planning and Implementation

Preparation and Administration

- Obtain specimens for culture and sensitivity tests and liver function studies and ensure that a physical examination for jaundice, liver tenderness, or enlargement has been performed before the first dose.
- Expect reduced dosage in patients with renal impairment.

• Question doses that exceed 35 mg/kg, which may cause liver damage.

Monitoring

• Monitor effectiveness by regularly assessing for improvement in infection and by evaluating culture and sensitivity results as prescribed.

• Closely monitor for jaundice, liver tenderness, or enlargement and changes in liver function tests.

• Monitor hematopoietic studies and serum uric acid level.

• Monitor patient for gout.

Supportive Care

• Notify doctor at once if patient develops signs of gout or hepatic impairment (loss of appetite, fatigue, malaise, jaundice, dark urine, and liver tenderness).

• Obtain an order for an antiemetic if GI reactions occur.

• Expect to adjust diabetic patient's treatment regimen because drug interferes with diabetes control.

Patient Teaching

• Stress the importance of patient taking the drug exactly as prescribed; warn against discontinuing drug without doctor's approval.

• Teach patient to watch for and immediately report signs of gout and hepatic impairment.

Evaluation

In patients receiving pyrazinamide, appropriate evaluation statements may include:

• Patient is free of infection.

• Patient's serum uric acid level remains normal throughout therapy.

• Patient and family state an understanding of pyrazinamide therapy.

pyrethrins

(pye ree´ thrinz)

A-200 Pyrinate◊, Barc◊, Pyrinyl◊, RID◊, TISIT◊, Triple X◊

• *Classification:* pediculocide (petroleum distillate)

• *Pregnancy Risk Category:* C

HOW SUPPLIED

Shampoo: pyrethrins 0.17% and piperonyl butoxide 2%; pyrethrins 0.3% and piperonyl butoxide 3%

Topical gel: pyrethrins 0.18% and piperonyl butoxide 2.2%; pyrethrins 0.33% and piperonyl butoxide 3%; pyrethrins 0.3% and piperonyl butoxide 4%

Topical solution: pyrethrins 0.18% and piperonyl butoxide 2%; pyrethrins 0.2%, piperonyl butoxide 2%, and deodorized kerosene 0.8%; pyrethrins 0.3% and piperonyl butoxide 3%

ACTION

Mechanism: Acts as contact poison that disrupts the parasite's nervous system, causing the parasite's paralysis and death.

Absorption: Absorbed through intact skin. Extent of absorption is unknown.

INDICATIONS & DOSAGE

Treatment of infestations of head, body, and pubic (crab) lice and their eggs—

Adults and children: apply to hair, scalp, or other infested area until entirely wet. Allow to remain for 10 minutes, but no longer. Wash thoroughly with warm water and soap, or shampoo. Remove dead lice and eggs with fine-toothed comb. Treatment may be repeated, if necessary, but don't exceed two applications within 24 hours. May repeat in 7 to 10 days to kill newly hatched lice.

CONTRAINDICATIONS & PRECAUTIONS

Contraindicated when skin is raw or inflammed and in patients allergic to ragweed. Use cautiously in infants and small children.

ADVERSE REACTIONS

Common reactions are in italics; life-threatening reactions are in bold italics.
Skin: *irritation with repeated use.*

INTERACTIONS

None significant.

EFFECTS ON DIAGNOSTIC TESTS

None reported.

NURSING CONSIDERATIONS

Besides those related universally to drug therapy (see "How to use this book"), consider the following specific recommendations:

Assessment

- Obtain a baseline assessment of the patient's head and body and pubic areas before therapy.
- Be alert for adverse reactions throughout therapy.
- Evaluate the patient's and family's knowledge about pyrethrins therapy.

Nursing Diagnoses

- Body image disturbance related to patient's underlying condition.
- High risk for impaired skin integrity related to pyrethrins-induced skin irritation.
- Knowledge deficit related to pyrethrins therapy.

Planning and Implementation

Preparation and Administration

- ***Topical use:*** Apply to hair, scalp, or other infected area until entirely wet. Allow to remain 10 minutes. Wash thoroughly with warm water and soap or shampoo. Remove dead lice and eggs with fine-toothed comb. Treatment may be repeated, if necessary, but don't exceed two applications within 24 hours. May repeat in 7 to 10 days to kill newly hatched lice.

Monitoring

- Monitor effectiveness by regularly checking patient's head and pubic area for lice.
- Observe for skin irritation, which may occur because product contains petroleum distillate.

Supportive Care

- Notify doctor immediately if skin irritation occurs.
- While assisting with self-care, encourage the patient to express fears and concerns about body image disturbance.
- Remember that topical corticosteroids or oral antihistamines may be needed for dermatitis that develops from scratching.
- According to some authorities, pyrethrins and lindane (Kwell) are equally effective for lice infestation, but pyrethrins is less hazardous.
- Know that drug is not effective against scabies.

Patient Teaching

- Instruct patient to apply medication.
- Teach patient not to apply to open areas or acutely inflamed skin or to face, eyes, mucous membranes, or urethral meatus. If accidental contact with eyes occurs, flush with water and notify the doctor.
- Inform patient that repeated use is discouraged because it can lead to skin irritation and possible systemic toxicity.
- Instruct patient to change and sterilize (boil, launder, dry clean, or apply very hot iron) all clothing and bed linen after drug is washed off.

Evaluation

In patients receiving pyrethrins, appropriate evaluation statements may include:

- Patient's body image disturbance has been resolved.
- Patient did not develop drug-induced irritation.
- Patient and family state an understanding of pyrethrins therapy.

pyridostigmine bromide

(peer id oh stig´ meen)
Mestinon*, Mestinon, Supraspan†, Mestinon Timespan, Regonol

- *Classification:* muscle stimulant (cholinesterase inhibitor)
- *Pregnancy risk category:* C

HOW SUPPLIED

Tablets: 60 mg
Tablets (timed-release): 180 mg
Syrup: 60 mg/5 ml
Injection: 5 mg/ml in 2-ml ampules or 5-ml vials

ACTION

Mechanism: Inhibits the destruction of acetylcholine released from the parasympathetic and somatic efferent nerves. Acetylcholine accumulates, promoting increased stimulation of the receptor.
Absorption: Poorly absorbed from the GI tract.
Distribution: Little is known; however, drug may cross the placenta, especially when administered in large doses. As a quaternary ammonium compound, drug is not expected to enter the CNS.
Metabolism: Exact metabolic fate is unknown; not hydrolyzed by cholinesterase.
Excretion: Drug and metabolites are excreted in urine.
Onset, peak, duration: Onset of action usually occurs 30 to 45 minutes after oral administration, 2 to 5 minutes after I.V., and 15 minutes after I.M. Duration of effect is usually 3 to 6 hours after oral dose and 2 to 3 hours after I.V. dose, depending on patient's physical and emotional status and disease severity.

INDICATIONS & DOSAGE

Antidote for nondepolarizing neuromuscular blocking agents–
Adults: 10 to 20 mg I.V. preceded by atropine sulfate 0.6 to 1.2 mg I.V.
Myasthenia gravis–
Adults: 60 to 120 mg P.O. q 3 or 4 hours. Usual dosage is 600 mg daily but higher dosage may be needed (up to 1,500 mg daily). Give 1/30 of oral dose I.M. or I.V. Dosage must be adjusted for each patient, depending on response and tolerance of adverse reactions. Alternatively, may give 180 to 540 mg timed-release tablets (1 to 3 tablets) b.i.d., with at least 6 hours between doses.

CONTRAINDICATIONS & PRECAUTIONS

Contraindicated in patients with intestinal or urinary tract obstruction because of drug's stimulatory effect on smooth muscle and in patients with bradycardia because drug may exacerbate this condition.

Administer with extreme caution to patients with bronchial asthma because drug may precipitate asthma attacks. Administer cautiously to patients with seizure disorders because drug may cause CNS stimulation; vagotonia, hyperthyroidism, or cardiac arrhythmias because drug may exacerbate these conditions; and with peptic ulcer disease because drug may increase gastric acid secretion.

ADVERSE REACTIONS

Common reactions are in italics; life-threatening reactions are in bold italics.
CNS: headache (with high doses), weakness, sweating, seizures.
CV: bradycardia, hypotension.
EENT: miosis.
GI: abdominal cramps, nausea, vomiting, diarrhea, excessive salivation.
Skin: rash.
Local: ***thrombophlebitis.***
Other: ***bronchospasm, bronchocon-***

striction, increased bronchial secretions, muscle cramps, muscle fasciculations.

INTERACTIONS

Atropine, anticholinergic agents, procainamide, quinidine: may reverse cholinergic effects. Observe for lack of drug effect.

EFFECTS ON DIAGNOSTIC TESTS

None reported.

NURSING CONSIDERATIONS

Besides those related universally to drug therapy (see "How to use this book"), consider the following specific recommendations:

Assessment

• Obtain a baseline assessment of the patient's underlying condition before therapy.
• Be alert for adverse reactions and drug interactions throughout therapy.
• Evaluate the patient's and family's knowledge about pyridostigmine therapy.

Nursing Diagnoses

• Altered health maintenance related to patient's underlying condition.
• Ineffective breathing pattern related to adverse reactions.
• Knowledge deficit related to pyridostigmine therapy.

Planning and Implementation

Preparation and Administration

• Know that optimum dosage is difficult to determine.
• Discontinue all other cholinergics before giving this drug.
• Be aware that drug has the longest duration of the cholinergics used for myasthenia gravis.
• Keep in mind that drug is used by the oral route in the treatment of senility associated with Alzheimer's disease.
• ***P.O. use:*** Do not crush the timed-release (Timespan or Supraspan) tablets.
• Give the syrup over ice to reduce sweetness if patients can't tolerate the taste.
• Store tablets in a tightly capped bottle, away from moisture.

Monitoring

• Monitor effectiveness by evaluating the reduction of symptoms of myasthenia gravis.
• Monitor for adverse reactions by frequently checking vital signs, especially respirations.
• Monitor and document the patient's response after each dose because it is difficult to determine optimum dosage.
• Monitor for diarrhea and other adverse GI reactions; if present, monitor hydration status.
• Monitor for abdominal or muscle cramping.

Supportive Care

• Have atropine injection readily available and be prepared to give as ordered to reverse toxicity.
• Position patient to make breathing easier and provide respiratory support as needed if adverse reactions occur.
• Report severe muscle weakness to doctor, who will determine if it reflects drug-induced toxicity or exacerbation of myasthenia gravis. Test dose of edrophonium I.V. will worsen drug-induced weakness but will temporarily relieve weakness caused by disease.

Patient Teaching

• Stress the importance of taking the drug exactly as ordered when the drug is used for the treatment of myasthenia gravis. Tell the patient to take it on time and in evenly spaced doses. If the doctor has ordered extended-release tablets, explain to the patient how these work and that he must take them at the same time each day, at least 6 hours apart.
• Explain to the patient that he may have to take this drug for the rest of his life.

Evaluation

In patients receiving pyridostigmine, appropriate evaluation statements may include:

• Patient can perform activities of daily living without assistance.

• Patient's respiratory pattern is unaffected by pyridostigmine therapy.

• Patient and family state an understanding of pyridostigmine therapy.

---

pyrimethamine

(peer i meth´ a meen)

Daraprim

pyrimethamine with sulfadoxine

Fansidar

• *Classification:* antimalarial (folic acid antagonist)

• *Pregnancy Risk Category:* C

HOW SUPPLIED

pyrimethamine

Tablets: 25 mg

pyrimethamine with sulfadoxine

Tablets: pyrimethamine 25 mg, sulfadoxine 500 mg

ACTION

Mechanism: Inhibits the enzyme dihydrofolate reductase, thereby impeding reduction of dihydrofolic acid to its active form, tetrahydrofolic acid.

Absorption: Well absorbed from the GI tract.

Distribution: Distributed to the kidneys, liver, spleen, and lungs; approximately 80% bound to plasma proteins.

Metabolism: Metabolized to several unidentified compounds.

Excretion: In the urine and in breast milk. Half-life: 2 to 6 days. Half-life not changed in end-stage renal disease.

Onset, peak, duration: Peak serum concentrations occur within 2 hours.

INDICATIONS & DOSAGE

Malaria prophylaxis and transmission control (pyrimethamine) –

Adults and children over 10 years: 25 mg P.O. weekly.

Children 4 to 10 years: 12.5 mg P.O. weekly.

Children under 4 years: 6.25 mg P.O. weekly.

Continue in all age groups at least 10 weeks after leaving endemic areas.

Acute attacks of malaria (Fansidar) –

Adults: 2 to 3 tablets as a single dose, either alone or in sequence with quinine or primaquine.

Children 9 to 14 years: 2 tablets.

Children 4 to 8 years: 1 tablet.

Children under 4 years: ½ tablet.

Malaria prophylaxis (Fansidar) –

Adults: 1 tablet weekly, or 2 tablets q 2 weeks.

Children 9 to 14 years: ¾ tablet weekly, or 1½ tablets q 2 weeks.

Children 4 to 8 years: ½ tablet weekly, or 1 tablet q 2 weeks.

Children under 4 years: ¼ tablet weekly, or ½ tablet q 2 weeks.

Acute attacks of malaria (pyrimethamine) –

Not recommended alone in nonimmune persons; use with faster-acting antimalarials, such as chloroquine, for 2 days to initiate transmission control and suppressive cure.

Adults and children over 15 years: 25 mg P.O. daily for 2 days.

Children under 15 years: 12.5 mg P.O. daily for 2 days.

Toxoplasmosis (pyrimethamine) –

Adults: initially, 100 mg P.O., then 25 mg P.O. daily for 4 to 5 weeks; during same time give 1 g sulfadiazine P.O. q 6 hours.

Children: initially, 1 mg/kg P.O., then 0.25 mg/kg daily for 4 to 5 weeks, along with 100 mg sulfadiazine/kg P.O. daily, divided q 6 hours.

CONTRAINDICATIONS & PRECAUTIONS

Contraindicated in patients with megaloblastic anemia from folate deficiency, because drug is a folate antagonist, and in patients with hypersensitivity to the drug or any of its components, and in those with chloroquine-resistant malaria (with pyrimethamine only). Use cautiously in patients with impaired renal function; in patients with possible folate deficiency including those with malabsorption syndrome, in alcoholism, or in pregnancy; and in patients receiving drugs such as phenytoin that affect folate levels. In patients with seizure disorders, reduce initial dosage for toxoplasmosis to avoid CNS toxicity. Use pyrimethamine with sulfadoxine cautiously in patients with severe allergy or bronchial asthma.

ADVERSE REACTIONS

Common reactions are in italics; life-threatening reactions are in bold italics.

Blood: ***agranulocytosis, aplastic anemia,*** megaloblastic anemia, bone marrow suppression, leukopenia, thrombocytopenia, pancytopenia.

CNS: stimulation and seizures (acute toxicity).

GI: anorexia, vomiting, diarrhea, atrophic glossitis.

Skin: rashes, ***erythema multiforme (Stevens-Johnson syndrome), toxic epidermal necrolysis.***

INTERACTIONS

Folic acid and para-aminobenzoic acid: decreased antitoxoplasmic effects. May require dosage adjustment.

Sulfonamides, co-trimoxazole: increased adverse effects. Use together cautiously.

EFFECTS ON DIAGNOSTIC TESTS

CBC: decreased WBC, RBC, and platelet counts.

NURSING CONSIDERATIONS

Besides those related universally to drug therapy (see "How to use this book"), consider the following specific recommendations:

Assessment

- Obtain a baseline assessment of infection before therapy.
- Be alert for adverse reactions and drug interactions throughout therapy.
- Evaluate the patient's and family's knowledge about pyrimethamine therapy.

Nursing Diagnoses

- High risk for injury related to ineffectiveness of pyrimethamine to eradicate the infection.
- High risk for impaired skin integrity related to adverse skin reactions to pyrimethamine.
- Knowledge deficit related to pyrimethamine therapy.

Planning and Implementation

Preparation and Administration

- ***P.O. use:*** Administer with meals to minimize GI distress.
- Be aware that because of the possibility of severe skin reactions, pyrimethamine with sulfadoxine should be used only in regions where chloroquine-resistant malaria is prevalent and only for travelers who plan to stay in the region longer than 3 weeks.

Monitoring

- Monitor effectiveness by regularly assessing the patient for improvement.
- If drug is used to treat toxoplasmosis, monitor blood counts, including platelets, twice weekly because dosages used approach toxic levels.
- Monitor patient for signs and symptoms of acute toxicity, such as stimulation and seizures, and for signs of folic or folinic acid deficiency.

Supportive Care

- Notify the doctor if the patient exhibits signs of folic or folinic acid deficiency, which may require reduction or discontinuation of the drug while

patient receives parenteral folinic acid until blood counts become normal.
• Withhold pyrimethamine with sulfadoxine and notify the doctor at the first sign of a skin rash.
• Institute seizure precautions throughout therapy.
• Obtain an order for an antiemetic or antidiarrheal, as needed.

Patient Teaching
• Tell patient to take the drug with meals to minimize GI distress.
• Instruct the patient who will receive prophylactic pyrimethamine with sulfadoxine to take the first dose 1 or 2 days before traveling to an endemic area.
• Warn the patient to discontinue pyrimethamine with sulfadoxine and notify doctor at first sign of skin rash.
• Stress the importance of receiving blood counts, including platelets, twice weekly if drug is used to treat toxoplasmosis.
• Teach patient to watch for and immediately report the signs of folic or folinic acid deficiency and acute toxicity.

Evaluation
In patients receiving pyrimethamine, appropriate evaluation statements may include:
• Patient is free of infection.
• Patient maintains intact skin integrity during therapy.
• Patient and family state an understanding of therapy.

QR

quazepam
(kway´ ze pam)
Doral

• Controlled Substance Schedule IV
• *Classification:* anxiolytic, sedative-hypnotic (benzodiazepine)
• *Pregnancy Risk Category:* X

HOW SUPPLIED

Tablets: 7.5 mg, 15 mg

ACTION

Mechanism: Acts on the limbic system and thalamus of the CNS by binding to specific benzodiazepine receptors.
Absorption: Well absorbed from the GI tract.
Distribution: Steady-state plasma levels of the parent drug appear after 7 days of once-daily administration. The drug is more than 95% bound to plasma proteins.
Metabolism: Hepatic; two active metabolites have been identified.
Excretion: 31% appears in the urine and 23% appears in the feces over a 5-day period. Only a trace amount of unchanged drug appears in the urine. Half-life: Mean elimination half-life of the parent drug and 2-oxo-quazepam, a metabolite, is 39 hours; of N-desalkyl-2-oxoquazepam, 733 hours.
Onset, peak, duration: Peak plasma levels of about 15 ng/ml occur within 2 hours.

INDICATIONS & DOSAGE

Insomnia –
Adults: 15 mg P.O. h.s. Some patients may respond to lower doses. Decrease dosage in elderly patients to 7.5 mg P.O. h.s. after 2 days of therapy.

CONTRAINDICATIONS & PRECAUTIONS

Contraindicated in patients allergic to the drug or other benzodiazepines, in pregnant patients, and in those with suspected or established sleep apnea. Patients who receive prolonged therapy with benzodiazepines may experience withdrawal symptoms if the drug is suddenly withdrawn (possibly after 6 weeks of continuous therapy).

ADVERSE REACTIONS

Common reactions are in italics; life-threatening reactions are in bold italics.
CNS: *fatigue, dizziness, daytime drowsiness, headache.*

INTERACTIONS

Alcohol or other CNS depressants, including antihistamines, opiate analgesics, and other benzodiazepines: increased CNS depression.

EFFECTS ON DIAGNOSTIC TESTS

None reported.

NURSING CONSIDERATIONS

Besides those related universally to drug therapy (see "How to use this book"), consider the following specific recommendations:
Assessment
• Obtain a baseline assessment of sleeping patterns and CNS status before therapy.
• Be alert for adverse reactions and drug interactions throughout therapy.
• Evaluate the patient's and family's knowledge about quazepam therapy.

Nursing Diagnoses
- Sleep pattern disturbance related to underlying patient problem.
- High risk for trauma related to adverse CNS reactions to quazepam.
- Knowledge deficit related to quazepam therapy.

Planning and Implementation
Preparation and Administration
- Before leaving the bedside, make sure the patient has swallowed the medication.

Monitoring
- Regularly monitor the effectiveness of quazepam by evaluating the patient's ability to sleep after administration.
- Monitor the patient's CNS status after initiating therapy for evidence of adverse reactions.
- After drug discontinuation, be alert for withdrawal symptoms.

Supportive Care
- After administration, institute safety precautions: remove cigarettes; keep bed rails up; and supervise or assist ambulation.
- Do not discontinue the drug abruptly. Patients who receive prolonged therapy with benzodiazepines may experience withdrawal symptoms if the drug is suddenly withdrawn (possible after 6 weeks of continuous therapy).
- Take precautions to prevent hoarding or self-overdosing, especially by the patient who is depressed or suicidal or has a history of drug abuse.

Patient Teaching
- Encourage the patient to report severe "hangover" or feeling oversedated so the doctor can be consulted for change of dose or drug.
- Warn the patient about the possible additive depressant effects that can occur with alcohol consumption. Additive effects can occur if alcohol is consumed on the day after the use of quazepam.
- Instruct the patient to remain in bed after taking drug and to call for assistance to use the bathroom.
- Warn the patient to avoid hazardous activities that require mental alertness, such as driving a car, until the adverse CNS reactions of the drug are known.
- Warn patients not to increase the drug dosage on their own, and to inform the doctor if they feel that the drug is no longer effective.

Evaluation
In patients receiving quazepam, appropriate evaluation statements may include:
- Patient states drug was effective in inducing sleep.
- Patient's safety maintained.
- Patient and family state an understanding of quazepam therapy.

---

quinacrine hydrochloride (mepacrine hydrochloride)
(kwin´ a kreen)
Atabrine

- *Classification:* anthelmintic, antiprotozoal, antimalarial (acridine derivative)
- *Pregnancy Risk Category:* C

HOW SUPPLIED
Tablets: 100 mg

ACTION
Mechanism: Antiprotozoal action against *Giardia* is unknown. Quinicrine alters DNA function in susceptible cestodes (tapeworms). Antimalarial action may be related to the inhibition of the digestion of hemoglobin by *Plasmodia.*
Absorption: Readily absorbed.
Distribution: Widely distributed to tissues, especially into the pancreas, lungs, liver, spleen, bone marrow, erythrocytes, and skeletal muscles; it crosses the placenta. The drug is highly protein-bound.

Metabolism: Drug appears to be metabolized slowly.
Excretion: Excreted slowly, primarily in urine; small amounts in feces, sweat, saliva, bile, and breast milk. Half-life: 5 days.
Onset, peak, duration: Peak serum concentrations usually occur within 8 hours.

INDICATIONS & DOSAGE

Treatment of giardiasis–
Adults: 300 mg P.O. in 3 divided doses for 5 to 7 days.
Children: 7 mg/kg/day P.O. given in 3 divided doses after meals for 5 days. Maximum 300 mg/day. Dosage may be repeated in 2 weeks.
Tapeworms (beef, pork, and fish)–
Adults and children over 14 years: 4 doses of 200 mg P.O. given 10 minutes apart (800 mg total).
Children 11 to 14 years: 600 mg P.O. total dosage, administered in 3 or 4 divided doses, 10 minutes apart.
Children 5 to 10 years: 400 mg P.O. total dosage, administered in 3 or 4 divided doses, 10 minutes apart.
Treatment of acute malaria attacks–
Adults and children over 8 years: 5 doses of 200 mg P.O. , followed by 100 mg P.O. t.i.d. for 6 days (2,800 mg total in 7 days).
Children age 4 to 8 years: 3 doses of 200 mg, followed by 100 mg b.i.d. for 6 days.
Children age 1 to 4 years: 3 doses of 100 mg, followed by 100 mg daily for 6 days.

CONTRAINDICATIONS & PRECLAUTIONS

Contraindicated in patients taking primaquine. Use cautiously in patients with: severe cardiac disease or G6PD deficiency; severe renal disease because the drug accumulates; hepatic or alcoholic illness or in those taking hepatotoxic drugs, because it concentrates in the liver; psoriasis or porphyria because it may exacerbate these conditions; and in psychotic patients because it can cause psychosis. Also use with caution in patients over age 60 and in infants under age 1.

ADVERSE REACTIONS

Common reactions are in italics; life-threatening reactions are in bold italics.
CNS: *headache, dizziness, nervousness, vertigo, mood shifts, nightmares,* ***seizures.***
GI: *diarrhea, anorexia, nausea, abdominal cramps,* vomiting.
GU: yellow urine.
Skin: pleomorphic skin eruptions, yellow discoloration.

INTERACTIONS

None significant.

EFFECTS ON DIAGNOSTIC TESTS

Cortisol: falsely elevated concentrations in urine and plasma.
Urinalysis: deep yellow discoloration of acid urine.

NURSING CONSIDERATIONS

Besides those related universally to drug therapy (see "How to use this book"), consider the following specific recommendations:

Assessment

- Obtain a baseline assessment of infection including appropriate specimens for analysis before therapy.
- Be alert for adverse reactions and drug interactions throughout therapy.
- Evaluate the patient's and family's knowledge about quinacrine therapy.

Nursing Diagnoses

- Altered health maintenance related to ineffectiveness of quinacrine.
- High risk for fluid volume deficit related to quinacrine-induced adverse GI reactions.
- Knowledge deficit related to quinacrine.

Planning and Implementation

Preparation and Administration

• Ensure that patient has been on a bland, nonfat, semisolid diet for 24 hours and has fasted after the evening meal before treatment.

• Administer drug after meals with large glass of water, tea, or fruit juice to reduce GI irritation. Bitter taste may be disguised by jam or honey.

Monitoring

• Monitor effectiveness by assessing for improvement of infection. Save all of patient's stool after treatment to look for the scolex (attachment organ), which will be stained yellow.

• Monitor patient's hydration status if adverse GI reactions occur.

Supportive Care

• Give a saline cathartic as prescribed 1 to 2 hours after drug is given to expel the worm. Collect all of patient's stool after treatment. Don't put toilet paper in bedpan.

• Administer sodium bicarbonate as prescribed with large doses of quinacrine to minimize nausea and vomiting.

• Obtain an order for an antiemetic or antidiarrheal agent as needed.

• Institute seizure precautions.

• Institute safety precautions if adverse CNS reactions occur.

Patient Teaching

• Instruct patient to eat a bland, nonfat, semisolid diet for 24 hours and fast after the evening meal before treatment.

• Tell patient to take the drug after meals with a large glass of water, tea, or fruit juice to reduce GI irritation. Suggest that the bitter taste may be disguised by jam or honey.

• Tell patient receiving large doses of quinacrine to take sodium bicarbonate with each dose if prescribed to minimize nausea and vomiting.

• Inform patient that a saline cathartic will be given 1 to 2 hours after drug to expel the worm.

• Stress the importance of saving all of stool after treatment. Tell patient not to put toilet paper in bedpan.

• Inform patient that temporary yellow color of skin and urine is not jaundice.

• Warn patient to avoid hazardous activities that require alertness until adverse CNS effects are known.

Evaluation

In patients receiving quinacrine, appropriate evaluation statements may include:

• Patient is free of infection and maintains normal health status.

• Patient maintains adequate hydration throughout therapy.

• Patient and family state an understanding of quinacrine therapy.

quinidine bisulfate

(kwin´ i deen)

(66.4% quinidine base)

Biquin Durules†, Kinidin Durules‡

quinidine gluconate

(62% quinidine base)

Duraquin, Quinaglute Dura-Tabs, Quinalan, Quinate†

quinidine polygalacturonate

(60.5% quinidine base)

Cardioquin

quinidine sulfate

(83% quinidine base)

Apo-Quinidine†, CinQuin, Novoquindin†, Quine, Quinidex Extentabs, Quinora

• *Classification:* ventricular, supraventricular antiarrhythmic; (cinchona alkaloid)

• *Pregnancy Risk Category:* C

HOW SUPPLIED

bisulfate

Tablets: 250 mg†‡

gluconate
Tablets (sustained-release): 324 mg, 325 mg†, 330 mg
Injection: 80 mg/ml
polygalacturonate
Tablets: 275 mg
sulfate
Tablets: 100 mg, 200 mg, 300 mg
Tablets (sustained-release): 300 mg
Capsules: 200 mg, 300 mg
Injection: 200 mg/ml

ACTION

Mechanism: A Class Ia antiarrhythmic that depresses phase O and prolongs the action potential. All Class I drugs have membrane-stabilizing (local anesthetic) effects.
Absorption: Although all quinidine salts are well absorbed from the GI tract, serum drug levels vary greatly. Although the drug can be given I.M., injection is painful and may increase plasma levels of creatinine kinase.
Distribution: Well distributed in all tissues except the brain; it concentrates in the heart, liver, kidneys, and skeletal muscle. Distribution volume decreases in patients with CHF, possibly requiring reduction in maintenance dosage. Approximately 80% of drug is bound to plasma proteins; the unbound (active) fraction may increase in patients with hypoalbuminemia from various causes, including hepatic insufficiency. Usual therapeutic serum levels depend on assay method and range as follows:
– Specific assay (EMIT, HPLC, fluorescence polarization): 2 to 5 mcg/ml
– Nonspecific assay (fluorometric): 4 to 8 mcg/ml.
Metabolism: About 60% to 80% of drug is metabolized in the liver to two metabolites that may have some pharmacologic activity.
Excretion: Approximately 10% to 30% of an administered dose is excreted in the urine within 24 hours as unchanged drug. Urine acidification increases quinidine excretion; alkalinization decreases excretion. Most of an administered dose is eliminated in the urine as metabolites. Half-life: Ranges from 5 to 12 hours (usual half-life is about 6½ hours).
Onset, peak, duration: Onset of action of quinidine sulfate is from 1 to 3 hours. For extended-release forms, onset of action may be slightly slower but duration of effect is longer, because this drug delivery system allows longer than usual dosing intervals. Peak plasma levels occur in 3 to 4 hours for quinidine gluconate and 6 hours for quinidine polygalacturonate. Duration of effect ranges from 6 to 8 hours.

INDICATIONS & DOSAGE

Atrial flutter or fibrillation–
Adults: 200 mg quinidine sulfate or equivalent base P.O. q 2 to 3 hours for 5 to 8 doses with subsequent daily increases until sinus rhythm is restored or toxic effects develop. Administer quinidine only after digitalization to avoid increasing AV conduction. Maximum dosage is 3 to 4 g daily.
Paroxysmal supraventricular tachycardia–
Adults: 400 to 600 mg I.M. gluconate q 2 to 3 hours until toxic adverse reactions develop or arrhythmia subsides.
Premature atrial and ventricular contractions; paroxysmal atrioventricular junctional rhythm; paroxysmal atrial tachycardia; paroxysmal ventricular tachycardia; maintenance after cardioversion of atrial fibrillation or flutter–
Adults: test dose is 50 to 200 mg P.O., then monitor vital signs before beginning therapy. Quinidine sulfate or equivalent base 200 to 400 mg P.O. q 4 to 6 hours; or initially, quinidine gluconate 600 mg I.M., then up to 400 mg q 2 hours, p.r.n.; or quinidine gluconate 800 mg (10 ml of the com-

mercially available solution) added to 40 ml dextrose 5% in water, infused I.V. at 16 mg (1 ml)/minute.
Children: test dose is 2 mg/kg; 3 to 6 mg/kg q 2 to 3 hours for 5 doses P.O. daily.

CONTRAINDICATIONS & PRECAUTIONS

Contraindicated in patients with complete AV block with an AV junctional or idioventricular pacemaker, because of potential for asystole; intraventricular conduction defects (especially with prolonged Q-T interval or QRS duration, or digitalis toxicity manifested by arrhythmias or AV conduction disorders), because quinidine in therapeutic concentration increases the Q-T interval and QRS duration through AV node and His-Purkinje effects; further prolongation would be detrimental in these conditions and complete heart block, ventricular tachycardia, ventricular fibrillation, or asystole may result; in patients with myasthenia gravis, because the drug's anticholinergic effects may exacerbate muscle weakness; and in patients with hypersensitivity to quinidine or related compounds.

Use cautiously in patients with incomplete AV block, because complete heart block may occur; in patients with CHF, because the drug's direct myocardial depressant effect may worsen heart failure; in patients with hypotension, because the drug causes alpha blockade, which exacerbates hypotension (especially when given I.V.); in patients with renal and hepatic dysfunction because toxic drug accumulation may result; and in patients with asthma, muscle weakness, or infection with fever, because these conditions may mask hypersensitivity reactions to the drug.

ADVERSE REACTIONS

Common reactions are in italics; life-threatening reactions are in bold italics.
Blood: ***hemolytic anemia, thrombocytopenia, agranulocytosis.***
CNS: *vertigo, headache, lightheadedness,* confusion, restlessness, cold sweat, pallor, fainting, dementia.
CV: *premature ventricular contractions;* ***severe hypotension; SA and AV block; ventricular fibrillation,*** *tachycardia;* ***aggravated CHF;*** *ECG changes (particularly widening of QRS complex, notched P waves, widened Q-T interval, ST segment depression).*
EENT: *tinnitus,* excessive salivation, blurred vision.
GI: *diarrhea, nausea, vomiting,* anorexia, abdominal pains.
Hepatic: hepatotoxicity including granulomatous hepatitis.
Skin: rash, petechial hemorrhage of buccal mucosa, pruritus.
Other: angioedema, acute asthmatic attack, ***respiratory arrest,*** *fever, cinchonism.*

INTERACTIONS

Acetazolamide, antacids, sodium bicarbonate: may increase quinidine blood levels due to alkaline urine. Monitor for increased effect.
Barbiturates, phenytoin, rifampin: may antagonize quinidine activity. Monitor for decreased quinidine effect.
Cimetidine: increased serum quinidine levels. Monitor for increased effect.
Digoxin: increased serum digoxin levels after initiating quinidine therapy. Monitor closely.
Nifedipine: may decrease quinidine blood levels. Monitor carefully.
Verapamil: may result in hypotension. Monitor blood pressure.
Warfarin: increased anticoagulant effect. Monitor closely.

EFFECTS ON DIAGNOSTIC TESTS

None reported.

NURSING CONSIDERATIONS

Besides those related universally to drug therapy (see "How to use this book"), consider the following specific recommendations:

Assessment

- Obtain a baseline assessment of the patient's heart rate and rhythm before quinidine therapy.
- Be alert for adverse reactions or drug interactions throughout therapy.
- Evaluate the patient's and family's knowledge about quinidine.

Nursing Diagnoses

- Decreased cardiac output related to ineffectiveness of quinidine therapy.
- Altered protection related to quinidine-induced proarrythmias.
- Knowledge deficit related to quinidine.

Planning and Implementation

Preparation and Administration

- Expect dosage to be decreased in patients with CHF and hepatic disease.
- Check apical pulse rate and blood pressure before starting therapy. If extemes in pulse rate are present, withhold drug and notify doctor at once.
- ***P.O. use:*** Administer drug with meals to minimize adverse GI reactions.
- ***I.V. use:*** Be aware that the I.V. route should only be used to treat acute arrhythmias. Mix 10 ml of quinidine gluconate with 40 ml dextrose 5% in water and infuse at 16 mg (1 ml)/minute. Never use discolored (brownish) quinidine solution.
- When changing route of administration, alter dosage as ordered to compensate for variations in quinidine base content.
- Store drug away from heat and direct light.

Monitoring

- Monitor effectiveness by regularly evaluating ECG recordings and heart rate and rhythm.
- Monitor adverse GI reactions, especially diarrhea, which are signs of toxicity.
- Monitor serum quinidine levels. Toxicity occurs when levels are greater than 8 mcg/ml.
- Monitor ECG for new arrhythmias.
- Monitor liver function tests during the first 4 to 8 weeks of therapy.
- Monitor CBC and platelet counts regularly.
- Monitor digoxin levels if drug is being administered concomitantly with digoxin.

Supportive Care

- If ECG disturbances occurs, withhold the drug, obtain a rhythm strip, and notify the doctor immediately.
- Have emergency equipment and drugs on hand to treat new arrhythmias. Be aware that lidocaine may be effective in treating quinidine-induced arrhythmias, because it increases AV conduction.
- Notify doctor immediately if patient develops adverse GI reactions, especially diarrhea, as these are signs of quinidine toxicity. Expect to draw blood sample for quinidine level to confirm toxicity.
- Be aware that after long-standing atrial fibrillation, restoration of normal sinus rhythm may result in thromboembolism due to dislodgement of thrombi from atrial wall. Anticoagulation often advised before restoration of normal atrial rhythm.
- Institute safety precautions if adverse CNS reactions occur.

Patient Teaching

- Stress importance of close follow-up care and frequent diagnostic studies to monitor effectiveness of quinidine and detect adverse reactions.
- Tell patient to take the drug with meals to minimize adverse GI reactions.
- Teach patient the signs of quinidine toxicity and tell the patient to report them immediately to the doctor if present.
- Instruct patient to ask for assis-

tance with activities if adverse CNS reactions occur.

Evaluation

In patients receiving quinidine, appropriate evaluation statements may include:

• Patient's ECG reveals arrhythmia has been corrected.
• Patient does not experience proarrythmias with quinidine use.
• Patient and family state an understanding of quinidine therapy.

quinine bisulfate (quinine bisulphate)

(kwye´ nine)

Bi-Chinine‡, Biquinate‡, Myoquin‡, Quinbisul‡

quinine sulfate (quinine sulphate)

Chinine‡, Legatrin, Novoquinine†, Quinamm, Quinate‡, Quindan, Quine-200◇, Quine-300, Quinoctal‡, Quiphile, Strema, Sulquin‡

• *Classification:* antimalarial (cinchona alkaloid)
• *Pregnancy Risk Category:* X

HOW SUPPLIED

bisulphate

Tablets: 100 mg, 300 mg

sulfate

Tablets: 260 mg, 325 mg◇

Capsules: 130 mg◇, 195 mg◇, 200 mg◇, 260 mg, 300 mg◇, 325 mg◇

ACTION

Mechanism: Mechanism of antiprotozoal action is unknown, but the drug is often referred to as a generalized protoplasmic poison. As a muscle relaxant, quinine appears to have a direct effect on muscle fibers that decreases their response to repetitive stimulation.

Absorption: Absorbed almost completely from the GI tract.

Distribution: Widely distributed into the liver, lungs, kidneys, and spleen; CSF levels reach 2% to 5% of serum levels. Quinine is about 70% bound to plasma proteins and readily crosses the placenta.

Metabolism: Metabolized in the liver.

Excretion: Less than 5% of a single dose is excreted unchanged in the urine; small amounts of metabolites appear in the feces, gastric juice, bile, saliva, and breast milk. Urine acidification hastens elimination. Half-life: 4 to 21 hours in healthy or convalescing persons; longer in patients with malaria.

Onset, peak, duration: Peak serum concentrations occur at 1 to 3 hours.

INDICATIONS & DOSAGE

Malaria due to Plasmodium falciparum *(chloroquine-resistant)–*

Adults: 650 mg P.O. q 8 hours for 10 days, with 25 mg pyrimethamine q 12 hours for 3 days, and with 500 mg sulfadiazine q.i.d. for 5 days.

Nocturnal leg cramps–

Adults: 260 to 300 mg P.O. at bedtime or after the evening meal.

CONTRAINDICATIONS & PRECAUTIONS

Contraindicated in pregnant patients and in patients with hypersensitivity to the drug, glucose-6-phosphate dehydrogenase (G6PD) deficiency, optic neuritis, or tinnitus; and in patients with a history of blackwater fever or of thrombocytopenic purpura associated with previous use of quinine ingestion. Use cautiously in patients with cardiac arrhythmias and in those taking sodium bicarbonate concomitantly.

ADVERSE REACTIONS

Common reactions are in italics; life-threatening reactions are in bold italics.

Blood: hemolytic anemia, thrombocytopenia, ***agranulocytosis,*** hypoprothrombinemia.

CNS: severe headache, apprehension, excitement, confusion, delirium, syncope, hypothermia, ***seizures*** (with toxic doses).
CV: hypotension, ***cardiovascular collapse*** with overdosage or rapid I.V. administration.
EENT: altered color perception, photophobia, blurred vision, night blindness, amblyopia, scotoma, diplopia, mydriasis, optic atrophy, tinnitus, impaired hearing.
GI: epigastric distress, diarrhea, nausea, vomiting.
GU: renal tubular damage, anuria.
Skin: rashes, pruritus.
Local: thrombosis at infusion site.
Other: asthma, flushing.

INTERACTIONS

Sodium bicarbonate: elevates quinine levels by decreasing quinine excretion. Use together cautiously.

EFFECTS ON DIAGNOSTIC TESTS

CBC: decreased platelets, and RBCs.
Glucose: hypoglycemia.
17-hydroxycorticosteroid and 17-ketogenic steroid tests: chemical interference.
Urinary catecholamines: false elevations.

NURSING CONSIDERATIONS

Besides those related universally to drug therapy (see "How to use this book"), consider the following specific recommendations:

Assessment

- Obtain a baseline assessment of infection before therapy.
- Be alert for adverse reactions and drug interactions throughout therapy.
- Evaluate the patient's and family's knowledge about quinine therapy.

Nursing Diagnoses

- High risk for injury related to ineffectiveness of quinine to eradicate infection.
- Altered protection related to quinine induced hematologic abnormalities.
- Knowledge deficit related to quinine.

Planning and Implementation

Preparation and Administration

- ***P.O. use:*** Administer after meals to minimize GI distress. Do not crush tablets, because drug is irritating to gastric mucosa.
- ***I.V. use:*** Be aware that I.V. quinine is no longer available. The Centers for Disease Control recommend the use of I.V. quinidine sulfate for treatment of severe cases of malaria.

Monitoring

- Monitor effectiveness by regularly assessing for improvement in infection.
- Monitor blood tests for abnormalities.
- Monitor for overdosage (to prevent cardiovascular collapse) or toxicity (CNS reactions).

Supportive Care

- Notify the doctor and discontinue the drug if any signs of idiosyncrasy or toxicity occur.
- Obtain an order for an analgesic if severe headache occurs.
- Institute safety precautions if visual disturbances or adverse CNS reactions occur.
- Obtain an order for an antiemetic or antidiarrheal agent as needed.

Patient Teaching

- Tell patient to take the drug after meals to minimize GI distress. Tell patient not to crush tablets, because drug is irritating to gastric mucosa.
- Teach patient to recognize and report signs and symptoms of toxicity or idiosyncrasy and to dicontinue the drug immediately if they occur.
- Warn patient to avoid hazardous activities if visual disturbances or adverse CNS reactions occur.

Evaluation

In patients receiving quinine, appropriate evaluation statements may include:

• Patient is free of infection.
• Patient's blood tests remain normal throughout therapy.
• Patient and family state an understanding of therapy.

rabies immune globulin, human
Hyperab, Imogam

• *Classification:* rabies prophylaxis agent (immune serum)
• *Pregnancy Risk Category:* C

HOW SUPPLIED
Injection: 150 IU/ml in 2-ml, 10-ml vials

ACTION
Mechanism: Provides passive immunity to rabies.
Absorption: Slow I.M. absorption.
Distribution: Rabies immune globulin probably crosses the placenta and distributes into breast milk.
Excretion: The serum half-life to rabies antibody titer is reportedly about 24 days.
Onset, peak, duration: Rabies antibody appears in serum within 24 hours and peaks within 2 to 13 days.

INDICATIONS & DOSAGE
Rabies exposure–
Adults and children: 20 IU/kg I.M. at time of first dose of rabies vaccine. Use half of dose to infiltrate wound area. Give remainder I.M. Don't give rabies vaccine and rabies immune globulin in same syringe or at same site.

CONTRAINDICATIONS & PRECAUTIONS
Contraindicated in patients with hypersensitivity to thimerosal, a component of this immune serum.

ADVERSE REACTIONS
Common reactions are in italics; life-threatening reactions are in bold italics.
Local: pain, redness, induration at injection site.
Other: slight fever, ***anaphylaxis,*** angioedema.

INTERACTIONS
Corticosteroids and immunosuppressive agents: interferes with response. Avoid during postexposure immunization period.
Live virus vaccines (measles, mumps, rubella, or polio): response to these vaccines may not be reliable because of antibodies present in rabies immune globulin. Don't administer live vaccines within 3 months of rabies immune globulin.

EFFECTS ON DIAGNOSTIC TESTS
None reported.

NURSING CONSIDERATIONS
Besides those related universally to drug therapy (see "How to use this book"), consider the following specific recommendations:

Assessment
• Obtain a baseline assessment of the patient's allergies, animal bites, and immunization reaction before therapy.
• Be alert for adverse reactions and drug interactions throughout therapy.
• Evaluate the patient's and family's knowledge about rabies immune globulin therapy.

Nursing Diagnoses
• Altered protection related to lack of immunity to rabies.
• Pain related to discomfort at injection site induced by immunization.
• Knowledge deficit related to rabies immune globulin.

Planning and Implementation
Preparation and Administration
• Check drug label. Do not confuse with rabies vaccine, which is a suspension of attenuated or killed microorganisms used to confer active

immunity. The two drugs are often given together prophylactically after exposure to known or suspected rabid animals.
• ***I.M. use:*** Do not administer more than 5 ml I.M. at one injection site; divide I.M. doses greater than 5 ml and administer at different sites.
• Do not give rabies vaccine and rabies immune globulin with the same syringe.
Monitoring
• Monitor effectiveness by checking the patient's antibody titers.
• Check vital signs.
• Observe injection site for local reaction to immunization (pain, redness, induration).
Supportive Care
• Treat fever with antipyretics.
• Apply ice or cold compress to injection site to relieve immunization-induced discomfort.
• Do not give repeated doses after rabies vaccine is started.
• Use only with rabies vaccine and local treatment of the wound. Give regardless of interval between exposure and initiation of therapy.
• This immune serum provides passive immunity.
Patient Teaching
• Inform the patient that a slight fever, pain, and redness at the injection site may follow immunization.
• Advise the patient that a tetanus booster may be necessary at this time.
Evaluation
In patients receiving rabies immune globulin, appropriate evaluation statements may include:
• Patient exhibits passive immunity to rabies.
• Patient is free of pain.
• Patient and family state an understanding of rabies immune globulin.

rabies vaccine, human diploid cell (HDCV)
Imovax

• *Classification:* viral vaccine
• *Pregnancy Risk Category:* C

HOW SUPPLIED
Intradermal injection: 0.25 IU rabies antigen/dose.
I.M. injection: 2.5 IU of rabies antigen/ml, in single-dose vial with diluent

ACTION
Mechanism: Promotes active immunity to rabies.
Pharmacokinetics: Unknown.
Onset, peak, duration: After intradermal injection, rabies antibodies appear in the serum within 7 to 10 days and peak at 30 to 60 days. Vaccine-induced immunity persists for about 1 year.

INDICATIONS & DOSAGE
Postexposure antirabies immunization–
Adults and children: five 1-ml doses of HDCV I.M. (for example, in the deltoid region). Give first dose as soon as possible after exposure; give an additional dose on each of days 3, 7, 14, and 28 after first dose.
Preexposure prophylaxis immunization for persons in high-risk groups–
Adults and children: three 1-ml injections administered I.M. Give first dose on day 0 (the first day of therapy), second dose on day 7, and third dose on either day 21 or 28. Alternatively, give 0.1 ml intradermally on the same dosage schedule.

CONTRAINDICATIONS & PRECAUTIONS
Rabies vaccine for preexposure prophylaxis should be postponed in pa-

tients with febrile illness. Use cautiously in persons with a history of hypersensitivity to neomycin or phenolsulfonphthalein, components of the vaccine.

ADVERSE REACTIONS

Common reactions are in italics; life-threatening reactions are in bold italics.
Systemic: headache, nausea, abdominal pain, muscle aches, dizziness, fever, diarrhea, ***anaphylaxis,*** *serum sickness.*
Local: *pain, erythema, swelling or itching at injection site.*

INTERACTIONS

Corticosteroids, immunosuppressive agents, antimalarial drugs: decreased response to rabies vaccine. Avoid concomitant use.

EFFECTS ON DIAGNOSTIC TESTS

None reported.

NURSING CONSIDERATIONS

Besides those related universally to drug therapy (see "How to use this book"), consider the following specific recommendations:

Assessment

- Obtain a baseline assessment of the patient's allergies, immunization history, and immunization reaction before therapy.
- Be alert for adverse reactions and drug interactions throughout therapy.
- Evaluate the patient's and family's knowledge about rabies vaccine therapy.

Nursing Diagnoses

- Altered protection related to lack of immunity to rabies virus.
- Ineffective breathing pattern related to vaccine-induced anaphylaxis.
- Knowledge deficit related to therapy.

Planning and Implementation

Preparation and Administration

- For I.M. and intradermal injection only. Do not give I.V.
- For preexposure prophylaxis give regimen of three 0.1-ml doses.
- For postexposure prophylaxis give only the 1-ml doses.

Monitoring

- Monitor effectiveness by checking the patient's antibody titers for rabies virus.
- Observe the patient for signs of anaphylaxis immediately after immunization.
- Check vital signs.
- Observe the injection site for local reaction (erythema, swelling).

Supportive Care

- Keep epinephrine 1:1000 available to treat possible anaphylaxis. Have oxygen and resuscitation equipment nearby.
- Stop corticosteroids during immunizing period.
- Use antihistamines to treat serum sickness–like allergic reactions to booster doses.
- The Centers for Disease Control recommends a booster dose with HDCV for all persons who have been potentially exposed to rabies virus since October 15, 1984, and who have received postexposure prophylaxis with Wyvac unless acceptable titers are proven.

Patient Teaching

- Instruct the patient to report respiratory difficulty or signs of serum sickness immediately.
- Advise the patient that redness, pain, swelling, and itching may occur at the injection site.
- Inform the patient that the vaccine is administered in divided doses over 28 days.

Evaluation

In patients receiving rabies vaccine, appropriate evaluation statements may include:

- Patient exhibits immunity to rabies virus.
- Patient demonstrates no signs of anaphylaxis or serum sickness.

• Patient and family state an understanding of HDCV therapy.

ramipril
(ra mi´ prill)
Altace

• *Classification:* antihypertensive (ACE inhibitor)
• *Pregnancy Risk Category:* D

HOW SUPPLIED
Capsules: 1.25 mg, 2.5 mg, 5 mg, 10 mg

ACTION
Mechanism: Inhibits angiotensin converting enzyme (ACE), preventing the pulmonary conversion of angiotensin I to angiotensin II, a potent vasoconstrictor. Reduced formation of angiotensin II decreases aldosterone secretion, reducing sodium and water retention and lowering blood pressure.
Absorption: At least 50% to 60%; not significantly influenced by the presence of food in the GI tract, although the rate of absorption is reduced.
Distribution: Ramipril is 73% serum protein-bound; ramiprilat, 58%.
Metabolism: Almost completely metabolized to ramiprilat, which has six times the ACE inhibitory activity of ramipril.
Excretion: After oral administration, about 60% of the parent drug and its metabolites are eliminated in the urine, the remainder in the feces. Half-life: After multiple daily doses of ramipril, the half-life of therapeutic ramiprilat concentrations is 13 to 17 hours.
Onset, peak, duration: After oral administration, peak plasma concentrations of ramipril are reached within 1 hour. Peak plasma levels of ramiprilat are reached in 2 to 4 hours.

INDICATIONS & DOSAGE
Treatment of essential hypertension (alone or in combination with diuretics) –
Adults: initially, 2.5 mg P.O. once daily. Increase dosage as necessary based on patient response. Maintenance dose is 2.5 to 20 mg daily as a single dose or in divided doses.

CONTRAINDICATIONS & PRECAUTIONS
Contraindicated in patients with hypersensitivity to the drug or with a history of angioneurotic edema. Use cautiously in patients with impaired renal or hepatic function and in situations conducive to hyperkalemia, including use of potassium-sparing diuretics, renal insufficiency, diabetes mellitus, potassium supplementation, and use of potassium-containing sodium substitutes.

ADVERSE REACTIONS
Common reactions are in italics; life-threatening reactions are in bold italics.
CNS: headache, dizziness, fatigue, asthenia.
GI: nausea, vomiting.
GU: impotence.
Other: cough.

INTERACTIONS
Diuretics: excessive hypotension, especially at the start of therapy. Before ramipril therapy begins, discontinue diuretic at least 3 days earlier, increase sodium intake, or reduce the starting dose of ramipril.
Lithium: increased serum lithium levels. Use together cautiously and monitor serum lithium levels.
Potassium supplements and potassium-sparing diuretics: increased risk of hyperkalemia because ramipril attenuates potassium loss. Avoid concomitant use or monitor plasma potassium closely.

EFFECTS ON DIAGNOSTIC TESTS

Blood glucose: increased levels.
BUN and serum creatinine: transiently increased levels.
Hemoglobin and hematocrit: decreased levels.
Serum bilirubin, liver enzymes, and uric acid: elevated levels.

NURSING CONSIDERATIONS

Besides those related universally to drug therapy (see "How to use this book"), consider the following specific recommendations:

Assessment

- Obtain a baseline assessment of the patient's blood pressure before beginning therapy.
- Be alert for adverse reactions and drug interactions throughout therapy.
- Evaluate the patient's and family's knowledge about ramipril therapy.

Nursing Diagnoses

- Altered tissue perfusion (renal, cerebral, cardiopulmonary, peripheral) related to the patient's underlying condition.
- High risk for injury related to adverse reactions to ramipril.
- Knowledge deficit related to ramipril therapy.

Planning and Implementation

Preparation and Administration

- Expect to start therapy at 1.25 mg P.O. daily in patients with renal insufficiency (creatinine clearance < 40 ml/min/1.73 m^2); subsequent dosage should be titrated gradually according to response. Maximum daily dosage is 5 mg.
- ***P.O. use:*** Patient may take this drug without regard for meals.

Monitoring

- Monitor effectiveness by frequently checking the patient's blood pressure and pulse rate.
- Monitor renal function (serum creatinine and BUN levels) in all patients receiving this drug but closely monitor renal function for the first few weeks of therapy in patients with severe CHF (have experienced acute renal failure) and in hypertensive patients with renal artery stenosis (have shown signs of worsening renal function at start of therapy).
- Monitor WBC counts in patients with impaired renal function or collagen vascular diseases (systemic lupus erythematosus or scleroderma) because such patients have developed agranulocytosis and bone marrow depression after therapy with other ACE inhibitors.
- Monitor for signs and symptoms of agranulocytosis and neutropenia.
- Monitor the patient for dizziness, fatigue, and other adverse reactions.

Supportive Care

- Institute safety measures such as continuous use of bed rails if adverse CNS reactions occur.

Patient Teaching

- Tell the patient to continue to take this drug even when feeling better.
- Instruct the patient to always check with the doctor or pharmacist before taking OTC medications.
- Advise the patient to avoid sudden position changes to prevent orthostatic hypotension, especially at the start of therapy.
- Tell the patient to report lightheadedness, sore throat, fever, or any sign of infection; difficulty breathing, signs of edema, or swelling; or any unusual bruising or bleeding. Explain that this drug may cause neutropenia or agranulocytosis.
- Tell the patient to avoid sodium substitutes containing potassium unless recommended by the doctor. Explain that excessive levels of potassium are dangerous.
- Teach the patient and family caregiver how to take blood pressure measurements. Tell them to notify the doctor if any significant change in blood pressure occurs.

Evaluation
In patients receiving ramipril, appropriate evaluation statements may include:
• Blood pressure is controlled within normal limits for this patient.
• Injury did not occur; patient did not experience adverse CNS reaction to ramipril therapy.
• Patient and family state an understanding of ramipril therapy.

ranitidine hydrochloride
(ra nye´ te deen)
Zantac*

• *Classification:* antiulcer agent (histamine$_2$-receptor antagonist)
• *Pregnancy Risk Category:* B

HOW SUPPLIED
Tablets: 150 mg, 300 mg
Dispersible tablets: 150 mg‡
Syrup: 15 mg/ml*
Injection: 25 mg/ml
Infusion: 0.5 mg/ml in 100-ml containers

ACTION
Mechanism: Competitively inhibits the action of histamine (H_2) at receptor sites of the parietal cells, decreasing gastric acid secretion.
Absorption: Approximately 50% to 60% of an oral dose is absorbed; food does not significantly affect absorption. After I.M. injection, drug is absorbed rapidly from parenteral sites.
Distribution: Well distributed to many body tissues and appears in CSF and breast milk. Drug is about 10% to 19% protein-bound.
Metabolism: In the liver.
Excretion: In urine and feces. Half-life: 2 to 3 hours.
Onset, peak, duration: Peak levels occur 1 to 3 hours after an oral dose; within 15 minutes after I.M. injection.

INDICATIONS & DOSAGE
Duodenal and gastric ulcer (short-term treatment); pathological hypersecretory conditions, such as Zollinger-Ellison syndrome–
Adults: 150 mg P.O. b.i.d. or 300 mg once daily h.s. Dosages up to 6 g/day may be prescribed in patients with Zollinger-Ellison syndrome. May also be administered parenterally: 50 mg I.V. or I.M. q 6 to 8 hours. When administering I.V. push, dilute to a total volume of 20 ml and inject over a period of 5 minutes. No dilution necessary when administering I.M. May also be administered by intermittent I.V. infusion. Dilute 50 mg ranitidine in 100 ml of dextrose 5% in water and infuse over 15 to 20 minutes.
Maintenance therapy of duodenal ulcer–
Adults: 150 mg P.O. h.s.
Gastroesophageal reflux disease (GERD)–
Adults: 150 mg P.O. b.i.d.

CONTRAINDICATIONS & PRECAUTIONS
Contraindicated in patients with ranitidine allergy. Use cautiously in patients with impaired hepatic function; dosage adjustment may be necessary in patients with impaired renal function.

ADVERSE REACTIONS
Common reactions are in italics; life-threatening reactions are in bold italics.
Blood: neutropenia, thrombocytopenia.
CNS: headache, malaise, dizziness, confusion.
CV: bradycardia.
GI: nausea, constipation.
Hepatic: elevated liver enzymes, jaundice.
Skin: rash.

Local: burning and itching at injection site.

INTERACTIONS

Antacids: may interfere with absorption of ranitidine (conflicting data). Stagger doses if possible.
Diazepam: decreased absorption when administered concomitantly with ranitidine.
Glipizide: possibly increased hypoglycemic effect. Dosage adjustment of glipizide may be necessary.
Procainamide: ranitidine may decrease renal clearance of procainamide (conflicting data).
Warfarin: ranitidine may interfere with warfarin clearance (conflicting data).

EFFECTS ON DIAGNOSTIC TESTS

CBC: decreased RBC, WBC and platelet counts.
Serum creatinine, lactic dehydrogenase, alkaline phosphatase, AST (SGOT), ALT (SGPT), GGT, and total bilirubin levels: increased.
Urine protein tests (Multistix): false-positive results.

NURSING CONSIDERATIONS

Besides those related universally to drug therapy (see "How to use this book"), consider the following specific recommendations:

Assessment

• Obtain a baseline assessment of the patient's GI pain before initiating ranitidine therapy.
• Be alert for adverse reactions and drug interactions throughout therapy.
• Evaluate the patient's and family's knowledge about ranitidine therapy.

Nursing Diagnoses

• Pain related to the patient's underlying condition.
• Constipation related to adverse GI reactions to ranitidine.
• Knowledge deficit related to ranitidine therapy.

Planning and Implementation

Preparation and Administration

• ***P.O. use:*** This drug can be taken without regard for meals. Absorption is not affected by food. If administered once a day, give at bedtime for best results.
• ***I.V. use:*** Solutions compatible for dilution with ranitidine are 0.9% sodium chloride solution, 5% and 10% dextrose injection, lactated Ringer's injection, and 5% sodium bicarbonate injection. To prepare I.V. injection, dilute 50 mg (2 ml) in 100 ml of compatible solution and infuse over 15 to 20 minutes.
• When administering premixed I.V. infusion, give by slow I.V. drip (over 15 to 20 minutes). Do not add other drugs to the solution. If used with a primary I.V. fluid system, the primary solution should be discontinued during the infusion.
• Expect dosage adjustment if the patient has impaired renal function.

Monitoring

• Monitor effectiveness by regularly assessing for relief of or decrease in the patient's GI pain.
• Monitor the patient for adverse drug reactions.
• Monitor the patient's stool for type, amount, and color.
• If administering drug I.V., frequently monitor I.V. site for signs of infiltration or phlebitis.
• Evaluate hematologic studies for abnormalities, such as neutropenia.
• Monitor blood chemistry results for changes in creatinine and hepatic enzymes, which may reflect changes in the patient's renal or hepatic function.

Supportive Care

• If I.V. injection site becomes infiltrated or shows signs of phlebitis, discontinue I.V. and restart in another site. Notify the doctor and, if indicated, apply warm compress to site.
• Take safety precautions if the patient develops dizziness, confusion,

or other mental status changes. For example, keep bed in low position, keep side rails up, and supervise the patient's activity.
• If the patient's stool becomes black and tarry, perform a test for occult blood and notify the doctor.
• Provide increased fluid intake, if not contraindicated, and notify the doctor if constipation occurs.
Patient Teaching
• Warn the patient to take drug as directed and to continue taking it even after pain subsides, to allow for adequate healing.
• Remind the patient who is taking ranitidine once daily to take it at bedtime for best results.
• Urge the patient to avoid smoking cigarettes, which may increase gastric acid secretion and worsen disease.
• Instruct the patient to avoid sources of GI irritation, such as alcohol, certain foods, and drugs containing aspirin.
• Instruct the patient to report immediately any signs of black, tarry stools; diarrhea; confusion; or rash.
Evaluation
In patients receiving ranitidine, appropriate evaluation statements may include:
• Patient has decrease in or relief of GI pain.
• Patient maintains normal bowel habits and does not experience constipation.
• Patient and family state an understanding of ranitidine therapy.

---

reserpine
(re ser´ peen)
Novoreserpine†, Serpalan, Serpasil*

• *Classification:* antihypertensive, antipsychotic (raawolfia alkaloid, peripherally acting anti-adrenergic agent)
• *Pregnancy Risk Category:* C

HOW SUPPLIED
Tablets: 0.1 mg, 0.25 mg, 1 mg

ACTION
Mechanism: A rauwolfia alkaloid that acts peripherally, inhibiting norepinephrine release and depleting norepinephrine stores in adrenergic nerve endings.
Absorption: Rapidly absorbed after oral administration.
Distribution: Widely distributed in the body; high concentrations in adipose tissue.
Metabolism: Extensively metabolized to inactive compounds.
Excretion: Slowly excreted as unchanged drug and metabolites in urine and feces. Half-life: Mean half-life is 33 hours.
Onset, peak, duration: Maximum antihypertensive effect does not occur for at least 2 to 3 weeks. Antihypertensive effects may persist for several days to weeks after discontinuation of drug therapy.

INDICATIONS & DOSAGE
Mild to moderate essential hypertension–
Adults: 0.1 to 0.25 mg P.O. daily.
Children: 5 to 20 mcg/kg P.O. daily.

CONTRAINDICATIONS & PRECAUTIONS
Contraindicated in patients with hypersensitivity to the drug; in patients receiving electroconvulsive therapy, because cerebral depletion of serotonin and catecholamines may predispose patient to seizures and extrapyramidal reactions; and in patients with depression, ulcerative colitis, or peptic ulcer disease, because drug may exacerbate these conditions.

Use cautiously in patients with seizure disorders or impaired renal function because the drug may worsen these conditions.

ADVERSE REACTIONS

Common reactions are in italics; life-threatening reactions are in bold italics.
CNS: mental confusion, *depression, drowsiness, nervousness, paradoxical anxiety, nightmares,* extrapyramidal symptoms, sedation.
CV: *orthostatic hypotension, bradycardia, syncope.*
EENT: *dry mouth, nasal stuffiness,* glaucoma.
GI: *hyperacidity, nausea, vomiting,* GI bleeding.
Skin: pruritus, rash.
Other: *impotence, weight gain.*

INTERACTIONS

MAO inhibitors: may cause excitability and hypertension. Use together cautiously.

EFFECTS ON DIAGNOSTIC TESTS

Urinary catecholamines and vanillylmandelic acid: decreased excretion.
Urinary corticosteroids: interference with detection by colorimetric assay.

NURSING CONSIDERATIONS

Besides those related universally to drug therapy (see "How to use this book"), consider the following specific recommendations:

Assessment
- Obtain a baseline assessment of the patient's blood pressure before beginning therapy.
- Be alert for adverse reactions and drug interactions throughout therapy.
- Evaluate the patient's and family's knowledge about reserpine therapy.

Nursing Diagnoses
- Altered tissue perfusion (renal, cerebral, cardiopulmonary, peripheral) related to the patient's underlying condition.
- High risk for injury related to adverse CV reactions to reserpine.
- Knowledge deficit related to reserpine therapy.

Planning and Implementation

Preparation and Administration
- ***P.O. use:*** Give this drug with meals.

Monitoring
- Monitor effectiveness by frequently checking the patient's blood pressure and pulse rate.
- Weigh the patient daily.
- Check the patient's blood pressure in the standing and supine position to monitor for orthostatic hypotension.
- Watch the patient closely for signs of mental depression.

Supportive Care
- Notify the doctor immediately if the patient reports nightmares.
- Keep in mind that the effects of this drug may last for 10 days after it's discontinued.

Patient Teaching
- Explain the importance of taking this drug as prescribed, even when feeling well.
- Tell the patient not to discontinue this drug suddenly even if unpleasant adverse reactions occur, but to discuss the problem with the doctor.
- Instruct the patient to check with the doctor or pharmacist before taking OTC medications.
- Warn that this drug can cause drowsiness. Tell the patient to avoid driving and other hazardous activities that require alertness and good coordination until CNS effects are known.
- Tell the patient to notify the doctor promptly if he experiences nightmares.
- Warn the female patient to notify the doctor promptly if she becomes pregnant.
- Tell the patient to weigh himself daily and to notify the doctor of any weight gain.
- Instruct the patient to minimize orthostatic hypotension by rising slowly and avoiding sudden position changes.
- Tell the patient to relieve dry mouth

with sugarless chewing gum, sour hard candy, or ice chips.

• Tell the patient to contact the doctor if he needs relief for nasal stuffiness.

• Recommend periodic eye examinations during therapy.

• Teach the patient and family caregiver to take blood pressure measurements. Tell them to notify the doctor of any significant change in blood pressure.

Evaluation

In patients receiving reserpine, appropriate evaluation statements may include:

• Blood pressure is controlled within normal limits for this patient.

• Injury did not occur; patient did not experience adverse CV reactions to reserpine.

• Patient and family state an understanding of reserpine therapy.

Rh_o(D) immune globulin, human

Gamulin Rh, HypRho-D, MICRhoGAM, Mini-Gamulin Rh, Rhesonativ, RhoGAM

• *Classification:* anti-Rh_o (D)-positive prophylaxis agent (immune serum)
• *Pregnancy Risk Category:* C

HOW SUPPLIED

Injection: 300 mcg of Rh_o(D) immune globulin/vial (standard dose); 50 mcg of Rh_o(D) immune globulin/vial (microdose)

ACTION

Mechanism: Suppresses the active antibody response and formation of anti-Rh_o(D) in Rh_o(D)-negative D^u-negative individuals exposed to Rh-positive blood.

Pharmacokinetics: Unknown.

INDICATIONS & DOSAGE

Rh exposure–

Women (postabortion, postmiscarriage, ectopic pregnancy, or postpartum): transfusion unit or blood bank determines fetal packed RBC volume entering woman's blood, then gives one vial I.M. if fetal packed RBC volume is less than 15 ml. More than one vial I.M. may be required if there is large fetomaternal hemorrhage. Must be given within 72 hours after delivery or miscarriage.

Transfusion accidents–

Adults and children: consult blood bank or transfusion unit at once. Must be given within 72 hours.

Postabortion or postmiscarriage to prevent Rh antibody formation–

Women: consult transfusion unit or blood bank. One microdose vial will suppress immune reaction to 2.5 ml Rh_o(D)-positive RBCs. Ideally should be given within 3 hours, but may be given up to 72 hours after abortion or miscarriage.

CONTRAINDICATIONS & PRECAUTIONS

Contraindicated in Rh_o(D)-positive or D^u-positive patients, in those previously immunized to Rh_o(D) blood factor, and in patients with hypersensitivity to thimerosal, a component of this immune serum. Rhesonativ is preservative-free and should be used for individuals sensitive to thimerosal.

ADVERSE REACTIONS

Common reactions are in italics; life-threatening reactions are in bold italics.

Local: discomfort at injection site.

Other: slight fever.

INTERACTIONS

Live virus vaccines: may interfere with response. Defer vaccination for 3 months after administration of Rh_o(D) immune globulin.

EFFECTS ON DIAGNOSTIC TESTS

None reported.

NURSING CONSIDERATIONS

Besides those related universally to drug therapy (see "How to use this book"), consider the following specific recommendations:

Assessment

- Obtain a baseline assessment of the patient's allergies and reaction to immunization before therapy.
- Be alert for adverse reactions or drug interactions during therapy.
- Evaluate the patient's and family's knowledge about $Rh_o(D)$ immune globulin.

Nursing Diagnoses

- Altered protection related to presence of active Rh antibodies.
- Pain related to local discomfort at injection site.
- Knowledge deficit related to $Rh_o(D)$ immune globulin.

Planning and Implementation

Preparation and Administration

- Immediately after delivery, send a sample of neonate's cord blood to laboratory for typing and crossmatching. Confirm if the mother is $Rh_o(D)$-negative and D^u-negative. Neonate must be $Rh_o(D)$-positive.
- Store at 36° to 46° F. (2° to 8° C.).

Monitoring

- Monitor effectiveness by checking the patient's antibody titers.
- Check vital signs.
- Observe injection site for local reaction.

Supportive Care

- MICRhoGAM is recommended for every woman after abortion or miscarriage up to 12 weeks' gestation unless she is $Rh_o(D)$-positive or D^u-positive, has Rh antibodies, or the father or the fetus (or both) is Rh-negative.
- This immune serum provides passive immunity to the woman exposed to Rh_o-positive fetal blood during pregnancy. Prevents formation of maternal antibodies (active immunity), which would endanger future Rh_o-positive pregnancies.
- Treat fever with antipyretics.
- Apply ice or cold compress to alleviate pain and redness at injection site.

Patient Teaching

- Explain to the patient how drug protects future Rh_o-positive infants.
- Inform the patient that a slight fever and discomfort at the injection site may follow immunization.

Evaluation

In patients receiving $Rh_o(D)$ immune globulin, appropriate evaluation statements may include:

- Patient exhibits suppression of active Rh_o antibody response.
- Patient is free of pain.
- Patient and family state an understanding of $Rh_o(D)$ immune globulin therapy.

---

ribavirin

(rye ba vye´ rin)

Virazole

- *Classification:* antiviral (synthetic nucleoside)
- *Pregnancy Risk Category:* X

HOW SUPPLIED

Powder to be reconstituted for inhalation: 6 g in 100-ml glass vial

ACTION

Mechanism: Inhibits viral activity by an unknown mechanism. May inhibit RNA and DNA synthesis by depleting intracellular nucleotide pools.

Absorption: Usually administered by aerosol for a local effect within the respiratory tract. Some drug is inadvertently absorbed; absorption varies with method of drug delivery during nebulization. Highest levels appear in patients given the drug via endotracheal tube using an aerosol genera-

tor; lower levels are found in patients given the drug via face mask. After oral administration, the drug is well absorbed.
Distribution: Concentrates in bronchial secretions; plasma levels are subtherapeutic. The drug appears to concentrate within RBCs.
Metabolism: Metabolized to 1, 2, 4-triazole-3-carboxamide (deribosylated ribavirin).
Excretion: Most of dose is excreted in the urine. Half-life: Following inhalation, first phase of plasma half-life is 9½ hours; second phase has extended half-life of 40 hours (from slow drug release from RBC binding sites. After oral administration, half-life is multiphasic, averaging 24 to 48 hours.
Onset, peak, duration: After aerosol treatment peak plasma concentrations are lower than those found in respiratory tract sections.

INDICATIONS & DOSAGE

Treatment of hospitalized infants and young children infected by respiratory syncytial virus (RSV)–
Infants and young children: solution in concentration of 20 mg/ml delivered via the Viratek Small Particle Aerosol Generator (SPAG-2). Treatment is carried out for 12 to 18 hours/day for at least 3, and no more than 7, days.

CONTRAINDICATIONS & PRECAUTIONS

Contraindicated in pregnant women and those who might become pregnant during therapy because of drug's potentially teratogenic or embryocidal effects.

Use with extreme caution in patients requiring ventilatory assistance because drug may precipitate in ventilatory apparatus, impairing ventilation.

ADVERSE REACTIONS

Common reactions are in italics; life-threatening reactions are in bold italics.
Blood: anemia, reticulocytosis.
EENT: conjunctivitis.
Respiratory: worsening of respiratory state.
Other: rash or erythema of eyelids.

INTERACTIONS

None significant.

EFFECTS ON DIAGNOSTIC TESTS

None reported.

NURSING CONSIDERATIONS

Besides those related universally to drug therapy (see "How to use this book"), consider the following specific recommendations:

Assessment

• Obtain a baseline assessment of infection before therapy.
• Be alert for adverse reactions and drug interactions throughout therapy.
• Evaluate the patient's and family's knowledge about ribavirin therapy.

Nursing Diagnoses

• High risk for injury related to ineffectiveness of ribavirin to eradicate the infection.
• Impaired gas exchange related to adverse respiratory reactions to ribavirin therapy.
• Knowledge deficit related to ribavirin.

Planning and Implementation

Preparation and Administration

• Obtain specimen for culture and sensitivity tests before administering first dose if possible. Treatment may begin pending results.
• ***Inhalation use:*** Drug must be administered by the Viratek Small Particle Aerosol Generator (SPAG-2). Don't use any other aerosol generating device. Use only sterile USP water for injection to mix drug. Discard solutions placed in the SPAG-2 unit at least every 24 hours before adding newly reconstituted solution.

Store reconstituted solutions at room temperature for 24 hours.

Monitoring

• Monitor effectiveness by regularly assessing for improvement in the infection process.

• Monitor patient's respiratory status closely.

Supportive Care

• Supplement treatment with supportive respiratory and fluid management.

• Be aware that ribavarin may precipitate in ventilator apparatus, possibly causing equipment malfunction with serious consequences; therefore drug is not recommended for ventilator-dependent patients.

Patient Teaching

• Instruct the parents about ribavirin, including the dose, frequency, action, and adverse reactions.

Evaluation

In patients receiving ribavirin, appropriate evaluation statements may include:

• Patient is free of infection.

• Patient's maintains adequate respiratory function throughout ribavirin therapy.

• Patient and family state an understanding of ribavirin therapy.

rifampin (rifampicin)

(rif´ am pin)

Rifadin, Rimactane, Rimycin‡, Rofact†

• *Classification:* antitubercular (rifamycin B derivative)

• *Pregnancy Risk Category:* C

HOW SUPPLIED

Capsules: 150 mg, 300 mg

Kit: 60 capsules, 300 mg

ACTION

Mechanism: Inhibits DNA-dependent RNA polymerase, thus impairing RNA synthesis.

Absorption: Completely absorbed from GI tract after oral administration.

Distribution: Widely distributed into body tissues and fluids, including ascitic, pleural, seminal, and cerebrospinal fluids, tears, and saliva; and into liver, prostate, lungs, and bone. Rifampin crosses the placenta; it is 84% to 91% protein-bound.

Metabolism: Metabolized extensively in the liver by deacetylation. The drug undergoes interohepatic circulation.

Excretion: Drug and metabolite are excreted primarily in bile; drug, but not metabolite, is reabsorbed. From 6% to 30% of rifampin and metabolite appears unchanged in urine in 24 hours; about 60% is excreted in feces. Some drug is excreted in breast milk. Half-life: 1½ to 5 hours.

Onset, peak, duration: Peak serum concentrations occur 1 to 4 hours after oral ingestion.

INDICATIONS & DOSAGE

Primary treatment in pulmonary tuberculosis–

Adults: 600 mg P.O. daily single dose 1 hour before or 2 hours after meals.

Children over 5 years: 10 to 20 mg/kg P.O. daily single dose 1 hour before or 2 hours after meals. Maximum dosage is 600 mg daily. Concomitant administration of other effective antitubercular drugs is recommended.

Meningococcal carriers–

Adults: 600 mg P.O. b.i.d. for 2 days.

Children 1 to 12 years: 10 mg/kg P.O. b.i.d. or 2 days, not to exceed 600 mg/dose.

Infants 3 months to 1 year: 5 mg/kg P.O. b.i.d. for 2 days.

Prophylaxis of Hemophilus influenza *type b–*

Adults and children: 20 mg/kg P.O. once daily for 4 days. Do not exceed 600 mg/day.

CONTRAINDICATIONS & PRECAUTIONS

Contraindicated in patients with hypersensitivity to any rifamycin. Use cautiously and at reduced dosages in patients with hepatic disease or alcoholism and in those taking other hepatotoxic drugs.

ADVERSE REACTIONS

Common reactions are in italics; life-threatening reactions are in bold italics.
Blood: thrombocytopenia, transient leukopenia, ***hemolytic anemia.***
CNS: headache, fatigue, *drowsiness,* ataxia, dizziness, mental confusion, generalized numbness.
GI: epigastric distress, anorexia, nausea, vomiting, abdominal pain, diarrhea, flatulence, sore mouth and tongue.
Metabolic: hyperuricemia.
Hepatic: ***serious hepatotoxicity*** *as well as transient abnormalities in liver function tests.*
Skin: pruritus, urticaria, rash.
Other: flu-like syndrome, discoloration of body fluids.

INTERACTIONS

Alcohol: may increase risk of hepatotoxicity.
Para-aminosalicylate sodium, ketoconazole: may interfere with absorption of rifampin. Give these drugs 8 to 12 hours apart.
Probenecid: may increase rifampin levels. Use cautiously.

EFFECTS ON DIAGNOSTIC TESTS

Gallbladder studies: interference with contrast material.
Liver excretion test: temporary retention of sulfobromophthalein.
Liver function tests: asymptomatic elevation in 14%.
Serum folate and vitamin B_{12}: interference with assays.
Serum uric acid: elevation.
Urinalysis: interference with spectrophotometric tests.
Vitamin D: reduced levels.

NURSING CONSIDERATIONS

Besides those related universally to drug therapy (see "How to use this book"), consider the following specific recommendations:

Assessment
- Obtain a baseline assessment of the infection before therapy.
- Be alert for adverse reactions and drug interactions throughout therapy.
- Evaluate the patient's and family's knowledge about rifampin therapy.

Nursing Diagnoses
- High risk for injury related to dosage regimen inadequate to eradicate the infection.
- Noncompliance (medication administration) related to prolonged therapy.
- Knowledge deficit related to rifampin.

Planning and Implementation

Preparation and Administration
- Obtain specimens for culture and sensitivity testing before first dose but do not delay therapy.
- ***P.O. use:*** Administer drug 1 hour before or 2 hours after meals for maximum absorption: capsule contents may be mixed with food or fluid to enhance swallowing.
- ***I.V. use:*** Follow manufacturer's instructions for reconstitution of I.V. rifampin. Infuse within 3 hours.
- Expect to administer at least one other antitubercular agent concomitantly.

Monitoring
- Monitor effectiveness by regularly assessing for improvement of the infection and by obtaining specimens for culture and sensitivity testing to detect drug resistance.
- Monitor hematologic, renal, and liver function studies and serum electrolytes as ordered.

Supportive Care
- When administered during the last few weeks of pregnancy, rifampin can

cause postnatal hemorrhage in the mother and infant, which may require treatment with vitamin K.
• Expect to adjust dosage of certain drugs (especially warfarin, corticosteroids, and oral hypoglycemics) if administered concomitantly because rifampin increases liver enzyme activity which inactivates these drugs.
• If patient is unable to comply with treatment regimen, discuss reasons and offer suggestions to improve compliance (For example, clues patient can use as a reminder to take medication).
Patient Teaching
• Tell the patient to take rifampin on an empty stomach, at least 1 hour before or 2 hours after a meal. If GI irritation occurs, the patient may need to take the drug with food.
• Urge the patient to comply with prescribed regimen, not to miss doses, not to double up on missed doses, and not to discontinue drug without checking with the doctor. Explain importance of follow-up appointments.
• Explain that drug turns all body fluids a red-orange color; advise the patient of possible permanent stains on clothes and soft contact lenses.
• Warn the female patient that this drug is potentially teratogenic. Recommend appropriate contraceptive measures during therapy.
• Advise users of oral contraceptive to substitute other methods; rifampin inactivates such drugs and may alter menstrual patterns.
• Advise the patient to avoid alcoholic beverages because alcohol may increase the risk of hepatotoxicity.
Evaluation
In patients receiving rifampin, appropriate evaluation statements may include:
• Patient is free of infection.
• Patient completes entire regimen of prescribed therapy.
• Patient and family state an understanding of rifampin therapy.

ritodrine hydrochloride
(ri´ toe dreen)
Yutopar

• *Classification:* tocolytic (beta-receptor agonist)
• *Pregnancy Risk Category:* B

HOW SUPPLIED
Tablets: 10 mg
Injection: 10-mg/ml, 15-mg/ml ampules

ACTION
Mechanism: Stimulates the beta$_2$-adrenergic receptors in uterine smooth muscle, inhibiting contractility.
Absorption: 30% absorbed by the oral route and 100% by the I.V. route. Food may inhibit the absorption and effectiveness of oral ritodrine.
Distribution: I.V. dose is distributed to the tissues within 6 to 9 minutes.
Metabolism: Hepatic; primarily to inactive sulfate and glucuronide conjugates.
Excretion: About 70% to 90% of an oral or I.V. dose is excreted in urine in 10 to 12 hours as unchanged drug and its conjugates. Ritodrine can be removed by dialysis.
Onset, peak, duration: Peak serum levels are 5 to 15 ng/ml after an oral dose and 32 to 50 ng/ml after an I.V. dose.

INDICATIONS & DOSAGE
Management of preterm labor–
I.V. therapy: dilute 150 mg (3 ampuls) in 500 ml of fluid, yielding a final concentration of 0.3 mg/ml. Usual initial dose is 0.1 mg/minute, to be gradually increased according to the results by 0.05 mg/minute q 10 minutes until desired result obtained. Ef-

fective dosage usually ranges from 0.15 and 0.35 mg/minute.

Note: I.V. infusion should be continued for 12 to 24 hours after contractions have stopped. Oral maintenance: 1 tablet (10 mg) may be given approximately 30 minutes before termination of I.V. therapy. Usual dosage for first 24 hours of oral maintenance is 10 mg q 2 hours. Thereafter, usual dosage is 10 to 20 mg q 4 to 6 hours. Total daily dosage should not exceed 120 mg.

CONTRAINDICATIONS & PRECAUTIONS

Contraindicated before the 20th week or after the 36th week of pregnancy; in patients with antepartum hemorrhage, preeclampsia or eclampsia, intrauterine infection, fetal death, chorioamnionitis, or conditions in which continuation of the pregnancy is hazardous; in those with maternal cardiac disease, pulmonary hypertension, uncontrolled cervical dilation, or maternal diabetes mellitus, because the drug may exacerbate these conditions; in patients with medical conditions that would be seriously affected by the drug, such as hypovolemia, cardiac arrhythmias associated with tachycardia or digitalis intoxication, and uncontrolled hypertension or bronchial asthma already treated with betamimetics or steroids; and in patients with hypersensitivity to any component of the preparation.

ADVERSE REACTIONS

Common reactions are in italics; life-threatening reactions are in bold italics.
CNS: nervousness, anxiety, headache.
CV: *dose-related alterations in blood pressure, palpitations,* ***pulmonary edema,*** *tachycardia,* ECG changes.
GI: nausea, vomiting.
Metabolic: *hyperglycemia,* hypokalemia.
Skin: rash (oral).
Other: erythema.

INTERACTIONS

Beta blockers: may inhibit ritodrine's action. Avoid concurrent administration.
Corticosteroids: may produce pulmonary edema in mother. When these drugs are used concomitantly, monitor closely.
Inhalational anesthetics: potentiated adverse cardiac effects, arrhythmias, hypotension.
Sympathomimetics: additive effects. Use together cautiously.

EFFECTS ON DIAGNOSTIC TESTS

Plasma insulin and glucose: elevated levels (with I.V. use).
Plasma potassium: decreased concentrations (values usually return to normal within 24 hours after drug is stopped).

NURSING CONSIDERATIONS

Besides those related universally to drug therapy (see "How to use this book"), consider the following specific recommendations:

Assessment

- Obtain a baseline assessment of labor patterns before therapy.
- Be alert for adverse reactions and drug interactions throughout therapy.
- Evaluate the patient's and family's knowledge about ritodrine therapy.

Nursing Diagnoses

- Anxiety related to the patient's underlying condition.
- Decreased cardiac output related to adverse reaction to drug.
- Knowledge deficit related to ritodrine hydrochloride therapy.

Planning and Implementation

Preparation and Administration

- Oral administration follows I.V. therapy.
- ***I.V. use:*** Dilute 150 mg in 500 ml of fluid to a concentration of 0.3 mg/ml. Increase initial dose according to results by 0.05 mg/minute every 10 minutes. Continue infusion for 12 to 24 hours after contractions have

stopped. Discard solution if it is discolored or contains a precipitate.
• ***Oral use:*** Administer 30 minutes before termination of I.V. Expect oral dose to be reduced after the first 24 hours.

Monitoring
• Monitor effectiveness by assessing for preterm labor contractions.
• Monitor the maternal and fetal cardiovascular status, especially during I.V. infusion. Cardiovascular effects including maternal pulse rate and blood pressure, and fetal heart rate should be closely monitored. A maternal tachycardia of over 140/minute or persistent respiratory rate of over 20/ minute may be a sign of impending pulmonary edema.
• Assess blood glucose levels especially in diabetic mothers.
• Measure intake and output carefully to avoid circulatory overload.

Supportive Care
• Notify the doctor of any changes in maternal or fetal cardiovascular condition.
• Discontinue drug if pulmonary edema develops.
• Offer the patient hard, sour candy to offset the dry mouth resulting from hard breathing during labor.
• Place the patient in a semi-Fowler's position.

Patient Teaching
• Explain to the mother the need to monitor blood glucose during use of this drug.
• Tell the patient to report any respiratory difficulties or shortness of breath.
• Explain that the I.V. infusion will be followed by the oral form of the drug.

Evaluation
In patients receiving ritodrine, appropriate evaluation statements may include:
• Patient reports absence of preterm labor.
• Patient is free of palpitations and ECG changes.
• Patient and family state an understanding of ritodrine hydrochloride therapy.

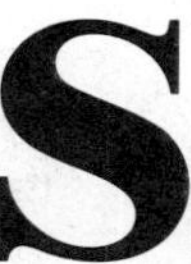

S

PHARMACOLOGIC CLASS

salicylates
aspirin
choline magnesium trisalicylate
choline salicylate
magnesium salicylate
salicylamide
salsalate
sodium salicylate
sodium thiosalicylate

OVERVIEW

Widely prescribed, these drugs are the standard of comparison and evaluation for other nonnarcotic analgesics, nonsteroidal anti-inflammatory drugs, and antipyretic drugs.

Salicylates may act peripherally by inhibiting the enzyme that decreases formation of the prostaglandins involved in pain and inflammation. These prostaglandins appear to sensitize pain receptors to mechanical stimulation or to other chemical mediators. These drugs may also act centrally, possibly in the hypothalamus. The anti-inflammatory action of the salicylates, also related to prostaglandin inhibition, may contribute to their analgesic effect. The exact mechanism of the latter effect is unknown.

Salicylates lower body temperature principally by inhibiting synthesis and release of the prostaglandins that mediate the effect of endogenous pyrogens on the hypothalamus. Also, salicylates produce a centrally mediated dilation of peripheral blood vessels, enhancing heat dissipation and sweating. Salicylates rarely decrease body temperature in afebrile patients.

CLINICAL INDICATIONS AND ACTIONS

Salicylates are used principally for the symptomatic relief of mild to moderate pain, inflammation, and fever.

Pain

Salicylates are most effective in treating low-intensity pain of headache, arthralgia, myalgia, and neuralgia. They may also relieve mild to moderate pain from dental and surgical procedures, dysmenorrhea, and rheumatic fever.

Inflammation

Salicylates are commonly used for initial long-term treatment of rheumatoid arthritis, juvenile arthritis, and osteoarthritis. It is important to note that in rheumatoid conditions, these agents offer only symptomatic relief, reducing pain, stiffness, swelling, and tenderness. They do not reverse or arrest the disease process.

Fever

Use of salicylates in fever is nonspecific and does not influence the course of the underlying disease.

OVERVIEW OF ADVERSE REACTIONS

Adverse reactions to salicylates involve mainly the GI tract, particularly gastric mucosa. Also, GI adverse reactions occur more frequently when aspirin is used than with other salicylates. Most common symptoms are dyspepsia, heartburn, epigastric distress, nausea, and abdominal pain. GI reactions usually occur in the first few days of therapy, often subside with continuous treatment, and can be minimized by administering salicylates with meals or food, antacids, or 8 oz of water or milk. The incidence and severity of GI bleeding are exposure-related.

Chronic salicylate intoxication (salicylism) may occur with prolonged therapy, at high doses. Signs and symptoms include tinnitus, hearing loss, hepatotoxicity, and adverse renal effects.

Salicylate-induced bronchospasm, with or without urticaria and angioedema, may occur in patients with hypersensitivity to these drugs, particularly those with the "triad" of aspirin sensitivity, rhinitis/nasal polyps, and asthma. A significant incidence of cross-reactivity has been observed with tartrazine.

REPRESENTATIVE COMBINATIONS

Aspirin with magnesium hydroxide, aluminum hydroxide, and caffeine: Accutrate, Anacin, Nervine, P.A.C. revised formula Paradol, 217; with phenacetin (acetophenetidin) and caffeine: APC, Pan-APC, Aspodyne; with phenacetin, caffeine, and phenolphthalein: Phenodyne, Gelsodyne; with butabarbital: Axotal; with caffeine and butabarbital: Fiorinal; with meprobomate: Equagesic, Equazine M, Meprogesic Q.

Salicylamide with phenacetin, caffeine, ascorbic acid, phenylephrine hydrochloride, and chlorpheniramine maleate: Genaid; with phenacetin, caffeine, ascorbic acid, phenylephrine hydrochloride, chlorpheniramine maleate, and dextromethorphan: Centuss; with phenacetin and chlorpheniramine maleate: Chlorphen.

Salicylic acid with sulfur: Sebulex, Fostex Medicated Cleansing, Meted.

See also: Opioids

salsalate

(sal´ sa late)

Arthra-G, Disalcid, Mono-Gesic, Salflex, Salgesic, Salsitab

- *Classification:* nonnarcotic analgesic, antipyretic, anti-inflammatory (salicylate)
- *Pregnancy Risk Category:* C

HOW SUPPLIED

Tablets: 500 mg, 750 mg
Capsules: 500 mg

ACTION

Mechanism: Each molecule of salsalate is hydrolyzed to two molecules of salicylate, which inhibit prostaglandin synthesis. Reduces fever by an action on the hypothalamus. Reduces inflammation by blocking prostaglandin synthesis. Produces analgesia by an ill-defined effect on the CNS, by its anti-inflammatory effect, and by blocking generation of pain impulses in the periphery.
Absorption: Rapidly and completely absorbed from the GI tract, chiefly the small intestine.
Distribution: Widely distributed to most body fluids and tissues. Protein-binding varies from 75% to 90%; it is concentration-dependent and decreases as serum concentrations increase.
Metabolism: Hydrolyzed in the liver, plasma, blood, and GI mucosa to salicylic acid.
Excretion: Metabolite and parent drug are excreted in urine. Half-life: Such capacity-limited biotransformation results in an increase in the half-life of salicylic acid from 3½ to 16 or more hours.
Onset, peak, duration: Peak effects occur at 2 hours.

INDICATIONS & DOSAGE

Arthritis–
Adults: 3 g P.O. daily, divided b.i.d. or t.i.d. Usual maintenance dose is 2 to 4 g daily.

CONTRAINDICATIONS & PRECAUTIONS

Contraindicated in patients with hypersensitivity to salicylamide and in the presence of GI ulcer or GI bleeding. Use cautiously in patients with hypoprothrombinemia, vitamin K deficiency, and bleeding disorders, because of the potential for bleeding; and in patients with decreased hepatic or renal function because the drug may accumulate.

Patients with known "triad" symptoms (aspirin hypersensitivity, rhinitis/nasal polyps, and asthma) are at high risk of bronchospasm. Salicylates may mask the signs and symptoms of acute infection (fever, myalgia, erythema); carefully evaluate patients with high risk for infection (such as those with diabetes).

ADVERSE REACTIONS

Common reactions are in italics; life-threatening reactions are in bold italics.

EENT: *tinnitus and hearing loss.*

GI: *nausea, vomiting, GI distress, occult bleeding.*

Hepatic: abnormal liver function studies, hepatitis.

Skin: *rash,* bruising.

Other: *hypersensitivity manifested by* ***anaphylaxis*** and asthma.

INTERACTIONS

Acetaminophen: increased plasma concentration of salsalate and acetaminophen.

Ammonium chloride (and other urine acidifiers): increased blood levels of salicylates. Monitor for salicylate toxicity.

Antacids in high doses (and other urine alkalinizers): decreased levels of salicylates. Monitor for decreased salicylate effect.

Corticosteroids: compete for binding sites. Monitor for decreased salicylate effect.

Oral anticoagulants: possible increased risk of bleeding. Avoid using together if possible.

EFFECTS ON DIAGNOSTIC TESTS

Serum AST (SGOT), ALT (SGPT), alkaline phosphatase and bilirubin: increased levels.

NURSING CONSIDERATIONS

Besides those related universally to drug therapy (see "How to use this book"), consider the following specific recommendations:

Assessment

- Obtain a baseline assessment of severity of pain before therapy.
- Be alert for adverse reactions and drug interactions throughout therapy.
- Evaluate the patient's and family's knowledge about salsalate therapy.

Nursing Diagnoses

- Pain related to the patient's underlying condition.
- High risk for fluid volume deficit related to adverse GI reactions to long-term, high-dose salicylate therapy.
- Knowledge deficit related to salsalate therapy.

Planning and Implementation

Preparation and Administration

- Give with food, milk, antacid, or large glass of water to reduce possible GI reactions.
- Avoid use in children or teenagers with chicken pox or influenza-like illness because of epidemiologic association with Reye's syndrome.

Monitoring

- Monitor effectiveness by regularly evaluating pain relief.
- Monitor the patient's blood salicylate level. Therapeutic blood salicylate level in arthritis is 10 to 30 mg/dl. With chronic therapy, mild toxicity may occur at plasma levels of 20 mg/dl. Tinnitus may occur at plasma levels of 30 mg/dl and above, but this is not a reliable indicator of toxicity, especially in very young patients and those over age 60.

• Observe patient on prolonged high-dose therapy for signs of GI bleeding. Watch for petechiae and bleeding gums.
• Ensure that patient maintains an adequate fluid intake.
• Observe the patient with nausea, vomiting, or bleeding for signs of fluid volume deficit including tachycardia, hypotension, decreased urine output and decreased electrolyte levels.
• Periodically review hemoglobin and prothrombin tests to help evaluate bleeding risk, especially during prolonged, high-dose therapy.

Supportive Care

• Keep in mind that this drug may cause an increase in serum levels of AST (SGOT), ALT (SGPT), alkaline phosphatase, and bilirubin and that abnormal liver function tests may also occur.
• Keep in mind that concomitant use of this drug with alcohol, steroids, or other NSAIDs may increase risk of GI bleeding.

Patient Teaching

• Advise the patient receiving prolonged treatment with large doses to watch for petechiae, bleeding gums, and signs of GI bleeding and to maintain adequate fluid intake. Encourage the use of a soft tooth brush.
• Explain that concomitant use with alcohol, steroids, or other NSAIDs may increase the risk of GI bleeding.
• Tell the patient to take the drug with food, milk, an antacid, or a large glass of water to reduce possible GI reactions.
• Tell the patient to notify the doctor promptly of GI reactions, tinnitus, or hearing loss.

Evaluation

In patients receiving salsalate, appropriate evaluation statements may include:
• Patient states salsalate has relieved pain.
• Patient exhibits no signs of fluid volume deficit.
• Patient and family state an understanding of salsalate therapy.

scopolamine (hyoscine)

(skoe pol´ a meen)

Transderm-Scōp, Transderm-V†

• *Classification:* antiemetic/antivertigo agent, anticholinergic)
• *Pregnancy Risk Category:* C

HOW SUPPLIED

Transdermal patch: 1.5 mg

ACTION

Mechanism: An anticholinergic that blocks muscarinic acetylcholine receptors. May affect neural pathways originating in the labyrinth to inhibit nausea and vomiting, but the exact mechanism of action is unknown.
Absorption: Well absorbed percutaneously from behind the ear; antiemetic effects begin several hours after application.
Distribution: Widely distributed throughout body tissues. It crosses the placenta and probably the blood-brain barrier.
Metabolism: Probably metabolized completely in the liver; however, its exact metabolic fate is unknown.
Excretion: Probably excreted in urine as metabolites. Half-life: About 8 hours.
Onset, peak, duration: Mydriatic and cycloplegic effects persist for 3 to 7 days.

INDICATIONS & DOSAGE

Prevention of nausea and vomiting associated with motion sickness–
Adults: One Transderm-Scōp system (a circular flat unit) programmed to deliver 0.5 mg scopolamine over 3 days (72 hours), applied to the skin

behind the ear several hours before the antiemetic is required.

Not recommended for children.

CONTRAINDICATIONS & PRECAUTIONS

Contraindicated in patients with glaucoma or a tendency toward glaucoma, because drug-induced cycloplegia and mydriasis may increase intraocular pressure; and obstructive uropathy, obstructive GI tract disease, asthma, chronic pulmonary disease, myasthenia gravis, paralytic ileus, intestinal atony, or toxic megacolon, because the drug may exacerbate these conditions.

Use cautiously in patients with autonomic neuropathy, hyperthyroidism, coronary artery disease, CHF, hypertension, or ulcerative colitis, because the drug may exacerbate these conditions; hepatic or renal disease, because toxic accumulation may occur; cardiac arrhythmias, because the drug may block vagal inhibition of the sinoatrial node pacemaker, worsening the arrhythmia; hiatal hernia associated with reflux esophagitis, because this drug may decrease lower esophageal sphincter tone; to patients over age 40, because the drug increases the glaucoma risk; to young children, because they may be more sensitive to drug effects; and in patients with hypersensitivity to belladonna alkaloids.

ADVERSE REACTIONS

Common reactions are in italics; life-threatening reactions are in bold italics.

CNS: *drowsiness,* restlessness, disorientation, confusion.

EENT: *dry mouth,* transient impairment of eye accommodation.

INTERACTIONS

None significant.

EFFECTS ON DIAGNOSTIC TESTS

None reported.

NURSING CONSIDERATIONS

Besides those related universally to drug therapy (see "How to use this book"), consider the following specific recommendations:

Assessment

- Obtain a baseline assessment of mental status and postauricular skin integrity before therapy.
- Be alert for adverse reactions and drug interactions throughout therapy.
- Evaluate the patient's and family's knowledge about scopolamine therapy.

Nursing Diagnoses

- High risk for fluid volume deficit related to nausea and vomiting induced by motion sickness.
- Altered thought processes related to scopolamine-induced confusion.
- Knowledge deficit related to scopolamine therapy.

Planning and Implementation

Preparation and Administration

- Wash and dry hands thoroughly before applying the system on dry skin behind the ear. After removing the system, discard it and wash both the hands and the application site thoroughly.
- If the system becomes displaced, remove it and replace it with another system on a fresh patch of skin in the postauricular area.

Monitoring

- Monitor effectiveness by monitoring for nausea and vomiting.
- Monitor fluid balance.
- Observe for signs of confusion, restlessness, and disorientation.
- Observe skin integrity at application site.

Supportive Care

- Be aware that the transdermal method of administration releases a controlled therapeutic amount of scopolamine.
- Use safety precautions in patients who develop adverse CNS reactions.

Patient Teaching
• Caution patient to wash hands after applying transdermal patch, particularly before touching eye. May cause pupil to dilate.
• Advise the patient to apply system the night before a planned trip because Transderm-Scop is most effective if used 12 hours before beginning to travel. It is also effective if applied 2 to 3 hours before experiencing motion.
• A patient brochure is available with the product; tell the patient to request it from the pharmacist.
• Warn the patient against driving and other activities that require alertness until CNS effects of drug are known.
• Advise the patient that sugarless hard candy may be helpful in minimizing dry mouth.
• Remind patient to remove old patch before applying new one.

Evaluation
In patients receiving scopolamine, appropriate evaluation statements may include:
• Patient exhibits no signs of fluid volume deficit.
• Patient demonstrates no signs of altered thought processes.
• Patient and family state an understanding of scopolamine therapy.

scopolamine butylbromide (hyoscine butylbromide)

(skoe pol′ a meen)
Buscopan†‡

scopolamine hydrobromide (hyoscine hydrobromide)

• *Classification:* antimuscarinic, antiemetic/antivertigo agent, antiparkenonian agent, (anticholinergic)
• *Pregnancy Risk Category:* C

HOW SUPPLIED

Capsules: 0.25 mg
Injection: 0.3, 0.4, 0.5, 0.6, and 1 mg/ml in 1-ml vials and ampules; 0.86 mg/ml in 0.5-ml ampules

ACTION

Mechanism: An anticholinergic that blocks the parasympathetic (muscarinic) actions of acetylcholine on organs innervated by postganglionic cholinergic neurons.
Absorption: Well absorbed percutaneously; antiemetic effects begin several hours after application. Also well absorbed from the GI tract; absorbed rapidly when administered I.M. or S.C.
Distribution: Widely distributed throughout body tissue. It crosses the placenta and the blood-brain barrier.
Metabolism: Probably metabolized completely in the liver; however, its exact metabolic fate is unknown. Antiemetic, mydriatic, and cycloplegic effects persist for 3 to 7 days.
Excretion: Probably excreted in urine as metabolites. Half-life: 8 hours.
Onset, peak, duration: Effects occur 15 to 30 minutes after I.M., S.C., or oral administration. Ophthalmic mydriatic effect peaks at 20 to 30 minutes after administration; cycloplegic effects peak 30 to 60 minutes after administration.

INDICATIONS & DOSAGE

Postencephalitic parkinsonism and other spastic states—
Adults: 0.5 to 1 mg P.O. t.i.d. to q.i.d.; 0.3 to 0.6 mg S.C., I.M., or I.V. (with suitable dilution) t.i.d. to q.i.d.
Children: 0.006 mg/kg P.O. or S.C. t.i.d. to q.i.d.; or 0.2 mg/m².
Preoperatively to reduce secretions and block cardiac vagal reflexes—
Adults: 0.4 to 0.6 mg S.C. 30 to 60 minutes before induction of anesthesia.

CONTRAINDICATIONS & PRECAUTIONS

Contraindicated in patients with glaucoma or a tendency toward glaucoma, because drug-induced cycloplegia and mydriasis may increase intraocular pressure; and in patients with obstructive uropathy, obstructive GI tract disease, asthma, chronic pulmonary disease, myasthenia gravis, paralytic ileus, intestinal atony, or toxic megacolon, because the drug may exacerbate these conditions.

Use cautiously in patients with autonomic neuropathy, hyperthyroidism, coronary artery disease, CHF, hypertension, or ulcerative colitis, because the drug may exacerbate these conditions; hepatic or renal disease, because toxic accumulation may occur; cardiac arrhythmias, because the drug may block vagal inhibition of the sinoatrial node pacemaker, worsening the arrhythmia; or hiatal hernia associated with reflux esophagitis, because this drug may decrease lower esophageal sphincter tone; to young children, because they may be more sensitive to drug effects; to patients with hypersensitivity to belladonna alkaloids; and to patients over age 40, because the drug increases the glaucoma risk.

ADVERSE REACTIONS

Common reactions are in italics; life-threatening reactions are in bold italics.

CNS: disorientation, restlessness, irritability, dizziness, drowsiness, headache.

CV: palpitations, tachycardia, paradoxical bradycardia.

EENT: dilated pupils, blurred vision, photophobia, increased intraocular pressure, difficulty swallowing.

GI: *constipation, dry mouth, nausea, vomiting, epigastric distress.*

GU: urinary hesitancy, urine retention.

Skin: rash, flushing, dryness.

Other: bronchial plugging, fever, ***depressed respirations.***

Adverse reactions may be caused by pending atropine-like toxicity and are dose related. Individual tolerance varies greatly.

INTERACTIONS

Alcohol, CNS depressants: increased CNS depression.

Centrally acting anticholinergics (tricyclic antidepressants, phenothiazines): increased adverse CNS reactions.

Digoxin: increased digoxin levels.

EFFECTS ON DIAGNOSTIC TESTS

None reported.

NURSING CONSIDERATIONS

Besides those related universally to drug therapy (see "How to use this book"), consider the following specific recommendations:

Assessment

- Obtain a baseline assessment of the patient's underlying condition before drug therapy.
- Be alert for adverse reactions and drug interactions throughout therapy.
- Evaluate the patient's and family's knowledge about scopolamine therapy.

Nursing Diagnoses

- Altered health maintenance related to the patient's underlying condition.
- Constipation related to adverse drug reaction.
- Knowledge deficit related to scopolamine butylbromide therapy.

Planning and Implementation

Preparation and Administration

- To determine body-surface area (m^2) for dosage calculation in children, use a nomogram.
- ***I.V. use:*** Intermittent and continuous infusions are not recommended. For direct injection, dilute with sterile water for injection and inject diluted drug at ordered rate through patent I.V. line. Protect I.V. solution

from freezing and light and store at room temperature.

Monitoring

• Monitor effectiveness by regularly assessing the patient's underlying condition.
• Monitor for adverse reactions or drug interactions to scopolamine butylbromide therapy by monitoring his intake and output.
• Monitor vital signs frequently for tachycardia, paroxysmal bradycardia, and decreased respirations.
• Monitor the patient's degree of dry mouth.
• Monitor the patient's bowel habits, because drug may cause constipation.
• Evaluate the patient's vision by asking about blurred vision.

Supportive Care

• Help the patient to get in and out of bed if he has dizziness or blurred vision.
• Institute safety precautions if he experiences dizziness or confusion and reorient the patient as necessary.
• Know that some patients become temporarily disoriented; symptoms disappear when the sedative effect is complete.
• Provide gum or sugarless hard candy to relieve dry mouth.
• If constipation occurs, obtain an order for a laxative.
• Provide additional fluids to help prevent constipation.
• Encourage the patient to void before taking this medication.
• Know that some of the adverse reactions (such as dry mouth, constipation) are an expected extension of the drug's pharmacologic activity.
• Know that tolerance to the drug may develop when given over a long period of time.

Patient Teaching

• Instruct the patient to avoid driving and other hazardous activities that require alertness if he is drowsy, dizzy, or has blurred vision.
• Encourage the patient to drink plenty of fluids to avoid constipation.
• Tell him to report any rash or skin eruptions.

Evaluation

In patients receiving scopolamine butylbromide, appropriate evaluation statements may include:
• The patient is able to perform activities of daily living without assistance.
• The patient does not develop constipation.
• Patient and family state an understanding of scopolamine butylbromide therapy.

scopolamine hydrobromide

(skoe pol´ a meen)
Isopto Hyoscine

• *Classification:* cycloplegic mydriatic (anticholinergic)
• *Pregnancy Risk Category:* C

HOW SUPPLIED

Ophthalmic solution: 0.25%

ACTION

Mechanism: Blocks muscarinic cholinergic receptors. Anticholinergic action leaves the pupil under unopposed adrenergic influence, causing it to dilate. A mydriatic and cycloplegic agent that has a more rapid onset but less pronounced effect than atropine.
Pharmacokinetics: Unknown.
Onset, peak, duration: Maximum mydriatic effect is seen within 15 minutes and usually lasts several days. Maximum cycloplegia is seen within 45 minutes and persists for up to 7 days.

INDICATIONS & DOSAGE

Cycloplegic refraction–
Adults: instill 1 to 2 drops of 0.25% solution in eye 1 hour before refraction.

Children: instill 1 drop of 0.25% solution or ointment b.i.d. for 2 days before refraction.
Iritis, uveitis–
Adults: instill 1 to 2 drops of 0.25% solution daily b.i.d. or t.i.d.
Children: instill 1 drop once daily to t.i.d.

ADVERSE REACTIONS

Common reactions are in italics; life-threatening reactions are in bold italics.
Eye: ocular congestion with prolonged use, conjunctivitis, *blurred vision,* eye dryness, increased intraocular pressure, *photophobia,* contact dermatitis.
Systemic: flushing, fever, dry skin and mouth, tachycardia, hallucinations, ataxia, irritability, confusion, delirium, somnolence, acute psychotic reactions.

INTERACTIONS

None significant.

EFFECTS ON DIAGNOSTIC TESTS

None reported.

NURSING CONSIDERATIONS

Besides those related universally to drug therapy (see "How to use this book"), consider the following specific recommendations:

Assessment

- Obtain a baseline assessment of the patient's vision and pupil size.
- Be alert for adverse reactions and drug interactions throughout therapy.
- Evaluate the patient's and family's knowledge about scopolamine hydrobromide therapy.

Nursing Diagnoses

- Sensory/perceptual alterations (visual) related to the patient's underlying condition.
- High risk for poisoning related to the drug's systemic adrenergic effects.
- Knowledge deficit related to scopolamine hydrobromide therapy.

Planning and Implementation

Preparation and Administration

- Instill in lacrimal sac: remove excess solution from around the eyes with a clean tissue or gauze and apply light finger pressure to lacrimal sac for 1 minute.
- May be used if patient is sensitive to atropine: has shorter duration and fewer adverse reactions.

Monitoring

- Monitor effectiveness by assessing the patient's visual status and pupil size.
- Monitor the patient for systemic effects, especially disorientation or delirium.

Supportive Care

- Notify the doctor immediately of changes in the patient's health status.

Patient Teaching

- Teach the patient how to instill the solution and advise him to wash his hands before and after administering the drug.

Evaluation

In patients receiving scopolamine hydrobromide, appropriate evaluation statements may include:

- Patient experiences therapeutic mydriasis.
- Patient remains free of systemic cholinergic effects.
- Patient and family state an understanding of scopolamine hydrobromide therapy.

---

secobarbital sodium

(see koe bar´ bi tal)
Novosecobarb†, Seconal Sodium

- Controlled Substance Schedule II
- *Classification:* sedative-hypnotic, anticonvulsant (barbiturate)
- *Pregnancy Risk Category:* D

HOW SUPPLIED

Tablets: 100 mg
Capsules: 50 mg, 100 mg
Injection: 50 mg/ml
Rectal injection: 50 mg/ml
Suppositories: 200 mg

ACTION

Mechanism: Probably interferes with transmission of impulses from the thalamus to the cortex of the brain. A barbiturate.
Absorption: After oral administration, 90% is absorbed rapidly. After I.M. or rectal administration, nearly 100% absorbed.
Distribution: Rapidly distributed throughout body tissues and fluids; approximately 30% to 45% is protein-bound.
Metabolism: Oxidized in the liver to inactive metabolites.
Excretion: 95% of a dose is eliminated as glucuronide conjugates and other metabolites in urine. Half-life: About 30 hours.
Onset, peak, duration: Peak serum concentration after oral or rectal administration occurs between 2 and 4 hours. The onset of action is rapid, occurring within 15 minutes when administered orally. Peak effects occur 15 to 30 minutes after oral and rectal administration, 7 to 10 minutes after I.M. administration, and 1 to 3 minutes after I.V. administration. Concentrations of 1 to 5 mcg/ml are needed to produce sedation; 5 to 15 mcg/ml are needed for hypnosis. Hypnosis lasts for 1 to 4 hours after oral doses of 100 to 150 mg. Duration of action is 3 to 4 hours.

INDICATIONS & DOSAGE

Sedation, preoperatively–
Adults: 200 to 300 mg P.O. 1 to 2 hours before surgery.
Children: 50 to 100 mg P.O. or 4 to 5 mg/kg rectally 1 to 2 hours before surgery.
Insomnia–
Adults: 100 to 200 mg P.O. or I.M.
Children: 3 to 5 mg/kg I.M., not to exceed 100 mg, with no more than 5 ml injected in any one site or 4 to 5 mg/kg rectally.
Acute tetanus seizure–
Adults and children: 5.5 mg/kg I.M. or slow I.V., repeated q 3 to 4 hours, if needed; I.V. injection rate not to exceed 50 mg per 15 seconds.
Acute psychotic agitation–
Adults: 50 mg/minute I.V. up to 250 mg I.V. initially, additional doses given cautiously after 5 minutes if desired response is not obtained. Not to exceed 500 mg total.
Status epilepticus–
Adults and children: 250 to 350 mg I.M. or I.V.

CONTRAINDICATIONS & PRECAUTIONS

Contraindicated in patients with hypersensitivity to barbiturates and in patients with bronchopneumonia, status asthmaticus, or other severe respiratory distress because of the potential for respiratory depression; depression or suicidal ideation, because the drug can worsen depression; uncontrolled acute or chronic pain, because exacerbation of pain and paradoxical excitement can occur; and porphyria, because this drug can trigger symptoms of this disease.

Use cautiously in patients who must perform hazardous tasks requiring mental alertness, because the drug causes drowsiness. Administer parenteral secobarbital slowly and with extreme caution to patients with hypotension or severe pulmonary or cardiovascular disease because of potential for adverse hemodynamic effects. Because tolerance and physical or psychological dependence may occur, prolonged use of high doses should be avoided.

Prenatal exposure to barbiturates is associated with an increased incidence of fetal abnormalities, and possibly brain tumors. Use of barbiturates in the third trimester may be associated with physical dependence in neonates. Risk-benefit must be considered.

ADVERSE REACTIONS

Common reactions are in italics; life-threatening reactions are in bold italics.
CNS: *drowsiness, lethargy, hangover,* paradoxical excitement in elderly patients.
GI: nausea, vomiting.
Skin: rash, urticaria.
Other: ***Stevens-Johnson syndrome,*** angioedema, exacerbation of porphyria.

INTERACTIONS

Alcohol or other CNS depressants, including narcotic analgesics: excessive CNS and respiratory depression. Use together cautiously.
Griseofulvin: decreased absorption of griseofulvin.
MAO inhibitors: inhibit metabolism of barbiturates; may cause prolonged CNS depression. Reduce barbiturate dosage.
Oral anticoagulants, estrogens and oral contraceptives, doxycycline, corticosteroids: secobarbital may enhance the metabolism of these drugs. Monitor for decreased effect.
Rifampin: may decrease barbiturate levels. Monitor for decreased effect.

EFFECTS ON DIAGNOSTIC TESTS

Cyanocobalamin: impaired absorption.
EEG patterns: changes in low-voltage, fast activity.
Phentolamine test: false-positive results.
Serum bilirubin: decreased concentrations in neonates, epileptics, and patients with congenital nonhemolytic unconjugated hyperbilirubinemia.

NURSING CONSIDERATIONS

Besides those related universally to drug therapy (see "How to use this book"), consider the following specific recommendations:

Assessment
- Obtain a baseline assessment of sleeping patterns and CNS status before therapy.
- Be alert for adverse reactions and drug interactions throughout therapy.
- Evaluate the patient's and family's knowledge about secobarbital therapy.

Nursing Diagnoses
- Sleep pattern disturbance related to underlying patient problem.
- High risk for trauma related to adverse CNS reactions caused by secobarbital.
- Knowledge deficit related to secobarbital therapy.

Planning and Implementation
Preparation and Administration
- Use injectable solution within 30 minutes after opening container to minimize deterioration. Don't use cloudy solution.
- Be aware that sterile secobarbital sodium is compatible with Ringer's injection and 0.9% sodium chloride solution; secobarbital sodium injection is not compatible with lactated Ringer's solution.
- To reconstitute, rotate ampule. Do not shake.
- Expect to reduce dosage during labor because barbiturates potentiate the effects of opiates.
- In renal insufficiency, use sterile drug reconstituted with sterile water for injection. Avoid commercial solution containing polyethylene glycol; it may irritate kidneys.
- Secobarbital in polyethylene glycol must be refrigerated.
- ***P.O. use:*** Before leaving the bedside, make sure the patient has swallowed tablet or capsule.
- ***I.V. use:*** Reserve I.V. use for emergency treatment and give under close

supervision. Be prepared to give artificial respiration.

• ***I.M. use:*** Give I.M. injection deeply. Superficial injection may cause pain, sterile abscess, and sloughing.

Monitoring

• Regularly monitor effectiveness by evaluating the patient's ability to sleep.

• Monitor the patient's CNS status for evidence of adverse reactions. Be aware that with I.V. barbiturates, the degree of CNS depression (from mild sedation to deep coma or death) depends on dosage, drug's pharmokinetics, patient's age and physical and emotional state, and concurrent use of other drugs.

• Closely monitor the elderly patient's responses to the drug as they are more sensitive to adverse CNS reactions.

• Monitor for signs of barbiturate toxicity: coma, pupillary constriction, cyanosis, clammy skin, and hypotension. Overdose can be fatal.

• Monitor the neonate's respiratory status closely if the mother received drug during labor because excessive dosage may cause neonatal respiratory depression.

• Monitor respiratory status closely after I.V. administration. Keep in mind that respiratory difficulty can occur 2 to 10 minutes after I.V. dose. Such reactions are cumulative and intensified with repeated administration.

• After drug discontinuation, be alert for withdrawal symptoms.

Supportive Care

• After administration, institute safety precautions: remove cigarettes, keep bed rails up, and supervise or assist ambulation.

• Withhold the drug if barbiturate toxicity is suspected.

• Do not discontinue the drug abruptly after prolonged use. The drug may cause dependence and severe withdrawal symptoms. Always withdraw barbiturates gradually.

• Take precautions to prevent hoarding or self-overdosing, especially by patients who are depressed, suicidal or have a history of drug abuse.

• Consult with the patient's doctor to obtain an analgesic order if the patient has pain. Barbiturates have no analgesic effect and may cause restlessness or delirium in presence of pain.

• ***With I.V use:*** Always keep resuscitation and mechanical ventilation equipment available. Maintain airway with ventilation and oxygen administration as needed; administer chest physiotherapy; administer a vasopressor, as ordered, for hypotension.

• Discontinue drug if skin eruptions occur; these may precede potentially fatal reactions.

Patient Teaching

• Explain that morning hangover is common after hypnotic dose. Encourage the patient to report severe hangover or oversedation so the doctor can be consulted for change of dose or drug.

• Explain that because hypnotic drugs suppress REM sleep, the patient may experience increased dreaming when drug is discontinued.

• Instruct the patient to remain in bed after taking drug and to call for assistance to use the bathroom.

• Warn the patient that drug may cause physical dependence.

• Warn the patient to avoid hazardous activities that require mental alertness if adverse CNS reactions are present after awakening.

• Advise the patient to avoid alcoholic beverages during therapy with secobarbital because this combination may cause excessive CNS depression.

• Tell the patient to notify the nurse or doctor if sleep pattern disturbances continue despite therapy.

Evaluation
In patients receiving secobarbital, appropriate evaluation statements may include:
• Patient states drug was effective in inducing sleep.
• Patient's safety maintained.
• Patient and family state an understanding of secobarbital therapy.

---

selegiline hydrochloride (L-deprenyl hydrochloride)
(sel ee´ jell een)
Eldepryl

• *Classification:* antiparkinsonian agent (MAO inhibitor)
• *Pregnancy Risk Category:* C

HOW SUPPLIED
Tablets: 5 mg

ACTION
Mechanism: Probably acts by selectively inhibiting monoamine oxidase (MAO) type B (found mostly in the brain). At higher-than-recommended doses, it is a nonselective inhibitor of MAO, including MAO type A (found in the GI tract). Also may directly increase dopaminergic activity by decreasing the reuptake of dopamine into nerve cells. Pharmacologically active metabolites (amphetamine and methamphetamine) may contribute to this effect.
Absorption: Well absorbed after oral administration.
Distribution: After a single dose, plasma levels are below detectable levels (less than 10 ng/ml).
Metabolism: Three metabolites have been detected in the serum and urine: N-desmethyldeprenyl, amphetamine, and methamphetamine.
Excretion: 45% of the drug appears as a metabolite in the urine after 48 hours.

INDICATIONS & DOSAGE
Adjunctive treatment to levodopa-carbidopa in the management of the symptoms associated with Parkinson's disease–
Adults: 10 mg P.O. daily, taken as 5 mg at breakfast and 5 mg at lunch. After 2 or 3 days of therapy, begin gradual decrease of carbidopa-levodopa dosage.

CONTRAINDICATIONS & PRECAUTIONS
Contraindicated in patients hypersensitive to the drug.

Some patients may experience an exacerbation of levodopa-induced adverse effects (including GI or CNS disturbances). Such effects may be ameliorated by decreasing the dosage of levodopa-carbidopa.

ADVERSE REACTIONS
Common reactions are in italics; life-threatening reactions are in bold italics.
CNS: *dizziness,* increased tremor, chorea, loss of balance, restlessness, blepharospasm, increased bradykinesia, facial grimace, stiff neck, dyskinesia, involuntary movements, increased apraxia, behavioral changes, tiredness, headache.
CV: orthostatic hypotension, hypertension, hypotension, arrhythmias, palpitations, new or increased anginal pain, tachycardia, peripheral edema, syncope.
GI: *nausea,* vomiting, constipation, weight loss, anorexia or poor appetite, dysphagia, diarrhea, heartburn, dry mouth, taste alteration.
GU: slow urination, transient nocturia, prostatic hypertrophy, urinary hesitancy, urinary frequency, urine retention, sexual dysfunction.
Skin: rash, hair loss, sweating.
Other: malaise.

INTERACTIONS
Adrenergic agents: possible increased pressor response, particularly in pa-

tients who have taken an overdose of selegiline.

EFFECTS ON DIAGNOSTIC TESTS

None reported.

NURSING CONSIDERATIONS

Besides those related universally to drug therapy (see "How to use this book"), consider the following specific recommendations:

Assessment

• Obtain a baseline assessment of the patient's parkinsonism signs and symptoms before therapy.
• Be alert for adverse reactions and drug interactions throughout therapy.
• Evaluate the patient's and family's knowledge about selegiline therapy.

Nursing Diagnoses

• Impaired physical mobility related to underlying parkinsonian syndrome.
• High risk for injury related to adverse CNS reactions to drug therapy.
• Knowledge deficit related to selegiline therapy.

Planning and Implementation

Preparation and Administration

• Do not exceed 10 mg total daily dosage.

Monitoring

• Monitor effectiveness by regularly checking the patient's body movements for signs of improvement.
• Monitor the patient for CNS and other adverse drug reactions.
• Monitor vital signs.

Supportive Care

• Notify the doctor if significant changes in vital signs or mental status occur.
• Institute safety precautions.
• Assist the patient with daily activities as needed.
• Keep in mind that some patients experience increased adverse reactions associated with levodopa (including muscle twitches) and require reduction of levodopa-carbidopa dosage; such patients commonly reduce dosage by 10% to 30%.

Patient Teaching

• Warn patients to move about cautiously at the start of therapy because they may experience dizziness and risk falling.
• Advise patient not to take more than 10 mg daily, because there is no evidence that a greater amount improves efficacy and it may increase adverse reactions.
• Instruct the patient's family to notify the doctor about changes in the patient's behavior or mental status.
• Inform patient about the possible interactions with tyramine-containing foods. Tell the patient to immediately report symptoms of hypertension, including severe headache. However, there is no evidence that this interaction occurs at recommended dosages; at 10 mg daily, the drug inhibits only MAO type B. No dietary restrictions appear necessary if the patient does not exceed the recommended dose.
• Advise the patient to avoid activities that could expose them to injury until adverse CNS and cardiovascular reactions are known.

Evaluation

In patients receiving selegiline, appropriate evaluation statements may include:

• Patient exhibits improved mobility with reduction of muscular rigidity and tremor.
• Patient's safety maintained; CNS and cardiovascular status unchanged as a result of drug therapy.
• Patient and family state an understanding of selegiline therapy.

---

senna

(sen´ a)

Black-Draught◇, Senokot◇, X-Prep Liquid*◇

• *Classification:* stimulant laxative (anthraquinone derivative)

• *Pregnancy Risk Category:* C

HOW SUPPLIED

Tablets: 187 mg◇, 217 mg◇, 600 mg◇
Granules: 326 mg/tsp◇, 1.65 g/½ tsp◇
Suppositories: 652 mg◇
Syrup: 218 mg/5 ml◇

ACTION

Mechanism: A stimulant laxative that increases peristalsis by direct effect on the smooth muscle of the intestine. Thought either to irritate the musculature or to stimulate the colonic intramural plexus. Also promotes fluid accumulation in the colon and small intestine.
Absorption: Minimally absorbed.
Distribution: In bile, saliva, the colonic mucosa, and breast milk.
Metabolism: Absorbed portion is metabolized in the liver.
Excretion: Unabsorbed senna is excreted mainly in feces; absorbed drug is excreted in urine and feces.
Onset, peak, duration: With oral administration, laxative effect occurs in 6 to 10 hours; with suppository, in 30 minutes to 2 hours.

INDICATIONS & DOSAGE

Acute constipation, preparation for bowel or rectal examination–
Adults: Dosage range for Senokot: 1 to 8 tablets P.O.; ½ to 4 teaspoonfuls of granules added to liquid; 1 to 2 suppositories h.s.; 1 to 4 teaspoonfuls syrup h.s. Black-Draught: 2 tablets or ¼ to ½ level teaspoonfuls of granules mixed with water.
Children over 27 kg: half adult dose of tablets, granules, or syrup (except Black-Draught tablets and granules not recommended for children).
Children 1 month to 1 year: 1.25 to 2.5 ml Senokot syrup P.O. h.s.

X-Prep Liquid used solely as single dose for preradiographic bowel evacuation. Give 20 g powder dissolved in juice or 75 ml liquid between 2 p.m. and 4 p.m. on day before X-ray procedure. May be given in divided doses for elderly or debilitated patients.

CONTRAINDICATIONS & PRECAUTIONS

Contraindicated in patients with fluid and electrolyte disturbances, appendicitis, abdominal pain, nausea or vomiting, fecal impaction, or intestinal obstruction or perforation, because the drug may worsen these conditions or symptoms.

ADVERSE REACTIONS

Common reactions are in italics; life-threatening reactions are in bold italics.
GI: *nausea;* vomiting; diarrhea; loss of normal bowel function in excessive use; *abdominal cramps,* especially in severe constipation; malabsorption of nutrients; "cathartic colon" (syndrome resembling ulcerative colitis radiologically) in chronic misuse; may cause constipation after catharsis; yellow, yellow-green cast to feces; diarrhea in nursing infants of mothers receiving senna; darkened pigmentation of rectal mucosa in long-term use, which is usually reversible within 4 to 12 months after stopping drug.
GU: red-pink discoloration in alkaline urine; yellow-brown color to acidic urine.
Metabolic: hypokalemia, protein-losing enteropathy, electrolyte imbalance with excessive use.
Other: laxative dependence in long-term or excessive use.

INTERACTIONS

None significant.

EFFECTS ON DIAGNOSTIC TESTS

None reported.

NURSING CONSIDERATIONS

Besides those related universally to drug therapy (see "How to use this

book"), consider the following specific recommendations:

Assessment

- Obtain a baseline assessment of history of bowel disorder, GI status, fluid intake, nutritional status, exercise habits, and normal pattern of elimination.
- Be alert for adverse reactions and drug interactions throughout therapy.
- Evaluate the patient's and family's knowledge about senna therapy.

Nursing Diagnoses

- Constipation related to interruption of normal pattern of elimination characterized by infrequent or absent stools.
- Pain related to senna-induced abdominal cramping.
- Knowledge deficit related to senna therapy.

Planning and Implementation

Preparation and Administration

- Avoid exposing to excessive heat or light.
- Schedule drug administration to avoid interference with scheduled activities or sleep. Be aware that senna acts 6 to 10 hours after ingestion.

Monitoring

- Monitor effectiveness by monitoring the frequency and characteristics of stools.
- Auscultate bowel sounds at least once a shift. Assess for pain and cramping.
- Monitor nutritional status and fluid intake.
- Monitor serum electrolytes in long-term use.

Supportive Care

- Do not give to patients with ulcerative bowel lesions; nausea, vomiting, abdominal pain, or other symptoms of appendicitis or acute surgical abdomen; fecal impaction; or intestinal obstruction or perforation.
- Be aware that senna is intended for short-term therapy and is more potent than cascara sagrada. Senna is one of the most effective laxatives for counteracting constipation caused by narcotic analgesics.
- Confine diet to clear liquids after X-Prep Liquid is taken.
- Provide privacy for elimination.
- Unless contraindicated, encourage fluid intake up to 2,500 ml a day.
- Consult with a dietitian to modify diet to increase fiber and bulk.

Patient Teaching

- Warn patient that senna may discolor alkaline urine red-pink and acidic urine yellow-brown.
- Discourage excessive use of laxatives.
- Teach the patient about the relationship between fluid intake, dietary fiber, exercise, and constipation.
- Teach patient that dietary sources of fiber include bran and other cereals, fresh fruit, and vegetables.
- Warn the patient that abdominal cramping may occur.

Evaluation

In patients receiving senna, appropriate evaluation statements may include:

- Patient reports return of normal pattern of elimination.
- Patient is free from abdominal cramping.
- Patient and family state an understanding of senna therapy.

silver nitrate 1%

- *Classification:* ophthalmic antiseptic; topical cauterizing agent (heavy metal)
- *Pregnancy Risk Category:* C

HOW SUPPLIED

Ophthalmic solution: 1%

ACTION

Mechanism: Silver ions readily combine with several reactive groups on proteins, causing denaturation. A

nonspecific bacteriostatic, germicidal, and astringent agent.
Pharmacokinetics: Unknown.

INDICATIONS & DOSAGE

Prevention of gonorrheal ophthalmia neonatorum–
Neonates: cleanse lids thoroughly; instill 1 drop of 1% solution into each eye.

CONTRAINDICATIONS & PRECAUTIONS

Contraindicated in patients with hypersensitivity to the preparation or any of its components. For ophthalmic use, the 1% solution is considered optimal but still must be used with caution, because cauterization of the cornea and blindness may result, especially with repeated applications. Solution should not be applied to wounds, cuts, or broken skin.

ADVERSE REACTIONS

Common reactions are in italics; life-threatening reactions are in bold italics.
Eye: periorbital edema, temporary staining of lids and surrounding tissue, conjunctivitis (with concentrations of 1% or greater).

INTERACTIONS

Bacitracin: inactivates silver nitrate. Don't use together.

EFFECTS ON DIAGNOSTIC TESTS

None reported.

NURSING CONSIDERATIONS

Besides those related universally to drug therapy (see "How to use this book"), consider the following specific recommendations:

Assessment

- Obtain a baseline assessment of neonate's general condition before therapy.
- Be alert for adverse reactions and drug interactions throughout therapy.
- Evaluate the patient's and family's knowledge about silver nitrate therapy.

Nursing Diagnoses

- Altered protection related to risk of gonorrheal ophthalmia.
- Impaired tissue integrity related to silver nitrate-induced periorbital edema.
- Knowledge deficit related to silver nitrate therapy.

Planning and Implementation

Preparation and Administration

- Store wax ampules away from heat and light.
- Wash hands before and after instillation of drops.
- Handle carefully; may stain skin and utensils.
- Do not irrigate eyes after instillation.

Monitoring

- Monitor effectiveness by observing the neonate for signs of gonorrheal ophthalmia.
- Monitor the extent of periorbital edema.

Supportive Care

- Do not use repeatedly.
- If 2% solution used accidentally in eye, prompt irrigation with normal saline is advised to prevent eye irritation.
- May delay instillation slightly to allow neonate to bond with mother.

Patient Teaching

- Advise the mother that periorbital edema and lid staining are temporary.
- Explain that silver nitrate is legally mandated in most states and given for the infant's protection.

Evaluation

In patients receiving silver nitrate, appropriate evaluation statements may include:

- Patient remains free from signs and symptoms of infection.
- Patient exhibits decrease or absence of periorbital edema.
- Patient and family state an understanding of silver nitrate therapy.

silver sulfadiazine

(sul fa dye´ a zeen)
Flamazine†, Flint SSD, Silvadene, Thermazene

- *Classification:* topical antibacterial
- *Pregnancy Risk Category:* C

HOW SUPPLIED

Cream: 1%

ACTION

Mechanism: Acts upon cell membrane and cell wall. Broad spectrum; bactericidal for many gram-positive and gram-negative organisms. Also effective against yeasts.
Absorption: Not absorbed; however, drug may release sulfadiazine, which is absorbed.
Excretion: In the urine.

INDICATIONS & DOSAGE

Prevention and treatment of wound infection especially for second- and third-degree burns–
Adults and children: apply 1/16" thickness of cream to cleansed and debrided burn wound, then apply daily or b.i.d.

CONTRAINDICATIONS & PRECAUTIONS

Contraindicated in pregnant women near term; in premature infants because drug has produced kernicterus in neonates; and in women of childbearing age unless benefits outweigh the possibility of fetal damage.

Use cautiously in patients with hypersensitivity to the drug. The possibility of cross-hypersensitivity with other sulfonamides should be kept in mind. Also use cautiously in patients with impaired hepatic or renal function.

ADVERSE REACTIONS

Common reactions are in italics; life-threatening reactions are in bold italics.
Blood: *neutropenia (in 3% to 5%) of those receiving extensive applications.*
Skin: pain, burning, rashes, itching.

INTERACTIONS

Topical proteolytic enzymes: inactivity of enzymes when used together. Do not use together.

EFFECTS ON DIAGNOSTIC TESTS

CBC: decreased neutrophil count possible after systemic absorption.

NURSING CONSIDERATIONS

Besides those related universally to drug therapy (see "How to use this book"), consider the following specific recommendations:

Assessment
- Obtain a baseline assessment of third-degree burn wounds before therapy.
- Be alert for adverse reactions and drug interactions throughout therapy.
- Evaluate the patient's and family's knowledge about silver sulfadiazine therapy.

Nursing Diagnoses
- Impaired skin integrity related to patient's underlying condition.
- High risk for infection related to silver sulfadiazine-induced neutropenia.
- Knowledge deficit related to silver sulfadiazine therapy.

Planning and Implementation
Preparation and Administration
- ***Topical use:*** Cleanse and debride burn wound prior to application. Use only on affected areas. Keep medicated at all times.
- Discard darkened cream.
- Bathe patient daily, if possible.

Monitoring
- Monitor effectiveness by inspecting patient's skin daily and noting any changes.

• Monitor for adverse reactions and drug interactions by frequently evaluating hepatic or renal function.
• Monitor serum sulfadiazine concentrations and renal function, and check urine for sulfa crystals.
• Monitor CBC and differential.
Supportive Care
• Be prepared to discontinue the drug and notify the doctor if hepatic or renal dysfunction occurs.
• Notify doctor if burning or excessive pain develops.
• Keep in mind that the drug is contraindicated in premature and newborn infants during the first month of life. (Drug may increase possibility of kernicterus.)
• Remember, reverse isolation and/or sterile application technique recommended to prevent wound contamination.
Patient Teaching
• Teach patient to apply medication, when appropriate.
• Instruct patient to report burning or pain.
Evaluation
In patients receiving silver sulfadiazine, appropriate evaluation statements may include:
• Burn wounds have healed.
• Neutropenia did not occur.
• Patient and family state an understanding of silver sulfadiazine therapy.

simethicone
(sye meth´ i kone)
Extra Strength Gas-X◇, Gas-X◇, Mylicon-80◇, Mylicon-125◇, Ovol-40†, Ovol-80†, Phazyme◇, Phazyme 55◇, Phazyme 95◇, Phazyme 125◇, Silain◇

• *Classification:* antiflatulent (dispersant)
• *Pregnancy Risk Category:* C

HOW SUPPLIED
Tablets◇: 40 mg, 50 mg, 60 mg, 80 mg, 95 mg, 125 mg
Capsules: 40 mg/0.6 ml◇

ACTION
Mechanism: By defoaming action, disperses or prevents formation of mucus-surrounded gas pockets in the GI tract.
Absorption: None.
Excretion: In feces.

INDICATIONS & DOSAGE
Flatulence, functional gastric bloating—
Adults and children over 12 years: 40 to 125 mg after each meal and h.s.

CONTRAINDICATIONS & PRECAUTIONS
None reported.

ADVERSE REACTIONS
Common reactions are in italics; life-threatening reactions are in bold italics.
GI: expulsion of excessive liberated gas as belching, rectal flatus.

INTERACTIONS
None significant.

EFFECTS ON DIAGNOSTIC TESTS
None reported.

NURSING CONSIDERATIONS
Besides those related universally to drug therapy (see "How to use this book"), consider the following specific recommendations:
Assessment
• Obtain a baseline assessment of the patient's pain or discomfort before beginning therapy.
• Be alert for adverse reactions and drug interactions throughout therapy.
• Evaluate the patient's and family's knowledge about simethicone therapy.
Nursing Diagnoses
• Pain related to excess gas in the digestive tract.

• Knowledge deficit related to simethicone therapy.

Planning and Implementation

Preparation and Administration

• ***P.O. use:*** Be sure patients chew tablets completely before swallowing. Administer after meals and at bedtime.

Monitoring

• Monitor effectiveness by asking the patient if pain and discomfort was relieved and noting passage of flatus and belching.

Supportive Care

• Encourage the patient to discuss any emotional factors or dietary habits that may be contributing to the patient's GI problems.

Patient Teaching

• Tell the patient to chew tablets thoroughly before swallowing and to take the medication after meals and at bedtime.

• Warn the patient not to take simethicone indiscriminately.

Evaluation

In patients receiving simethicone, appropriate evaluation statements may include:

• Patient's pain subsides or is relieved.

• Patient and family state an understanding of simethicone therapy.

sodium bicarbonate◇

• *Classification:* systemic and urinary alkalinizer, systemic hydrogen ion buffer, oral antacid (electrolyte)
• *Pregnancy Risk Category:* C

HOW SUPPLIED

Tablets: 300 mg◇, 325 mg◇, 600 mg◇, 650 mg◇
Injection: 4% (2.4 mEq/5 ml), 4.2% (5 mEq/10 ml), 5% (297.5 mEq/500 ml), 7.5% (8.92 mEq/10 ml and 44.6 mEq/50 ml), 8.4% (10 mEq/10 ml and 50 mEq/50 ml)

ACTION

Mechanism: A systemic alkalinizing agent that increases plasma bicarbonate concentration. Restores buffering capacity of the body and neutralizes excess acid.
Absorption: Well absorbed after oral administration as sodium and bicarbonate ions.
Distribution: Throughout the extracellular fluid; probably crosses the placenta.
Metabolism: When it combines with hydrogen ions, bicarbonate is converted to carbonic acid, then dissociates to carbon dioxide and water.
Excretion: Bicarbonate is filtered and reabsorbed by the kidney; less than 1% of filtered bicarbonate is excreted.

INDICATIONS & DOSAGE

Cardiac arrest–
Adults and children: as a 7.5% or 8.4% solution, 1 mEq/kg I.V. followed by 0.5 mEq/kg I.V. every 10 minutes depending on blood gases. Further dosages based on blood gases. If blood gases unavailable, use 0.5 mEq/kg I.V. q 10 minutes until spontaneous circulation returns.
Infants up to 2 years: 4.2% solution, I.V. infusion. Rate not to exceed 8 mEq/kg daily.
Metabolic acidosis–
Adults and children: dosage depends on blood CO_2 content, pH, and patient's clinical condition. Generally, 2 to 5 mEq/kg I.V. infused over 4- to 8-hour period.
Systemic or urinary alkalinization–
Adults: 325 mg to 2 g P.O. q.i.d.
Children: 12 to 120 mg/kg P.O. daily.
Antacid–
Adults: 300 mg to 2 g P.O. chewed and taken with glass of water.

CONTRAINDICATIONS & PRECAUTIONS

Contraindicated in patients with metabolic or respiratory alkalosis; hypochloremic alkalosis from diuretics, vomiting, or nasogastric suction; hypocalcemia because alkalosis may produce tetany; and in prolonged therapy because it may cause sodium overload or metabolic acidosis.

Use cautiously in patients with CHF, pulmonary disease, ascites, or other fluid-retaining states because of the large sodium load; in patients with potassium depletion because alkalosis may lower serum potassium levels, predisposing the patient to cardiac arrhythmias; and in neonates and children under age 2 because rapid injection of hypertonic sodium may cause hypernatremia.

ADVERSE REACTIONS

Common reactions are in italics; life-threatening reactions are in bold italics.

GI: gastric distention, belching, flatulence.

GU: renal calculi or crystals.

Metabolic: (with overdose) alkalosis, hypernatremia, hyperkalemia, hyperosmolarity.

INTERACTIONS

None significant.

EFFECTS ON DIAGNOSTIC TESTS

Serum electrolytes: altered levels.
Serum lactate: increased levels.

NURSING CONSIDERATIONS

Besides those related universally to drug therapy (see "How to use this book"), consider the following specific recommendations:

Assessment

• Obtain a baseline assessment of arterial blood gases, serum electrolytes, and urine pH and output before initiating sodium bicarbonate therapy.
• Be alert for adverse reactions and drug interactions throughout therapy.
• Evaluate the patient's and family's knowledge about sodium bicarbonate therapy.

Nursing Diagnoses

• High risk for injury related to acid-base imbalance.
• Altered protection related to sodium bicarbonate overdose.
• Knowledge deficit related to sodium bicarbonate therapy.

Plannning and Implementation

Preparation and Administration

• ***I.V. use:*** Sodium bicarbonate may be mixed with other I.V. solutions except those containing dopamine or norepinephrine. Dose is usually administered in I.V. bolus form q 10 minutes as needed.
• ***P.O. use:*** Give oral preparation with a full glass of water. Do not administer oral sodium bicarbonate with milk or other alkaline solutions.

Monitoring

• Monitor effectiveness by regularly checking arterial blood gases, serum electrolytes, and urine pH and output.
• Monitor vital signs: tachycardia, hypotension, dyspnea, and fever may indicate fluid volume deficit.
• Monitor skin turgor and mucous membranes to indicate fluid volume deficit.
• Monitor for signs of metabolic alkalosis (indicates overdose).
• Monitor mental and neurologic status.
• Monitor patient's weight daily.

Supportive Care

• Hold dose and notify the doctor if drug overdose occurs.
• Frequently check I.V. site and patency; if infiltration results in extravasation of sodium bicarbonate to surrounding tissues, elevate the extremity, apply heat, and consult the doctor for additional orders.
• Maintain accurate record of intake and output.
• Provide frequent skin and mouth care to relieve skin and mucous membrane dryness.
• Encourage oral intake of fluids if the patient is alert.

• Institute safety precautions due to potential weakness and altered thought processes.
• Reorient the patient to person, place, and time as needed.

Patient Teaching

• Teach the patient and family to identify and report signs of metabolic alkalosis (overdose).
• Teach the patient and family to monitor the patient's fluid volume by weighing the patient daily and recording his fluid intake and urine output.
• Advise the patient not to take oral sodium bicarbonate with milk or other alkaline solutions.
• Discourage use of sodium bicarbonate as an antacid or with the use of other antacid preparations containing sodium.
• Teach the patient to avoid high-sodium food.

Evaluation

In patients receiving sodium bicarbonate, appropriate evaluation statements may include:
• Patient's metabolic acidosis is resolved without serious patient injury.
• Patient does not experience signs and symptoms of sodium bicarbonate overdose.
• Patient and family state an understanding of sodium bicarbonate therapy.

---

sodium cellulose phosphate

Calcibind

• *Classification:* antiurolithic (ion exchange resin)
• *Pregnancy Risk Category:* C

HOW SUPPLIED

Powder: 2.5-g packets or 300-g bulk. Inorganic phosphate content approximately 34%; sodium content approximately 11%.

ACTION

Mechanism: Binds calcium in the GI tract and decreases the amount absorbed.
Absorption: Not absorbed from the GI tract.
Distribution: None significant.
Metabolism: Undergoes partial (7% to 30%) hydrolysis in the intestine, which causes release of phosphorus ions. The resin undergoes cationic modification in the intestine, exchanging calcium and magnesium for sodium.
Excretion: The nonabsorbable cationically modified resin and unchanged resin are excreted in feces.

INDICATIONS & DOSAGE

Treatment of absorptive hypercalciuria type I with recurrent calcium oxalate or calcium phosphate renal stones–

Adults: 15 g/day P.O. (5 g with each meal) in patients with urine calcium greater than 300 mg/day. When urine calcium declines to less than 150 mg/day, reduce dosage to 10 g/day (5 g with dinner, 2.5 g with two remaining meals).

CONTRAINDICATIONS & PRECAUTIONS

Contraindicated in patients with primary or secondary hyperthyroidism, including renal hypercalciuria (renal calcium leak); hypomagnesemic states (serum magnesium less than 1.5 mg/dl); bone disease (such as osteoporosis, osteomalacia, and osteitis); hypocalcemic states (such as hypoparathyroidism and intestinal malabsorption); normal or low intestinal absorption and renal excretion of calcium; and enteric hyperoxaluria.

Use with caution to avoid parathyroid bone disease caused by inhibiting intestinal calcium absorption; in patients with Type I hypercalciuria, dosage should be just sufficient to restore normal calcium absorption.

Use cautiously, if at all, in patients with CHF or ascites. Safe use in pregnancy has not been established.

Use only while monitoring serum calcium, magnesium, copper, zinc, iron, parathyroid hormone, and complete blood count every 3 to 6 months. Hyperoxaluria and hypomagnesuria may negate the beneficial effects of hypocalciuria on new stone formation.

ADVERSE REACTIONS

Common reactions are in italics; life-threatening reactions are in bold italics.
CNS: drowsiness, mood or mental changes, ***seizures,*** trembling.
GI: anorexia, nausea, vomiting, discomfort, diarrhea, dyspepsia.
GU: hyperoxaluria, hypomagnesuria.
Other: acute arthralgias.

INTERACTIONS

Magnesium-containing products: may bind drug. Separate doses by at least 1 hour.

EFFECTS ON DIAGNOSTIC TESTS

None reported.

NURSING CONSIDERATIONS

Besides those related universally to drug therapy (see "How to use this book"), consider the following specific recommendations:

Assessment
- Obtain a baseline assessment of serum and urine calcium, magnesium, and oxalate levels before therapy.
- Be alert for adverse reactions and drug interactions throughout therapy.
- Evaluate the patient's and family's knowledge about sodium cellulose phosphate therapy.

Nursing Diagnoses
- Altered renal tissue perfusion related to absorptive hypercalciuria.
- Altered thought processes related to drug-induced mood or mental changes.
- Knowledge deficit related to sodium cellulose phosphate therapy.

Planning and Implementation

Preparation and Administration
- ***P.O. use:*** Administer drug with meals to facilitate absorption.
- Dosage may be decreased as urinary calcium levels decrease.

Monitoring
- Monitor effectiveness by monitoring urine calcium levels.
- Monitor fluid and electrolyte balance.
- Monitor urine oxalate and magnesium levels.
- Observe for signs of CNS adverse reaction (seizure, drowsiness, mood or mental changes).

Supportive Care
- Do not give in primary or secondary hyperparathyroidism—including renal hypercalciuria, hypomagnesemic states, bone disease, hypocalcemic states, normal or low intestinal absorption, renal excretion of calcium, or enteric hyperoxaluria.
- Be aware that drug is recommended only for the type of absorptive hypercalciuria in which both intestinal calcium absorption and urine calcium remain abnormally high even with a calcium-restricted diet. Inappropriate use can cause hypocalciuria, which can stimulate parathyroid function and lead to bone disease.
- Because of the difficulty involved in managing sodium cellulose phosphate therapy, many doctors prefer to treat hypercalciuria with a low-calcium diet, high fluid intake, and thiazides when necessary.
- Use seizure and safety precautions for patients who develop CNS adverse reactions.
- Strain all urine to detect passage of renal calculi.
- Arrange for consultation with dietitian.

Patient Teaching
- Advise patient to maintain a calcium-restricted diet and avoid all dairy products.
- Advise patient to restrict dietary intake of oxalate (found in spinach, rhubarb, chocolate and tea) because of risk of developing drug-induced hyperoxaluria and hypomagnesuria which may predispose to stone formation.
- Instruct patient to avoid Vitamin C which may increase urine oxalate.
- Encourage fluid intake to maintain urine output at least 2 liters/day.
- Encourage a low sodium diet. Instruct the patient to avoid salty foods and to avoid adding salt at the table.

Evaluation

In patients receiving sodium cellulose phosphate, appropriate evaluation statements may include:
- Patient is free from signs of impaired renal tissue perfusion.
- Patient remains free from drug induced altered thought processes.
- Patient and family state an understanding of sodium cellulose phosphate therapy.

sodium chloride, hypertonic

Adsorbonac Ophthalmic Solution, Muro-128 Ointment, Sodium Chloride Ointment 5%

- *Classification:* osmotic ophthalmic anti-edema agent (electrolyte solution)
- *Pregnancy Risk Category:* C

HOW SUPPLIED

Ophthalmic ointment: 5%
Ophthalmic solution: 2%, 5%

ACTION

Mechanism: Removes excess fluid from the cornea by an osmotic action.
Pharmacokinetics: Unknown.

INDICATIONS & DOSAGE

Corneal edema (postoperative) after cataract extraction or corneal transplantation; also in trauma or bullous keratopathy–
Adults and children: instill 1 to 2 drops q 3 to 4 hours, or apply ointment at bedtime.

CONTRAINDICATIONS & PRECAUTIONS

Contraindicated in patients with hypersensitivity to the drug or any of its components.

ADVERSE REACTIONS

Common reactions are in italics; life-threatening reactions are in bold italics.
Eye: slight stinging.
Other: hypersensitivity.

INTERACTIONS

None significant.

EFFECTS ON DIAGNOSTIC TESTS

None reported.

NURSING CONSIDERATIONS

Besides those related universally to drug therapy (see "How to use this book"), consider the following specific recommendations.

Assessment
- Obtain a baseline assessment of the patient's visual status and corneal appearance.
- Be alert for adverse reactions and drug interactions throughout therapy.
- Evaluate the patient's and family's knowledge about hypertonic sodium chloride therapy.

Nursing Diagnoses
- Sensory/perceptual alterations (visual) related to the patient's underlying condition.
- Pain related to drug-induced ocular irritation.
- Knowledge deficit related to hypertonic sodium chloride therapy.

Planning and Implementation
Preparation and Administration
• Instill solution in lacrimal sac; remove excess fluid from around eyes with a clean tissue or gauze, and apply light finger pressure to lacrimal sac for one minute.
• Apply thin strip of ointment to conjunctival sac; avoid touching applicator tip to any surface.
• Store solution in tightly closed container.
Monitoring
• Monitor effectiveness by assessing the patient's visual status and corneal appearance.
• Monitor for vision changes such as diplopia, photophobia, and appearance of floating spots. Inspect the eyes for redness and irritation.
Supportive Care
• Notify doctor immediately of any vision changes or signs of ocular irritation.
Patient Teaching
• Teach patient how to instill ointment or solution, and advise him to wash his hands before and after administering the drug.
• Advise the patient that a few drops of sterile irrigating solution may be used inside the bottle cap to prevent caking of solution on dropper tip.
• Warn the patient that ointment may cause blurred vision, and advise him to avoid hazardous activities, such as driving, while vision is affected.
Evaluation
In patients receiving hypertonic sodium chloride, appropriate evaluation statements include:
• Patient experiences a therapeutic reduction in corneal edema.
• Patient remains free of adverse ocular effects.
• Patient and family state an understanding of hypertonic sodium chloride therapy.

sodium fluoride
Fluor-A-Day†, Fluoritab, Flura, Flura-Drops, Karidium, Luride, Pediaflor, Phos-Flur

sodium fluoride, topical
ACT◇, Checkmate, Fluorigard◇, Fluorinse, Flura-Drops, Gel II, Gel-Kam, Gel-Tin, Home Treatment Fluoride Gelution, Karigel, Karigel-N, Listermint with Fluoride◇, Minute-Gel, Point-Two, PreviDent, Stop, Thera-Flur, Thera-Flur N

• *Classification:* dental caries prophylactic (trace mineral)
• *Pregnancy Risk Category:* C

HOW SUPPLIED
sodium fluoride
Tablets: 0.5 mg, 1 mg (sugar-free)
Tablets (chewable): 0.25 mg (sugar-free)
Drops: 0.125 mg/drop (30 ml), 0.125 mg/drop (60 ml, sugar-free), 0.25 mg/drop (19 ml), 0.25 mg/drop (24 ml, sugar-free), 0.5 mg/ml (50 ml)
Rinse: 0.01%◇ (180 ml, 260 ml, 540 ml, 720 ml); 0.02%◇ (180 ml, 300 ml, 360 ml, 480 ml)
sodium fluoride, topical
Gel: 0.5% (24 g, 30 g, 60 g, 120 g, 125 g, 130 g), 0.5% (250 g, sugar-free), 1.23% (480 g)
Gel drops: 0.5% (24 ml, 60 ml)
Rinse: 0.02%◇ (250 ml, 480 ml, 500 ml), 0.09% (250 ml, 480 ml), 0.09% (480 ml, sugar-free)

ACTION
Mechanism: Increases tooth resistance to the cariogenic microbial process and resistance to acid dissolution. May catalyze bone remineralization.
Absorption: Readily and almost completely absorbed from the GI tract. A large amount may be absorbed in the

stomach, and the rate of absorption may depend on the gastric pH. Also acts topically on teeth.
Distribution: Stored in bones and developing teeth after absorption. Skeletal tissue also has a high storage capacity for fluoride ions. Because of the storage-mobilization mechanism in skeletal tissue, a constant fluoride supply may be provided. Although teeth have a small mass, they also serve as storage sites. Fluoride deposited in teeth is not released readily. Fluoride has been found in all organs and tissues, with a low accumulation in noncalcified tissues, and is distributed into sweat, tears, hair, and saliva. Crosses the placenta and is distributed into breast milk. Fluoride concentrations in milk range from approximately 0.05 to 0.13 ppm and remain fairly constant.
Metabolism: None.
Excretion: Rapidly excreted, mainly in the feces. About 90% of fluoride is filtered by the glomerulus and reabsorbed by the renal tubules.

INDICATIONS & DOSAGE

Aid in the prevention of dental caries–
Children over 3 years: 1 mg P.O. daily.
Children under 3 years: 0.5 mg P.O. daily.
Topical: use once daily after thoroughly brushing teeth and rinsing mouth. Rinse around and between teeth for 1 minute, then spit out.
Adults and children over 12 years: 10 ml of 0.01% to 0.02% solution.
Children 6 to 12 years: 5 ml of 0.2% solution.

CONTRAINDICATIONS & PRECAUTIONS

Contraindicated in patients with hypersensitivity to the fluoride ion and when the fluoride content of drinking water exceeds 0.7 ppm. Patients on a low-sodium or sodium-free diet should avoid sodium fluoride. If the fluoride content of drinking water is 0.3 ppm or more, 1-mg tablets or rinse must not be used in children under age 3. The 1-mg rinse should not be used in children under age 6 because young children cannot perform the necessary rinse correctly. Some formulations contain tartrazine, which may cause an allergic reaction in certain individuals.

ADVERSE REACTIONS

Common reactions are in italics; life-threatening reactions are in bold italics.
CNS: headaches, weakness.
GI: gastric distress.
Other: hypersensitivity.

INTERACTIONS

None significant.

EFFECTS ON DIAGNOSTIC TESTS

None reported.

NURSING CONSIDERATIONS

Besides those related universally to drug therapy (see "How to use this book"), consider the following specific recommendations:
Assessment
- Obtain a baseline assessment of patient's underlying condition before therapy.
- Be alert for adverse reactions and drug interactions throughout therapy.
- Evaluate the patient's and family's knowledge about sodium fluoride therapy.

Nursing Diagnoses
- Impaired skin integrity related to adverse drug reactions.
- Pain related to drug-induced headache.
- Knowledge deficit related to sodium fluoride therapy.

Planning and Implementation
Preparation and Administration
- Tablets may be dissolved in mouth, chewed, or swallowed whole.
- Drops may be administered orally

*Liquid form contains alcohol. **May contain tartrazine.

undiluted or mixed with fluids or food.
• Topical forms (rinses and gels) should not be swallowed. Most effective when used immediately after brushing the teeth.
Monitoring
• Monitor effectiveness by observing for reduction of dental caries.
• Monitor for adverse reactions and drug interactions by assessing the patient's skin for atopic dermatitis, eczema, and urticaria.
• Monitor the patient for drug-induced headache.
Supportive Care
• Chronic toxicity (florosis) may result from prolonged use of higher-than-recommended doses.
• Used investigationally in treating osteoporosis.
• The presence of fluoride in prenatal vitamins has been shown to produce healthier teeth in infants.
• Obtain an order for a mild analgesic if the patient develops a drug-induced headache.
Patient Teaching
• Advise patient to notify dentist if tooth mottling occurs.
• Tell the patient that the tablets may be dissolved in mouth, chewed, or swallowed whole.
• Advise the patient not to swallow the topical forms (rinses and gels) and that they are best used immediately after brushing the teeth.
• Tell the patient to dilute drops or rinses in plastic containers rather than glass.

Evaluation

In patients receiving sodium fluoride, appropriate evaluation statements may include:
• Patient does not develop a drug-induced headache.
• Patient does not develop impaired skin integrity.
• Patient and family state an understanding of sodium fluoride therapy.

sodium phosphates
Fleet Phospho-Soda◇

• *Classification:* saline laxative (acid salt)
• *Pregnancy Risk Category:* C

HOW SUPPLIED
Liquid: 2.4 g sodium phosphate and 900 mg sodium biphosphate/5 ml◇
Enema: 160 mg/ml sodium phosphate and 60 mg/ml sodium biphosphate◇

ACTION
Mechanism: A saline laxative that produces an osmotic effect in the small intestine by drawing water into the intestinal lumen.
Absorption: About 1% to 20% of sodium and phosphate is absorbed; the extent of absorption is unknown.
Excretion: Mostly in the feces. Absorbed phosphate and sodium are excreted in the urine.
Onset, peak, duration: With oral administration, action begins in 3 to 6 hours; with enema administration, in 2 to 5 minutes.

INDICATIONS & DOSAGE
Constipation–
Adults: 5 to 20 ml liquid P.O. with water; or 4 g powder dissolved in warm water P.O.; or 20 to 30 ml solution mixed with 120 ml cold water P.O.; or 60 to 135 ml enema.

CONTRAINDICATIONS & PRECAUTIONS
Contraindicated in patients with fluid and electrolyte disturbances, impaired renal function, edema, or CHF and in other patients required to limit sodium intake; and in patients with appendicitis, abdominal pain, nausea or vomiting, fecal impaction, or intestinal obstruction or perforation, because the drug may

worsen the symptoms of these disorders.

Use cautiously in patients with large hemorrhoids or anal excoriation because of the potential for irritation.

ADVERSE REACTIONS

Common reactions are in italics; life-threatening reactions are in bold italics.
GI: *abdominal cramping.*
Metabolic: fluid and electrolyte disturbances (hypernatremia, hyperphosphatemia) if used daily.
Other: laxative dependence in long-term or excessive use.

INTERACTIONS

None significant.

EFFECTS ON DIAGNOSTIC TESTS

None reported.

NURSING CONSIDERATIONS

Besides those related universally to drug therapy (see "How to use this book"), consider the following specific recommendations:

Assessment

- Obtain a baseline assessment of history of bowel disorder, GI status, fluid intake, nutritional status, exercise habits, renal function, cardiovascular status, and normal pattern of elimination.
- Be alert for adverse reactions and drug interactions throughout therapy.
- Evaluate the patient's and family's knowledge about sodium phosphates therapy.

Nursing Diagnoses

- Constipation related to interruption of normal pattern of elimination characterized by infrequent or absent stools.
- Pain related to abdominal cramping caused by sodium phosphates.
- Knowledge deficit related to sodium phosphates therapy.

Planning and Implementation

Preparation and Administration

- Check order, and read drug label carefully.
- Available in oral or rectal forms.
- Mix powder with warm water.

Monitoring

- Monitor effectiveness by checking the frequency and characteristics of stools.
- Auscultate bowel sounds at least once a shift. Assess for pain and cramping.
- Monitor serum electrolytes with long-term use.
- Weigh patient daily while receiving sodium phosphates to detect fluid loss or retention.
- Monitor nutritional status and fluid balance.

Supportive Care

- Be aware that sodium phosphates is a saline laxative and up to 10% of the sodium content may be absorbed.
- Used in preparation for barium enema, sigmoidoscopy, and for the treatment of fecal impaction. Also prescribed to treat hypercalcemia or as a phosphate replacement.
- Provide privacy for elimination.
- Unless contraindicated, encourage fluid intake up to 2,500 ml a day.
- Consult with a dietitian to modify diet to increase fiber and bulk.

Patient Teaching

- Discourage excessive use of laxatives.
- Teach the patient about the relationship between fluid intake, dietary fiber, exercise, and constipation.
- Teach patient that dietary sources of fiber include bran and other cereals, fresh fruit, and vegetables.
- Warn patient that sodium phosphates may cause abdominal cramping.

Evaluation

In patients receiving sodium phosphates, appropriate evaluation statements may include:

• Patient reports return of normal pattern of elimination.
• Patient is free from abdominal cramping.
• Patient and family state an understanding of sodium phosphates therapy.

sodium polystyrene sulfonate
(pol ee stye´ reen)
Kayexalate, Resonium A, SPS

• *Classification:* potassium-removing resin (cation-exchange resin)
• *Pregnancy Risk Category:* C

HOW SUPPLIED
Oral powder: 1.25 g/5 ml suspension
Rectal: 1.25 g/5 ml suspension

ACTION
Mechanism: The potassium-removing resin exchanges sodium ions for potassium ions in the intestine: 1 g of sodium polystyrene sulfonate is exchanged for 0.5 to 1 mEq of potassium. The resin is then eliminated. Much of the exchange capacity is used for cations other than potassium (calcium and magnesium) and possibly for fats and proteins.
Absorption: Not absorbed.
Distribution: Drug remains in the intestine.
Metabolism: None.
Excretion: Unchanged in feces.
Onset, peak, duration: Onset of action varies from hours to days.

INDICATIONS & DOSAGE
Hyperkalemia –
Adults: 15 g P.O. daily to q.i.d. in water or sorbitol (3 to 4 ml/g of resin).

For rectal administration, 30 to 50 g/100 ml of sorbitol q 6 hours as warm emulsion deep into sigmoid colon (20 cm). In persistent vomiting or paralytic ileus, high retention enema of sodium polystyrene sulfonate (30 g) suspended in 200 ml of 10% methylcellulose, 10% dextrose, or 25% sorbitol solution.
Children: 1 g of resin P.O. for each mEq of potassium to be removed.

Oral administration preferred since drug should remain in intestine for at least 6 hours; otherwise, consider nasogastric administration.

For nasogastric administration, mix dose with appropriate medium–aqueous suspension or diet appropriate for renal failure; instill in plastic tube.

CONTRAINDICATIONS & PRECAUTIONS
Contraindicated in patients whose sodium intake must be restricted. Use cautiously in elderly patients; and those on digitalis therapy; with severe CHF, severe hypertension, or marked edema.

ADVERSE REACTIONS
Common reactions are in italics; life-threatening reactions are in bold italics.
GI: *constipation,* fecal impaction (in elderly patients), anorexia, gastric irritation, nausea, vomiting, *diarrhea (with sorbitol emulsions).*
Other: *hypokalemia,* hypocalcemia, hypomagnesemia, sodium retention.

INTERACTIONS
Antacids and laxatives (nonabsorbable cation-donating type, including magnesium hydroxide): systemic alkalosis, reduced potassium exchange capability. Don't use together.

EFFECTS ON DIAGNOSTIC TESTS
Serum magnesium and calcium: altered levels.

NURSING CONSIDERATIONS
Besides those related universally to drug therapy (see "How to use this

book"), consider the following specific recommendations:

Assessment

• Obtain a baseline assessment of serum potassium level, electrolytes, and ECG before therapy.

• Be alert for adverse reactions and drug interactions throughout therapy.

• Evaluate the patient's and family's knowledge about sodium polystyrene sulfonate therapy.

Nursing Diagnoses

• High risk for injury related to hyperkalemia.

• Altered GI tissue perfusion related to drug-induced fecal impaction.

• Knowledge deficit related to sodium polystyrene sulfonate therapy.

Planning and Implementation

Preparation and Administration

• Premixed forms are available (SPS and other).

• Do not heat resin. This will impair effectiveness of the drug.

• ***P.O. use:*** Mix resin only with water or sorbitol. Above all, *never* mix drug with orange juice (high potassium content) to disguise taste.

• Chill oral suspension for greater palatability.

• ***Rectal use:*** Give cleansing enema first. Mix drug only with water or sorbitol. Prepare at room temperature and stir gently during administration. Do not use other vehicles (mineral oil) for rectal administration to prevent impactions. Ion exchange requires aqueous medium. Sorbitol content prevents impaction.

• Use #28 French rubber tube for rectal dose; insert 20 cm into sigmoid colon. Tape tube in place. Alternatively, consider an indwelling urinary catheter with a 30-ml balloon inflated distal to anal sphincter to aid retention. This is especially helpful in patients with poor sphincter control, such as those who've had a CVA. Use gravity flow. Drain returns constantly through Y-tube connection. Place patient in knee-chest position or with hips up on pillows during administration to minimize back leakage.

• After rectal administration, flush tubing with 50 to 100 ml of nonsodium fluid to ensure delivery of all medication.

Monitoring

• Monitor effectiveness by checking serum potassium level at least once a day.

• Observe patient for signs of hypokalemia: irritability, confusion, cardiac arrhythmias, ECG changes, muscle weakness, some paralysis, and digitalis toxicity in some digitalized patients.

• Monitor blood pressure, fluid and electrolyte balance regularly.

• Monitor serum calcium in patients receiving sodium polystyrene therapy for more than 3 days. Supplementary calcium may be needed.

• Observe for signs of sodium overload (edema,decreased urine output); about one-third of resin's sodium content is retained.

• Check perianal skin for breakdown, especially where tube was taped in place.

• Observe for constipation in patients receiving oral or nasogastric administration.

Supportive Care

• Treat constipation with sorbitol (10 to 20 ml of 70% syrup every 2 hours as needed) to produce one to two watery stools per day.

• Provide good skin care, especially in the perianal area.

• Flush rectum to remove resin when therapy is completed.

• Consider solid form of resin. Resin cookie and candy recipes are available; consult pharmacist or dietitian.

• If hyperkalemia is severe, more drastic treatment should be added: for example, dextrose 50% with regular insulin I.V. push. Do not depend solely on polystyrene resin to lower serum potassium in severe hyperkalemia.

Patient Teaching
- Explain necessity of retaining the enema for at least 30 to 60 minutes and preferably for 6 to 10 hours.
- Advise patient that chilling the drug may make it more palatable, but stress importance of not mixing it with orange juice or any other fluid to mask taste.

Evaluation
In patients receiving sodium polystyrene sulfonate, evaluation statements may include:
- Patient is free from injury related to hyperkalemia.
- Patient is free from signs of fluid volume deficit.
- Patient and family state an understanding of sodium polystyrene sulfonate therapy.

sodium salicylate
(sal i´ sill ate)
Uracel-5◇

- *Classification:* nonnarcotic analgesic, antipyretic, anti-inflammatory (salicylate)
- *Pregnancy Risk Category:* C

HOW SUPPLIED
Tablets: 325 mg◇, 650 mg◇
Tablets (enteric-coated): 324 mg◇, 325 mg◇, 650 mg◇
Injection: 1 g/10 ml

ACTION
Mechanism: Inhibits prostaglandin synthesis. Reduces fever by an action on the hypothalamus. Reduces inflammation by blocking prostaglandin synthesis. Produces analgesia by an ill-defined effect on the CNS, by its anti-inflammatory effect, and by blocking generation of pain impulses in the periphery.
Absorption: Rapidly and almost completely absorbed (85% to 100%) from the GI tract.
Distribution: Widely distributed into most body tissues and fluids. Protein-binding is concentration-dependent, varies from 75% to 90%, and decreases as serum concentrations increase. Severe toxic side effects may occur at serum concentrations > 400 mcg/ml. Therapeutic blood salicylate concentrations for arthritis are 20 to 30 mg/100 ml.
Metabolism: Hydrolyzed in the liver.
Excretion: Excreted in urine.
Onset, peak, duration: Peak serum levels are seen after 4 to 6 hours.

INDICATIONS & DOSAGE
Minor pain or fever–
Adults: 325 to 650 mg P.O. q 4 to 6 hours, p.r.n., or 500 mg slow I.V. infusion over 4 to 8 hours. Maximum dosage is 1 g daily.
Arthritis–
Adults: 3.5 to 5.4 g P.O. daily in divided doses.

CONTRAINDICATIONS & PRECAUTIONS
Contraindicated in patients with GI ulcer, GI bleeding, or hypersensitivity to the drug or other nonsteroidal anti-inflammatory drugs (NSAIDs).

Use cautiously in patients with renal impairment, hypoprothrombinemia, vitamin K deficiency, and bleeding disorders; and in patients with CHF and hypertension because of the drug's sodium content.

Patients with known "triad" symptoms (aspirin hypersensitivity, rhinitis/nasal polyps, and asthma) are at high risk of bronchospasm because of cross-sensitivity to salicylates.

ADVERSE REACTIONS
Common reactions are in italics; life-threatening reactions are in bold italics.
EENT: *tinnitus, hearing loss.*
GI: *nausea, vomiting, GI distress.*
Hepatic: abnormal liver function studies, hepatitis.
Skin: *rash.*

Local: thrombophlebitis (from I.V.).
Other: *hypersensitivity manifested by **anaphylaxis*** or asthma.

INTERACTIONS

Ammonium chloride (and other urine acidifiers): increased blood levels of salicylates. Monitor for salicylate toxicity.
Antacids in large doses (and other urine alkalinizers): decreased levels of salicylates. Monitor for decreased salicylate effect.
Corticosteroids: enhance salicylate elimination. Monitor for decreased salicylate effect.
Oral anticoagulants: increased risk of bleeding. Avoid using together if possible.

EFFECTS ON DIAGNOSTIC TESTS

Serum uric acid: falsely increased levels.
Urinary vanillylmandelic acid or aceto-acetic acid (Gerhardt test): test interference.
Urine glucose with copper sulfate: false-positive results with high-dose (2.4 g/day) therapy; false-negative results with glucose enzymatic method.

NURSING CONSIDERATIONS

Besides those related universally to drug therapy (see "How to use this book"), consider the following specific recommendations:

Assessment

- Obtain a baseline assessment of pain before therapy.
- Be alert for adverse reactions and drug interactions throughout therapy.
- Evaluate the patient's and family's knowledge about sodium salicylate therapy.

Nursing Diagnoses

- Pain related to the patient's underlying condition.
- Altered nutrition: Less than body requirements, related to adverse GI reactions to sodium salicylate therapy.
- Knowledge deficit related to sodium salicylate therapy.

Planning and Implementation

Preparation and Administration

P.O. use: Give with food, milk, antacid, or large glass of water to reduce possible GI reactions.

- ***I.V. use:*** Infuse diluted drug *slowly* or over ordered time (usually 4 to 8 hours) through patent I.V. line, usually the primary line. Rapid infusion may cause thrombophlebitis and extravasation.
- Avoid use in children or teenagers with chicken pox or influenza-like illness as recommended by the Centers for Disease Control because of epidemiologic association with Reye's syndrome.
- Keep in mind that comcomitant use with alcohol, steroids, or other NSAIDs may increase risk of GI bleeding.

Monitoring

- Monitor effectiveness by regularly evaluating the patient's pain relief.
- Monitor the patient's blood salicylate level. Therapeutic level in arthritis is 10 to 30 mg/dl. With chronic therapy, mild toxicity may occur at plasma levels of 20 mg/dl. Tinnitus may occur at plasma levels of 30 mg/dl and above, but is not a reliable indicator of toxicity, especially in very young patients and those over age 60.
- Obtain hemoglobin and prothrombin tests periodically to help evaluate bleeding risk, especially during prolonged, high-dose therapy.
- Monitor the patient for toxicity. Febrile, dehydrated children can develop toxicity rapidly.

Supportive Care

- Keep in mind that this drug may cause an increase in serum levels of AST (SGOT), ALT (SGPT), alkaline phosphatase, and bilirubin and that abnormal liver function tests may also occur.
- Remember that, unlike aspirin, so-

dium salicylate does not inhibit platelet aggregation.

• Offer frequent small meals and encourage between-meal snacks if adverse GI reactions interfere with adequate nutrition.

Patient Teaching

• Advise the patient receiving prolonged treatment with large doses to watch for petechiae, bleeding gums, and signs of GI bleeding and to maintain adequate fluid intake. Encourage the use of a soft toothbrush.

• Explain that concomitant use with alcohol, steroids, or other NSAIDs may increase the risk of GI bleeding.

• Tell the patient taking the drug orally to take it with food, milk, an antacid, or a large glass of water to reduce possible GI reactions.

• Tell the patient to notify the doctor of GI reactions, tinnitus, or hearing loss.

Evaluation

In patients receiving sodium salicylate, appropriate evaluation statements may include:

• Patient states that sodium salicylate has relieved pain.

• Patient's nutitional status is unaffected by adverse GI reactions.

• Patient and family state an understanding of sodium salicylate therapy.

somatrem

(soe´ ma trem)

Protropin

• *Classification:* human growth hormone (anterior pituitary hormone)

• *Pregnancy Risk Category:* C

HOW SUPPLIED

Injectable lyophilized powder: 5 mg (10 IU)/vial

ACTION

Mechanism: Human growth hormone of recombinant DNA origin that stimulates linear, skeletal muscle, and organ growth.

Metabolism: Approximately 90% of a dose is metabolized in the liver.

Excretion: Approximately 0.1% of a dose is excreted in urine unchanged. Half-life: 20 to 30 minutes; however, tissue effects are long lasting.

INDICATIONS & DOSAGE

Long-term treatment of children who have growth failure because of lack of adequate endogenous growth hormone secretion–

Children (prepuberty): 0.1 mg/kg I.M. or S.C. given three times weekly.

CONTRAINDICATIONS & PRECAUTIONS

Contraindicated in patients with hypersensitivity to the drug or to benzyl alcohol, closed epiphyses (because the drug stimulates bone growth), or an intracranial lesion actively growing within the previous 12 months.

The drug's diabetogenic action requires that it be used cautiously in patients with a family history of diabetes. Untreated hypothyroidism may interfere with growth response to somatrem.

ADVERSE REACTIONS

Common reactions are in italics; life-threatening reactions are in bold italics.

Endocrine: *hypothyroidism, hyperglycemia.*

Other: *antibodies to growth hormone.*

INTERACTIONS

Glucocorticoids: may inhibit growth-promoting action of somatrem. Glucocorticoid dose may need to be adjusted.

EFFECTS ON DIAGNOSTIC TESTS

Glucose tolerance test: reduced with high doses.

Thyroid function tests: thyroxine-binding capacity and radioactive iodine uptake.

Total protein: altered results.

NURSING CONSIDERATIONS

Besides those related universally to drug therapy (see "How to use this book"), consider the following specific recommendations:

Assessment

• Obtain a baseline assessment of the child's growth pattern before initiating somatrem therapy.

• Be alert for adverse reactions and drug interactions throughout therapy.

• Evaluate the patient's and family's knowledge about somatrem therapy.

Nursing Diagnoses

• Altered growth and development related to lack of adequate endogenous growth hormone secretion.

• Altered health maintenance related to metabolic dysfunction caused by somatrem therapy.

• Knowledge deficit related to somatrem therapy.

Planning and Implementation

Preparation and Administration

• To prepare the solution, inject the bacteriostatic water for injection (which is supplied) into the vial containing the drug. Then swirl the vial with a gently rotary motion until the contents are completely dissolved. Don't shake the vial.

• After reconstitution, vial solution should be clear. Don't inject into the patient if the solution is cloudy or contains any particles.

• Store reconstituted vial in refrigerator. Must use within 7 days. Be sure to check the drug's expiration date before using.

Monitoring

• Monitor effectiveness through regular checkups of height and of blood and radiologic studies as ordered.

• Monitor patient for signs of glucose intolerance and hyperglycemia.

• Monitor periodic thyroid function tests for hypothyroidism, which may require treatment with a thyroid hormone.

Supportive Care

• Notify doctor if metabolic abnormalities occur and be prepared to provide supportive care.

Patient Teaching

• Stress importance of regular checkups.

• Inform patient and parents that drug is of no value for enhancing athletic performance.

• Teach patient and parents to watch for signs of glucose intolerance, hyperglycemia, and hypothyroidism and to notify doctor if they occur.

• Reassure patient and family that somatrem is pure and safe.

Evaluation

In patients receiving somatrem, appropriate evaluation statements may include:

• Patient demonstrates growth.

• Patient does not develop a metabolic abnormality.

• Patient and family state an understanding of somatrem therapy.

spectinomycin dihydrochloride

(spek ti noe mye´ sin)

Trobicin

• *Classification:* antibiotic (aminocyclitol)

• *Pregnancy Risk Category:* B

HOW SUPPLIED

Injection: 2-g vial with 3.2-ml diluent; 4-g vial with 6.2-ml diluent

Powder for injection: 2 g, 4 g

ACTION

Mechanism: Inhibits protein synthesis by binding to the 30S subunit of the ribosome.

Absorption: Not absorbed from the GI tract; rapidly absorbed following I.M. injection.

Distribution: Largely unknown. Drug is apparently not bound to plasma proteins.

Excretion: Most of dose is excreted unchanged in the urine. Half-life: Ranges from 1 to 3 hours. Drug dosage is unchanged in renal failure.
Onset, peak, duration: Peak concentrations occur in 1 and 2 hours for 2-g and 4-g doses, respectively.

INDICATIONS & DOSAGE

Gonorrhea –
Adults: 2 to 4 g I.M. single dose injected deeply into the upper outer quadrant of the buttock.

CONTRAINDICATIONS & PRECAUTIONS

Contraindicated in patients with hypersensitivity to the drug. Use cautiously in patients with strong history of drug allergies.

ADVERSE REACTIONS

Common reactions are in italics; life-threatening reactions are in bold italics.
CNS: insomnia, dizziness.
GI: nausea.
GU: decreased urine output.
Skin: urticaria.
Local: pain at injection site.
Other: fever, chills (may mask or delay symptoms of incubating syphilis).

INTERACTIONS

None significant.

EFFECTS ON DIAGNOSTIC TESTS

BUN, AST (SGOT), and serum alkaline phosphatase: increased levels.
Hemoglobin, hematocrit, and creatinine clearance: decreased levels.

NURSING CONSIDERATIONS

Besides those related universally to drug therapy (see "How to use this book"), consider the following specific recommendations:

Assessment
- Obtain a baseline assessment of infection before therapy.
- Be alert for adverse reactions and drug interactions throughout therapy.
- Evaluate the patient's and family's knowledge about spectinomycin therapy.

Nursing Diagnoses
- High risk for injury related to ineffectiveness of spectinomycin in eradicating the infection.
- High risk for fluid volume deficit related to spectinomycin-induced nausea.
- Knowledge deficit related to spectinomycin therapy.

Planning and Implementation
Preparation and Administration
- Obtain specimen for culture and sensitivity tests before first dose. Therapy may begin pending test results.
- Obtain serologic test for syphilis before administering first dose because drug may mask or delay symptoms of incubating syphilis.
- ***I.M. use:*** use a 20G needle to administer drug. The 4-g dose (10 ml) should be divided into two 5-ml injections – one in each buttock. Shake vial vigorously after reconstitution according to manufacturer's instructions and again before withdrawing the dose. Store at room temperature after reconstitution and use within 24 hours.

Monitoring
- Monitor effectiveness by regularly assessing for improvement in the infection.
- Monitor patient's hydration status if nausea occurs.

Supportive Care
- Obtain an order for an antiemetic as needed.

Patient Teaching
- Instruct the patient and family about spectinomycin, including the dose, frequency, action, and adverse reactions.

Evaluation
In patients receiving spectinomycin, appropriate evaluation statements may include:
- Patient is free from infection.

• Patient's maintains adequate hydration throughout therapy.
• Patient and family state an understanding of spectinomycin therapy.

spironolactone
(speer on oh lak´ tone)
Aldactone, Novospiroton†, Sincomen†, Spirotone‡

• *Classification:* antihypertensive, management of edema, diagnosis of primary hyperaldosteronism, treatment of diuretic-induced hypokalemia (potassium-sparing diuretic)
• *Pregnancy Risk Category:* D

HOW SUPPLIED
Tablets: 25 mg, 50 mg, 100 mg

ACTION
Mechanism: A potassium-sparing diuretic that antagonizes aldosterone in the distal tubule, increasing excretion of sodium and water but sparing potassium.
Absorption: About 90% is absorbed after oral administration.
Distribution: Spironolactone and its major active metabolite, canrenone, are more than 90% plasma protein-bound.
Metabolism: Rapidly and extensively metabolized to canrenone.
Excretion: Primarily in urine, and a small amount is excreted in feces via the biliary tract. Half-life: Of canrenone, 13 to 24 hours.
Onset, peak, duration: Gradual onset of action; maximum effect occurs on 3rd day of therapy.

INDICATIONS & DOSAGE
Edema –
Adults: 25 to 200 mg P.O. daily in divided doses.
Children: initially, 3.3 mg/kg P.O. daily in divided doses.
Hypertension –
Adults: 50 to 100 mg P.O. daily in divided doses.
Treatment of diuretic-induced hypokalemia –
Adults: 25 to 100 mg P.O. daily when oral potassium supplements are considered inappropriate.
Detection of primary hyperaldosteronism –
Adults: 400 mg P.O. daily for 4 days (short test) or 3 to 4 weeks (long test). If hypokalemia and hypertension are corrected, a presumptive diagnosis of primary hyperaldosteronism is made.

CONTRAINDICATIONS & PRECAUTIONS
Contraindicated in patients with serum potassium levels above 5.5 mEq/liter; in those who are receiving other potassium-sparing diuretics or potassium supplements because these drugs conserve potassium and can cause severe hyperkalemias; in patients with anuria, acute or chronic renal insufficiency, or diabetic nephropathy because of risk of hyperkalemia; and in patients with hypersensitivity to the drug.

Use cautiously in patients with severe hepatic insufficiency because electrolyte imbalance may precipitate hepatic encephalopathy and in patients with diabetes, who are at increased risk of hyperkalemia.

ADVERSE REACTIONS
Common reactions are in italics; life-threatening reactions are in bold italics.
CNS: headache.
GI: anorexia, nausea, diarrhea.
Metabolic: *hyperkalemia,* dehydration, hyponatremia, transient elevation in BUN, acidosis.
Skin: urticaria.
Other: gynecomastia in men, breast soreness and menstrual disturbances in women.

INTERACTIONS

ACE inhibitors, potassium supplements: concomitant use may result in hyperkalemia. Don't use together.
Aspirin: possible blocked spironolactone effect. Watch for diminished spironolactone response.
Digoxin: may alter digoxin clearance and increase risk of toxicity. Monitor digoxin levels.

EFFECTS ON DIAGNOSTIC TESTS

Plasma and urinary 17-hydroxycorticosteroids: altered levels with fluorometric determinations.
Serum digoxin: false elevations on radioimmunoassay.

NURSING CONSIDERATIONS

Besides those related universally to drug therapy (see "How to use this book"), consider the following specific recommendations:

Assessment

- Obtain a baseline assessment of blood pressure, urine output, weight, serum electrolytes, and peripheral edema before initiating spironolactone therapy.
- Be alert for adverse reactions and drug interactions throughout therapy.
- Evaluate the patient's and family's knowledge about spironolactone therapy.

Nursing Diagnoses

- Fluid volume excess related to sodium and fluid retention.
- High risk for injury related to hyperkalemia due to spironolactone therapy.
- Knowledge deficit related to spironolactone therapy.

Planning and Implementation

Preparation and Administration

- ***P.O. use:*** Give spironolactone with meals to enhance absorption.

Monitoring

- Monitor effectiveness by regularly checking urine output, blood pressure, weight, and evidence of edema.
- Monitor BUN levels and serum electrolytes, especially potassium.
- Monitor for signs of hyperkalemia: muscle weakness and cramps, paresthesia, diarrhea, and cardiac arrhythmias.
- Monitor skin turgor and mucous membranes for signs of fluid volume depletion.

Supportive Care

- Hold drug and notify the doctor if hyperkalemia or dehydration occurs.
- Keep accurate record of intake and output, and blood pressure.
- Weigh the patient daily.
- Provide frequent skin and mouth care to relieve dryness due to diuretic therapy.
- Answer the patient's call bells promptly; make sure patient's bathroom or bedpan is easily accessible.
- Use safety precautions to prevent the risk of injury due to falls.
- Elevate the patient's legs to reduce peripheral edema.

Patient Teaching

- Teach the patient and family to identify and report signs of hyperkalemia.
- Teach the patient and family to monitor the patient's fluid volume by recording daily weight and intake and output.
- Advise the patient to avoid excessive intake of high-potassium foods and potassium-containing sodium substitutes.
- Instruct the patient to avoid concomitant use of potassium supplements.
- Advise the patient to change positions slowly, especially when rising to a standing position, to avoid dizziness and fainting due to orthostatic hypotension.
- Tell the patient to take spironolactone with meals and, if possible, early in the day to avoid interruption of sleep due to nocturia.

Evaluation

In patients receiving spironolactone, appropriate evaluation statements may include:
- Patient is free of edema.
- Patient's serum potassium remains within normal range.
- Patient and family state an understanding of spironolactone therapy.

stanozolol

(stan oh´ zoe lole)
Winstrol

- Controlled Substance Schedule III
- *Classification:* angioedema prophylactic (anabolic steroid)
- *Pregnancy Risk Category:* X

HOW SUPPLIED

Tablets: 2 mg

ACTION

Mechanism: An anabolic steroid that stimulates cytosol steroid receptors in tissues to effect protein synthesis. Also stimulates erythropoiesis.
Pharmacokinetics: Unknown.

INDICATIONS & DOSAGE

Prevention of hereditary angioedema –
Adults: 2 mg P.O. t.i.d. to 4 mg P.O. q.i.d for 5 days initially. Dosage is gradually reduced at intervals of 1 to 3 months to a dosage of 2 mg daily.
Children age 6 to 12: Administer up to 2 mg P.O. daily.
Children under age 6: 1 mg. P.O. daily

Note: Stanozolol should be used in children only during an acute attack.

CONTRAINDICATIONS & PRECAUTIONS

Contraindicated in patients with severe renal or cardiac disease, which may be worsened by the fluid and electrolyte retention this drug may cause; hepatic disease, because impaired elimination may cause toxic accumulation of the drug; in male patients with breast cancer, benign prostatic hypertrophy with obstruction, or undiagnosed abnormal genital bleeding, because this drug can stimulate the growth of cancerous breast or prostate tissue in males; and in pregnant women because animal studies have shown that administration of anabolic steroids during pregnancy causes masculinization of the fetus. Because of its hypercholesterolemic effects, administer cautiously in patients with a history of coronary artery disease.

ADVERSE REACTIONS

Common reactions are in italics; life-threatening reactions are in bold italics.
Androgenic: in women – *acne, edema, oily skin, weight gain, hirsutism, hoarseness,* clitoral enlargement, decreased or increased libido. In men – prepubertal: premature epiphyseal closure, acne, priapism, growth of body and facial hair, phallic enlargement; postpubertal: testicular atrophy, oligospermia, decreased ejaculatory volume, impotence, gynecomastia, epididymitis.
CV: edema.
GI: gastroenteritis, nausea, vomiting, constipation, diarrhea, change in appetite.
GU: bladder irritability.
Hepatic: reversible jaundice, hepatotoxicity.
Hypoestrogenic: in women – flushing; sweating; vaginitis with itching, drying, burning or bleeding; menstrual irregularities.
Other: hypercalcemia.

INTERACTIONS

None significant.

EFFECTS ON DIAGNOSTIC TESTS

Fasting plasma glucose, glucose tolerance test, and metyrapone test: abnormal results.
17-ketosteroid levels: may decrease.
Liver function tests and serum creatinine levels: results may be elevated.
Prothrombin time (especially during anticoagulant therapy): prolonged.
Serum sodium, potassium, calcium, phosphate, and cholesterol: elevated levels.
Sulfobromophthalein retention: increased.
Thyroid function test results (protein-bound iodine, radioactive iodine uptake, thyroid-binding capacity): possibly decreased.

NURSING CONSIDERATIONS

Besides those related universally to drug therapy (see "How to use this book"), consider the following specific recommendations:

Assessment

• Obtain a baseline assessment of the patient's history of hereditary angioedema before initiating stanozolol therapy.
• Be alert for adverse reactions and drug interactions throughout therapy.
• Evaluate the patient's and family's knowledge about stanozolol therapy.

Nursing Diagnoses

• High risk for injury related to the patient's underlying condition.
• Body image disturbance related to adverse androgenic reactions associated with stanozolol.
• Knowledge deficit related to stanozolol therapy.

Planning and Implementation

Preparation and Administration

• Check that in children, therapy is preceded by X-ray of wrist bones to establish level of bone maturation. During treatment, bone maturation may proceed more rapidly than linear growth; dosage should be intermittent and X-rays taken periodically.
• Be aware that a lower dosage is recommended in younger women (2 mg b.i.d.) to avoid virilization.
• Be aware that stanozolol should be used in children only during an acute attack.
• ***P.O. use:*** Administer with food or meals if GI upset occurs.

Monitoring

• Monitor effectiveness by regularly assessing severity and incidence of angioedema attacks.
• Monitor female patients for signs of virilization and menstrual irregularities.
• Monitor for jaundice, which may be reversed by dosage adjustment. Periodic liver function tests should be performed.
• Monitor the patient receiving concomitant anticoagulant therapy for ecchymotic areas, petechiae, or abnormal bleeding. Monitor prothrombin time.
• Monitor boys under age 7 for precocious sexual development.
• Monitor the patient's weight routinely for fluid retention.
• Monitor for symptoms of hypoglycemia in patients with diabetes. Check blood glucose levels regularly.
• Monitor serum cholesterol in cardiac patients.

Supportive Care

• Promptly report signs of menstrual irregularities and virilization in females. They require re-evaluation of therapy. Be aware that virilization effects may be irreversible despite prompt discontinuation of the drug.
• Give the patient a diet high in calories and protein, unless contraindicated. Give small frequent feedings. Also implement salt restriction if edema occurs; expect to administer a diuretic concurrently, if needed.
• Carefully evaluate results of laboratory studies. Many laboratory results may be altered during therapy and for 2 to 3 weeks after therapy ends.
• Obtain an order for an antiemetic,

antidiarrheal, or laxative, as indicated.
• Prepare patient for altered body image if androgenic adverse reactions occur.
• Be prepared to treat hypoglycemia in diabetic patients and notify doctor because it may require adjustments in the patient's antidiabetic regimen.
Patient Teaching
• Tell the patient to take drug with food or meals if GI upset occurs.
• Tell female patients to report menstrual irregularities; therapy should be discontinued pending etiologic determination.
• Explain to female patients that virilization may occur. Tell them to report it immediately.
• Stress importance of not abusing drug to enhance athletic performance.
• Instruct patient to eat a diet high in calories and protein and low in sodium, if not contraindicated, and to eat small frequent meals.
• Advise the diabetic patient about increased risk of hypoglycemia; instruct him how to manage symptoms if present and to notify doctor.
Evaluation
In patients receiving stanozolol, appropriate evaluation statements may include:
• Patient does not experience an angioedema attack.
• Patient states acceptance of body image changes caused by stanozolol therapy.
• Patient and family state an understanding of stanozolol therapy.

streptokinase
(strep toe kye´ nase)
Kabikinase, Streptase

• *Classification:* thrombolytic enzyme (plasminogen activator)
• *Pregnancy Risk Category:* C

HOW SUPPLIED
Injection: 100,000 IU, 250,000 IU, 600,000 IU, 750,000 IU, 1,500,000 IU in vials for reconstitution

ACTION
Mechanism: Activates plasminogen in two steps: Plasminogen and streptokinase form a complex that exposes the plasminogen-activating site. Plasminogen is converted to plasmin by cleavage of the peptide bond. Plasmin catalyzes the dissolution of the fibrin clot.
Distribution: Forms a plasminogen-streptokinase complex within the plasma.
Metabolism: Partially inactivated by antistreptococcal antibodies.
Excretion: Half-life: About 23 minutes.
Onset, peak, duration: Most patients experience reperfusion within 2 hours of the start of an infusion.

INDICATIONS & DOSAGE
Arteriovenous cannula occlusion—
Adults: 250,000 IU in 2 ml I.V. solution by I.V. pump infusion into each occluded limb of the cannula over 25 to 35 minutes. Clamp off cannula for 2 hours. Then aspirate contents of cannula; flush with saline solution and reconnect.
Venous thrombosis, pulmonary embolism, and arterial thrombosis and embolism—
Adults: loading dose is 250,000 IU I.V. infusion over 30 minutes. Sustaining dose is 100,000 IU/hour I.V. infusion for 72 hours for deep vein thrombosis and 100,000 IU/hour over 24 to 72 hours by I.V. infusion pump for pulmonary embolism.
Lysis of coronary artery thrombi following acute myocardial infarction—
Adults: loading dose is 20,000 IU via coronary catheter, followed by a

maintenance dose. Maintenance dose is 2,000 IU/minute for 60 minutes as an infusion. Alternatively, may be administered as an I.V. infusion. Usual adult dose is 1.5 million units infused over 60 minutes.

CONTRAINDICATIONS & PRECAUTIONS

Contraindicated in patients with ulcerative wounds, active internal bleeding, recent trauma with possible internal injuries, visceral or intracranial malignancy, ulcerative colitis, diverticulitis, severe hypertension, acute or chronic hepatic or renal insufficiency, uncontrolled hypocoagulation, chronic pulmonary disease with cavitation, subacute bacterial endocarditis or rheumatic valvular disease, recent cerebral embolism, thrombosis or hemorrhage, and diabetic hemorrhagic retinopathy because excessive bleeding may occur.

Use with extreme caution during pregnancy or 10 days postpartum and for 10 days after any intracranial, intraspinal, or intra-arterial diagnostic procedure or any surgery, including liver or kidney biopsy, lumbar puncture, thoracentesis, paracentesis, or extensive or multiple cutdowns. Use reasonable caution when treating patients with arterial emboli originating from left side of heart because of risk of cerebral infarction.

ADVERSE REACTIONS

Common reactions are in italics; life-threatening reactions are in bold italics.
Blood: bleeding, low hematocrit.
CV: transient lowering or elevation of blood pressure.
EENT: periorbital edema.
Skin: urticaria.
Local: phlebitis at injection site.
Other: ***hypersensitivity to drug,*** *fever,* ***anaphylaxis,*** musculoskeletal pain, minor breathing difficulty, bronchospasms, angioneurotic edema.

INTERACTIONS

Anticoagulants: concurrent use with streptokinase is not recommended. Reversing the effects of oral anticoagulants must be considered before beginning therapy; heparin may be stopped and its effect allowed to diminish.
Aspirin, dipyridamole, indomethacin, phenylbutazone, drugs affecting platelet activity: increased risk of bleeding. Combined therapy with low-dose aspirin (162.5 mg) or dipyridamole has improved acute and long-term results.

EFFECTS ON DIAGNOSTIC TESTS

Hematocrit: moderately decreased.
Thrombin time, activated partial thromboplastin time (APTT), and prothrombin time (PT): increased.

NURSING CONSIDERATIONS

Besides those related universally to drug therapy (see "How to use this book"), consider the following specific recommendations:

Assessment
- Obtain a baseline assessment of ECG, vital signs, PT, and APTT before therapy.
- Be alert for adverse reactions and drug interactions throughout therapy.
- Evaluate the patient's and family's knowledge about streptokinase therapy.

Nursing Diagnoses
- Altered tissue perfusion related to the patient's underlying condition.
- Fluid volume deficit related to the adverse effects of streptokinase therapy.
- Knowledge deficit related to streptokinase therapy.

Planning and Implementation
Preparation and Administration
- ***Direct injection:*** To clear arteriovenous cannula obstruction, reconstitute using 2 ml of 0.9% sodium chloride injection or dextrose 5% injection for each 250,000 IU of streptoki-

nase. Add diluent slowly, directed at the side of the vial (rather than onto the powder). Roll and tilt the vial gently; avoid shaking, which may cause foaming and an increase in flocculation. Slight flocculation doesn't interfere with safe use; however, solutions containing many particles should be discarded. Use an infusion pump to slowly deliver 250,000 IU of reconstituted drug into each occluded cannula over 25 to 35 minutes. Then clamp off the cannula(s) for 2 hours. After 2 hours, aspirate contents of the cannula(s) and flush with 0.9% sodium chloride. Reconnect cannula.

• ***Continuous infusion:*** Reconstitute with 0.9% sodium chloride injection or dextrose 5% injection. Further dilute generally to a volume of 45 ml (loading dose infusion) or to a multiple of 45 ml to a maximum of 500 ml (continuous maintenance infusion), with the same solution used for reconstitution. Infusions should be administered through a 0.22- or 0.45-micron filter. Use volumetric or syringe pumps because reconstituted streptokinase solution may alter drop size, influencing the accuracy of drop counting infusion devices. For loading dose in pulmonary embolism, deep vein thronbosis, or arterial embolism or thrombosis, give diluted drug through a peripheral I.V. line, using an infusion pump to deliver 250,000 IU over 30 minutes. Set rate at 30 ml/hour (for 750,000 IU vial) or 90 ml/hour (for 250,000 IU vial) with dilution equaling 45 ml. For maintenance dose, set infusion pump to deliver 100,000 IU/hour. Continue infusion for 24 to 72 hours for arterial embolism or thrombosis, and 72 hours for deep vein thrombosis. For coronary artery thrombi, give diluted drug through a peripheral I.V. line, using an infusion pump with the rate set at 1.5 million IU/hour for 1 hour. No maintenance dose required.

• ***Intermittent infusion:*** Not recommended.

Monitoring

• Monitor effectiveness by carefully checking vital signs and clotting status.

• Monitor the patient's percutaneous puncture sites and cuts for oozing because streptokinase may lyse fibrin deposits at these sites. Watch carefully and frequently for any bleeding.

Supportive Care

• Remember to avoid I.M. injections. Perform venipunctures carefully and infrequently if possible. Avoid invasive arterial procedures before and during therapy. Use an upper extremity if necessary.

• Keep in mind that the loading dose is used to neutralize the antibodies present in many patients because exposure to streptococci (source of streptokinase) is common. Determine patient resistance to streptokinase to help establish dose. Don't give loading dose greater than 1 million IU.

• Remember that heparin isn't recommended during streptokinase therapy but may be used soon afterward to minimize the risk of recurrent thrombosis and pulmonary emboli.

• Be aware that blood pressure should not be taken in the lower extremities to avoid dislodging deep venous thrombi.

• Try to avoid excessive moving and handling of the patient; pad the side rails since bruising is more likely during therapy.

Patient Teaching

• Tell the patient to report any oozing or bleeding immediately.

• Teach the patient to report any changes in heart rate or rhythm, dyspnea, headache, hematuria, hematemesis, nausea, back pain, abdominal pain, muscle pain, rash, or swelling.

Evaluation

In patients receiving streptokinase, appropriate evaluation statements may include:

• Patient has improved or stabilized cardiovascular status.
• Patient has not experienced injury from excessive blood loss related to the adverse effects of streptokinase.
• Patient and family state an understanding of streptokinase therapy.

streptomycin sulfate
(strep toe mye´ sin)

• *Classification:* antibiotic (aminoglycoside)
• *Pregnancy Risk Category:* D

HOW SUPPLIED
Injection: 400 mg/ml, 500 mg/ml, 1-g vial, 5-g vial

ACTION
Mechanism: Inhibits protein synthesis by binding directly to the 30S ribosomal subunit of susceptible bacteria. Generally bactericidal.
Absorption: Poorly absorbed after oral administration and is given parenterally. Peak blood levels occur within 2 hours of I.M. administration.
Distribution: Widely distributed after parenteral administration; intraocular penetration is poor. CSF penetration is low, even in patients with inflamed meninges. Streptomycin crosses the placenta; it is 36% protein-bound.
Metabolism: Not metabolized.
Excretion: Primarily excreted in urine by glomerular filtration; small amounts may be excreted in bile and breast milk. Half-life: 2 to 3 hours in adults; extends to 110 hours in severe renal damage.
Onset, peak, duration: Peak serum concentration occurs 1 to 2 hours after I.M. administrtion.

INDICATIONS & DOSAGE
Streptococcal endocarditis–
Adults: 10 mg/kg I.M. (maximum 0.5 g) q 12 hours for 2 weeks with penicillin.
Primary and adjunctive treatment in tuberculosis–
Adults: with normal renal function, 1 g I.M. daily for 2 to 3 months, then 1 g 2 or 3 times a week. Inject deeply into upper outer quadrant of buttocks.
Children: with normal renal function, 20 mg/kg daily in divided doses injected deeply into large muscle mass. Give concurrently with other antitubercular agents, but *not* with capreomycin, and continue until sputum specimen becomes negative.
Patients with impaired renal function: initial dose is same as for those with normal renal function. Subsequent doses and frequency determined by renal function study results.
Enterococcal endocarditis–
Adults: 1 g I.M. q 12 hours for 2 weeks, then 500 mg I.M. q 12 hours for 4 weeks with penicillin.
Tularemia–
Adults: 1 to 2 g I.M. daily in divided doses injected deep into upper outer quadrant of buttocks. Continue until patient is afebrile for 5 to 7 days.

CONTRAINDICATIONS & PRECAUTIONS
Contraindicated in patients with hypersensitivity to streptomycin or any aminoglycoside. Use cautiously in patients with: decreased renal function; tinnitus, vertigo, and high-frequency hearing loss who are susceptible to ototoxicity; dehydration, myasthenia gravis, parkinsonism, and hypocalcemia; and in neonates and other infants, and elderly patients.

ADVERSE REACTIONS
Common reactions are in italics; life-threatening reactions are in bold italics.
CNS: ***neuromuscular blockade.***

EENT: *ototoxicity (tinnitus, vertigo, hearing loss).*
GU: some nephrotoxicity (not nearly as frequent as with other aminoglycosides).
Local: pain, irritation, and sterile abscesses at injection site.
Skin: ***exfoliative dermatitis.***
Other: ***hypersensitivity*** (rash, fever, urticaria, and angioneurotic edema), headache, ***transient agranulocytosis.***

INTERACTIONS

Cephalothin: increases nephrotoxicity. Use together cautiously.
Dimenhydrinate: may mask symptoms of streptomycin-induced ototoxicity. Use together cautiously.
General anesthetics, neuromuscular blocking agents: may potentiate neuromuscular blockade.
I.V. loop diuretics (e.g. furosemide): increased ototoxicity. Use cautiously.

EFFECTS ON DIAGNOSTIC TESTS

BUN, nonprotein nitrogen, or serum creatinine levels: elevated levels and increased excretion of casts.
Urine glucose: false-positive reaction with copper sulfate (Benedict's reagent or Clinitest).

NURSING CONSIDERATIONS

Besides those related universally to drug therapy (see "How to use this book"), consider the following specific recommendations:

Assessment
- Obtain a baseline assessment of infection before therapy.
- Be alert for adverse reactions and drug interactions throughout therapy.
- Evaluate the patient's and family's knowledge about streptomycin therapy.

Nursing Diagnoses
- High risk for injury related to ineffectiveness of streptomycin in eradicating the infection.
- Sensory/perceptual alterations (auditory) related to streptomycin-induced ototoxicity.
- Knowledge deficit related to streptomycin.

Planning and Implementation
Preparation and Administration
- Obtain specimen for culture and sensitivity tests before first dose except when treating tuberculosis. Therapy may begin pending test results.
- Evaluate patient's hearing before therapy begins.
- Protect hands when preparing. Drug is irritating.
- ***I.M. use:*** Administer drug deep I.M. into upper outer quadrant of buttocks.
- When used to treat primary tuberculosis expect to discontinue streptomycin when sputum is negative.

Monitoring
- Monitor effectiveness by regularly assessing patient for improvement of infection.
- To monitor serum streptomycin level, draw blood for peak streptomycin level 1 to 2 hours after I.M. injection; for trough levels, just before next dose. Don't use a heparinized tube because heparin is incompatible with aminoglycosides.
- Monitor patient's hearing during therapy and for 6 months after therapy.

Supportive Care
- Notify doctor if patient complains of roaring noises, fullness in ears or hearing loss.
- Encourage patient to consume 2,000 ml of fluid daily (if not contraindicated) during therapy to minimize chemical irritation of the renal tubules.

Patient Teaching
- Emphasize the need to drink 2,000 ml of fluid each day, not including coffee, tea, or other caffeinated beverages.
- Instruct the patient to notify the doctor immediately if hearing loss,

roaring noises, or fullness in ears occurs.
• Tell the patient to alert the doctor if infection worsens or does not improve.
• Stress the importance of recommended blood tests to monitor streptomycin level and determine the effectiveness of therapy.
• Teach patient to recognize and promptly report the signs and symptoms of superinfection (continued fever and other signs of new infection, especially if upper respiratory tract).

Evaluation
In patients receiving streptomycin, appropriate evaluation statements may include:
• Patient is free of infection.
• Patient's auditory function remains normal throughout therapy.
• Patient and family state an understanding of streptomycin therapy.

streptozocin
(strep toe zoe´ sin)
Zanosar

• *Classification:* antineoplastic (alkylating agent, nitrosourea)
• *Pregnancy Risk Category:* C

HOW SUPPLIED
Injection: 1-g vials

ACTION
Mechanism: An alkylating agent that cross-links strands of cellular DNA and interferes with RNA transcription, causing an imbalance of growth that leads to cell death. Cell cycle–nonspecific.
Absorption: Not active orally and must be given I.V.
Distribution: Parent drug and metabolites distribute mainly into the liver, kidneys, intestines, and pancreas. The drug has not been shown to cross the blood-brain barrier; however, its metabolites achieve CSF concentrations equivalent to the plasmaconcentration.
Metabolism: Extensively metabolized in the liver and kidneys. Chemical structures of the metabolites are not known, and it is not known if the metabolites are pharmacologically active.
Excretion: The drug and its metabolites are primarily excreted in urine. A small amount of a dose may also be excreted in expired air. Half-life: Biphasic; elimination: initial half-life, 5 minutes; terminal elimination half-life, 35 to 40 minutes. Metabolites exhibit triphasic elimination: initial half-life is about 5 minutes; second phase, about 3½ hours; and terminal elimination half-life, over 40 hours.

INDICATIONS & DOSAGE
Treatment of metastatic islet cell carcinoma of the pancreas; colon cancer; exocrine pancreatic tumors; and carcinoid tumors–
Adults and children: 500 mg/m² I.V. for 5 consecutive days q 6 weeks until maximum benefit or until toxicity is observed. Alternatively, 1,000 mg/m² at weekly intervals for the first 2 weeks. Don't exceed a single dose of 1,500 mg/m².

CONTRAINDICATIONS & PRECAUTIONS
No contraindications known. Use cautiously in patients with renal or hepatic dysfunction or hematologic compromise. Dosage adjustments are necessary.

ADVERSE REACTIONS
Common reactions are in italics; life-threatening reactions are in bold italics.
Blood: *leukopenia,* ***thrombocytopenia.***
GI: *nausea, vomiting,* diarrhea.
Hepatic: elevated liver enzymes.
Metabolic: hyperglycemia and hypoglycemia.
Renal: ***renal toxicity*** *(evidenced by*

azotemia, glycosuria, and renal tubular acidosis), mild proteinuria.
Local: *sloughing, severe irritation if extravasation occurs.*

INTERACTIONS

Doxorubicin: prolonged elimination half-life of doxorubicin if administered with streptozocin. Dose of doxorubicin should be reduced.
Other potentially nephrotoxic drugs such as aminoglycosides: increased risk of renal toxicity. Use cautiously.
Phenytoin: may decrease the effects of streptozocin. Monitor carefully.

EFFECTS ON DIAGNOSTIC TESTS

Blood glucose: decreased levels because of a sudden release of insulin.
BUN and serum creatinine: increased levels.
Liver function tests: increased values.
Serum albumin: decreased.

NURSING CONSIDERATIONS

Besides those related universally to drug therapy (see "How to use this book"), consider the following specific recommendations:

Assessment
- Obtain a baseline assessment of the patient's underlying condition and CBC, BUN, creatinine, electrolytes, glucose and liver enzyme levels, urinalysis results and creatinine clearance test results.
- Be alert for adverse reactions and drug interactions throughout therapy.
- Evaluate the patient's and family's knowledge about streptozocin therapy.

Nursing Diagnoses
- Impaired tissue perfusion related to streptozocin-induced adverse drug reactions.
- High risk for injury related to nephrotoxic adverse reactions.
- Knowledge deficit related to streptozocin therapy.

Planning and Implementation
Preparation and Administration
- Expect to administer lower doses in renal, hepatic, or hematopoietic impairment.
- Antiemetics may be given preceding or during infusion of this drug to decrease severe nausea and vomiting.
- Keep I.V. dextrose available, especially with the first dose of streptozocin, because of the risk of hypoglycemia.
- ***I.V. use:*** Exercise caution when preparing and administering this drug to avoid mutagenic, teratogenic, and carcinogenic risks. Use a biological containment cabinet, wear gloves and mask, and avoid contaminating work surfaces. Reconstitute with 0.9% sodium chloride to make a pale gold solution. It's best to use the reconstituted drug within 12 hours after reconstitution. However, the drug will remain stable for at least 48 hours if refrigerated. Avoid drug contact with skin. If contact occurs, wash the area liberally with soap and water.

For direct infusion, rapidly inject reconstituted drug through port of primary I.V. line containing a free-flowing compatible solution. For intermittent infusion, infuse the diluted drug over ordered duration (usually 15 minutes to 6 hours) via I.V. line containing a free-flowing compatible solution.

For continuous infusion, infuse diluted drug over ordered duration. Continuous 5 day I.V. infusions have been given, but prolonged continuous administration may cause CNS toxicity.

Monitoring
- Monitor for nephrotoxicity by noting results of follow-up diagnostic tests and overall physicall status.
- Monitor renal function test results for 4 weeks after each course of drug therapy. Mild proteinuria seems to be the earliest sign of streptozocin-induced nephrotoxicity.

• Monitor daily serum glucose levels to identify occurrence of hypoglycemia.
• Monitor for signs of bleeding (hematuria, ecchymosis, petechia, epistaxis, melena).
• Monitor for signs of infection (temperature elevation, sore throat, malaise).
• Monitor CBC and hepatic function weekly during and after the therapy.
• Monitor intake and output during drug therapy.
• Monitor urine for protein and glucose each shift. Report proteinuria to doctor.

Supportive Care

• If extravasation occurs, immediately stop the infusion, apply cold compresses to the area and elevate the arm. In some cases, administration of the drug is completed in another vein.
• Encourage fluid intake to aid clearance of active metabolites.
• Avoid giving the patient anticoagulants and aspirin products, if possible. If one of these products must be used, administer with extreme caution.
• Administer antiemetic as required. Nausea and vomiting occur in almost all patients.
• Remember that therapeutic effects are often accompanied by toxicity. Renal toxicity is dose-related and cumulative.
• Do not give any I.M. injections when the platelet count is less than $100,000/mm^3$.

Patient Teaching

• Warn patients to watch for signs of infection (sore throat, fever, fatigue) and for signs of bleeding (easy bruising, nosebleeds, bleeding gums). Tell him to take his temperature daily.
• Teach patient to avoid the use of all OTC products containing aspirin.
• Review all possible adverse reactions with the patient. Explain how to prevent or decrease their severity and when to notify the doctor.

Evaluation

In patients receiving streptozocin, appropriate evaluation statements may include:

• Tissue perfusion was adequate during drug therapy.
• Adequate renal function was maintained throughout streptozocin therapy.
• Patient and family state an understanding of streptozocin therapy.

succinylcholine chloride (suxamethonium chloride)

(suk sin ill koe´ leen)

Anectine, Anectine Flo-Pack, Quelicin, Scoline‡, Sucostrin

• *Classification:* skeletal muscle relaxant (depolarizing neuromuscular blocking agent)
• *Pregnancy Risk Category:* C

HOW SUPPLIED

Injection: 20 mg/ml, 50 mg/ml, 100 mg/ml; 100 mg/vial, 500 mg/vial, 1 g/vial

ACTION

Mechanism: A depolarizing agent that activates nicotinic receptors at the muscle end plate. Prolonged depolarization leads to paralysis.
Absorption: Rapidly absorbed after I.M. injection. Drug is usually administered I.V.
Distribution: After I.V. administration, it is distributed in extracellular fluid and rapidly reaches its site of action. It crosses the placenta.
Metabolism: Rapidly hydrolyzed by plasma pseudocholinesterase to choline and succinylmonocholine, which has nondepolarizing activity and is only 5% as active as succinylcholine.
Excretion: About 10% is excreted unchanged in urine.

Onset, peak, duration: After I.V. bolus administration, succinylcholine has a rapid onset of action (30 seconds), reaches its peak within 1 minute, and persists for 2 to 3 minutes, gradually dissipating within 10 minutes.

INDICATIONS & DOSAGE

Adjunct to anesthesia to induce skeletal muscle relaxation; facilitate intubation and assist with mechanical ventilation or orthopedic manipulations (drug of choice); lessen muscle contractions in pharmacologically or electrically induced seizures–

Dosage depends on anesthetic used, individual needs, and response. Dosages are representative and must be adjusted.

Adults: 25 to 75 mg I.V., then 2.5 mg/minute, p.r.n., or 2.5 mg/kg I.M. up to maximum of 150 mg I.M. in deltoid muscle.

Children: 1 to 2 mg/kg I.M. or I.V. Maximum I.M. dosage is 150 mg. (Children may be less sensitive to succinylcholine than adults.)

CONTRAINDICATIONS & PRECAUTIONS

Contraindicated in patients with abnormally low plasma pseudocholinesterase. Use cautiously in patients with personal or family history of malignant hypertension or hyperthermia; hepatic, renal, or pulmonary impairment; or respiratory depression, severe burns or trauma, electrolyte imbalances, and in patients receiving quinidine or digitalis therapy. Also use cautiously in patients with hyperkalemia, paraplegia, spinal neuraxis injury, degenerative or dystrophic neuromuscular disease, myasthenia gravis, myasthenic syndrome of lung cancer or bronchogenic carcinoma, dehydration, thyroid disorders, collagen diseases, porphyria, fractures, muscle spasms, glaucoma, eye surgery or penetrating eye wounds, pheochromocytoma, and (in large doses) cesarean section; and in elderly or debilitated patients.

ADVERSE REACTIONS

Common reactions are in italics; life-threatening reactions are in bold italics.

CV: bradycardia, tachycardia, hypertension, hypotension, arrhythmias.

EENT: increased intraocular pressure.

Other: ***prolonged respiratory depression, apnea, malignant hyperthermia,*** muscle fasciculation, *postoperative muscle pain,* myoglobinemia, excessive salivation, ***allergic or idiosyncratic hypersensitivity reactions.***

INTERACTIONS

Aminoglycoside antibiotics (including amikacin, gentamicin, kanamycin, neomycin, streptomycin); polymyxin antibiotics (polymyxin B sulfate, colistin); cholinesterase inhibitors such as neostigmine, pyridostigmine, edrophonium, physostigmine, or echothiophate; general anesthetics (such as halothane, enflurane, isoflurane): potentiated neuromuscular blockade, leading to increased skeletal muscle relaxation and possible respiratory paralysis. Use cautiously during surgical and postoperative periods.

Digitalis glycosides: possible cardiac arrhythmias. Use together cautiously.

Magnesium sulfate (parenterally): potentiated neuromuscular blockade, increased skeletal muscle relaxation, and possible respiratory paralysis. Use with caution, preferably with reduced doses.

MAO inhibitors, lithium, cyclophosphamide: prolonged apnea. Use with caution.

Narcotic analgesics, methotrimeprazine: potentiated neuromuscular blockade, leading to increased skeletal muscle relaxation and possible respiratory paralysis. Use with extreme caution.

EFFECTS ON DIAGNOSTIC TESTS

Serum potassium: may increase levels.

NURSING CONSIDERATIONS

Besides those related universally to drug therapy (see "How to use this book"), consider the following specific recommendations:

Assessment

- Obtain a baseline assessment of the patient's skeletal muscle function and respiratory pattern before drug therapy.
- Be alert for adverse reactions and drug interactions throughout therapy.
- Evaluate the patient's and family's knowledge about succinylcholine therapy.

Nursing Diagnoses

- Ineffective breathing pattern related to adverse drug reaction.
- Knowledge deficit related to succinylcholine therapy.

Planning and Implementation

Preparation and Administration

- Succinylcholine should only be used by personnel experienced in airway management.
- Know that this drug is the drug of choice for short procedures (less than 3 minutes) and for orthopedic manipulations. Use caution in fractures or dislocations.
- Duration of action prolonged to 20 minutes by continuous I.V. infusion.
- ***I.V. use:*** Repeated or continuous infusions of succinylcholine alone are not advised; may cause reduced response or prolonged muscle relaxation and apnea.
- If given I.M., give deep I.M., preferably high into the deltoid muscle.
- Give test dose (10 mg I.M. or I.V.) after patient has been anesthetized. Normal response (no respiratory depression or transient depression for up to 5 minutes) indicates drug may be given. Do not give if patient develops respiratory paralysis sufficient to permit endotrachael intubation. (Recovery within 30 to 60 minutes.)
- Store injectable form in the refrigerator. Store powder form at room tempedrature, tightly closed. Use immediately after reconstitution. Do not mix with alkaline solutions (thiopental, sodium bicarbonate, barbiturates).

Monitoring

- Monitor baseline electrolyte determinations.
- Monitor effectiveness by checking the patient's degree of skeletal muscle function.
- Monitior for adverse reactions and drug interactions by checking respirations every 5 to 10 minutes during the infusion for respiratory depression and apnea.
- Monitor the patient's heart rate for bradycardia or tachycardia, blood pressure for hypotension or hypertension, and ECG for arrythmias.
- Monitor the patient's temperature for malignant hyperthermia.
- Monitor the patient's respirations closely until patient is fully recovered from neuromuscular blockade as evidenced by tests of muscle strength (hand grip, head lift, and ability to cough).

Supportive Care

- Have respiratory support equipment (endotracheal equipment, ventilator, oxygen, atropine, and epinephrine) on hand.
- Do not use reversing agents with this drug. Unlike nondepolarizing agents, neostigmine or edrophonium may worsen neuromuscular blockade.

Patient Teaching

- Tell the patient that this drug will be given as a part of anesthesia.
- Tell the patient that he may experience some residual muscle weakness.
- Reassure patient that postoperative stiffness is normal and will soon subside.

Evaluation
In patients receiving succinylcholine, appropriate evaluation statements may include:
• Patient's breathing pattern remains normal.
• Patient and family state an understanding of succinylcholine therapy.

sucralfate
(soo kral' fate)
Carafate, Sulcrate†

• *Classification:* antiulcer agent (pepsin inhibitor)
• *Pregnancy Risk Category:* B

HOW SUPPLIED
Tablets: 1 g

ACTION
Mechanism: Adheres to and protects the ulcer surface by forming a barrier.
Absorption: Only about 3% to 5% of a dose is absorbed.
Distribution: Acts locally, at the ulcer site. Absorbed drug is distributed to many body tissues, including the liver and kidneys.
Metabolism: None.
Excretion: About 90% of a dose is excreted in feces; absorbed drug is excreted unchanged in urine.
Onset, peak, duration: Duration of effect is 5 hours.

INDICATIONS & DOSAGE
Short-term (up to 8 weeks) treatment of duodenal ulcer–
Adults: 1 g P.O. q.i.d. 1 hour before meals and h.s.

CONTRAINDICATIONS & PRECAUTIONS
Contraindicated in patients with sucralfate allergy.

ADVERSE REACTIONS
Common reactions are in italics; life-threatening reactions are in bold italics.
CNS: dizziness, sleepiness.
GI: *constipation,* nausea, gastric discomfort, diarrhea, bezoar formation.

INTERACTIONS
Antacids: may decrease binding of drug to gastroduodenal mucosa, impairing effectiveness. Don't give within 30 minutes of each other.

EFFECTS ON DIAGNOSTIC TESTS
None reported.

NURSING CONSIDERATIONS
Besides those related universally to drug therapy (see "How to use this book"), consider the following specific recommendations:
Assessment
• Obtain a baseline assessment of the patient's GI pain before initiating sucralfate therapy.
• Be alert for adverse reactions and drug interactions throughout therapy.
• Evaluate the patient's and family's knowledge about sucralfate therapy.
Nursing Diagnoses
• Pain related to the patient's underlying condition.
• Constipation related to adverse GI effects of sucralfate.
• Knowledge deficit related to sucralfate therapy.
Planning and Implementation
Preparation and Administration
• ***P.O. use:*** Sucralfate may inhibit absorption of other drugs. Schedule other medications 2 hours before or after sucralfate. A patient who has difficulty swallowing a tablet may place it in 15 to 30 ml of water at room temperature, allow it to disintegrate, and then ingest the resulting suspension. This is particularly useful for the patient with esophagitis and painful swallowing. Administer drug on an empty stomach (1 hour before each meal and at bedtime).

• Do not administer this drug within 30 minutes of an antacid. An antacid may interfere with the drug's binding effect.
• Sucralfate is poorly water-soluble. For administration by nasogastric tube, have the pharmacist prepare water-sorbitol suspension of sucralfate. Alternatively, place tablet in 60-ml syringe; add 20 ml water. Let stand with tip up for about 5 minutes, occasionally shaking gently. A suspension will form that may be administered from the syringe. After administration, tube should be flushed several times to ensure that the patient receives the entire dose.
• Therapy exceeding 8 weeks is not recommended.
• Some experts believe that 2 g b.i.d. is as effective as standard regimen.

Monitoring
• Monitor effectiveness by regularly assessing relief of or decrease in the patient's GI pain.
• Monitor the patient's bowel habits for signs and symptoms of constipation. Monitor the patient's stool for amount, type, and color.

Supportive Care
• If the patient develops constipation, notify the doctor and obtain an order for a laxative. Also advise the patient about dietary and other measures he may take to prevent constipation.
• If the patient's stool becomes black and tarry, perform a test for occult blood and notify the doctor of the results.

Patient Teaching
• Remind the patient to take the drug on an empty stomach at least 1 hour before meals.
• Advise the patient to continue taking drug as directed, even after pain begins to subside, to ensure adequate healing.
• Tell the patient that he may take an antacid 1 hour before or 1 hour after sucralfate.
• Warn the patient not to take drug longer than 8 weeks.
• Urge the patient to avoid smoking because it may increase gastric acid secretion and worsen disease.
• Instruct the patient to avoid sources of GI irritation, such as alcohol, certain foods, and drugs containing aspirin.
• Instruct the patient to immediately report any signs of black, tarry stools; diarrhea; confusion; or rash.

Evaluation
In patients receiving sucralfate, appropriate evaluation statements may include:
• Patient experiences complete or partial relief of GI pain.
• Patient does not experience constipation.
• Patient and family state an understanding of sucralfate therapy.

sufentanil citrate
(soo fen´ ta nil)
Sufenta

• Controlled Substance Schedule II
• *Classification:* anesthetic adjunct to anesthesia (opioid)
• *Pregnancy Risk Category:* C (D for prolonged use or use of high doses at term)

HOW SUPPLIED
Injection: 50 mcg/ml

ACTION
Mechanism: Binds with opiate receptors at many sites in the CNS (brain, brain stem, and spinal cord), altering both perception of and emotional response to pain through an unknown mechanism.
Distribution: Highly lipophilic, drug is rapidly and extensively distributed in animals. It is highly protein-bound ($>90\%$) and redistributed rapidly.

Metabolism: Mainly in the liver. Relatively little accumulation occurs.
Excretion: Sufentanil and its metabolites are excreted primarily in urine. Half-life: Elimination half-life of about 2½ hours.
Onset, peak, duration: After I.V. administration, sufentanil has a more rapid onset of action (1½ to 3 minutes) than does morphine or fentanyl.

INDICATIONS & DOSAGE

Adjunct to general anesthetic –
Adults: 1 to 8 mcg/kg I.V. administered with nitrous oxide/oxygen.
As a primary anesthetic –
Adults: 8 to 30 mcg/kg I.V. administered with 100% oxygen and a muscle relaxant.

CONTRAINDICATIONS & PRECAUTIONS

Contraindicated in patients with hypersensitivity to the drug or any phenylpiperidine opiate (alfentanil, diphenoxylate, fentanyl, or meperidine).

Administer with extreme caution to patients with supraventricular arrhythmias; avoid or use with caution in patients with head injury or increased intracranial pressure, because drug obscures neurologic parameters; and during pregnancy and labor, because drug readily crosses placenta (premature infants are especially sensitive to the drug's respiratory and CNS depressant effects).

Administer cautiously to patients with renal or hepatic dysfunction, because drug accumulation or prolonged duration of action may occur; asthma or chronic obstructive pulmonary disease, because drug depresses respiration and suppresses cough reflex; seizure disorders, because drug may precipitate seizures; to patients undergoing biliary tract surgery, because drug may cause biliary spasm; to elderly or debilitated patients, who are more sensitive to drug's effects; and to patients prone to physical or psychic addiction, because of the drug's high abuse potential.

ADVERSE REACTIONS

Common reactions are in italics; life-threatening reactions are in bold italics.
CNS: chills.
CV: *hypotension,* hypertension, bradycardia, tachycardia.
GI: nausea, vomiting.
Skin: itching.
Other: *chest wall rigidity,* intraoperative muscle movement, ***respiratory depression.***

INTERACTIONS

Alcohol, CNS depressants: additive effects. Use together cautiously.

EFFECTS ON DIAGNOSTIC TESTS

Plasma amylase and lipase: increased levels.
Serum prolactin: increased levels.

NURSING CONSIDERATIONS

Besides those related universally to drug therapy (see "How to use this book"), consider the following specific recommendations:

Assessment
• Obtain a baseline assessment of the patient's respiratory and cardiovascular status before therapy.
• Be alert for adverse reactions and drug interactions throughout therapy.
• Evaluate the patient's and family's knowledge about sufentanil therapy.

Nursing Diagnoses
• Decreased cardiac output related to adverse cardiac effects of therapy.
• Ineffective breathing pattern related to sufentanil-induced respiratory depression or chest wall rigidity.
• Knowledge deficit related to sufentanil therapy.

Planning and Implementation
Preparation and Administration
• Should only be administered by persons specifically trained in the use of I.V. anesthetics.

• Keep patient supine during administration to minimize hypotension.
• Reduce dose in elderly and debilitated patients.

Monitoring

• Monitor patient's rate and pattern of breathing for evidence of respiratory depression during therapy for at least 1 hour after dose.
• With high doses, monitor for muscle rigidity, especially involving the chest wall.
• Monitor patient's cardiovascular status closely during surgery. Frequently monitor postoperative vital signs.
• Closely monitor for signs of withdrawal when discontinuing sufentanil after prolonged use.

Supportive Care

• If respiratory rate drops below 8 breaths/minute, arouse patient to stimulate breathing and notify the doctor.
• During therapy with sufentanil, keep narcotic antagonist (naloxone) and resuscitative equipment available.
• ***Treatment of overdose:*** Maintain airway patency and provide respiratory support. Give naloxone as needed to reverse respiratory depression. Also administer I.V. fluids and vasopressors, as ordered, to maintain blood pressure and neuromuscular blockers to relieve muscle rigidity.
• Keep in mind that when sufentanil is used at doses greater than 8 mcg/kg, postoperative mechanical ventilation and observation are essential because of extended postoperative respiratory depression.
• Be aware that compared to fentanyl, sufentanil has a more rapid onset and shorter duration of action. Sufentanil is five to seven times more potent than fentanyl.
• Be aware that physical dependence is possible.

Patient Teaching

• Explain the anesthetic effect of sufentanil, as well as preoperative and postoperative care.
• Tell the patient to rise slowly after I.V. administration to reduce faintness and dizziness.

Evaluation

In patients receiving sufentanil, appropriate evaluation statements include:

• Cardiac status is within normal limits.
• Respiratory status is within normal limits.
• Patient and family state an understanding of sufentanil therapy.

sulconazole nitrate

(sul kon´ a zole)
Exelderm

• *Classification:* antifungal agent (imidazole derivative)
• *Pregnancy Risk Category:* C

HOW SUPPLIED

Topical solution: 1%

ACTION

Mechanism: Unknown. An imidazole derivative that inhibits the growth of both fungi and yeast.

INDICATIONS & DOSAGE

Treatment of tinea cruris and tinea corporis caused by Trichophyton mentagrophytes, Epidermophyton floccosum, *and* Microsporum canis; *treatment of tinea versicolor (caused by* Malassezia furfur*)* –
Adults: massage a small amount of solution into affected area daily to b.i.d.

CONTRAINDICATIONS & PRECAUTIONS

Contraindicated in patients hypersensitive to any component of the product.

ADVERSE REACTIONS

Common reactions are in italics; life-threatening reactions are in bold italics.
Local: itching, burning, stinging.

INTERACTIONS

None reported.

EFFECTS ON DIAGNOSTIC TESTS

None reported.

NURSING CONSIDERATIONS

Besides those related universally to drug therapy (see "How to use this book"), consider the following specific recommendations:

Assessment

- Obtain a baseline assessment of skin lesions before therapy.
- Be alert for adverse reactions and drug interactions throughout therapy.
- Evaluate the patient's and family's knowledge about sulconazole therapy.

Nursing Diagnoses

- Impaired skin integrity related to patient's underlying condition.
- High risk for impaired skin integrity related to sulconazole-induced pruritus and burning.
- Knowledge deficit related to sulconazole nitrate therapy.

Planning and Implementation

Preparation and Administration

- ***Topical use:*** Clean affected area, then apply a small amount.

Monitoring

- Monitor effectiveness by regularly examining the skin of the affected area.
- Monitor the patient for adverse reactions and drug interactions by frequently observing for irritation.
- Monitor condition for improvement; if no improvement occurs in 4 weeks, diagnoses should be reconsidered.

Supportive Care

- Treatment should continue for at least 3 weeks.
- Be prepared to discontinue treatment and notify the doctor if irritation develops during treatment.
- Efficacy against athlete's foot (tinea pedis) has not been proven.

Patient Teaching

- Teach patient to apply medication.
- Inform patient that clinical improvement is usually apparent within a week, with symptomatic relief in just a few days. Explain to the patient that he should complete the full course of therapy, even after symptoms subside, to prevent recurrence.
- Instruct patient to avoid contact with the eyes and to wash hands thoroughly after applying.

Evaluation

In patients receiving sulconazole nitrate, appropriate evaluation statements may include:

- Patient's superficial lesions have healed.
- Patient did not develop drug-induced itching and burning.
- Patient and family state an understanding of sulconazole therapy.

---

sulfacetamide sodium 10%

(sul fa see´ ta mide)

Bleph-10 Liquifilm Ophthalmic, Cetamide Ophthalmic, Sodium Sulamyd 10% Ophthalmic, Sulf-10 Ophthalmic

sulfacetamide sodium 15%

Isopto Cetamide Ophthalmic, Sulfacel-15 Ophthalmic

sulfacetamide sodium 30%

Sodium Sulamyd 30% Ophthalmic

- *Classification:* antibiotic (sulfonamide)
- *Pregnancy Risk Category:* C

HOW SUPPLIED

Ophthalmic ointment: 10%
Ophthalmic solution: 10%, 15%, 30%

ACTION

Mechanism: Prevents the conversion of para-aminobenzoic acid to folic acid in susceptible bacteria, preventing cell growth. Usually bacteriostatic, but may be bactericidal.
Absorption: No evidence that sulfacetamide is absorbed from the eye.

INDICATIONS & DOSAGE

Inclusion conjunctivitis, corneal ulcers, trachoma, chlamydial infection–
Adults and children: instill 1 to 2 drops of 10% solution into lower conjunctival sac q 2 to 3 hours during day, less often at night; or instill 1 to 2 drops of 15% solution into lower conjunctival sac q 1 to 2 hours initially, increasing interval as condition responds; or instill 1 drop of 30% solution into lower conjunctival sac q 2 hours. Instill ½″ to 1″ of 10% ointment into conjunctival sac q.i.d. and h.s. May use ointment at night along with drops during the day.

CONTRAINDICATIONS & PRECAUTIONS

Contraindicated in patients with suspected hypersensitivity to sulfonamides or to any ingredients of the preparation. Use cautiously to avoid overgrowth of nonsusceptible organisms during prolonged therapy.

ADVERSE REACTIONS

Common reactions are in italics; life-threatening reactions are in bold italics.
Eye: slowed corneal wound healing (ointment), *pain on instilling eyedrop,* headache or brow pain, photophobia.
Other: hypersensitivity (including itching or burning), overgrowth of nonsusceptible organisms, ***Stevens-Johnson syndrome,*** sensitivity to light.

INTERACTIONS

Local anesthetics (procaine, tetracaine), para-aminobenzoic acid derivatives: decreased sulfacetamide sodium action. Wait 30 minutes to 1 hour after instilling anesthetic or para-aminobenzoic acid derivative before instilling sulfacetamide.
Silver preparations: precipitate formation. Avoid using together.

EFFECTS ON DIAGNOSTIC TESTS

None reported.

NURSING CONSIDERATIONS

Besides those related universally to drug therapy (see "How to use this book"), consider the following specific recommendations:

Assessment

- Obtain a baseline assessment of the patient's allergies to other current eye medications before therapy.
- Be alert for adverse reactions and drug interactions throughout therapy.
- Evaluate the patient's and family's knowledge about sulfacetamide sodium therapy.

Nursing Diagnoses

- Altered protection related to ocular infection.
- Pain related to burning and stinging induced by instillation of sulfacetamide drops.
- Knowledge deficit related to sulfacetamide sodium therapy.

Planning and Implementation

Preparation and Administration

- Store away from heat in tightly sealed, light-resistant container.
- Wash hands before and after administration.
- Check dosage; three strengths available.
- Remove as much purulent exudate from lids as possible before instillation; exudate interferes with sulfacetamide action.
- Do not use discolored (dark brown) solution.

• Wait at least 5 minutes before administering other eye medications.

Monitoring

• Monitor the effectiveness of sulfacetamide sodium therapy by culturing the eye to check for the presence of microorganisms.
• Observe color, amount, and consistency of exudate.
• Observe for signs of hypersensitivity.

Supportive Care

• Obtain order for medication to relieve drug-induced headache.
• Apply warm moist compresses to eye area to aid in removal of dried exudate.
• Often used with systemic tetracycline in treating trachoma and inclusion conjunctivitis.
• Primarily used in minor ocular infections.

Patient Teaching

• Teach the patient how to instill. Advise him to wash hands before and after instillation. Warn him not to touch tip of the dropper to the eye or surrounding tissue.
• Instruct the patient to apply light finger pressure to the lacrimal sac for 1 minute after the drops have been instilled. Caution him to avoid scratching or rubbing the eyes.
• Warn the patient that the eyedrops may cause burning or stinging and that the solution may stain clothing.
• Advise the patient to wear sunglasses to minimize photophobia and avoid prolonged exposure to sunlight.
• Instruct the patient to watch for signs of hypersensitivity (itching lids, swelling, constant burning). If it occurs, stop the drug and notify the doctor immediately.
• Stress the importance of compliance with the recommended therapy.
• Instruct the patient not to share eye medication with family members. If a family member develops the same symptoms, contact the doctor.

Evaluation

In patients receiving sulfacetamide sodium, appropriate evaluation statements may include:

• Patient remains free from signs and symptoms of infection.
• Patient reports decrease or absence of pain.
• Patient and family state an understanding of sulfacetamide therapy.

sulfadiazine

(sul fa dye´ a zeen)
Microsulfon

• *Classification:* antibiotic (sulfonamide)
• *Pregnancy Risk Category:* B (D if near term)

HOW SUPPLIED

Tablets: 500 mg

ACTION

Mechanism: Inhibits formation of dihydrofolic acid from para-aminobenzoic acid (PABA), decreasing bacterial folic acid synthesis.
Absorption: Readily absorbed from the GI tract after oral administration.
Distribution: Widely distributed into most body tissues and fluids, including synovial, pleural, amniotic, prostatic, peritoneal, and seminal fluids. CSF penetration is poor. Sulfadiazine crosses the placenta; it is 32% to 56% protein-bound.
Metabolism: Partially metabolized in the liver.
Excretion: Both unchanged drug and metabolite are excreted primarily in urine by glomerular filtration and, to a lesser extent, by renal tubular secretion; some is excreted in breast milk. Urine solubility of unchanged drug increases as urine pH increases. Half-life: About 24 hours.
Onset, peak, duration: Peak serum levels occur at 2 hours.

INDICATIONS & DOSAGE

Urinary tract infection–
Adults: initially, 2 to 4 g P.O., then 500 mg to 1 g P.O. q 6 hours.
Children: initially, 75 mg/kg or 2 g/m² P.O., then 150 mg/kg or 4 g/m² P.O. in 4 to 6 divided doses daily. Maximum daily dosage is 6 g.
Rheumatic fever prophylaxis, as an alternative to penicillin–
Children over 30 kg: 1 g P.O. daily.
Children under 30 kg: 500 mg P.O. daily.
Adjunctive treatment in toxoplasmosis–
Adults: 4 g P.O. in divided doses q 6 hours for 3 to 4 weeks, discontinued for 1 week; given with pyrimethamine 25 mg P.O. daily for 3 to 4 weeks.
Children: 100 mg/kg P.O. in divided doses q 6 hours for 3 to 4 weeks; given with pyrimethamine 2 mg/kg daily for 3 days, then 1 mg/kg daily for 3 to 4 weeks.

CONTRAINDICATIONS & PRECAUTIONS

Contraindicated in patients with hypersensitivity to sulfonamides or to any other drug containing sulfur (thiazides, furosemide, or oral sulfonylureas); and in patients with severe renal or hepatic dysfunction, or porphyria; during pregnancy, at term, and during lactation; and in infants under age 2 months.

Administer cautiously to patients with mild to moderate renal or hepatic impairment, urinary obstruction (because of the risk of drug accumulation), severe allergies, asthma, blood dyscrasias, or glucose-6-phosphate dehydrogenase (G6PD) deficiency.

ADVERSE REACTIONS

Common reactions are in italics; life-threatening reactions are in bold italics.
Blood: ***agranulocytosis, aplastic anemia,*** megaloblastic anemia, thrombocytopenia, leukopenia, ***hemolytic anemia.***
CNS: headache, mental depression, convulsions, hallucinations.
GI: *nausea, vomiting, diarrhea,* abdominal pain, anorexia, stomatitis.
GU: ***toxic nephrosis with oliguria and anuria,*** crystalluria, hematuria.
Hepatic: jaundice.
Skin: ***erythema multiforme (Stevens-Johnson syndrome),*** generalized skin eruption, ***epidermal necrolysis, exfoliative dermatitis,*** photosensitivity, urticaria, pruritus.
Local: irritation, extravasation.
Other: *hypersensitivity, serum sickness, drug fever,* ***anaphylaxis.***

INTERACTIONS

Ammonium chloride, ascorbic acid: doses sufficient to acidify urine may cause precipitation of sulfonamide and crystalluria. Don't use together.
Oral anticoagulants: increased anticoagulant effect.
Oral contraceptives: decreased contraceptive effectiveness and increased risk of breakthrough bleeding.
Oral hypoglycemic agents: increased hypoglycemic effect.
PABA-containing drugs: inhibit antibacterial action. Don't use together.

EFFECTS ON DIAGNOSTIC TESTS

CBC: decreased RBC, WBC, and platelet counts.
Liver function tests: elevated results.
Urine glucose tests with copper sulfate (Benedict's reagent or Clinitest): altered results.

NURSING CONSIDERATIONS

Besides those related universally to drug therapy (see "How to use this book"), consider the following specific recommendations:

Assessment

- Obtain a baseline assessment of infection before therapy.
- Be alert for adverse reactions and drug interactions throughout therapy.

• Evaluate the patient's and family's knowledge about sulfadiazine therapy.

Nursing Diagnoses

• High risk for injury related to ineffectiveness of sulfadiazine to eradicate the infection.
• High risk for fluid volume deficit related to adverse GI reactions caused by sulfadiazine.
• Knowledge deficit related to sulfadiazine.

Planning and Implementation

Preparation and Administration

• Obtain specimen for culture and sensitivity tests before first dose. Therapy may begin pending test results. Also obtain specimens for CBC and urinalysis before therapy begins.
• Give drug on schedule to maintain constant blood level.
• Protect drug from light.
• ***P.O. use:*** Administer with a full glass (8 oz or 240 ml) of water.

Monitoring

• Monitor effectiveness by regularly assessing for improvement of infection.
• Monitor intake and output. Urine output should be at least 1,500 ml/day to ensure adequate hydration. Inadequate urine output can lead to crystalluria or tubular deposits of the drug.
• Monitor hydration status if GI reactions occur.
• Monitor urine pH daily; urine cultures, CBCs and urinalysis throughout therapy.
• Monitor for signs of blood dyscrasias (purpura, ecchymosis, sore throat, fever, and pallor).

Supportive Care

• Force fluid intake to 3,000 to 4,000 ml/day. (Patient's output should be at least 1,500 ml/day).
• To aid prevention of crystalluria, sodium bicarbonate may be administered to alkalinize urine.
• Report any signs of blood dyscrasias immediately.
• Be aware that folic or folinic acid may be used during rest periods in toxoplasmosis therapy to reverse hematopoietic depression and anemia associated with drug.
• Obtain an order for an antiemetic or antidiarrheal agent if needed.

Patient Teaching

• Tell the patient to take medication exactly as prescribed, even if feeling better, and to take entire amount prescribed.
• Tell patient to protect drug from light and to take drug on schedule to maintain constant blood level.
• Advise diabetic patients that drug may increase effects of oral hypoglycemic agents.
• Advise the patient to avoid exposure to direct sunlight because of risk of photosensitivity reaction.
• Tell the patient to take drug with a full glass of water and to drink at least 3,000 to 4,000 ml/day of water daily.
• Teach patient how to measure intake and output and urine pH.
• Instruct patient to be alert for signs of blood dyscrasias and if present to report them immediately.

Evaluation

In patients receiving sulfadiazine, appropriate evaluation statements may include:

• Patient is free of infection.
• Patient maintains adequate hydration throughout therapy.
• Patient and family state an understanding of therapy.

sulfamethoxazole (sulphamethoxazole)

(sul fa meth ox´ a zole)

Apo-Sulfamethoxazole†, Gantanol, Gantanol DS

• *Classification:* antibiotic (sulfonamide)
• *Pregnancy Risk Category:* B (D if near term)

• *Pregnancy Risk Category:* B (D if near term)

HOW SUPPLIED

Tablets: 500 mg, 1,000 mg
Oral suspension: 500 mg/5 ml

ACTION

Mechanism: Inhibits formation of dihydrofolic acid from para-aminobenzoic acid (PABA), decreasing bacterial folic acid synthesis.
Absorption: Readily absorbed from the GI tract after oral administration.
Distribution: Widely distributed into most body tissues and fluids, including cerebrospinal, synovial, pleural, amniotic, prostatic, peritoneal, and seminal fluids. Sulfamethoxazole crosses the placenta; it is 50% to 70% protein-bound.
Metabolism: Partially metabolized in the liver.
Excretion: Both unchanged drug and metabolites are excreted primarily in urine by glomerular filtration and, to a lesser extent, by renal tubular secretion; some is excreted in breast milk. Urinary solubility of unchanged drug increases as urine pH increases. Half-life: 7 to 12 hours in patients with normal renal function.
Onset, peak, duration: Peak serum levels after oral administration occur at 2 hours.

INDICATIONS & DOSAGE

Urinary tract and systemic infections–
Adults: initially, 2 g P.O., then 1 g P.O. b.i.d. up to t.i.d. for severe infections.
Children and infants over 2 months: initially, 50 to 60 mg/kg P.O., then 25 to 30 mg/kg b.i.d. Maximum dosage should not exceed 75 mg/kg daily.
Lymphogranuloma venereum (genital, inguinal, or anorectal infection)–
Adults: 1 g P.O. daily for at least 3 weeks.

CONTRAINDICATIONS & PRECAUTIONS

Contraindicated in patients with hypersensitivity to sulfonamides or to any other drug containing sulfur (thiazides, furosemide, or oral sulfonylureas); in patients with severe renal or hepatic dysfunction, or porphyria; during pregnancy, at term, and during lactation; and in infants under age 2 months.

Use cautiously in patients with mild to moderate renal or hepatic impairment, urinary obstruction (because of the risk of drug accumulation), severe allergies, asthma, blood dyscrasias, or glucose-6-phosphate dehydrogenase deficiency.

ADVERSE REACTIONS

Common reactions are in italics; life-threatening reactions are in bold italics.
Blood: *agranulocytosis, aplastic anemia,* megaloblastic anemia, thrombocytopenia, leukopenia, hemolytic anemia.
CNS: headache, mental depression, seizures, hallucinations.
GI: *nausea, vomiting, diarrhea,* abdominal pain, anorexia, stomatitis.
GU: toxic nephrosis with oliguria and anuria, crystalluria, hematuria.
Hepatic: jaundice.
Skin: *erythema multiforme (Stevens-Johnson syndrome), generalized skin eruption, epidermal necrolysis, exfoliative dermatitis,* photosensitivity, urticaria, pruritus.
Other: *hypersensitivity, serum sickness, drug fever, anaphylaxis.*

INTERACTIONS

Ammonium chloride, ascorbic acid: doses sufficient to acidify urine may cause precipitation of sulfonamide and crystalluria. Don't use together.
Oral anticoagulants: increased anticoagulant effect.
Oral contraceptives: decreased contraceptive effectiveness and increased risk of breakthrough bleeding.

Oral hypoglycemic agents: increased hypoglycemic effect.
PABA-containing drugs: inhibit antibacterial action. Don't use together.

EFFECTS ON DIAGNOSTIC TESTS

CBC: decreased RBC, WBC, and platelet counts.
Liver function tests: elevated results.
Urine glucose tests with copper sulfate (Benedict's reagent or Clinitest): altered results.

NURSING CONSIDERATIONS

Besides those related universally to drug therapy (see "How to use this book"), consider the following specific recommendations:

Assessment

- Obtain a baseline assessment of infection before therapy.
- Be alert for adverse reactions and drug interactions throughout therapy.
- Evaluate the patient's and family's knowledge about sulfamethoxazole therapy.

Nursing Diagnoses

- High risk for injury related to ineffectiveness of sulfamethoxazole in eradicating the infection.
- High risk for fluid volume deficit related to adverse GI reactions caused by sulfamethoxazole.
- Knowledge deficit related to sulfamethoxazole.

Planning and Implementation

Preparation and Administration

- Obtain specimen for culture and sensitivity tests before first dose. Therapy may begin pending test results. Also obtain specimens for CBC and urinalysis before therapy begins.
- Give drug on schedule to maintain constant blood level.
- ***P.O. use:*** Administer with a full glass (8 oz or 240 ml) of water.

Monitoring

- Monitor effectiveness by regularly assessing for improvement of infection.
- Monitor intake and output. Urine output should be at least 1,500 ml/day to ensure adequate hydration. Inadequate urine output can lead to crystalluria or tubular deposits of the drug.
- Monitor urine pH daily; urine cultures, CBCs, and urinalysis regularly throughout therapy.
- Monitor hydration status if GI reactions occur.
- Monitor for signs of blood dyscrasias (purpura, ecchymosis, sore throat, fever, and pallor).

Supportive Care

- Force fluid intake of 3,000 to 4,000 ml/day. (Patient's output should be at least 1,500 ml/day).
- To aid prevention of crystalluria, sodium bicarbonate may be administered to alkalinize urine.
- Report any signs of blood dyscrasias immediately.
- Obtain an order for an antiemetic or antidiarrheal agent if needed.

Patient Teaching

- Tell the patient to take medication exactly as prescribed, even if he feels better, and to take entire amount prescribed.
- Tell patient to take drug on schedule to maintain constant blood level.
- Inform diabetic patients that drug may increase effects of oral hypoglycemic agents.
- Advise patient to avoid exposure to direct sunlight because of risk of photosensitivity reaction.
- Tell patient to take drug with a full glass of water and to drink at least 3,000 to 4,000 ml of water daily.
- Teach patient how to measure intake and output and urine pH.
- Instruct patient to be alert for signs of blood dyscrasias and, if present, to report them immediately.

Evaluation

In patients receiving sulfamethoxazole, appropriate evaluation statements may include:

- Patient is free of infection.

• Patient maintains adequate hydration throughout therapy.
• Patient and family state an understanding of sulfamethoxazole therapy.

sulfasalazine (salazosulfapyridine, sulphasalazine)

(sul fa sal´ a zeen)
Azulfidine, Azulfidine EN-Tabs, PMS Sulfasalazine E.C.†, Salazopyrin†‡, Salazopyrin EN-Tabs†‡, S.A.S., S.A.S.-Enteric

• *Classification:* antibiotic (sulfonamide)
• *Pregnancy Risk Category:* B (D if near term)

HOW SUPPLIED

Tablets: 500 mg with or without enteric coating
Oral suspension: 250 mg/5 ml

ACTION

Mechanism: Sulfasalazine is cleaved within the colon to sulfapyridine and mesalamine (5-aminosalicylic acid). Sulfapyridine may exhibit some antibacterial activity by decreasing bacterial folic acid synthesis. Mesalamine, an anti-inflammatory agent, acts locally to decrease irritation.
Absorption: Poorly absorbed from the GI tract after oral administration; about 80% is transported to the colon, where intestinal flora metabolize the drug to its active components. Sulfapyridine is absorbed from the colon, but 5-aminosalicylic acid is not.
Distribution: Human data unavailable; animal studies have identified drug and metabolites in sera, liver, and intestinal walls. Parent drug and metabolites cross the placenta.
Metabolism: Cleaved by intestinal flora in the colon.
Excretion: Systemically absorbed drug is excreted chiefly in urine; some parent drug and metabolites are excreted in breast milk. Half-life: About 6 to 8 hours.
Onset, peak, duration: peak serum concentrations occur within 1.5 to 6 hours after oral administration; sulfapyridine levels peak within 6 to 24 hours.

INDICATIONS & DOSAGE

Mild to moderate ulcerative colitis, adjunctive therapy in severe ulcerative colitis–
Adults: initially, 3 to 4 g P.O. daily in evenly divided doses; usual maintenance dosage is 1.5 to 2 g P.O. daily in divided doses q 6 hours. May need to start with 1 to 2 g initially, with a gradual increase in dosage to minimize adverse effects.
Children over 2 years: initially, 40 to 60 mg/kg P.O. daily, divided into 3 to 6 doses; then 30 mg/kg daily in 4 doses. May need to start at lower dose if GI intolerance occurs.

CONTRAINDICATIONS & PRECAUTIONS

Contraindicated in patients with hypersensitivity to sulfonamides or to any other drug containing sulfur (thiazides, furosemide, or oral sulfonylureas); hypersensitivity to salicylates; severe renal or hepatic dysfunction, or porphyria; during pregnancy, at term, and during lactation; and in infants and children under age 2. Also contraindicated in patients with intestinal or urinary tract obstructions because of the risk of local GI irritation and of crystalluria.

Use cautiously in patients with mild to moderate renal or hepatic impairment, severe allergies, asthma, blood dyscrasias, or glucose-6-phosphate dehydrogenase deficiency.

ADVERSE REACTIONS

Common reactions are in italics; life-threatening reactions are in bold italics.

Blood: ***agranulocytosis, aplastic anemia,*** megaloblastic anemia, thrombocytopenia, leukopenia, hemolytic anemia.
CNS: headache, mental depression, ***seizures,*** hallucinations.
GI: *nausea, vomiting, diarrhea,* abdominal pain, anorexia, stomatitis.
GU: toxic nephrosis with oliguria and anuria, crystalluria, hematuria.
Hepatic: jaundice, hepatoxicity.
Skin: ***erythema multiforme (Stevens-Johnson syndrome),*** *generalized skin eruption,* ***epidermal necrolysis, exfoliative dermatitis,*** photosensitivity, urticaria, pruritus.
Other: *hypersensitivity, serum sickness, drug fever,* ***anaphylaxis,*** oligospermia, infertility.

INTERACTIONS

Folic acid: absorption may be decreased.
Oral anticoagulants: increased anticoagulant effect.
Oral contraceptives: decreased contraceptive effectiveness and increased risk of breakthrough bleeding.
Oral hypoglycemic agents: increased hypoglycemic effect.

EFFECTS ON DIAGNOSTIC TESTS

Urine glucose tests with cupric sulfate (Benedict's reagent or Clinitest): altered results.
Liver function tests: elevated results.
CBC: decreased RBCs, WBCs, and platelets.

NURSING CONSIDERATIONS

Besides those related universally to drug therapy (see "How to use this book"), consider the following specific recommendations:

Assessment

- Obtain a baseline assessment of infection before therapy.
- Be alert for adverse reactions and drug interactions throughout therapy.
- Evaluate the patient's and family's knowledge about sulfasalazine therapy.

Nursing Diagnoses

- High risk for injury related to ineffectiveness of sulfasalazine in eradicating the infection.
- High risk for fluid volume deficit related to adverse GI reactions to sulfasalazine.
- Knowledge deficit related to sulfasalazine therapy.

Planning and Implementation

Preparation and Administration

- Obtain specimen for culture and sensitivity tests before first dose. Therapy may begin pending test results.
- Give drug on schedule to maintain constant blood level.
- ***P.O. use:*** Administer after food and space doses evenly to minimize adverse GI effects.

Monitoring

- Monitor effectiveness by regularly assessing for improvement of infection.
- Monitor hydration status if GI reactions occur.

Supportive Care

- Obtain an order for an antiemetic or antidiarrheal agent if needed.

Patient Teaching

- Tell the patient to take medication exactly as prescribed, even if he feels better, and to take entire amount prescribed.
- Tell patient to take drug after food to minimize adverse GI reactions.
- Warn patient that drug colors alkaline urine orange-yellow.
- Advise diabetic patients that drug may increase effects of oral hypoglycemic agents.
- Advise patient to avoid exposure to direct sunlight because of risk of photosensitivity reaction.

Evaluation

In patients receiving sulfasalazine, appropriate evaluation statements may include:

- Patient is free of infection.

• Patient maintains adequate hydration throughout therapy.
• Patient and family state an understanding of sulfasalazine therapy.

sulfinpyrazone
(sul fin peer´ a zone)
Anturan†, Anturane

• *Classification:* renal tubular-blocking agent, platelet aggregation inhibitor (uricosuric agent)
• *Pregnancy Risk Category:* C

HOW SUPPLIED
Tablets: 100 mg
Capsules: 200 mg

ACTION
Mechanism: Blocks renal tubular reabsorption of uric acid, increasing excretion. Also inhibits platelet aggregation.
Absorption: Completely absorbed after oral administration.
Distribution: 98% to 99% protein-bound.
Metabolism: Rapidly metabolized in the liver.
Excretion: Drug and its metabolites are eliminated in urine; about 50% is excreted unchanged.
Onset, peak, duration: Peak plasma levels occur in 2 hours. Effects usually last 4 to 6 hours but may persist up to 10 hours.

INDICATIONS & DOSAGE
Inhibition of platelet aggregation, increase of platelet survival time in treatment of thromboembolic disorders, angina, myocardial infarction, transient cerebral ischemic attacks, peripheral arterial atherosclerosis–
Adults: 200 mg P.O. q.i.d.
Maintenance therapy for common gout: reduction, prevention of joint changes and tophi formation–
Adults: 100 to 200 mg P.O. b.i.d. first week, then 200 to 400 mg P.O. b.i.d. Maximum dosage is 800 mg daily.

CONTRAINDICATIONS & PRECAUTIONS
Contraindicated in patients with hypersensitivity to the drug or to other prazolone derivatives, such as phenylbutazone; in patients with active peptic ulcer disease, gouty nephropathy, bone-marrow depression, or azotemia; in patients with elevated uric acid levels from radiation, chemotherapy, or myeloproliferative disease; or in patients with history of an acute attack (within 2 weeks).

Use cautiously in patients with a history of peptic ulcer disease and in patients with impaired renal or hepatic function, because drug may worsen these conditions.

ADVERSE REACTIONS
Common reactions are in italics; life-threatening reactions are in bold italics.
Blood: ***agranulocytosis,*** blood dyscrasias (rare).
CNS: dizziness, vertigo, tinnitus.
GI: *nausea, dyspepsia,* epigastric pain, blood loss, reactivation of peptic ulcers.
Skin: rash.

INTERACTIONS
Oral anticoagulants: increased anticoagulant effect and risk of bleeding. Use together cautiously.
Oral antidiabetic agents: increased effects. Monitor closely.
Probenecid: inhibits renal excretion of sulfinpyrazone. Use together cautiously.
Salicylates: inhibits uricosuric effect of sulfinpyrazone. Do not use together.

EFFECTS ON DIAGNOSTIC TESTS
Renal function tests: altered results.
Urinary aminohippuric acid and phenolsulfonphthalein: decreased excretion.

NURSING CONSIDERATIONS

Besides those related universally to drug therapy (see "How to use this book"), consider the following specific recommendations:

Assessment

- Obtain a baseline assessment of patient's joint stiffness and pain as well as his uric acid levels before therapy.
- Be alert for adverse reactions and drug interactions throughout therapy.
- Evaluate the patient's and family's knowledge about sulfinpyrazone therapy.

Nursing Diagnoses

- Pain (joint) related to patient's underlying condition.
- High risk for infection related to sulfinpyrazone-induced agranulocytosis.
- Knowledge deficit related to sulfinpyrazone therapy.

Planning and Implementation

Preparation and Administration

- Force fluids to maintain minimum daily output of 2 to 3 liters. Alkalinize urine with sodium bicarbonate or other agent as ordered.
- Give with milk, food, or antacids to minimize GI disturbances.
- Administer prophylactic colchicine during the first 3 to 6 months of sulfinpyrazone therapy, as ordered, because sulfinpyrazone may increase frequency, severity, and duration of acute gout attacks during the first 6 to 12 months of therapy.

Monitoring

- Monitor effectiveness by assessing pain level, uric acid levels, and renal status.
- Periodic monitoring of BUN, CBC, and renal function studies is advised during prolonged use.
- Monitor for symptoms of agranulocytosis such as an elevated temperature and necrotic ulcerations in the mouth, rectum and vagina, as well as exhaustion.
- Monitor intake and output, particularly at the start of therapy. Sulfinpyrazone may lead to renal colic and formation of uric acid stones. Intake and output should be monitored until acid levels are normal (about 6 mg/100 ml).

Supportive Care

- Be aware that sulfinpyrazone decreases urinary excretion of aminohippuric acid, interfering with laboratory test results.
- Lifelong therapy may be required in patients with hyperuricemia.
- Notify doctor if fever develops and administer antipyretics as ordered.
- Remember, sulfinpyrazone contains no analgesic or anti-inflammatory agent and is of no value during acute gout attacks.

Patient Teaching

- Warn patients to avoid any aspirin-containing medications because they may precipitate gout. Acetaminophen may be used for pain.
- Instruct the patient and family that drug must be taken regularly so blood levels can be monitored and dosage adjusted if necessary.
- Advise patients with gout to restrict foods high in purine: anchovies, liver, sardines, kidneys, sweetbreads, peas, and lentils.
- Alkalinizing agents are used therapeutically to increase sulfinpyrazone activity.

Evaluation

In patients receiving sulfinpyrazone, appropriate evaluation statements may include:

- Patient expresses relief of gout pain.
- Patient does not develop infection.
- Patient and family state an understanding of sulfinpyrazone therapy.

---

sulfisoxazole (sulfafurazole, sulphafurazole)

(sul fi sox´ a zole)

Azo-Sulfisoxazole†‡, Gantrisin, Novosoxazole†

sulfisoxazole acetyl

Gantrisin Pediatric Syrup, Gantrisin Pediatric Suspension

• *Classification:* antibiotic (sulfonamide)
• *Pregnancy Risk Category:* B (D if near term)

HOW SUPPLIED

sulfisoxazole
Tablets: 500 mg
sulfisoxazole acetyl
Oral solution: 500 mg/5 ml
Oral suspension: 500 mg/5 ml

ACTION

Mechanism: Inhibits formation of dihydrofolic acid from para-aminobenzoic acid (PABA), decreasing bacterial folic acid synthesis.
Absorption: Readily absorbed from the GI tract after oral administration.
Distribution: Distributed into extracellular compartments; CSF penetration is good, with levels reaching 8% to 57% of plasma levels. Sulfisoxazole crosses the placenta; it is 85% protein-bound.
Metabolism: Partially metabolized in the liver.
Excretion: Both unchanged drug and metabolites are excreted primarily in urine by glomerular filtration and, to a lesser extent, renal tubular secretion; some drug is excreted in breast milk. Urinary solubility of unchanged drug increases as urine pH increases. Half-life: About 4½ to 8 hours in patients with normal renal function.
Onset, peak, duration: Peak serum levels occur at 2 to 4 hours after oral administration.

INDICATIONS & DOSAGE

Urinary tract and systemic infections–
Adults: initially, 2 to 4 g P.O., then 1 to 2 g P.O. q.i.d.
Children over 2 months: initially, 75 mg/kg P.O. daily or 2 g/m² P.O. daily in divided doses q 6 hours, then 150 mg/kg or 4 g/m² P.O. daily in divided doses q 6 hours.

CONTRAINDICATIONS & PRECAUTIONS

Contraindicated in patients with hypersensitivity to sulfonamides or to any other drug containing sulfur (thiazides, furosemide, or oral hypoglycemics); in patients with severe renal or hepatic dysfunction, or porphyria; during pregnancy, at term, and during lactation; and in infants under age 2 months.

Administer sulfonamides cautiously to patients with mild to moderate renal or hepatic impairment, urinary obstruction (because of hazard of drug accumulation), severe allergies, asthma, blood dyscrasias, or glucose-6-phosphate dehydrogenase (G6PD) deficiency.

Ophthalmic preparations are incompatible with silver preparations. Opthamic ointments may impair corneal healing. Nonsusceptible organisms and fungi may proliferate. Paraaminobenzoic acid, present in purulent exudate, will inactivate sulfonamides.

ADVERSE REACTIONS

Common reactions are in italics; life-threatening reactions are in bold italics.
Blood: ***agranulocytosis, aplastic anemia,*** megaloblastic anemia, thrombocytopenia, leukopenia, ***hemolytic anemia.***
CNS: headache, mental depression, seizures, hallucinations.
GI: *nausea, vomiting, diarrhea,* abdominal pain, anorexia, stomatitis.
GU: ***toxic nephrosis with oliguria and anuria,*** crystalluria, hematuria.
Hepatic: jaundice.
Skin: ***erythema multiforme (Stevens-Johnson syndrome),*** generalized skin eruption, ***epidermal necrolysis, exfoliative dermatitis,*** photosensitivity, urticaria, pruritus.

Other: *hypersensitivity, serum sickness, drug fever,* ***anaphylaxis.***

INTERACTIONS

Ammonium chloride, ascorbic acid: doses sufficient to acidify urine may cause crystalluria and precipitation of sulfonamide. Don't use together.
Oral anticoagulants: increased anticoagulant effect.
Oral contraceptives: decreased contraceptive effectiveness and increased risk of breakthrough bleeding.
Oral hypoglycemic agents: increased hypoglycemic effect.
PABA-containing drugs: inhibit antibacterial action. Don't use together.

EFFECTS ON DIAGNOSTIC TESTS

CBC: decreased RBCs, WBCs, or platelets.
Liver function tests: elevated results.
Urine glucose tests with copper sulfate (Benedict's reagent or Clinitest): altered results.

NURSING CONSIDERATIONS

Besides those related universally to drug therapy (see "How to use this book"), consider the following specific recommendations:

Assessment

- Obtain a baseline assessment of infection before therapy.
- Be alert for adverse reactions and drug interactions throughout therapy.
- Evaluate the patient's and family's knowledge about sulfisoxazole therapy.

Nursing Diagnoses

- High risk for injury related to ineffectiveness of sulfisoxazole to eradicate the infection.
- High risk for fluid volume deficit related to adverse GI reactions caused by sulfisoxazole.
- Knowledge deficit related to sulfisoxazole.

Planning and Implementation

Preparation and Administration

- Obtain specimen for culture and sensitivity tests before first dose. Therapy may begin pending test results. Also obtain specimens for CBC, prothrombin time, and urinalysis before therapy begins.
- Give drug on schedule to maintain constant blood level.
- ***P.O. use:*** Administer with a full glass (8 oz or 240 ml) of water.

Monitoring

- Monitor effectiveness by regularly assessing for improvement of infectious process.
- Monitor intake and output. Urine output should be at least 1,500 ml/day to ensure proper hydration. Inadequate urine output can lead to crystalluria or tubular deposits of the drug.
- Monitor urine pH daily; urine cultures, CBCs, prothrombin times, and urinalysis throughout therapy.
- Monitor hydration status if GI reactions occur.
- Monitor for signs of blood dyscrasias (purpura, ecchymosis, sore throat, fever, and pallor).

Supportive Care

- Force fluid intake to 3,000 to 4,000 ml/day. (Patient's output should be at least 1,500 ml/day).
- To aid prevention of crystalluria, sodium bicarbonate may be administered to alkalinize urine.
- Report any signs of blood dyscrasias immediately.
- Obtain an order for an antiemetic or antidiarrheal agent if needed.
- When drug is given preoperatively, the patient should receive a low-residue diet and a minimal number of enemas and cathartics.

Patient Teaching

- Tell the patient to take medication exactly as prescribed, even if feeling better, and to take entire amount prescribed.

• Tell patient to take drug on schedule to maintain constant blood level.
• Advise diabetic patients that drug may increase effects of oral hypoglycemic agents.
• Advise the patient to avoid exposure to direct sunlight because of risk of photosensitivity reaction.
• Tell the patient to take drug with a full glass of water and to drink at least 3,000 to 4,000 ml/day of water daily.
• Teach patient how to measure intake and output and urine pH.
• Instruct patient to be alert for signs of blood dyscrasias and if present to report them immediately.

Evaluation

In patients receiving sulfisoxazole, appropriate evaluation statements may include:
• Patient is free of infection.
• Patient maintains adequate hydration throughout therapy.
• Patient and family state an understanding of sulfisoxazole therapy.

PHARMACOLOGIC CLASS

sulfonamides

co-trimoxazole (trimethoprim-sulfamethoxazole)
sulfacetamide
sulfacytine
sulfadiazine
sulfamethizole
sulfamethoxazole
sulfapyridine
sulfasalazine
sulfisoxazole

OVERVIEW

Sulfonamides were the first effective drugs used to treat systemic bacterial infections. The prototype, sulfanilamide, was discovered in 1908 and first used clinically in 1933. Since then, many derivatives have been synthesized, and many therapeutic milestones have been reached, including improved solubility of sulfonamides in urine (which reduces renal toxicity) and discovery of the advantages of combinations such as triple sulfa and, especially, of combined trimethoprim and sulfamethoxazole (co-trimoxazole). Development of other major antibiotics has reduced the clinical impact of sulfonamides; however, introduction of the combination agent co-trimoxazole has increased their use in certain infections.

Sulfonamides are bacteriostatic. They inhibit biosynthesis of folic acid, which is needed for cell growth; susceptible bacteria are those that synthesize folic acid.

Sulfonamides are well absorbed from the GI tract after oral administration, except for sulfasalazine, which is absorbed minimally by the oral route which contributes to its therapeutic usefulness in treating inflammatory bowel disease. Sulfonamides are distributed widely into tissues and fluids, including pleural, peritoneal, synovial, and ocular fluids; some, including sulfisoxazole, penetrate CSF. Sulfonamides readily cross the placenta and are found in breast milk. Sulfonamides are metabolized by the liver and excreted in urine by glomerular filtration. Hemodialysis removes both sulfamethoxazole and sulfisoxazole, but peritoneal dialysis removes only sulfisoxazole.

CLINICAL INDICATIONS AND ACTIONS

Bacterial infections

When first introduced, sulfonamides were active against many gram-positive and gram-negative organisms; over time, many bacteria have become resistant. Currently, sulfonamides are active against some strains of staphylococci, streptococci, *Nocardia asteroides* and *brasiliensis, Clostridium tetani* and *perfringens, Bacillus anthracis, Escherichia coli,* and *Neisseria gonorrhoeae* and *meningitidis.* Resistance to sulfonamides is common if therapy continues beyond 2 weeks; resistance to one sulfonamide usually means cross-resistance to others.

Sulfonamides are used to treat urinary tract infections caused by *E. coli, Proteus mirabilis* and *vulgaris, Klebsiella, Enterobacter,* and *Staphylococcus aureus,* and genital lesions caused by *Haemophilus ducreyi* (chancroid). They are the drugs of choice in nocardiosis, usually with surgical drainage and/or combined with other antibiotics, including ampicillin, erythromycin, cycloserine, or minocycline. Sulfonamides also are used to treat otitis media and may be used as alternative therapy against *Chlamydia trachomatis.* Sulfadiazine is used to eradicate meningococci from the nasopharynx of carriers of *N. meningitidis.*

Co-trimoxazole is used to treat infections of the urinary tract, respiratory tract, and ear; to treat chronic bacterial prostatitis; and to prevent recurrent urinary tract infection in women, and "traveler's diarrhea."

Parasitic infections

Sulfonamides combined with pyrimethamine are used to treat toxoplasmosis; certain sulfonamides are combined with quinine and pyrimethamine to treat chloroquine-resistant *Plasmodium falciparum* malaria.

Co-trimoxazole is also used to treat *Pneumocystis carinii* pneumonia.

Inflammations

Sulfasalazine, used to treat inflammatory bowel disease, is cleaved in the intestine to sulfapyridine and 5-aminosalicylic acid. Sulfapyridine is used to treat dermatitis herpetiformis.

OVERVIEW OF ADVERSE REACTIONS

Sulfonamides cause adverse reactions affecting many organs and systems. Many are considered caused by hypersensitivity, including the following: rash, fever, pruritus, erythema multiforme, erythema nodosum, Stevens-Johnson syndrome, Lyell's syndrome, exfoliative dermatitis, photosensitivity, joint pain, conjunctivitis, leukopenia, and bronchospasm. Hematologic reactions include granulocytopenia, thrombocytopenia, agranulocytosis, hypoprothrombinemia, and, in glucose-6-phosphate dehydrogenase (G6PD) deficiency, hemolytic anemia. Renal effects usually result from crystalluria (precipitation of the sulfonamide in the renal system). GI reactions include anorexia, stomatitis, pancreatitis, diarrhea, and folic acid malabsorption. Oral therapy commonly causes nausea and vomiting. Hepatotoxicity and CNS reactions (dizziness, confusion, headache, ataxia, drowsiness, and insomnia) are rare.

REPRESENTATIVE COMBINATIONS

Sulfadiazine with sulfamerazine: Triple-Sulfa; with sulfamerazine and sulfacetamide: Acet-Dia-Mer-Sulfonamides, Coco-Diazine, Chero-Trisulfa; with sulfamerazine and sulfathiazole: Dia-Mer-Sulfonamides.

Sulfamethizole with sulfacetamide and phenazopyridine: Triurisil, Urotrol; with phenazopyridine and oxytetracycline: Azotrex, Urobiotic; with sulfathiazole, sulfacetamide, sulfabenzomide, and urea: Triple Sulfa, Sulfagyn, V.V.S., Trysul, Gyne-Sulf, Sultrin, Femguard.

Sulfamethoxazole with phenazopyridine hydrochloride: Azo Gantanol, Azo Sulfamethoxazole; with trimethoprim: Bactrim, Cotrim, Co-trimoxazole, Novotrimel*, Septra.

Sulfisoxazole with phenylazodiaminopyridine hydrochloride: Azo-sulfisoxazole, Azo-Sulfizin, Velmatrol-A; with erythromycin ethyl succinate: Pediazole; with phenazopyridine hydrochloride: Azo-

Gantrisin, Axo-Sulfisoxazole, Azo-Urizole, Thiosulfil-A, Thiosulfil-A Forte, Rosoxol-Azo.

PHARMACOLOGIC CLASS

sulfonylureas

acetohexamide
chlorpropamide
glipizide
glyburide
tolazamide
tolbutamide

OVERVIEW

In 1942, a sulfonamide, an antibacterial agent, was discovered to have hypoglycemic effects. Subsequent experiments showed that this drug did not exert similar effects in pancreatectomized animals. Later, tolbutamide was introduced and soon became popular for managing certain diabetic patients. The sulfonylurea hypoglycemic agents are sulfonamide derivatives that exert no antibacterial activity.

Sulfonylureas lower blood glucose levels by stimulating insulin release from the pancreas. These agents work only in the presence of functioning beta cells in the islet tissue of the pancreas.

The sulfonylureas are divided into first-generation agents (acetohexamide, chlorpropamide, tolbutamide, and tolazamide) and second-generation agents (glyburide and glipizide). Clinically, their most important differences are their durations of action.

CLINICAL INDICATIONS AND ACTIONS

Diabetes mellitus, non-insulin-dependent

Sulfonylureas are used to manage mild to moderately severe, stable, nonketotic NIDDM that cannot be controlled by diet alone. Sulfonyl-

COMPARING ORAL HYPOGLYCEMICS

Typically, sulfonylureas have similar actions and produce similar effects. They differ mainly in duration of action and dosage.

SULFONYLUREAS	EQUIVALENT DAILY DOSAGE	ONSET	ACTION PEAK	DURATION
First generation				
acetohexamide (Dymelor)	500 mg once daily or b.i.d.	1 hr	2 hr	12 to 24 hr
chlorpropamide (Diabenase)	250 mg once daily	1 hr	3 to 6 hr	60 hr
tolazamide (Tolinase)	250 mg once daily or b.i.d.	4 to 6 hr	6 to 10 hr	12 to 24 hr
tolbutamide (Orinase)	1,000 mg b.i.d. or t.i.d.	½ to 1 hr	4 to 8 hr	6 to 12 hr
Second generation				
glipizide (Glucotrol)	5 mg once daily	1 to 1½ hr	2 to 3 hr	10 to 24 hr
glyburide (DiaβBeta)	5 mg once daily	2 hr	3 to 4 hr	24 hr

ureas stimulate insulin release from the pancreas. After long-term therapy, extrapancreatic hypoglycemic effects include reduced hepatic glucose production, an increased number of insulin receptors, and changes in insulin binding.
Neurogenic diabetes insipidus
Although an unlabelled indication, chlorpropamide has been used in selected patients to treat neurogenic diabetes insipidus. The drug appears to potentiate the effect of minimal levels of antidiuretic hormone.

OVERVIEW OF ADVERSE REACTIONS

Dose-related side effects, which are usually not serious and respond to decreased dosage, include headache, nausea, vomiting, anorexia, heartburn, weakness, and paresthesia. Hypoglycemia may follow excessive dosage, increased exercise, decreased food intake, or consumption of alcohol. Signs and symptoms of overdose include anxiety, chills, cold sweats, confusion, cool pale skin, difficulty in concentration, drowsiness, excessive hunger, headache, nausea, nervousness, rapid heartbeat, shakiness, unsteady gait, weakness, and unusual fatigue. Administration of oral hypoglycemics has been associated with increased cardiovascular mortality compared with treatment by diet alone or diet plus insulin, according to a long-term prospective clinical trial conducted by the University Group Diabetes Program.

REPRESENTATIVE COMBINATIONS

None.

---

sulindac

(sul in´ dak)
Clinoril

• *Classification:* nonnarcotic analgesic, antipyretic, anti-inflammatory (nonsteroidal anti-inflammatory)
• *Pregnancy Risk Category:* B (D in 3rd trimester)

HOW SUPPLIED

Tablets: 100 mg◇, 150 mg, 200 mg

ACTION

Mechanism: Produces anti-inflammatory, analgesic, and antipyretic effects, possibly through inhibition of prostaglandin synthesis.
Absorption: About 90% of a dose is absorbed from the GI tract. The active metabolite undergoes considerable enterohepatic recirculation.
Distribution: Highly protein-bound.
Metabolism: Inactive; is metabolized hepatically to the active sulfide metabolite.
Excretion: In urine. Half-life: Of the parent drug, about 8 hours; of the active metabolite about 16 hours.
Onset, peak, duration: Peak plasma levels of the active metabolite are seen in about 2 hours.

INDICATIONS & DOSAGE

Osteoarthritis, rheumatoid arthritis, ankylosing spondylitis—
Adults: 150 mg P.O. b.i.d. initially; may increase to 200 mg P.O. b.i.d.
Acute subacromial bursitis or supraspinatus tendinitis, acute gouty arthritis—
Adults: 200 mg P.O. b.i.d. for 7 to 14 days. Dose may be reduced as symptoms subside.

CONTRAINDICATIONS & PRECAUTIONS

Contraindicated in patients with hypersensitivity to the drug and in patients in whom aspirin or other nonsteroidal anti-inflammatory drugs (NSAIDs) induce symptoms of asthma, urticaria, or rhinitis. Patients with known "triad" symptoms (aspirin hypersensitivity, rhinitis/nasal polyps, and asthma) are at high risk of bronchospasm because of cross-sensitivity to sulindac.

Serious GI toxicity, especially ulceration and hemorrhage, can occur at any time in patients on chronic NSAID therapy. Use cautiously in patients with a history of GI bleeding, hepatic or renal disease, cardiac decompensation, or hypertension.

Drug may mask the signs and symptoms of acute infection (fever, myalgias, erythema). Carefully evaluate patients with high infection risk (such as those with diabetes).

ADVERSE REACTIONS

Common reactions are in italics; life-threatening reactions are in bold italics.

Blood: prolonged bleeding time, ***aplastic anemia.***

CNS: dizziness, headache, nervousness.

EENT: tinnitus, transient visual disturbances.

GI: *epigastric distress, peptic ulceration, occult blood loss, nausea.*

Hepatic: elevated enzymes.

Skin: rash, pruritus.

Other: edema.

INTERACTIONS

None significant.

EFFECTS ON DIAGNOSTIC TESTS

Bleeding time: prolonged.

BUN, serum creatinine, and potassium: increased levels.

Serum alkaline phosphatase and transaminase: increased concentrations.

NURSING CONSIDERATIONS

Besides those related universally to drug therapy (see "How to use this book"), consider the following specific recommendations:

Assessment

• Obtain a baseline assessment of the patient's pain before therapy.

• Be alert for adverse reactions and drug interactions throughout therapy.

• Evaluate the patient's and family's knowledge about sulindac therapy.

Nursing Diagnoses

• Pain related to the patient's underlying condition.

• Sensory or perception alteration (visual) related to transient adverse effect of sulindac therapy.

• Knowledge deficit related to sulindac therapy.

Planning and Implementation

Preparation and Administration

• Give drug with meals, milk, or antacids to reduce adverse GI reactions.

Monitoring

• Regularly monitor the patient for relief of pain.

• Monitor the patient for visual disturbances and other adverse reactions, such as GI toxicity.

• Monitor the patient for fluid retention; sulindac causes sodium retention. However, it has the least effect on the kidneys.

Supportive Care

• Notify the doctor if the patient's pain persists or worsens.

Patient Teaching

• Advise the patient to notify the doctor if pain persists or becomes worse.

• Tell the patient to notify the doctor immediately if prolonged bleeding occurs.

• Tell the patient to take the drug with food or milk.

• Because serious GI toxicity can occur at any time in chronic NSAID therapy, teach the patient signs and symptoms of GI bleeding. Tell the patient to report these to the doctor immediately.

• Tell the patient to notify the doctor of any visual disturbances and to have a complete visual examination.

• Tell the patient to report edema and have blood pressure checked monthly.

Evaluation

In patients receiving sulindac, appropriate evaluation statements include:

• Patient states pain is relieved.
• Patient does not develop sensory or perceptual alteration (visual).
• Patient and family state an understanding of sulindac therapy.

T

tamoxifen citrate
(ta mox´ i fen)
Nolvadex, Nolvadex D†‡, Tamofen†

• *Classification:* antineoplastic (nonsteroidal antiestrogen)
• *Pregnancy Risk Category:* D

HOW SUPPLIED
Tablets: 10 mg, 15.2 mg†
Tablets (film-coated): 30.4 mg†

ACTION
Mechanism: A nonteroidal antiestrogen that is structurally related to clomiphene. Competes with estradiol for binding to cytoplasmic estrogen receptors.
Absorption: Well absorbed across the GI tract after oral administration.
Distribution: Widely distributed into total body water.
Metabolism: Extensively metabolized in the liver to several metabolites.
Excretion: Tamoxifen and its metabolites are excreted primarily in feces, mostly as metabolites. Half-life: Distribution phase half-life of 7 to 14 hours. Secondary peak plasma levels occur 4 days after a dose, probably because of enterohepatic circulation. Terminal elimination half-life is more than 7 days.

INDICATIONS & DOSAGE
Advanced premenopausal and postmenopausal breast cancer–
Women: 10 mg P.O. b.i.d.

CONTRAINDICATIONS & PRECAUTIONS
Contraindicated in the first 4 months of pregnancy because of the potential for fetal harm.

ADVERSE REACTIONS
Common reactions are in italics; life-threatening reactions are in bold italics.
Blood: transient fall in WBC or platelets.
GI: nausea in 10% of patients, vomiting, anorexia.
GU: vaginal discharge and bleeding.
Metabolic: hypercalcemia.
Skin: rash.
Other: temporary bone or tumor pain, hot flashes in 7% of patients. Brief exacerbation of pain from osseous metastases.

INTERACTIONS
None significant.

EFFECTS ON DIAGNOSTIC TESTS
Serum calcium: increased concentrations usually in patients with bone metastases.

NURSING CONSIDERATIONS
Besides those related univerally to drug therapy (see "How to use this book"), consider the following specific recommendations:
Assessment
• Obtain a baseline assessment of the patient's underlying condition before initiating therapy.
• Be alert for adverse reactions and drug interactions throughout therapy.
• Evaluate the patient's and family's knowledge about tamoxifen therapy.
Nursing Diagnoses
• Altered protection related to adverse drug reactions.

• High risk for fluid volume deficit related to adverse drug reactions.
• Knowledge deficit related to tamoxifen therapy.

Planning and Implementation

Preparation and Administration

• Administer medication on time despite nausea; if vomiting becomes a problem, premedicate patient with an antiemetic.

Monitoring

• Monitor effectiveness by noting results of follow-up diagnostic tests and overall physical status.
• Monitor the patient for adverse drug reactions and interactions by frequently receiving CBC and differential and platelet counts for evidence of immunosuppression.
• Monitor the patient's weight, hydration, and nutritional status if GI adverse reactions occur.
• Monitor serum calcium level. Tamoxifen may compound hypercalcemia related to bone metastases.
• Monitor the patient for infection if leukopenia occurs; observe for fever, chills, or purulent drainage or sputum.
• Monitor for bleeding (bruising, epistaxis, or hematuria) if the patient's platelet count drops.
• Monitor for bone or tumor pain.
• Monitor for hot flashes

Supportive Care

• Obtain an order for mild analgesics to control bone or tumor pain as indicated.
• Provide comfort measures to relieve hot flashes: environmental temperature control, skin care, and adequate intake of oral fluids.
• Institute infection and bleeding precautions if immunosuppression occurs.
• Provide the patient with an adequate diet and encourage him to eat if anorexia is a problem.
• Provide the patient with fluids if nausea and vomiting occur.
• Know that drug has been used to stimulate ovulation in women with ogilomenorrhea or amenorrhea who may have previously used oral contraceptives.

Patient Teaching

• Advise the patient that short-term therapy with tamoxifen induces ovulation. Recommend barrier contraception.
• Reassure the patient that bone pain during therapy usually indicates that the drug will produce a good response; tell the patient to request an analgesic from doctor.
• Instruct patient and family in comfort measures to relieve hot flashes: controlling environmental temperature, avoiding alcohol and tobacco, maintaining oral fluid intake, and dressing in layers of clothing to accommodate perceived changes in body temperature.
• Teach the patient and family protective measures to conserve the patient's energy and prevent infection or bleeding: allowing adequate rest, avoiding fatigue, and avoiding exposure to people with colds or other infections.
• Instruct the patient to eat a high-caloric diet and how to manage nausea, anorexia, and vomiting; stress importance of continuing medication despite GI adverse reactions. Tell the patient to notify doctor if vomiting occurs shortly after a dose is taken.

Evaluation

In patient receiving tamoxifen, appropriate evaluation statements may include:

• Patient's tumor size is decreasing with tamoxifen therapy.
• Patient demonstrates no visual alterations.
• Patient and family state an understanding of tamoxifen therapy.

temazepam

(te maz´ e pam)
Restoril, Temaz

• Controlled Substance Schedule IV
• *Classification:* sedative-hypnotic (benzodiazepine)
• *Pregnancy Risk Category:* X

HOW SUPPLIED

Capsules: 15 mg, 30 mg

ACTION

Mechanism: Acts on the limbic system, thalamus, and hypothalamus of the CNS to produce hypnotic effects. A benzodiazepine.
Absorption: Well absorbed through the GI tract.
Distribution: Widely distributed throughout the body. Drug is 98% protein-bound.
Metabolism: In the liver primarily to inactive metabolites.
Excretion: Metabolites are excreted in urine as glucuronide conjugates. Half-life: Ranges from 10 to 17 hours.
Onset, peak, duration: Peak levels occur in 1 to 3 hours. Onset of action occurs at 30 to 60 minutes.

INDICATIONS & DOSAGE

Insomnia –
Adults: 15 to 30 mg P.O. h.s.
Adults over 65 years: 15 mg P.O. h.s.

CONTRAINDICATIONS & PRECAUTIONS

Contraindicated in patients with hypersensitivity to the drug; in patients with acute narrow-angle glaucoma or untreated open-angle glaucoma because of possible anticholinergic effects; in coma, because the drug's hypnotic or hypotensive effect may be prolonged or intensified; in patients with acute alcohol intoxication who have depressed vital signs, because the drug will worsen CNS depression; in patients with a history of drug abuse or suicidal tendencies, and in pregnant patients.

Use cautiously in patients with psychoses, because the drug is rarely beneficial in such patients and may induce paradoxical reactions; myasthenia gravis, Parkinson's disease, or chronic obstructive pulmonary disease, because it may exacerbate these disorders; or impaired hepatic or renal function, which prolongs elimination of the drug; and in elderly or debilitated patients, who are usually more sensitive to the drug's CNS effects.

ADVERSE REACTIONS

Common reactions are in italics; life-threatening reactions are in bold italics.
CNS: *drowsiness, dizziness, lethargy,* disturbed coordination, daytime sedation, confusion.
GI: anorexia, diarrhea.

INTERACTIONS

Alcohol or CNS depressants, including narcotic analgesics: increased CNS depression. Use together cautiously.

EFFECTS ON DIAGNOSTIC TESTS

EEG: minor changes (usually low-voltage, fast activity) during and after therapy.
Liver function tests: elevated results.

NURSING CONSIDERATIONS

Besides those related universally to drug therapy (see "How to use this book"), consider the following specific recommendations:

Assessment

• Obtain a baseline assessment of sleeping patterns and CNS status before therapy.
• Be alert for adverse reactions and drug interactions throughout therapy.
• Evaluate the patient's and family's knowledge about temazepam therapy.

Nursing Diagnoses
• Sleep pattern disturbance related to underlying patient problem.
• High risk for trauma related to adverse CNS reactions to temazepam.
• Knowledge deficit related to temazepam therapy.

Planning and Implementation
Preparation and Administration
• Before leaving the bedside, make sure the patient has swallowed the medication.
Monitoring
• Regularly monitor effectiveness by evaluating the patient's ability to sleep.
• Monitor for evidence of CNS and other adverse reactions. Keep in mind that elderly patients are more sensitive to the drug's adverse CNS effects.
Supportive Care
• After administration, institute safety precautions: remove cigarettes, keep bed rails up, and supervise or assist ambulation.
• Take precautions to prevent hoarding or self-overdosing, especially by the patient who is depressed or suicidal or has a history of drug abuse.
Patient Teaching
• Encourage the patient to report severe hangover or oversedation so the doctor can be consulted for change of dose or drug. However keep in mind that this relatively short-acting drug causes less severe next day hangover than flurazepam on diazepam.
• Instruct the patient to remain in bed after taking drug and to call for assistance to use the bathroom.
• Warn the patient to avoid hazardous activities that require mental alertness until adverse CNS reactions are known.
• Tell the patient to notify the nurse or doctor if sleep pattern disturbances continue despite therapy, if adverse reactions develop, or if questions arise about temazepam.
• Explain that onset of action may take as long as 2 to 2 ½ hours.
• Warn about the additive depressant effects that can follow alcohol consumption.

Evaluation
In patients receiving temazepam, appropriate evaluation statements may include:
• Patient states drug was effective in inducing sleep.
• Patient's safety maintained.
• Patient and family state an understanding of temazepam therapy.

terazosin hydrochloride
(ter ay´ zoe sin)
Hytrin

• *Classification:* antihypertensive (selective $alpha_1$ blocker)
• *Pregnancy Risk Category:* C

HOW SUPPLIED
Tablets: 1 mg, 2 mg, 5 mg

ACTION
Mechanism: Decreases blood pressure by vasodilation produced in response to blockade of $alpha_1$-adrenergic receptors.
Absorption: Rapidly absorbed after oral administration. Approximately 90% of the oral dose is bioavailable.
Distribution: About 90% to 94% is plasma protein-bound.
Metabolism: Hepatic.
Excretion: About 40% is excreted in urine, 60% in feces, mostly as metabolites. Up to 30% may be excreted unchanged. Half-life: Approximately 12 hours.
Onset, peak, duration: Peak plasma concentrations in 1 to 2 hours.

INDICATIONS & DOSAGE
Hypertension—
Adults: initial dose is 1 mg P.O. h.s., gradually increased according to pa-

tient response. Usual dosage range is 1 to 5 mg daily. Maximum recommended dosage is 20 mg/day.

CONTRAINDICATIONS & PRECAUTIONS

Contraindicated in patients with hypersensitivity to terazosin.

ADVERSE REACTIONS

Common reactions are in italics; life-threatening reactions are in bold italics.
CNS: asthenia, *dizziness,* headache, nervousness, paresthesia, somnolence, decreased libido.
CV: *palpitations,* postural hypotension, tachycardia, *peripheral edema.*
EENT: *nasal congestion,* sinusitis, blurred vision.
GI: *nausea.*
Respiratory: dyspnea.
Other: back pain, muscle pain, weight gain, impotence.

INTERACTIONS

Antihypertensives: excessive hypotension. Use together cautiously.

EFFECTS ON DIAGNOSTIC TESTS

Hematocrit and hemoglobin: decreased levels.
Total protein and albumin: decreased levels.
WBC: decreased count.

NURSING CONSIDERATIONS

Besides those related universally to drug therapy (see "How to use this book"), consider the following specific recommendations:

Assessment

- Obtain a baseline assessment of the patient's blood pressure before beginning therapy.
- Be alert for adverse reactions and drug interactions throughout therapy.
- Evaluate the patient's and family's knowledge about terazosin hydrochloride therapy.

Nursing Diagnoses

- Altered tissue perfusion (renal, cerebral, cardiopulmonary, peripheral) related to the patient's underlying condition.
- High risk for injury related to adverse reactions.
- Knowledge deficit related to terazosin therapy.

Planning and Implementation

Preparation and Administration

- ***P.O. use:*** Do not exceed initial dose of 1 mg.
- If this drug is discontinued for several days, patient will require retitration from initial dosing regimen (1 mg. P.O. at bedtime).

Monitoring

- Monitor effectiveness by frequently checking the patient's blood pressure and pulse rate.
- Monitor for orthostatic hypotension by checking the patient's supine and standing blood pressure.

Supportive Care

- Institute safety measures such as continuous use of bed rails if dizziness occurs.

Patient Teaching

- Explain the importance of taking this drug as prescribed, even when feeling well.
- Tell the patient not to discontinue this drug suddenly even if unpleasant adverse reactions occur but to discuss the problem with the doctor.
- Instruct the patient to check with the doctor or pharmacist before taking any OTC medications.
- Instruct the patient to avoid driving and other hazardous activities that require mental alertness for 12 hours after the first dose.
- Teach the patient and family caregiver to take blood pressure measurements. Tell the patient to notify the doctor if significant changes in blood pressure occur.

Evaluation
In patients receiving terazosin, appropriate evaluation statements may include:
• Blood pressure controlled within normal limits for this patient.
• Injury did not occur; patient did not experience dizziness.
• Patient and family state an understanding of terazosin therapy.

terbutaline sulfate
(ter byoo´ ta leen)
Brethaire, Brethine, Bricanyl

• *Classification:* bronchodilator, tocolytic (adrenergic [beta$_2$-agonist])
• *Pregnancy Risk Category:* B

HOW SUPPLIED
Tablets: 2.5 mg, 5 mg
Aerosol inhaler: 200 mcg/metered spray
Injection: 1 mg/ml

ACTION
Mechanism: Relaxes bronchial smooth muscle by acting on beta$_2$-adrenergic receptors. Also relaxes uterine muscle.
Absorption: 33% to 50% of an oral dose is absorbed through the GI tract; also well absorbed after S.C. administration.
Distribution: Widely distributed; less than 1% of a dose appears in breast milk.
Metabolism: Partially metabolized in liver to inactive compounds.
Excretion: After parenteral administration, 60% is excreted unchanged in urine, 3% in feces via bile, and the remainder in urine as metabolites. After oral administration, most is excreted as metabolites.
Onset, peak, duration: Onset of action occurs within 30 minutes, peaks within 2 to 3 hours, and persists for 4 to 8 hours. After S.C. injection, onset occurs within 15 minutes, peaks within 30 to 60 minutes, and persists for 1½ to 4 hours. After oral inhalation, onset of action occurs within 5 to 30 minutes, peaks within 1 to 2 hours, and persists for 3 to 4 hours.

INDICATIONS & DOSAGE
Relief of bronchospasm in patients with reversible obstructive airway disease–
Adults and children over 11 years: 2 inhalations separated by a 60-second interval, repeated q 4 to 6 hours. May also administer 2.5 to 5 mg P.O. q 8 hours or 0.25 mg S.C.
Treatment of premature labor–
Women: 0.01 mg/minute by I.V. infusion. Increase by 0.005 mg q 10 minutes up to 0.025 mg/minute or until contractions cease. Or, give 0.25 mg S.C. hourly until contractions cease. Maintenance dosage is 5 mg P.O. q 4 hours for 48 hours, then 5 mg q 6 hours.

CONTRAINDICATIONS & PRECAUTIONS
Contraindicated in patients with hypersensitivity to the drug or to other sympathomimetics. Use cautiously in patients with diabetes, hypertension, hyperthyroidism, or cardiac disease (especially when associated with arrhythmias).

ADVERSE REACTIONS
Common reactions are in italics; life-threatening reactions are in bold italics.
CNS: *nervousness, tremors, headache,* drowsiness, sweating.
CV: palpitations, increased heart rate.
EENT: drying and irritation of nose and throat (with inhaled form).
GI: vomiting, nausea.

INTERACTIONS
MAO inhibitors: when given with sympathomimetics, may cause severe hypertension (hypertensive crisis). Don't use together.

Propranolol and other beta blockers: blocked bronchodilating effects of terbutaline.

EFFECTS ON DIAGNOSTIC TESTS

Spirometry: reduced sensitivity for diagnosis of bronchospasm.

NURSING CONSIDERATIONS

Besides those related universally to drug therapy (see "How to use this book"), consider the following specific recomendations:

Assessment

- Obtain a baseline assessment of cardiopulmonary status before therapy by taking vital signs, obtaining an ECG (if ordered) and auscultating the heart and lung fields.
- Be alert for adverse reactions and drug interactions throughout therapy.
- Evaluate the patient's and family's knowledge about terbutaline sulfate therapy.

Nursing Diagnoses

- Ineffective airway clearance related to patient's underlying condition.
- High risk for injury related to adverse CNS reactions to terbutaline.
- Knowledge deficit related to terbutaline therapy.

Planning and Implementation

Preparation and Administration

- ***S.C. use:*** Protect injection from light. Do not use if discolored. Give S.C. injections in lateral deltoid area.

Monitoring

- Monitor effectiveness by monitoring respiratory rate, auscultating lung fields, and following laboratory studies such as arterial blood gases.
- Monitor for adverse CNS reactions such as nervousness, tremors, or headache.
- Monitor neonates for hypoglycemia when used as a treatment for preterm labor. Although not approved by the FDA for such use, it is considered an effective treatment of preterm labor and is used in many hospitals.
- Monitor for toxicity, particularly when aerosol and tablets are used concomitantly.

Supportive Care

- Notify the doctor if you notice that the patient is developing a tolerance to the drug.
- Institute safety measures such as assisting the patient when out of bed and using side rails continuously if adverse CNS reactions develop.

Patient Teaching

- Inform the patient that a tolerance may develop with prolonged use.
- Warn the patient about possible paradoxical bronchospasm. If this occurs, the drug should be discontinued immediately.
- Tell the patient that he may use tablets and aerosol concomitantly.
- Teach patient to perform oral inhalation correctly. Give the following instructions for using a metered-dose inhaler:
  – Clear nasal passages and throat.
  – Breathe out, expelling as much air from lungs as possible.
  – Place mouthpiece well into mouth as inhaler is released, and inhale deeply.
  – Hold breath for several seconds, remove mouthpiece, and exhale slowly.
- Tell the patient to wait at least 2 minutes before repeating procedure for a second dose if more than one inhalation is ordered. Tell the patient who is also using a steroid inhaler to use the bronchodilator first, then wait about 5 minutes before using the steroid. This allows the bronchodilator to open passages for maximum effectiveness.

Evaluation

In patients receiving terbutaline, appropriate evaluation statements may include:

- Patient experiences improved respiratory status.
- Patient does not experience CNS adverse reactions to terbutaline.
- Patient and family state an understanding of terbutaline therapy.

terconazole

(ter kone´ a zole)

Terazol 3 Vaginal Suppositories, Terazol 7 Vaginal Cream

• *Classification:* antifungal (triazole derivative)
• *Pregnancy Risk Category:* C

HOW SUPPLIED

Vaginal cream: 0.4%
Vaginal suppositories: 80 mg

ACTION

Mechanism: Exact mechanism unknown; may increase fungal cell membrane permeability (*Candida* species only).
Absorption: Minimal; absorption may range from 5% to 16%.
Distribution: Effect is mainly local.
Excretion: Half-life: 52.2 hours.
Onset, peak, duration: After daily intravaginal administration of 0.8% terconazole 40 mg for 7 days, low plasma concentrations gradually rose to a daily peak at 6.6 hours.

INDICATIONS & DOSAGE

Local treatment of vulvovaginal candidiasis–
Adults: insert 1 applicatorful of cream into vagina h.s. for 7 days; or 1 suppository intravaginally h.s. for 3 days; may repeat course if necessary after reconfirmation by smear and/or culture

CONTRAINDICATIONS & PRECAUTIONS

Contraindicated in patients who are allergic to the drug or to any of its components. If irritation or sensitization occurs, drug should be discontinued.

ADVERSE REACTIONS

Common reactions are in italics; life-threatening reactions are in bold italics.
CNS: headache.
Skin: vulvovaginal burning, irritation.
Other: fever, chills, body aches.

INTERACTIONS

None.

EFFECTS ON DIAGNOSTIC TESTS

None reported.

NURSING CONSIDERATIONS

Besides those related universally to drug therapy (see "How to use this book"), consider the following specific recommendations:

Assessment

• Obtain a baseline assessment of vulvovaginal infection before therapy.
• Be alert for adverse reactions and drug interactions throughout therapy.
• Evaluate the patient's and family's knowledge about terconazole therapy.

Nursing Diagnoses

• Impaired tissue integrity related to patient's underlying condition.
• High risk for altered body temperature related to terconazole-induced fever.
• Knowledge deficit related to terconazole therapy.

Planning and Implementation

Preparation and Administration

• ***Intravaginal use:*** Insert cream using enclosed applicator.
• If vaginal suppository is used, have patient remain supine for about 30 minutes after inserting the suppository.

Monitoring

• Monitor effectiveness by regularly checking for vaginal drainage, burning and itching.
• Monitor for adverse reactions and interactions by frequently assessing vital signs especially temperature.
• Monitor for drug-induced headache.
• Monitor for local skin irritation and burning.

Supportive Care
- Obtain an order for a mild analgesic if the patient develops a drug-induced headache.
- Be prepared to discontinue use and do not retreat if patient develops fever, chills, other flu-like symptoms or sensitivity.
- Be aware drug is contraindicated in patients with sensitivity to terconazole or any inactive ingredients in formulations.
- Some photosensitivity reactions were observed after dermal use; more with vaginal use.
- Remember, vaginal burning or itching is reported less frequently with terconazole than with miconazole or clotrimazole.

Patient Teaching
- Teach patient application of medication.
- Inform patient that therapeutic effect of terconazole is unaffected by menstruation. However, patient should not use tampons during treatment.
- Tell patient to use for full treatment period prescribed.
- Explain how to prevent reinfection.
- Tell the patient to take a mild analgesic if she develops a drug-induced headache.

Evaluation

In patients receiving terconazole, appropriate evaluation statements may include:
- Vulvovaginal infection has resolved.
- Patient did not develop a drug-induced fever.
- Patient and family state an understanding of terconazole therapy.

---

terfenadine

(ter fen´ a deen)

Seldane, Teldane‡

- *Classification:* antihistamine, (H_1-receptor antagonist (butyrophenone derivative)
- *Pregnancy Risk Category:* C

HOW SUPPLIED

Tablets: 60 mg

ACTION

Mechanism: Competes with histamine for H_1-receptor sites on effector cells. Prevents but does not reverse histamine-mediated responses. Considered a nonsedating antihistamine because the drug's chemical structure limits entry into the CNS.

Absorption: Well absorbed from the GI tract.

Distribution: Mainly distributed into the lungs, liver, GI tract, spleen, and bile; lower concentrations have been detected in the blood, kidneys, and heart. Terfenadine is extensively (97%) protein-bound; it does not cross the blood-brain barrier, and it is unknown if the drug crosses the placenta or is distributed into breast milk.

Metabolism: Almost completely metabolized in the GI tract and liver (first-pass effect).

Excretion: Only 1% of drug is excreted unchanged; about 60% of drug and metabolites is excreted in feces, with the remaining 40% excreted in urine. Half-life: Elimination half-life is about 16 to 23 hours.

Onset, peak, duration: Action begins within 1 to 2 hours and peaks in 3 to 6 hours.

INDICATIONS & DOSAGE

Rhinitis, allergy symptoms–

Adults and children over 12 years: 60 mg P.O. b.i.d.

Children 6 to 12 years: 30 to 60 mg P.O. b.i.d.

Children 3 to 5 years: 15 mg P.O. b.i.d.

CONTRAINDICATIONS & PRECAUTIONS

Contraindicated in patients with hypersensitivity to the drug. Use with caution in patients with asthma or other lower respiratory diseases, because its mild anticholinergic effects might aggravate these conditions.

ADVERSE REACTIONS

Common reactions are in italics; life-threatening reactions are in bold italics.

CNS: fatigue, dizziness, *headache*, sedation.

GI: abdominal distress, nausea.

EENT: dry throat and mouth, nasal stuffiness.

INTERACTIONS

None significant.

EFFECTS ON DIAGNOSTIC TESTS

Diagnostic skin tests: test interference.

NURSING CONSIDERATIONS

Besides those related universally to drug therapy (see "How to use this book"), consider the following specific recommendations.

Assessment

- Obtain a baseline assessment of the patient's rhinitis or allergy symptoms before terfenadine therapy.
- Be alert for adverse reactions and drug interactions throughout therapy.
- Evaluate the patient's and family's knowledge about terfenadine therapy.

Nursing Diagnoses

- Ineffective airway clearance related to the patient's underlying condition.
- Pain related to terfenadine-induced headache.
- Knowledge deficit related to terfenadine therapy.

Planning and Implementation

Preparation and Administration

- ***P.O. use:*** Break tablets for childrens' dosages.

Monitoring

- Monitor effectiveness by noting relief of allergy symptoms and evaluating respiratory status.
- Periodically ask the patient if headache occurs.

Supportive Care

- Expect the drug to relieve symptoms about 1 hour after the drug is taken.
- Keep patients well hydrated, because terfenadine may cause a mild anticholinergic drying effect, especially if the patient has a lower airway disease, such as asthma.
- Remember that terfenadine does not cause the degree of drowsiness and sedation associated with other antihistamines because the drug does not cross the blood-brain barrier. In addition, its anticholinergic and antiserotonin effects are mild.

Patient Teaching

- Explain to parents that the tablet can be broken to give children the prescribed dosage.
- Instruct the patient not to exceed prescribed dose and tell him that relief of symptoms should occur about 1 hour after the drug is given.
- Tell the patient that a mild analgesic can be taken if headache occurs. Tell the patient to notify the doctor if headache is severe.

Evaluation

In patients receiving terfenadine, appropriate evaluation statements may include:

- Patient's allergy symptoms are relieved with terfenadine.
- Patient tolerates therapy without painful headache.
- Patient and family state an understanding of terfenadine therapy.

terpin hydrate* ◇
(ter´ pin)

- *Classification:* expectorant (oliphotic alcohol)
- *Pregnancy Risk Category:* C

HOW SUPPLIED
Elixir: 85 mg/5 ml (43% alcohol)* ◇

ACTION
Mechanism: Increases production of respiratory tract fluids to help liquefy and reduce the viscosity of thick secretions.
Pharmacokinetics: Unknown.

INDICATIONS & DOSAGE
Excessive bronchial secretions–
Adults: 5 to 10 ml P.O. of elixir q 4 to 6 hours.

CONTRAINDICATIONS & PRECAUTIONS
Contraindicated in patients with peptic ulcer; not recommended in children under age 12, because of its high alcohol content. Use with caution in patients taking other CNS depressants and during pregnancy; alcohol crosses the placental barrier, and excessive use may cause congenital anomalies from its high alcohol content.

ADVERSE REACTIONS
Common reactions are in italics; life-threatening reactions are in bold italics.
GI: nausea, vomiting.

INTERACTIONS
None significant.

EFFECTS ON DIAGNOSTIC TESTS
None reported.

NURSING CONSIDERATIONS
Besides those related universally to drug therapy (see "How to use this book"), consider the following specific recommendations:
Assessment
- Obtain a baseline assessment of the patient's cough and sputum production before initiating therapy.
- Be alert for adverse reactions and drug interactions throughout therapy.
- Evaluate the patient's and family's knowledge about terpin hydrate.

Nursing Diagnoses
- Ineffective airway clearance related to the patient's underlying condition.
- High risk for fluid volume deficit related to adverse effects of terpin hydrate.
- Knowledge deficit related to terpin hydrate therapy.

Planning and Implementation
Preparation and Administration
- Do not give in large doses because of high alcohol content of elixir (86 proof).

Monitoring
- Monitor effectiveness by regularly evaluating the patient's cough and sputum production.
- Monitor hydration status; record intake and output.

Supportive Care
- Provide the necessary tissues and waste receptacles for disposing of expectorated respiratory secretions.
- Provide good oral hygiene for the patient receiving terpin hydrate.
- Obtain an order for an antiemetic, as needed.

Patient Teaching
- Tell the patient to avoid sources of respiratory irritants such as fumes, smoke, and dust.
- Encourage deep-breathing exercises.

Evaluation
In patients receiving terpin hydrate, appropriate evaluation statements may include:
- Patient's lungs are clear and respiratory secretions and cough are decreased.
- Patient does not experience fluid volume deficit.

• Patient and family state an understanding of terpin hydrate therapy.

testolactone

(tess toe lak′ tone)
Teslac

• Controlled Substance Schedule III
• *Classification:* antineoplastic (androgen)
• *Pregnancy Risk Category:* C

HOW SUPPLIED

Tablets: 50 mg

ACTION

Mechanism: A synthetic agent chemically related to androgens that may block pituitary gonadotropin synthesis or block the effects of progestins. Changes the tumor's hormonal environment and alters the neoplastic process.
Absorption: Well absorbed across the GI tract after oral administration.
Distribution: Widely distributed.
Metabolism: Extensively metabolized in the liver.
Excretion: Drug and metabolites are excreted primarily in urine.

INDICATIONS & DOSAGE

Advanced postmenopausal breast cancer–
Women: 250 mg P.O. q.i.d.

CONTRAINDICATIONS & PRECAUTIONS

Contraindicated in the treatment of breast cancer in men and in premenopausal women because of the potential for adverse hormonal effects. Use cautiously in patients with hypercalcemia and cardiovascular disease.

ADVERSE REACTIONS

Common reactions are in italics; life-threatening reactions are in bold italics.
CNS: paresthesias.
CV: increased blood pressure, edema.
GI: nausea, vomiting, diarrhea.
Metabolic: hypercalcemia.
Other: alopecia.

INTERACTIONS

Oral anticoagulants: increased pharmacologic effects. Monitor carefully.

EFFECTS ON DIAGNOSTIC TESTS

Serum calcium, urinary creatinine, and urinary 17-ketosteroids: increased concentrations.

NURSING CONSIDERATIONS

Besides those related universally to drug therapy (see "How to use this book"), consider the following specific recommendations:

Assessment
• Obtain a baseline assessment of patient's underlying condition before initiating therapy.
• Be alert for adverse reactions and drug interactions throughout therapy.
• Evaluate the patient's and family's knowledge about testolactone therapy.

Nursing Diagnoses
• Body image disturbance related to adverse drug reactions.
• High risk for fluid volume deficit related to adverse reactions.
• Knowledge deficit related to testolactone therapy.

Planning and Implementation
Preparation and Administration
• ***P.O. use:*** Dosage may be decreased if patient is also on anticoagulants.
• Obtain serum calcium and electrolytes before initiating therapy.
Monitoring
• Monitor effectiveness by noting results of follow-up diagnostic tests and overall physical status.
• Monitor effectiveness by regularly checking tumor size and rate of growth through appropriate studies.
• Monitor hydration status if patient develops nausea, vomiting, and diarrhea.

• Monitor serum calcium level and electrolytes throughout treatment.
• Monitor the patient's vital signs–drug may cause hypertension.
• Monotor for CNS effects. Drug may cause parasthesias.

Supportive Care
• Know that testolactone is an androgen.
• Provide immobilized patients who are prone to hypercalcemia with alternate methods to exercise to prevent complications.
• Know that higher-than-recommended doses do not increase incidence of remission.
• Provide the patient with fluids if he develops nausea, vomiting, and diarrhea.

Patient Teaching
• Assure patient that this drug causes less virilization than testosterone.
• Encourage patient to increase daily fluid intake to 3,000 ml daily.
• Suggest that the patient obtain a wig or a hairpiece if hair loss is a problem.

Evaluation
In patients receiving testolactone, appropriate evaluation statements may include:
• Patient's body image is not disturbed.
• Patient does not develop fluid volume deficit.
• Patient and family state an understanding of testolactone therapy.

---

testosterone
(tess toss´ ter one)
Andro, Andronaq, Histerone, Malogen, Testaqua, Testoject

testosterone cypionate
Andro-Cyp, Andronaq-LA, Andronate, dep Andro, Depotest, Depo-Testosterone, Duratest, T-Cypionate, Tesionate, Testa-C, Testoject-LA, Testred Cypionate, Virilon IM

testosterone enanthate
Android-T, Andro-LA, Andryl, Delatestryl, Durathate, Everone, Malogex†, Testone LA, Testrin PA

testosterone propionate
Malogen†, Testex

• Controlled Substance Schedule III
• *Classification:* androgen replacement, antineoplastic (androgen)
• *Pregnancy Risk Category:* X

HOW SUPPLIED
testosterone
Injection (aqueous suspension): 25 mg/ml, 50 mg/ml, 100 mg/ml
Pellets (sterile) for subcutaneous implantation: 75 mg
testosterone cypionate
Injection (in oil): 50 mg/ml, 100 mg/ml, 200 mg/ml
testosterone enanthate
Injection (in oil): 100 mg/ml, 200 mg/ml
testosterone propionate
Injection (in oil): 25 mg/ml, 50 mg/ml, 100 mg/ml

ACTION
Mechanism: An androgen that stimulates cytosol steroid receptors in tissues to effect protein synthesis. Stimulates target tissues to develop normally in androgen-deficient males.
Absorption: Must be administered parenterally because inactivated rapidly by the liver or GI mucosa when given orally. The esters are less polar, and therefore are absorbed slowly from the I.M. injection site. Because they can irritate the tissues, absorption may be erratic.
Distribution: Normally 98% to 99% plasma-protein bound, primarily to sex hormone binding globulin.
Metabolism: Extensively metabolized to several 17-ketosteroids by two main pathways in the liver. A large

portion of these metabolites then form glucuronide and sulfate conjugates.
Excretion: Very little unchanged testosterone appears in urine or feces. Approximately 90% of metabolized testosterone is excreted in urine in the form of sulfate and glucuronide conjugates. Half-life: Ranges from 10 to 100 minutes.
Onset, peak, duration: The duration of action of testosterone cypionate and enanthate is 2 to 4 weeks; the duration of action of testosterone propionate is somewhat shorter.

INDICATIONS & DOSAGE

Eunuchoidism, eunuchism, male climacteric symptoms–
Adults: 10 to 25 mg (base) I.M. 2 to 5 times weekly.
Breast engorgement of nonnursing mothers–
25 to 50 mg (base) I.M. daily for 3 to 4 days, starting at delivery.
Breast cancer in women 1 to 5 years postmenopausal–
100 mg (base) I.M. 3 times weekly as long as improvement maintained.
Eunuchism, eunuchoidism, deficiency after castration and male climacteric–
Adults: 200 to 400 mg (cypionate or enanthate) I.M. q 4 weeks.
Oligospermia–
Adults: 100 to 200 mg (cypionate or enanthate) I.M. q 4 to 6 weeks for development and maintenance of testicular function.
Eunuchism and eunuchoidism, male climacteric, impotence–
Adults: 10 to 25 mg (propionate) I.M. 2 to 4 times weekly.
Metastatic breast cancer in women–
50 to 100 mg (propionate) I.M. 3 times weekly. 200 to 400 mg (cypionate or enanthate) I.M. q 2 to 4 weeks.
Postmenopausal or primary osteoporosis–
Adults: 200 to 400 mg (enanthate) I.M. q 4 weeks.

CONTRAINDICATIONS & PRECAUTIONS

Contraindicated in patients with severe renal or cardiac disease, which may be worsened by the fluid and electrolyte retention caused by this drug; hepatic disease, because impaired elimination of the drug may cause toxic accumulation; in male patients with prostatic or breast cancer, benign prostatic hypertrophy with obstruction, or undiagnosed abnormal genital bleeding, because the drug can stimulate the growth of cancerous breast or prostate tissue; and in pregnant or breast-feeding women, because animal studies have shown that administration of androgens during pregnancy causes masculinization of the fetus.

ADVERSE REACTIONS

Common reactions are in italics; life-threatening reactions are in bold italics.
Androgenic: in women–*acne, edema, oily skin, weight gain, hirsutism, hoarseness,* clitoral enlargement, decreased or increased libido. In men–prepubertal: premature epiphyseal closure, acne, priapism, growth of body and facial hair, phallic enlargement; postpubertal: testicular atrophy, oligospermia, decreased ejaculatory volume, impotence, gynecomastia, epididymitis.
CV: edema.
GI: gastroenteritis, nausea, vomiting, constipation, diarrhea, change in appetite.
GU: bladder irritability.
Hepatic: reversible jaundice.
Hypoestrogenic: in women–flushing; sweating; vaginitis with itching, drying, burning, or bleeding; menstrual irregularities.
Local: pain at injection site, indura-

tion, irritation and sloughing with pellet implantation, edema.
Other: hypercalcemia.

INTERACTIONS

None significant.

EFFECTS ON DIAGNOSTIC TESTS

Glucose tolerance tests: abnormal results.
Liver function test results and serum creatinine levels: may be elevated.
Prothrombin time (especially in patients on anticoagulant therapy): prolonged.
Serum 17-ketosteroids: decreased levels.
Serum sodium, potassium, calcium, phosphate, and cholesterol: increased levels.
Thyroid function test results (protein-bound iodine, radioactive iodine uptake, thyroid-binding capacity): possibly decreased.

NURSING CONSIDERATIONS

Besides those related universally to drug therapy (see "How to use this book"), consider the following specific recommendations:

Assessment
- Obtain a baseline assessment of the patient's underlying condition being treated with testosterone before initiating therapy.
- Be alert for adverse reactions and drug interactions throughout therapy.
- Evaluate the patient's and family's knowledge about testosterone therapy.

Nursing Diagnoses
- Sexual dysfunction related to the patient's hormonal deficiency.
- Body image disturbance related to adverse androgenic reactions associated with testosterone.
- Knowledge deficit related to testosterone therapy.

Planning and Implementation
Preparation and Administration
- ***I.M. use:*** Inject deep into upper outer quadrant of gluteal muscle. Rotate injection sites to prevent muscle atrophy.
- Store I.M. preparations at room temperature. If crystals appear, warming and shaking the bottle will usually disperse them.
- ***S.C. use:*** Follow doctor's instructions when pellets are used for subcutaneous implantation.

Monitoring
- Monitor the patient with metastatic breast cancer for hypercalcemia, which usually indicates progression of bone metastases.
- Monitor liver function studies regularly.
- Monitor prepubertal boys by X-ray for rate of bone maturation.
- Monitor for ecchymotic areas, petechiae, or abnormal bleeding in patients receiving concomitant anticoagulant therapy. Monitor prothrombin time.
- Monitor the patient's weight routinely for fluid retention.
- Monitor the injection site for soreness; because of possibility of postinjection furunculosis.
- Monitor patient for hypoglycemia, because drug enhances this effect.

Supportive Care
- Report signs of virilization in females so doctor can reevaluate treatment.
- Give the patient a diet high in calories and protein, unless contraindicated. Give small, frequent feedings. Also implement salt restriction if edema occurs and expect to administer a diuretic concurrently, if needed.
- Carefully evaluate results of laboratory studies, because many laboratory results may be altered during therapy and for 2 to 3 weeks after therapy ends.
- Obtain an order for an antiemetic, antidiarrheal, or laxative, as indicated.
- Prepare patient for altered body image, which may result from potential androgenic adverse reaction.

Patient Teaching
• Explain to female patients that virilization may occur. Tell these patients to report androgenic effects immediately. Discontinuation of drug will prevent further androgenic changes, but will probably not reverse those already present.
• Advise male patients to report priapism, reduced ejaculatory volume, and gynecomastia. These effects require discontinuation of drug.
• Instruct patient to eat a diet high in calories and protein, unless contraindicated, and to restrict sodium intake if edema occurs.
• Teach patient how to recognize signs of hypoglycemia and tell the patient to report them immediately.
• Instruct patient to report soreness at injection site.
• Advise the patient to report persistent GI distress, diarrhea, or the onset of jaundice.

Evaluation
In patients receiving testosterone, appropriate evaluation statements may include:
• Patient's underlying condition being treated with testosterone shows improvement.
• Patient states acceptance of altered body image as a result of testosterone therapy.
• Patient and family state an understanding of testosterone therapy.

---

tetanus antitoxin (TAT), equine
(tet´ nus)

• *Classification:* tetanus antitoxin
• *Pregnancy Risk Category:* D

HOW SUPPLIED
Injection: not less than 400 units/ml in 1,500-unit and 20,000-unit vials

ACTION
Mechanism: Neutralizes and binds tetanus toxin.
Pharmacokinetics: Unknown.

INDICATIONS & DOSAGE
Tetanus prophylaxis–
Patients over 30 kg: 3,000 to 5,000 units I.M. or S.C.
Patients under 30 kg: 1,500 to 3,000 units I.M. or S.C.
Tetanus treatment–
All patients: 10,000 to 20,000 units injected into wound. Give additional 40,000 to 100,000 units I.V. Start tetanus toxoid at same time but at different site and with a different syringe.

CONTRAINDICATIONS & PRECAUTIONS
Use TAT with caution in patients allergic to equine-derived preparations.

ADVERSE REACTIONS
Common reactions are in italics; life-threatening reactions are in bold italics.
Systemic: joint pain, hypersensitivity,
Local: pain, numbness, skin rash.
anaphylaxis, *serum sickness.*

INTERACTIONS
None significant.

EFFECTS ON DIAGNOSTIC TESTS
None reported.

NURSING CONSIDERATIONS
Besides those related universally to drug therapy (see "How to use this book"), consider the following specific recommendations:

Assessment
• Obtain a baseline assessment of the patient's allergies (especially to horses) and immunization reaction before therapy.
• Be alert for adverse reactions and drug interactions throughout therapy.
• Evaluate the patient's and family's knowledge about tetanus antitoxin therapy.

Nursing Diagnoses
- Altered protection related to neurotoxic effects of tetanus toxin.
- Impaired physical mobility related to antitoxin-induced joint pain.
- Knowledge deficit related to tetanus antitoxin.

Planning and Implementation

Preparation and Administration
- Test for sensitivity before giving. Give 0.1 ml as a 1:1000 dilution in normal saline solution intradermally.
- ***I.V. use:*** Give I.V. tetanus antitoxin in addition to antitoxin injected into the wound.

Monitoring
- Monitor effectiveness by observing for the absence of signs of tetany, indicating that the toxin has been successfully neutralized.
- Observe the patient for signs of anaphylaxis immediately after injecting antitoxin.
- Monitor joint mobility and range of motion.

Supportive Care
- Keep epinephrine 1:1000 available in case of anaphylaxis. Have oxygen and resuscitation equipment nearby.
- Obtain order for medication to relieve joint pain. Provide comfort measures, such as padding, support, and positioning. Assist with range of motion and ambulation.
- Use only when tetanus immune globulin (human) not available.
- Give preventive dose to those who have had two or fewer injections of tetanus toxoid and who have had tetanus-prone injuries that are more than 24 hours old.

Patient Teaching
- Instruct the patient to report respiratory difficulty immediately.
- Advise the patient that pain, rash, and numbness may occur at the injection site.
- Inform the patient that a tetanus toxoid booster is necessary every 10 years.

Evaluation

In patients receiving tetanus antitoxin, appropriate evaluation statements may include:
- Patient exhibits decrease or absence of signs of tetany.
- Patient is pain free.
- Patient and family state an understanding of tetanus antitoxin.

tetanus toxoid, adsorbed

tetanus toxoid, fluid
(tet´ nus)

- *Classification:* tetanus prophylaxis agent (toxoid)
- *Pregnancy Risk Category:* C

HOW SUPPLIED
adsorbed

Injection: 5 to 10 Lf units of inactivated tetanus/0.5-ml dose, in 0.5-ml syringes and 5-ml vials

fluid

Injection: 4 to 5 Lf units of inactivated tetanus/0.5-ml dose, in 0.5-ml syringes and 7.5-ml vials

ACTION
Mechanism: Promotes immunity to tetanus by inducing production of antitoxin.

Pharmacokinetics: Unknown.

Onset, peak, duration: Active immunity usually persists for 10 years. Adsorbed tetanus toxoid usually produces more persistent antitoxin titers than tetanus toxoid fluid.

INDICATIONS & DOSAGE
Primary immunization—

Adults and children: 0.5 ml (adsorbed) I.M. 4 to 6 weeks apart for two doses, then third dose 1 year after the second; 0.5 ml (fluid) I.M. or S.C. 4 to 8 weeks apart for three doses, then fourth dose of 0.5 ml 6 to

12 months after third dose. Booster is 0.5 ml I.M. at 10-year intervals.

CONTRAINDICATIONS & PRECAUTIONS

Contraindicated in patients with a history of neurologic or severe hypersensitivity reaction following a previous dose.

ADVERSE REACTIONS

Common reactions are in italics; life-threatening reactions are in bold italics.

Systemic: slight fever, chills, malaise, aches and pains, flushing, urticaria, pruritus, tachycardia, hypotension, ***anaphylaxis.***

Local: erythema, induration, nodule.

INTERACTIONS

Chloramphenicol: may interfere with response to tetanus toxoid.

EFFECTS ON DIAGNOSTIC TESTS

None reported.

NURSING CONSIDERATIONS

Besides those related universally to drug therapy (see "How to use this book"), consider the following specific recommendations:

Assessment

- Obtain a baseline assessment of the patient's allergies, immunization history, and immunization reaction before therapy.
- Be alert for adverse reactions and drug interactions throughout therapy.
- Evaluate the patient's and family's knowledge about tetanus toxoid therapy.

Nursing Diagnoses

- Altered protection related to lack of immunity to tetanus.
- Ineffective breathing pattern related to vaccine-induced anaphylaxis.
- Knowledge deficit related to tetanus toxoid.

Planning and Implementation

Preparation and Administration

- Determine the date of last tetanus immunization.
- Do not confuse this drug with tetanus immune globulin, human.
- ***I.M. or S.C. use only.*** Do not give I.V.

Monitoring

- Monitor effectiveness by checking the patient's antibody titers to tetanus.
- Observe the patient for signs of anaphylaxis immediately after injection.
- Check vital signs.
- Observe the injection site for local reaction to the vaccine (redness, nodule, induration).

Supportive Care

- Keep epinephrine 1:1000 available to treat possible anaphylaxis. Have oxygen and resuscitation equipment nearby.
- Treat fever with antipyretics.
- Do not give vaccine to patients with immunosuppression or immunoglobulin abnormalities.
- Defer immunization in acute illness, polio outbreaks, except in emergencies.
- Do not use hot or cold compresses; may increase severity of local reaction.
- Adsorbed form produces longer duration of immunity. Fluid form produces quicker booster effect in patients previously actively immunized.

Patient Teaching

- Instruct the patient to report respiratory difficulty immediately.
- Advise the patient that tetanus toxoid boosters are necessary every 10 years.
- Inform the patient that a slight fever, malaise, aches, and pains may follow immunization.
- Advise the patient to avoid applying hot or cold compresses to the injection site.

Evaluation
In patients receiving tetanus toxoid, appropriate evaluation statements may include:
- Patient exhibits immunity to tetanus.
- Patient demonstrates no signs of anaphylaxis.
- Patient and family state an understanding of tetanus toxoid.

tetracaine (ophthalmic)
(tet´ ra kane)
Pontocaine Eye

tetracaine hydrochloride
Pontocaine

- *Classification:* local anesthetic (para-amino benzoic acid derivative)
- *Pregnancy Risk Category:* C

HOW SUPPLIED
tetracaine
Ophthalmic ointment: 0.5%
tetracaine hydrochloride
Ophthalmic solution: 0.5%

ACTION
Mechanism: An ester-type local anesthetic that produces anesthesia by preventing initiation and transmission of impulses at the nerve-cell membrane. Probably acts by blocking sodium channels.
Pharmacokinetics: Unknown.
Onset, peak, duration: Onset of action is rapid, and the duration prolonged (2 or 3 hours or longer of surgical anesthesia).

INDICATIONS & DOSAGE
Anesthesia for tonometry, gonioscopy; removal of corneal foreign bodies, suture removal from cornea; other diagnostic and minor surgical procedures–
Adults and children: instill 1 to 2 drops of 0.5% solution or a small strip of ointment in eye just before procedure.

CONTRAINDICATIONS & PRECAUTIONS
Contraindicated in patients hypersensitive to ester-type local anesthetics. Also contraindicated in patients hypersensitive to para-amino benzoic acid (PABA) because the drug is probably metabolized to PABA by pseudocholinesterase. This drug is for short-term use only. Chronic use of ophthalmic anesthetics can result in delayed wound healing or corneal epithelial erosions.

ADVERSE REACTIONS
Common reactions are in italics; life-threatening reactions are in bold italics.
Eye: transient stinging in eye 30 seconds after initial instillation, epithelial damage in excessive or long-term use.

INTERACTIONS
Cholinesterase inhibitors: prolonged ocular anesthesia and increased risk of toxicity.
Sulfonamides: interference with sulfonamide antibacterial activity. Wait 30 minutes after anesthesia before instilling sulfonamide.

EFFECTS ON DIAGNOSTIC TESTS
None reported.

NURSING CONSIDERATIONS
Besides those related universally to drug therapy (see "How to use this book"), consider the following specific recommendations:

Assessment
- Obtain a baseline assessment of the patient's vision and ocular appearance.
- Be alert for adverse reactions and drug interactions throughout therapy.
- Evaluate the patient's and family's knowledge about tetracaine hydrochloride therapy.

Nursing Diagnoses
- Sensory/perceptual alterations (visual) related to the patient's underlying condition.
- Pain related to tetracaine hydrochloride-induced irritation or accidental abrasion.
- Knowledge deficit related to tetracaine hydrochloride therapy.

Planning and Implementation
Preparation and Administration
- Do not use solution that is discolored.
- Store solution in a tightly closed container.
- Avoid repeated use or exceeding the recommended dosage.

Monitoring
- Monitor effectiveness by assessing the patient's visual status and degree of anesthesia.
- Monitor for drug-induced eye and skin irritation.

Supportive Care
- Notify doctor immediately of any changes in the patient's visual status.

Patient Teaching
- Warn the patient not to touch or rub his eye while it is anesthetized, as he may unknowingly irritate the eye or abrade the cornea.
- Tell the patient he may experience transient stinging in his eye about 30 seconds after instillation of the drug.

Evaluation
In patients receiving tetracaine, appropriate evaluation statements may include:
- Patient experiences therapeutic anesthesia.
- Patient remains free of drug-related irritation and injury.
- Patient and family state an understanding of tetracaine therapy.

tetracaine hydrochloride (systemic)
(tet´ ra kane)
Pontocaine

- *Classification:* local anesthetic (para-amino benzoic acid derivative)
- *Pregnancy Risk Category:* C

HOW SUPPLIED
Injection: 1%
Injection (with dextrose, 6%): 0.2%, 0.3%
Powder for reconstitution: 20 mg/ampule

ACTION
Mechanism: An ester-type local anestetic that blocks depolarization by interfering with sodium-potassium exchange across the nerve cell membrane, preventing generation and conduction of the nerve impulse.
Absorption: Slowly absorbed into the vasculature. Addition of epinephrine or similar vasoconstrictor retards absorption.
Distribution: Widely distributed; drug crosses the placenta.
Metabolism: In the plasma, by pseudocholinesterase, to para-amino benzoic acid (PABA) which undergoes further degredation in the liver. Slowest route of hydrolysis as compared to other ester-type anesthetics.
Excretion: In the urine as PABA and metabolites.
Onset, peak, duration: Variable, but average onset is 15 minutes; duration of action about 1.5 to 3 hours.

INDICATIONS & DOSAGE
Low spinal (saddle block) in vaginal delivery–
give 2 to 5 mg as hyperbaric solution (in 10% dextrose).

Perineum and lower extremities: give 5 to 10 mg.
Up to costal margin: give 15 to 20 mg.

CONTRAINDICATIONS & PRECAUTIONS

Contraindicated in patients hypersensitive to the drug or its components; for caudal or epidural anesthesia in patients with serious diseases of the CNS; use cautiously in severely debilitated patients and in those with liver disease.

ADVERSE REACTIONS

Common reactions are in italics; life-threatening reactions are in bold italics.
Skin: dermatologic reactions.
Other: edema, ***status asthmaticus, anaphylaxis,*** anaphylactoid reactions.

The following systemic effects may result from high blood levels of the drug:
CNS: anxiety, nervousness, seizures followed by drowsiness, unconsciousness, tremors, twitches, shivering, and ***respiratory arrest.***
CV: myocardial depression, ***arrhythmias, cardiac arrest.***
EENT: blurred vision, tinnitus.
GI: nausea, vomiting.

INTERACTIONS

None significant.

EFFECTS ON DIAGNOSTIC TESTS

None reported.

NURSING CONSIDERATIONS

Besides those related universally to drug therapy (see "How to use this book"), consider the following specific recommendations:

Assessment

- Obtain a baseline assessment of the patient's sensory status before therapy.
- Be alert for adverse reactions and drug interactions throughout therapy.
- Evaluate the patient's and family's knowledge about tetracaine therapy.

Nursing Diagnoses

- Pain related to inadequate block.
- Decreased cardiac output related to adverse reaction to tetracaine.
- Knowledge deficit related to tetracaine therapy.

Planning and Implementation

Preparation and Administration

- Don't use cloudy, discolored, or crystallized solutions.
- Spinal anesthesia use: Keep in mind that when cerebrospinal fluid is added to powdered drug or drug solution during spinal anesthesia, solution may be cloudy.
- Protect from light. Store refrigerated.

Monitoring

- Monitor effectiveness by evaluating pain relief. Continue to monitor sensory level every 15 minutes after completion of surgery or delivery until sympathetic innervation return.
- Monitor for signs of anaphylaxis following administration of drug. Drug contains sulfites.
- Monitor for signs of myocardial depression as well as unconsciousness, seizures, and other adverse reactions, including respiratory and cardiac arrest, which may result from high blood levels of the drug.

Supportive Care

- Keep resuscitative equipment and drugs available.
- Consult with the doctor if pain relief is ineffective.
- Be aware that onset occurs in 15 minutes; duration up to 3 hours.
- Notify the doctor immediately if the patient's CNS, cardiac or respiratory status deteriorates.
- Keep patient flat until sympathetic return has been established to prevent hypotension.
- Keep in mind that tetracaine hydrochloride is 10 times as strong as procaine hydrochloride.

Patient Teaching
• Explain that the drug will cause a local loss of sensation providing pain relief in the selected body area, but unlike general anesthesia will not cause unconsciousness.
• Describe the route of administration, such as low spinal (saddle block).

Evaluation
In patients receiving tetracaine, appropriate evaluation statements may include:
• Effective sensory block is achieved.
• Cardiac status is within normal limits.
• Patient and family state an understanding of tetracaine therapy.

tetracycline (ophthalmic)
(tet ra sye´ kleen)
Achryomycin Ophthalmic

tetracycline hydrochloride
Achromycin

• *Classification:* antibiotic (tetracycline)
• *Pregnancy Risk Category:* D

HOW SUPPLIED
tetracycline
Ophthalmic suspension: 10 mg/ml
tetracycline hydrochloride
Ophthalmic ointment: 10 mg/g

ACTION
Mechanism: Binds to the 30S ribosomal subunit within susceptible bacteria, inhibiting protein synthesis. Usually bacteriostatic.
Absorption: After topical ophthalmic administration of ointment or solution, trace amounts of drug appear within the aqueous humor.
Distribution: Bacteriostatic levels are present in tears for 2 hours following application of solution and 6 hours after ointment.

INDICATIONS & DOSAGE
Superficial ocular infections and inclusion conjunctivitis–
Adults and children: instill 1 to 2 drops in eye b.i.d., q.i.d., or more often, depending on severity of infection.
Trachoma–
Adults and children: instill 2 drops in each eye b.i.d., t.i.d., or q.i.d. Continue for 1 to 2 months or longer, or use 1% ointment t.i.d. or q.i.d. for 30 days.
Prophylaxis of ophthalmia neonatorum–
Neonates: 1 to 2 drops into each eye shortly after delivery.

CONTRAINDICATIONS & PRECAUTIONS
Contraindicated in patients with hypersensitivity to any tetracycline; during the second half of pregnancy; and in children under age 8 because of the risk of permanent discoloration of teeth, enamel defects, and retardation of bone growth.

Use cautiously in patients with decreased renal function because it may elevate BUN levels and exacerbate renal dysfunction; and in patients apt to be exposed to direct sunlight or ultraviolet light, because of the risk of photosensitivity reactions.

ADVERSE REACTIONS
Common reactions are in italics; life-threatening reactions are in bold italics.
Eye: itching, blurred vision (with ointment).
Other: hypersensitivity (eye itching and dermatitis), overgrowth of nonsusceptible organisms with long-term use.

INTERACTIONS
None significant.

EFFECTS ON DIAGNOSTIC TESTS
BUN: elevated levels in decreased renal function.

Urine catecholamines: false elevations in fluorometric tests.
Urine glucose test: false-negative results with oxidase reagent (Clinistix or Tes-Tape).

NURSING CONSIDERATIONS

Besides those related universally to drug therapy (see "How to use this book"), consider the following specific recommendations:

Assessment

- Obtain a baseline assessment of the patient's allergies before therapy.
- Be alert for adverse reactions and drug interactions throughout therapy.
- Evaluate the patient's and family's knowledge about tetracycline therapy.

Nursing Diagnoses

- Altered protection related to ocular infection.
- Sensory/perceptual alteration–visual, related to tetracycline ointment-induced visual blurring.
- Knowledge deficit related to tetracycline therapy.

Planning and Implementation

Preparation and Administration

- Store in tightly sealed, light-resistant container.
- Wash hands before and after administration.
- Clean eye area of excess exudate before administration.
- Shake suspension well before use.
- For prophylaxis of ophthalmia neonatorum, apply ointment no later than 1 hour after birth.

Monitoring

- Monitor effectiveness by culturing the eye to check for microorganisms.
- Observe color, amount, and consistency of exudate.
- Monitor for hypersensitivity reaction.
- Check patient's vision.

Supportive Care

- Apply warm, moist compresses to eye area to aid removal of dried exudate.
- Use safety precautions if vision is impaired. Assist with activities.
- Ophthalmic ointment may be used with suspension to provide drug contact with affected area at night.

Patient Teaching

- Teach the patient to instill. Advise him to wash hands before and after administration. Warn him not to touch tip of applicator to eye or surrounding tissues. Remind the patient to shake the suspension well before use.
- Instruct the patient to apply light finger pressure to the lacrimal sac for 1 minute after instillation. Caution him to avoid scratching or rubbing the eye area.
- Instruct the patient to watch for signs of hypersensitivity (itching lids, swelling, constant burning). If these develop, stop the drug and notify the doctor immediately.
- Inform the patient or family that trachoma therapy should continue for 1 to 2 months or longer. Stress the importance of compliance with recommended therapy. Untreated trachoma may result in blindness.
- Advise the patient and family that gnats and flies are vectors of *Chlamydia trachomatis.* Warn the patient not to let them settle around the eye area. Explain that infection is spread by direct contact, so hand washing is essential to prevent the spread.
- Severe trachoma may require oral therapy as well.
- Warn patient to avoid sharing washcloths and towels with other family members during infection.
- Instruct the patient not to share eye medications with family members. A family member who develops the same symptoms should contact the doctor.

Evaluation

In patients receiving tetracycline, appropriate evaluation statements may include:

• Patient remains free from signs and symptoms of infection.
• Patient reports a decrease or absence in visual blurring.
• Patient and family state an understanding of tetracycline therapy.

tetracycline hydrochloride (topical)

(tet ra sye´ kleen)
Topicycline

- *Classification:* antibiotic (tetracyline)
- *Pregnancy Risk Category:* D

HOW SUPPLIED

Ointment: 3%
Topical solution: 2.2 mg/ml

ACTION

Mechanism: Binds to the 30S subunit of bacterial ribosomes and disrupts protein synthesis.
Absorption: 2% hydroalcoholic solutions are not absorbed; however, when n-decyl methyl sulfoxide is added, the drug penetrates into adjacent tissues.

INDICATIONS & DOSAGE

Acne vulgaris–
Adults and children over 12 years: apply generously to affected areas b.i.d. until skin is thoroughly covered.

CONTRAINDICATIONS & PRECAUTIONS

Contraindicated in patients with hypersensitivity to any tetracycline; during the second half of pregnancy; and in children under age 8 because of the risk of permanent discoloration of teeth, enamel defects, and retardation of bone growth.

Because of the risk of systemic absorption of the drug, use cautiously in patients with decreased renal function.

ADVERSE REACTIONS

Common reactions are in italics; life-threatening reactions are in bold italics.
Skin: *temporary stinging or burning on application;* slight yellowing of treated skin, especially in patients with light complexions; severe dermatitis; treated skin areas fluoresce under black lights.

INTERACTIONS

None significant.

EFFECTS ON DIAGNOSTIC TESTS

None reported.

NURSING CONSIDERATIONS

Besides those related universally to drug therapy (see "How to use this book"), consider the following specific recommendations:

Assessment
• Obtain a baseline assessment of acne before therapy.
• Be alert for adverse reactions and drug interactions throughout therapy.
• Evaluate the patient's and family's knowledge about tetracycline therapy.

Nursing Diagnoses
• Impaired skin integrity related to patient's underlying condition.
• High risk for impaired skin integrity related to tetracycline-induced dermatitis.
• Knowledge deficit related to tetracycline therapy.

Planning and Implementation
Preparation and Administration
• ***Topical use:*** Apply generously to affected areas. Apply in morning and evening.
• Store at room temperature, away from excessive heat.
Monitoring
• Monitor effectiveness by regularly assessing acne lesions.
• Monitor condition, if no improvement or condition worsens, stop using and notify doctor.
• Monitor for adverse reactions and interactions by frequently assessing

the patient's skin for slight yellowing or stinging or burning on application.

Supportive Care

• Keep in mind that prolonged use may result in overgrowth of nonsusceptible organisms.

• Notify doctor if adverse reactions occur.

• Be aware, serum levels with topical tetracycline hydrochloride are much lower than those for orally administered drug, so significant systemic effects are unlikely.

Patient Teaching

• Inform patient that normal use of cosmetics is permitted during therapy.

• Tell patient not to share drug with family members. Medication is to be used by one person only.

• Warn patient that drug should be used or discarded within 2 months.

• Explain that floating plug in bottle of topicycline is an inert and harmless result of reconstitution of the preparation – shouldn't be removed.

• Inform patient to control flow rate of solution by increasing or decreasing pressure of the applicator against the skin.

Evaluation

In patients receiving tetracyline, appropriate evaluation statements may include:

• Patient's acne vulgaris has resolved.

• Patient did not develop drug-induced dermatitis.

• Patient and family state an understanding of tetracycline therapy.

tetracycline hydrochloride (systemic)

(tet ra sye´ kleen)

Achromycin, Achromycin V, Apo-Tetra†, Austramycin V‡, Bristacycline, Cyclopar, Hostacycline P‡, Kesso-Tetra, Nor-Tet, Novotetra†, Panmycin**, Panmycin P‡, Robitet, Sarocycline, Sumycin, Tetracap, Tetracyn, Tetralan, Tetralean†

• *Classification:* antibiotic (tetracycline)
• *Pregnancy Risk Category:* D

HOW SUPPLIED

Tablets: 250 mg, 500 mg
Capsules: 250 mg, 500 mg
Oral suspension: 125 mg/5 ml

ACTION

Mechanism: Exerts bacteriostatic effect by binding to the 30S ribosomal subunit of microorganisms, thus inhibiting protein synthesis.

Absorption: 75% to 80% is absorbed after oral administration. Food or milk products significantly reduce oral absorption.

Distribution: Widely distributed into body tissues and fluids, including synovial, pleural, prostatic, and seminal fluids, bronchial secretions, saliva, and aqueous humor; CSF penetration is poor. Tetracycline crosses the placenta; it is 20% to 67% protein-bound.

Metabolism: Not metabolized.

Excretion: Primarily excreted unchanged in urine by glomerular filtration; some of the drug is excreted in breast milk. Half-life: 6 to 12 hours in adults with normal renal function.

Onset, peak, duration: Peak serum levels occur at 2 to 4 hours after oral administration.

INDICATIONS & DOSAGE

Infections caused by sensitive gram-negative and gram-positive organisms, trachoma, rickettsiae, Mycoplasma, *and* Chlamydia –

Adults: 250 to 500 mg P.O. q 6 hours.

Children over 8 years: 25 to 50 mg/kg P.O. daily, divided q 6 hours.

Uncomplicated urethral, endocervical, or rectal infection caused by Chlamydia trachomatis –

Adults: 500 mg P.O. q.i.d. for at least 7 days.

Brucellosis–
Adults: 500 mg P.O. q 6 hours for 3 weeks with streptomycin 1 g I.M. q 12 hours week 1 and daily week 2.
Gonorrhea in patients sensitive to penicillin–
Adults: initially, 1.5 g P.O., then 500 mg q 6 hours for 7 days.
Syphilis in patients sensitive to penicillin–
Adults: 30 to 40 g P.O. total in equally divided doses over 10 to 15 days.
Acne–
Adults and adolescents: initially, 250 mg P.O. q 6 hours, then 125 to 500 mg P.O. daily or every other day.
Shigellosis–
Adults: 2.5 g P.O. in 1 dose.

CONTRAINDICATIONS & PRECAUTIONS

Contraindicated in patients with hypersensitivity to any tetracycline; during the second half of pregnancy; and in children under age 8 because of the risk of permanent discoloration of teeth, enamel defects, and retardation of bone growth. Use cautiously in patients with decreased renal function because it may elevate BUN levels and exacerbate renal dysfunction; and in patients apt to be exposed to direct sunlight or ultraviolet light, because of the risk of photosensitivity reactions.

ADVERSE REACTIONS

Common reactions are in italics; life-threatening reactions are in bold italics.
Blood: neutropenia, eosinophilia.
CNS: dizziness, headache, ***intracranial hypertension.***
CV: ***pericarditis.***
EENT: sore throat, glossitis, dysphagia.
GI: anorexia, *epigastric distress, nausea,* vomiting, *diarrhea,* stomatitis, enterocolitis, inflammatory lesions in anogenital region.
Metabolic: *increased BUN.*
Skin: *maculopapular and erythematous rashes, urticaria, photosensitivity, increased pigmentation.*

INTERACTIONS

Antacids (including sodium bicarbonate) and laxatives containing aluminum, magnesium, or calcium; food, milk, or other dairy products: decrease antibiotic absorption. Give antibiotic 1 hour before or 2 hours after any of the above.
Ferrous sulfate and other iron products, zinc: decrease antibiotic absorption. Give tetracyclines 3 hours after or 2 hours before iron administration.
Lithium carbonate: may alter serum lithium levels.
Methoxyflurane: may cause severe nephrotoxicity with tetracyclines.
Oral contraceptives: decreased contraceptive effectiveness and increased risk of breakthrough bleeding.

EFFECTS ON DIAGNOSTIC TESTS

BUN: elevated levels in patients with decreased renal function.
Urine catecholamines: false elevations in fluorometric tests.
Urine tests with glucose enzymatic reagent (Clinistix or Tes-Tape): false-negative results.

NURSING CONSIDERATIONS

Besides those related universally to drug therapy (see "How to use this book"), consider the following specific recommendations:

Assessment
- Obtain a baseline assessment of infection before therapy.
- Be alert for adverse reactions and drug interactions throughout therapy.
- Evaluate the patient's and family's knowledge about tetracycline therapy.

Nursing Diagnoses
- Altered protection related to ineffectiveness of tetracycline to eradicate the infection.
- High risk for infection related to

development of superinfection caused by tetracycline therapy.
• Knowledge deficit related to tetracycline.

Planning and Implementation

Preparation and Administration

• Obtain specimen for culture and sensitivity tests before first dose. Therapy may begin pending test results.
• Check expiration date. Outdated or deteriorated tetracyclines have been associated with reversible nephrotoxicity (Fanconi's syndrome).
• Be aware that use of tetracycline during the last half of pregnancy and in children under 8 years may cause permanent discoloration of teeth, enamel defects, and retardation of bone growth. Question an order for tetracycline in these patients before administering the first dose.
• Do not expose drug to light or heat.
• ***P.O. use:*** Taking drug with food, milk or other dairy products, antacids, sodium bicarbonate, or iron products reduces it effectiveness. Administer with a full glass of water on an empty stomach, at least 1 hour before meals or 2 hours afterward. Give at least 1 hour before bedtime to prevent esophagitis. Shake liquid preparation before administering. Do not administer within 1 to 3 hours of other medications.
• ***I.V. use:*** Reconstitute 100-mg and 250-mg powder for injection with 5 ml sterile water, 500 mg with 10 ml. Further dilute in 100 to 1,000 ml volume of dextrose 5% in 0.9% sodium chloride solution. Refrigerate diluted solution for I.V. use and use within 24 hours. Do not mix tetracycline solution with any other I.V. additive.
• Be aware that tetracycline may be used as a pleural sclerosing agent in malignant pleural effusion. The drug is instilled through a chest tube by a doctor familiar with the technique.

Monitoring

• Monitor effectiveness by regularly assessing for improvement of infectious process.
• Monitor for signs and symptoms of superinfections.
• Monitor hydration status if adverse GI reactions occur.
• Monitor I.V. site for phlebitis.

Supportive Care

• If the patient develops a superinfection, or new infection, notify the doctor. Prepare to discontinue the drug and subsitute another antibiotic, as prescribed. If the patient develops oral thrush, provide good mouth care.
• If the patient develops diarrhea, nausea, or vomiting, request an antiemetic or antidiarrheal agent, if needed. Expect to substitute a parenteral form of tetracycline or another antibiotic as prescribed.
• Rotate I.V. site to minimize irritation.

Patient Teaching

• Advise the patient to avoid direct exposure to sunlight and ultraviolet light and to use a sunscreen with a sun protection factor of 15 or higher to help prevent photosensitivity reactions. Remind the patient that photosensitivity persists for up to 2 days after discontinuation of drug.
• Tell patient to take oral tetracycline with a full glass of water (To facilitate passage to the stomach), 1 hour before or 2 hours after meals for maximum absorption, and not less than 1 hour before bedtime (to prevent irritation from esophageal reflux).
• Tell patient not to take the drug with food, milk or other dairy products, antacids, sodium bicarbonate, or iron compounds as it may interfere with absorption. Tell the patient to take antacids 3 hours after tetracycline.
• Emphasize the importance of completing prescribed regimen exactly as

ordered and keeping follow-up appointments.
• Tell patient to check expiration dates and discard any outdated tetracycline as it may become toxic.
• Teach patient to report signs of superinfection (furry overgrowth on tongue, vaginal itch or discharge, foul-smelling stool). Stress good oral hygiene.
• Advise female patient taking an oral contraceptive to use an alternative means of contraception during tetracycline therapy and for 1 week after it is discontinued.

Evaluation
In patients receiving tetracycline, appropriate evaluation statements may include:
• Patient is free of infection.
• Patient does not develop a superinfection during therapy.
• Patient and family state an understanding of therapy.

tetrahydrozoline hydrochloride (ophthalmic)
(tet ra hye drozz´ a leen)
Murine Plus◇, Optigene◇, Soothe◇, Tetrasine◇, Visine◇

• *Classification:* ophthalmic decongestant (sympathomimetic)
• *Pregnancy Risk Category:* C

HOW SUPPLIED
Ophthalmic solution: 0.05%◇

ACTION
Mechanism: Produces vasoconstriction by activating alpha receptors on the blood vessels and arterioles of the conjunctiva.
Pharmacokinetics: Unknown.

INDICATIONS & DOSAGE
Ocular congestion, irritation, and allergic conditions–
Adults and children over 2 years: instill 1 to 2 drops of 0.05% solution in eye b.i.d. or t.i.d., or as directed by doctor.

CONTRAINDICATIONS & PRECAUTIONS
Contraindicated in patients with narrow-angle glaucoma, because it may increase intraocular pressure; in those receiving MAO inhibitors, because it may precipitate a hypertensive crisis; and in those hypersensitive to any component of the preparation. Use cautiously in patients with hyperthyroidism, hypertension, heart disease, or diabetes mellitus.

ADVERSE REACTIONS
Eye: transient stinging, pupillary dilation, increased intraocular pressure, irritation, iris floaters in elderly.
Systemic: drowsiness, CNS depression, cardiac irregularities, headache, dizziness, tremors, insomnia.

INTERACTIONS
Tricyclic antidepressants, guanethidine, MAO inhibitors: hypertensive crisis if tetrahydrozoline is systemically absorbed. Don't use together.

EFFECTS ON DIAGNOSTIC TESTS
None reported.

NURSING CONSIDERATIONS
Besides those related universally to drug therapy (see "How to use this book"), consider the following specific recommendations:

Assessment
• Obtain a baseline assessment of the patient's vision and ocular appearance.
• Be alert for adverse reactions and drug interactions throughout therapy.
• Evaluate the patient's and family's

knowledge about tetrahydrozoline hydrochloride therapy.

Nursing Diagnoses

• Sensory/perceptual alterations (visual) related to the patient's underlying condition.
• High risk for poisoning related to possible systemic effects of the drug.
• Knowledge deficit related to tetrahydrozoline hydrochloride

Planning and Implementation

Preparation and Administration

• Instill in lacrimal sac: remove excess solution from around the eyes with a clean tissue or gauze and apply light fingure pressure to lacrimal sac for 1 minute.

Monitoring

• Monitor effectiveness by assessing the patient's visual status and conjunctival appearance.
• Monitor for systemic effects.
• Monitor for persistent irritation or rebound congestion.

Supportive Care

• Notify the doctor immediately if changes in the patient's health or visual status occur.

Patient Teaching

• Teach the patient how to instill the solution and advise him to wash his hands before and after administering the drug.
• Warn the patient that the drug may cause brief, transient stinging when instilled.
• Warn the patient not to exceed the recommended dosage or use the drug for more than 48 hours: rebound congestion may develop with prolonged or overuse.

Evaluation

In patients receiving tetrahydrozoline, appropriate evaluation statements may include:

• Patient experiences relief of ocular irritation.
• Patient remains free of systemic effects.
• Patient and family state an understanding of tetrahydrozoline therapy.

tetrahydrozoline hydrochloride (nasal)

(tet ra hye drozz´ a leen)

Tyzine Drops, Tyzine Pediatric Drops

• *Classification:* nasal decongestant (sympathomimetic)
• *Pregnancy Risk Category:* C

HOW SUPPLIED

Nasal solution: 0.05%, 0.1%

ACTION

Mechanism: An alpha-adrenergic agonist that produces local vasoconstriction of dilated arterioles to reduce blood flow and nasal congestion.

Pharmacokinetics: Unknown.

Onset, peak, duration: Onset is less than 15 minutes; duration of effect is usually 4 to 8 hours.

INDICATIONS & DOSAGE

Nasal congestion–

Adults and children over 6 years: apply 2 to 4 drops of 0.1% solution or spray to nasal mucosa q 4 to 6 hours, p.r.n.

Children 2 to 6 years: apply 2 to 3 drops of 0.05% solution to nasal mucosa q 4 to 6 hours, p.r.n.

CONTRAINDICATIONS & PRECAUTIONS

Contraindicated in patients with narrow-angle glaucoma, because it may increase intraocular pressure; in those receiving MAO inhibitors, because it may precipitate a hypertensive crisis; and in those hypersensitive to any component of the preparation. Use cautiously in patients with hyperthyroidism, hypertension, heart disease, or diabetes mellitus.

ADVERSE REACTIONS

Common reactions are in italics; life-threatening reactions are in bold italics.

EENT: *transient burning, stinging;*

sneezing, rebound nasal congestion in excessive or long-term use.

INTERACTIONS
None significant.

EFFECTS ON DIAGNOSTIC TESTS
None reported.

NURSING CONSIDERATIONS
Besides those related universally to drug therapy (see "How to use this book"), consider the following specific recommendations:

Assessment
- Obtain a baseline assessment of the patient's breathing pattern and degree of nasal congestion.
- Be alert for adverse reactions and drug interactions throughout therapy.
- Evaluate the patient's and family's knowledge about tetrahydrozoline therapy.

Nursing Diagnoses
- Ineffective airway clearance related to the patient's underlying condition.
- Ineffective airway clearance related to rebound congestion with excessive use.
- Knowledge deficit related to tetrahydrozoline hydrochloride therapy.

Planning and Implementation

Preparation and Administration
- Do not use 0.1% solution in children under 6 years.
- ***Topical use:*** Have patient clear nasal passage by blowing nose gently before application. Then have the patient tilt the head back and instill the ordered amount of drops. Tell the patient to try to hold this position for 5 minutes to allow distribution of the drug throughout the nose. If a nasal spray is used, have the patient hold the head upright and then spray into the nostril quickly. Have the patient wait 3 to 5 minutes and then blow his nose. Then repeat the procedure.

Monitoring
- Monitor effectiveness by assessing the patient's breathing pattern and degree of nasal congestion.
- Monitor usage and signs of rebound.

Supportive Care
- Notify the doctor immediately of any changes in the patient's health status.

Patient Teaching
- Teach the patient how to administer the drug, and tell him it should be used by one person only.
- Warn the patient not to exceed the recommended dose and to use the drug only as needed. Tell him excessive or long-term use may result in rebound congestion.
- Warn the patient he may experience transient burning or stinging upon administration.

Evaluation

In patients receiving tetrahydrozoline hydrochloride, appropriate evaluation statements may include:
- Patient obtains relief from nasal congestion.
- Patient remains free of rebound congestion.
- Patient and family state an understanding of tetrahydrozoline hydrochloride therapy.

---

theophylline
(thee off′ lin)

Immediate-release liquids: Accurbron*, Aerolate, Aquaphyllin, Asmalix*, Bronkodyl*, Elixicon, Elixomin*, Elixophyllin*, Lanophyllin*, Lixolin, Slo-Phyllin, Theolair, Theon*, Theophyl*

Immediate-release tablets and capsules: Bronkodyl, Elixophyllin, Nuelin‡, Slo-Phyllin, Somophyllin-T

Timed-release tablets: Constant-T, Duraphyl, Quibron-T/SR, Respbid, Sustaire, Theo-Dur, Theolair-SR, Theo-Time, Uniphyl

*Liquid form contains alcohol. **May contain tartrazine.

Timed-release capsules: Aerolate, Bronkodyl S-R, Elixophyllin SR, Lodrane, Nuelin-SR‡, Slo-bid Gyrocaps, Slo-Phyllin, Somophyllin-CRT, Theo-24, Theobid Duracaps, Theobid Jr., Theochron, Theo-Dur Sprinkle, Theophyl-SR, Theospan SR, Theovent Long-acting

theophylline sodium glycinate
Acet-Am†, Synophylate

- *Classification:* bronchodilator (xanthine derivative)
- *Pregnancy Risk Category:* C

HOW SUPPLIED

theophylline
Tablets: 100 mg, 125 mg, 200 mg, 225 mg, 250 mg, 300 mg
Tablets (chewable): 100 mg
Tablets (extended-release): 100 mg, 200 mg, 250 mg, 300 mg, 400 mg, 500 mg
Capsules: 50 mg, 100 mg, 200 mg, 250 mg
Capsules (extended-release): 50 mg, 60 mg, 65 mg, 75 mg, 100 mg, 125 mg, 130 mg, 200 mg, 250 mg, 260 mg, 300 mg
Elixir: 27 mg/5 ml, 50 mg/5 ml*
Oral solution: 27 mg/5 ml, 53 mg/5 ml
Oral suspension: 100 mg/5 ml
Syrup: 27 mg/5 ml, 50 mg/5 ml
Dextrose 5% injection: 200 mg in 50 ml or 100 ml; 400 mg in 100 ml, 250 ml, 500 ml, or 1,000 ml; 800 mg in 500 ml or 1,000 ml
theophylline sodium glycinate
Elixir: 110 mg/5 ml (equivalent to 55 mg anhydrous theophylline/5 ml)

ACTION

Mechanism: Inhibits phosphodiesterase, the enzyme that degrades cyclic 3′, 5′ adenosine monophosphate (cyclic AMP). Cyclic AMP alters intracellular calcium levels, resulting in relaxation of smooth muscle of the bronchial airways and pulmonary blood vessels.
Absorption: Well absorbed after oral administration. Food alters the rate, but not the extent, of absorption.
Distribution: In all tissues and extracellular fluids except fatty tissue.
Metabolism: Metabolized to inactive compounds.
Excretion: Small amounts (8% to 12%) are excreted in the urine; only about 10% is excreted in the feces unchanged. Half-life: Variable; averages 7 to 9 hours in healthy adults, 1.5 to 9.5 hours in children, and 15 to 58 hours in neonates. The half-life in smoking adults is shorter (4 to 5 hours); longer in adults with CHF, cor pulmonale, COPD, or liver disease.
Onset, peak, duration: Dependent on serum concentration of drug; serum theophylline concentrations of 10 to 20 mcg/ml are usually required for optimum response.

INDICATIONS & DOSAGE

Prophylaxis and symptomatic relief of bronchial asthma, bronchospasm of chronic bronchitis and emphysema –
Adults: 6 mg/kg P.O. followed by 2 to 3 mg/kg q 4 hours for 2 doses. Maintenance dosage is 1 to 3 mg/kg q 8 to 12 hours.
Children 9 to 16 years: 6 mg/kg P.O. followed by 3 mg/kg q 4 hours for 3 doses. Maintenance dosage is 3 mg/kg q 6 hours.
Children 6 months to 9 years: 6 mg/kg P.O. followed by 4 mg/kg q 4 hours for 3 doses. Maintenance dosage is 4 mg/kg q 6 hours.

Most oral timed-release forms are given q 8 to 12 hours. Several products, however, may be given q 24 hours.

Symptomatic relief of bronchial asthma, pulmonary emphysema, and chronic bronchitis–
Adults: 330 to 660 mg (sodium glycinate) P.O. q 6 to 8 hours, after meals.
Children over 12 years: 220 to 330 mg (sodium glycinate) P.O. q 6 to 8 hours.
Children 6 to 12 years: 330 mg (sodium glycinate) P.O. q 6 to 8 hours.
Children 3 to 6 years: 110 to 165 mg (sodium glycinate) P.O. q 6 to 8 hours.
Children 1 to 3 years: 55 to 110 mg (sodium glycinate) P.O. q 6 to 8 hours.
Parenteral theophylline for patients not currently receiving theophylline–
Loading dose: 4.7 mg/kg I.V. slowly; then maintenance infusion.
Adults (nonsmokers): 0.55 mg/kg/hour for 12 hours, then 0.39 mg/kg/hour.
Otherwise-healthy adult smokers: 0.79 mg/kg/hour for 12 hours; then 0.63 mg/kg/hour.
Older adults with cor pulmonale: 0.47 mg/kg/hour for 12 hours; then 0.24 mg/kg/hour.
Adults with CHF or liver disease: 0.38 mg/kg/hour for 12 hours; then 0.08 to 0.16 mg/kg/hour.
Children 9 to 16 years: 0.79 mg/kg/hour for 12 hours; then 0.63 mg/kg/hour.
Children 6 months to 9 years: 0.95 mg/kg/hour for 12 hours; then 0.79 mg/kg/hour.

Switch to oral theophylline as soon as patient shows adequate improvement.

Symptomatic relief of bronchospasm in patients currently receiving theophylline–
Adults and children: each 0.5 mg/kg I.V. or P.O. (loading dose) will increase plasma levels by 1 mcg/ml. Ideally, dose is based upon current theophylline level. In emergency situations, some clinicians recommend a 2.5 mg/kg P.O. dose of rapidly absorbed form if no obvious signs of theophylline toxicity are present.

CONTRAINDICATIONS & PRECAUTIONS

Contraindicated in patients with hypersensitivity to xanthines. Use cautiously in patients with compromised cardiac or circulatory function, diabetes, glaucoma, hypertension, hyperthyroidism, peptic ulcer, or gastroesophageal reflux.

ADVERSE REACTIONS

Common reactions are in italics; life-threatening reactions are in bold italics.
CNS: *restlessness, dizziness,* headache, *insomnia,* light-headedness, ***seizures,*** muscle twitching.
CV: *palpitations, sinus tachycardia,* extrasystoles, flushing, marked hypotension, increase in respiratory rate.
GI: *nausea, vomiting, anorexia,* bitter aftertaste, dyspepsia, heavy feeling in stomach, diarrhea.
Skin: urticaria.

INTERACTIONS

Barbiturates, phenytoin, rifampin: enhanced metabolism and decreased theophylline blood levels. Monitor for decreased effect.
Beta-adrenergic blockers: antagonism. Propranolol and nadolol, especially, may cause bronchospasms in sensitive patients. Use together cautiously.
Erythromycin, troleandomycin, cimetidine, influenza virus vaccine, oral contraceptives: decreased hepatic clearance of theophylline; increased plasma levels. Monitor for signs of toxicity.

EFFECTS ON DIAGNOSTIC TESTS

Plasma-free fatty acids: increased.
Theophylline: falsely elevated levels in the presence of furosemide, phenylbutazone, probenecid, theobromine, caffeine, tea, chocolate, cola beverages, and acetaminophen.
Urinary catecholamines: increased.

NURSING CONSIDERATIONS

Besides those related universally to drug therapy (see "How to use this book"), consider the following specific recommendations:

Assessment

• Obtain a baseline assessment of the patient's cardiopulmonary status by taking vital signs, performing an ECG (if ordered), auscultating heart and lung fields.

• Be alert for adverse reactions and drug interactions throughout therapy.

• Evaluate the patient's and family's knowledge about theophylline therapy.

Nursing Diagnoses

• Ineffective airway clearance related to patient's underlying condition.

• Fluid volume deficit related to theophylline-induced nausea and vomiting.

• Knowledge deficit related to theophylline therapy.

Planning and Implementation

Preparation and Administration

• ***P.O. use:*** Give drug around the clock, using sustained-release product at bedtime as prescribed. For the patient experiencing GI symptoms, administer with a full glass of water after meals, even though food in stomach delays absorption.

• Administer Theo-24 brand of theophylline on an empty stomach because food accelerates this drug's absorption.

• Do not confuse sustained-release dosage forms with standard-release dosage forms.

• ***I.V. use:*** Administer theophylline exactly as prescribed; use infusion pump when administering continuous infusions.

• Be aware that habitual cigarette or marijuana smokers may require increased drug dosage because smoking causes the drug to be metabolized faster. Decreased daily dosages may be necessary in patients with CHF, hepatic disease, or in elderly patients because metabolism and excretion may be decreased.

Monitoring

• Monitor effectiveness by regularly assessing the patient's respiratory status, especially to evaluate if bronchospasms have been relieved. Keep in mind that dosage is determined by monitoring patient response, tolerance, and pulmonary function and serum theophylline levels. Serum theophylline concentrations should range fron 10 to 20 mcg/ml; toxicity has been reported with levels above 20 mcg/ml. Serum theophylline levels are checked approximately every 6 months.

• Monitor vital signs; measure and record intake and output. Expected clinical effects include improvement in quality of pulse and respiration.

• Monitor hydration status if the patient develops GI reactions.

• Monitor for signs of theophylline toxicity: nausea, vomiting, insomnia, irritability, tachycardia, extrasystoles, tachypnea, or tonic-clonic seizures. The onset of toxicity may be sudden and severe, with arrhythmias and seizures as the first signs.

Supportive Care

• Notify the doctor if the patient's respiratory status does not improve with theophylline therapy.

• Institute safety and seizure precautions if adverse CNS reactions occur.

• Obtain an order for an antiemetic or antidiarrheal if GI reactions occur.

• Help the patient identify nonpharmacologic ways to manage insomnia; if ineffective, obtain an order for a hypnotic.

• Administer a mild analgesic as prescribed for theophylline-induced headache.

• Be prepared to treat theophylline toxicity. Treatment may include induction of emesis except in patients experiencing seizures, then use of activated charcoal and cathartics; treatment of arrhythmias with I.V. lidocaine; treatment of seizures with I.V. diazepam; and supportive respiratory care as needed.

Patient Teaching

- Instruct the patient regarding medication and dosage schedule; if a dose is missed, tell the patient to take it as soon as possible, but not to double up on doses.
- Advise the patient of possible signs of toxicity.
- Tell the patient to take the drug at regular intervals as instructed and around the clock. Patients tend to want to take extra "breathing pills."
- Warn patient not to dissolve, crush, or chew extended-release products. Small children unable to swallow these can ingest (without chewing) the contents of bead-filled capsules sprinkled over soft food.
- Warn elderly patients of dizziness, a common adverse reaction at start of therapy.
- Tell the patient to avoid eating and drinking large quantities of xanthine-containing foods and beverages.
- Warn the patient that OTC remedies may contain ephedrine in combination with theophylline salts; excessive CNS stimulation may result. Tell the patient to check with the doctor or pharmacist before taking any other medications.
- Supply instructions for home care and dosage schedule. Stress the importance of follow-up care and of having theophylline levels checked regularly.

Evaluation

In patients receiving theophylline, appropriate evaluation statements may include:

- Patient's respiratory status is improved with theophylline therapy.
- Patient does not experience adverse GI reactions and maintains adequate hydration.
- Patient and family state an understanding of theophylline therapy.

thiabendazole

(thye a ben´ da zole)
Mintezol

- *Classification:* anthelmintic (benzimidazole)
- *Pregnancy Risk Category:* C

HOW SUPPLIED

Tablets (chewable): 500 mg
Oral suspension: 500 mg/5 ml

ACTION

Mechanism: Unknown.
Absorption: Readily absorbed from the GI tract; also absorbed through intact skin.
Distribution: Little is known about the distribution of thiabendazole. Most of the drug is cleared from the plasma within 8 hours of administration.
Metabolism: Almost completely metabolized in the liver.
Excretion: Approximately 90% of a thiabendazole dose is excreted in urine as metabolites within 48 hours; about 5% is excreted in feces. More than half of a dose is excreted within 24 hours.
Onset, peak, duration: Peak serum concentration occurs at 1 to 2 hours.

INDICATIONS & DOSAGE

Systemic infection with pinworm, roundworm, threadworm, whipworm, cutaneous larva migrans, and trichinosis–
Adults or children: 25 mg/kg P.O. in two doses daily for 2 successive days. Maximum dosage is 3 g daily.
Cutaneous infestations with larva migrans (creeping eruption)–
Adults and children: 25 mg/kg P.O. b.i.d. for 2 to 5 days. Maximum 3 g daily. If lesions persist after 2 days, repeat course.

Pinworm—two doses daily for 1 day; repeat in 7 days.
Roundworm, threadworm, whipworm—two doses daily for 2 successive days.
Trichinosis—two doses daily for 2 to 4 successive days.

CONTRAINDICATIONS & PRECAUTIONS

Contraindicated in patients with hypersensitivity to the drug. Use with caution in patients with compromised renal or hepatic function, malnutrition or anemia, and in patients in whom vomiting would be hazardous.

ADVERSE REACTIONS

Common reactions are in italics; life-threatening reactions are in bold italics.
CNS: impaired mental alertness, impaired physical coordination, *drowsiness, giddiness,* headache, dizziness.
GI: *anorexia, nausea, vomiting,* diarrhea, epigastric distress.
Skin: rash, pruritus, ***erythema multiforme.***
Other: lymphadenopathy, fever, flushing, chills.

INTERACTIONS

None significant.

EFFECTS ON DIAGNOSTIC TESTS

AST (SGOT): Transient elevations.

NURSING CONSIDERATIONS

Besides those related universally to drug therapy (see "How to use this book"), consider the following specific recommendations:

Assessment

- Obtain a baseline assessment of infection, including appropriate specimens for analysis before therapy.
- Be alert for adverse reactions and drug interactions throughout therapy.
- Evaluate the patient's and family's knowledge about thiabendazole therapy.

Nursing Diagnoses

- Altered health maintenance related to ineffectiveness of thiabendazole.
- High risk for fluid volume deficit related to adverse GI reactions caused by thiabendazole therapy.
- Knowledge deficit related to thiabendazole.

Planning and Implementation

Preparation and Administration

- ***P.O. use:*** Administer drug after meals. Shake suspension before measuring dose. Ensure that patient has chewed tablets before swallowing.

Monitoring

- Monitor effectiveness by assessing for improvement of infections and by obtaining appropriate specimens for analysis.

Supportive Care

- Provide supportive care as indicated and prescribed for patients who are anemic, dehydrated or malnourished.
- Institute safety precautions if adverse CNS reactions occur.
- Ensure that all family members and suspected contacts also receive treatment to prevent reinfection.
- Obtain an order for an antiemetic or antidiarrheal agent as needed.

Patient Teaching

- Tell patient to take the drug after meals and to chew tablets before swallowing, and to shake the suspension before measuring the dose.
- Warn that medication may cause drowsiness, dizziness and other adverse CNS reactions. Advise patient to avoid hazardous activities that require alertness during therapy.
- Inform patient that no dietary restrictions, laxatives, or enemas are necessary with treatment.
- Emphasize the need for good personal hygiene, especially careful hand washing.
- To avoid reinfection, tell patient to wash perianal area daily, change undergarments and bedclothes daily, and wash hands and clean fingernails

before meals and after bowel movements.
• Advise patient to avoid preparing food during infestation.
• Inform patient that all family members and suspected contacts will require treatment to prevent reinfection.
Evaluation
In patients receiving thiabendazole, appropriate evaluation statements may include:
• Patient is free of infection and maintains normal health status.
• Patient maintains adequate hydration throughout therapy.
• Patient and family state an understanding of therapy.

---

thiethylperazine maleate
(thye eth il per´ a zeen)
Norzine, Torecan**

• *Classification:* antiemetic, antivertigo agent, (piperazine derivative)
• *Pregnancy Risk Category:* C

HOW SUPPLIED
Tablets: 10 mg
Injection: 5 mg/ml
Suppositories: 10 mg

ACTION
Mechanism: A phenothiazine derivative that blocks dopamine receptors. Acts on the chemoreceptor trigger zone to inhibit nausea and vomiting.
Pharmacokinetics: Unknown.

INDICATIONS & DOSAGE
Nausea and vomiting–
Adults: 10 mg P.O., I.M., or rectally daily, b.i.d., or t.i.d.

CONTRAINDICATIONS & PRECAUTIONS
Contraindicated in severe CNS depression, hepatic disease, coma, phenothiazine hypersensitivity and in pregnancy.

ADVERSE REACTIONS
Common reactions are in italics; life-threatening reactions are in bold italics.
Blood: *transient leukopenia,* ***agranulocytosis.***
CNS: *extrapyramidal reactions (high incidence),* sedation (low incidence), pseudoparkinsonism, EEG changes, dizziness.
CV: *orthostatic hypotension,* tachycardia, EKG changes.
EENT: *ocular changes, blurred vision.*
GI: *dry mouth, constipation.*
GU: *urine retention,* dark urine, menstrual irregularities, gyneocmastia, inhibited ejaculation.
Hepatic: *cholestatic jaundice.*
Metabolic: hyperprolactinemia.
Skin: *mild photosensitivity,* dermal allergic reactions.
Other: weight gain, increased appetite.

INTERACTIONS
Antacids: inhibited absorption of oral phenothiazines. Separate antacid and phenothiazine dosage by at least 2 hours.
Anticholinergics, including antidepressants and antiparkinsonian agents: increased anticholinergic activity, aggravated parkinson-like symptoms. Use together cautiously.
Barbiturates: may decrease thiethylperazine effect. Monitor for decreased antiemetic effect.

EFFECTS ON DIAGNOSTIC TESTS
None reported.

NURSING CONSIDERATIONS
Besides those related universally to drug therapy (see "How to use this book"), consider the following specific recommendations:
Assessment
• Obtain a baseline assessment of allergies, mental status, vision and eye

condition, blood pressure, and liver function studies before therapy.
• Be alert for adverse reactions and drug interactions throughout therapy.
• Evaluate the patient's and family's knowledge about thiethylperazine maleate therapy.

Nursing Diagnoses

• High risk for fluid volume deficit related to nausea and vomiting.
• Sensory/perceptual alterations (visual), related to thiethylperazine-induced ocular changes and blurred vision.
• Knowledge deficit related to thiethylperazine maleate therapy.

Planning and Implementation

Preparation and Administration

• Store suppositories tightly covered and at a temperature below 77° F (25° C).
• ***I.M. use:*** Give deep I.M. injection on or shortly before terminating anesthesia to prevent nausea and vomiting associated with anesthesia and surgery.
• Do not give I.V. because it may cause severe hypotension.
• Avoid getting drug on skin to prevent contact dermatitis.

Monitoring

• Monitor effectiveness by observing the patient for nausea and vomiting.
• Monitor blood pressure and pulse regularly; be alert for tachycardia and hypotension.
• Observe for extrapyramidal reactions.
• Check CBC, platelet count, differential, and liver function studies in long-term use.
• Observe for changes in visual acuity.
• Monitor fluid balance.

Supportive Care

• Do not give in severe CNS depression, hepatic disease, coma, or phenothiazine hypersensitivity.
• Use only when vomiting cannot be controlled by other measures or when only a few doses are required. Be aware that the drug is possibly effective in dizziness; not effective in motion sickness.
• After anesthesia, position patient on side and have airway and suction equipment nearby.

Patient Teaching

• Warn patient about hypotension; advise him to stay in bed for 1 hour after drug is given.
• Instruct patient to report decreased urine output, visual changes, and any CNS effects immediately.

Evaluation

In patients receiving thiethylperazine, appropriate evaluation statements may include:
• Patient exhibits no signs of fluid volume deficit.
• Patient does not have blurred vision.
• Patient and family state an understanding of thiethylperazine therapy.

thioguanine (6-thioguanine, 6-TG)

(thye oh gwah´ neen)
Lanvis†

• *Classification:* antineoplastic (antimetabolite)
• *Pregnancy Risk Category:* D

HOW SUPPLIED

Tablets (scored): 40 mg

ACTION

Mechanism: An antimetabolite purine antagonist that is a chemical analog of the naturally occurring purines hypoxanthine and guanine. Drug is converted intracellularly to a ribonucleotides which blocks the synthesis and use of purines. May also be incorporated into DNA and RNA. Also has some immunosuppressant activity.
Absorption: After an oral dose, absorption is incomplete and variable. The average bioavailability is 30%.

Distribution: Rapidly incorporated into the RNA and DNA of bone marrow cells; after five daily doses; it may replace 50% to 100% of the guanine in DNA. The drug does not cross the blood-brain barrier to any appreciable extent.
Metabolism: Rapidly and extensively metabolized in the liver and other tissues to less active metabolites.
Excretion: In the urine, mainly as metabolites. Only trace amounts of parent drug are found. Half-life: Biphasic; elimination: initial half-life is 15 minutes, and terminal half-life is 11 hours.

INDICATIONS & DOSAGE

Acute leukemia, chronic granulocytic leukemia –
Adults and children: initially, 2 mg/kg daily P.O. (usually calculated to nearest 20 mg); then increased gradually to 3 mg/kg daily if no toxic effects occur.

CONTRAINDICATIONS & PRECAUTIONS

Contraindicated in patients with a history of resistance to previous therapy with the drug. Use cautiously in renal or hepatic dysfunction because of the potential for drug accumulation.

ADVERSE REACTIONS

Blood: *leukopenia,* anemia, ***thrombocytopenia*** (occurs slowly over 2 to 4 weeks).
GI: nausea, vomiting, stomatitis, diarrhea, anorexia.
Hepatic: hepatotoxicity, jaundice.
Metabolic: hyperuricemia.

INTERACTIONS

None significant.

EFFECTS ON DIAGNOSTIC TESTS

Blood and urine: increased uric acid levels.

NURSING CONSIDERATIONS

Besides those related universally to drug therapy (see "How to use this book"), consider the following specific recommendations:

Assessment
- Obtain a baseline assessment of patient's overall physical status, CBC, serum uric acid, and hepatic profile before initiating therapy.
- Be alert for adverse reactions and drug interactions throughout therapy.
- Evaluate the patient's and family's knowledge about thioguanine therapy.

Nursing Diagnoses
- Altered protection related to thioguanine-induced myelosuppression and immunosuppression.
- Altered oral mucous membrane related to thioguanine-induced stomatitis.
- Knowledge deficit related to thioguanine therapy.

Planning and Implementation

Preparation and Administration
- Keep in mind that this drug is sometimes ordered as 6-thioguanine. The numeral 6 is part of the drug name and does not signify dosage units.
- Be aware that dosage modification may be necessary in renal or hepatic dysfunction.

Monitoring
- Monitor effectiveness by noting results of follow-up diagnostic tests and patient's overall physical status.
- Monitor serum urine uric acid levels.
- Monitor for hepatotoxicity. Watch for tenderness over the liver and jaundice.
- Monitor for signs of infection (cough, fever, sore throat) and bleeding (easy bruising, nosebleeds, bleeding gums).
- Monitor CBC daily during induction, then weekly during maintenance therapy.
- Monitor for GI reactions, such as stomatitis, nausea, vomiting, and diarrhea.

Supportive Care
• Keep in mind that hepatotoxic effects may be reversible if treatment is discontinued promptly on discovery of symptoms.
• To help prevent infection, maintain the patient's optimal health and protect him from undue exposure to environmental contagions. If signs of infection occur, notify doctor promptly; administer antibiotics, as ordered.
• Encourage increased fluid intake of 3,000 cc daily.
• Avoid all I.M. injections if the platelet count falls below 100,000/mm³.
• Provide frequent mouth care.
• Provide a safe environment to minimize risk of bleeding.

Patient Teaching
• Instruct patient about need for protective measures, including conservation of energy, balanced diet, adequate rest, personal cleanliness, clean environment, and avoidance of exposure to persons with infections.
• Teach patient to avoid the use of all OTC products containing aspirin. Instruct patient about safety precautions to reduce risks of bleeding from falls, cuts, or other injuries.
• Instruct patient about the need for frequent oral hygiene. Tell the patient to use a soft-bristled toothbrush and nonalcoholic mouthwash. If oral lesions are present, tell the patient to avoid alcohol, smoking, and extremely hot or spicy foods. If lesions are painful, tell the patient to consult with the doctor about using a topical oral anesthetic.
• Warn patients to watch for signs of infection (sore throat, fever, fatigue), and for signs of bleeding (easy bruising, nosebleeds, bleeding gums). Tell patient to take temperature daily and to report signs of infection or bleeding.
• Encourage the patient to drink at least 3 liters of fluids daily, and to void as often as possible.

Evaluation

In patients receiving thioguanine, appropriate evaluation statements may include:
• Patient does not demonstrate signs and symptoms of infection or bleeding.
• Oral lesions are absent, or if present, complications are avoided or minimized.
• Patient and family state an understanding of thioguanine therapy.

thiopental sodium (thiopentone sodium)

(thye oh pen´ tal)

Intraval Sodium‡, Pentothal Sodium

• Controlled Substance Schedule III
• *Classification:* anesthetic (barbiturate)
• *Pregnancy Risk Category:* C

HOW SUPPLIED

Injection: 250-mg, 400-mg, 500-mg syringes; 500-mg/1-g vial with diluent; 1-g (2.5%), 2.5-g (2.5%), 5-g (2.5%), 2.5-g (2%), and 5-g (2%) kits
Rectal suspension: 2-g disposable syringe (400 mg/g of suspension)

ACTION

Mechanism: Inhibits the firing rate of neurons within the ascending reticular-activating system.
Absorption: Thiopental is given I.V. only.
Distribution: Throughout the body; highest initial concentration occurs in vascular areas of the brain, primarily gray matter; drug is 80% protein-bound. Redistribution of the drug is primarily responsible for its short duration of action.
Metabolism: Extensively metabolized but slowly in the liver.

Excretion: Unchanged thiopental is not excreted in significant amounts.
Onset, peak, duration: Duration of action depends on tissue redistribution. Peak brain concentrations are reached in 10 to 20 seconds. Depth of anesthesia may increase for up to 40 seconds. Consciousness returns in 20 to 30 minutes.

INDICATIONS & DOSAGE

Induce anesthesia before administering other anesthetics–
Adults: 210 to 280 mg (3 to 4 ml/kg) usually required for average adult (70 kg).
General anesthetic for short-term procedures–
Adults: 2 to 3 ml 2.5% solution (50 to 75 mg) administered I.V. only at intervals of 20 to 40 seconds, depending on reaction. Dose may be repeated with caution, if necessary.
Seizures following anesthesia–
Adults: 75 to 125 mg (3 to 5 ml of 2.5% solution) immediately.
Psychiatric disorders (narcoanalysis, narcosynthesis)–
Adults: 100 mg/minute (4 ml/minute 2.5% solution) until confusion occurs and before sleep.
Basal anesthesia by rectal administration–
Adults and children: administer up to 1 g/22.5 kg (50 lb) body weight, or 0.5 ml 10% solution/kg body weight. Maximum 1 to 1.5 g (children weighing 34 kg or more) and 3 to 4 g (adults weighing 91 kg or more).

Note: Thiopental is rarely administered rectally for basal sedation or anesthesia because of variable absorption from the rectum.

CONTRAINDICATIONS & PRECAUTIONS

Contraindicated in patients with acute intermittent or variegate porphyria but not in other porphyrias; in patients with hypersensitivity to the drug; and whenever general anesthesia is contraindicated.

Use cautiously in patients with respiratory, cardiac, circulatory, renal, or hepatic dysfunction; severe anemia; shock; myxedema; and status asthmaticus (use *extreme* caution), because drug may worsen these conditions.

ADVERSE REACTIONS

Common reactions are in italics; life-threatening reactions are in bold italics.
CNS: *prolonged somnolence,* retrograde amnesia.
CV: ***myocardial depression,*** *arrhythmias.*
Skin: tissue necrosis with extravasation.
Respiratory: ***respiratory depression*** *(momentary apnea following each injection is typical),* ***bronchospasm, laryngospasm.***
Local: pain at injection site.
Other: sneezing, coughing, *shivering.*

INTERACTIONS

None significant.

EFFECTS ON DIAGNOSTIC TESTS

EEG: alteration in patterns (dose-dependent)

NURSING CONSIDERATIONS

Besides those related universally to drug therapy (see "How to use this book"), consider the following specific recommendations:

Assessment

- Obtain a baseline assessment of the patient's vital signs, CNS status, and overall physical condition before therapy.
- Be alert for adverse reactions or drug interactions throughout therapy.
- Evaluate the patient's and family's knowledge about thiopental sodium therapy.

Nursing Diagnoses

- High risk for injury related to thiopental sodium-induced CNS effects.

• Ineffective breathing pattern related to possible thiopental sodium-induced respiratory depression.
• Knowledge deficit related to thiopental sodium therapy.

Planning and Implementation

Preparation and Administration

• ***I.V. use:*** Keep in mind that drug should be administered only by staff specially trained to give anesthetics and to manage their adverse effects. Avoid extravasation.
• Do not heat solutions for sterilization. Solutions should be used within 24 hours.
• Give test dose (1 to 3 ml 2.5% solution) to assess reaction to the drug.

Monitoring

• Monitor effectiveness by evaluating CNS depression of level of consciousness after administration of thiopental sodium.
• Monitor respiratory rate, pattern, and other vital signs before, during, and after anesthesia. Keep in mind that thiopental sodium can cause respiratory depression, laringospasm, and bronchospasm.

Supportive Care

• Notify the doctor immediately if vital signs change, or if any other adverse reaction develops.
• Have resuscitative equipment and oxygen ready. Maintain airway.
• Implement safety measures to protect the unconscious patient.
• When used as general anesthetic, give atropine sulfate as premedication to diminish laryngeal reflexes and to prevent laryngeal spasm.
• Be aware that solutions of atropine sulfate, d-tubocurarine, or succinylcholine may be given concurrently.
• Remember that this drug has potential for abuse.

Patient Teaching

• Explain that drug may be used to induce anesthesia or provide anesthesia for short-term procedures. The patient will lose consciousness and will not experience pain during surgery.
• Tell the patient what to expect during induction of anesthesia and during recovery from general anesthesia. As needed, clarify any other information provided by the anesthesiologist, including risks.
• After administration, warn the patient to avoid alcohol or other CNS depressants and that psychomotor skills may be impaired for 24 hours.

Evaluation

In patients receiving thiopental sodium, appropriate evaluation statements may include:
• Central depression of level of consciousness achieved; patient safety is maintained.
• Patent airway and adequate ventilatory status is maintained.
• Patient and family state an understanding of thiopental sodium therapy.

thioridazine hydrochloride

(thye oh rid´ a zeen)

Aldazine‡, Apo-Thioridazine†, Mellaril*, Mellaril-S, Novoridazine†, PMS Thioridazine†

• *Classification:* antipsychotic (phenothiazine)
• *Pregnancy Risk Category:* C

HOW SUPPLIED

Tablets: 10 mg, 15 mg, 25 mg, 50 mg, 100 mg, 200 mg
Oral suspension: 25 mg/5 ml, 100 mg/5 ml
Oral concentrate: 30 mg/ml, 100 mg/ml (3% to 4.2% alcohol)
Syrup: 10 mg/5 ml

ACTION

Mechanism: Blocks postsynaptic dopamine receptors in the brain. A piperidine phenothiazine.
Absorption: Rate and extent of absorption vary with administration

route. Oral tablet absorption is erratic and variable; absorption of oral concentrates and syrups is much more predictable.
Distribution: Widely distributed into the body, including breast milk. Drug is 91% to 99% protein-bound.
Metabolism: Extensively metabolized by the liver and forms the active metabolite mesoridazine.
Excretion: Most is excreted as metabolites in urine; some in feces via the biliary tract.
Onset, peak, duration: With oral tablets, onset ranges from 30 minutes to 1 hour. Peak effects occur at 2 to 4 hours; steady-state serum level is achieved within 4 to 7 days. Duration of action is 4 to 6 hours.

INDICATIONS & DOSAGE

Psychosis–
Adults: initially, 25 to 100 mg P.O. t.i.d., with gradual increments up to 800 mg daily in divided doses, if needed. Dosage varies.
Adults over 65 years: initial dose, 25 mg P.O. t.i.d.
Depressive neurosis, alcohol withdrawal, dementia in geriatric patients, behavioral problems in children–
Adults: initially, 25 mg P.O. t.i.d. Maintenance dosage is 20 to 200 mg daily.
Children over 2 years: 0.5 to 3 mg/kg P.O. daily in divided doses.

CONTRAINDICATIONS & PRECAUTIONS

Contraindicated in patients with hypersensitivity to phenothiazines and related compounds, including allergic reactions involving hepatic function; or those with blood dyscrasias or bone marrow depression because of its adverse hematologic effects; in patients with disorders accompanied by coma, brain damage, CNS depression, circulatory collapse, or cerebrovascular disease because of the drug's additive CNS depression and adverse effects on blood pressure; and in patients receiving adrenergic-blocking agents or spinal or epidural anesthetics because of the risk of excessive respiratory, cardiac, and CNS depression.

Use cautiously in patients with cardiac disease (arrhythmias, CHF, angina pectoris, valvular disease, or heart block), encephalitis, Reye's syndrome, head injury, respiratory disease, seizure disorders, glaucoma, prostatic hypertrophy, urine retention, Parkinson's disease, of pheochromocytoma, because drug may exacerbate these conditions; and in hypocalcemia, because it increases the risk of extrapyramidal reactions.

ADVERSE REACTIONS

Common reactions are in italics; life-threatening reactions are in bold italics.
Blood: transient leukopenia, ***agranulocytosis.***
CNS: extrapyramidal reactions (low incidence), *tardive dyskinesia, sedation (high incidence),* EEG changes, dizziness.
CV: *orthostatic hypotension,* tachycardia, ECG changes.
EENT: *ocular changes, blurred vision,* pigmentary retinopathy.
GI: *dry mouth, constipation.*
GU: *urine retention,* dark urine, menstrual irregularities, gynecomastia, inhibited ejaculation.
Hepatic: cholestatic jaundice.
Metabolic: hyperprolactinemia.
Skin: *mild photosensitivity,* dermal allergic reactions.
Other: weight gain; increased appetite; rarely, ***neuroleptic malignant syndrome*** (fever, tachycardia, tachypnea, profuse diaphoresis).
After abrupt withdrawal of long-term therapy: gastritis, nausea, vomiting, dizziness, tremors, feeling of warmth or cold, sweating, tachycardia, headache, insomnia.

INTERACTIONS

Alcohol, other CNS depressants: increased CNS depression. Avoid concomitant use.
Antacids: inhibit absorption of oral phenothiazines. Separate antacid and phenothiazine doses by at least 2 hours.
Barbiturates, lithium: may decrease phenothiazine effect. Observe patient.
Centrally acting antihypertensives: decreased antihypertensive effect.

EFFECTS ON DIAGNOSTIC TESTS

ECG: quinidine-like effects.
Liver function test: elevated results.
Protein-bound iodine: elevated levels.
Urine porphyrins, urobilinogen, amylase, and 5-HIAA: false-positive results because of darkening of urine by metabolites.
Urine pregnancy tests using human chorionic gonadotropin: false-positive results.

NURSING CONSIDERATIONS

Besides those related universally to drug therapy (see "How to use this book"), consider the following specific recommendations:

Assessment

• Obtain baseline assessment of patient's mental status, including psychotic symptoms, before therapy.
• Be alert for adverse reactions and drug interactions throughout thioridazine hydrochloride therapy.
• Evaluate the patient's and family's knowledge about thioridazine hydrochloride therapy.

Nursing Diagnoses

• Impaired thought processes related to patient's underlying condition.
• Urinary retention related to adverse drug reaction.
• Knowledge deficit related to thioridazine therapy.

Planning and Implementation

Preparation and Administration

• Protect medication from light. Slight yellowing of injection or concentrate is common and does not affect potency. Discard markedly discolored solutions.
• Dose of 100 mg is therapeutic equivalent of 100 mg of chlorpromazine.
• Dosage above 800 mg may be associated with ocular toxicity (pigmentary retinopathy).
• *Caution:* Note different concentrations of liquid formulations.
• Not available in the injectable form. Mesoridazine is prescribed when parenteral form of a thioridazine-like drug is desired.
• Shake suspension well before using.
• ***P.O. use:*** Dilute liquid concentrate with 60 ml tomato or fruit juice, carbonated beverages, coffee, tea, milk, water, or semisolid food just before giving.
• Avoid skin contact with the liquid because it may cause a rash.

Monitoring

• Monitor effectiveness by regularly observing the patient's behavior for changes in psychotic symptoms.
• Monitor for extrapyramidal and anticholinergic effects (blurred vision, dry mouth, constipation, urine retention), and tardive dyskinesia during prolonged therapy.
• Frequently check the patient's blood pressure for orthostatic hypotension, especially after parenteral administration.
• Monitor therapy by weekly bilirubin tests during the first month; periodic blood tests (CBC and liver function); and ophthalmic tests (long-term use).
• Monitor for neuroleptic malignant syndrome. This rare, potentially fatal reaction is not necessarily related to type of neuroleptic or duration of drug therapy, but usually occurs in men (60% of affected patients).

Supportive Care
• Keep the patient supine for 1 hour after I.M. administration. Then assist patient to get up slowly to avoid orthostatic hypotension.
• Do not discontinue drug abruptly unless required by severe adverse reactions.
• Increase the patient's fluid and fiber intake—if not contraindicated—to prevent constipation. If necessary, request doctor's order for a laxative.
• Give the patient sugarless gum, sour hard candy, ice chips or mouthwash rinse to relieve dryness.
• Treat acute dystonic reactions with I.V. diphenhydramine, as ordered.
• Hold dose if patient develops jaundice, symptoms of blood dyscrasias (fever, sore throat, infection, cellulitis, weakness), persistent (longer than a few hours) extrapyramidal reactions, or any such reactions during pregnancy.

Patient Teaching
• Tell the patient to avoid exposure to direct sunlight and to use a sunscreen when going outdoors to prevent photosensitivity reactions. (*Note:* Sun lamps and tanning beds may cause burning of the skin or skin discoloration.)
• Tell the patient not to stop taking the drug suddenly.
• Encourage the patient to report difficult urination, sore throat, dizziness, or fainting.
• Advise the patient to increase fluid and fiber in the diet, if appropriate.
• Tell the patient to avoid driving and other hazardous activities that require alertness until the effect of the drug is established. Tell the patient that excessive sedative effects tend to subside after several weeks.
• Explain which fluids are appropriate for diluting the concentrate and show the dropper technique for measuring dose. Warn the patient not to spill liquid preparation on skin because rash and irritation may occur.
• Tell the patient that sugarless hard candy, chewing gum, or ice chips can alleviate dry mouth.
• Tell the patient to notify the doctor if he develops blurred vision.

Evaluation
In patients receiving thioridazine, appropriate evaluation statements may include:
• Patient demonstrates a decrease in psychotic behavior.
• Patient voids without difficulty.
• Patient and family state an understanding of thioridazine therapy.

thiotepa
(thy oh tep´ a)

• *Classification:* antineoplastic (alkylating agent)
• *Pregnancy Risk Category:* D

HOW SUPPLIED
Injection: 15-mg vials

ACTION
Mechanism: An alkylating agent that cross-links strands of cellular DNA and interferes with RNA transcription, causing an imbalance of growth that leads to cell death. Also exhibits some immunosuppressant activity. Cell cycle–nonspecific.
Absorption: Absorption across the GI tract is incomplete. Absorption from the bladder is variable, ranging from 10% to 100% of an instilled dose. Absorption is increased by certain pathologic conditions, such as extensive tumor infiltration or mucosal irritation. Intramuscular and pleural membrane absorption of thiotepa is also variable.
Distribution: Crosses the blood-brain barrier; unknown if drug enters breast milk.
Metabolism: Extensively metabolized in the liver.
Excretion: Metabolites and traces of

parent drug are excreted in urine. About 60% of a dose is excreted within 24 to 72 hours.

INDICATIONS & DOSAGE

Breast and ovarian cancer; lymphomas and bronchogenic carcinomas–
Adults and children over 12 years: 0.2 mg/kg I.V. daily for 4 to 5 days at intervals of 2 to 4 weeks.
Bladder tumor–
Adults and children over 12 years: 60 mg in 60 ml water instilled in bladder for 2 hours once weekly for 4 weeks.
Neoplastic effusions–
Adults and children over 12 years: 0.6 to 0.8 mg/kg intracavitarily, p.r.n. Stop drug or decrease dosage if WBC is below 4,000/mm³ or if platelets are below 150,000/mm³.
Malignant meningeal neoplasms–
Adults: 1 to 10 mg/m² intrathecally once or twice weekly.

CONTRAINDICATIONS & PRECAUTIONS

Contraindicated in patients with a history of hypersensitivity to the drug and in patients with preexisting hepatic, renal, or bone marrow impairment because of the potential for additive toxicity.

ADVERSE REACTIONS

Common reactions are in italics; life-threatening reactions are in bold italics.
Blood: *leukopenia begins within 5 to 30 days;* ***thrombocytopenia; neutropenia.***
GI: *nausea, vomiting.*
GU: amenorrhea, decreased spermatogenesis.
Metabolic: hyperuricemia.
Skin: hives, rash.
Local: intense pain at administration site.
Other: headache, fever, tightness of throat, dizziness.

INTERACTIONS

Succinylcholine: prolonged neuromuscular blockade.

EFFECTS ON DIAGNOSTIC TESTS

Blood and urine: increased uric acid levels.
Plasma pseudocholinesterase: decreased concentrations.

NURSING CONSIDERATIONS

Besides those related universally to drug therapy (see "How to use this book"), consider the following specific recommendations:

Assessment

- Obtain a baseline assessment of the patient's underlying condition and CBC, platelet, and uric acid levels before initiating therapy.
- Be alert for adverse reactions and drug interactions throughout therapy.
- Evaluate the patient's and family's knowledge about thiotepa therapy.

Nursing Diagnoses

- High risk for infection related to the immunosuppressant effects of the drug.
- Alteration in nutrition: Less than body requirements related to GI adverse effects as evidenced by nausea and vomiting.
- Knowledge deficit related to thiotepa therapy.

Planning and Implementation

Preparation and Administration

- Expect to administer lower doses in renal, hepatic, or hematopoietic impairment.
- Keep in mind that this drug may be given by all parenteral routes, including direct injection into tumor.
- ***I.V. use:*** Refrigerate and protect dry powder from direct sunlight to avoid possible drug breakdown. Exercise caution when preparing and administering this drug to avoid mutagenic, teratogenic, and carcinogenic risks. Use a biological containment cabinet, gloves, and mask, and avoid contaminating work surfaces. Reconstitute

with sterile water for injection only. Discard refrigerated solution after 5 days. When administerineg the drug, if pain occurs at the insertion site, dilute the drug further or use a local anesthetic to reduce pain at infusion site. Make sure drug does not infiltrate.
• ***Bladder instillation:*** Dehydrate patient 8 to 10 hours prior to therapy. Instill 30 to 60 ml of drug into bladder by catheter; ask patient to retain solution for 2 hours. Reposition every 15 minutes for maximal area contact.

Monitoring
• Monitor effectiveness by noting results of follow-up diagnostic tests and overall physical status.
• Monitor CBC and uric acid levels before and during therapy. White blood cell counts are used as guide to indicate drug's effectiveness to aid dosage titration.
• Monitor CBC level weekly for at least 3 weeks after last dose.
• Monitor for signs of infection and bleeding.

Supportive Care
• As ordered, give transfusions of whole blood, platelets, or WBCs, which may relieve hematopoietic toxicity.
• Avoid giving the patient anticoagulants and aspirin products, if possible.
• Give antiemetics as ordered. Nausea and vomiting occurs in almost all patients.
• Give antiiotics as ordered if infection develops.
• Encourage fluid intake to help prevent hyperuricemia with resulting uric acid nephropathy. Keep in mind that allopurinol may be administered to help prevent hyperurecemia.
• Keep in mind that therapeutic effects are often accompanied by toxicity. It is usually delayed and prolonged because drug binds to tissues and stays in body several hours.
• Expect the doctor to stop therapy with this drug if WBC count is less than 4,000/mm³ and platelets are less than 150,000/mm³. The drug is contraindicated when blood counts drop to this level.
• Do not give any I.M. injections when the platelet count is below 100,000/mm³.

Patient Teaching
• Explain all possible adverse effects to the patient. Tell the patient how to help prevent and alleviate the severity of the adverse reactions and when to notify the doctor. Also explain that the drug is highly toxic with a low therapeutic index and that many adverse effects are unavoidable.
• Be sure to stress the importance of adequate fluid intake.
• Warn patients to watch for signs of even minor infection (sore throat, fever, fatigue), and for signs of bleeding (easy bruising, nosebleeds, bleeding gums). Take temperature daily.
• Teach patient to avoid the use of all OTC products containing aspirin.

Evaluation

In patients receiving thiotepa, appropriate evaluation statements may include:
• Patient is free of infections during thiotepa therapy.
• Patient maintains nutritional status during thiotepa therapy.
• Patient and family state an understanding of thiotepa therapy.

thiothixene
(thye oh thix´ een)
Navane

thiothixene hydrochloride
Navane*

• *Classification:* antipsychotic (thioxanthine)
• *Pregnancy Risk Category:* C

*Liquid form contains alcohol. **May contain tartrazine.

HOW SUPPLIED

thiothixene
Capsules: 1 mg, 2 mg, 5 mg, 10 mg, 20 mg
thiothixene hydrochloride
Oral concentrate: 5 mg/ml (7% alcohol)
Injection: 2 mg, 5 mg/ml

ACTION

Mechanism: Blocks postsynaptic dopamine receptors in the brain. A thioxanthene.
Absorption: Rapidly absorbed.
Distribution: Widely distributed into the body. Drug is 91% to 99% protein-bound.
Metabolism: Minimally metabolized.
Excretion: Most is excreted as parent drug in feces via the biliary tract.
Onset, peak, duration: I.M. onset of action is 10 to 30 minutes. Peak serum levels occur at 1 to 6 hours after I.M. administration. Peak therapeutic effects may not be seen for several weeks.

INDICATIONS & DOSAGE

Acute agitation–
Adults: 4 mg I.M. b.i.d. to q.i.d. Maximum dosage is 30 mg daily I.M. Change to P.O. as soon as possible.
Mild to moderate psychosis–
Adults: initially, 2 mg P.O. t.i.d. May increase gradually to 15 mg daily.
Severe psychosis–
Adults: initially, 5 mg P.O. b.i.d. May increase gradually to 15 to 30 mg daily. Maximum recommended daily dose is 60 mg. Not recommended in children under 12 years.

CONTRAINDICATIONS & PRECAUTIONS

Contraindicated in patients with hypersensitivity to thioxanthenes, phenothiazines, and related compounds, including that evidenced by jaundice and other allergic symptoms; or those with blood dyscrasias and bone marrow depression because of its adverse hematologic effects; and disorders accompanied by coma, brain damage, CNS depression, circulatory collapse, or cerebrovascular disease because of the drug's additive CNS depression and adverse effects on blood pressure.

Use cautiously in patients with cardiac disease (arrhythmias, CHF, angina pectoris, valvular disease, or heart block), encephalitis, Reye's syndrome, head injury, respiratory disease, seizure disorders, glaucoma, prostatic hypertrophy, urine retention, Parkinson's disease, or pheochromocytoma, because it may exacerbate these conditions; in patients with hypocalcemia because it increases the risk of extrapyramidal reactions; and in patients with hepatic or renal impairment because diminished metabolism and excretion cause drug to accumulate.

ADVERSE REACTIONS

Common reactions are in italics; life-threatening reactions are in bold italics.
Blood: transient leukopenia, ***agranulocytosis.***
CNS: *extrapyramidal reactions (high incidence), tardive dyskinesia,* sedation (low incidence), pseudoparkinsonism, EEG changes, dizziness.
CV: *orthostatic hypotension,* tachycardia, ECG changes.
EENT: ocular changes, *blurred vision.*
GI: *dry mouth, constipation.*
GU: *urine retention,* dark urine, menstrual irregularities, gynecomastia, inhibited ejaculation.
Hepatic: cholestatic jaundice.
Metabolic: hyperprolactinemia.
Skin: *mild photosensitivity,* dermal allergic reactions.
Local: pain at I.M. injection site, sterile abscess.
Other: weight gain; increased appetite; rarely, ***neuroleptic malignant syndrome*** (fever, tachycardia, tachypnea, profuse diaphoresis).
After abrupt withdrawal of long-term

therapy: gastritis, nausea, vomiting, dizziness, tremors, feeling of warmth or cold, sweating, tachycardia, headache, insomnia.

INTERACTIONS

Alcohol, other CNS depressants: increased CNS depression. Avoid concomitant use.

EFFECTS ON DIAGNOSTIC TESTS

ECG: quinidine-like effects.
Liver function tests: elevated results.
Protein-bound iodine: elevated levels.
Urine porphyrins, urobilinogen, amylase, and 5-HIAA: false-positive results because of darkening of urine by metabolites.
Urine pregnancy tests using human chorionic gonadotropin: false-positive results.

NURSING CONSIDERATIONS

Besides those related universally to drug therapy (see "How to use this book"), consider the following specific recommendations:

Assessment

- Obtain baseline assessment of patient's mental status, including psychotic symptoms, before therapy.
- Be alert for adverse reactions and drug interactions throughout thiothixene or thiothixene hydrochloride therapy.

Nursing Diagnoses

- Impaired thought processes related to patient's underlying condition.
- Urine retention related to adverse drug reaction.
- Knowledge deficit related to thiothixene or thiothixene hydrochloride therapy.

Planning and Implementation

Preparation and Administration

- Protect medication from light. Slight yellowing of injection or concentrate is common and does not affect potency. Discard markedly discolored solutions.
- Dose of 4 mg is therapeutic equivalent of 100 mg of chlorpromazine.
- ***P.O. use:*** Dilute liquid concentrate with 60 ml tomato or fruit juice, carbonated beverages, coffee, tea, milk, water, or semisolid food just before giving.
- ***I.M. use:*** Give injection deeply only in upper outer quadrant of buttocks. Massage slowly afterward to prevent sterile abscess.
- Store I.M. form in refrigerator.
- Avoid skin contact with the injectable or liquid form because it may cause a rash.

Monitoring

- Monitor effectiveness by regularly observing the patient's behavior for changes in psychotic symptoms.
- Monitor for extrapyramidal and anticholinergic effects (blurred vision, dry mouth, constipation, urine retention), and tardive dyskinesia, during prolonged therapy.
- Frequently check the patient's blood pressure for orthostatic hypotension, especially after parenteral administration.
- Monitor therapy by weekly bilirubin tests during the first month; periodic blood tests (CBC and liver function); and ophthalmic tests (long-term use).
- Monitor for neuroleptic malignant syndrome. This rare, potentially fatal reaction is not necessarily related to type of neuroleptic or duration of drug therapy, but usually occurs in men (60% of affected patients).

Supportive Care

- Keep the patient supine for 1 hour after I.M. administration. Then assist patient to get up slowly to avoid orthostatic hypotension.
- Do not discontinue drug abruptly unless required by severe adverse reactions.
- Increase the patient's fluid and fiber intake—if not contraindicated—to prevent constipation. If necessary, request doctor's order for a laxative.
- Give the patient sugarless gum, sour

hard candy, ice chips, or mouthwash rinse to relieve dry mouth.
• Treat acute dystonic reactions with I.V. diphenhydramine, as ordered.
• Hold the dose if patient develops jaundice, symptoms of blood dyscrasias (fever, sore throat, infection, cellulitis, weakness), persistent (longer than a few hours) extrapyramidal reactions, or any such reactions during pregnancy.

Patient Teaching

• Tell the patient to avoid exposure to direct sunlight and to use a sunscreen when going outdoors to prevent photosensitivity reactions. (*Note:* Sun lamps and tanning beds may cause burning of the skin or skin discoloration.)
• Tell the patient not to stop taking the drug suddenly.
• Encourage the patient to report difficult urination, sore throat, dizziness, or fainting.
• Advise the patient to increase fluid and fiber in the diet, if appropriate.
• Tell the patient to avoid driving and other hazardous activities that require alertness until the effect of the drug is established. Tell the patient that excessive sedative effects tend to subside after several weeks.
• Explain which fluids are appropriate for diluting the concentrate and show the dropper technique for measuring dose. Warn the patient to avoid spilling liquid preparation on skin because it may cause a rash and irritation.
• Tell the patient that sugarless hard candy, chewing gum, or ice chips can alleviate dry mouth.

Evaluation

In patients receiving thiothixene or thiothixene hydrochloride, appropriate evaluation statements may include:
• Patient demonstrates a decrease in psychotic behavior.
• Patient voids without difficulty.
• Patient and family state an understanding of thiothixene or thiothixene hydrochloride therapy.

PHARMACOLOGIC CLASS

thrombolytic enzymes

alteplase
anistreplase
streptokinase
urokinase

OVERVIEW

When a thrombus obstructs a blood vessel, permanent damage to the ischemic area may occur before the body can dissolve the clot. Thrombolytic agents were developed in the hope that speeding lysis of the clot would prevent permanent ischemic damage.

Thrombolytic enzymes act chiefly by converting plasminogen to plasmin; in contrast, anticoagulants act by preventing thrombi from developing. Thrombolytics are more likely to produce clinical bleeding than are oral anticoagulants. Streptokinase is a protein-like substance produced by group C beta-hemolytic streptococci; urokinase is an enzyme isolated from human kidney tissue cultures. Alteplase is a tissue-type plasminogen activator synthesized by recombinant DNA technology. Anistreplase is anisoylated streptokinase-plasminogen activated complex (APSAC).

CLINICAL INDICATIONS AND ACTIONS

Thrombosis, thromboembolism

Alteplase, streptokinase, and urokinase are used to treat acute pulmonary thromboembolism; streptokinase and urokinase are used to treat deep vein thrombosis, acute arterial thromboembolism, or acute coronary arterial thrombosis and to clear arteriovenous cannula occlusion and venous catheter obstruction. Anistreplase is used, with alteplase, streptokinase, and urokinase, to manage

COMPARING THROMBOLYTIC ENZYMES

Thrombolytic enzymes dissolve clots by accelerating the formation of plasmin by activated plasminogen. Plasminogen activators, found in most tissues and body fluids, help plasminogen (an inactive enzyme) convert to plasmin (an active enzyme), which dissolves the clot.

Two thrombolytic enzymes—streptokinase and urokinase—have been widely used; two enzymes—tissue plasminogen activator (TPA or alteplase) and anistreplase—have recently been added to current use. Doses of these enzymes may vary according to the patient's condition.

DRUG	ACTION	INITIAL DOSE	MAINTENANCE THERAPY
alteplase	Directly converts plasminogen to plasmin	I.V. bolus: 6 to 10 mg over 1 to 2 min	I.V. infusion: 50 to 54 mg/hr over 1st hour; 20 mg (20 ml)/hr over next 2 hr, then discontinue
anistreplase	Directly converts plasminogen to plasmin	I.V. push: 30 units over 2 to 3 min	Not necessary
streptokinase	Indirectly activates plasminogen, which converts to plasmin	Intracoronary bolus: 15,000 to 20,000 IU	Intracoronary infusion: 2,000 to 4,000 IU/min over 60 min
		I.V. bolus: none needed	I.V. infusion: 1,500,000 units over 60 min
urokinase	Directly converts plasminogen to plasmin	Intracoronary bolus: none needed	Intracoronary infusion: 2,000 units/lb/hr (4,400 units/kg/hr); rate of 15 ml of solution/hr for total of 12 hr (total volume shouldn't exceed 200 ml)

acute myocardial infarction. These agents are administered in an attempt to lyse coronary artery thrombi, which may result in improved ventricular function and decreased risk of CHF.

OVERVIEW OF ADVERSE REACTIONS

Adverse reactions to these agents are essentially an extension of their actions; hemorrhage is the most common adverse effect. These agents cause bleeding twice as often as does heparin, and, although both may cause allergic reactions, streptokinase is more likely to do so than urokinase. Information regarding hypersensitivity to alteplase is limited.

REPRESENTATIVE COMBINATIONS

None.

thyroglobulin

(thye roe glob´ yoo lin)
Proloid

- *Classification:* thyroid replacement (thyroid hormone)
- *Pregnancy Risk Category:* A

HOW SUPPLIED

Tablets: 32 mg, 65 mg, 100 mg, 130 mg, 200 mg

ACTION

Mechanism: Stimulates the metabolism of all body tissues by accelerating the rate of cellular metabolism.
Pharmacokinetics: Not fully understood. Drug is absorbed from the GI tract and is highly bound to plasma proteins.

INDICATIONS & DOSAGE

Cretinism and juvenile hypothyroidism–
Children 1 year and older: dosage may approach adult dosage (60 to 180 mg P.O. daily), depending on response.
Children 4 to 12 months: 60 to 80 mg P.O. daily.
Children 1 to 4 months: initially, 15 to 30 mg P.O. daily, increased at 2-week intervals. Usual maintenance dosage is 30 to 45 mg P.O. daily.
Hypothyroidism or myxedema–
Adults: initially, 15 to 30 mg P.O. daily, increased by 15 to 30 mg at 2-week intervals until desired response. Usual maintenance dosage is 60 to 180 mg P.O. daily, as a single dose.
Adults over 65 years: initially, 7.5 to 15 mg P.O. daily; dosage is doubled at 6- to 8-week intervals until desired response is obtained.

CONTRAINDICATIONS & PRECAUTIONS

Contraindicated in patients with hypersensitivity to beef or pork and in patients with thyrotoxicosis, acute myocardial infarction, and uncorrected adrenal insufficiency because thyroid hormones increase tissue metabolic demands. Thyroglobulin is also contraindicated for treating obesity because it is ineffective and can cause life-threatening adverse reactions.

Use cautiously in patients with angina or other cardiovascular disease because of the risk of increased metabolic demands; diabetes mellitus because of reduced glucose tolerance; malabsorption states; and long-standing hypothyroidism or myxedema because they may be more sensitive to the effects of thyroid hormones.

ADVERSE REACTIONS

Common reactions are in italics; life-threatening reactions are in bold italics.

Adverse reactions of thyroid hormones are extensions of their pharmacologic properties and reflect patient sensitivity to them.
CNS: hyperirritability, *nervousness, insomnia,* twitching, *tremors,* headache.
CV: increased cardiac output, *tachycardia,* cardiac arrhythmias, *angina pectoris,* increased blood pressure, ***cardiac decompensation and collapse.***
GI: diarrhea, abdominal cramps, vomiting.
Other: weight loss, heat intolerance, hyperhidrosis, menstrual irregularities; in infants and children–accelerated rate of bone maturation.

INTERACTIONS

Cholestyramine and colestipol: thyroglobulin absorption impaired. Separate doses by 4 to 5 hours.
I.V. phenytoin: free thyroid released. Monitor for tachycardia.

EFFECTS ON DIAGNOSTIC TESTS

^{131}I thyroid uptake, protein-bound iodine levels, and liothyronine uptake: altered results.

NURSING CONSIDERATIONS

Besides those related universally to drug therapy (see "How to use this book"), consider the following specific recommendations:

Assessment
- Obtain a baseline assessment of the patient's thyroid status before initiating thyroglobulin therapy.
- Be alert for adverse reactions and drug interactions throughout therapy.
- Evaluate the patient's and family's knowledge about thyroglobulin therapy.

Nursing Diagnoses
- High risk for activity intolerance related to the patient's underlying condition.
- Decreased myocardial tissue perfusion related to thyroglobulin-induced angina pectoris.
- Knowledge deficit related to thyroglobulin therapy.

Planning and Implementation
Preparation and Administration
- ***P.O. use:*** Administer daily dose in morning to prevent insomnia.

Monitoring
- Monitor effectiveness by regularly checking thyroid function studies and assessing the patient for signs and symptoms of thyroid dysfunction.
- Monitor the patient for signs of overdosage.
- Monitor the patient's temperature, pulse rate, and blood pressure regularly for alterations such as fever, tachycardia, or hypertension.
- Monitor patients with cornonary artery disease who must receive thyroid hormones carefully for possible coronary insufficiency if catecholamines must be given.
- Monitor patients with myxedema closely because they are unusually sensitive to thyroid hormone.

Supportive Care
- Withhold drug and notify the doctor if the patient develops signs of overdosage. Be prepared to treat overdosage with antithyroid drugs.
- Assist the patient with activities, as needed, until a euthyroid state is achieved.
- Obtain an order for an antiemetic or antidiarrheal agent, as needed.
- Keep the patient dry if profuse sweating occurs.
- Be aware that thyroid hormones alter thyroid function tests.

Patient Teaching
- Instruct the patient to take the medication at the same time each day; encourage morning dosing to avoid insomnia.
- Tell the patient to notify doctor if he experiences headache, diarrhea, nervousness, excessive sweating, heat intolerance, chest pain, increased pulse rate, or palpitations. Also tell patient to notify doctor immediately if any signs of aggravated cardiovascular disease develop.
- Tell the patient who has achieved a stable response not to change product brands because they are not all bioequivalent.
- Stress the importance of taking the drug exactly as prescribed and of receiving follow-up care.

Evaluation
In patients receiving thyroglobulin, appropriate evaluation statements may include:
- Patient is able to perform activities without overtiring.
- Patient does not exhibit signs and symptoms of anginia pectoris.
- Patient and family state an understanding of thyroglobulin therapy.

thyroid dessicated
(thye´ roid)
Armour Thyroid, S-P-T, Thyrar, Thyroid Strong, Thyroid USP Enseals, Thyro-Teric

- *Classification:* thyroid replacement (thyroid hormone)
- *Pregnancy Risk Category:* A

HOW SUPPLIED
Tablets: 16 mg, 32 mg, 65 mg, 98 mg, 130 mg, 195 mg, 260 mg, 325 mg

Tablets (bovine origin): 32 mg, 65 mg, 130 mg
Tablets (enteric-coated): 32 mg, 65 mg, 130 mg
Strong tablets (50% stronger than thyroid USP, and containing 0.3% iodine): 32 mg, 65 mg, 130 mg, 195 mg
Capsules (porcine origin): 65 mg, 130 mg, 195 mg, 325 mg

ACTION

Mechanism: Stimulates the metabolism of all body tissues by accelerating the rate of cellular metabolism.
Absorption: From the GI tract.
Distribution: Highly bound to plasma proteins.

INDICATIONS & DOSAGE

Adult hypothyroidism–
Adults: initially, 60 mg P.O. daily, increased by 60 mg q 30 days until desired response. Usual maintenance dosage is 60 to 180 mg P.O. daily, as a single dose.
Adults over 65 years: 7.5 to 15 mg P.O. daily; dosage is doubled at 6- to 8-week intervals.
Adult myxedema–
Adults: 16 mg P.O. daily. May double dosage q 2 weeks to maximum 120 mg.
Cretinism and juvenile hypothyroidism–
Children 1 year and older: dosage may approach adult dosage (60 to 180 mg P.O.) daily, depending on response.
Children 4 to 12 months: 30 to 60 mg P.O. daily.
Children 1 to 4 months: initially, 15 to 30 mg P.O. daily, increased at 2-week intervals. Usual maintenance dosage is 30 to 45 mg P.O. daily.

CONTRAINDICATIONS & PRECAUTIONS

Contraindicated in patients with hypersensitivity to beef or pork; in those with thyrotoxicosis, acute myocardial infarction, or uncorrected adrenal insufficiency (thyroid increases tissue metabolic demands); and for treating obesity because it is ineffective and can cause life-threatening adverse reactions.

Use cautiously in patients with angina or other cardiovascular disease because of the risk of increased metabolic demands; diabetes mellitus because of reduced glucose tolerance; malabsorption states; and chronic hypothyroidism or myxedema because they may be more sensitive to the effects of thyroid.

ADVERSE REACTIONS

Common reactions are in italics; life-threatening reactions are in bold italics.

Adverse reactions of thyroid hormones are extensions of their pharmacologic properties and reflect patient sensitivity to them.
CNS: *hyperirritability, nervousness, insomnia,* twitching, tremors, headache.
CV: increased cardiac output, *tachycardia,* cardiac arrhythmias, *angina pectoris,* increased blood pressure, ***cardiac decompensation and collapse.***
GI: diarrhea, abdominal cramps, vomiting.
Other: weight loss, heat intolerance, hyperhidrosis, menstrual irregularities; in infants and children–accelerated rate of bone maturation.

INTERACTIONS

Cholestyramine: thyroid absorption impaired. Separate doses by 4 to 5 hours.
I.V. phenytoin: free thyroid released. Monitor for tachycardia.

EFFECTS ON DIAGNOSTIC TESTS

^{131}I thyroid uptake, protein-bound iodine levels, and liothyronine uptake: altered results.

NURSING CONSIDERATIONS

Besides those related universally to drug therapy (see "How to use this

book"), consider the following specific recommendations:

Assessment

• Obtain a baseline assessment of the patient's thyroid status before initiating thyroid dessicated therapy.

• Be alert for adverse reactions and drug interactions throughout therapy.

• Evaluate the patient's and family's knowledge about thyroid dessicated therapy.

Nursing Diagnoses

• High risk for activity intolerance related to the patient's underlying condition.

• Decreased myocardial tissue perfusion related to thyroid dessicated-induced angina pectoris.

• Knowledge deficit related to thyroid dessicated therapy.

Planning and Implementation

Preparation and Administration

• ***P.O. use:*** Administer daily dose in morning to prevent insomnia.

Monitoring

• Monitor effectiveness by regularly checking thyroid function studies and assessing the patient for signs and symptoms of thyroid dysfunction. Be aware that response in children is monitored by checking sleeping pulse rate and basal morning temperatures.

• Monitor the patient for signs of overdosage.

• Monitor the patient's temperature, pulse rate, and blood pressure regularly for alterations such as fever, tachycardia, or hypertension.

• Monitor patients with cornonary artery disease who must receive thyroid hormones carefully for possible coronary insufficiency if catecholamines must be given.

• Monitor patients with myxedema closely as these patients are unusually sensitive to thyroid hormone.

Supportive Care

• Withhold drug and notify the doctor if the patient develops signs of overdosage. Be prepared to treat overdosage with antithyroid drugs.

• Assist the patient with activities, as needed, until a euthyroid state is achieved.

• Obtain an order for an antiemetic or antidiarrheal agent, as needed.

• Keep the patient dry if profuse sweating occurs.

• Be aware that thyroid hormones alter thyroid function tests.

Patient Teaching

• Instruct the patient to take the medication at the same time each day; encourage morning dosing to avoid insomnia.

• Tell the patient to notify doctor if he experiences headache, diarrhea, nervousness, excessive sweating, heat intolerance, chest pain, increased pulse rate, or palpitations. Also tell patient to notify doctor immediately if any signs of aggravated cardiovascular disease develop.

• Tell the patient who has achieved a stable response not to change product brands because they are not all bioequivalent.

• Stress the importance of taking the drug exactly as prescribed and of receiving follow-up care.

Evaluation

In patients receiving thyroid dessicated, appropriate evaluation statements may include:

• Patient is able to perform activities without overtiring.

• Patient does not exhibit signs and symptoms of anginia pectoris.

• Patient and family state an understanding of thyroid dessicated therapy.

PHARMACOLOGIC CLASS

thyroid hormone antagonists

methimazole
propylthiouracil (PTU)
radioactive iodine (^{131}I)

OVERVIEW

Studies on the developmental mechanism of goiter began in the 1920s.

Two goitrogens were found in the 1940s that were the prototypes of two different classes of thyroid hormones, one of which contains thiourеylene.

Methimazole and PTU inhibit oxidation of iodine in the thyroid gland by blocking iodine's ability to combine with tyrosine to form thyroxine. PTU also inhibits the peripheral conversion of thyroxine (T_4) to triiodothyronine (T_3). PTU is theoretically preferred over methimazole in thyroid storm because of its peripheral activity.

^{131}I is deposited rapidly into the colloid of the follicles of the thyroid gland. The beta rays originate within the follicle and destroy parenchymal cells of the thyroid but very little surrounding tissue.

CLINICAL INDICATIONS AND ACTIONS

Hyperthyroidism

Thyroid hormone antagonists inhibit the synthesis of thyroid hormone by interfering with the incorporation of iodine into thyroglobulin. These drugs also inhibit the formation of iodothyronine. Clinical effects of these drugs become evident only when the preformed hormone is depleted and circulating hormone levels decline. PTU, besides blocking hormone synthesis, inhibits the peripheral deiodination of levothyroxine to liothyronine.

Preparation for thyroidectomy

By inhibiting synthesis of thyroid hormone and causing a euthyroid state, these drugs help reduce surgical problems during thyroidectomy; as a result, the mortality for a single-stage thyroidectomy is very low. Iodide reduces the vascularity of the gland and makes it less friable. Sodium iodide or potassium iodide also exert long-term antagonism to the release of preformed thyroid hormones and can be used if the patient needs surgery but is allergic to either methimazole or propylthiouracil.

Thyrotoxic crisis

PTU inhibits peripheral deiodination of levothyroxine to liothyronine.

Thyroid carcinoma

^{131}I is trapped rapidly by the thyroid and deposited in the colloid of the follicles. The destructive beta rays originate within the follicle and act almost exclusively on the parenchymal cells of the thyroid, with little damage to surrounding tissue. However, with large doses of ^{131}I, characteristic cytotoxic effects of ionizing radiation occur.

OVERVIEW OF ADVERSE REACTIONS

Therapeutic doses can cause fever, chills, sore throat, weakness, backache, swelling of feet, joint pain, and unusual bleeding or bruising. Toxic doses can cause constipation, cold intolerance, dry puffy skin, headache, sleepiness, muscle aches, and unusual weight gain.

REPRESENTATIVE COMBINATIONS

None.

PHARMACOLOGIC CLASS

thyroid hormones

levothyroxine sodium (T_4)
liothyronine sodium (T_3)
liotrix
thyroglobulin
thyroid USP (desiccated)
thyrotropin (TSH)

OVERVIEW

The thyroid gland was first described by Wharton in 1656. In 1891, Murray was the first to treat hypothyroidism by injecting an extract of the thyroid gland. The next year, the extract was found to be effective orally. Thyroid hormones are now used for treating hypothyroidism (myxedema and cretinism), nontoxic goiter, and (with antithyroid drugs) thyrotoxicosis and as a diagnostic aid.

Thyroid hormone synthesis is regulated by thyroid-stimulating hormone (TSH) secreted by the anterior pituitary. TSH secretion is controlled by a feedback mechanism and by thyrotropin-releasing hormone (TRH) from the hypothalamus. Thyroid hormone, which contains triiodothyronine (T_3) and thyroxine (T_4), is stored in the thyroid as thyroglobulin. The amounts of T_3 and T_4 released into circulation are regulated by TSH. T_4 is the major component of normal secretions of the thyroid gland and is the major determinant of normal thyroid function.

Thyroid hormones include natural (thyroid USP and thyroglobulin) and synthetic (levothyroxine, liothyronine, and liotrix) derivatives. The thyroid hormones have catabolic and anabolic effects and influence normal metabolism, growth, and development. Thyroid hormones influence every organ system and are vital to normal central nervous system (CNS) function.

TSH increases iodine uptake by the thyroid and increases formation and release of thyroid hormone. TSH is isolated from bovine anterior pituitary glands.

CLINICAL INDICATIONS AND ACTIONS

Hypothyroidism (myxedema, cretinism, or replacement therapy)

All drugs in this class (except TSH) are used to treat hypothyroidism but the drug of choice is levothyroxine (T_4). Dessicated thyroid is rarely used today. These hormones affect protein and carbohydrate metabolism, promote gluconeogenesis, increase the utilization and mobilization of glycogen stores, stimulate protein synthesis, and regulate cell growth and differentiation. The major effect of exogenous thyroid hormones is to increase the metabolic rate of tissue.

Nontoxic goiter

Levothyroxine, liotrix, liothyronine, and thyroid USP are used to suppress TSH secretion in the management of simple goiter.

Diagnostic uses

Liothyronine is used in the T_3 suppression test to differentiate suspected hyperthyroidism from euthyroidism in patients with borderline or high ^{131}I uptake values. TSH increases iodine uptake by the thyroid and increases formation and release of thyroid hormone.

Thyrotoxicosis

Levothyroxine, liotrix, and thyroid USP are used with antithyroid agents to prevent goitrogenesis and hypothyroidism.

Because thyroid hormones have wide-ranging metabolic effects and are potentially dangerous, they are not indicated for relief of vague symptoms, such as mental and physical sluggishness, irritability, depression, nervousness and ill-defined pains; to treat obesity in patients with normal thyroid function; to treat metabolic insufficiency not associated with thyroid insufficiency; or to treat menstrual disorders or male infertility not associated with hypothyroidism.

OVERVIEW OF ADVERSE REACTIONS

Adverse reactions to thyroid hormones are extensions of their pharmacologic properties. Signs of overdose include nervousness, insomnia, tremor, tachycardia, palpitations, nausea, headache, fever, and sweating.

REPRESENTATIVE COMBINATIONS

Thyroid dessicated powder with vitamin B_1, vitamin B_2, vitamin B_6, and niacinamide: Henydin-M, Hendyin-R.
Thyroid with iodized calcium and peptone: Thycal.

ticarcillin disodium

(tye kar sill′ in)
Ticar, Ticillin‡

- *Classification:* antibiotic (extended-spectrum penicillin, alpha-carboxypenicillin)
- *Pregnancy Risk Category:* B

HOW SUPPLIED

Injection: 1 g, 3 g, 6 g
I.V. infusion: 3 g
Pharmacy bulk package: 20 g, 30 g

ACTION

Mechanism: Bactericidal against microorganisms by inhibiting cell wall synthesis during active multiplication. Bacteria resist ticarcillin by producing penicillinases—enzymes that convert penicillin to inactive penicilloic acid.
Absorption: Ticarcillin is not absorbed from the GI tract and must be administered parenterally. The drug is readily absorbed from I.M. injection sites, but peak serum levels are higher after I.V. administrations.
Distribution: Ticarcillin disodium is distributed widely. It penetrates minimally into CSF with uninflamed meninges. Ticarcillin crosses the placenta; it is 45% to 65% protein-bound.
Metabolism: About 13% of a dose is metabolized by hydrolysis to inactive compounds.
Excretion: Ticarcillin is excreted primarily (80% to 93%) in urine by renal tubular secretion and glomerular filtration; it is also excreted in bile and in breast milk. Half-life: Elimination half-life in adults is about 1 hour; in severe renal impairment, half-life is extended to about 3 hours.
Onset, peak, duration: Peak plasma concentrations occur 30 to 75 minutes after I.M. dose and immediately after the completion of an I.V. infusion.

INDICATIONS & DOSAGE

Severe systemic infections caused by susceptible strains of gram-positive and especially gram-negative organisms (including Pseudomonas, Proteus) –
Adults: 18 g I.V. or I.M. daily, divided into doses given q 4 to 6 hours.
Children: 200 to 300 mg/kg I.V. or I.M. daily, divided into doses given q 4 to 6 hours.

CONTRAINDICATIONS & PRECAUTIONS

Contraindicated in patients with hypersensitivity to any penicillin or cephalosporin. Use cautiously in patients with renal impairment because drug is excreted by kidneys; decreased dosage is required in moderate-to-severe renal failure. Also use cautiously in patients with bleeding tendencies, hypokalemia, or sodium restriction.

ADVERSE REACTIONS

Common reactions are in italics; life-threatening reactions are in bold italics.
Blood: leukopenia, neutropenia, eosinophilia, ***thrombocytopenia, hemolytic anemia.***
CNS: ***seizures,*** neuromuscular excitability.
GI: nausea, diarrhea.
Metabolic: *hypokalemia.*
Local: pain at injection site, vein irritation, phlebitis.
Other: *hypersensitivity (rash, pruritus, urticaria, chills, fever, edema,* ***anaphylaxis),*** overgrowth of nonsusceptible organisms.

INTERACTIONS

Aminoglycoside antibiotics (e.g., gentamicin, tobramycin): chemically incompatible. Don't mix together in I.V.
Probenecid: increases blood levels of ticarcillin and other penicillins. Pro-

benecid may be used for this purpose.

EFFECTS ON DIAGNOSTIC TESTS

Aminoglycoside serum levels: falsely decreased concentrations.
CBC: transient reductions in RBCs, WBCs, and platelet counts.
Coombs' test: positive results.
Electrolytes: hypokalemia and hypernatremia.
Liver function studies: transient elevations.
Prothrombin time: prolonged.
Urine or serum proteins: interference with methods that use sulfosalicylic acid, trichloroacetic acid, acetic acid, or nitric acid; not with tests using bromophenol blue (Albustix, Albutest, MultiStix).

NURSING CONSIDERATIONS

Besides those related universally to drug therapy (see "How to use this book"), consider the following specific recommendations:

Assessment

- Obtain a baseline assessment of infection before therapy.
- Be alert for adverse reactions and drug interactions throughout therapy.
- Evaluate the patient's and family's knowledge about ticarcillin therapy.

Nursing Diagnoses

- High risk for injury related to ineffectiveness of ticarcillin to eradicate the infection.
- Fluid volume excess related to administration of the drug.
- Knowledge deficit related to ticarcillin therapy.

Planning and Implementation

Preparation and Administration

- Obtain specimen for culture and sensitivity tests before first dose. Therapy may begin pending test results.
- Before first dose ask the patient about previous allergic reactions to this drug or other penicillin. However, a negative history of penicillin allergy does not guarantee future safety.
- Give ticarcillin at least 1 hour before bacteriostatic antibiotics.
- Expect to reduce dosage regimen of ticarcillin for a patient with impaired renal function. Because ticarcillin is dialyzable, the patient undergoing hemodialysis may need dosage adjustments.
- Be aware that ticarcillin is almost always used with another antibiotic, such as an aminoglycoside in life-threatening situations.
- ***I.M. use:*** Administer drug deep I.M. into large muscle.
- ***I.V. use:*** Infuse I.V. drug intermittently (over 30 minutes) to prevent vein irritation. Mix with dextrose 5% in water or other suitable I.V. fluids.

Monitoring

- Monitor effectiveness by regularly assessing for improvement of infectious process.
- Allergic reactions are the major adverse reactions to penicillin, especially with large doses, parenteral administration, or prolonged therapy. Keep in mind that the previously nonallergic patient may become sensitized to penicillin during therapy.
- Monitor the patient's fluid balance (intake and output, weight) as ticarcillin contains 5.2 mEq of sodium per gram of drug. Also monitor patient's serum electrolytes as prescribed.

Supportive Care

- Discontinue the drug at once if the patient develops anaphylactic shock (exhibited by rapidly developing dyspnea and hypotension). Notify the doctor and prepare to administer immediate treatment, such as epinephrine, corticosteroids, antihistamines, and other resuscitative measures as indicated.
- Change I.V. site every 48 hours.
- If the patient develops signs of excess fluid volume (e.g., edema, weight gain), notify the doctor.

Patient Teaching
• Advise the patient who becomes allergic to ticarcillin to wear medical alert identification stating this information.

Evaluation
In patients receiving ticarcillin, appropriate evaluation statements may include:
• Patient is free of infection.
• Patient maintains normal fluid volume balance throughout therapy.
• Patient and family state an understanding of ticarcillin therapy.

ticarcillin disodium/clavulanate potassium

(tye kar sill´ in/klav´ yoo la nate)
Timentin

• *Classification:* antibiotic (extended-spectrum penicillin, beta-lactamase inhibitor)
• *Pregnancy Risk Category:* B

HOW SUPPLIED

Injection: 3 g ticarcillin and 100 mg clavulanic acid

ACTION

Mechanism: Clavulanic acid increases ticarcillin's effectiveness by inactivating beta lactamases, which destroy ticarcillin.
Absorption: Clavulanate is well absorbed from the GI tract, but ticarcillin is not. This combination drug is administered intravenously.
Distribution: Ticarcillin disodium is distributed widely. It penetrates minimally into CSF with uninflamed meninges; clavulanic acid penetrates into pleural fluid, lungs, and peritoneal fluid. Ticarcillin disodium achieves high concentrations in urine, protein-binding is 45% to 65% for ticarcillin and 22% to 30% for clavulanic acid; both drugs cross the placenta.
Metabolism: About 13% of a ticarcillin dose is metabolized by hydrolysis to inactive compounds; clavulanic acid is thought to undergo extensive metabolism, but its fate is as yet unknown.
Excretion: Ticarcillin is excreted primarily (83% to 90%) in urine by renal tubular secretion and glomerular filtration; it is also excreted in bile and in breast milk. Clavulanate metabolites are excreted in urine by glomerular filtration and in breast milk. Half-life: Of ticarcillin in normal adults is about 1 hour and that of clavulanate is about 1 hour; in severe renal impairment, ticarcillin's half-life is extended to about 3 hours and clavulanate to about 4½ hours.
Onset, peak, duration: Peak plasma concentration occurs immediately after infusion.

INDICATIONS & DOSAGE

Treatment of infections of the lower respiratory tract, urinary tract, bones and joints, skin and skin structure, and septicemia when caused by beta-lactamase–producing strains of bacteria or by ticarcillin-susceptible organisms—
Adults: 1 vial (ticarcillin 3 g and clavulanate potassium 0.1 g) administered by I.V. infusion q 4 to 6 hours.

CONTRAINDICATIONS & PRECAUTIONS

Contraindicated in patients with hypersensitivity to any penicillin or cephalosporin. Use cautiously in patients with renal impairment because drug is excreted by the kidney; decreased dosage is required in moderate-to-severe renal failure.

ADVERSE REACTIONS

Common reactions are in italics; life-threatening reactions are in bold italics.
Blood: leukopenia, neutropenia, eosinophilia, ***thrombocytopenia, hemolytic anemia.***

CNS: ***seizures,*** neuromuscular excitability.
GI: nausea, diarrhea.
Metabolic: *hypokalemia.*
Local: pain at injection site, vein irritation, phlebitis.
Other: *hypersensitivity (rash, pruritus, urticaria, chills, fever, edema,* ***anaphylaxis),*** overgrowth of nonsusceptible organisms.

INTERACTIONS

Aminoglycoside antibiotics (e.g., gentamicin, tobramycin): chemically incompatible. Don't mix together in I.V.
Probenecid: increases blood levels of ticarcillin. Probenecid may be used for this purpose.

EFFECTS ON DIAGNOSTIC TESTS

Aminoglycoside serum levels: falsely decreased concentration.
Coombs' test: positive results.
Electrolytes: hypokalemia and hypernatremia.
Liver function studies: transient elevations and transient reductions in RBCs, WBCs, and platelet counts.
Prothrombin time: prolonged.
Urine or serum proteins: interference with methods that use sulfosalicylic acid, trichloroacetic acid, acetic acid, or nitric acid; not with tests using bromophenol blue (Albustix, Albutest, MultiStix).

NURSING CONSIDERATIONS

Besides those related universally to drug therapy (see "How to use this book"), consider the following specific recommendations:

Assessment

- Obtain a baseline assessment of infection before therapy.
- Be alert for adverse reactions and drug interactions throughout therapy.
- Evaluate the patient's and family's knowledge about ticarcillin/clavulanate therapy.

Nursing Diagnoses

- High risk for injury related to ineffectiveness of ticarcillin/clavulanate to eradicate the infection.
- Altered protection related to ticarcillin/clavulanate–induced allergic reaction.
- Knowledge deficit related to ticarcillin/clavulanate therapy.

Planning and Implementation

Preparation and Administration

- Obtain specimen for culture and sensitivity tests before first dose. Therapy may begin pending test results.
- Before first dose, ask about previous allergic reactions to this drug or other penicillins. However, a negative history of penicillin allergy does not guarantee future safety.
- Give ticarcillin/clavulanate at least 1 hour before bacteriostatic antibiotics.
- Expect to reduce dosage of ticarcillin/clavulanate for a patient with impaired renal function. Because drug is dialyzable, the dialysis patient may need dosage adjustments.
- ***I.V. use:*** Infuse I.V. drug intermittently (over 30 minutes) to prevent vein irritation.

Monitoring

- Monitor effectiveness by regularly assessing for improvement of infection.
- Allergic reactions especially with large doses, parenteral administration, or prolonged therapy. Keep in mind that the previously nonallergic patient may become sensitized to penicillin during therapy.
- Monitor for bacterial or fungal superinfections during high-dose or prolonged therapy, especially in elderly, debilitated, or immunosuppressed patients.
- Monitor CBC, platelets, and serum potassium level.

Supportive Care

- Discontinue the drug immediately if the patient develops signs of ana-

phylactic shock (rapidly developing dyspnea and hypotension). Notify the doctor and prepare to administer immediate treatment, such as epinephrine, corticosteroids, antihistamines, and other resuscitative measures as indicated.
• Change I.V. site every 48 hours.
Patient Teaching
• Advise the patient who becomes allergic to ticarcillin/clavulanate to wear medical alert identification stating this information.
Evaluation
In patients receiving ticarcillin/clavulanate, appropriate evaluation statements may include:
• Patient is free of infection.
• Patient does not experience an allergic reaction to ticarcillin/clavulanate.
• Patient and family state an understanding of therapy.

timolol maleate (systemic)
(tye´ moe lole)
Apo-Timol†, Blocadren

• *Classification:* antihypertensive adjunct in MI (beta-adrenergic blocking agent)
• *Pregnancy Risk Category:* C

HOW SUPPLIED
Tablets: 5 mg, 10 mg, 20 mg

ACTION
Mechanism: Blocks response to beta stimulation and depresses renin secretion.
Absorption: About 90% of an oral dose is absorbed from the GI tract.
Distribution: Throughout the body; depending on assay method, drug is 10% to 60% protein-bound.
Metabolism: About 80% of a given dose is metabolized in the liver to inactive metabolites.
Excretion: Drug and metabolites are excreted primarily in urine. Half-life: Approximately 4 hours.
Onset, peak, duration: Peak plasma concentration occurs in 1 to 2 hours.

INDICATIONS & DOSAGE
Hypertension–
Adults: initially 10 mg P.O. b.i.d. Usual daily maintenance dosage is 20 to 40 mg. Maximum daily dosage is 60 mg. Drug is used either alone or in combination with diuretics.
Myocardial infarction (long-term prophylaxis in patients who have survived acute phase)–
Adults: Recommended dosage for long-term prophylaxis in survivors of acute myocardial infarction is 10 mg P.O. b.i.d.

CONTRAINDICATIONS & PRECAUTIONS
Contraindicated in patients with hypersensitivity to the drug; severe bradycardia, overt cardiac failure, second- or third-degree atrioventricular block, or cardiogenic shock, because the drug may worsen these conditions; and bronchial asthma, allergic bronchospasm, or severe chronic obstructive pulmonary disease.

Use cautiously in patients with impaired hepatic or renal function because of potential for impaired metabolism and excretion; cardiomyopathy because beta-adrenergic blockade may precipitate CHF; diabetes mellitus because it may mask some signs of hypoglycemia; and emphysema or other pulmonary disease because the drug may inhibit bronchodilating effects of endogenous catecholamines.

ADVERSE REACTIONS
Common reactions are in italics; life-threatening reactions are in bold italics.
CNS: fatigue, lethargy, vivid dreams.
CV: *bradycardia, hypotension,* ***CHF,*** peripheral vascular disease.
GI: nausea, vomiting, diarrhea.

Metabolic: hypoglycemia without tachycardia.
Respiratory: dyspnea, ***bronchospasm.***
Skin: rash.
Other: ***increased airway resistance,*** fever.

INTERACTIONS

Digitalis glycosides: excessive bradycardia and increased depressant effect on myocardium. Use together cautiously.
Indomethacin: decrease in antihypertensive effect. Monitor blood pressure and adjust dosage.
Insulin, oral hypoglycemic drugs: can alter requirements for these drugs in previously stabilized diabetics. Monitor for hypoglycemia.

EFFECTS ON DIAGNOSTIC TESTS

Blood glucose: slightly increased levels.
BUN, serum potassium, uric acid: slightly increased levels.
Hemoglobin and hematocrit: slightly decreased.

NURSING CONSIDERATIONS

Besides those related universally to drug therapy (see "How to use this book"), consider the following specific recommendations:

Assessment

- Obtain a baseline assessment of the patient's blood pressure before beginning therapy.
- Be alert for adverse reactions and drug interactions throughout therapy.
- Evaluate the patient's and family's knowledge about timolol maleate therapy.

Nursing Diagnoses

- Altered tissue perfusion (renal, cerebral, cardiopulmonary, peripheral) related to the patient's underlying condition.
- Decreased cardiac output related to adverse CV reactions to timolol.
- Knowledge deficit related to timolol maleate therapy.

Planning and Implementation

Preparation and Administration

- Always check the patient's apical pulse rate before giving this drug. If you detect extremes in pulse rates, withhold drug and call the doctor immediately.
- Remember that at least 7 days should intervene between increases in dosage.

Monitoring

- Monitor effectiveness by frequently checking the patient's blood pressure and pulse rate.
- Monitor for signs of decreased cardiac output (dependent edema, jugular vein distention, fatigue, weakness, breathlessness, crackles) and other adverse reactions.

Supportive Care

- Keep in mind that this drug masks the common signs of shock and hypoglycemia.
- Position the patient with signs of decreased cardiac output in semi- to high Fowler's position and frequently encourage coughing and deep breathing.
- Keep in mind that timolol therapy should not be discontinued abruptly, but gradually reduce over 1 to 2 weeks.

Patient Teaching

- Explain the importance of taking this drug as prescribed, even when feeling well.
- Tell the patient not to discontinue this drug suddenly even if unpleasant adverse reactions occur but to discuss the problem with the doctor. Explain that abrupt discontinuation of the drug can exacerbate angina and myocardial infarction.
- Instruct the patient to check with the doctor or pharmacist before taking OTC medications.
- Warn the patient who's taking this medication for hypertension not to increase the dosage without first consulting the doctor.
- Teach the patient and family care-

giver to take blood pressure measurements. Tell them to notify the doctor of significant changes in blood pressure.

Evaluation

In patients receiving timolol, appropriate evaluation statements may include:

• Blood pressure is controlled within normal limits for this patient.
• Patient did not experience signs and symptoms of decreased cardiac output.
• Patient and family state an understanding of timolol therapy.

timolol maleate (ophthalmic)

(tye´ moe lole)

Timoptic Solution

• *Classification:* antiglaucoma agent (beta-adrenergic blocking agent)
• *Pregnancy Risk Category:* C

HOW SUPPLIED

Ophthalmic solution: 0.25%, 0.5%

ACTION

Mechanism: A nonselective beta adrenergic blocking agent. Reduces intraocular pressure by decreasing aqueous humor formation and possibly increases aqueous outflow.
Absorption: Some systemic absorption across the conjunctival mucosa.
Onset, peak, duration: Onset occurs in 15 to 30 minutes, peaks in 1 to 5 hours, and lasts about 24 hours.

INDICATIONS & DOSAGE

Chronic open-angle glaucoma, secondary glaucoma, aphakic glaucoma, ocular hypertension–
Adults: initially, instill 1 drop of 0.25% solution in each eye b.i.d.; reduce to 1 drop daily for maintenance. If patient doesn't respond, instill 1 drop of 0.5% solution in each eye b.i.d. If intraocular pressure is controlled, dosage may be reduced to 1 drop in each eye daily.

CONTRAINDICATIONS & PRECAUTIONS

Contraindicated in patients with hypersensitivity to the drug; in patients with severe bradycardia, overt cardiac failure, second- or third-degree atrioventricular block, or cardiogenic shock, because the drug may worsen these conditions; and in patients with bronchial asthma, allergic bronchospasm, or severe chronic obstructive pulmonary disease.

Use cautiously in patients with impaired hepatic or renal function because of potential for impaired metabolism and excretion; cardiomyopathy because beta-adrenergic blockade may precipitate CHF; diabetes mellitus because it may mask some signs of hypoglycemia; and emphysema or other pulmonary disease because the drug may inhibit bronchodilating effects of endogenous catecholamines. Some clinicians may need to discontinue the drug 48 hours before surgery because systemic absorption of the drug does occur. However, this practice remains controversial.

ADVERSE REACTIONS

Common reactions are in italics; life-threatening reactions are in bold italics.
CNS: headache, depression, fatigue.
CV: slight reduction in resting heart rate.
Eye: minor irritation. Long-term use may decrease corneal sensitivity.
GI: anorexia.
Other: apnea in infants, *evidence of beta blockade and systemic absorption (hypotension, bradycardia, syncope, exacerbation of asthma, and* ***CHF****).*

INTERACTIONS

General anesthetics, fentanyl: excessive hypotension.
Propranolol, metoprolol tartrate,

other oral beta-adrenergic blocking agents: increased ocular and systemic effect. Use together cautiously.

EFFECTS ON DIAGNOSTIC TESTS

BUN, serum potassium, uric acid, and blood glucose: slightly increased levels.
Hemoglobin and hematocrit: slightly decreased levels.

NURSING CONSIDERATIONS

Besides those related universally to drug therapy (see "How to use this book"), consider the following specific recommendations:

Assessment
- Obtain a baseline assessment of the patient's visual status, ocular pressure, and vital signs.
- Be alert for adverse reactions and drug interactions throughout therapy.
- Evaluate the patient's and family's knowledge about timolol maleate therapy.

Nursing Diagnoses
- Sensory/perceptual alterations (visual) related to the patient's underlying condition.
- Decreased cardiac output related to drug-induced systemic beta-blockade.
- Knowledge deficit related to timolol maleate therapy.

Planning and Implementation
Preparation and Administration
- Instill in lacrimal sac; remove excess solution from around eyes with a clean tissue or gauze and apply light finger pressure to lacrimal sac for 1 minute to decrease systemic absorption.

Monitoring
- Monitor effectiveness by assessing the patient's visual status and intraocular pressure.
- In some patients, stabilization of response may take a few weeks. You should determine intraocular pressure 4 weeks after initiating therapy.
- Closely monitor BP and apical rate for drug-induced hypotension or bradycardia; obtain ECG as indicated.
- Monitor patients with underlying cardiac or pulmonary disease closely.

Supportive Care
- Notify the doctor immediately of any changes in the patient's health status.
- Obtain an order for a mild analgesic if the patient experiences headache.

Patient Teaching
- Teach patient how to instill and advise him to wash his hands before and after administering the drug, and avoid touching the dropper to any surface.
- Tell the patient the drug can safely be used with conventional (PMMA) hard contact lenses.
- Warn diabetic patients that the drug may mask signs of hypoglycemia.

Evaluation
In patients receiving timolol maleate, appropriate evaluation statements may include:
- Patient experiences a therapeutic reduction in intraocular pressure.
- Patient remains free of systemic beta-blockade.
- Patient and family state an understanding of timolol maleate therapy.

tioconazole

(tye oh kone´ a zole)
Vagistat

- *Classification:* antifungal (imidazole derivative)
- *Pregnancy Risk Category:* C

HOW SUPPLIED

Vaginal ointment: 6.5%

ACTION

Mechanism: A fungicidal imidazole that alters cell wall permeability.
Pharmacokinetics: Unknown.

INDICATIONS & DOSAGE

Treatment of vulvovaginal candidiasis–

Women: insert 1 applicatorful (about 4.6 g) intravaginally h.s.

CONTRAINDICATIONS & PRECAUTIONS

Contraindicated in patients hypersensitive to the drug. Patients should discontinue use of the drug if irritation occurs.

ADVERSE REACTIONS

Common reactions are in italics; life-threatening reactions are in bold italics.

GU: *burning, itching,* discharge, vulvar edema and swelling, irritation.

INTERACTIONS

None reported.

EFFECTS ON DIAGNOSTIC TESTS

None reported.

NURSING CONSIDERATIONS

Besides those related universally to drug therapy (see "How to use this book"), consider the following specific recommendations:

Assessment

- Obtain a baseline assessment of vulvovaginal infection before therapy.
- Be alert for adverse reactions and drug interactions throughout therapy.
- Evaluate the patient's and family's knowledge about ticonazole therapy.

Nursing Diagnoses

- Impaired skin integrity related to patient's underlying condition.
- High risk for impaired skin integrity related to ticonazole-induced burning and itching.
- Knowledge deficit related to ticonazole therapy.

Planning and Implementation

Preparation and Administration

- ***Intravaginal use:*** Insert one applicatorful into the vagina.
- To avoid contamination of the ointment, open the applicator just before using it.

Monitoring

- Monitor effectiveness by regularly examining vaginal area for inflammation and drainage.
- Monitor the patient for adverse reactions and interactions by assessing the patient for burning, itching, and discharge.

Supportive Care

- Resistant infections could result from reinfection. Evaluate patients with persistent infections for sources of reinfection.
- Note that intractable candidiasis may be a sign of diabetes mellitus. If patient does not respond to therapy, urine and blood glucose tests should be performed.
- Be prepared to discontinue drug and notify doctor if adverse reactions occur.

Patient Teaching

- Review correct use of the drug with the patient. Instruct the patient to insert drug high into the vagina. Offer written instructions for the patient, which are available with the product.
- Emphasize the need to complete the full course of therapy, even after symptoms have improved.
- Instruct patient to use a sanitary napkin to avoid staining of clothing.
- Inform patient to avoid sexual intercourse during therapy or advise partner to use a condom to prevent reinfection.

Evaluation

In patients receiving ticonazole, appropriate evaluation statements may include:

- Patient states vulvovaginal infection is improving.
- Patient did not develop drug-induced burning and itching.
- Patient and family state an understanding of ticonazole therapy.

tobramycin

(toe bra mye´ sin)
Tobrex

- *Classification:* antibiotic (aminoglycoside)
- *Pregnancy Risk Category:* B

HOW SUPPLIED

Ophthalmic ointment: 0.3%
Ophthalmic solution: 0.3%

ACTION

Mechanism: An aminoglycoside antibiotic that blocks protein synthesis in susceptible bacteria by binding to the 30S ribosomal subunit.
Absorption: Animal studies indicate that the drug is absorbed into the aqueous humor after topical ophthalmic administration. Absorption is enhanced when the cornea is abraded.
Excretion: Cleared from the surface of the eye within 15 to 30 minutes of application.
Onset, peak, duration: Peak levels are seen within the cornea and aquaeous humor within 1 to 2 hours of instillation.

INDICATIONS & DOSAGE

Treatment of external ocular infections caused by susceptible gram-negative bacteria –
Adults and children: In mild to moderate infections, instill 1 or 2 drops into the affected eye q 4 hours or a thin strip of ointment q 8 to 12 hours. In severe infections, instill 2 drops into the infected eye hourly until condition improves; then reduce frequency. Or, apply thin strip of ointment q 3 to 4 hours until improvement then reduce frequency.

CONTRAINDICATIONS & PRECAUTIONS

Contraindicated in patients with hypersensitivity to tobramycin or any other aminoglycoside.

Use cautiously in patients with decreased renal function; in patients with tinnitus, vertigo, and high-frequency hearing loss who are susceptible to ototoxicity; in patients with dehydration, myasthenia gravis, parkinsonism, and hypocalcemia; in neonates and other infants; and in elderly patients.

ADVERSE REACTIONS

Common reactions are in italics; life-threatening reactions are in bold italics.
Eye: burning or stinging upon instillation, lid itching, lid swelling, blurred vision (with ointment).
Other: hypersensitivity.

INTERACTIONS

Tetracycline-containing eye preparations: incompatible with tyloxapol, an ingredient in Tobrex. Don't use together.

EFFECTS ON DIAGNOSTIC TESTS

BUN, nonprotein nitrogen, or serum creatinine: elevated levels.
Urinary excretion of casts: increased.

NURSING CONSIDERATIONS

Besides those related universally to drug therapy (see "How to use this book"), consider the following specific recommendations:
Assessment
- Obtain a baseline assessment of the patient's allergies before therapy.
- Be alert for adverse reactions and drug interactions throughout therapy.
- Evaluate the patient's and family's knowledge about tobramycin therapy.

Nursing Diagnoses
- Altered protection related to ocular infection.
- Pain related to burning and stinging upon instillation of medication.

• Knowledge deficit related to tobramycin therapy.

Planning and Implementation

Preparation and Administration

• Wash hands before and after administration.
• Cleanse eye area of excessive exudate before administration.
• Allow at least a 5-minute interval before instilling a second eye medication.

Monitoring

• Monitor effectiveness by culturing the eye to check for microorganisms.
• Observe amount, color, and consistency of exudate.
• Observe for signs of hypersensitivity reaction.
• Monitor serum tobramycin levels if ophthalmic preparation given concomitantly with systemic tobramycin.
• Observe for clinical symptoms of tobramycin overdose (keratitis, erythema, increased lacrimation, edema, and lid itching).

Supportive Care

• Apply warm, moist compresses to eye area to aid in removal of dried exudate.
• Stop drug and notify doctor if signs of tobramycin overdose develop.
• Avoid prolonged use; may result in overgrowth of nonsusceptible organisms, including fungi.

Patient Teaching

• Warn the patient that tobramycin eyedrops may cause burning and stinging on instillation.
• Teach the patient how to instill. Advise him to wash hands before and after administration. Warn him not to let tip of dropper touch eye or surrounding tissue.
• Instruct the patient to apply light finger pressure to the lacrimal sac for 1 minute after instillation of drops. Caution him to avoid rubbing or scratching eye area.
• Instruct the patient to watch for signs of hypersensitivity (itching lids, swelling, constant burning). If hypersensitivity develops, stop drug and notify doctor immediately.
• Warn the patient to avoid sharing washcloths and towels with family members during infection.
• Instruct the patient not to share eye medications with family members. A family member who develops the same symptoms should contact the doctor.

Evaluation

In patients receiving tobramycin, appropriate evaluation statements may include:

• Patient remains free from signs and symptoms of infection.
• Patient reports decrease or absence of pain on instillation.
• Patient and family state an understanding of tobramycin therapy.

tobramycin sulfate

(toe bra mye´ sin)

Nebcin

• *Classification:* antibiotic (aminoglycoside)
• *Pregnancy Risk Category:* D

HOW SUPPLIED

Injection: 40 mg/ml, 10 mg/ml (pediatric)

ACTION

Mechanism: Inhibits protein synthesis by binding directly to the 30S ribosomal subunit of susceptible bacteria. Generally bactericidal.

Absorption: Poorly absorbed after oral administration and is given parenterally. Peak plasma levels are similar following I.M. or I.V. administration.

Distribution: Widely distributed after parenteral administration; intraocular penetration is poor. CSF penetration is low, even in patients with inflamed meninges. Protein binding is minimal. Tobramycin crosses the placenta.

Metabolism: Not metabolized.
Excretion: Primarily excreted in urine by glomerular filtration; small amounts may be excreted in bile and breast milk. Half-life: 2 to 3 hours in adults; 24 to 60 hours in severe renal damage.
Onset, peak, duration: Peak serum concentrations occur 30 to 90 minutes after I.M. administration, and immediately following an I.V. infusion.

INDICATIONS & DOSAGE

Serious infections caused by sensitive strains of Escherichia coli, Proteus, Klebsiella, Enterobacter, Serratia, Staphylococcus aureus, Pseudomonas, Citrobacter, Providencia –
Adults and children with normal renal function: 3 mg/kg I.M. or I.V. daily divided q 8 hours. Up to 5 mg/kg I.M. or I.V. daily divided q 6 to 8 hours for life-threatening infections.
Neonates under 1 week: up to 4 mg/kg I.M. or I.V. daily divided q 12 hours. For I.V. use, dilute in 50 to 100 ml normal saline solution or dextrose 5% in water for adults and in less volume for children. Infuse over 20 to 60 minutes.
Patients with impaired renal function: initial dose is same as for those with normal renal function. Subsequent doses and frequency determined by renal function and serum concentrations of tobramycin.

CONTRAINDICATIONS & PRECAUTIONS

Contraindicated in patients with hypersensitivity to tobramycin or any aminoglycoside. Use cautiously in patients with: decreased renal function; tinnitus, vertigo, and high-frequency hearing loss who are susceptible to ototoxicity; dehydration, myasthenia gravis, parkinsonism, and hypocalcemia; and in neonates and other infants, and elderly patients.

ADVERSE REACTIONS

Common reactions are in italics; life-threatening reactions are in bold italics.
CNS: headache, lethargy, ***neuromuscular blockade.***
EENT: *ototoxicity (tinnitus, vertigo, hearing loss).*
GU: ***nephrotoxicity*** *(cells or casts in the urine, oliguria, proteinuria, decreased creatinine clearance, increased BUN and serum creatinine levels).*
Other: ***hypersensitivity.***

INTERACTIONS

Cephalothin: increase nephrotoxicity. Use together cautiously.
Dimenhydrinate: may mask symptoms of ototoxicity. Use with caution.
General anesthetics, neuromuscular blocking agents: may potentiate neuromuscular blockade.
I.V. loop diuretics (e.g., furosemide): increase ototoxicity. Use cautiously.
Other aminoglycosides, amphotericin B, cisplatin, methoxyflurane: increases nephrotoxicity. Use together cautiously.
Parenteral penicillins (e.g., carbenicillin and ticarcillin): tobramycin inactivation in vitro. Don't combine in I.V.

EFFECTS ON DIAGNOSTIC TESTS

BUN, nonprotein nitrogen, or serum creatinine: elevated levels and increased urinary excretion of casts.

NURSING CONSIDERATIONS

Besides those related universally to drug therapy (see "How to use this book"), consider the following specific recommendations:
Assessment
- Obtain a baseline assessment of infection before therapy.
- Be alert for adverse reactions and drug interactions throughout therapy.
- Evaluate the patient's and family's knowledge about tobramycin therapy.

Nursing Diagnoses

• High risk for injury related to ineffectiveness of tobramycin to eradicate the infection.

• Altered urinary elimination related to tobramycin induced nephrotoxicity.

• Knowledge deficit related to tobramycin.

Planning and Implementation

Preparation and Administration

• Obtain specimen for culture and sensitivity tests before first dose is administered. Therapy may begin pending test results.

• Weigh patient and obtain baseline renal function studies before therapy.

• ***I.V. use:*** Dilute in 50 to 100 ml normal saline solution or dextrose 5% in water for adults and in less volume for children. Infuse over 20 to 60 minutes. After I.V. infusion, flush line with normal saline solution or dextrose 5% in water.

Monitoring

• Monitor effectiveness by regularly assessing patient for improvement of infection.

• To monitor serum tobramycin level, draw blood for peak level 1 hour after I.M. injection and 30 minutes to 1 hour after infusion ends; for trough level just before next dose. Don't collect blood in a heparinized tube because heparin is incompatible with aminoglycosides. Peak blood levels over 12 mcg/ml and trough levels above 2 mcg/ml may be associated with increased toxicity.

• Monitor renal function (intake and output, specific gravity, urinalysis, BUN, and creatinine levels, and creatinine clearance).

Supportive Care

• Notify doctor if signs of decreased renal function occur or patient complains of tinnitus, vertigo, or hearing loss.

• Encourage patient to consume 2,000 ml of fluid daily (if not contraindicated) during therapy to minimize chemical irritation of the renal tubules.

Patient Teaching

• Emphasize the need to drink 2,000 ml of fluid each day, not including coffee, tea, or other caffeinated beverages.

• Instruct the patient to promptly report changes in urinary elimination patterns or disturbances or loss of hearing.

• Tell the patient to alert the doctor if infection worsens or does not improve.

• Stress the importance of recommended blood tests to monitor drug level and renal function, to determine the effectiveness of therapy, or to detect increased risk of adverse reactions.

• Teach patient to watch for and promptly report the signs and symptoms of superinfection (continued fever and other signs of new infection, especially of upper respiratory tract).

• Inform patient that usual duration of therapy is 7 to 10 days.

Evaluation

In patients receiving tobramycin, appropriate evaluation statements may include:

• Patient is free of infection.

• Patient's renal function studies remain normal throughout therapy.

• Patient and family state an understanding of therapy.

tocainide hydrochloride

(toe kay´ nide)

Tonocard

• *Classification:* ventricular antiarrhythmic (local anesthetic [amide])

• *Pregnancy Risk Category:* C

HOW SUPPLIED

Tablets: 400 mg, 600 mg

ACTION

Mechanism: A Class Ib antiarrhythmic that depresses phase O and shortens the action potential. All Class I drugs have membrane-stabilizing effects.
Absorption: Rapidly and completely absorbed from the GI tract; unlike lidocaine, it undergoes negligible first-pass effect in the liver.
Distribution: Distributed widely and apparently crosses the blood–brain barrier and placenta in animals (however, it is less lipophilic than lidocaine). Only about 10% to 20% of the drug is bound to plasma protein.
Metabolism: Apparently in the liver to inactive metabolites.
Excretion: In the urine as unchanged drug and inactive metabolites. About 30% to 50% of an orally administered dose is excreted in the urine as metabolites. Half-life: Elimination half-life is approximately 11 to 23 hours, with an initial biphasic plasma concentration decline similar to that of lidocaine. Half-life may be prolonged in patients with renal or hepatic insufficiency. Urine alkalinization may substantially decrease the excretion of unchanged drug in the urine.
Onset, peak, duration: Peak serum levels occur in 30 minutes to 2 hours after oral administration. Bioavailability is nearly 100%.

INDICATIONS & DOSAGE

Suppression of symptomatic ventricular arrhythmias, including frequent premature ventricular contractions and ventricular tachycardia –
Adults: initially, 400 mg P.O. q 8 hours. Usual dosage is between 1,200 and 1,800 mg daily in three divided doses.

CONTRAINDICATIONS & PRECAUTIONS

Contraindicated in patients with second- or third-degree heart block who do not have an artificial pacemaker, because the drug may further decrease conduction; and in patients with hypersensitivity to amide-type anesthetic agents, including lidocaine. Tocainide appears to have less effect on conduction than quinidine and procainamide.

Use with caution in patients with CHF, because the drug has a mild negative inotropic action and may slightly increase systemic vascular resistance, thereby exacerbating heart failure; atrial flutter or ventricular fibrillation, because the drug may accelerate the ventricular rate; preexisting bone marrow failure or cytopenia, because the drug may cause adverse hematologic effects; and severe renal or hepatic dysfunction, because the drug may accumulate and cause toxicity.

ADVERSE REACTIONS

Common reactions are in italics; life-threatening reactions are in bold italics.
Blood: ***aplastic anemia.***
CNS: *light-headedness, tremors,* restlessness, paresthesias, confusion, dizziness.
CV: hypotension, arrhythmias, *CHF.*
EENT: blurred vision.
GI: *nausea, vomiting, epigastric pain,* constipation, diarrhea, anorexia.
Hepatic: hepatitis.
Respiratory: ***respiratory arrest,*** pulmonary fibrosis, pneumonitis, ***pulmonary edema.***
Skin: rash.

INTERACTIONS

Beta blockers: decreased myocardial contractility; increased CNS toxicity.

EFFECTS ON DIAGNOSTIC TESTS

None reported.

NURSING CONSIDERATIONS

Besides those related universally to drug therapy (see "How to use this

book"), consider the following specific recommendations:

Assessment

• Obtain a baseline assessment of the patient's heart rate and rhythm before tocainide therapy.
• Be alert for adverse reactions and drug interactions throughout therapy.
• Evaluate the patient's and family's knowledge about tocainide therapy.

Nursing Diagnoses

• Decreased cardiac output related to ineffectiveness of tocainide therapy.
• Altered protection related to tocainide-induced proarrhythmias.
• Knowledge deficit related to tocainide.

Planning and Implementation

Preparation and Administration

• ***P.O. use:*** Administer the drug with food to minimize adverse GI reactions.

Monitoring

• Monitor effectiveness by regularly evaluating ECG recordings and heart rate and rhythm.
• Monitor therapeutic blood levels of tocainide. Therapeutic blood levels range from 4 to 10 mcg/ml.
• Monitor patient for tremor, which may indicate approaching maximum dose.
• Monitor ECG for new arrhythmias.

Supportive Care

• If ECG disturbances occurs, withhold the drug, obtain a rhythm strip, and notify the doctor immediately.
• Have emergency equipment and drugs on hand to treat new arrhythmias.
• Institute safety precautions if adverse CNS reactions occur.
• Obtain an order for an antiemetic, antidiarrheal, or laxative, as needed.

Patient Teaching

• Tell patient to take drug with food to minimize adverse GI reactions.
• Reassure patient that adverse reactions are generally mild, transient, and reversible by reducing dosage.
• Instruct patient to ask for assistance with activities if adverse CNS reactions occur.

Evaluation

In patients receiving tocainide, appropriate evaluation statements may include:

• Patient's ECG reveals arrhythmia has been corrected.
• Patient does not experience proarrhythmias with tocainide use.
• Patient and family state an understanding of tocainide therapy.

tolazamide

(tole az´ a mide)
Ronase, Tolamide, Tolinase

• *Classification:* antidiabetic agent (sulfonylurea)
• *Pregnancy Risk Category:* C

HOW SUPPLIED

Tablets: 100 mg, 250 mg, 500 mg

ACTION

Mechanism: A sulfonylurea that lowers blood glucose by stimulating insulin release from the pancreatic beta cells and reducing glucose output by the liver. An extrapancreatic effect increases peripheral sensitivity to insulin.
Absorption: Slowly absorbed from the GI tract.
Distribution: Probably distributed into the extracellular fluid.
Metabolism: Metabolized to several mildly active metabolites.
Excretion: Primarily in urine as metabolites, with small amounts excreted as unchanged drug. Half-life: 7 hours.
Onset, peak, duration: Onset of action within 4 to 6 hours, with maximum hypoglycemic effect within 10 hours; duration of action is 12 to 24 hours.

INDICATIONS & DOSAGE

Adjunct to diet to lower the blood glucose in patients with non-insulin-dependent diabetes mellitus (type II)–

Adults: initially, 100 mg P.O. daily with breakfast if fasting blood sugar (FBS) under 200 mg/dl; or 250 mg if FBS is over 200 mg/dl. May adjust dosage at weekly intervals by 100 to 250 mg. Maximum dosage is 500 mg b.i.d. before meals.

Adults over 65: 100 mg P.O. once daily.

To change from insulin to oral therapy–

Adults: if insulin dosage is under 20 units daily, insulin may be stopped and oral therapy started at 100 mg P.O. daily with breakfast. If insulin dosage is 20 to 40 units daily, insulin may be stopped and oral therapy started at 250 mg P.O. daily with breakfast. If insulin dosage is over 40 units daily, decrease insulin 50% and start oral therapy at 250 mg P.O. daily with breakfast. Increase dosages as above.

CONTRAINDICATIONS & PRECAUTIONS

Contraindicated in patients with hypersensitivity to sulfonylureas or thiazides and in patients with nonfunctioning pancreatic beta cells; and burns, acidosis, diabetic coma, severe infection, ketosis, or severe trauma or in those who are undergoing major surgery because such conditions of severe physiologic stress require insulin for adequate blood glucose control.

Use cautiously in patients with hepatic or renal insufficiency because of the important roles of the liver in metabolism and the kidneys in elimination; and in patients with impaired adrenal, pituitary, and thyroid function.

ADVERSE REACTIONS

Common reactions are in italics; life-threatening reactions are in bold italics.

GI: nausea, vomiting.

Metabolic: hypoglycemia.

Skin: rash, urticaria, facial flushing.

Other: hypersensitivity reactions.

INTERACTIONS

Anabolic steroids, chloramphenicol, clofibrate, guanethidine, MAO inhibitors, oral anticoagulants, phenylbutazone, salicylates, sulfonamides: increased hypoglycemic activity. Monitor blood glucose level.

Beta blockers, clonidine: prolonged hypoglycemic effect and masked symptoms of hypoglycemia. Use together cautiously.

Corticosteroids, glucagon, rifampin, thiazide diuretics: decreased hypoglycemic response. Monitor blood glucose level.

EFFECTS ON DIAGNOSTIC TESTS

Alkaline phosphatase and cholesterol: altered levels.

NURSING CONSIDERATIONS

Besides those related universally to drug therapy (see "How to use this book"), consider the following specific recommendations:

Assessment

- Obtain a baseline assessment of the patient's blood glucose level before initiating tolazamide therapy.
- Be alert for adverse reactions and drug interactions throughout therapy.
- Evaluate the patient's and family's knowledge about tolazamide therapy.

Nursing Diagnoses

- Altered nutrition: More than body requirements, related to the patient's inability to release sufficient insulin to maintain normal blood glucose levels.
- High risk for injury related to tolazamide-induced hypoglycemia.
- Knowledge deficit related to tolazamide therapy.

Planning and Implementation

Preparation and Administration

• Consider that some patients taking drug may be controlled effectively on a once-daily regimen, whereas others show better response with divided dosing.

• ***P.O. use:*** Administer once-daily doses with breakfast; divided doses are usually given before the morning and evening meals.

Monitoring

• Monitor effectiveness by regularly checking patient's blood glucose levels. Monitor blood glucose levels more frequently if the patient is under stress, having difficulty controlling blood glucose levels, or is newly diagnosed.

• Monitor the patient for signs and symptoms of both hyperglycemia and hypoglycemia; note time and circumstances of each reaction.

• Monitor the patient's hemoglobin A_1C regularly, as ordered.

• Monitor the patient for cardiovascular dysfunction because sulfonylureas have been associated with an increased risk of cardiovascular mortality as compared to diet or diet and insulin therapy.

• Monitor elderly patients closely because they may be more sensitive to drug's adverse reactions.

Supportive Care

• Notify the doctor if blood glucose levels remain elevated or frequent episodes of hypoglycemia occur.

• Treat a hypoglycemic reaction with an oral form of rapid-acting glucose if the patient is awake or with glucagon or I.V. glucose if the patient cannot be aroused. Follow up treatment with a complex carbohydrate snack when patient is awake, and determine cause of reaction.

• Be sure ancillary treatment measures, such as diet and exercise programs, are being used appropriately.

• Discuss with the doctor how to deal with noncompliance issues.

• Patient transferring from insulin therapy to an oral antidiabetic requires blood glucose monitoring at least t.i.d. before meals. Patient may require hospitalization during transition.

Patient Teaching

• Emphasize to the patient the importance of following the prescribed diet, exercise, and medical regimens.

• Tell the patient to take the medication at the same time each day. If a dose is missed, it should be taken immediately, unless it's almost time to take the next dose. Instruct the patient not to take double doses.

• Advise the patient to avoid alcohol while taking drug. Remind him that many foods and nonprescription medications contain alcohol.

• Encourage the patient to wear a medical alert bracelet or necklace.

• Tell the patient to take drug with food; once-daily dosage should be taken with breakfast.

• Teach the patient how to monitor blood glucose levels as prescribed.

• Teach the patient how to recognize the signs and symptoms of hyperglycemia and hypoglycemia and what to do if they occur.

• Stress the importance of compliance and close follow-up with drug therapy. Be sure patient knows that therapy relieves symptoms but doesn't cure disease.

Evaluation

In patients receiving tolazamide, appropriate evaluation statements may include:

• Patient's blood glucose level is normal.

• Patient recognizes hypoglycemia early and treats hypoglycemic episodes effectively before injury occurs.

• Patient and family state an understanding of tolazamide therapy.

tolazoline hydrochloride

(tole az´ oh leen)
Priscoline

• *Classification:* antihypertensive (peripheral vasodilator, alpha-adrenergic blocking agent)
• *Pregnancy Risk Category:* C

HOW SUPPLIED

Injection: 25 mg/ml

ACTION

Mechanism: Direct-acting vasodilator. May have some alpha-receptor blocking effects.
Absorption: Rapidly and almost completely after I.M. administration.
Distribution: Concentrates primarily in kidneys and liver.
Metabolism: None.
Excretion: In urine, primarily as unchanged drug. Half-life: Inversely related to urine output and can range from 1.5 to 41 hours.
Onset, peak, duration: When administered I.V., onset of effect is very rapid and peaks within 30 minutes.

INDICATIONS & DOSAGE

Persistent pulmonary hypertension of the newborn–
Neonates: initially, 1 to 2 mg/kg I.V. over 10 minutes, followed by infusion of 1 to 2 mg/kg/hour.
Peripheral vasospastic disorders–
Adults: 10 to 50 mg I.M. or I.V. q.i.d.

CONTRAINDICATIONS & PRECAUTIONS

Contraindicated in patients with hypersensitivity to the drug and in patients with known or suspected coronary artery disease or after a cerebrovascular accident.

Use cautiously in patients with gastritis or peptic ulcer disease because the drug can stimulate gastric secretion; and in patients with mitral stenosis because the drug can increase or decrease pulmonary artery pressure and total pulmonary resistance. Tolazoline may activate stress ulcers.

ADVERSE REACTIONS

Common reactions are in italics; life-threatening reactions are in bold italics.
CV: *arrhythmias, anginal pain, hypertension, flushing,* transient postural vertigo, palpitations, *orthostatic hypotension.*
GI: *nausea, vomiting, diarrhea, epigastric discomfort, exacerbation of peptic ulcer.*
Local: burning at injection site.
Other: weakness, paradoxical response in seriously damaged limbs, increased pilomotor activity, tingling, chilliness, apprehension, ***pulmonary hemorrhage.***

INTERACTIONS

Ethyl alcohol: possible disulfiram reaction from accumulation of acetaldehyde. Use together cautiously.
Vasopressors (epinephrine, norepinephrine): may cause a paradoxical fall in blood pressure.

EFFECTS ON DIAGNOSTIC TESTS

None reported.

NURSING CONSIDERATIONS

Besides those related universally to drug therapy (see "How to use this book"), consider the following specific recommendations:
Assessment
• Obtain a baseline assessment of the patient's cardiopulmonary or cardiovascular status before drug therapy.
• Be alert for adverse reactions and drug interactions throughout therapy.
• Evaluate the patient's and family's knowledge about tolazoline therapy.
Nursing Diagnoses
• Altered tissue perfusion (cardiopulmonary) related to the patient's underlying condition.

• High risk for injury related to adverse drug reaction.
• Knowledge deficit related to tolazoline therapy.

Planning and Implementation

Preparation and Administration

• ***I.V. use:*** Patient should be supine during administration.
• Response should be evident within 30 minutes for treatment of persistent pulmonary hypertension of the newborn. Little information is available regarding infusions lasting longer than 48 hours.
• Drug is often used to distinguish between functional (vasospastic) and organic (obstructive) forms of peripheral vascular disease.
• Appearance of flushing usually indicates maximum tolerable dosage.

Monitoring

• Monitor the patient's vital signs. Watch especially for blood pressure changes and arrhythmias.

Supportive Care

• Keep patient warm during parenteral administration to increase response.
• Assist the patient to get in and out of bed if orthostatic hypotension occurs.
• Provide the patient with fluids if nausea, vomiting, and diarrhea occur.

Patient Teaching

• Warn patient against exposure to cold, which can aggravate tissue damage.
• Instruct the patient to avoid alcohol; chills and flushing may occur.
• Instruct patient to minimize orthostatic hypotension by avoiding sudden posture change.

Evaluation

In patients receiving tolazoline, appropriate evaluation statements may include:

• Patient maintains tissue perfusion and cellular oxygenation.
• The patient does not sustain any injuries.
• Patient and family state an understanding of tolazoline therapy.

tolbutamide

(tole byoo´ ta mide)

Apo-Tolbutamide, Mobenol†, Novobutamide†, Oramide, Orinase

• *Classification:* antidiabetic agent (sulfonylurea)
• *Pregnancy Risk Category:* C

HOW SUPPLIED

Tablets: 250 mg, 500 mg

ACTION

Mechanism: A sulfonylurea that lowers blood glucose levels by stimulating insulin release from the pancreatic beta cells and reducing glucose output by the liver. An extrapancreatic effect increases peripheral sensitivity to insulin.
Absorption: Readily absorbed from the GI tract.
Distribution: Probably distributed into the extracellular fluid. It is 95% protein-bound.
Metabolism: In the liver to inactive metabolites.
Excretion: Drug and metabolites are excreted in urine and feces. Half-life: 4 to 5 hours.
Onset, peak, duration: Onset of action within 1 hour. The maximum hypoglycemic activity occurs within 8 hours; duration of action is 6 to 12 hours.

INDICATIONS & DOSAGE

Stable, maturity-onset (Type II) nonketotic diabetes mellitus uncontrolled by diet alone and previously untreated—
Adults: initially, 1 to 2 g P.O. daily as single dose or divided b.i.d. to t.i.d. May adjust dosage to maximum of 3 g daily.

To change from insulin to oral therapy–
Adults: if insulin dosage is under 20 units daily, insulin may be stopped and oral therapy started at 1 to 2 g P.O. daily. If insulin dosage is 20 to 40 units daily, insulin is reduced 30% to 50% and oral therapy started as above. If insulin dosage is over 40 units daily, insulin is decreased 20% and oral therapy started as above. Further reductions in insulin are based on patient's response to oral therapy.

CONTRAINDICATIONS & PRECAUTIONS

Contraindicated in patients with hypersensitivity to sulfonylureas or thiazides and in patients with nonfunctioning pancreatic beta cells; and in patients with burns, acidosis, diabetic coma, severe infection, ketosis, or severe trauma or in those who require major surgery because such conditions of physiologic stress require insulin for adequate control of glucose levels.

Use cautiously in patients with hepatic or renal insufficiency because of the important roles of the liver in metabolism and the kidneys in elimination; and in patients with impaired adrenal, pituitary, or thyroid function.

ADVERSE REACTIONS

Common reactions are in italics; life-threatening reactions are in bold italics.
GI: nausea, heartburn.
Metabolic: hypoglycemia, dilutional hyponatremia.
Skin: rash, pruritus, facial flushing.
Other: hypersensitivity reactions.

INTERACTIONS

Anabolic steroids, chloramphenicol, clofibrate, guanethidine, MAO inhibitors, oral anticoagulants, phenylbutazone, salicylates, sulfonamides: increased hypoglycemic activity. Monitor blood glucose level.
Beta blockers, clonidine: prolonged hypoglycemic effect and masked symptoms of hypoglycemia. Use together cautiously.
Corticosteroids, glucagon, rifampin, thiazide diuretics: decreased hypoglycemic response. Monitor blood glucose level.

EFFECTS ON DIAGNOSTIC TESTS

Alkaline phosphatase, bilirubin, cholesterol, total protein: altered results.
Cephalin flocculation (thymol turbidity) and ^{131}I thyroid uptake: altered results.
Urine porphyrins and protein: altered levels.

NURSING CONSIDERATIONS

Besides those related universally to drug therapy (see "How to use this book"), consider the following specific recommendations:

Assessment

- Obtain a baseline assessment of the patient's blood glucose level before initiating tolbutamide therapy.
- Be alert for adverse reactions and drug interactions throughout therapy.
- Evaluate the patient's and family's knowledge about tolbutamide therapy.

Nursing Diagnoses

- Altered nutrition: More than body requirements, related to inability to produce sufficient insulin to maintain normal blood glucose levels.
- High risk for injury related to tolbutamide-induced hypoglycemia.
- Knowledge deficit related to tolbutamide therapy.

Planning and Implementation

Preparation and Administration

- Consider that some patients taking drug may be controlled effectively on a once-daily regimen, whereas others show better response with divided dosing.
- ***P.O. use:*** Administer with meals. Once daily dosing should be administered with breakfast.

Monitoring
• Monitor effectiveness by regularly checking patient's blood glucose levels. Monitor blood glucose levels more frequently if the patient is under stress, having difficulty controlling blood glucose levels, or is newly diagnosed.
• Monitor the patient for signs and symptoms of both hyperglycemia and hypoglycemia; note time and circumstances of each reaction.
• Monitor the patient's hemoglobin A_1C regularly, as ordered.
• Monitor the patient for cardiovascular dysfunction because sulfonylureas have been associated with an increased risk of cardiovascular mortality as compared to diet or diet and insulin therapy.
• Monitor elderly patients closely because they may be more sensitive to this drug's adverse reactions.

Supportive Care
• Notify the doctor if blood glucose levels remain elevated or frequent episodes of hypoglycemia occur.
• Treat a hypoglycemic reaction with an oral form of rapid-acting glucose if the patient is awake or with glucagon or I.V. glucose if the patient cannot be aroused. Follow up treatment with a complex carbohydrate snack when patient is awake, and determine cause of reaction.
• Be sure ancillary treatment measures, such as diet and exercise programs, are being used appropriately.
• Discuss with the doctor how to approach noncompliance issues.
• Patients transferring from insulin therapy to an oral antidiabetic requires blood glucose monitoring at least t.i.d. before meals. Patient may require hospitalization during transition.

Patient Teaching
• Emphasize the importance of following the prescribed diet, exercise, and medical regimens.
• Tell the patient to take the medication at the same time each day. If a dose is missed, it should be taken immediately, unless it's almost time to take the next dose. Instruct the patient not to take double doses.
• Advise the patient to avoid alcohol while taking drug. Remind him that many foods and nonprescription medications contain alcohol.
• Encourage the patient to wear a medical alert bracelet or necklace.
• Tell the patient to take drug with food; once-daily dosage should be taken with breakfast.
• Teach the patient how to monitor blood glucose levels as prescribed.
• Teach the patient how to recognize the signs and symptoms of hyperglycemia and hypoglycemia and what to do if they occur.
• Stress the importance of compliance and close follow-up with drug therapy. Be sure patient knows that therapy relieves symptoms but doesn't cure disease.

Evaluation

In patients receiving tolbutamide, appropriate evaluation statements may include:
• Patient's blood glucose level is normal.
• Patient recognizes hypoglycemia early and treats hypoglycemic episodes effectively before injury occurs.
• Patient and family state an understanding of tolbutamide therapy.

tolmetin sodium

(tole´ met in)
Tolectin, Tolectin DS

• *Classification:* nonnarcotic analgesic, antipyretic, anti-inflammatory (nonsteroidal anti-inflammatory)
• *Pregnancy Risk Category:* B (D in 3rd trimester)

HOW SUPPLIED

Tablets: 200 mg
Capsules: 400 mg

ACTION

Mechanism: Produces anti-inflammatory, analgesic, and antipyretic effects, possibly through inhibition of prostaglandin synthesis.
Absorption: Rapidly absorbed from the GI tract.
Distribution: Highly protein-bound.
Metabolism: Hepatic.
Excretion: In urine. Half-life: About 1 hour.
Onset, peak, duration: Peak plasma levels are seen in 30 to 60 minutes.

INDICATIONS & DOSAGE

Rheumatoid arthritis, osteoarthritis, gout, dysmenorrhea, juvenile rheumatoid arthritis–
Adults: 400 mg P.O. t.i.d. or q.i.d. Maximum dosage is 2 g daily.
Children 2 years or older: 15 to 30 mg/kg P.O. daily in divided doses.

CONTRAINDICATIONS & PRECAUTIONS

Contraindicated in patients with hypersensitivity to tolmetin or zomepirac, or in patients in whom aspirin or other nonsteroidal anti-inflammatory drugs (NSAIDs) induce symptoms of asthma, urticaria, or rhinitis. Patients with known "triad" symptoms (aspirin hypersensitivity, rhinitis/nasal polyps, and asthma) are at high risk of bronchospasm because of cross-sensitivity to tolmetin.

Serious GI toxicity, especially ulceration or hemorrhage, can occur at any time in patients on chronic NSAID therapy. Use cautiously in patients with a history of GI bleeding or GI ulcer because the drug may irritate the GI tract; in patients with renal disease because the drug may be nephrotoxic; or in patients with cardiac disease because it may cause peripheral edema, sodium retention, and hypertension.

Drug may mask the signs and symptoms of acute infection (fever, myalgias, erythema). Evaluate patients with high risk of infection (such as those with diabetes) carefully.

ADVERSE REACTIONS

Common reactions are in italics; life-threatening reactions are in bold italics.
Blood: prolonged bleeding time.
CNS: headache, dizziness, drowsiness.
GI: *epigastric distress, peptic ulceration, occult blood loss, nausea.*
GU: nephrotoxicity, pseudoproteinuria.
Skin: rash, urticaria, pruritus.
Other: sodium retention, edema.

INTERACTIONS

Oral anticoagulants: increased risk of bleeding. Monitor patient closely.

EFFECTS ON DIAGNOSTIC TESTS

Bleeding time: prolonged.
BUN, serum potassium and transaminase: increased levels.
Hemoglobin and hematocrit: decreased levels.
Urinary protein assays with tests using sulfusalicylic acid (not Albustix or Unistix): falsely elevated results (pseudoproteinuria).

NURSING CONSIDERATIONS

Besides those related universally to drug therapy (see "How to use this book"), consider the following specific recommendations:

Assessment

• Obtain a baseline assessment of the patient's pain before therapy.
• Be alert for adverse reactions and drug interactions throughout therapy.
• Evaluate the patient's and family's knowledge about tolmetin therapy.

Nursing Diagnoses

• Pain related to the patient's underlying condition.

*Liquid form contains alcohol. **May contain tartrazine.

• Impaired tissue integrity related to peptic ulceration, a possible adverse reaction to therapy.
• Knowledge deficit related to tolmetin therapy.

Planning and Implementation

Preparation and Administration
• Give with food, milk, or antacids to reduce adverse GI reactions.

Monitoring
• Regularly monitor for relief of pain, keeping in mind that full therapeutic effects may be delayed 2 to 4 weeks.
• Monitor for signs and symptoms of peptic ulceration and other adverse drug reactions.
• Test the patient's stool for occult blood.
• Regularly monitor the patient's renal and hepatic function and recommend eye examinations during long-term therapy.

Supportive Care
• Notify the doctor if the pain is not relieved or worsens.
• Anticipate that tolmetin may falsely elevate urinary protein, causing pseudoproteinuria. This drug is the only NSAID reported to do so.
• Hold dose and notify the doctor if the patient develops nausea, vomiting, or epigastric distress that is not relieved by taking drug with food or milk, or if renal or hepatic abnormalities occur.

Patient Teaching
• Tell the patient that therapeutic effect should begin in 1 week, but full effect may take 2 to 4 weeks.
• Advise the patient to notify the doctor if pain persists or becomes worse.
• Tell the patient to take the drug with food, milk, or antacids.
• Tell the patient to report nausea, vomiting, epigastric pain, anorexia, or weight loss, which may be due to peptic ulceration, a possible adverse reaction.
• Because serious GI toxicity can occur at any time in chronic NSAID therapy, teach the patient signs and symptoms of GI bleeding. Tell the patient to report these to the doctor immediately.

Evaluation

In the patient receiving tolmetin, appropriate evaluation statements include:
• Patient states pain is relieved.
• Patient's tissue integrity remains intact.
• Patient and family state an understanding of tolmetin therapy.

tolnaftate

(tole naf′ tate)

Aftate for Athlete's Foot◇, Aftate for Jock Itch◇, Footwork◇, Fungatin◇, Genaspor◇, NP-27◇, Tinactin◇, Zeasorb-AF◇

• *Classification:* topical antifungal
• *Pregnancy Risk Category:* C

HOW SUPPLIED

Aerosol liquid: 1% (with 36% alcohol)◇
Aerosol powder: 1% (with 14% alcohol)◇
Cream: 1%◇
Gel: 1%◇
Powder: 1%◇
Pump spray liquid: 1% (with 36% alcohol)◇
Topical solution: 1%◇

ACTION

Mechanism: Unknown; drug exhibits fungistatic and fungicidal activity.
Pharmacokinetics: Unknown.

INDICATIONS & DOSAGE

Superficial fungal infections of the skin, infections due to common pathogenic fungi, tinea pedis, tinea cruris, tinea corporis, tinea versicolor–
Adults and children: ¼″ to ½″ ribbon of cream or 3 drops of lotion to

cover about the size of one hand; same amount of cream or 3 drops of lotion to cover the toes and interdigital webs of one foot; or an amount of gel, powder, or spray to cover affected area. Apply and massage gently into skin b.i.d. for 2 to 6 weeks.

CONTRAINDICATIONS & PRECAUTIONS

Contraindicated in patients hypersensitive to the drug. Discontinue therapy if sensitization occurs. If no improvement is seen after 4 weeks of therapy, the patient should contact the doctor.

When treating nail or scalp infections, tolnaftate should only be used in conjunction with other drugs.

ADVERSE REACTIONS

None significant.

INTERACTIONS

None significant.

EFFECTS ON DIAGNOSTIC TESTS

None reported.

NURSING CONSIDERATIONS

Besides those related universally to drug therapy (see "How to use this book"), consider the following specific recommendations:

Assessment

- Obtain a baseline assessment of skin infection before therapy.
- Be alert for adverse reactions and drug interactions throughout therapy.
- Evaluate the patient's and family's knowledge about tolnaftate therapy.

Nursing Diagnoses

- Impaired skin integrity related to patient's underlying condition.
- Body image disturbance related to patient's underlying condition.
- Knowledge deficit related to tolnaftate therapy.

Planning and Implementation

Preparation and Administration

- ***Topical use:*** Apply ¼″ to ½″ ribbon of cream or 3 drops of lotion to cover about the size of one hand. Apply and massage gently into skin.

Monitoring

- Monitor effectiveness by regularly checking skin infection.
- Monitor condition; if it worsens, discontinue use and notify doctor.

Supportive Care

- Remember that it is commonly used to treat athlete's foot (tinea pedis). If no improvement after 10 days, consult doctor.
- Don't use to treat hair or nail infections. Will not eradicate fungus from these structures.
- Powder or aerosol may continue to be used inside socks and shoes of persons susceptible to tinea infections.

Patient Teaching

- Teach patient how to apply medication.
- Tell patient the drug is odorless and greaseless. Won't stain or discolor skin, hair, nails, or clothing.
- Inform patient to continue using for full treatment period prescribed, even if condition has improved.

Evaluation

In patients receiving tolnaftate, appropriate evaluation statements may include:

- Skin infection is resolved.
- Patient did not develop body image disturbance
- Patient and family state an understanding of tolnaftate therapy.

---

tranylcypromine sulfate

(tran ill sip´ roe meen)

Parnate

- *Classification:* antidepressant (MAO inhibitor)

• *Pregnancy Risk Category:* C

HOW SUPPLIED

Tablets: 10 mg

ACTION

Mechanism: Promotes accumulation of neurotransmitters by inhibiting MAO.
Absorption: Rapidly and completely from the GI tract.
Distribution: Not fully understood. Dosage adjustments are determined by therapeutic response and adverse reaction profile.
Metabolism: Hepatic.
Excretion: Primarily in urine within 24 hours; some drug is excreted in feces via the biliary tract. Half-life: 2½ hours; enzyme inhibition is prolonged and unrelated to half-life.
Onset, peak, duration: Peak serum levels occur at 1 to 3 hours; onset of therapeutic activity may not occur until patient has had 3 to 4 weeks of daily therapy.

INDICATIONS & DOSAGE

Treatment of depression–
Adults: 10 mg P.O. b.i.d. Increase to maximum of 30 mg daily, if necessary, after 2 weeks. Not recommended for children under 16 years.

CONTRAINDICATIONS & PRECAUTIONS

Contraindicated in patients with uncontrolled hypertension, because it may precipitate hypertensive crisis; and in patients with seizure disorders because it lowers the seizure threshold, even in patients controlled on anticonvulsant therapy.

Use cautiously in patients with angina pectoris and other cardiovascular disease, diabetes Types I and II, Parkinson's disease and other motor disorders, hyperthyroidism, or pheochromocytoma because drug may worsen these conditions; renal or hepatic insufficiency because reduced metabolism and excretion may cause drug to accumulate; and bipolar disorder because drug may provoke or worsen manic phase; reduce dosage during manic phase.

ADVERSE REACTIONS

Common reactions are in italics; life-threatening reactions are in bold italics.
CNS: *dizziness,* vertigo, headache, overactivity, hyperreflexia, tremors, muscle twitching, mania, jitters, confusion, memory impairment, fatigue.
CV: *orthostatic hypotension,* arrhythmias, ***paradoxical hypertension.***
EENT: blurred vision.
GI: dry mouth, *anorexia,* nausea, diarrhea, constipation, abdominal pain.
GU: impotence.
Skin: rash.
Other: peripheral edema, sweating, weight changes, chills, altered libido.

INTERACTIONS

Alcohol, barbiturates, and other sedatives; narcotics; dextromethorphan; tricyclic antidepressants: use with caution and in reduced dosage.
Amphetamines, antihistamines, ephedrine, levodopa, meperidine, metaraminol, methotrimeprazine, methylphenidate, phenylephrine, phenylpropanolamine: pressor effects of these drugs are enhanced by tranylcypromine. Use together cautiously.
Insulin, oral hypoglycemic agents: tranylcypromine may alter requirements of antidiabetic medications.

EFFECTS ON DIAGNOSTIC TESTS

Liver function tests: elevated results.
Urinary catecholamines: elevated levels.

NURSING CONSIDERATIONS

Besides those related universally to drug therapy (see "How to use this book"), consider the following specific recommendations:

Assessment
- Obtain a baseline assessment of the patient's degree of depression and blood pressure, CBC levels, and liver function test results before beginning therapy with this drug.
- Be alert for adverse reactions and drug interactions throughout therapy.
- Evaluate the patient's and family's knowledge about tranylcypromine therapy.

Nursing Diagnoses
- Ineffective individual coping related to the patient's underlying condition.
- High risk for injury related to tranylcypromine-induced dizziness or orthostatic hypotension.
- Knowledge deficit related to tranylcypromine therapy.

Planning and Implementation

Preparation and Administration
- Ask the patient about recent ingestion of tyramine-rich foods before administering drug.
- Administer the drug at bedtime when possible to minimize discomfort from CNS and anticholinergic reactions.
- Expect this drug to be used only when TCA or electroconvulsive therapy is ineffective or contraindicated.
- Dosage is usually reduced to maintenance level as soon as possible.

Monitoring
- Monitor effectiveness by having the patient discuss his feelings (ask broad, open-ended questions) and by evaluating his behavior.
- Monitor nutritional status and weight if anorexia occurs.
- Monitor blood pressure readings, CBC, and liver function test results throughout treatment. Watch blood pressure readings for paradoxical hypertension.
- Monitor for suicidal tendencies.

Supportive Care
- Institute safety measures, such as assisting with activities, if adverse CNS reactions or orthostatic hypotension occur. Advise the patient to change positions slowly to minimize orthostatic hypotension.
- Hold dose and notify the doctor if the patient develops symptoms of overdose (palpitations, severe hypotension, or frequent headaches).
- Do not withdraw drug abruptly.
- Have phentolamine (Regitine) available to combat severe hypertension.
- If anorexia develops, encourage the patient to eat highly nutritious foods and more frequent smaller meals.

Patient Teaching
- Tell the patient therapy must continue for 2 weeks or more before noticeable effect, and 4 weeks or more for full effect.
- MAO inhibitors are most often reported to cause hypertensive crisis with high-tyramine ingestion; warn the patient to avoid foods high in tyramine or tryptophan (aged cheese, Chianti wine, beer, avocados, chicken livers, chocolate, bananas, soy sauce, meat tenderizers, salami, bologna) and self-medication with OTC cold, hay fever, or weight-loss preparations. (Give patient a list of foods to avoid when taking MAO inhibitors.)
- Tell the patient to avoid combining drug with alcohol or other CNS depressants.
- Advise the patient how to overcome anorexia.
- Warn the patient to avoid driving and other hazardous activities that require mental alertness if adverse CNS reactions occur.
- Tell the diabetic patient to monitor blood glucose level closely because drug may alter levels.
- Instruct the patient to continue safety precautions for 7 days after discontinuing the drug because of residual effects.

Evaluation

In patients receiving tranylcypromine, appropriate evaluation statements include:
- Patient reports improved feelings about himself and life.

• Patient is not injured as a result of adverse reactions to tranylcypromine.
• Patient and family state an understanding of tranylcypromine therapy.

trazodone hydrochloride

(traz´ oh done)
Desyrel, Trazon, Trialodine

• *Classification:* antidepressant (triazolopyridine)
• *Pregnancy Risk Category:* C

HOW SUPPLIED

Tablets: 50 mg, 100 mg, 150 mg

ACTION

Mechanism: Inhibits serotonin reuptake into presynaptic neurons of the CNS.
Absorption: Nearly complete after oral administration. Absorption is enhanced in the presence of food.
Distribution: Widely distributed; drug does not concentrate in any tissue. Small amounts may appear in breast milk. Drug is 90% protein-bound.
Metabolism: Hepatic.
Excretion: Most (75%) is excreted in urine within 3 days; the rest in feces. Half-life: Terminal elimination half-life is 5 to 9 hours.
Onset, peak, duration: Peak levels are seen in 1 hour. Concomitant ingestion of food delays absorption, extends peak effect of drug to 2 hours, and increases amount of drug absorbed by 20%. Steady-state plasma levels are reached in 3 to 7 days of daily administration.

INDICATIONS & DOSAGE

Treatment of depression–
Adults: initial dosage is 150 mg P.O. daily in divided doses, which can be increased by 50 mg daily q 3 to 4 days. Average dosage ranges from 150 mg to 400 mg daily. Maximum dosage is 600 mg.

CONTRAINDICATIONS & PRECAUTIONS

Contraindicated in patients with known hypersensitivity to tricyclic antidepressants, trazodone, and related compounds; and in the acute recovery phase of MI. Use with great caution in patients with other cardiac disease (arrhythmias, CHF, angina pectoris, valvular disease, or heart block) because similar drugs have adversely affected cardiac function. Also use cautiously in patients with priapism or ejaculatory disorders because drug may cause or exacerbate such disorders; surgical correction is necessary (and not always successful) in as many as 30% of patients who experience priapism or prolonged, painful erections; and also in patients receiving electroconvulsive therapy and those with hepatic or renal dysfunction.

ADVERSE REACTIONS

Common reactions are in italics; life-threatening reactions are in bold italics.
CNS: *drowsiness, dizziness,* nervousness, fatigue, confusion, tremors, weakness.
CV: orthostatic hypotension, tachycardia.
EENT: blurred vision, tinnitus.
GI: dry mouth, constipation, nausea, vomiting, anorexia.
GU: urine retention, priapism possibly leading to impotence.
Skin: rash, urticaria.
Other: sweating.

INTERACTIONS

Alcohol, CNS depressants: enhanced CNS depression.
Antihypertensives: added hypotensive effect of trazodone. Antihypertensive dosage may have to be decreased.
Digoxin, phenytoin: trazodone may increase serum levels of these drugs. Monitor for toxicity.
MAO inhibitors: No clinical experience. Use together very cautiously.

EFFECTS ON DIAGNOSTIC TESTS

CBC: decreased WBC counts.
ECG: elongated Q-T and PR intervals, flattened T waves.
Liver function tests: elevated results.
Serum glucose: altered levels.

NURSING CONSIDERATIONS

Besides those related universally to drug therapy (see "How to use this book"), consider the following specific recommendations:

Assessment
- Obtain a baseline assessment of depression before therapy.
- Be alert for adverse reactions and drug interactions throughout therapy.
- Evaluate the patient's and family's knowledge about trazodone hydrochloride therapy.

Nursing Diagnoses
- Ineffective individual coping related to the patient's underlying condition.
- High risk for injury related to CNS adverse reactions to trazodone.
- Knowledge deficit related to trazodone therapy.

Planning and Implementation
Preparation and Administration
- Administer after meals or a light snack for optimal absorption and to decrease incidence of dizziness.

Monitoring
- Monitor effectiveness by having the patient discuss his feelings (ask broad, open-ended questions) and by evaluating his behavior.
- Monitor for mood changes and suicidal tendencies.

Supportive Care
- Take note if patient complains of prolonged and painful erection. Priapism is a potential problem in men taking trazodone; it may require surgical intervention.
- Note mood changes and monitor patient for suicidal tendencies.
- Institute safety precautions if adverse CNS reactions occur.

Patient Teaching
- Teach family the signs of suicidal tendency or ideation.
- Warn the patient to avoid driving and other hazardous activities that require alertness and good psychomotor coordination until CNS effects of the drug are known. Tell the patient that drowsiness and dizziness usually subside after first few weeks.
- Tell the patient that treatment must continue for 2 weeks or more before noticeable effect, and 4 weeks or more before full effect. Encourage the patient to continue taking medication until it achieves full therapeutic effect.

Evaluation
In patients receiving trazodone, appropriate evaluation statements may include:
- Patient behavior and communication indicate improvement of depression.
- Patient has not experienced injury from adverse CNS reactions.
- Patient and family state an understanding of trazodone therapy.

---

tretinoin (vitamin A acid, retinoic acid)

(tret´ i noyn)
Retin-A, StieVAA†

- *Classification:* antiacne agent (vitamin A derivative)
- *Pregnancy Risk Category:* B

HOW SUPPLIED

Cream: 0.025%, 0.05%, 0.1%
Gel: 0.025%, 0.01%
Solution: 0.05%

ACTION

Mechanism: Inhibits comedones by increasing epidermal cell mitosis and turnover.
Absorption: Minimally absorbed after topical application. Only 9% to

18% penetrates into the horny layer of the skin; lesser amounts penetrate into the dermis. Only 0.1% to 6% of a dose reaches the systemic circulation.
Excretion: In urine.

INDICATIONS & DOSAGE

Acne vulgaris (especially grades I, II, and III), treatment of fine wrinkles from photodamaged skin–
Adults and children: cleanse affected area and lightly apply solution once daily h.s.

CONTRAINDICATIONS & PRECAUTIONS

Contraindicated in patients with hypersensitivity to vitamin A/retinoic acid. It should be used cautiously in patients with eczema. Avoid contact of drug with eyes, mouth, angles of the nose, mucous membranes, or open wounds. Use of topical preparations containing high concentrations of alcohol, menthol, spices, or lime should be avoided, as they may cause skin irritation. Avoid use of medicated cosmetics on treated skin.

ADVERSE REACTIONS

Common reactions are in italics; life-threatening reactions are in bold italics.
Skin: *feeling of warmth, slight stinging, local erythema, peeling,* chapping, swelling, blistering, crusting, temporary hyperpigmentation or hypopigmentation.

INTERACTIONS

Topical preparations containing sulfur, resorcinol, or salicylic acid: increased risk of skin irritation. Don't use together.

EFFECTS ON DIAGNOSTIC TESTS

None reported.

NURSING CONSIDERATIONS

Besides those related universally to drug therapy (see "How to use this book"), consider the following specific recommendations:

Assessment
- Obtain a baseline assessment of skin condition before therapy.
- Be alert for adverse reactions and drug interactions throughout therapy.
- Evaluate the patient's and family's knowledge about tretinoin.

Nursing Diagnoses
- Impaired skin integrity due to underlying condition.
- Pain related to drug application.
- Knowledge deficit related to tretinoin therapy.

Planning and Implementation

Preparation and Administration
- Use with caution in eczema.
- ***Topical use:*** Cleanse affected area before application. Apply drug in a thin layer once daily h.s. Avoid application around eyes and lips.
- Expect dosage to be adjusted if local irritation develops.
- Avoid contact of the drug with eyes, mouth, and mucous membranes.

Monitoring
- Monitor effectiveness by assessing severity and frequency of dermal lesions.
- Assess the skin for excessive dryness and scaling. Remember that some dryness and scaling are normal reactions.

Supportive Care
- Provide emotional support to the patient experiencing severe acne.
- Administer mild analgesics as ordered.
- Keep in mind that relapses generally occur within 3 to 6 weeks after treatment.

Patient Teaching
- Tell the patient to expect some redness and scaling at the beginning of therapy or with increase in dosage.
- Teach the patient to cleanse area thoroughly with nonmedicated or nonperfumed soaps before application of medication.
- Reassure the patient that beneficial

effects occur within 3 to 6 weeks after initiation of treatment.
• Warn the patient to protect area from direct sunlight. Explain that if the patient becomes sunburned, therapy will be delayed until the sunburn subsides. Instruct the patient to use SPF 15 sunblock and protective clothing if unable to avoid sun exposure.
• Tell the patient who develops sunburn to hold therapy until the sunburn subsides.
• Explain that increased sensitivity to wind or cold temperatures may be experienced while on this drug.
• Tell the patient to avoid using topical products containing alcohol, astringents, spices, and lime because these may interfere with drug action.
• Tell the patient not to use any medicated cosmetics during therapy.

Evaluation

In patients receiving tretinoin, appropriate evaluation statements may include:
• Patient reports a decrease in skin lesions.
• Patient reports decrease in discomfort with medication application.
• Patient and family state an understanding of tretinoin therapy.

triamcinolone (systemic)

(trye am sin´ oh lone)

Aristocort, Atolone, Kenacort**, Tricilone

triamcinolone acetonide

Cenocort A, Cinonide, Kenaject, Kenalog, Kenalone, Tac-3, Tramacort, Triam-A, Triamonide, Tri-Kort, Trilog

triamcinolone diacetate

Amcort, Aristocort Forte, Aristocort Intralesional, Articulose-L.A., Cenocort Forte, Cinalone, Kenacort, Triam-Forte, Trilone, Tristoject

triamcinolone hexacetonide

Aristospan Intra-articular, Aristospan Intralesional

• *Classification:* anti-inflammatory, immunosuppressant (glucocorticoid)
• *Pregnancy Risk Category:* C

HOW SUPPLIED

triamcinolone
Tablets: 1 mg, 2 mg, 4 mg, 8 mg
Syrup: 2 mg/ml, 4 mg/ml
triamcinolone acetonide
Injection (suspension): 3 mg/ml, 10 mg/ml, 40 mg/ml
triamcinolone diacetate
Injection (suspension): 25 mg/ml, 40 mg/ml
triamcinolone hexacetonide
Injection (suspension): 5 mg/ml, 20 mg/ml
Oral inhalation aerosol: 100 mcg/metered spray, 240 doses/inhaler

ACTION

Mechanism: Decreases inflammation, mainly by stabilizing leukocyte lysosomal membranes. Also suppresses the immune response, stimulates bone marrow, and influences protein, fat, and carbohydrate metabolism.
Absorption: Readily absorbed after oral administration.
Distribution: Rapidly removed from the blood and distributed to muscle, liver, skin, intestines, and kidneys; extensively bound to plasma proteins (transcortin and albumin). Only the unbound portion is active. Distributed into breast milk and crosses the placenta.
Metabolism: In the liver to inactive glucuronide and sulfate metabolites.
Excretion: Inactive metabolites and small amounts of unmetabolized drug are excreted by the kidneys. Insignificant amounts are also excreted in feces. Half-life: 18 to 36 hours.
Onset, peak, duration: After oral and I.V. administration, peak effects occur in about 1 to 2 hours. The suspen-

*Liquid form contains alcohol. **May contain tartrazine.

sions for injection have variable onset and duration of action, depending on the site of injection (intra-articular space, muscle, or blood supply to that muscle).

INDICATIONS & DOSAGE

Severe inflammation or immunosuppression–
Adults: 4 to 48 mg P.O. daily divided b.i.d., t.i.d., or q.i.d., or 40 mg I.M. (diacetate or acetonide) weekly; or 5 to 48 mg (diacetate or acetonide) into lesions; or 2 to 40 mg (diacetate or acetonide) into joints and soft tissue; or up to 0.5 mg (hexacetonide) per square inch of affected skin intralesional; or 2 to 20 mg (hexacetonide) intra-articular or intrasynovial into soft tissue or into joint or lesion. Often, a local anesthetic is injected into the joint with triamcinolone.
Steroid-dependent asthma–
Adults: 2 inhalations t.i.d. to q.i.d. Maximum 16 inhalations daily.
Children 6 to 12 years: 1 to 2 inhalations t.i.d. to q.i.d. Maximum 12 inhalations daily.

CONTRAINDICATIONS & PRECAUTIONS

Contraindicated in patients with hypersensitivity to ingredients of adrenocorticoid preparations and in patients with systemic fungal infections (except in adrenal insufficiency). Patients receiving triamcinolone should not be given live virus vaccines because triamcinolone suppresses the immune response.

Use with extreme caution in patients with GI ulceration, renal disease, hypertension, osteoporosis, diabetes mellitus, thromboembolic disorders, seizures, myasthenia gravis, CHF, tuberculosis, hypoalbuminemia, hypothyroidism, cirrhosis of the liver, emotional instability, psychotic tendencies, hyperlipidemias, glaucoma, or cataracts because the drug may exacerbate these conditions.

Because adrenocorticoids increase susceptibility to and mask symptoms of infection, triamcinolone should not be used (except in life-threatening situations) in patients with viral infections or bacterial infections not controlled by anti-infective agents.

ADVERSE REACTIONS

Common reactions are in italics; life-threatening reactions are in bold italics.

Most adverse reactions of corticosteroids are dose- or duration-dependent.
CNS: *euphoria, insomnia,* psychotic behavior, pseudotumor cerebri.
CV: ***CHF,*** hypertension, edema.
EENT: cataracts, glaucoma.
GI: *peptic ulcer,* GI irritation, increased appetite.
Metabolic: *possible hypokalemia, hyperglycemia and carbohydrate intolerance,* growth suppression in children.
Skin: delayed wound healing, acne, various skin eruptions.
Other: muscle weakness, pancreatitis, hirsutism, susceptibility to infections. Acute adrenal insufficiency may occur with increased stress (infection, surgery, or trauma) or abrupt withdrawal after long-term therapy.
Withdrawal symptoms: rebound inflammation, fatigue, weakness, arthralgia, fever, dizziness, lethargy, depression, fainting, orthostatic hypotension, dyspnea, anorexia, hypoglycemia. ***Sudden withdrawal may be fatal.***
Inhalation:
EENT: hoarseness, fungal infections of mouth and throat.
GI: dry mouth.

INTERACTIONS

Barbiturates, phenytoin, rifampin: decreased corticosteroid effect. Triamcinolone dose may need to be increased.
Indomethacin, aspirin: increased risk

of GI distress and bleeding. Give together cautiously.

EFFECTS ON DIAGNOSTIC TESTS

Diagnostic skin tests: suppressed reactions.
Nitroblue tetrazolium test for systemic bacterial infections: decreased.
Serum glucose and cholesterol: increased levels.
Serum potassium, calcium, thyroxine, and triiodothyronine: decreased levels.
Thyroid function tests (^{131}I uptake and protein-bound iodine concentrations): decreased.
Urine glucose and calcium: increased levels.

NURSING CONSIDERATIONS

Besides those related universally to drug therapy (see "How to use this book"), consider the following specific recommendations:

Assessment

• Obtain a baseline assessment of the patient's underlying condition before initiating drug therapy.
• Be alert for adverse reactions and drug interactions throughout therapy.
• Evaluate the patient's and family's knowledge about triamcinolone therapy.

Nursing Diagnoses

• Impaired tissue integrity related to inflammation caused by the patient's underlying condition.
• High risk for injury related to adverse reactions to triamcinolone.
• Knowledge deficit related to triamcinolone therapy.

Planning and Implementation

Preparation and Administration

• Do not use for alternate-day therapy.
• Gradually reduce dosage after prolonged therapy. Never discontinue therapy abruptly, because sudden withdrawal can be fatal.
• Always titrate to lowest effective dose as prescribed.
• Give a daily dosage in the morning for better results and less toxicity.
• Expect to increase dosage as prescribed during times of physiologic stress (surgery, trauma, or infection).
• ***P.O. use:*** Give with food when possible to avoid GI upset.
• ***I.M. use:*** Give injection deep into gluteal muscle. Rotate injection sites to prevent muscle atrophy. Don't use diluents that contain preservatives. Flocculation may occur.
• Parenteral form is not for I.V. use.
• ***Inhalation use:*** Administer bronchodilator therapy several minutes before triamcinolone therapy. When administering have patient hold breath for a few seconds to enhance action of drug and allow 1 minute to elapse before repeat inhalations. Never administer for relief of emergency asthma attacks.

Monitoring

• Monitor for adverse reactions, because drug can cause serious or life-threatening multisystem dysfunction.
• Monitor the patient's weight, blood pressure, blood glucose level, and serum electrolyte levels regularly.
• Monitor the patient for infection. Drug may mask or exacerbate infections.
• Monitor the patient's stress level. Stress (fever, trauma, surgery, or emotional problems) may increase adrenal insufficiency. Dose may have to be increased.
• Monitor the patient's mental status for depression or psychotic episodes, especially in high-dose therapy.
• Monitor patients receiving immunizations for decreased antibody response.
• Monitor the patient for early signs of adrenal insufficiency or cushingoid symptoms.

Supportive Care

• Notify the doctor immediately if serious adverse drug reactions occur and be prepared to administer supportive care.

• Unless contraindicated, give the patient a low-sodium diet high in potassium and protein. Potassium supplement may be needed.
• Be aware that diabetic patients may have increased insulin requirements.
• Have patient taking inhaled form of drug drink a glass of water after inhalation therapy to help prevent fungal infections.
• Keep inhaler clean by washing with warm water and drying thoroughly after use.

Patient Teaching
• Be sure that the patient understands the need to take the drug as prescribed. Give the patient instructions on what to do if a dose is inadvertently missed.
• Warn the patient not to discontinue the drug abruptly or without the doctor's approval.
• Advise the patient to take oral form with meals to minimize adverse GI reactions.
• Teach patient how to administer inhaled form and to care for inhaler.
• Inform the patient of the possible therapeutic and adverse effects of the drug, so that he may report complications to the doctor as soon as possible.
• Tell the patient to carry a medical alert card indicating the need for supplemental adrenocorticoids during stress.
• Teach the patient to recognize signs of early adrenal insufficiency (fatigue, muscular weakness, joint pain, fever, anorexia, nausea, dyspnea, dizziness, and fainting) and to notify the doctor promptly if they occur.
• Warn patients on long-term therapy about cushingoid symptoms, which may develop regardless of route of administration.
• Tell patient to eat a low-sodium diet that is high in potassium and protein unless contraindicated.

Evaluation
In patients receiving triamcinolone, appropriate evaluation statements may include:
• Patient's condition being treated with triamcinolone therapy shows improvement.
• Patient does not experience serious adverse reactions associated with triamcinolone.
• Patient and family state an understanding of triamcinolone therapy.

triamcinolone acetonide (topical)
(try am sin´ oh lone)
Aristocort, Kenalog, Kenalone‡

• *Classification:* topical anti-inflammatory (glucocorticoid)
• *Pregnancy Risk Category:* C

HOW SUPPLIED
Aerosol: 0.2 mg/2-second spray
Cream: 0.02%‡, 0.025%, 0.1%, 0.5%
Lotion: 0.025%, 0.1%
Ointment: 0.02%‡, 0.025%, 0.1%, 0.5%

ACTION
Mechanism: Produces local anti-inflammatory, vasoconstrictor, and antipruritic actions. Diffuses across cell membranes to form complexes with specific cytoplasmic receptors, influencing cellular metabolism. Corticosteroids stabilize leukocyte lysosomal membranes, inhibit local actions and accumulation of macrophages, decrease local edema, and reduce the formation of scar tissue.
Absorption: Depends on the potency of the preparation, the amount applied, and the nature of the skin at the application site. It is lowest in areas with a thick stratum corneum (on the palms, soles, elbows, and knees) and higher in thinner areas (face, eyelids, and genitals). Absorp-

tion increases in areas of skin damage, inflammation, or occlusion. Some systemic absorption occurs, especially through the oral mucosa.
Distribution: After topical application, distributed throughout the local skin layer. Any drug absorbed into circulation is rapidly distributed to muscle, liver, skin, intestines, and kidneys.
Metabolism: After topical administration, metabolized primarily in the skin. The small amount absorbed into systemic circulation is metabolized primarily in the liver to inactive compounds.
Excretion: Inactive metabolites are excreted by the kidneys, primarily as glucuronides and sulfates, but also as unconjugated products. Small amounts of the metabolites are also excreted in feces.

INDICATIONS & DOSAGE

Inflammation of corticosteroid-responsive dermatoses–
Adults and children: clean area; apply aerosol, cream, lotion, or ointment sparingly b.i.d. to q.i.d.
Aerosol–shake can well. Direct spray onto affected area from a distance of approximately 6″ (15 cm) and apply for only 3 seconds.

CONTRAINDICATIONS & PRECAUTIONS

Contraindicated in patients who are hypersensitive to any component of the preparation. Use cautiously in patients with viral, fungal, or tubercular skin lesions, and with extreme caution in patients with impaired circulation because the drug may increase the risk of skin ulceration.

ADVERSE REACTIONS

Common reactions are in italics; life-threatening reactions are in bold italics.
Skin: burning, itching, irritation, dryness, folliculitis, hypertrichosis, hypopigmentation, acneiform eruptions, perioral dermatitis, allergic contact dermatitis. With occlusive dressings: *maceration of skin, secondary infection, atrophy, striae, miliaria.*

INTERACTIONS

None significant.

EFFECTS ON DIAGNOSTIC TESTS

None reported.

NURSING CONSIDERATIONS

Besides those related universally to drug therapy (see "How to use this book"), consider the following specific recommendations:

Assessment
- Obtain a baseline assessment of the patient's skin integrity before triamcinolone therapy.
- Be alert for adverse reactions and drug interactions throughout therapy.
- Evaluate the patient's and family's knowledge about topical triamcinolone therapy.

Nursing Diagnoses
- Impaired skin integrity related to the patient's underlying condition.
- High risk for infection related to adverse drug reactions.
- Knowledge deficit related to topical triamcinolone therapy.

Planning and Implementation
Preparation and Administration
- Avoid applications near eyes, mucous membranes, or in the ear canal.
- Read order and drug labels carefully.
- Wear gloves when administering drug.
- Before applying, gently wash the patient's skin. Apply a thin layer of medication and rub in gently.
- When treating hairy sites, part hair and apply directly to lesion.
- To apply an occlusive dressing (only if ordered by doctor), apply cream heavily, then cover with a thin, pliable, nonflammable plastic film; seal to adjacent normal skin with hypoallergenic tape.

• Know that the aerosol preparation contains alcohol and may produce irritation or burning in open lesions. When using on the face, cover the patient's eyes and warn against inhalation of the spray. To avoid freezing tissues, do not spray longer than 3 seconds or closer than 6″ (15 cm).
• Treatment should be continued for a few days after clearing of lesions to prevent recurrence.

Monitoring

• Monitor effectiveness by regularly assessing skin for extent and severity of inflammation.
• Monitor for hypersensitivity reaction to triamcinolone.
• Monitor for signs of secondary infection.
• Frequently assess the patient's skin for burning, itching, and dryness.
• Monitor patients who must use occlusive dressings for maceration of the skin and secondary infection.

Supportive Care

• To minimize adverse reactions, use occlusive dressing intermittently. Don't use occlusive dressings in the presence of infection or on weeping or exudative lesions. Do not leave in place longer than 16 hours each day.
• For patients with eczematous dermatitis who may develop irritation with adhesive material, hold dressing in place with gauze, elastic bandage, or stockings.
• Notify the doctor and remove occlusive dressing if fever develops.
• Withhold the drug and notify the doctor if hypersensitivity reaction or infection occurs.
• Have the patient's fingernails cut short to minimize skin trauma from scratching.
• Apply cool, moist compresses to involved areas to relieve itching and burning.
• When used on diaper area in young children, avoid tight-fitting diapers or plastic pants.

Patient Teaching

• Instruct the patient to cleanse involved area before applying triamcinolone in a thin layer to cover the entire surface.
• Teach the patient how to apply an occlusive dressing.
• Instruct the patient to complete the entire treatment regimen as prescribed, even if the lesions appear to have healed.
• Tell the patient and family not to share the prescription with others.

Evaluation

In patients receiving topical triamcinolone, appropriate evaluation statements may include:

• Patient's skin maintains integrity.
• Patient does not develop secondary infection.
• Patient and family state an understanding of topical triamcinolone therapy.

triamterene

(trye am´ ter een)
Dyrenium, Dytac‡

• *Classification:* diuretic (potassium-sparing diuretic)
• *Pregnancy Risk Category:* D

HOW SUPPLIED

Tablets: 50 mg, 100 mg

ACTION

Mechanism: A potassium-sparing diuretic that inhibits sodium reabsorption and potassium excretion by direct action on the distal tubule.
Absorption: Rapidly absorbed after oral administration, but the extent varies.
Distribution: About 67% protein-bound.
Metabolism: Metabolized by hydroxylation and sulfation.
Excretion: Drug and metabolites are

excreted in urine. Half-life: 100 to 150 minutes.
Onset, peak, duration: Diuresis usually begins in 2 to 4 hours. Diuretic effect may be delayed 2 to 3 days if drug is used alone; maximum antihypertensive effect may be delayed 2 to 3 weeks.

INDICATIONS & DOSAGE

Diuresis–
Adults: initially, 100 mg P.O. b.i.d. after meals. Total daily dosage should not exceed 300 mg.

CONTRAINDICATIONS & PRECAUTIONS

Contraindicated in patients with serum potassium levels above 5.5 mEq/liter; anuria, acute or chronic renal insufficiency, or diabetic nephropathy because drug may worsen the signs and symptoms of these conditions; hypersensitivity to the drug; and in those who are receiving other potassium-sparing diuretics or potassium supplements because of the potential for hyperkalemia.

Use cautiously in patients with severe hepatic insufficiency because electrolyte imbalance may precipitate hepatic encephalopathy, and in patients with diabetes, who are at increased risk of hyperkalemia.

ADVERSE REACTIONS

Common reactions are in italics; life-threatening reactions are in bold italics.
Blood: megaloblastic anemia related to low folic acid levels.
CNS: dizziness.
CV: hypotension.
EENT: sore throat.
GI: dry mouth, nausea, vomiting.
Metabolic: *hyperkalemia,* dehydration, hyponatremia, transient elevation in BUN, acidosis.
Skin: photosensitivity, rash.
Other: ***anaphylaxis,*** muscle cramps.

INTERACTIONS

ACE inhibitors, potassium supplements: increased risk of hyperkalemia. Don't use together.
Indomethacin, NSAIDs: may enhance the risk of nephrotoxicity. Avoid concomitant use.
Quinidine: may interfere with some laboratory tests that measure quinidine levels. Inform laboratory that patient is taking triamterene.

EFFECTS ON DIAGNOSTIC TESTS

Serum quinidine determinations: interference with fluorometric enzyme assay.

NURSING CONSIDERATIONS

Besides those related universally to drug therapy (see "How to use this book"), consider the following specific recommendations:

Assessment
- Obtain a baseline assessment of blood pressure, urine output, weight, serum electrolytes, and peripheral edema before initiating triamterene therapy.
- Be alert for adverse reactions and drug interactions throughout therapy.
- Evaluate the patient's and family's knowledge about triamterene therapy.

Nursing Diagnoses
- Fluid volume excess related to sodium and fluid retention.
- High risk for injury related to hyperkalemia due to triamterene therapy.
- Knowledge deficit related to triamterene therapy.

Planning and Implementation
Preparation and Administration
- ***P.O. use:*** Give drugs after meals to prevent nausea and, if possible, early in the day to prevent nocturia.
- Be aware that full diuretic effects are delayed 2 to 3 days when used alone.

Monitoring
• Monitor effectiveness by regularly checking urine output, blood pressure, weight, and evidence of edema.
• Monitor for blood dyscrasias.
• Monitor BUN levels and serum electrolytes, especially potassium.
• Monitor for signs of hyperkalemia: muscle weakness and cramps, paresthesia, diarrhea, and cardiac arrhythmias.
• Monitor skin turgor and mucous membranes for signs of fluid volume depletion.
Supportive Care
• Hold drug and notify the doctor if hyperkalemia or dehydration occurs.
• Keep accurate record of intake and output, and blood pressure.
• Provide frequent skin and mouth care to relieve dryness due to diuretic therapy.
• Answer the patient's call bells promptly; make sure patient's bathroom or bedpan is easily accessible.
• Use safety precautions to prevent the risk of injury due to falls.
• Elevate the patient's legs to reduce peripheral edema.
Patient Teaching
• Teach the patient and family to identify and report signs of hyperkalemia.
• Teach the patient and family to monitor the patient's fluid volume by recording daily weight and intake and output.
• Advise the patient to avoid excessive intake of foods high in potassium and of potassium-containing sodium substitutes.
• Instruct the patient to avoid concomitant use of potassium supplements.
• Advise the patient to change positions slowly, especially when rising to a standing position, to avoid dizziness and fainting due to orthostatic hypotension.
• Tell the patient to take drug after meals and, if possible, early in the day to avoid interruption of sleep due to nocturia.
Evaluation
In patients receiving triamterene, appropriate evaluation statements may include:
• Patient is free of edema.
• Patient's serum potassium remains within normal range.
• Patient and family state an understanding of triamterene therapy.

triazolam
(trye ay´ zoe lam)
Halcion

• Controlled Substance Schedule IV
• *Classification:* sedative-hypnotic (benzodiazepine)
• *Pregnancy Risk Category:* X

HOW SUPPLIED
Tablets: 0.125 mg, 0.25 mg

ACTION
Mechanism: Acts on the limbic system, thalamus, and hypothalamus of the CNS to produce hypnotic effects. A benzodiazepine.
Absorption: Well absorbed through the GI tract after oral administration.
Distribution: Widely distributed throughout the body. Drug is 90% protein-bound.
Metabolism: In the liver primarily to inactive metabolites.
Excretion: Metabolites are excreted in urine. Half-life: Ranges from approximately 1½ to 5½ hours.
Onset, peak, duration: Peak levels occur in 1 to 2 hours. Onset of action occurs at 15 to 30 minutes.

INDICATIONS & DOSAGE
Insomnia –
Adults: 0.125 to 0.25 mg P.O.
Adults over 65: 0.125 mg P.O. h.s.; increase as needed to 0.25 mg P.O. h.s.

CONTRAINDICATIONS & PRECAUTIONS

Contraindicated in patients with hypersensitivity to the drug; acute narrow-angle glaucoma or untreated open-angle glaucoma, because of the drug's possible anticholinergic effect; in coma, because the drug's hypnotic or hypotensive effect may be prolonged or intensified; in pregnant patients, because it may be fetotoxic; and in patients with acute alcohol intoxication with depressed vital signs, because the drug will worsen CNS depression.

Use cautiously in patients with psychoses, because the drug is rarely beneficial in such patients and may induce paradoxical reactions; myasthenia gravis or Parkinson's disease, because it may exacerbate the disorder; impaired hepatic function, which prolongs elimination of the drug; in elderly or debilitated patients, who are usually more sensitive to the drug's CNS effects; and in individuals prone to addiction or drug abuse.

ADVERSE REACTIONS

Common reactions are in italics; life-threatening reactions are in bold italics.

CNS: *drowsiness, dizziness, headache,* rebound insomnia, amnesia, lightheadedness, lack of coordination, mental confusion.

GI: nausea, vomiting.

INTERACTIONS

Alcohol or other CNS depressants, including narcotic analgesics: excessive CNS depression. Use together cautiously.

Cimetidine, erythromycin: may cause prolonged triazolam blood levels. Monitor for increased sedation.

EFFECTS ON DIAGNOSTIC TESTS

EEG patterns: minor changes (low-voltage, fast activity) during and after therapy.

Liver function tests: elevated results.

NURSING CONSIDERATIONS

Besides those related universally to drug therapy (see "How to use this book"), consider the following specific recommendations:

Assessment

- Obtain a baseline assessment of sleeping patterns and CNS status before therapy.
- Be alert for adverse reactions and drug interactions throughout therapy.
- Evaluate the patient's and family's knowledge about triazolam therapy.

Nursing Diagnoses

- Sleep pattern disturbance related to underlying patient problem.
- High risk for trauma related to adverse CNS reactions to triazolam.
- Knowledge deficit related to triazolam therapy.

Planning and Implementation

Preparation and Administration

- Before leaving the bedside, make sure the patient has swallowed the medication.

Monitoring

- Regularly monitor effectiveness by evaluating the patient's ability to sleep.
- Monitor CNS status for evidence of adverse reactions. Keep in mind that elderly patients are more sensitive to adverse CNS reactions.

Supportive Care

- After administration, institute safety precautions: remove cigarettes, keep bed rails up, and supervise or assist ambulation.
- Take precautions to prevent hoarding or self-overdosing, especially by a patient who is depressed or suicidal or has a history of drug abuse.
- Keep in mind that this drug is faster acting than temazepam, another derivative.

Patient Teaching

- Encourage the patient to report severe hangover or oversedation so the doctor can be consulted for change of dose or drug. Keep in mind that triazolam is very short-acting and has less tendency to cause morning drowsiness.

- Instruct the patient to remain in bed after taking drug and to call for assistance to use the bathroom.
- Warn the patient that drug may cause physical dependence with long-term use.
- Warn the patient to avoid hazardous activities that require mental alertness if adverse CNS reactions are present after awakening.
- Tell the patient that rebound insomnia may occur for one or two nights after stopping therapy.
- Warn the patient not to take more than the prescribed amount because overdosage can occur at a total daily dose of 2 mg (four times the highest recommended amount).
- Tell the patient to notify the nurse or doctor if sleep pattern disturbances continue despite therapy.

Evaluation

In the patient receiving triazolam, appropriate evaluation statements include:

- Patient states drug was effective in inducing sleep.
- Patient's safety maintained.
- Patient and family state an understanding of triazolam therapy.

PHARMACOLOGIC CLASS

tricyclic antidepressants

amitriptyline hydrochloride
amoxapine
clomipramine hydrochloride
desipramine hydrochloride
doxepin hydrochloride
imipramine hydrochloride
imipramine pamoate
maprotiline hydrochloride
nortriptyline hydrochloride
protriptyline hydrochloride
trimipramine maleate

OVERVIEW

The inherent mood-elevating activity of tricyclic antidepressants (TCAs) was discovered during research with iminodibenzyl, a compound originally investigated for sedative, analgesic, antihistaminic, and antiparkinsonian effects. Clinical trials in 1958 with the class prototype, imipramine, found no antipsychotic activity, but clearly demonstrated marked mood-elevating effects.

Although the precise mechanism of their CNS effects is not established, tricyclic antidepressants may exert their effects by inhibiting reuptake of the neurotransmitters norepinephrine and serotonin in the CNS. TCAs also have antihistaminic, sedative, anticholinergic, vasodilatory, and quinidine-like effects; the drugs are structurally similar to phenothiazines and share similar adverse reactions.

All of the currently available TCAs have equal clinical efficacy when given in equivalent therapeutic doses; choice of specific therapy is determined primarily by pharmacokinetic properties and the patient's adverse reaction profile. Patients may respond to some TCAs and not others; if a patient does not respond to one drug, another should be tried.

CLINICAL INDICATIONS AND ACTIONS

Depression

TCAs are used to treat major depression and dysthymic disorder. Depressed patients who are also anxious are helped most by the more sedating agents – doxepin, imipramine, and trimipramine. Protriptyline has a stimulant effect that evokes a favorable response in withdrawn depressed patients; only maprotiline has Food and Drug Administration approval for use in depression mixed with anxiety.

Obsessive-compulsive disorder (OCD)

Clomipramine is used in the treatment of OCD.

Enuresis
Imipramine is used to treat enuresis in children over age 6.
Severe, chronic pain
TCAs, especially amitriptyline, desipramine, doxepin, imipramine, and nortriptyline, are useful in the management of severe chronic pain.

OVERVIEW OF ADVERSE REACTIONS

Adverse reactions to TCAs are similar to those seen with phenothiazine antipsychotic agents, including varying degrees of sedation, anticholinergic effects, and orthostatic hypotension. The tertiary amines have the strongest sedative effects; tolerance to these effects usually develops in a few weeks. Protriptyline has the least sedative effect (and may be stimulatory), but shares with the tertiary amines the most pronounced effects on blood pressure and cardiac tissue. Maprotiline and amoxapine are most likely to cause seizures, especially in overdose situations. Desipramine has a greater margin of safety in patients with prostatic hypertrophy, paralytic ileus, glaucoma, and urinary retention, because of its relatively low level of anticholinergic activity.

REPRESENTATIVE COMBINATIONS

Amitriptyline hydrochloride with perphenazine: Etrafon, Triavil; with chlordiazepoxide: Limbitrol.

---

trifluoperazine hydrochloride

(trye floo oh per´ a zeen)
Apo-Trifluoperazine†, Calmazine‡, Novo-Flurazine†, Solazine†, Stelazine, Suprazine, Terfluzine†

- *Classification:* antipsychotic, antiemetic (phenothiazine)
- *Pregnancy Risk Category:* C

HOW SUPPLIED

Tablets (regular and film-coated): 1 mg, 2 mg, 5 mg, 10 mg
Oral concentrate: 10 mg/ml
Injection: 2 mg/ml

ACTION

Mechanism: Blocks postsynaptic dopamine receptors in the brain. A piperazine phenothiazine.
Absorption: Rate and extent vary with route of administration. Oral tablet absorption is erratic and variable; absorption of oral concentrate is more predictable. I.M. drug is absorbed rapidly.
Distribution: Widely distributed in the body, including breast milk. Drug is 91% to 99% protein-bound.
Metabolism: Extensively metabolized by the liver, but no active metabolites are formed.
Excretion: Most of drug is excreted in urine via the kidneys; some in feces via the biliary tract.
Onset, peak, duration: With oral tablet onset of action ranges from 30 minutes to 1 hour. Duration of action is about 4 to 6 hours. Peak therapeutic effect may not be seen for several weeks of therapy.

INDICATIONS & DOSAGE

Anxiety states–
Adults: 1 to 2 mg P.O. b.i.d.
Schizophrenia and other psychotic disorders–
Adults: *outpatients*–1 to 2 mg P.O. b.i.d., up to 4 mg daily; *hospitalized*–2 to 5 mg P.O. b.i.d.; may gradually increase to 40 mg daily. 1 to 2 mg I.M. q 4 to 6 hours, p.r.n.
Children 6 to 12 years (hospitalized or under close supervision): 1 mg P.O. daily or b.i.d.; may increase gradually to 15 mg daily.

CONTRAINDICATIONS & PRECAUTIONS

Contraindicated in patients with hypersensitivity to phenothiazines and related compounds, including allergic reactions involving hepatic function; blood dyscrasias and bone marrow depression because of the drug's adverse hematologic effects; disorders accompanied by coma, brain damage, CNS depression, circulatory collapse, or cerebrovascular disease because of additive CNS depression and adverse blood pressure effects; and in patients taking adrenergic-blocking agents or spinal or epidural anesthetics because of risk of excessive respiratory, cardiac, and CNS depression.

Use cautiously in patients with cardiac disease (arrhythmias, CHF, angina pectoris, valvular disease, or heart block), encephalitis, Reye's syndrome, head injury, respiratory disease, seizure disorders, glaucoma, prostatic hypertrophy, urine retention, Parkinson's disease, and pheochromocytoma, because it may exacerbate these conditions; hypocalcemia because it increases the risk of extrapyramidal reactions; and hepatic or renal dysfunction because diminished metabolism and excretion cause the drug to accumulate.

ADVERSE REACTIONS

Common reactions are in italics; life-threatening reactions are in bold italics.

Blood: transient leukopenia, ***agranulocytosis.***

CNS: *extrapyramidal reactions (high incidence), tardive dyskinesia,* sedation (low incidence), pseudoparkinsonism, EEG changes, dizziness.

CV: *orthostatic hypotension,* tachycardia, ECG changes.

EENT: ocular changes, *blurred vision.*

GI: *dry mouth, constipation.*

GU: *urine retention,* dark urine, menstrual irregularities, gynecomastia, inhibited ejaculation.

Hepatic: cholestatic jaundice.

Metabolic: hyperprolactinemia.

Skin: *mild photosensitivity,* dermal allergic reactions.

Local: pain at I.M. injection site, sterile abscess.

Other: weight gain; increased appetite; rarely, ***neuroleptic malignant syndrome*** (fever, tachycardia, tachypnea, profuse diaphoresis).

After abrupt withdrawal of long-term therapy: gastritis, nausea, vomiting, dizziness, tremors, feeling of warmth or cold, sweating, tachycardia, headache, insomnia.

INTERACTIONS

Alcohol, other CNS depressants: increased CNS depression. Avoid concomitant use.

Antacids: inhibit absorption of oral phenothiazines. Separate antacid and phenothiazine doses by at least 2 hours.

Barbiturates, lithium: may decrease phenothiazine effect. Observe patient.

Centrally acting antihypertensives: decreased antihypertensive effect.

EFFECTS ON DIAGNOSTIC TESTS

ECG: quinidine-like effects.

Liver function tests: elevated results.

Protein-bound iodine: elevated levels.

Urine porphyrins, urobilinogen, amylase, and 5-HIAA: false-positive results from darkening of urine by metabolites.

Urine pregnancy tests using human chorionic gonadotropin: false-positive results.

NURSING CONSIDERATIONS

Besides those related universally to drug therapy (see "How to use this book"), consider the following specific recommendations:

Assessment

- Obtain baseline assessment of patient's mental status, including psychotic symptoms, before therapy.
- Be alert for adverse reactions and drug interactions throughout therapy.
- Evaluate the patient's and family's

knowledge about trifluoperazine therapy.

Nursing Diagnoses

• Impaired thought processes related to patient's underlying condition.

• Urinary retention related to adverse drug reaction.

• Knowledge deficit related to trifluoperazine therapy.

Planning and Implementation

Preparation and Administration

• Protect medication from light. Slight yellowing of injection or concentrate is common and does not affect potency. Discard markedly discolored solutions.

• Dose of 5 mg is therapeutic equivalent of 100 mg of chlorpromazine.

• ***I.M. use:*** Give injection deeply only in upper outer quadrant of buttocks. Massage slowly afterward to prevent sterile abscess.

• ***P.O. use:*** Dilute liquid concentrate with 60 ml tomato or fruit juice, carbonated beverages, coffee, tea, milk, water, or semisolid food just before giving.

• Drug is a prototype piperazine phenothiazine.

• Avoid skin contact with the injectable or liquid form because it may cause a rash.

Monitoring

• Monitor effectiveness by regularly observing the patient's behavior for changes in psychotic symptoms.

• Monitor for extrapyramidal and anticholinergic effects (blurred vision, dry mouth, constipation, urine retention), and tardive dyskinesia during prolonged therapy.

• Frequently check the patient's blood pressure for orthostatic hypotension, especially after parenteral administration.

• Monitor therapy by weekly bilirubin tests during the first month; periodic blood tests (CBC and liver function); and ophthalmic tests (long-term use).

• Monitor for neuroleptic malignant syndrome. This rare, potentially fatal reaction is not necessarily related to type of neuroleptic or duration of drug therapy, but usually occurs in men (60% of affected patients).

Supportive Care

• Keep the patient supine for 1 hour after I.M. administration. Then assist patient to get up slowly to avoid orthostatic hypotension.

• Do not discontinue drug abruptly unless required by severe adverse reactions.

• Increase the patient's fluid and fiber intake – if not contraindicated – to prevent constipation. If necessary, request doctor's order for a laxative.

• Give the patient sugarless gum, sour hard candy, or a mouthwash rinse to relieve dry mouth.

Patient Teaching

• Tell the patient to avoid exposure to the sun and to use a sunscreen when going outdoors to prevent photosensitivity reactions. (*Note:* Sun lamps and tanning beds may cause burning of the skin or skin discoloration.)

• Tell the patient not to stop taking the drug suddenly.

• Encourage the patient to report difficult urination, sore throat, dizziness, or fainting.

• Advise the patient to increase fluid and fiber in the diet, if appropriate.

• Tell the patient to avoid driving and other hazardous activities that require alertness until the effect of the drug is established. Excessive sedative effects tend to subside after several weeks.

• Explain which fluids are appropriate for diluting the concentrate and show the dropper technique for measuring dose. Warn the patient to avoid spilling liquid on skin because rash and irritation may occur.

• Tell the patient that sugarless hard candy, chewing gum, or ice chips can alleviate dry mouth.

Evaluation
In patients receiving trifluoperazine, appropriate evaluation statements may include:
• Patient demonstrates a decrease in psychotic behavior.
• Patient voids without difficulty.
• Patient and family state an understanding of trifluoperazine therapy.

trifluridine
(trye flure´ i deen)
Viroptic Ophthalmic Solution 1%

• *Classification:* antiviral (pyrimidine nucleoside)
• *Pregnancy Risk Category:* C

HOW SUPPLIED
Ophthalmic solution: 1%

ACTION
Mechanism: A pyrimidine nucleoside chemically related to idoxuride. Interferes with viral replication, probably by blocking DNA synthesis.
Absorption: After topical ophthalmic administration, drug penetrates the cornea and can be found in aqueous humor. Intraocular penetration is enhanced in patients with corneal epithelial defects, such as inflammation, ulceration, or abrasion. Systemic absorption does not occur.
Metabolism: The major metabolite, 5-carboxy-2′-deoxyridine, has less antiviral activity than trifluridine. It is formed on the epithelial side of the cornea.

INDICATIONS & DOSAGE
Primary keratoconjunctivitis and recurrent epithelial keratitis caused by herpes simplex virus, types I and II–
Adults: 1 drop of solution q 2 hours while patient is awake, to a maximum of 9 drops daily until re-epithelialization of the corneal ulcer occurs; then 1 drop q 4 hours (minimum 5 drops daily) for an additional 7 days.

CONTRAINDICATIONS & PRECAUTIONS
Contraindicated in patients with hypersensitivity reactions or chemical intolerance to trifluridine. Use cautiously during long-term therapy; the possibility of viral resistance after multiple exposures must be considered.

ADVERSE REACTIONS
Common reactions are in italics; life-threatening reactions are in bold italics.
Eye: *stinging upon instillation,* edema of eyelids, increased intraocular pressure.
Other: hypersensitivity.

INTERACTIONS
None significant.

EFFECTS ON DIAGNOSTIC TESTS
None reported.

NURSING CONSIDERATIONS
Besides those related universally to drug therapy (see "How to use this book"), consider the following specific recommendations:
Assessment
• Obtain a baseline assessment of the patient's allergies before therapy.
• Be alert for adverse reactions and drug interactions throughout therapy.
• Evaluate the patient's and family's knowledge about trifluridine therapy.
Nursing Diagnoses
• Altered protection related to ocular infection.
• Pain related to trifluridine-induced stinging on instillation.
• Knowledge deficit related to trifluridine therapy.
Planning and Implementation
Preparation and Administration
• Give only to patients with diagnosis of herpetic keratitis.

• Wash hands before and after administration.
• Check expiration dates; store in refrigerator.
• Cleanse eye area of excess exudate before administration.
• Do not use for longer than 21 consecutive days because of the potential risk of ocular toxicity.

Monitoring
• Monitor effectiveness by culturing the eye to check for microorganisms.
• Observe amount, color, and consistency of exudate.
• Monitor for signs of increased intraocular pressure.
• Observe for signs of ocular toxicity or hypersensitivity.

Supportive Care
• Apply warm, moist compresses to eye area to aid in removal of dried exudate.
• Notify doctor if no improvement is seen after 7 days of treatment or complete re-epithelization is not seen after 14 days of treatment; another form of therapy should be considered.
• More effective than idoxuridine or vidarabine with fewer adverse reactions.

Patient Teaching
• Warn the patient the solution may cause burning and stinging on instillation.
• Reassure the patient that mild local irritation of the conjunctiva and cornea follows instillation.
• Teach the patient how to instill. Advise him to wash hands before and after instillation. Advise him to avoid touching tip of applicator to eye or surrounding tissues.
• Instruct the patient to apply light finger pressure to the lacrimal sac for 1 minute after instillation. Caution him to avoid rubbing or scratching eye area.
• Warn the patient not to share washcloths or towels with family members during infection.
• Instruct the patient not to share eye medications with family members. A family member who develops the same symptoms should contact the doctor.

Evaluation
In patients receiving trifluridine, appropriate evaluation statements may include:
• Patient remains free from signs and symptoms of infection.
• Patient reports decrease or absence of pain induced by trifluridine instillation.
• Patient and family state an understanding of trifluridine therapy.

trihexyphenidyl hydrochloride
(trye hex ee fen´ i dill)
Aparkane†, Apo-Trihex†, Artane*, Artane Sequels, Novohexidyl†, Trihexane, Trihexy-2, Trihexy-5

• *Classification:* antiparkinsonian agent (anticholinergic)
• *Pregnancy Risk Category:* C

HOW SUPPLIED
Tablets: 2 mg, 5 mg
Capsules (sustained-release): 5 mg
Elixir: 2 mg/5 ml

ACTION
Mechanism: Blocks central cholinergic receptors, helping to restore balance of cholinergic activity in the basal ganglia.
Absorption: Rapidly absorbed after oral administration.
Distribution: Crosses the blood-brain barrier; little else is known about its distribution.
Excretion: In the urine as unchanged drug and metabolites.
Onset, peak, duration: Onset of action occurs within 1 hour. Duration of effect is 6 to 12 hours.

INDICATIONS & DOSAGE

Drug-induced parkinsonism–
Adults: 1 mg P.O. 1st day, 2 mg 2nd day, then increases by 2 mg q 3 to 5 days until total of 6 to 10 mg is given daily. Usually given t.i.d. with meals and, if needed, q.i.d. (last dose should be before bedtime) or may switch to extended-release form b.i.d. Postencephalitic parkinsonism may require 12 to 15 mg total daily dosage.

CONTRAINDICATIONS & PRECAUTIONS

Contraindicated in patients with a history of sensitivity to the drug. Administer cautiously to patients with narrow-angle glaucoma, because drug-induced cycloplegia and mydriasis may increase intraocular pressure, or cardiac disorders, arteriosclerosis, renal disorders, hepatic disorders, hypertension, obstructive GI or GU tract disease, or suspected prostatic hypertrophy, because the drug may exacerbate these conditions.

ADVERSE REACTIONS

Common reactions are in italics; life-threatening reactions are in bold italics.
CNS: nervousness, dizziness, headache, restlessness, agitation, hallucinations, euphoria, delusion, amnesia.
CV: tachycardia.
EENT: blurred vision, mydriasis, increased intraocular pressure.
GI: constipation, *dry mouth, nausea.*
GU: urinary hesitancy, urine retention.

Adverse reactions are dose-related.

INTERACTIONS

Amantadine: additive anticholinergic adverse reactions, such as confusion and hallucinations. Reduce dosage before administering amantadine.

EFFECTS ON DIAGNOSTIC TESTS

None reported.

NURSING CONSIDERATIONS

Besides those related universally to drug therapy (see "How to use this book"), consider the following specific recommendations:

Assessment

- Obtain a baseline assessment of the patient's parkinsonian signs and symptoms before therapy.
- Be alert for adverse reactions and drug interactions throughout therapy.
- Evaluate the patient's and family's knowledge about trihexyphenidyl therapy.

Nursing Diagnoses

- Impaired physical mobility related to underlying parkinsonism.
- Altered oral mucous membrane related to trihexyphenidyl-induced dry mouth.
- Knowledge deficit related to trihexyphenidyl therapy.

Planning and Implementation

Preparation and Administration

- Administer with or after meals to decrease adverse GI reactions.
- Keep in mind that patient may develop a tolerence to this drug, so gradually increased dosage may be needed.

Monitoring

- Monitor effectiveness by regularly checking the patient's body movements for signs of improvement.
- Regularly check the patient's oral mucous membranes for dryness.
- Monitor the patient's GU status for urinary hesitancy or urine retention.
- Make certain that patient receives gonioscopic evaluation and close monitoring of intraocular pressure, esepcially if over age 40.

Supportive Care

- Give the patient cool drinks, ice chips, or sugarless gum or hard candy to relieve dry mouth.
- Assist the patient with activities and institute safety precautions, if needed.

Patient Teaching

- Warn the patient to avoid hazardous activities that require alertness

until CNS effects of the drug are known.
• Advise the patient to report signs of urinary hesitancy or urine retention.
• Suggest measures for relieving dry mouth.
• Tell the patient to take the drug with or after meals to minimize GI discomfort.
• Explain the importance of having intraocular pressure monitored at regular intervals, especially if patient is over age 40.

Evaluation

In patients receiving trihexyphenidyl, appropriate evaluation statements include:
• Patient exhibits improved mobility.
• Patient maintains integrity of oral mucous membranes.
• Patient and family state an understanding of trihexyphenidyl therapy.

trilostane
(trye´ loe stane)
Modrastane

• *Classification:* adrenocortical steroidogenesis inhibitor (testosterone derivative)
• *Pregnancy Risk Category:* X

HOW SUPPLIED
Capsules: 30 mg, 60 mg

ACTION
Mechanism: Reversibly lowers elevated circulating levels of glucocorticoids by inhibiting the enzyme system essential for their production in the adrenal gland.
Pharmacokinetics: Unknown.

INDICATIONS & DOSAGE
Adrenal cortical hyperfunction in Cushing's syndrome–
Adults: 30 mg P.O. q.i.d. initially. May be increased at intervals of 3 to 4 days to maximum of 480 mg daily.

CONTRAINDICATIONS & PRECAUTIONS
Contraindicated in patients with adrenal insufficiency and in patients hypersensitive to the drug. Use with extreme caution in patients with hepatic or renal disease. Because of the risk of teratogenic effects, this drug should not be used in women of childbearing age unless the possibility of pregnancy has been excluded and an effective nonhormonal means of contraception is started. Although in some cases the drug has been used for longer periods, the manufacturer warns that the drug should not be used for periods longer than 3 months. Because it can alter aldosterone secretion, monitor blood pressure and serum potassium levels periodically.

ADVERSE REACTIONS
Common reactions are in italics; life-threatening reactions are in bold italics.
CNS: headache.
CV: *orthostatic hypotension.*
EENT: burning of oral and nasal membranes.
GI: *diarrhea, upset stomach,* nausea, flatulence, bloating.
Metabolic: hyperkalemia.
Skin: flushing, rash.
Other: fever, fatigue.

INTERACTIONS
Aminoglutethimide, mitotane: may cause severe adrenocortical hypofunction.
Thiazides, loop diuretics: decreased potassium loss because trilostane inhibits aldosterone production.

EFFECTS ON DIAGNOSTIC TESTS

Plasma testosterone: falsely elevated levels.
Urine and serum 11-hydroxy and other corticosteroids: falsely elevated levels.
Urine and serum estrogen: may interfere with radioimmunoassay results.

NURSING CONSIDERATIONS

Besides those related universally to drug therapy (see "How to use this book"), consider the following specific recommendations:

Assessment

- Obtain a baseline assessment of the patient's underlying condition before initiating therapy.
- Be alert for adverse reactions and drug interactions throughout therapy.
- Evaluate the patient's and family's knowledge about trilostane therapy.

Nursing Diagnoses

- High risk for fluid volume deficit related to adverse drug reactions.
- High risk for injury related to drug-induced adverse reactions.
- Knowledge deficit related to trilostane therapy.

Planning and Implementation

Preparation and Administration

- ***P.O. use:*** Therapy should be started in the hospital setting to establish a dosage routine.

Monitoring

- Monitor effectiveness by noting results of follow-up diagnostic tests and by regularly checking tumor size and rate of growth through appropriate studies.
- Monitor corticosteroid levels and serum electrolytes.
- Monitor blood pressure regularly in all patients; the drug may cause orthostatic hypotension by suppressing aldosterone production.

Supportive Care

- Obtain baseline liver and kidney function, electrolyte levels, and temperature before initiating therapy.
- Trilostane is prescribed when surgery or pituitary radiation is inappropriate or must be delayed.
- Know that patients should show response within 2 weeks of initiation of therapy.
- Be prepared to discontinue the drug if no response has occurred.
- Provide the patient with fluids if diarrhea is severe.
- Obtain an order for a mild analgesic if the patient develops a drug-induced headache.
- Institute safety precautions and assist the patient with ambulation if he develops orthostatic hypotension.

Patient Teaching

- Explain that the drug does not cure the underlying disease.
- Instruct the patient to minimize orthostatic hypotension by slowly rising from a sitting or supine position.
- Tell the patient to expect a response in 2 weeks.

Evaluation

In patients receiving trilostane, appropriate evaluation statements may include:

- Patient does not develop fluid volume loss.
- Patients remains free of injury related to adverse drug reactions.
- Patient and family state an understanding of trilostane therapy.

---

trimeprazine tartrate

(trye mep´ ra zeen)
Panectyl†, Temaril*

- *Classification:* antipruritic (phenothiazine-derivative antihistamine)
- *Pregnancy Risk Category:* C

HOW SUPPLIED

Tablets: 2.5 mg
Spansule capsules (sustained-release): 5 mg
Syrup: 2.5 mg/5 ml (5.7% alcohol)*

ACTION

Mechanism: Competes with histamine for H_1-receptor sites on effector cells. Prevents but does not reverse histamine-mediated responses.
Absorption: Well absorbed.
Metabolism: Hepatic.
Excretion: Renal.
Onset, peak, duration: After oral administration, onset of action in 15 to 60 minutes with peak effect in 1 to 2 hours and duration of 3 to 6 hours.

INDICATIONS & DOSAGE

Pruritus–
Adults: 2.5 mg P.O. q.i.d.; or (timed-release) 5 mg P.O. b.i.d.
Children 3 to 12 years: 2.5 mg P.O. at bedtime or t.i.d., p.r.n.
Children 6 months to 3 years: 1.25 mg P.O. at bedtime or t.i.d., p.r.n.

Note: Children under 12 years should use only as directed by a doctor.

CONTRAINDICATIONS & PRECAUTIONS

Contraindicated in patients with hypersensitivity to trimeprazine or to phenothiazines; bone marrow depression, because the drug may exacerbate this syndrome; or seizure disorders, because the drug may increase the incidence of seizures; during acute asthma attacks, because it thickens bronchial secretions; in acutely ill or dehydrated children, because they are at increased risk of developing dystonias; and in comatose patients and newborns.

Because of its significant anticholinergic activity, use with caution in patients with narrow-angle glaucoma; pyloroduodenal obstruction or urinary bladder obstruction from prostatic hypertrophy or narrowing of the bladder neck; cardiovascular disease or hypertension, because of the hazard of palpitations and tachycardia; acute or chronic respiratory dysfunction (especially in children) because trimeprazine may suppress the cough reflex; and in children with a history of sleep apnea or a family history of sudden infant death syndrome. The relationship between these conditions and trimeprazine has not been studied; however, death has occurred in children who received usual doses of phenothiazine antihistamines.

ADVERSE REACTIONS

Common reactions are in italics; life-threatening reactions are in bold italics.
Blood: ***agranulocytosis,*** leukopenia.
CNS: (especially in elderly patients) drowsiness, dizziness, confusion, headache, restlessness, tremors, irritability, insomnia; (in children) paradoxical excitation.
CV: hypotension, palpitations, tachycardia.
GI: anorexia, nausea, vomiting, *dry mouth and throat.*
GU: urinary frequency, urine retention.
Skin: urticaria, rash, *photosensitivity.*

INTERACTIONS

CNS depressants: increased sedation. Use together cautiously.
MAO inhibitors: increased anticholinergic effects. Don't use together.
Phenothiazines: increased effects. Don't use together.

EFFECTS ON DIAGNOSTIC TESTS

Diagnostic skin tests: test interference.
Urine pregnancy tests: false-positive or false-negative results.

NURSING CONSIDERATIONS

Besides those related universally to drug therapy (see "How to use this book"), consider the following specific recommendations:

Assessment

• Obtain a baseline assessment of the patient's pruritus before beginning therapy.

• Be alert for adverse reactions and drug interactions throughout therapy.
• Evaluate the patient's and family's knowledge about trimeprazine tartrate therapy.

Nursing Diagnoses

• High risk for impaired skin integrity related to pruritus.
• High risk for infection related to trimeprazine-induced agranulocytosis.
• Knowledge deficit related to trimeprazine therapy.

Planning and Implementation

Preparation and Administration

• *P.O. use:* Give with food or milk to reduce GI distress.

Monitoring

• Monitor effectiveness by frequently checking irritated areas of the skin and questioning the patient about the relief of pruritus.
• During long-term therapy, monitor blood counts for leukopenia and agranulocytosis.
• Monitor carefully for infection, especially if the patient's WBC count is decreased.

Supportive Care

• Notify the doctor if the patient shows signs of an infection.

Patient Teaching

• Suggest that patient drink coffee or tea to reduce drowsiness.
• Tell the patient that sugarless gum, sour hard candy, or ice chips may relieve dry mouth.
• Warn patient about the risk of photosensitivity. Recommend use of a sunscreen. Tell the patient to notify the doctor and stop taking the drug if photosensitivity occurs.
• Warn patient to avoid alcoholic beverages during therapy and to avoid driving and other hazardous activities that require alertness until adverse CNS effects are known.
• Warn patient to discontinue trimeprazine tartrate 4 days before allergy skin testing to preserve the accuracy of the tests.

Evaluation

In patients receiving trimeprazine, appropriate evaluation statements may include:

• Pruritus is relieved.
• Infection did not occur.
• Patient and family state an understanding of trimeprazine therapy.

trimethobenzamide hydrochloride

(trye meth oh ben´ za mide)

Tebamide, Tegamide, Ticon, Tigan, Tiject-20

• *Classification:* antiemetic (ethanolamine-related antihistamine)
• *Pregnancy Risk Category:* C

HOW SUPPLIED

Capsules: 100 mg, 250 mg
Injection: 100 mg/ml
Suppositories: 100 mg, 200 mg

ACTION

Mechanism: A phenothiazine derivative that blocks dopamine receptors. Acts on the chemoreceptor trigger zone to inhibit nausea and vomiting.
Absorption: Approximately 60% of an oral dose is absorbed.
Distribution: Unknown.
Metabolism: Approximately 50% to 70% of a dose is metabolized, probably in the liver.
Excretion: In urine and feces.
Onset, peak, duration: After oral administration, action begins in 10 to 40 minutes; after I.M. administration, in 15 to 35 minutes. After oral administration, duration of effect is 3 to 4 hours; after I.M. administration, 2 to 3 hours.

INDICATIONS & DOSAGE

Nausea and vomiting (treatment) – **Adults:** 250 mg P.O. t.i.d. or q.i.d.; or 200 mg I.M. or rectally t.i.d. or q.i.d.

Postoperative nausea and vomiting (prevention) –
Adults: 200 mg I.M. or rectally (single dose) before or during surgery; may repeat 3 hours after termination of anesthesia, p.r.n.
Children 13 to 40 kg: 100 to 200 mg P.O. or rectally t.i.d. or q.i.d.
Children under 13 kg: 100 mg rectally t.i.d. or q.i.d. Limited to prolonged vomiting of known etiology.

CONTRAINDICATIONS & PRECAUTIONS

Contraindicated in patients with hypersensitivity to this drug, benzocaine, or other local anesthetics. The injectable form is contraindicated in children; suppositories are contraindicated in neonates and premature infants. Some clinicians consider the use of centrally acting antiemetics a contributing factor in the development of Reye's syndrome.

Use cautiously in patients with acute febrile illness, encephalitis, Reye's syndrome, encephalopathy, gastroenteritis, dehydration, or electrolyte imbalance, because the drug may mask the symptoms of these conditions.

ADVERSE REACTIONS

Common reactions are in italics; life-threatening reactions are in bold italics.
CNS: *drowsiness,* dizziness (in large doses).
CV: hypotension.
GI: diarrhea, exaggeration of preexisting nausea (in large doses).
Hepatic: ***liver toxicity.***
Skin: skin hypersensitivity reactions.
Local: pain, stinging, burning, redness, swelling at I.M. injection site.
Other: antiemetic effect may mask signs of overdosage of toxic agents, or intestinal obstruction, brain tumor, or other conditions.

INTERACTIONS

None significant.

EFFECTS ON DIAGNOSTIC TESTS

None reported.

NURSING CONSIDERATIONS

Besides those related universally to drug therapy (see "How to use this book"), consider the following specific recommendations:

Assessment

- Obtain a baseline assessment of blood pressure, liver function, and allergies.
- Be alert for adverse reactions and drug interactions throughout therapy.
- Evaluate the patient's and family's knowledge about trimethobenzamide therapy.

Nursing Diagnoses

- High risk for fluid volume deficit related to nausea and vomiting.
- Pain related to trimethobenzamide-induced stinging and burning at injection site.
- Knowledge deficit related to trimethobenzamide therapy.

Planning and Implementation

Preparation and Administration

- Read order carefully, because three forms of the drug are available.
- ***I.M. use:*** Administer by deep I.M. injection into upper outer quadrant of gluteal region to reduce pain and local irritation.
- Store suppositories in the refrigerator.

Monitoring

- Monitor effectiveness by observing the patient for nausea and vomiting.
- Monitor blood pressure and fluid balance.
- Observe for signs of hypersensitivity.
- Observe injection site for local reaction.
- Monitor liver function studies with long-term use.
- Observe for drowsiness and dizziness.

Supportive Care

- Do not give to children with a viral disease (a possible cause of vomiting

*Liquid form contains alcohol. **May contain tartrazine.

in children); may contribute to the development of Reye's syndrome, a potentially fatal acute childhood encephalopathy, characterized by fatty degeneration of the liver.
• Discontinue drug if allergic skin reaction occurs. Suppositories are contraindicated in hypersensitivity to benzocaine or similar local anesthetic.
• Encourage sufficient fluid intake to prevent fluid volume deficit.
• Be aware that drug has little if no value in preventing motion sickness and limited value as an antiemetic.

Patient Teaching
• Warn patient of possible drowsiness and dizziness. Tell him to avoid driving and other hazardous activities requiring alertness until CNS effects of drug are known.
• Advise the patient that burning, swelling, and redness may occur at the injection site.

Evaluation
In patients receiving trimethobenzamide, appropriate evaluation statements may include:
• Patient exhibits no signs of fluid volume deficit.
• Patient remains free from pain at injection site.
• Patient and family state an understanding of trimethobenzamide therapy.

trimethoprim
(trye meth´ oh prim)
Alprin‡, Proloprim, Trimpex, Triprim‡

• *Classification:* antibiotic (synthetic folate antagonist)
• *Pregnancy Risk Category:* C

HOW SUPPLIED
Tablets: 100 mg, 200 mg

ACTION
Mechanism: Interferes with the action of dihydrofolate reductase, inhibiting bacterial synthesis of folic acid. Because resistance to this agent develops rapidly when used alone, trimethoprim is usually given in combination with other drugs.
Absorption: Absorbed quickly and completely.
Distribution: Widely distributed. Approximately 42% to 46% of dose is plasma protein-bound.
Metabolism: Less than 20% of dose is metabolized in the liver.
Excretion: Most of dose is excreted in the urine via filtration and secretion. Half-life: 8 to 11 hours in adults with normal renal function; prolonged in impaired renal function. Serum half-life is shorter in children, ranging from 5.5 hours in children age 1 to 10 to 7.7 hours in children under age 1.
Onset, peak, duration: Peak serum levels reached in 1 to 4 hours.

INDICATIONS & DOSAGE
Treatment of uncomplicated urinary tract infections caused by susceptible strains of Escherichia coli, Proteus mirabilis, Klebsiella, *and* Enterobacter–
Adults: 100 mg P.O. every 12 hours for 10 days.
Note: Not recommended for children under age 12.

CONTRAINDICATIONS & PRECAUTIONS
Contraindicated in patients who are hypersensitive to the drug and in patients with megaloblastic anemia resulting from folate deficiency because drug may worsen this condition.
Drug is not recommended in patients with creatinine clearance below 15 ml/minute because of potential for increased renal toxicity. Administer cautiously to patients with renal or hepatic dysfunction because drug ac-

cumulation may occur and cause dose-related toxic effects.

ADVERSE REACTIONS

Common reactions are in italics; life-threatening reactions are in bold italics.
Blood: thrombocytopenia, leukopenia, megaloblastic anemia, methemoglobinemia.
GI: *epigastric distress, nausea, vomiting,* glossitis.
Skin: *rash, pruritus,* ***exfoliative dermatitis.***
Other: fever.

INTERACTIONS

Phenytoin: may decrease phenytoin metabolism and increase serum levels of phenytoin.

EFFECTS ON DIAGNOSTIC TESTS

BUN and serum creatinine: increased levels.
Liver enzymes: increased levels.

NURSING CONSIDERATIONS

Besides those related universally to drug therapy (see "How to use this book"), consider the following specific recommendations:

Assessment

- Obtain a baseline assessment of infection before therapy.
- Be alert for adverse reactions and drug interactions throughout therapy.
- Evaluate the patient's and family's knowledge about trimethoprim therapy.

Nursing Diagnoses

- High risk for injury related to ineffectiveness of trimethoprim to eradicate the infection.
- High risk for fluid volume deficit related to trimethoprim-induced adverse GI reactions.
- Knowledge deficit related to trimethoprim.

Planning and Implementation

Preparation and Administration

- Obtain specimen for culture and sensitivity tests before first dose. Therapy may begin pending test results.
- Expect reduced dosage in patients with severely impaired renal function.

Monitoring

- Monitor the effectiveness of trimethoprim therapy by regularly assessing for improvement in the infectious process.
- Monitor CBC routinely and check patient for clinical signs such as sore throat, fever, pallor, or purpura, because these may be early signs of serious blood disorders.
- Monitor hydration status if adverse GI reactions occur.

Supportive Care

- Obtain an order for an antiemetic or antidiarrheal agent as needed.
- Be aware that prolonged use of trimethoprim at high doses may cause bone marrow suppression. Notify doctor immediately of sore throat, fever, pallor, purpura, or change in CBC.

Patient Teaching

- Stress importance of frequent blood tests to detect adverse reactions.
- Instruct patient to continue taking the drug, even if feeling better, and to take entire amount prescribed.

Evaluation

In patients receiving trimethoprim, appropriate evaluation statements may include:

- Patient is free from infection.
- Patient's maintains adequate hydration throughout therapy.
- Patient and family state an understanding of trimethoprim therapy.

trimipramine maleate

(trye mi´ pra meen)
Apo-Trimip†, Surmontil

- *Classification:* antidepressant (tricyclic antidepressant)
- *Pregnancy Risk Category:* C

HOW SUPPLIED

Tablets: 25 mg‡
Capsules: 25 mg, 50 mg, 100 mg

ACTION

Mechanism: Increases the amount of norepinephrine or serotonin, or both, in the CNS by blocking their reuptake by the presynaptic neurons. This allows these neurotransmitters to accumulate.
Absorption: Rapidly absorbed from the GI tract after oral administration.
Distribution: Widely distributed in the body. Drug is 90% protein-bound.
Metabolism: By the liver; a significant first-pass effect may explain variability of serum levels in different patients taking the same dosage.
Excretion: In urine; some in feces via the biliary tract. Half-life: 9.1 hours.
Onset, peak, duration: Peak effect occurs in 2 hours; steady state within 7 days.

INDICATIONS & DOSAGE

Treatment of depression–
Adults: 75 mg P.O. daily in divided doses, increased to 200 mg daily. Dosages over 300 mg daily not recommended.
Enuresis–
Children over 6 years: initial dosage 25 mg P.O. 1 hour before bedtime; if no response, increase dosage to 50 mg in children under 12 years, and to 75 mg in children over 12 years.

CONTRAINDICATIONS & PRECAUTIONS

Contraindicated in patients with hypersensitivity to tricyclic antidepressants, trazodone, and related compounds; in the acute recovery phase of MI because drug depresses cardiac function and causes arrhythmia; coma or severe respiratory depression because of additive CNS and respiratory depression; and during or within 14 days of therapy with MAO inhibitors.

Use cautiously in patients with other cardiac disease (arrhythmias, CHF, angina pectoris, valvular disease, or heart block), respiratory disorders, seizure disorders, bipolar disease, glaucoma, hyperthyroidism, and parkinsonism; thyroid replacement therapy; diabetes Types I and II; prostatic hypertrophy, paralytic ileus, or urine retention, because drug may worsen these conditions; hepatic or renal dysfunction because diminished metabolism and excretion cause the drug to accumulate; in patients undergoing electroconvulsive therapy, and in patients undergoing surgery using general anesthesia because drug may increase cardiac sensitivity to the effects of general anesthetics or pressor agents.

ADVERSE REACTIONS

Common reactions are in italics; life-threatening reactions are in bold italics.
CNS: *drowsiness, dizziness,* excitation, seizures, tremors, weakness, confusion, headache, nervousness.
CV: *orthostatic hypotension, tachycardia, ECG changes,* hypertension.
EENT: *blurred vision,* tinnitus, mydriasis.
GI: *dry mouth, constipation,* nausea, vomiting, anorexia, paralytic ileus.
GU: *urine retention.*
Skin: rash, urticaria.
Other: *sweating,* allergy.
After abrupt withdrawal of long-term therapy: nausea, headache, malaise. (Does not indicate addiction.)

INTERACTIONS

Barbiturates: decrease TCA blood levels. Monitor for decreased antidepressant effect.
Cimetidine: may increase trimipramine serum levels. Monitor for increased adverse reactions.
Epinephrine, norepinephrine: in-

crease hypertensive effect. Use with caution.
MAO inhibitors: may cause severe excitation, hyperpyrexia, or seizures, usually with high dose. Use together cautiously.
Methylphenidate: increases TCA blood levels. Monitor for enhanced antidepressant effects.

EFFECTS ON DIAGNOSTIC TESTS

CBC: decreased WBC count.
ECG: prolonged conduction time (elongation of Q-T and PR intervals, flattened T waves).
Liver function tests: elevated levels.
Prothrombin time: altered.

NURSING CONSIDERATIONS

Besides those related universally to drug therapy (see "How to use this book"), consider the following specific recommendations:

Assessment

- Obtain a baseline assessment of depression before therapy.
- Be alert for adverse reactions and drug interactions throughout therapy.
- Evaluate the patient's and family's knowledge about trimipramine therapy.

Nursing Diagnoses

- Ineffective individual coping related to the patient's underlying condition.
- High risk for injury related to adverse reactions to trimipramine.
- Knowledge deficit related to trimipramine therapy.

Planning and Implementation

Preparation and Administration

- Whenever possible, patient should take full dose at bedtime to avoid daytime sedation.
- Expect reduced dosage in elderly or debilitated patients and adolescents.

Monitoring

- Monitor effectiveness by having the patient discuss his feelings (ask broad, open-ended questions) and by evaluating his behavior.
- Monitor blood pressure (supine and standing), ECG for changes, and heart rate for tachycardia.
- Monitor bowel patterns for constipation and check for urine retention.
- Monitor for mood changes and suicidal tendencies.

Supportive Care

- Institute safety precautions if adverse CNS reactions occur.
- Do not withdraw drug abruptly.
- If psychotic signs increase, notify doctor and expect dosage to be reduced. Allow only a minimum supply of tablets to lessen suicide risk.
- If not contraindicated, increase the patient's fluid and fiber intake to prevent constipation; if needed, obtain an order for a laxative.
- Assist the patient in changing positions slowly to minimize orthostatic hypotension.

Patient Teaching

- Tell the patient to relieve dry mouth with sugarless hard candy or chewing gum, but explain that saliva substitutes may be necessary.
- Teach the patient to increase fluids to minimize constipation. Suggest stool softener or high-fiber diet, if needed.
- Warn the patient to avoid driving and other hazardous activities that require alertness and good psychomotor coordination until CNS effects of the drug are known. Tell the patient that drowsiness and dizziness usually subside after first few weeks. Inform the patient that drug has strong sedative effects. Warn against combining drug with alcohol or other CNS depressants.
- Tell the patient that therapy must continue for 2 weeks or more before noticeable effect, and for 4 weeks or more before full effect. Encourage the patient to continue to take medication until it achieves full therapeutic effect.
- Advise the patient not to take any other drugs (prescription or OTC) without first consulting the doctor.

• Warn the patient about the possibility of morning orthostatic hypotension. Instruct the patient to rise slowly and to sit for several minutes before standing up.

Evaluation

In the patient receiving trimipramine, appropriate evaluation statements include:

• Patient behavior and communication indicate improvement of depression.

• Patient has not experienced injury from adverse reactions to trimipramine.

• Patient and family state an understanding of trimipramine therapy.

---

tripelennamine citrate

(tri pel enn´ a meen)

PBZ*

tripelennamine hydrochloride

PBZ, PBZ-SR, Pelamine, Pyribenzamine

• *Classification:* antihistamine, H_1-receptor antagonist (ethylenediamine derivative antihistamine)

• *Pregnancy Risk Category:* B

HOW SUPPLIED

citrate

Elixir: 37.5 mg/5 ml (equivalent to 25 mg/5 ml tripelennamine hydrochloride)*

hydrochloride

Tablets: 25 mg, 50 mg

Tablets (sustained-release): 100 mg.

ACTION

Mechanism: Competes with histamine for H_1-receptor sites on effector cells. Prevents but does not reverse histamine-mediated responses.

Absorption: Well absorbed from GI tract; drug is also absorbed topically, but a topical form is no longer available in the U.S.

Distribution: High concentrations are found in the liver; drug crosses the placenta.

Metabolism: Probably hepatic; drug is extensively metabolized.

Excretion: Metabolites appear in the urine.

Onset, peak, duration: Peak plasma levels occur 2 to 3 hours after oral administration.

INDICATIONS & DOSAGE

Rhinitis, allergy symptoms–

Adults: 25 to 50 mg P.O. q 4 to 6 hours; or (timed-release) 100 mg b.i.d. or t.i.d. Maximum dosage is 600 mg daily.

Children: 5 mg/kg P.O. daily in four to six divided doses. Maximum dosage is 300 mg daily.

CONTRAINDICATIONS & PRECAUTIONS

Contraindicated in patients with hypersensitivity to this drug or antihistamines with a similar chemical structure, such as pyrilamine; in neonates, other infants, and breast-feeding women, because young children may be more susceptible to the toxic effects of antihistamines; during asthma attacks because it thickens bronchial secretions; and in patients who have taken MAO inhibitors within the preceding 2 weeks.

Because of significant anticholinergic effects, use with caution in patients with narrow-angle glaucoma; pyloroduodenal obstruction or urinary bladder obstruction from prostatic hypertrophy or narrowing of the bladder neck; and cardiovascular disease or hypertension, because drug may cause palpitations.

ADVERSE REACTIONS

Common reactions are in italics; life-threatening reactions are in bold italics.

CNS: (especially in elderly patients) *drowsiness,* dizziness, confusion, restlessness, tremors, irritability, insomnia.

CV: palpitations.
GI: anorexia, diarrhea or constipation, *nausea, vomiting, dry mouth.*
GU: urinary frequency, urine retention.
Skin: urticaria, rash.
Other: thick bronchial secretions.

INTERACTIONS

CNS depressants: increased sedation. Use together cautiously.
MAO inhibitors: increased anticholinergic effects. Don't use together.

EFFECTS ON DIAGNOSTIC TESTS

Diagnostic skin tests: test interference.

NURSING CONSIDERATIONS

Besides those related universally to drug therapy (see "How to use this book"), consider the following specific recommendations.

Assessment

- Obtain a baseline assessment of the patient's respiratory symptoms before beginning tripelennamine citrate therapy.
- Be alert for adverse reactions and drug interactions throughout therapy.
- Evaluate the patient's and family's knowledge about tripelennamine therapy.

Nursing Diagnoses

- Ineffective airway clearance related to patient's underlying condition.
- High risk for fluid volume loss related to adverse GI effects of tripelennamine.
- Knowledge deficit related to tripelennamine therapy.

Planning and Implementation

Preparation and Administration

- ***P.O. use:*** Give with food or milk to reduce GI distress.

Monitoring

- Monitor effectiveness by evaluating patient's relief of symptoms and respiratory status.
- Monitor the patient for adverse GI reactions, especially nausea and vomiting.

Supportive Care

- Notify the doctor if nausea or vomiting occur.
- Expect the doctor to substitute another antihistamine if tolerance develops.

Patient Teaching

- Suggest that patient drink coffee or tea to reduce drowsiness.
- Tell the patient that sugarless gum, sour hard candy, or ice chips may relieve dry mouth.
- Warn patient to avoid drinking alcoholic beverages during therapy and to avoid hazardous activities such as driving that require alertness until adverse CNS effects are known.
- Warn patient to discontinue tripelennamine 4 days before allergy skin testing to preserve the accuracy of the tests.

Evaluation

In patients receiving tripelennamine, appropriate evaluation statements may include:

- Patient's respiratory symptoms are relieved with tripelennamine therapy.
- Patient does not experience fluid volume deficit; adverse GI reactions did not occur.
- Patient and family state an understanding of tripelennamine therapy.

---

triprolidine hydrochloride

(trye proe´ li deen)
Actidil*◇, Myidyl

- *Classification:* antihistamine, H_1-receptor antagonist (alkylamine)
- *Pregnancy Risk Category:* C

HOW SUPPLIED

Tablets: 2.5 mg◇
Syrup: 1.25 mg/5 ml◇

ACTION

Mechanism: Competes with histamine for H_1-receptor sites on effector cells. Prevents but does not reverse histamine-mediated responses.
Absorption: Well absorbed from the GI tract.
Distribution: Not fully known; drug is distributed to the lungs, spleen, and kidneys.
Metabolism: By the liver.
Excretion: Drug and metabolites are excreted in the urine. Half-life: About 2 to 6 hours.
Onset, peak, duration: Rapid onset of action, with peak effects occurring in about 3½ hours, and a duration of about 12 hours.

INDICATIONS & DOSAGE

Colds and allergy symptoms–
Adults: 2.5 mg P.O. q 4 to 6 hours. Maximum dosage is 10 mg/day.
Children over 6 years: 1.25 mg P.O. q 4 to 6 hours. Maximum dosage is 5 mg/day.
Children 4 to 6 years: 0.9 mg P.O. q 4 to 6 hours. Maximum dosage is 3.75 mg/day.
Children 2 to 4 years: 0.6 mg P.O. q 4 to 6 hours. Maximum dosage is 2.5 mg/day.
Children 4 months to 2 years: 0.3 mg P.O. q 4 to 6 hours. Maximum dosage is 1.25 mg/day.

Note: Children under 12 years should use only as directed by a doctor.

CONTRAINDICATIONS & PRECAUTIONS

Contraindicated in patients with hypersensitivity to this drug or other antihistamines with similar chemical structures (brompheniramine, chlorpheniramine, and dexchlorpheniramine); during asthma attacks, because triprolidine thickens bronchial secretions; and in patients who have taken MAO inhibitors within the previous 2 weeks.

Use cautiously in patients with narrow-angle glaucoma; pyloroduodenal obstruction or urinary bladder obstruction from prostatic hypertrophy or narrowing of the bladder neck, because of its marked anticholinergic effects; cardiovascular disease, hypertension, or hyperthyroidism, because of the risk of palpitations and tachycardia; or renal disease, diabetes, bronchial asthma, urine retention, or stenosing peptic ulcers.

Pregnant women, especially in the third trimester, and those who are breast-feeding should avoid triprolidine. Most antihistamines have not been studied in such patients, but seizures and other severe reactions have occurred in neonates, especially premature infants.

ADVERSE REACTIONS

Common reactions are in italics; life-threatening reactions are in bold italics.
CNS: (especially in elderly patients) *drowsiness,* dizziness, confusion, restlessness, insomnia, *stimulation.*
GI: anorexia, diarrhea or constipation, nausea, vomiting, *dry mouth.*
GU: urinary frequency, urine retention.
Skin: urticaria, rash.

INTERACTIONS

CNS depressants: increased sedation.
MAO inhibitors: increased anticholinergic effects. Don't use together.

EFFECTS ON DIAGNOSTIC TESTS

Diagnostic skin tests: test interference.

NURSING CONSIDERATIONS

Besides those related universally to drug therapy (see "How to use this book"), consider the following specific recommendations:

Assessment
• Obtain a baseline assessment of the patient's respiratory symptoms before beginning triprolidine therapy.
• Be alert for adverse reactions and drug interactions throughout therapy.
• Evaluate the patient's and family's knowledge about triprolidine therapy.
Nursing Diagnoses
• Ineffective airway clearance related to the patient's underlying condition.
• High risk for injury related to adverse CNS reactions to triprolidine.
• Knowledge deficit related to triprolidine therapy.
Planning and Implementation
Preparation and Administration
• ***P.O. use:*** Give with food or milk to reduce GI distress.
Monitoring
• Monitor effectiveness by frequently checking the patient's respiratory symptoms and noting the patient's relief of cold and allergy symptoms.
• Monitor for adverse CNS reactions. Drowsiness is common, especially in elderly patients.
Supportive Care
• Institute safety measures, such as the continuous use of side rails if the patient is hospitalized, if drowsiness occurs. Notify the doctor if drowsiness is incapacitating for the patient.
Patient Teaching
• Tell the patient to take this drug with food or milk to reduce GI distress.
• Tell the patient that drinking coffee or tea can reduce drowsiness and that sugarless gum, sour hard candy, or ice chips may relieve dry mouth.
• Warn patient to avoid drinking alcoholic beverages during therapy and to avoid hazardous activities, such as driving, that require alertness until adverse CNS effects are known.
• Warn patient to discontinue triprolidine 4 days before allergy skin testing to preserve the accuracy of the tests.

Evaluation
In patients receiving triprolidine, appropriate evaluation statements may include:
• Patient's cold and allergy symptoms are relieved with triprolidine therapy.
• Injury did not occur; patient has not experienced adverse CNS reactions.
• Patient and family state an understanding of triprolidine therapy.

tromethamine
(troe meth´ a meen)
Tham

• *Classification:* systemic alkalinizer (sodium-free organic amine)
• *Pregnancy Risk Category:* C

HOW SUPPLIED
Injection: 18 g/500 ml

ACTION
Mechanism: Combines with hydrogen ions and associated acid anions; the resulting salts are excreted.
Distribution: At pH of 7.4, about 25% of drug is not ionized; this portion may enter cells to neutralize acidic ions of intracellular fluid.
Metabolism: None.
Excretion: Rapidly excreted by the kidneys.

INDICATIONS & DOSAGE
Metabolic acidosis (associated with cardiac bypass surgery or with cardiac arrest) –
Adults: dosage depends on bicarbonate deficit. Calculate as follows: ml of 0.3 M tromethamine solution required = wt in kg × bicarbonate deficit (mEq/liter). Additional therapy based on serial determinations of existing bicarbonate deficit.
Children: calculate dosage as above. Give slowly over 3 to 6 hours. Additional therapy based on degree of aci-

dosis. Total 24-hour dosage should not exceed 33 to 40 ml/kg.

CONTRAINDICATIONS & PRECAUTIONS

Contraindicated in patients with uremia or anuria because of renal excretion; in patients with chronic respiratory acidosis because it decreases serum carbon dioxide levels and may cause respiratory failure; in pregnant patients; or when used longer than 24 hours, except in life-threatening emergencies.

Use cautiously in neonates and other infants, and in patients with renal disease and poor urine output because drug may accumulate in patients with decreased renal function.

ADVERSE REACTIONS

Common reactions are in italics; life-threatening reactions are in bold italics.
CNS: ***respiratory depression.***
Metabolic: hypoglycemia, hyperkalemia (with decreased urine output).
Local: venospasm; I.V. thrombosis; inflammation, necrosis, and sloughing if extravasation occurs.

INTERACTIONS

None significant.

EFFECTS ON DIAGNOSTIC TESTS

Blood glucose: transiently decreased concentrations.
Serum electrolytes: altered levels.

NURSING CONSIDERATIONS

Besides those related universally to drug therapy (see "How to use this book"), consider the following specific recommendations:

Assessment
- Obtain a baseline assessment of arterial blood gases, serum electrolytes, bicarbonate, and glucose levels before initiating therapy.
- Be alert for adverse reactions and drug interactions throughout therapy.
- Evaluate the patient's and family's knowledge about tromethamine therapy.

Nursing Diagnoses
- High risk for injury related to acid-base imbalance.
- Altered protection related to tromethamine-induced hypoglycemia or hyperkalemia.
- Knowledge deficit related to tromethamine therapy.

Planning and Implementation

Preparation and Administration
- ***I.V. use:*** Administer only as an intermittent infusion over 1 hour (not exceeding 5 ml/minute) through an 18G needle into a central line or an antecubital vein. Use an infusion pump if possible. In children, infuse over 6 hours.
- Except in life-threatening situations, expect the drug not to be administered longer than 1 day.

Monitoring
- Monitor effectiveness by regularly checking arterial blood gases, serum electrolytes, bicarbonate, and glucose levels.
- Monitor patient's respiratory status closely for evidence of respiratory depression.
- Monitor I.V. site closely for infiltration.

Supportive Care
- Hold dose and notify the doctor if respiratory depression or other metabolic abnormalities occur.
- If infiltration results in extravasation of tromethamine to surrounding tissues, infiltrate area with 1% procaine and hyaluronidase 150 units and consult the doctor for additional orders.
- Maintain accurate record of intake and output.
- Institute safety precautions due to potential weakness and altered thought processes.
- Reorient the patient to person, place, and time as needed.
- Have mechanical ventilation readily

available when giving drug to patient with associated respiratory acidosis.

Patient Teaching

• Tell patient to report any pain or discomfort in area of I.V. site immediately.

• Instruct patient on the signs and symptoms of hypoglycemia and hyperkalemia and to notify health professionals if any occur.

Evaluation

In patients receiving tromethamine, appropriate evaluation statements may include:

• Patients metabolic acidosis is resolved.

• Patient does not experience hypoglycemia or hyperkalemia.

• Patient and family state an understanding of tromethamine therapy.

---

tropicamide

(troe pik´ a mide)

Mydriacyl, Tropicacyl

• *Classification:* cycloplegic, mydriatic (anticholinergic agent)

• *Pregnancy Risk Category:* C

HOW SUPPLIED

Ophthalmic solution: 0.5%, 1%

ACTION

Mechanism: A mydriatic and cycloplegic agent that blocks muscarinic cholinergic receptors in the eye. Anticholinergic action leaves the pupil under unopposed adrenergic influence, causing it to dilate.

Pharmacokinetics: Unknown.

Onset, peak, duration: Peak effect usually occurs in 20 to 40 minutes. Recovery from cycloplegic and mydriatic effects usually occurs in about 6 hours.

INDICATIONS & DOSAGE

Cycloplegic refractions–

Adults: instill 1 drop of 1% solution; repeat in 5 minutes. Additional drop may be instilled in 20 to 30 minutes.

Children: instill 1 drop of 0.5% to 1% solution; may repeat in 5 minutes.

Fundus examinations–

Adults and children: instill 1 to 2 drops of 0.5% solution in each eye 15 to 20 minutes before examination.

CONTRAINDICATIONS & PRECAUTIONS

Contraindicated in patients with narrow-angle glaucoma and in patients hypersensitive to any component of the preparation. Use cautiously in patients in whom increased intraocular pressure may occur and in children because of increased risk of cardiovascular and CNS effects.

ADVERSE REACTIONS

Common reactions are in italics; life-threatening reactions are in bold italics.

Eye: *transient stinging on instillation,* increased intraocular pressure (less than with other mydriatic agents because of shorter duration of action), *blurred vision, photophobia.*

Systemic: flushing, fever, dry skin, dry mouth and throat, ataxia, irritability, confusion, somnolence, hallucinations, behavioral disturbances in children.

INTERACTIONS

None significant.

EFFECTS ON DIAGNOSTIC TESTS

None reported.

NURSING CONSIDERATIONS

Besides those related universally to drug therapy (see "How to use this book"), consider the following specific recommendations:

Assessment
• Obtain a baseline assessment of the patient's vision and pupil size.
• Be alert for adverse reactions and drug interactions throughout therapy.
• Evaluate the patient's and family's knowledge about tropicamide therapy.
Nursing Diagnoses
• Sensory/perceptual alterations (visual) related to the patient's underlying condition.
• High risk for poisoning related to the drug's systemic adrenergic effects.
• Knowledge deficit related to tropicamide therapy.
Planning and Implementation
Preparation and Administration
• Instill in lacrimal sac; remove excess solution from around eyes with clean tissue or gauze and apply light finger pressure to lacrimal sac for 1 minute.
Monitoring
• Monitor effectiveness by assessing the patient's visual status and pupil size.
• Monitor the patient for systemic adrenergic effects.
Supportive Care
• Notify the doctor immediately of any changes in the patient's health status.
• Keep physostigmine on hand (antidote of choice).
Patient Teaching
• Teach the patient how to instill the solution and advise him to wash his hands before and after administering the drug.
• Warn the patient that the drug causes transient stinging when instilled.
• Warn the patient to avoid hazardous activities such as driving until temporary blurring of vision subsides.
• Advise the patient that dark glasses should be worn to ease any discomfort from photophobia (lasts about 2 hours).

Evaluation
In patients receiving tropicamide, appropriate evaluation statements may include:
• Patient experiences therapeutic mydriasis.
• Patient remains free of systemic cholingeric effects.
• Patient and family state an understanding of tropicamide therapy.

tuberculin purified protein derivative (PPD)
Aplisol, PPD-stabilized Solution (Mantoux test), Tubersol

• *Classification:* diagnostic skin test (*Mycobacterium tuberculosis* and *M. bovis* antigen)
• *Pregnancy Risk Category:* C

HOW SUPPLIED
Injection (intradermal): 1 tuberculin unit (TU)/0.1 ml, 5 TU/0.1 ml, 250 TU/0.1 ml

ACTION
Mechanism: Causes a cell-mediated immune response.
Pharmacokinetics: Unknown.
Onset, peak, duration: Test site should be examined in 48 to 72 hours.

INDICATIONS & DOSAGE
Diagnosis of tuberculosis, evaluation of immunocompetence in patients with cancer, malnutrition–
Adults and children: initially, 1 TU (0.1 ml of appropriate solution) intradermally into flexor surface of the forearm. Use tuberculin syringe with 26G or 27G ⅝″ to ½″ needle. Retest with 5 TU and, if negative, 250 TU. If still no response, the individual is nonreactive.

CONTRAINDICATIONS & PRECAUTIONS

Severe reactions to tuberculin PPD are rare and usually result from extreme sensitivity to the tuberculin.

Inadvertent subcutaneous administration of PPD may result in a febrile reaction in highly sensitized patients. Old tubercular lesions are not activated by administration of PPD.

ADVERSE REACTIONS

Common reactions are in italics; life-threatening reactions are in bold italics.
Local: pain, pruritus, vesiculation, ulceration, necrosis.
Other: ***anaphylaxis,*** Arthus reaction.

INTERACTIONS

None significant.

EFFECTS ON DIAGNOSTIC TESTS

None reported.

NURSING CONSIDERATIONS

Besides those related universally to drug therapy (see "How to use this book"), consider the following specific recommendations:

Assessment

• Obtain a baseline assessment of the patient's general health status before therapy.
• Be alert for adverse reactions or drug interactions throughout therapy.
• Evaluate the patient's and family's knowledge about PPD skin test.

Nursing Diagnoses

• Ineffective airway clearance related to possible anaphylactoid reaction to PPD.
• High risk for impaired skin integrity related to local hypersensitivity reaction to PPD.
• Knowledge deficit related to PPD skin test.

Planning and Implementation

Preparation and Administration

• Keep in mind that S.C. injection invalidates test results. Bleb (6 to 10 mm in diameter) must form on skin upon intradermal injection.
• Never give initial test with second test strength (250 tuberculin units). Use only when a patient has negative response to a 5-tuberculin unit PPD but has the clinical signs and symptoms of tuberculosis.

Monitoring

• Read test results within 48 to 72 hours. An induration of 10 mm or more indicates a significant reaction (formerly called positive reaction). Significance of a reaction is determined not only by the size of the reaction but by circumstances. For example, a reaction of 5 mm or more may be considered significant in a close relative of a person with known tuberculosis. A reaction of 2 mm or more may be considered significant in infants and children. The amount of induration at the site—not erythema—determines the significance of the reaction.
• Monitor skin for signs of hypersensitivity reactions, such as vesiculation, ulceration, and necrosis.
• Watch for possible dyspnea, bronchospasm, stridor, and other indications of anaphylaxis following administration of PPD.

Supportive Care

• Obtain history of allergies and reactions to skin tests.
• If reaction is positive, further testing is needed to confirm diagnosis. Report all known cases of tuberculosis to the appropriate public health agency.
• Keep epinephrine 1:1,000 available.
• Keep in mind that reactivity to this test may be depressed or suppressed for as long as 4 to 6 weeks in individuals who have received concurrent or recent immunization with certain viral vaccines (for example, measles or influenza), in those who are receiving corticosteroid or immunosuppressive agents, in malnourished patients, and in those who have had

viral infections (rubeola, influenza, mumps, and probably others).
• Report signs of allergic reaction immediately.
• Be aware that strongly positive tests can result in scarring at the site.
• Apply cold packs or topical corticosteroids, as ordered, to relieve pain and itching if severe local reaction occurs.

Patient Teaching
• Explain the intradermal testing procedure.
• Tell the patient not to wash off the circle marked on the skin, because it aids the reading of test results.
• Instruct the patient to notify the doctor about manifestations of allergic reactions immediately.

Evaluation

In patients receiving PPD, appropriate evaluation statements may include:
• Patent airway maintained; no evidence of anaphylactoid reaction.
• Skin integrity maintained.
• Patient and family state an understanding of PPD skin test.

tuberculosis multiple-puncture tests

Aplitest (dried purified protein derivative [PPD]), Mono-Vacc Test (liquid Old Tuberculin [OT]), Sclavo Test (dried PPD), Tine Test (dried OT, dried PPD)

• *Classification:* diagnostic skin test (*Mycobacterium tuberculosis* and *M. bovis* antigen)

• *Pregnancy Risk Category:* C

HOW SUPPLIED

Test: 25 devices/pack, 5 tuberculin units/device

ACTION

Mechanism: Causes a cell-mediated immune response.
Pharmacokinetics: Unknown.
Onset, peak, duration: A delayed hypersensitivity reaction is evident in 5 to 6 hours and peaks in 48 to 72 hours.

INDICATIONS & DOSAGE

Screening for tuberculosis–
Adults and children: cleanse skin thoroughly with alcohol; make skin taut on flexor surface of forearm and press points firmly into selected site. Hold device at injection site for about 3 seconds to ensure stabilizing the dried tuberculin B in tissue lymph.

CONTRAINDICATIONS & PRECAUTIONS

Severe reactions to tuberculin are rare and usually result from extreme sensitivity to the tuberculin.
Old tubercular lesions are not activated by the drug.

ADVERSE REACTIONS

Common reactions are in italics; life-threatening reactions are in bold italics.
Local: hypersensitivity (vesiculation, ulceration, necrosis).
Other: ***anaphylaxis.***

INTERACTIONS

Virus vaccine: tuberculosis skin-test reaction may be suppressed if test is given within 4 to 6 weeks after immunization with live or attenuated virus.

EFFECTS ON DIAGNOSTIC TESTS

None reported.

NURSING CONSIDERATIONS

Besides those related universally to drug therapy (see "How to use this book"), consider the following specific recommendations:

Assessment
• Obtain a baseline assessment of the patient's general health status before therapy.
• Be alert for adverse reactions or drug interactions throughout testing.
• Evaluate the patient's and family's knowledge about tuberculosis multiple-puncture tests.
Nursing Diagnoses
• Ineffective airway clearance related to possible anaphylactoid reaction to test.
• High risk for impaired skin integrity related to local hypersensitivity reaction to drug.
• Knowledge deficit related to tuberculosis multiple-puncture tests.
Planning and Implementation
Preparation and Administration
• When administering tuberculosis multiple-puncture tests, be sure to press points firmly into selected site.
Monitoring
• Read test results within 48 to 72 hours. Questionable or positive reactions must be verified by the Mantoux test. Induration—not erythema—at the site determines significance of the reaction. Induration of 1 to 2 mm is significant. Keep in mind that false-positive reaction can occur in sensitive patients.
• Monitor skin for signs of hypersensitivity reactions, such as ulceration or necrosis.
• Keep in mind that if vesiculation is present, the test may be interpreted as positive.
• Watch for possible dyspnea, bronchospasm, stridor, and other indications of anaphylaxis following administration of skin test.
Supportive Care
• Obtain history of allergies, especially to acacia (a stabilizer in the Tine Test), and reactions to skin tests.
• Report all cases of tuberculosis to appropriate public health agency.
• Keep epinephrine 1:1,000 available.
• Keep in mind that reactivity to this test may be depressed or suppressed for as long as 4 to 6 weeks in individuals who have received concurrent or recent immunization with certain viral vaccines (for example, measles or influenza), in those who are receiving corticosteroid or immunosuppressive agents, in malnourished patients, and in those who have had recent viral infections (rubeola, influenza, mumps, and probably others) or miliary tuberculosis.
• Report signs of allergic reaction immediately.
• Apply cold packs or topical corticosteroids, as ordered, to relieve pain and itching if severe local reaction occurs.
• Rarely, minimal bleeding can occur at the puncture site. It does not interfere with interpretation of the test results.
Patient Teaching
• Explain the skin testing procedure.
• Tell the patient not to wash off the circle marked on the skin, because this aids reading of the test results.
• Instruct the patient to notify the doctor about signs of allergic reactions immediately.
Evaluation
In patients receiving a tuberculosis multiple-puncture test, appropriate evaluation statements include:
• Patent airway maintained; no evidence of anaphylactoid reaction.
• Skin integrity maintained.
• Patient and family state an understanding of tuberculosis multiple-puncture test.

tubocurarine chloride
(too boo kyoor ar´ een)
Tubarine†

• *Classification:* skeletal muscle relaxant (nondepolarizing neuromuscular blocking agent)

• *Pregnancy Risk Category:* C

HOW SUPPLIED

Injection: 3 mg (20 units)/ml; 10 mg/ml‡

ACTION

Mechanism: Prevents acetylcholine from binding to the receptors on the muscle end plate, thus blocking depolarization. Nondepolarizing agent.
Absorption: Unpredictable following I.M. injection; drug is usually given I.V.
Distribution: Into extracellular fluid and rapidly reaches its site of action. Drug is 40% to 45% bound to plasma proteins; redistribution to tissues is responsible for termination of drug effect.
Metabolism: Tubocurarine undergoes N-demethylation in the liver.
Excretion: Approximately 33% to 75% of a dose is excreted unchanged in urine in 24 hours; up to 11% is excreted in bile.
Onset, peak, duration: After I.V. injection, onset of muscle relaxation is rapid and peaks within 2 to 5 minutes. Duration is dose-related; effects usually begin to subside in 20 to 30 minutes. Paralysis may persist for 25 to 90 minutes. Subsequent doses have longer durations. After I.M. injection, the onset of paralysis is unpredictable (10 to 25 minutes); duration is dose-related. After tissue compartment is saturated, the drug may persist in tissues for up to 24 hours; 40% to 45% is bound to plasma proteins, mainly globulins.

INDICATIONS & DOSAGE

Adjunct to anesthesia to induce skeletal muscle relaxation; facilitate intubation, orthopedic manipulations– Dosage depends on anesthetic used, individual needs, and response. Dosages listed are representative and must be adjusted.
Adults: 1 unit/kg or 0.15 mg/kg I.V. slowly over 60 to 90 seconds. Average, initially, 40 to 60 units I.V. May give 20 to 30 units in 3 to 5 minutes. For longer procedures, give 20 units, p.r.n.
Children: 1 unit/kg or 0.15 mg/kg.
Assist with mechanical ventilation–
Adults and children: initially, 0.0165 mg/kg I.V. (average 1 mg or 7 units), then adjust subsequent doses to patient's response.
Lessen muscle contractions in pharmacologically or electrically induced seizures–
Adults and children: 1 unit/kg or 0.15 mg/kg slowly over 60 to 90 seconds. Initial dose is 20 units (3 mg) less than calculated dose.

CONTRAINDICATIONS & PRECAUTIONS

Contraindicated in patients with hypersensitivity to the drug and in whom histamine release may be hazardous, and in patients with known sensitivity to sulfites.

Administer cautiously to patients with bronchogenic carcinoma; cardiovascular, renal, hepatic, or pulmonary function impairment; dehydration or electrolyte imbalance; hyperthermia; hypothermia; hypotension; myasthenia gravis; shock; or sensitivity to sulfites.

ADVERSE REACTIONS

Common reactions are in italics; life-threatening reactions are in bold italics.
CV: hypotension, circulatory depression.
Other: profound and prolonged muscle relaxation, ***respiratory depression to the point of apnea, hypersensitivity, idiosyncrasy,*** residual muscle weakness, increased salivation, ***bronchospasm.***

INTERACTIONS

Aminoglycoside antibiotics (including amikacin, gentamicin, kanamycin, neomycin, streptomycin), polymyxin

antibiotics (polymyxin B sulfate, colistin), general anesthetics (such as halothane, enflurane, isoflurane): potentiated neuromuscular blockade, leading to increased skeletal muscle relaxation and possible respiratory paralysis. Use cautiously during surgical and postoperative periods.
Quinidine: prolonged neuromuscular blockade. Use together with caution. Monitor closely.
Thiazide diuretics, furosemide, ethacrynic acid, amphotericin B, propranolol, methotrimeprazine, narcotic analgesics: potentiated neuromuscular blockade, leading to increased respiratory paralysis. Use with extreme caution during surgical and postoperative periods.

EFFECTS ON DIAGNOSTIC TESTS

None significant.

NURSING CONSIDERATIONS

Besides those related universally to drug therapy (see "How to use this book"), consider the following specific recommendations:

Assessment

- Obtain a baseline assessment of skeletal muscle function and respiratory pattern before drug therapy.
- Be alert for adverse reactions and drug interactions throughout therapy.
- Evaluate the patient's and family's knowledge about tubocurarine therapy.

Nursing Diagnoses

- Ineffective breathing pattern related to the patient's underlying condition.
- Impaired verbal communication related to drug-induced paralysis.
- Knowledge deficit related to tubocurarine therapy.

Planning and Implementation

Preparation and Administration

- Tubocurarine should be administered only by personnel experienced in airway management.
- Have emergency respiratory support equipment (endotracheal equipment, ventilator, oxygen, atropine, edrophonium, epinephrine, and neostigmine) on hand before administration.
- ***I.V. use:*** Give I.V. slowly (60 to 90 seconds).
- ***I.M. use:*** Give deep I.M. in deltoid muscle.
- Do not mix with barbiturate solutions (precipitate will form); use only fresh solutions.
- Usually administered with a cholinergic blocker (such as atropine or glycopyrrolate).
- If succinylcholine is used, allow effects to subside before giving pancuronium.
- ***I.V. use:*** Continuous and intermittent infusions are not recommended.

Monitoring

- Monitor effectiveness by regularly checking relaxation of the patient's skeletal muscles; close observation of the patient is mandatory.
- Closely monitor baseline electrolyte determinations (electrolyte imbalance can potentiate neuromuscular effects) and vital signs (watch respiration and heart rate).
- Measure intake and output. Renal dysfunction may prolong duration of action, because much of the drug is unchanged before excretion.
- Monitor respirations and respiratory status closely until patient recovers fully from neuromuscular blockade, as evidenced by tests of muscle strength (hand grip, head lift, and ability to cough).
- Monitor for adverse reactions or drug interactions by frequently checking vital signs (every 15 minutes) for hypotension and respiratory depression.

Supportive Care

- Maintain adequate ventilation through respiratory support equipment throughout drug therapy and provide pulmonary care as indicated.
- Once spontaneous recovery starts, tubocurarine-induced neuromuscular blockade may be reversed with an an-

ticholinesterase agent (such as neostigmine or edrophonium).

• Provide emotional support for the intubated patient who is awake.

• Administer pain medication regularly (as condition dictates) because the patient will be unable to communicate that pain is present.

• Anticipate the patient's needs and try to meet them. Explain everything thoroughly before performing any procedure. Use nonverbal communication, especially eye contact.

• Protect the patient from injury when moving him in bed.

• Provide meticulous eye care because blink reflex will be absent.

Patient Teaching

• Reassure the patient that necessary pain management will be provided regularly.

• Inform the patient that drug-induced paralysis will inhibit his ability to communicate but that he will receive continuous monitoring and care.

• Reassure the patient that as soon as the need for neuromuscular blockade is no longer necessary, the drug-induced paralysis will be reversed.

Evaluation

In the patient receiving tubocurarine, appropriate evaluation statements may include:

• Patient maintains adequate ventilation.

• Patient's basic needs are anticipated and met.

• Patient and family state an understanding of tubocurarine therapy.

UVW

uracil mustard

(yoor´ a sill)
Uracil Mustard Capsules**

• *Classification:* antineoplastic (alkylating agent)
• *Pregnancy Risk Category:* X

HOW SUPPLIED

Capsules: 1 mg

ACTION

Mechanism: An alkylating agent that cross-links strands of cellular DNA and interferes with RNA transcription, causing an imbalance of growth that leads to cell death. Cell-cycle–nonspecific.
Absorption: Animal studies report rapid but incomplete absorption after oral administration.
Excretion: Animal studies report rapid elimination from the plasma with no drug detected 2 hours after administration. Less than 1% of a dose is excreted in urine.

INDICATIONS & DOSAGE

Chronic lymphocytic and myelocytic leukemia; Hodgkin's disease; non-Hodgkin's lymphomas of the histiocytic and lymphocytic types; reticulum cell sarcoma; lymphomas; mycosis fungoides; polycythemia vera; cancer of ovaries, cervix, and lungs—
Adults: 1 to 2 mg P.O. daily for 3 months or until desired response or toxicity; maintenance dosage is 1 mg daily for 3 out of 4 weeks until optimum response or relapse; or 3 to 5 mg P.O. for 7 days not to exceed total dosage of 0.5 mg/kg, then 1 mg daily until response, then 1 mg daily 3 out of 4 weeks.

CONTRAINDICATIONS & PRECAUTIONS

Contraindicated in patients with a history of hypersensitivity to tartrazine, a dye contained in the capsules. The incidence of hypersensitivity is low, but it seems to occur frequently in patients allergic to aspirin.

Use cautiously in patients whose bone marrow shows infiltration with malignant cells because hematopoietic toxicity may be increased.

ADVERSE REACTIONS

Common reactions are in italics; life-threatening reactions are in bold italics.
Blood: bone marrow suppression, delayed 2 to 4 weeks; ***thrombocytopenia;*** *leukopenia;* anemia.
CNS: irritability, nervousness, mental cloudiness, and depression.
GI: *nausea, vomiting, diarrhea, epigastric distress,* abdominal pain, anorexia.
Metabolic: hyperuricemia.
Skin: pruritus, dermatitis, hyperpigmentation, alopecia.

INTERACTIONS

None significant.

EFFECTS ON DIAGNOSTIC TESTS

Blood and urine uric acid: increased levels.

NURSING CONSIDERATIONS

Besides those related universally to drug therapy (see "How to use this book"), consider the following specific recommendations:

*Liquid form contains alcohol.

**May contain tartrazine.

Assessment
• Obtain a baseline assessment of the patient's underlying condition, CBC, and platelet count before therapy.
• Be alert for adverse reactions throughout therapy.
• Evaluate the patient's and family's knowledge about uracil mustard therapy.
Nursing Diagnoses
• High risk for infection related to immunosuppressant effects of uracil mustard.
• Altered nutrition: Less than body requirements related to GI adverse effects as evidenced by nausea and vomiting.
• Knowledge deficit related to uracil mustard therapy.
Planning and Implementation
Preparation and Administration
• ***P.O. use:*** Give at bedtime to reduce nausea. Expect dosage modification in severe thrombocytopenia, aplastic anemia, leukopenia, or acute leukemia.
Monitoring
• Monitor effectiveness by noting results of follow-up diagnostic tests and overall physical status.
• Monitor biweekly CBC for 4 weeks, then note results again 4 weeks after the end of therapy.
• Monitor serum uric acid levels.
• Monitor patient for signs of infection (fever, sore throat, fatigue) and bleeding (easy bruising, nosebleeds, bleeding gums, melena).
• Monitor platelet count closely.
Supportive Care
• Avoid giving anticoagulants and aspirin products if possible. If they must be given, use with extreme caution.
• Administer antiemetics as ordered. Nausea and vomiting occur in almost all patients.
• Provide adequate fluid intake and give allopurinol as ordered to prevent hyperuricemia and resulting hyperuricemia.
• Do not give any I.M. injections when platelet count is less than 100,000/mm^3.
Patient Teaching
• Warn patients to watch for signs of infection (sore throat, fever, fatigue), and for signs of bleeding (easy bruising, nosebleeds, bleeding gums).
• Tell the patient to take his temperature daily.
• Teach patient to avoid the use of all OTC products containing aspirin.
• Encourage the patient to maintain an adequate fluid intake and be sure that the patient understands the importance of fluid intake.
• Explain all the potential reactions. Tell the patient how to try to avoid them and when to notify the doctor. Be sure that the patient understands that most patients do experience some adverse reactions because of the drug's toxicity.
Evaluation
In patients receiving uracil mustard, appropriate evaluation statements may include:
• Patient does not experience infection during therapy.
• Patient maintains adequate nutrition during therapy.
• Patient and family state an understanding of uracil mustard therapy.

urokinase
(yoor oh kin´ ase)
Abbokinase, Ukidan‡, Win-Kinase

• *Classification:* thrombolytic enzyme
• *Pregnancy Risk Category:* B

HOW SUPPLIED
Injection: 5,000 IU/ml unit-dose vial; 250,000-IU vial

ACTION
Mechanism: Activates plasminogen by directly cleaving peptide bonds at two different sites.

Metabolism: Probably hepatic; drug is cleared rapidly from the plasma by the liver.
Excretion: In bile and urine. Half-life: About 20 minutes.
Onset, peak, duration: Most patients experience reperfusion within 2 hours.

INDICATIONS & DOSAGE

Lysis of acute massive pulmonary emboli and lysis of pulmonary emboli accompanied by unstable hemodynamics–
Adults: for I.V. infusion only by constant infusion pump that will deliver a total volume of 195 ml.
Priming dose: 4,400 IU/kg of urokinase–normal saline solution admixture given over 10 minutes. Follow with 4,400 IU/kg hourly for 12 to 24 hours. Total volume should not exceed 200 ml. Follow therapy with continuous I.V. infusion of heparin, then oral anticoagulants.
Coronary artery thrombosis–
Adults: following a bolus dose of heparin ranging from 2,500 to 10,000 units, infuse 6,000 IU/minute of urokinase into the occluded artery for up to 2 hours. Average total dosage is 500,000 IU.
Venous catheter occlusion–
Instill 5,000 IU into occluded line, wait 5 minutes, then aspirate. Repeat aspiration attempts q 5 minutes for 30 minutes. If not patent after 30 minutes, cap line and let urokinase work for 30 to 60 minutes before aspirating. May require second instillation.

CONTRAINDICATIONS & PRECAUTIONS

Contraindicated in patients with ulcerative wounds, active internal bleeding and recent trauma with possible internal injuries, pregnancy and first 10 days postpartum, ulcerative colitis, diverticulitis, severe hypertension, acute or chronic hepatic or renal insufficiency, uncontrolled hypocoagulation, chronic pulmonary disease with cavitation, subacute bacterial endocarditis or rheumatic valvular disease and recent cerebral embolism, thrombosis or hemorrhage, or diabetic hemorrhagic retinopathy because of the potential for excessive bleeding.

Use with extreme caution for 10 days after intracranial, intraspinal, or intra-arterial diagnostic procedure or after any surgery, including liver or kidney biopsy, lumbar puncture, thoracentesis, paracentesis, or extensive or multiple cutdowns.

ADVERSE REACTIONS

Common reactions are in italics; life-threatening reactions are in bold italics.
Blood: bleeding, low hematocrit.
Local: phlebitis at injection site.
Other: hypersensitivity (not as frequent as streptokinase), musculoskeletal pain, ***bronchospasm, anaphylaxis.***

INTERACTIONS

Anticoagulants: concurrent use with urokinase is not recommended. Consider reversing the effects of oral anticoagulants before beginning therapy; heparin must be stopped and its effect allowed to diminish.
Aspirin, dipyridamole, indomethacin, phenylbutazone, other drugs affecting platelet activity: increased risk of bleeding.

EFFECTS ON DIAGNOSTIC TESTS

Hematocrit: moderately decreased.
Thrombin time, activated partial thromboplastin time (PTT) and prothrombin time (PT): increased.

NURSING CONSIDERATIONS

Besides those related universally to drug therapy (see "How to use this book"), consider the following specific recommendations:

Assessment
- Obtain a baseline assessment of vital signs, hemoglobin, hematocrit, PT, and PTT before therapy.
- Be alert for adverse reactions and drug interactions throughout therapy.
- Evaluate the patient's and family's knowledge about urokinase therapy.

Nursing Diagnoses
- Altered tissue perfusion (cardiopulmonary) related to the patient's underlying condition.
- Fluid volume deficit related to the adverse effects of urokinase.
- Knowledge deficit related to urokinase therapy.

Planning and Implementation
Preparation and Administration
- Supplied as a lyophilized white powder in vials containing 250,000 units. Reconstitute with 5.2 ml of sterile water for injection (without preservatives) for a solution of 50,000 IU/ml. Don't use bacteriostatic water; it contains preservatives. Dilute solution further with 0.9% sodium chloride or dextrose 5% in water. Total volume administered shouldn't exceed 200 ml. Refrigerate vials at 35° to 47° F (2° to 8° C). Reconstitute immediately before use and discard unused portion. Don't use highly colored solutions and don't add other drugs to the solution. Reconstituted solution should be clear, practically colorless, and without particulate matter. To avoid filament formation, roll and tilt vial during reconstitution; avoid shaking. Solution may be filtered through a 0.45 micron or smaller cellulose filter.
- ***Direct injection:*** To clear a venous catheter occlusion, slowly inject solution into occluded line, wait 5 minutes, then aspirate. Repeat aspiration attempts q 5 minutes for 30 minutes. If not patent after 30 minutes, cap line and let urokinase work for 30 minutes to 1 hour before aspirating. May require second injection.
- ***Continuous infusion:*** Administer initial dose of diluted solution over 10 minutes, using an infusion pump. Infuse subsequent doses, as ordered, over 12 hours.
- ***Intermittent infusion:*** Not recommended.

Monitoring
- Monitor effectiveness by regularly checking vital signs, hemoglobin, hematocrit, PT and PTT.
- Monitor pulses, color, and sensitivity of extremities every hour.
- Check percutaneous puncture sites and cuts for oozing, bruising, and hematoma formation because urokinase may lyse fibrin deposits.
- Monitor for bleeding every 15 minutes for the first hour, every 30 minutes for the next 7 hours, and then once each shift.
- Monitor for signs of hypersensitivity and have corticosteroids available to treat allergic reactions.

Supportive Care
- Remember to have typed and crossmatched RBCs and whole blood available to treat hemorrhage.
- Maintain alignment of involved extremity to prevent bleeding at infusion site.
- Avoid I.M. injections, unnecessary handling of the patient, and arterial invasive procedures. If arterial puncture is necessary, use an upper extremity, apply pressure at the site for 30 minutes, and apply a pressure dressing. Check the site frequently for bleeding. Also avoid venipuncture or perform as infrequently as possible.
- Keep in mind that urokinase may be followed by heparin usually within 1 hour after discontinuation to prevent recurrent thrombosis.
- Keep in mind that hematocrit, plasma fibrinogen, and plasminogen levels may decrease for 12 to 24 hours after therapy stops. Fibrin split products increase similarly. Monitor these levels.

Patient Teaching
• Instruct the patient to report symptoms of bleeding.
• Explain to the patient that bruising may occur during therapy and that he should try to avoid bumping his arms and legs on bed side rails.

Evaluation
In patients receiving urokinase, appropriate evaluation statements may include:
• Patient's cardiopulmonary status is improved.
• Patient has not experienced excessive blood loss.
• Patient and family state an understanding of urokinase therapy.

valproate sodium
(val proe´ ate)
Depakene Syrup, Epilim‡, Myproic Acid Syrup

valproic acid
(val proe´ ik)
Dalpro, Depa, Depakene, Myproic Acid

divalproex sodium
(dye val´ proe ex)
Depakote, Epival†, Valcote‡

• *Classification:* anticonvulsant (carboxylic acid derivative)
• *Pregnancy Risk Category:* D

HOW SUPPLIED
valproate sodium
Syrup: 250 mg/ml‡
valproic acid
Tablets (enteric-coated): 200 mg‡, 500 mg‡
Crushable tablets: 100 mg‡
Capsules: 250 mg
Syrup: 200 mg/5 ml‡
divalproex sodium
Tablets (enteric-coated): 125 mg, 250 mg, 500 mg

ACTION
Mechanism: Increases brain levels of gamma-aminobutyric acid (GABA), which transmits inhibitory nerve impulses in the CNS. Valproic acid may also decrease GABA's enzymatic catabolism.
Absorption: Valproate sodium and divalproex sodium quickly convert to valproic acid after administration of oral dose; valproic acid is rapidly and completely absorbed. Bioavailability is the same for both forms of the drug.
Distribution: Rapidly distributed throughout the body; drug is 80% to 95% protein-bound.
Metabolism: Valproic acid is metabolized by the liver.
Excretion: Valproic acid is excreted in urine; some drug is excreted in feces and exhaled air. Breast milk levels are 1% to 10% of serum levels. Half-life: Averages about 10 hours, but may be longer with high plasma levels.
Onset, peak, duration: Peak plasma concentrations occur in 1 to 4 hours (with uncoated tablets) and 3 to 5 hours (with enteric-coated tablets).

INDICATIONS & DOSAGE
Simple and complex absence seizures, mixed seizure types (including absence seizures), investigationally in generalized, tonic-clonic seizures—
Adults and children: initially, 15 mg/kg P.O. daily divided b.i.d. or t.i.d.; then may increase by 5 to 10 mg/kg daily at weekly intervals up to maximum of 60 mg/kg daily, divided b.i.d. or t.i.d.

CONTRAINDICATIONS & PRECAUTIONS
Contraindicated in patients with hypersensitivity to valproic acid and in patients with a history of hepatic disease because valproic acid may be hepatotoxic. Use with caution in patients taking oral anticoagulants or

multiple anticonvulsants. Patients with congenital metabolic or seizure disorders with mental retardation, especially children under age 2, appear to be at increased risk of adverse effects.

ADVERSE REACTIONS

Common reactions are in italics; life-threatening reactions are in bold italics.

Because drug usually used in combination with other anticonvulsants, adverse reactions reported may not be caused by valproic acid alone.

Blood: *inhibited platelet aggregation,* ***thrombocytopenia,*** increased bleeding time.

CNS: *sedation,* emotional upset, depression, psychosis, aggression, hyperactivity, behavioral deterioration, muscle weakness, tremor.

EENT: stomatitis.

GI: *nausea, vomiting,* indigestion, diarrhea, abdominal cramps, constipation, increased appetite and weight gain, *anorexia,* pancreatitis. (*Note:* lower incidence of GI effects with divalproex.)

Hepatic: *elevated enzymes,* ***toxic hepatitis.***

Metabolic: *elevated serum ammonia.*

Other: alopecia.

INTERACTIONS

Antacids, aspirin: may cause valproic acid toxicity. Use together cautiously and monitor blood levels.

Phenobarbital: increased phenobarbital levels.

Phenytoin: increased or decreased.

EFFECTS ON DIAGNOSTIC TESTS

Liver function tests: abnormal results.

Urine ketones: false-positive results.

NURSING CONSIDERATIONS

Besides those related universally to drug therapy (see "How to use this book"), consider the following specific recommendations:

Assessment

- Obtain a baseline assessment of patient's seizure activities before therapy.
- Be alert for adverse reactions and drug interactions throughout therapy.
- Evaluate the patient's and family's knowledge about valproic acid or its derivatives.

Nursing Diagnoses

- High risk for injury related to patient's underlying seizure disorder.
- Altered protection related to drug-induced bleeding.
- Knowledge deficit related to drug therapy.

Planning and Implementation

Preparation and Administration

- Give drug with food or milk to reduce adverse GI reactions. Advise against chewing capsules, which causes irritation of mouth and throat.
- Available as pleasant-tasting red syrup. Keep out of reach of children.
- Syrup is rapidly absorbed, reaching peak effect within 15 minutes.
- Syrup shouldn't be mixed with carbonated beverages because it may be irritating to mouth and throat.
- Don't administer syrup to the patient who needs sodium restriction. Consult the doctor to provide alternative drug form.
- Know that syrup is rapidly absorbed and achieves peak effect within 15 minutes.
- Expect lower dosage in elderly patients.

Monitoring

- Regularly monitor effectiveness by evaluating seizure activity.
- Obtain liver function studies, platelet count, and prothrombin time, before starting drug and monitor periodically thereafter.
- Monitor for nonspecific symptoms, such as malaise, fever, and lethargy, which may precede serious or fatal hepatotoxicity.
- Monitor for bleeding tendencies,

such as easy bruising and spontaneous epistaxis.
• If monitoring urine ketones, keep in mind that this drug may produce false-positive test results.
• Know that therapeutic drug level is 50 to 100 mcg/ml.

Supportive Care
• Maintain seizure precautions.
• Institute safety precautions until sedative effects of the drug are known; assist the patient with activities as needed.
• Institute bleeding precautions. Advise the patient to use an electric shaver and soft toothbrush, and to avoid cuts and bruises.
• Expect dosage reduction if the patient develops tremor.
• Know that valproic acid has been used investigationally to prevent febrile seizures in children.

Patient Teaching
• Warn the patient to avoid hazardous activities that require alertness and good psychomotor coordination until CNS effects of the drug are known.
• Instruct the patient to take bleeding precautions.
• Warn the patient not to discontinue the drug suddenly, and to call the doctor at once if adverse reactions develop.
• Inform the diabetic patient that drug may produce false-positive test results for ketones in urine.
• Stress importance of follow-up care and periodic diagnostic tests.
• Tell the patient to report nonspecific symptoms, such as malaise, fever, lethargy, and bleeding, immediately.
• Advise the patient to take drug with food or milk to reduce adverse GI reactions. Warn against chewing capsules or mixing syrup with carbonated beverages because it may cause mouth and throat irritation and an unpleasant taste.
• Emphasize the importance of storing pleasant-tasting red syrup form out of the reach of children.
• Warn the patient to avoid alcohol during therapy; it may decrease drug's effectiveness and may increase adverse CNS effects.
• Encourage the patient to wear identification listing drug and presence of seizure disorder.

Evaluation
In patients receiving valproic acid or its derivatives, appropriate evaluation statements include:
• Patient is free of seizure activity.
• Patient does not experience bleeding throughout valproic acid therapy.
• Patient and family state an understanding of therapy with valproic acid or its derivatives.

vancomycin hydrochloride
(van koe mye´ sin)
Vancocin

• *Classification:* antibiotic (glycopeptide)
• *Pregnancy Risk Category:* C

HOW SUPPLIED
Powder for oral solution: 1-g, 10-g bottles
Powder for injection: 500-mg, 1-g vials

ACTION
Mechanism: Hinders bacterial cell wall synthesis, damaging the bacterial plasma membrane and making the cell more vulnerable to osmotic pressure.
Absorption: Minimal systemic absorption after oral administration makes it useful to treat enterocolitis or antibiotic-associated pseudomembraneous colitis. However, substantial absorption can occur in patients with colitis, especially those with renal

failure. For treatment of systemic infections, the drug must be given intravenously.
Distribution: After I.V. administration, vancomycin is distributed widely in body fluids, including pericardial, pleural, ascitic, synovial, and placental fluid; it achieves therapeutic levels in CSF in patients with inflamed meninges.
Excretion: When administered parenterally, vancomycin is excreted renally, mainly by filtration. When administered orally, drug is excreted in feces. Half-life: 6 hours in patients with normal renal function; about 36 hours in patients with creatinine clearance ranging from 10 to 30 ml/minute, 146 hours if creatinine clearance is below 10 ml/minute.
Onset, peak, duration: Plasma levels peak after the completion of an I.V. infusion.

INDICATIONS & DOSAGE

Severe staphylococcal infections when other antibiotics ineffective or contraindicated–
Adults: 500 mg I.V. q 6 hours, or 1 g q 12 hours.
Children: 44 mg/kg I.V. daily, divided q 6 hours.
Neonates: 10 mg/kg I.V. daily, divided q 6 to 12 hours.
Antibiotic-associated pseudomembranous and staphylococcal enterocolitis–
Adults: 125 to 500 mg P.O. q 6 hours for 7 to 10 days.
Children: 44 mg/kg P.O. daily, divided q 6 hours.
Endocarditis prophylaxis for dental procedures–
Adults: 1 g I.V. slowly over 1 hour, starting 1 hour before procedure.

CONTRAINDICATIONS & PRECAUTIONS

Contraindicated in patients with hypersensitivity to the drug. Administer cautiously to patients with hearing loss because of its ototoxic effect (especially at high serum levels).

ADVERSE REACTIONS

Common reactions are in italics; life-threatening reactions are in bold italics.
Blood: transient eosinophilia, leukopenia.
EENT: tinnitus, ototoxicity.
GI: nausea.
GU: nephrotoxicity.
Skin: "red-neck" syndrome with rapid I.V. infusion (maculopapular rash on face, neck, trunk, and extremities).
Local: pain or thrombophlebitis with I.V. administration, necrosis.
Other: chills, fever, ***anaphylaxis,*** superinfection.

INTERACTIONS

Aminoglycosides, amphotericin B, cisplatin, pentamidine: increased risk of nephrotoxicity.

EFFECTS ON DIAGNOSTIC TESTS

BUN and serum creatinine levels: may increase.
CBC: neutropenia and eosinophilia.

NURSING CONSIDERATIONS

Besides those related universally to drug therapy (see "How to use this book"), consider the following specific recommendations:

Assessment
- Obtain a baseline assessment of infection before therapy.
- Be alert for adverse reactions and drug interactions throughout therapy.
- Evaluate the patient's and family's knowledge about vancomycin therapy.

Nursing Diagnoses
- High risk for injury related to ineffectiveness of vancomycin to eradicate the infection.
- Sensory-perceptual alterations (auditory) related to vancomycin induced ototoxicity.
- Knowledge deficit related to vancomycin.

Planning and Implementation
Preparation and Administration
• Obtain specimen for culture and sensitivity tests before first dose. Therapy may begin pending test results.
• Assess patient's renal status before beginning vancomycine therapy. Patients with impaired renal function may require dosage reduction. Be aware that patient receiving hemodialysis and peritoneal dialysis requires usual dose only once every 5 to 7 days.
• ***P.O. use:*** To prepare drug for oral administration, reconstitute as directed in manufacturer's instructions. Reconstituted solution is stable for 2 weeks when refrigerated.
• ***I.V. use:*** To prepare drug for I.V. injection, reconstitute 500-mg or 1-g vial with 10 ml of sterile water for injection to yield 50 mg/ml or 100 mg/ml respectively. Withdraw desired dose and further dilute to 100 to 250 ml with 0.9% sodium chloride solution or 5% dextrose in water. Infuse over at least 60 minutes to avoid adverse reactions related to rapid infusion rate. Reconstituted solution remains stable for 96 hours when refrigerated. Do not mix drug with other drugs in the same I.V. solution. Avoid extravasation, which can cause severe irritation and necrosis.
Monitoring
• Monitor effectiveness by regularly assessing for improvement in the infection.
• Monitor closely for signs of ototoxicity, especially in the patients with renal impairment and in those who are receiving long-term I.V. therapy with high doses of vancomycin.
• Monitor renal function regularly as ordered.
• If the patient is receiving concurrent treatment with another ototoxic or nephrotoxic drug, vancomycin serum concentrations (peak and trough levels) and the serum creatinine level.
Supportive Care
• Withhold vancomycin and notify the doctor if tinnitus or hearing loss occurs. Expect to discontinue drug and initiate another antibiotic, as prescribed.
• If the patient develops maculopapular rash on face, neck, trunk, and upper extremities, stop the infusion and report this reaction promptly.
Patient Teaching
• Tell patient to take the drug exactly as directed, even after feeling better, and to take entire amount prescribed. Tell the patient that treatment of staphylococcal endocarditis will continue for at least for 4 weeks
• Tell the patient to report fullness or ringing in ears immediately. This reaction requires discontinuation of the drug.
• Advise patient to tell the nurse promptly about pain or discomfort at the I.V. site.
Evaluation
In patients receiving vancomycin, appropriate evaluation statements may include:
• Patient is free from infection.
• Patient maintains adequate hydration throughout therapy.
• Patient and family state an understanding of therapy.

varicella-zoster immune globulin (VZIG)
(var ah sel´ ah zah´ ster)

• *Classification:* varicella-zoster prophylaxis agent (immune serum)
• *Pregnancy Risk Category:* C

HOW SUPPLIED
Injection: 10% to 18% solution of the globulin fraction of human plasma containing 125 units of

*Liquid form contains alcohol. **May contain tartrazine.

varicella-zoster virus antibody (volume is about 1.25 ml)

ACTION

Mechanism: Provides passive immunity to varicella-zoster virus.
Pharmacokinetics: Unknown.
Onset, peak, duration: After I.M. absorption, the persistence of antibodies is unknown, but protection should last at least 3 weeks. Protection is sufficient to prevent or reduce the severity of varicella infections.

INDICATIONS & DOSAGE

Passive immunization of susceptible immunodeficient patients after exposure to varicella (chicken pox or herpes zoster) –
Children to 10 kg: 125 units I.M.
Children 10.1 to 20 kg: 250 units I.M.
Children 20.1 to 30 kg: 375 units I.M.
Children 30.1 to 40 kg: 500 units I.M.
Adults and children over 40 kg: 625 units I.M.

CONTRAINDICATIONS & PRECAUTIONS

Use cautiously in patients with hypersensitivity to thimerosal, a component of this immune serum.

ADVERSE REACTIONS

Common reactions are in italics; life-threatening reactions are in bold italics.
Systemic: gastrointestinal distress, malaise, headache, ***respiratory distress, anaphylaxis.***
Local: discomfort at injection site, rash.

INTERACTIONS

Live virus vaccines: may interfere with response. Defer vaccination for 3 months after administration of VZIG.

EFFECTS ON DIAGNOSTIC TESTS

None reported.

NURSING CONSIDERATIONS

Besides those related universally to drug therapy (see "How to use this book"), consider the following specific recommendations:

Assessment
- Obtain a baseline assessment of the patient's allergies and immunization reaction before therapy.
- Be alert for adverse reactions and drug interactions throughout therapy.
- Evaluate the patient's and family's knowledge about varicella-zoster immune globulin.

Nursing Diagnoses
- Altered protection related to lack of immunity to varicella-zoster virus.
- Altered nutrition: Less than body requirements related to immunization-induced GI distress.
- Knowledge deficit related to varicella-zoster immune globulin immunization.

Planning and Implementation
Preparation and Administration
- Store vial in refrigerator.
- ***I.M. use:*** Administer by deep I.M. injection only. Do not give I.V.
- Give as soon as possible after presumed exposure for maximum benefit.

Monitoring
- Monitor effectiveness by checking the patient's antibody titers.
- Observe the patient for signs of anaphylaxis immediately after injection.
- Check vital signs.

Supportive Care
- Keep epinepherine 1:1000 available in case of anaphylaxis. Have oxygen and resuscitation equipment nearby.
- Obtain order for medication to relieve immunization-induced headache and GI distress.
- Encourage patient to have small, frequent, bland meals as tolerated.
- Do not give to patients with a his-

tory of severe reaction to human immune serum globulin or sever thrombocytopenia.
• VZIG is not recommended for nonimmunosuppressed patients.
• Administer VZIG carefully and with discretion because supplies are limited.
• Although usually restricted to children under 15 years, VZIG may be administered to adolescents and adults if necessary.
• Not commercially distributed. Available only from 20 regional distribution centers throughout the United States. These centers will distribute to Canada and overseas. Call the Centers for Disease Control for the distribution center in your area: Monday to Friday, 8 a.m. to 4:30 p.m. (EST), (404) 329-3670; weekends, nights, and holidays (emergencies only), (404) 329-2888.

Patient Teaching
• Tell the patient that it is important to administer the drug as soon as possible after presumed exposure to permit development of immunity.
• Explain that in most cases this drug's use in restricted to children under 15 years.

Evaluation
In patients receiving varicella-zoster immune globulin (VZIG), appropriate evaluation statements may include:
• Patient develops immunity to varicella-zoster virus.
• Patient did not develop GI disorders.
• Patient and family state an understanding of varicella-zoster immune globulin therapy.

vasopressin (antidiuretic hormone)
(vay soe press´ in)
Pitressin

vasopressin tannate
Pitressin Tannate

• *Classification:* antidiuretic hormone, peristaltic stimulant, hemostatic agent (posterior pituitary hormone)
• *Pregnancy Risk Category:* B

HOW SUPPLIED
vasopressin
Injection: 0.5-ml and 1-ml ampules, 20 units/ml
vasopressin tannate
Injection: 1-ml ampules, 5 units/ml

ACTION
Mechanism: Promotes reabsorption of water through the renal tubular epithelium and produces a concentrated urine (antidiuretic hormone effect).
Absorption: Because drug is destroyed by trypsin in the GI tract, it must be administered intranasally or parenterally.
Distribution: Throughout the extracellular fluid, with no evidence of protein-binding.
Metabolism: Most of a dose is destroyed rapidly in the liver and kidneys.
Excretion: Approximately 5% is excreted unchanged in urine after 4 hours. Half-life: 10 to 20 minutes.
Onset, peak, duration: Duration of action after I.M. or S.C. administration is 2 to 8 hours.

INDICATIONS & DOSAGE
Nonnephrogenic, nonpsychogenic diabetes insipidus–
Adults: 5 to 10 units I.M. or S.C. b.i.d. to q.i.d., p.r.n.; or intranasally (aqueous solution used as spray or applied to cotton balls) in individualized doses, based on response. For chronic therapy, inject 2.5 to 5 units Pitressin Tannate in oil suspension I.M. or S.C. q 2 to 3 days.
Children: 2.5 to 10 units I.M. or S.C. b.i.d. to q.i.d., p.r.n.; or intranasally

(aqueous solution used as spray or applied to cotton balls) in individualized doses. For chronic therapy, inject 1.25 to 2.5 units Pitressin Tannate in oil suspension I.M. or S.C. q 2 to 3 days.
Postoperative abdominal distention–
Adults: 5 units (aqueous) I.M. initially, then q 3 to 4 hours, increasing dose to 10 units, if needed. Reduce dose proportionately for children.
To expel gas before abdominal X-ray–
Adults: inject 10 units S.C. at 2 hours, then again at 30 minutes before X-ray. Enema before first dose may also help to eliminate gas.
Upper GI tract hemorrhage–
Adults: 0.2 to 0.4 units/minute by intraarterial injection. Do not use tannate in oil suspension.

CONTRAINDICATIONS & PRECAUTIONS

Contraindicated in patients with chronic nephritis accompanied by nitrogen retention or hypersensitivity to the drug. Use cautiously in patients with seizure disorders, migraines, asthma, or heart failure (because rapid addition of extracellular water may be hazardous) and in those with vascular disease, angina pectoris, coronary thrombosis, or arteriosclerosis (because large doses may precipitate myocardial infarction). Preoperative and postoperative polyuric patients may have considerably reduced hormone requirements.

ADVERSE REACTIONS

Common reactions are in italics; life-threatening reactions are in bold italics.
CNS: tremor, dizziness, headache.
CV: *angina in patients with vascular disease,* vasoconstriction. Large doses may cause hypertension, electrocardiographic changes. ***(With intra-arterial infusion: bradycardia, cardiac arrhythmias, pulmonary edema.)***
GI: abdominal cramps, nausea, vomiting, diarrhea, intestinal hyperactivity.
GU: uterine cramps, anuria.
Skin: circumoral pallor.
Other: water intoxication (drowsiness, listlessness, headache, confusion, weight gain), hypersensitivity reactions (urticaria, angioneurotic edema, bronchoconstriction, fever, rash, wheezing, dyspnea, ***anaphylaxis),*** sweating.

INTERACTIONS

Chlorpropamide: increased antidiuretic response. Use together cautiously.
Lithium, demeclocycline: reduced antidiuretic activity. Use together cautiously.

EFFECTS ON DIAGNOSTIC TESTS

None reported.

NURSING CONSIDERATIONS

Besides those related universally to drug therapy (see "How to use this book"), consider the following specific recommendations:

Assessment
- Obtain a baseline assessment of the patient's underlying condition before initiating vasopressin therapy.
- Be alert for adverse reactions and drug interactions throughout therapy.
- Evaluate the patient's and family's knowledge about vasopressin therapy.

Nursing Diagnoses
- Fluid volume deficit related to a compromised regulatory system causing excretion of large volumes of urine.
- Pain related to vasopressin-induced angina in patients with vascular disease.
- Knowledge deficit related to vasopressin therapy.

Planning and Implementation
Preparation and Administration
- Check expiration date before administering.

• Never inject drug during first stage of labor; may cause ruptured uterus.
• ***I.M. use:*** Place tannate in oil in warm water for 10 to 15 minutes. Then shake thoroughly to make suspension uniform before withdrawing I.M. injection dose. Small brown particles must be seen in suspension. Use absolutely dry syringe to avoid dilution.
• Rotate both S.C. and I.M. injection sites to prevent tissue damage.
• Give with one to two glasses of water, if appropriate to reduce adverse reactions and to improve therapeutic response.

Monitoring
• Monitor effectiveness by regularly monitoring the patient's intake and output, serum and urine osmolality, and urine specific gravity for treatment of diabetes insipidus or alleviation of symptoms of other disorders.
• Monitor for early signs of water intoxication (drowsiness, listlessness, headache, confusion, anuria, and weight gain) to prevent seizures, coma, and death. Overhydration more likely with long-acting tannate oil suspension than with aqueous vasopressin solution.
• Monitor the patient's weight daily and observe for edema.
• Monitor patient's blood pressure on vasopressin twice daily. Watch for excessively elevated blood pressure or lack of response to drug, which may be indicated by hypotension.

Supportive Care
• Adjust the patient's fluid intake to reduce risk of water intoxication and of sodium depletion, especially in young or elderly patients.
• Overdose may cause oxytocic or vasopressor activity. Withhold drug as prescribed until effects subside.
• Administer a mild analgesic for drug-induced headache, if not contraindicated.
• Offer patient ice chips or frequent sips of water if nausea occurs. If nausea persists or becomes severe, obtain an order for an antiemetic.
• Be aware that a rectal tube will facilitate gas expulsion following vasopressin injection.

Patient Teaching
• Teach patient how to administer drug.
• Emphasize that the patient should not increase or decrease dosage unless instructed by doctor.
• Review fluid intake measurement and methods for measuring fluid output with patient.
• Tell the patient to contact doctor if signs of water intoxication (drowsiness, listlessness, headache, or shortness of breath) develop.
• Advise the patient to wear medical alert identification.
• Teach patients to rotate injection sites to prevent tissue damage.

Evaluation
In patients receiving vasopressin, appropriate evaluation statements may include:
• Patient achieves normal fluid and electrolyte balance.
• Patient with vascular disease does not experience angina.
• Patient and family state an understanding of vasopressin therapy.

vecuronium bromide
(ve kyoo´ roe ni um)
Norcuron

• *Classification:* skeletal muscle relaxant (nondepolarizing neuromuscular blocking agent)
• *Pregnancy Risk Category:* C

HOW SUPPLIED
Injection: 10 mg/vial

ACTION
Mechanism: Prevents acetylcholine from binding to the receptors on the

muscle end plate, thus blocking depolarization. Nondepolarizing agent.
Distribution: After I.V. administration, distributed in extracellular fluid and rapidly reaches its site of action. It is 60% to 90% plasma protein-bound. The volume of distribution is decreased in children under age 1 and may be decreased in elderly patients.
Metabolism: Undergoes rapid and extensive hepatic metabolism.
Excretion: Drug and metabolites appear to be primarily excreted in feces by biliary elimination; drug and its metabolites are also excreted in urine. Half-life: Terminal elimination half-life ranges from 31 to 60 minutes.
Onset, peak, duration: After I.V. administration, onset of action occurs within 1 minute; action peaks at 3 to 5 minutes. The duration is about 25 to 40 minutes depending on anesthetic used, dose, and number of doses given.

INDICATIONS & DOSAGE

Adjunct to general anesthesia, to facilitate endotracheal intubation and to provide skeletal muscle relaxation during surgery or mechanical ventilation–
Dosage depends on anesthetic used, individual needs, and response. Dosages are representative and must be adjusted.
Adults and children over 9 years: Initially, 0.08 to 0.10 mg/kg I.V. bolus. Maintenance doses of 0.010 to 0.015 mg/kg within 25 to 40 minutes of initial dose should be administered during prolonged surgical procedures. Maintenance doses may be given q 12 to 15 minutes in patients receiving balanced anesthesia.

Children under 10 years may require a slightly higher initial dose and may also require supplementation slightly more often than adults.

CONTRAINDICATIONS & PRECAUTIONS

Contraindicated in patients with hypersensitivity to the drug. Administer with extreme caution to patients with myasthenia gravis, neuromuscular diseases, or bronchogenic carcinoma because of the potential for prolonged neuromuscular blockade; and to patients with severe electrolyte disorders or dehydration. Administer cautiously to elderly or debilitated patients; patients with cardiovascular, hepatic, pulmonary, or renal function impairment; or in pregnant women receiving magnesium sulfate because lower doses may be required. In severely obese patients, maintenance of airway and ventilation support may require special attention.

ADVERSE REACTIONS

Common reactions are in italics; life-threatening reactions are in bold italics.
CV: transient increases in heart rate.
Local: redness, itching, induration.
Other: ***prolonged dose-related apnea.***

INTERACTIONS

Aminoglycoside antibiotics (including amikacin, gentamicin, kanamycin, neomycin, streptomycin); polymyxin antibiotics (polymyxin B sulfate, colistin); clindamycin; quinidine; general anesthetics (such as halothane, enflurane, isoflurane): potentiated neuromuscular blockade, leading to increased skeletal muscle relaxation and possible respiratory paralysis. Use cautiously during surgical and postoperative periods.
Narcotic analgesics: potentiated neuromuscular blockade, leading to increased skeletal muscle relaxation and possible respiratory paralysis. Use with extreme caution, and reduce dose of vecuronium.

EFFECTS ON DIAGNOSTIC TESTS

None significant.

NURSING CONSIDERATIONS

Besides those related universally to drug therapy (see "How to use this book"), consider the following specific recommendations:

Assessment

- Obtain a baseline assessment of skeletal muscle function and respiratory pattern before drug therapy.
- Be alert for adverse reactions and drug interactions throughout therapy.
- Evaluate the patient's and family's knowledge about vecuronium bromide therapy.

Nursing Diagnoses

- Ineffective breathing pattern related to the patient's underlying condition.
- Impaired verbal communication related to drug-induced paralysis.
- Knowledge deficit related to vecuronium therapy.

Planning and Implementation

Preparation and Administration

- Vecuronium should be administered only by personnel experienced in airway management.
- Have emergency respiratory support equipment (endotracheal equipment, ventilator, oxygen, atropine, edrophonium, epinephrine, and neostigmine) on hand before administration.
- Store in refrigerator. Discard after 24 hours.
- Usually administered together with a cholinergic blocker (such as atropine or glycopyrrolate).
- ***I.V. use:*** Intermittent infusion is not recommended.
- Vecuronium provides conditions for intubation within 2½ to 3 minutes. The duration of effect is 25 to 40 minutes.

Monitoring

- Monitor effectiveness by regularly checking relaxation state of the patient's skeletal muscles; close observation of the patient is mandatory.
- Monitor respirations and respiratory status closely until patient recovers fully from neuromuscular blockade, as evidenced by tests of muscle strength (hand grip, head lift, and ability to cough).
- Monitor for drug interactions and adverse reactions by frequently checking the patient's vital signs for transient increases in heart rate.
- Know that the drug is well tolerated in renal failure.
- Know that unlike other nodepolarizing neuromuscular blockers, vecuronium has no effect on the cardiovascular system. Also, the drug causes no histamine release and therefore no histamine-related hypersensitivity reactions such as bronchospasm, hypertension, or tachycardia.
- Remember that prior administration of succinylcholine may enhance the neuromuscular blocking effect and duration of action.

Supportive Care

- Maintain adequate ventilation through respiratory support equipment throughout drug therapy and provide pulmonary care as indicated.
- Once spontaneous recovery starts, vecuronium-induced neuromuscular blockade may be reversed with an anticholinesterase agent (such as neostigmine or edrophonium).
- Provide emotional support for the intubated patient who is awake.
- Administer pain medication on regular basis (as condition dictates) because the patient will be unable to communicate that pain is present.
- Anticipate the patient's needs and try to meet them. Explain everything thoroughly before performing any procedure. Use nonverbal communication, especially eye contact.
- Protect the patient from injury when moving him in bed.
- Provide eye care since blink reflex will be absent.

Patient Teaching

- Reassure the patient that necessary pain management will be provided regularly.
- Inform the patient that drug-induced paralysis will inhibit his abil-

ity to communicate but that he will receive continuous monitoring and care.

• Reassure the patient that as soon as the need for neuromuscular blockade is no longer necessary, the drug-induced paralysis will be reversed.

Evaluation

In patients receiving vecuronium, appropriate evaluation statements may include:

• Patient maintains adequate ventilation.

• Patient's basic needs are anticipated and met.

• Patient and family state an understanding of vecuronium therapy.

verapamil hydrochloride

(ver ap´ a mill)

Calan, Calan SR, Cordilox Oral‡, Isoptin, Isoptin SR, Veradil‡

• *Classification:* antianginal, antihypertensive, antiarrhythmic (calcium channel blocker)

• *Pregnancy Risk Category:* C

HOW SUPPLIED

Tablets: 40 mg, 80 mg, 120 mg

Tablets (sustained-release): 240 mg

Injection: 2.5 mg/ml

ACTION

Mechanism: Inhibits calcium ion influx across cardiac and smooth muscle cells, thus decreasing myocardial contractility and oxygen demand, and dilates coronary arteries and arterioles.

Absorption: Rapidly and completely absorbed from the GI tract after oral administration; however, only about 20% to 35% of the drug reaches systemic circulation because of first-pass effect.

Distribution: Steady-state distribution volume in healthy adults ranges from about 4.5 to 7 liters/kg but may increase to 12 liters/kg in patients with hepatic cirrhosis. Approximately 90% of circulating drug is bound to plasma proteins.

Metabolism: Hepatic.

Excretion: In the urine as unchanged drug and active metabolites. Half-life: Elimination half-life is normally 6 to 12 hours and increases to 16 hours in hepatic cirrhosis. In infants, elimination half-life may be 5 to 7 hours.

Onset, peak, duration: When administered I.V., effects occur within minutes after injection and usually persist for 30 to 60 minutes (possibly up to 6 hours). Therapeutic serum levels are 80 to 300 ng/ml.

INDICATIONS & DOSAGE

Management of vasospastic (also called Prinzmetal's or variant) angina and classic chronic, stable angina pectoris; chronic atrial fibrillation–

Adults: starting dose is 80 mg P.O. t.i.d. or q.i.d. Dosage may be increased at weekly intervals. Some patients may require up to 480 mg daily.

Treatment of supraventricular arrhythmias–

Adults: 0.075 to 0.15 mg/kg (5 to 10 mg) I.V. push over 2 minutes with ECG and blood pressure monitoring. Repeat dose in 30 minutes if no response.

Children 1 to 15 years: 0.1 to 0.3 mg/kg as I.V. bolus over 2 minutes.

Children less than 1 year: 0.1 to 0.2 mg/kg as I.V. bolus over 2 minutes under continuous ECG monitoring.

Dose can be repeated in 30 minutes if no response.

Migraine headache prophylaxis–

Adults: 80 mg P.O. q.i.d.

Treatment of hypertension–

Adults: 240-mg sustained-release tablet once daily in the morning. If response is not adequate, may give an additional half tablet in the evening or one tablet q 12 hours. Alternatively, may give 80-mg immediate-release tablet t.i.d. or q.i.d.

CONTRAINDICATIONS & PRECAUTIONS

Contraindicated in patients with severe hypotension (systolic blood pressure below 90 mm Hg) or cardiogenic shock, because of the drug's hypotensive effect; second- or third-degree AV block or sick sinus syndrome (unless a functioning artificial ventricular pacemaker is in place), because of the drug's effects on the cardiac conduction system; severe left ventricular dysfunction (indicated by pulmonary wedge pressure above 20 mm Hg and left ventricular ejection fraction below 20%), unless heart failure results from supraventricular tachycardia, because the drug may worsen the condition; ventricular dysfunction or AV abnormalities in patients who are receiving beta-adrenergic blockers, because of the drug's negative inotropic effect and inhibition of the cardiac conduction system; and hypersensitivity to the drug.

Use with caution in patients with moderately severe ventricular dysfunction or heart failure, because the drug may precipitate or worsen the condition; hypertrophic cardiomyopathy, because the drug may cause serious and sometimes fatal adverse cardiovascular effects (such as pulmonary edema, hypotension, heart block, or sinus arrest); hepatic or renal impairment, because the drug may accumulate (generally, the dose should be reduced and the patient carefully monitored); sick sinus syndrome or atrial flutter or fibrillation with an accessory bypass tract (such as Wolff-Parkinson-White or Lown-Ganong-Levine syndrome), because the drug may precipitate life-threatening adverse effects (for example, ventricular fibrillation or cardiac arrest); or wide-complex ventricular tachycardia, because the drug may cause marked hemodynamic deterioration and ventricular fibrillation; and in those patients receiving the drug I.V., because of possible adverse hemodynamic effects (hypotension) and adverse ECG effects (such as bradycardia and heart block).

ADVERSE REACTIONS

Common reactions are in italics; life-threatening reactions are in bold italics.
CNS: dizziness, headache, fatigue.
CV: *transient hypotension,* ***CHF,*** bradycardia, AV block, ***ventricular asystole,*** peripheral edema.
GI: *constipation,* nausea (primarily from oral form).
Hepatic: elevated liver enzymes.

INTERACTIONS

Carbamazepine, digitalis glycosides: verapamil may increase the serum levels of these drugs. Monitor patient for toxicity.
Lithium: verapamil may decrease serum lithium levels. Monitor patient closely.
Propranolol (and other beta blockers, including ophthalmic timolol), disopyramide: may cause heart failure. Use together cautiously.
Quinidine, antihypertensives: may result in hypotension. Monitor blood pressure.
Rifampin: may decrease oral bioavailability of verapamil. Monitor patient for lack of effect.

EFFECTS ON DIAGNOSTIC TESTS

None reported.

NURSING CONSIDERATIONS

Besides those related universally to drug therapy (see "How to use this book"), consider the following specific recommendations:

Assessment

- Obtain a baseline assessment of the patient's angina status before verapamil therapy.
- Be alert for adverse reactions and

*Liquid form contains alcohol. **May contain tartrazine.

drug interactions throughout verapamil therapy.
• Evaluate the patient's and family's knowledge about verapamil therapy.
Nursing Diagnoses
• Pain related to ineffectiveness of verapamil therapy.
• Altered tissue perfusion (cerebral) related to adverse reactions to therapy.
• Knowledge deficit related to verapamil.
Planning and Implementation
Preparation and Administration
• Expect patients with severely compromised cardiac function or those receiving beta blockers to receive a lower dose of verapamil.
• ***P.O. use:*** Administer extended-release tablets on an empty stomach. Taking extended-release tablets with food may decrease rate and extent of absorption.
• ***I.V. use:*** Administer undiluted drug at a rate of 5 to 10 mg over at least 2 minutes. Inject directly into vein or into an I.V. line containing a free-flowing compatible solution. In elderly patients, give over at least 3 minutes to reduce adverse effects.
Monitoring
• Monitor effectiveness by regularly evaluating pain relief obtained by patient.
• Monitor blood pressure and ECG regularly.
• Monitor liver function studies during prolonged treatment.
Supportive Care
• Notify the doctor if pain relief is not obtained with verapamil therapy.
• Institute safety precautions if CNS reactions or hypotension occurs.
• Keep emergency equipment nearby and be prepared to treat arrhythmias such as AV block or ventricular asystole.
• Encourage patient to increase fiber content of diet (if not contraindicated) to prevent constipation, or obtain an order for a laxative if constipation occurs.
• Assist the patient with daily activities if fatigue occurs.
• Obtain an order for a mild analgesic if a headache occurs.
Patient Teaching
• Stress importance of taking the drug exactly as prescribed even when feeling well.
• Tell the patient to schedule activities to allow adequate rest if fatigue becomes troublesome.
• Explain to the patient that if verapamil is being used to terminate a supraventricualr tachycardia, the doctor may instruct the patient to perform vagal maneuvers after receiving the drug.
• If the patient continues nitrate therapy during titration of oral verapamil dosage, urge continued compliance. Sublingual nitroglycerin, especially, may be taken as needed when anginal symptoms are acute.
• Warn the patient to avoid hazardous activities that require alertness if adverse CNS effects occur.
• Instruct patient to increase dietary fiber content and fluid (if not contraindicated) to prevent constipation.
Evaluation
In patients receiving verapamil, appropriate evaluation statements may include:
• Patient states anginal pain is relieved with verapamil therapy.
• Patient maintains adequate cerebral tissue perfusion throughout verapamil therapy.
• Patient and family state an understanding of verapamil therapy.

vidarabine
(vye dare´ a been)
Vira-A Ophthalmic

• *Classification:* antiviral (purine nucleoside)

• *Pregnancy Risk Category:* C

HOW SUPPLIED

Ophthalmic ointment: 3% in 3.5-g tube (equivalent to 2.8% vidarabine)

ACTION

Mechanism: A purine nucleoside that blocks viral DNA synthesis, probably by blocking the enzyme DNA polymerase.
Absorption: After topical ophthalmic administration, systemic absorption is not expected to occur.
Distribution: Trace amounts of the drug and its major metabolite can be found in the aqueous humor.
Metabolism: Rapidly deaminated within the cornea to ara-hypoxanthine, which has less antiviral activity.

INDICATIONS & DOSAGE

Acute keratoconjunctivitis, superficial keratitis, and recurrent epithelial keratitis resulting from herpes simplex types I and II–
Adults and children: instill ½" ointment into lower conjunctival sac 5 times daily at 3-hour intervals.

CONTRAINDICATIONS & PRECAUTIONS

Contraindicated in patients with hypersensitivity to the drug. Use cautiously in patients with hepatic or renal dysfunction because they may be more susceptible to dose-related adverse reactions, and in patients with restricted fluid intake because they may not tolerate the large fluid volumes needed for drug administration.

ADVERSE REACTIONS

Common reactions are in italics; life-threatening reactions are in bold italics.
Eye: temporary burning, itching, mild irritation, pain, lacrimation, foreign body sensation, conjunctival injection, superficial punctate keratitis, photophobia.
Other: hypersensitivity.

INTERACTIONS

None significant.

EFFECTS ON DIAGNOSTIC TESTS

Leukocytes, platelet count, reticulocyte count, hemoglobin and hematocrit levels: decreased values.
Serum bilirubin and AST (SGOT): levels may increase.

NURSING CONSIDERATIONS

Besides those related universally to drug therapy (see "How to use this book"), consider the following specific recommendations:

Assessment

• Obtain a baseline assessment of the patient's allergies before therapy.
• Be alert for adverse reactions and drug interactions throughout therapy.
• Evaluate the patient's and family's knowledge about vidarabine therapy.

Nursing Diagnoses

• Altered protection related to ocular infection.
• Pain related to burning and irritation induced by vidarabine instillation.
• Knowledge deficit related to vidarabine therapy.

Planning and Implementation

Preparation and Administration

• Store in tightly sealed, light-resistant container.
• Wash hands before and after administration.
• Clean excess exudate from eye area before administration.
• Do not give for longer tham 21 days, or 3 to 5 days after healing.

Monitoring

• Monitor effectiveness by culturing the eye to check for microorganism.
• Observe amount, color, and consistency of exudate.
• Monitor for signs of hypersensitivity.

Supportive Care
• Apply warm, moist compresses to eye area to aid in removal of dried exudate.
• Continue vidarabine therapy for several days after steroid therapy.
• Not effective against RNA virus, adenoviral ocular infection, or bacterial, fungal, or chlamydial infections.
Patient Teaching
• Warn patient not to exceed recommended frequency or duration of dosage.
• Teach the patient to instill. Advise him to wash hands before and after administration. Avoid touching the tip of the applicator to the eye or surrounding tissue.
• Instruct him to apply light finger pressure to the lacrimal sac for 1 minute after instillation. Caution him to avoid scratching or rubbing the eye area.
• Warn the patient not to share towels and washcloths with family members during infection.
• Instruct the patient not to share eye medications with family members. A family member who develops the same symptoms should contact the doctor.
Evaluation
In patients receiving vidarabine, appropriate evaluation statements may include:
• Patient remains free from signs and symptoms of infection.
• Patient reports decrease in or absence of pain induced by instillation.
• Patient and family state an understanding of vidarabine therapy.

vidarabine monohydrate (adenine arabinoside, ara-A)
(vye dare´ a been)
Vira-A

• *Classification:* antiviral (purine nucleoside)
• *Pregnancy Risk Category:* C

HOW SUPPLIED
Concentrate for I.V. infusion:
200 mg/ml in 5-ml vial (equivalent to 187.4 mg vidarabine)

ACTION
Mechanism: Becomes incorporated into viral DNA and inhibits viral multiplication.
Absorption: Poorly absorbed poorly when administered orally, I.M. or S.C. and must be given I.V.
Distribution: Vidarabine and arabinosyl-hypoxanthine (ara-Hx), its active metabolite, are distributed widely in body tissues and fluids. CSF concentration equals about 30% of serum levels. Parent compound is 20% to 30% plasma protein-bound; arabinosyl-hypoxanthine is 1% to 3% plasma protein-bound.
Metabolism: Most (75% to 87%) of a dose of vidarabine is rapidly deaminated to the active metabolite, ara-Hx.
Excretion: Within 24 hours, 1% to 3% of the drug appears in the urine as parent drug and 41% to 53% as ara-Hx. Half-life: Half-lives of parent compound and active metabolite are 1½ and 3½ hours, respectively.
Onset, peak, duration: In adults peak ara-Hx and vidarabine plasma levels ranging from 3 to 6 mcg/ml and 0.2 to 0.4 mcg/ml, respectively, are attained after slow intravenous infusion of vira-A doses of 10 mg/kg of body weight.

INDICATIONS & DOSAGE
Herpes simplex virus encephalitis–
Adults and children: (including neonates): 15 mg/kg I.V. daily for 10 days. Slowly infuse the total daily dose by I.V. infusion at a constant rate over 12- to 24-hour period. Avoid rapid or bolus injection.

CONTRAINDICATIONS & PRECAUTIONS

Contraindicated in patients with hypersensitivity to the drug. Administer cautiously to patients with hepatic or renal dysfunction because they may be more susceptible to dose-related adverse effects, and to patients with restricted fluid intake because they may not tolerate the large fluid volumes needed for drug administration.

ADVERSE REACTIONS

Common reactions are in italics; life-threatening reactions are in bold italics.
Blood: anemia, neutropenia, ***thrombocytopenia.***
CNS: tremor, dizziness, hallucinations, confusion, psychosis, ataxia.
GI: *anorexia, nausea,* vomiting, diarrhea.
Hepatic: elevated AST (SGOT), bilirubin.
Skin: pruritus, rash.
Local: pain at injection site.
Other: weight loss.

INTERACTIONS

Allopurinol: concurrent therapy reduces metabolism of vidarabine and increases risk of CNS adverse effects.

EFFECTS ON DIAGNOSTIC TESTS

AST (SGOT) and serum bilirubin: may increase levels.
CBC: decreased leukocytes, platelets, and reticulocytes.
Hemoglobin and hematocrit: decreased values.

NURSING CONSIDERATIONS

Besides those related universally to drug therapy (see "How to use this book"), consider the following specific recommendations:

Assessment
- Obtain a baseline assessment of infection before therapy.
- Be alert for adverse reactions and drug interactions throughout therapy.
- Evaluate the patient's and family's knowledge about vidarabine therapy.

Nursing Diagnoses
- High risk for injury related to ineffectiveness of vidarabine to eradicate the infection.
- High risk for fluid volume deficit related to vidarabine-induced adverse GI reactions.
- Knowledge deficit related to vidarabine therapy.

Planning and Implementation

Preparation and Administration
- Be aware that patients with renal impairment may need dosage adjustment.
- ***I.V. use:*** Must be diluted to a concentration of less than 0.5 mg/ml. Any I.V. solution is suitable as a diluent. Administer with an I.V. filter of 0.45 μm or smaller and an infusion pump. Infuse the diluted daily dose over 12 to 24 hours.
- Once in solution, vidarabine is stable at room temperature for at least 2 weeks.

Monitoring
- Monitor effectiveness by regularly assessing for improvement in the infection.
- Monitor hematologic tests, such as hemoglobin, hematocrit, WBC, and platelets during therapy. Also monitor renal and liver function studies.
- Monitor hydration status if adverse GI reactions occur.

Supportive Care
- Obtain an order for an antiemetic or antidiarrheal agent as needed.
- Institute safety precautions if adverse CNS reactions occur.

Patient Teaching
- Advise patient to tell the nurse promptly about pain or discomfort at the I.V. site.

Evaluation

In patients receiving vidarabine, appropriate evaluation statements may include:
- Patient is free of infection.

• Patient's maintains adequate hydration throughout therapy.
• Patient and family state an understanding of vidarabine therapy.

vinblastine sulfate (VLB)

(vin blas´ teen)

Alkaban-AQ, Velban, Velbe†‡, Velsar

• *Classification:* antineoplastic (vinca alkaloid)
• *Pregnancy Risk Category:* D

HOW SUPPLIED

Injection: 10-mg vials (lyophilized powder), 10-mg/10-ml vials

ACTION

Mechanism: A vinca alkaloid that arrests mitosis in metaphase, blocking cell division. Binds to or crystallizes critical microtubule proteins of the mitotic spindle.
Absorption: Unpredictably absorbed from the GI tract; usually given I.V.
Distribution: Widely distributed into body tissues. The drug crosses the blood-brain barrier but does not achieve therapeutic concentrations in the CSF.
Metabolism: Partially metabolized in the liver to desacetylvinblastine, which is more active than the parent compound.
Excretion: Primarily in feces via the bile as unchanged drug. A smaller portion is excreted in urine. Half-life: Elimination is triphasic, with half-lives of 35 minutes, 53 minutes, and 19 hours for the alpha, beta, and terminal phases, respectively.

INDICATIONS & DOSAGE

Breast or testicular cancer, Hodgkin's and non-Hodgkin's lymphomas, choriocarcinoma, lymphosarcoma, neuroblastoma, mycosis fungoides, histiocytosis–
Adults and children: 0.1 mg/kg or 3.7 mg/m² I.V. weekly or q 2 weeks. May be increased to maximum dosage (adults) of 0.5 mg/kg or 18.5 mg/m² I.V. weekly according to response. Dosage should not be repeated if WBC less than 4,000/mm³.

CONTRAINDICATIONS & PRECAUTIONS

Contraindicated in patients with severe leukopenia or bacterial infections because treatment with myelosuppressive drugs such as vinblastine causes an increased frequency of infections. Instruct patients to report any symptoms of sore throat and fever and of unusual bruising or bleeding. Leukocyte, erythrocyte, and platelet counts, and hemoglobin should be monitored weekly during therapy. Vinblastine can impair fertility; aspermia has occurred after treatment with vinblastine.

ADVERSE REACTIONS

Common reactions are in italics; life-threatening reactions are in bold italics.
Blood: *leukopenia* (nadir days 4 to 10 and lasts another 7 to 14 days), ***thrombocytopenia.***
CNS: depression, *paresthesias, peripheral neuropathy and neuritis, numbness, loss of deep tendon reflexes, muscle pain and weakness.*
CV: hypertension.
EENT: pharyngitis.
GI: *nausea, vomiting, stomatitis,* ulcer and bleeding, *constipation, ileus, anorexia, weight loss,* abdominal pain.
GU: oligospermia, aspermia, urine retention.
Skin: dermatitis, vesiculation.
Local: *irritation, phlebitis,* cellulitis, necrosis if I.V. extravasates.
Other: ***acute bronchospasm,*** reversible alopecia in 5% to 10% of patients, *pain in tumor site,* low fever.

INTERACTIONS

Mitomycin: increased risk of bronchospasm and shortness of breath.

Phenytoin: decreased plasma phenytoin levels.

EFFECTS ON DIAGNOSTIC TESTS

Blood and urine: increased uric acid concentrations.

NURSING CONSIDERATIONS

Besides those related universally to drug therapy (see "How to use this book"), consider the following specific recommendations:

Assessment

• Obtain baseline assessment of the patient's underlying condition before initiating therapy.
• Be alert for adverse reactions and drug interactions throughout therapy.
• Evaluate the patient's and family's knowledge about vinblastine therapy.

Nursing Diagnoses

• High risk for impaired skin integrity related to adverse drug reactions.
• Body image disturbance related to adverse drug reactions.
• Knowledge deficit related to vinblastine therapy.

Planning and Implementation

Preparation and Administration

• Read order and drug label carefully before administration of drug. Use extreme caution to avoid confusing vinblastine with vincristine.
• Exercise caution when preparing and administering this drug to avoid mutagenic, teratogenic, and carcinogenic risks. Use a biological containment cabinet, gloves, and mask and avoid contaminating work surfaces.
• Reconstitute 5-mg vial with 5 ml sterile sodium chloride injection. This yields 1 mg/ml. Maximum single dose is 2 mg. Refrigerate all vials.
• Label all syringes containing vincristine "FOR I.V. USE ONLY." Never give vinblastine I.M. or S.C.
• Check I.V. site and patency of line before administration.
• ***I.V. use:*** Drug may be injected directly into a vein or into a running I.V. infusion slowly over 1 minute or may also be added to 50 ml of dextrose 5% in water or 0.9% sodium chloride solution and infused over 15 minutes.

Monitoring

• Monitor effectiveness by noting the results of follow-up diagnostic tests and overall physical status by regularly checking CBC and differential, and tumor size and rate of growth with appropriate studies.
• Monitor for the effectiveness of drug therapy by frequently checking CBC and differential, and tumor size and rate of growth with appropriate studies.
• Monitor for presence of petechiae, epistaxis, melena, or hematuria if platelet count drops.
• Monitor respiratory status; be alert for life-threatening bronchospasm. This reaction is most likely to occur in patients also receiving mitomycin.
• Monitor bowel sounds regularly; monitor bowel function.
• Monitor urine output, noting decreased or absent urine flow suggestive of urine retention.
• Monitor for depression of Achilles tendon reflex, numbness, tingling, footdrop or wristdrop, difficulty in walking alone, slapping gait, or difficulty walking on heels. Neurotoxicity is less than with vincristine therapy.
• Monitor weight, nutritional status, and hydration status if GI adverse reactions occur.
• Monitor the injection site for possible extravasation.

Supportive Care

• Administer an antiemetic, as ordered, if the patient develops nausea.
• Give stool softeners or laxatives, if necessary.
• Be prepared to discontinue drug and notify doctor if serious adverse reactions occur.
• If infiltration of I.V. results in extravasation of vinblastine, stop infusion, apply ice packs to the site every 2 hours for 24 hours, and notify doc-

tor. Be prepared to dilute the drug with 0.9% sodium chloride injection and/or local injection of hydrocortisone. However, some doctors prefer a local injection of hyaluronidase and mild heat.

- Provide a private room and reverse isolation for patients with compromised immune systems.
- Institute safety precautions to minimize risk of injury due to impaired mobility and sensory alterations.
- Provide frequent mouth care. Use a soft toothbrush and mild mouthwash to avoid injury to oral mucous membranes.
- Provide assistance with ambulation.
- Administer an antiemetic as needed.
- Provide emotional support and opportunities for the patient to express fears and concerns.

Patient Teaching

- Advise the patient that burning or stinging at I.V. site during administration is common.
- Advise the patient that alopecia may occur, but is usually reversible.
- Instruct patient about need for protective measures, including conservation of energy, balanced diet, adequate rest, personal cleanliness, clean environment, avoidance of exposure to persons with infections, and using support while walking to avoid risk of injury due to falls.
- Encourage adequate fluid intake to increase urine output.

Evaluation

In patients receiving vinblastine, appropriate evaluation statements may include:

- Patient does not develop impaired skin intergity from drug-induced extravasation.
- Patient states feelings about changes in body image and demonstrates coping behaviors.
- Patient and family state an understanding of vinblastine therapy.

vincristine sulfate

(vin kris´ teen)
Oncovin, Vincasar PFS

- *Classification:* antineoplastic (vinca alkaloid)
- *Pregnancy Risk Category:* D

HOW SUPPLIED

Injection: 1-mg/ml, 2-mg/2-ml, 5-mg/5-ml multiple-dose vials; 1-mg/1-ml, 2-mg/2-ml preservative-free vials

ACTION

Mechanism: A vinca alkaloid that arrests mitosis in metaphase, blocking cell division. Binds to or crystallizes critical microtubule proteins of the mitotic spindle.
Absorption: Unpredictably absorbed from the GI tract; usually given I.V.
Distribution: Rapidly and widely distributed into body tissues and is bound to erythrocytes and platelets. The drug crosses the blood-brain barrier but does not achieve therapeutic concentrations in CSF.
Metabolism: Extensively metabolized in the liver.
Excretion: Drug and metabolites are primarily excreted into feces via the bile; a smaller portion is eliminated in urine. Half-life: Elimination is triphasic, with half-lives of about 4 minutes, 2¼ hours, and 85 hours for the distribution, second, and terminal phases, respectively.

INDICATIONS & DOSAGE

Acute lymphoblastic and other leukemias, Hodgkin's disease, lymphosarcoma, reticulum cell sarcoma, neuroblastoma, rhabdomyosarcoma, Wilms' tumor, osteogenic and other sarcomas, lung and breast cancer–
Adults: 1 to 2 mg/m^2 I.V. weekly.
Children: 1.5 to 2 mg/m^2 I.V. weekly. Maximum single dosage (adults and children) is 2 mg.

CONTRAINDICATIONS & PRECAUTIONS

Contraindicated in patients with the demyelinating form of Charcot-Marie-Tooth syndrome because of the drug's neurotoxic effects. Use with caution in patients with preexisting neuromuscular disease, closely monitoring for neurotoxicity. Leukocyte count and hemoglobin should be checked before each dose. Also use cautiously in patients with jaundice or hepatic dysfunction.

ADVERSE REACTIONS

Common reactions are in italics; life-threatening reactions are in bold italics.
Blood: rapidly reversible mild anemia and leukopenia.
CNS: *peripheral neuropathy,* sensory loss, *loss of deep tendon reflexes, paresthesias, wristdrop and footdrop,* ataxia, cranial nerve palsies (headache, *jaw pain,* hoarseness, vocal cord paralysis, visual disturbances), *muscle weakness and cramps,* depression, agitation, insomnia; some neurotoxicities may be permanent.
EENT: diplopia, optic and extraocular neuropathy, ptosis.
GI: *constipation, cramps,* ileus that mimics surgical abdomen, *nausea, vomiting,* anorexia, *stomatitis,* weight loss, dysphagia.
GU: urine retention, syndrome of inappropriate antidiuretic hormone (SIADH).
Local: severe local reaction when extravasated, *phlebitis,* cellulitis.
Other: ***acute bronchospasm,*** *reversible alopecia (up to 71% of patients).*

INTERACTIONS

Asparaginase: decreased hepatic clearance of vincristine.
Calcium channel blockers: enhanced vincristine accumulation in cells.
Digoxin: decreased digoxin effects. Monitor serum digoxin.
Mitomycin: possibly increased frequency of bronchospasm and acute pulmonary reactions.

EFFECTS ON DIAGNOSTIC TESTS

Blood and urine: increased uric acid concentrations.
Serum potassium: increased concentrations.

NURSING CONSIDERATIONS

Besides those related universally to drug therapy (see "How to use this book"), consider the following specific recommendations:

Assessment
- Obtain a baseline assessment of the patient's underlying condition before initiating therapy.
- Be alert for adverse reactions and drug interactions throughout therapy.
- Evaluate the patient's and family's knowledge about vincristine therapy.

Nursing Diagnoses
- High risk for fluid volume deficit related to adverse drug reactions.
- Body image disturbance related to adverse drug reactions.
- Knowledge deficit related to vincristine therapy.

Planning and Implementation

Preparation and Administration
- Read order and drug label carefully before administration of drug. Use extreme caution to avoid confusing vincristine with vinblastine.
- Follow institutional policy for handling hazardous materials to minimize risk to personnel.
- All vials contain 1 mg/ml solution and should be refrigerated. The 5-ml vials are for multiple-dose use only. Don't administer entire vial to a patient as a single dose.
- Check opened vials for discoloration and particles.
- Label all syringes containing vincristine "FOR I.V. USE ONLY." Never give vincristine I.M. or S.C.
- Check patient's I.D. band and ask patient's name before administration.

• Check I.V. site and patency of line before administration.
• ***I.V. use:*** Vincristine may be injected directly into a vein or into a running I.V. infusion slowly over 1 minute.
• Vincristine may also be added to 50 ml of dextrose 5% in water or 0.9% sodium chloride solution and infused over 15 minutes.
• If infiltration of I.V. results in extravasation of vincristine, stop infusion, apply ice packs to the site every 2 hours for 24 hours, and notify doctor.

Monitoring

• Obtain baseline CBC and differential, muscle tone and reflexes, bowel and bladder elimination patterns, nutritional status, vital signs, and patient's underlying cancerous state before initiating therapy.
• Monitor effectiveness by noting the results of follow-up diagnostic tests and overall physical status and by regularly checking CBC and differential, and tumor size and rate of growth with appropriate studies.
• Monitor for presence of petechiae, epistaxis, melena, or hematuria if platelet count drops.
• Monitor respiratory status; be alert for life-threatening bronchospasm.
• Monitor bowel sounds regularly; monitor bowel function.
• Monitor urine output, noting decreased or absent urine flow suggestive of urine retention.
• Monitor for depression of Achilles tendon reflex, numbness, tingling, footdrop or wristdrop, difficulty in walking alone, slapping gait, or difficulty walking on heels.
• Monitor for visual changes.
• Monitor weight, nutritional status, and hydration status if GI adverse reactions occur.
• Monitor electrolyte levels and urine output for evidence of SIADH.
• Monitor the I.V. site for extravasation.
• Monitor the patient for drug interactions.

Supportive Care

• Be prepared to discontinue drug and notify doctor if serious adverse reactions occur.
• Provide a private room and reverse isolation for patients with compromised immune systems.
• Institute safety precautions to minimize risk of injury due to impaired mobility and sensory alterations.
• Help patient to turn every 2 hours and provide skin care, especially over areas with bony prominences, as needed.
• Provide frequent mouth care. Use a soft toothbrush and mild mouthwash to avoid injury to oral mucous membranes.
• Give stool softeners or laxatives and encourage fluid intake to treat constipation.
• Provide support while patient is walking.
• Administer an antiemetic as needed.
• Provide the patient emotional support and opportunities to express feelings about body image.
• If local extravasation occurs, be prepared to treat (according to manufacturer's directions) with a local injection of hyaluronidase and the application of moderate heat. However, some doctors prefer the application of cold compresses, dilution with 0.9% sodium chloride injection or infiltration of sodium bicarbonate (5 ml of 8.4% injection), and/or local injection of hydrocortisone.
• Provide the patient with fluid if nausea and vomiting are severe.

Patient Teaching

• Advise the patient that burning or stinging at I.V. site during administration is common.
• Advise the patient that alopecia may occur, but is usually reversible.
• Teach the patient and family protective measures to consume energy and prevent infections: getting adequate

rest, avoiding fatigue, maintaining a balanced diet and adequate fluid intake, avoiding exposure to people with colds or other infections, and using support while walking to avoid risk of injury due to falls.

• Encourage adequate fluid intake to increase urine output and facilitate excretion of uric acid.

Evaluation

In patients receiving vincristine, appropriate evaluation statements may include:

• Patient does not develop fluid volume deficit.

• Patient states feelings about changes in body image and demonstrates coping behaviors.

• Patient and family state an understanding of vincristine therapy.

vitamin A (retinol)

(ret´ i nole)

Acon, Aquasol A

• *Classification:* nutritional agent (vitamin)

• *Pregnancy Risk Category:* A (X if > RDA)

HOW SUPPLIED

Tablets: 10,000 IU

Capsules: 10,000 IU◇, 25,000 IU, 50,000 IU

Drops: 30 ml with dropper (5,000 IU/0.1 ml)

Injection: 2-ml vials (5,000 IU/ml with 0.5% chlorobutanol, polysorbate 80, butylated hydroxyanisol, and butylated hydroxytoluene)

ACTION

Mechanism: Coenzyme necessary for retinal function, bone growth, and differentiation of epithelial tissues. Combines with opsin, a retinal pigment, to form rhodopsin, which is necessary for adaptation of vision to darkness.

Absorption: Normal doses are absorbed readily and completely if fat absorption is normal. Larger doses, or regular doses in patients with fat malabsorption, low protein intake, or hepatic or pancreatic disease, may be absorbed incompletely. Because vitamin A is fat-soluble, absorption requires bile salts, pancreatic lipase, and dietary fat.

Distribution: Stored (primarily as palmitate) in Kupffer's cells of the liver. Normal adult liver stores are sufficient to provide vitamin A requirements for 2 years. Lesser amounts of retinyl palmitate are stored in the kidneys, lungs, adrenal glands, retinas, and intraperitoneal fat. Circulates bound to a specific $alpha_1$ protein, retinol-binding protein (RBP). Blood level assays may not reflect liver storage because serum levels depend partly on circulating RBP. Liver storage should be adequate before discontinuing therapy. Is distributed into breast milk and does not readily cross the placenta.

Metabolism: In the liver.

Excretion: Conjugated with glucuronic acid and then further metabolized to retinal and retinoic acid. Retinoic acid is excreted in feces via biliary elimination. Retinal, retinoic acid, and other water-soluble metabolites are excreted in urine and feces. Normally, no unchanged retinol is excreted in urine, except in patients with pneumonia or chronic nephritis.

INDICATIONS & DOSAGE

Recommended daily allowance (RDA)–

Note: RDAs have been converted to IU for convenience. Vitamin A activity is expressed as retinol equivalents (RE).

1 RE = 1 mcg retinol or 3.33 IU

1 RE = 6 mcg beta carotene or 10 IU

An average equivalent of 1 RE is 5 IU.
Neonates and infants to 1 year: 1,875 IU.
Children over 1 year to 3 years: 2,000 IU.
Children 4 to 6 years: 2,500 IU.
Children 7 to 10 years: 3,500 IU.
Males over 11 years: 5,000 IU.
Females over 11 years: 4,000 IU.
Pregnant women: 4,000 IU.
Lactating women (first 6 months): 6,500 IU.
Lactating women (second 6 months): 6,000 IU.
Severe vitamin A deficiency with xerophthalmia –
Adults and children over 8 years: 500,000 IU P.O. daily for 3 days, then 50,000 IU P.O. daily for 14 days, then maintenance with 10,000 to 20,000 IU P.O. daily for 2 months, followed by adequate dietary nutrition and RDA vitamin A supplements.
Severe vitamin A deficiency–
Adults and children over 8 years: 100,000 IU P.O. or I.M. daily for 3 days, then 50,000 IU P.O. or I.M. daily for 14 days, then maintenance with 10,000 to 20,000 IU P.O. daily for 2 months, followed by adequate dietary nutrition and RDA vitamin A supplements.
Children 1 to 8 years: 17,500 to 35,000 IU I.M. daily for 10 days.
Infants under 1 year: 7,500 to 15,000 IU I.M. daily for 10 days.
Maintenance only–
Children 4 to 8 years: 15,000 IU I.M. daily for 2 months, then adequate dietary nutrition and RDA vitamin A supplements.
Children under 4 years: 10,000 IU I.M. daily for 2 months, then adequate dietary nutrition and RDA vitamin A supplements.

CONTRAINDICATIONS & PRECAUTIONS

Contraindicated in patients with hypervitaminosis A; in those with sensitivity to vitamin A or other ingredients in commercially available preparations; I.V. use is contraindicated because it may cause fatal anaphylaxis. The efficacy of large systemic doses of vitamin A in treating acne has not been established; this use should be avoided because of the potential for toxicity.

Vitamin A intake from fortified foods, dietary supplements, self-prescribed drugs, and prescription drug sources should be evaluated. Prolonged administration of dosages that exceed 25,000 IU/day requires close supervision.

ADVERSE REACTIONS

Common reactions are in italics; life-threatening reactions are in bold italics. Adverse effects are usually seen only with toxicity (hypervitaminosis A).
Blood: hypoplastic anemia, leukopenia.
CNS: irritability, headache, ***increased intracranial pressure,*** fatigue, lethargy, malaise.
EENT: miosis, papilledema, exophthalmos.
GI: anorexia, epigastric pain, diarrhea.
GU: hypomenorrhea.
Hepatic: jaundice, hepatomegaly.
Skin: alopecia; drying, cracking, scaling of skin; pruritus; lip fissures; ***massive desquamation;*** increased pigmentation; night sweating.
Other: skeletal–slow growth, decalcification of bone, fractures, hyperostosis, painful periostitis, premature closure of epiphyses, migratory arthralgia, cortical thickening over the radius and tibia, bulging fontanelles; splenomegaly. ***Fatal anaphylaxis with I.V. use.***

INTERACTIONS

Mineral oil, cholestyramine resin: reduced GI absorption of fat-soluble vitamins. If needed, give mineral oil at bedtime.

EFFECTS ON DIAGNOSTIC TESTS

Bilirubin: falsely elevated determinations.
Serum cholesterol: falsely increased levels (interference with the Zlatkis-Zak reaction).

NURSING CONSIDERATIONS

Besides those related universally to drug therapy (see "How to use this book"), consider the following specific recommendations:

Assessment

- Obtain a baseline assessment of patient's underlying condition before therapy.
- Be alert for adverse reactions and drug interactions throughout therapy.
- Evaluate the patient's and family's knowledge about vitamin A therapy.

Nursing Diagnoses

- Sensory/perceptual alterations (visual) related to the patient's underlying condition.
- High risk for impaired skin integrity related to adverse drug reactions.
- Knowledge deficit related to vitamin A therapy.

Planning and Implementation

Preparation and Administration

- Liquid preparations are available if nasogastric administration is necessary. May be mixed with cereal or fruit juice.
- Protect from light and heat.
- In pregnant women, avoid doses exceeding RDA.

Monitoring

- Monitor effectiveness by frequently assessing the patient's visual perception.
- Monitor for adverse reactions and interactions by assessing the patient's skin for drying, cracking, scaling, pruritus, and lip fissures.
- Monitor for CNS effects by assessing for headache, irritability, fatigue, lethargy, and malaise.
- Monitor the patient's eating and bowel patterns; drug may cause anorexia and diarrhea.
- Monitor CBC; drug may cause hypoplastic anemia and leukopenia.
- Evaluate the patient's intake of vitamin A from fortified foods, dietary supplements, self-administered drugs, and prescription drug sources.

Supportive Care

- Know that chronic toxicity in infants has resulted from doses of 18,500 IU daily for 1 to 3 months. In adults, chronic toxicity has resulted from doses of 50,000 IU daily for over 8 months; 500,000 IU daily for 2 months; and 1 million IU daily for 1 day.
- Know that acute toxicity has resulted from single doses of 25,000 IU/kg of body weight; 350,000 IU in infants and over 2 million IU in adults have also proved acutely toxic.
- Know that adequate vitamin A absorption requires suitable protein intake, bile (give supplemental salts if necessary), concurrent RDA doses of vitamin E, and zinc (multivitamins usually supply zinc, but supplements may be necessary in long-term parenteral therapy).
- Know that absorption is fastest and most complete with water-miscible preparations, immediate with emulsions, and slowest with oil suspensions.
- In severe hepatic dysfunction, diabetes, and hypothyroidism, use vitamin A rather than carotene because the vitamin itself is more easily absorbed and the diseases adversely affect conversion of carotenes into vitamin A. If carotenes are prescribed, dosage should be doubled.

Patient Teaching
• Discourage self-administration of megavitamin doses without specific indications to avoid toxicity.
• Emphasize that patient should not share the prescribed vitamins with family members or others. Other family members who need vitamin therapy should contact doctor.

Evaluation
In patients receiving vitamin A, appropriate evaluation statements may include:
• Patient states his night blindness has improved.
• Patient does not develop drug-induced impaired skin integrity.
• Patient and family state an understanding of vitamin A therapy.

vitamin B_1 (thiamine hydrochloride)

(thye´ a min)
Apatate Drops, Betalin S◇, Betamin‡, Beta-Sol‡, Biamine, Thia

• *Classification:* nutritional agent (vitamin)
• *Pregnancy Risk Category:* A (C if > RDA)

HOW SUPPLIED

Tablets◇: 5 mg, 10 mg, 25 mg, 50 mg, 100 mg, 250 mg, 500 mg
Elixir: 2.25 mg/5 ml (with alcohol 10%)◇
Injection: 100 mg/ml

ACTION

Mechanism: Combines with adenosine triphosphate to form a coenzyme, thiamine pyrophosphate, which is necessary for carbohydrate metabolism.
Absorption: Readily absorbed after oral administration of small doses; after oral administration of a large dose, the total amount absorbed is limited to 8 to 15 mg. In alcoholics and in patients with cirrhosis or malabsorption, GI absorption is decreased. When given with meals, GI rate of absorption decreases, but total absorption remains the same. Absorbed rapidly and completely after I.M. administration.
Distribution: Widely distributed into body tissues. When intake exceeds the minimal requirements, tissue stores become saturated. About 100 to 200 mcg/day is distributed into the milk of breast-feeding women on a normal diet.
Metabolism: In the liver.
Excretion: Excess is excreted in the urine. After large doses (more than 10 mg), both unchanged thiamine and metabolites are excreted in urine after tissue stores become saturated.

INDICATIONS & DOSAGE

Recommended daily allowance (RDA)–
Neonates and infants to 6 months: 0.3 mg.
Infants 6 months to 1 year: 0.4 mg.
Children over 1 year to 3 years: 0.7 mg.
Children 4 to 6 years: 0.9 mg.
Children 7 to 10 years: 1 mg.
Males 11 to 14 years: 1.3 mg.
Males 15 to 50 years: 1.5 mg.
Males 51 years and over: 1.2 mg.
Females 11 to 50 years: 1.1 mg.
Females 51 years and over: 1 mg.
Pregnant women: 1.5 mg.
Lactating women: 1.6 mg.
Beriberi–
Adults: 10 to 500 mg, depending on severity, I.M. t.i.d. for 2 weeks, followed by dietary correction and multivitamin supplement containing 5 to 10 mg thiamine daily for 1 month.
Children: 10 to 50 mg, depending on severity, I.M. daily for several weeks with adequate dietary intake.
Anemia secondary to thiamine deficiency; polyneuritis secondary to alcoholism, pregnancy, or pellagra–
Adults: 100 mg P.O. daily.

Children: 10 to 50 mg P.O. daily in divided doses.
Wernicke's encephalopathy–
Adults: up to 500 mg to 1 g I.V. for crisis therapy, followed by 100 mg b.i.d. for maintenance.
"Wet beriberi," with myocardial failure–
Adults and children: 100 to 500 mg I.V. for emergency treatment.

CONTRAINDICATIONS & PRECAUTIONS

Contraindicated in patients with suspected vitamin B_1 sensitivity (an intradermal test dose is recommended before parenteral administration); and in patients hypersensitive to the drug or to any ingredient in thiamine preparations. Thiamine-deficient patients may experience a sudden onset or worsening of Wernicke's encephalopathy (nystagmus, bilateral sixth nerve palsy, ataxia, and confusion) after I.V. glucose administration. In suspected thiamine deficiency, administer thiamine before a glucose load is given.

ADVERSE REACTIONS

Common reactions are in italics; life-threatening reactions are in bold italics.
CNS: restlessness.
CV: *hypotension after rapid I.V. injection,* angioneurotic edema, cyanosis.
EENT: ***tightness of throat (allergic reaction).***
GI: nausea, hemorrhage, diarrhea.
Skin: feeling of warmth, pruritus, urticaria, sweating.
Other: *anaphylactoid reactions,* weakness, ***pulmonary edema.***

INTERACTIONS

None significant.

EFFECTS ON DIAGNOSTIC TESTS

Serum theophylline concentrations: interference with the Schack and Waxler spectrophotometric determination with high doses.
Uric acid: false-positive results in the phosphotungstate method.
Urobilinogen: false-positive results with Ehrlich's reagent spot tests.

NURSING CONSIDERATIONS

Besides those related universally to drug therapy (see "How to use this book"), consider the following specific recommendations:

Assessment
- Obtain a baseline assessment of patient's underlying condition before therapy.
- Be alert for adverse reactions and drug interactions throughout therapy.
- Evaluate the patient's and family's knowledge about vitamin B_1 therapy.

Nursing Diagnoses
- Fatigue related to the patient's underlying condition.
- Altered tissue perfusion (cardiovascular) related to adverse drug reaction.
- Knowledge deficit related to vitamin B_1 therapy.

Planning and Implementation
Preparation and Administration
- ***I.V. use:*** Direct injection is not recommended. Administer by intermittent or continuous infusion at a rate not to exceed 20 mg/minute.
- Perform a skin test before therapy if patient has a history of hypersensitivity.
- Use parenteral administration only when P.O. route is not feasible.
- Unstable in alkaline solutions; should not be used with materials that yield alkaline solutions.

Monitoring
- Monitor effectiveness by assessing the patient's level of fatigue.
- Monitor for adverse reactions by monitoring the patient's vital signs, especially blood pressure; drug may cause hypotension after rapid I.V. injection.
- Monitor for cyanosis.
- Monitor CNS effects by assessing the patient for restlessness.

• Monitor the patient for allergic reactions by asking about any feelings of tightness in the throat.
• Monitor for skin reactions (feeling of warmth, pruritus, urticaria, or sweating).
• Monitor hydration status if nausea and diarrhea occur.
• Monitor patients with alcoholism, cirrhosis, or GI disease closely for thiamine malabsorption, which is most likely to occur with these diseases.

Supportive Care

• Clinically significant deficiency can follow approximately 3 weeks of totally thiamine-free diet. Thiamine deficiency usually requires concurrent treatment for multiple deficiencies.
• Doses over 30 mg t.i.d may not be fully used. After tissue saturation with thiamine, it is excreted in urine as pyridimine.
• If beriberi occurs in a breast-fed infant, both mother and child should be treated with vitamin B_1.
• Be prepared to give epinephrine to treat anaphylaxis that may occur after parenteral doses.

Patient Teaching

• Inform the mother of a breast-fed infant with beriberi that she and her child will need treatment with vitamin B_1.

Evaluation

In patients receiving vitamin B_1, appropriate evaluation statements may include:

• Patient states a reduction in level of fatigue.
• Patient does not develop drug-induced hypotension.
• Patient and family state an understanding of vitamin B_1 therapy.

vitamin B_2 (riboflavin)◊
(rye´ boe flay vin)

• *Classification:* nutritional agent (vitamin)
• *Pregnancy Risk Category:* A (C if > RDA)

HOW SUPPLIED

Tablets: 5 mg◊, 10 mg◊, 25 mg◊
Tablets (sugar-free): 50 mg◊, 100 mg◊

ACTION

Mechanism: Acts as a coenzyme necessary for tissue respiration. Functions in the body as flavin adenine dinucleotide (FAD) and flavin mononucleotide (FMN).
Absorption: Readily absorbed from the GI tract, but the extent of absorption is limited. Absorption occurs at a specialized segment of the mucosa; and is limited by the duration of the drug's contact with this area. Before being absorbed, riboflavin-5-phosphate is rapidly dephosphorylated in the GI lumen. GI absorption increases when the drug is administered with food and decreases when hepatitis, cirrhosis, biliary obstruction, or probenecid administration is present.
Distribution: Widely distributed to body tissues. Free riboflavin is present in the retina. Riboflavin is stored in limited amounts in the liver, spleen, kidneys, and heart, mainly in the form of FAD. FAD and FMN are approximately 60% protein-bound in blood. Riboflavin crosses the placenta, and breast milk contains about 400 ng/ml.
Metabolism: Metabolized to FMN in erythrocytes, GI mucosal cells, and the liver; FMN is converted to FAD in the liver.
Excretion: Approximately 9% is excreted unchanged in the urine after normal ingestion. Excretion involves

renal tubular secretion and glomerular filtration. The amount excreted unchanged is directly proportional to the dose. Removal by hemodialysis is slower than by natural renal excretion.
Half life: Approximately 66 to 84 minutes in healthy individuals.

INDICATIONS & DOSAGE

Recommended daily allowance (RDA) –
Neonates and infants to 6 months: 0.4 mg.
Infants 6 months to 1 year: 0.5 mg.
Children over 1 year to 3 years: 0.8 mg.
Children 4 to 6 years: 1.1 mg.
Children 7 to 10 years: 1.2 mg.
Males 11 to 14 years: 1.5 mg.
Males 15 to 18 years: 1.8 mg.
Males 19 to 50 years: 1.7 mg.
Males 51 years and over: 1.4 mg.
Females 11 to 50 years: 1.3 mg.
Females 51 years and over: 1.2 mg.
Pregnant women: 1.6 mg.
Lactating women (first 6 months): 1.8 mg.
Lactating women (second 6 months): 1.7 mg.
Riboflavin deficiency or adjunct to thiamine treatment for polyneuritis or cheilosis secondary to pellagra –
Adults and children over 12 years: 5 to 50 mg P.O. daily, depending on severity.
Children under 12 years: 2 to 10 mg P.O. daily, depending on severity.

For maintenance, increase nutritional intake and supplement with vitamin B complex.

CONTRAINDICATIONS & PRECAUTIONS

None reported.

ADVERSE REACTIONS

Common reactions are in italics; life-threatening reactions are in bold italics.
GU: high doses turn urine bright yellow.

INTERACTIONS

None significant.

EFFECTS ON DIAGNOSTIC TESTS

Catecholamines and urobilinogen: false elevations of fluorometric determinations.
Urinalysis: altered results of spectrophotometry or color reactions. Large doses can cause bright yellow urine.

NURSING CONSIDERATIONS

Besides those related universally to drug therapy (see "How to use this book"), consider the following specific recommendations:

Assessment
- Obtain a baseline assessment of patient's underlying condition before therapy.
- Be alert for adverse reactions and drug interactions throughout therapy.
- Evaluate the patient's and family's knowledge about vitamin B_2 therapy.

Nursing Diagnoses
- Sensory/perceptual alteration (visual) related to the patient's underlying condition.
- Altered nutrition: Less than body requirements.
- Knowledge deficit related to vitamin B_2 therapy.

Planning and Implementation

Preparation and Administration
- Drug may be given I.M. or I.V. as a component of multiple vitamins.
- Protect from light.

Monitoring
- Monitor effectiveness by assessing the patient's visual ability.
- Monitor for adverse reactions by observing the patient's urine for change in color.

Supportive Care
- Encourage the patient to take this drug with meals because food increases absorption.
- Know that riboflavin deficiency usually accompanies other vitamin B–complex deficiencies and may require multivitamin therapy.

Patient Teaching
• Emphasize proper nutritional habits to prevent recurrence of deficiency.
• Tell the patient that this drug may turn his urine bright yellow.

Evaluation
In patients receiving vitamin B$_2$, appropriate evaluation statements may include:
• Patient states an improvement of his visual ability.
• Patient's nutritional status shows improvement.
• Patient and family state an understanding of vitamin B$_2$ therapy.

vitamin B$_3$ derivatives

niacin (nicotinic acid)
(nye´ a sin)
Niac, Nico-400, Nicobid◇, Nicolar**, Ni-Span◇

niacinamide (nicotinamide)◇
(nye a sin´ a mide)

• *Classification:* nutritional agent (vitamin)
• *Pregnancy Risk Category:* A (C if > RDA)

HOW SUPPLIED
niacin
Tablets: 20 mg◇, 25 mg◇, 50 mg◇, 100 mg◇, 500 mg
Tablets (timed-release): 150 mg
Capsules (timed-release): 125 mg◇, 250 mg◇, 300 mg◇, 400 mg◇, 500 mg
Elixir: 50 mg/5 ml◇
Injection: 30-ml vials, 100 mg/ml
niacinamide
Tablets: 50 mg◇, 100 mg◇, 500 mg◇
Tablets (timed-release): 1,000 mg◇
Injection: 100 mg/ml

ACTION
Mechanism: Niacin or vitamin B$_3$ is the common name for nicotinic acid. It functions as a component of two important coenzymes necessary for cellular respiration, nicotinamide adenine dinucleotide (NAD or coenzyme I) and nicotinamide adenine dinucleotide phosphate (NADP or coenzyme II). Necessary for lipid metabolism, tissue respiration, and glycogenolysis. Also (niacin only) decreases synthesis of low-density lipoproteins and inhibits lipolysis in adipose tissue.
Absorption: Rapidly absorbed from the GI tract.
Distribution: Widely distributed in body tissues; niacin is distributed in breast milk.
Metabolism: By the liver.
Excretion: In urine. About 50% of a dose is excreted unchanged. Half life: 45 minutes.
Onset, peak, duration: Peak plasma levels occur in 45 minutes.

INDICATIONS & DOSAGE
Recommended daily allowance (RDA)–
Neonates and infants to 6 months: 5 mg.
Infants 6 months to 1 year: 6 mg.
Children 1 to 3 years: 9 mg.
Children 4 to 6 years: 12 mg.
Children 7 to 10 years: 13 mg.
Males 11 to 14 years: 17 mg.
Males 15 to 18 years: 20 mg.
Males 19 to 50 years: 19 mg.
Males 51 years and over: 15 mg.
Females 11 to 50 years: 15 mg.
Females 51 years and over: 13 mg.
Pregnant women: 17 mg.
Lactating women: 20 mg.
Pellagra–
Adults: 10 to 20 mg P.O., S.C., I.M., or I.V. infusion daily, depending on severity of niacin deficiency. Maximum daily dosage recommended is 500 mg; should be divided into 10 doses, 50 mg each.
Children: up to 300 mg P.O. or 100 mg I.V. infusion daily, depending on severity of niacin deficiency.

After symptoms subside, advise ad-

equate nutrition and RDA supplements to prevent recurrence.
Peripheral vascular disease and circulatory disorders–
Adults: 250 to 800 mg P.O. daily in divided doses.
Adjunctive treatment of hyperlipidemias, especially with hypercholesterolemia–
Adults: 1.5 to 3 g P.O. daily in three divided doses with or after meals, increased at intervals to 6 g daily.

CONTRAINDICATIONS & PRECAUTIONS

Contraindicated in patients with hypersensitivity to the drug and in those with liver disease because large doses may cause liver damage; in patients with peptic ulcer, which niacin may activate; and in patients with arterial hemorrhage, severe hypotension, or niacin hypersensitivity.

Use cautiously in patients with gout, diabetes mellitus, or gallbladder disease because it may exacerbate the symptoms of these disorders.

ADVERSE REACTIONS

Common reactions are in italics; life-threatening reactions are in bold italics. Most adverse reactions are dose-dependent.
CNS: dizziness, transient headache.
CV: *excessive peripheral vasodilation (especially niacin).*
GI: *nausea, vomiting, diarrhea,* possible activation of peptic ulcer, epigastric or substernal pain.
Hepatic: ***hepatic toxicity.***
Metabolic: hyperglycemia, hyperuricemia.
Skin: *flushing,* pruritus, dryness.

INTERACTIONS

Antihypertensive drugs (sympathetic blocking type): may have an additive vasodilating effect and cause postural hypotension. Use together cautiously. Warn patient about postural hypotension.

EFFECTS ON DIAGNOSTIC TESTS

Urine catecholamines: altered results of fluorometric tests.
Urine glucose: altered results with copper sulfate (Benedict's reagent).

NURSING CONSIDERATIONS

Besides those related universally to drug therapy (see "How to use this book"), consider the following specific recommendations:

Assessment
- Obtain a baseline assessment of patient's underlying condition before therapy.
- Be alert for adverse reactions and drug interactions throughout therapy.
- Evaluate the patient's and family's knowledge about vitamin B_3 therapy.

Nursing Diagnoses
- Altered tissue perfusion (peripheral) related to the patient's underlying condition.
- High risk for fluid volume deficit related to adverse drug reaction.
- Knowledge deficit related to vitamin B_3 therapy.

Planning and Implementation

Preparation and Administration
- Give with meals to minimize GI reactions.
- Aspirin (80 to 325 mg P.O. given 30 minutes before niacin dose) may reduce the flushing response to niacin.
- ***I.V. use:*** Give slow I.V. (no faster than 2 mg/minute). May be given by direct injection, or by intermittent or continuous infusion.

Monitoring
- Monitor effectiveness by assessing the patient's circulation.
- Assess laboratory values for possible hyperglycemia and hyperuricemia.
- Monitor hydration status if nausea, vomiting, and diarrhea occurs.
- Monitor for epigastric or substernal pain.
- Monitor hepatic studies and blood glucose level early in therapy.
- Monitor for drug-induced headache.

Supportive Care
• Provide additional fluids if nausea, vomiting, and diarrhea become severe.
• Obtain an order for a mild analgesic if the patient develops a drug-induced headache.
• Time-released niacin or niacinamide may avoid excessive flushing effects with large doses. However, know that time-released niacin has been associated with hepatic failure even at doses as low as 1 g per day.
Patient Teaching
• Explain to the patient that he may experience flushing with administration. Reassure patient that this is harmless.
• Stress that medication used to treat hyperlipoproteinemia or to dilate peripheral vessels is not "just a vitamin."
• Explain the importance of adhering to therapeutic regimen.
• Advise patient against self-medicating for hyperlipidemia.
Evaluation
In patients receiving vitamin B_3, appropriate evaluation statements may include:
• Patient states an improvement of peripheral circulation.
• Patient does not develop drug-induced fluid volume deficit.
• Patient and family state an understanding of vitamin B_3 therapy.

vitamin B_6 (pyridoxine hydrochloride)

(peer i dox´ een)
Beesix, Hexa-Betalin, Hexacrest, Nestrex◇

• *Classification:* nutritional agent (vitamin)
• *Pregnancy Risk Category:* A (C if > RDA)

HOW SUPPLIED

Tablets◇*:* 10 mg, 25 mg, 50 mg, 100 mg, 200 mg, 250 mg, 500 mg
Tablets (timed-release): 500 mg
Injection: 100 mg/ml.

ACTION

Mechanism: Acts as coenzyme for the metabolism of carbohydrates, fat, and proteins.
Absorption: Readily absorbed from the GI tract after oral administration. GI absorption may be diminished in patients with malabsorption syndromes or after gastric resection. Normal serum levels are 30 to 80 ng/ml.
Distribution: Stored mainly in the liver. The total body store is approximately 16 to 27 mg. Pyridoxal and pyridoxal phosphate, the most common forms found in the blood, are highly protein-bound. Pyridoxal crosses the placenta; fetal plasma concentrations are five times greater than maternal plasma concentrations. After maternal intake of 2.5 to 5 mg/day, concentration in breast milk is approximately 240 ng/ml.
Metabolism: Degraded to 4-pyridoxic acid in the liver.
Excretion: In erythrocytes, pyridoxine is converted to pyridoxal phosphate, and pyridoxamine is converted to pyridoxamine phosphate. The phosphorylated form of pyridoxine is transaminated to pyridoxal and pyridoxamine. Pyridoxal is oxidized in the liver and excreted in urine. Half-life: 15 to 20 days.

INDICATIONS & DOSAGE

Recommended daily allowance (RDA)–
Neonates and infants to 6 months: 0.3 mg.
Infants 6 months to 1 year: 0.6 mg.
Children over 1 year to 3 years: 1 mg.
Children 4 to 6 years: 1.1 mg.
Children 7 to 10 years: 1.4 mg.

Males 11 to 14 years: 1.7 mg.
Males 15 years and over: 2 mg.
Females 11 to 14 years: 1.4 mg.
Females 15 to 18 years: 1.5 mg.
Females 19 years and over: 1.6 mg.
Pregnant women: 2.2 mg.
Lactating women: 2.1 mg.
Dietary vitamin B_6 deficiency–
Adults: 10 to 20 mg P.O., I.M., or I.V. daily for 3 weeks, then 2 to 5 mg daily as a supplement to a proper diet.
Children: 100 mg P.O., I.M., or I.V. to correct deficiency, then an adequate diet with supplementary RDA doses to prevent recurrence.
Seizures related to vitamin B_6 deficiency or dependency–
Adults and children: 100 mg I.M. or I.V. in single dose.
Vitamin B_6–responsive anemias or dependency syndrome (inborn errors of metabolism)–
Adults: up to 600 mg P.O., I.M., or I.V. daily until symptoms subside, then 50 mg daily for life.
Children: 100 mg I.M. or I.V., then 2 to 10 mg I.M. or 10 to 100 mg P.O. daily.
Prevention of vitamin B_6 deficiency during isoniazid therapy–
Adults: 25 to 50 mg P.O. daily.
Children: at least 0.5 to 1.5 mg P.O. daily.
Infants: at least 0.1 to 0.5 mg P.O. daily.
If neurologic symptoms develop in pediatric patients, increase dosage as necessary.
Treatment of vitamin B_6 deficiency secondary to isoniazid–
Adults: 100 mg P.O. daily for 3 weeks, then 50 mg daily.

CONTRAINDICATIONS & PRECAUTIONS

Contraindicated in patients with a history of pyridoxine sensitivity and for I.V. administration to patients with heart disease. The use of large doses of vitamin B_6 during pregnancy may cause pyridoxine-dependent seizures in infants.

ADVERSE REACTIONS

Common reactions are in italics; life-threatening reactions are in bold italics.
CNS: drowsiness, paresthesias.

INTERACTIONS

None significant.

EFFECTS ON DIAGNOSTIC TESTS

Urobilinogen: false-positive reaction with spot test using Ehrlich's reagent.

NURSING CONSIDERATIONS

Besides those related universally to drug therapy (see "How to use this book"), consider the following specific recommendations:

Assessment

- Obtain a baseline assessment of patient's underlying condition before therapy.
- Be alert for adverse reactions and drug interactions throughout therapy.
- Evaluate the patient's and family's knowledge about vitamin B_6 therapy.

Nursing Diagnoses

- Impaired skin integrity related to the patient's underlying condition.
- High risk for injury related to drowsiness caused by vitamin B_6 therapy.
- Knowledge deficit related to vitamin B_6 therapy.

Planning and Implementation

Preparation and Administration

- Protect from light. Do not use injection solution if it contains a precipitate. Slight darkening is acceptable.
- Do not mix vitamin B_6 in the same syringe as sodium bicarbonate if it is required to control acidosis in isoniazid toxicity.
- ***I.V. use:*** Direct injection is accomplished by injecting the undiluted drug into I.V. line containing a free-flowing compatible solution. Intermit-

tent infusion is also permitted. Continuous infusion is not used.

Monitoring

• Monitor by frequently assessing the patient's skin for relief of symptoms.

• Assess patient for drowsiness and paresthesias.

Supportive Care

• Patients receiving levodopa alone (not with carbidopa) should not take vitamin B_6.

• Know that this drug is used to treat seizures and coma as a result of isoniazid overdose. Dosage is equal to the amount of isonazid ingested.

Patient Teaching

• Explain that pyridoxine in combination therapy with isoniazid has a specific therapeutic purpose and is not "just a vitamin."

• If drug is prescribed for maintenance therapy, emphasize the importance of compliance and of good nutrition.

Evaluation

In patients receiving vitamin B_6, appropriate evaluation statements may include:

• Patient states an improvement of impaired skin integrity.

• Patient does not experience injury related to drug-induced drowsiness.

• Patient and family state an understanding of vitamin B_6 therapy.

vitamin B_9 (folic acid)

(foe´ lik)

Folvite, Novofolacid†

• *Classification:* nutritional agent (vitamin)

• *Pregnancy Risk Category:* A (C if > RDA)

HOW SUPPLIED

Tablets: 0.1 mg, 0.4 mg, 0.8 mg, 1 mg

Injection: 10-ml vials (5 mg/ml with 1.5% benzyl alcohol or 10 mg/ml with 1.5% benzyl alcohol and 0.2% EDTA)

ACTION

Mechanism: Necessary for normal erythropoiesis and nucleoprotein synthesis.

Absorption: Rapidly absorbed from the GI tract, mainly from the proximal part of the small intestine.

Distribution: The active metabolite tetrahydrofolic acid and its derivatives are distributed into all body tissues; liver contains about half of the total body folate stores. Folate is actively concentrated in the CSF. Folic acid is distributed into breast milk.

Metabolism: In the liver to N^5-methyltetrahydrofolic acid, the main form of folate storage and transport.

Excretion: A single 0.1- to 0.2-mg dose of folic acid usually results in only a trace amount of the drug in the urine. After large doses, excessive folate is excreted unchanged in the urine. Small amounts have been recovered in feces. About 0.05 mg/day of normal body folate stores is lost by a combination of urinary and fecal excretion and oxidative cleavage of the molecule.

Onset, peak, duration: Peak activity in blood occurs within 30 minutes to 1 hour after oral administration. Normal serum folate concentrations range from 0.0005 to 0.015 mcg/ml. Usually, serum levels below 0.005 mcg/ml indicate folate deficiency; those below 0.002 mcg/ml usually result in megaloblastic anemia.

INDICATIONS & DOSAGE

Recommended daily allowance (RDA)–

Neonates and infants to 6 months: 25 mcg.

Infants 6 months to 1 year: 35 mcg.

Children over 1 year to 3 years: 50 mcg.

Children 4 to 6 years: 75 mcg.

Children 7 to 11 years: 100 mcg.
Children 11 to 14 years: 150 mcg
Males 15 years and over: 200 mcg.
Females 15 years and over: 180 mcg.
Pregnant women: 400 mcg.
Lactating women (first 6 months): 280 mcg.
Lactating women (second 6 months): 260 mcg.
Megaloblastic or macrocytic anemia secondary to folic acid or other nutritional deficiency, hepatic disease, alcoholism, intestinal obstruction, excessive hemolysis–
Pregnant and lactating women: 0.8 mg P.O., S.C., or I.M. daily.
Adults and children over 4 years: 1 mg P.O., S.C., or I.M. daily for 4 to 5 days. After anemia secondary to folic acid deficiency is corrected, proper diet and RDA supplements are necessary to prevent recurrence.
Children under 4 years: up to 0.3 mg P.O., S.C., or I.M. daily.
Prevention of megaloblastic anemia of pregnancy and fetal damage–
Women: 1 mg P.O., S.C., or I.M. daily throughout pregnancy.
Nutritional supplement–
Adults: 0.1 mg P.O., S.C., or I.M. daily.
Children: 0.05 mg P.O. daily.
Treatment of tropical sprue–
Adults: 3 to 15 mg P.O. daily.
Test of megaloblastic anemia patients to detect folic acid deficiency without masking pernicious anemia–
Adults and children: 0.1 to 0.2 mg P.O. or I.M. for 10 days while maintaining a diet low in folate and vitamin B_{12}.
(Reticulosis, reversion to normoblastic hematopoiesis, and return to normal hemoglobin indicate folic acid deficiency.)

CONTRAINDICATIONS & PRECAUTIONS

Contraindicated in patients with pernicious, aplastic, or normocytic anemias. Folic acid may obscure the diagnosis of pernicious anemia, which can cause disabling neurologic complications.

ADVERSE REACTIONS

Common reactions are in italics; life-threatening reactions are in bold italics.
Skin: allergic reactions (rash, pruritus, erythema).
Other: ***allergic bronchospasms,*** general malaise.

INTERACTIONS

Chloramphenicol: antagonism of vitamin B_9. Monitor for decreased vitamin B_9 effect. Use together cautiously.

EFFECTS ON DIAGNOSTIC TESTS

Serum and erythrocyte folate: altered results; falsely low levels with the *Lactobacillus* case assay method in patients receiving antibiotics, such as tetracycline, which suppress the growth of this organism.

NURSING CONSIDERATIONS

Besides those related universally to drug therapy (see "How to use this book"), consider the following specific recommendations:

Assessment

- Obtain a baseline assessment of patient's underlying condition before therapy.
- Be alert for adverse reactions and drug interactions throughout therapy.
- Evaluate the patient's and family's knowledge about vitamin B_9 therapy.

Nursing Diagnoses

- Altered oral mucous membranes related to the patient's underlying condition.
- Ineffective breathing pattern related to adverse respiratory reaction to vitamin B_9 therapy.
- Knowledge deficit related to vitamin B_9 therapy.

Planning and Implementation
Preparation and Administration
• Patients with small-bowel resection and intestinal malabsorption may require parenteral administration routes.
• Don't mix with other medication in the same syringe for I.M. injections.
• Protect from light and heat.
• ***I.V. use:*** Continuous and intermittent infusion is not recommended. Slowly inject dose directly into vein or into the tubing of a free-flowing compatible I.V. solution.
Monitoring
• Monitor effectiveness by assessing the oral mucous membranes.
• Monitor for adverse reactions and interactions by assessing the patient's skin for rash, pruritus, and erythema.
• Monitor the hematologic response to vitamin B_9 in patients receiving chloramphenicol concurrently.
Supportive Care
• Know that peak folate activity occurs in the blood in 30 minutes to 1 hour.
• Know that adequate nutrition is necessary to prevent recurrence of anemia.
• May use concurrent vitamin B_9 and vitamin B_{12} therapy if appropriate for diagnosis.
Patient Teaching
• Advise patients with pernicious anemia to avoid multivitamins containing vitamin B_9.
• Teach the patient how proper nutrition can prevent the recurrence of anemia.
Evaluation
In patients receiving vitamin B_9, appropriate evaluation statements may include:
• Patient's sore mouth shows improvement.
• Patient does not develop allergic bronchospasm.
• Patient and family state an understanding of vitamin B_9 therapy.

vitamin B_{12} derivatives

cyanocobalamin (vitamin B_{12})
(sye an oh koe bal′ a min)
Anacobin†, Bedoce, Bedoz†, Betalin 12, Bioglan B_{12} Plus‡, Crystamine, Cyanabin†, Cyanocobalamin, Cyano-Gel, Dodex, Kaybovite, Poyamin, Redisol, Rubesol-1000, Rubion†, Rubramin, Sigamine

hydroxocobalamin (vitamin B_{12a})
(hye drox o koe bal′ a min)
Alpha-Ruvite, Codroxomin, Droxomin, Rubesol-L.A.

• *Classification:* nutritional agent (vitamin)
• *Pregnancy Risk Category:* A (C if > RDA)

HOW SUPPLIED
Tablets: 25 mcg◇, 50 mcg◇, 100 mcg◇, 250 mcg◇, 500 mcg, 1,000 mcg
Injection: 30-ml vials (30 mcg/ml, 100 mcg/ml, 120 mcg/ml with benzyl alcohol, 1,000 mcg/ml, 1,000 mcg/ml with benzyl alcohol), 10-ml vials (100 mcg/ml, 100 mcg/ml with benzyl alcohol, 1,000 mcg/ml, 1,000 mcg/ml with benzyl alcohol, 1,000 mcg/ml with methyl and propyl parabens), 5-ml vials (1,000 mcg/ml with benzyl alcohol), 1-ml vials (1,000 mcg/ml with benzyl alcohol), 1-ml unimatic (1,000 mcg/ml with benzyl alcohol)

ACTION
Mechanism: A coenzyme necessary for cell growth and replication, hematopoiesis, nucleoprotein and myelin synthesis. Activates folic acid coenzymes used in the formation of red blood cells.
Absorption: After oral administration, is absorbed irregularly from the distal small intestine. Protein-bound

to intrinsic factor in the stomach, and this bond must be split by proteolysis and gastric acid before absorption can occur. Absorption depends on sufficient intrinsic factor and calcium. Oral form is not absorbed in malabsorptive states, achlorhydria, and pernicious anemia; however, is absorbed rapidly from I.M. and S.C. injection sites.
Distribution: Into the liver, bone marrow, and other tissues, including the placenta. At birth, the vitamin B concentration in neonates is three to five times that in the mother. Distributed into breast milk in concentrations approximately equal to the maternal concentration. Unlike cyanocobalamin, hydroxocobalamin is absorbed more slowly parenterally and may be taken up by the liver in larger quantities; it also produces a greater increase in serum cobalamin levels and less urinary excretion. Vitamin B_{12} is stored in the liver.
Metabolism: In the liver.
Excretion: In healthy persons receiving only dietary vitamin B_{12}, approximately 3 to 8 mcg of the vitamin is secreted into the GI tract daily, mainly from bile, and all but about 1 mcg is reabsorbed; less than 0.25 mcg is usually excreted in the urine daily. When administered in amounts that exceed the binding capacity of plasma, the liver, and other tissues, it is free in the blood for urinary excretion.
Onset, peak, duration: After I.M. or S.C. injection, the plasma level peaks within 1 hour; after oral administration of doses below 3 mcg, peak plasma levels are not reached for 8 to 12 hours.

INDICATIONS & DOSAGE

Recommended daily allowance (RDA) for cyanocobalamin–
Neonates and infants to 6 months: 0.3 mcg.
Infants 6 months to 1 year: 0.5 mcg.
Children over 1 year to 3 years: 0.7 mcg.
Children 4 to 6 years: 1 mcg.
Adults and children 11 years and over: 2 mcg.
Pregnant women: 2.2 mcg.
Lactating women: 2.6 mcg.
Vitamin B_{12} deficiency caused by inadequate diet, subtotal gastrectomy, or any other condition, disorder, or disease except malabsorption related to pernicious anemia or other GI disease–
Adults: 25 mcg P.O. daily as dietary supplement, or 30 to 100 mcg S.C. or I.M. daily for 5 to 10 days, depending on severity of deficiency. Maintenance dosage is 100 to 200 mcg I.M. once monthly. For subsequent prophylaxis, advise adequate nutrition and daily RDA vitamin B_{12} supplements.
Children: 30 to 100 mcg S.C. or I.M. daily for 5 to 10 days, depending on severity of deficiency. Maintenance dosage is at least 60 mcg/month I.M. or S.C. For subsequent prophylaxis, advise adequate nutrition and daily RDA vitamin B_{12} supplements.
Pernicious anemia or vitamin B_{12} malabsorption–
Adults: initially, 100 to 1,000 mcg I.M. daily for 2 weeks, then 100 to 1,000 mcg I.M. once monthly for life. If neurologic complications are present, follow initial therapy with 100 to 1,000 mcg I.M. once q 2 weeks before starting monthly regimen.
Children: 1,000 to 5,000 mcg I.M. or S.C. given over 2 or more weeks in 100-mcg increments; then 60 mcg I.M. or S.C. monthly for life.
Methylmalonic aciduria–
Neonates: 1,000 mcg I.M. daily for 11 days with a protein-restricted diet.
Schilling test flushing dose–
Adults and children: 1,000 mcg I.M. in a single dose.

CONTRAINDICATIONS & PRECAUTIONS

Contraindicated in patients with known hypersensitivity to cobalt, vitamin B_{12}, or any component of these medications; in patients with hereditary optic nerve atrophy (Leber's disease) because rapid optic nerve atrophy has been reported as an adverse effect. An intradermal test dose is recommended. After starting vitamin B_{12} therapy, serum potassium concentrations should be monitored to avoid fatal hypokalemia. Use cautiously in persons who are susceptible to gout (because of the potential for increased nucleic acid degeneration) and those with heart disease (because of the potential for increased blood volume).

ADVERSE REACTIONS

Common reactions are in italics; life-threatening reactions are in bold italics.

CV: peripheral vascular thrombosis.

GI: transient diarrhea.

Skin: itching, transitory exanthema, urticaria.

Local: pain, burning at S.C. or I.M. injection sites.

Other: ***anaphylaxis,*** anaphylactoid reactions with parenteral administration.

INTERACTIONS

Aminoglycosides, colchicine, para-aminosalicylic acid and salts, chloramphenicol: malabsorption of vitamin B_{12}. Don't use together.

EFFECTS ON DIAGNOSTIC TESTS

Intrinsic factor antibodies: false-positive results (present in the blood of half of all patients with pernicious anemia).

NURSING CONSIDERATIONS

Besides those related universally to drug therapy (see "How to use this book"), consider the following specific recommendations:

Assessment

- Obtain a baseline assessment of patient's underlying condition before therapy.
- Be alert for adverse reactions and drug interactions throughout therapy.
- Evaluate the patient's and family's knowledge about vitamin B_{12} therapy.

Nursing Diagnoses

- Altered oral mucous membranes related to the patient's underlying condition.
- Diarrhea related to adverse drug reaction.
- Knowledge deficit related to vitamin B_{12} therapy.

Planning and Implementation

Preparation and Administration

- Use I.V. administration only if other routes are ruled out. Anaphylactoid reactions may be caused by I.V administration.
- Don't mix parenteral liquids in the same syringe with other medications.
- Protect from light and heat.
- Drug is physically incompatible with dextrose solutions, alkaline or strongly acidic solutions, oxidizing and reducing agents, and many other drugs.
- Hydroxocobalamin is approved for I.M. use only. Advantage of hydroxocobalamin over cyanocobalamin is longer duration.

Monitoring

- Monitor effectiveness by assessing the patient's oral mucous membranes.
- Assess the patient's bowel habits, because drug may cause transient diarrhea.
- Monitor the patient's skin for urticaria and itching.
- Monitor for anaphylactoid reactions with parenteral administration.
- Monitor for pain and burning at the injection site with I.M. or S.C. injections.
- Closely monitor serum potassium for first 48 hours.
- Monitor patients with infection, tumors, or with renal, hepatic, and

other debilitating diseases for reduced therapeutic response.

Supportive Care

- Know that drug may cause false-positive intrinsic factor antibody test.
- Know that 50% to 98% of injected dose may appear in urine within 48 hours. Major portion of drug is excreted within first 8 hours after injection.
- Know that deficiencies are more common in strict vegetarians and their breast-fed infants.

Patient Teaching

- For patients with pernicious anemia, emphasize the importance of returning for monthly injections. Although total body stores may last 3 to 6 years, anemia will recur if not treated monthly.

Evaluation

In patients receiving vitamin B_{12}, appropriate evaluation statements may include:

- Patient's sore mouth and tongue has healed.
- Patient does not develop diarrhea.
- Patient and family state an understanding of vitamin B_{12} therapy.

vitamin C (ascorbic acid)

(a skor´ bik)

Ascorbicap◇, Cebid Timecelles◇, Cetane, Cevalin◇, Cevi-Bid, Ce-Vi-Sol*, Cevita◇, C-Span◇, Dull-C◇, Flavettes‡, Redoxon†, Solucap C, Vita C Crystals◇

- *Classification:* nutritional agent (vitamin)
- *Pregnancy Risk Category:* A (C if > RDA)

HOW SUPPLIED

Tablets◇: 25 mg, 50 mg, 100 mg, 250 mg, 500 mg, 1,000 mg, 1,500 mg
Tablets (chewable): 100 mg◇, 250 mg◇, 500 mg◇
Tablets (effervescent): 1,000 mg sugar-free◇
Tablets (timed-release): 500 mg◇, 750 mg◇, 1,000 mg◇, 1,500 mg
Capsules (timed-release): 500 mg◇
Crystals: 100 g (4 g/tsp)◇, 1,000 g (4 g/tsp, sugar-free)◇
Oral liquid: 50 ml (35 mg/0.6 ml)*◇
Oral solution: 50 ml (100 mg/ml)◇
Powder: 100 g (4 g/tsp)◇, 500 g (4 g/tsp)◇, 1,000 g (4 g/tsp, sugar-free)◇
Syrup: 20 mg/ml in 120 ml and 480 ml◇; 500 mg/5ml in 5 ml◇, 10 ml◇, 120 ml◇, 473 ml◇
Injection: 100 mg/ml in 2-ml, 10-ml ampules; 250 mg/ml in 10-ml ampules and 10-ml, 30-ml, 50-ml vials; 500 mg/ml in 2-ml, 5-ml ampules and 50-ml vials; 500 mg/ml (with monothioglycerol) in 1-ml ampules

ACTION

Mechanism: Necessary for collagen formation and tissue repair; involved in oxidation-reduction reactions throughout the body.
Absorption: Readily absorbed from the GI tract.
Excretion: In the urine. Doses in excess of 2 g/day will acidify the urine.

INDICATIONS & DOSAGE

Recommended daily allowance (RDA)–
Neonates and infants to 6 months: 30 mg.
Infants 6 months to 1 year: 35 mg.
Children 1 to 3 years: 40 mg.
Children 4 to 10 years: 45 mg.
Children 11 to 14 years: 50 mg.
Children 15 years and over and adults: 60 mg.
Pregnant women: 70 mg.
Lactating women (first 6 months): 95 mg.
Lactating women (second 6 months): 90 mg.
Frank and subclinical scurvy–
Adults: 100 mg to 2 g, depending on severity, P.O., S.C., I.M., or I.V. daily,

*Liquid form contains alcohol. **May contain tartrazine.

then at least 50 mg daily for maintenance.
Children: 100 to 300 mg, depending on severity, P.O., S.C., I.M., or I.V. daily, then at least 35 mg daily for maintenance.
Infants: 50 to 100 mg P.O., I.M., I.V., or S.C. daily.
Extensive burns, delayed fracture or wound healing, postoperative wound healing, severe febrile or chronic disease states–
Adults: 200 to 500 mg S.C., I.M., or I.V. daily.
Children: 100 to 200 mg P.O., S.C., I.M., or I.V. daily.
Prevention of vitamin C deficiency in those with poor nutritional habits or increased requirements–
Adults: at least 45 mg P.O., S.C., I.M., or I.V. daily.
Pregnant and lactating women: at least 60 mg P.O., S.C., I.M., or I.V. daily.
Children: at least 40 mg P.O., S.C., I.M., or I.V. daily.
Infants: at least 35 mg P.O., S.C., I.M., or I.V. daily.
Potentiation of methenamine in urine acidification–
Adults: 4 to 12 g P.O. daily in divided doses.

CONTRAINDICATIONS & PRECAUTIONS

Ascorbic acid products containing tartrazine can cause allergic reactions, including bronchial asthma, in susceptible individuals (many are also allergic to aspirin). Prolonged use of large doses of ascorbic acid may increase its metabolism. If intake is then reduced to normal levels, rebound scurvy may occur. Use of large doses during pregnancy has caused scurvy in neonates.

Patients on salt-restricted diets must consider that each gram of sodium ascorbate contains approximately 5 mEq of sodium.

ADVERSE REACTIONS

Common reactions are in italics; life-threatening reactions are in bold italics.
CNS: faintness or dizziness with fast I.V. administration.
GI: diarrhea, epigastric burning.
GU: acid urine, oxaluria, renal calculi, ***renal failure.***
Skin: discomfort at injection site.

INTERACTIONS

None significant.

EFFECTS ON DIAGNOSTIC TESTS

Occult blood in stool: false-negative results if administered less than 48 to 72 hours after ascorbic acid.
Urine glucose: false-positive determinations with glucose enzymatic method with large doses (more than 500 mg); false-positive results with copper reduction method (Benedict's reagent).

NURSING CONSIDERATIONS

Besides those related universally to drug therapy (see "How to use this book"), consider the following specific recommendations:

Assessment
- Obtain a baseline assessment of patient's underlying condition before therapy.
- Be alert for adverse reactions and drug interactions throughout therapy.
- Evaluate the patient's and family's knowledge about vitamin C therapy.

Nursing Diagnoses
- Altered nutrition: Less than body requirements, related to the patient's underlying condition.
- Diarrhea related to adverse drug reaction.
- Knowledge deficit related to vitamin C therapy.

Planning and Implementation
Preparation and Administration
- ***I.V. use:*** Avoid rapid I.V. administration. Direct injection should be administered slowly over 2 to 3 minutes. Intermittent infusion may be admin-

istered by infusion of the diluted drug over 20 to 30 minutes. Continuous infusion may also be used.
• Protect the solution from light.
Monitoring
• Check urine pH to ensure efficacy when administering for urine acidification.
• Monitor effectiveness by evaluating the reduction of symptoms of deficiency.
• Monitor for adverse reactions and interactions by monitoring the patient's bowel pattern; drug may cause diarrhea.
• Monitor for faintness and dizziness if the drug is administered rapidly by the I.V. route.
• Monitor the patient's urinary elimination pattern; drug may cause renal failure.
Supportive Care
• Know that this drug should be used cautiously in patients with G6PD deficiency.
• Know that I.V. administration requires extreme caution in patients with renal insufficiency.
Patient Teaching
• Advise the patient that rapid I.V. administration may cause faintness or dizziness.
• Tell the patient that he may experience discomfort at the injection site.
Evaluation
In patients receiving vitamin C, appropriate evaluation statements may include:
• Patient states a reduction of symptoms related to deficiency.
• Patient does not develop diarrhea.
• Patient and family state an understanding of vitamin C therapy.

vitamin D derivatives

cholecalciferol (vitamin D_3)
(kole e kal si´ fer ole)
Delta-D◇, Vitamin D_3◇

ergocalciferol (vitamin D_2)
(er goe kal sif´ e role)
Calciferol, Drisdol, Radiostol†, Radiostol Forte†, Vitamin D

• *Classification:* nutritional agent (vitamin)
• *Pregnancy Risk Category:* A (D if > RDA)

HOW SUPPLIED
Tablets: 1.25 mg (50,000 IU)
Capsules: 0.625 mg (25,000 IU), 1.25 mg (50,000 IU)
Oral liquid: 8,000 IU/ml in 60-ml dropper bottle
Injection: 12.5 mg (500,000 IU)/ml

ACTION
Mechanism: Promotes absorption and utilization of calcium and phosphate; helps to regulate serum calcium concentration.
Absorption: From the small intestine.
Distribution: Widely distributed and bound to proteins stored in the liver.
Metabolism: In the liver and kidneys. Half-life: Average, 24 hours.
Excretion: Bile (feces) is the primary excretion route. A small percentage is excreted in urine.
Onset, peak, duration: Onset of action is 10 to 24 hours. Duration of action is up to 6 months.

INDICATIONS & DOSAGE
Recommended daily allowance (RDA) for cholecalciferol–
Neonates and infants to 6 months: 300 IU.
Infants 6 months to adults 24 years: 400 IU.
Adults 25 years and over: 200 IU.
Pregnant or lactating women: 400 IU.
Rickets and other vitamin D deficiency diseases; renal osteodystrophy–
Adults: initially, 12,000 IU P.O. or I.M. daily, increased as indicated by

response up to 500,000 IU daily in most cases and up to 800,000 IU daily for vitamin D–resistant rickets.
Children: 1,500 to 5,000 IU P.O. or I.M. daily for 2 to 4 weeks, repeated after 2 weeks, if necessary. Alternatively, a single dose of 600,000 IU may be given.

Monitor serum calcium daily to guide dosage. After correction of deficiency, maintenance includes adequate dietary nutrition and RDA supplements.

Hypoparathyroidism–
Adults and children: 50,000 to 200,000 IU P.O. or I.M. daily, with 4-g calcium supplement.

CONTRAINDICATIONS & PRECAUTIONS

Contraindicated in patients with hypercalcemia or vitamin D toxicity, malabsorption syndrome, or abnormal sensitivity to vitamin D effects.

Use with extreme caution in patients with impaired renal function, heart disease, renal stones, or arteriosclerosis; and in patients receiving digitalis glycosides.

ADVERSE REACTIONS

Common reactions are in italics; life-threatening reactions are in bold italics.

Side effects listed are usually seen in vitamin D toxicity only.

CNS: headache, dizziness, ataxia, weakness, somnolence, decreased libido, overt psychosis, ***seizures.***
CV: calcifications of soft tissues, including the heart.
EENT: dry mouth, metallic taste, rhinorrhea, conjunctivitis (calcific), photophobia, tinnitus.
GI: anorexia, nausea, constipation, diarrhea.
GU: polyuria, albuminuria, hypercalciuria, nocturia, impaired renal function, renal calculi.
Metabolic: hypercalcemia, hyperphosphatemia.
Skin: pruritus.
Other: bone and muscle pain, bone demineralization, weight loss.

INTERACTIONS

Mineral oil, cholestyramine resin: inhibited GI absorption of oral vitamin D. Space doses. Use together cautiously.

EFFECTS ON DIAGNOSTIC TESTS

AST (SGOT) and ALT (SGPT): elevated levels.
Serum cholesterol: falsely increases levels.

NURSING CONSIDERATIONS

Besides those related universally to drug therapy (see "How to use this book"), consider the following specific recommendations:

Assessment
- Obtain a baseline assessment of patient's underlying condition before therapy.
- Be alert for adverse reactions and drug interactions throughout therapy.
- Evaluate the patient's and family's knowledge about vitamin D therapy.

Nursing Diagnoses
- Altered nutrition: Less than body requirements, related to the patient's underlying condition.
- Altered oral mucous membranes related to adverse drug reaction.
- Knowledge deficit related to vitamin D therapy.

Planning and Implementation
Preparation and Administration
- I.M. injection of vitamin D dispersed in oil is preferable in patients who are unable to absorb the oral form.
- If I.V. use is necessary, use only water-miscible solutions intended for dilution in large-volume parenterals.

Monitoring
- Monitor for adverse reactions and interactions by checking the patient's eating and bowel habits; dry mouth, nausea, vomiting, metallic taste, and

constipation may be early signs and symptoms of toxicity.

• Monitor effectiveness by assessing for reduced symptoms of the underlying condition.
• Monitor for CNS effects, such as headache, dizziness, ataxia, weakness, and seizures.
• Monitor serum and urine calcium, potassium, and urea if high therapeutic doses are used.
• Monitor the patient's skin for dryness.
• Monitor renal studies for polyuria, albuminuria, hypercalciuria, and signs of impaired renal function.

Supportive Care

• Patients with hyperphosphatemia require dietary phosphate restrictions and binding agents to avoid metastatic calcifications and renal calculi.
• Malabsorption from inadaquate bile or hepatic dysfunction may require the addition of exogenous bile salts to oral vitamin D.
• Know that this vitamin is fat-soluble.
• Know that doses of 60,000 IU/day can cause hypercalcemia.

Patient Teaching

• Warn patient of the dangers of increasing dosage without consulting the doctor.
• Advise patient to restrict daily intake of magnesium-containing antacids.

Evaluation

In patients receiving vitamin D, appropriate evaluation statements may include:

• Patient's nutritional status is improving.
• Patient does not develop drug-induced dry mouth.
• Patient and family state an understanding of vitamin D therapy.

vitamin E (alpha tocopherol)

Aquasol E◇, Eprolin◇, Pertropin◇, Solucap E◇, Tocopher◇

• *Classification:* nutritional agent (vitamin)
• *Pregnancy Risk Category:* A (C if > RDA)

HOW SUPPLIED

Tablets◇: 100 IU, 200 IU, 400 IU, 500 IU, 600 IU, 1,000 IU
Tablets (chewable): 100 IU◇, 200 IU◇, 400 IU◇
Capsules◇: 50 IU, 100 IU, 200 IU, 400 IU, 600 IU, 1,000 IU
Oral solution: 50 IU/ml◇

ACTION

Mechanism: Acts as a cofactor and an antioxidant.
Absorption: GI absorption depends on the presence of bile. Only 20% to 60% of the vitamin obtained from dietary sources is absorbed. As dosage increases, the fraction absorbed decreases.
Distribution: To all tissues. Storage in adipose tissue.
Metabolism: In the liver by glucuronidation.
Excretion: Primarily in bile. Some enterohepatic circulation may occur. Small amounts of the metabolites are excreted in urine.

INDICATIONS & DOSAGE

Recommended daily allowance (RDA) –
Neonates and infants to 6 months: 4 IU.
Infants 6 months to 1 year: 6 IU.
Children over 1 year to 3 years: 9 IU.
Children 4 to 10 years: 10 IU.
Males 11 years and over: 15 IU.
Females 11 years and over: 12 IU.
Pregnant women: 15 IU.
Lactating women (first 6 months): 18 IU.

Lactating women (second 6 months): 16 IU.
Vitamin E deficiency in premature infants and in patients with impaired fat absorption–
Adults: 60 to 75 IU, depending on severity, P.O. or I.M. daily.
Children: 1 mg equivalent/0.6 g of dietary unsaturated fat P.O. or I.M. daily.

CONTRAINDICATIONS & PRECAUTIONS

Vitamin E is usually nontoxic. A complex and potentially fatal syndrome has occurred in several premature infants who received I.V. therapy with vitamin E; however, this form of the drug is no longer available.

ADVERSE REACTIONS

None reported.

INTERACTIONS

Mineral oil, cholestyramine resin: inhibited GI absorption of oral vitamin E. Space doses. Use together cautiously.

EFFECTS ON DIAGNOSTIC TESTS

None reported.

NURSING CONSIDERATIONS

Besides those related universally to drug therapy (see "How to use this book"), consider the following specific recommendations:

Assessment
- Obtain a baseline assessment of patient's underlying condition before therapy.
- Be alert for adverse reactions and drug interactions throughout therapy.
- Evaluate the patient's and family's knowledge about vitamin E therapy.

Nursing Diagnoses
- Impaired skin integrity related to the patient's lack of vitamin E.
- Altered nutrition: Less than body requirements, related to the patient's underlying condition.
- Knowledge deficit related to vitamin E therapy.

Planning and Implementation
Preparation and Administration
- Use cautiously with mineral oil and cholestyramine resin. May be necessary to space the doses.

Monitoring
- Monitor effectiveness by assessing the patient's skin for reduced symptoms of underlying condition.
- Monitor for thrombophlebitis with megadoses.

Supportive Care
- Know that water-miscible forms are more completely absorbed in GI tract than other forms.
- Adequate bile is essential for absorption.
- Requirements increase with rise in dietary polyunsaturated acids.
- May protect other vitamins against oxidation.

Patient Teaching
- Discourage self-medication with megadoses.

Evaluation
In patients receiving vitamin E, appropriate evaluation statements may include:
- Patient states an improvement of impaired skin integrity.
- Patient's nutritional status is improving.
- Patient and family state an understanding of vitamin E therapy.

vitamin K derivatives

phytonadione (vitamin K_1)

(fye toe na dye´ one)
AquaMEPHYTON, Konakion, Mephyton

menadione (vitamin K_3)

(men a dye´ one)

menadiol sodium diphosphate

(men a dye´ ole)

Synkavite†, Synkayvite

• *Classification:* nutritional agent (vitamin)
• *Pregnancy Risk Category:* C

HOW SUPPLIED

phytonadione
Tablets: 5 mg
Injection (aqueous colloidal solution): 2 mg/ml, 10 mg/ml
Injection (aqueous dispersion): 2 mg/ml, 10 mg/ml
menadione
Powder
menadiol sodium
Tablets: 5 mg
Injection: 5 mg/ml, 10 mg/ml, 37.5 mg/ml

ACTION

Mechanism: Vitamin K is required for synthesis of blood coagulation factors; drug is involved in carboxylation of the inactive precursors of these factors.
Absorption: Requires bile salts for absorption from the GI tract. Absorbed directly into blood stream.
Distribution: To all tissues.
Excretion: High fecal concentration.

INDICATIONS & DOSAGE

Hypoprothrombinemia secondary to vitamin K malabsorption, drug therapy, or excess vitamin A–
Adults: 2.5 to 25 mg phytonadione, depending on severity, P.O. or parenterally, repeated and increased up to 50 mg, if necessary. Or 5 to 15 mg P.O. or parenterally, titrated to patient's requirements.
Children: 5 to 10 mg P.O. or parenterally.
Infants: 2 mg P.O. or parenterally.
I.V. injection rate for children and infants should not exceed 3 mg/m²/minute or a total of 5 mg.
Hypoprothrombinemia secondary to effect of oral anticoagulants–
Adults: 2.5 to 10 mg P.O., S.C., or I.M., based on prothrombin time, repeated, if necessary, within 12 to 48 hours after oral dose or within 6 to 8 hours after parenteral dose. In emergency, give 10 to 50 mg slow I.V., rate not to exceed 1 mg/minute, repeated q 4 hours, p.r.n.
Prevention of hemorrhagic disease in neonates–
Neonates: 0.5 to 1 mg S.C. or I.M. immediately after birth, repeated within 6 to 8 hours, if needed, especially if mother received oral anticoagulants or long-term anticonvulsant therapy during pregnancy.
Differentiation between hepatocellular disease or biliary obstruction as source of hypoprothrombinemia–
Adults and children: 10 mg I.M. or S.C.
Prevention of hypoprothrombinemia related to vitamin K deficiency in long-term parenteral nutrition–
Adults: 5 to 10 mg S.C. or I.M. weekly.
Children: 2 to 5 mg S.C. or I.M. weekly.
Prevention of hypoprothrombinemia in infants receiving less than 0.1 mg/liter vitamin K in breast milk or milk substitutes–
Infants: 1 mg S.C. or I.M. monthly.

CONTRAINDICATIONS & PRECAUTIONS

Contraindicated in patients hypersensitive to any of its analogues; during the last few weeks of pregnancy or labor, because menadiol sodium diphosphate has caused toxic reactions in neonates; and in infants.

Use cautiously in patients with impaired hepatic function, because large doses may further decrease hepatic function. Menadiol sodium diphosphate may induce erythrocyte hemolysis in patients with glucose-6-phosphate dehydrogenase deficiency.

ADVERSE REACTIONS

Common reactions are in italics; life-threatening reactions are in bold italics.
CNS: dizziness, seizure-like movements.
CV: transient hypotension after I.V. administration, rapid and weak pulse, ***cardiac irregularities.***
GI: nausea, vomiting.
Skin: sweating, flushing, erythema.
Local: pain, swelling, and hematoma at injection site.
Other: ***bronchospasms,*** dyspnea, cramp-like pain, ***anaphylaxis*** *and anaphylactoid reactions (usually after rapid I.V. administration).*

INTERACTIONS

Mineral oil, cholestyramine resin: inhibited GI absorption of oral vitamin K. Space doses. Use together cautiously.

EFFECTS ON DIAGNOSTIC TESTS

Urine steroids: falsely elevated levels.

NURSING CONSIDERATIONS

Besides those related universally to drug therapy (see "How to use this book"), consider the following specific recommendations:

Assessment

- Obtain a baseline assessment of patient's underlying condition before therapy.
- Be alert for adverse reactions and drug interactions throughout therapy.
- Evaluate the patient's and family's knowledge about vitamin K therapy.

Nursing Diagnoses

- High risk for fluid volume deficit related to adverse reactions.
- Altered tissue perfusion related to drug-induced hypotension.
- Knowledge deficit related to vitamin K therapy.

Planning and Implementation

Preparation and Administration

- Protect parenteral products from light. Wrap infusion container with aluminum foil.
- Weekly addition of phytonadione 5 to 10 mg to TPN solutions may be ordered.
- Check manufacturer's labels for administration route restrictions.
- Use caution in handling bulk menadione powder. It is irritating to the skin and the respiratory tract.
- ***I.V. use:*** Administer phytonadione I.V. by slow infusion (over 2 to 3 hours). Mix in 0.9% sodium chloride solution, dextrose 5% in water, or dextrose 5% in 0.9% sodium chloride solution. Observe patient closely for flushing, weakness, tachycardia, and hypotension; may progress to shock.

When administering menadione, I.V. rate should not exceed 1 mg/minute. Never inject more than 10 mg at once. Drug may be administered by direct injection, intermittent infusion, or continuous infusion.

Monitoring

- Monitor effectiveness by assessing prothrombin time.
- Assess the patient's vital signs for transient hypotension, especially after I.V. administration, as well as for rapid weak pulse and cardiac irregularities.
- Monitor respiratory status; drug may cause bronchospasm, dyspnea, anaphylaxis, and anaphylactoid reactions.
- Monitor the injection site for pain, swelling, and hemotoma.
- Monitor hydration status if nausea and vomiting become severe.

Supportive Care

- Never use menadione in neonates (especially in premature neonates) because it can cause hemolytic anemia, hyperbilirubinemia, kernicterus, brain damage, and death.
- Do not use menadione to treat hy-

poprothrombinemia induced by oral anticoagulant. Phytonadione is the drug of choice.
• Excessive use of menadione may temporarily defeat oral anticoagulant therapy. Higher doses of oral anticoagulant or interim use of heparin may be required.
• Provide additional fluids if nausea and vomiting become severe.
• Failure to respond to vitamin K may indicate coagulation defects.
• In severe bleeding, don't delay other measures, such as fresh frozen plasma or whole blood.
• This vitamin is fat-soluble.
• I.V. injections produce more rapid but shorter-lived effects than S.C. or I.M. injections.

Patient Teaching
• Tell the patient to report any discomfort at the injection site.

Evaluation
In patients receiving vitamin K therapy, appropriate evaluation statements may include:
• Patient does not develop nausea and vomiting.
• Patient does not develop drug-induced hypotension.
• Patient and family state an understanding of vitamin K therapy.

PHARMACOLOGIC CLASS

vitamins

Fat-soluble
vitamin A_1 (retinol)
vitamin A_2 (dehydroretinol)
vitamin A acid (retinoic acid)
provitamin A (carotene)
vitamin D
vitamin D_2 (ergocalciferol)
vitamin D_3 (cholecalciferol)
vitamin E
tocopherol and tocotrienols: alpha, beta, gamma, delta
vitamin K (menadione, phytonadione)

Water-soluble
vitamin B_1 (thiamine)
vitamin B_2 (riboflavin)
vitamin B_3 (niacin)
vitamin B_5 (pantothenic acid)
vitamin B_6 (pyridoxine)
vitamin B_9 (folic acid, folacin)
vitamin B_{12} (cyanocobalamin)
vitamin C (ascorbic acid)
biotin

OVERVIEW
Vitamins are chemically unrelated organic compounds which are required for normal growth and maintenance of metabolic functions. Since the body is unable to synthesize many vitamins, it must obtain them from exogenous sources. Vitamins do not furnish energy and are not essential building blocks for the body; however, they are essential for the transformation of energy and for the regulation of metabolic processes.

Vitamins are classified as fat-soluble or water-soluble, and the Food and Nutrition Board of the National Research Council determines the recommended dietary allowances (RDAs) for each. These allowances represent amounts that will provide adequate nutrition in most healthy persons; they are not minimum requirements. Note that a diet which includes ample intake of the four basic food groups will provide sufficient quantities of vitamins. If needed, vitamins should be used as an adjunct to a regular diet and not as a food substitute.

Controversy has existed for years over the vitamin issue. Some argue that vitamin supplementation is unnecessary; some recommend moderate supplementation for everyone; still others advocate the use of megavitamins. The public should be warned against self-medication with vitamins, as the safety and efficacy of their chronic use for relief of mild or

RECOMMENDED DAILY ALLOWANCES FOR ADULTS AGES 23 TO 50

VITAMIN	MALES	FEMALES	PREGNANT FEMALES	LACTATING FEMALES*
A	1,000 mcg	800 mcg	800 mcg	1,300 mcg
B_1	1.5 mg	1.1 mg	1.5 mg	1.6 mg
B_2	1.7 mg	1.3 mg	1.6 mg	1.8 mg
B_6	2 mg	1.6 mg	2.2 mg	2.1 mg
B_{12}	2 mcg	2 mcg	2.2 mcg	2.6 mcg
C	60 mg	60 mg	70 mg	95 mg
D	200 IU	200 IU	400 IU	400 IU
E	10 IU	8 IU	10 IU	12 IU
K	80 mcg	65 mcg	65 mcg	65 mcg
Folic acid	200 mcg	180 mcg	400 mcg	280 mcg
Niacin	19 mg	15 mg	17 mg	20 mg

*first 6 months

self-limiting conditions has not been established.

Vitamins are available as single drugs or in combination with several other vitamins with or without minerals, trace elements, iron, fluoride, or other nutritional supplements. Frequently, diets deficient in one vitamin are also deficient in other vitamins of similar dietary source. Malabsorption syndromes also affect the usage of several vitamins as do certain disease states which increase metabolic rates. Therefore, multiple vitamin therapy may prove rational and useful in these situations.

Fat-soluble vitamins are absorbed with dietary fats and stored in the body in moderate amounts. They are not normally excreted in urine. Chronic ingestion of therapeutic amounts can result in excessive build-up of these agents and lead to toxicity.

Water-soluble vitamins are not stored in the body in any appreciable amounts and are excreted in urine. These agents seldom cause toxicity in patients with normal renal function.

Both fat-soluble and water-soluble vitamins are essential for the maintenance of normal structure and normal metabolic functions of the body.

CLINICAL INDICATIONS AND ACTIONS

Vitamin deficiency or malabsorption; conditions of metabolic stress

Vitamin supplementation is required when deficiencies exist, in malabsorption syndrome, in hypermetabolic disease states, during pregnancy and lactation, and in the elderly, alcoholics, or dieters. Multiple vitamins may be indicated for patients taking oral contraceptives, estrogens, prolonged antibiotic therapy, isoniazid, or for patients receiving prolonged I.V. hyperalimentation (IVH).

Persons with increased metabolic requirements, such as infants, and those suffering severe injury, trauma, major surgery, or severe infection also require supplementation. Prolonged diarrhea, severe GI disorders, malignancy, surgical removal or sections of GI tract, obstructive jaundice, cystic fibrosis, and other conditions leading to reduced or poor absorption are included indications for multiple vitamin therapy. Refer to individual agents for specific indications.

OVERVIEW OF ADVERSE REACTIONS

The most frequent adverse reactions seen with both types of vitamins include nausea, vomiting, diarrhea, tiredness, weakness, headache, loss of appetite, skin rash, and itching.

REPRESENTATIVE COMBINATIONS

The following list includes selected combinations that are available only by prescription.

B vitamins (oral) niacin (B_3), pantothenic acid (B_5), pyridoxine (B_6), and cyanocobalamin (B_{12}), with folic acid (B_9), iron, manganese, zinc, and 13% alcohol: Megaton Elixir; with thiamine (B_1), riboflavin (B_2), ferric pyrophosphate, and 15% alcohol: Senilizol Elixir; with thiamine (B_1), riboflavin (B_2), ascorbic acid, and folic acid: Berocca, B Plex, Strovite, BC with folic acid; with thiamine (B_1), riboflavin (B_2), ascorbic acid, folic acid, and biotin: Nephrocaps.

B vitamins (parenteral) thiamine (B_1) and cyanocobalamin (B_{12}): Bexibee injection; with riboflavin (B_2), niacin (B_3), pantothenic acid (B_5), pyridoxine (B_6), and ascorbic acid: Becomject/C, Kay Plex, Vicam, Scorbex/12.

Multivitamins (oral) vitamins A, D, E, thiamine (B_1), riboflavin (B_2), niacin (B_3), pantothenic acid (B_5), pyridoxine (B_6), cyanocobalamin (B_{12}), and ascorbic acid: Theracebrin, Al-Vite; vitamins E, thiamine (B_1), riboflavin (B_2), niacin (B_3), pantothenic acid (B_5), pyridoxine (B_6), cyanocobalamin (B_{12}), ascorbic acid, and folic acid: Cefol Filmtabs; vitamins E, thiamine (B_1), niacin (B_3), pyridoxine (B_6), cyanocobalamin (B_{12}), ascorbic acid, folic acid, and iron: Vicef; vitamins A, E, thiamine (B_1), riboflavin (B_2), niacin (B_3), pantothenic acid (B_5), pyridoxine (B_6), cyanocobalamin (B_{12}), ascorbic acid, folic acid, iron, iodine, and calcium: Eldec.

Multivitamins (parenteral) vitamins A, D, E, thiamine (B_1), riboflavin (B_2), thiamine (B_3), pantothenic acid (B_5), pyridoxine (B_6), cyanocobalamin (B_{12}), ascorbic acid, biotin, and folic acid: Berocca parenteral nutrition, MVI, MVC.

Multivitamins with fluoride (oral) vitamins A, D, thiamine (B_1), riboflavin (B_2), niacin (B_3), pantothenic acid (B_5), pyridoxine (B_6), cyanocobalamin (B_{12}), ascorbic acid, folic acid, and fluoride: Aldeflor, Polyvitamins with fluoride, Mulvidren, Polytabs-F; vitamins A, D, E, thiamine (B_1), riboflavin (B_2), niacin (B_3), pyridoxine (B_6), cyanocobalamin (B_{12}), ascorbic acid, folic acid, and fluoride: Poly-Vi-Flor, Florvite, Vidaylin F.

---

warfarin sodium

(war´ far in)

Coumadin, Panwarfin**, Warfilone Sodium†

• *Classification:* anticoagulant (coumarin derivative)
• *Pregnancy Risk Category:* D

HOW SUPPLIED

Tablets: 2 mg, 2.5 mg, 5 mg, 7.5 mg, 10 mg
Injection: 50 mg/vial

*Liquid form contains alcohol. **May contain tartrazine.

ACTION

Mechanism: Inhibits vitamin K–dependent activation of clotting factors II, VII, IX, and X, which are formed in the liver.
Absorption: Rapidly and completely absorbed from the GI tract.
Distribution: Highly bound to plasma protein, especially albumin; drug crosses placenta but does not appear to accumulate in breast milk.
Metabolism: Hydroxylated by liver into inactive metabolites.
Excretion: Metabolites are reabsorbed from bile and excreted in urine. Half-life: Of parent drug, 1 to 3 days.
Onset, peak, duration: Because therapeutic effect is relatively more dependent on clotting factor depletion (factor X has half-life of 40 hours), prothrombin time (PT) will not peak for 1½ to 3 days despite use of a loading dose. Duration of action is 2 to 5 days.

INDICATIONS & DOSAGE

Treatment of pulmonary emboli; prevention and treatment of deep vein thrombosis, myocardial infarction, rheumatic heart disease with heart valve damage, atrial arrhythmias–
Adults: 10 to 15 mg P.O. for 3 days, then dosage based on daily prothrombin (PT) times. Usual maintenance dosage is 2 to 10 mg P.O. daily. Alternate regimen: initially, 40 to 60 mg P.O. daily; then 2 to 10 mg daily based on PT determinations.

Warfarin sodium also available for I.V. use (50 mg/vial). Reconstitute with sterile water for injection. I.V. form rarely used and may be in periodic short supply.

CONTRAINDICATIONS & PRECAUTIONS

Contraindicated in patients with bleeding or hemorrhagic tendencies caused by open wounds, visceral cancer, GI ulcers, severe hepatic or renal disease, severe or uncontrolled hypertension (diastolic pressure over 110 mm Hg), subacute bacterial endocarditis, or vitamin K deficiency, or after recent brain, eye, or spinal cord surgery because excessive bleeding can occur.

Use cautiously in patients with diverticulitis, colitis, mild-to-moderate hypertension, or mild-to-moderate hepatic or renal disease; during lactation; in patients with any drainage tubes; in conjunction with regional or lumbar block anesthesia; or in patients with any condition that increases risk of hemorrhage.

ADVERSE REACTIONS

Common reactions are in italics; life-threatening reactions are in bold italics.
Blood: ***hemorrhage with excessive dosage,*** leukopenia.
GI: paralytic ileus, intestinal obstruction (both resulting from hemorrhage), diarrhea, vomiting, cramps, nausea.
GU: excessive uterine bleeding.
Skin: dermatitis, urticaria, *rash,* necrosis, alopecia.
Other: *fever.*

INTERACTIONS

Acetaminophen: increased bleeding possible with chronic (greater than 2 weeks) therapy with acetaminophen. Monitor very carefully.
Amiodarone, chloramphenicol, clofibrate, diflunisal, thyroid drugs, heparin, anabolic steroids, cimetidine, disulfiram, glucagon, inhalation anesthetics, metronidazole, quinidine, influenza vaccine, sulindac, sulfinpyrazone, sulfonamides: increased prothrombin time. Monitor patient carefully for bleeding. Consider anticoagulant dosage reduction.
Barbiturates: inhibition of hypoprothrombinemic effect of anticoagulants. If barbiturates are withdrawn, reduce anticoagulant dose; inhibition may last weeks after barbiturate is

withdrawn, but fatal hemorrhage can occur when inhibition disappears.
Cholestyramine: decreased response when used too close together. Administer 6 hours after oral anticoagulants.
Ethacrynic acid, indomethacin, mefenamic acid, oxyphenbutazone, phenylbutazone, salicylates: increased prothrombin time; ulcerogenic effects. Don't use together.
Glutethimide, chloral hydrate, triclofos sodium: increased or decreased prothrombin time. Avoid use if possible, or monitor patient carefully.
Griseofulvin, haloperidol, ethchlorvynol, carbamazepine, paraldehyde, rifampin: decreased prothrombin time with reduced anticoagulant effect. Monitor patient carefully.

EFFECTS ON DIAGNOSTIC TESTS

Lactic dehydrogenase: increased activity.
PT and partial thromboplastin time: prolonged.
Serum transaminase: elevated levels.
Serum theophylline: falsely negative levels.
Uric acid excretion: increased.

NURSING CONSIDERATIONS

Besides those related universally to drug therapy (see "How to use this book"), consider the following specific recommendations:

Assessment

- Obtain a baseline assessment of PT before therapy.
- Be alert for adverse reactions and drug interactions throughout therapy.
- Evaluate the patient's and family's knowledge about warfarin sodium therapy.

Nursing Diagnoses

- Altered tissue perfusion (cardiopulmonary, peripheral) related to the patient's underlying condition.
- High risk for injury related to the adverse effects of warfarin sodium.
- Knowledge deficit related to warfarin sodium therapy.

Planning and Implementation

Preparation and Administration

- ***I.V. use:*** Available as a powder in a 50-mg vial. Protect from light and store at room temperature. Reconstitute by adding 2 ml of sterile water for injection for a solution of 25 mg/ml. Use immediately after reconstitution; solution contains no preservatives. Inject desired dose into I.V. tubing containing a free-flowing compatible solution. Compatible I.V. solutions include: dextran 6% and 0.9% sodium chloride, dextrose 2.5% in half-strength Ringers injection, dextrose 2.5% in water, Ionosol B with dextrose 5%, Ionosol D-CM, Ionosol MB with dextrose 5%, Ionosol PSL, Ringers injection, 0.45% sodium chloride, 0.9% sodium chloride, and ⅙ M sodium lactate. Intermittent infusion and continuous infusion are not recommended.
- ***P.O. use:*** Because onset of action is delayed, heparin sodium is often given during the first few days of treatment. When heparin sodium is being given simultaneously, don't draw blood for PT within 5 hours of intermittent I.V. heparin administration. However blood for PT may be drawn at any time during continuous heparin infusion. Daily dose is based on PT. Usual maintenance dose is 2 to 10 mg P.O. daily. Initially, the patient may receive 10 to 15 mg P.O. for 3 days or alternately 40 to 60 mg P.O. daily followed by the 2 to 10 mg maintenance dose based on PT determinations. Drug should be given at the same time daily. The half-life of warfarin's anticoagulant effect is 36 to 44 hours. Effect can be neutralized by vitamin K injections.

Monitoring

- Monitor effectiveness by regularly checking the patient's PT. Keep in mind that changes in diet, environment, physical condition, and concur-

rent drug use may alter response to warfarin.
• Monitor the patient closely for signs of bleeding. Test all exudates for microscopic blood and observe bleeding precautions.
• Monitor the patient for fever and skin rash since these may signal a severe reaction; notify the doctor immediately and withhold the drug.
• Observe nursing infants of mothers on the drug for unexpected bleeding.

Supportive Care
• Remember that patients with renal or hepatic failure and elderly patients are especially sensitive to warfarin effect.
• Keep in mind that food and enteral feedings that contain vitamin K may impair anticoagulation. Labels should be read carefully.
• Avoid abrupt discontinuation. Taper the dose gradually over 3 to 4 weeks.

Patient Teaching
• Tell the patient to report bleeding gums, bruising on the arms or legs, petechiae, nosebleeds, melena, tarry stools, hematuria, hematemesis, or excessive menstrual bleeding immediately.
• Tell the patient to avoid OTC products containing aspirin, other salicylates, or drugs that interact with warfarin. He should take his dose the same time daily.
• Tell the patient to use an electric shaver and brush his teeth with a soft toothbrush. If he needs dental work or surgery, his warfarin will need to be adjusted. He should also carry a card that alerts those concerned to his potential for bleeding and his anticoagulant therapy.
• Tell the patient to eat consistent amounts of leafy green vegetables, which contain vitamin K, since varying amounts may alter anticoagulant effects.

Evaluation

In patients receiving warfarin sodium, appropriate evaluation statements may include:
• Patient's PT reflects the goals of the anticoagulant therapy (1.5 to 2 times normal).
• Patient has not experienced injury from abnormal or excessive bleeding related to the adverse effects of warfarin.
• Patient and family state an understanding of warfarin sodium therapy.

XYZ

PHARMACOLOGIC CLASS

xanthine derivatives
aminophylline
caffeine
dyphylline
oxtriphylline
theophylline

OVERVIEW

The xanthines have been used in beverages for their stimulant action for many centuries. Theophylline and its salts and analogs were first found to relax smooth muscle. These drugs have extensive therapeutic use, especially in management of chronic respiratory disorders. Numerous dosage forms are available to assist in patient compliance and help control the toxicities associated with these agents.

The xanthines (caffeine, theobromine, and theophylline) are structurally related; they directly relax smooth muscle, stimulate the CNS, induce diuresis, increase gastric acid secretion, inhibit uterine contractions, and have weak inotropic and chronotropic effects on the heart. Their physiologic effect is a relaxation of all smooth muscle, with respiratory smooth muscle the most sensitive to this effect at nontoxic doses. Of these agents, theophylline exerts the greatest effect on smooth muscle.

CLINICAL INDICATIONS AND ACTIONS

Treatment of respiratory disorders
Xanthines are indicated in the symptomatic treatment of asthma and bronchospasm associated with emphysema and chronic bronchitis. By relaxing the smooth muscle of the respiratory tract, they increase air flow and vital capacity. Additionally, they slow the onset of diaphragmatic fatigue and stimulate the respiratory center in the CNS.

COMPARING XANTHINE DERIVATIVES

The table below compares the varying theophylline content of several common xanthine derivatives. (Dyphylline is not included because although it has the same pharmacologic action as theophylline, it is a chemical derivative and not a true theophylline salt.)

DRUG	APPROXIMATE THEOPHYLLINE CONTENT	EQUIVALENT DOSE
theophylline anhydrous	100%	100 mg
theophylline monohydrate	90.7% (±1.1%)	110 mg
aminophylline anhydrous	85.7% (±1.7%)	116 mg
aminophylline dehydrate	78.9% (±1.6%)	127 mg
oxytriphylline	63.6% (±1.9%)	156 mg
theophylline sodium glycinate	45.9% (±1.4%)	217 mg

*Liquid form contains alcohol. **May contain tartrazine.

OVERVIEW OF ADVERSE REACTIONS

The xanthines stimulate the CNS and heart while relaxing smooth muscle. This produces such reactions as hypotension, palpitations, arrhythmias, restlessness, irritability, nausea, vomiting, urinary retention, and headache. Adverse effects are dose-related, except for hypersensitivity, and can be controlled by dosage adjustment and monitored via serum levels.

REPRESENTATIVE COMBINATIONS

Dyphylline with chlorpheniramine maleate, guaifenesin, dextromethorphan hydrobromide and phenylephrine: Dilor-G. *Oxtriphylline* with guaifenesin: Brondecon. *Theophylline* with phenobarbital: Bronkolixir, Bronkotab, with ephedrine and phenobarbital: Quadrinal, Azma-Aid, Phedral, Primatene "P" Formula, Tedral, Tedrigen, Theofedral; with guaifenesin: Asbron G, Quibron; with hydroxyzine hydrochloride and ephedrine: Marax, Marax D.F.

---

xylometazoline hydrochloride

(zye loe met az´ oh leen)

4-Way Long Acting, Neo-Synephrine II, Otrivin, Sine-Off Nasal Spray, Sinex-L.A.

- *Classification:* nasal decongestant (alpha-adrenergic agonist)
- *Pregnancy Risk Category:* C

HOW SUPPLIED

Nasal solution: 0.05%, 0.1%

ACTION

Mechanism: Produces local vasoconstriction of dilated arterioles to reduce blood flow and nasal congestion.

Pharmacokinetics: Unknown.

Onset, peak, duration: Onset is about 10 minutes; duration of effect, 5 to 6 hours.

INDICATIONS & DOSAGE

Nasal congestion–

Adults and children over 12 years: apply 2 to 3 drops or 1 to 2 sprays of 0.1% solution to nasal mucosa q 8 to 10 hours.

Children under 12 years: apply 2 to 3 drops or 1 spray of 0.05% solution to nasal mucosa q 8 to 10 hours.

CONTRAINDICATIONS & PRECAUTIONS

Contraindicated in patients with narrow-angle glaucoma, because the drug may increase intraocular pressure; in patients receiving tricyclic antidepressants, because of the potential for adverse cardiovascular effects; and in those hypersensitive to any components of the preparation.

Use cautiously in patients with hyperthyroidism, cardiac disease, hypertension, diabetes mellitus, or advanced arteriosclerosis.

ADVERSE REACTIONS

Common reactions are in italics; life-threatening reactions are in bold italics.

EENT: rebound nasal congestion or irritation with excessive or long-term use; transient burning, stinging; dryness or ulceration of nasal mucosa; sneezing.

INTERACTIONS

None significant.

EFFECTS ON DIAGNOSTIC TESTS

None reported.

NURSING CONSIDERATIONS

Besides those related universally to drug therapy (see "How to use this book"), consider the following specific recommendations.

Assessment

• Obtain a baseline assessment of the patient's breathing pattern and degree of nasal congestion.

• Be alert for adverse reactions or drug interactions throughout therapy.

• Evaluate the patient's and family's knowledge about xylometazoline hydrochloride therapy.

Nursing Diagnoses

• Ineffective airway clearance related to the patient's underlying condition.

• Ineffective airway clearance related to rebound congestion from excessive use.

• Knowledge deficit related to xylometazoline hydrochloride

Planning and Implementation

Preparation and Administration

• ***Topical use:*** Have patient clear the nasal passages by gently blowing his nose. To administer nasal drops, have the patient tilt his head back and then instill the medication. Have the patient try to maintain this position for 5 minutes after instillation to permit the medication to permit distribution throughout the nasal passage. If nasal spray is used, have the patient hold his head upright and quickly spray the nostril. Have the patient wait 3 to 5 minutes and then blow his nose.

Monitoring

• Monitor effectiveness by assessing the patient's breathing pattern and degree of nasal congestion.

• Monitor usage and signs of rebound congestion.

Supportive Care

• Notify the doctor of any changes in the patient's health status.

Patient Teaching

• Teach the patient how to administer the solution and tell him it should be used by one person only.

• Warn the patient not to exceed the recommended dose; explain that exceesive use may result in rebound congestion.

• Warn the patient he may experience transient burning or stinging upon administration.

Evaluation

In patients receiving xylometazoline hydrochloride, appropriate evaluation statements may include:

• Patient obtains relief from nasal congestion.

• Patient remains free of rebound congestion.

• Patient and family state an understanding of xylometazoline hydrochloride therapy.

zidovudine (azidothymidine, AZT)

(zye doe´ vue deen)

Retrovir

• *Classification:* antiviral (thymidine analogue)

• *Pregnancy Risk Category:* C

HOW SUPPLIED

Capsules: 100 mg

Syrup: 50 mg/5 ml

Injection: 20 mg/ml

ACTION

Mechanism: Prevents replication of the human immunodeficiency virus (HIV) by inhibiting the enzyme reverse transcriptase.

Absorption: Rapidly absorbed from the GI tract, but average systemic bioavailability is 65% because of first-pass metabolism.

Distribution: Preliminary data reveal good CSF penetration. Approximately 36% of zidovudine dose is plasma protein-bound.

Metabolism: Rapidly metabolized to an inactive compound.

Excretion: Parent drug and metabolite are excreted by glomerular filtration and tubular secretion in the kidneys. Urine recovery of parent drug and metabolite is 14% and 74% respectively. Half-life: Elimination half-

life of parent drug and metabolite is 1 hour.
Onset, peak, duration: After oral dosing, peak serum concentrations occur within 0.5 to 1.5 hours.

INDICATIONS & DOSAGE

Patients with AIDS or advanced AIDS-related complex (ARC) who have a history of Pneumocystis carinii *pneumonia or a CD_4 lymphocyte count below 200 cells/mm² –*
Adults: initially, 200 mg P.O. q 4 hours around the clock for 1 month, then 100 mg P.O. q 4 hours around the clock.
Children: dosage is individualized and will vary according to treatment IND protocol. Early studies have employed doses between 0.9 and 1.4 mg/kg/hour by continuous I.V. infusion; others have used 100 mg/m² I.V. or P.O. q 6 hours.
Postexposure prophylaxis–
Adults: dosage will vary according to study protocol, but most studies use 200 mg P.O. q 4 hours around the clock for 6 to 8 weeks. Some investigators attempt to initiate therapy within 1 hour of exposure.
Asymptomatic HIV infection–
Adults: 100 mg P.O. q 4 hours while awake (500 mg daily).
Children 3 months to 12 years: 180 mg/m² P.O. q 6 hours (720 mg/m²/day) not to exceed 200 mg q 6 hours.

CONTRAINDICATIONS & PRECAUTIONS

Use cautiously in patients with compromised bone marrow function. Significant anemia may occur after 2 to 6 weeks of therapy, possibly necessitating dosage adjustment, drug discontinuation, or transfusions.

ADVERSE REACTIONS

Common reactions are in italics; life-threatening reactions are in bold italics.
Blood: ***Severe bone marrow depression (resulting in anemia), granulocytopenia, thrombocytopenia.***
CNS: *headache,* agitation, restlessness, insomnia, confusion, anxiety.
GI: nausea, anorexia.
Skin: rash, itching.
Other: myalgia.

INTERACTIONS

Acyclovir: possible lethargy and fatigue. Use together cautiously.
Co-trimoxazole, acetaminophen: may impair hepatic metabolism of zidovudine, increasing the drug's toxicity.
Other cytotoxic drugs: additive adverse effects on the bone marrow.
Pentamidine, dapsone, flucytosine, amphotericin B: increased risk of nephrotoxicity.
Probenecid: may decrease the renal clearance of zidovidine.

EFFECTS ON DIAGNOSTIC TESTS

CBC: decreased RBCs, WBCs, and platelets.

NURSING CONSIDERATIONS

Besides those related universally to drug therapy (see "How to use this book"), consider the following specific recommendations:

Assessment
- Obtain a baseline assessment of infection before therapy.
- Be alert for adverse reactions and drug interactions throughout therapy.
- Evaluate the patient's and family's knowledge about zidovudine therapy.

Nursing Diagnoses
- High risk for injury related to ineffectiveness of zidovudine to prevent or erradicate the infection.
- Noncompliance (medication administration) related to prolonged therapy.
- Knowledge deficit related to zidovudine.

Planning and Implementation
Preparation and Administration
- ***P.O. use:*** Administer q 4 hours around the clock.

• ***I.V. use:*** Dilute before administration. Remove the calculated dose from the vial; add to dextrose 5% injection to achieve a concentration that does not exceed 4 mg/ml. Administer 1 to 2 mg/kg infused over 1 hour at a constant rate; administer every 4 hours around the clock. Avoid rapid infusion or bolus injection. Adding mixture to biological or colloidal fluids (e.g., blood products, protein solutions) is not recommended. After drug is diluted, the solution is physically and chemically stable for 24 hours at room temperature and for 48 hours if refrigerated at 35.6°F to 46.4°F to minimize the risk of microbial contamination. Store undiluted vials at 59°F to 77°F and protect them from light.

Monitoring

• Monitor effectiveness by regularly assessing for progression of infection.
• Monitor CBC and platelet counts for signs of anemia or granulocytopenia.
• Monitor for signs and symptoms of opportunistic infection (including pneumonia, meningitis, and sepsis).

Supportive Care

• If the patient develops significant anemia (hemoglobin level below 7.5 mg/dl or reduction by more that 25% of baseline value) and/or significant granulocytopenia (granulocyte count below 750/mm^3 or reduction by more than 50% of baseline value), notify the doctor; interruption of therapy may be necessary. For less significant anemia or granulocytopenia, a reduction in daily dose, and possibly blood transfusions may be indicated.
• If the patient develops anemia, provide supportive care; for example, schedule the patient's activities to provide frequent rest periods.
• If signs of an opportunistic infection occur, notify the doctor immediately.
• Administer a mild analgesic, as prescribed, if the patient experiences a headache. If the patient develops other adverse reactions, notify the doctor for appropriate treatment and provide supportive care as appropriate. For example, take safety precautions if the patient experiences adverse CNS reactions, such as dizziness; administer a mild sedative for insomnia as prescribed; or monitor hydration if the patient experiences adverse GI reactions.

Patient Teaching

• Inform patient that drug does not cure HIV infection or AIDS but may reduce morbidity resulting from opportunistic infections and thus prolong the patient's life. However, the optimum dosage and duration of treatment are not yet known.
• Instruct the patient to take the drug every 4 hours around the clock even though it means interrupting sleep. Suggest ways to avoid missing doses.
• Inform the patient that drug does not reduce the risk of transmitting the virus to others through sexual contact or blood contamination.
• Warn patient to avoid OTC medications or other drugs not medically approved to treat HIV infection without first checking with the doctor, pharmacist, or nurse.
• Inform patient about the importance of follow-up medical visits to evaluate for adverse reactions and to monitor clinical status. Emphasize that frequent (at least every 2 weeks) blood counts are strongly recommended.
• Advise the breast-feeding patient that the manufacturer recommends discontinuation of breastfeeding during therapy with zidovudine.
• Warn patient to avoid hazardous activities that require alertness if such adverse CNS reactions as dizziness occur.
• Tell the patient to store the drug at room temperature and to protect it from light.

Evaluation
In patients receiving zidovudine, appropriate evaluation statements may include:
• Patient is free of infection.
• Patient complies with prescribed therapy regimen.
• Patient and family state an understanding of therapy.

zinc sulfate
(zink)
Bufopto Zinc Sulfate◇, Eye-Sed Ophthalmic◇, Op-Thal-Zin◇

• *Classification:* ophthalmic decongestant (trace element)
• *Pregnancy Risk Category:* C

HOW SUPPLIED
Ophthalmic solution: 0.2%◇

ACTION
Mechanism: Produces astringent action on the conjunctiva.
Pharmacokinetics: Unknown.

INDICATIONS & DOSAGE
Ocular congestion, irritation–
Adults and children: instill 1 to 2 drops of 0.2% solution in eye b.i.d. or t.i.d.

CONTRAINDICATIONS & PRECAUTIONS
Contraindicated in patients hypersensitive to any component in the preparation, including boric acid or benzalkonium chloride. Use cautiously in patients with glaucoma.

If patients experience eye pain or visual disturbances, they should discontinue the drug and contact a physician. If ocular irriation or redness continues, or the condition treated persists for more than 3 days, they should discontinue the drug and contact a physician.

ADVERSE REACTIONS
Common reactions are in italics; life-threatening reactions are in bold italics.
Eye: irritation.

INTERACTIONS
Opthalmic solutions containing sodium borate, methylcellulose, or acacia: may cause a precipitate to form.

EFFECTS ON DIAGNOSTIC TESTS
None reported.

NURSING CONSIDERATIONS
Besides those related universally to drug therapy, (see "How to use this book"), consider the following recommendations.
Assessment
• Obtain a baseline assessment of the patient's vision and ocular appearance.
• Be alert for adverse reactions or drug interactions during therapy.
• Evaluate the patient's and family's knowledge about zinc sulfate therapy.
Nursing Diagnoses
• Sensory/perceptual alterations (visual) related to the patient's underlying condition.
• Pain related to zinc sulfate-induced irritation.
• Knowledge deficit related to zinc sulfate therapy.
Planning and Implementation
Preparation and Administration
• Instill in lacrimal sac; remove excess solution from around eyes with a clean tissue or gauze and apply light finger pressure to lacrimal sac for 1 minute.
• Store solution in a tightly closed container.
Monitoring
• Monitor the effectiveness of zinc sulfate therapy by assessing the patient's visual status and conjunctival appearance.
• Monitor for drug-induced ocular irritation.

Supportive Care
• Notify the doctor if changes in the patient's visual status occur.
Patient Teaching
• Teach the patient how to instill the solution and advise him to wash his hands before and after administering the drug.
• Tell the patient to report any persistent or increased irritation.

Evaluation

In patients receiving zinc sulfate, appropriate evaluation statements may include:
• Patient experiences relief of ocular irritation.
• Patient remains free of drug-induced discomfort.
• Patient and family state an understanding of zinc sulfate therapy.

INDEX

Generic drug names are listed alphabetically throughout the book.

A

B

C

D

E

F

G

H

I

J

K

L

M

O

P

Q

R